DAVIS ADVANTAGE
PATHOPHYSIOLOGY

Your
PERSONALIZED LEARNING PLAN
is waiting for you!

1. Scratch off the shiny surface you'll find on the inside front cover to reveal your unique access code.*

2. Go to: **www.DavisAdvantage.com**

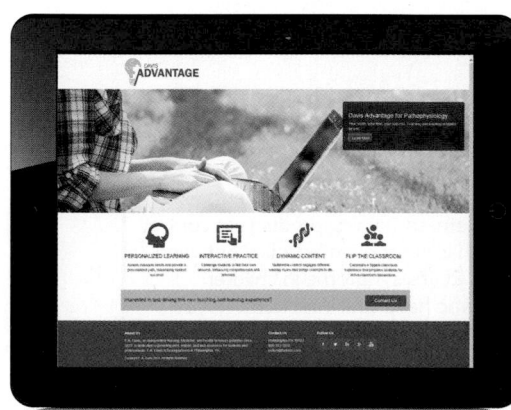

3. Click the "LOGIN/JOIN" button at the top of the page.

4. Enter your access code.

Note: Before activating your code, you will be asked to create a new student account or log into your account with your DavisPlus credentials. If you are using Davis Advantage Pathophysiology in a class, you will have the option to enter your Class ID when registering. Your instructor will provide you with your Class ID.

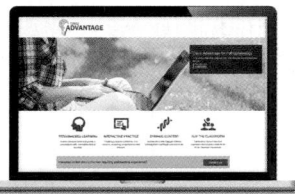

DAVIS ADVANTAGE
PATHOPHYSIOLOGY

YOUR NEEDS.
YOUR TIME.
YOUR SUCCESS!

GET THE DAVIS ADVANTAGE!
Combine the power to create your own Personalized Learning Plan online with

PATHOPHYSIOLOGY: Introductory Concepts and Clinical Perspectives

Activate your Access Code today!

1. Scratch off the shiny surface below to reveal your unique access code.

2. Go to: **www.DavisAdvantage.com**

3. Click the "LOGIN/JOIN" button at the top of the page.

4. Enter your access code.

Note: Before activating your code, you will be asked to create a new student account or log into your account with your DavisPlus credentials. If you are using Davis Advantage Pathophysiology in a class, you will have the option to enter your Class ID when registering. Your instructor will provide you with your Class ID.

SCRATCH OFF
shiny surface with care!

*Each access code may only be redeemed one time. If your access code has already been used, visit www.DavisAdvantage.com

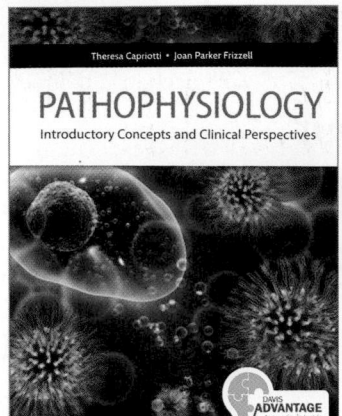

PATHOPHYSIOLOGY for the REAL-WORD

Real-world perspectives bridge the gap between the science of disease and clinical patient care. You'll clearly see "how" to interpret assessment findings and "why" to choose interventions.

Chapters organized by body systems help you understand the relationships between the underlying pathology and the patient assessment data, laboratory findings, and diagnostic testing results.

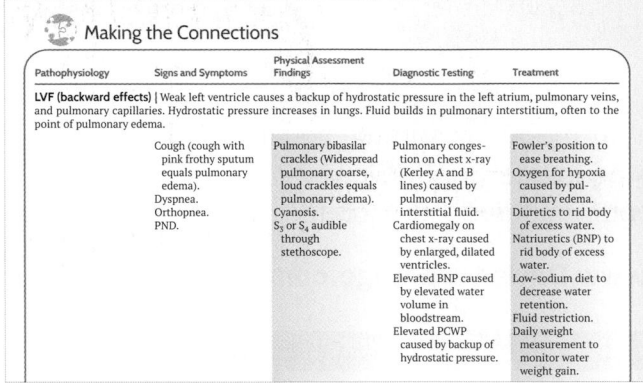

Making the Connections boxes demonstrate the relationship between a disease state, the diagnosis, and nursing care.

 CLINICAL CONCEPT

Fever, although advantageous to the immune system, can reach levels high enough to cause seizures and brain damage. Therefore, it is recommended to keep fever below 102°F through the use of antipyretic medications such as aspirin, ibuprofen, or acetaminophen. These medications inhibit prostaglandin formation and, thus, reduce fever.

Clinical Concept boxes explain how key concepts apply to clinical practice.

ALERT! Never give children or adolescents aspirin or any salicylate-containing products to control a fever. Research has demonstrated a link between salicylate use and Reye's syndrome in children and adolescents who have viral infections. Reye's syndrome is a life-threatening disorder in which mitochondrial failure leads to liver failure and encephalopathy.

Alerts, highlighted in red, warn you of potential problems or complications that can arise in patients based on the underlying pathophysiology.

Chapter Summary

- Inflammation is an essential process for protecting the body during injury or infection.
- In the initial phase, WBCs are attracted to the site of the injury in a process called chemotaxis.
- Blood vessel walls become more permeable so fluid and WBCs can move out of the bloodstream to the site of injury.
- Types of WBCs include neutrophils, eosinophils, basophils, lymphocytes, and monocytes, which turn into macrophages.
- The five cardinal signs of inflammation are rubor (redness), tumor (swelling), calor (heat), dolor (pain), and loss of function.

- C-reactive protein and erythrocyte sedimentation rates increase in acute inflammation.
- Inflammation can undergo healing and resolution or persist as chronic inflammation.
- Healing involves one of three processes: primary, secondary, or tertiary intention.
- Nutrition status, oxygen supply, steroid use, diabetes, and immunosuppression affect the process of healing.
- There are many possible complications of wound healing including keloid formation, contracture, stricture and fistula formation, wound dehiscence, and evisceration.

Chapter Summaries make it easy to review the most important concepts.

Get the DAVIS ADVANTAGE

PATHOPHYSIOLOGY and your PERSONALIZED LEARNING PLAN
work together to provide everything you need to succeed!

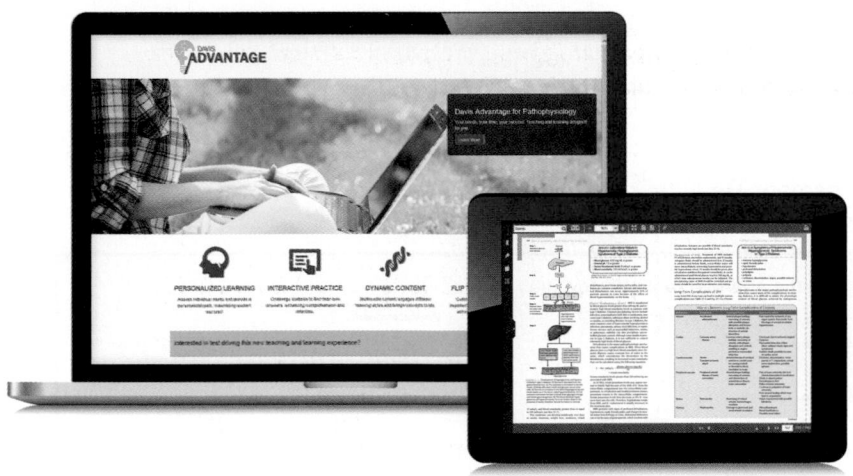

Study anytime, anywhere.
Desktop, laptop, tablet, or mobile phone. An integrated e-book version of your text lets you study wherever there's an internet connection.

Davis Advantage for Pathophysiology

combines your text with an online program that makes this challenging, but must-know content easier to master.

www.DavisAdvantage.com

#1 ASSIGNMENTS

The first screen you see when you log in lists the assignments made by your instructor.

Each assignment is mapped to a specific chapter in the text. You can either read your printed text or click on the ebook link to be taken directly to that chapter in the ebook.

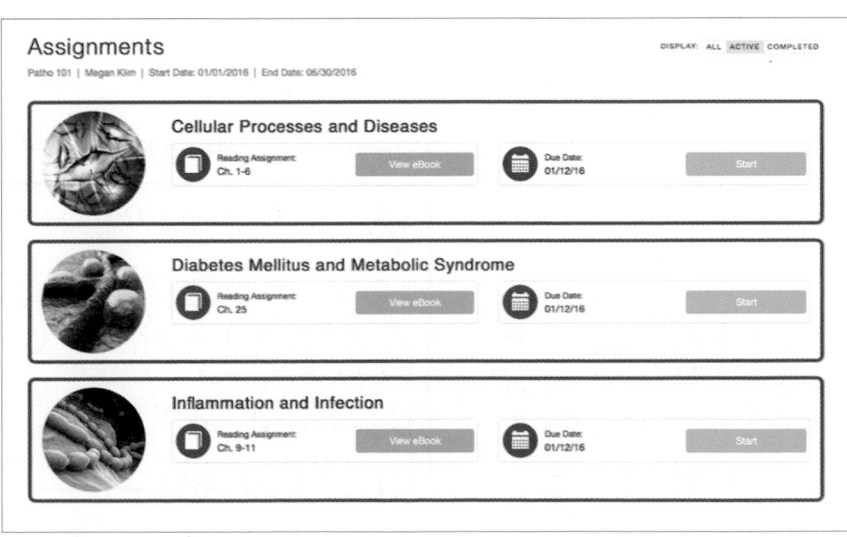

#2 PRE-ASSESSMENTS

Pre-Assessments drive your Personalized Learning Plan. Each assignment begins with a pre-assessment quiz that evaluates your comprehension and retention of the content and concepts within that module.

Pre-Assessment Results identify your strengths with thumbs up to indicate competency and thumbs down for areas of weakness that require more study.

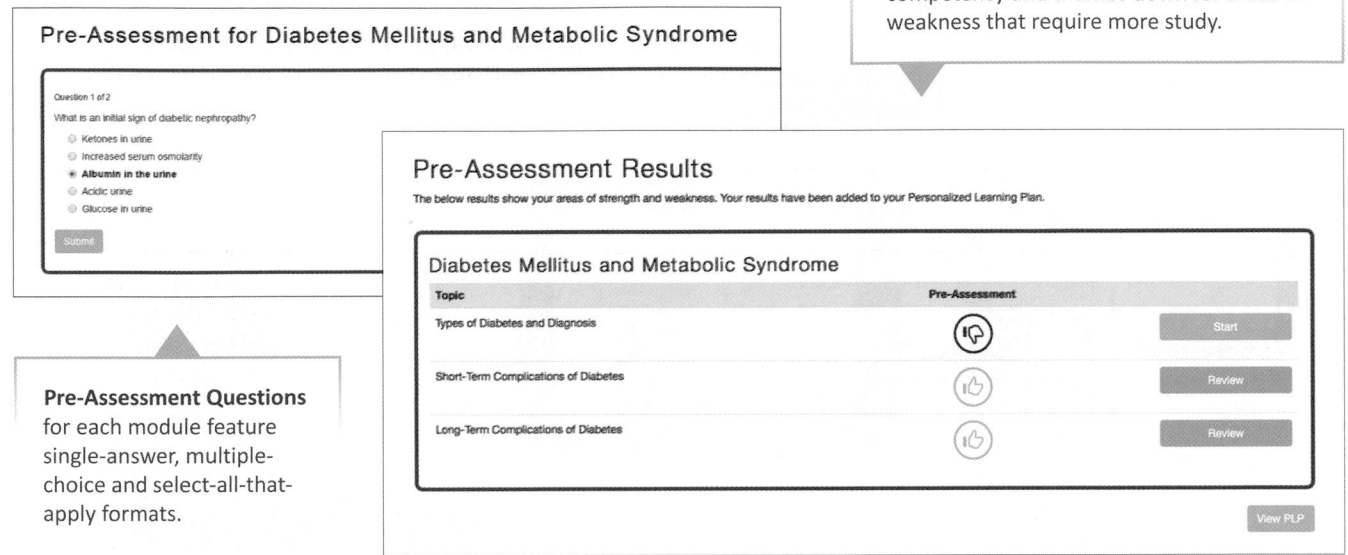

Pre-Assessment Questions for each module feature single-answer, multiple-choice and select-all-that-apply formats.

#3 PERSONALIZED LEARNING PLANS

The results of the Pre-Assessment create your Personalized Learning Plan which is mapped to your individual needs to create a path to success. It provides an overview of what topics you need to work through to enhance your understanding and achieve mastery.

Personalized Learning Plans identify the topics on which you need to focus your study time and the activities to be completed.

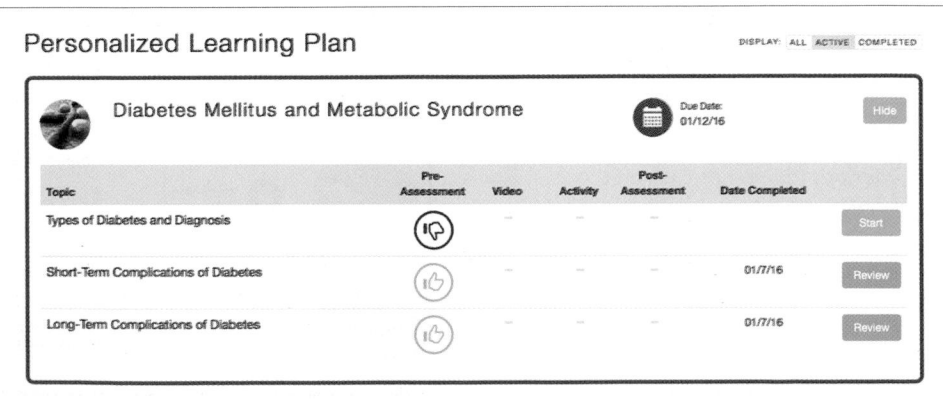

#4 INTERACTIVE LEARNING

Your Personalized Learning Plan for each topic guides you through an animated mini-lecture to reinforce key concepts; creates an interactive exercise that lets you apply your knowledge; and produces a post-assessment to confirm comprehension.

Brand-new videos (over 45 in all) are animated mini-lectures that present key concepts for each topic, connecting with all learning styles.

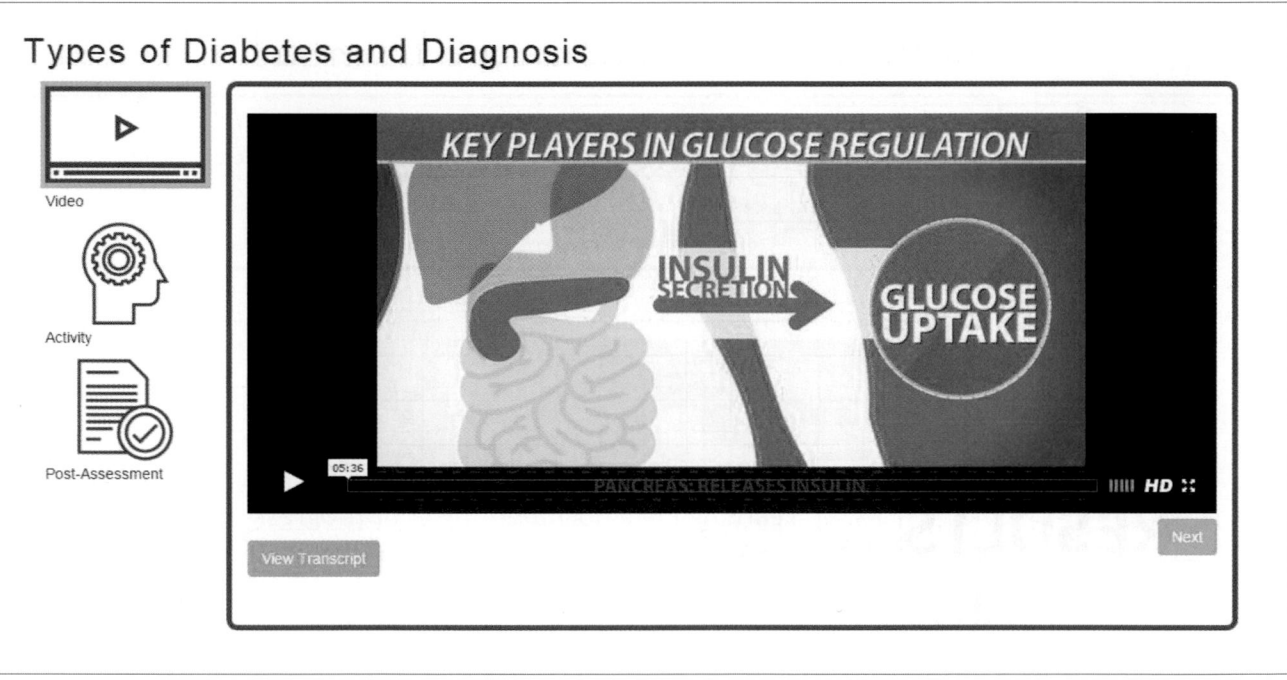

Exploratory learning and interactive exercises, including case studies and activities, check your understanding and expand your knowledge.

Rationales for correct and incorrect answers help you understand why you got a question right or wrong.

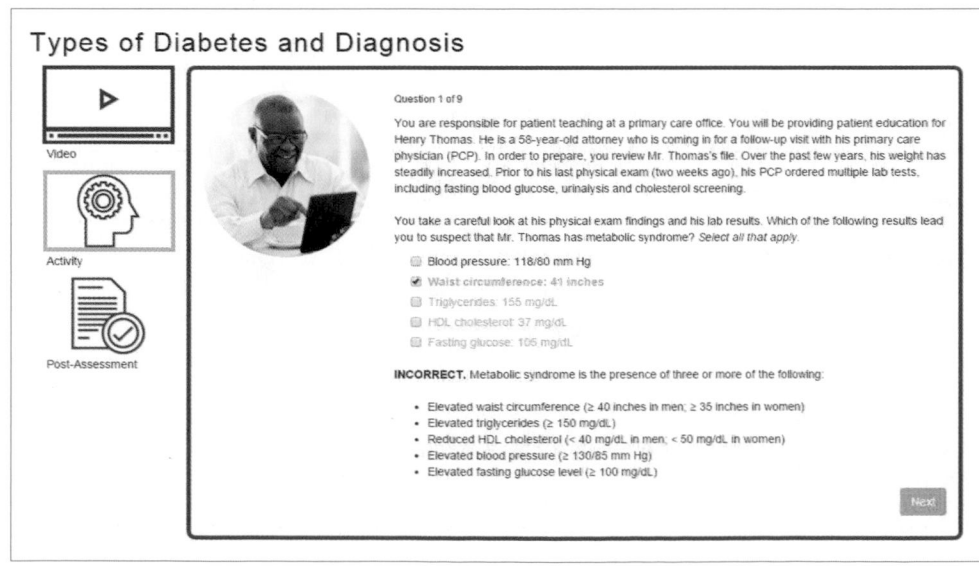

#5 POST-ASSESSMENT

After completing each section, a post-assessment quiz unlocks to assess your mastery of the content within the topic.

Post-Assessment for Types of Diabetes and Diagnosis

Question 1 of 5

Which hormone released by the pancreas causes the liver to release glucose in the blood to counteract hypoglycemia?

- ○ cortisol
- ○ epinephrine
- ● **glucagon**
- ○ insulin
- ○ growth hormone

Submit

Post-Assessment results provide you with immediate feedback.

Post-Assessment for Types of Diabetes and Diagnosis

Results

Congratulations! You answered 5 out of 5 questions correctly. You have completed this topic.

View PLP

#6 RESULTS

Your post-assessment results feed into your Personalized Learning Plan, documenting your progress through each activity for each topic. Even after you complete each section successfully, you can return to review any topic for additional practice and exam prep.

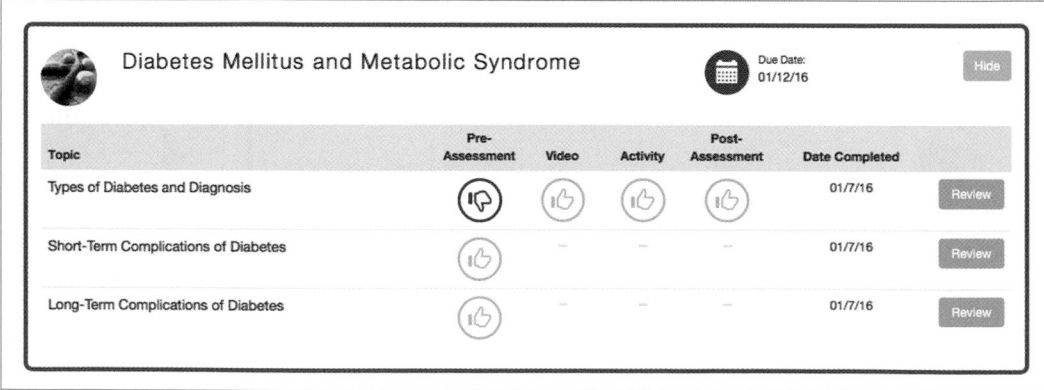

Topic	Pre-Assessment	Video	Activity	Post-Assessment	Date Completed	
Types of Diabetes and Diagnosis	👍	👍	👍	👍	01/7/16	Review
Short-Term Complications of Diabetes	👍	–	–	–	01/7/16	Review
Long-Term Complications of Diabetes	👍	–	–	–	01/7/16	Review

Diabetes Mellitus and Metabolic Syndrome — Due Date: 01/12/16 — Hide

Your Personalized Learning Plan presents a snapshot of your progress through each step in the learning process, making it easy for you to identify areas for additional study.

PATHOPHYSIOLOGY

Introductory Concepts and Clinical Perspectives

Theresa Capriotti, DO, MSN, CRNP, RN
Clinical Associate Professor
Villanova University
Villanova, Pennsylvania

Joan Parker Frizzell, PhD, CRNP, ANP-BC
Associate Professor
School of Nursing & Health Sciences
La Salle University
Philadelphia, Pennsylvania
Nurse Practitioner
Roxborough Memorial Hospital
Philadelphia, Pennsylvania

F.A. Davis Company • Philadelphia

F.A. Davis Company
1915 Arch Street
Philadelphia, PA 19103
www.fadavis.com

Printed in the United States of America

Last digit indicates print number: 10 9 8 7 6 5 4

Acquisitions Editor, Nursing: Megan E. Klim
Manager of Content Development: William F. Welsh
Content Project Manager: Jacalyn C. Clay
Electronic Project Editor: Katherine E. Crowley
Design and Illustration Manager: Carolyn O'Brien

As new scientific information becomes available through basic and clinical research, recommended treatments and drug therapies undergo changes. The author(s) and publisher have done everything possible to make this book accurate, up-to-date, and in accord with accepted standards at the time of publication. The author(s), editors, and publisher are not responsible for errors or omissions or for consequences from application of the book, and make no warranty, expressed or implied, in regard to the contents of the book. Any practice described in this book should be applied by the reader in accordance with professional standards of care used in regard to the unique circumstances that may apply in each situation. The reader is advised always to check product information (package inserts) for changes and new information regarding dose and contraindications before administering any drug. Caution is especially urged when using new or infrequently ordered drugs.

Library of Congress Cataloging-in-Publication Data

Library of Congress Cataloging-in-Publication Data

Capriotti, Theresa, author.
 Pathophysiology : introductory concepts and clinical perspectives / Theresa Capriotti, Joan Parker Frizzell.
  p. ; cm.
 Includes bibliographical references and index.
 ISBN 978-0-8036-1571-7 — ISBN 0-8036-1571-X
 I. Frizzell, Joan Parker, author. II. Title.
 [DNLM: 1. Disease—Nurses' Instruction. QZ 140]
 RB113
 616.07—dc23
                2015002590

I would like to thank the following people who have inspired me to write this book . . . my mother, Johanna Capriotti, for being the first person to show me a biology book . . . my father, Vincent Capriotti, for teaching me how to draw and trudge through all the challenges of life . . . Dr. Robert Benjamin, who saved my life . . . Dr. Louise Fitzpatrick, who hired me to do what I love . . . my three sons, David, Michael, and Peter Wolinsky, who give me so much happiness . . . and Rocco, who sat right next to me with each word I typed. . . .

–Teri Capriotti

The completion of a project such as this requires encouragement and support from family, friends, and colleagues. I would like to thank all of them for enabling me to attain this professional goal. Dr. Zane Robinson Wolf, who recruited me to La Salle University so that I could teach my favorite courses–Pathophysiology & Pharmacology . . . Joanne DaCunha, for introducing me to Teri Capriotti so that I could be a part of this book . . . my parents, Edwin and Virginia Parker, for their love and devotion to family . . . Penny Lind, a true friend and confidante . . . my daughter, Virginia Joan Scharf, and my grandchildren–Peter, Melissa, Stephen, and Samantha–who fill my life with joy . . . HollyBerry, who makes me laugh . . . my students, who make teaching a worthwhile profession . . .

–Joan Parker Frizzell

CONTRIBUTORS

Elise M. Alverson, DNP, RN, FNP-BC, CNE
Associate Professor
Valparaiso University
Valparaiso, Indiana

Kenya Beard, EdD, GNP-BC, NP-C, ACNP-BC, CNE
Associate Professor, Macy Faculty Scholar
Director, Center for Multicultural Education & Health
   Disparities
Hunter College
New York, New York

Linda Brandon
Heart Failure Care Manager
New England Quality Care Alliance
Braintree, Massachusetts

Dona Rinaldi Carpenter, RN, EdD
Undergraduate Program Director
Scranton University
Scranton, Pennsylvania

Linda A. Carrick, PhD, RN, CNAA
Adjunct Assistant Professor of Nursing
University of Pennsylvania, School of Nursing
Philadelphia, Pennsylvania

Deborah W. Chapa, PhD, ACNP-BC
Assistant Professor, Director, Doctor of Nursing
   Practice
George Washington University, School of Nursing
Washington, District of Columbia

Michael Clinton, RN, PhD
Professor
American University of Beirut, Hariri School of Nursing
Beirut, Lebanon

Ferne M. Cohen, EdD, CRNA
Assistant Chair, Nurse Anesthesia Program
Drexel University
Philadelphia, Pennsylvania

Denise Coppa, PhD, RNP
Associate Professor
University of Rhode Island, School of Nursing
Kingston, Rhode Island

Darleen Crisileo, RN
Staff RN, Post-Anesthesia Care Unit
Massachusetts General Hospital
Canton, Massachusetts

Renee Crossman, BN, RN, MHS
Lecturer
Memorial University School of Nursing
St. John's, Newfoundland
Canada

Angela J. Daniel, MSN, MBA, RN
Associate Editor, Animations
Elsevier Publishing
Atlanta, Georgia

Stephanie Denninghoff, MSN, CNOR
Instructor
Riverside School of Professional Nursing
Newport News, Virginia

Elaine K. Diegmann, CNM, ND, FACNM
Program Director, Nurse Midwifery
University of Medicine and Dentistry of New Jersey,
   School of Nursing
Newark, New Jersey

Sr. Rosemary Donley, PhD, APRN, FAAN
Professor, Jacques Laval Chair for Social Justice
Duquesne University School of Nursing
Pittsburgh, Pennsylvania

Patricia A. Dunn, PhD, RNC
Associate Professor
Holy Family University
Philadelphia, Pennsylvania

Claire Faust, MSN, APN
Nursing Program Coordinator, College of Nursing & Allied
   Health
Burlington County College
Pemberton, New Jersey

Cynthia M. Finn, RN, BS, CCRN
Staff RN, Cardiac Surgical ICU
Massachusetts General Hospital
Boston, Massachusetts

Elizabeth Galik, PhD, CRNP
Associate Professor
University of Maryland School of Nursing
Baltimore, Maryland

Diane M. Gay, RN
Massachusetts General Hospital
Boston, Massachusetts

Catherine A. Griffith, PhD, RN, ACNP-BC
Clinical Research Nurse
Harvard Catalyst Clinical & Translational Science
   Center at Massachusetts General Hospital MGH
   Clinical Research Center
Boston, Massachusetts

Kathie Judy Guth, MS, RN
Instructor and Clinical Nurse Specialist
Johns Hopkins University, School of Nursing
Baltimore, Maryland

Patricia Hindin, PhD, CNM
Assistant Professor
Rutgers, The State University of New Jersey
Newark, New Jersey

Joanna F. Hofmann, EdD, RN, ANP/GNP-C
Adjunct Professor
Nyack Christian College
Nyack, New York

Janice J. Hoffman, PhD, RN, ANEF
Associate Professor, Assistant Dean of the Baccalaureate
   Nursing Program
University of Maryland School of Nursing
Baltimore, Maryland

Susan H. Jones, RN, BSN, MS, EdD
Associate Professor, Nursing (Retired)
Hampton University School of Nursing
Hampton, Virginia

Julie A. Koch, DNP, RN, FNP-BC
Assistant Professor, FNP Program Coordinator
Valparaiso University College of Nursing and Health
   Professions
Valparaiso, Indiana

Marianne Kraemer, RN, EdM, MPA, CCRN
Chief Nursing Officer
Kennedy Health System
Stratford, New Jersey

Ginette Lange, PhD, CNM, RN
Associate Professor
University of Medicine and Dentistry of New Jersey,
   School of Nursing
Newark, New Jersey

Ciara Levine, MSN, RN
Assistant Professor of Nursing
La Salle University
Philadelphia, Pennsylvania

Claude Lieber, MD, FACS
Clinical Associate Professor of Surgery, Thomas Jefferson
   Medical College, Philadelphia, Retired
Chief of Surgery, Wilmington VA Medical Center, Retired
Adjunct, Department of Nursing, Florida Gulf Coast
   University, Retired

Sandra MacDonald, RN, BN, MN, PhD
Professor
Memorial University of Newfoundland School of Nursing
St. John's, Newfoundland
Canada

Carol Isaac MacKusick, PhD, MSN, RN, CNN
Assistant Professor
West Carolina University
Cullowhee, North Carolina

Dr. April Manuel, PhD, BN
Assistant Professor
Memorial University School of Nursing
St. John's, Newfoundland
Canada

Kimberly Meyer, MSN, CNRN, ACNP-BC
Neurosurgery Nurse Practitioner
University of Louisville Medical Center Trauma Institute
Louisville, Kentucky

Helen Miley, RN, PhD, CCRN, AG-ACNP
Specialty Director, Adult Geriatric Acute Care Nurse
   Practitioner Program
Rutgers University
Newark, New Jersey

Judy I. Murphy, PhD, RN, CNE, CHSE
Simulation Coordinator, Nurse Researcher
Rhode Island College School of Nursing
Assistant Professor of Clinical Medicine
Alpert Medical School Brown University
Providence, Rhode Island

Margie Pierce, MS, RRT, CPFT
Director of Respiratory and Neurophysiology Services
Pennsylvania Hospital
Philadelphia, Pennsylvania

Susan Padham Porterfield, PhD, FNP-c
Assistant Dean for Graduate Programs, College
   of Nursing
Florida State University
Tallahassee, Florida

Alicemarie S. Poyss, PhD, CNL, APRN-BC
Associate Clinical Professor, CNL Track Director
Drexel University College of Nursing and Health
    Professions
Philadelphia, Pennsylvania

Ingrid Pretzer-Aboff, PhD, RN
Associate Professor, Co-Director of The Nurse Managed
    Health Center, Parkinson's Clinic
University of Delaware
Newark, Delaware

Francia I. Reed, MS, RN, FNP-C
Clinical Assistant Professor
State University of New York, Institute of Technology
Utica, New York

Kimberly D. Ryan-Nicholls, RPN, RN, BScN, MDE
Associate Professor, Psychiatric Nursing
Brandon University, School of Health Studies
Brandon, Manitoba
Canada

Mary Clare A. Schafer, MS, RN, ONC, CRRN
Orthopaedic Day Rehabilitation Coordinator
Magee Rehabilitation Hospital
Philadelphia, Pennsylvania

Deborah Schiavone, PhD, PMHCNS-BC, CNE
Program Director
Stratford University
Woodbridge, Virginia

Emily Karwacki Sheff, MS, RN, CMSRN, FNP, BC
Assistant Professor
MGH Institute of Health Professions
Charlestown, Massachusetts

Susan K. Smith, DNP, RN, CEN, CCRN
SK Smith Consulting
Warriors Mark, Pennsylvania

Julia Spinolo, DNP, APRN-BC, LNC
Assistant Professor of Nursing
Clayton State University
Morrow, Georgia

Angela Starkweather, PhD, MSN, CCRN, CNRN
Assistant Professor
Washington State University, College of Nursing
Spokane, Washington

Dr. Kimberly Subasic, PhD, MS, BSN
Assistant Professor
University of Scranton
Scranton, Pennsylvania

Patricia A. Thompson, BSN, MSN, FNP-BC
Family Nurse Practitioner
Hattiesburg Clinic, Wiggins Clinic
Hattiesburg, Mississippi

Ann Tritak, RN, EdD
Professor and Director, DNP Program
Saint Peter's University School of Nursing
Jersey City, New Jersey

Kathleen O'Rourke Vito, PhD, PHCNS-BC, RN
Associate Professor of Nursing
Felician College
Lodi, New Jersey

Diane M. Wieland, PhD, MSN, RN, PMHCNS-BC, CNE
Associate Professor
La Salle University, School of Nursing and Health
    Sciences
Philadelphia, Pennsylvania

Mary Wilby, PhD, MSN, RN
Assistant Professor of Nursing
La Salle University
Philadelphia, Pennsylvania

Joyce S. Willens, PhD, RN, BC
Assistant Professor
Villanova University
Villanova, Pennsylvania

Erin Winterhalter, MPH, RD, LDN, CDE
Director, MacDonald Center for Obesity Prevention
    and Education
Villanova University College of Nursing
Villanova, Pennsylvania

Tamara L. Zurakowski, PhD, GNP-BC
Adjunct Associate Professor
University of Pennsylvania
Philadelphia, Pennsylvania

REVIEWERS

Christina Amidei, RN, MSN, CRN, CCRN, FAAN
Instructor
University of Central Florida
Orlando, Florida

Susan Apold, PhD, RN, ANP-BC
Dean, Division of Nursing
Concordia College
Bronxville, New York

Judith L. Bateman, RN, MSN
Instructor
Black Hawk College
Moline, Illinois

(Pricilla) Diane Benson, RN, EdD, MSN, MEd
Associate Professor of Nursing
Texas A&M Health Science Center College of Nursing
Brian, Texas

Elizabeth A. Berro, MA, RN, PNP, CHSE
Clinical Assistant Professor, Co-Director
    for Undergraduate Simulation
Pace University
Pleasantville, New York

Jane Blood-Siegfried, RN, CPNP, DNSc
Assistant Clinical Professor
Duke University, School of Nursing
Durham, North Carolina

Carol Botwinski, EdD, ARNP, NNP-BC
Associate Professor and Associate Director, Nursing
University of Tampa
Tampa, Florida

Kevin Branch
Professor
Cambrian College
Sudbury, Ontario
Canada

Jacqueline Burchum, DNSc, APRN, BC
Assistant Professor
The University of Memphis, Loewenberg School
    of Nursing
Memphis, Tennessee

Mary C. Butash, MSN, RN, CRNP, CRRN
Nursing Instructor
Roxborough Memorial Hospital, School of Nursing
Philadelphia, Pennsylvania

Sheryl Oakes Caddy, RN, BSN, JD
Faculty
Linn-Benton Community College
Albany, Oregon

Christine L. Candenhouten, MSN, RN, CNOR
Associate Professor of Nursing
Bellin College of Nursing
Green Bay, Wisconsin

Sharon Carroll, RN, BN, MN(c)
Instructor, Nursing Program
Medicine Hat College
Medicine Hat, Alberta
Canada

Ava Chase, DNP, FNP-C
Clinical Professor of Nursing
Graceland University
Independence, Missouri

Maureen M. Covelli, PhD, RN
Associate Professor
University of Central Florida
Orlando, Florida

Janet Czermak, BSN, MS, MA, CNS
Associate Professor
Essex County College
Newark, New Jersey

Jenny L. D'Agostino, RN, MSN
Assistant Professor of Nursing
University of Central Missouri
Warrensburg, Missouri

Michelle M. De Lima, MSN, RN, CNOR
Instructor
Delgado Community College, Charity School of Nursing
New Orleans, Louisiana

Patricia Delmoe, RN, MN, ACLS, PALS
Nursing Instructor
Maricopa Community College, Boswell Campus
Sun City, Arizona

Loretta H. Diehl, RN, MSN
College Associate Professor
New Mexico State University at Alamogordo
Alamogordo, New Mexico

Dare Domico, RN, DSN
Professor
Georgia Baptist College of Nursing of Mercer University
Atlanta, Georgia

Evelyn G. Duffy, DNP, AGPCNP-BC, FAANP
Associate Professor, Director of the Adult-Gerontology
    Nurse Practitioner Program, Associate Director of the
    University Center on Aging and Health
Case Western Reserve University, Frances Payne Bolton
    School of Nursing
Cleveland, Ohio

Julie Eggert, PhD, GNP-BC, AOCN
Associate Professor, Doctoral Program Coordinator
Clemson University
Clemson, South Carolina

Betty Elder, PhD, RN
Associate Professor
Wichita State University, School of Nursing
Wichita, Kansas

Heather Ferrillo, APRN, MSN, FNP-BC
Clinical Assistant Professor
Sacred Heart University
Fairfield, Connecticut

Diane M. Ford, RN, MS, APRN, BC
Assistant Professor of Nursing
Andrews University
Berrien Springs, Missouri

Dorothy Fraser, MSN, FNP
Faculty
California State University, Fresno
Fresno, California

Martha Gainer, MS, APN-CFNP, APN-CNS
Lecturer
Governors State University, College of Health
    Professions
University Park, Illinois

Masoud Ghaffari, PhD, MSN/RN, MEd, MT (ASCP), CMA
Associate Professor, College of Nursing
East Tennessee State University
Johnson City, Tennessee

Kathleen A. Goei, RN, MSN, PhD
Adjunct Professor
University of the Incarnate Word, School of Physical
    Therapy
San Antonio, Texas

Carol J. Green, PhD, CNS, RN, CNE
Professor of Nursing
Graceland University School of Nursing
Independence, Missouri

G. Lynn Green, APNP-BC, NP-C, MSN, CHC, CLNC
Nurse Practitioner, Adjunct Faculty
Bellin College of Nursing
Green Bay, Wisconsin

Carole L. Gutterman, Ph.D., CURN
Professor Division of Nursing
Coordinator Masters in Nursing Education Track
Molloy College
Rockville Centre, NY

Pamela G. Harrison, EdD, RN, CNE
Professor of Nursing
Indiana Wesleyan University
Marion, Indiana

Judy R. Hembd, RN, MSN
Instructor
MSU-Northern Department of Nursing
Havre, Montana

Lori Hendrickx, RN, EdD, CCRN
Professor
South Dakota State University
Brookings, South Dakota

Dr. Jennifer Hill, DNP, ARNP
Nurse Practitioner and Clinical Instructor
Blank Children's Health Center
Des Moines, Iowa

Nancy Hutton-Haynes, RN, PhD, CCRN
Assistant Professor
Saint Luke's College
Kansas City, Missouri

Saundra E. Hyman, BSN, RN
Adjunct Clinical Faculty
La Salle University
Philadelphia, Pennsylvania

Robert L. Ismeurt, PhD, RN
Associate Professor
Arizona State University, College of Nursing
    and Healthcare Innovation
Phoenix, Arizona

Marilyn Nelsen Pase, RN, MSN, BSN, BS Biology, CEL Online Graduate Teaching Certificate,
NMSU Department of Education
Associate Professor, School of Nursing
New Mexico State University
Las Cruces, New Mexico

Cathy Penn, MS, RN, CRRN
Associate Professor of Nursing
Mount Mercy University
Cedar Rapids, Iowa

Jack Pennington, PhD
Professor
Barnes-Jewish College
St. Louis, Missouri

Katherine C. Pereira, DNP, RN, FNP-BC, ADM-BC, FAAN, FAANP
Associate Professor
Duke University
Durham, North Carolina

Carrie L. Pucino, DEd, RN, CCRN
Assistant Professor
York College of Pennsylvania
York, Pennsylvania

Donna Rawlin, RN, BScN, MSc (T), PhD (student)
Professor and Coordinator, Learning Resource Center
Mohawk College
Hamilton, Ontario
Canada

Illa Reeve, RN, MS
BSN Program Director
Presentation College
Aberdeen, South Dakota

Maela Rizon-Babate, RN, MAN
Assistant Professor
Notre Dame of Dadiangas University, College of Health Sciences
General Santos City, Philippines

Jan Rodd, RN, MN
Assistant Professor, Department of Nursing
Albany State University
Albany, Georgia

Elizabeth Ruddick, MSN
Professor of Nursing
Central Methodist University
Fayette, Missouri

Anne C. Russell, PhD, RN, CNS-BC
Associate Professor
Associate Director, Adult-Gerontology Clinical Nurse Specialist Concentration
Wright State University-Miami Valley, College of Nursing & Health
Dayton, Ohio

Bedelia H. Russell, PhD (c), MSN, RN, CPNP-PC, CNE
Interim Dean, Assistant Professor
Whitson-Hester School of Nursing, Tennessee Tech University
Cookeville, Tennessee

Hazel Sanderson-Marcoux, EdD, RN
Associate Dean, School of Nursing
Long Island University, Brooklyn Campus
Brooklyn, New York

Dr. Maura C. Schlairet, RN, MSN, EdD
Assistant Professor
Valdosta State University, College of Nursing
Valdosta, Georgia

Jane P. Shelby, RN, MSN
Associate Professor, Director of Undergraduate Studies
Belmont University School of Nursing
Nashville, Tennessee

Gayle H. Shiba, DNSc
Associate Professor
University of Memphis
Cordova, Tennessee

John Silver, PhD, RN, MBAC
Fellow–Institute of Nursing Leadership
Nova Southeastern University
Ft. Lauderdale, Florida

Melissa S. Smith, DNP, FNP-BC
Assistant Professor
UMKC-SON
Kansas City, Missouri

Traci Snedden, MSN, PNP
Clinical Instructor
University of Colorado
Denver, Colorado

Margaret Stinner, RN, MS
Instructor, Pathophysiology
Mount Carmel College of Nursing
Columbus, Ohio

CONTENTS IN BRIEF

CONTENTS

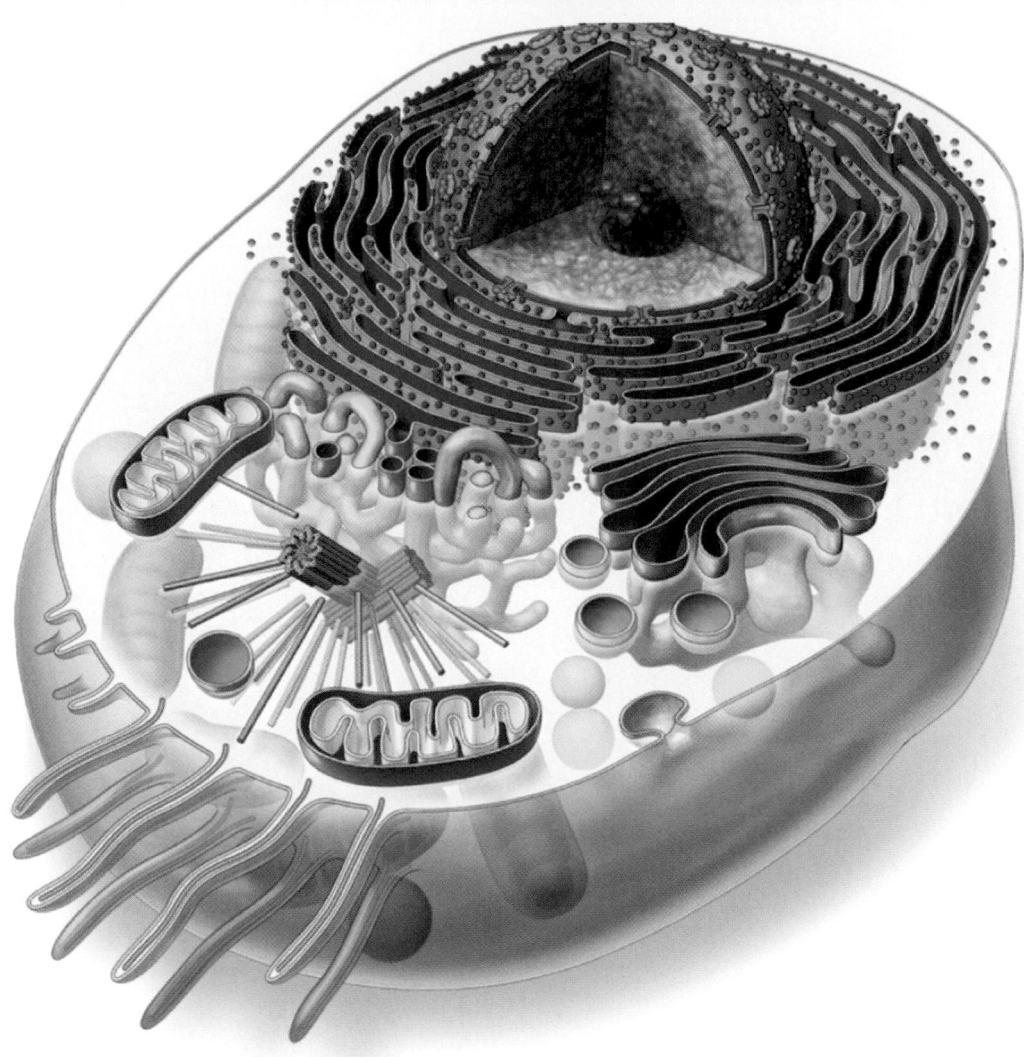

Chapters

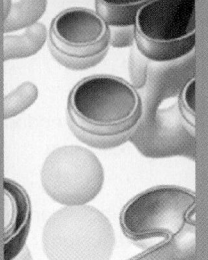

The Cell in Health and Illness

Key Terms

Aerobic metabolism

Anaerobic metabolism

Autolysis

Cellular dehydration

Cellular edema

Cellular hypoxia

Codon

Deoxyribonucleic acid (DNA)

Free radicals

Glycoproteins

Heterolysis

Lysosomes

Mitochondria

Na$^+$/K$^+$ ATPase pump

Nucleotide

Plasma membrane

Purine base

Pyrimidine base

Ribosomes

Transcription

Translation

All forms of disease start with disruptions of normal cellular structure and function, which is why tissues and their cellular components need to be examined when studying illness. Biochemical diagnostic studies provide insight into these physiologic changes. Because disease is initiated at the cellular level, it is first necessary to understand the cell's basic internal microenvironment.

Cell Structure and Function

All body tissues and organs are composed of cells—the basic unit in which all structural, functional, and environmental alterations occur in disease processes. Each cell performs internal processes vital for the body's normal physiologic function. Specialized intracellular structures, called organelles, carry out specific activities to sustain life. At the same time, cells sense and respond to their external environment while freely exchanging materials and energy with their surroundings. Through these actions, cells ensure homeostasis, regulating the internal environment to maintain balance and equilibrium in response to internal and external changes. When these responses are compromised, illness occurs. In other words, an illness of the whole organism is the macroscopic presentation of what is occurring at a microscopic level within the cell.

The cell is bounded by a **plasma membrane** and composed of cytoplasm, organelles, and a nucleus. Cytoplasm is a colloidal internal fluid environment that contains water, ions, proteins, carbohydrates, and lipids; it is a gel-like substance that suspends the cellular organelles within it (see Fig. 1-1). The nucleus contains genetic material, otherwise known as **deoxyribonucleic acid (DNA),** that ultimately regulates cellular activity.

Normal cell function, including the cell's major functions of growth, energy production and metabolism, replication, and protein synthesis, requires synchronized organelle function, biochemical processes, and specific environmental conditions. Disease most commonly arises from dysfunction of one or more of the cellular organelles, proteins, or biochemical processes. This chapter will review concepts regarding the structure and function of the major cellular organelles and clinical consequences of their dysfunction from a clinical perspective.

The Plasma Membrane

The plasma membrane acts as a barrier from the cell's external environment and protects the internal organelles from injury. The cell's outside layer separates the intracellular and extracellular environments (see Fig. 1-1). Its major component is a phospholipid bilayer that contains proteins and cholesterol. The protein structures have varied functions, some of which include ion channels for exchange with the extracellular environment (see Fig. 1-2). The plasma membrane is semipermeable, which means it selectively allows substances in or out.

Extracellular and intracellular fluid, ions, and other molecules can diffuse back and forth through the pores of the semipermeable plasma membrane. The core lipid region remains impermeable to water and water-soluble substances while at the same time allowing lipid-soluble substances such as oxygen and carbon dioxide to diffuse across. When disease alters the plasma membrane's configuration, excess fluid can enter the cell's internal environment, causing swelling; this is referred to as **cellular edema.** Conversely, intracellular fluid can leak out of the cell through the pores, causing cell shrinkage; this is termed **cellular dehydration.** Either

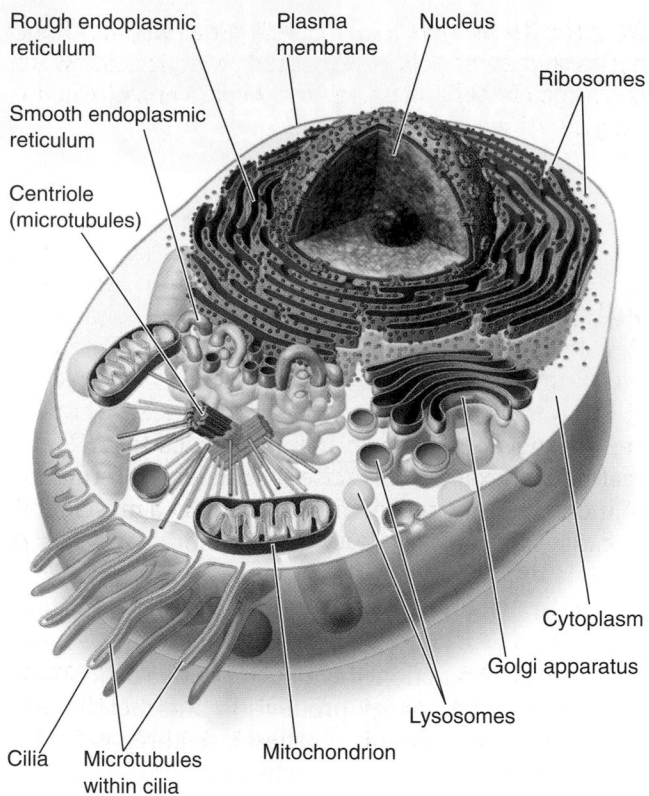

FIGURE 1-1. The cell is the body's basic structural unit. It contains a nucleus, which houses the DNA. It also contains organelles, which are surrounded by cytoplasm.

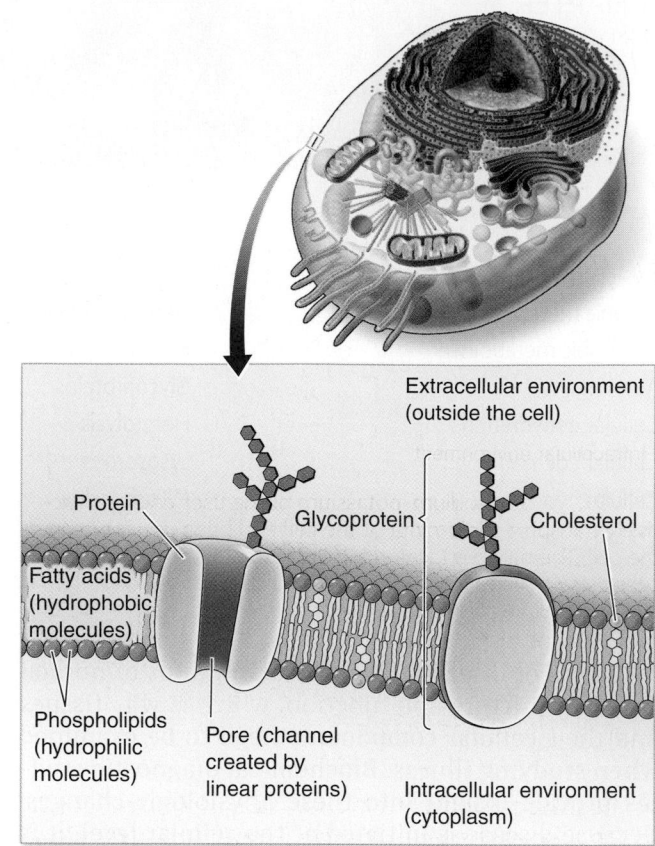

FIGURE 1-2. The plasma membrane consists mainly of lipids and proteins. The membrane's fundamental structure is the phospholipid bilayer, which forms a stable barrier between the extracellular compartment, which is the outside of the cell, and the intracellular compartment, which is the inside of the cell. Proteins embedded within the phospholipid bilayer carry out the specific functions of the plasma membrane, which include active transport of molecules.

cellular edema or dehydration can disrupt organelle function.

On the plasma membrane's outer surface, carbohydrates attach to cell surface protein molecules; these structures are called **glycoproteins** (see Fig. 1-2). Glycoproteins are surface markers, also called antigens, that identify cells as part of the individual's own tissues. For example, a red blood cell contains glycoprotein surface markers that identify the individual's blood type as A, B, O, or AB. When any of these cellular surface markers are altered, the immune system will recognize them as foreign and provoke an attack on the cell. Identifying "self" from "non-self" substances is a major function of the immune system. The provocation of the immune system is the basis for allergies, autoimmune disorders, transplant rejection, and transfusion reactions.

Damage to the plasma membrane causes a breach in the security of the cell's interior environment. A damaged plasma membrane leaves all organelles open to injurious agents. It is particularly dangerous to leave the nucleus, which contains the DNA, vulnerable to injury.

The Sodium-Potassium Pump

For optimal cell function, it is necessary for potassium (K^+) ions to be at a higher concentration inside the cell compartment and for sodium (Na^+) to be at higher concentration outside the cell. The plasma membrane is more soluble to K^+ ions and less soluble to Na^+ ions, so K^+ ions tend to leak out of the cell and Na^+ ions are

retained. Also, because of osmosis, water tends to travel from outside the cell to inside it. This causes a gradient of more positivity outside the cell than inside the cell.

The maintenance of the cellular movement of Na^+ outside and K^+ inside requires energy. The sodium-potassium pump uses adenosine triphosphate (ATP) to constantly move these two ions in opposite directions across the plasma membrane (see Fig. 1-3). The mechanism is called active transport by Na^+/K^+ ATPase. In active transport, for every three sodium ions pumped out, two potassium ions are pumped in. In this way, the **Na^+/K^+ ATPase pump** helps maintain resting potential and cellular fluid volume. For most animal cells, the Na^+/K^+ ATPase pump is responsible for one-third of the cell's energy expenditure. For neurons, the Na^+/K^+ ATPase pump is responsible for two-thirds of the cell's energy expenditure.

The Na^+/K^+ ATPase pump can be pharmacologically altered through the administration of certain drugs. For instance, the Na^+/K^+ ATPase pump found in the membrane of heart cells is an important target for cardiac glycosides, which are drugs used to improve the force of the heart's contraction. In heart muscle cells, the Na^+/K^+ ATPase pump works to pump calcium out

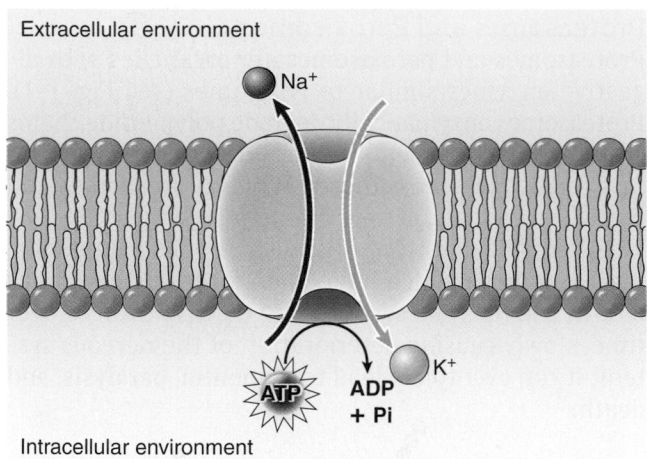

Extracellular environment

Intracellular environment

FIGURE 1-3. The sodium-potassium pump uses energy to actively transport sodium out of the cell and bring potassium into the cell. The pump is located in the plasma membrane of all cells. Active transport is responsible for the intracellular compartment containing relatively high concentrations of potassium ions but low concentrations of sodium ions. The pump moves these two ions in opposite directions across the plasma membrane. For every three sodium ions pumped out, two potassium ions are pumped in.

of the internal environment of the heart muscle cells, which relaxes the heart muscle. Pharmacological slowdown of the Na^+/K^+ ATPase pump keeps more calcium inside the heart muscle cell, strengthening its force of contraction.

Mitochondria

Mitochondria are the cell's energy producers. Cell types differ in their number of mitochondria according to their energy needs. For example, muscle cells have abundant numbers of mitochondria because they require a high amount of energy to function, whereas bone cells have fewer mitochondria. The mitochondria's primary function is to convert organic nutrients into cell energy in the form of ATP. Mitochondria accomplish this through the process of **aerobic metabolism,** which requires oxygen. When no oxygen is available for cells, a situation called **cellular hypoxia,** the cell converts to another form of metabolism: **anaerobic metabolism.** Anaerobic metabolism, also referred to as glycolysis, occurs outside the mitochondria. In anaerobic metabolism, glucose is used to create energy.

Energy Metabolism
Aerobic metabolism requires oxygen and provides the maximum amount of energy for cellular function: a net yield of 34 ATP. When oxygen is not available, anaerobic metabolism produces significantly less cellular energy: a net yield of 2 ATP as well as pyruvic acid.

Pyruvic acid is converted into acetyl-coenzyme A, which triggers a series of reactions known as the Krebs cycle, also called the citric acid cycle. With the use of oxygen, mitochondria produce a net yield of 34 ATP

from the Krebs cycle (see Fig. 1-4). However, in cellular hypoxia, pyruvic acid is converted to lactic acid, which is noxious to cells, causing muscle pain and biochemical alterations such as acidosis.

Mitochondrial DNA
Mitochondria are unique because they are the only cellular organelles that have their own distinctive DNA. Cell biologists speculate that mitochondria were self-sustaining, independent-living, bacteria-like organisms that, over the course of evolution, became incorporated into human cells. However, because they contain their own DNA, they are also able to reproduce within the cell whenever there is an increased need for ATP formation. For example, exercise stimulates the formation of increased numbers of mitochondria in a muscle cell. Because of this, the muscle uses more oxygen and yields more energy.

During human fertilization, the sperm provides minimal mitochondria, which results in almost all the mitochondrial DNA being derived maternally. Because of this unique characteristic of mitochondrial DNA, geneticists use it to study an individual's maternal hereditary lineage.

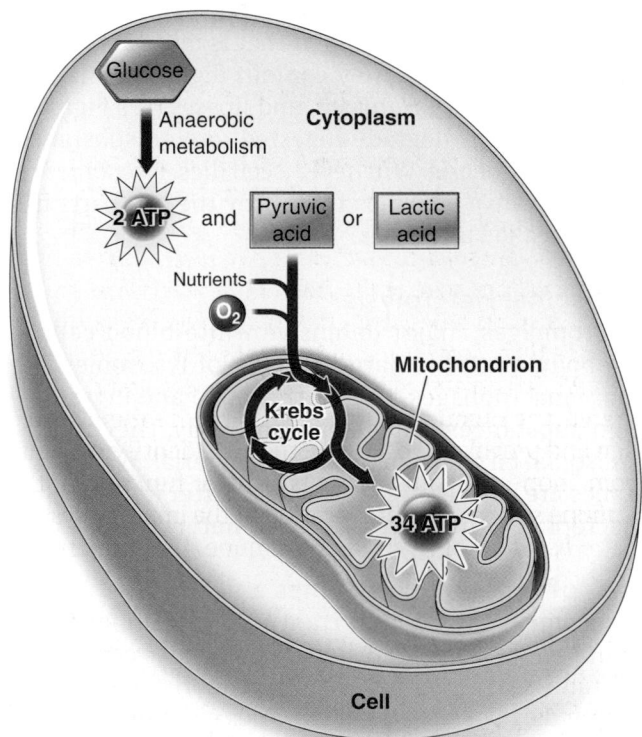

FIGURE 1-4. Cellular energy production. The mitochondrion uses oxygen to produce a net yield of 34 ATP through the process of aerobic metabolism. When no oxygen is available, the cell enters anaerobic metabolism to convert glucose to 2 ATP and pyruvic acid, which occurs outside the mitochondria in the cytoplasm. In the presence of oxygen, pyruvic acid is converted into acetyl coenzyme A, which triggers the Krebs cycle, also called the citric acid cycle. However, in cellular hypoxia, pyruvic acid is converted to lactic acid, which is noxious to cells, causing muscle pain and biochemical alterations such as acidosis.

Mitochondrial DNA is subject to mutation by oxygen-derived **free radicals,** also called reactive oxygen species. It is theorized that in aging and in disorders such as diabetes, cancer, and heart failure, mitochondrial DNA undergoes mutations and the mitochondrial damage is partly responsible for the cellular impairment observed in the diseases. There are also diseases that target mitochondria specifically. Injury of mitochondria can occur in the cells of different organs, and mitochondrial disease causes a wide array of problems, including energy depletion and severe muscle weakness (see Chapter 3: Genetic Basis of Disease).

 CLINICAL CONCEPT

Mitochondrial diseases are worse when the defective mitochondria are present in the muscles, cerebrum, or nerves, because these cells use more energy than most other cells in the body.

Lysosomes

Lysosomes are small, membrane-enclosed organelles with an internal environment that is more acidic than the rest of the cell. They contain digestive enzymes such as lysozyme, proteases, and lipases (see Fig. 1-1). These enzymes degrade ingested foreign substances and cellular debris. Whenever a cell dies, lysosomes release digestive enzymes to destroy the cell parts in a process called **autolysis.**

Lysosomal Heterolysis

Macrophages, major defensive white blood cells of the body, contain a large number of lysosomes. Because macrophages constantly engulf and ingest foreign substances that invade the body, they rely on lysosomal enzymes to digest the material. When lysosomes are used to digest foreign matter ingested by a macrophage, the process is called **heterolysis.**

Lack of Lysosomal Enzymes and Disease

Lysosomes play an important part in cellular metabolic processes. Lysosomal enzymes constantly degrade waste products, cellular debris, and foreign matter. Lack of lysosomal enzymes can cause a harmful accumulation of a nondegraded substance. For example, Tay Sachs disease is a lipid storage disease resulting from a deficiency in a lysosomal enzyme. This causes the accumulation of ganglioside, a specific type of lipid found in the central nervous system. Ganglioside then accumulates in the cells of the liver, heart, nervous system, retina, and spleen, causing organ dysfunction and widespread systemic illness.

Proteasomes and Peroxisomes

Proteasomes and peroxisomes are organelles with digestive enzymes similar to lysosomes (see Fig. 1-1). Proteasomes enzymatically degrade polypeptide chains and proteins while peroxisomes break down long chain fatty acids and free radicals. When proteasomes and peroxisomes malfunction, disease can occur.

Adrenoleukodystrophy is a disorder of dysfunctional peroxisomes in which long chain fatty acids accumulate in the nervous system. The disease evolves over time, slowly causing deterioration of the nervous system; it can eventually lead to dementia, paralysis, and death.

 CLINICAL CONCEPT

Accelerated cellular proteasome activity occurs in cachexia (wasting of body mass) associated with cancer.

Endoplasmic Reticulum

The endoplasmic reticulum (ER) is a network of tubules within the cell that act as a transport system. There are two main types of ER: smooth and rough. The smooth ER is the location for lipid production, which includes corticosteroids, oils, and phospholipids. The rough ER is a tubular network with attached ribosomes that synthesize proteins. During ER stress, proteins cannot travel to their proper intracellular locations and are rapidly degraded. Increasing numbers of studies suggest that ER stress is involved in the pathogenesis of a number of diseases, including neurodegenerative diseases, cancer, obesity, diabetes, and atherosclerosis.

Ribosomes

Ribosomes are small, spherical organelles composed of ribosomal ribonucleic acid (rRNA). Some are free-standing within the cytoplasm and some are attached to rough ER. Ribosomes can be likened to cellular "protein factories" (see Fig. 1-1). Proteins manufactured by ribosomes are destined to become parts of the cell, enzymes, or exported protein secretions. Different types of cells manufacture different proteins. For example, ribosomes in pancreatic beta islet cells synthesize the proteins that make up insulin, whereas thyroid cell ribosomes manufacture proteins that build thyroxine. In all cells, protein synthesis by the ribosomes is directed by specific information received from the nucleus. Messenger RNA (mRNA) from the nucleus acts as a blueprint for the construction of proteins. Transfer RNA (tRNA) plays a key role in the assembly of proteins. During severe hypoxic states, ribosomal protein synthesis ceases.

Golgi Apparatus

Once protein synthesis has been completed by ribosomes, the proteins are transported via ER to the Golgi apparatus to be processed, packaged, and secreted (see Fig. 1-1).

An example of this process is seen in the formation of hormones such as insulin and adrenocorticotropic hormone (ACTH). The initial protein is manufactured in the ribosome and referred to as a preprohormone. The preprohormone contains a signal peptide that directs its transfer to the ER. As the preprohormone is transferred from the ribosome to the ER, the signal peptide is removed. At this point it is referred to as a prohormone and is transported to the Golgi apparatus. Within the Golgi apparatus, further processing converts the prohormone into the actual hormone that will be secreted by the endocrine gland's cells. This processing may include dividing the prohormone into smaller units or the addition of carbohydrate units. The completed hormone is stored in a secretory granule within the Golgi apparatus until it leaves the cell to be secreted by the gland.

Secretory Vesicles

Secretory vesicles, which are formed by the endoplasmic reticulum-Golgi apparatus system, store substances that are secreted by cells prior to their release. Secretory vesicles move to the cell's periphery, waiting for the release of their contents into the extracellular space.

Microtubules and Microfilaments

Microtubules are hollow filaments composed of protein subunits called tubulin. They have a dynamic structure, meaning that they are constantly being formed, broken down, and reformed. Microtubules comprise structures involved in cell division such as centrioles and the mitotic spindle. They also provide a pathway for transporting secretory vesicles to the cell's perimeter. For example, microtubules form tunnel-like pathways for the movement of neurotransmitters down the axon of a neuron to the synapse.

Cilia are cellular projections that contain microtubules. The movement of cilia propels substances along the outside of the cells. An example of this is seen in the mucociliary apparatus of the respiratory tract. The ciliated respiratory epithelial cells propel mucous and inhaled debris out of the lung through a sweeping motion.

Microfilaments are solid, flexible fibers, sometimes referred to as actin filaments. Microfilaments help the cell change shape as seen in the amoeboid movements of macrophages and contraction of muscles. Actin and myosin are the key proteins in the contractile units of muscle cells. During contraction, one end of the actin filament elongates while the other end contracts.

The Nucleus

The nucleus is the cell's master mind. It contains the body's genetic material, DNA, which regulates all cell structure and function. DNA consists of extremely long, double-stranded helical chains containing variable sequences of **nucleotides,** known as the DNA double helix. The DNA nucleotides consist of nitrogenous bases and a phosphate bound to a pentose (five-carbon sugar) called deoxyribose. The nitrogenous bases are either **purine bases,** consisting of adenine and guanine, or **pyrimidine bases,** consisting of thymine and cytosine. The DNA molecule resembles a twisted ladder with phosphate-pentose backbone and the purine–pyrimidine base pairs represented by the individual steps on the ladder (see Fig. 1-5). These uniquely sequenced base pairs form the individual's genetic code.

Within the helical structure of DNA, there is a precise pairing of purine and pyrimidine bases: Adenine always binds with thymine and guanine always binds with cytosine. This precise pairing of the nitrogenous bases provides DNA with the unique molecular ability to replicate.

DNA Replication

When DNA reproduces or replicates itself, both strands are duplicated, resulting in two identical DNA helices. However, as a result of the replication process, each DNA helix contains one original strand and one newly formed daughter strand.

Specific enzymes called DNA polymerase are involved in the process of DNA replication. First, the DNA strand uncoils and begins to split into two separate strands. One strand becomes a template and the new nucleotides begin to pair up in an orderly fashion with the DNA template strand. As the purine bases pair up with the pyrimidine bases, hydrogen bonds are formed. This bonding enables the newly created daughter strand to be formed alongside the original strand. At the completion of the process, there are two identical strands of DNA.

Transcription and Translation

Protein synthesis is a requirement for normal physiologic function. DNA directs the cell to carry out protein synthesis through a two-step process known as **transcription,** which occurs in the nucleus, and **translation,** which occurs in the ribosome.

During transcription, the two strands of the helical DNA structure uncoil and separate. One of the strands

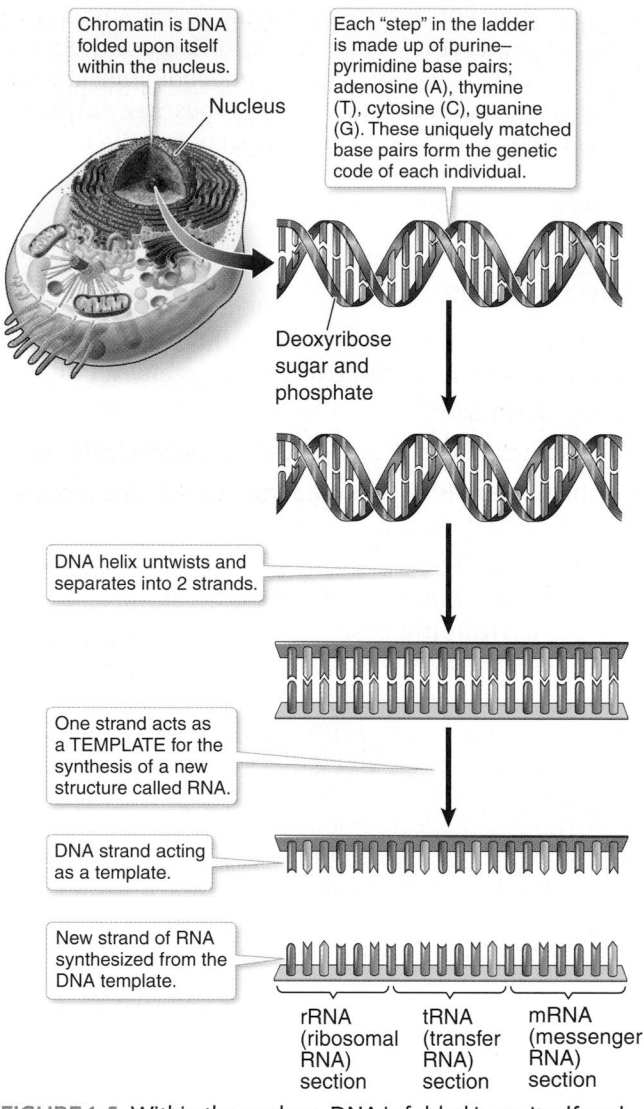

Chromatin is DNA folded upon itself within the nucleus.

Nucleus

Each "step" in the ladder is made up of purine–pyrimidine base pairs; adenosine (A), thymine (T), cytosine (C), guanine (G). These uniquely matched base pairs form the genetic code of each individual.

Deoxyribose sugar and phosphate

DNA helix untwists and separates into 2 strands.

One strand acts as a TEMPLATE for the synthesis of a new structure called RNA.

DNA strand acting as a template.

New strand of RNA synthesized from the DNA template.

rRNA (ribosomal RNA) section tRNA (transfer RNA) section mRNA (messenger RNA) section

FIGURE 1-5. Within the nucleus, DNA is folded in on itself and is known as chromatin. When DNA is stretched out, it forms a double helix that resembles a twisted ladder with purine-pyrimidine nitrogenous base pairs represented by the individual steps on the ladder. The purine-pyrimidine nitrogenous base pairs consist of amino acids adenosine, cytosine, thymine, and guanine. These are matched in a unique sequence to form an individual's distinctive genetic code.

acts as a template for the synthesis of RNA. RNA differs from DNA in some important ways; for example, it is single stranded and can travel to sites outside of the nucleus. The pentose sugar in RNA is ribose, and the pyrimidine base thymine is replaced with uracil.

The RNA molecule copies genetic information from the main DNA molecule and then leaves the nucleus. The RNA molecule is composed of three types of RNA (see Fig. 1-6):

1. mRNA
2. tRNA
3. Ribosomal RNA (rRNA).

Protein Synthesis

The single RNA strand transports the genetic information for protein synthesis from the nuclear DNA to the

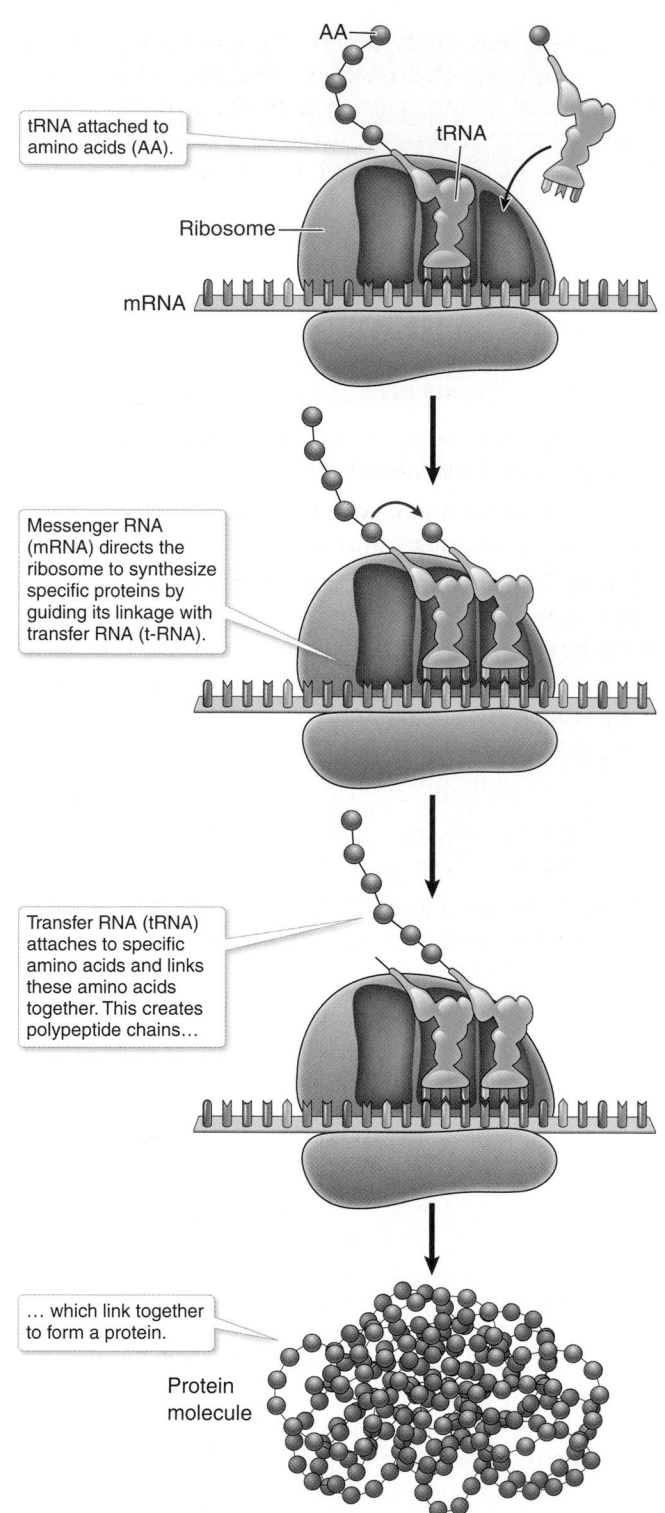

AA

tRNA attached to amino acids (AA).

tRNA

Ribosome

mRNA

Messenger RNA (mRNA) directs the ribosome to synthesize specific proteins by guiding its linkage with transfer RNA (t-RNA).

Transfer RNA (tRNA) attaches to specific amino acids and links these amino acids together. This creates polypeptide chains…

… which link together to form a protein.

Protein molecule

FIGURE 1-6. Translation. Following the process of transcription, the process of translation occurs at the ribosome. This is how RNA transfers genetic information to the ribosome for the synthesis of specific cellular proteins.

ribosomes. At the ribosomes, RNA begins the next process called translation. During translation, ribosomes interpret the message from mRNA in order to manufacture proteins. tRNA gathers and joins the exact amino acids that will form the protein designated by mRNA (see Fig. 1-6). Ribosomal RNA is mainly involved in the formation of the ribosome itself.

There is specificity within the combination of nitrogenous bases that enables selection of the correct sequence of amino acids to form the desired protein. Three nitrogenous bases form a **codon** that is interpreted by the ribosome. Each codon has a specific link to an exact amino acid. One codon signals the start of protein synthesis, other codons link to specific amino acids, and another codon signals the end of the protein synthesis. By interpreting the codons, specific proteins are formed to meet the cell's needs.

Chapter Summary

- The plasma membrane is a semipermeable barrier.
- A defect in the plasma membrane's integrity allows organelles to be vulnerable to injury.
- Glycoproteins are surface markers that identify cells as part of the individual's own tissues.
- The sodium-potassium pump, which maintains the cellular movement of Na^+ outside and K^+ inside the cell, requires energy.
- Aerobic metabolism occurs at the mitochondria and yields 34 ATP.
- Anaerobic metabolism occurs outside the mitochondria within the cell and yields 2 ATP, as well as lactic acid.
- The mitochondria have their own DNA that is solely inherited from the individual's mother.
- Lysosomes are small spherical organelles that contain digestive enzymes and perform autolysis or heterolysis.
- Proteosomes break down proteins and peroxisomes break down lipids.
- Ribosomes can be likened to cellular protein factories.
- In the nucleus, RNA is formed from DNA in the process called transcription.
- At the ribosomes, messenger RNA provides the direction for specific protein synthesis.
- DNA is composed of purine bases, consisting of adenine and guanine, and pyrimidine bases, consisting of thymine and cytosine.
- RNA is composed of purine bases consisting of adenine and guanine, and pyrimidine bases, consisting of uracil and cytosine.

Bibliography

Barrett, K., Barman, S., Boitano, S., & Brooks, H. (2012). *Ganong's review of medical physiology.* 24th ed. New York, NY: McGraw-Hill.

Hall, J. (2011). *Guyton & Hall textbook of medical physiology.* 12th ed. Philadelphia, PA: Elsevier.

Harvey, R. A., & Ferrier, D. R. (2013). *Lippincott's illustrated reviews: biochemistry.* 6th ed. Philadelphia, PA: Wolters Kluwer.

Katzung, B. G., Masters, S., & Trevor, A. (2012). *Basic and clinical pharmacology.* 12th ed. New York, NY: Lange Medical Books/McGraw-Hill Companies.

Kumar, V., Abbas, A. K., & Aster, J. C. (2014). *Robbins & Cotran pathologic basis of disease.* 9th ed. Philadelphia, PA: Elsevier Saunders.

National Institutes of Health. (2014). Stem cell basics. Retrieved from http://stemcells.nih.gov/info/basics/Pages/Default.aspx

National Library of Medicine. (2012). What is mitochondrial DNA? Retrieved from http://ghr.nlm.nih.gov/handbook/basics/mtdna

Nature. (2014a). Human genome collection. Retrieved from http://www.nature.com/nature/supplements/collections/humangenome/

Nature. (2014b). Senescence, ageing and cancer. Retrieved from http://www.nature.com/nature/focus/senescence/

The 1000 Genomes Project Consortium. (2011). A map of human genome variation from population-scale sequencing. Retrieved from http://www.nature.com/nature/journal/v467/n7319/full/nature09534.html

U.S. Department of Energy. (2014). Human Genome Project information. Retrieved from http://web.ornl.gov/sci/techresources/Human_Genome/index.shtml

United Mitochondrial Disease Foundation. (2014). What is mitochondrial disease? Retrieved from http://www.umdf.org/site/pp.aspx?c=8qKOJ0MvF7LUG&b=7934627

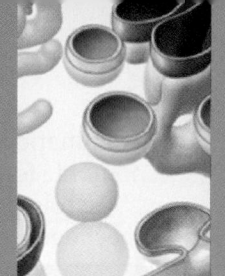

Cellular Injury, Adaptations, and Maladaptive Changes

Key Terms

Aneurysm

Angiogenesis

Apoptosis

Atherogenesis

Atrophy

Benign

Biopsy

Dysplasia

Etiology

Gangrene

Histology

Hyperplasia

Hypertrophy

Infarction

Ischemia

Malignant

Metaplasia

Neoplasia

Oxidative stress

Pathognomonic changes

Pathological hypertrophy

Physiologic hypertrophy

The human body's intricate processes are vulnerable to many kinds of insults and stresses that can cause cells to take on distinctive changes and put the body's normal function and structure at risk for either temporary or permanent injury.

Injurious agents are also known as etiologic agents; an **etiology** is the original cause of a cellular alteration or disease. For example, the etiology of a sore throat is commonly streptococcus, a bacterial organism. On microscopic examination, cells infected with streptococcus demonstrate distinctive alterations associated with the infection, including inflammation and swelling.

In general, cells exhibit characteristic changes associated with specific etiologic agents or changes in their environment. Different etiologic agents create distinctive cellular changes, for example:

- Exposure to extreme cold temperatures will cause localized frostbite and tissue necrosis.
- Exposure to electrical current can burn tissue and cause cardiac rhythm disturbances.
- Alcohol abuse can cause the liver to take on characteristic fatty changes.

Cells are capable of maintaining homeostasis in the face of temporary stressors, insults, or changes in their environment. However, prolonged or severe insults can cause homeostasis to be disrupted. Therefore, under the influence of different etiologic agents, cells can do one of two things:

1. Develop adaptive, compensatory changes in an attempt to maintain homeostasis.
2. Develop maladaptive changes, which are derangements of structure or function.

In circumstances of overwhelming insult, cell injury or cell death can occur. Cell injury can be reversible, but if the injurious agent is persistent or severe enough, cell injury can lead to cell death.

> ## CLINICAL CONCEPT
>
> The point at which cells can no longer achieve reversible changes varies according to type of cell. For example, brain cells cannot withstand low oxygen delivery (hypoxia) for more than 6 minutes, whereas skeletal muscle can tolerate hypoxia for prolonged periods of time.

Basic Concepts of Cellular Adaptations, and Maladaptive Changes

Cellular adaptations and maladaptive changes occur as a result of specific disease processes, altered cell function, or environmental influences. Cells that undergo these changes develop distinctive structural or functional characteristics. The study of specific cell alterations can assist clinicians in identifying the etiology and predicting the consequences of cell changes.

Histology is the microscopic study of tissues and cells, and it yields important diagnostic information for the clinician. A **biopsy** extracts a cell sample from an organ or mass of tissue to allow for histological examination. Identifiable histological findings can assist clinicians in identifying the etiology of cellular changes. Unique histological findings that represent distinct disease processes are referred to as **pathognomonic changes.** For example, an inflamed, craterlike breach in the gastrointestinal mucosa, as seen on an endoscopic examination of the stomach and duodenum, is pathognomonic for peptic ulcer disease.

Histological changes are also examined on autopsy specimens. An autopsy is an examination of the tissues and organs of a deceased individual that allows for a study of the cause of death. Clinicians can learn significant details about cellular adaptations, maladaptations, cell injury, and cell death from autopsy specimens. The following sections detail the most common adaptive and maladaptive cellular changes encountered in patients in the clinical setting.

Atrophy

Atrophy is a cellular adaptation in which cells revert to a smaller size in response to changes in metabolic requirements or their environment. Atrophy occurs when a cell's environment cannot support its metabolic requirements. The cell's smaller size allows for less metabolic demand and more efficient functioning that is compatible with survival.

Atrophy is best exemplified by the shrinking of skeletal muscle cells in an individual with lower extremity paralysis (see Fig. 2-1). Paralysis causes lack of muscle contraction, loss of nerve stimulation, and decreased workload of leg muscles. Gradually, the size of skeletal muscle cells decreases and they undergo diminished metabolic activity. Other causes of cellular atrophy include:

- Disuse or diminished workload
- Lack of nerve stimulation (paralysis)
- Loss of hormonal stimulation
- Inadequate nutrition
- Decreased blood flow (ischemia)
- Aging.

Hypertrophy

Hypertrophy is an increase in individual cell size that results in an enlargement of functioning tissue mass (see Fig. 2-1). In hypertrophy, each individual cell becomes larger. Hypertrophy increases the cell's functional components, which leads to greater metabolic demand and energy needs.

Physiologic Hypertrophy vs. Pathological Hypertrophy

Hypertrophy can occur as a result of normal physiologic stimuli or abnormal pathological conditions. Normal physiologic stimuli include exercise, which increases muscle mass. Exercise stimulates physiologic hypertrophy of muscle cells, enhances the functional components of each cell, and increases the number of blood vessels that perfuse the enlarged muscle. Exercise stimulates **angiogenesis,** which is the growth of new blood vessel branches. Exercise also increases the number of mitochondria in each muscle cell, which in turn increases energy production. For example, a weightlifter

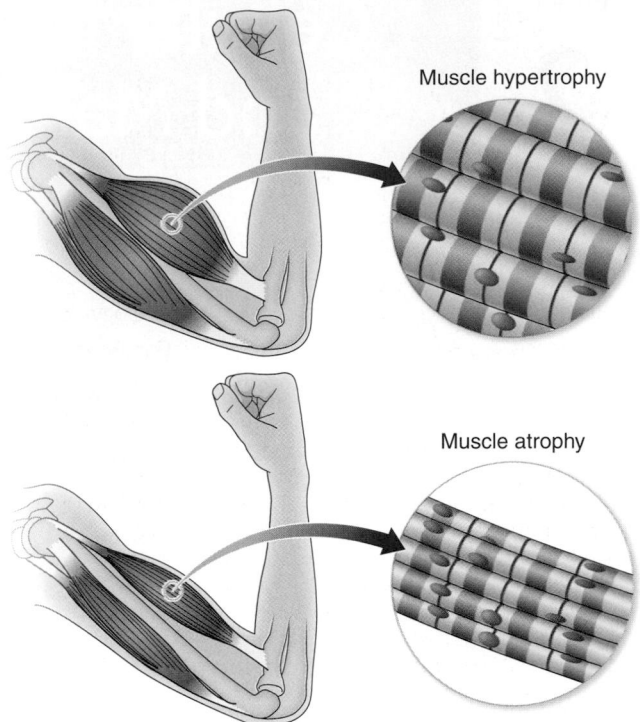

FIGURE 2-1. Skeletal muscle cell atrophy versus hypertrophy. Atrophy of the arm muscle occurs when skeletal muscle cells revert to a smaller size in response to changes in their environment, such as lack of circulation, diminished workload (disuse), or decreased neural stimulation. Conversely, hypertrophy of the arm muscle occurs when skeletal muscle cells enlarge in size in response to increased workload.

who wants to develop stronger biceps lifts weights to increase workload on the biceps muscles. The increased workload stimulates increased size of each skeletal muscle cell within each biceps muscle. The stimulus for hypertrophy increases the muscle cell's actin and myosin filaments, enzymes, mitochondria, blood vessel growth, and adenosine triphosphate (ATP) production.

In **physiologic hypertrophy,** the enlarged muscle is adequately perfused and supplied with blood flow, oxygen, and nutrients because of angiogenesis. In well-trained athletes, the heart physiologically hypertrophies because of the enlargement of each individual myocardial cell. There is a proportional increase in myocardial cell size and enhancement of coronary blood supply of the myocardial cells. Therefore, the enlarged heart in an athlete is supplied with abundant coronary artery blood flow, which delivers large amounts of oxygen and nutrients (see Fig. 2-2).

Pathological hypertrophy occurs when there is an increase in cellular size without an increase in the supportive structures necessary for the enlarged cell's increased metabolic needs. Pathological hypertrophy of cells can occur in disease processes or may be a compensatory maladaptation to changed environmental conditions. For example, in hypertension, blood pressure within the aorta and systemic arterial circulation is elevated. High aortic blood pressure creates a higher workload for the left ventricle; in response, each cardiac

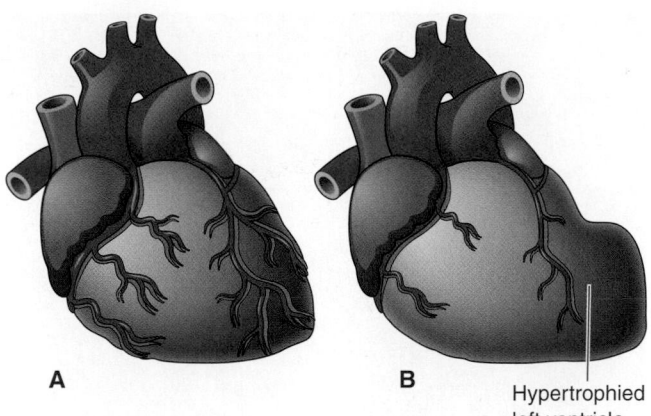

A   **B**

Hypertrophied
left ventricle

FIGURE 2-2. Physiologic versus pathological hypertrophy of heart muscle. (A) In physiologic hypertrophy, the heart muscle is proportionately enlarged and significant coronary blood vessel growth occurs, allowing for sufficient coronary blood flow. (B) In this figure, there is disproportionate enlargement of the left ventricle compared with the remainder of the heart muscle. This is pathological hypertrophy of the left ventricle, which occurs in long-standing hypertension. In pathological hypertrophy, there is lack of growth of coronary vasculature to supply the enlarged cardiac muscle.

muscle cell undergoes pathological hypertrophy. Although each cardiac muscle cell increases in size, in pathological hypertrophy there is no corresponding increase in blood vessel growth to supply these muscle cells. As each cardiac muscle cell in the left ventricle undergoes hypertrophy, the whole left ventricle eventually hypertrophies. This resulting enlarged left ventricular muscle mass has an increased need for oxygen and blood flow; however, without concurrent growth of blood vessels it outgrows its supply of coronary blood flow and is susceptible to effects of inadequate blood flow, also called **ischemia.**

Hyperplasia

Hyperplasia is the increase in the number of cells in a tissue or organ. It only occurs in tissues with cells that are capable of mitotic division, such as the epithelium and glandular tissue. Although new research suggests that nerves and cardiac cells may be able to divide, it is generally thought that those cells, along with brain and skeletal muscle cells, do not undergo mitosis and are not capable of hyperplasia.

Hyperplasia is stimulated by hormonal or compensatory cellular mechanisms. An example of hormonal stimulation of hyperplasia occurs in pregnancy, when estrogen stimulation results in mitotic division of breast gland cells.

Hyperplasia can also occur as a maladaptive compensatory mechanism when it overcompensates by exceeding the cell mass necessary for regeneration. Excessive numbers of cells in a specific tissue or organ can have detrimental effects. For example, a keloid is a maladaptive hyperplastic accumulation of epithelial cells and connective tissue that can occur in wound healing. It creates an elevated, disfiguring scar that requires cosmetic surgery (see Fig. 2-3).

Metaplasia

Metaplasia is the replacement of one cell type by another cell type. It is likely a result of the cell's genetic reprogramming in response to a change in environmental conditions. Commonly, metaplasia occurs in response to chronic inflammation, and the substitution of cells enables the tissue's survival.

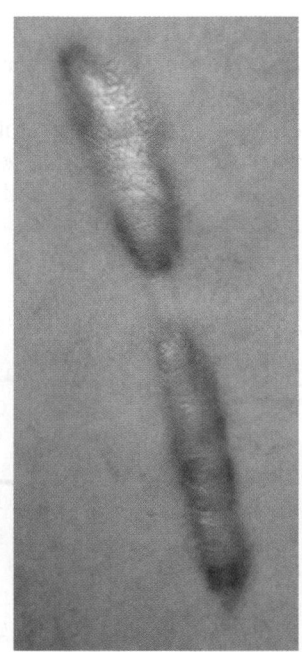

FIGURE 2-3. Keloid. (From Nugent & Vitale. (2014). *Fundamentals of nursing: content review plus practice questions.* 1st ed. Philadelphia, PA: F.A. Davis Company, with permission.)

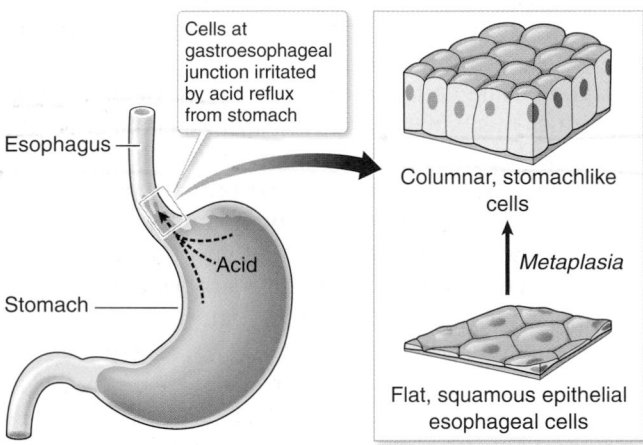

FIGURE 2-4. Metaplasia can occur in gastroesophageal reflux disease (GERD). In GERD, cells in the gastroesophageal junction are chronically irritated because of exposure to stomach acid. Lower esophageal squamous epithelial cells can undergo a metaplastic change into columnar stomachlike cells. When this condition develops, it is called Barrett's esophagus.

ALERT The metaplastic change that occurs in GERD is a condition referred to as Barrett's esophagus, which requires periodic examination and aggressive treatment because it can deteriorate into cancer of the esophagus (see Fig. 2-5).

Dysplasia

Dysplasia is deranged cellular growth within a specific tissue, often as a result of chronic inflammation or a precancerous condition. On histological examination, dysplastic cells vary in size, shape, and architectural organization compared with healthy cells. Cervical dysplasia, often detected on a Papanicolaou (Pap) test, is a common example of this cellular change (see Fig. 2-6). When discovered, frequent examinations are necessary because dysplasia is the classic precursor to cancer of the cervix.

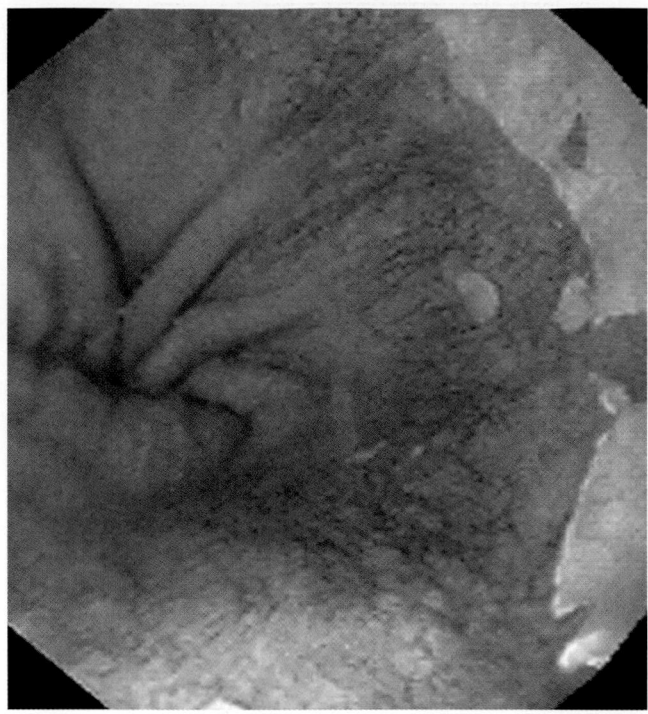

FIGURE 2-5. Metaplastic lower esophageal cells visualized on endoscopic examination. Lower esophageal cells, which are normal squamous epithelium type cells, as shown in pale pink, change into cells that are columnar stomachlike cells in response to acid reflux, as shown in dark pink. This condition is called Barrett's esophagus. *(Courtesy of H. Worth Boyce, MD.)*

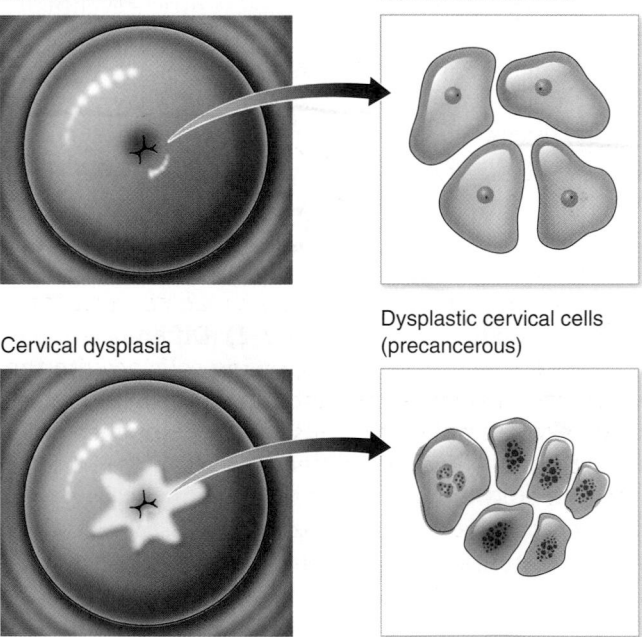

FIGURE 2-6. Normal cervix and cervical cells versus cervical dysplasia and dysplastic cells.

Neoplasia

Neoplasia means new growth and usually refers to disorganized, uncoordinated, uncontrolled proliferative cell growth that is cancerous. The words *tumor* and *neoplasm* are often used interchangeably, and both indicate new cells growing within a specific tissue or organ.

BOX 2-1. Cellular Differentiation: Benign and Malignant Neoplasms

Cellular differentiation is a characteristic used to designate a neoplasm as benign or malignant. Neoplastic cells that resemble the normal, healthy cells within the tissue where they are found are termed *well-differentiated*. Benign neoplasms contain well-differentiated cells, or cells that resemble the healthy cells of the tissue of origin. Another characteristic of benign neoplasms is that the cells do not metastasize or break loose from the tissue of origin.

Conversely, neoplastic cells can appear very different from the healthy cells within their tissue of origin, in which case the cells are termed *poorly differentiated*. Malignant neoplasms contain fewer well-differentiated cells and have a tendency to break away, enter the lymphatic or circulatory systems, and metastasize to distant sites to form secondary neoplasms.

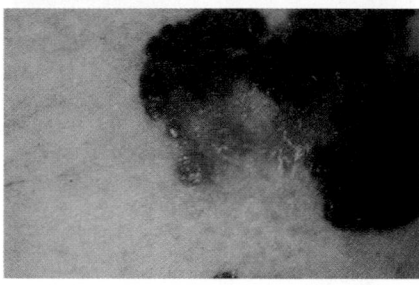

FIGURE 2-7. Normal skin vs. malignant melanoma. In normal skin, skin cells are lined up in an orderly fashion. In malignant melanoma, skin cells are numerous and disorderly in architecture. (From Goldsmith and Tharp. [1997]. *Adult and pediatric dermatology: a color guide to diagnosis and treatment.* Philadelphia, PA: F.A. Davis Company, with permission.)

Neoplasms can be classified as **benign** or **malignant,** depending on an important cell characteristic called differentiation (see Box 2-1). Differentiation is the process whereby newly growing cells acquire the specialized structure and function of the cells they replace. For example, skin cells that are sloughed daily are replaced by normally differentiated epithelial cells. The new epithelial cells are structurally and functionally exact copies of the sloughed cells. However, in cases of malignant melanoma (skin cancer), poorly differentiated, neoplastic epithelial cells, which do not look or act like normal skin cells, replace normal epithelial cells. Additionally, the cells are arranged in a disorganized fashion so that when viewed with a microscope, the normal cellular arrangement or tissue architecture is altered (see Fig. 2-7).

Basic Concepts of Cellular Injury

Cell injury occurs when cells are exposed to a severe stress that no longer allows them to maintain homeostasis,

which results in structural and functional changes. The basic changes of cell injury include dysfunction of the sodium-potassium pump, loss of plasma membrane integrity, mitochondrial dysfunction, defects in protein synthesis, intracellular accumulations, cellular swelling, and DNA damage. If the damaging stimulus is removed, cellular injury may be reversible. If the stress is prolonged, the cells may reach a critical point, which is variable for different cells, when recovery is not possible, resulting in organelle disruption and irreversible cell injury.

Dysfunction of the Sodium-Potassium Pump

When the cell is unable to produce sufficient ATP, a high energy compound, cellular physiologic functions are reduced. Lack of sufficient ATP contributes to failure of active transport mechanisms such as the sodium-potassium pump (Na^+/K^+ ATPase).

Under normal, healthy circumstances, Na^+/K^+ ATPase expels three sodium ions from the intracellular environment and pumps in two potassium ions. This contributes to the development of membrane polarity in excitable tissues such as muscle cells and neurons. It also maintains the normal osmotic relationships between ions, with sodium being the major extracellular ion and potassium the major intracellular ion.

However, when this active transport system is not functioning, the normal osmotic balance is altered. The intracellular sodium ion concentration is increased because it is not being adequately removed from the cell. This increase in intracellular sodium draws in water, leading to cellular swelling.

With a lack of ATP, an energy-dependent calcium pump—which maintains intracellular calcium at extremely low levels—also becomes dysfunctional. As a result, calcium accumulates within the cell and disrupts numerous biochemical processes. Calcium also activates a number of enzymes that further deplete ATP, damage the plasma membrane, disrupt DNA, and induce cell degeneration. Pathological calcification, the deposition of calcium and other minerals within tissues, occurs in a variety of conditions. Calcifications often accumulate in areas of cell injury and cell death (see Box 2-2).

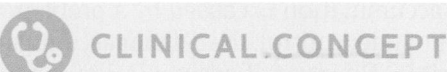

CLINICAL CONCEPT

On mammography, microcalcifications often indicate that the tissue has cancerous changes.

Loss of Plasma Membrane Integrity

The plasma membrane surrounds the whole perimeter of the cell and acts as a guardian of internal organelles. With a breach of membrane integrity, injurious agents can affect any of the organelles. In addition, water can enter the intracellular compartment, causing cellular

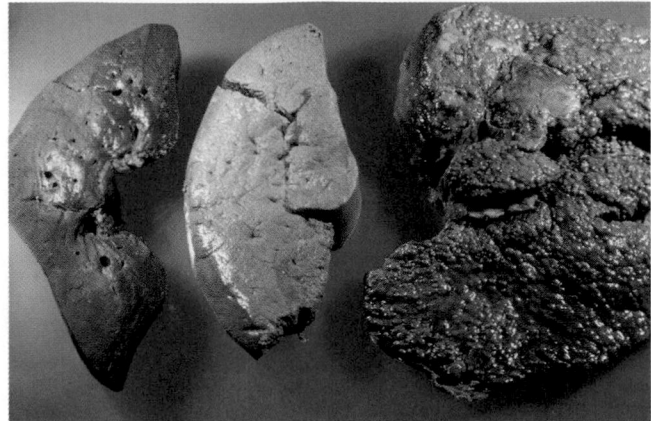

FIGURE 2-8. Normal liver versus fatty liver. *(From Arthur Glauberman/ Photo Researchers, Inc. Enhancement by: Mary Martin/Science Source.)*

swelling. The mitochondria can be damaged, which would halt the cell's ability to produce energy. Organelles can swell and deteriorate. The nucleus, which contains the DNA, would be left vulnerable to injury and the cell will be left without regeneration ability.

Defects in Protein Synthesis Ability

When the cell is low in energy because of hypoxia or mitochondrial dysfunction, there is decreasing ATP. With dwindling ATP availability, the critical cellular process of protein synthesis begins to fail. The cells cannot manufacture proteins, which are crucial constituents for their own regeneration and many different kinds of body processes. Lack of protein synthesis can begin the process of cell degeneration or cell death.

Intracellular Accumulations

Cells can accumulate excessive amounts of various substances, such as cellular constituents, environmentally acquired substances, or cell breakdown products, because of abnormal metabolic function, exposure to high amounts of environmental material, or aging. Accumulated substances may be harmless or toxic to the cell and can be transient or permanently imbedded in the cell.

If the accumulation is caused by a problem that can be brought under control, the cellular accumulation may be reversible. However, if accumulation is progressive and continual, cellular injury can occur. For example, intracellular accumulation can occur in the liver when exposed to excessive amounts of alcohol. Hepatocytes, which are integrally involved in lipid metabolism, can sustain toxic injury from alcohol and accumulate large quantities of intracellular fat. Fatty liver is a distinctive histological change associated with alcoholism that causes the liver to enlarge and become dysfunctional (see Fig. 2-8).

Another intracellular accumulation occurs in familial hypercholesterolemia, a condition that causes defective

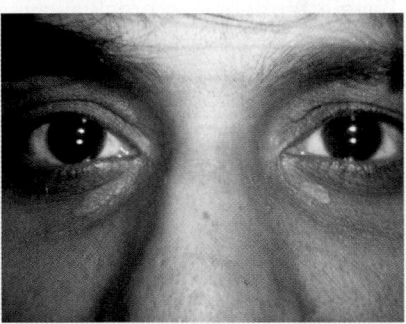

FIGURE 2-9. Xanthelasma is an intracellular accumulation of cholesterol within skin cells around the eyelids. This condition is seen in individuals with familial hypercholesterolemia. *(Courtesy of Wills Eye Hospital, Philadelphia, PA.)*

cholesterol metabolism. Xanthomas and xanthelasma are yellow, raised skin lesions that develop because of intracellular accumulation of excess cholesterol within epithelial cells (see Fig. 2-9).

An example of an environmentally derived cellular accumulation occurs in anthracosis, otherwise known as coal miner's lung disease. Individuals who chronically inhale coal dust demonstrate accumulations of this substance within respiratory tract epithelial cells, which leads to blackening of the lung tissues (see Fig. 2-10).

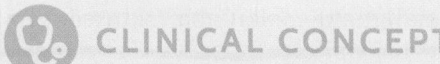

CLINICAL CONCEPT

A transient accumulation of the cell breakdown product, bilirubin, occurs in jaundice. Bilirubin, a breakdown product of hemoglobin, can accumulate in the body in liver disorders or conditions of excess hemolysis (red blood cell breakdown). Bilirubin, a yellow-pigmented substance, has high affinity for elastin, a constituent of the sclera of the eye and skin (see Fig. 2-11). Jaundice, the yellow hue of the skin and sclera, diminishes when bilirubin levels are reduced.

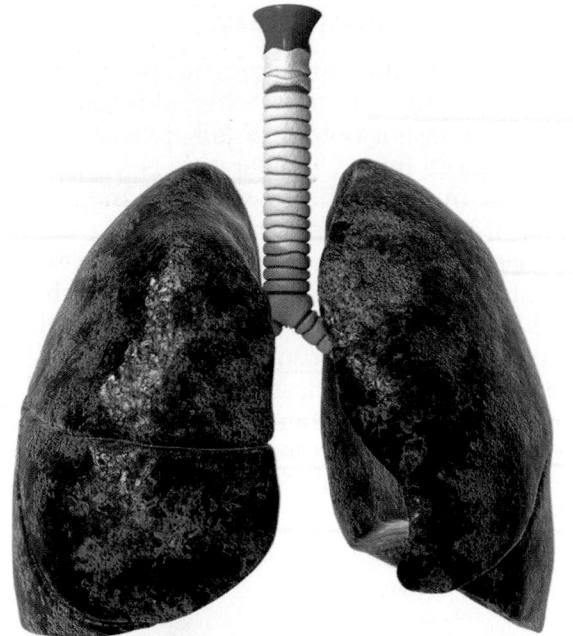

FIGURE 2-10. Anthracosis, also known as coal miner's lung and black lung. *(From David Mack/Science Source.)*

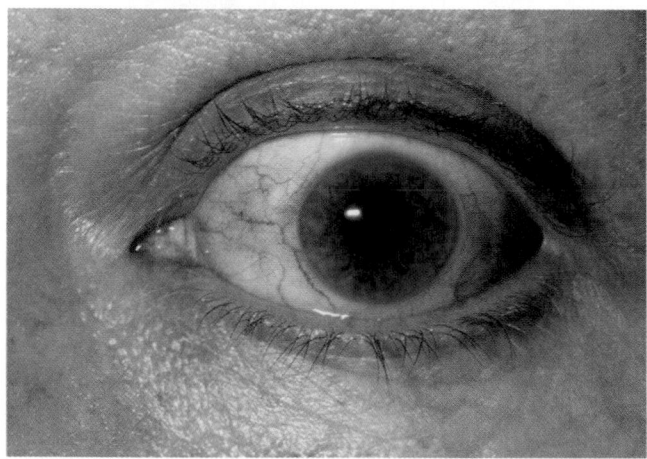

FIGURE 2-11. Jaundice of the sclera. Jaundice is caused by bilirubin, a yellow pigment that can accumulate in the sclera and skin in liver disease and other disorders. *(From Dr. P. Marazzi/Science Source.)*

↳ pancreatic cancer

Genetic Damage

Injury to the cell's DNA can cause mutations, which, in turn, initiate changes in cell structure and function. Mutated DNA will be transcribed in the nucleus to produce mutated RNA. The abnormal RNA will, in turn, direct the cell's ribosomes to produce abnormal proteins. The abnormal proteins then rebuild the cell in an abnormal fashion and manufacture abnormal secretions.

Changes in the cell's structure and function often will be incompatible with life. Commonly, changes in the cell's DNA will initiate changes that bring about genetically programmed cell degeneration, also called apoptosis.

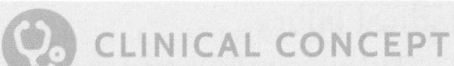

CLINICAL CONCEPT

DNA mutations are common with exposure to high doses of radiation. With radiation damage, genes can mutate into oncogenes, which trigger cancerous cell changes. The cancerous cells manufacture cancerous proteins, also called oncoproteins.

Causes of Cell Injury

There are many stressors and injurious agents that can cause cellular injury. Causes of cell injury can be categorized as follows:

- Hypoxic cell injury
- Free radical injury (oxidative stress)
- Physical agents of injury
- Chemical injury
- Infectious agent injury
- Injurious immunological reactions
- Genetic defects
- Nutritional imbalances.

Hypoxic Cell Injury

Oxygen deprivation, also known as hypoxia, is the most common cause of cell injury. Cellular hypoxia commonly results when the blood cannot deliver enough oxygen to the cells. The most common cause of cellular hypoxia is diminished circulation, also called ischemia. Ischemia occurs most often because of obstruction of arterial blood flow. The obstruction is commonly atherosclerotic plaque and clot formation, which blocks circulation downstream from the clot.

Another cause of cellular hypoxia is anemia. In anemia, the blood lacks sufficient hemoglobin (Hgb), which is the molecule in the red blood cell that carries oxygen. Inadequate Hgb results in insufficient oxygen carried by the blood, which, in turn, results in the cells not receiving fully oxygenated blood. This results in hypoxia.

Hypoxia causes the cell to enter anaerobic metabolism, during which it generates 2 ATP; a low amount of energy, and pyruvic acid. Pyruvic acid changes into lactic acid. The inadequate cell energy slows down all metabolic functions of the cell, and the lactic acid alters cellular biochemical activity. Lactic acid is particularly irritating to muscle cells. Anaerobic metabolism cannot sustain cell life for a prolonged time.

Other causes of hypoxia include exposure to low concentrations of oxygen in the environment, such as occurs at high altitudes; inadequate oxygen diffusion at the alveoli, as in pneumonia; suffocation injury; or airway obstruction caused by a foreign body or inflammation of oropharyngeal tissues.

Free Radical Injury

Cells generate energy in the mitochondria through a process called oxidative phosphorylation. During this process, often described as a respiratory burst, small amounts of reactive oxygen molecules are produced as by-products. These reactive oxygen molecules are referred to as free radicals or reactive oxygen species. Free radicals are also present in many environmental substances, such as cigarette smoke, pesticides, and other toxins.

Free radicals have a single, unpaired electron in an outer orbit that creates instability and reactivity with adjacent molecules; they react with constituents of the cell's plasma membrane and organelle membranes, causing oxidative degradation. Free radicals are oxidizing agents with the ability to penetrate the cell's plasma membrane, disrupt internal organelles, and damage the nucleus and its DNA.

Cells have multiple mechanisms to remove free radicals and thereby minimize injury. These mechanisms involve a series of enzymes referred to as superoxide dismutases. However, free radical generation can overwhelm the mechanisms of removal, in which case a form of cell injury known as **oxidative stress** occurs.

CLINICAL CONCEPT

Individuals can counteract free radical injury through consumption of antioxidants such as vitamin A, E, C, and beta-carotene.

Oxidative stress commonly occurs in cells that undergo transient ischemia and subsequent resumption of circulation, also known as ischemic-reperfusion injury. Depending on the ischemic insult's intensity and duration, variable numbers of cells may proceed to die after blood flow is restored to tissues. During the reperfusion phase, new damaging forces are activated by reactive free radicals, causing the death of cells that might have recovered otherwise.

CLINICAL CONCEPT

In the clinical setting, heart disease commonly involves ischemic-reperfusion injury, which commonly occurs when a blood clot that obstructs a coronary artery causes cardiac muscle ischemia. After this occurs, the region undergoes reperfusion with clot dissolution. The mitochondria in the region undergo interrupted oxidative phosphorylation because of the temporary hypoxia and release of free radicals as by-products, which cause injury to surrounding tissue.

Physical Agents of Injury

There are many different physical agents of cell injury. Mechanical trauma from an external force such as a laceration, gunshot wound, or fall are obvious causes of physical cell injury. Temperature extremes, which can result in such injuries as burns and frostbite; radiation; electrical shock; and extreme changes in atmospheric pressure can also cause cell injury. Sunburn, brought upon by excessive exposure to sunlight, is an observable example of cell injury caused by a physical agent. Excessive noise is considered a mechanical stressor of the inner ear's delicate organs.

In addition to direct trauma to the cells and tissues, physiologic responses to trauma often include the initiation of the inflammatory response, which can lead to healing or further cell damage (see Chapter 9: Inflammation and Dysfunctional Wound Healing).

CLINICAL CONCEPT

Hypertension, high pressure within the arteries, acts as a physical force against the endothelial lining of the vasculature. The constant stress of the pulsatile force of blood flow against the arterial endothelium causes a shearing injury. Endothelial injury caused by the forces of hypertension initiates the development of atherosclerosis throughout the arterial system.

Chemical Injury

Chemical injury can be caused by either endogenous, biological substances or exogenous, synthetic substances that influence the cell. Chemical agents commonly injure the plasma membrane and gain access to the cell's interior to cause dysfunction of organelles.

Imbalances of the body's biological chemical constituents, such as electrolytes, can cause cell injury. For example, high sodium levels in the bloodstream, termed *hypernatremia,* cause intracellular fluid depletion (cellular dehydration) and reversible cell shrinkage. The symptoms associated with this include lethargy, weakness, irritability, and confusion (see Chapter 7: Fluid and Electrolyte Imbalances).

In uncontrolled diabetes mellitus (DM), high glucose levels in the bloodstream, termed *hyperglycemia,* cause chemical injury of the endothelial cells that line the arteries. High levels of blood glucose react with endothelial membrane constituents to yield substances called advanced glycation end-products, which can damage the coronary and cerebral arteries, arteries of the kidneys, vessels of the lower extremity, and the retina of the eyes. The altered metabolic processes associated with DM initiate the process of atherosclerosis. Consequently, individuals with chronically uncontrolled diabetes are susceptible to diseases associated with atherosclerosis: coronary artery disease, peripheral arterial disease, and cerebrovascular disease (see Chapter 25: Diabetes and Metabolic Syndrome).

Alternatively, exogenous chemical substances such as drugs, environmental pollutants, or poisons can cause cellular injury in various ways. Many drugs, such as nonsteroidal anti-inflammatory drugs (NSAIDs) and antibiotics such as aminoglycosides, can have nephrotoxic side effects. Nephrotoxic drugs have chemically damaging effects on the cells of the kidney's nephron tubules.

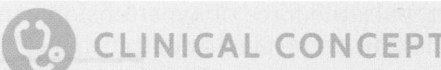

> ## CLINICAL CONCEPT
>
> Carbon monoxide (CO) binds very tightly to the hemoglobin molecule, decreasing its oxygen-carrying capacity. This is why the amount of oxygen delivered to the tissues is decreased in carbon monoxide poisoning.

Infectious Agents of Injury

A wide variety of microorganisms, including bacteria, viruses, fungi, and parasites, can cause cellular injury. Each type of microorganism carries out injurious cell processes in a distinctive manner. An example is the human papilloma virus (HPV), a sexually transmitted infectious agent that can cause cancerous cell changes within the cervix. Another example is *Helicobacteria pylori,* which causes peptic ulcer disease. *H. pylori* is a bacterium that erodes the gastrointestinal mucosal lining and allows gastric acids to penetrate and damage underlying cells (see Fig. 2-12). The constant acid irritation leads to ulceration of the gastrointestinal cells, also termed peptic ulcer (see Chapter 29: Disorders of the Esophagus, Stomach, and Small Intestine).

Injurious Immunological Reactions

The immune system is the body's major defense mechanism against infectious agents. In some instances, however, the immune system can overreact and attack the body's own cells, causing cell injury and creating disease. For example, allergies are adverse immune reactions in response to contact with an environmental substance known as an antigen. In allergy, the immune system is triggered to synthesize antibodies that cause inflammatory changes in the body.

Another example of immunological cell injury occurs in autoimmune diseases such as rheumatoid arthritis (RA). In RA, immune system cells, such as T cells and B cells, are triggered by an unknown antigen to attack the body's own joints.

Genetic Defects

Genetic disorders can damage and mutate DNA, resulting in the initiation of events that can cause cell injury.

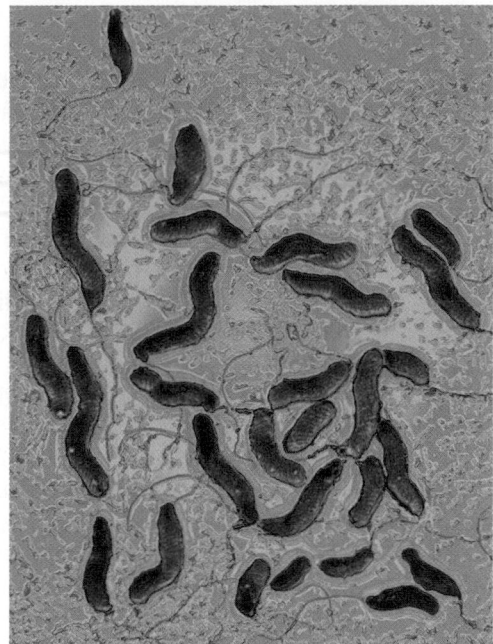

FIGURE 2-12. Histological view of *Helicobacteria pylori*, which is a bacterial organism that erodes the gastric mucosa to cause peptic ulcer disease. *(From James Cavallini/Science Source.)*

Damaged DNA is transcribed as defective RNA, which transmits flawed instructions to the ribosomes. At the ribosomes, the defective RNA causes synthesis of abnormal cellular proteins, which can initiate disease.

Nutritional Imbalances

Undernutrition, overnutrition, and malnutrition are all capable of causing cell injury. Starvation can cause inadequate supply of the nutrients necessary for proper cell function. Without sufficient proteins, carbohydrates, vitamins, and minerals, cell dysfunction can occur. An example of the effects of protein starvation can be seen in disorders such as marasmus and kwashiorkor, which are conditions seen in individuals suffering from severe protein starvation.

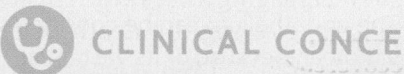

> ## CLINICAL CONCEPT
>
> Protein starvation causes low levels of albumin in the bloodstream, which leads to fluid shifting from the blood into the interstitial spaces. Excess fluid accumulation within the peritoneal cavity is most apparent in these starving individuals. The individuals demonstrate wasting of the trunk, bony extremities, and protuberant abdominal swelling.

Obesity, or excessive nutrition, can also cause cell injury. Excessive fat stores can place stress on the heart and pancreas, resulting in heart disease and diabetes. Excess body weight increases the heart's workload because of the obese body's increased metabolic requirements.

Excess body weight also places strain on joints, which predisposes to arthritis.

Malnutrition, the inadequate daily intake of carbohydrates, fats, protein, vitamins, and minerals, can also adversely affect cell function. Optimal cellular function requires daily ingestion of sufficient quantities of essential amino acids, glucose, fats, vitamins, and trace amounts of minerals for enzymatic reactions. Carbohydrates are needed for all cellular functions, particularly brain cell metabolism. Fat is necessary in the diet for the storage of fat-soluble vitamins A, D, E, and K; synthesis of hormones; and formation of all cell membranes. Proteins are the basic building blocks of all cells in the body.

Many persons have difficulty obtaining the daily requirement of vitamins, minerals, and nutrients from diet alone. For this reason, many nutritionists recommend adding a daily multivitamin to the diet.

Significance of Endothelial Cell Injury

The arterial blood vessels are lined by a continuous layer of endothelium that plays a key role in vascular function. Endothelial cells constitute a large area of responsive and secretory tissue that is influenced by blood flow changes, shear stress forces, inflammatory mediators, and various circulating substances. One of the substances secreted by endothelium is angiogenesis growth factor, also called vascular endothelial growth factor (VEGF), which stimulates the synthesis of collateral blood vessel branches. The endothelial cells also secrete vasodilating substances, such as nitric oxide (NO), and vasoconstricting substances, such as endothelin. Blood constituents such as glucose, lipids, platelets, norepinephrine, epinephrine, acetylcholine, vasopressin, natriuretic peptides, and angiotensin II act on the endothelium; each constituent affects the vasculature's function differently and may have detrimental effects.

> **ALERT** The endothelium can be considered the body's largest organ because of its vast area. When it is injured, there are widespread effects. Recognition that the arterial endothelium is an extensive, body-wide, active tissue that is highly vulnerable to injury is key to understanding cardiovascular disease.

Endothelial cell injury acts as an initiator of arteriosclerosis and the fundamental cell change that causes cardiovascular disease. The most significant injurious agents of the endothelial cells are hypertension, diabetic hyperglycemia, free radicals, persistent secretion of angiotensin II, and low density lipoprotein cholesterol (LDL-C). These are the most common insults that lay the foundation for cardiovascular disease. It is important for clinicians to understand all the etiologies

of endothelial injury, because cardiovascular disease is currently the most common disease among Americans. ✳

Hypertension

Hypertension exerts a shearing force against the endothelial cell membranes, creating multiple areas of injury on the interior walls of arteries. The high blood pressure force of hypertension can also weaken the integrity of the smooth muscle within the arterial walls. A weakened area in an arterial wall is called an **aneurysm.** After the formation of an aneurysm, the persistent, pulsatile force of hypertension can further weaken the wall of the aneurysm, causing rupture and hemorrhage. For example, a berry aneurysm is an example of a cerebral aneurysm located on the Circle of Willis within the brain (see Fig. 2-13). A surge in blood pressure can rupture this aneurysm and cause a fatal cerebral hemorrhage.

Diabetic Hyperglycemia

In uncontrolled diabetes, high blood glucose levels chemically injure the membranes of endothelial cells. Glucose reacts with the constituents of the endothelial membrane and creates advanced glycation end-products, which further undermine the endothelial cells' integrity. High-circulating glucose also stimulates the endothelium to secrete endothelin, a potent vasoconstrictor, thereby causing arterial narrowing. Diabetes provokes the combined effects of endothelial injury and vasoconstriction, which stimulates arterial vessel narrowing and accelerates the development of arteriosclerosis throughout the body.

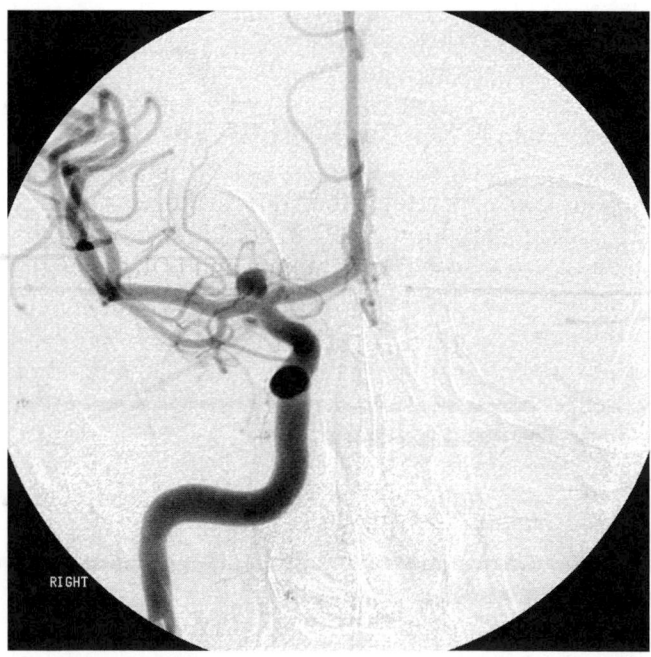

FIGURE 2-13. A weakening in an arterial wall is referred to as an aneurysm. An aneurysm of a cerebral artery is often called a berry aneurysm because of its resemblance to a berry hanging from a vine. *(From Living Art Enterprises/Science Source.)*

Free Radicals

Free radicals are highly reactive oxidizing molecules found within the environment and generated by certain cellular processes in the body. Cigarettes are a major source of free radicals, which injure the endothelium, and nicotine, which provokes vasoconstriction, both of which potentiate arterial dysfunction.

Persistent Secretion of Angiotensin II

Angiotensin II, a product of the renin-angiotensin-aldosterone cascade, acts as a potent arterial vasoconstrictor. In heart disease, constant secretion of angiotensin II is a persistent stimulus for arterial narrowing, which raises blood pressure. High blood pressure and vasoconstriction create detrimental resistance and high workload for the heart. Persistent secretion of angiotensin II worsens heart disease. For this reason, angiotensin-converting enzyme (ACE) inhibitors and angiotensin II receptor blockers (ARBs) are the antihypertensive medications commonly prescribed in heart disease.

Low-Density Lipoprotein (LDL) Cholesterol

Atherogenesis is the gradual and progressive development of atherosclerotic plaque within the arteries that is initiated by endothelial injury. Areas of endothelial injury undergo inflammation, which attracts white blood cells and platelets to the region. These inflammatory changes cause diminished vasodilatory capacity of the artery and set up conditions for the LDL cholesterol deposition and clot formation. LDL cholesterol accumulates within macrophages to form foam cells, which form the foundation for large spans of atherosclerotic plaque along the artery walls.

During the formation of atherosclerosis, endothelial nitric oxide is depleted, which inhibits the dilatory capacity of arteries. Vasodilatory capacity is crucial to sustain coronary artery blood flow to the heart muscle. Therefore, depletion of NO in addition to inflammatory changes of the endothelium and LDL deposition create arterial vasoconstriction and atherosclerosis—a highly detrimental combination for coronary arteries (see Fig. 2-14).

Cell Degeneration and Death

Apoptosis and necrosis are the two major forms of cell death. In **apoptosis,** cells degenerate at a specific time period with no adverse effects on the body. Cellular necrosis, however, is cell death caused by injury. The cell is overcome by an insult, cannot maintain homeostasis, becomes severely dysfunctional, and may adversely affect neighboring tissues or the organ as a whole.

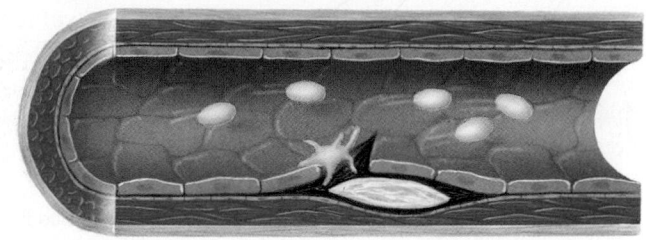
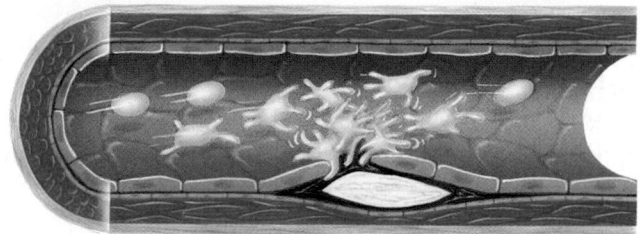
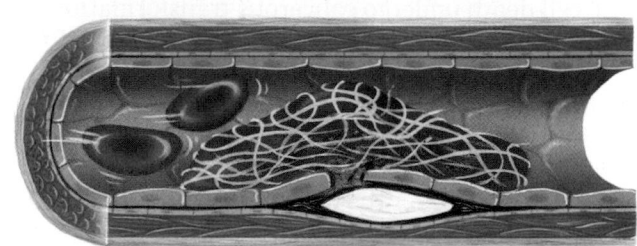

FIGURE 2-14. Endothelial injury and development of atherosclerosis. *(From BSIP/Science Source.)*

Apoptosis

Apoptosis is a genetically programmed degenerative change that results in cell death. It is an organized process that eliminates unwanted, unnecessary, or damaged cells without inflammation or any adverse effects on surrounding tissue (see Fig. 2-15). It can occur as a normal physiologic process or may be involved in a disease process.

An example of physiologic apoptosis occurs during the hand's embryonic development, which originates as a paddle-shaped structure. Apoptosis of select cells occurs within the paddle-shaped hand plate to form indentations to shape the individual fingers. The apoptotic cells disintegrate in a stepwise manner without disrupting other cells.

Physiologic apoptosis also occurs in female adult ovaries during menopause. During this time, the ovaries become dysfunctional and degenerate according to a genetically determined life span. Cells that have completed their function and need elimination also undergo apoptosis. For example, white blood cells that become exhausted after participation in immune reactions undergo apoptosis.

Some disorders are associated with the dysfunction of cellular apoptosis; as a consequence, cellular life

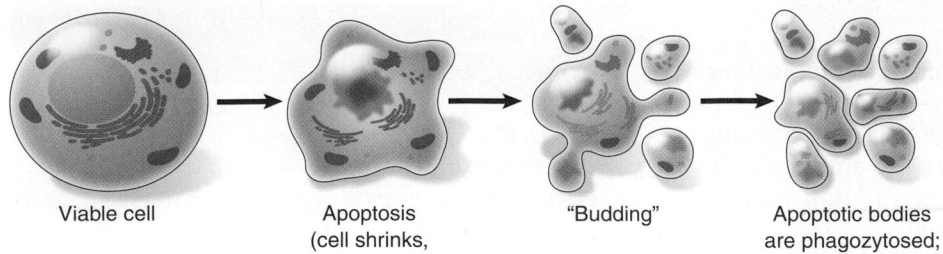

FIGURE 2-15. Apoptosis is a genetically programmed step-by-step involutional cellular process. The cell shrinks, deoxyribonucleic acid undergoes orderly fragmentation, and organelles degenerate. The degenerated cells are phagocytosed by white blood cells, do not stimulate inflammation, and do not have adverse effects on the body.

Viable cell

Apoptosis (cell shrinks, chromatin condenses)

"Budding"

Apoptotic bodies are phagozytosed; no inflammation

span is prolonged. In these disorders, cells have an abnormally long survival, accumulate, and become disadvantageous to the body. Cells that fail to undergo apoptosis can give rise to certain cancers, tumors, and detrimental hyperplastic cell changes. Prostate cancer is theorized to arise from cells that lose their apoptotic function. In elderly males, the prostate gland enlarges because apoptosis fails and cells continually multiply. Some of the prostate cells that fail to experience apoptotic cell death undergo cancerous transformation.

Alternatively, some disorders are associated with increased cellular apoptosis, which results in excessive cell death rates. Certain degenerative neurological diseases, such as spinal muscular atrophy, are thought to arise from nerve cells that undergo increased apoptotic rates and, consequently, die prematurely. In another example, accelerated apoptosis of thyroid epithelial cells results in thyroid gland dysfunction. Hashimoto's thyroiditis is a common autoimmune disease that causes gradual failure of the thyroid gland because of increased apoptotic cell death.

Cell Necrosis

Cell necrosis occurs when cells die because of stressors or insults that overwhelm the cell's ability to survive. Necrosis is an irreversible process whereby the cell undergoes a series of changes, including membrane disintegration, chromatin fragmentation, lysosomal activation, and lysis. With cell necrosis, lysosomes break open and release digestive enzymes, initiating autolysis. The body initiates an inflammatory reaction against the necrotic cells, and necrotic cell bodies are left as remnants (see Fig. 2-16). The enzymes and other cellular chemicals that are released from the dead cells enter the systemic circulation and can be measured as indicators of cell death.

Infarction, also called ischemic necrosis, is the death of tissue as a consequence of prolonged ischemia. For example, when there is a lack of sufficient coronary artery blood supply to the myocardial muscle, ischemia occurs. If ischemia is prolonged without resumption of circulation to the region of myocardial muscle, infarction occurs. When infarction occurs, lysosomal enzymes and proteins from dead cardiac cells are released into the bloodstream. Blood levels of the lysosomal enzyme, CPKmb, and the cardiac protein, troponin, are measured to confirm myocardial infarction (see Fig. 2-17).

Any tissue that sustains prolonged ischemia is susceptible to infarction, but individual cell types have different tolerance levels. For example, in ischemic conditions, brain and myocardial cells undergo infarction and cell death within minutes, whereas skeletal muscle cells can tolerate lack of circulation for hours.

Gangrene

After cells die, necrosis of tissue develops. Dead tissue is a medium for certain types of bacteria, a condition known as **gangrene.** Gangrene can occur when tissues endure prolonged ischemia, undergo infarction and necrosis, and then are exposed to bacteria that thrive

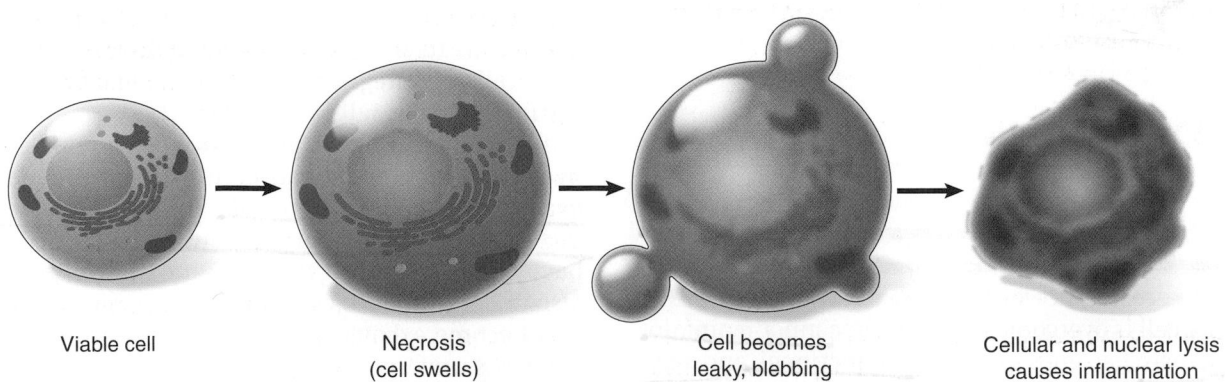

Viable cell

Necrosis (cell swells)

Cell becomes leaky, blebbing

Cellular and nuclear lysis causes inflammation

FIGURE 2-16. The stages of cellular necrosis. In cellular necrosis, the cell swells, loses cellular integrity, and stimulates inflammation.

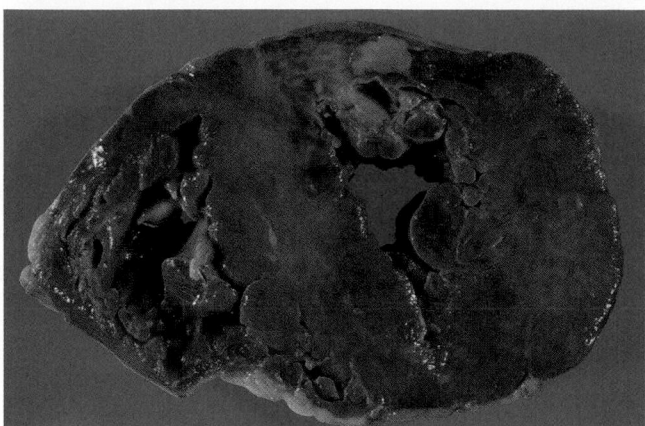

FIGURE 2-17. Cross section of the heart showing an enlarged left ventricle with myocardial infarction. *(From Dr. E. Walker/Science Source.)*

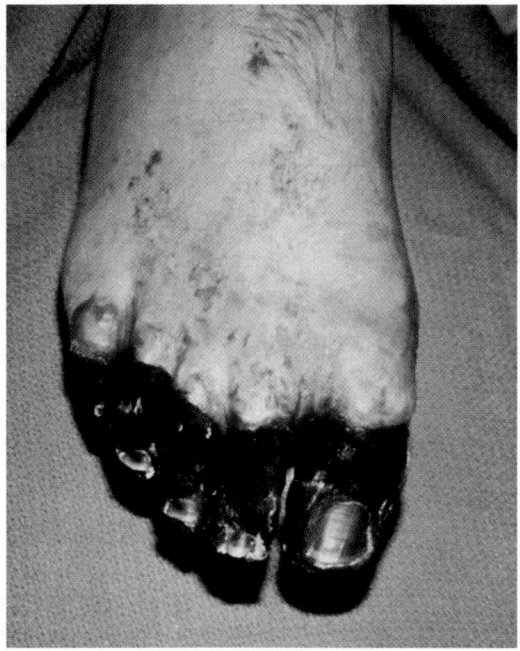

FIGURE 2-18. Gangrene. *(Courtesy of CDC/William Archibald.)*

on the decaying tissue. *Clostridium perfringens* is an anaerobic bacteria that proliferates in exposed necrotic tissue and emits a gas identifiable as a foul odor associated with gangrene. In clinical settings, gangrene is most often seen in patients with peripheral arterial obstructive disease of the lower extremities. Prolonged ischemia of the lower extremities leads to infarction, followed by necrosis of tissue and superimposed gangrenous infection (see Fig. 2-18).

Clinical Interventions to Reverse Cell Injury

Clinical interventions can reverse the effects of cell injury and death through various medical and surgical treatment modalities. In some cases, injured cells can be treated to reverse the damage so that cellular regeneration can take

place. Different types of cellular changes require specific types of therapy.

Removal of injurious stimuli can reverse muscle atrophy. If the atrophy is caused by lack of circulation or nerve stimulation, restoration of these processes can allow for rehabilitation of normal cell size. With hyperplasia, metaplasia, and hypertrophy, the eradication of injurious stimuli can allow for the resumption of normal growth patterns in some cases.

CLINICAL CONCEPT

Hyperplasia of the uterine endometrium can resolve with appropriate hormone therapy that counteracts the effects of excessive estrogen. Acid suppression treatment can resolve the metaplasia of Barrett's esophagus. Treatment of hypertension can cause some regression of left ventricular hypertrophy.

Neoplastic growths usually require surgical removal. If neoplasia is malignant, more intense treatment modalities, such as radiation and chemotherapy, may need to be employed to completely eliminate all tumor cells.

Intracellular accumulations can usually be eradicated by resolving the etiology of the metabolic derangement. If the etiology is irreversible, then only palliative or supportive treatments for the disease's effects are available.

Interventions to Treat Permanent Cell Injury

Treatments to reverse permanent cell injury are limited. For example, in myocardial infarction, the heart muscle cells die and are permanently dysfunctional and nonregenerated. This leaves a segment of the heart muscle as a noncontracting unit, which weakens the heart pump overall. If a large region of cardiac muscle is damaged, heart failure is inevitable.

In neurodegenerative diseases, such as Parkinson's disease, specific brain cells undergo degeneration and progressively die, causing the patient to endure gradual, progressive neurological deterioration. For Parkinson's and most other neurodegenerative diseases, there are limited therapeutic options. Most patients must endure the effects of the progressive deterioration.

Permanent, irreversible cell injury may be tolerable and the patient may be able to survive with limited organ function. However, when life-sustaining organs are irreversibly damaged, transplantation and other modes of cellular regeneration need to be considered. Transplantation, a surgical intervention that replaces irreversibly injured cells, tissues, and organs with viable donor tissue, has historically proven successful for many patients. However, donor organs are always in short supply and the transplant recipients often experience organ rejection. Research in biotechnology and genetic engineering has introduced new modalities of cellular regeneration involving embryonic stem cells and therapeutic cloning techniques. These are controversial new techniques that offer promise but are still in their infancy stages of development.

Transplantation

Transplantation is the most prevalent method to replace permanently injured tissues or organs. The field of transplantation is complex and involves the solicitation of donors, harvesting of organs, matching of donor organs and recipients, surgical implantation, and interventions to prevent organ rejection. It has proven successful for resolution of many conditions, such as kidney failure, heart failure, and pancreatic and liver disease. Bone marrow transplants have also demonstrated various levels of success for different types of cancers and hematologic disorders. Umbilical cord blood has become an alternative source for cells to treat hematologic disorders.

Transplantation therapy, however, is associated with many obstacles: Short supply of donor organs, exact tissue matching of donor and recipient organs, and transplant rejection are just some of the obstacles within this form of therapy. Researchers are continuing to search for better methods to restore depleted cells, dead tissues, and dysfunctional organs.

Restoration With Stem Cells

Cell biologists have been studying the effects of cell death, particularly the death of cells that are incapable of regeneration, such as brain, neuron, and heart muscle cells. Other than through transplantation, these cells are not capable of functional restoration; therefore, cell biologists have been investigating methods to regenerate these kinds of cells. Researchers are currently involved in stem cell research using stem cells derived from embryonic tissues. Human embryonic stem cells are derived from fertilized eggs in the blastocyst stage, a phase of primitive cell division that occurs shortly after fertilization. These primitive cells are at an undifferentiated stage and are capable of developing into any specialized tissue or organ. Research has introduced the prospect of utilizing human embryonic stem cells for tissue repair and cell regeneration.

Stem cells have also been obtained from amniotic fluid and the umbilical cord during the birthing process. These pluripotential stem cells are capable of developing into other cell types. Adult stem cells, which have been harvested from skeletal and cardiac muscle, are under investigation for their potential to generate new skeletal and cardiac muscle tissue.

Reproductive Cloning

Research into the therapeutic use of embryonic stem cells has coincided with another field of investigation called cloning. Cloning is a new and controversial biotechnological field that involves manipulation of genetic material, which is called genetic engineering. In 1996, a group of scientists in Edinburgh, Scotland, experimented with a process termed nuclear transfer for reproductive cloning. After many attempts, the scientists accomplished a nuclear transfer procedure that succeeded. They extracted the nucleus of a mammary cell from an adult sheep and placed it in a donated unfertilized egg, which had its nucleus removed. They then implanted the egg containing the new nucleus into the uterus of a "foster mother" sheep. After the appropriate period of development within the uterus, the foster mother sheep gave birth to a lamb named Dolly, the first cloned sheep. Dolly was an identical newborn version of the original donor sheep. After reaching adulthood, breeders successfully enabled Dolly to give birth to offspring of her own. Unfortunately, after 6 years of adulthood, Dolly died an early death caused by multiple health problems, a common occurrence in animal clones.

Since the 1980s, scientists have been experimenting with the reproductive cloning of farm animals with varying success rates, with published data showing that on average 1% to 3% of cloned embryos lead to live births. Many cloned offspring die late in pregnancy or soon after birth, and investigations demonstrate that clones that live into adulthood commonly have abnormalities. Currently, reproductive cloning is performed among livestock, such as cattle, pigs, and goats. Clones of rabbits, mice, rats, mules, and cats have also been created.

Presently there is an international debate regarding the scientific use of reproductive cloning technology, as there are many ethical issues surrounding its use. However, breakthroughs in research continue to occur and cannot be rescinded. The debate regarding the use of this biotechnology will likely continue for quite some time.

Therapeutic Cloning

At present, cloning technology and embryonic stem cell research are under investigation for the creation of transplant organs. Therapeutic cloning is a field that involves harvesting of embryonic stem cells and performing nuclear transfer on these cells. The procedure involves taking an embryonic stem cell and extracting its nucleus. This is followed by injecting the embryonic stem cell with the DNA from the cell of a patient in need of a transplant, thereby creating an embryonic stem cell with the exact DNA match of the patient. The stem cell then is coaxed to develop into the tissue or organ that is needed. This technology has created a proposed method by which individuals in need of transplant can obtain exact tissue matches of organs

For example, an individual with diabetes could theoretically obtain an exact match of his or her own pancreatic cells through the method of therapeutic cloning. An embryonic stem cell could be infused with the diabetic individual's DNA to generate new genetically identical pancreatic tissue. The newly generated pancreatic tissue could be implanted into the diabetic individual and produce natural insulin. Theoretically, newly generated insulin-secreting pancreatic tissue derived from embryonic stem cells could cure diabetes. However, at present, this type of research is in its infancy stages and most of the assertions are speculative (see Box 2-3).

BOX 2-3. The Promise of Embryonic Stem Cell Therapy

Embryonic stem cells are undifferentiated cells with an unlimited capacity for self-renewal and potential for new tissue formation. However, there are supply limitations and ethical issues involved in using embryonic stem cells for scientific research. In the past few years, researchers have found that stem cells can be harvested from other sources such as umbilical cord blood, amniotic membranes, and fetal and some adult tissue. These discoveries have incited a revolution in regenerative medicine and cancer therapies by providing the possibility of generating multiple therapeutically useful cell types. Stem cells could be used for treating numerous pathological conditions such as cancer, hematopoietic and immune system disorders, heart failure, chronic liver disease, stroke, diabetes, Parkinson's and Alzheimer's disease, and arthritis.

Umbilical cord blood (UCB) is a rich source of stem cells and can be supplied by placentae, which were previously discarded after childbirth. The value of UCB has provoked the establishment of UCB banks throughout the world. Transplant of UCB stem cells has shown great promise for children with hematologic cancers. Current research is comparing bone marrow stem-cell transplants with UCB transplants in patients with cancer. Investigations demonstrate comparable results between the two kinds of transplants for pediatric hematologic cancer patients. However, bone marrow stem-cell transplants require a donor-recipient match, which can be an arduous search. Because UCB transplants can be derived from any woman during childbirth, the supply of donors is almost limitless.

Investigators are also examining fetal and amniotic membrane cells for their therapeutic potential. Like UCB, these cells may also have the potential for generation of multiple types of tissue. Investigators have confirmed that some stem cells are contained in adult organs, although quantities and capacity to regenerate are much more limited than those of the embryo or fetal-related cells. Adult mesenchymal stem cells are under investigation for their potential in the treatment of heart failure and stroke. As experimental treatments, researchers are attempting to transplant mesenchymal stem cells into the injured regions of the heart and brain to replace nonfunctional cells.

Several clinical trials have begun to evaluate the efficacy and safety of these treatments. Because of the immense potential of stem cell-based therapies, it is certain that future researchers will continue to explore the therapeutic uses of UCB, fetal, adult, and amniotic membrane cells.

Chapter Summary

- Cells are vulnerable to many kinds of injurious agents that can cause adaptations, maladaptive changes, and reversible or irreversible damage.

- Physical trauma, temperature extremes, electrical injury, radiation, free radicals, high circulating glucose in diabetes, and high blood pressure can all damage the plasma membrane and leave cellular organelles vulnerable to injury.

- Atrophy is the diminished size and growth of tissue, whereas hypertrophy is an increase in the size of each individual cell of an organ or tissue.

- The most common organ damaged by injurious agents is the endothelium. Endothelial injury initiates arteriosclerosis, which leads to circulatory obstruction.

- Hypertension, high cholesterol levels, hyperglycemia, and free radicals are major injurious agents of the endothelium.

- Ischemia is the lack of adequate blood flow to tissues. Ischemia leads to cellular hypoxia, the most common form of cell injury. Prolonged ischemia leads to infarction or death of tissue.

- Apoptosis is the cell's genetically programmed degeneration.

- Transplantation may not be the only remedy for nonregenerative organs.

- Cellular regeneration is under investigation, and stem cells and therapeutic cloning are the methods under intense scrutiny.

Bibliography

Barrett, K., Barman, S., Boitano, S., & Brooks, H. (2012). *Ganong's review of medical physiology.* 24th ed. New York, NY: McGraw-Hill.

Boström, P., & Frisén, J. (2013). New cells in old hearts. *N Engl J Med, 368*(14), 1358–1360. doi: 10.1056/NEJMcibr1300157.

Eltzschig, H. K., & Carmeliet, P. (2011). Hypoxia and inflammation. *N Engl J Med, 364*(7), 656–665. doi: 10.1056/NEJMra0910283.

Ferroni, P., Basili, S., Paoletti, V., & Davi, G. (2006). Endothelial dysfunction and oxidative stress in arterial hypertension. *Nutr, Met, Card Dis, 16*(3), 222–233.

Galkina, E., & Ley, K. (2009). Immune and inflammatory mechanisms of atherosclerosis. *Ann Rev Imm, 27,* 165–197. doi: 10.1146/annurev.immunol.021908.132620.

Hall, J. (2011). *Guyton & Hall textbook of medical physiology.* 12th ed. Philadelphia, PA: Elsevier.

Harvey, R. A., & Ferrier, D. R. (2011). *Lippincott's illustrated reviews: biochemistry.* 5th ed. Philadelphia, PA: Wolters Kluwer.

Ilancheran, S., Michalska, A., S. Peh, et al. (2007, May 9). Stem cells derived from human fetal membranes display multi-lineage differentiation potential. *Biol Rep*, 577–588.

Iwasa, J. (2012). HMS cell biology visualization: proteosome structure and function. Retrieved from http://biochem.web.utah.edu/iwasa/projects/proteasome.html

Jaenisch, R. (2004). Human cloning—the science and ethics of nuclear transplantation. *N Engl J Med*, 351(27), 2787–2791.

Jegathesan, J., Liebenthal, J. A., Arnett, M., et al. (2004). Apoptosis: understanding the new molecular pathway. *MEDSURG Nurs*, 13(6), 371–376.

Katzung, B. G., Masters, S., & Trevor, A. (2012). *Basic and clinical pharmacology.* 12th ed. New York: Lange Medical Books/McGraw-Hill Companies.

Kerbel, R. S. (2008). Tumor angiogenesis. *N Engl J Med*, 358(19), 2039–2049. doi: 10.1056/NEJMra0706596.

Kim, S. U. (2014, May 21). Lysosomal storage diseases: stem cell-based cell- and gene-therapy. *Cell Trans.* Epub ahead of print.

Kolata, G. (1997, February 24). With cloning of a sheep, the ethical ground shift. *The New York Times*, p. 1, B8.

Kumar, V., Abbas, A. K., Fausto, N., & Aster, J. C (2014). *Robbins & Cotran pathologic basis of disease.* 9th ed. Philadelphia, PA: Elsevier Saunders.

Li, J., Flammer, A. J., Lennon, R. J., et al. (2012, October). Comparison of the effect of the metabolic syndrome and multiple traditional cardiovascular risk factors on vascular function. *Mayo Clin Proceed,* 87(10), 968–975. doi: 10.1016/j.mayocp.2012.07.004.

Lerou, P. H., & Daley, G. Q. (2005). Therapeutic potential of embryonic stem cells. *Blood Rev,* 19(6), 321–331.

Longo, D. L., Kasper, D. L., Fauci, A. S., et al. (Eds.). (2012). *Harrison's principles of internal medicine.* 18th ed. New York: McGraw-Hill.

McPhee, S. J., & Hammer, G. (2014). *Pathophysiology of disease: an introduction to clinical medicine.* 7th ed. New York: McGraw-Hill.

Mimeault, M., Hauke, R., & Batra, S. K. (2007, August 1). Stem cells: a revolution in therapeutics—recent advances in stem cell biology and their therapeutic applications in regenerative medicine and cancer therapies. *Clin Pharm Ther.* Sep vol 82 issue (3) pgs. 252- 264.

Nachman, R. L., & Rafii, S. (2008). Platelets, petechiae, and preservation of the vascular wall. *N Engl J Med,* 359(12), 1261–1270. doi: 10.1056/NEJMra0800887.

Nash, D. T. (2000, July). Endothelial dysfunction: why it belongs in general practice. *Consultant*, 1525–1529.

National Institutes of Health. (2009). Stem cell basics. Retrieved from http://stemcells.nih.gov/info/basics/basics3.asp

Nature. (2015). Human genome collection. Retrieved from http://www.nature.com/nature/supplements/collections/humangenome/

Ohnishi, S., Ohgushi, H., Kitamura, S., & Nagaya, N. (2007). Mesenchymal stem cells for the treatment of heart failure. *Int J Hem*, 86(1), 17–21.

O'Shea, P. (2012, April 18). Future medicine shaped by an interdisciplinary new biology. *Lancet*, 379(9825), 1544–1550. doi: 10.1016/S0140-6736(12)60476-0.

Papadakis, M., McPhee, S. J., & Rabow, M. W. (2014). *Current medical diagnosis and treatment.* New York: Lange Medical Books.

Polovina, M. M., & Potpara, T. S. (2014). Endothelial dysfunction in metabolic and vascular disorders. *Postgrad Med,* 126(2), 38–53. doi: 10.3810/pgm.2014.03.2739.

Radisic, M., & Christman, K. L. (2013). Materials science and tissue engineering: repairing the heart. *Mayo Clin Proceed*, 88(8), 884–898. doi: 10.1016/j.mayocp.2013.05.003.

Sedlak, T. W., & Snyder, S. (2006). Messenger molecules and cell death: therapeutic implications. *JAMA*, 295(1), 81–89.

Sharpless, N. E., & DePinho, R. A. (2005). Cancer: crime and punishment. *Nature,* 436, 636–637. doi: 10.1038/436636a.

Smith, A. R., & Wagner, J. E. (2009). Alternative haematopoietic stem cell sources for transplantation: place of umbilical cord blood. *Brit J Haem*, 14(2), 246–261.

Tan, K. C., Chow, W. S., Ai, V. H., et al. (2002). Advanced glycation end products and endothelial dysfunction in type 2 diabetes. *Diabetes Care,* 25(6), 1055–1059.

Tang, Y., Yashura, T., Hara, M. et al. (2007). Transplantation of bone marrow-derived stem cells: a promising therapy for stroke. *Cell Trans*, 16(2), 159–169.

Terzic, A., Folmes, C. D., Martinez-Fernandez, A., & Behfar, A. (2011). Regenerative medicine: on the vanguard of health care. *Mayo Clin Proceed*, 86(7), 600–602. doi: 10.4065/mcp.2011.0325.

Thomson, J. A., Itskovitz-Eldor, J., Shapiro, S. S., et al. (1998). Embryonic stem cell lines derived from human blastocysts. *Science*, 282(5391), 1145–1171.

Vermeulen, L., de Sousa, E., Melo, F., Richel, D. J., & Medema, J. P. (2012). The developing cancer stem-cell model: clinical challenges and opportunities. *Lancet Oncol*, 13(2), e83–89. doi: 10.1016/S1470-2045(11)70257-1.

Vogel, R. A. (2000). The Mediterranean diet and endothelial function: why some dietary fats may be healthy. *Cleveland Clin J Med*, 67(4), 232, 235–236. Erratum in: *Cleveland Clin J Med,* 67(7), 467.

Watt, S. M., & Contreras, M. (2005). Stem cell medicine: umbilical cord blood and its stem cell potential. *Sem Fetal Neonat Med*, 10(3), 209–220.

Zacharias, D. G., Nelson, T. J., Mueller, P. S., & Hook, C. C. (2011). The science and ethics of induced pluripotency: what will become of embryonic stem cells? *Mayo Clin Proceed*, 86(7), 634–640. doi: 10.4065/mcp.2011.0054.

Zweier, J. L., & Talukder, M. A. (2006). The role of oxidants and free radicals in reperfusion injury. *Cardio Res,* 70(2), 181–190.

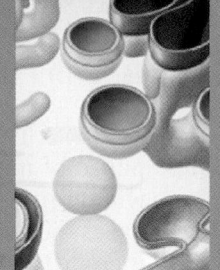

Genetic Basis of Disease

Key Terms

Allele

Aneuploidy

Autosomal

Carrier

Dominant

Gene locus

Genomics

Genotype

Heterozygous

Homozygous

Karyotype

Mutation

Oncogene

Oncoproteins

Pharmacogenomics

Phenotype

Recessive

Single nucleotide polymorphisms (SNP)

Translocation

Tumor suppressor gene

Many disease processes are the result of abnormal cellular activity that occurs from alterations in the cell's genetic control (see deoxyribonucleic acid [DNA] in Chapter 1). When there is a change in the sequence of DNA nucleotides, there are resultant changes in cellular physiology. Specific changes in DNA are linked to specific diseases, and clinicians can identify precise changes in DNA that are related to specific diseases. Also, because DNA is passed on to subsequent generations, specific inheritance patterns can be identified. These changes in DNA, inheritance patterns, and their associated illnesses compose the genetic basis of disease.

The fundamental unit of DNA is the gene, which is located on a chromosome. A genome refers to the collection of all of an organism's genes. The Human Genome Project was established by the National Institutes of Health and other research organizations to study all of the human body's genes. It was a major 13-year research study from 1990 through 2003, and its results have enabled researchers to identify tens of thousands of genes linked to specific disorders and traits. The project revolutionized the understanding of DNA and continues to provide increasing knowledge regarding gene mapping and disease predisposition. As a result of this knowledge, current health-care treatments and research encompass the fields of genomics and pharmacogenomics.

Genomics is the study of an organism's multiple genes and their interactions. **Pharmacogenomics** is the study of how genes influence an individual's response to medications.

Basic Concepts of Genetics

DNA Components

DNA is a double helical structure that can be broken down into nucleotides. A nucleotide is a combination of a pentose sugar molecule, phosphate, and a purine or pyrimidine nitrogen base. The nitrogen bases are adenine (A), thymine (T), guanine (G), and cytosine (C) (see Fig. 3-1). The nitrogenous base pairs combine in specific ways in DNA: adenine and thymine (A)–(T) or guanine and cytosine (G)–(C). In ribonucleic acid (RNA), there is one different nitrogen base called uracil. In RNA, uracil replaces thymine, which means that RNA base pairs combine like so: adenine and uracil (A)–(U) or (G)–(C).

Genes

Each DNA molecule contains many genes—the basic units of heredity. A gene is a specific arrangement of nucleotide bases, which carry a code for constructing

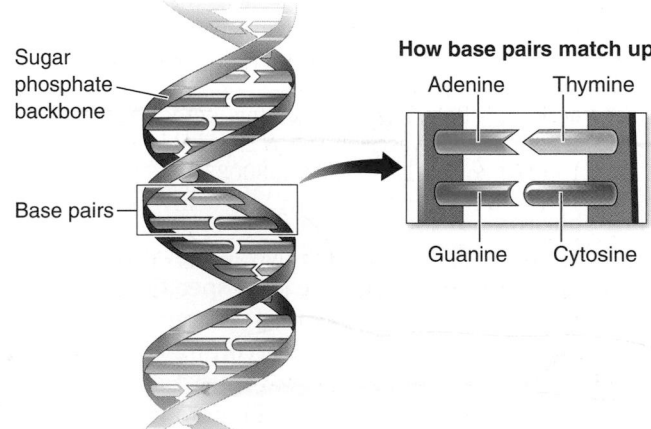

FIGURE 3-1. The nitrogenous bases of deoxyribonucleic acid (DNA). When DNA is stretched out, it forms a double helix that resembles a twisted ladder with purine-pyrimidine nitrogenous pairs represented by individual steps on the ladder. The purine-pyrimidine nitrogenous pairs consist of the amino acids adenosine, cytosine, thymine, and guanine. These are matched in a unique sequence to form an individual's genetic code.

proteins. The human genome is estimated to be composed of more than 30,000 genes. Human genes vary widely in length, often extending over thousands of bases, but only about 10% of the genome is known to include the protein-coding sequences called exons. Interspersed within many genes are intron sequences, which have no coding function.

Within a gene, an arrangement of three specific DNA bases is called a codon. Codons hold the directions for synthesis of a specific amino acid; for example, the base sequence ATG codes for the amino acid methionine. An average-sized gene is made of 3,000 nitrogenous base pairs. Because three bases code for one amino acid, an average gene can code for 1,000 amino acids. These amino acids link together to form the proteins synthesized by the cell; this means that the genetic code is a series of codons that specify which amino acids are required to make up specific proteins.

Mutations

Genes can undergo **mutation,** which can cause disease. A mutation occurs when a gene is damaged or changed in such a way as to alter the genetic code carried by that gene. A mutation can be inherited from parents or can occur sporadically because of environmental influences. Gametes, also referred to as germ cells, include the sperm and the ovum. Mutations that affect the gamete genes, otherwise known as germ cell mutations, can be passed down to future offspring. Mutations that arise in body cells, also called somatic cells, can have mutations, but these are not passed down to offspring and do not cause hereditary diseases.

Mutations usually involve a whole gene or chromosome. However, some mutations can cause partial or complete deletion of a gene or a single nucleotide base; these are called point mutations.

Gene Nomenclature

As researchers have discovered the various genes in the human genome, each has been given a label. Some genes have been given names that are acronyms of diseases or names that identify their effect. For example, the gene that is associated with breast cancer is called the BRCA gene, and the gene that is associated with retinoblastoma is the Rb gene. These are names associated with the disease caused by the mutation.

Not all genes, however, have such specific names. To identify any gene, a specific type of nomenclature is followed. All genes can be identified according to their **gene locus,** or their location on a chromosome. Understanding a gene locus requires knowledge of chromosomal structure. Each chromosome pair takes on the formation of an "X" because of the position of their central point, called the centromere. This centromere creates upper arm and lower arm portions of the chromosome pair.

Commonly, chromosome pairs have short upper arms and long lower arms. The upper arm portion of the chromosome is referred to as the "p" arm. The lower arm portion is referred to as the "q" arm. Chromosomes

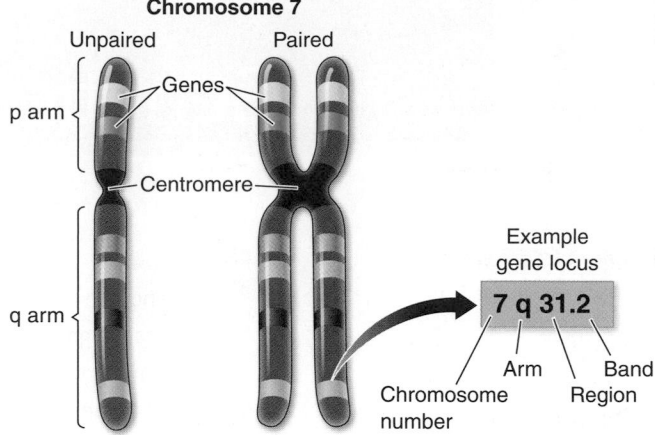

FIGURE 3-2. A gene locus is the gene's location on the chromosome. The central region of a pair of chromosomes is called the centromere, which divides the chromosome into a short arm (p) and a long arm (q). A gene is named by listing the chromosome number, followed by the arm it sits on, p or q. The numbered region on the p or q arm is listed and can be further broken down into band and sub-band, for example: 7 q 31.2.

are further divided into zones called regions, bands, and subbands (see Fig. 3-2).

When indicating a specific gene locus, the chromosome number, arm, and region are designated. For example, the gene linked to Duchenne muscular dystrophy has been located at Xp21, the short arm ("p") of the X chromosome in the 21st region. Cystic fibrosis (CF) is associated with a defect in the gene locus 7 q 31.2. This indicates that the gene is located on the long arm ("q") of the seventh chromosome in a region designated as 31.2.

As previously stated, some genes have been given specific names. These genes have two names; for example, the gene associated with breast cancer can be referred to as the BRCA gene or 17q21. This indicates that the BRCA gene is located on the 17th chromosome's long arm in the 21st region. Table 3-1 identifies the gene locus for different genetic diseases.

The Human Karyotype

A **karyotype** refers to a picture of the chromosomes that are contained within the DNA of a species. The human karyotype contains 23 pairs of chromosomes. During a specific stage of cell division, the helical DNA molecule stretches out and separates into 23 pairs of chromosomes. During this stage, geneticists can study individual chromosomes and genes by obtaining a picture of the 23 chromosome pairs. Each individual has a unique karyotype—a distinct picture of their 23 pairs of chromosomes (see Fig. 3-3). A karyotype can be used to identify an individual, similar to how fingerprints are used.

The human karyotype can be assembled from any human cell with a nucleus. Karyotype testing is commonly performed on an individual's white blood cells (WBCs) or swabbed cheek cells.

TABLE 3-1. Genetic Diseases and Their Gene Locus	
Disease	**Gene Locus**
Huntington disease	4p16
Cystic fibrosis	7q31
Hemophilia type A	Xq28
Marfan syndrome	15q15–15q21
Sickle cell anemia	11p15
Breast cancer BRCA1	17q21
Breast cancer BRCA2	13q
Fragile X syndrome	Xq27
Phenylketonuria	12q21
Duchenne muscular dystrophy	Xp21
Retinoblastoma	13q14
Hemochromatosis	6p21
Familial hypercholesterolemia	19p13
Polycystic kidney disease	16p4
Alpha 1 antitrypsin deficiency	14q31 and 14q32
Familial Alzheimer disease	21q11
Cleft palate	Xq13
Tay Sachs disease	15q22
Familial adenomatous polyposis	5q21 and 5q22
Neurofibromatosis type 1	17q11

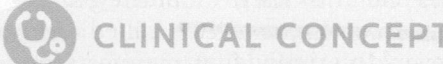

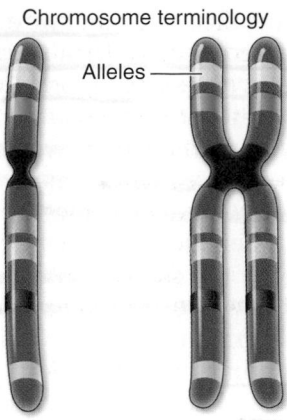

Chromosome terminology

Alleles

FIGURE 3-4. On every pair of chromosomes there are genes that determine the same characteristic. Each individual gene is called an allele. They occupy the same position on each chromosome. One allele is inherited from the mother and the other allele is inherited from the father.

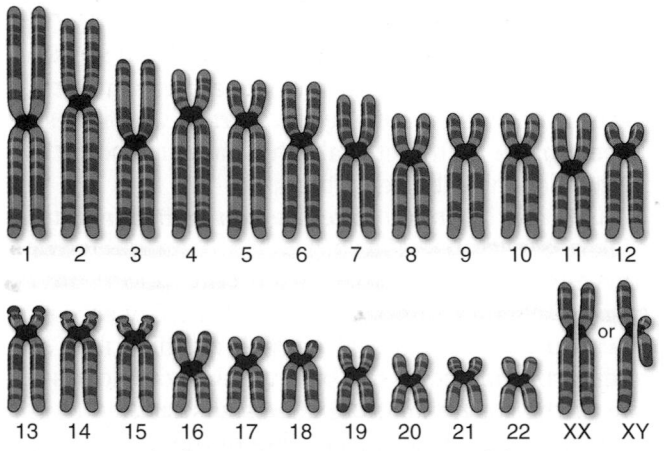

FIGURE 3-3. The human karyotype is a picture of the 23 pairs of chromosomes. Each pair of chromosomes is numbered 1 to 23. The 23rd pair contains the sex chromosomes. The 1st to 22nd pairs are called autosomes, which determine the body's genetic characteristics. Each person has a unique karyotype, which is why a karyotype can be used to identify a specific individual.

Of the 23 chromosome pairs, 22 pairs carry genes related to body traits, called somatic chromosomes or autosomes. One pair carries genes related to gender, called the sex chromosome pair. Females possess the XX sex chromosome pair and males possess the XY pair. The Y chromosome is much smaller than the X and contains the sex determining region. Every chromosome contains individual genes that contain traits of inheritance that transmit information from one generation to another. Each chromosome in a pair contains corresponding genes, known as **alleles.** Each allele is inherited from each parent (see Fig. 3-4).

CLINICAL CONCEPT

The normal human karyotype contains 22 pairs of autosomal chromosomes and one pair of sex chromosomes. Normal female karyotypes are 46,XX; males are 46,XY.

Regulation of Gene Expression

Daily cellular function involves the production of proteins and other substances that are responsible for maintaining physiologic homeostasis. DNA is transcribed into RNA in the nucleus in a process known as transcription. RNA then leaves the nucleus and directs the cell to carry out a specific kind of protein synthesis at the ribosomes in a process known as translation. Although every cell in the body contains identical DNA with its accompanying genetic information, not all of the genes are active. Some genes are silenced. The active genes are only those necessary for the particular tissue's function. For example, all pancreatic beta cells contain all of an individual's DNA. However, because the pancreatic beta cells need to specifically produce insulin, those genes needed for synthesis of insulin are turned on, and the genes for synthesis of other hormones are turned off. There are regulatory regions on a gene that determine whether or not it is active or inactive. Also, there are specific transcription factors that interact with these regulatory regions in turning protein synthesis on or off.

Inheritance Patterns

The transmission of genetic information from parents to children begins with the formation of the gametes (sperm and ova). During the process of meiosis, gametes are formed that contain DNA derived from the parents. When the gametes fuse to form a zygote, chromosome pairs are formed. One chromosome of the pair comes from the mother and the other chromosome comes from the father. The genes that carry specific traits on corresponding sites of both chromosomes are the alleles, and these alleles are paired according to specific traits. The two allelic combinations determine inheritance of certain traits. Alleles can be either heterozygous or homozygous for a certain trait, which has implications for how the trait will be manifested in the individual. **Heterozygous** alleles have different codes for genetic traits; **homozygous** alleles have identical codes for genetic traits.

Genetic traits can be either **dominant** or **recessive**, with the dominant trait being expressed or visible in heterozygous individuals. When letters are used to diagram the genetic trait, capital letters are used for dominant characteristics. Small letters represent recessive characteristics. For example, a person with heterozygous alleles for brown eyes has two different alleles inherited from the two parents—a "B" allele for brown eyes and a "b" allele for blue eyes. This individual's technical genetic makeup, called a **genotype,** is Bb. However, this individual manifests brown eyes, which is the **phenotype.** A phenotype is defined as how genetic traits manifest themselves in the individual; it is the actual, physical, or somatic expression of the genotype. The reason the individual manifests brown eyes, despite having two different alleles, is because the "B" allele is dominant. The dominant allele is expressed in a heterozygous individual.

Homozygous alleles are genes with the identical trait inherited from the individual's two parents. As an example, a brown-eyed person can have a "B" allele from one parent and a "B" allele from the other parent. This homozygous individual's genotype is BB and his or her phenotype displays brown eyes, because B is dominant.

Homozygous alleles can contain the genetic code for recessive traits and can cause manifestation of these traits. As an example, if an individual inherits a "b" allele for eye color from one parent and inherits another "b" allele from the other parent, this results in a "bb" combination. This is a recessive combination of alleles (each "b" representing blue eyes), and the person manifests blue eye color. A recessive trait is usually expressed in an individual if there are corresponding recessive alleles on each chromosome, otherwise known as a homozygous pair (see Fig. 3-5).

A dominant trait is usually expressed if corresponding alleles are homozygous or heterozygous. In a heterozygous state, the dominant allele silences the recessive allele. A **carrier** is a person who is heterozygous for a recessive trait and does not manifest it; in other words, a carrier possesses a recessive allele, but the dominant allele silences it. The carrier does not externally demonstrate the recessive trait but can pass it on to his or her offspring. For example, an individual can carry the trait for blue eyes but have the phenotype of brown eyes. That individual would have a "Bb" genotype.

The inheritance of some genetic traits is considered to be sex linked. As stated earlier, the female genotype is XX, whereas the male genotype is XY. Because the Y chromosome is smaller than the X chromosome, it does not have comparable alleles for many of the X chromosome traits. Therefore, genetic traits on the X chromosome are dominant in males. However, they may be either dominant or recessive in females. Traits that are not sex linked are referred to as **autosomal** traits.

Mendelian Inheritance

The basic concepts of genetics were initially developed through the work of Gregor Mendel, a 19th century Augustinian monk. As a high school science teacher, he began to study inheritance patterns by examining the characteristics of pea plants in his garden. His descriptions of inheritance patterns of dominant and recessive traits have been used to introduce the concepts of heredity. However, some genetic traits and illnesses have a more multifactorial inheritance pattern than Mendelian inheritance patterns.

In Mendelian inheritance, the Punnet Square is used to depict the chance of dominant versus recessive traits. This method is used to configure possible combinations of gene traits in offspring. The allelic traits of each parent are used to configure all possible combinations. The alleles contributed by one parent are placed across the top of the square, and the alleles contributed by the other parent are placed on the left of the square.

Autosomal Inheritance. If a mother and a father are heterozygous for brown eyes (Bb) and they want to know the chances of their offspring having brown versus blue eyes, the Punnett Square method can be used (see Fig. 3-6).

The results of the Punnett Square depicted in Figure 3-6 demonstrate that there is a 25% chance that the offspring will be homozygous for brown eyes (BB), a 50% chance that offspring will be heterozygous for brown eyes (Bb), and a 25% chance that offspring will be homozygous for blue eyes (bb). Therefore, in this case, brown eyes would be considered an autosomal dominant trait because it is evident in all individuals with the B or brown eye gene. The B gene is dominant and silences the b gene, which is recessive.

Parents who possess the sickle cell anemia trait often need information about the chances that their

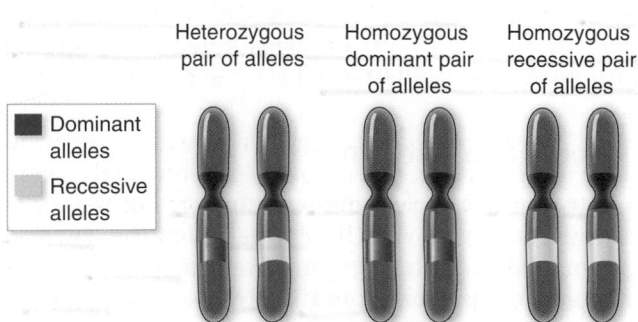

FIGURE 3-5. Genetic traits can be either dominant or recessive, with the dominant trait usually being expressed over the recessive genetic trait. Individuals can be homozygous or heterozygous with regard to genetic traits. Homozygous individuals have both alleles expressing the same trait. Heterozygous individuals have both alleles expressing different traits.

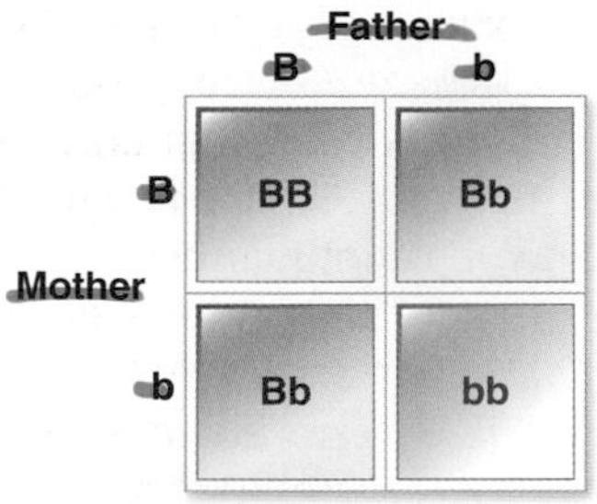

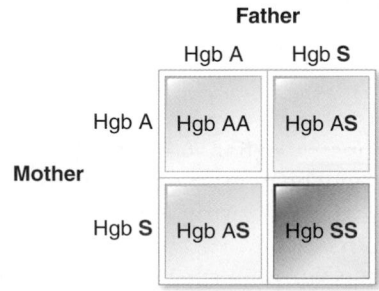

Father

	B	b
B	BB	Bb
b	Bb	bb

Mother

FIGURE 3-6. Using a Punnett Square to determine eye color. In this Punnett Square, the mother is Bb genotype and brown eyes phenotype (Brown [B] eyes are dominant; blue [b] is recessive). The father is Bb genotype and brown eyes phenotype (Brown [B] eyes are dominant; blue [b] is recessive). There is a 25% chance of homozygous brown eye color, genotype BB; a 25% chance of homozygous blue recessive eye color, genotype bb; and a 50% chance a child will be heterozygous for Bb, brown eyes.

offspring will have sickle cell anemia. An individual with sickle cell trait is heterozygous for sickle cell anemia. This can also be referred to as a "carrier" state, because he or she can transmit the gene for sickle cell anemia to children. A Punnett Square can be used to configure the possible genetic combinations of offspring (see Fig. 3-7).

The results of the Punnett Square in Figure 3-7 demonstrate that there is a 25% chance that this couple's offspring will be homozygous for sickle cell anemia (Hgb S–Hgb S), a 50% chance that their offspring will be heterozygous for sickle cell anemia (Hgb S–Hgb normal), and a 25% chance that their offspring will not have sickle cell anemia (Hgb normal–Hgb normal). Therefore, there is a 25% chance that the parents with sickle cell trait will have an offspring who will suffer from sickle cell anemia. In this case, sickle cell anemia is considered an autosomal recessive disorder.

Sex-Linked Inheritance

If the gene is located on the X chromosome, the inheritance pattern is considered to be sex-linked, or X-linked. Because the X chromosome has no corresponding allele

on the Y chromosome, the X allele is dominant. The X alleles will dominate over the lack of Y alleles. Therefore, the X allele will always show up in male offspring. However, for female offspring, it will follow a similar pattern to autosomal dominant or recessive.

The classic example to explain this is the inheritance pattern of hemophilia. The gene responsible for hemophilia is carried on the X chromosome. There is no corresponding allele on the Y chromosome. Females can have one X chromosome with the hemophilia allele and one normal X chromosome. The normal X chromosome allele silences the allele with hemophilia. Therefore, females can be carriers of hemophilia but not express the disease. Because the allelic trait is on the X chromosome in the male and the male Y chromosome has no corresponding allele, hemophilia is expressed in the male. There is no Y allele to silence the hemophilia allele on the X chromosome. Therefore, males express the allele on the X chromosome and suffer from the disease (see Fig. 3-8).

Penetrance and Expressivity

Despite the fact that two individuals might have the same genotype, their phenotypic characteristics might be different. This difference is the result of varying penetrance of the genetic characteristic. Penetrance is determined by whether the disorder's symptoms are clearly evident. Expressivity is based on the symptoms' severity. Based on these two concepts, the severity of a genetic disorder may vary from one individual to another.

Genetic penetrance is described by a ratio of the number of people who have the phenotype as compared with the number of people who have the genotype. A gene is considered to be highly penetrant if almost all of the individuals with the gene develop the characteristics. For example, in breast cancer, there is an increased risk of developing this disorder in women who inherit the BRCA1 or BRCA2 gene. Thus, the penetrance of these genes is based on the likelihood or lifetime risk of developing cancer. In women who inherit BRCA1, the penetrance is about 85%; for BRCA2, it is about 20%. This is important information that must be considered in deciding whether or not to be tested for the presence of the BRCA1 and BRCA2 genes.

Variations in genetic expressivity can be seen in several genetic disorders. For some individuals, there is evidence of the disorder without some of the more serious characteristics. This can be observed in familial hypercholesterolemia (FH), a genetic disorder with an alteration in the low density lipoprotein receptor. With an altered receptor, individuals develop high blood cholesterol levels. However, among individuals with this genetic alteration, there are different severities of disease. The disease's severity is based on the severity of the alteration in the lipoprotein receptor. Therefore, cholesterol levels in affected individuals can range

Father

	Hgb A	Hgb S
Hgb A	Hgb AA	Hgb AS
Hgb S	Hgb AS	Hgb SS

Mother

FIGURE 3-7. Using a Punnett Square to determine sickle cell disease. In this Punnett Square, the mother is heterozygous and the father is heterozygous. Mother and father, who are both carriers of sickle cell anemia, have a 25% chance of having a child with full sickle cell disease, a 25% chance of having a child with no trait at all, and a 50% chance of having a heterozygous child.

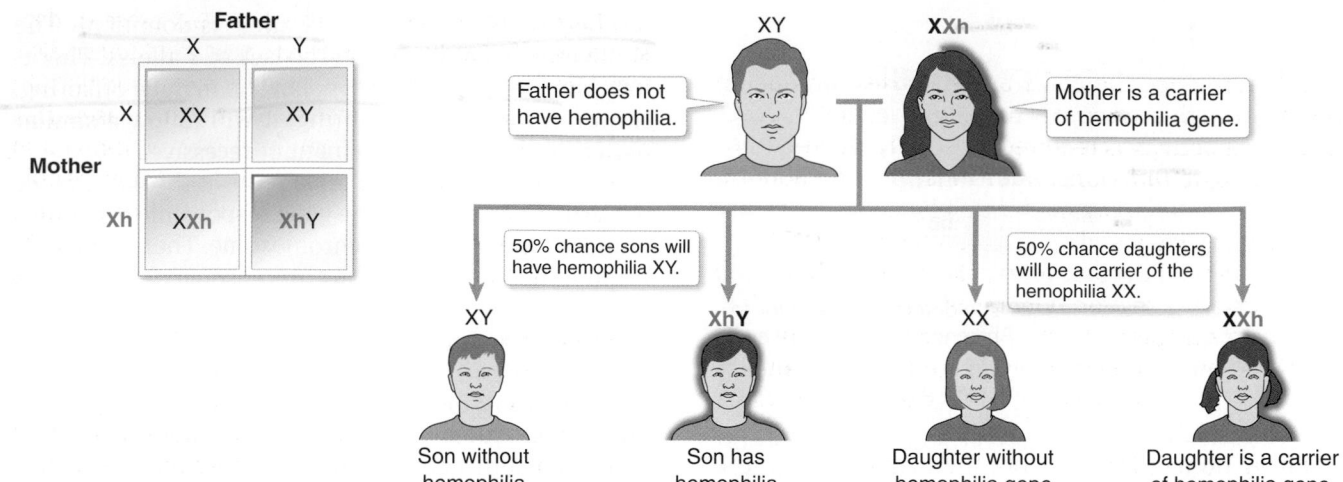

FIGURE 3-8. The following Punnett Square and genogram show how hemophilia, which is an X-linked genetic disorder, is inherited. The X chromosome, which is dominant over the Y chromosome, determines the trait's heredity in an X-linked disorder. The X chromosome is a full chromosome, whereas the Y chromosome is a piece of chromosomal material. In this genogram, the mother is a carrier of hemophilia; therefore, her genotype is XXh. The father does not have hemophilia and his genotype is XY. A Punnett Square can be used to determine the chances of the child having hemophilia or carrying the trait. There is a 25% chance that the parents will have a daughter who is a carrier of hemophilia, a 25% chance of having a son with hemophilia, a 25% chance of having a son without the disorder, and a 25% chance of having a daughter who is not a carrier.

from moderately elevated to extremely high. Affected individuals have varying severity of the disease.

Multifactorial Inheritance

Single gene inherited disorders or single mutations are quite rare. In fact, the majority of diseases are the result of multifactorial genetic influences. Diseases such as hypertension, heart disease, diabetes mellitus (DM), and cancer are caused by multifactorial gene mutations. In these diseases, an individual inherits one or more genes that predispose to a disorder and then environmental triggers, diet, and exercise contribute to disease development. For example, multifactorial inheritance factors are involved in the development of type 1 and type 2 DM:

- In type 1 DM, there are several genes on chromosomes 6, 7, and 11 that increase the risk of developing the disorder. However, type 1 DM has an autoimmune component that may be trigged by exposure to the Coxsackie virus or bovine serum albumin from cow's milk.
- In type 2 DM, obesity and increased abdominal fat distribution patterns are associated with insulin resistance, which characterizes the disorder. There is also a strong family history of type 2 DM in affected individuals. Both these factors contribute to the development of Type 2 DM.

An interesting aspect of multifactorial inheritance relates to variation in the genes that are associated with increased risk of developing a disorder. These variations are referred to as **single nucleotide polymorphisms (SNP)**. These are changes in one nucleotide of a gene sequence. A nucleotide contains a purine or pyrimidine, pentose (sugar), and phosphate (see Fig. 3-9). For example, for the healthy population a nucleotide for a certain trait may contain the sequence AACGT—adenine, adenine, cytosine, guanine, and thymine. However, it may be found that in a group of people with a certain disease there is a variation in the sequence such as ATCGT—adenine, thymine, cytosine, guanine, and thymine. This alteration is a SNP that can be researched to further study the disease.

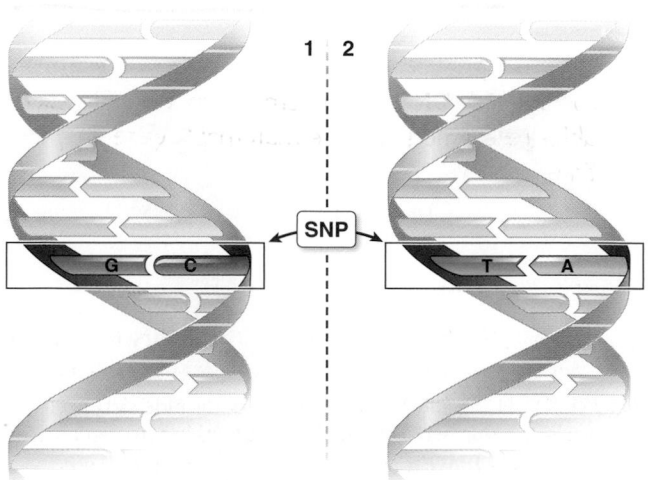

FIGURE 3-9. A single-nucleotide polymorphism is a variation in a DNA sequence occurring when a single nucleotide–A, T, C, or G–in the genome differs between a pair of chromosomes.

Mitochondria and Inherited Diseases

Mitochondria are the cell's powerhouses, producing energy through a series of complex biochemical reactions. Their activity is required for supplying energy for all physiologic functions. Additionally, mitochondria are the only cellular organelles that have their own distinctive ribosomes and DNA. Mitochondrial DNA is a double-stranded circular molecule responsible for the formation of the key components of energy production. Cell biologists speculate that mitochondria were self-sustaining, independent-living, bacteria-like organisms that, over the course of evolution, became incorporated into human cells.

During human fertilization, the ovum destroys the sperm's mitochondria, which results in all mitochondrial DNA being derived from the mother. Because mitochondrial DNA is unique, geneticists can use mitochondrial DNA to study an individual's maternal hereditary lineage.

Alterations in nutrient delivery to the cell can damage mitochondria. In addition, mitochondrial DNA can be subject to impairment or mutation by free radicals. Although there is a repair process for DNA within the cell's nucleus, this does not usually happen for mitochondrial DNA. Cumulative damage of mitochondrial DNA can be implicated in the aging process and in diseases such as diabetes, cancer, and heart failure.

Inherited mitochondrial disorders include neurogenerative disorders, hypertrophic cardiomyopathy, ophthalmoplegia, and maternally inherited deafness. This inheritance pattern is passed on from the mother to all offspring. Other inherited mitochondrial diseases include disorders of balance and sensation, classified as ataxia-neuropathy syndromes. It is theorized that the cellular damage and symptoms are related to the progressive decrease in cellular mitochondrial activity. The symptoms are more evident when the altered mitochondrial function affects the muscles and the nerves.

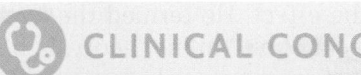

CLINICAL CONCEPT

Mitochondrial DNA is maternally inherited, which enables researchers to trace maternal lineage far back in time.

Pharmacogenomics

There are individual differences in the ability to respond and metabolize certain medications. An inherited autosomal recessive trait called slow acetylator phenotype occurs in about 50% of blacks and whites in the United States. Individuals with this recessive trait produce less of an enzyme necessary to metabolize certain medications. They are also at an increased risk of developing drug-induced lupus erythematosus.

Pharmacogenomics has also provided more understanding of individual responses to warfarin (Coumadin), which is used to decrease the formation of blood clots in patients with irregular heartbeats and increased risk of myocardial infarction or stroke. However, individual responses to this medication are variable. Some people obtain therapeutic effects fairly quickly, whereas others require higher dosages and multiple blood tests to achieve the same effects. This variability in response has been linked to the presence of a gene that reduces the metabolism and elimination of warfarin. People with the reduced metabolism and elimination of warfarin need a lower dose to achieve a therapeutic effect. Testing for the enzymes produced by this gene provides information that enables health-care providers to prescribe the correct dose of medication with less risk of adverse effects.

Alterations in DNA

The DNA within the nucleus must be protected because it contains the vital information for heredity and all cellular activity in the body. DNA is vulnerable to damage if a breech occurs in the nuclear membrane or an injurious agent penetrates the nucleus. However, there are internal repair processes that attempt to restore DNA to its normal state. If the change in DNA involves an altered nitrogenous base sequence in one strand of the DNA, its complementary strand can be a template for repair. The mismatched base sequence is removed from the altered strand. The DNA replication process then uses the complementary strand to match up the appropriate bases, completing the repair process.

Defective DNA can be inherited, which means that it was present at birth or acquired in the course of an individual's life span. Therefore, genetic mutations are referred to as either hereditary or acquired, also called sporadic. A hereditary alteration would be evident in prior and present generations, whereas an acquired alteration would be seen in the individual as well as in his or her offspring.

Regardless of the cause, if DNA is damaged, vital genetic material can be defective or mutated. If vital genetic "blueprints" are damaged, there is consequent misdirection of all cellular activity.

In cases of DNA injury, damaged genes are defective and, in turn, transcribed as defective m-RNA. Defective m-RNA will then carry defective directions to the ribosomes, which in turn manufacture defective proteins. Defective proteins synthesized by the cell can be the cause of a disease process.

DNA alterations or mutations are changes in nucleotide sequences, deletions, or insertions of nucleotides. These changes can represent the change of base sequences in a codon, leading to a change in the protein structure. For example, a nucleotide base substitution results in a different amino acid being included in hemoglobin formation, leading to the development of sickle cell anemia. The normal nucleotide base sequence is GAG (guanine–adenine–guanine), which codes for glutamic acid. In sickle cell disease, the sequence is GTG (guanine–thymine–guanine), which codes for valine. This change in amino acid alters the hemoglobin structure, forming the sickle cell HgbS.

Deletion of a nucleotide may cause its specific gene to be nonfunctional. This is the case with individuals with phenylketonuria. Affected individuals are unable to produce a specific enzyme, phenylalanine hydroxylase, which converts phenylalanine to tyrosine. Lack of phenylalanine hydroxylase leads to a buildup of phenylalanine in the systemic circulation. The accumulation of phenylalanine can cause phenylketonuria (PKU), a disease that includes growth retardation, hypopigmentation, and mental retardation.

CLINICAL CONCEPT

Most newborns in developed countries are screened for PKU soon after birth. A sign of PKU is a musty odor of the urine and sweat.

Oncogenes and Tumor Suppressor Genes

An individual can possess a genetic mutation called an activated **oncogene.** Proto-oncogenes are normal genes that control cell proliferation. Mutation of proto-oncogenes leads to activated oncogenes. This mutation causes uncontrolled cellular proliferation or insuppressible cancerous growth.

Activated oncogenes can be inherited or acquired. When the cell that possesses this activated oncogene undergoes transcription, the RNA will carry the defective message of the activated oncogene onto the ribosomes. The ribosomes, in turn, will synthesize defective proteins called **oncoproteins.** These oncoproteins will direct the cell to undergo uncontrolled proliferation, persistent mitotic divisions, or persistent cancerous growth, which is why activated oncogenes can be considered cancer-causing genes.

Another genetic defect associated with cancer involves **tumor suppressor genes,** which are genes that inhibit uncontrolled cellular mitosis and persistent proliferation. An example is the p53 tumor suppressor gene, which stops the mitotic cell division cycle. When defective, tumor suppressor genes do not suppress cancerous transformation of cells and cancer growth occurs uninhibited.

Another way that cancer occurs is through viral insertion of an oncogene. For example, the human papilloma virus (HPV) inserts its DNA into the DNA of tissue cells. When activated, this DNA stimulates the abnormal growth cycle associated with cancer cells. Additionally, it inhibits the action of p53, a tumor suppressor gene. This is the mechanism for the development of cervical cancer from HPV infection.

There is also the multistage theory of cancer development. According to this theory, there must be an initial exposure to a carcinogen that mutates the gene. The next step involves continued exposure to that carcinogen or another carcinogen with similar effects. Finally, the alterations lead to tumor development. Small cell lung cancer in smokers is believed to develop in this way.

CLINICAL CONCEPT

An activated oncogene can lead to formation of oncoproteins and a cancerous change in the cell. A defective tumor suppressor gene can also lead to a cancerous change in the cell.

Knudson's "Two Hit" Hypothesis

Pairs of alleles make up an individual's genotype. If one of the pair's alleles becomes damaged or mutated, the normal corresponding allele can counteract the effect in most cases. In 1971, Alfred Knudson proposed the "two hit" hypothesis to explain the genetic mechanisms in the initiation of certain cancers. He was studying retinoblastoma, a cancer of the retina, which can occur spontaneously or as a hereditary disorder.

It had been observed that retinoblastoma occurred in a younger age in patients with a hereditary predisposition for the cancer than in patients without a hereditary predisposition. Additionally, children with retinoblastoma were more likely to develop the cancer in both eyes than those adults who developed it spontaneously. Knudson tried to understand why cancer developed in only some persons with hereditary predisposition and not others with the same hereditary risk. He studied individuals born with a genetic mutation in one allele for retinoblastoma. In order for actual cancer to develop, Knudson noted that a mutation of one allele was not sufficient because the normal allele counteracted the effect. He termed the initial allelic mutation as the "first hit" in his theory. In his investigations, he noted that cancer only developed in persons who acquired a second allelic mutation. Persons who developed cancer possessed a hereditary mutation on one allele and acquired a second mutation on their normal allele sometime in the course of their lifetime. Therefore, he hypothesized that for many cancers to develop, both corresponding alleles on a chromosome must be mutated. Hence, Knudson called this the "two hit" hypothesis, which has been found to hold true as the required initiating events for many diseases as well as many types of cancer.

For example, if an individual discovers his or her personal inheritance of the BRCA1 or BRCA2 gene, this does not mean that the individual is 100% likely to develop cancer. The individual has a heightened risk of cancer because of the allelic mutation, but this is not the only factor involved in development of cancer. A second allelic mutation would need to be acquired, perhaps through carcinogen exposure, for the disease to actually develop.

Many tumors are examined to determine whether or not one mutation is accompanied by a second mutation. This information has been helpful in cancer research. In terms of hereditary cancer syndromes, it is important to note that an additional mutation is often needed for tumor development.

This model of the "two hit hypothesis" has been applied to the development of other illnesses as well. For example, the tendency to develop schizophrenia can be linked to specific genes related to neurological development. Once the "at risk" gene has been transmitted to offspring (first hit), an environmental factor during the nervous system's development (second hit) alters formation of neural networks, leading to the development of schizophrenia.

As Knudson proposed, in many diseases both alleles must be mutated for a disease to manifest in an individual. This holds true unless a disease is notably autosomal dominant, meaning only one allele needs to be mutated for the disease to come to fruition. Hereditary familial adenomatous polyposis (FAP) is an autosomal dominant disorder, and in these individuals only one allele needs to be mutated in order for the disease to manifest itself.

Chromosomal Alterations

Genetic disorders also occur as a result of changes in the number or structure of chromosomes. Alterations in chromosome division during meiosis result in a different number of chromosomes. This condition is known as **aneuploidy.** This usually occurs when a chromosomal pair does not separate in the anaphase stage of meiosis, a condition known as nondisjunction and anaphase lag. The gamete will have one additional or one fewer chromosome. Other chromosomal alterations can occur when a piece of one chromosome breaks off and joins another. This is referred to as **translocation.** A chromosome can also break and lose a portion of genetic material; this is called a deletion.

The most common chromosomal alteration is Down syndrome, a major cause of intellectual disability. About 95% of individuals with Down syndrome have trisomy, or an additional chromosome, giving them a total of 47 chromosomes. A common replication occurs with chromosome 21, so that there are three copies of this chromosome. This is referred to as trisomy 21, also called Down syndrome. Some individuals have a translocation of chromosomal material from chromosome 21 to either chromosome 22 or 14; this is another form of Down's syndrome.

Turner syndrome, a disorder that affects females, causes hypogonadism and physical characteristics such as a webbed neck, broad chest, and short stature. Instead of 46 chromosomes, females with Turner syndrome have

45 chromosomes—and instead of two X chromosomes, they only have one, giving them a designation of 45,X.

Errors of the mitosis of cells in early embryonic development can give rise to a condition known as mosaicism. Mosaicism occurs when there are cells with different numbers of chromosomes within the same individual. Mosaicism that affects the sex chromosomes is fairly common. In the division of a fertilized ovum, an error can develop where one cell has 45,X and another cell has 47,XXX. All descendent cells from these abnormal cells will have either 45,X or 47,XXX. The individual will exhibit a variation of Turner syndrome.

Many more structural and numerical errors of chromosomes can occur that result in abnormal karyotypes. Those discussed here are major types of chromosomal errors. It is estimated that 7.5% of all conceived embryos have a chromosomal abnormality. Often these types of chromosomal abnormalities are not compatible with life, resulting in fetal or embryonic death.

Genetic Assessment

When dealing with inheritable disorders, assessment includes a family history with multigenerational patterns of illness as well as ethnic, cultural, and social practices. The multigenerational history should include, at a minimum, three generations of a family. This information is then displayed in a genogram (see Fig. 3-10).

Gathering assessment data may require a tactful approach from the health-care professional because some families are reluctant to divulge all of this information during an initial visit. However, certain illness patterns are seen in specific ethnic groups. For example, Tay Sachs disease is associated with people who have an ethnic heritage of Ashkenazi Jewish ancestry. Thalassemia anemia is more prevalent in people of Mediterranean or East Asian descent. Asians often exhibit G6PD deficiency. Cultural practices and shared dietary patterns may increase the risk of developing multifactorial disorders such type 2 DM and cardiovascular disease. This aspect of history taking can provide important clues in evaluating the risk of developing certain inheritable disorders.

Molecular Analysis of Genetic Disorders

It is possible to identify mutations at the DNA level and offer diagnostic tests for an increasing number of genetic disorders. Acquired genetic alterations, inherited disorders, and infectious disease can be detected using molecular analysis techniques such as polymerase chain reaction (PCR) and fluorescence in situ hybridization (FISH).

Karyotyping

A karyotype analysis involves staining the condensed chromosomes of mitotic cells with Giemsa dye. It is an overall picture of an individual's chromosome pairs.

Family History by Genogram

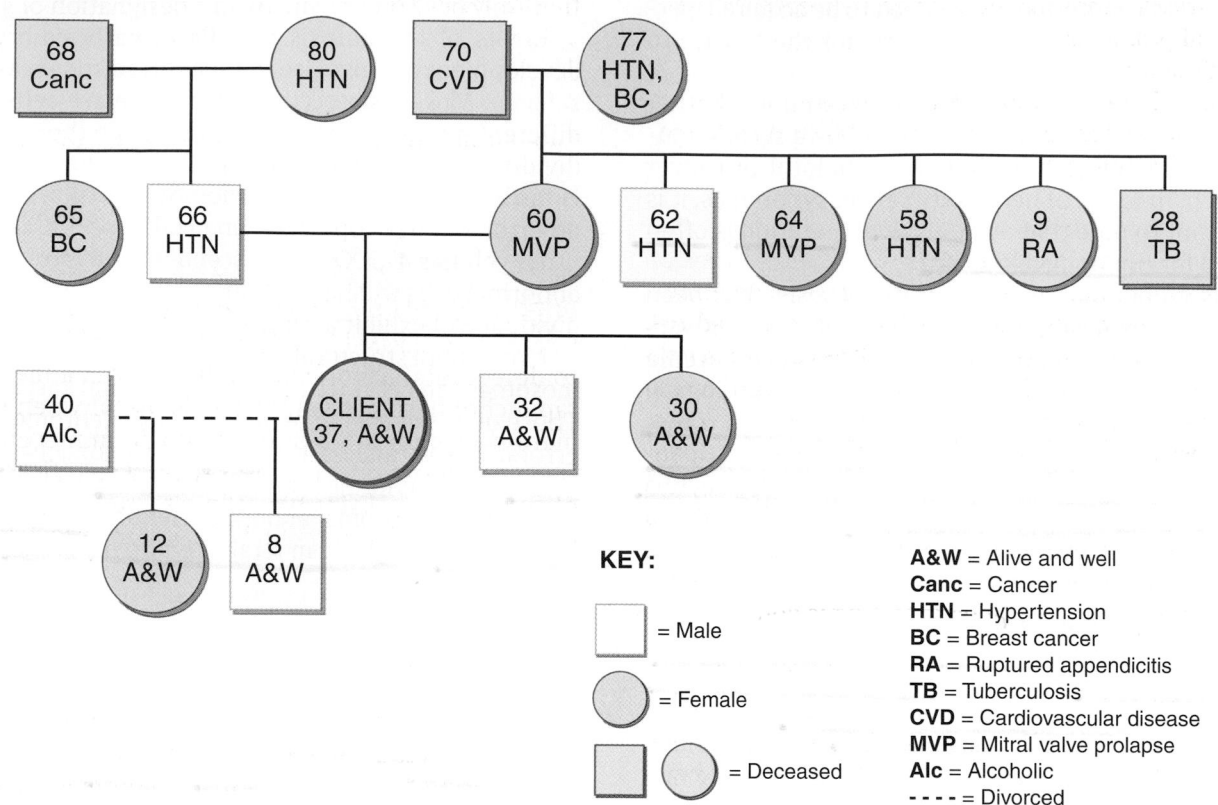

FIGURE 3-10. Example of a genogram. *(From Dillon, P. (2007). Nursing health assessment.* 2nd ed. Philadelphia: F.A. Davis Company, with permission.)*

The dye stains regions of chromosomes that are rich in the base pairs adenine (A) and thymine (T), producing a dark band. A common misconception is that bands represent single genes, but in fact the thinnest bands contain over a million base pairs and potentially hundreds of genes. The analysis allows for comparisons of chromosomes for their length, the placement of centromeres, and the location and sizes of bands.

Polymerase Chain Reaction
PCR is a procedure that produces multiple copies of a short segment of DNA and amplifies the segment for further study in the laboratory. The PCR procedure can be applied to a very small sample of DNA and be used for diagnostic testing. It does not require mitotic cells as does karyotyping. It is commonly used for genetic analysis in cancer and infectious disease detection, forensics, and research.

Fluorescence in Situ Hybridization
FISH is a procedure used to map the genetic material in an individual's cells. It has been used for detection of numeric abnormalities of chromosomes, subtle chromosomal microdeletions, and translocations not detectable by routine karyotyping. It does not require mitotic cells as does karyotyping.

Southern Blotting
Southern blotting is a molecular genetic testing technique used to detect DNA fragments, which can vary because of various types of mutations; these include gene insertions, gene deletions, expanded trinucleotide repeats, and single nitrogenous base changes. For example, Southern blotting could be used to locate a particular gene or DNA fragment within an entire genome.

Prenatal Diagnosis of Genetic Disorders
Prenatal diagnosis or prenatal screening is used for early detection of birth defects and genetic diseases in a fetus or embryo in utero. This diagnosis can identify disorders such as neural tube defects, Down syndrome, chromosome abnormalities, spina bifida, cleft palate, Tay Sachs disease, sickle cell anemia, thalassemia, CF, and fragile X syndrome. Screening can also be used for prenatal sex discernment. Common testing procedures include CVS, amniocentesis, and percutaneous umbilical cord blood sampling (PUBS). In general, genetic testing is offered to couples or individuals identified as being at risk for a particular genetic problem. Some of the risk factors that health-care providers consider in deciding who should be offered testing include family history, medical history, and ethnicity. Examples include:

- Women 35 years or older who are pregnant or are planning to become pregnant
- Abnormal ultrasound findings
- Couples who are close blood relatives, such as first cousins

- Women who have a condition, such as diabetes, that can be associated with an increased risk of fetal problems
- Ethnicity
- Unexplained or multiple miscarriages
- Family history of an inherited condition, intellectual disability, or birth defects.

Maternal Serum Screening

Maternal serum screening refers to tests performed on a pregnant woman's blood for the purpose of determining if her developing fetus may have an increased risk of having an open neural tube defect (ONTD), Down syndrome, or trisomy 18. Proteins that are produced by the developing placenta and fetus enter the mother's blood. The most commonly tested proteins are AFP (alpha-fetoprotein), hCG (human chorionic gonadotropin), uE3 (unconjugated estriol), and DIA (dimeric inhibin A). If a maternal serum screening test is positive, it indicates an increased chance for a fetal problem. In this case, additional, more specific diagnostic testing is done.

Chorionic Villus Sampling

CVS is a diagnostic procedure performed during pregnancy to diagnose chromosome abnormalities, some inherited disorders, and certain birth defects in a fetus. CVS is most commonly offered when a woman is at an advanced maternal age (35 years and older at time of delivery) because of the increased chance of a fetal chromosome problem. CVS may also be offered if an inherited genetic problem is identified in the family. CVS is performed between 10 and 12 weeks of pregnancy. Under the visualization of ultrasound, a thin needle is either inserted through the abdomen or a specially designed catheter is passed through the vagina and a small sample of placenta is removed. The placenta contains cells generated by the fetus. Approximately 99% of fetal chromosome abnormalities can be diagnosed from CVS.

(**ALERT!** CVS is contraindicated in pregnant women with vaginal bleeding, uterine fibroids, retroverted uterus, and those carrying twins.)

Amniocentesis

Amniocentesis is a test primarily used to diagnose fetal chromosome problems. It can also help diagnose fetal defects, such as spina bifida, abdominal wall defects, and some inherited disorders. Amniocentesis is performed on amniotic fluid, usually between 16 and 18 weeks of pregnancy. As the fetus grows and sheds cells, those cells can be found in the amniotic fluid and used to study the fetal chromosomes.

Amniocentesis detects about 99% of fetal chromosome abnormalities. A thin needle is inserted through the mother's abdomen (under ultrasound guidance) into the amniotic sac, and a small amount of amniotic fluid is removed.

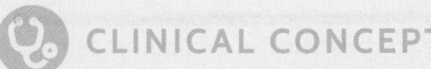

CLINICAL CONCEPT

Amniocentesis is recommended for pregnant women older than age 35 years.

Percutaneous Umbilical Cord Blood Sampling

PUBS, also called cordocentesis, is a diagnostic genetic test that examines blood from the fetal umbilical cord to detect fetal abnormalities. It provides a means of rapid chromosome analysis and is useful when information cannot be obtained through amniocentesis, CVS, or ultrasound. This test carries a significant risk of complication and is typically reserved for pregnancies determined to be at high risk for genetic defects.

Gene Therapy

Gene therapy is an experimental technique that uses genes to treat or prevent disease. The future goal for this type of treatment is to treat a disorder by inserting a gene into a patient's cells instead of using drugs or surgery. Researchers are testing several approaches to gene therapy. The most promising procedure being investigated is the insertion of a normal gene into the genome of a target cell to replace a nonfunctional or mutated gene.

In most gene therapy studies, a "normal" gene is inserted into a patient's genome to replace an "abnormal," disease-causing gene. This is accomplished using a carrier molecule called a vector. The vector carries and delivers the therapeutic gene to the patient's target cells that exhibit the disorder. Currently, the most common vector is a virus that has been genetically altered to carry normal human DNA. The adenovirus (cold virus) is commonly used as a viral vector in many research studies. For example, the adenovirus has been used to deliver "corrected" DNA to respiratory cells that contain the gene that codes for CF. The viral vector enters the target cells and inserts its "correct" genetic material. The target cells then start to manufacture cells with the "corrected" genetic code. The corrected target cells then proceed to synthesize the correct cellular proteins to restore health.

There are some nonviral options for gene delivery under investigation. Researchers have created an artificial lipid molecule, called a liposome, that can carry therapeutic DNA. The liposome can pass through a target cell's plasma membrane and replace the target cell DNA. This procedure is still experimental but offers promise.

Researchers also are experimenting with the insertion of a "47th" artificial human chromosome into target cells. This artificial normal chromosome would exist along with the standard 46 chromosomes and not affect their function. The artificial 47th chromosome would be a large vector capable of carrying substantial amounts of correct genetic code into cells. Scientists are trying to construct such a chromosome that could avoid being attacked by the body's immune system. Currently, genetic therapy is under investigation and not used in any FDA-approved treatments.

Ethical Concerns

Health-care professionals have to be able to counsel patients about what the results of genetic testing mean for them. Patients need to know all of the treatment options. Because this is a relatively new area of health care, health-care professionals are exploring the best approaches to use in each instance of testing for inheritable disorders. This area needs further research.

Pathophysiology of Selected Genetic and Chromosomal Disorders

Familial Hypercholesterolemia

FH is an autosomal dominant disorder that causes severe elevations in total cholesterol and low-density lipoprotein (LDL) cholesterol. Although hypercholesterolemia is a common finding in many individuals, heterozygous FH occurs in approximately 1 per 500 persons in the United States. Homozygous FH, which is a more severe disease than the heterozygous form, occurs in approximately one in 1 million individuals in the United States. FH is a disorder of absent or dysfunctional LDL receptors. The LDL receptor gene is located on the short arm of chromosome 19.

In FH, the liver, which normally processes cholesterol, lacks the receptors for LDL cholesterol, causing the liver to not take up LDL. This increases blood LDL levels. Normally, the uptake of LDL by the hepatocytes will suppress the liver's synthesis of cholesterol. However, when LDL is not taken up by hepatocytes, hepatic synthesis of cholesterol is not suppressed. This leads to further cholesterol production despite high levels of circulating cholesterol. The total cholesterol levels of infants and children with homozygous FH are higher than 600 mg/dL. In patients with heterozygous FH, half the LDL receptors are normal and half are rendered ineffective by the mutation. These patients' total cholesterol and LDL cholesterol levels are twice as high as the recommended level of LDL (fewer than 100 mg/dL). LDL cholesterol levels of 200 to 400 mg/dL are common in heterozygous FH.

In homozygous FH, severe and widespread atherosclerosis occurs early in life. Children are at risk for early acute myocardial infarction. In heterozygous FH, early adulthood coronary artery disease is the most serious clinical manifestation. Untreated men are likely to develop symptoms by the fourth decade of life and women in the fifth decade. Early manifestations include xanthomas and xanthelasma, which are deposits of cholesterol under the skin. Xanthelasma specifically occurs in the skin around the eyes. Corneal arcus is a light colored ring that is obvious in the iris of the eye. Cholesterol-lowering drugs, a low fat diet, and daily exercise are the treatment recommendations.

CLINICAL CONCEPT

A family history of early cardiovascular disease, such as myocardial infarction of a first-degree relative younger than age 55 years, is indicative of FH.

Familial Adenomatous Polyposis

FAP is an autosomal dominant inherited disorder characterized by the early onset of hundreds to thousands of adenomatous polyps throughout the colon. If left untreated, patients with this syndrome develop colon cancer by age 40 years. In addition, an increased risk exists for the development of other malignancies.

FAP is caused by a mutated gene at 5q21 called the APC gene. Under normal conditions, the APC gene is a tumor suppressor gene that triggers apoptosis in colon cells. The mutation of this gene prevents its function as a tumor suppressor and allows uncontrolled growth of colonic tumors called polyps. The polyps have a high likelihood of becoming malignant tumors and colorectal cancer can develop.

This is an autosomal dominant disorder; every colonic cell in patients with FAP has one mutated APC allele. Inactivation of the other normal allele of the APC gene removes the tumor suppressive function of APC, thus allowing uncontrolled growth of adenomatous polyps.

Incidence varies from 1 case in 6,850 persons to 1 case in 31,250 persons worldwide. The cause of death is colorectal cancer, which develops in all patients unless they prevent disease. The mean age at which colorectal cancer develops in patients with classic FAP is 39 years. Patients can be asymptomatic until cancer has already metastasized. In patients with FAP, 75% to 80% have a family history of polyps or colorectal cancer at age 40 years or younger. If symptoms are present, they include unexplained rectal bleeding (hematochezia), diarrhea, or abdominal pain. To prevent disease, patients with family history should have a colonoscopy every 1 to 2 years beginning at age 10 to 12 years.

Surgical treatment to excise and biopsy polyps is necessary. The patient may require removal of the colon (colectomy). The patient with FAP is also susceptible to other types of cancer, such as thyroid, liver, adrenal, pancreatic, or gastric cancer, as well as medulloblastoma.

Marfan Syndrome

Marfan syndrome is an inherited connective-tissue disorder transmitted as an autosomal dominant trait. It affects about 1 in 10,000 individuals, and perhaps as many as 1 in 3,000 to 5,000. About 75% of affected individuals have an affected parent. Sporadic mutation accounts for the remaining 25%.

Marfan syndrome results from mutations in the fibrillin-1 (FBN1) gene on chromosome 15, which contains the code for the glycoprotein fibrillin. Fibrillin is a major building block of microfibrils, which constitute the structural components of the aorta and other heart valves, airways of the lung, suspensory ligament of the lens, dura mater of the spinal cord, and other connective tissues of the body. The mitral, tricuspid, and aortic heart valves are commonly affected. Cardiovascular disease, mainly aortic dilatation and dissection, is the major cause of morbidity and mortality. Death after infancy usually involves ascending aortic dissection and chronic aortic regurgitation. Dissection generally occurs at the aortic root and is uncommon in childhood and adolescence.

If untreated, Marfan syndrome is highly lethal; the average age at death is 30 to 40 years. There are many clinical signs and symptoms such as:

- Tall stature with elongated arms and fingers
- Kyphoscoliosis
- Ligament hypermobility of the hips, knees, ankles, arches, wrists, and fingers
- Heart murmur from aortic regurgitation or mitral prolapse
- Dysrhythmia
- Abrupt onset of thoracic pain, which occurs in more than 90% of patients with aortic dissection
- Syncope
- Shock
- Pallor
- Pulselessness
- Paresthesia or paralysis in the extremities
- Low back pain near the tailbone
- Burning sensation and numbness or weakness in the legs caused by dura mater defects
- Joint pain (adult patients)
- Dyspnea, severe palpitations, and substernal pain in severe pectus excavatum (concave sternum)
- Breathlessness, often with chest pain, in spontaneous pneumothorax
- Visual problems, including loss of vision, from lens dislocation or retinal detachment.

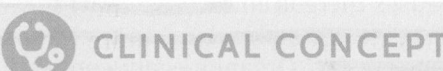

CLINICAL CONCEPT

In Marfan's syndrome, sudden onset of hypotension may indicate aortic rupture.

Genetic testing, chest x-ray, aortic angiogram, echocardiogram, CT, and MRI are needed to diagnose Marfan syndrome. Heart valve problems are a priority in treatment. Preventive procedures for cardiovascular disease are necessary, such as valve replacement and medications to prevent dysrhythmias. Scoliosis may require orthopedic surgery. Pneumothorax needs to be treated with a chest tube to suction. Pectus excavatum may require surgery. Ophthalmological consultation is needed as well. Genetic counseling is important to inform patients and families and to assist with family planning and reproductive decisions.

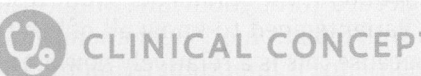

CLINICAL CONCEPT

Individuals with Marfan syndrome are at increased risk of spontaneous pneumothorax, aortic dissection, and heart valve abnormalities.

Neurofibromatosis

Neurofibromatosis (NF) is a genetic disorder with cutaneous, neurological, and orthopedic manifestations. There are two types of disease: NF type 1 (NF1) and NF type 2 (NF2). NF1 is more common than NF2, and there is less cutaneous involvement in NF2 compared with NF1. The manifestations of NF1 result from a mutation in the NF1 gene, which is a tumor suppressor gene that codes for the protein neurofibromin. Decreased production of this protein results in various clinical features. The NF1 gene has been localized to the long arm of chromosome 17. The estimated incidence of NF1 is 1 in 3,000. NF1 and NF2 are autosomal dominant conditions, but approximately half of the cases are caused by a new, sporadic genetic mutation.

The NF2 gene is located on the long arm of chromosome 22. The NF2 gene product, known as merlin, serves as a tumor suppressor; decreased production of this protein results in a predisposition to develop tumors of the central and peripheral nervous systems. The estimated incidence of NF2 is 1 in 37,000 per year. Although the genetic change causing NF2 is present at conception, as with NF1, the clinical manifestations occur over the course of many years. The typical age of onset of symptoms is in the late teens to early 20s. Many of the problems associated with NF do not appear until adolescence; therefore, the diagnosis is often delayed. The clinical criteria used to diagnose NF are as follows:

- Six or more café-au-lait spots (hyperpigmented macules)
- Axillary or inguinal freckles
- Two or more typical neurofibromas or one large neurofibroma
- Optic nerve tumor
- Two or more tumors in the iris (Lisch nodules), often only identified by an ophthalmologist

- Long-bone abnormalities
- First-degree relative (e.g., mother, father, sister, brother) with NF1.

The earliest clinical findings in childhood are café-au-lait spots. These are darkly pigmented, flat macules. Cutaneous neurofibromas, which are irregularly shaped, darkly pigmented, raised lesions, appear over time in older children, adolescents, and adults. Other signs include optic and acoustic nerve tumors, scoliosis, bowing of the legs, tumors of the meninges and spinal cord, and macrocephaly. Diagnosis requires genetic testing, CT, MRI, neurological evaluation, and acoustic and ophthalmological examinations. Periodic neurological examination is needed throughout life. Surgical treatment of tumors with radiation or chemotherapy is common. Genetic counseling is important to inform patients and families and to assist with family planning and reproductive decisions.

Ehlers-Danlos Syndrome

Ehlers-Danlos syndrome (EDS) is a group of disorders that characteristically involve diminished strength and integrity of the skin, joints, and other connective tissues. The patient's skin is highly elastic and joints are hypermobile. EDS is caused by abnormalities in the synthesis of collagen and other connective tissue proteins. Collagen is composed of the most abundant protein in the body. A minimum of 29 genes contribute to the collagen protein structure, and the genes are located on 15 of the 23 pairs of human chromosomes. The classic form of EDS occurs because of a mutation on the 9q34.2 and 9q34.3 genes, also called the COL3A1 and COL3A2 genes.

The prevalence of EDS has been reported as 1 in 5,000 to 10,000 persons, but the exact figure is unknown. The clinical manifestations include skin hyperelasticity, hypermobility of joints, easy bruising, and poor wound healing. Persons may also have mitral valve prolapse (MVP), arterial aneurysms, dissections, and occlusions. Genetic testing, MRI, CT, and echocardiogram are used in diagnosis. Skin biopsy is inconclusive.

The patient should not place undue stress on joints as they can dislocate. Periodic cardiovascular examination may be necessary for those with MVP, aneurysm, or aortic dissection. Treatment is symptomatic and high dose vitamin C has been used.

Cystic Fibrosis

Cystic fibrosis (CF) is the most common lethal inherited disease in the Caucasian population. The incidence of CF varies according to ethnicity. The incidence is 1 in 3,500 in persons of Caucasian European ancestry, 1 per 9,500 in Hispanic Americans, 1 per 15,000 in African Americans, and 1 in 31,000 among Asian Americans.

CF is an autosomal recessive disease caused by defects in the cystic fibrosis transmembrane conductance regulator (CFTR) gene, which encodes for a protein that functions as a chloride channel and also regulates the flow of other ions across the surface of epithelial cells. The CFTR gene locus is 7q31.

CF involves multiple organ systems, but chiefly the respiratory system and pancreas. Pancreatic enzyme insufficiency with associated complications occurs in patients. There is a reduced water content of secretions, which causes thick mucus plugging of the pancreas's ductules. The clogged ducts prevent pancreatic enzymes from reaching the intestine. This often causes malabsorption and failure to thrive in infants. Pancreatitis, cholelithiasis, and cirrhosis of the liver occur in many patients. Pulmonary involvement occurs in 90% of patients. The respiratory epithelium produces excess amounts of thick mucus that blocks airways and causes a high susceptibility to pulmonary infection for the patient's lifetime. Signs and symptoms include pulmonary wheezes, rhonchi, excess mucus in sputum, sinusitis, nasal polyps, abdominal pain caused by pancreatitis and cholecystitis, cirrhosis of liver, and rectal prolapse.

A patient is usually diagnosed by age 1 year. Newborn screening for CF is universally required in the United States. Diagnostic testing involves screening for immunoreactive trypsinogen (IRT), a pancreatic protein typically elevated in infants with CF. If that test is positive, repeat IRT testing and DNA testing are done. A sweat test called the quantitative pilocarpine iontophoresis test (QPIT) is used to collect sweat and analyze its chloride content. However, the sweat test is not always reliable. Chest x-ray, abdominal x-ray, chest CT, and abdominal ultrasound are used in the diagnosis as well. Genetic testing is recommended for individuals with a positive family history who are planning a pregnancy. Treatment for affected individuals includes pancreatic enzyme supplements, bronchodilators, mucolytics, nebulizer treatments, antibiotics, and anti-inflammatory medications. Patients may require nutritional supplements and insulin.

A new agent, ivacaftor (Kalydeco), was approved by the U.S. Food and Drug Administration (FDA) in January 2012. Ivacaftor is a CFTR potentiator. End-stage lung disease is the principal cause of death in many individuals. With treatment, an individual with CF born in the United States today is expected to survive longer than 40 years.

Lysosomal Storage Disease

Lysosomes are cellular organelles that contain digestive enzymes used to break down cellular debris. Lysosomal storage diseases are rare inherited disorders characterized by the failure of lysosomal function. In these diseases there is an accumulation of undigested or partially digested molecules, which ultimately cause cellular dysfunction. Organomegaly, connective-tissue problems, ocular pathology, and central nervous system (CNS) dysfunction are known to occur in these disorders.

More than 50 lysosomal storage diseases have been discovered. Lysosomal storage diseases are classified according to the accumulated substances, which include the sphingolipidoses, oligosaccharidoses, mucolipidoses, mucopolysaccharidoses (MPSs), lipoprotein storage disorders, lysosomal transport defects, and others. Each lysosomal storage disease presents differently according to the undigested substance that accumulates within the cells and according to which major organ is affected.

Tay Sachs Disease

Tay Sachs disease is a lysosomal storage disease that results from a mutation on chromosome 15. The lysosomal enzyme, hexosaminidase A, is severely deficient. The disease is prevalent among Ashkenazi Jews in whom a carrier rate of 1 in 30 persons has been found. The enzyme that is deficient ordinarily breaks down ganglioside, which is abundant in many organs, including the heart, liver, spleen, and brain. Ganglioside accumulates in the cells, particularly the CNS. The accumulation of ganglioside causes progressive destruction of neurons and brain cells. The cerebellum, basal ganglia, brainstem, spinal cord, and autonomic nervous system are notably affected.

Infants born with Tay Sachs appear normal until approximately age 6 months. As the infant matures, motor incoordination, lethargy, muscle flaccidity, and increasing cognitive impairment become apparent. A characteristic that is diagnostic of Tay Sachs is a "cherry red spot" seen on the retina on ophthalmological examination. The nervous system becomes increasingly impaired throughout the first year of life. Death usually occurs by age 3 years. Prenatal diagnosis and carrier detection of Tay Sachs disease is possible. Genetic counseling is important to inform patients and families and to assist with family planning and reproductive decisions.

Niemann-Pick Disease

Neimann-Pick disease results from an accumulation of sphingomyelin in cells because of an inherited deficiency of the lysosomal enzyme sphingomyelinase. There are two forms of the disease: type A and type B. Type A is a severe deficiency that causes widespread neurological involvement and visceral accumulation of sphingomyelin. Type B is similar except for the lack of CNS involvement. Individuals affected by type A usually die by age 3, whereas those with type B live into adulthood.

As with Tay Sachs disease, Niemann-Pick disease occurs largely in Ashkenazi Jews. There is a defect in the gene at 11p15.4. Sphingomyelin is present in practically all cell membranes throughout the body. Cells accumulate the lipid substance in the brain, spleen, liver, lymph nodes, bone marrow, gastrointestinal tract, and lungs. There is usually massive enlargement of the spleen. Clinical manifestations in type A are apparent by age 6 months. A protuberant abdomen, progressive gastrointestinal problems, fever, and generalized lymphadenopathy are present. The infant exhibits progressive motor dysfunction. The diagnosis is made by biochemical assays for sphingomyelinase in a biopsy of the liver or bone marrow. Carriers can be detected by DNA testing. Genetic counseling is important to inform patients and families and to assist with family planning and reproductive decisions.

Gaucher Disease

Gaucher disease is an autosomal recessive disorder caused by a mutation in the gene 1q21 that codes for the enzyme glucocerebrosidase. This disease is the most common lysosomal storage disease. As a result of the missing enzyme, the glycolipid glucocerebroside accumulates in macrophages and the CNS. The disease most commonly occurs in Ashkenazi Jews. The carrier frequency in these individuals is approximately 1 per 15 population, whereas the disease frequency is 1 per 855 population. There are several types of disease, but type I Gaucher disease is present in 99% of affected individuals.

More than 150 gene mutations can cause Gaucher disease, and it is not possible to diagnose the disease based on one single genetic test. The CNS, spleen, skeleton, and WBCs are affected in type 1 disease. Type II Gaucher disease affects neurons, is apparent in infants, and does not have a predilection for Jews. Progressive CNS involvement occurs with death at an early age.

In the cellular analysis of Gaucher disease, cells that have accumulated glucocerebroside are called Gaucher cells. They are found throughout the body in the spleen, liver, bone marrow, lymph nodes, tonsils, thymus, and Peyer's patches in the GI tract.

Type I Gaucher disease may not become apparent until adulthood. Symptoms are related to splenomegaly or bone marrow involvement. Thrombocytopenia and bone fractures can occur. Replacement enzyme therapy is possible and so a fairly long life expectancy is seen. Bone marrow transplantation is also done.

Wilson Disease

Wilson disease is a rare, autosomal recessive, inherited disorder of copper metabolism. The condition is characterized by excessive deposition of copper in the liver, brain, and other tissues. The major physiologic problem is excessive absorption of copper from the small intestine and decreased excretion of copper by the liver. The genetic defect is at 13q14, which is the copper-transporting adenosine triphosphatase gene (ATP7B) in the liver. The predominant route of copper excretion (approximately 95%) in the body is in the bile synthesized by the liver. However, in Wilson disease excretion of excess copper into bile is impaired. Initially, the excess copper accumulates in the liver, leading to damage to hepatocytes. Eventually, as liver copper levels increase, it increases in the circulation and is deposited in other organs.

The prevalence of Wilson disease is 1 per 30,000 individuals in the United States. It commonly presents as hepatic dysfunction in more than half of patients, with the most common initial presentation being cirrhosis. Another common presenting symptom is tremor, occurring in approximately half of individuals. Characteristic corneal Kayser-Fleischer rings are seen in the eyes of at least 98% of patients. Frequent early symptoms include difficulty speaking, excessive salivation, ataxia, mask-like facies, clumsiness with the hands, and personality changes. Late manifestations include dystonia, spasticity, grand mal seizures, rigidity, and flexion contractures. Psychiatric symptoms may be present. Skeletal involvement is a common feature of Wilson disease, with more than half of patients exhibiting osteopenia on radiological examination and an arthropathy that is similar to osteoarthritis. The arthropathy generally involves the spine and large appendicular joints, such as knees, wrists, and hips. Hemolytic anemia is a rare (10% to 15%) complication of the disease. Urolithiasis, hematuria, nephrocalcinosis, and proteinuria are common signs of kidney involvement.

Diagnosis is made by measuring serum ceruloplasmin levels and urine copper levels, and well as through liver biopsy. CT and MRI scans can show lesions in the brain. The main treatment for Wilson disease is pharmacological treatment with chelating agents. Liver transplantation may be necessary.

G6PD Deficiency

Glucose-6-phosphate dehydrogenase (G6PD) deficiency is the most common enzyme disorder in humans. Inherited as a recessive X-linked disorder, G6PD deficiency affects 400 million people worldwide. Like sickle cell anemia, G6PD deficiency confers protection against malaria, which probably accounts for its continual presence from generation to generation within the population.

G6PD deficiency is an X-linked inherited disease that primarily affects men. The highest prevalence rates of 5% to 25% occur in Africa, the Middle East, Asia, and the Mediterranean. All mutations that cause G6PD deficiency are found at the gene locus Xq28.

The disorder is characterized by abnormally low levels of G6PD, a metabolic enzyme involved in the pentose phosphate pathway that produces nicotinamide adenine dinucleotide phosphate (NADPH), which is especially important in red blood cell (RBC) metabolism. NADPH protects the RBCs against oxidative stresses that can destroy them. People deficient in G6PD have RBCs that undergo hemolysis under stresses such as infection or exposure to certain medications or chemicals. Interestingly, individuals with G6PD deficiency can undergo hemolysis in response to ingestion of fava beans; because of this, some refer to this disorder as favism. Individuals can have a mild case of G6PD deficiency, in which they are asymptomatic, or a severe case of the disorder, in which they often exhibit hemolysis. Hemolysis most often is exhibited as jaundice, yellowing of the skin and sclera. Symptomatic patients can present at birth with neonatal jaundice and acute hemolytic anemia.

Diagnostic tests include complete blood count, reticulocyte count, and blood smear analysis of RBCs for Heinz bodies, which are accumulations of degraded hemoglobin in RBCs. When a macrophage in the spleen identifies an RBC with a Heinz body, it takes in the Heinz body and a small piece of the RBC membrane. The RBC's phagocytosis by the macrophage leads to characteristic misshapen RBCs called bite cells that can be seen on RBC analysis. Diagnosis requires measurement of liver enzymes, bilirubin levels, lactate dehydrogenase, haptoglobin, and a direct antiglobulin test (Coombs' test). Other tests include direct DNA testing and sequencing of the G6PD gene. The Beutler fluorescent spot test performed on the blood can visually identify abnormal NADPH produced by G6PD under ultraviolet light. When the blood spot does not fluoresce, the test is positive.

Prevention is the most important measure in G6PD deficiency. Patients should avoid drugs and foods that cause hemolysis. If hemolysis is severe, blood transfusions may be necessary. Transfused RBCs are not G6PD deficient and will live a normal life span in the recipient's circulation. Some patients require removal of the spleen because this is a site of red cell destruction. Folic acid should be given because the body is in a state of high RBC synthesis.

Klinefelter Syndrome

Klinefelter syndrome is one of the most common male chromosomal genetic diseases. Approximately 1 in 500 to 1,000 males is born with this disease, and approximately 250,000 men in the United States are affected. Males commonly have a 47,XXY karyotype; however, an extra X or Y can be present in some variants of the disease. The error occurs in the separation of chromosomes during meiosis. The X chromosome carries genes that code for testis function, brain development, and growth. The addition of more than one extra X or Y chromosome to a male karyotype results in variable physical and cognitive abnormalities.

The consequences of an extra sex chromosome are numerous. Lack of development of the testes, gynecomastia, and skeletal and cardiovascular abnormalities are common. Mental ability diminishes with extra chromosomes. All major areas of cognitive development, including expressive and receptive language, are affected by extra X chromosome material. However, not all individuals are cognitively impaired. Testosterone deficiency causes tall, lanky body proportions; sparse or absent facial, axillary, and pubic hair; decreased muscle mass and strength; feminine distribution of adipose tissue; decreased physical endurance; and osteoporosis. These patients are at a higher risk of autoimmune diseases, DM, MVP, osteopenia and osteoporosis, breast and testicular tumors, systemic lupus erythematosus, and rheumatoid arthritis.

Klinefelter syndrome can be diagnosed prenatally in amniocentesis; however, it may not be suspected until adolescence. Genetic testing and hormone analysis can be done to confirm the diagnosis. Echocardiogram and bone density testing should be done with diagnosis because of the high prevalence of MVP and osteoporosis.

Testosterone replacement should begin at puberty, around age 12 years, and the dose should increase until it is sufficient to raise all sex hormones to normal levels. Psychoeducational evaluation and support is necessary. Physical therapy may be needed to build and tone muscles. Infertility treatment is possible since not all patients are completely sterile. Microsurgical sperm extraction for in vitro fertilization is possible in some cases.

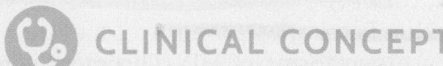

CLINICAL CONCEPT

In Klinefelter syndrome, XXY males commonly have weaker muscles and reduced strength. As they grow older, they tend to become taller than average and lack changes associated with puberty.

Turner Syndrome

Turner syndrome results from a complete or partially missing X chromosome in the female, so that karyotype is 45,X. It affects 1 in 2,000 births. As many as 15% of spontaneous abortions, also referred to as miscarriages, have a 45,X karyotype. There are many variations of the abnormal karyotype that makes this disease more severe in some than others. Some affected individuals have a mosaic chromosome pattern. At birth, the infant commonly has lymphedema of the feet and neck. The lymphedema subsides, leaving an elastic skin of the neck, later referred to as webbed neck. More than 95% of adult women with Turner syndrome exhibit short stature and infertility. Lack of breast development and amenorrhea at puberty occurs in many of those affected, though pubic hair distribution is often normal. An abundance of pigmented nevi, a broad shield-shaped chest, and small hips are common. Cardiovascular problems include hypertension, coarctation of the aorta, aortic valve abnormalities, and an underdeveloped left side of the heart. Scoliosis may be present, and the arms may have a deformity called cubitus valgus, which is a skeletal abnormality of the arm's carrying angle. Hypothyroidism is common, as are visual problems such as strabismus, cataract, and amblyopia. The

patient presents with ovarian failure at puberty and the oocytes are often degenerated.

Patients with suspected Turner syndrome require genetic testing and hormone level evaluation. Echocardiogram, bone density, and bone age testing are necessary. Treatment involves estrogen therapy and growth hormone administration. The patient should be treated symptomatically for all other effects of the disease.

Fragile X Syndrome

Fragile X syndrome, also termed Martin-Bell syndrome, is the most common cause of inherited cognitive impairment and is the second most common cause of genetically associated mental deficiencies after trisomy 21. It is a disorder of the X chromosome at Xq27.3, characterized by long repeating sequences of the three nucleotides cytosine (C), guanine (G), and guanine (G). The Xq27.3 gene is also called the familial mental retardation (FMR) 1 gene. The incidence is 1 in 1,550 for affected males and 1 in 8,000 for affected females. Problems include mild-to-moderate autistic-like behavior (most notably, hand flapping and avoidance of eye contact), shyness, sensory integration difficulties, attention deficits, hyperactivity, impulsivity, depressed affect, anxiety, mathematical learning disabilities, aggressive tendencies, deficiency in abstract thinking, developmental delays particularly in language, and decreasing IQ with increasing age.

In addition to the cognitive, behavioral, and neuropsychological findings, the organ systems most frequently involved include the craniofacial, genital, and musculoskeletal systems. Males have a long face with large mandible, large everted ears, and large testicles. Hypermobile joints, high arched palate, scoliosis, and MVP are also common.

The standard diagnostic test involves molecular genetic techniques. The exact number of CGG triplet repeats can be determined by Southern blot and PCR. Treatment is symptomatic according to the patient's various health problems. Genetic counseling is important to inform patients and families and to assist with family planning and reproductive decisions.

Down Syndrome

Down syndrome is the most common chromosomal disorder in humans and the most common cause of intellectual disability. It is characterized by cognitive impairment, dysmorphic facial features, and other distinctive traits. Down syndrome is primarily caused by trisomy of chromosome 21: three chromosomes at chromosome number 21. The term *mongolism* was once commonly used to describe this condition but is now considered obsolete. Trisomy 21 causes multiple systemic complications, but not all defects occur in each patient, as there is a wide variation in the severity of the disorder.

The frequency is about 1 case in 800 live births. Each year, approximately 6,000 children are born with Down syndrome. It can be diagnosed prenatally with amniocentesis, PUBS, CVS, and extraction of fetal cells from the maternal circulation. It is often diagnosed shortly after birth by recognition of the characteristic features, though they are most obvious in children older than age 1 year.

The disorder's occurrence is strongly dependent on maternal age. It varies from an incidence of 1 in 1,500 births in a mother aged 15 to 29 years to an incidence of 1 in 50 births to mothers older than 45 years.

The clinical features of Down syndrome include flat facial profile, oblique palpebral fissures, and epicanthic folds around the eyes. Approximately 80% of children have an IQ of 25 to 50. The remaining 20% have normal or near normal intelligence. Approximately 40% of children with Down syndrome have congenital heart disease and esophageal and intestinal malformation. Children have a 10- to 20-fold increased risk of developing leukemia. The immune system is weak, which makes children with Down syndrome susceptible to infection.

Currently, technological advances in medicine have lengthened the lives of adults with Down syndrome to an average of 47 years. Many affected adults can become employed and lead normal lives with assistance. Almost all long-living adults with Down syndrome eventually develop a dementia that is similar to Alzheimer disease.

Prader-Willi Syndrome

Prader-Willi syndrome (PWS), also called Angelman syndrome, is a disorder caused by a deletion or disruption of genes in the proximal arm of chromosome 15. The mutation usually occurs on the paternal chromosome of pair number 15. Most cases of PWS occur because of a sporadic genetic mutation. Incidence of this disease is unclear. Some researchers report an incidence of 1 in 16,000, whereas others report 1 in 52,000. Most manifestations of PWS are attributable to hypothalamic dysfunction. Consequently, multiple body systems are involved. Commonly associated characteristics include severe obesity, hypotonia, low IQ, short stature, hypogonadotropic hypogonadism, strabismus, small hands and feet, ataxic gait, behavioral problems, and seizures. Persons with PWS overeat and do not have the normal sensation of satiety. The person endures constant hunger because of dysfunction of the hypothalmus. Individuals need monitoring for development of morbid obesity, diabetes, and thyroid problems.

Complications from hypogonadism, such as osteoporosis and fracture, behavioral issues such as psychoses, type 2 DM, and heart failure may shorten life expectancy. Prader-Willi syndrome causes many lifelong, multisystem problems, though patients frequently reach adulthood and are able to function in a group home setting.

Huntington Disease

Huntington disease (HD) is an adult-onset, autosomal dominant inherited disorder associated with degeneration of specific neurons in the basal ganglia and cortex. The estimated prevalence of HD in the United States ranges from 4.1 to 8.4 per 100,000 people. The average age of onset of HD ranges from 35 to 44 years, whereas the average age of death of an individual with HD ranges from 51 to 57 years. Most patients survive between 10 and 25 years after the onset of illness.

HD is caused by a genetic defect at 4p16.3 called the Huntington gene (also called the HTT or HD gene). The gene defect causes a part of DNA, called a CAG repeat sequence, to repeat many more times than it should and form the Huntingtin protein.

There are two forms of HD. The most common is adult-onset; persons with this form usually develop symptoms in their mid-30s and 40s. An early onset form of HD accounts for a small number of cases and begins in childhood or adolescence.

The clinical presentation of HD includes a movement disorder, a cognitive disorder, and a behavioral disorder. Patients may present with one or all disorders in varying degrees. Chorea is the most common movement disorder seen in HD. Initially, mild chorea causes dancelike movements or tics. Severe chorea occurs later and can cause uncontrollable flailing of the extremities, termed ballism. As the disease progresses, chorea is replaced by parkinsonian features, such as slowed up movements, muscle rigidity, and postural instability. In advanced disease, patients develop an akinetic-rigid syndrome, without movement at all. Other late features are spasticity, dysarthria (the inability to speak), and dysphagia, which is difficulty with swallowing. Slowed cognition to dementia occurs gradually. Severe depression and suicidal ideation is common.

No specific imaging study can be used to diagnose HD. Patients who have HD and predominant features of bradykinesia and rigidity may benefit from Parkinson type treatment of levodopa or dopamine agonists. Antidepressants, antipsychotic medications, and anticonvulsants may be necessary. Genetic testing can show the defect of HD, and family members need counseling. More research is needed for treatments of this disease.

Chapter Summary

- A genome refers to the collection of all of an organism's genes.
- A nucleotide is a combination of a pentose sugar molecule, phosphate, and purine or pyrimidine nitrogen base. The nitrogen bases are adenine (A), thymine (T), guanine (G), and cytosine (C) in DNA. Instead of thymine, uracil is the nitrogen base in RNA.
- Transcription is the synthesis of RNA from DNA in the nucleus and translation is the synthesis of proteins from RNA at the ribosomes.
- Single nucleotide polymorphisms (SNP) are changes in one nucleotide of a gene sequence.
- A gene locus is the gene's position on a specific chromosome. The upper arm of a chromosome is the "p" arm and the lower arm is called the "q" arm.
- A karyotype is an overall picture of all an individual's chromosome pairs. The dye stains regions of chromosomes that are rich in the base pairs adenine (A) and thymine (T), producing a dark band.
- A genotype is the technical allelic makeup of a trait. A phenotype is the physical expression of the genotype.
- An individual can possess allelic traits that are homozygous or heterozygous.
- A Punnett Square can be used to predict single gene inheritance patterns.

- A carrier is a person who is heterozygous for a recessive trait but does not manifest it; the dominant allele silences it.
- If a gene is located on the X chromosome, the inheritance pattern is considered to be sex linked, or X-linked.
- Genetic mutations are hereditary or acquired.
- Oncogenes and tumor suppressor genes are involved in carcinogenesis.
- Mitochondria have their own DNA, which is maternally inherited.
- The severity of a genetic disorder may vary from one individual to another based on penetrance and expressivity.
- In an individual with a mosaic genetic pattern, some cells contain the gene mutation and some do not.
- Aneuploidy refers to a disorder related to chromosome number. Genes can be translocated from one chromosome to another or deleted from chromosomes.
- Polymerase chain reaction and fluorescent in situ hybridization are molecular techniques for identifying genes.
- Chorionic villus sampling and amniocentesis are common procedures used for prenatal diagnosis.

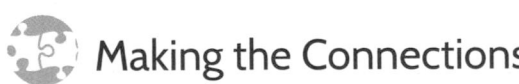 Making the Connections

Disorder and Pathophysiology	Signs and Symptoms	Physical Assessment Findings	Diagnostic Testing	Treatment
Familial Hypercholesterolemia | Defect of gene that codes for the LDL receptor in the liver; liver processing of cholesterol cannot occur; liver produces excessive cholesterol.				
	Premature arteriosclerosis. Premature coronary artery disease. Premature myocardial infarction.	Cholesterol deposits under the skin called xanthoma and xanthelasma.	Extremely high serum cholesterol and LDL. Genetic testing.	Antilipidemia medications.
Familial Adenomatous Polyposis | Mutation at gene locus; 5p21; the APC gene which causes numerous intestinal polyps and susceptibility to colon cancer.				
	Melena, diarrhea, hematochezia, abdominal pain, and malabsorption.	None.	Colonoscopy reveals hundreds of polyps. Biopsies needed to rule out colon cancer. Genetic testing.	Removal of the colon may be necessary.

Continued

Making the Connections—cont'd

Disorder and Pathophysiology	Signs and Symptoms	Physical Assessment Findings	Diagnostic Testing	Treatment
Marfan Syndrome | Mutation in the fibrillin-1 gene on chromosome 15, which contains the code for the glycoprotein fibrillin. Fibrillin is normally found in heart valves, airways, and other tissue. Fibrillin is deficient in Marfan syndrome.				
	Sudden dyspnea with pneumothorax. Sudden chest pain with aortic dissection. Lower back pain in tailbone with spinal dura involvement.	Tall, lanky appearance. Elongated arms and fingers. Heart murmur, pectus excavatum, ligament hypermobility, and kyphoscoliosis.	Genetic testing. Echocardiogram, chest x-ray, aortic angiogram, and others that diagnose various conditions associated with genetic defects.	Treatment is for symptoms and multiple conditions that result from the genetic defect.
Neurofibromatosis | Mutation in the NF1 gene or NF2 gene. The NF gene is a tumor suppressor gene that codes for the protein neurofibromin; decreased production of this protein results in tumors of various organs.				
	Vision and hearing defects. Back pain caused by scoliosis and spinal cord tumors.	Characteristic café-au-lait spots. Scoliosis, bowing of the legs, tumors of the meninges, spinal cord, and skin. Macrocephaly.	Genetic testing. CT, MRI, neurological evaluation, acoustic and ophthalmological examinations because of various tumors.	Treatment is for symptoms and multiple conditions that result from the genetic defect.
Ehlers-Danlos Syndrome | Mutation on the 9q34.2 and 9q34.3 genes; also called the COL3A1 and COL3A2 genes, that code for collagen. Results in collagen deficiency.				
	Skin hyperelasticity. Hypermobility of joints. Easy bruising and poor wound healing.	Skin and joint hyperelasticity. Heart murmur of MVP.	Genetic testing, MRI, CT, angiograms, and echocardiograms are used in diagnosis.	Treatment is for symptoms and multiple conditions that result from the genetic defect.
Cystic Fibrosis | Defects in the CFTR gene, which encodes for a protein that functions as a chloride channel and also regulates the flow of other ions across the surface of epithelial cells. The CFTR gene locus is 7q31. Chiefly affected organs are the respiratory system and pancreas. Excessive mucus and thickened secretions form plugs.				
	Chronic cough, upper respiratory infections, and gastrointestinal disturbances caused by pancreatitis, cirrhosis of liver, and gallstones.	Pulmonary wheezes, rhonchi, and excess mucus in sputum. Sinusitis, nasal polyps, abdominal pain caused by pancreatitis and cholesystitis, and cirrhosis of the liver. Rectal prolapse.	Genetic testing. IRT, a pancreatic protein typically elevated in infants with CF. A sweat test called QPIT is used to collect sweat and analyze its chloride content. Chest x-ray, abdominal x-ray, chest CT and abdominal ultrasound.	Pancreatic enzyme supplements, bronchodilators, mucolytics, nebulizer treatments, antibiotics, and anti-inflammatory medications.
Tay Sachs Disease | Mutation on chromosome 15. The lysosomal enzyme, hexosaminidase A, is severely deficient, which allows ganglioside to accumulate in tissues particularly the brain and spinal cord.				
	Motor incoordination. Lethargy, muscle flaccidity, and cognitive impairment.	Lethargy, muscle flaccidity, poor suck reflex in infant. Lack of completing developmental milestones.	Genetic testing. A characteristic "cherry red spot" is seen on the retina on ophthalmological examination.	Treatment is for symptoms and multiple conditions that result from the genetic defect.

Continued

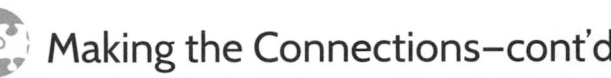

Making the Connections–cont'd

Disorder and Pathophysiology	Signs and Symptoms	Physical Assessment Findings	Diagnostic Testing	Treatment
Neimann-Pick Disease | Defect at gene at 11p15.4 that causes deficiency of the lysosomal enzyme sphingomyelinase. Cells of various organs such as the brain, spleen, lymph nodes, lungs, and liver accumulate sphingomyelin.				
	Fever, gastrointestinal problems, enlarged abdomen, generalized lymphadenopathy, and motor dysfunction.	Splenomegaly, protuberant abdomen, progressive gastrointestinal problems, fever, and generalized lymphadenopathy are present. The infant exhibits progressive motor dysfunction.	The diagnosis is made by biochemical assays for sphingomyelinase in a biopsy of the liver or bone marrow. Carriers can be detected by DNA testing.	Treatment is for symptoms and multiple conditions that result from the genetic defect.
Gaucher Disease | An autosomal, recessive disorder caused by a mutation in the gene 1q21 that codes for the enzyme glucocerebrosidase. Accumulation of glucocerebroside protein in the CNS, spleen, skeleton, and WBCs.				
	Enlarged spleen and liver. Bone lesions that may be painful. Weakness, numbness, and parethesias. Swelling of lymph nodes and adjacent joints. Distended abdomen. Brownish tint to the skin. Easy bruising. Susceptibility to infection.	Splenomegaly and hepatomegaly. Weakness of extremities. Lymphadenopathy, arthropathy, and distended abdomen. Brownish tint to the skin. Yellow fatty deposits on the sclera.	Cellular analysis of Gaucher disease: cells that have accumulated glucocerebroside are called Gaucher cells. They are found throughout the body in the spleen, liver, bone marrow, lymph nodes, tonsils, thymus, and Peyer's patches in the GI tract.	Replacement enzyme therapy is possible, and so a fairly long life expectancy is seen. Bone marrow transplantation is also done.
Wilson Disease | Autosomal recessive inherited disorder of copper metabolism. Genetic defect is at 13q 14, which is the copper-transporting adenosine triphosphatase gene (abbreviated ATP7B) in the liver, causing excessive deposition of copper in the liver, brain, and other tissues.				
	Jaundice caused by liver dysfunction. Tremor, difficulty speaking, excessive salivation, ataxia, masklike facies, and clumsiness. Spasticity and grand mal seizures. Rigidity, flexion contractures, and psychiatric symptoms may be present. Joint pain and abdominal pain caused by kidney stones.	Jaundice. Difficulty speaking. Excessive salivation. Ataxia, masklike facies, clumsiness, muscle spasticity, rigidity, and flexion contractures. Joint pain of spine and large appendicular joints, such as knees, wrists, and hips.	Kayser-Fleisher rings in the eye. Liver enzymes may be elevated. Osteopenia on radiological examination. Urolithiasis, hematuria, nephrocalcinosis, and proteinuria are common signs of kidney involvement. Serum ceruloplasmin levels, urine copper levels elevated, and liver biopsy shows copper. CT and MRI scans can show lesions in the brain.	Chelating agents that bind copper. Liver transplantation.

Continued

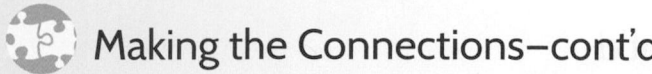

Making the Connections—cont'd

Disorder and Pathophysiology	Signs and Symptoms	Physical Assessment Findings	Diagnostic Testing	Treatment
G6PD Deficiency | All mutations that cause G6PD deficiency are found at the gene locus Xq28. A metabolic enzyme involved in RBC metabolism. Some of the RBCs undergo hemolysis when the body is under stress.				
	Jaundice with stresses to the body.	Jaundice with stresses to the body.	Misshapen RBCs called "bite cells" seen on blood smear. Liver enzymes normal. Lactate dehydrogenase, bilirubin elevation, haptoglobin, and direct antiglobulin test. Other tests include direct DNA testing and sequencing of the G6PD gene, as well as the Beutler fluorescent spot test.	Periods of hemolysis and jaundice do not require treatment and resolve on their own.
Klinefelter Syndrome | Males commonly have a 47,XXY karyotype; however, an extra X or Y can be present in some variants of the disease.				
	Tall, lanky body proportions. Sparse or absent facial, axillary, and pubic hair. Decreased muscle mass and strength. Feminine distribution of adipose tissue. Decreased physical endurance. Osteoporosis.	Tall, lanky body proportions. Sparse or absent facial, axillary, and pubic hair. Decreased muscle mass and strength. Feminine distribution of adipose tissue. Decreased physical endurance. Osteoporosis. These patients are at a higher risk of autoimmune diseases, DM, MVP, osteopenia and osteoporosis, breast and testicular tumors, systemic lupus erythematosus, and rheumatoid arthritis.	Genetic testing and hormone analysis can be done to confirm the diagnosis. Echocardiogram and bone density testing should be done with diagnosis caused by high prevalence of MVP and osteoporosis.	Testosterone therapy and other treatment for symptoms and multiple conditions that result from the genetic defect.
Turner Syndrome | A combination of disorders that results from a complete or partially missing X chromosome in the female so that the karyotype is 45,X.				
	At birth, the infant commonly has lymphedema of the feet and neck. The lymphedema subsides, leaving an elastic skin of the neck, later referred to as a webbed neck. Heart problems can cause cyanosis and dyspnea.	Hypertension, coarctation of the aorta, and aortic valve abnormalities can cause heart murmur. Underdeveloped left side of the heart can cause dyspnea or cyanosis. Short stature. Infertility.	Genetic testing and hormone level evaluation. Echocardiogram, bone density, and bone age testing.	Estrogen therapy and growth hormone administration. Surgery may be necessary for cardiac defects. Patient should be treated symptomatically for all other effects of the disease.

Continued

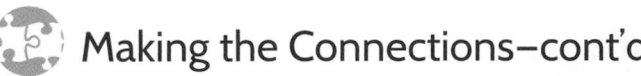

Making the Connections—cont'd

Disorder and Pathophysiology	Signs and Symptoms	Physical Assessment Findings	Diagnostic Testing	Treatment
	Short stature. Vision problems. Lack of energy, obesity, and fatigue caused by hypothyroidism. Lack of breast development.	Lack of breast development. Amenorrhea. Abundance of pigmented nevi. Broad shield-shaped chest. Small hips. Scoliosis cubitus valgus. Hypothyroidism. Strabismus. Cataract. Amblyopia.		

Down Syndrome | Chromosomal abnormality that involves three copies of chromosome 21; this abnormality causes multiple organ system problems.

Disorder and Pathophysiology	Signs and Symptoms	Physical Assessment Findings	Diagnostic Testing	Treatment
	Infant has facial features that are distinctive for Down syndrome. Delay in developmental milestones. Congenital heart defects are common: dyspnea, cyanosis, and syncope (fainting) can result. Esophageal and intestinal complications are also common, which can cause problems with swallowing and malabsorption.	Flat facial profile. Oblique palpebral fissures and epicanthic folds around the eyes. Heart murmur. Cyanosis. Dyspnea. Approximately 80% of children have IQ of 25 to 50. The remaining 20% have normal or near normal intelligence.	Genetic testing. Echocardiogram, ECG, and chest and abdominal x-rays to test for common problems with the heart, lungs, and intestine.	Treatment is for symptoms and multiple conditions that result from the genetic defect.

Fragile X Syndrome | Disorder of the X chromosome at Xq27.3, characterized by long repeating sequences of the three nucleotides: cytosine (C), guanine (G), and guanine (G).

Disorder and Pathophysiology	Signs and Symptoms	Physical Assessment Findings	Diagnostic Testing	Treatment
	Mild-to-moderate autisticlike behavior (most notably, hand flapping and avoidance of eye contact). Shyness. Attention deficits. Hyperactivity. Impulsivity. Anxiety. Cognitive difficulties.	Males have a long face with large mandible, large everted ears, and large testicles. Hypermobile joints. High arched palate. Scoliosis. MVP.	Genetic testing. The exact number of CGG triplet repeats can be determined by Southern blot and PCR.	Treatment is for symptoms and multiple conditions that result from the genetic defect.

Continued

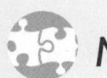 ## Making the Connections—cont'd

Disorder and Pathophysiology	Signs and Symptoms	Physical Assessment Findings	Diagnostic Testing	Treatment
Prader-Willi Syndrome | Deletion or disruption of genes in the proximal arm of chromosome 15. The mutation usually occurs on the paternal chromosome of pair number 15.				
	Severe obesity. Hypotonia. Low IQ. Short stature. Hypogonadotropic hypogonadism. Strabismus. Small hands and feet. Ataxic gait. Behavioral problems. Seizures.	Severe obesity. Hypotonia. Low IQ. Short stature. Hypogonadotropic hypogonadism. Strabismus. Small hands and feet. Ataxic gait. Behavioral problems. Seizures.	Genetic testing. A number of diagnostic tests, depending on disease manifestations.	Treatment is for symptoms and multiple conditions that result from the genetic defect.
Huntington Disease | Genetic defect at 4p16.3, called the huntingtin gene. The gene defect causes a part of DNA called a CAG repeat sequence to repeat many more times than it should and form the huntingtin protein. Autosomal dominant inherited disorder associated with degeneration of specific neurons in the basal ganglia and cortex.				
	Lack of control of movements called chorea, gradually deteriorating to lack of movement, blank facies, tremor, and rigidty. Cognitive decline. Depression and psychosis possible.	Muscle spasticity. Difficulty with speech and swallowing. Subtle tic-like movements may progress to flailing type movements. Eventually akinesia or lack of any movement occurs. Dementia is late in course of disease.	No imaging studies can show deterioration well. Genetic testing and clinical picture makes diagnosis.	May benefit from Parkinson type treatment of levodopa or dopamine agonists. Antidepressants, antipsychotic medications, and anticonvulsants may be necessary. Genetic testing can show the defect of HD, and family members need counseling.

Bibliography

Bancroft, E. K. (2013). How advances in genomics are changing patient care. *Nurs Clin N Am, 48*(4), 557–569. doi: 10.1016/j.cnur.2013.08.002.

Cho, M. H., McDonald, M. L., Zhou, X., et al. (2014). Risk loci for chronic obstructive pulmonary disease: a genome-wide association study and meta-analysis. *Lancet Respir Med, 2*(3), 14–25. doi: 10.1016/S2213-2600(14)70002-5.

Codier, E., & Codier, D. (2014). Understanding mitochondrial disease and goals for its treatment. *Brit J Nurs, 23*(5), 254–258.

Dewey, F. E., Grove, M. E., Pan, C., et al. (2014). Clinical interpretation and implications of whole-genome sequencing. *JAMA, 311*(10), 1035–1045. doi: 10.1001/jama.2014.1717.

Falcone, G. J., Malik, R., Dichgans, M., & Rosand, J. (2014). Current concepts and clinical applications of stroke genetics. *Lancet Neurol, 13*(4), 405–418. doi: 10.1016/S1474-4422(14)70029-8.

Feero, W. G., Guttmacher, A. E., & Collins, F. S. (2010). Genomic medicine—an updated primer. *N Engl J Med, 362*(21), 2001–2011. doi: 10.1056/NEJMra0907175.

Hegele, R. A., Ginsberg, H. N., Chapman, M. J., et al. (2013, December 23). The polygenic nature of hypertriglyceridemia: implications for definition, diagnosis, and management. *Lancet Diabetes Endocrinol*, pii: S2213-8587(13)70191-8. doi: 10.1016/S2213-8587(13)70191-8.

Hirsch, F. R., & Bunn, P. A., Jr. (2014). Progress in research on screening and genetics in lung cancer. *Lancet Resp Med, 2*(1), 19–21. doi: 10.1016/S2213-2600(13)70264-9.

Jeffers, L., Morrison, P. J., McCaughan, E., & Fitzsimons, D. (2014, April 11). Maximising survival: the main concern of women with hereditary breast and ovarian cancer who undergo genetic testing for BRCA1/2. *Eur J Oncol Nurs*, pii: S1462-3889(14)00039-8. doi: 10.1016/j.ejon.2014.03.007.

Kamali, F., & Wynne, H. (2010). Pharmacogenetics of warfarin. *Ann Rev Med, 61*, 63–75.

Klein, E. L. (2014). The increasing role of genetics and genomics in women's health. *Nurs Women's Health, 18*(2), 149–153. doi: 10.1111/1751-486X.12111.

Knudson, A. G. (1971). Mutation and cancer: statistical study of retinoblastoma. *Proceed Nat Acad Sci, USA, 68*, 820–823.

Kumar, V., Abbas, A. K., & Aster, J. C. (2014). *Robbins and Cotran pathologic basis of disease*. 9th ed. Philadelphia, PA: Elsevier Publishing Co.

Lee, B. I., & Heo, K. (2014, January). Epilepsy: new genes, new technologies, new insights. *Lancet Neurol,* 13(1), 7–9. doi: 10.1016/S1474-4422(13)70240-0.

Manace, L. C., & Babyatsky, M. W. (2012). Putting genome analysis to good use: lessons from C-reactive protein and cardiovascular disease. *Cleveland Clin J Med,* 79(3), 182–191. doi: 10.3949/ccjm.79a.09169.

Mandell, B. F. (2012). Exploring the human genome, and re-learning genetics by necessity. *Cleveland Clin J Med,* 79(3), 162. doi: 10.3949/ccjm.79b.12003.

McCormack, R. T., Armstrong, J., & Leonard, D. (2014). Codevelopment of genome-based therapeutics and companion diagnostics: insights from an Institute of Medicine roundtable. *JAMA,* 311(14), 1395–1396. doi: 10.1001/jama.2014.1508. No abstract available. Erratum in: *JAMA.* 2014 Apr 9; 311(14):1396.

McPhee, S. J., & Hammer, J. (2010). *Pathophysiology of disease.* 6th ed. New York: Lange Medical Books/McGraw-Hill Medical Publishing Division.

Mester, J. L., Schreiber, A. H., & Moran, R. T. (2012). Genetic counselors: your partners in clinical practice. *Cleveland Clin J Med,* 79(8), 560–568. doi: 10.3949/ccjm.79a.11091.

National Human Genome Research Institute. National Institutes of Health. (2014a). Fact sheets on science, research, ethics and the Institute. Retrieved from http://www.genome.gov/27527637

National Human Genome Research Institute. National Institutes of Health. (2014b). Genetics, genomics and patient management. Retrieved from http://www.genome.gov/27527637

National Human Genome Research Institute. National Institutes of Health. (2014c). Genetics 101 for health care professionals. Retrieved from http://www.genome.gov/27527637

National Human Genome Research Institute. National Institutes of Health. (2014d). Guidelines and tools to assess history of common diseases. Retrieved from http://www.genome.gov/27527637

National Human Genome Research Institute. National Institutes of Health. (2014e). The talking glossary of genetics. Retrieved from http://www.genome.gov/Glossary/

Schaefer, G. B., & Thompson, J. N. (2013). *Medical genetics: an integrated approach.* New York: McGraw-Hill.

Solomon, B. D., & Muenke, M. (2012). When to suspect a genetic syndrome. *Am Fam Phys,* 86(9), 826–833.

Stoessl, A. J. (2014, March 29). Gene therapy for Parkinson's disease: a step closer? *Lancet,* 383(9923), 1107–1109. doi: 10.1016/S0140-6736(13)62108-X.

Taylor, C., Kavanagh, P., & Zuckerman, B. (2014). Sickle cell trait—neglected opportunities in the era of genomic medicine. *JAMA,* 311(15), 1495–1496. doi: 10.1001/jama.2014.2157.

Zaslav, A. L., Marino, M. A., Jurgens, C. Y., & Mercado, T. (2013). Cytogenetic evaluation: a primer for pediatric nurse practitioners. *J Pediatr Health Care,* 27(6), 426–433. doi: 10.1016/j.pedhc.2012.04.006.

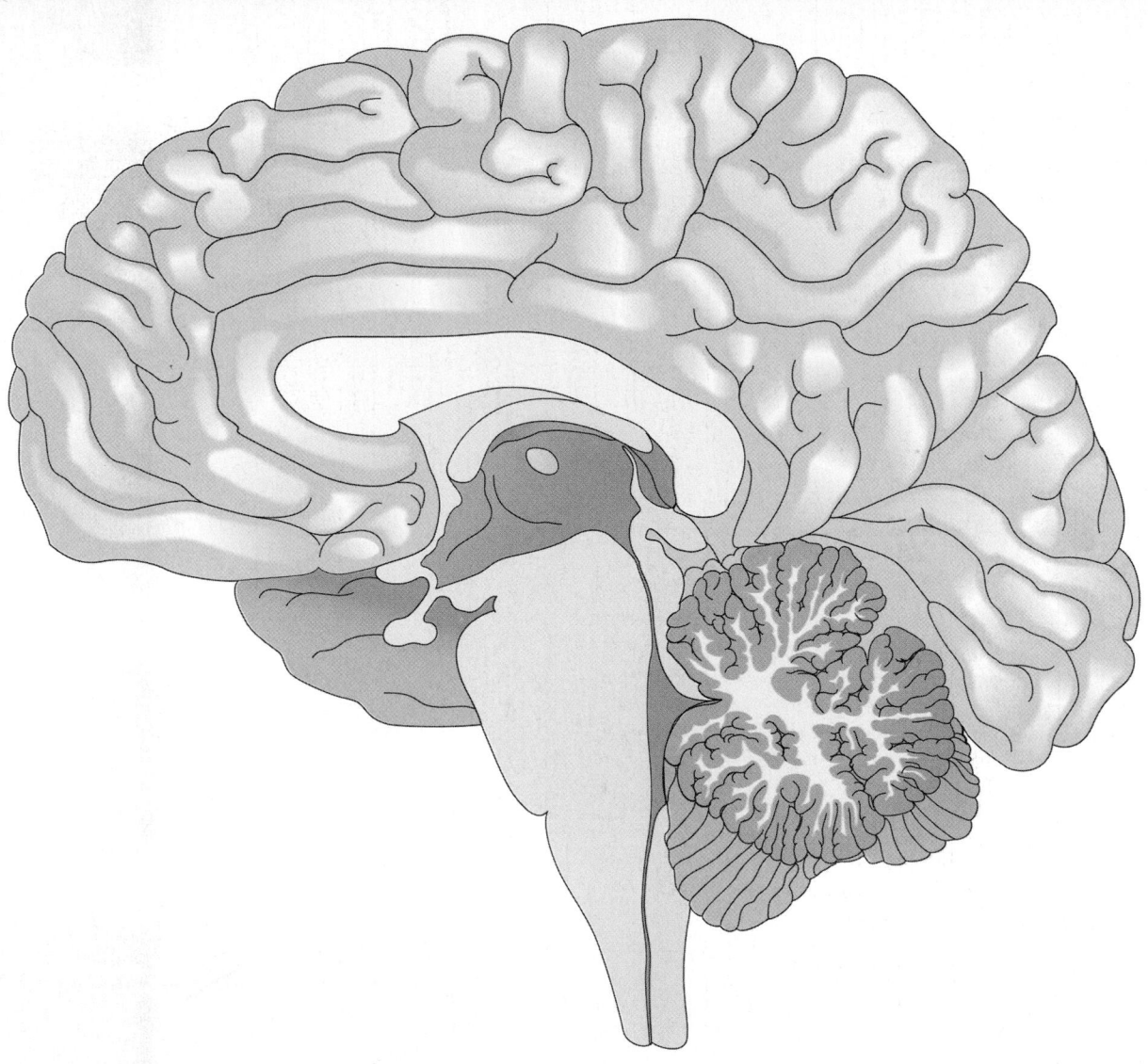

Chapters

Stress, Exercise, and Immobility

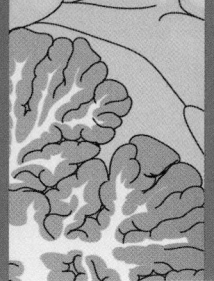

Key Terms

Adaptive ability

Allostasis

Allostatic load

Allostatic overload

Contracture

Decubitus ulcer

Distress

Eustress

Fight-or-flight reaction

General adaptation syndrome

Homeostasis

Immunosuppression

Natriuresis

Negative nitrogen balance

Orthostatic hypotension

Pathological fracture

Polysomnography

REM sleep

Trabecular bone

Stress can be a physical or psychological experience that disturbs comfort, threatens safety, or imperils life. It can develop because of physical injury, such as fracture of a bone, or because of feelings related to work, school, social, or family issues.

A certain amount of psychological stress is advantageous in that it can motivate an individual. **Eustress** describes stress that stimulates a person positively, such as when a job promotion provokes positive feelings and reaction. However, **distress** describes stress that evokes negative feelings and adverse reactions. For many in society, psychological stress can rise to overwhelming levels, which can lead to disruption of normal functioning and major health problems.

Any type of stress triggers a primal physical response from the body. This response can be useful, in that it excites the nervous, endocrine, and musculoskeletal systems and allows one to quickly react to an emergent situation. During acute stress, the body automatically initiates a set of involuntary responses; heart rate speeds up and myocardial contractile function strengthens. The bronchioles dilate, allowing more air to enter the lungs. Chemical mediators provoke stress hormones that are released into the bloodstream, priming the body to be alert. Concentration becomes more focused, reaction time is faster, and strength and agility increase. When the stressful situation ends, hormonal signals switch off the stress response and the body returns to normal. Primitive man depended on this stress response for survival. In prehistoric times, stress was an intermittent experience and its intensity varied according to environmental factors. The stress response was evoked infrequently and ended after the threat was avoided.

However, in our modern society, stress is often a frequent, constant, or long-term experience. Electronic forms of communication have created a sense of urgency in personal interactions, employer-employee relationships are less permanent than in the past, relocation for employment is expected, social support is often lacking for individuals, many persons lack time for leisure activities, citizens are asked to be vigilant about threats of terrorism on a daily basis, and acts of violence have become commonplace in U.S. society. Stress has become part of our daily culture and coping with stressors has become necessary in today's society.

This constant stress puts great strain on the body. Frequent or long-term stressors cause stress hormones to continually pulsate through the system in high levels, causing them to never leave the blood and tissues. Research shows that such long-term activation of the stress response can have a hazardous effect on the body, diminishing immunity and increasing the risk of autoimmune disease, cancer, heart disease, depression, and a variety of other illnesses.

The Effects of Stress

There is a human mind-body connection that significantly impacts the individual's total well-being. Emotions and psychological conditions can cause biological responses that can lead to physical illness. This is seen when an anxious individual develops physical symptoms of chest pain, hyperventilation, tachycardia, and diaphoresis; this individual feels physically ill despite the emotional etiology of the condition.

Conversely, physiologic disorders can influence a person's state of mind and cause emotional consequences: an individual enduring the chest pain of myocardial infarction commonly experiences anxiety, a psychological reaction to the physical disturbance.

The mind-body connection has provoked much investigation into stress and stress-related illnesses. The body's reaction to an acute stress has been well researched; less is known about the cumulative effects of prolonged stress. At present, theories devised by physiologists Hans Selye, Walter Cannon, and Bruce McEwen are well-accepted explanations of the effects of stress on the body.

Selye's Stress Response Theory

Hans Selye, a scientist who studied physiologic reactions to stress in the 1930s and 1940s, first described the body's reaction to acute stress. According to Selye, a stressor is a challenging demand on the body that arouses a response from multiple organ systems. Stressors can be positive or negative experiences for the individual and have potential to cause adverse health effects. Fear, bereavement, promotion, new role assumption, home relocation, trauma of any type, infection, surgery, debilitating illness, and exposure to intense heat or cold are examples of stressful experiences.

In addition to the stressor, the individual's adaptive ability is an important element in the body's stress reaction. **Adaptive ability** is the way in which the individual manages the stress and reduces the stressor's effect on his or her life. Effective adaptive ability allows an individual to maintain homeostasis. **Homeostasis** is a condition of equilibrium when various physiologic parameters such as blood pressure, respirations, heart rate, oxygen tension, blood pH, blood glucose, body temperature, and white blood cell (WBC) count are within normal, narrow ranges.

An individual's adaptive ability depends on coping mechanisms and conditioning factors. Coping mechanisms are the emotional and behavioral responses used to manage threats to physiologic and psychological homeostasis. How a person copes with stressful events depends on how he or she perceives and interprets the event. For example, an individual can perceive an employment promotion as a positive new challenge or a negative added burden. The mind's interpretation of the stressful event influences the stressor's physiologic effects.

An individual's reaction to a stressor is also influenced by conditioning factors, such as age, gender, genetic predisposition, pre-existing health conditions, life experiences, developmental level, educational level, and social support. For example, how an individual copes with a diagnosis of cancer is greatly influenced by his or her past experiences with the disease. An individual may fear the diagnosis if he or she observed the suffering of another with the same diagnosis. Alternatively, the individual may not fear the diagnosis if he or she is encouraged by others who conquered and survived the disease.

Neuroendocrine and Immune Responses

The physiologic reaction to stress can have protective, restorative effects or damaging, injurious consequences on the body. In the short term, there is a protective activation of the neurological, endocrine, and immune systems, the major organ systems affected by stress, as the body increases its defenses to cope with the acute threat. However, prolonged exposure to stress and long-term activation of the neuroendocrine and immune systems eventually has a negative effect on the body.

According to Selye, regardless of the source, stress is a threat to homeostasis that provokes a coordinated, adaptive reaction called the **general adaptation syndrome.** Selye developed this theory as an attempt to scientifically analyze the body's reaction to stress. In 1936, his research involved exposing animals to unpleasant or harmful stimuli such as physical trauma and extreme cold and examining the physiologic responses. He found that all animals showed a similar set of reactions that involved three stages:

1. alarm
2. resistance
3. exhaustion.

Alarm Stage. The alarm stage is a state of arousal characterized by the central nervous system, sympathetic nervous system (SNS), and adrenal gland stimulation. The SNS, also known as the adrenergic nervous system, releases the catecholamine norepinephrine, which increases alertness and stimulates cardiorespiratory and vascular responses. Norepinephrine also causes vasoconstriction of the arterial blood vessels that bring blood to the heart muscle, lungs, and skeletal muscles. Heart and respiratory rate increase as peripheral circulation decreases in the extremities. Decreased circulation of the hands and feet create cold, clammy extremities. Sweat gland activity increases to disperse excess heat generated by a surge in energy. The pupils dilate, which increases visual acuity, and the bronchioles dilate to enhance respiratory capacity. Blood flow to the gastrointestinal (GI) and genitourinary systems diminishes, which slows activity in these areas.

Discharge of the SNS provides the temporary ability to endure a stressor. This neurological discharge also occurs in the **fight-or-flight reaction,** first described by Walter B. Cannon in the 1920s. The fight-or-flight reaction is a basic survival response to an acute, severe stressor that incites involuntary neuroendocrine physiologic changes. The effects of the alarm stage in Selye's theory of stress are the same as those described in Cannon's fight-or-flight reaction theory (see Fig. 4-1).

Also during the alarm stage of Selye's stress response, the hypothalamus of the brain releases corticotropin-releasing factor, which stimulates the anterior pituitary gland to secrete adrenocorticotropic hormone (ACTH). ACTH acts on the adrenal cortex to secrete the glucocorticoid cortisol, which raises blood glucose levels, enhances muscle strength, and potentiates sympathetic activity. Cortisol powerfully enhances the body's ability to resist stress by mobilizing glucose, amino acids, and fat stores for cellular energy production (see Fig. 4-1).

In acute stress, cortisol also causes an increase in WBC response and counteracts inflammation. Immunity is enhanced for the initial 3 to 5 days, but if stress is prolonged, cortisol will cause **immunosuppression.** The activity of WBCs is diminished by long-term, elevated cortisol levels.

The adrenal medulla is also stimulated to secrete the catecholamine epinephrine and the mineralocorticoid aldosterone. Epinephrine potentiates the sympathetic reaction and aldosterone acts at the kidney's nephrons to increase sodium and water reabsorption into the bloodstream. Concurrently, the posterior pituitary gland secretes antidiuretic hormone (ADH), also called vasopressin, which further enhances water reabsorption from the kidney nephrons into the

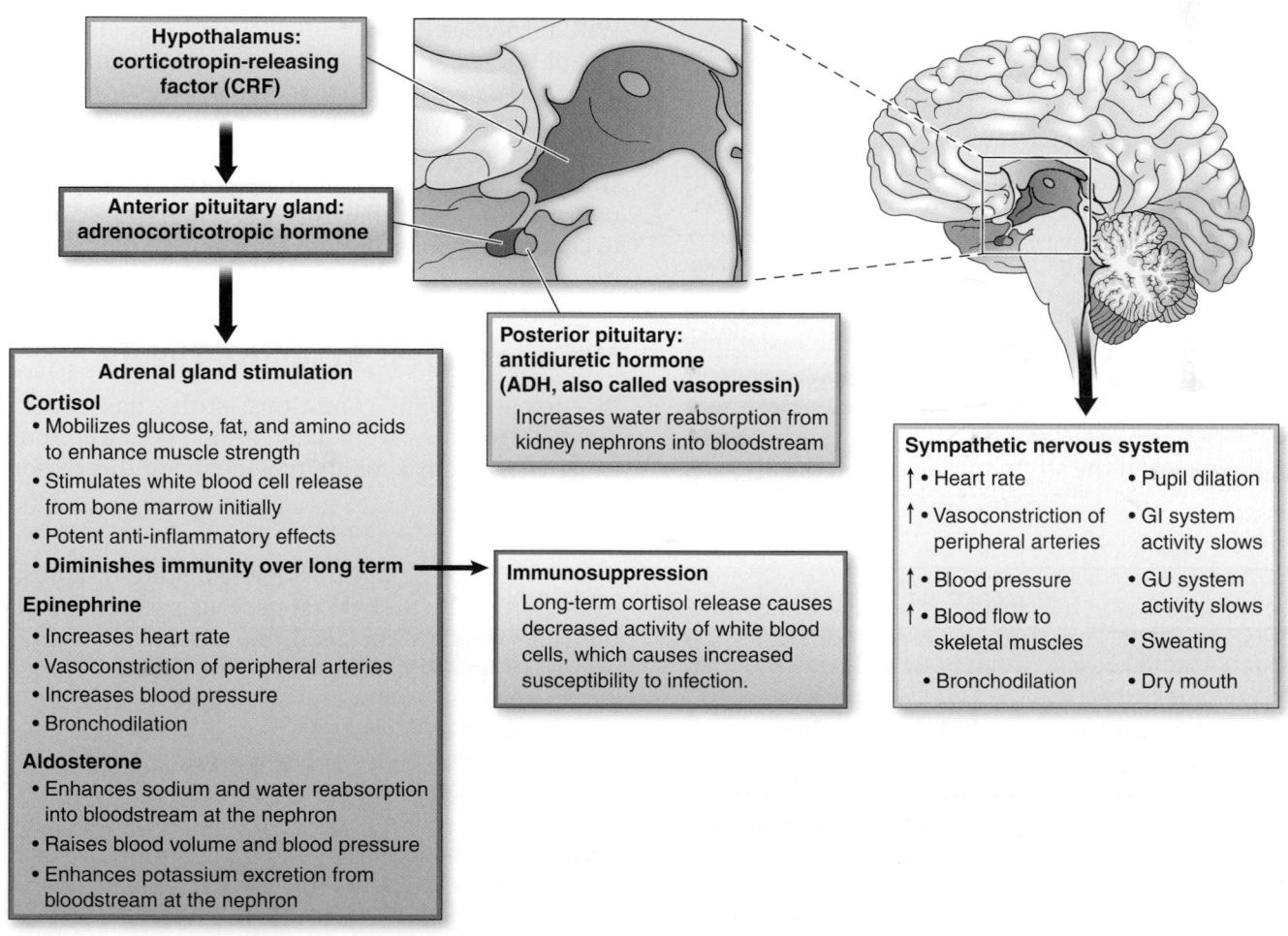

FIGURE 4-1. The fight-or-flight reaction is a basic survival response to an acute, severe stressor that incites involuntary neuroendocrine physiologic changes. The fight-or-flight reaction causes the same effects as those described in the alarm stage of Selye's theory of stress. During severe stress, the hypothalamus of the brain releases corticotropin-releasing factor, which in turn stimulates the anterior pituitary to secrete ACTH. ACTH stimulates the adrenal gland to secrete cortisol, epinephrine, and aldosterone. Concurrently, the posterior pituitary secretes antidiuretic hormone, also called vasopressin. Long-term stimulation of cortisol causes diminished activity of WBCs, which causes immunosuppression.

bloodstream. The extra sodium and water in the bloodstream and vasoconstrictive effects of norepinephrine and epinephrine increase blood pressure (see Fig. 4-1).

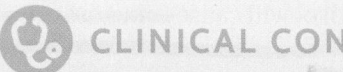

CLINICAL CONCEPT

A potent anti-inflammatory effect occurs with the administration of the pharmacological form of cortisone, also called prednisone or dexamethasone. However, long-term use of pharmacological cortisone will send negative feedback to the pituitary gland and shut off secretion of ACTH. Lack of ACTH will decrease stimulation of the adrenal gland and reduce natural corticosteroid secretion. Eventually this leads to atrophy of the adrenal gland and resultant immunosuppression. For this reason, pharmacological cortisone should only be used for short-term treatment.

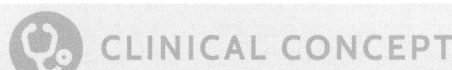

CLINICAL CONCEPT

Some studies show that stress-induced cortisol secretion may contribute to central fat accumulation.

Resistance Stage. Selye termed the second phase of the general adaptation syndrome as the resistance stage. During this stage the body attempts to stave off the effects of stress through continual hormone and catecholamine secretion. However, this is a time-limited stage; if the stress subsides, then the SNS and adrenal stimulation abate, and the parasympathetic nervous system (PSNS) responses resume a state of relaxation. Activation of the PSNS, also known as the cholinergic nervous system, causes the opposite effects of the SNS. The PSNS slows heart rate, constricts the bronchioles, decreases pupil size, and enhances GI and genitourinary activity (see Table 4-1). Under the influence of the PSNS, the body is in a relaxed, quiet state.

Exhaustion Stage. If the stressor does not subside and the stress is prolonged, the high levels of hormone and catecholamine secretion cannot be sustained and the exhaustion stage ensues. During this stage, stress overwhelms the body's ability to defend itself: The body's resources are depleted and signs of systemic dysfunction occur. During this stage, an individual commonly feels rundown, unable to cope, depressed, anxious, and physically ill.

Chronic stress can have a cumulative, negative impact on physical health and mental well-being. Long-term secretion of cortisol suppresses immunity, and WBC responses become sluggish and less efficient—one of the major adverse effects of prolonged stress. Selye also demonstrated that chronic stress caused atrophy of the thymus gland and a consequent decline in T lymphocytes, another cause of immunosuppression. Immunosuppression predisposes the individual to infection and other diseases; therefore, illness is commonly experienced at times of prolonged or severe stress.

McEwen's Stress Response Theory

In current societal conditions, stress has become more of a routine part of daily life and not an episodic experience or crisis for an individual. For this reason,

	Sympathetic Nervous System (Adrenergic)	Parasympathetic Nervous System (Cholinergic)
Neurotransmitter	Norepinephrine	Acetylcholine
Heart	Increased heart rate	Decreased heart rate
Vascular	Vasoconstriction of peripheral arteries Increased blood pressure	Vasodilation of peripheral arteries Decreased blood pressure
Lungs	Bronchodilation	Bronchoconstriction
Pupils	Pupil dilation (mydriasis)	Pupil constriction (miosis)
Gastrointestinal system	Decreased blood flow to GI system slows activity	Increased blood flow to GI system normalizes activity
Genitourinary system	Decreased blood flow to GU system slows activity	Increased blood flow to GU system normalizes activity
Other	Sweating (diaphoresis) Dry mouth Feelings of nervousness Tremors possible	Feeling of relaxation

TABLE 4-1. Effects of the Autonomic Nervous System

another theoretical model, devised by Bruce McEwen in the 1990s, has become accepted as an explanation of the cumulative adverse health effects of frequent, recurring stress. Selye's theory explains the body's reaction to intermittent, infrequent episodes of stress, whereas McEwen's theory attempts to explain long-term stress.

Allostasis and Allostatic Load

McEwen's theory of allostasis and allostatic load attempts to explain how the body adapts to frequent stressors and how stressors can change the body's set points of homeostasis. McEwen coined the term **allostasis** to describe a dynamic state of balance that changes according to exposure to stressors (see Fig. 4-2). In contrast, homeostasis is a set state of balance with strict, unchanging parameters or set points. According to past stress theory, the body's reactions to stress occur with the intent to reestablish homeostasis with definite set points of normal. McEwen theorizes that frequent stressors change the body's physiologic balance and create new set points. For example, individuals exposed to job stress on a daily basis may develop high blood pressure while in the work environment. If this stress becomes chronic, it can drive the individual's physiologic blood pressure to high levels that persist in and out of the work environment.

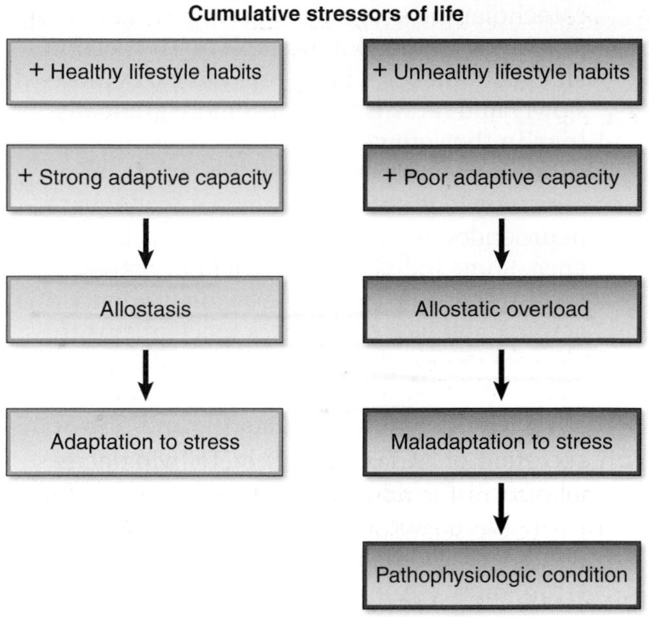

Cumulative stressors of life

+ Healthy lifestyle habits	+ Unhealthy lifestyle habits
+ Strong adaptive capacity	+ Poor adaptive capacity
Allostasis	Allostatic overload
Adaptation to stress	Maladaptation to stress
	Pathophysiologic condition

FIGURE 4-2. McEwen's theory of allostasis and allostatic load. Frequent, cumulative stressors exert an allostatic load. The individual's lifestyle and adaptive capacity influence the reaction to the cumulative stress. An individual with a healthy lifestyle and strong adaptive capability will be able to balance and adapt successfully to stressors, a state called allostasis. An individual with an unhealthy lifestyle and poor adaptive capability will experience allostatic overload, which results in a pathophysiologic state.

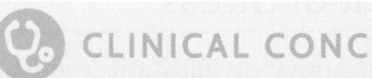

> ### CLINICAL CONCEPT
>
> Long-term high blood pressure causes endothelial damage and accelerates development of atherosclerosis over time; in this way, atherosclerosis caused by hypertension is a stress-related disease.

Allostatic load can be defined as the wear and tear on body systems caused by stress reactions. In prolonged stress, hormones and catecholamines have a cumulative, noxious effect and are part of the allostatic load on the body (see Fig. 4-2). For example, chronic secretion of the hormone epinephrine causes arterial vasoconstriction and raises blood pressure. Chronic cortisol secretion causes immunosuppression and sleep disruption.

According to McEwen, allostatic load can accumulate because of any of the four following mechanisms:

1. **Repeated stressful experiences:** This mechanism of allostatic load can occur when, for example, a person experiences multiple stresses consecutively or simultaneously. Death of a loved one, illness, moving to another home, and divorce are common types of stresses for an individual. If a person has to deal with all of these at once, the neuro-endocrine stress reaction is provoked multiple times and the body isn't given sufficient time to recover and reestablish homeostasis.

2. **Inability of the individual to adapt to stress:** Every individual differs in his or her adaptive ability to deal with stress. Some have fewer coping mechanisms than others or insufficient social support. For example, those who relocate to live in a new region that is unfamiliar to them may experience diminished adaptive ability to handle stress because of lack of support from friends and family.

3. **Prolonged reaction to a stressor:** This mechanism of allostatic load occurs when an individual has an inappropriately prolonged reaction to a stressor. When a person is called upon to take an examination, he or she experiences the neuroendocrine stress response before and during the examination. Many individuals also experience the stress for a lengthy time after the termination of the experience. For such persons, the stress reaction begins before the stressful event and does not shut down in a timely manner, creating an inappropriately detrimental, lengthened exposure to the stress hormones and catecholamines. Interestingly, studies show that after the conclusion of a stressful event, stress-induced hormones and

catecholamines return to baseline values more slowly with aging. For example, with exertion, an elderly person's heart rate increases more slowly and returns to normal more gradually than in the younger adult.

4. **Inadequate response to a stressor:** Lastly, allostatic load can result from an inadequate neuroendocrine response to a stressful experience. Some individuals have a faulty stress response that causes imbalanced neuroendocrine activity and lack of feedback mechanisms to shut off the reaction. The individual has inappropriate hypoactivity and hyperactivity of different systems involved in the stress response. Lab animals that secrete inadequate amounts of cortisol during stress demonstrate inadequate shutdown of localized inflammatory mediators. These lab animals, in turn, demonstrate more autoimmune and inflammatory diseases. These studies have led to theories that many autoimmune and inflammatory diseases are stress-related in etiology.

According to McEwen, allostatic load is not only determined by the stressor, but also by how well the individual adapts to the stressor. The individual's adaptive ability is influenced by genetic makeup, cognitive ability, developmental level, socioeconomic status, lifestyle choices, diet, exercise, pre-existing conditions, past life experiences, and support of others. When stress exceeds the body's ability to adapt, **allostatic overload** results, initiating pathophysiologic disorders (see Fig. 4-2.). For example, an obese, sedentary individual who overeats has a high risk of developing insulin resistance and type 2 diabetes. The excess fat and insulin resistance are stressors to the body, and the individual's adaptive ability is hindered by sedentary behavior and poor eating habits. The stressors and lack of adaptive ability contribute to the allostatic load. In the individual who develops insulin resistance and type 2 diabetes, the allostatic load overwhelms the individual's ability to return the body to homeostasis and causes a state of pathological imbalance. The body can resume an allostatic state of stability with treatment for diabetes and reduce allostatic load through exercise and weight loss. If allostatic load is reduced significantly, the body may be able to reestablish homeostasis and diabetes can subside.

Stress is an increasingly significant consideration in diagnosis and treatment of many common illnesses (see Box 4-1). Clinicians frequently recommend stress management, weight reduction, smoking cessation, and exercise in addition to medical, pharmacological, and surgical treatments. These recommendations aim to lessen lifestyle-related stressors on the body, thereby reducing allostatic load. Stress reduction can boost immunity and reverse many of the negative effects of illness.

BOX 4-1. Common Stress-Related Disorders

- Asthma
- Atherosclerosis
- Autoimmune diseases
- Cardiac rhythm disturbances
- Cerebrovascular disease
- Coronary artery disease
- Diabetes
- General anxiety disorder
- Hypertension
- Irritable bowel disease
- Migraine headache
- Peptic ulcer disease
- Skin disorders such as urticaria (hives)
- Substance abuse

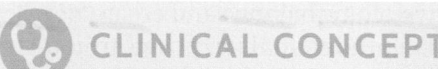

CLINICAL CONCEPT

Elderly individuals have less resiliency against stress, as the body requires more time for recovery from a stressful event.

Treatment of Stress

Overwhelming stress or allostatic overload occurs when the individual's adaptive ability is exceeded. Symptoms such as nervousness, irritability, headaches, lack of concentration ability, insomnia, changes in appetite, depression, and panic attacks are often the result of allostatic overload. When stress interferes with normal daily functioning, many persons seek treatment from clinicians or counselors. Lifestyle modifications, stress management programs, psychotherapy, alternative medical practices, and pharmacological treatments are often recommended for excessive stress.

Lifestyle Practices

Many lifestyle factors affect how our body deals with stress. Adequate sleep, exercise, and nutrition are necessary elements for resiliency against stress.

Reducing Caffeine Intake

Caffeine is a stimulant contained in coffee, tea, cola, chocolate, and many appetite suppressants. Nine out of 10 Americans consume some type of caffeine regularly. For most people, moderate doses of caffeine (200 to 300 mg, or about two to three cups of brewed coffee a day) aren't harmful.

Caffeine readily crosses the blood–brain barrier and acts as an antagonist of adenosine receptors found in the brain. The reduction in adenosine activity results in increased activity of the neurotransmitter dopamine, which causes mental alertness. Caffeine can also increase levels of epinephrine and serotonin. Epinephrine stimulates the SNS, leading to increased heart rate, blood pressure, and blood flow to muscles and vasoconstriction of arterioles, which perfuse the skin and inner organs. Biochemically, it stimulates glycogenolysis, inhibits glycolysis, and stimulates gluconeogenesis to produce more glucose for the muscles and release of glucose into the bloodstream from the liver. Also, caffeine stimulates serotonin in the brain, which produces positive changes in mood.

Side effects of excessive caffeine intake include nervousness, tremulousness, and increased heart rate and blood pressure. Many studies have been done to investigate an association between caffeine, coffee drinking, and coronary artery disease. Caffeine can stimulate occasional premature atrial contractions in the heart, which can be perceived as palpitations by an individual. However, research studies have not established a link between caffeine and development of coronary artery disease.

 CLINICAL CONCEPT

In individuals experiencing a high level of stress, even moderate coffee drinking can cause increased jitteriness, nervousness, insomnia, and heart palpitations. These individuals should either decrease or eliminate their caffeine intake.

 CLINICAL CONCEPT

Caffeine tolerance develops very quickly, especially among heavy coffee drinkers. Caffeine-habituated individuals can experience caffeine withdrawal 12 to 24 hours after the last dose of caffeine. It resolves within 24 to 48 hours. The most prominent symptoms are headache, irritability, anxiety, fatigue, and drowsiness.

Ensuring Restorative Sleep

For the body to cope with daily stress, restorative sleep is necessary. Studies show that restorative sleep is a heightened anabolic state, when there is growth and rejuvenation of the immune, nervous, skeletal, and muscular systems. Restorative sleep requires a sufficient length of time devoted to sleep so that the body can enter the five different stages of sleep that begin after the body is relaxed and preparing for sleep (see Box 4-2).

 CLINICAL CONCEPT

To examine sleep patterns, a diagnostic test called **polysomnography** is performed. Sensors are placed on the patient to monitor electrical activity of the brain, eye movement, muscle contraction, and cardiac and respiratory function during sleep.

Lack of Sufficient Sleep. Generally, sleep disorders affect the quality, duration, and onset of sleep. Sleep deprivation, frequently changing sleep schedule, stress, and environment all affect the progression of the sleep cycle.

 CLINICAL CONCEPT

According to the National Sleep Foundation (NSF) (1999–2004), at least 60% of adults report having sleep problems a few nights a week or more; most persons go undiagnosed and untreated. More than 40% of adults experience daytime sleepiness severe enough to interfere with their daily activities.

Irritability and moodiness are the first symptoms a person experiences from lack of sleep. Sleep deprivation can cause apathy, slowed speech, flattened emotional responses, impaired memory, poor judgment, and an inability to multitask. Extreme sleep deprivation causes a person to fall into microsleeps (5 to 10 seconds) that result in lapses of attention and possible hallucinations.

Everyone's individual sleep needs vary. In general, most healthy adults function best with 8 to 10 hours of sleep a night. However, some individuals are able to function without sleepiness or drowsiness after as little as 6 hours of sleep. The need for sleep doesn't decline with age; however, the ability to sleep for 6 to 8 hours at one time may be reduced.

 CLINICAL CONCEPT

Obstructive sleep apnea (OSA) is a common cause of nonrestorative sleep. OSA is caused by the relaxation of pharyngeal soft tissue that collapses over the airways during sleep. The hallmark symptom of OSA is excessive daytime sleepiness; the patient may also report snoring and repetitive pauses in breathing.

BOX 4-2. The Five Stages of Sleep

STAGE 1

Stage 1 sleep, or drowsiness, is first in the sequence. On polysomnography, brain waves show a 50% reduction in activity between wakefulness and stage 1 sleep. The eyes are closed. This stage usually lasts between 5 and 10 minutes.

STAGE 2

Stage 2 is a period of light sleep during which polysomnographic readings show spontaneous periods of muscle tone mixed with periods of muscle relaxation. The heart rate slows, and body temperature decreases. At this point, the body prepares to enter deep sleep.

STAGE 3 AND STAGE 4

In stage 3, slow brain waves called *delta waves* begin to appear, interspersed with smaller, faster waves. By stage 4, the brain produces delta waves almost exclusively. It is very difficult to wake someone during stages 3 and 4, which together are called deep sleep. There is no eye movement or muscle activity. People awakened during deep sleep do not adjust immediately and often feel groggy and disoriented for several minutes after they wake up.

STAGE 5

Stage 5 is referred to as **REM sleep** because rapid eye movement (REM) occurs during this stage. Although REM sleep is not completely understood, some physiologic changes are distinguishable during this stage. Breathing becomes more rapid, irregular, and shallow, and the eyes jerk rapidly in various directions. There is a decrease in the activity of the monoamine neurotransmitters, such as norepinephrine, in the brain. Muscles of the extremities become temporarily paralyzed, heart rate increases, and blood pressure rises. Uniquely, dreaming occurs during REM sleep.

Although REM sleep is not well understood, many theories exist about the function and significance of this stage of sleep. Theories have stated REM sleep is important because it:

- allows for consolidation of procedural and spatial memories
- helps the monoamine receptors in the brain to recover to regain full sensitivity
- provides the neurological stimulation needed to form mature neural connections for proper central nervous system development in newborns.

Experts agree that there seem to be no ill effects from lack of REM sleep, but it appears to be necessary for restorative sleep. Researchers have found that suppressing REM sleep greatly increases the number of attempts an individual will make to enter REM sleep. Also, once the suppression ceases, the proportion of time spent in REM sleep will increase significantly, an event known as REM rebound.

THE SLEEP CYCLE

When people sleep, they cycle through the stages of sleep in a repetitive manner. A complete sleep cycle takes approximately 90 to 110 minutes and is composed of stages 1 through 5, with stage 2 and 3 repeated before stage 5. A normal sleep cycle has the following pattern: restful wakefulness, stage 1, 2, 3, 4, repeat of stage 3, repeat of stage 2, and then stage 5 REM sleep. A person may complete five cycles in a typical night's sleep.

Improving Nutrition

Stress can affect eating patterns and nutritional status of an individual. Conversely, nutritional status can affect the ability to deal with stress. Individual eating patterns vary in response to stress. Many persons report that, when under stress, they eat excessively; others complain of a loss of appetite because of stress. Six small nutritious meals instead of three large meals is often recommended as a strategy for those under stress. Also, slowing down, taking a seated position, and relaxing while eating is recommended.

Persons under stress commonly skip meals, which is an unhealthy practice. Skipping meals can lead to hypoglycemia, which causes dizziness, tachycardia, diaphoresis, poor concentration ability, possible syncope, and poor intake of daily recommended vitamins and minerals. Conversely, some persons under stress overeat or increase intake of fast food. These are unhealthy practices that can lead to obesity, sluggishness, and indigestion.

Many persons under stress endure indigestion, heartburn, constipation, diarrhea, nausea, and vomiting. Conditions such as inflammatory bowel disease and irritable bowel syndrome are exacerbated by stress. Considerable research has been done that confirms a brain–gut axis, which is a neurological connection between the central nervous system, autonomic nervous system, and GI tract.

The Role of Serotonin and Tryptophan. Research is focusing on the role of serotonin in GI disorders. Serotonin is an important neurotransmitter found in both the brain and GI tract. In the GI system, cells of the small intestine called enterochromaffin cells release serotonin, which stimulates peristaltic, secretory, vasodilatory, and parasympathetic activity. Serotonin allows for full, complete, and relaxed function of the GI system. During stress there is a deficit of serotonin; this causes decreased GI function and higher susceptibility to indigestion.

It is theorized that serotonin levels in the brain also become depleted during stress. Studies with humans and animals show that serotonin in the brain promotes feelings of calm, personal security, relaxation, confidence, and concentration, whereas lack of serotonin in the brain causes a lack of feelings of well-being.

Tryptophan, one of the essential amino acids obtained from dietary sources, is the precursor to serotonin. Some dietary sources of tryptophan include meats, soy products, some kinds of cheese, milk, brown rice, and peanuts. Many protein sources contain the essential amino acids, with a small percentage in the form of tryptophan. In order to form serotonin, tryptophan must cross the blood–brain barrier and compete with the other ingested amino acids. Insulin is a carrier molecule that facilitates transport of glucose, some amino acids, and fatty acids into muscle and liver cells. In the presence of insulin, most competing amino acids are absorbed into muscle cells, whereas tryptophan remains behind in the circulation. By facilitating absorption of competing amino acids into muscle, insulin frees tryptophan so that it can enter the brain.

Ingestion of carbohydrates is the greatest dietary stimulus for release of insulin; carbohydrates, which stimulate insulin, enhance the uptake of competing amino acids into muscle and allow the brain to absorb tryptophan. Once inside the brain, tryptophan is converted into serotonin. At the pineal gland of the brain, some serotonin is converted to melatonin, an enhancer of sleep, which is why tryptophan has earned a reputation as having calming, relaxing effects over individuals. Anecdotally, many persons claim that some carbohydrate-rich foods are comforting; these individuals report increased intake of carbohydrates when under stress. Occasional indulgence in this type of food is probably useful to relieve anxiety in the short-term, but habitually, foods rich in carbohydrate are likely to cause obesity.

Balancing Work and Leisure Activities

Working persons need to balance their lives with sufficient time for recreation and leisure. Initially, increased stress produces increased performance. However, after a certain point prolonged stress results in decreased performance, as efforts to work harder become either unproductive or even counterproductive.

One of the first symptoms of distress is fatigue and irritability. These symptoms are signals that the individual's adaptive ability is reaching its threshold and stress relief is necessary or exhaustion can result.

Utilizing Social Support

Persons under stress often need to talk about their problems with a supportive, active listener. Social support from friends, coworkers, or relatives can provide some relief of stress. Supportive others can offer feedback, validation, encouragement, and advice. Many times, simply allowing the individual to voice his or her feelings enables stress relief.

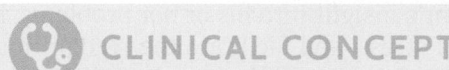

CLINICAL CONCEPT

Journaling is another form of expression that can be useful for relieving stress. Although not a social medium, writing affords the person a private place to express feelings, work out problems, and organize thoughts about specific issues, much as he or she would with a supportive listener.

Using Humor

Humor can be used as a coping mechanism to reduce stress and promote general wellness. Studies show that among cancer patients, various types of humorous material lessened anxiety and discomfort and provoked open discussion of concerns and fears. Researchers also found that humor has a positive effect on the immune system. Humor is associated with an increased pain threshold and enhanced function of specific WBCs, called natural killer cells. In addition, research shows that patients demonstrate specific neuroendocrine changes associated with improved physical stress responses and increased feelings of well-being after humorous interventions.

Exercising

Exercise can reduce stress, alleviate depression and anxiety, enhance coping mechanisms, and boost self-confidence. It stimulates blood flow to the brain, which enhances secretion of the neurotransmitters serotonin, norepinephrine, and dopamine, which counteract depression and anxiety.

Over the long term, exercise reduces the effect of neuroendocrine excitation that is provoked by stress. The long-term effect of regular exercise is likened to meditation in that it can activate the PSNS and endow the individual with a relaxation effect.

Utilizing Psychotherapy

Individual psychotherapy involves regularly scheduled counseling sessions between the patient and a mental health professional such as a psychologist, psychiatrist, social worker, or psychiatric clinician. The sessions may focus on current or past problems, sources of anxiety, and current thoughts, feelings, or relationships. Sharing these experiences with an objective mental health professional allows a patient to ventilate and come to understand how to manage stress and anxiety.

Cognitive-behavioral therapy and interpersonal psychotherapy are the major types of psychotherapeutic techniques used. Cognitive-behavioral therapy explores the patient's beliefs, expectations, and cognitive appraisals of self, the world, and the nature of personal problems. The therapist attempts to explore the patient's sources of anxiety and give recommendations regarding coping behaviors to manage the stress. In interpersonal therapy, the therapist attempts to enhance the patient's insight into his or her problems, identify sources of stress, and facilitate the recognition of the patient's own coping abilities or disabilities.

Stress Management Programs

Stress management programs assist an individual in coping with various types of stress through education, counseling, and support group interaction. These types of programs are commonly available within hospitals or other clinical settings. Usually directed by a psychologist or psychiatrist, patients are able to verbalize their problems and anxieties, explore their sources of stress, and receive advice for coping from others in the support group and a mental health professional.

Alternative Practices to Reduce Stress

Alternative medical practices and complementary therapies have been increasingly used by individuals who want natural remedies for disorders. Research studies have shown that meditation and yoga are techniques that can reduce stress.

Meditation

Meditation is a state of concentrated attention. It involves turning the attention inward to a single point of reference. Different meditative disciplines encompass a wide range of spiritual and psychophysical practices that can emphasize development of either a high degree of mental concentration or mental quiescence.

Many persons who meditate retreat to a quiet area and focus intently on one word or concept for a daily prearranged time period with the body in a resting state in order to free the mind. Research demonstrates that daily periods devoted to quiet, restful meditation can alleviate stress.

Yoga

Yoga is an exercise technique that uses different poses to induce relaxation, body alignment, muscle strength, stamina, flexibility, and stress reduction. The person's own body weight provides the resistance needed to strengthen muscles from head to toe.

Yoga enables a person to stretch tight muscles, increase range of motion, enhance balance, and improve alignment. It also boosts energy, calms the person, and enhances awareness, focus, and patience. Research shows that a set period devoted to yoga in a quiet environment combined with meditation relieves stress.

Pharmacological Treatments to Reduce Stress

There are some pharmacological agents that can be prescribed for stress. These include sedatives, sleep aids, and antidepressants. Keep in mind that pharmacological agents should be used in combination with professional counseling or psychotherapy.

Sedatives

A sedative is a substance that depresses the central nervous system, resulting in relaxation, anxiety relief, drowsiness, and slowed breathing. A sedative can also cause slurred speech, unstable gait, poor judgment, and slowed reflexes. Sedatives may be referred to as tranquilizers, depressants, anxiolytics, soporifics, sleeping pills, "downers" (slang), or sedative-hypnotics. When a patient experiences extreme stress or an anxiety attack, sedatives are most often the prescribed medication for rapid relief. However, sedatives can be abused to produce an overly calming effect; alcohol is the most common sedating substance used within the population. At high doses, or when abused, many of these drugs can cause unconsciousness and death.

Antidepressants

Antidepressants are often the treatment of choice for adults with moderate or severe depression and anxiety. Sadness, anxiety, depression-related sleep and appetite disorders, concentration, and energy levels all can improve with antidepressant medications. They achieve their effect by modulating the neurotransmitters in the brain—serotonin, norepinephrine, or dopamine. Dozens of antidepressants are available and each affects brain neurotransmitters in a different way. Patients often must try different medications to find the particular one that is effective and suitable for them.

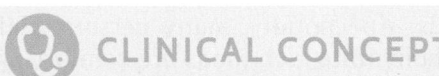

CLINICAL CONCEPT

Antidepressants usually require at least 3 weeks to reach therapeutic blood levels.

Sleep Hygiene

Stress can cause insomnia, and patients may require sleep aids or substances to help them sleep. There are several types of prescribed sleep medications, but the most utilized is the over-the-counter sleep aid diphenhydramine (Benadryl[R]).

It is recommended that a person develop a sleep routine using natural techniques such as quiet time, reading, warm milk, or chamomile tea to induce sleep. It is advisable to avoid caffeine, alcohol, and any stimulant medications such as phenylephrine or pseudoephedrine, as these can interfere with sleep.

The Beneficial Effects of Exercise

Daily physical activity is a necessary component of health promotion and disease prevention. Regular exercise is associated with cardiovascular health, respiratory fitness, decreased risk of chronic disease, bone strengthening, regulation of blood sugar, emotional well-being, and greater longevity (see Box 4-3).

BOX 4-3. Therapeutic Effects of Exercise

- Increases number of mitochondria in muscle cells
- Raises HDL-C
- Stimulates angiogenesis
- Enhances glucose entry into muscle cells
- Improves cardiovascular conditioning: increases perfusion of myocardium and cardiac output, enhances vascular dilation capacity, increases venous return, increases efficiency of heart, decreases blood pressure and pulse rate over long term
- Stimulates osteoblastic activity
- Decreases body fat
- Builds muscle mass
- Creates positive psychological effects on mood and stress relief

---

BOX 4-4. Obesity-Related Disorders

- Cardiovascular disease
- Deep venous thrombosis
- Degenerative joint disease
- Diabetes mellitus
- Gallbladder disease
- Higher risk for breast, prostate, colon, and uterine cancer
- Poor wound healing
- Sleep apnea
- Venous insufficiency

In general, most people can participate in some form of exercise. However, individuals with cardiovascular disease, chronic respiratory illnesses, diabetes, or disabling conditions should consult a physician before beginning an exercise regimen. As a rule, persons younger than age 35 years in good health do not need a medical examination before starting an exercise program.

The basic types of exercise include those that facilitate stretching and flexibility, aerobic fitness, muscular strength, and endurance. In general, the public health recommendation is moderate-intensity physical activity for 40 minutes 3 to 4 days per week. It is suggested that persons alternate between flexibility, aerobic, and isometric exercise in order to target all muscle groups.

Weight

Physical activity is important to prevent obesity, a significant public health problem in the United States among adults, adolescents, and children. Obesity is defined as excess body fat resulting from consumption of calories in excess of those expended. Exercise requires energy and expends the calories consumed by the individual. As one exercises, energy is derived from the breakdown of glycogen and fat stores; this process can decrease obesity.

Heredity, sociocultural factors, and environmental influences also play a role in the development of obesity. Obesity is associated with multiple disease processes including cancers (see Box 4-4).

Cardiovascular System

There is an inverse relationship between the level of physical activity and the incidence of cardiovascular disease. Individuals who exercise regularly demonstrate less atherosclerosis, coronary artery disease, and acute cardiac events. Exercise improves coronary blood flow and vascular endothelial function. The vascular endothelium or lining of arterial blood vessels respond to exercise by producing vasodilator compounds such as prostacyclin and nitric oxide. These vasodilator compounds widen the arterial blood vessels, allowing more blood flow to various regions of the body. Specifically, nitric-oxide dependent vasodilation of the coronary arteries increases myocardial perfusion and prevents endothelial inflammation, platelet activation, and thrombus formation.

Individuals who exercise are found to have lower levels of fibrinogen, an indicator of active clot formation, and C-reactive protein, an inflammatory mediator. For this reason, it is theorized that exercise has an antiatherogenic effect on the endothelium, which prevents endothelial injury and arteriosclerotic plaque and clot formation.

In addition, exercise stimulates angiogenesis, which is the growth of collateral blood vessels. Physical activity stimulates vascular endothelial growth factor secretion, which provokes synthesis of new blood vessels by the endothelial cells. Within the heart muscle, the growth of collateral coronary artery branches provides extra circulatory routes for blood flow to the myocardium. Within the extremities, growth of collateral arterial blood vessels provides new routes of blood flow to the leg muscles. For this reason, walking is recommended to counteract peripheral arterial occlusive disease. Walking stimulates the development of new vascular branches off existing arterial vessels which, in turn, increases routes of circulation in the extremities.

Regular exercise also lowers blood pressure and pulse rate over time. It enhances the heart's efficiency by increasing cardiac muscle mass and growth of coronary vessel branches. A muscular, well-perfused heart contracts more efficiently and requires fewer contractions to yield cardiac output. The efficient heart beats at a slower pace and has adequate time for cardiac filling during diastole. The athletic heart can beat at a slower pace to eject sufficient blood from the ventricles for the body's metabolic requirements. Exercise also stimulates peripheral arterial vasodilation, which opens blood vessels throughout the body, diminishes resistance, and decreases resting systemic blood pressure. Peripheral vasodilation decreases the aortic resistance against the left ventricle and eases the heart's workload.

Venous return is greatly enhanced during aerobic exercise. Contraction of the large leg muscles, in particular, creates a pumping action to facilitate upward flow of venous blood back to the heart. The contractile muscle action and blood flow counteracts venous stasis and clot formation in the legs. Increased amounts of venous blood returns to the right side of the heart, lungs, and into the left side of the heart. Greater venous return raises stroke volume and cardiac output in the healthy heart.

Exercise also increases the formation of high-density lipoprotein cholesterol (HDL-C). The total cholesterol in the body is derived from foods and synthesized by the liver. Total cholesterol is composed of low-density lipoprotein (LDL-C) and HDL-C. The body metabolizes cholesterol to yield either form of cholesterol. LDL-C is deposited within the endothelium to become atherosclerotic plaque, and the HDL-C component is excreted. It is advantageous for more of the total cholesterol in the body to become HDL-C versus LDL-C. Exercise stimulates the body to form more HDL-C than LDL-C. Persons who exercise demonstrate lower total cholesterol levels and higher levels of HDL-C compared with sedentary individuals.

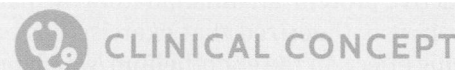

CLINICAL CONCEPT

Exercise stimulates angiogenesis, increases the number of mitochondria in the muscles, and raises HDL cholesterol.

Cardiac Exercise Stress Testing

Exercise stress testing is used to evaluate the cardiovascular status of patients by measuring their energy expenditure and physiologic responses while walking or running on a treadmill. Changing the speed and incline of the treadmill can vary the exercise workload on the body. The patient's heart rate, blood pressure, and electrocardiogram are continuously monitored during the stress test. The patient is challenged to exercise at various levels until maximal heart rate is reached, which is estimated by age.

As a general rule, the predicted maximal heart rate can be estimated by subtracting age from 220. For example, the target heart rate for a 70-year-old person would be: 220 – 70 or 150 beats/minute. For optimal exercise effects, persons are encouraged to reach at least 85% of their maximal heart rate.

Exercise capacity assessed by a cardiac stress test is a strong predictor of risk of death from cardiovascular disease. During a stress test, the patient is gradually challenged to exercise to peak capacity on a treadmill so clinicians can assess cardiovascular status. Along with physiologic monitoring, the individual's feelings

during exertion are monitored as the treadmill speed and incline increase. Research shows that as an individual's exercise capacity increases, risk of death from cardiovascular disease decreases. Research also shows that less fit or less active persons can improve their survival if they increase their level of physical activity. A program of regular exercise can improve fitness by 15% to 30% within 3 to 6 months. Exercise levels must be maintained or else the benefits wane with discontinued activity.

Pulmonary System

Exercise increases the depth and rate of breathing, ventilatory capacity of the lungs, and oxygen and carbon dioxide diffusion at the alveolar-capillary membranes. Enhanced cardiac output creates a greater volume of blood delivered to the pulmonary vasculature and pulmonary perfusion increases. Greater depth and rate of breathing increases the blood's oxygenation.

As exercise continues and a person tires, increased levels of carbon dioxide, decreased oxygen, and decreased blood pH stimulate chemoreceptors in the medulla, aorta, and carotid arteries to increase breathing rate. How long a person is able to exercise depends on the ability of the cardiovascular system and lungs to deliver oxygenated blood to the contracting muscles.

Muscles work most efficiently when using oxygen to perform aerobic metabolism. Muscles that do not receive adequate oxygen eventually enter into anaerobic metabolism, which can only support the exercising body for a short period of time.

Musculoskeletal System

Isometric exercise can build muscle strength; it enlarges muscle size by contracting muscles against increasing levels of workload. Weight lifters typically perform isometric exercises to build muscle mass. Aerobic exercise is both an endurance and isometric type of activity. Walking or running are aerobic exercises that increase efficiency of the muscles, build muscle mass, increase the number of mitochondria, and enhance blood supply.

With isometric exercise, muscles can hypertrophy and double in size. Muscle fibers enlarge, the number of mitochondrial enzymes increase substantially, and there is an increase in stored glycogen and triglycerides. Increased glycogen and triglycerides enhance the potential for anaerobic metabolic activity in the muscles, whereas the increase in mitochondrial enzymes augments the aerobic metabolic capacity of the muscles.

Both aerobic and isometric types of exercise can increase metabolic rate or the amount of energy used by the body during rest. Metabolic rate is directly proportional to lean body mass; the more muscle mass, the greater the metabolic rate. Muscles expend more calories than fat. For example, a pound of muscle can burn up to 50 more calories a day than a pound of fat. Therefore, an exercise program that combines aerobic and isometric activities appears to be the best approach for increasing muscle efficiency, raising metabolic rate, and controlling body weight.

Bone

Bone is a dynamic organ continually undergoing remodeling by osteoblast and osteoclastic activity. Osteoblasts continually deposit new bone, and osteoclasts actively absorb bone. Normally, except in growing bones, the rates of bone deposition and absorption are equal to each other so that total mass of bone remains constant. Bone is deposited according to compressional loads and remodels according to load stress patterns.

Physical activity stimulates increases in bone diameter and strength throughout the life span. Exercise-stimulated bone strengthening and remodeling diminishes the risk of fracture by counteracting the development of osteoporosis.

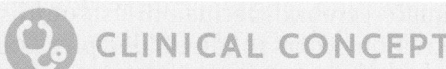

CLINICAL CONCEPT

Weight-bearing exercises stimulate osteoblastic activity and calcification of bone.

Glucose Tolerance

Exercise enhances cellular glucose uptake and reduces glucose intolerance. For reasons not clearly understood, muscle cells become more permeable to glucose even in the absence of insulin during the process of contraction. In diabetes, exercise is recommended as an adjunct to dietary restrictions and weight control, as these therapies combined can often reverse the disease process.

ALERT! Persons with diabetes mellitus must be vigilant of hypoglycemia during periods of intense exercise.

Gastrointestinal System

During intense exercise, blood is shunted away from the GI tract toward active skeletal muscles and the cardiorespiratory system. However, over the long term, regular exercise is known to assist peristaltic activity, counteract constipation, and reduce risk of colon cancer, diverticulosis, and inflammatory bowel disease.

Psychological Effects

Regular exercise increases oxygen delivery to the brain and stimulates neurotransmitters such as dopamine, serotonin, and norepinephrine, which can elevate mood. There is also evidence that endorphins, which are natural pain relievers, rise in the bloodstream after exercise. High endorphin levels in the brain endow an individual with a feeling of well-being. Lastly, exercise is hypothesized to have a detoxification effect on the body, as it may increase metabolism sufficiently to allow the body to excrete stress hormones more rapidly.

The Harmful Effects of Physical Inactivity and Immobility

Lack of physical activity has become a public health problem in the United States. Immobility may be a consequence of severe neuromuscular injury, as experienced by paralyzed individuals; a prerequisite for healing, as in stabilization of a fractured bone; or it can be a lifestyle choice. Regardless of the cause, immobility is a risk factor for obesity, cardiovascular deconditioning, muscular atrophy, osteoporosis, and other disease processes (see Box 4-5).

BOX 4-5. Effects of Immobility

- Atelectasis
- Bone demineralization
- Deconditioning of the heart and muscles
- Decreased pulmonary ventilation, including vital capacity, tidal volume, and functional residual capacity
- Decubitus ulcers
- Depression
- Diminished peristalsis and constipation
- Disorientation
- Gait and balance disturbance
- Gastroesophageal reflux
- Increased susceptibility to aspiration
- Increased susceptibility to orthostatic hypotension
- Joint contractures
- Kidney stones
- Loss of appetite
- Muscle atrophy
- Reduced cough effectiveness
- Stasis of pulmonary secretions and increased risk of pneumonia
- Urinary stasis
- Urinary tract infection
- Venous stasis
- Venous thromboembolism

Lack of regular physical activity causes a characteristic pattern of suboptimal systemic function. It reduces stimulation of the cardiovascular, pulmonary, GI, genitourinary, and musculoskeletal systems. Prolonged inactivity can cause electrolyte imbalances, glucose intolerance, circulatory dysfunction, skin breakdown, and altered sensory perception.

Circulatory System Changes

With immobility, there are changes that occur in the arteries and veins. Veins are weak-walled structures with valves that often fail to direct blood flow upward to the heart. Arteries, although muscular structures, do not vasoconstrict rapidly with position changes, causing a condition called orthostatic hypotension.

Venous Stasis

When walking, the leg muscles contract against the force of gravity and exert a positive pressure force on the veins of the legs. The gastrocnemius muscle of the lower leg, in particular, keeps blood pumping up toward the heart. In the supine position, the body cannot counteract the forces of gravity. With immobility, there is stagnation of venous blood in the lower extremities—a condition called venous stasis. The stasis of venous blood increases hydrostatic pressure within the veins of the legs, which is then transmitted into the capillaries. With this increase in pressure, fluid is displaced from the blood into the interstitial tissue, forming edema. Ankle edema is common in persons with venous insufficiency.

Because the blood is stagnant in venous stasis, there is a susceptibility of the blood to clot. A clot that forms in the venous circulation of the legs is called deep vein thrombosis (DVT).

Pulmonary Embolism

The risk of pulmonary embolism (PE) increases with immobility and venous insufficiency. A venous clot can form in the stagnant blood of a deep vein of the lower extremity. The venous clot then can travel into the inferior vena cava and into the right side of the heart. When a clot travels, it is referred to as an embolism. From the right ventricle the clot is pumped into the pulmonary artery and can lodge and obstruct pulmonary circulation. The clot is then referred to as a PE—a potentially fatal condition because it blocks the perfusion of lung tissue.

CLINICAL CONCEPT

Patients on bedrest can develop venous stasis, which can lead to DVT and, eventually, PE. A PE can be fatal and prevention is the most effective strategy. Thromboembolic dressing (TED) stockings, sequential pneumatic compression devices, and anticoagulant medications are often used to decrease risk of DVT in patients on bedrest.

Orthostatic Hypotension

Orthostatic hypotension occurs when a patient attempts to resume the upright position after a prolonged period of bedrest. After an extended period in the supine position, an individual's arterial baroreceptors (pressure sensors that stimulate the SNS to vasoconstrict the arterial blood vessels) require time to readjust to the upright position. Under normal conditions, as a person changes from the lying to standing position, the arterial blood vessels experience a drop in blood pressure that stimulates the baroreceptors inside the walls of the arteries. The baroreceptors then stimulate the SNS to vasoconstrict arteries and increase heart rate in response to the drop in blood pressure. Blood pressure then readjusts to ensure cerebral perfusion.

When the patient with orthostatic hypotension attempts to rise to a standing position, he or she commonly experiences a delay in arterial vasoconstriction, and the patient's blood pressure temporarily falls as he or she stands. During this episode, the patient experiences a temporary interval of inadequate cerebral perfusion. Patients often feel faint, dizzy, or weak; they may also be unable to stand and may experience syncope, or loss of consciousness. This transient episode of inadequate cerebral perfusion lasts until arterial vasoconstriction occurs to raise blood pressure.

ALERT! A supine patient who attempts to assume the standing position quickly can experience symptoms of orthostatic hypotension. These symptoms include dizziness, tachycardia, diaphoresis, and possibly syncope. Clinicians need to be vigilant of this syndrome to prevent falls in patients and should assist patients in assuming a sitting position for a short time before standing.

ALERT! Elderly individuals and individuals on antihypertensive medications have increased susceptibility to orthostatic hypotension.

Natriuresis

In the first few days of bedrest, body fluid volume redistribution causes a temporary natural diuretic effect called **natriuresis,** which is water loss from the body. Initially, when the body assumes the supine position, heightened centralized blood volume, which inhibits ADH and aldosterone, suppresses the baroreceptors. The suppression of ADH and aldosterone inhibits water reabsorption from the nephron tubules into the bloodstream and enhances natriuresis. Plasma volume becomes more concentrated with the initial water loss, but after a few days fluid volume stabilizes.

Cardiovascular System Changes

With prolonged inactivity or immobility, the cardiovascular system becomes deconditioned and the heart has to work harder and beat faster in order to eject sufficient ventricular blood to supply the organs with adequate circulation. Cardiac output initially increases in the supine position because of the redistribution of blood volume to the centralized region of the body. With extended periods of bedrest, however, venous return decreases, which diminishes cardiac filling. Left ventricular end diastolic volume decreases, stroke volume decreases, and reduced cardiac output results. To compensate for the decreased cardiac output, heart rate increases. A rapid heart rate compromises the amount of diastolic filling time in the ventricles.

Pulmonary System Changes

Bedrest and immobility cause pulmonary changes in lung volumes and breathing mechanics because the supine position is not conducive to full ventilation and lung expansion. In the upright position, breathing is facilitated by the rib cage, intercostal muscles, and diaphragm. In the supine condition, the abdominal muscles cannot optimally facilitate pulmonary expansion.

 CLINICAL CONCEPT

Individuals must exert more energy to breathe in the supine position; because of this, they tend to have shallow ventilations. Clinicians must recognize that the ideal position to facilitate the patient's breathing is in the upright, seated position.

Patients on bedrest have diminished ability to expand the lungs, decreased strength of cough, and consequent susceptibility to atelectasis, or collapse of the alveoli. Atelectasis causes areas of submaximal oxygenation within the lungs and consequent hypoxemia, or low oxygen in the bloodstream. Because of the lack of strength of the cough reflex and shallow ventilation, pulmonary secretions tend to accumulate and pool. Pooled pulmonary secretions create conditions conducive to pneumonia.

Bedridden patients are commonly at risk for aspiration or choking. Aspiration occurs when gastric contents or food particles are swallowed into the lungs versus the esophagus. Because of weakened muscles, pulmonary inefficiency, weakened cough, and possibly a weak gag reflex, the patient may not be able to adequately coordinate swallowing to prevent choking. The bedridden patient may also be at increased risk of gastroesophageal reflux, which can cause gastric contents to enter the lungs and lead to aspiration pneumonia.

Musculoskeletal System Changes

To function efficiently, muscles need periodic contraction and relaxation. The sliding actin and myosin subunits within a muscle require activation. Similarly, bones require weight-bearing conditions to stimulate their growth and remodeling. With immobility, muscle and bone experience negative effects.

Effects on Muscle

Unstimulated, noncontracting muscle fibers have fewer metabolic requirements and adapt by decreasing in size, which is why muscles undergo disuse atrophy when an individual is immobilized or on bedrest.

Muscles also weaken in strength and shorten in length with disuse. **Contractures** occur when muscles shorten over joints that are inactive for prolonged periods of time. An inactive joint contracts and constricts and becomes increasingly limited in range of motion. The connective tissue around inactive joints also undergoes shortening and degeneration, which contributes to the contracture. This is most apparent in paralyzed individuals who do not receive range of motion exercises.

 CLINICAL CONCEPT

Without activity, the joints naturally assume positions of flexion contractures—fingers clench and wrists flex inward, arms flex at the elbows, hips and legs flex toward the medial aspect of the body, and the neck flexes forward to bring the chin to the chest. The immobilized, inactive body will assume a fetal position if joints are allowed to develop contractures (see Fig. 4-3). For this reason, clinicians need to ensure proper body alignment, turn immobile patients, and perform daily passive range of motion exercises on those with limited mobility.

Effects on Bone

Bone also begins to degenerate with lack of weight-bearing activity or exercises. **Trabecular bones,** which

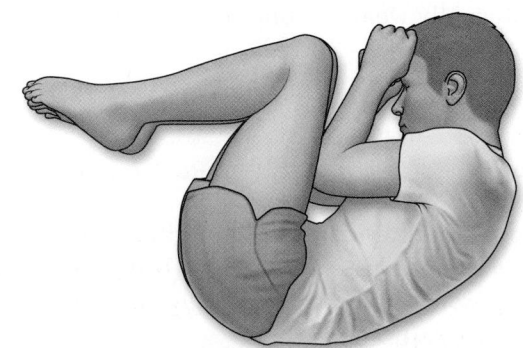

FIGURE 4-3. The fetal position.

have a nonsolid, latticelike interior, are the first to undergo degeneration because of inactivity. Cortical bone, which has a solid interior, degenerates more slowly.

The hip joint (femur head and neck), wrist, and vertebrae are areas that contain a high amount of trabecular bone. In individuals with osteoporosis, fracture is common in these areas. Vertebral compression fractures are also a major cause of disability in the elderly population. These fractures are often subtle, painful, and lead to the spinal deformities that cause the patient to assume a hunched posture.

> **ALERT!** Hip fracture is a major cause of morbidity, disability, and mortality within the elderly population. Between 25% and 75% of elderly individuals who suffer hip fracture can neither walk independently nor achieve their previous level of independent living within 1 year following their fracture. Between 18% and 33% of older hip fracture patients die within 1 year of their fracture.

Bone metabolism is a function of the opposing actions of the osteoblasts and osteoclasts. With lack of physical activity, osteoblasts are not sufficiently stimulated to keep producing bone; osteoclasts, however, continue to absorb bone unopposed. Osteoclastic activity overtakes osteoblastic activity, causing bone demineralization and osteoporosis.

Calcium and phosphorus leach out of deteriorating bones into the bloodstream and then into the urine. The urinary calcium can increase susceptibility to kidney stone formation, particularly if the patient is dehydrated. In immobile patients, replacement of calcium without weight-bearing exercise is of no value and adds to the calcium excreted in the urine.

Osteoporosis from inactivity can weaken bones to the point of pathological fracture. A **pathological fracture** is a break in the bone's integrity caused by extreme stress from a nontraumatic etiology. The bone is internally weakened by a pre-existing condition and fractures easily without trauma or with only slight trauma. Osteoporosis, neoplasms or cancerous tumors within bone, and metabolic conditions that internally weaken bones can cause pathological fracture.

 CLINICAL CONCEPT

Osteoporosis often causes pathological fracture of the hip or vertebrae because these are composed of trabecular, nonsolid bone that undergoes deterioration earlier than cortical, solid bone.

Renal and Urological System Changes

The renal system functions optimally when gravitational forces assist urine flow downward from the kidneys, into the ureters and bladder, and then into the urethra. For this reason, the supine position does not facilitate urine drainage as efficiently as the upright position. Because of this, urinary stasis, or pooling of urine in the bladder, is more common when the patient is in the supine position.

 CLINICAL CONCEPT

Urinary stasis, which occurs with prolonged immobility, predisposes to urinary tract infections because urine is a medium for bacteria.

> **ALERT!** Prolonged bedrest places the individual at greater risk for kidney stone formation, as the excess protein and calcium from the deterioration of muscle and bone are excreted in the urine.

Gastrointestinal System Changes

The supine position is not conducive to efficient digestive processes and peristaltic activity. Peristaltic wave activity significantly diminishes, and the lack of physical activity inhibits movement of intestinal contents and gas. Patients on bedrest also tend to have diminished appetite, slowed peristalsis, and decreased rate of intestinal absorption. The muscle atrophy that occurs also causes diminished strength of the diaphragm and abdominal and pelvic muscles, which are needed for defecation. Constipation is a frequent consequence of physical inactivity. In addition, the supine position increases susceptibility to gastroesophageal reflux.

CLINICAL CONCEPT

In the upright position, gravitational forces pull gastric contents downward and oppose the regurgitation of fluids or food particles into the esophagus and pharynx. Elevation of the head and chest of the patient on bedrest can counteract the risk of reflux and possible aspiration.

Metabolic and Endocrine System Changes

Inactive people have lower energy requirements than those who exercise, but they also have lower metabolic rates. Lack of physical activity leads to muscle protein breakdown, catabolic activity, and negative nitrogen balance. Catabolism is the breakdown of cells and production of waste products from the degeneration. During catabolism, proteins derived from different body tissues break down into amino acids. Amino acids are nitrogen-rich compounds that keep the body supplied with a source of nitrogen. As proteins break down, amino acids released into the bloodstream are then excreted in the urine. The loss of amino acids diminishes the amount of nitrogen in the body, a state referred to as **negative nitrogen balance.**

Carbohydrate or glucose intolerance also begins to develop with prolonged physical inactivity. After two weeks of bedrest, peripheral cellular glucose uptake decreases by 50% and blood glucose levels rise. Pancreatic insulin secretion is forced to increase to maintain normal blood glucose levels.

Parathyroid hormone levels increase in response to immobility, which stimulates osteoclastic activity and bone degeneration and facilitates the leaching of calcium from bones. Calcium then increases in the bloodstream and enters the kidney. In the kidney an excess of calcium can precipitate in the urine and form kidney stones.

Thyroid hormone, growth hormone, and epinephrine levels change with immobility as well. Circadian rhythm peak and trough levels of these hormones change, which may be why persons on bedrest experience changes in appetite, sleep, and mood.

Integumentary System Changes

During bedrest, a large surface area of the skin is in contact with the bed and under constant pressure; this pressure is particularly transmitted to skin that lies over bony prominences, including the occiput of the skull, shoulders, elbows, sacrum, ankles, and heels of the feet. The constant pressure irritates the epithelium, impairs blood flow to the area under pressure, and interferes with tissue–blood exchange of nutrients, oxygen, and waste products. Also, body moisture and shear force from bed linens contribute to skin breakdown.

Decubitus Ulcers

Skin breakdown and tissue ischemia can lead to the development of **decubitus ulcers,** also known as pressure ulcers or bedsores. There are four stages of decubitus ulcers. These stages are categorized according to depth of tissue involvement (see Fig. 4-4):

- **Stage I:** Skin exhibits persistent redness and irritation.
- **Stage II:** There is loss of skin in the epidermal or dermal layers.
- **Stage III:** Ulcers show deterioration of epidermis, dermis, and deeper layers of subcutaneous tissue.
- **Stage IV:** There is loss of full thickness of tissue down into the fascia, muscle, and bone.

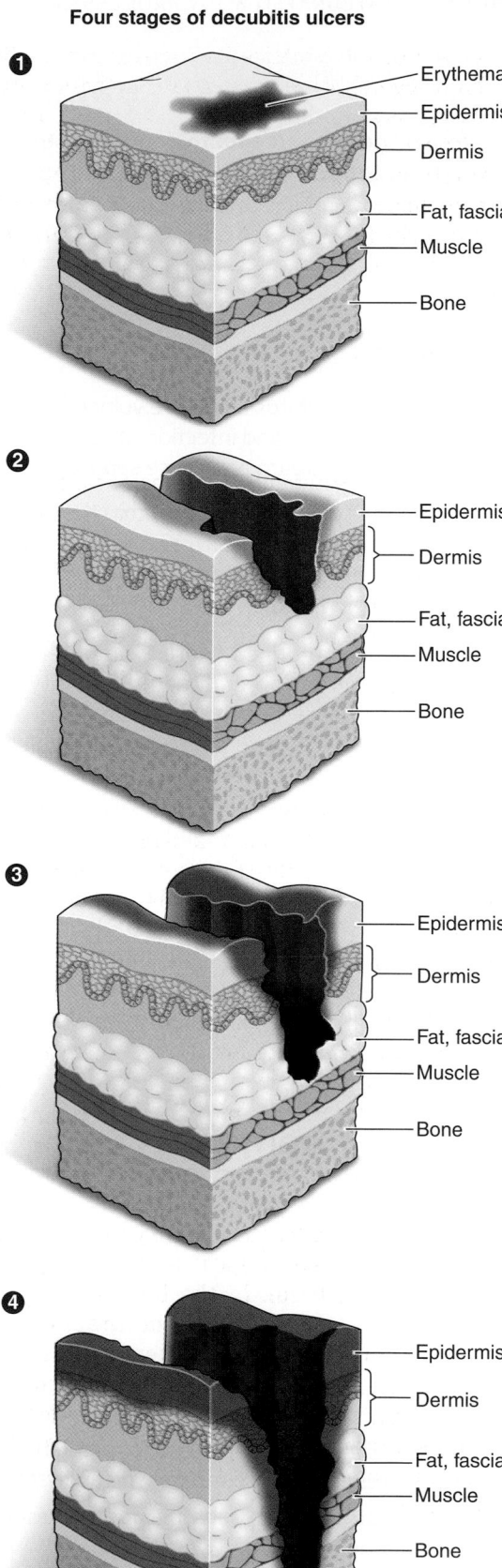

Four stages of decubitis ulcers

FIGURE 4-4. The four stages of decubitus ulcers. Stage I: Epidermis has an area of persistent erythema over the region of skin subjected to pressure. Stage II: Area of skin loss and ulceration or blistering through epidermis and dermis. Stage III: Area of deep ulceration through dermis down through fat to fascia. Stage IV: Area of extensive destruction of tissue down through fascia, muscle, tendons, and exposing bones.

CLINICAL CONCEPT

Clinicians need to frequently reposition immobilized patients in bed and keep skin dry and free from irritation to prevent decubiti. Once decubiti form, extensive measures of wound care are necessary. Common sites for decubitus ulcers are shown in Figure 4-5.

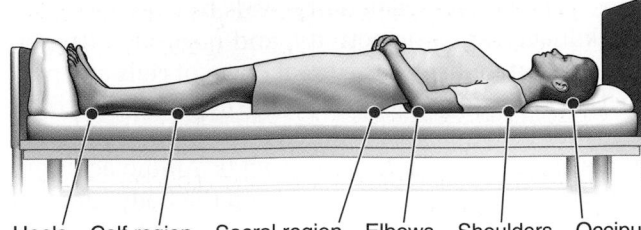

Heels   Calf region   Sacral region   Elbows   Shoulders   Occiput

FIGURE 4-5. Sites at risk for decubitus ulcers for patients in supine position.

ALERT! Decubitus ulcers are vulnerable to bacterial contamination and infection; these can extend into the bloodstream and cause septicemia, which is a bloodstream infection.

Psychosocial Changes

Inactivity and prolonged bedrest can alter an individual's mood, orientation, and cognitive ability. Social isolation and sensory deprivation may also occur with prolonged inactivity and bedrest. Research shows that individuals exhibit heightened anxiety, depression, restlessness, fear, and mood swings when enduring isolation. Individuals can also experience decreased levels of concentration, decreased problem-solving ability, disorientation, hallucinations, vivid dreams, ineffective thought processes, and altered tactile responses. Elderly persons who are subjected to prolonged bedrest and social isolation commonly exhibit episodes of acute delirium, clinical depression, and cognitive decline.

Interventions to Counteract Effects of Immobility

Rehabilitative interventions are necessary to counteract the many systemic consequences of inactivity and prolonged bedrest. Active and passive range of motion exercises and early mobilization of hospitalized patients are necessary measures to prevent complications of inactivity. Isometric and aerobic exercise regimens can rebuild muscle, improve cardiac and pulmonary function, enhance GI activity, strengthen bones, and counteract venous stasis. Regular exercise is recommended to counteract depression and relieve mental stress.

To prevent skin breakdown and decubitus ulcers, patients on bedrest should assume positional changes at least every 2 hours. Immobile patients need to be turned onto their side periodically. In general, the prone position is avoided because it hinders chest excursion for optimal respiratory function. When possible, patients should be seated in a chair for part of the day and ambulate small distances. Provide cushioning to the areas of the body where bony prominences irritate skin to relieve pressure. Special mattresses and padding are available for this purpose. Health-care providers need to assess the patient's skin for areas of erythema and irritation periodically to prevent development of decubitus ulcers. Dependent areas, particularly the sacral region, need to be assessed frequently. TED stockings are used to facilitate venous return from the distal areas of the limbs upward.

Chapter Summary

- A stressor is a challenging demand on the body that arouses a response from multiple organ systems.
- Eustress is stress that results in a positive response.
- Adaptive ability is the way in which the individual manages the stress and reduces the effect of the stressor on his or her life.
- Selye's general adaptation syndrome of stress consists of three stages: alarm, resistance, and exhaustion.
- Stimulation of the SNS causes a fight-or-flight reaction.
- Cortisol powerfully enhances the body's ability to resist stress by mobilizing glucose, amino acids, and fat stores for cellular energy production.

- Long-term secretion of cortisol or prolonged use of pharmacological cortisone causes immunosuppression.
- According to McEwen, allostatic load can be defined as the wear and tear on body systems caused by stress reactions. In prolonged stress, hormones and catecholamines have a cumulative, noxious effect and are part of the allostatic load on the body.
- When stress exceeds the body's ability to adapt, allostatic overload results, which initiates pathophysiologic disorders.

- There are five stages of sleep that begin after the body is relaxed and preparing for sleep. Stage 5, REM sleep, is necessary for restorative sleep.
- Exercise stimulates blood flow to the brain; this enhances secretion of the neurotransmitters serotonin, norepinephrine, and dopamine, which counteract depression and anxiety.
- Exercise has many systemwide therapeutic effects, including stimulation of vascular endothelial growth factor, elevation of HDL, and stimulation of osteoblastic activity.

- Immobility has widespread negative effects on the body, including susceptibility to skin breakdown, pulmonary infection, muscle atrophy, contractures, orthostatic hypotension, urolithiasis, osteoporosis, deep vein thrombosis, and PE.
- Skin breakdown in the form of decubitus ulcers can occur over the bony prominences of the body when in the supine position for long intervals.
- Infection of decubitus ulcers is common and can lead to septicemia (systemwide infection).

Bibliography

Alpert, J. S. (2010). Balancing work, family and friends, and lifestyle. *Am J of Med*, 123(9), 775–776. doi: 10.1016/j.amjmed.2010.04.018.

AUTHOR. (2008). Preventing bedsores. *Am Fam Phys*, 78(10), 1195–1196.

Andrews, R. C., Cooper, A. R., Montgomery, A. A., et al. (2011). Diet or diet plus physical activity versus usual care in patients with newly diagnosed type 2 diabetes: the early ACTID randomised controlled trial. *Lancet*, 378(9786), 129–139. Epub 2011 Jun 24.

Barnes, J. N., & Joyner, M. J. (2013). Physical activity and cardiovascular risk: 10 metabolic equivalents or bust. *Mayo Clin Proc*, 88(12), 1353–1355. doi: 10.1016/j.mayocp.2013.10.015.

Barrett, K. E., Barman, S. M., Boitano, S., & Brooks, H. L. (2012). *Ganong's review of medical physiology.* 24th ed. New York: McGraw-Hill.

Bauman, A. E., Reis, R. S., Sallis, J. F., et al. (2012). Correlates of physical activity: why are some people physically active and others not? *Lancet*, 380(9838), 258–271. doi: 10.1016/S0140-6736(12)60735-1.

Benoit, R., & Mion, L. (2012). Risk factors for pressure ulcer development in critically ill patients: a conceptual model to guide research. *Research in Nursing and Health*, Apr 17. doi: 10.1002/nur.21481.

Borrell, L. N., Dallo, F. J., & Nguyen, N. (2010). Racial/ethnic disparities in all-cause mortality in U.S. adults: the effect of allostatic load. *Public Health Reports*, 125(6), 810–816.

Brame, A. L., & Singer, M. (2010). Stressing the obvious? An allostatic look at critical illness. *Crit Care Med*, 38(10 Suppl), S600–S607.

Cecchini, M., Sassi, F., Lauer, J. A., et al. (2010). Tackling of unhealthy diets, physical inactivity, and obesity: health effects and cost-effectiveness. *Lancet*, 376(9754), 1775–1784. Epub 2010 Nov 10.

Chen, P. H., Kuo, H. Y., & Chueh, K. H. (2010). Sleep hygiene education: efficacy on sleep quality in working women. *J Nurs Res*, 18(4), 283–289.

Chyu, L., & Upchurch, D. M. (2011). Racial and ethnic patterns of allostatic load among adult women in the United States: findings from the National Health and Nutrition Examination Survey 1999–2004. *J Womens Health*, 20(4), 575–583. Epub 2011 Mar 23.

Cicchetti, D. (2011). Allostatic load. *Dev Psych*, 23(3), 723–724.

Costedio, M. M., Hyman, N., & Mawe, G. M. (2007). Serotonin and its role in colonic function and in gastrointestinal disorders. *Dis Colon Rectum*, 50(3), 376–388.

Dang, S. L. (2013). ABCDEs of ICU: early mobility. *Crit Care Nurs Q*, 36(2), 63–68. doi: 10.1097/CNQ.0b013e318283cf45.

Das, P., & Horton, R. (2012). Rethinking our approach to physical activity. *Lancet*, 380(9838), 189–190. doi: 10.1016/S0140-6736(12)61024-1.

de Souto Barreto, P. (2013a). Exercise for depression in elderly people. *Lancet*, 382(9901), 1325. doi: 10.1016/S0140-6736(13)62131-5.

de Souto Barreto, P. (2013b). Prescription of physical activity. *Lancet*, 381(9878), 1623. doi: 10.1016/S0140-6736(13)61019-3.

Dubnov-Raz, G., & Berry, E. M. (2011). The dietary treatment of obesity. *Med Clin N America*, 95(5), 939–952.

Elsawy, B., & Higgins, K. E. (2010). Physical activity guidelines for older adults. *Am Fam Phys*, 81(1), 55–59.

Epel, E. S., McEwen, B., Seeman, T., et al. (2000). Stress and body shape: stress-induced cortisol secretion is consistently greater among women with central fat. *Psych Med*, 62(5), 623–632.

Figueredo, V. M. (2009). The time has come for physicians to take notice: the impact of psychosocial stressors on the heart. *Am J Med*, 122(8), 704–712. doi: 10.1016/j.amjmed.2009.05.001.

Floyd, J. A., Janisse, J. J., Jenuwine, E. S., & Ager, J. W. (2007). Changes in REM-sleep percentage over the adult lifespan, *Sleep*, 30(7), 829–836.

Frey, D. J., Fleshner, M., & Wright, K. P. (2007). The effects of 40 hours of total sleep deprivation on inflammatory markers in healthy young adults. *Brain, Behavior & Immunity*, May 22. Epub ahead of print.

Galasko, C. S. (2012). Physical activity for people with disabilities. *Lancet*, 380(9851), 1384–1385. doi: 10.1016/S0140-6736(12)61799-.

Gavin, T. P., Robinson, C. B., Yeager, R. C., et al. (2004). Angiogenic growth factor response to acute systemic exercise in human skeletal muscle. *J App Phys*, 96(1), 19–24.

Goldstein, D. S. (2010). Adrenal responses to stress. *Cell Mol Neurobiology*, 30(8), 1433–1440.

Grief, S. N., & Miranda, R. L. (2010). Weight loss maintenance. *Am Fam Phys*, 82(6), 630–634.

Guyton, A. C., & Hall, J. E. (2010). *Textbook of medical physiology.* 12th ed. Philadelphia, PA: W.B. Saunders Publishing Co.

Hallal, P. C., Bauman, A. E., Heath, G. W., et al. (2012). Physical activity: more of the same is not enough. *Lancet*, 380(9838), 190–191. doi: 10.1016/S0140-6736(12)61027-7.

Halpin, D. J., & Rencic, J. J. (2012). A real exercise stress test. *Am J Med*, 125(8), 761–763. doi: 10.1016/j.amjmed.2012.06.003.

Hambrecht, R., Wolf, A., Gielen, S., et al. (2000). Effect of exercise on coronary endothelial function in patients with coronary artery disease. *N Engl J Med, 342*(7), 454–460.

Hassan, M., York, K. M., Li, H., et al. (2007). Mental stress-induced myocardial ischemia in coronary artery disease patients with left ventricular dysfunction. *J Nuclear Card, 14*(3), 269–271.

Heath, G. W., Parra, D. C., Sarmiento, O. L., et al. (2012). Evidence-based intervention in physical activity: lessons from around the world. *Lancet, 380*(9838), 272–281. doi: 10.1016/S0140-6736(12)60816-2.

Jackson, M. (2014). The stress of life: a modern complaint? *Lancet, 383*(9914), 300–301.

Juster, R. P., Bizik, G., Picard, M., et al. (2011). A transdisciplinary perspective of chronic stress in relation to psychopathology throughout life span development. *Dev Psych, 23*(3), 725–776. Review.

Juster, R. P., Marin, M. F., Sindi, S., et al. (2011). Allostatic load associations to acute, 3-year and 6-year prospective depressive symptoms in healthy older adults. *Physiol Behav, 104*(2), 360–364. Epub 2011 Feb 23.

Kalisch, B. J., Lee, S., & Dabney, B. W. (2014). Outcomes of inpatient mobilization: a literature review. *J Clin Nurs, 23*(11-12), 1486–1501. doi: 10.1111/jocn.12315. Epub 2013 Sep 13.

Khan, K. M., Thompson, A. M., Blair, S. N., et al. (2012). Sport and exercise as contributors to the health of nations. *Lancet, 380*(9836), 59–64. doi: 10.1016.

Karatsoreos, I. N., & McEwen, B. S. (2011). Psychobiological allostasis: resistance, resilience and vulnerability. *Trends Cog Sci, 15*(12), 576–584. Epub 2011 Nov 9.

Kavan, M. G., Elsasser, G. N., & Barone, E. J. (2012). The physician's role in managing acute stress disorder. *Am Fam Phys, 86*(7), 643–649.

Kivimäki, M., Nyberg, S. T., Batty, G. D., et al. (2012). Job strain as a risk factor for coronary heart disease: a collaborative meta-analysis of individual participant data. *Lancet, 380*(9852), 1491–1497. doi: 10.1016/S0140-6736(12)60994-5. Epub 2012 Sep 14.

Kohl, H. W., 3rd, Craig, C. L., Lambert, E. V., et al. (2012). The pandemic of physical inactivity: global action for public health. *Lancet, 380*(9838), 294–305. doi: 10.1016/S0140-6736(12)60898-8.

Kripke, C. (2009). Aerobic activity for cognitive function. *Am Fam Phys, 79*(7), 562.

Kyrou, I., Chrousos, G. P., & Tsigos, C. (2006). Stress, visceral obesity, and metabolic complications. *Ann NY Acad of Sci, 1083*, 77–110.

Lach, H. W., Lorenz, R. A., & L'Ecuyer, K. M. (2014). Aging muscles and joints: mobilization. *Crit Care Nurs Clin N America, 26*(1), 105–113. doi: 10.1016/j.ccell.2013.10.005. Epub 2013 Nov 11.

Latimer-Cheung, A. E., Toll, B. A., & Salovey, P. (2013). Promoting increased physical activity and reduced inactivity. *Lancet, 381*(9861), 114. doi: 10.1016/S0140-6736(13)60045-8.

Lee, I. M., Bauman, A. E., Blair, S. N., et al. (2013). Annual deaths attributable to physical inactivity: whither the missing 2 million? *Lancet, 381*(9871), 992–993. doi: 10.1016/S0140-6736(13)60705-9. Epub 2013 Mar 22.

Lee, I. M., Shiroma, E. J., Lobelo, F., et al. (2012). Effect of physical inactivity on major non-communicable diseases worldwide: an analysis of burden of disease and life expectancy. *Lancet, 380*(9838), 219–229. doi: 10.1016/S0140-6736(12)61031-9.

Lin, J. S. (2010). Encouraging physical activity among frail older adults. *Am Fam Phys, 82*(3), 230.

Madhavan, S. M., & Sappati Biyyani, R. S. (2009). No symptoms, no stress. *Am J Med, 122*(5), 432–434. doi: 10.1016/j.amjmed.2008.10.011.

Markus, C. R. (2007). Effects of carbohydrates on brain tryptophan availability and stress performance. *Biol Psych,* Jun 30. Epub ahead of print.

McEwen, B. S. (1998). Protective and damaging effects of stress mediators. *N Engl J Med, 338*(3), 171–179.

McEwen, B. S. (2005). Stressed or stressed out: what is the difference? *J Psych Neuro, 30*(5), 315–318.

McEwen, B. S. (2006). Sleep deprivation as a neurobiologic and physiologic stressor: allostasis and allostatic load. *Metabolism, 55*(10 Suppl 2), S20–S23.

McEwen, B. S. (2007). Physiology and neurobiology of stress and adaptation: central role of the brain. *Phys Rev, 87*(3), 873–904.

McEwen, B. S., & Gianaros, P. J. (2011). Stress- and allostasis-induced brain plasticity. *Ann Rev Med, 62*, 431–445.

McPhee, S. J., & Papadakis, M. A. (2012). *Current medical diagnosis and treatment.* 51st ed. New York: McGraw-Hill.

Milani, R. V., & Lavie, C. J. (2009). Reducing psychosocial stress: a novel mechanism of improving survival from exercise training. *Am J Med, 122*(10), 931–938. doi: 10.1016/j.amjmed.2009.03.028. Epub 2009 Aug 13.

Moore, P. K., Marzec, L. N., & Krantz, M. J. (2013). Signs of stress: deep symmetric T-wave inversions. *Am J Med, 26*(8), 682–684. doi: 10.1016/j.amjmed.2013.03.005. Epub 2013 Jun 10.

National Institutes of Health (NIH), National Heart, Lung, and Blood Institute (NHLBI), NHLBI Obesity Prevention Initiative, North American Association for the Study of Obesity. (2000). *The practical guide to identification, evaluation, and treatment of overweight and obesity in adults.* Retrieved from http://www.nhlbi.nih.gov./guidelines/obesity/prctgd_c.pdf

Netterstrøm, B. (2012). Job strain as a measure of exposure to psychological strain. *Lancet, 380*(9852), 1455–1456. doi: 10.1016/S0140-6736(12)61512-8. Epub 2012 Sep 14.

Nigam, A., & Juneau, M. (2011). Survival benefit associated with low-level physical activity. *Lancet, 378*(9798), 1202–1203. Epub 2011 Aug 16.

Panagiotakos, D., Kokkinos, P., Manios, Y., & Pitsavos, C. (2004). Physical activity and markers of inflammation and thrombosis related to coronary heart disease. *Prevent Card,* Fall 2004 (7), 190–194.

Peix, A., Trapaga, A., Asen, L., et al. (2006). Mental stress-induced myocardial ischemia in women with angina and normal coronary angiograms. *J Nucl Card, 14*(4), 507–513.

Pelliccia, F., Greco, C., Vitale, C., et al. (2014). Takotsubo syndrome (stress cardiomyopathy): an intriguing clinical condition in search of its identity. *Am J Med,* Apr 19. pii: S0002-9343 (14)00309-X. doi: 10.1016/j.amjmed.2014.04.004. Epub ahead of print.

Porcelli, P., & Todarello, O. (2007). Psychological factors affecting functional gastrointestinal disorders. *Advan Psych Med, 28*, 24, 34–56.

Pugliese, G., & Balducci, S. (2014). NAVIGATOR: physical activity for cardiovascular health? *Lancet, 383*(9922), 1022–1023. doi: 10.1016/S0140-6736(13)62551-9. Epub 2013 Dec 20.

Quinlan, J. D., Guaron, M. R., Deschere, B. R., & Stephens, M. B. (2010). Care of the returning veteran. *Am Fam Phys, 82*(1), 43–49.

Ramachandruni, S., Fillingim, R., McGorray, S. P., et al. (2011). Allostatic processes in the family. *Dev Psych, 23*(3), 921–938.

Rimmer, J. H., & Marques, A. C. (2012). Physical activity for people with disabilities. *Lancet*, 380(9838), 193–195. doi: 10.1016/S0140-6736(12)61028-9.

Romero, D. V., Treston, J., & O'Sullivan, A. L. (2006). Raising awareness of pressure ulcer prevention and treatment. *Adv Skin Wound Care*, 9(7), 398–405.

Samuriwo, R. (2012). Pressure ulcer prevention: the role of the multidisciplinary team. *Brit J Nurs*, 21(5), S4, S6, S8.

Schmid, S. M., Hallschmid, M., & Schultes, B. (2014). The metabolic burden of sleep loss. *Lancet Diabetes Endocrinol*, Mar 25. pii: S2213-8587(14)70012-9. doi: 10.1016/S2213-8587(14)70012-9. Epub ahead of print.

Schofield, R. S., & Sheps, D. S. (2006). Mental stress provokes ischemia in coronary artery disease subjects without exercise- or adenosine-induced ischemia. *J Am College of Card*, 47, 987–991.

Sowers, J. R. (2003). Obesity as a cardiovascular risk factor. *Am J Med*, 115(8A), 37S–41S.

Spear, M. (2013). Pressure ulcer staging-revisited. *Plast Surg Nurs*, 33(4), 192–194. doi: 10.1097/PSN.0000000000000015.

Swinburn, B. A., Sacks, G., Hall, K. D., et al. (2011). The global obesity pandemic: shaped by global drivers and local environments. *Lancet*, 378(9793), 804–814.

Takata, S., & Yasui, N. (2001). Disuse osteoporosis. *J Med Invest*, 48(3-4), 147–156.

Takeda, E., Terao, J., Nakaya, Y., et al. (2004). Stress control and human nutrition. *J Med Invest*, 52, 139–145.

Theisen, S., Drabik, A., & Stock, S. (2012). Pressure ulcers in older hospitalised patients and its impact on length of stay: a retrospective observational study. *J Clin Nurs*, 21(3-4), 380–387. doi: 10.1111/j.1365-2702.2011.03915.x. Epub 2011 Dec 9.

Touma, C., & Pannain, S. (2011). Does lack of sleep cause diabetes? *Cleveland Clin J Med*, 78(8), 549–558. doi: 10.3949/ccjm.78a.10165.

Tsigos, C., & Chrousos, G. P. (2002). Hypothalamic-pituitary-adrenal axis, neuroendocrine factors and stress. *J Psych Res*, 53(4), 865–871.

Underwood, M., Lamb, S. E., Eldridge, S., et al. (2013). Exercise for depression in elderly residents of care homes: a cluster-randomised controlled trial. *Lancet*, 382(9886), 41–49. doi: 10.1016/S0140-6736(13)60649-2. Epub 2013 May 2.

Wadden, T. A., Webb, V. L., Moran, C. H., & Bailer, B. A. (2012). Lifestyle modification for obesity: new developments in diet, physical activity, and behavior therapy. *Circulation*, 125(9), 1157–1170. doi: 10.1161/CIRCULATIONAHA.111.039453.

Wen, C. P., Wai, J. P., Tsai, M. K., et al. (2011). Minimum amount of physical activity for reduced mortality and extended life expectancy: a prospective cohort study. *Lancet*, 378(9798), 1244–1253. Epub 2011 Aug 16.

Wilczweski, P., Grimm, D., Gianakis, A., et al. (2012). Risk factors associated with pressure ulcer development in critically ill traumatic spinal cord injury patients. *J Trauma Nurs*, 19(1), 5–10.

Winkelman, C. (2007). Inactivity and inflammation in the critically ill patient. *Crit Care Clin*, 23(1), 21–34.

Zeller, J. M., Rosenberg, L., & McCann, J. (2003). The effect of mirthful laughter on stress and natural killer cell activity. *Alt Ther Health Med*, 9(2), 38–45.

Obesity and Nutritional Imbalances

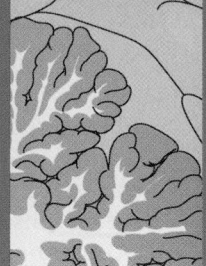

Key Terms

Adipokine
Adiponectin
Adiposity
Anorexia nervosa
Bariatric surgery
Basal metabolic rate (BMR)

Binge eating
Body mass index (BMI)
Bulimia nervosa
Dumping syndrome
Gastric banding
Gastric bypass

Ghrelin
Leptin
Lipolysis
Night eating syndrome (NES)
Purging disorder
Resistin

Few issues impact individuals in such a comprehensive way as their weight. Many people in the United States and other industrialized nations struggle to maintain their weight within normal weight parameters. Once individuals exceed their ideal weight by 20% they are considered overweight. When that level rises to 30%, they meet the criteria of obesity, which is defined as increased body weight related to excess fat accumulation. Obesity is particularly problematic because it predisposes an individual to multiple conditions, including cardiovascular disease, arthritis, diabetes, and hyperlipidemia. It also exerts an effect on the whole body, including psychological well-being.

Epidemiology

There are a disproportionate number of obese individuals in the United States as compared with the rest of the world. According to the latest reports from the National Institute of Diabetes and Digestive and Kidney Diseases, greater than 65% of Americans are overweight or obese; in addition, 1 in 20 adults is morbidly obese. The National Heart Lung and Blood Institute rates obesity at epidemic proportions, and the problem is steadily worsening.

The United States doesn't stand alone when dealing with this health issue. Most industrialized nations have seen a tremendous increase in the rate of obese individuals. Over the last 20 years, the percentage of overweight adults worldwide has increased by 300%. In the United States, obesity prevalence rates have progressively risen, from 19.4% in 1997 to 24.5% in 2004 and 26.6% in 2007. It is projected that by the year 2020, 40% of the U.S. population will be obese.

Age

Once thought of as a problem of aging caused by more sedentary lifestyles, obesity is becoming more of a problem among younger individuals; recent studies have shown that more than 20% of children between the ages of 6 and 11 years old are obese. Childhood obesity, already at levels that are alarmingly high, continues to rise.

ALERT Childhood obesity is a direct contributor to adult obesity and predisposes to an earlier onset of a myriad of health problems.

Gender

According to the Centers for Disease Control and Prevention, 32% of adult men and 35% of adult women in the United States are obese. If you combine the two categories of overweight and obesity, the prevalence estimates are 72% for men and 64% for women. Therefore, more than two-thirds of the U.S. male and female population require intervention for weight loss and management.

Race

There are large disparities in obesity prevalence by race-ethnic group among women. Non-Hispanic black and Mexican American women have greater prevalence rates of obesity than white women. Approximately 53% of non-Hispanic black women and 51% of Mexican American women 40 to 59 years of age are obese, compared with 39% of non-Hispanic white women of the same age. Such distinctive ethnic disparities in obesity are not observed in men. Asian Americans have lower rates of obesity than all of the other ethnic groups.

Socioeconomic Status

Obesity is linked to both affluence and poverty. Affluent individuals may overindulge and intake excessive calories—and in some developing nations, being overweight or obese may be viewed as a status symbol and a public representation of a person's wealth. By contrast, in the United States, obesity is associated with poverty and lack of appropriate food choices. Many people who live in lower socioeconomic areas have little or no access to nutrient-rich, low-calorie foods or fresh produce. Many in the lower socioeconomic areas rely on fast food, which is inexpensive and commonly rich in fat, sodium, and sugar.

Etiology

Obesity results when energy intake exceeds energy expenditure. If the body doesn't expend all the energy it takes in, it stores this energy as fat. However, individuals vary widely in their propensity to gain weight and accrue fat mass. People differ in their susceptibility to gain weight even at identical levels of caloric input and activity. This indicates that there are factors, other than excess food intake and inadequate activity, involved in the accumulation of excess body fat. A science of obesity is emerging and current research is broadening our understanding, but there are still many unanswered questions.

Obesity is a metabolic disorder caused by changes in cellular insulin sensitivity, glucose utilization, fat accumulation, hepatic glucose production, and fluid balance. Fat cells, also called adipocytes, are considered endocrine cells. They secrete **adipokines,** which are hormones and proteins that affect body metabolism. Adipocytes can increase in number and each cell can hypertrophy to cause fat mass.

The subcutaneous tissue and omentum, which is the membranous covering over the intestine, are major areas of fat storage in the body. Visceral fat can be found surrounding organs as well. Adipokines affect cellular insulin sensitivity, fat breakdown, blood lipid levels, and hepatic glucose production. They also influence appetite, hunger, and satiety. The more adipose tissue there is, the greater the influence of adipokines. Obesity itself increases susceptibility to additional accumulation of adipose tissue.

Genetics is another etiologic factor of obesity, though the link between genetics and obesity is not well understood. Only a small number of genetic disorders are known to cause obesity. Data suggest that 5% of children who are obese have mutations at 2p23

and 18q21.3. Persons who lack the leptin gene or have leptin receptor gene mutations at 7q31 are found to be obese. Some patients with enzyme alterations caused by a mutation at 5q15-21 have significant obesity. Severe obesity is seen in individuals with a mutation in an adipocyte transcription factor gene at 3p25. Many different gene loci are being investigated as potential "obesity genes."

It is currently thought that a combination of genes and environmental influences are the cause for obesity. In addition, familial influences, traditions, and culture significantly contribute to the way individual eating habits develop.

Various disorders cause obesity as a secondary effect. Hypothyroidism, Cushing's syndrome, and polycystic ovarian syndrome are three diseases that cause body fat accumulation, but there are many others. When the primary disorder is remedied, obesity is no longer a problem.

Pathophysiology

Adipose tissue provides insulation, warmth, and cushioning for body organs and serves as a storage depot for excess energy. However, fat is not simply a repository of triglycerides that break down into fatty acids. Adipocytes are metabolically active and secrete a wide variety of repetitive adipokines. Adipokines include the inflammatory mediators, tumor necrosis factor alpha (TNF-alpha) and interleukin-6 (IL-6), as well as the vascular activators, angiotensinogen (AGT) and plasminogen activator inhibitor (PAI). Other adipokines, called adiponectin, leptin, and resistin, regulate glucose, insulin, and lipid metabolism, respectively (see Fig. 5-1). Therefore, adipose tissue influences many metabolic processes in the body.

Adipokines

Adiponectin is a plasma protein that enhances cellular sensitivity to insulin, exerts anti-inflammatory effects, and is protective against the formation of arteriosclerosis; it has an inverse relationship with the fat content, or **adiposity,** of the body. The lower the adiposity, the greater amount of adiponectin produced. The greater the adiposity, the fewer adiponectin produced.

High adiposity with resulting lower adiponectin decreases cellular sensitivity to insulin which, in turn, leads to glucose intolerance and subsequent elevations in blood glucose levels; this situation is also correlated with low high-density lipoprotein (HDL) levels and high triglyceride levels. Because of the beneficial effects, some researchers have referred to adiponectin as a "good" adipokine. However, obese individuals produce less adiponectin and cannot reap the benefits.

Leptin, another "good" adipokine, is a hormone produced by adipocytes that affects body weight, appetite, and energy expenditure. As the amount of fat

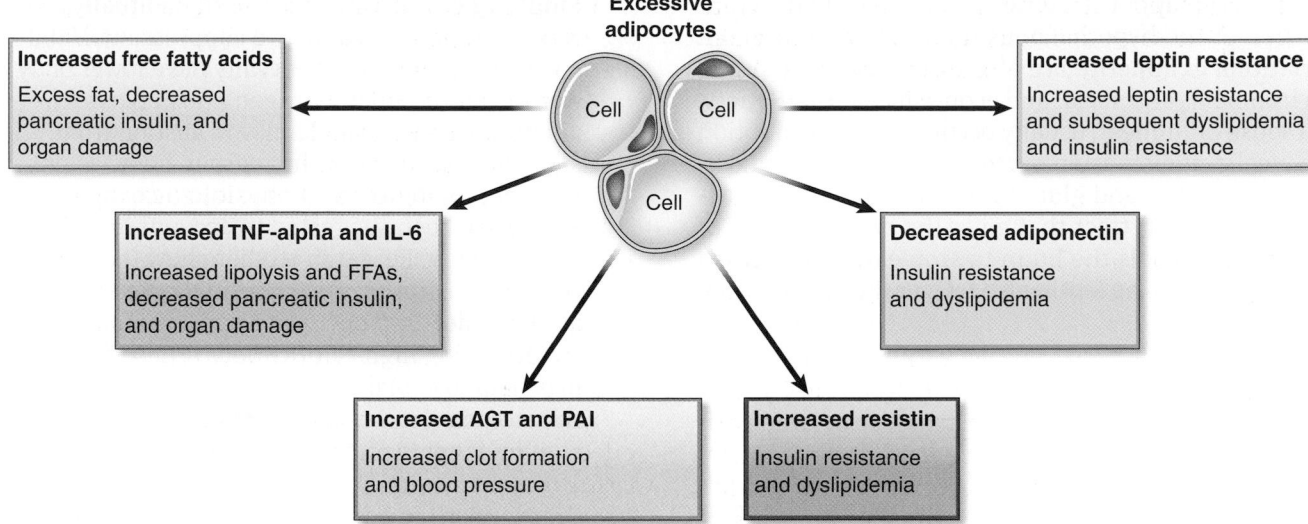

FIGURE 5-1. Adipocytes and released adipokines and their effects.

stored in adipocytes rises, leptin is released into the blood and sends signals to the brain that the body has had enough to eat. Research shows that obese individuals have high levels of leptin but are resistant to its effects, resulting in leptin desensitization. This results in the individual not receiving a feeling of satiety following a meal. Leptin also works with adiponectin to enhance cellular sensitivity to insulin, reduce triglyceride levels, and inhibit fat accumulation.

Resistin is another adipokine that is found in the blood of individuals with obesity. It is known to interfere with the actions of insulin, causing insulin resistance in mice. Resistin also enhances hepatic glucose production, raises triglyceride levels, reduces HDL levels, and causes endothelial dysfunction that predisposes to early arteriosclerotic lesion formation. Whether resistin activity in mice can be ascribed to a similar role in humans is controversial. However, because of its actions, resistin has been called a "bad" adipokine.

Vascular Mediators as Adipokines

Angiotensinogen (AGT) is a precursor to angiotensin II, a major vasoconstrictor that raises blood pressure. Adipocytes release AGT, which has led to an association between excess adipose tissue and increased vascular tone. Studies have shown a correlation between high circulating levels of AGT, hypertension, and preliminary vascular changes of arteriosclerosis.

Tissue plasminogen activator (tPA) is one of the body's natural fibrinolytic substances that dissolves clots. Plasminogen activator inhibitor (PAI), a product of adipocytes, blocks the action of tPA. Because obesity produces PAI and blocks fibrinolysis, obesity increases susceptibility to clot formation. The combination of AGT and PAI is associated with clot formation, hypertension, and arteriosclerosis; therefore, these are "bad" adipokines. The greater the number of fat cells, the greater the risk of cardiovascular disease because of adipose tissue secretion of adipokines, AGT, and PAI.

Inflammatory Mediators as Adipokines

Tumor necrosis factor alpha (TNF-alpha) and interleukin-6 (IL-6) are inflammatory mediators that reduce cellular insulin sensitivity, blunt the beneficial effect of adiponectin, and promote lipolysis. **Lipolysis** causes formation of free fatty acids (FFA), which have negative effects on the body.

FFAs are highly destructive to tissues, causing damage to intracellular membranes through lipid oxidation and injury to mitochondria. Excess FFAs in the bloodstream are deposited in various organs, causing organ dysfunction. An excess of FFA overwhelms the pancreas, leading to reduced secretion of insulin and resulting glucose intolerance. Excess FFAs are also deposited in the liver, causing nonalcoholic steatosis of hepatocytes, which leads to cirrhosis. The myocardium is also affected by excess FFAs, decreasing the efficiency of the heart muscle. Therefore, excess adipose tissue, which secretes inflammatory mediators and indirectly stimulates formation of FFAs, can lead to pancreatic, liver, and myocardial dysfunction.

Intestinal Peptides and Food Intake

Food intake is influenced by hunger and satiety, which are regulated by the hypothalamus. Low blood glucose triggers the hunger center of the hypothalamus. The empty stomach also generates impulses interpreted as hunger pangs that transmit signals to the hypothalamus. **Ghrelin** is a peptide secreted in the stomach that stimulates hunger and regulates short-term food intake; it is also theorized to regulate long-term body weight and adiposity because it stimulates secretion of growth hormone.

Appetite is distinguished from hunger in that it is primarily the result of visual, olfactory, and emotional triggers. The appetite center is in a slightly different location of the hypothalamus than the hunger center. Variations in appetite are also influenced by culture, environment, and social and economic factors. Satiety, or a sense of fullness, usually occurs after consumption of a meal. Gut distension causes the release of peptides, cholecystokinin, and glucagonlike peptide in the gastrointestinal (GI) tract that gives the body a feeling of satiety and signals the brain to stop eating. Increased levels of circulating leptin also trigger the brain to stop eating.

Risk Factors

Each individual needs a certain number of calories to meet the needs of daily energy expenditure. Approximately 70% of required calories are utilized for energy by the body at rest. About 10% of caloric expenditure is used for the metabolic processing of food. The remaining 20% of calories are used for energy required for activity and exercise. As discussed earlier, weight gain occurs when caloric intake exceeds caloric expenditure, which is why risk factors for obesity include excess calorie ingestion and sedentary behavior. Other risk factors include poverty, female gender, age, smoking cessation, disorders that cause obesity as a secondary effect, and genetic susceptibility.

- **Excess calorie ingestion:** Poor food choices, such as fast foods that are high-caloric and nutrient-poor, put individuals at risk for obesity. Unlike home-cooked meals, fast food meals are typically large in quantity and high in calories, salt, and fat.
- **Sedentary behavior:** Lack of physical activity is a major risk factor for obesity. Activity stimulates the use of glucose by the muscles and subsequent activation of fat stores.
- **Poverty:** Poverty is a risk factor because of the fact that impoverished communities usually have fewer healthy food choices and fewer recreational areas for exercise.
- **Female gender:** On average, men have more muscle than women. Because muscle burns more calories than other types of tissue, men use more calories than women, even at rest, which is why women are more likely than men to gain weight with the same calorie intake. Pregnancy is also a risk factor for obesity. Women tend to weigh an average of 4 to 6 pounds more after a pregnancy than before the pregnancy. Weight gain often compounds with each pregnancy, and this weight gain contributes to obesity in women.
- **Age:** People tend to lose muscle and gain fat as they age, and they also experience a slowing of their metabolic rate. These consequences of aging lower calorie requirements; if older individuals don't change their eating habits or increase their activity level, they will then put on weight.

- **Smoking cessation:** When used habitually, cigarettes can act as an appetite suppressant. Habitual cigarette smokers generally have lower body weight than comparably aged nonsmokers. In addition, habitual smokers who abstain from smoking often have an increase in body weight. Both psychological and physiologic explanations have been suggested to account for this phenomenon. Research studies show that nicotine administration and cigarette smoking are accompanied by a decreased consumption of sweet-tasting high caloric foods. These findings may help to explain the changes in body weight that accompany smoking cessation. Persons who stop smoking report an average weight gain of 10 pounds.
- **Disorders that cause obesity as a secondary effect:** There are many disorders that cause obesity as a secondary effect. For example, persons affected by hypothyroidism are susceptible to obesity because of a lack of thyroid hormone. Cushing's syndrome, caused by the overactivity of the adrenal gland, also causes weight gain. Many disorders increase the risk of obesity; usually, if the major pathological condition is remedied, the accumulation of fat can be alleviated (see Box 5-1).
- **Genetic susceptibility:** Genetic susceptibility to obesity is a subject that requires more research. Only a few genetic disorders are known to directly cause obesity, but there is a wide spectrum of ways in which genes can favor fat accumulation in a given environment. Genes can influence the body in the following ways:
  - drive to overeat
  - tendency to be sedentary
  - diminished ability to use dietary fats as fuel
  - enlarged, easily stimulated capacity to store body fat.

Not all people living in industrialized countries with abundant food and reduced physical activity become

---

BOX 5-1. Disorders and Conditions That Cause Obesity

Cushing's syndrome
Prader-Willi syndrome
Growth hormone deficiency
Hypogonadism
Hypothalamic obesity
Hypothyroidism
Insulinoma
Polycystic ovarian syndrome
Pregnancy
Pseudohypoparathyroidism
Tube-feeding related obesity

obese, nor do all obese people have the same body fat distribution or suffer the same health issues. This diversity occurs among groups of the same racial or ethnic background and even within families living in the same environment. The variation in how people respond to the same environmental conditions is an additional indication that genes play a role in the development of obesity.

Clinical Manifestations

Body weight consists of lean body mass and fat. Obese individuals have an excess amount of fat on their body. Overweight individuals have a body weight that is approximately 20% over ideal weight. Obesity occurs when a patient's body weight is approximately 30% over the ideal. Morbid obesity is diagnosed when an individual's body weight is 40% greater than ideal or more.

The location of fat accumulation on an individual's body often can be categorized as apple-shaped or pear-shaped. In apple-shaped or central obesity, fat accumulates around the abdomen. In pear-shaped obesity, fat accumulates around the hips and buttocks. Central obesity has a higher associated risk of health problems.

In obese persons, fat accumulation is not limited to the subcutaneous region. On autopsy, it is apparent that organs become covered in visceral fat and the heart and arteries collect fat within the interior walls and outer walls.

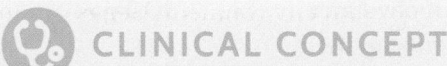

CLINICAL CONCEPT

Central obesity is associated with cardiovascular disease risk. A waist measurement that exceeds 35 inches in women or 40 inches in men is considered a cardiovascular risk factor.

Diagnosis

Two key factors in determining obesity are amount of body fat and location of body fat. Typically, the amount of body fat is difficult to measure. The main techniques that have been adopted for this purpose are categorized as follows:

- **Density-based:** hydrodensitometry and air displacement plethysmography
- **Scanning:** computerized tomography, magnetic resonance imaging, and dual-energy x-ray absorptiometry
- **Bioelectrical impedance and anthropometric:** skinfold, waist circumference, and waist-hip ratio.

The majority of these methods are not practical for patient use and are limited to research settings. Anthropometric measures using skinfold calipers are most

---

BOX 5-2. Calculating Percentage of Body Fat

The formula for men is:

$$\%Fat = 495/(1.0324 - 0.19077(\log(waist - neck)) + 0.15456(\log(height))) - 450$$

The formula for women is:

$$\%Fat = 495/(1.29579 - 0.35004(\log(waist + hip - neck)) + 0.22100(\log(height))) - 450$$

The American Council on Exercise uses the following categories based on percentage of body fat:

	Women	Men
Essential fat	10% to 12%	2% to 4%
Athletes	14% to 20%	6% to 13%
Fitness	21% to 24%	14% to 17%
Acceptable	25% to 31%	18% to 25%
Obese	32% or more	26% or more

Lean Body Mass or **Fat-Free Mass.** This is derived by subtracting the calculated value of body fat from the total weight.

Lean Body Mass = Weight x (100 − %Body Fat)

---

commonly used to estimate an individual's percentage of body fat. It is recommended that three specific sites be measured on the body:

- **Men:** chest, abdomen, and thigh
- **Women:** triceps, suprailiac, and thigh.

It is recommended that the three sites be measured three different times to get as near an accurate result as possible. Mathematical equations have been developed to yield percentage of body fat based on skinfold measurements (see Box 5-2).

Lean body mass is determined by multiplying body fat percentage by weight; the result is an estimate of how many pounds of fat make up the body. Subtract that number from weight, and this yields lean body mass. It is generally recommended that females have no more than 30% and males have no more than 25% body fat.

The most common method used to compare a patient's body weight to the ideal standard is the calculation of **body mass index (BMI).** BMI makes a comparison of height to weight and gives a score in relationship to ranges (see Box 5-3). The formula for BMI is:

Weight in pounds × 703 / height in inches / height in inches

Weight in pounds × 703 divided by height in inches and then divided by height in inches again.

BOX 5-3. Body Mass Index Values

- Underweight: < 18.5
- Normal weight: 18.5–24.9
- Overweight: 25–29.9
- Obesity: ≥ 30
- Morbid obesity: ≥ 40

CLINICAL CONCEPT

BMI charts are not accurate in individuals with increased weight because of high muscle mass.

CLINICAL CONCEPT

Weight cycling, also known as yo-yo dieting, has been associated with increased cardiovascular disease in some research studies. Weight fluctuation is also a risk factor for gallbladder disease.

Treatment

Diet

Nutrient balance is achieved by consuming foods from each of the three major categories: carbohydrates, proteins, and lipids, as well as vitamins and minerals. The United States Department of Agriculture (USDA) provides guidelines for nutritional intake in the website My Plate.gov, which aims to guide consumers in healthy food choices by detailing approximately the amount of different food types that should appear on a plate of food (see Fig. 5-2). In addition, the USDA publishes recommended daily allowances for all nutrients (see Table 5-1).

Dietary approaches to treat obesity involve calorie restriction. Adjustments made to the diet must create a negative caloric balance. Total calories consumed daily have to be fewer than calories expended daily. The recommended method begins by calculating an individual's **basal metabolic rate (BMR),** which is the minimum caloric requirement needed to sustain metabolic processes in a resting state (see Box 5-4). This calculation is based on age, sex, and size. BMR is responsible for burning up to 70% of total calories expended per day. The remaining 30% of calories are used for activity.

According to exercise physiologists McArdle and Katch, the average maintenance level for women in the United States is 2,000 to 2,100 calories per day and the average for men is 2,700 to 2,900 per day. These are

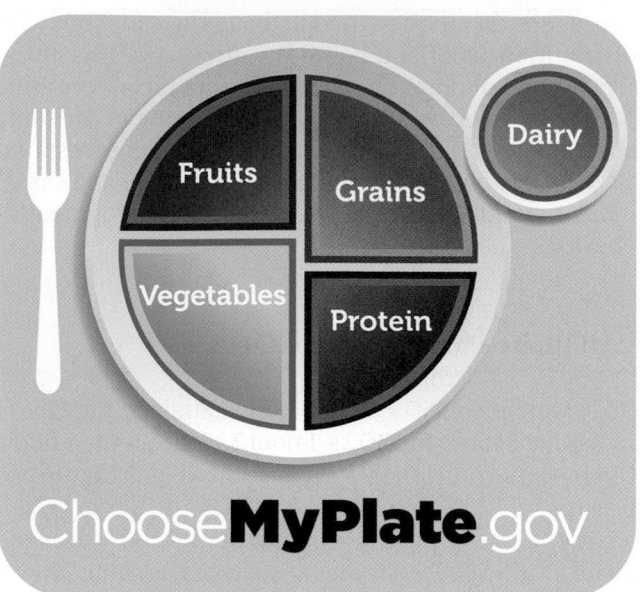

FIGURE 5-2. USDA MyPlate. *(Courtesy of the USDA's Center for Nutrition Policy and Promotion.)*

TABLE 5-1. Daily Recommended Allowances*	
Nutrient	**Daily Values**
Total fat	65 g
Saturated fatty acids	20 g
Cholesterol	300 mg
Sodium	2,400 mg
Potassium	3,500 mg
Total carbohydrates	300 g
Fiber	25 g
Protein	50 g
VITAMINS	
Calcium	1,000 mg
Folate	400 µg
Iron	18 mg
Niacin	20 mg
Riboflavin	1.7 mg
Thiamin	1.5 mg
Vitamin A	5,000 IU
Vitamin B$_6$	2.0 mg
Vitamin B$_{12}$	6.0 µg
Vitamin C	60 mg
Vitamin D	400 IU
Vitamin E	30 IU
Vitamin K	80 µg

*Based on a 2,000 calorie intake; for adults and children 4 or more years of age. (Courtesy of the U.S. Food and Drug Administration.)

only averages; caloric expenditure varies widely among individuals and is higher for athletes and lower for sedentary individuals.

A low-calorie diet creates a caloric deficit of 500 to 1,000 Cal/day, which will yield a weight loss of 1 to

BOX 5-4. Calculating Basal Metabolic Rate

To calculate BMR, use the following formulas. Keep in mind that 1 inch equals 2.54 centimeters and 1 kilogram equals 2.2 pounds.

- **Men**: BMR = 66 + (13.7 x wt in kg) + (5 x ht in cm) – (6.8 x age in years)
- **Women**: BMR = 655 + (9.6 x wt in kg) + (1.8 x ht in cm) – (4.7 x age in years)
- **Example**: You are a 30-year-old woman, who is 5'6" (167.6 cm) tall and weighs 120 lbs (54.5 kilos). Your BMR = 655 + (9.6 x 54.5) + (1.8 x 167.6) – (4.7 x 30) = 655 + 523 +302 – 141 = 1,339 calories/day.

Now that you know your BMR, you can calculate total daily energy expenditure by multiplying your BMR by your activity multiplier:

- **Sedentary**: BMR x 1.2 (little or no exercise)
- **Lightly active**: BMR x 1.375 (light exercise/sports 1–3 days/wk)
- **Moderately active**: BMR x 1.55 (moderate exercise/sports 3–5 days/wk)
- **Very active**: BMR x 1.725 (hard exercise/sports 6–7 days/wk)
- **Extra active**: BMR x 1.9 (hard daily exercise/sports, a physical job, or 2X day training [i.e., marathon, contest])
- **Example**: Your BMR is 1,339 calories per day. You work out 3 to 4 times per week, so your activity level is moderately active. Your activity factor is 1.55. Your total daily energy expenditure = 1.55 x 1,339 = 2,075 calories/day.

2 pounds per week. These diets, which allow approximately 1,000 to 1,500 Cal/day, may be balanced in nutrient intake or may be restrictive of certain food groups. These diets are best used for individuals with a BMI of 35 or greater.

Very low-calorie diets allow 800 calories or fewer per day and are reserved for people with a BMI greater than 30 who need to achieve rapid weight loss. Individuals can lose about 3 to 5 pounds per week. Long-term results may not be any more effective than those achieved with less restrictive plans. This diet regimen should be used under the supervision of a health-care provider.

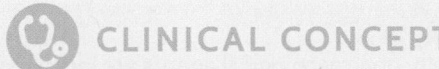 CLINICAL CONCEPT

Benefits of weight loss, such as decreased blood pressure in hypertension and improved glycemic control in diabetes, are seen with even a small reduction in weight.

Activity

Activity is related to weight management by causing caloric expenditures. Moderate levels of physical activity help to maintain the balance of caloric intake and expenditure, and therefore weight. Increases in physical activity, especially aerobic activity, stimulates the use of glucose and subsequent activation of glycogen stores. After utilization of glycogen stores, fat becomes mobilized and reduced. Walking is a simple activity recommended by most clinicians. Different kinds of physical activity allow for different amounts of calorie expenditure (see Table 5-2).

Pharmacology

Pharmacological interventions are designed for short-term use to augment a plan of weight reduction. Individuals need to also employ behavior modifications, dietary adjustments, and engage in some physical activity. Medications offer a possible adjunct, but their effect is modest. They are limited by side effects, and the weight loss is usually short term; as soon as treatment is stopped, the weight is regained in a large number of patients.

According to the National Institute of Health, pharmaceutical interventions should be reserved for

TABLE 5-2. Exercise and Calorie Expenditure

This table shows calories used in common physical activities at both moderate and vigorous levels.

Moderate Physical Activity	Approximate Calories/ 30 Minutes for a 154 lb Person[1]	Approximate Calories/ Hr for a 154 lb Person[1]
Hiking	185	370
Light gardening/yard work	165	330
Dancing	165	330
Golf (walking and carrying clubs)	165	330
Bicycling (<10 mph)	145	290
Walking (3.5 mph)	140	280
Weight lifting (general light workout)	110	220
Stretching	90	180

[1]Calories burned per hour will be higher for persons who weigh more than 154 lbs (70 kg) and lower for persons who weigh less.
(Adapted from U.S. Department of Health and Human Services, U.S. Department of Agriculture. *Dietary Guidelines for Americans 2005.*)

individuals who have increased medical risks related to obesity. Appetite suppressants are for short-term use and require health-care provider prescription. Over-the-counter appetite suppressants, however, are generally not recommended by most clinicians because of their sympathomimetic side effects.

 CLINICAL CONCEPT

Antiobesity pharmacological agents are indicated for individuals with a BMI ≥ 30 or a BMI ≥ 27 with concurrent obesity-related medical problems. Individuals should be under a physician's care while on the agent.

Surgical Options

Liposuction is considered a minor procedure that focuses on a specific site of fat reduction. For individuals with severe obesity, bariatric surgery is recommended. The two categories of surgery are gastric bypass and gastric restrictive procedures.

Liposuction

Liposuction is the most commonly performed cosmetic procedure in the United States. The ideal candidate is physically fit and eats well-balanced meals but is unable to reduce a fatty deposit that is well localized. Liposuction is performed on an outpatient basis, requiring only several hours. A small incision and tunnel is formed at the site of subcutaneous fat accumulation. Anesthetic and a suction catheter are used to remove fat. Compression garments and absorptive pads are applied for the immediate postoperative period. Return to physical activities may be within a few days depending on the patient's comfort. Complications are minimal, with the most significant complications attributed to anesthesia or fluid shifts secondary to large volume liposuction. To maintain weight loss, individuals must adhere to behavior modification guidelines.

ALERT Liposuction performed in one session for persons who are morbidly obese is associated with high risk of mortality from fluid shifts.

Bariatric Surgery

Surgical therapy to decrease obesity is termed **bariatric surgery.** This is appropriate for persons with a BMI of 40 or greater and individuals with a BMI of between 35 and 40 who have medical problems related to their obesity. To determine eligibility for surgical procedures, patients must undergo a thorough assessment. Two general categories of the procedures are gastric bypass and gastric restrictive procedures.

Gastric Bypass. **Gastric bypass** is done by surgically restructuring the upper portion of the stomach to leave an extremely small pouch available for digesting food. The surgeon then alters the connection of the stomach to the small bowel. The jejunum is cut and connected to the newly created pouch in the superior portion of the stomach. The lower portion of the stomach and the duodenum are bypassed.

The procedure promotes weight loss in two ways. First, it limits the volume of food consumed to ½ to 1 ounce and the individual experiences satiety sooner. Second, it alters the ability of the stomach and small bowel to absorb calories and nutrients, while simultaneously preserving the health of the remaining distal portion of the stomach.

Gastric bypass usually results in significant weight loss in a short period of time. It is not without possible complications and surgical risks. To maintain weight loss, individuals must adhere to behavior modification guidelines.

Gastric Banding. **Gastric banding,** such as vertical banding and lap-band procedures, are done by surgically separating a smaller upper portion of the stomach from the lower portion, while maintaining a small opening between the two sections. The banding process keeps the opening from enlarging. The anatomical attachment of the duodenum to the distal portion of the stomach is undisturbed. This procedure promotes weight loss by limiting the amount of food that can be consumed and producing early satiety.

Surgical Complications

Although the previous procedures can be performed by laparoscopy, they carry all of the typical operative risks. In addition to those risks, gastric procedures may cause vitamin and mineral deficiency, especially of B_{12}, calcium, and iron. Herniation of the proximal stomach pouch may also occur, as well as a rupture of the suture line. Other possible complications are vomiting and a malabsorption disorder called dumping syndrome.

Also called rapid gastric emptying, **dumping syndrome** occurs when the undigested contents of the stomach are transported or "dumped" into the small intestine too rapidly. Dumping syndrome causes malabsorption of important nutrients, vitamins, and minerals. Symptoms that occur shortly after eating include abdominal cramps, nausea, and diarrhea. Diarrhea, sweating, tachycardia, and severe hypotension can occur hours after eating. Some people also experience hypoglycemia, related to excessive levels of insulin delivered to the bloodstream, as part of the syndrome. Most cases of dumping syndrome improve as the patient learns to eat better and the digestive system adjusts. Alternatively, clinicians can prescribe medications that slow the passage of food out of the stomach, such as Acarbose or Octreotide.

Nutritional Imbalances

Nutritional imbalances include vitamin and mineral deficiencies and excesses. Both types of disorders have serious adverse effects on the body.

Vitamin and Mineral Deficiencies

Vitamin deficiency can have serious effects on overall health (see Table 5-3). B vitamins and vitamin C are water-soluble and are not stored in the body. Deficiencies of B vitamins are related to beriberi (thiamine), pellagra (Niacin), irritability and depression (B_6), and megaloblastic anemia (folic acid and B_{12}). Insufficient vitamin C leads to scurvy.

Fat-soluble vitamins, A, D, E, and K, can be stored in the liver and fat tissue; as such, they are less likely to be related to deficits. Although labeled a vitamin, vitamin D is a hormone produced in the body as a result of exposure to sunshine. Vitamin D works in close correlation with parathyroid hormones to regulate the absorption of calcium. Individuals with little opportunity for sun exposure, such as home-bound persons or those living in northern climates, may need to take vitamin D supplements.

Minerals are as essential as vitamins in maintaining normal physiologic functioning. Mineral deficits can be reflected in diminished capacity to maintain water balance, conduct nerve impulses, and contract muscle fibers. For example:

- Calcium deficit is related to decreased bone formation and altered nerve conduction.
- Iron deficit is related to fatigue and anemia.

- Potassium deficit is related to muscle weakness, especially of cardiac muscle.
- Sodium deficit can be associated with weakness and GI disturbances.
- Zinc deficits are related to inadequate growth, especially secondary sex characteristics.

Vitamin and Mineral Excesses

Vitamin and mineral excesses, which occur when an individual consumes large quantities of vitamins and minerals over short periods of time, can lead to toxicity. Medical problems triggered by excess vitamins, or hypervitaminosis, are as serious as those caused by vitamin deficits. Overdoses of fat-soluble vitamins are more dangerous than water-soluble vitamins. For example, extremely large doses of vitamin A may cause nausea, vomiting, abdominal pain, hair loss, and headaches. Excess vitamin D can lead to nausea, vomiting, loss of appetite, and confusion. Among water-soluble vitamins, excesses of vitamin C can cause diarrhea and nausea. Excess vitamin B_6 is related to irreversible nerve damage.

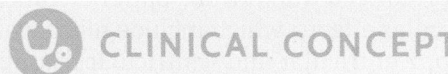

CLINICAL CONCEPT

Excessive amounts of vitamins are generally defined as 10 times the recommended level.

Eating Disorders

Eating disorders include anorexia nervosa, bulimia nervosa, and binge eating. Some persons with eating disorders also engage in purging. Purging includes self-induced vomiting, laxative abuse, inappropriate diuretic use, and excessive exercising.

Anorexia Nervosa

Anorexia nervosa is an eating disorder characterized by an individual who refuses to maintain body weight within minimal normal standards. Although individual weights may vary, weights that fall below the 85th percentile, or a BMI of less than 17.5, may indicate anorexia nervosa.

The term *anorexia* is a bit of a misnomer: by pure definition, it actually describes a loss of appetite. The individual with anorexia nervosa does not lose appetite; instead, he or she intentionally undertakes starvation practices. Individuals often have a disturbed body image, imagining their body as fat. The individual achieves weight loss by a number of means such as severely restricting diet, binging and purging, misusing laxatives and diuretics, and exercising excessively.

Patients with anorexia nervosa often display other personality traits such as a desire for perfection, academic

TABLE 5-3. Nutrient Deficiency Table	
Nutrient	**Clinical Disorder Related to Deficiency**
Folate	Megaloblastic anemia
Niacin	Pellagra: pigmented rash on sun-exposed areas
Riboflavin	Cheilosis: fissures and irritation at edges of mouth
Thiamine	Beriberi: neuropathy, muscle weakness, and wasting
Vitamin A	Nightblindness
Vitamin B_6	Neuropathy, depression, microcytic anemia
Vitamin B_{12}	Megaloblastic anemia
Vitamin C	Scurvy: petechiae, ecchymosis, inflamed and bleeding gums
Vitamin D	Rickets: skeletal deformities, osteomalacia
Vitamin E	Peripheral neuropathy, retinopathy, skeletal muscle atrophy
Vitamin K	Bleeding, elevated prothrombin time

success, and a denial of hunger in the face of starvation. Psychiatric characteristics include excessive dependency needs, developmental immaturity, social isolation, obsessive-compulsive behavior, and constriction of affect. Many patients also have comorbid mood disorders, with depression being most prevalent.

In the United States, prevalence of anorexia nervosa is 0.3% to 1%; however, some studies have shown rates as high as 4% among women. The rates among men are estimated at 0.1%. As many as 13% of adolescent girls exhibit symptoms of anorexia but do not meet full diagnostic criteria. Anorexia nervosa is found in all developed countries and in all socioeconomic classes. Eighty-five percent of patients have onset between the ages of 13 and 18.

In any eating disorder, malnutrition can lead to protein deficiency, hypoglycemia, anemia, and vitamin deficiencies. Thyroid function can become suppressed and electrolyte disturbances are common. Delayed puberty, amenorrhea, anovulation, low estrogen states, increased growth hormone, decreased antidiuretic hormone, hypercarotenemia, and hypothermia can occur. Decreased gonadotropin levels and hypogonadism may occur among males who are affected.

With prolonged starvation, patients can develop cardiovascular effects, which include mitral valve prolapse, supraventricular and ventricular dysrhythmias, long QT syndrome, bradycardia, orthostatic hypotension, and congestive heart failure.

Renal disturbances include decreased glomerular filtration rate, elevated blood urea nitrogen (BUN), edema, acidosis with dehydration, hypokalemia, hypochloremic alkalosis with vomiting, hypoalbuminemia, and hyperaldosteronism.

Gastrointestinal findings include constipation, delayed gastric emptying, and gastric dilation and rupture when binge eating. Patients who induce vomiting develop dental enamel erosion, palatal trauma, enlarged parotids, esophagitis, Mallory-Weiss lesions, and elevated liver enzymes.

Studies show that with psychiatric treatment, 47% of patients with anorexia show complete recovery, 33% show some improvement, but 20% of patients develop chronic, relapsing anorexia. Mortality rates are from 4% to 18% and suicide is a common cause of death.

Bulimia Nervosa

Bulimia nervosa is an eating disorder characterized by two key features:

1. An individual eats a very large quantity of food in a short period of time. This is considered binging and usually takes place in a specified amount of time, often in minutes and usually fewer than 2 hours. For diagnostic purposes, these binges must occur at least twice weekly for 3 months or longer. Generally, the type of food consumed is high in calories and sugar. This binging is usually associated with a sense of loss of control perceived by the individual.

2. The individual will rid himself or herself of the food just eaten to avoid any associated weight gain. The individual may utilize similar inappropriate behaviors as the anorexic, including vomiting, laxative abuse, or excessive exercise. The person who suffers from bulimia is usually within the normal weight range, or may be slightly higher or lower than his or her expected weight. This disorder is also associated with increased symptoms of depression or mood disorders.

Bulimia nervosa is thought to be significantly under-recognized because most persons do not report it. In the United States, the prevalence of bulimia nervosa is estimated at 1%. From those who report the syndrome, lifetime prevalence is 0.5% for males and 1.5% for females. Approximately 65.3% of patients with bulimia have a normal BMI between 18.5 and 29.9 and only 3.5% have a BMI less than 18.5. Bulimia nervosa is prevalent in all ethnic, racial, and socioeconomic groups. It is mainly a disease of young women, with average age of onset at 19 years old. It is estimated to be prevalent in as many as 20% of certain male population groups that require specific body weight such as competitive athletes.

Signs and symptoms are related to the activities an individual uses to avoid weight gain, such as vomiting or the use of laxatives. Typical problems include electrolyte imbalances, sore throat, lymph node enlargement, worn tooth enamel, tooth decay, gastroesophageal reflux disease, severe dehydration, and renal complications related to diuretic abuse. Diagnostic studies include electrolyte levels, liver enzymes, serum albumin, BUN, electrocardiogram (ECG), and serum creatinine. With malnutrition and if weight drops to severely low levels, there are similar metabolic consequences as in anorexia nervosa.

Binge Eating

Binge eating is a disorder that resembles bulimia. A person with this disorder will eat a large quantity of food in a small period of time, or may eat continuously for the entire day. The eating is not triggered by hunger and is not discontinued with signs of satiety. The individual may continue to eat despite the fact that he or she is physically uncomfortable from being full.

Outwardly, these individuals may show no signs of having problems, except that some may be obese or overweight. In addition to the previously noted symptoms, these individuals may hoard food, frequently eat alone, make repeated unsuccessful attempts at dieting, and may feel depressed about their size. Unlike people suffering from bulimia, binge-eaters do not engage in inappropriate compensatory behaviors to prevent weight gain or promote weight loss. Severe obesity is a common consequence of binge eating.

Complications are similar to those experienced by obese individuals, such as cardiovascular issues, including hypertension. Additionally, binge eating is closely linked to psychiatric disorders of anxiety and depression.

Purging Disorders

Individuals with **purging disorder** regularly use self-induced vomiting, laxatives, diuretics, or other extreme methods to control their weight or shape. Some engage in excessive bouts of exercise. Usually the individual is not significantly underweight or overweight; however, he or she is commonly obsessed about weight control. Individuals with purging disorder usually do not have large, out-of-control binge eating episodes. They do not engage in restricted eating. They eat normal meals but have certain times when they feel obliged to purge in order to control weight. Individuals who purge, like those with anorexia or bulimia, have significant body image disturbances and high incidence of anxiety and depression. If weight drops to severely low levels, there are similar metabolic consequences as those found in anorexia nervosa.

Night Eating Syndrome

Night eating syndrome (NES), also known as nocturnal eating syndrome, is an eating disorder characterized by a persistent pattern of late-night binge eating. Affected individuals claim to be unaware of eating while asleep. The diagnosis is controversial. It affects between 1% and 2% of the population and can affect all ages and both sexes. However, most cases are not reported. NES is commonly associated with depression. It has been proposed that individuals have low nocturnal levels of the hormones melatonin and leptin.

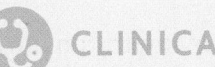 **CLINICAL CONCEPT**

A combination of psychotherapy, behavior modification, and treatment of underlying mental health disorders is necessary for successful treatment of eating disorders.

Chapter Summary

- Over the last 20 years, the percentage of overweight adults worldwide has increased by 300%. Obesity results when energy intake exceeds energy expenditure; fat is a form of stored energy. Individuals vary widely in their propensity to gain weight and accrue fat mass, even at identical levels of caloric input and activity.

- BMI is the current method used to measure body weight; however, it doesn't accurately reflect adiposity and it is inaccurate in highly muscular individuals.

- Adipose tissue is an endocrine organ that secretes adipokines such as adiponectin, leptin, and resistin.

- Adipokines are hormones, thrombogenic substances, inflammatory mediators, and proteins that exert influence on glucose and lipid metabolism, hunger, and satiety.

- Adiponectin enhances cellular sensitivity to insulin, exerts anti-inflammatory effects, and is protective against the formation of arteriosclerosis; it has an inverse relationship with the fat content, or adiposity, of the body.

- As the amount of fat stored in adipocytes rises, leptin is released into the blood and sends signals to the brain that the body has had enough to eat. Obese individuals have high levels of leptin but are resistant to its effects, resulting in leptin desensitization.

- Disorders associated with obesity include cardiovascular disease, diabetes mellitus, osteoarthritis, sleep apnea, and gallbladder and liver disease.

- Diet and exercise are the recommended treatment for excess body fat.

- In persons with severe obesity, bariatric surgery procedures can reverse detrimental health problems.

- Vitamin and mineral deficiencies often occur in individuals with poor diet.

- Persons on diets that restrict certain foods, such as vegetarians, need to be particularly aware of sources of iron and vitamin B_{12}.

- Food intake can be an emotional issue that is involved in mental health problems such anorexia, bulimia, and purging.

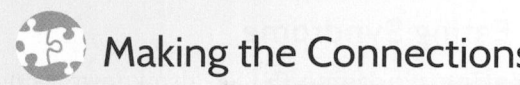

Making the Connections

Disorder and Pathophysiology	Signs and Symptoms	Physical Assessment Findings	Diagnostic Testing	Treatment
Obesity	A metabolic disorder that involves excess fat accumulation caused by lack of sufficient activity and excess caloric intake. Obesity is a metabolic disorder that involves changes in cellular insulin sensitivity, satiety, glucose utilization, fat accumulation, hepatic glucose production, and fluid balance.			
	Lethargy. Indigestion caused by GERD. Osteoarthritis caused by excessive weight on knees and hips.	Apple-shaped or pear-shaped excess fat accumulation. Waist circumference in males > 40 inches; in females >35 inches.	BMI ≥ 30. Skinfold fat measurement >25% in males, >30% in females. Dyslipidemia: low HDL, high LDL, high triglycerides. Elevated blood glucose. Elevated blood pressure.	Diet. Exercise. Pharmacological agents: appetite suppressors. Liposuction. Bariatric surgery.
Anorexia Nervosa	Intentional self-restriction of food, causing severe weight loss.			
	Patient usually denies any problems. Individual sees self as overweight and is obsessed with taking off body weight through not eating or purging. Disturbed self body image Refusal to put on weight.	BMI < 17.5. Multiple system disturbances; lack of body fat, hair loss, cold intolerance, delayed puberty, orthostatic hypotension, amenorrhea, heart murmur of mitral valve prolapse. Abnormal heart rhythm. Edema.	Electrolyte imbalances such as hypokalemia. Complete blood count abnormalities showing anemia. Increased BUN showing dehydration. ECG abnormalities. Elevated liver enzymes. Low thyroid function. Iron deficiency Low estrogen.	Psychiatric treatment Nasogastric tube feedings. Rehydration and correction of any complications.
Bulimia Nervosa	An illness in which a person binges on food or has regular episodes of overeating and feels a loss of control. The person then uses different methods—such as self-induced vomiting or abusing laxatives—to prevent weight gain. Some with bulimia also have anorexia nervosa.			
	Patient usually denies problems.	Patient may be of normal body weight. Typical problems include electrolyte imbalances, sore throat, lymph node enlargement, worn tooth enamel, tooth decay, gastroesophageal reflux disease, severe dehydration, and renal complications related to diuretic abuse.	Diagnostic studies for electrolyte levels, liver enzymes, serum albumin, BUN, ECG, and serum creatinine.	Psychiatric treatment. Correction of any side effects.

Continued

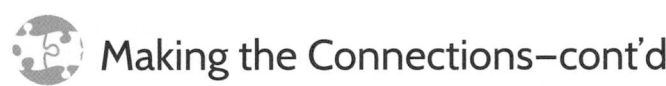

Making the Connections—cont'd

Disorder and Pathophysiology	Signs and Symptoms	Physical Assessment Findings	Diagnostic Testing	Treatment
Binge Eating | Eating a large quantity of food in a small period of time, or eating continuously for the entire day. The eating is not triggered by hunger and is not discontinued with signs of satiety or feeling uncomfortably full.				
	Patient usually denies problems.	Obesity is common. Patient may hoard food, eat alone, or try numerous diets.	None.	Psychiatric treatment Treatment for obesity, including diet and activity.
Purging Disorder | Individuals with purging disorder regularly use self-induced vomiting, laxatives, diuretics, or other extreme methods to control their weight or shape. Some engage in excessive bouts of exercise. Usually the individual is not significantly underweight or overweight, but commonly obsessed about weight control.				
	Patient usually denies problems.	Normal weight is common.	None.	Psychiatric treatment.
Night Eating Syndrome | Characterized by a persistent pattern of late-night binge eating. Affected individuals claim to be unaware of eating while asleep.				
	Obesity.	Obesity.	None.	Psychiatric treatment.

Bibliography

Appel, L. J., Clark, J. M., Yeh, H. C., et al. (2011). Comparative effectiveness of weight-loss interventions in clinical practice. *N Engl J Med, 365*(21), 1959–1968.

Arner, E., Rydén, M., & Arner, P. (2010). Tumor necrosis factor alpha and regulation of adipose tissue. *N Engl J Med, 362*(12), 1151–1153.

Astrup, A. (2010). Drug management of obesity—efficacy versus safety. *N Engl J Med, 363*(3), 288–290.

Bally, C., Blackburn, P., & Brown, N. (2010). Care of the bariatric patient. Health concerns after surgery. *Adv Nurse Pract, 18*(6), 37–39.

Batsis, J. A., Romero-Corral, A., Collazo-Clavell, M. L., et al. (2008). Effect of bariatric surgery on the metabolic syndrome: a population-based, long-term controlled study. *Mayo Clinic Proceedings, 83*(8), 897–907.

Berrington de Gonzalez, A., Hartge, P., Cerhan, J. R., et al. (2010). Body-mass index and mortality among 1.46 million white adults. *N Engl J Med, 363*(23), 2211–2219.

Bhattacharyya, S., & Kaddoura, S. (2009). Perioperative safety and bariatric surgery. *N Engl J Med, 361*(19), 1911.

Bleich, S.N. & Rutkow, L. (2013). Improving obesity prevention at the local level-emerging opportunities. *NEngU Med, 368* (19), 1761–1763.

Boelsen-Robinson, T., Gearon, E., & Peeters, A. (2014). Incidence of childhood obesity in the United States. *N Engl J Med, 370*(17), 1659–1660. doi: 10.1056/NEJMc1402397#SA2.

Boggs, D. A., Rosenberg, L., Cozier, Y. C., et al. (2011). General and abdominal obesity and risk of death among black women. *N Engl J Med, 365*(10), 901–908.

Boling, C. L., Westman, E. C., & Yancy, W. S. (2009). Comparison of weight-loss diets. *N Engl J Med, 360*(21), 2247–2248.

Bray, G. A. (2010). Let's treat obesity seriously. *Am Fam Phys, 81*(12), 1406–1408.

Bucholz, E. M., Rathore, S. S., Reid, K. J., et al. (2012). Body mass index and mortality in acute myocardial infarction patients. *Am J Med, 125*(8), 796–803. doi: 10.1016/j.amjmed.2012.01 .018. Epub 2012 Apr 5.

Buchwald, H., Ikramuddin, S., Dorman, R. B., et al. (2011). Management of the metabolic/bariatric surgery patient. *Am J Med, 124*(12), 1099–1105. doi: 10.1016/j.amjmed.2011.05.035. Epub 2011 Oct 18.

Carlsson, L. M., Peltonen, M., Ahlin, S., et al. (2012). Bariatric surgery and prevention of type 2 diabetes in Swedish obese subjects. *N Engl J Med, 367*(8), 695–704. doi: 10.1056/ NEJMoa1112082.

Casazza, K., Fontaine, K. R., Astrup, A., et al. (2013). Myths, presumptions, and facts about obesity. *N Engl J Med, 368*(5), 446–454. doi: 10.1056/NEJMsa1208051.

Chang, H. J. (2010). Scientists probe brain's role in obesity. *JAMA, 303*(1), 19.

Chang, S. H., Stoll, C. R., Song, J., et al. (2014). The effectiveness and risks of bariatric surgery: an updated systematic review and meta-analysis, 2003–2012. *J Am Med Assoc Surg, 149*(3), 275–287. doi: 10.1001/jamasurg .2013.3654.

Compston, J. E., Watts, N. B., Chapurlat, R., et al. (2011). Obesity is not protective against fracture in postmenopausal women: GLOW. *Am J Med, 124*(11), 1043–1050. doi: 10.1016/j.amjmed .2011.06.013.

Courcoulas, A. P., Christian, N. J., Belle, S. H., et al. (2013). Weight change and health outcomes at 3 years after bariatric surgery among individuals with severe obesity. *JAMA, 310*(22), 2416–2425. doi: 10.1001/jama.2013 .280928.

Croswell, J., & Luger, S. (2012). Screening for and management of obesity in adults. *Am Fam Phys, 86*(10), 947–948.

Cummings, D. E., & Cohen, R. V. (2014). Beyond BMI: The need for new guidelines governing the use of bariatric and metabolic surgery. *Lancet Diabetes Endocrinol*, 2(2), 175–181. doi: 10.1016/S2213-8587(13)70198-0.

Cunningham, S. A., Kramer, M. R., & Narayan, K. M. (2014a). Incidence of childhood obesity in the United States. *N Engl J Med*, 370(5), 403–411.

Cunningham, S. A., Kramer, M. R., & Narayan, K. M. (2014). Incidence of childhood obesity in the United States. *N Engl J Med*, 370(17), 1660–1661. doi: 10.1056/NEJMc1402397.

Curfman, G. D., Morrissey, S., & Drazen, J. M. (2010). Sibutramine—another flawed diet pill. *N Engl J Med*, 363(10), 972–974.

Department of Health and Human Services (HHS) and the Department of Agriculture (USDA). (2010). *Dietary guidelines for Americans*, Washington, DC. 2010. Retrieved from: http://www.health.gov/dietaryguidelines/2010.asp

Dixon, J. B., & Kral, J. G. (2014). BMI and mortality among adults with incident type 2 diabetes. *N Engl J Med*, 370(14), 1362–1363. doi: 10.1056/NEJMc1401876#SA4.

Dixon, J. B., le Roux, C. W., Rubino, F., & Zimmet, P. (2012). Bariatric surgery for type 2 diabetes. *Lancet*, 379(9833), 2300–2311 .doi: 10.1016/S0140-6736(12)60401-2. Epub 2012 Jun 9.

Drolet, R., Richard, C., Sniderman, A. D., et al. (2008). Hypertrophy and hyperplasia of abdominal adipose tissues in women. *Int J Obesity*, 32, 283–291.

Field, A. E., Malspies, S. M., & Willet, W. C. (2009). Weight cycling and mortality among middle-aged or older women. *Arch Int Med*, 169(9), 881–886.

Flegal, K. M., Carroll, M. D., Ogden, C. L., & Curtin, L. R. (2010). Prevalence and trends in obesity among US adults, 1999–2008. *JAMA*, 303(3), 235–241.

Gillman, M. W., & Ludwig, D. S. (2013). How early should obesity prevention start? *N Engl J Med*, 369(23), 2173–2175. doi: 10.1056/NEJMp1310577. Epub 2013 Nov 13.

Glandt, M., & Raz, I. (2011). Present and future: pharmacologic treatment of obesity. *J Obes, 2011*, 636181. Epub 2011 Feb 8.

Global Burden of Metabolic Risk Factors for Chronic Diseases Collaboration (BMI Mediated Effects), Lu, Y., Hajifathalian, K., et al. (2014). Metabolic mediators of the effects of body-mass index, overweight, and obesity on coronary heart disease and stroke: a pooled analysis of 97 prospective cohorts with 1·8 million participants. *Lancet*, 383(9921), 970–983. doi: 10.1016/S0140-6736(13)61836-X. Epub 2013 Nov 22.

Goldfine, A. B., Vernon, A., & Zinner, M. (2014). Where are the health care cost savings with bariatric surgery in obesity management? *J Am Med Assoc Surg*, 149(1), 5–6. doi: 10.1001/jamasurg.2013.3060.

Gondoni, L. A., & Liuzzi, A. (2011). Diet and physical activity interventions in severely obese adults, *JAMA*, 305(6), 563.

Grief, S. N. (2010). Strategies to facilitate weight loss in patients who are obese. *Am Fam Phys*, vol 82 issue 12, page 1434.

Grief, S. N., & Miranda, R. L. (2010). Weight loss maintenance. *Am Fam Phys*, 82(6), 630–634.

Hennekens, C. H., & Andreotti, F. (2013). Leading avoidable cause of premature deaths worldwide: case for obesity. *Am J Med*, 126(2), 97–98. doi: 10.1016/j.amjmed .2012.06.018.

Hossain, P., Kawar, B., & El Nahas, M. (2007, Jan 18). Obesity and diabetes in the developing world—a growing challenge. *N Engl J Med*, 356(3), 213–215.

Ikramuddin, S., & Livingston, E. H. (2013). New insights on bariatric surgery outcomes. *JAMA*, 310(22), 2401–2402. doi: 10.1001/jama.2013.280927.

Jacobs, D. O. (2012). Bariatric surgery—from treatment of disease to prevention? *N Engl J Med*, 367(8), 764–765. doi: 10.1056/NEJMe1207860.

Jackson, C. L., & Stampfer, M. J. (2014). Maintaining a healthy body weight is paramount. *J Am Med Assoc Intern Med*, 74(1), 23–24. doi: 10.1001/jamainternmed.2013.8298.

James, W. P., Caterson, I. D., Coutinho, W., et al. (2010). Effect of sibutramine on cardiovascular outcomes in overweight and obese subjects. *N Engl J Med*, 363(10), 905–917.

Jensen, M. D., & Ryan, D. H. (2014). New obesity guidelines: promise and potential. *JAMA*, 311(1), 23–24. doi: 10.1001/jama.2013.282546.

Johnson, W. D., Brashear, M. M., Gupta, A. K., et al. (2011). Incremental weight loss improves cardiometabolic risk in extremely obese adults. *Am J Med*, 124(10), 931–938. doi: 10.1016/j.amjmed.2011.04.033.

Kadowaki, T., Yamauchi, T., Okada-Iwabu, M., & Iwabu, M. (2014). Adiponectin and its receptors: implications for obesity-associated diseases and longevity. *Lancet Diabetes Endocrinol*, (1), 8–9. doi: 10.1016/S2213-8587(13)70120-7. Epub 2013 Dec 3.

Kaplan, L. M. (2010). Pharmacologic therapies for obesity. *Gastr Clin N America*, 39(1), 69–79.

Kashyap, S. R., Gatmaitan, P., Brethauer, S., & Schauer, P. (2010). Bariatric surgery for type 2 diabetes: weighing the impact for obese patients. *Cleveland Clin J Med*, 77(7), 468–476.

Katan, M. B., & Ludwig, D. S. (2010). Extra calories cause weight gain—but how much? *JAMA*, 303(1), 65–66.

Klok, M. D., Jakobsdottir, S., & Drent, M. L. (2007). The role of leptin and ghrelin in the regulation of food intake and body weight in humans: a review. *Obesity Rev*, 8(1), 21–34.

Kumar, V., Abbas, A. K., Fausto, N., & Aster, J. (2010). *Robbins & Cotran pathologic basis of disease*. 8th ed. Philadelphia, PA: WB Saunders.

Ladabaum, U., Mannalithara, A., Myer, P. A., & Singh, G. (2014). Obesity, abdominal obesity, physical activity, and caloric intake in U.S. adults: 1988–2010. *Am J Med*, Mar 10. pii: S0002-9343(14)00191-0. doi: 10.1016/j.amjmed.2014.02 .026. Epub ahead of print.

Lavie, C. J., Milani, R. V., Ventura, H. O., & Romero-Corral, A. (2010). Body composition and heart failure prevalence and prognosis: getting to the fat of the matter in the "obesity paradox." *Mayo Clinic Proceedings*, 85(7), 605–608.

Leibel, R. L. (2008). Energy in, energy out, and the effects of obesity-related genes. *N Engl J Med*, 359(24), 2603–2604.

Lenhard, J. M. (2011). Lipogenic enzymes as therapeutic targets for obesity and diabetes. *Curr Pharm Design*, 17(4), 325–331.

Longitudinal Assessment of Bariatric Surgery (LABS) Consortium, Flum, D. R., Belle, S. H., et al. (2009). Perioperative safety in the longitudinal assessment of bariatric surgery. *N Engl J Med*, 361(5), 445–454.

Longo, D., Fauci, A., Braunwald, E., et al. (2012). *Harrison's principles of internal medicine*. 18th ed. New York: McGraw-Hill.

Madsbad, S., Dirksen, C., & Holst, J. J. (2014). Mechanisms of changes in glucose metabolism and bodyweight after bariatric surgery. *Lancet Diabetes Endocrinol*, 2(2), 152–164. doi: 10.1016/S2213-8587(13)70218-3. Epub 2014 Feb 3.

Main, M. L., Rao, S. C., & O'Keefe, J. H. (2010). Trends in obesity and extreme obesity among US adults. *JAMA*, 303(17), 1695.

Mayo Foundation for Medical Education and Research. (2012). Obesity complications. Retrieved from http://www.mayoclinic.com/health/obesity/DS00314/DSECTION=complications

McAuley, P. A., Artero, E. G., Sui, X., et al. (2012). The obesity paradox, cardiorespiratory fitness, and coronary heart disease. *Mayo Clinic Proceedings*, 87(5), 443–451. doi: 10.1016/j.mayocp.2012.01.013. Epub 2012 Apr 12.

McCarthy, M. I. (2010). Genomics, type 2 diabetes and obesity. *N Engl J Med,* 363(23), 2339–2350.

Mingrone, G., Panunzi, S., De Gaetano, A., et al. (2012). Bariatric surgery versus conventional medical therapy for type 2 diabetes. *N Engl J Med,* 366(17), 1577–1585.

Mozaffarian, D., Hao, T., Rimm, E. B., Willett, W. C., & Hu, F. B. (2011). Changes in diet and lifestyle and long-term weight gain in women and men. *N Engl J Med,* 364(25), 2392–2404.

Myers, J., Lata, K., Chowdhury, S., et al. (2011). The obesity paradox and weight loss. *Am J Med,* 124(10), 924–930. doi: 10.1016/j.amjmed.2011.04.018. Epub 2011 Jul 26.

National Institute of Diabetes and Digestive and Kidney Diseases. *Understanding adult overweight and obesity* from NIH publication no. 06-3680, 2008, updated Dec 2012. Retrieved from http://win.niddk.nih.gov/publications/understanding.htm

National Institute of Diabetes and Digestive and Kidney Diseases. Weight-control information network. *Understanding adult overweight and obesity* from NIH publication no. 06-3680, 2008, updated Dec 2012. Retrieved from http://win.niddk.nih.gov

National Institute of Mental Health, National Institute of Health. *Eating disorders.* Retrieved from http://www.nimh.nih.gov/health/topics/eating-disorders/index.shtml. NIH publication no. TR14-4901. 2014.

Ogden, C. L., Carroll, M. D., Kit, B. K., & Flegal, K. M. (2014). Prevalence of childhood and adult obesity in the United States, 2011–2012. *JAMA,* 311(8), 806–814. doi: 10.1001/jama.2014.732.

O'Hare, J. D., Zielinski, E., Cheng, B., Scherer, T., & Buettner, C. (2011). Central endocannabinoid signaling regulates hepatic glucose production and systemic lipolysis. *Diabetes,* 60(4), 1055–1062.

Park, S. K., Chen, Y., Shen, C. Y., et al. (2011). Association between body-mass index and risk of death in more than 1 million Asians. *N Engl J Med,* 364(8), 719–729.

Phillips, S. A., & Kung, J. T. (2010). Mechanisms of adiponectin regulation and use as a pharmacological target. *Curr Opin Pharm,* 10(6), 676–683.

Rao, G. (2010). Office-based strategies for the management of obesity. *Am Fam Phys,* 81(12), 1449–1456.

Rejeski, W. J., Ip, E. H., Bertoni, A. G., et al. (2012). Lifestyle change and mobility in obese adults with type 2 diabetes. *N Engl J Med,* 366(13), 1209–1217.

Richardson, L. A. (2010). Laparoscopic gastric banding vs lifestyle intervention in severely obese adolescents. *JAMA,* 303(23), 2356.

Rondinone, C. M. (2006). Adipocyte-derived hormones, cytokines, and mediators. *Endocrine,* 29(1), 81–90.

Salazar, M. R., Carbajal, H. A., Espeche, W. G., et al. (2014). Identification of cardiometabolic risk: visceral adiposity index versus triglyceride/HDL cholesterol ratio. *Am J Med,* 127(2), 152–157. doi: 10.1016/j.amjmed.2013.10.012. Epub 2013 Nov 1.

Sallis, J. F., & Hinckson, E. A. (2014). Reversing the obesity epidemic in young people: building up the physical activity side of energy balance. *Lancet Diabetes Endocrinol,* 2(3), 190–191. doi: 10.1016/S2213-8587(13)70193-1.

Schauer, P. R., Kashyap, S. R., Wolski, K., et al. (2012). Bariatric surgery versus intensive medical therapy in obese patients with diabetes. *N Engl J Med,* 366(17), 1567–1576.

Silk, A. W., & McTigue, K. M. (2011). Reexamining the physical examination for obese patients. *JAMA,* 305(2), 193–194.

Slawson, D. (2014). Long-term results of drug treatment for obesity. *Am Fam Phys,* 89(5), 389–390.

Smith, S. R., Weissman, N. J., Anderson, C. M., et al. (2010). Multicenter, placebo-controlled trial of lorcaserin for weight management. *N Engl J Med,* 363(3), 245–256.

Stefan, N., Häring, H. U., Hu, F. B., & Schulze, M. B. (2013). Metabolically healthy obesity: epidemiology, mechanisms, and clinical implications. *Lancet Diabetes Endocrinol,* 1(2), 152–162. doi: 10.1016/S2213-8587(13)70062-7. Epub 2013 Aug 30.

Thorogood, A., Mottillo, S., Shimony, A., et al. (2011). Isolated aerobic exercise and weight loss: a systematic review and meta-analysis of randomized controlled trials. *Am J Med,* 124(8), 747–755. doi: 10.1016/j.amjmed.2011.02.037.

Tobias, D., Pan, A., & Hu, F. B. (2014). BMI and mortality among adults with incident type 2 diabetes. *N Engl J Med,* 370(14), 1363–1364. doi: 10.1056/NEJMc1401876.

Tobias, D. K., Pan, A., Jackson, C. L., et al. (2014). Body-mass index and mortality among adults with incident type 2 diabetes. *N Engl J Med,* 370(3), 233–244. doi: 10.1056/NEJMoa1304501. Erratum in: *N Engl J Med.* 2014 Apr 3;370(14):1368.

Torpy, J. M., Lynm, C., & Glass, R. M. (2010). JAMA patient page. Bariatric surgery. *JAMA,* 303(6), 576.

Unick, J. L., Beavers, D., Bond, D. S., et al. (2013). The long-term effectiveness of a lifestyle intervention in severely obese individuals. *Am J Med,* 126(3), 236–242, 242.e1-2. doi: 10.1016/j.amjmed.2012.10.010.

Van Gaal, L. F., & Maggioni, A. P. (2014). Overweight, obesity, and outcomes: fat mass and beyond. *Lancet,* 383(9921), 935–936. doi: 10.1016/S0140-6736(13)62076-0. Epub 2013 Nov 22.

Villareal, D. T., Chode, S., Parimi, N., et al. (2011). Weight loss, Exercise or both and physical function in obese adults. *N Engl J Med,* 364(13), 1218–1229.

Wadden, T. A., Volger, S., Sarwer, D. B., et al. (2011). A two-year randomized trial of obesity treatment in primary care practice. *N Engl J Med,* 365(21), 1969–1979.

Wentworth, J. M., Playfair, J., Laurie, C., et al. (2014). Multidisciplinary diabetes care with and without bariatric surgery in overweight people: a randomised controlled trial. *Lancet Diabetes Endocrinol,* Apr 7. pii: S2213-8587(14)70066-X. doi: 10.1016/S2213-8587(14)70066-X. Epub ahead of print.

Wing, R. R. (2010). Treatment options for obesity: do commercial weight loss programs have a role? *JAMA,* 304(16), 1837–1838.

Yanovski, S. Z., & Yanovski, J. A. (2011). Obesity prevalence in the United States—up, down, or sideways? *N Engl J Med,* 364(11), 987–989.

Yanovski, S. Z., & Yanovski, J. A. (2014). Long-term drug treatment for obesity: a systematic and clinical review. *JAMA,* 311(1), 74–86. doi: 10.1001/jama.2013.281361.

Yanovski, S. Z. (2011). Obesity treatment in primary care—are we there yet? *N Engl J Med,* 365(21), 2030–2031.

Zheng, W., McLerran, D. F., Rolland, B., et al. (2011). Association between body-mass index and risk of death in more than 1 million Asians. *N Engl J Med,* 364(8), 719–729.

Zimmet, P., & Alberti, K. G. (2012). Surgery or medical therapy for obese patients with type 2 diabetes? *N Engl J Med,* 366(17), 1635–1636.

Pain

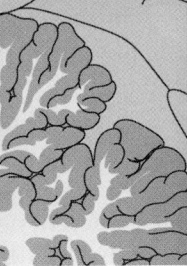

Key Terms

Addiction
Afferent neuron
Catastrophize
Colic
Efferent neuron
Gate control theory

Modulation
Neuromatrix theory
Neuropathic pain
Nociceptors
OLDCART
Paresthesia

Perception
Phantom limb pain
Referred pain
Simple reflex arc
Transduction
Transmission

Pain has been recognized as a source of human suffering since ancient times, when our ancestors believed evil spirits and sin to be its cause. Later, pain was associated with apparent tissue damage, whereas pain without apparent cause was thought to be unreal, psychosomatic, or caused by patient malingering. In the last decade, there have been changes in the assessment and treatment of pain. Clinicians have given the patient's perception of pain greater credibility than in the past and now ask patients to describe and quantify their pain regardless of evident pathology, with the knowledge that pain is a subjective experience. The International Association for the Study of Pain defines pain as an unpleasant sensory and emotional experience associated with actual or potential tissue damage.

Although unpleasant, it is important to remember that pain is a protective mechanism; it allows the body to detect injury while also enabling the body to protect itself from more serious injury.

Epidemiology

Numerous research studies have identified the detrimental effects of uncontrolled pain on morbidity and mortality, quality of life, and health-care costs. Optimal pain management is associated with a quicker rate of recovery, better functioning, and fewer postoperative complications. Pain is the most common symptom that prompts people to seek medical attention, accounting for over 70 million office visits per year in the United States. It is also the second leading reason for work absenteeism, resulting in over 50 million lost workdays per year and an estimated $3 billion in lost wages. Pain costs employers an estimated $80 billion per year because of lost productivity, health-care costs, and compensation.

Basic Concepts Related to Pain

An understanding of how pain sensation is interpreted by the body involves the spinal cord and brain. At times, pain triggers an immediate response without interpretation by the brain through a simple reflex. At other times, pain signals travel from the periphery to an ascending tract in the spinal cord up to the brain for interpretation.

Nociceptors, which are specialized pain nerve fibers, and neurotransmitters, which can have an enhancing or inhibitory effect on pain, are involved in the travel of pain sensation in the spinal cord. The brain can inhibit the experience of pain through natural neurochemicals called endogenous opioids. Endorphins are examples of these natural opioids. The assessment of pain requires knowledge of areas on the body represented by sensory and motor nerves called dermatomes and myotomes. Localizing pain to specific dermatomes or myotomes can give clinicians diagnostic clues regarding the source of pain.

The Central Nervous System and Pain

The brain and spinal cord are integral components in the experience of pain perception. Within the center of the spinal cord there is an "H"-shaped region called the substantia gelatinosa. Spinal nerves enter the spinal cord at the posterior region of the substantia gelatinosa called the dorsal horn. The neurons that enter the dorsal horn are called afferent neurons. **Afferent neurons** are sensory nerves that carry pain, temperature, touch, proprioception, vibration, and pressure sensations into the spinal cord. **Efferent neurons** are motor nerves; these neurons exit the spinal cord through the ventral horn and extend to the muscles of the body.

Simple Reflex Arc

A simple reflex occurs in the body without need for interpretation by the brain. In a **simple reflex arc,** an afferent neuron carries sensory impulses into the dorsal horn of the spinal cord. The afferent neuron connects with an interneuron in the substantia gelatinosa. The interneuron connects to an efferent neuron that exits via the ventral horn and enacts motor activity.

The simple reflex is protective: It allows for immediate action by the body without time for interpretation by the brain. For example, when touching a hot stove, the finger senses the heat and afferent neurons bring the sensory impulses into the spinal cord via the dorsal horn. It connects with an interneuron, which connects with an efferent neuron that enacts the motor activity of pulling the finger away immediately. A protective response is elicited before the brain has a chance to interpret the event (see Fig. 6-1).

A simple reflex arc is also seen when a clinician tests a patient for deep tendon reflexes. For example, the clinician tests the patellar reflex when tapping the tendon of the quadriceps muscle at the knee. The reflex hammer taps the tendon, and afferent neurons carry the signal into the spinal cord, where they connect with interneurons. An interneuron then connects to an efferent motor neuron and the reflexive kick motion of the quadriceps muscle occurs.

The brain can also interpret pain in the pain sensory experience. The afferent neuron carries sensory information from the periphery into the dorsal horn of the spinal cord, where it synapses with an interneuron in the substantia gelatinosa. The interneuron then synapses with another neuron that is within an ascending tract called the spinothalamic tract. The spinothalamic tract directs sensory neuronal impulses from the spinal cord up through the brainstem to the hypothalamus and upper regions of the brain cortex. The axons of the spinothalamic tract cross over to the other side of the spinal cord before their arrival in the brain. From the somatosensory portion of the brain, motor neurons descend downward in the spinal cord and cross over at the medulla to control the opposite side of the body. These motor neurons, known as the corticospinal tract, exit via the ventral horn of the spinal cord to control muscles of the body (see Fig. 6-2).

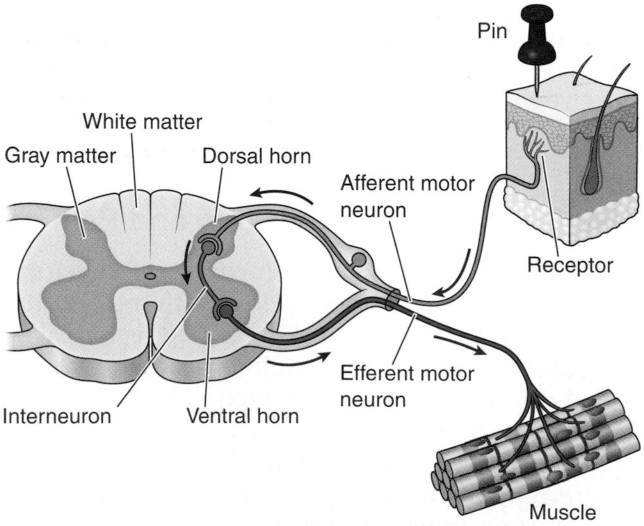

Nociception

Nociception is the response of the nervous system to painful stimuli. Nerve fibers that respond to noxious stimuli are termed **nociceptors.** Nociceptors are found in the skin, muscle, connective tissue, bone, circulatory system, and abdominal, pelvic, and thoracic viscera. Afferent neurons, which are nociceptors, carry the sensations of touch, temperature, vibration, proprioception, and pain into the dorsal horn of the spinal cord.

Afferent neurons can be categorized as A-delta and C fibers. A-delta fibers are large in diameter and myelinated. These fibers conduct impulses rapidly and cause the first, short-lived acute experience of pain, such as occurs when a finger senses a burn and pulls away from the heat source. C fibers are smaller in diameter and unmyelinated. These fibers conduct impulses slowly and cause longer lasting, persistent dull pain, such as the pain that occurs after a burn has taken place.

Neurotransmitters

Neurotransmitters are excitatory or inhibitory chemical mediators that are released from one neuron to stimulate another (see Table 6-1). There are approximately 50 neurotransmitters, including acetylcholine, norepinephrine, dopamine, serotonin, and gamma aminobutyric acid (GABA). Acetylcholine and norepinephrine are excitatory neurotransmitters, whereas dopamine, serotonin, and GABA are inhibitory. A nerve impulse travels down a neuron from dendrites to the cell body into the axon and eventually the presynaptic membrane, which contains vesicles that release neurotransmitters into a synaptic cleft. In the postsynaptic membrane, receptors on the adjoining neuron pick up freely flowing neurotransmitters. Once the neurotransmitter is picked up by receptors in the postsynaptic membrane, the molecule is internalized in the neuron and the impulse continues. Within the dorsal horn of the spinal cord and brain, communication of nociceptive information between various neurons occurs via neurotransmitters. Some neurotransmitters are manipulated for pharmacological management of pain. For example, the neurotransmitter serotonin is stimulated by the pharmacological agent sumatriptan as a remedy for migraine headache.

FIGURE 6-1. In a simple reflex arc, a sensation is felt and transmitted via a nerve impulse that travels via the afferent neuron into the dorsal horn of the spinal cord. It connects with an interneuron located in the spinal cord, which connects with an efferent neuron that travels out the ventral horn of the spinal cord and stimulates a motor activity. A simple reflex arc enables a quick action response before the brain has a chance to interpret the event.

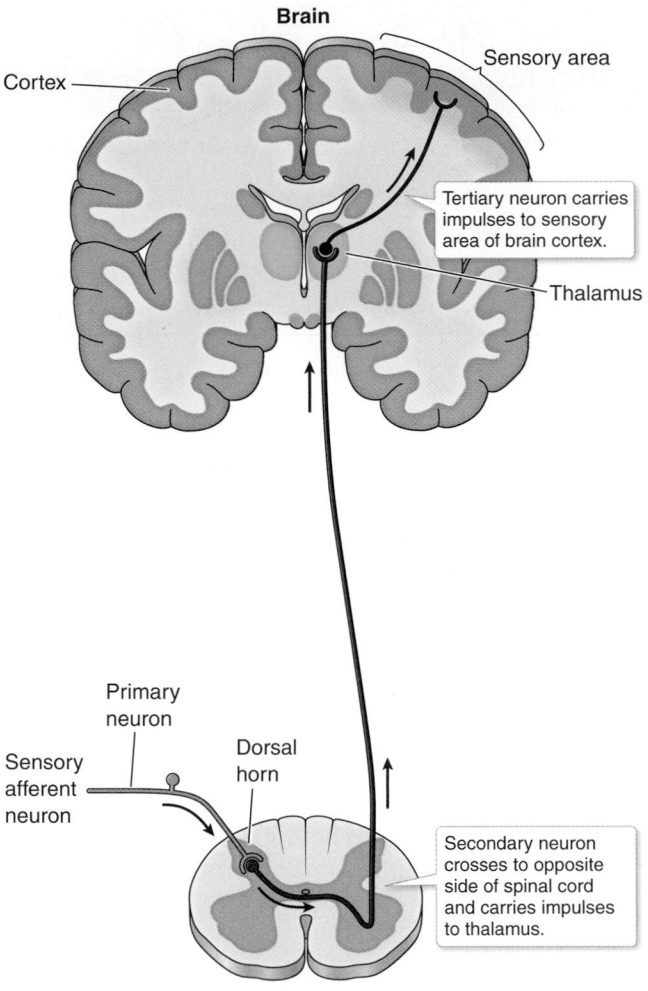

FIGURE 6-2a. The spinothalamic tract directs afferent sensory impulses from the periphery into the dorsal horn of the spinal cord (primary neuron). It connects with an interneuron in the spinal cord that crosses over to the opposite side of the spinal cord (secondary neuron) to the thalamus. The interneuron then connects with another neuron (tertiary neuron) that directs impulses to the upper regions of the brain sensory cortex.

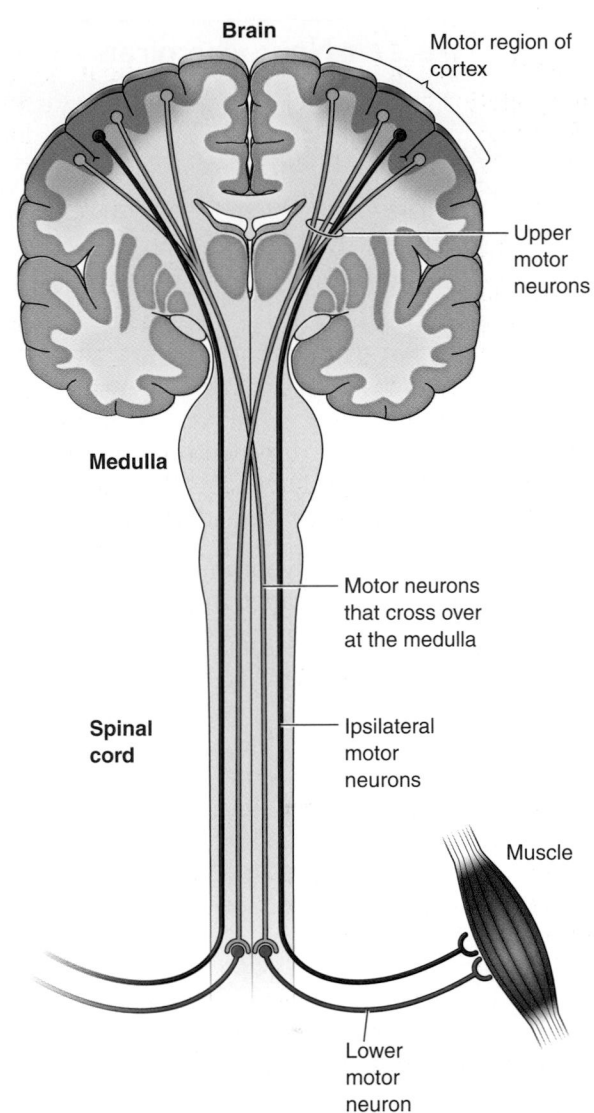

FIGURE 6-2b. From the motor region of the brain, corticospinal tract neurons descend down into the medulla where the majority of neurons cross over to the opposite side of the spinal cord. The area of crossover in the medulla is called the area of decussation. Some corticospinal tract neurons do not cross over and remain ipsilateral. The motor neurons descend via the spinal cord and exit via the ventral horn of the spinal cord, then connect to a lower motor neuron to stimulate muscle activity.

TABLE 6-1. Neurochemicals and Neurotransmitters Influence on Pain	
Neurochemicals	**Action**
Prostaglandins (from COX 1 enzymatic pathway)	Enhances inflammation, pain, edema
Interleukins	Enhances inflammation, pain, edema
Tumor necrosis factor	Enhances inflammation, edema, pain, and decreases appetite
Leukotrienes	Enhances inflammation, edema, and bronchospasm, particularly in asthma and allergy
Bradykinins	Enhances inflammation
Glutamate	Amplifies pain signal
Substance P	Amplifies pain signal
Enkephalins, endorphins	Inhibitory influence on pain; natural opioid

Continued

TABLE 6-1. Neurochemicals and Neurotransmitters Influence on Pain–cont'd

Neurotransmitters	Action
Acetylcholine	Inhibitory action on pain in spinal cord
Gamma-aminobutyric acid	Inhibitory action on pain in the spinal cord and brain
Norepinephrine	Inhibitory action on pain in the spinal cord
Dopamine	Inhibitory action on pain in spinal cord and brain
Serotonin	Conveys analgesic signals from the PAG area to the NRM of the brain (serotonin is diminished in migraine headache)

Endogenous Opioids

Endogenous opioids, which are natural analgesic neurochemicals that inhibit pain sensation, are similar to neurotransmitters. Endogenous opioids include endorphins, enkephalins, and dynorphins. Major areas of the midbrain and brainstem called the periaqueductal gray matter (PAG) and nucleus raphe magnus (NRM) are particularly influential in pain inhibition (see Fig. 6-3).

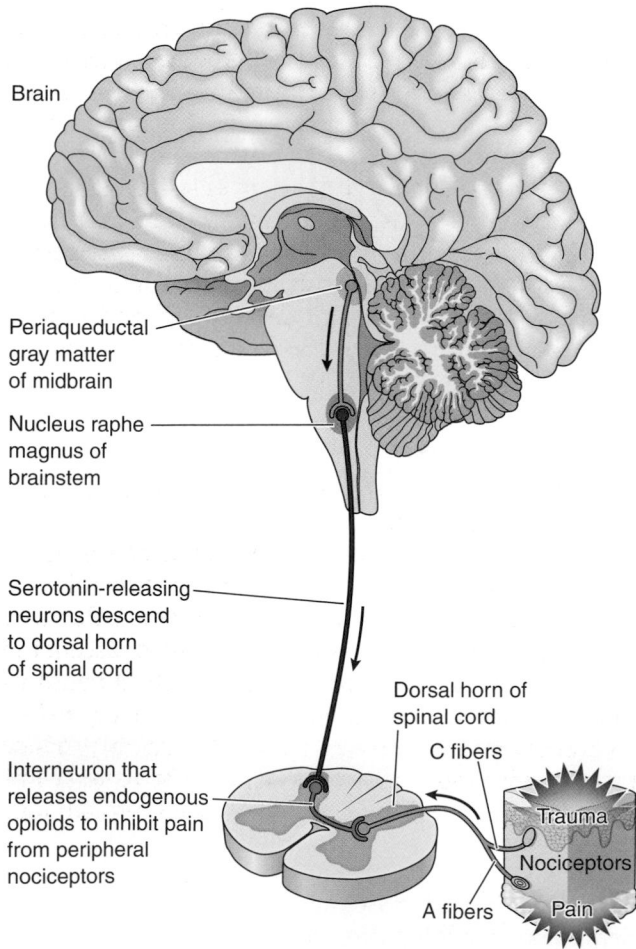

FIGURE 6-3. Pain inhibition by natural opioids. Stimulation of the PAG matter of the midbrain activates encephalin-releasing neurons that project to the NRM in the brainstem. Serotonin released from the NRM descends to the dorsal horn of the spinal cord, where it forms connections with inhibitory interneurons that release endogenous opioids. The endogenous opioids bind to opioid receptors in the axons of incoming C and A-delta fibers carrying pain signals from nociceptors activated in the periphery.

Stimulation of the PAG activates enkephalin-releasing neurons that project to the NRM in the brainstem.

From the NRM, serotonin-releasing neurons descend to the dorsal horn of the spinal cord, where there is a connection with interneurons in the spinal cord that release endogenous opioids. The natural opioids bind to and inhibit receptors in the axons of incoming C and A-delta fibers, which carry pain signals of nociceptors from the periphery.

The NRM is also specifically involved in migraine headaches, which are theorized to evolve from a serotonin deficiency that causes abnormal cerebral vasodilation and vasoconstriction. Migraine medications work by stimulating NRM neurons to release serotonin which, in turn, stimulate interneurons to release endogenous opioids.

Sensitization

The pain mechanism may be altered in some individuals, as well as in some diseases and conditions. For instance, some neurons may increase the rate or intensity of firing at the level of the dorsal root ganglion. Repeated or excessive stimulation of C fibers, a process known as wind-up, sensitizes the afferent neurons so that even mild stimulation may be perceived as painful. Sensitization exaggerates excitement of nerve fibers and impairs inhibitory (analgesic) interneuron influences at the level of the dorsal horn, brainstem, or both. An example of sensitization occurs when an individual lightly rubs a certain area of skin over and over. At first this is sensed as slight tactile contact. However, with continual light rubbing the skin becomes hypersensitive. The afferent neurons are repeatedly stimulated until eventually they become extremely sensitive to any kind of tactile contact.

Dermatomes and Myotomes

Spinal nerves have motor fibers and sensory fibers. The motor fibers innervate certain muscles, whereas the sensory fibers innervate certain areas of skin. A dermatome is a skin area innervated by the sensory fibers of a single nerve root; a myotome is a group of muscles primarily innervated by the motor fibers of a single nerve root. Dermatome and myotome patterns of distribution are relatively consistent from person to person (see Fig. 6-4). Dermatomes are named according to the spinal nerve roots that supply them and can be

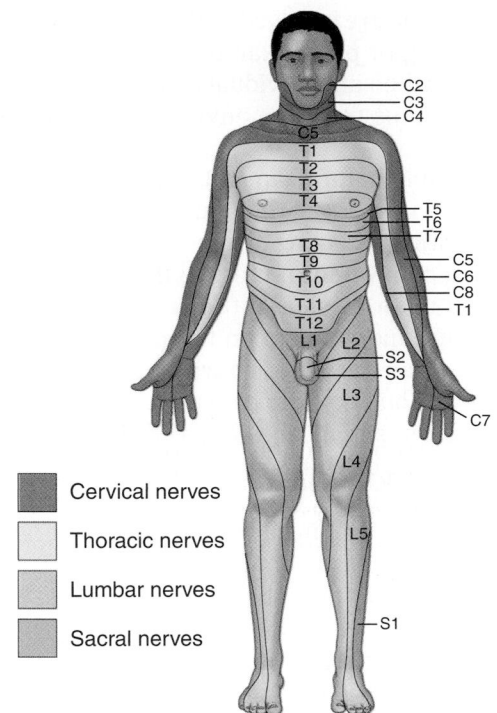

Figure 6-4. Sensory dermatomes. A dermatome is the area of skin supplied by nerves originated from a spinal nerve. (From Thompson, G. S. (2013). *Understanding anatomy and physiology.* Philadelphia: F.A. Davis Company, with permission.)

correlated with spinal nerve dysfunction. For example, with impingement of the 5th cervical spinal nerve (C5), the patient complains of pain in the area of the C5 dermatome, which encompasses the shoulder and upper arm. A clinician can correlate the dermatome of the patient's pain with the specific spinal nerve that is involved in the disorder.

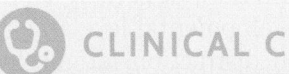 CLINICAL CONCEPT

Sciatica, a cause of low back pain, is a common reason for individuals to seek primary health care. The pain arises from sciatic nerve impingement. The patient complains of pain in the region of the dermatome, which originates in the L4–S1 region of the back and radiates down the posterior leg.

Basic Pathophysiologic Concepts Related to Pain

The mechanism of pain is complex and theories have provided a framework for our understanding. Pain diminishes the quality of life and patients look to the clinician for relief. In order to implement interventions that can alleviate pain, the source and process need to be understood.

Pain Theories

In 1965, researchers Melzack and Wall developed the landmark **gate control theory,** which revolutionized our understanding of pain and changed how clinicians treat pain. According to this theory, there are two major points:

1. Pain is not necessarily proportional to the amount of tissue injury.
2. Sensation travels both to and from the brain.

Before the development of this theory, only the central nervous system, spinal cord, and brain were recognized as integral parts of the pain experience. The gate control theory proposed that tissue injury and inflammation stimulates specific pain fibers in peripheral nerves and sends signals to the spinal cord. In the spinal cord, the neural signals are influenced by other neurons, where the pain signal can become dampened or amplified. The signals then continue up to the brain, where interpretation occurs. Signals can also come down from the brain to the neurons in the spinal cord and modulate the pain.

Further research, however, demonstrated that the gate control theory was not a complete explanation of the pain experience, as it did not explain chronic pain syndromes, phantom limb pain, and other types of pain without an obvious cause. This prompted Melzack to develop the **neuromatrix theory** of pain, which emphasizes the brain's influence in experiences of pain. According to this theory, pain is not simply a sensory experience but one that involves our thoughts, past experiences, emotions, and stress. Our understanding of pain now involves both of these theories—and there is still further research needed.

Gate Control Theory

The gate control theory involves impulse conduction of pain through a three-neuron chain. The first neuron is an afferent neuron, which is stimulated by pain in the periphery, and an impulse travels into the spinal cord. The second neuron is an interneuron that is influenced by descending nerve tracts from the brain or ascending nerve tracts from the spinal cord. The third neuron's impulse projects upward into the brain (see Fig. 6-5).

According to the gate control theory, to produce pain, A-delta and C fiber afferent nociceptive nerve impulses within the three-neuron chain go through four processes:

1. transduction
2. transmission
3. modulation
4. perception.

Transduction is the initial process of converting painful stimuli into neuronal impulses. Transduction occurs after direct tissue injury or inflammation. In traumatic tissue injury, nociceptors are directly stimulated. In tissue inflammation, chemical mediators such

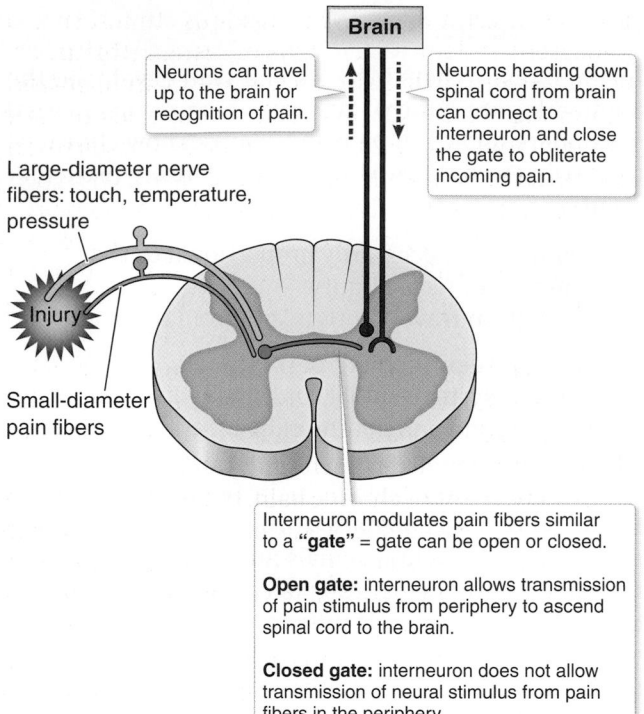

FIGURE 6-5. Gate control mechanism. When large nerve fibers from the periphery are stimulated, small diameter pain fibers cannot get through the interneuron gate. The gate is closed. Therefore, when injury occurs, rubbing, cold treatment, or shaking off pain can dull or obliterate the pain. When pain nerve fibers from the periphery are stimulated and the interneuron gate is open, the neural stimulus is transmitted up the spinal cord to the brain for recognition. Pain can also be influenced by descending spinal nerves from the brain down into the spinal cord to the interneuron. The descending neural pathway can close the interneuron gate. This is how distraction and endorphins can obliterate pain.

as prostaglandins (PGs) stimulate the nociceptor. After the nociceptor is stimulated, impulses are produced along the nerve's axon to enter the dorsal horn of the spinal cord. The travel of the impulse along the axon is **transmission.** In the dorsal horn of the spinal cord, synaptic connections occur between the incoming afferent neuron and an interneuron, which can be influenced by ascending and descending nerve tracts from the brain. The influence on the afferent neuron by other neurons in the spinal cord is **modulation.** The spinothalamic tract, which travels from the spinal cord up to the brain, is the most prominent nociceptive pathway in the spinal cord.

Modulation is the effect of the interneuron on the afferent neuron; the effect can be amplification or dampening of pain. According to the gate control theory, the afferent neuron encounters a "gate" when it connects with an interneuron in the spinal cord. The gate is the interneuron's influence on the afferent neuron, which can be negative or positive. The interneuron can be influenced by descending pathways from the brain or ascending pathways from the spinal cord. If the gate is opened, pain is amplified; if the gate is closed, pain may be dampened. Neurotransmitters released by

the interneuron are involved in the gate's amplification or dampening of pain. Examples of pain modulation can be seen when an individual experiences an obvious painful stimulus from the environment but does not feel the pain.

For example, neurotransmitters called endorphins are negative influences that dampen an afferent neuron's pain stimulus. Long distance runners, who do not experience pain when running to the point of exhaustion, often report a pleasant feeling due to the effect of endorphin modulation on the pain stimulus. Pain modulation can also be seen when a person walks on hot coals without experiencing pain. The afferent neuron brings the signal of pain from the feet into the spinal cord, but the influence of an interneuron modulates the pain signal, in essence closing the gate. The interneuron is influenced by descending nerve pathways from the brain that conduct impulses from thoughts that distract the person from feeling the pain.

Conversely, a person can experience a minor pain stimulus but perceive it as extremely painful. In this case, the afferent nociceptive stimulus is minor but the interneuron is open to the influence of descending pathways from the brain that augment the experience of pain. The person cognitively perceives the pain is extreme, and this influences the pain experience. This often occurs in persons who overreact when receiving an intramuscular injection. The injection in reality is a minor pinching sensation; however, many persons perceive it as severe because of cognitive influences on the experience.

Perception of pain is the conscious awareness of the experience of pain. Perception results from impulse transmission up to the thalamus, limbic system, midbrain, cerebral cortex, and reticular system. This is where the individual interprets the pain. An individual's perception of pain is influenced by a multitude of factors, including developmental level, memory, past experiences, attention, distraction, fatigue, fear, stress, and mood states such as anxiety and depression.

The Neuromatrix Theory

The neuromatrix theory of pain developed by Melzack in 1990 highlights the brain's role in pain sensation. Melzack developed the theory mainly because the gate control theory cannot explain pain experienced with no apparent pathological source. For example, **phantom limb pain** commonly occurs after a patient undergoes an amputation—burning, cramping, and shooting pains are experienced by 70% of amputees long after the amputation has occurred. Patients experience pain in the absent extremity as though the extremity is still part of the body, and the pain is often intractable with no effective treatment. Phantom limb pain, particularly, illustrates the complex role of the brain in modulating the body's sensation of pain.

The neuromatrix theory proposes that pain is a multidimensional experience produced from characteristic neurosignature patterns arising from nerve impulses generated by a widely distributed neural network, called the body-self neuromatrix, located in the brain. Similar to the gate control theory, the brain can be triggered by sensory input from nociceptors in the periphery, but in the neuromatrix theory the brain can also generate painful sensations independently. Nociceptive stimulation is not a prerequisite for pain sensation.

The neuromatrix is genetically determined and shaped by sensory input during the individual's life. The neuromatrix is the brain's perception of the body. It consists of complex neural networks that are built into the brain from birth and develop throughout life. With time, all sensory input from the body undergoes repeated processing so that characteristic patterns of input, known as a neurosignature, are impressed on the brain.

With these principles in mind, phantom limb pain can be understood. The absence of sensory input does not stop the brain from generating messages about missing body parts. The body's extremities are part of the neurosignature impressed upon the neuromatrix. Well-developed neurological pathways involving the extremities have been present in the brain since before birth. The extremities are part of the neurosignature and the brain still perceives the extremities and their pain.

Types of Pain

The major types of pain include acute, chronic, and neuropathic pain. Acute pain is experienced immediately after tissue injury. Chronic pain is a prolonged pain sensation that may or may not be related to tissue injury. Neuropathic pain is often difficult for the patient to describe; it is a feeling of pain perpetuated by dysfunctional neurons. Neuropathic pain is reported by the patient in many different ways, from numbness to sharp, piercing pain.

Acute Pain

Acute pain results from new onset of tissue injury or inflammation. Acute pain is sudden, lasts hours to days, and resolves with healing of the disorder. Acute pain plays a biologically protective role because it facilitates tissue repair and healing by making the injured area and surrounding tissue hypersensitive to all kinds of stimuli. This, in turn, makes the injured individual avoid exposing the area to external stimuli, thereby allowing for an undisturbed healing process. Acute pain occurs following surgery and in disorders such as myocardial infarction, fracture, and appendicitis.

Chronic Pain

Chronic pain persists beyond the expected time for a given disease process or injury and is defined as having a duration greater than 6 months. Chronic pain may arise as a result of sustained noxious stimuli such as persistent inflammation. Cancer, osteoarthritis, and rheumatological diseases such as rheumatoid arthritis commonly cause chronic pain. Unlike acute pain, chronic pain is debilitating and does not serve any biological or protective function. It is pain that initially occurs because of a pathological condition; however, it is not relieved. Chronic pain continues because of a long-lasting pathological condition, although it may not have an apparent associated pathological condition. In chronic pain, the pain eventually becomes the patient's focus. For example, fibromyalgia is an example of a syndrome of chronic musculoskeletal pain with no readily apparent pathological tissue; yet, it is defined as a condition of chronic pain.

In some cases of chronic pain, the neuromatrix theory is well illustrated. Chronic pain can begin as acute pain caused by acute pathology. After the acute pathology resolves, chronic pain can persist and continue to be perceived by the brain. This is a complex condition that is difficult to treat but can be explained by the neuromatrix theory. The pain continues because its neural network evolves into a neurosignature that becomes imprinted onto the brain. There is no pathological condition, yet the pain is still perceived. Commonly, chronic pain does not respond to conventional analgesic treatments.

Neuropathic Pain

Neuropathic pain is caused by injury or malfunction of the spinal cord and/or peripheral nerves. Neuropathic pain is typically a burning, tingling, shooting, stinging, or pins and needles sensation, often referred to as **paresthesia**. Some people also complain of a stabbing, piercing, cutting, and drilling pain.

Neuropathic pain is a unique kind of pain because it cannot be described as either acute or chronic. It can occur within days, weeks, or months of an injury and tends to occur in waves of frequency and intensity. Neuropathic pain is diffuse and occurs at the level or below the level of injury, most often in the legs, back, feet, thighs, and toes, although it can also occur in the upper body. Some disorders that cause neuropathic pain include postherpetic neuralgias, spinal nerve radiculopathy, diabetic polyneuropathy, postsurgical pain syndromes, and complex regional pain syndrome. Neuropathic pain is very difficult to treat. Often alternate therapies such as transcutaneous electrical neural stimulation (TENS), antidepressants, or acupuncture are needed to provide relief.

Sources of Pain

There are various sources of pain; some sources are obvious, such as traumatic body injury. However, some sources of pain may not be readily apparent, yet they are clearly perceived by the brain. Pain from areas rich in nociceptors is easy to locate. However, some areas of the body can be painful because of damage to an internal organ that sends neural impulses far from the origin of injury; this is called referred pain.

Cutaneous Pain

Injury to the skin or superficial tissues causes cutaneous pain. Cutaneous nociceptors terminate just below the skin, where a high concentration of nerve endings exists. Cutaneous nerve endings produce a well-defined, localized pain of short duration. Examples of injuries that produce cutaneous pain include minor cuts and bruises, first-degree burns, and lacerations.

Deep Somatic Pain

Deep somatic pain originates from ligaments, tendons, bones, blood vessels, and nerves themselves. These areas contain small numbers of somatic nociceptors. The scarcity of pain receptors in these areas produces a dull, poorly localized pain of longer duration than cutaneous pain; examples include sprains and broken bones. Myofascial pain is a type of somatic pain that is usually caused by tender points in muscles, tendons, and fascia; it may be localized or referred.

Visceral Pain

Visceral pain is defined as pain emanating from deep organs, usually resulting from disease processes. It is much different than cutaneous nociception because of the small number of nociceptors. Visceral pain can be vague and not well localized and is usually described as pressurelike, deep squeezing, dull, or diffuse. Most visceral pain occurs because of distension of hollow muscular walled organs such as the gastrointestinal tract, genitourinary tract, and gallbladder. The nerves within an organ are stretched with distention, and this signal is interpreted as pain by the brain.

Inflammation, as in cystitis or pancreatitis, is also a cause of visceral pain. This type of visceral pain commonly occurs because of PGs and other inflammatory mediators that are produced by tissues in inflammation. PGs cause edema, pain, and fever, as well as continually stimulate inflammation. Visceral pain can also be associated with systemic symptoms such as malaise, weakness, and nausea.

Referred Pain

Referred pain occurs when the pain response occurs at a distance from the actual pathology. It is a hallmark of visceral pain (see Fig. 6-6). Referred pain occurs when nerve fibers from regions of high sensory input, such as the skin, and nerve fibers from regions of normally low sensory input, such as the internal organs, converge on the same levels of the spinal cord.

The best known example of referred pain is pain experienced during myocardial infarction. Nerves from damaged heart tissue convey pain signals to spinal cord levels C4–T4 on the left side, which happen to be the same levels that receive sensation from the left side of the chest and part of the left arm. The brain doesn't have a strong neurosignature of the heart but it does have a strong impression from the adjoining thoracic skin and muscles, so it interprets the signals from the heart as pain in the chest and left arm.

Referred pain often occurs at the shoulder from irritation of the diaphragm muscle. A ruptured organ beneath the diaphragm gives off escaped air that stays beneath the diaphragm and acts as an irritant. An inflamed organ can enlarge and also irritate the diaphragm. There is not a strong neurosignature of the diaphragm muscle in the brain. If the diaphragm is irritated, the patient feels shoulder pain. This occurs because the diaphragm is innervated by the sensory

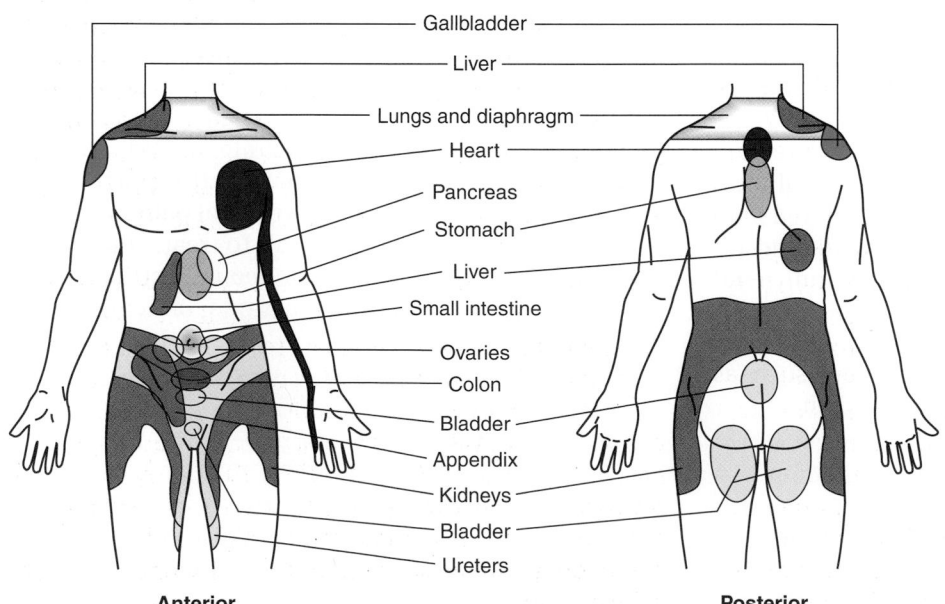

Anterior **Posterior**

— Gallbladder —
— Liver —
— Lungs and diaphragm —
— Heart —
— Pancreas
— Stomach
— Liver —
— Small intestine —
— Ovaries —
— Colon —
— Bladder —
— Appendix —
— Kidneys —
— Bladder —
— Ureters —

FIGURE 6-6. Sites of referred pain. (From Williams, L., & Hopper, P. (2011). *Understanding medical-surgical nursing* (4th ed.). Philadelphia: F.A. Davis Company, with permission.)

fibers of the cervical spinal nerves C3 through C5. These nerves also innervate the shoulder muscles and skin. When there are pain signals from C3 through C5, the brain interprets the signals as coming from the shoulder because it has a better neurosignature of the shoulder muscles and skin compared with the diaphragm.

Phantom Pain

Phantom pain is the sensation of pain originating in an amputated part of the body. Patients describe a burning, stinging, or cramping pain, or they may describe a feeling that the missing body part is positioned awkwardly or painfully. Phantom pain is constant and is most intense right after the amputation. The pain usually develops within the first month after amputation and most often develops in patients who had a high degree of pain preamputation. The pain becomes intermittent and resolves with time, although some patients can still experience phantom pain years after the amputation. Phantom pain is usually worse at night, after the extremity has been in a dependent position, and it can be worsened by anxiety and stress. The neuromatrix theory explains the reason for phantom limb pain best. The body's extremities are part of the neurosignature impressed upon the neuromatrix since birth. Well-developed neurological pathways are part of the neurosignature and the brain still perceives the extremities despite their amputation.

Pain Assessment

It is important for the clinician to listen to the patient's complaint of pain, including its quality, duration, associated features, and alleviating factors. Pain is referred to as the fifth vital sign because its assessment is so important to the patient's health. A thorough history is necessary, as is careful physical assessment. The clinician should allow the patient to point to the area of pain before the physical exam; this area should always be examined last.

Clinical Presentation

Pain is subjective, and pain behaviors differ from person to person. Some clients are stoic and suppressed in their expression, whereas others can exaggerate their pain. Nonverbal and behavioral expressions are not consistent or reliable indicators of pain intensity or quality, and they should not be used to determine the presence or absence of pain. However, because pain is a subjective feeling, the clinician cannot assume the client is inaccurate in his or her description, which is why assessment relies heavily on the client report.

Pain is often accompanied by symptoms and physiologic conditions that offer diagnostic clues of

---

BOX 6-1. OLDCART

Use the OLDCART mnemonic to assess pain, its features, and its treatment.

- **O**nset: When did the pain begin?
- **L**ocation: Where does it hurt? Can you point to where it hurts?
- **D**uration: How long does it last?
- **C**haracteristics: What does it feel like?
- **A**ggravating factors/Does anything make it worse?
- **R**elieving factors: Does anything make it better?
- **T**reatment: Did anything make it better (pain medication, ice, heat)?

---

the complete clinical picture, including tachycardia, hypertension, tachypnea, mydriasis, diaphoresis, hypervigilance, anxiety, and increased muscle tone. To assess the pain and accompanying symptoms, the initial history can be obtained by using the **OLDCART** mnemonic, which prompts essential questions (see Box 6-1). OLDCART stands for onset, location, duration, characteristics, aggravating or relieving factors and associated symptoms, and treatment.

If a patient cannot find words to describe the character of pain, the clinician should prompt the patient by asking if the pain is throbbing, aching, stabbing, crushing, or piercing. It is common for the clinician to use a 0 to 10 scale, and ask the patient for a number that describes the pain's severity: 1 being mild to 10 being the worst pain ever experienced. The clinician should also ask about associated symptoms such as depression, anxiety, anorexia, nausea, and insomnia, which may affect the treatment plan.

Distinguishing Features of Pain
Pain can have certain characteristics and associated symptoms. When seeking a diagnosis, it is necessary to obtain a complete clinical picture of the problem by searching for additional distinguishing features of the pain. For example, myocardial pain can present like epigastric pain of esophagitis. However, distinguishing features that characterize the pain as cardiac include associated dyspnea, pallor, and diaphoresis. These associated features enable the clinician to make the specific diagnosis of cardiac chest pain (see Table 6-2).

Another example is colicky pain. **Colic** is a pain that occurs in waves; it builds to a peak and then declines. Spasmodic pain within hollow organs, such as the hyperperistalsis of gastroenteritis, can cause colicky pain. If the hollow organ is the intestine, its muscular walls can spasm to cause colicky pain. Other abdominal organs can also cause colicky pain, particularly the gallbladder in cholecystitis. A gallstone can develop in cholelithiasis. The muscular walls of the gallbladder or cystic duct can spasm around the gallstone, causing colicky pain.

TABLE 6-2. Distinguishing Features of Pain

Disorder	Pain	Associated Features
Myocardial infarction	Squeezing, crushing chest pain	Radiation into left arm Radiation possible up to jaw Radiation to back Dyspnea Diaphoresis Pallor Hypotension Levine's sign (fist to chest)
Peripheral arterial disease	Intermittent claudication of lower extremity	Cramping in the leg that occurs with a similar distance each time it is sensed Associated with pallor, paresthesias, cooler leg temperature Caused by lack of sufficient arterial flow
Pleuritis/Pneumonia/Pleurisy	Chest pain with coughing or deep breathing	Pleural friction rub heard on auscultation with stethoscope; squeaking or grating sounds of the pleural linings rubbing together that can be described as the sound made by treading on fresh snow
Cholecystitis/Cholelithiasis (inflammation of gallbladder with gallstone)	Biliary colic; intense pain comes on in waves	Nausea Vomiting Eructation (belching) Full feeling of stomach Tenderness of the right upper quadrant of the abdomen with palpation; called Murphy's sign
Appendicitis	Pain starts in the umbilical area then gradually becomes localized to right lower quadrant of abdomen; called McBurney's point	Extreme tenderness of right lower quadrant Signs of peritoneal inflammation include: • Patient wanting to remain stationary • Jumping, coughing that hurts abdomen • Psoas sign • Rebound tenderness • Guarding • Rovsing's sign • Rectal pain
Nephrolithiasis (kidney stone)	Colicky pain from costovertebral region around body into the groin	Patient cannot find a comfortable position; intense pain and hematuria
Uterine/Ovarian/Fallopian disorders	Pelvic or abdominal pain radiates down leg to inner thigh obturator nerve	Air can collect under the diaphragm, causing referred shoulder pain
Stomach/Duodenum Peptic Ulcer	Gnawing, burning pain	Pain occurs between meals; food soothes pain
Ruptured peptic ulcer/ Pancreatitis	Pain in umbilical area straight into the back	Tachycardia Nausea Vomiting Anxiety
Aortic aneurysm/Aortic dissection	Tearing, midthoracic pain	Pallor Hypotension Anxiety

Cholecystitis, appendicitis, pancreatitis, and diverticulitis are often referred to as disorders of the acute abdomen. The pain of the acute abdomen is unique because organs of the gastrointestinal tract that lie within the peritoneal cavity can cause inflammation of the peritoneal membrane. Peritoneal inflammation is intense and exhibited by abdominal muscle rigidity, a phenomenon called guarding. Rebound tenderness also occurs in peritoneal inflammation; pain occurs when the examiner palpates and lifts the hand from the abdomen. The patient with peritoneal inflammation usually cannot tolerate movement because it aggravates the peritoneal membrane. With this in mind, asking the patient to jump or cough usually makes the pain worse.

Interestingly, when there is rupture of an organ beneath the diaphragm, free air can escape from the organ and irritate the diaphragm. The diaphragm's irritation refers pain to the shoulder; it is necessary that the clinician recognize patterns of referred pain (see Fig. 6-6).

Some people who suffer from chronic pain conditions **catastrophize,** which is defined as an exaggerated negative orientation toward actual or anticipated pain experiences. These misinterpretations of pain can lead to a cycle of avoidance of activity, disuse, and disability.

In the face of continuing pain, people may have pain-related anxiety and feel they have no control over the pain. Depression is also common in patients with chronic pain. Prolonged pain is difficult to endure and, as a result, people undergo major affective and behavior changes, including increased or decreased appetite, restricted activity levels, social withdrawal, life role changes, poor sleep, chronic fatigue, and decreased concentration.

Physical Assessment

Following the history, a thorough examination should be conducted to detect sensory, motor, and coordination abnormalities. Patients with pain may have changes in the way they respond to touch. The motor exam may reveal increased or decreased muscle tone, weakened muscles, tremor, paralysis, hyporeflexia, or hyperreflexia. The patient's gait should be observed; abnormalities may be seen with musculoskeletal pathology, altered balance, or incoordination. Some types of pain, such as peritoneal irritation, decrease when the patient is stationary. When observing the patient, the examiner should note whether a position change lessens or worsens the pain. Other types of pain, such as pain associated with peristalsis, gallstones, and kidney stones, decrease when the patient moves.

The physical exam will also provide clues as to the amount of physical disability the patient experiences because of the pain. The clinician should be aware of

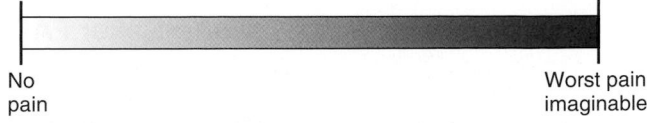

No pain   Worst pain imaginable

FIGURE 6-7. Visual analog scale. *(From Wilkinson, J., & Treas, L. (2011). Fundamentals of nursing, Volume 2 (2nd ed.).* Philadelphia. F.A. Davis Company, with permission.)

sensory dermatomes and myotomes, as these can assist in the localization of pain.

Diagnosis

Pain severity may be assessed by one of several reliable and valid tools for measuring pain, such as the McGill Pain Scale, which assesses the quality and severity of the patient's pain, and the visual analog scale (VAS), which assesses pain on a sliding scale. Clinicians commonly use the VAS by asking the patient to quantify his or her pain on a scale of 0 to 10, with 0 being no pain and 10 being most severe pain (see Fig. 6-7). The Wong-Baker FACES scale, which is commonly used for children and adults with cognitive impairment, is a variation of the VAS that is also valid and reliable (see Fig. 6-8).

Diagnostic tests may be employed based on clinical findings, patient disorders, or to guide treatment approaches. Various imaging techniques or nerve studies may also be helpful (see Box 6-2).

🩺 CLINICAL CONCEPT

Normal results on studies should not deter the clinician from diagnosing and treating the patient if the clinical exam is consistent with a certain type of pain. In fact, allowing the pain to continue without treatment may be associated with the initiation of chronic pain pathways.

Treatment

The World Health Organization's (WHO) Step Analgesic Ladder provides an approach to the pharmacological management of pain. Although it was initially created to treat cancer pain, this tool has been proposed as an excellent model for all types of pain (see Fig. 6-9). Some researchers have recently recommended modifications regarding the inclusion of a 4th step that describes procedures for intractable pain. The modification also adds opioids—tramadol, oxycodone, hydromorphone, and buprenorphine—and new ways of administering them, such as patient-controlled analgesia, epidural administration, and transdermal patch.

Wong-Baker FACES® Pain Rating Scale

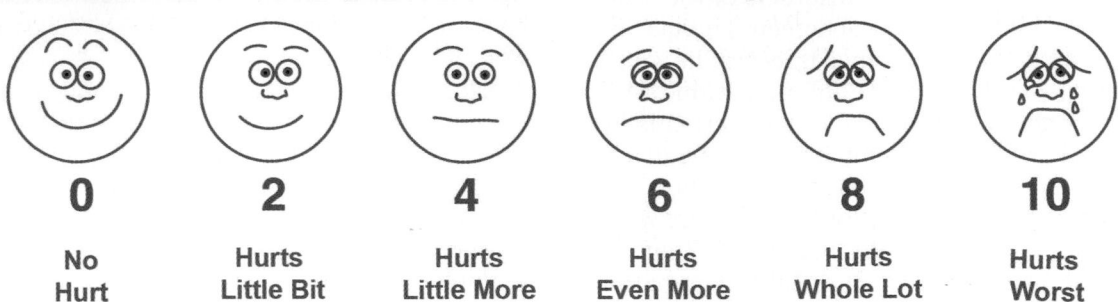

0	2	4	6	8	10
No Hurt	Hurts Little Bit	Hurts Little More	Hurts Even More	Hurts Whole Lot	Hurts Worst

FIGURE 6-8. Wong-Baker FACES Pain Rating Scale. *(www.wongbakerFACES.org. © 1983. Wong-Baker FACES Foundation. Used with permission.)*

BOX 6-2. Diagnostic Studies for Pain

There are a wide variety of diagnostic studies for pain because of the many different possible causes. The etiology of pain influences the manner of treatment.

- **Blood tests:** Detect diabetes, vitamin deficiencies, and liver, kidney, or immune problems.
- **Nerve conduction study:** Shows how fast nerves are able to transmit impulses as well as the strength of those signals. Can determine whether or not muscle function is a problem or whether other neurological conditions are present, such as multiple sclerosis.
- **Electromyography:** Measures the electrical activity of one or more muscles while being flexed. Shows how well muscles are receiving impulses from nerves.
- **Nerve injection:** Injection of the nerve with lidocaine or bupivacaine (Marcaine) just above the site of involvement can be the most valuable diagnostic tool. The patient can define the extent of relief obtained from such an injection, which can be helpful in defining the zone of injury and expected relief from surgical release or excision.
- **Myelogram:** Contrast medium is injected into the subarachnoid space to visualize the spinal cord.
- **Ultrasound, computed tomography scan, or magnetic resonance imaging:** Checks whether cysts, tumors, blood vessels, or bones are compressing nerves.

WHO analgesic (pain relief) ladder

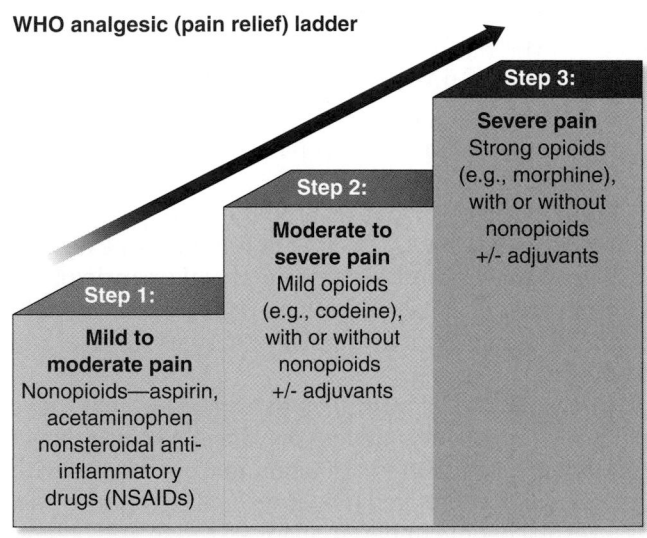

Step 1:
Mild to moderate pain
Nonopioids—aspirin, acetaminophen nonsteroidal anti-inflammatory drugs (NSAIDs)

Step 2:
Moderate to severe pain
Mild opioids (e.g., codeine), with or without nonopioids +/- adjuvants

Step 3:
Severe pain
Strong opioids (e.g., morphine), with or without nonopioids +/- adjuvants

FIGURE 6-9. WHO step ladder approach to analgesic treatment. The "pain ladder" is a term coined by the WHO to describe its guidelines for the use of drugs in pain management. Originally applied to the management of cancer pain, it is now widely used for the management of all types of pain. The general principle is to start with first step drugs and then to climb the ladder if pain is still present. The medications range from over-the-counter drugs with minimal side effects at the lowest rung to more powerful opioids at the highest rung. *(Adapted from WHO, http://www.who.int/cancer/palliative/painladder/en/ July 8, 2015)*

There are three major classes of pharmacological pain relievers: opioid, nonopioid, and adjuvant medications. The analgesic ladder proposes that treatment of pain should begin with a nonopioid medication such as a nonsteroidal anti-inflammatory drug (NSAID). If the pain is not properly controlled, a weak opioid should be introduced. If the use of this medication is insufficient to treat the pain, a more powerful opioid can be used instead. Two products belonging to the same category should not be used simultaneously, as they would not offer any different pain control while also increasing risk of adverse effects. When using multiple pain relievers, each drug should have a different mode of action. The WHO analgesic ladder recommends the use of adjuvant treatments such as antidepressants for neuropathic pain or for unrelieved pain associated with cancer.

The analgesic ladder can be used in a bidirectional fashion: the slower upward pathway for chronic pain and cancer pain and the faster downward direction for intense acute pain and uncontrolled chronic pain. The ladder can be used to ascend slowly one step at a time in the case of chronic pain and, if necessary, increase the rate of climb according to the intensity of the pain. Once pain is controlled, the WHO recommends that the patient "step down" on the ladder.

Opioids

Opioids are powerful medications that may be used alone or in conjunction with other analgesics. Table 6-3 displays the names and uses of some of the most commonly prescribed opioids.

Morphine is the prototypical opioid and can be administered in many forms. It can produce analgesia, euphoria, and sedation. Side effects include diminished concentration ability, nausea, vomiting, feelings of bodily warmth, heaviness of the extremities, dry mouth, pruritus, and respiratory depression. It is effective against pain from skeletal muscles, joints, viscera, and skin structures.

Morphine is most effective when given before the painful stimulus; this approach plays a protective role by preventing sensitization. In general, controlled-release opioids given on a scheduled basis are recommended for patients with persistent or continuous pain to promote constant levels of analgesia, prevent fluctuations in blood levels, and avoid adverse events associated with high peak opioid levels.

ALERT! Opioids have high abuse potential. Addiction, tolerance, and physical dependence can occur.

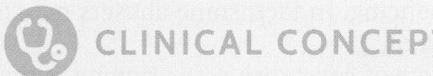
CLINICAL CONCEPT

Morphine can cause respiratory depression, particularly in patients with lung disease. It is commonly administered to patients in hospice who need palliative care.

TABLE 6-3. Commonly Used Opioid Analgesics		
Drug	**Indication**	**Side Effects**
Morphine	Severe pain Prototypical opioid medication	Drowsiness Euphoria Respiratory depression
Codeine	Moderate pain 10% of people lack the enzyme needed to make codeine active (CYP2D6)	Greater amounts of nausea and vomiting compared with other opioids Drowsiness Euphoria Respiratory depression
Hydromorphone	Severe pain Duration of action is slightly less than morphine	Drowsiness Euphoria Respiratory depression
Meperidine	Severe pain	Repeated dosing not recommended as accumulation of meperidine metabolites can cause central nervous system excitation and high risk of seizures
Methadone	Severe pain Weaning off heroin in a detoxification program Good oral potency with a long plasma half-life (24–36 hours)	Drowsiness Dizziness Nausea Vomiting Hypotension Constipation
Oxycodone	Severe pain	Drowsiness Euphoria Respiratory depression
Oxymorphone	Severe pain	Drowsiness Euphoria Respiratory depression
Fentanyl	Severe pain May be administered via IV, SQ, transmucosal, epidural, and intrathecal route Short duration of action compared with morphine	Diarrhea Drowsiness Urinary retention Weakness Dyspnea Indigestion Dry mouth

Complications of Opioid Use

Complications of opioid use include substance abuse, tolerance, withdrawal, and physical dependence. For this reason, opioids should be used sparingly in the lowest dose that can alleviate the pain.

Substance Abuse. Substance abuse refers to the dysfunctional use of a substance in amounts or methods not condoned by health-care professionals. Patients with problems of substance abuse may suffer from pain, but many abusers feign the amount of pain they are experiencing. In fact, some abusers may not have any pain at all.

Predictors of substance abuse among patients with chronic pain include a familial or personal history of substance abuse; history of legal problems or criminal activity; regular contact with high-risk people; problems with past employers, family, or friends; medication craving; risk-taking or thrill-seeking behavior; heavy tobacco use; and history of severe depression or anxiety. There are many psychosocial and behavioral factors involved in substance abuse, and patients require a consultation with an addiction specialist who can provide ongoing care.

 CLINICAL CONCEPT

Patients who are prescribed opioid medications have the potential for abuse. Appropriate screening should take place with the Screener Opioid Assessment for Patients with Pain before initiating drug therapy.

Opioid Withdrawal, Tolerance and Physical Dependence. **Addiction** is a primary, chronic, neurological disease with genetic, psychosocial, and environmental factors influencing its development and manifestations. It is characterized by behavior that includes one or more of the following:

- impaired control over drug use
- compulsive use of drug
- continued use despite harm from using the drug
- craving of the drug.

Tolerance is a state of adaptation in which chronic exposure to a drug causes gradual decreasing results over time. As a person takes opioids for an extended period of time, he or she becomes less sensitive to it and requires higher dosages to achieve the same effect. Receptors in the brain become less sensitive with continued use of opioids. This means that patients need more opioid to achieve the same effect with continued use. When the body can no longer make enough natural opioids to satisfy the less sensitive receptors, the body becomes dependent on the external source. This is physical dependence, a state of adaptation that is

manifested by a drug withdrawal syndrome that can be produced by abrupt cessation, rapid dose reduction, decreasing blood level of the drug, or administration of an antagonist.

For patients who have been on long-term opioid agonists such as morphine, there is a normal physiologic tolerance to the drug. The patient becomes habituated to a certain dosage of opioid and reliant on the drug. Withdrawal occurs when the patient develops systemic symptoms in response to a lack of adequate opioid dosage needed by the body. Symptoms of withdrawal can be seen within hours of missing a regular dose, including nausea, vomiting, tachycardia, sweating, restlessness, irritability, insomnia, lacrimation, and rhinorrhea. The extent of symptoms will depend upon the drug dose and how long it has been taken. Tapering the medication slowly over several weeks can help minimize the intensity of symptoms. Clonidine may also be used to treat withdrawal.

Naloxone is a drug that helps to counter the effects of opiate overdose because it has an extremely high affinity for opioid receptors in the central nervous system. Naloxone is a competitive antagonist that blocks opioid attachment to neural receptors. It is specifically used to counteract life-threatening depression of the central nervous system and respiratory system.

ALERT! Naloxone will cause rapid onset of withdrawal symptoms in patients who use opioids.

 CLINICAL CONCEPT

Patients with opioid addiction require rehabilitation where a multidisciplinary approach to care can be delivered. Methadone, a synthetic opioid, is commonly administered to prevent the symptoms of opioid withdrawal. Methadone does not have the euphoric effects of opioids such as heroin. It is commonly administered in decreasing dosages to slowly wean the patient off opioids and diminish effects of withdrawal.

Nonopioid Analgesics

Nonopioid analgesics include acetaminophen (Tylenol) and NSAIDs such as aspirin, ibuprofen, naproxen sodium, and celecoxib. All of these agents except for acetaminophen work by blocking cyclooxygenase enzymes (COX 1 and 2) that prevent the release of prostaglandins (PGs) from white blood cells and inflammatory tissue. PGs are chemical mediators involved in physiologic processes and the inflammation reaction. Some PGs are necessary for gastric mucus production, renal perfusion, and thrombus formation; these PGs utilize the COX 1 enzyme pathway. Other PGs cause edema, pain, inflammation, and dysmenorrheal uterine contractions; these PGs utilize the COX 2 enzyme pathway (see Fig. 6-10). NSAIDs are nonselective cyclooxygenase pathway inhibitors that block both COX 1 and 2 enzymes. Because the NSAIDs are nonselective, they can cause some adverse physiologic effects, including diminished gastric mucus and ulceration, decreased renal perfusion, and diminished clotting. Patients who routinely use NSAIDs should be counseled about the side effects of gastric irritation, clotting deficit, and renal insufficiency (see Fig. 6-10).

Celecoxib is a selective COX 2 enzyme inhibitor. Specific inhibition of the COX 2 enzyme pathway blocks PGs that cause edema, inflammation, and pain. COX 2 inhibitors were developed so that the selectivity of the drug would avoid the adverse side effects of the nonselective NSAIDs. However, recent research and clinical experience has shown that those who used the COX 2 inhibitor rofecoxib (Vioxx®) had an increased risk of myocardial infarction, strokes, and deep vein thrombosis. Rofecoxib was taken off the market, but celecoxib (Celebrex®) is a COX 2 agent that is still available and prescribed.

Adjuvant Medications

Adjuvant medications are used to amplify the analgesic effect of pain medication. Antidepressants and anticonvulsants are often used as adjuvant medications, but their exact mechanism in pain relief is not clear. Local anesthetic agents and corticosteroids can also assist in pain relief.

Antidepressants

Antidepressants can increase synaptic serotonin, norepinephrine, and dopamine levels. They also have been found to enhance the effect of analgesics in some types of neuropathic pain. Tricyclic antidepressants (TCAs), however, have many unpleasant and potentially dangerous side effects, limiting their use in some patients. Older adults, for example, are prone to toxic effects from TCAs.

Serotonin-norepinephrine reuptake inhibitors have also proven to be effective for treating some types of neuropathic pain. They are safer to use than TCAs and are a better option for patients with cardiac disease. The relative risk for withdrawal because of side effects is low and there is no need for drug level monitoring. Side effects include sedation, confusion, hypertension, nausea, vomiting, constipation, loss of appetite, and weakness.

ALERT! Overdose of tricyclic antidepressants is often fatal.

Local Anesthetics

Local anesthetics produce anesthesia by inhibiting excitation of nerve endings or by blocking conduction in peripheral nerves. This is achieved by anesthetics reversibly binding to and inactivating sodium channels. Sodium influx through these channels is necessary for the depolarization of nerve cell membranes and subsequent propagation of impulses along the course of the nerve. When a nerve loses depolarization and capacity to propagate an impulse, the individual loses sensation in the area supplied by the nerve. Commonly used agents include lidocaine, mepivacaine, prilocaine, cocaine, procaine, and benzocaine.

Injected Corticosteroids

Steroids are the most potent anti-inflammatory agents available and are used to reduce inflammation of the

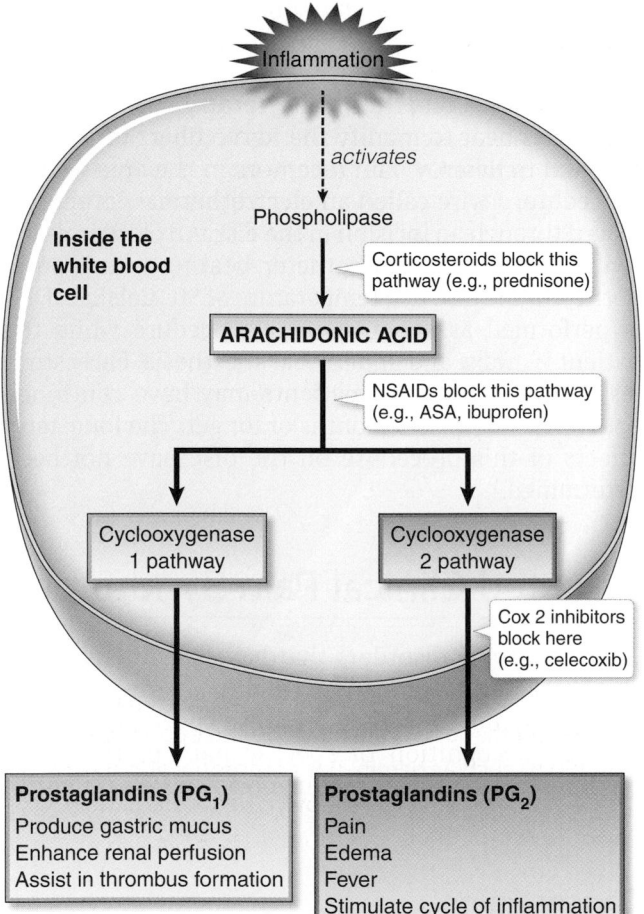

FIGURE 6-10. Inflammation pathways of PGs and sites of anti-inflammatory drug action. After inflammation stimulates the inflammatory reaction, white blood cells produce PGs via the cyclooxygenase pathways. The cyclooxygenase 1 pathway produces prostaglandins (PG1s) that assist the body in performing significant functions. The cyclooxygenase 2 pathway produces prostaglandins (PG2s) that cause uncomfortable side effects of inflammation. Anti-inflammatory drugs block the formation of PGs at the sites shown. Corticosteroids and NSAIDs block the formation of both types of PGs. Therefore, corticosteroids and NSAIDs block gastric mucus production, decrease renal perfusion, and inhibit thrombus formation. COX 2 inhibitors can specifically block the PG2s that cause the uncomfortable side effects of inflammation.

tissue compressing the affected nerves, as well as to reduce neuronal edema. Corticosteroids can be injected into joints to treat musculoskeletal disorders, as well as into the epidural space to reduce spinal nerve root impingement from spinal degenerative conditions such as disc herniation. Prolotherapy, an injection of lidocaine and a corticosteroid into affected muscles and joints, can be used to treat mechanical low back pain and fibromyalgia.

 CLINICAL CONCEPT

Epidural administration of local anesthetic and corticosteroid is often used for intractable back pain.

Anticonvulsants

A trial of antiepileptic medication may be beneficial for a wide range of neuropathic symptoms, including trigeminal neuralgia, painful diabetic neuropathy, and postherpetic neuralgia. Carbamazepine, gabapentin, and lamotrigine are anticonvulsant agents that are effective in neuropathic pain. The exact physiologic mechanism by which these drugs work is not clearly understood.

Nonpharmacological Pain Management

Nonpharmacological methods may be used alone or in conjunction with pharmacological agents for pain relief. Nonpharmacological activities usually have a low-risk profile. Some are thought to be effective because the treatment activates the body's own endorphins and enkephalins. Therapies include acupuncture, TENS, and intradiscal electrothermal therapy (IDET).

Acupuncture

Acupuncture is an ancient Chinese medical intervention that involves the stimulation of the body using thin, solid metallic needles that are inserted by hand. The aim of the procedure is to improve levels of qi (pronounced chi), which practitioners believe is the energy force behind all life, and to restore balance in the opposing forces of yin and yang. The needles are placed along specific, invisible energy channels called meridians that run along the length of the body.

Research studies have shown acupuncture can help relieve neuropathic pain associated with spinal cord injury, chronic pelvic pain, hot flashes associated with menopause, breathlessness associated with chronic obstructive pulmonary disease, and postchemotherapy fatigue. More research is needed to investigate acupuncture's benefits for other disorders.

Transcutaneous Electrical Nerve Stimulation

TENS is the use of low voltage electrical current to help relieve pain. In TENS therapy, a small, battery-operated device delivers electrical current through the skin via electrodes placed near the source of pain. It is theorized that the electricity stimulates nerves in the affected area and sends signals to the brain that scramble normal pain perception. TENS has been shown to be helpful to relieve pain of diabetic neuropathy, degenerative disk disease, and dysmenorrhea.

Guided Imagery

Guided imagery is a program of directed thoughts and suggestions that guide the imagination toward a relaxed, focused state. Instructors, videos, or scripts assist the patient through this process. Guided imagery is based on the concept that the body and mind are connected. Using all the senses, the body can respond as though the imagined scenario is real. Guided imagery promotes relaxation, which can lower blood pressure and reduce other problems related to stress. It has been used for weight loss, smoking cessation, and pain management.

Intradiscal Electrothermal Therapy

IDET uses heat to modify the nerve fibers of a spinal disc and to destroy pain receptors in the area. In this procedure, a wire called an electrothermal catheter is placed through an incision in the disc. An electrical current passes through the catheter, heating a small outer portion of the disc to a temperature of 90° Celsius. IDET is performed as an outpatient procedure while the patient is awake and under local anesthesia. Early studies indicate that some patients may have continued pain relief for up to 6 months or longer. The long-term effects of this procedure on the disc have not been determined.

Selected Clinical Pain Syndromes

There are some disorders that have specific patterns and characteristics of pain. The clinician needs to recognize the manifestations of these specific pain syndromes. Recognition of specific pain patterns and qualities can assist in the diagnosis and treatment of these disorders.

Cancer Pain

One out of every three persons suffering from cancer endures pain. Cancer pain can be dull, aching, or sharp. It can be intermittent or constant and result from the cancerous lesion or the treatment.

Tumors can cause pain by putting pressure on or destroying adjacent tissue. Cancer cells secrete enzymes and inflammatory mediators that penetrate and irritate tissues. Enzymatic destruction of adjoining tissues is also common in cancer. Pain can come from the primary tumor itself or from other areas in the body where the cancer has metastasized. Tumors secrete chemical mediators such as endothelin-1, which is a strong vasoconstrictor that decreases circulation to certain areas. Tumors also secrete PGs and substance P, which can cause pain, edema, and constant inflammation.

Some cancer treatments, such as chemotherapy, can cause painful side effects such as mouth sores, diarrhea, and nerve damage. Radiation treatment in cancer can leave a burning sensation in the region that is radiated. Surgery can leave painful scars along with a burning sensation.

Bone pain is a debilitating form of pain that is often caused by the metastasis of cancer. The outer periosteal layer of bone tissue is highly pain-sensitive and a frequent cause of pain. Tumors within the center of bone involve the endosteal and haversian nerve supply. Interior tumors secrete enzymes and inflammatory mediators that stimulate nociceptors and produce dull, diffuse pain. When the cancer cells have established themselves within bone, the mechanical dynamics of the bone matrix become weaker as skeletal strength decreases. This leads to several other complications throughout the body, including pain, that decrease the patient's quality of life.

Spinal Nerve Radiculopathy

Spinal nerve radiculopathy, also called radiculitis, is spinal nerve impingement, which is a common cause of low back pain when the sciatic nerve is entrapped by a herniated vertebral disk. Often this is caused by a traumatic twisting of the lower back or from cumulative trauma on the vertebrae. The pain of sciatic nerve radiculopathy, commonly called sciatica, occurs at the lumbosacral region with radiation down the leg. The patient may also report numbness and tingling in the foot and may have decreased motion and weight-bearing ability in the leg.

Cervical radiculopathy is another common site of spinal nerve impingement. This is often caused by herniation of a cervical disc that places pressure on the spinal cord. There is pain in the neck that radiates down the arm. The patient may report numbness in the hand or fingers and may have weakness in the extremity.

Diabetic Peripheral Neuropathy

Diabetic peripheral neuropathy affects both sensory and motor nerves in the extremities. In uncontrolled diabetes, hyperglycemia causes increased levels of intracellular glucose in nerves. This leads to biochemical changes that cause impaired axonal transport and structural breakdown of nerves. The deleterious effects cause abnormal action potential propagation in both sensory and motor nerves. The individual loses sensation in the feet and suffers from imbalance because of a lack of motor control.

The reaction of excess glucose with nerve cell membranes results in advanced glycation end (ACE) products

that disrupt neuronal integrity. ACE products also cause endothelial injury, which predisposes the individual to arteriosclerotic plaque accumulation in arterial blood vessels. Arteriosclerosis in the small vessels of the lower extremities causes diminished circulation. The lack of neural sensation, decreased motor control, and diminished circulation in the lower extremities increases susceptibility to trauma and wound formation. The individual with diabetes often loses sensation in the feet and cannot perceive injury of the foot. In this case, a minor injury can become severe in the numb foot. Without a pain stimulus to warn the individual of the injury, the injury often worsens and becomes infected. Poor wound healing because of dysfunction of white blood cells in diabetes increases susceptibility to infection and pain. Together, all the conditions in uncontrolled diabetes increase the risk of lower extremity amputation.

Complex Regional Pain Syndrome

Complex regional pain syndrome (CRPS) is a chronic, progressive disorder characterized by severe pain, edema, discoloration, and changes in the skin. The cause of this syndrome is currently unknown. Precipitating factors include injury and surgery, although there are cases that have no injury associated with the site of pain. CRPS often affects an arm or a leg and may spread to another part of the body. It is associated with dysfunction of the autonomic nervous system, resulting in impairment and disability. Treatment is often unsatisfactory, but early multidisciplinary therapy such as combined physical therapy, pain medications, and occupational therapy can bring improvement in some patients. There are two types of CRPS:

1. Type I CRPS has been formerly called many different names, including reflex sympathetic dystrophy, Sudeck's atrophy, reflex neurovascular dystrophy, and algoneurodystrophy. In Type I CRPS there is no demonstrable nerve lesion.
2. Type II CRPS, formerly known as causalgia, has evidence of obvious nerve damage.

Postherpetic Neuralgia

Varicella zoster is a viral infection that presents in childhood as "chicken pox." The virus produces a characteristic pruritic, vesicular rash that often starts on the trunk and spreads out to the extremities, face, and head. Following the acute phase, the virus enters the sensory nervous system, where it remains dormant within the dorsal root of the spinal nerves throughout adulthood. When dormant, there are no symptoms. With advancing age or immunocompromised states, the virus reactivates along a nerve and an eruption called "shingles" occurs.

Shingles is the reactivation of varicella zoster, but it is renamed herpes zoster when it develops in the adult.

Even though the rash might appear the same, shingles does not have the same effect on the body as chicken pox. It is commonly an acute, vesicular and linear rash along a nerve dermatome that causes excruciating pain. The pain develops as the acute rash subsides; sharp pain can persist in shingles-affected areas for months. This is a common pain syndrome known as postherpetic neuralgia.

Fibromyalgia

Fibromyalgia is a common syndrome in which people experience long-term, bodywide pain, as well as pain in joints, muscles, tendons, and other soft tissues. The disorder has also been linked to fatigue, sleep problems, headaches, depression, anxiety, and other symptoms. Its cause is unknown. Men and women of all ages can contract fibromyalgia, but the disorder is most common among women aged 20 to 50 years.

The primary symptom of fibromyalgia is pain, and the exact locations of the pain are called tender points. Tender points are found in the soft tissue on the back of the neck, shoulders, sternum, lower back, hips, shins, elbows, and knees and can include fibrous tissue or muscles of specific body areas (see Fig. 6-11). The pain, which is described as deep-aching, radiating, gnawing, shooting, or burning, spreads out from these

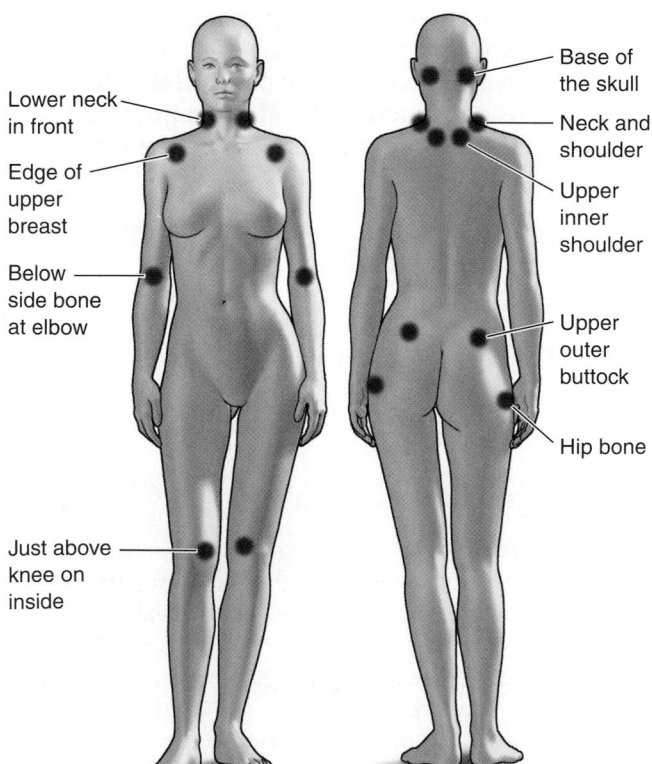

FIGURE 6-11. Trigger points, or tender points, are used to diagnose fibromyalgia. Individuals who have fibromyalgia experience abnormal sensitivity when light pressure is applied to the areas delineated in the diagram.

areas and ranges from mild to severe. The joints are not affected, although the pain may feel like it is coming from them.

People with fibromyalgia tend to wake up with body aches and stiffness. For some patients, pain improves during the day and increases again during the evening, though many patients have daylong, non-stop pain. Pain can increase with activity, cold or damp weather, anxiety, and stress. Fatigue and problems with sleep are seen in almost all patients with fibromyalgia.

Diagnosis requires a history of at least 3 months of widespread pain, and pain and tenderness in at least 11 of 18 tender-point sites (see Fig. 6-11). Sometimes, laboratory tests and x-rays are done to help confirm the diagnosis by ruling out other conditions that may have similar symptoms. Treatment should focus on not only relieving symptoms, but also on helping patients learn how to cope with their symptoms. Patients may start with physical therapy, exercise, and methods for reducing stress. If these methods fail to improve symptoms, an antidepressant or muscle relaxant may be added to the treatment.

Trigeminal Neuralgia

Trigeminal neuralgia, also called Tic Douloureux, is a nerve disorder that causes a stabbing or electric-shock-like pain in parts of the face. The pain arises from the trigeminal nerve, cranial nerve V, which carries pain and sensation to the face. It can affect part or all of the face, as well as the surface of the eye. The condition usually affects older adults; often, no specific cause is found, though pressure on the trigeminal nerve from a swollen blood vessel or tumor or multiple sclerosis may be a cause. The patient feels very painful, sharp, electriclike spasms that usually last a few seconds or minutes, but can become constant. Pain is usually only on one side of the face, often around the eye, cheek, and lower part of the face. It can be triggered by touch, sounds, or common activities, such as brushing teeth, chewing, drinking, eating, or shaving. Diagnosis includes a neurological examination, which is usually normal. Tests performed to look for the problem's cause include blood tests, magnetic resonance imaging of the head, and trigeminal reflex testing.

Certain medications such as anticonvulsants, muscle relaxers, and tricyclic antidepressants can help reduce the pain and the rate of attacks. Patients may need surgery to relieve pressure on the nerve.

Headache

Headache, also called cephalalgia, is one of the most common causes of pain and one of the most common reasons that patients seek health care. Headache interferes with functions needed for daily living, such as concentration ability, vision, hearing, appetite, and exercise ability. There are various causes of headache and most are innocuous, but headache can be a warning sign of a serious condition such as brain tumor or subarachnoid hemorrhage. Different kinds of headache have distinctive pain patterns, characteristics, and associated symptoms. The clinician needs to understand the features of different types of headache in order to rule out critical, life-threatening conditions and underlying pathology that causes headache. The most common types of headache are:

- tension
- cluster
- migraine.

Tension Headache

Tension headaches are the most common type of headache, occurring episodically because of stress. The pain is gradual in onset and presents as a pressure or bandlike sensation in the head. Pain is often bifrontal or occipitofrontal. This headache is often associated with muscular tightness in the neck, shoulders, and occipital area of the head. The individual's vital signs and neurological examination are normal. Nonopioid medications provide relief.

Cluster Headache

A cluster headache is a neurovascular disorder characterized by severe, unilateral, periorbital pain. The underlying pathophysiology is not understood. It commonly occurs in early morning hours or during sleep. Pain is described as sharp, stabbing, and unilateral with radiation to the cheek, jaw, occipital region, or neck. The hallmark of the cluster headache is the accompanying symptoms of tearing of the eyes, conjunctival injection, rhinorrhea, eyelid edema, ptosis, and miosis. The patient is commonly restless and cannot find a comfortable position.

Alcohol, tobacco, stress, allergy, and weather changes can provoke a cluster headache. The patient's vital signs and neurological examination are normal. Nonopioid or a weak opioid medication can relieve the pain.

Migraine Headache

Migraine headache is a disabling, recurrent headache disorder that affects 30 million persons a year, with 75% of the sufferers being women. It is a neurogenic process with secondary changes in cerebral perfusion. The pathology of migraine headaches is not totally understood. It is theorized that they originate in the raphe nucleus in the brainstem, where ascending serotonergic fibers travel to the thalamus. Low serotonin levels in the brain lead to constriction and dilation of blood vessels, triggering a migraine. Medications that are serotonin stimulants can block the vascular dysfunction of migraine headache.

Without treatment, a migraine headache can last 4 to 72 hours. Classically, the headache is a unilateral, vascular, throbbing headache with associated symptoms of nausea, vomiting, and sensitivity to light and sound. It is often preceded by an aura, a visual or sensory experience that occurs before the headache. Often the aura consists of scotomas (blind spots within the visual field), visual scintillations (flashing lights in the visual field), or paresthesias. Migraines are commonly precipitated by stress, hormones, smoking, weather changes, food additives, caffeine, alcohol, or excessive fatigue. Acute migraine treatment involves selective serotonin receptor agonists such as sumatriptan. Preventive medications include beta blockers and tricyclic antidepressants.

Chapter Summary

- Pain is a subjective experience that has always been difficult to understand.
- The gate control theory focuses on peripheral tissue damage and acute stimulation of the spinal cord neurons.
- The neuromatrix theory emphasizes the role of the brain and the significant impression of chronic pain in the brain's neural network.
- Pain is regarded as the fifth vital sign and specific assessment tools are used to evaluate severity.
- To assess pain and its accompanying symptoms, the initial history can be obtained by using the 'OLDCART' mnemonic: onset; location; duration; character; alleviating, aggravating, and accompanying factors; relieving factors; and treatment.
- When performing physical assessment, examine the area of pain last.
- It is difficult to quantify pain, but treating acute pain completely is advised in order to avoid development of intractable or chronic pain.
- The WHO recommends a step ladder approach for prescribing opioid, nonopioid, and adjuvant medications.
- Opioids have a high potential for abuse, tolerance, and physical dependence.
- Antidepressants and local anesthetics are commonly used as adjuvant pain treatment.
- Nonpharmacological treatment such as acupuncture and transdermal electrical nerve stimulation have shown effectiveness for some kinds of pain.

Bibliography

Arnold, L. M., Clauw, D. J., Dunegan, L. J., Turk, D. C., & FibroCollaborative. (2012). A framework for fibromyalgia management for primary care providers. *Mayo Clinic Proceedings*, 87(5), 488–496.

Anonymous. (2012). Pain control—a basic kindness. *Lancet*, 379(9831), 2024.

Baumblatt, J. A., Wiedeman, C., Dunn, J. R., et al. (2014). High-risk use by patients prescribed opioids for pain and its role in overdose deaths. *J Am Med Assoc Intern Med*, Mar 3. doi: 10.1001/jamainternmed.2013.12711. Epub ahead of print.

Berman, B. M., Langevin, H. M., Witt, C. M., & Dubner, R. (2010). Acupuncture for chronic low back pain. *N Engl J Med*, 363(5), 454–461.

Blondell, R. D., Azadfard, M., & Wisniewski, A. M. (2013). Pharmacologic therapy for acute pain. *Am Fam Phys*, 87(11), 766–772.

Casazza, B. A. (2012). Diagnosis and treatment of acute low back pain. *Am Fam Phys*, 85(4), 343–350.

Chon, T. Y., & Lee, M. C. (2013). Acupuncture. *Mayo Clinic Proceedings*, 88(10), 1141–1146. doi: 10.1016/j.mayocp.2013.06.009.

Clauw, D. J. (2014). Fibromyalgia: a clinical review. *JAMA*, 311(15), 1547–1555. doi: 10.1001/jama.2014.3266.

Culpepper, L. (2010). Recognizing and diagnosing fibromyalgia. *J Clin Psych*, 71(1), E30.

Daffner, R. H. (2010). Radiologic evaluation of chronic neck pain. *Am Fam Phys*, 82(8), 959–964.

Delany, P. A. (2010). Acupuncture for chronic back pain: what level of evidence? *Am Fam Phys*, 82(8), 869.

de Leon-Casasola, O. A. (2013). Opioids for chronic pain: new evidence, new strategies, safe prescribing. *Am J Med*, 126 (3 Suppl 1), S3–11. doi: 10.1016/j.amjmed.2012.11.011.

Dworkin, R. H., O'Connor, A. B., Audette, J., et al. (2010). Recommendations for the pharmacological management of neuropathic pain: an overview and literature update. *Mayo Clinic Proceedings*, 85(3 Suppl), S3–S14.

Eubanks, J. D. (2010). Cervical radiculopathy: nonoperative management of neck pain and radicular symptoms. *Am Fam Phys*, 81(1), 33–40.

Friedrich, M. J. (2012). Research yields new insights into mechanisms and treatment of pain. *JAMA*, 307(3), 239–241.

Gilron, I., Bailey, J. M., Tu, D., et al. (2009). Nortriptyline and gabapentin, alone and in combination for neuropathic pain: a double-blind, randomised controlled crossover trial. *Lancet*, 374(9697), 1252–1261.

Gilron, I., Jensen, T. S., & Dickenson, A. H. (2013). Combination pharmacotherapy for management of chronic pain: from bench to bedside. *Lancet Neurol*, 12(11), 1084–1095. doi: 10.1016/S1474-4422(13)70193-5. Epub 2013 Sep 25.

Gloth, F. M. 3rd. (2013). Opioids in chronic pain: evolving best practice strategies. Introduction. *Am J Med*, 126(3 Suppl 1), S1–S2. doi: 10.1016/j.amjmed.2012.11.010. Epub 2012 Dec 6.

Goldberg, D. S. (2012). The lived experiences of chronic pain. *Am J Med*, 125(8), 836–837. doi: 10.1016/j.amjmed.2012.01.032.

Gordh, T. E., Jensen, T. S., & Kalso, E. (2010). Reporting of trials of gabapentin. *N Engl J Med*, 362(17), 1641.

Gregory, D. S., Seto, C. K., Wortley, G. C., & Shugart, C. M. (2008). Pain. *Am Fam Phys*, 78(7), 835–842.

Groninger, H., & Vijayan, J. (2014). Pharmacologic management of pain at the end of life. *Am Fam Phys*, 90(1), 26–32.

Haanpää, M. L., Gourlay, G. K., Kent, J. L., et al. (2010). Treatment considerations for patients with neuropathic pain and other medical comorbidities. *Mayo Clinic Proceedings*, 85(3 Suppl), S15–S25. Review.

Harris, P. F., Arnold, R. M., Braun, U. K., et al. (2012). Update in palliative care—2011. *J Gen Int Med*, (5), 582–587.

Hitzeman, N., & Athale, N. (2010). Opioids for osteoarthritis of the knee or hip. *Am Fam Phys*, 81(9), 1094.

Iannetti, G. D., & Mouraux, A. (2010). From the neuromatrix to the pain matrix (and back). *Experiments in Brain Research*, 205(1), 1–12.

Johnston, S. (2010). Effectiveness and safety of high-dose opioids for chronic pain. *Am Fam Phys*, 15;81(6), 693–696.

Kaasa, S. (2013). Interview: cancer pain management: the last decade and looking forward. *Pain Management*, 3(6), 431–434. doi: 10.2217/pmt.13.56.

Kabani, R., & Brassard, A. (2014). Dermatological findings in early detection of complex regional pain syndrome. *JAMA Dermatol*, Apr 23. doi: 10.1001/jamadermatol.2013.7459. Epub ahead of print.

Koes, B. (2011). Management of low back pain in primary care: a new approach. *Lancet*, 378(9802), 1530–1532.

Krafft, R. M. (2008). Trigeminal neuralgia. *Am Fam Phys*, 77(9), 1291–1296.

Kumar, V., Abbas, A. K., Fausto, N., & Aster, J. (2014). *Robbins & Cotran pathologic basis of disease*. 9th ed. Philadelphia, PA: WB Saunders. Affiliations.

Last, A. R., & Hulbert, K. (2009). Chronic low back pain: evaluation and management. *Am Fam Phys*, 79(12), 1067–1074.

Latham, J. L., & Martin, S. N. (2014). Infiltrative anesthesia in office practice. *Am Fam Phys*, 89(12), 956–962.

Latremoliere, A., & Woolf, C. (2009). Central sensitization: a generator of pain hypersensitivity by central neural plasticity. *J Pain*, 10(9), 895–926.

Lindsay, T. J., Rodgers, B. C., Savath, V., & Hettinger, K. (2010). Treating diabetic peripheral neuropathic pain. *Am Fam Phys*, 82(2), 151–158.

Loder, E. (2010). Triptan therapy in migraine. *N Engl J Med*, 363(1), 63–70.

Longo, D., Fauci, A., Braunwald, E., et al. (2011). *Harrison's principles of internal medicine*. 18th ed. New York: McGraw-Hill.

Makris, U. E., Abrams, R. C., Gurland, B., & Reid, M. C. (2014). Management of persistent pain in the older patient: a clinical review. *JAMA*, 312(8), 825–836. doi: 10.1001/jama.2014.9405.

Melzack, R. (1989). Labat lecture. Phantom limbs. *Reg Anesthesia*, 14(5), 208–211.

Melzack, R. (1990). Phantom limbs and the concept of a neuromatrix. *Trends in Neuroscience*, 13(3), 88–92.

Melzack, R. (1996). Gate control theory: on the evolution of pain concepts. *Pain Forum*, 5, 128–138.

Melzack, R. (1999). From the gate to the neuromatrix. *Pain*, Aug Suppl 6, S121–S126.

Melzack, R. (2001). Pain and the neuromatrix in the brain. *J Dental Ed*, 65(12), 1378–1382.

Melzack, R. (2005). Evolution of the neuromatrix theory of pain. The Prithvi Raj Lecture: presented at the Third World Congress of World Institute of Pain, Barcelona 2004. *Pain Practitioner*, 5(2), 85–94.

Melzack, R., & Wall, P. (1965). Pain mechanisms: a new theory. *Science*, 150(3699), 971–979.

Mendell, L. M. (2014). Constructing and deconstructing the gate theory of pain. *Pain*, 155(2), 210–216. doi: 10.1016/j.pain.2013.12.010. Epub 2013 Dec 12.

Moayedi, M., & Davis, K. D. (2013). Theories of pain: from specificity to gate control. *J Neurophysiol,* 109(1), 5–12. doi: 10.1152/jn.00457.2012. Epub 2012 Oct 3.

Mohari, M., & Burger, H. (2010). Effect of transcutaneous electrical nerve stimulation on sensation thresholds in patients with painful diabetic neuropathy: an observational study. *Int J Rehab Res*, 33(3), 211–217.

Moore, A., Wiffen, P., & Kalso, E. (2014). Antiepileptic drugs for neuropathic pain and fibromyalgia. *JAMA,* 312(2), 182–183. doi: 10.1001/jama.2014.6336.

Passik, S. D. (2009). Issues in long-term opioid therapy: unmet needs, risks, and solutions. *Mayo Clinic Proceedings*, 84(7), 593–601.

Pizzo, P. A., & Clark, N. M. (2012). Alleviating suffering 101—pain relief in the United States. *N Engl J Med*, 366(3), 197–199.

Portenoy, R. K. (2011). Treatment of cancer pain. *Lancet,* 377(9784), 2236–2247.

Schmader, K. E., Baron, R., Haanpää, M. L., et al. (2010). Treatment considerations for elderly and frail patients with neuropathic pain. *Mayo Clinic Proceedings*, 85(3 Suppl), S26–S32.

Schug, S. A., & Pogatzki-Zahn, E. M. (2011). Pain: clinical updates: volume XIX, issue 1. *Nonspecific Treatment Effects in Pain Medicine*. Retrieved from http://www.iasp-pain.org

Seehusen, D. A. (2010). Opioid therapy for chronic non-cancer pain. *Am Fam Phys*, 82(1), 40–45.

Towards better control of chronic pain. (2010). *Lancet,* 375(9728), 1754–1755.

Turk, D. C., Audette, J., Levy, R. M., Mackey, S. C., & Stanos, S. (2010). Assessment and treatment of psychosocial comorbidities in patients with neuropathic pain. *Mayo Clinic Proceedings*, 85(3 Suppl), S42–S50.

Turk, D. C., Wilson, H. D., & Cahana, A. (2011). Treatment of chronic non-cancer pain. *Lancet,* 377(9784), 226–235.

Vargas-Schaffer, G. (2010). Is the WHO analgesic ladder still valid?: Twenty-four years of experience. *Can Fam Phys*. Retrieved from http://www.cfp.ca/content/56/6/514.full.

Vickers, A. J., & Linde, K. (2014). Acupuncture for chronic pain. *JAMA,* 311(9), 955–956. doi: 10.1001/jama.2013.285478.

Weaver-Agostoni, J. (2013). Cluster headache. *Am Fam Phys*, 88(2), 122–128.

Webster, L. R. (2011). Opioids and deaths. *N Engl J Med*, 364(7), 687.

Wu, C. L., & Raja, S. N. (2011). Treatment of acute postoperative pain. *Lancet*, 377(9784), 2215–2225.

Yancey, J. R., Sheridan, R., & Koren, K. G. (2014). Chronic daily headache: diagnosis and management. *Am Fam Phys*, 89(8), 642–648.

Yeh, G. Y., Kaptchuk, T. J., & Shmerling, R. H. (2010). Prescribing tai chi for fibromyalgia—are we there yet? *N Engl J Med*, 363(8), 783–784.

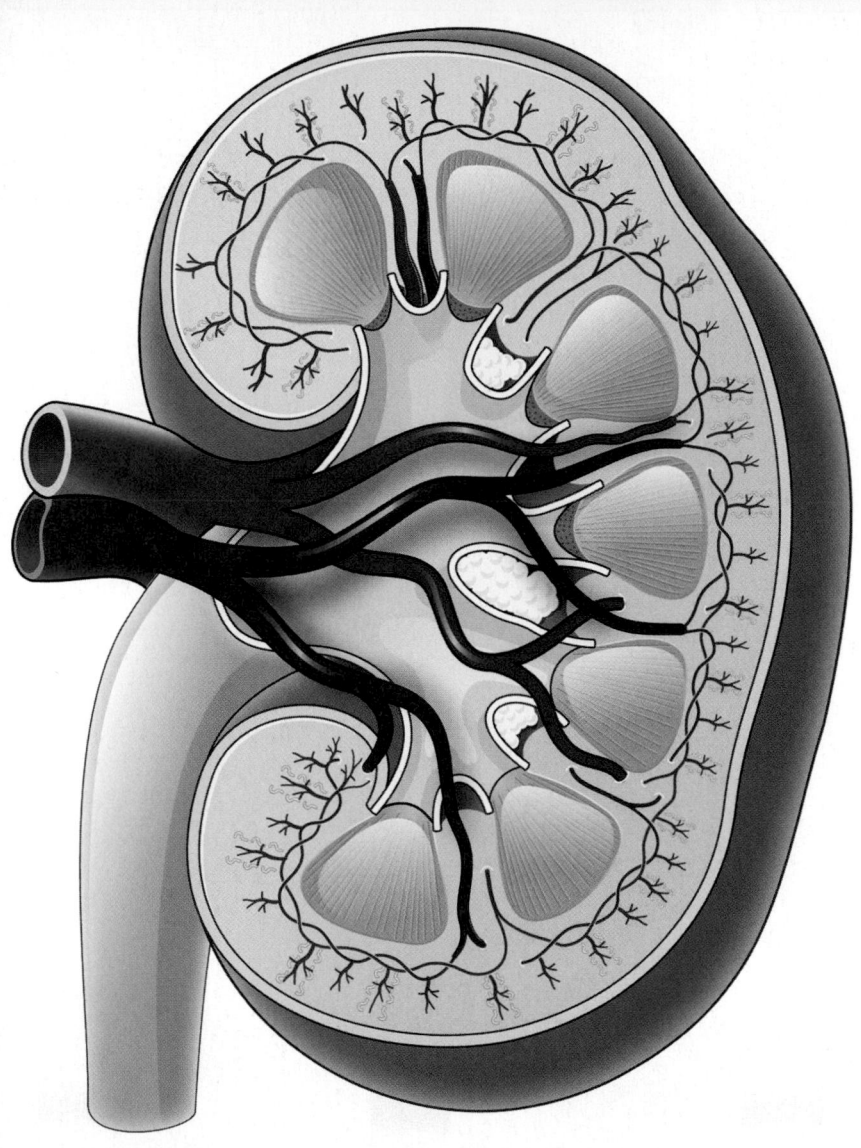

Chapters

Fluid and Electrolyte Imbalances

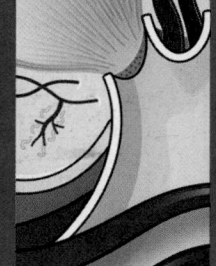

Key Terms

Effusion

Electrolyte

Extracellular fluid (ECF)

Hydrostatic pressure

Hypercalcemia

Hyperkalemia

Hypermagnesemia

Hypernatremia

Hyperphosphatemia

Hypocalcemia

Hypokalemia

Hypomagnesemia

Hyponatremia

Hypophosphatemia

Interstitial fluid (ISF)

Intracellular fluid (ICF)

Oncotic pressure

Osmolality

Osmolarity

Osmotic pressure

Tonicity

The human body is composed of approximately 60% water. It is the major constituent of the cells and bloodstream and acts as the body's solvent. **Electrolytes,** which are positively and negatively charged ions, are the body's solutes. Protein, specifically albumin, is the major solute in the bloodstream; body fluid, which is a solution largely composed of water, is the solvent. Electrolytes and protein, the solutes, have two main functions:

1. deliver nutrients and electrolytes to cells
2. carry away waste products from cellular metabolism.

Basic Concepts of Fluid and Electrolyte Balance

Water is found in three different fluid compartments (see Fig. 7-1):

1. **intracellular fluid (ICF)**
2. **extracellular fluid (ECF)**
3. **interstitial fluid (ISF).**

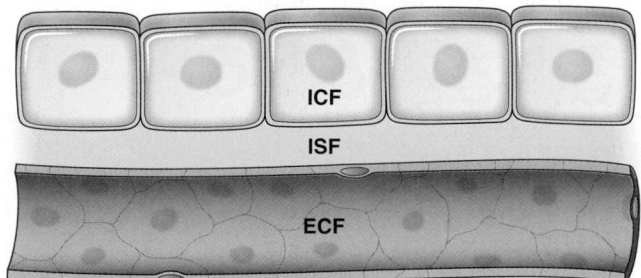

FIGURE 7-1. There are three basic fluid compartments in the body where water is located. The ICF compartment is inside of the cells. The ECF compartment is within the bloodstream. The ISF compartment is between the intracellular and extracellular compartments.

A constant state of fluid and electrolyte exchange occurs between the cell and its environment—mainly between the ICF and ECF. Two-thirds of the body's water content is mainly contained within the ICF and one-third is within the ECF. Each cell is enveloped by a plasma membrane. This is a semipermeable membrane that allows passive movement of fluid and electrolytes back and forth, but restricts larger particles. Table 7-1 describes the different transport mechanisms that maintain the concentration differences between ICF and ECF.

Fluid Balance

Intracellular Fluid Compartment

In the adult, 40% of total body weight is the water contained within the ICF compartment. Water can diffuse out of the ICF and cause cell shrinkage or cellular dehydration. Conversely, water can enter the ICF and cause cell swelling or cellular edema.

Extracellular Fluid Compartment

In the adult, 20% of total body weight is the water contained within the ECF compartment. Most of the ECF is found within the intravascular compartment or blood vessels. The ECF contains electrolytes, oxygen, glucose, and other nutrients to be delivered to cells, as well as cellular waste products designated for excretion.

Interstitial Fluid Compartment

ISF, which is a filtrate of the blood, is located between the cells and between the cells and capillaries. Like blood, it contains water and electrolytes, mainly sodium (Na^+). ISF lacks proteins because they are too large to diffuse out of the blood vessels into the interstitial spaces. However, during inflammation, capillary membranes become extrapermeable; the pores enlarge, allowing proteins such as white blood cells out to the tissues.

TABLE 7-1. Transport Mechanisms

Transport Mechanism	Description	Illustration
Diffusion	The process by which molecules passively spread from areas of high concentration to areas of low concentration. Water and electrolytes diffuse from high concentration to lower concentration until an equilibrium is reached.	
Osmosis	The tendency of molecules of a solvent to pass through a semipermeable membrane from a less concentrated solution into a more concentrated one, equalizing the concentrations on each side of the membrane. Electrolytes and water move through the cell's semi-permeable plasma membrane, but large proteins such as albumin cannot pass through the membrane. A semi-permeable membrane selectively allows some molecules through its pores and obstructs others according to size.	
Facilitated transport	The passing of certain molecules through the plasma membrane with assistance from carrier proteins. Glucose undergoes facilitated transport into the cell by the carrier protein insulin.	

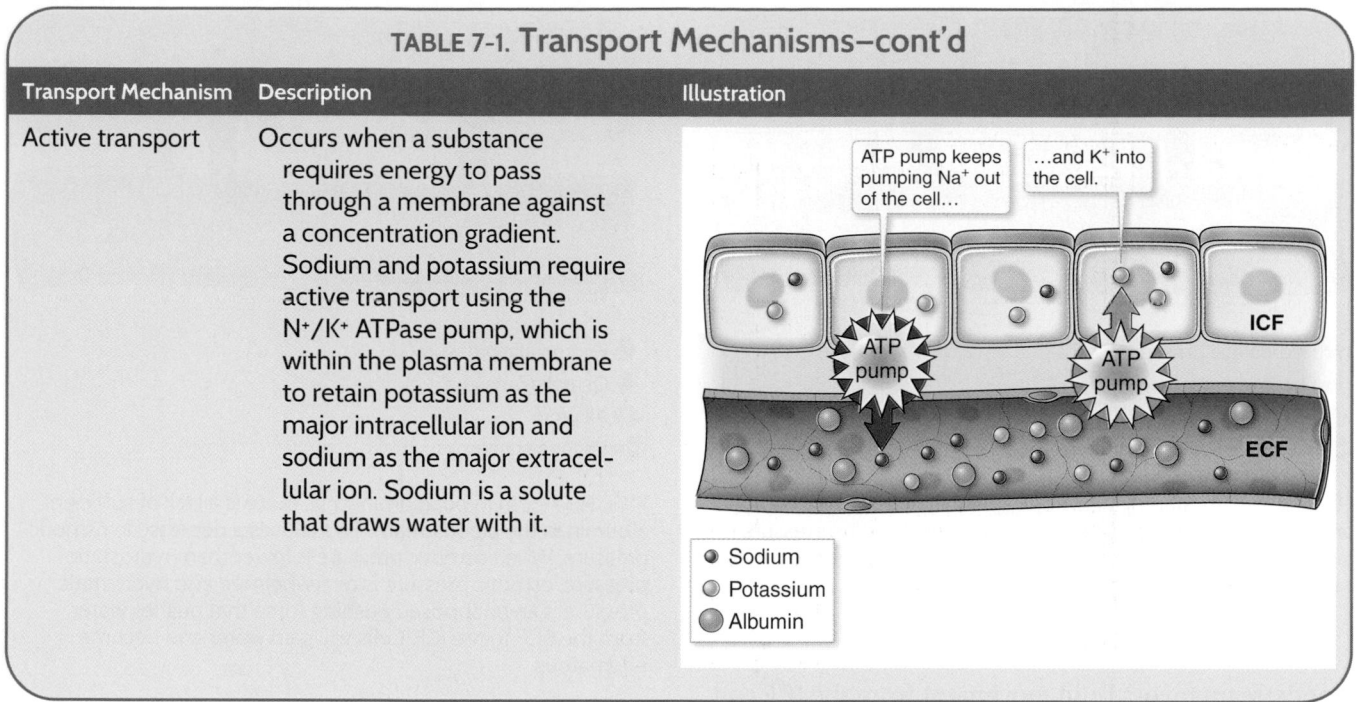

TABLE 7-1. Transport Mechanisms–cont'd		
Transport Mechanism	**Description**	**Illustration**
Active transport	Occurs when a substance requires energy to pass through a membrane against a concentration gradient. Sodium and potassium require active transport using the N⁺/K⁺ ATPase pump, which is within the plasma membrane to retain potassium as the major intracellular ion and sodium as the major extracellular ion. Sodium is a solute that draws water with it.	

Hydrostatic Pressure

Hydrostatic pressure is the pushing force exerted by water in the bloodstream. The heart's pulsatile pumping action is the source of hydrostatic pressure, which exerts an outward force that pushes water through the capillary membrane pores into the ISF and ICF compartments (see Fig. 7-2). Osmotic pressure opposes hydrostatic pressure at all capillary membranes.

Osmotic Pressure

Osmotic pressure is the pressure exerted by the solutes in solution. In the bloodstream, osmotic pressure is exerted by electrolytes, mainly sodium ions and plasma proteins. Osmotic pressure is a force that pulls water into the bloodstream from the ICF and ISF and opposes hydrostatic pressure (see Fig. 7-3). Osmotic

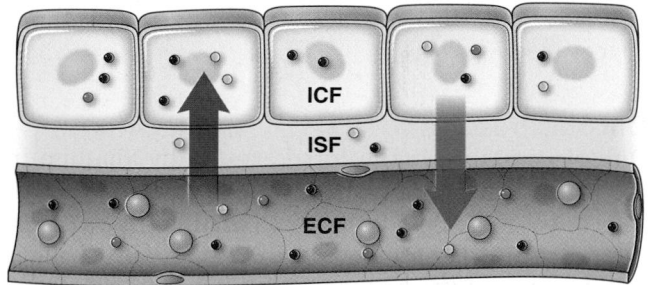

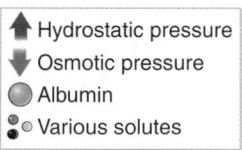

FIGURE 7-3. In Starling's Law of Capillary Forces, osmotic pressure pulls water from the ICF into the ECF at every cell-capillary interface. The osmotic pressure opposes the hydrostatic pressure; in healthy conditions, each force balances out the other.

pressure is determined by the number of particles or their concentration within the solution. A solution with a greater number of particles has a higher osmotic pressure. **Oncotic pressure,** also called colloidal oncotic pressure, refers to the force exerted specifically by albumin in the bloodstream. Albumin is the main colloidal protein in the bloodstream and is essential for maintaining the oncotic pressure in the vascular system. Albumin attracts water and helps keep it inside the blood vessel.

When a membrane such as a cell membrane separates two solutions with different osmotic pressures, fluid will move from the solution with lower osmotic pressure into the solution that has the higher osmotic pressure, which is why a high osmotic pressure in the

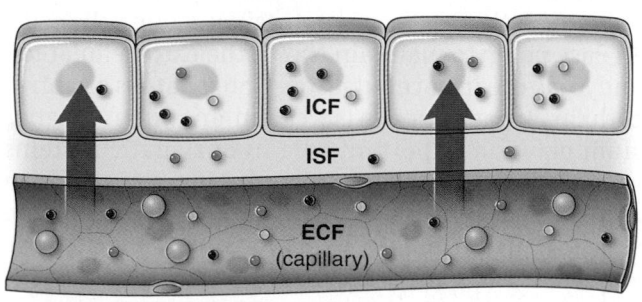

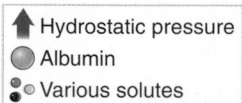

FIGURE 7-2. In Starling's Law of Capillary Forces, hydrostatic pressure pushes water outward from the ECF to the ICF at the capillary-cell interface.

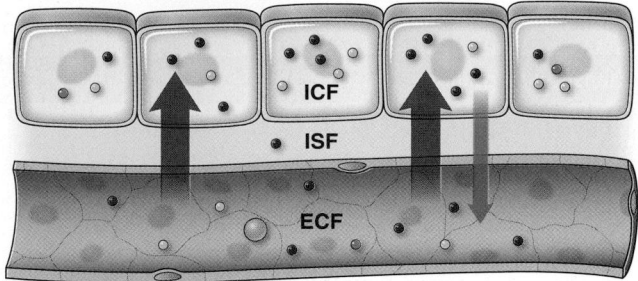

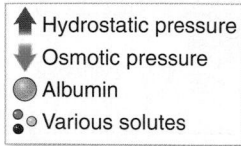

FIGURE 7-4. In Starling's Law of Capillary Forces, when osmotic pressure is lower than hydrostatic pressure, osmotic pressure is overwhelmed and hydrostatic pressure is an unopposed force, causing water to flow from the ECF to the ICF.

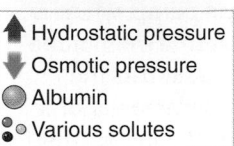

FIGURE 7-5. In hypoalbuminemia, there is a lack of sufficient albumin in the bloodstream. This causes a decrease in osmotic pressure. When osmotic pressure is lower than hydrostatic pressure, osmotic pressure is overwhelmed and hydrostatic pressure is an unopposed pushing force that pushes water from the ECF to the ICF. Cells will gain water and become edematous.

bloodstream favors fluid movement from the ICF and ISF into the bloodstream. Conversely, when the osmotic pressure is reduced, fluid moves out of the bloodstream and into interstitial and intracellular spaces (see Fig. 7-4).

Oncotic Pressure

Oncotic pressure is the force exerted by albumin in the bloodstream. Total albumin in the bloodstream is indicative of the body's protein nutritional status. The normal serum albumin level is 3.1 to 4.3 g/dL. Changes in this albumin level alter oncotic pressure. For example, in hypoalbuminemia (lack of sufficient albumin in the bloodstream), there is a reduced oncotic pressure. Hypoalbuminemia causes an imbalance in the oncotic pressure versus hydrostatic pressure forces. With reduced albumin, the oncotic pressure is low and the force exerted by hydrostatic pressure overwhelms the oncotic pressure. This causes water in the bloodstream to push outward from the capillary pores toward the ISF and ICF (see Fig. 7-5).

Osmolality

Osmolality is a measurement of the concentration of solutes per kg of solvent. It is based on 1 mole (or gram molecular weight equivalent) of a substance dissolved in 1 kilogram of water. In clinical practice, osmolality can be used to evaluate the body's hydration status based on the concentration of fluid and particles in solution. Normal plasma osmolality is 282 to 295 milliOsmoles per kilogram of water. Low osmolality indicates fewer amounts of solutes in solution, whereas high osmolality indicates greater amount of solutes. If the bloodstream is well hydrated, serum osmolality is 282 milliOsmoles per kg of water or fewer. If the bloodstream is concentrated and has low water, the serum osmolality will be 295 milliOsmoles per kg of water

or greater. Serum osmolality can be calculated using the following mathematical formula: milliOsmoles of solute /kg of water = 2 x serum sodium + serum glucose /18 + BUN / 2.4.

Osmolarity

Osmolarity is the number of osmoles of solute per liter of solution; it is dependent on the number of particles suspended in a solution. In the body, the major solutes are albumin, sodium (Na^+), potassium (K^+), phosphate (PO_4-), magnesium (Mg^{++}), calcium (Ca^{++}), bicarbonate (HCO_3-), and glucose. The major protein within the bloodstream is albumin, which is the solute in the ECF that exerts the most osmotic pressure. Sodium, the main determinant of osmolarity, is a positive ion, also called a cation; it is found mostly in the ECF and assists in the maintenance of fluid balance and osmotic pressure. Potassium is the main intracellular cation; it assists in the maintenance of neuromuscular excitability and acid-base balance. Both sodium and potassium require the cell's ATPase pump to maintain Na^+ as the extracellular ion and K^+ as the intracellular ion. Phosphate is an intracellular negative ion, also called an anion. Magnesium plays an important role in enzymatic systems within the body. Calcium plays an important role in neuromuscular irritability, blood clotting, and bone structure. Bicarbonate is responsible for acid-base balance.

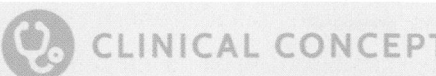

CLINICAL CONCEPT

The serum albumin level is used to evaluate an individual's nutritional status.

Tonicity

Tonicity refers to the amount of solutes in solution compared with the bloodstream. The term is also used to describe the various intravenous solutions used in the clinical setting. There are three types of intravenous (IV) solutions:

1. **isotonic solution**: This has the same tonicity as blood; when infused as an intravenous solution, it does not cause fluid shifts or alter body cell size. It has a concentration of particles and fluid that is similar to blood and body fluids. A standard isotonic intravenous solution is 0.9% NaCl solution, also called normal saline. It is used frequently as a bloodstream volume expander. Often an isotonic solution is used to keep an open connection to the intravenous route for medication administration or a blood transfusion.

2. **hypotonic solution**: This has fewer particles and more water than blood and body fluids. When a hypotonic solution is infused, it adds water to the bloodstream and causes a fluid shift from ECF to ICF, to deliver water to the body as in dehydration treatment. A standard hypotonic solution is 0.45% NaCl, and is also referred to a half normal saline.

3. **hypertonic solution**: This contains more particles and less water than blood and body fluids. When a hypertonic solution is infused into the bloodstream, this adds solutes to the bloodstream and causes fluids to shift from ICF to ECF, causing body cells to shrink. A commonly used hypertonic IV solution is mannitol. It can be used to diminish cell swelling, particularly in cerebral edema. Another hypertonic solution that is used less often is 3.0% NaCl.

 CLINICAL CONCEPT

A solution often used as a temporary replacement for blood, called Ringer's lactate, consists of similar physiologic constituents as those found in blood.

Starling's Law of Capillary Forces

Starling's Law of Capillary Forces explains the movement of fluid that occurs at every capillary bed in the body. There are two major opposing forces at every capillary membrane:

1. hydrostatic pressure
2. osmotic pressure (includes oncotic pressure).

Within every capillary, the blood contains electrolytes and proteins that exert osmotic pressure. The fluid within the capillary exerts hydrostatic pressure. These pressure forces oppose each other and attempt to

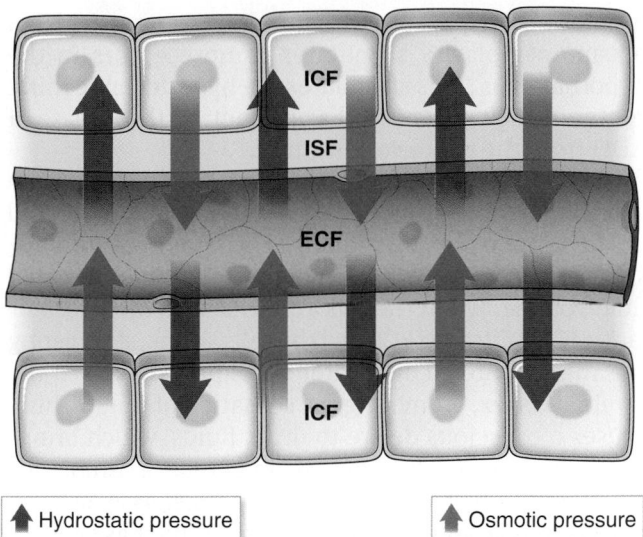

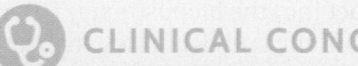

▲ Hydrostatic pressure	▲ Osmotic pressure
Symbolizes the pushing outward force of hydrostatic pressure pushing water from ECF (capillary) into ICF.	Symbolizes the pulling force of osmotic (oncotic) pressure created by solutes (albumin), which favors fluid movement from the ICF into the ECF (capillary).

FIGURE 7-6. In Starling's Law of Capillary Forces, when hydrostatic and osmotic pressures are equal at every capillary-cell interface, homeostasis exists.

balance each other out at every capillary membrane, thereby creating a state of homeostasis (see Fig. 7-6).

CLINICAL CONCEPT

Principles of Starling's Law can be applied in the clinical setting. For example, swelling can be reduced using an Epsom salt bath, which is a hypertonic magnesium salt solution. For example, placing a swollen finger in an Epsom salt bath will draw ICF from the finger into the Epsom salt solution, thereby reducing the finger's swelling.

Fluid Homeostasis

Various physiologic mechanisms work together in order to maintain fluid homeostasis. In terms of fluid volume, both fluid intake and output must be regulated to prevent fluid volume overload, also known as edema, and fluid volume deficit, also known as dehydration. However, in addition to fluid volume status, the relative composition of body fluids, including electrolyte and acid or base concentrations, needs to be consistent. The kidney, RAAS, osmoreceptors, thirst sensation, antidiuretic hormone, and natriuretic peptides work together to maintain fluid homeostasis in the body.

Osmoreceptors, Antidiuretic Hormone, and Thirst.
Changes in plasma osmolarity are responsible for both the sensation of thirst and the release of antidiuretic

hormone (ADH), also called arginine vasopressin. High plasma osmolarity stimulates osmoreceptors in the hypothalamus. This stimulates the hypothalamic thirst center of the brain as well as promoting the release of ADH from the posterior pituitary.

Thirst is a conscious desire to drink fluids. It is triggered by a response in the thirst center, which is located in the anterior hypothalamus. The osmoreceptors respond to changes in both blood osmolarity and blood fluid volume. When there is an increase in blood osmolarity, ICF shifts into ECF and the cells shrink, stimulating the thirst center. This center transmits signals to the cerebral cortex, promoting the sensation of thirst. Thirst causes a conscious desire to drink fluids, which brings water into the body's bloodstream to reduce osmolarity. Massive loss of blood and fluid volume, as is seen in severe trauma, will trigger the sense of thirst as well.

In a healthy person, osmoreceptors, ADH, and thirst responses work together. ADH is produced by the hypothalamus. Once the ADH is synthesized, it travels by an axonal transport mechanism to the posterior pituitary gland. When the bloodstream lacks sufficient water, plasma osmolarity is increased and the osmoreceptors shrink. This stimulates the ADH neurons to depolarize, releasing ADH from the posterior pituitary. In addition to changes in osmolarity, other factors such as pain, trauma, and medications also stimulate the release of ADH.

After release into the bloodstream, ADH stimulates water reabsorption from the nephron tubule fluid at the collecting duct into the bloodstream. This raises the blood's water content and decreases the water in the tubule fluid, which eventually becomes concentrated urine. When there is enough water in the bloodstream, plasma osmolarity decreases, and ADH secretion is inhibited.

Renin-Angiotensin-Aldosterone System. Hypotension, hypovolemia, dehydration, and low cardiac output cause low circulation throughout the body. Reduced circulation causes low renal perfusion, which stimulates renin secretion by the kidney's juxtaglomerular apparatus. Renin initiates the RAAS, a compensatory mechanism used to replenish blood volume and raise blood pressure (see Fig. 7-7).

Renin is an enzyme released from the kidney in response to decreased renal perfusion. Renin converts angiotensinogen, a large protein produced by the liver, to angiotensin I. In the lungs, angiotensin-converting enzyme (ACE) changes angiotensin I into angiotensin II, a powerful vasoconstrictor. Angiotensin II binds to receptors in the adrenal cortex, stimulating the synthesis and secretion of aldosterone, which is a mineralocorticoid that increases sodium and water reabsorption into the bloodstream at the distal tubule of the nephrons. Aldosterone also stimulates the excretion of potassium into the nephron tubules, which eventually becomes urine. When blood volume decreases, aldosterone begins the reabsorption of sodium from the distal tubules into the bloodstream, and this brings

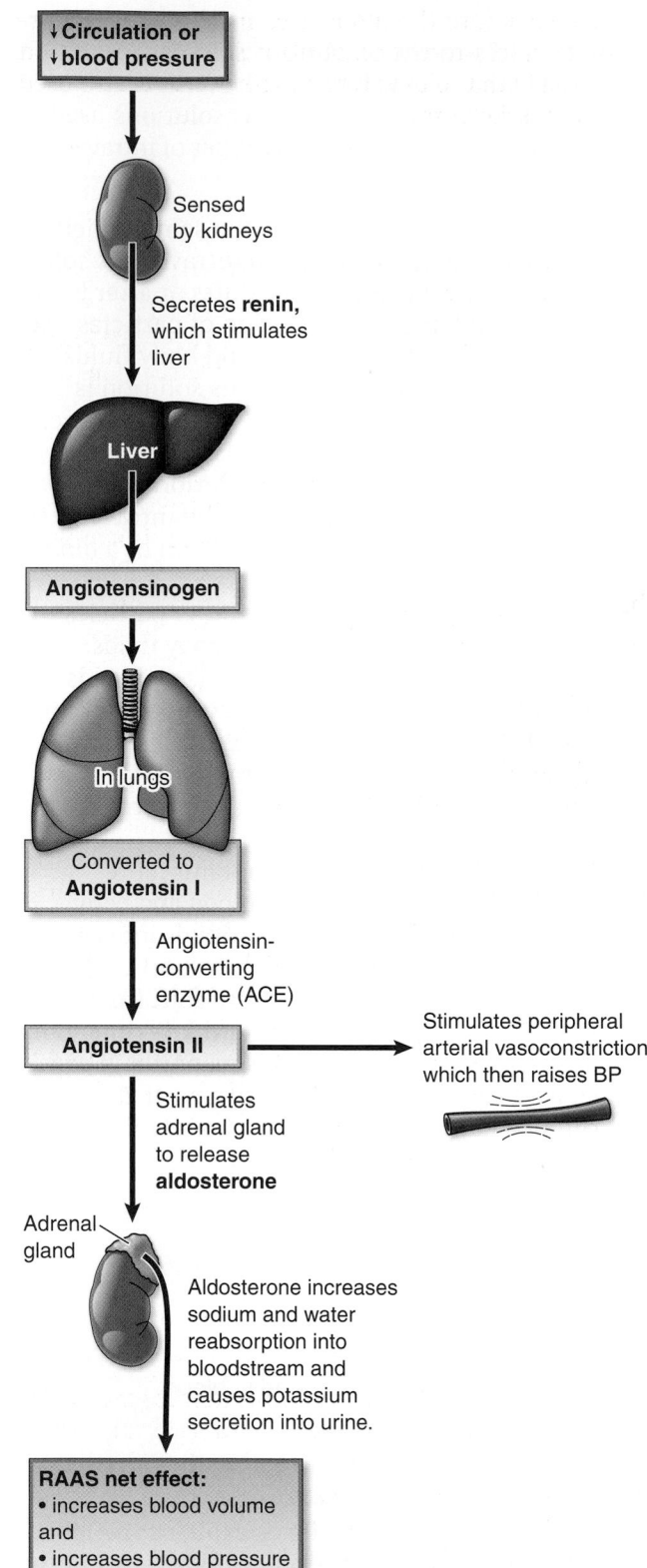

FIGURE 7-7. The RAAS. When there is a decrease in circulation or drop in blood pressure, the kidney senses decreased perfusion and releases renin. Renin stimulates the liver to release a protein called angiotensinogen. Angiotensinogen reaches the lungs and is transformed into angiotensin I. In the lungs, ACE transforms angiotensin I into angiotensin II. Angiotensin II is a potent arterial vasoconstrictor; it also stimulates the adrenal gland to release aldosterone. Aldosterone increases sodium and water reabsorption into the bloodstream at the nephron. It also causes potassium excretion from the bloodstream into the urine. The net effect of the RAAS is to raise blood volume and increase blood pressure.

sodium back into the bloodstream. This causes more absorption of water, and blood volume will increase. When the blood volume returns to normal, aldosterone secretion is reduced.

 CLINICAL CONCEPT

Spironolactone is an aldosterone antagonist that causes retention of potassium in the bloodstream. It works at the distal tubule by interfering with the reabsorption of sodium. Sodium is excreted but potassium is spared.

Natriuretic Peptides. Natriuresis is the excretion of a large amount of both sodium and water by the kidneys in response to excess ECF volume. It is a process of natural diuresis initiated by the body. There are three major peptides that promote natriuresis: atrial natriuretic peptide (ANP), brain natriuretic peptide (BNP), and C-type natriuretic peptide (CNP). ANP is produced by the heart's atria and is secreted in response to excess ECF volume that stretches the heart's atrial chambers. CNP is produced by endothelial cells of the arteries and ventricular cells of the heart.

BNP is produced in the heart's ventricles and, to a lesser extent, in the brain. It is excreted in response to fluid volume overload stretching the heart's ventricles—the more the ventricle is stretched by blood volume, the more BNP is secreted. Both ANP and BNP promote natriuresis at the glomerulus by increasing glomerular filtration rate. CNP has limited diuretic and natriuretic effects compared with ANP and BNP, but it has only been recently identified and is not completely understood.

Basic Pathophysiologic Concepts of Fluid and Electrolyte Imbalance

Regulation of fluid balance is important for maintaining the body's normal homeostatic functioning. Alterations in fluid balance occur for a variety of reasons and can be related to illness or exposure to extreme heat. Because sodium is the major extracellular ion, it has a key role in fluid balance. Fluid volume deficit or excess fluid volume has ancillary effects on different systems of the body.

Edema

Edema occurs when there is an excess of fluid in the ISF and ICF compartments. It can occur because of elevated hydrostatic pressure created by excess water in the bloodstream or diminished osmotic force created by a low amount of solutes in the bloodstream. Edema can also occur because of inflammation, which causes increased capillary permeability; the capillary pores enlarge to allow fluid and cells out of the bloodstream to reach the site of injury. The fluid that moves into the ISF and ICF causes the edema.

When edema occurs because of high hydrostatic pressure in the bloodstream, the osmotic pressure force is overwhelmed and does not balance out the hydrostatic force. Consequently, according to Starling's Law of Capillary Forces, hydrostatic pressure pushes fluid out of the capillary membrane pores into the ISF and ICF. An example of this occurs in left-sided heart failure, where high hydrostatic pressure develops in the pulmonary bloodstream. The high hydrostatic pressure forces fluid out of the pulmonary blood vessels and into the alveolar spaces and the interstitial tissue. This is known as pulmonary edema. Edema can also occur in the peritoneal cavity as ascites, the pleural cavity as pleural effusion, and in the lower extremities as ankle edema.

Edema can also occur because of a low amount of solute in the bloodstream. Low albumin in the blood, also called hypoalbuminemia, causes an imbalance in capillary forces. Because albumin is the major source of oncotic pressure, hypoalbuminemia will cause low oncotic pressure in the bloodstream. According to Starling's Law of Capillary Forces, for homeostasis to occur, oncotic pressure needs to equal hydrostatic pressure. When oncotic pressure is low, hydrostatic pressure will be the overriding force and push fluid out of the capillary into the ISF and ICF compartments, thereby creating an edematous state.

An example of edema caused by hypoalbuminemia occurs in severe protein starvation. Without sufficient nutritional protein, blood albumin levels become extremely low and, consequently, oncotic pressure is diminished. There is an imbalance between oncotic pressure and hydrostatic pressure at every capillary-cell interface. Hydrostatic pressure overwhelms oncotic pressure and it pushes water out of the capillary into the ISF and ICF. Edema occurs throughout the body at every capillary-cell interface, and this is often most apparent in the peritoneal cavity as a swollen abdomen. In persons who are starving, the disorder is known as kwashiorkor.

A specific kind of edema, called dependent edema, often forms in the lower extremities. Under healthy conditions, venous return to the heart from the lower extremities is assisted by venous valves and muscle contractions. A weakened venous valve system, lack of muscle contractions, and gravitational forces can allow venous blood to collect in the lower extremities. When an individual stands or sits in one position for an extended period of time, venous blood can pool in the lower extremities. Increased hydrostatic pressure in the veins allows fluid to flow out of the capillary into interstitial tissues. Fluid accumulates in the ankles and feet, which are the dependent parts of the body. To avoid dependent edema, brisk venous circulation back to the heart and vigorous muscle activity need to be maintained in the lower extremities.

CLINICAL CONCEPT

Thromboembolic stockings (TEDS) and pneumatic compression devices that surround the lower leg attempt to enhance venous return from the lower extremities up to the heart in patients on bedrest.

Sodium retention caused by illness or consumption of salty foods can also contribute to edema. Excess sodium in the ECF pulls fluid from the ICF into the ECF, causing cellular dehydration. Dehydration causes thirst which, in turn, encourages the individual to drink water or other liquids. This ingestion and the movement of water from the ICF into the ECF causes an excess of water in the bloodstream, which increases hydrostatic pressure. As a result, hydrostatic pressure rises and overcomes osmotic pressure with resulting edema. This is also seen whenever there is increased activation of the RAAS. With increased cycling of the RAAS, enhanced sodium and water reabsorption into the bloodstream occurs, which raises blood volume and blood pressure.

 CLINICAL CONCEPT

Pitting edema occurs when pressure is applied to a small area and an indentation persists for some time after the release of the pressure. Depending on the severity, an individual can have +1, +2, or +3 pitting edema (see Fig. 7-8).

Sequestered Fluids

During illness, fluids can become sequestered in body cavities that are normally free of fluids, such as the

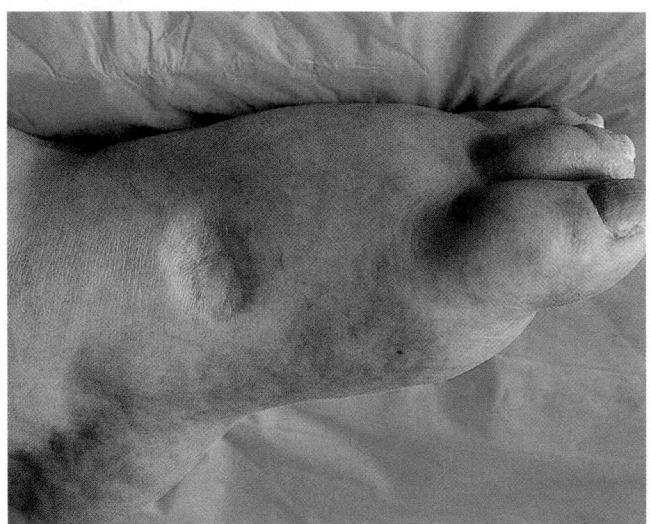

FIGURE 7-8. Pitting edema. Application of pressure over a bony area displaces the excess fluid, leaving an indentation or pit. (From Williams, L., & Hopper, P. (2011), *Understanding medical-surgical nursing.* 4th ed. Philadelphia, PA: F.A. Davis Company, with permission.)

pericardial sac, peritoneal cavity, and pleural space. When this occurs, it is referred to as third space accumulation of fluids. The fluid that accumulates in these cavities is commonly called an **effusion.** An effusion can be a transudate, which is a serous filtrate of blood, or an exudate, which contains material such as blood, lymph, proteins, pathogens, and inflammatory cells. Either type of effusion can surround organs and interfere with function. For example, a pleural effusion interferes with full lung expansion and ventilation, whereas a pericardial effusion can constrict the heart and prevent maximal filling of blood in the atria and ventricles.

 CLINICAL CONCEPT

A pericardial effusion can lead to cardiac tamponade, a disorder in which the heart's pumping action is restricted because of an accumulation of fluid surrounding it.

Fluid Volume Overload

Fluid volume overload occurs when the bloodstream has an excessive amount of water. One of the most common causes of fluid volume overload is heart failure. In heart failure, the RAAS is constantly cycling, which brings an excessive amount of water into the bloodstream. Blood volume increases, which increases the hydrostatic pressure. High hydrostatic pressure overwhelms osmotic pressure at every capillary bed, leading to edema in various places in the body. Ankle edema, peritoneal edema, and pulmonary edema occur in heart failure.

Fluid volume overload can also be seen in certain cancers that secrete ADH, causing a disorder known as syndrome of inappropriate ADH (SIADH). Other causes of ADH-related fluid volume overload include cirrhosis of the liver, polycystic kidney disease, and some forms of hypertension. Disorders that cause constant secretion of ADH promote excess water reabsorption from the collecting duct of the nephrons into the bloodstream. Water reabsorption into the blood causes fluid volume overload. Without concomitant absorption of sodium, water overload leads to dilution of electrolytes. Dilutional hyponatremia occurs because of the excess water in the bloodstream.

CLINICAL CONCEPT

SIADH can occur in certain cancers, brain disorders, and after brain surgery.

Dehydration

Dehydration is a state of diminished water volume in the body. In dehydration, there is a deficit of intracellular fluid, which causes body cells to shrink. There is also a decreased amount of water in the extracellular fluid. Dehydration has many causes, including reduced fluid intake and excessive fluid loss caused by illness. Lack of sufficient ADH production or lack of renal stimulation by ADH can also lead to excessive fluid loss and dehydration, as can certain gastrointestinal disorders such as prolonged diarrhea. Burns, fever, and perspiration also commonly cause large fluid loss. Regardless of cause, dehydration causes hypovolemia, a diminished level of circulating blood volume that increases the osmolarity of the blood.

For example, in uncontrolled diabetes, glucose rises to high levels and acts as a solute in the blood. The high amount of solute in the blood raises osmotic pressure, which imbalances the capillary forces. If osmotic pressure rises to exceed hydrostatic pressure inside the capillary, then water from the ICF and ISF move into the capillary and the cells lose water. This causes cells to shrink in a process known as cellular dehydration. The fluid shift into the circulation delivers more water to the kidneys, which is then excreted as excess urine or polyuria. Because of fluid shifts, the key symptoms of uncontrolled diabetes mellitus are thirst and polyuria.

Cellular dehydration can also occur because of hypernatremia (high sodium content of blood), which raises solute content and, in turn, raises osmotic pressure. High osmotic pressure causes water to shift from the ICF into the ECF. Cellular dehydration occurs with loss of ICF, causing the cells to shrink. The ECF gains fluid, which is excreted via the kidney; this leads to further dehydration. This situation continues until water is replenished.

> **ALERT!** There is a risk of renal dysfunction if the adult patient develops oliguria, which is urine output of fewer than 400 mL/day or fewer than 20 to 30 mL/hour. The kidney needs to yield a minimum of 400 mL of fluid daily to sufficiently excrete waste products.

The physiologic response to dehydration is multifaceted. Osmoreceptors respond to the blood's high osmotic content and stimulate the thirst center in the hypothalamus. Thirst occurs, which makes the person drink fluid to replace fluid lost from the cells. The blood vessel baroreceptors sense a decreased blood pressure in dehydration. This, in turn, stimulates the sympathetic nervous system, which vasoconstricts arterial vessels and increases heart rate to compensate. Additionally, osmoreceptors stimulate ADH secretion from the posterior pituitary gland. The ADH works at the nephron to increase water reabsorption into the bloodstream. Simultaneously, because there is low blood volume in dehydration, there is decreased circulation to the kidneys. Decreased kidney perfusion provokes renin secretion, which activates the RAAS, resulting in increased sodium and water in the bloodstream, raising blood volume. Additionally, angiotensin II acts as a potent vasoconstrictor, which raises blood pressure. These compensatory mechanisms restore fluid balance and maintain blood pressure in states of dehydration (see Fig. 7-9).

Assessment of Fluid Volume Status

Fluid losses and gains can be clinically assessed in many ways. A basic method to clinically assess an individual's fluid volume status is daily weight. When using daily weight to assess fluid volume status, it is important to take the measurement using the same scale, at the same time of day every day. A weight change of 2 pounds from one day to the next is likely caused by water gained or lost.

A record of the patient's 24-hour intake and output (I&O) is another common way to monitor fluid status. The amount of fluid intake necessary for the adult patient with normal heart and renal function is 1,500 mL/m^2 of body surface per day. On average, this is approximately 2 liters of fluid per day.

All fluids, including oral, intravenous, and tube feedings, are recorded as intake. All measurements should be recorded in milliliters (mL), so it is important to understand how to convert ounces to mL: 1 ounce of fluid is equal to 30 mL. Water from ingested food can be estimated at approximately 500 to 1,000 mL/day. Output includes urine, vomitus, wound or ostomy drainage, and insensible water losses through the lungs, sweat, and feces. Wound or ostomy drainage and vomitus must be estimated. Insensible water loss is usually 1,000 mL/day, but it may be more if fever is present. Water requirements increase during specific conditions; for example, water requirements increase by 100 to 150 mL per day for each Celsius degree of body temperature elevation (see Box 7-1). I&O should be approximately equal over a 24-hour period. The daily I&O record can indicate fluid retention, which is a positive fluid balance, or fluid deficit, which is a negative fluid balance (see Fig. 7-10).

Another clinical assessment of fluid status involves the patient's vital signs. The patient who is dehydrated may have tachycardia and hypotension, particularly postural hypotension. To assess for postural hypotension, measure the blood pressure in the lying and standing positions.

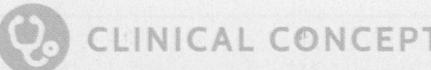

CLINICAL CONCEPT

Orthostatic hypotension, which occurs in dehydration, is a systolic blood pressure decrease of at least 20 mm Hg or a diastolic blood pressure decrease of at least 10 mm Hg within 3 minutes when going from a lying to a standing position.

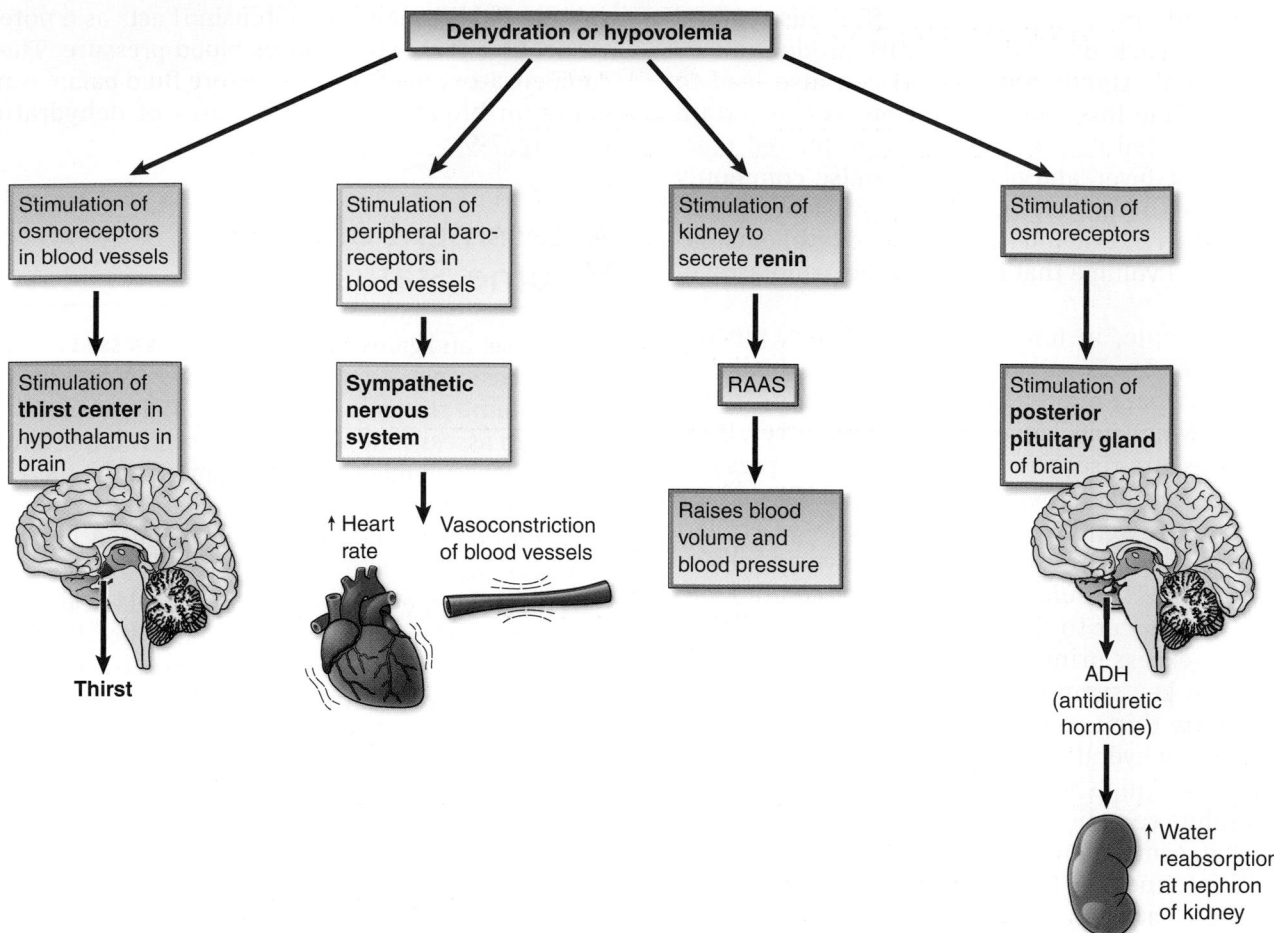

FIGURE 7-9. Physiologic responses to dehydration. The following pathways exhibit the ways the body compensates in dehydration and hypovolemia (low blood volume).

BOX 7-1. Conditions That Cause Dehydration and Increase Water Requirements

Bleeding
Breastfeeding
Burns
Fever
GI fluid loss
Hypotension
Nephrolithiasis
Polyuria
Surgical drains
Sweating
Tachypnea

Finally, a patient with a fluid volume deficit will have a number of symptoms of dehydration, including thirst, dry mucous membranes, poor skin turgor, hypotension, low urine output, and dark colored urine. Poor skin turgor is demonstrated through nonelasticity of the skin.

When the skin is pinched, a small tent of the skin remains.

A patient who has fluid volume excess will have edema, moist mucous membranes, and may have hypertension. With fluid excess, weight gain can occur and possibly ascites, as well as pitting edema. In severe fluid volume excess, dyspnea may also be present because of pulmonary edema. Box 7-2 presents the different signs and symptoms of fluid volume deficit and excess.

Electrolyte Imbalances

For a cell to function properly, serum electrolytes must be within normal range. Sodium is the main extracellular electrolyte, whereas potassium is the main intracellular electrolyte. The cellular Na^+/K^+ ATPase pump is constantly at work to try to retain K^+ in the intracellular compartment and move Na^+ to the extracellular environment.

Many enzymatic, hormonal, and chemically mediated mechanisms are dependent on normal levels of serum electrolytes. They are involved in the generation of ATP, transcription and translation of deoxyribonucleic acid (DNA) and ribonucleic acid (RNA), neural transmission, and muscular contraction.

INTAKE AND OUTPUT SHEET

Hospital # _____ Patient's name _____

Date _____ Room # _____

	INTAKE			OUTPUT			
				Urine		Gastric	
	By Mouth	Tube	Parenteral	Voided	Catheter	Emesis	Suction
Time 7–3	6 oz tea		IV mL DsW in NaCl 0.9%	500 mL			
Time 3–11	6 oz tea		IV mL DsW in NaCl 0.9%	500 mL			
Time 11–7	8 oz water			200 mL			
24-hour total	600 mL		1,000 mL				
24-hour grand total • Intake 1,600 mL				24-hour grand total • Output 1,100 mL			

FIGURE 7-10. Sample I&O record.

BOX 7-2. Signs and Symptoms of Fluid Volume Deficit and Excess

FLUID VOLUME DEFICIT
Dark urine with high specific gravity
Depressed fontanelles (infant)
Dry mucous membranes
Low urine output
Orthostatic hypotension
Poor skin turgor
Thirst
Weight loss

FLUID VOLUME EXCESS
Ascites
Crackles in lungs
Dyspnea caused by pulmonary fluid accumulation
Edema, either ankle or sacral
Weight gain (2 lbs = 1 liter of fluid)

Alterations in sodium, potassium, and calcium ion levels have a major effect on neurotransmission and muscular contraction. Changes in nerve and muscle excitability are particularly important in cardiac muscle where rhythm disruption and conduction disturbances can be life-threatening.

Most cells maintain an electrochemical gradient because of the effect of intracellular and extracellular sodium and potassium. This is most apparent in cell-to-cell impulse propagation in neurotransmission. Without stimulation, cells maintain a resting membrane potential created by a set ratio of intracellular and extracellular sodium and potassium ions. Action potentials, which are the impulses generated along neuronal axons, are created by changes in sodium and potassium ions in ICF and ECF. During an action potential, sodium ion channels open in the plasma membrane, allowing the entry of sodium ions into the cell. This is followed by the opening of potassium ion channels that permit the exit of potassium ions from the cell. The inward flow of sodium ions increases the concentration of positively charged cations in the cell and causes depolarization, where the potential of the cell is higher than the cell's resting potential. The sodium channels close at the peak of the action potential, whereas potassium continues to leave the cell. The efflux of potassium ions decreases the membrane potential in the repolarization phase (see Fig. 7-11). With imbalances of sodium and potassium in the body, neural transmission in the body is widely

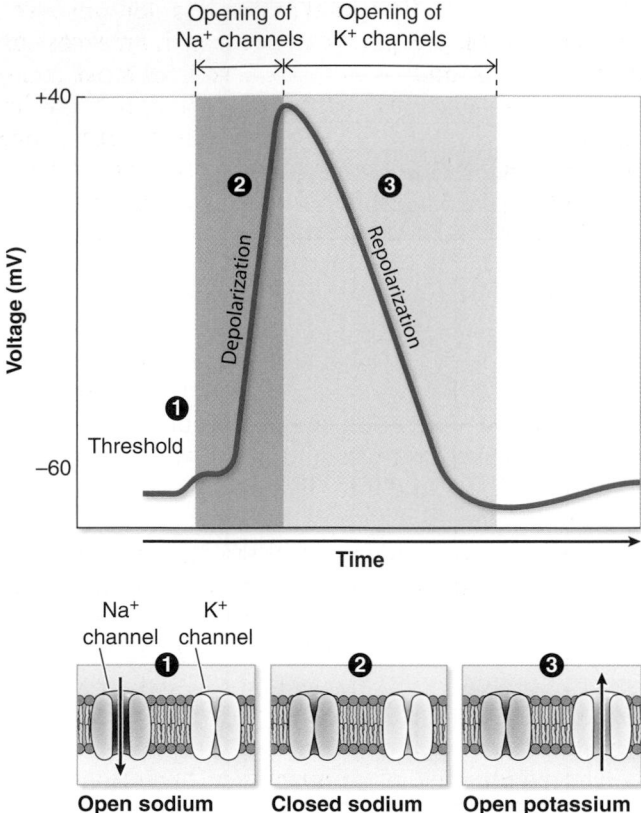

FIGURE 7-11. Nerve impulses are generated by action potentials within the neuron plasma membrane. Action potentials are generated by special types of ion channels embedded in a cell's plasma membrane. These channels are shut when the membrane potential is near the resting potential of the cell. (1) When the channels open, they allow an inward flow of sodium ions, which produces a rise in the membrane potential known as depolarization. This then causes more channels to open, and the process proceeds until all of the available sodium ion channels are open, resulting in a large upswing in the membrane potential. (2) The ion channels then close and sodium ions can no longer enter the neuron. (3). Potassium channels are then activated, and there is an outward current of potassium ions, returning the electrochemical gradient to the resting state. This is called repolarization.

disrupted. There is body-wide muscular weakness and changes in sensation such as paresthesias. The muscles of the gastrointestinal system dysfunction, causing nausea, constipation, and abdominal distention. Confusion and disorientation are common symptoms of CNS dysfunction. Cardiac dysfunction is particularly apparent with potassium level disruption. ECG changes, rhythm disturbances, and postural hypotension occur.

Cardiac muscle contractility is largely dependent on calcium ions. Like neurons and other muscles, a given cardiac muscle cell has a resting membrane potential. A notable difference between skeletal and cardiac muscle is how each depolarizes the muscle cells. When skeletal muscle is stimulated by motor nerves, an influx of Na+ quickly depolarizes the skeletal muscle cell. In cardiac muscle cells, calcium influx through voltage-gated calcium channels on the plasma membrane causes muscle contraction. Changes in serum calcium levels can cause hypotension, cardiac dysrhythmias, heart failure, and diminished responsiveness to cardiac drugs.

Sodium Imbalances

Sodium is the main electrolyte in the ECF and is the primary determinant of the ECF's osmolarity and volume. It must constantly be pumped out of the cell into the bloodstream. Sodium has many important physiologic roles. It controls the distribution of water, helps maintain normal fluid balance, and contributes to osmotic pressure. Sodium is also important to maintain the electrical gradient of neural membranes. However, because it is an extracellular ion, alterations in fluid balance can adversely affect its levels, which is why serum sodium levels need to be interpreted based on hydration status. The average diet contains 1 to 3 grams of sodium per day.

> ### 🫧 CLINICAL CONCEPT
>
> A low sodium diet consists of fewer than 1,500 mg of sodium per day. Low sodium diets are recommended in hypertension and heart failure.

Hyponatremia. **Hyponatremia** is a sodium serum level of less than 135 mEq/L. The clinical picture of hyponatremia centers around water. When dehydration occurs because the body has lost sodium and fluid together, it is known as hypovolemic hyponatremia; its cause is either renal or nonrenal.

The causes of renal hypovolemic hyponatremia include adrenal insufficiency, osmotic diuresis, diuretic use, and salt-losing nephritis. The causes of nonrenal hypovolemic hyponatremia include diarrhea, vomiting, excessive sweating, cystic fibrosis, gastric lavage, fistulas, burns, and wounds. In cases of dehydration caused by hypovolemic hyponatremia, the symptoms are thirst, dry mouth, orthostatic hypotension, tachycardia, azotemia (high blood urea nitrogen concentration), and oliguria.

Conversely, hyponatremia can occur in the presence of hypervolemia, which is excess water. In this case, hyponatremia develops because it is diluted within an excess of water, which is why it is a dilutional hyponatremia; symptoms include headache, lethargy, apathy, confusion, nausea, vomiting, diarrhea, muscle cramps, and muscle spasms.

Hyponatremia most commonly occurs when water excretion is impaired and it is diluted within a large volume of water in the bloodstream. This is clinically significant when hyponatremia is part of a drop in the serum total osmolality, which is measured by the calculation: 2(Na) mEq/L + serum glucose (mg/dL)/18 + BUN (mg/dL)/2.8.

When there is an acute drop in the serum osmolality, neuronal cell swelling occurs because of the water shift from the extracellular space to the intracellular space. Swelling of the brain cells results in two consequences:

- It inhibits ADH secretion from neurons in the hypothalamus and hypothalamic thirst center, which leads to excess water elimination as dilute urine.
- There is an immediate cellular adaptation with loss of electrolytes, and over the next few days there is a more gradual loss of organic intracellular solutes.

Severe hyponatremia can cause seizures, coma, and irreversible neurological damage because of brain swelling.

Treatment of hyponatremia is based on its etiology. If the patient is dehydrated, slow replacement of sodium with adequate fluid intake is the easiest method. Slow treatment is necessary as rapid correction of serum sodium can precipitate severe neurological complications. If that does not help, more aggressive measures will need to be taken, such as replacement with normal saline or hypertonic saline solution.

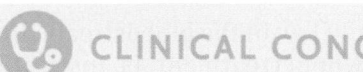

CLINICAL CONCEPT

A patient who receives normal saline or hypertonic saline needs to be watched carefully for edema, particularly for pulmonary edema or other signs of fluid overload.

If the etiology of hyponatremia is SIADH, treatment requires restriction of water intake and investigating the source of ADH. If the etiology of hyponatremia is fluid overload, then diuretics will be used to remove excess water. Knowing the etiology of the patient's low sodium is critical for choosing appropriate treatment.

Tolvaptan is a medication indicated for the treatment of clinically significant hypervolemic hyponatremia, which is indicated by a serum sodium of 125 mEq/L or less marked hyponatremia that is symptomatic and has resisted correction with fluid restriction.

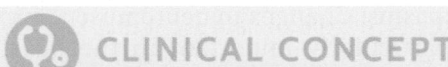

CLINICAL CONCEPT

Severe hyponatremia (less than 125 mEq/L) has a high mortality rate. In instances when the serum sodium level is lower than 105 mEq/L, the mortality is over 50%. Postoperative and elderly patients have the highest incidence of hyponatremia.

Hypernatremia. **Hypernatremia** is a sodium level greater than 145 mEq/L. It can occur with an excess of or decrease in body water (see Box 7-3). Most commonly, it is caused by water loss, although it can be caused by salt loading. With kidney dysfunction, there are other factors that may be involved, such as the inability of the renal tubule to react to ADH, causing the kidneys to not reabsorb water. With an inadequate amount of water in the blood, sodium is more concentrated and presents as a high serum level. Also, if the kidneys have a decreased glomerular filtration rate, there is low sodium and water reabsorption into the bloodstream, which stimulates the adrenal gland's secretion of aldosterone. Aldosterone causes reabsorption of sodium and water from the nephron tubule fluid into the circulation, raising the sodium level.

When hypernatremia of any etiology occurs, cells become dehydrated. The high osmotic load of the increased sodium acts to extract water from the cells. Dehydrated cells shrink from water extraction. Cells immediately respond to combat this shrinkage and osmotic force by transporting electrolytes across the cell membrane, thus altering rest potentials of electrically active membranes. After an hour of hypernatremia, intracellular organic solutes are generated in an effort to restore cell volume and to avoid structural damage. This protective mechanism is important to remember when treating a patient with hypernatremia. Cerebral edema ensues if water replacement proceeds at a rate that does not allow for excretion or metabolism of accumulated solutes.

The effects of cellular dehydration are seen principally in the central nervous system (CNS), where stretching of shrunken neurons and alteration of membrane potentials from electrolyte flux lead to ineffective functioning. If shrinkage is severe enough, stretching and rupture of bridging veins may cause intracranial hemorrhage.

The clinical manifestations of hypernatremia can be divided into two distinct patterns, one with fluid overload and one without fluid overload. If hypernatremia causes water retention, then the picture is one of an edematous state: weight gain and hypertension. With severe edematous states, there may also be mental changes and pulmonary edema causing dyspnea. If the hypernatremia is that of sodium retention and water loss, the patient will appear to be dehydrated and demonstrate thirst, irritability, tachycardia, flushed skin, dry mucous membranes, and oliguria.

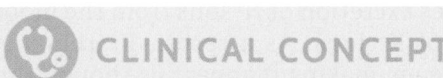

CLINICAL CONCEPT

Hypernatremia risk is highest in breastfed infants and the elderly.

BOX 7-3. Causes of Hyponatremia and Hypernatremia

Causes of Hyponatremia	Causes of Hypernatremia
• Adrenal insufficiency • Burns • Cirrhosis • Congestive heart failure • Diaphoresis with more salt lost than water • Diarrhea • Diuretic therapy • Excess hypotonic fluid administration (called *dilutional hyponatremia*) • Hyperglycemia • Hypoaldosteronism • Laxatives • Nasogastric suction • Psychogenic polydipsia • Renal disease • Syndrome of inappropriate antidiuretic hormone, which causes excess reabsorption of water into the bloodstream at the nephron	• Certain medications such as osmotic diuretics, sodium bicarbonate, and sodium chloride • Cushing's syndrome • Diabetes insipidus (lack of antidiuretic hormone) • Diarrhea • Excess sodium administration • Excessive adrenocortical secretion • Hypercalcemia • Impaired thirst • Increased aldosterone • Potassium depletion • Profuse diaphoresis • Tube feedings with lack of adequate water administration • Uncontrolled diabetes mellitus • Water deprivation

Treatment of hypernatremia depends on the underlying cause. Replacement fluids can be given orally or parenterally if it is caused by fluid depletion. Oral glucose-electrolyte replacement solutions are available for infants and children. If excess water is present, diuretic therapy may be necessary.

The mortality rate from hypernatremia is high, especially among elderly patients. Mortality rates of 42% to 75% have been reported for acute changes and 10% to 60% for chronic hypernatremia.

Potassium Imbalances

Potassium is the main electrolyte of the ICF; adults require 40 to 60 mEq/L/day of K^+. Fluid shifts between the ICF and ECF can cause temporary changes in plasma potassium levels. Additionally, potassium levels should be assessed in relation to acid-base balance. Potassium will move from the ICF to the ECF based on changes in the hydrogen ion $[H^+]$ concentration in the bloodstream. When H^+ is high in the bloodstream, H^+ excretion takes precedence over K^+ excretion at the kidney. In acidosis, aldosterone stimulates excretion of H^+ ions from the bloodstream instead of K^+ ions. As a result, K^+ remains in the bloodstream, making it appear as though there is an excess of K^+ in the blood, but this is not true hyperkalemia. When the acidosis is treated, K^+ will move into the ICF compartment, which will demonstrate that K^+ is actually low in the bloodstream. In diabetic ketoacidosis, when treatment is instituted using insulin, K^+ moves into the intracellular compartment. This movement of K^+ into the cells leaves an actual low K^+ level in the blood, thereby requiring administration of supplemental potassium.

Potassium is involved in a wide range of body functions, including conduction of nerve impulses in skeletal, cardiac, and smooth muscle; acid-base balance; synthesis of adenosine-5'-triphosphate; osmotic balance; and the kidney's ability to concentrate urine. The nephron regulates potassium because of the action of aldosterone, which absorbs sodium and water and excretes potassium at the distal tubule.

Muscle contains the bulk of the body's potassium, and alterations in potassium levels have neuromuscular effects. A decrease in serum potassium causes decreased neuromuscular excitability, resulting in muscle weakness. An increase in potassium causes increased neuromuscular excitability, resulting in muscle spasms. Changes in neuromuscular excitability are particularly important in the heart, where alterations in serum potassium can produce serious cardiac arrhythmias.

Hypokalemia. **Hypokalemia** refers to a plasma concentration of potassium below 3.5 mEq/L. Diuretic therapy is the most common cause of hypokalemia; it is present in 20% to 50% of patients on nonpotassium-sparing diuretics. African Americans and females are more susceptible. Risk is enhanced by concomitant illness such as heart failure or nephrotic syndrome. Both thiazide and loop diuretics increase the loss of K^+ in the urine.

Inadequate intake is also a frequent cause of hypokalemia. Patients who are NPO, alcoholics, patients who have undergone bariatric surgery, and those who suffer eating disorders are at greatest risk. A daily potassium intake of at least 10 to 30 mEq is required for optimal cell function.

The body can also lose approximately 80% to 90% of potassium via the kidneys, with the remainder lost through sweat and feces. Renal losses are increased by stress, trauma, metabolic alkalosis, and increased levels of aldosterone. Skin and gastrointestinal losses of K^+ can become excessive in burns, vomiting, nasogastric suctioning, and diarrhea. Severe diarrheal illness can cause a loss of potassium of 40 to 60 mEq/L.

The major signs and symptoms associated with hypokalemia include anorexia, nausea, vomiting, sluggish bowel, cardiac arrhythmias, postural hypotension, muscle fatigue, and weakness. Leg cramps are particularly common. Also, respiratory muscles can be weakened in severe hypokalemia. There can be decreased or absent deep tendon reflexes on physical examination. On ECG, there is a prolonged PR interval, flattened T wave, and prominent U wave (see Fig. 7-12).

There are specific clinical conditions that can decrease potassium levels in the bloodstream. When large amounts of IV dextrose solution are administered to patients, excessive secretion of insulin is released by the pancreas; this can cause hypokalemia. The administration of adrenergic agents, such as epinephrine or albuterol, can also cause a drop in blood potassium levels. Commonly, diuretics also cause a loss of potassium from the bloodstream.

Digitalis toxicity often occurs when the patient is in the state of hypokalemia. Digitalis is a drug used when a patient is in heart failure. Heart failure often causes a loss of potassium because of the cycling of the RAAS when the heart is weakened. When digitalis is administered to a patient, potassium and digitalis compete for binding sites in the heart. In hypokalemia, there are open binding sites for potassium in the heart and digitalis binds to these sites. When a high number of binding sites become occupied by digitalis, there is an increased potential for digitalis toxicity.

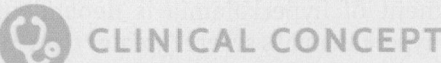
CLINICAL CONCEPT

Diuretics and digitalis are often prescribed together in heart failure. Diuretics commonly cause urinary loss of potassium leading to hypokalemia. Hypokalemia causes increased binding of digitalis in the heart, which increases susceptibility of digitalis toxicity, commonly demonstrated as arrhythmias. Potassium blood level and digitalis level need to be frequently monitored in heart failure.

Treatment of hypokalemia is accomplished by replacement of potassium with foods such as orange juice, bananas, dried fruits, meats, and oral or parenteral K^+ preparations. Potassium can also be prescribed intravenously; commonly 20 mEq of potassium chloride (KCl) per liter of intravenous solution is administered to NPO patients, not to exceed a total of 60 mEq/day.

ALERT! Rapid administration of K^+ can cause cardiac arrest. IV potassium must always be diluted, and never given as an IV bolus. It is excoriating to the skin and blood vessels in large doses. In emergency cases, up to 40 mEq of potassium can be administered through a central venous line.

Hyperkalemia

Hyperkalemia is a blood K^+ level greater than 5.2 mEq/dL. Normal kidney function is important in the regulation of potassium. Any decrease in renal perfusion, such as decreased cardiac output, will diminish the kidney's ability to excrete K^+, thus increasing the amount of potassium in the body.

The clinical presentation of a patient with hyperkalemia will depend on the level of the potassium imbalance and if it is chronically elevated or acutely elevated. Early symptoms of hyperkalemia include numbness or tingling of the extremities, muscle cramping, diarrhea, apathy, and mental confusion. The ECG will show wide QRS complexes and tall, peaked T waves; as the potassium level rises, the ECG will show bradycardia, irregular pulse rate, and, ultimately, cardiac arrest (see Fig. 7-13).

Hypokalemia

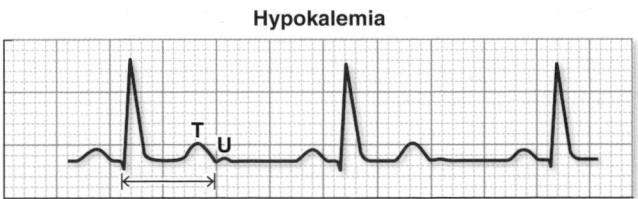

FIGURE 7-12. Electrocardiogram changes indicative of hypokalemia.

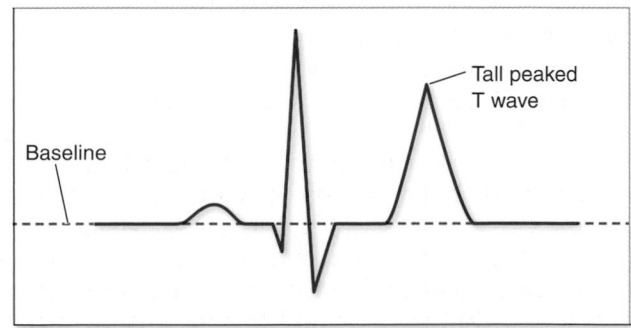

FIGURE 7-13. Electrocardiogram changes indicative of hyperkalemia.

Treatment of hyperkalemia is dependent on the cause. If hyperkalemia is severe (greater than 7.0 mEq/L), rapid treatment is needed to move K^+ from ECF to ICF. Continuous ECG monitoring is necessary. An infusion of 50% dextrose, 10 units of regular insulin, and 75 mEq of sodium bicarbonate can be administered. If K^+ levels continue to be elevated and the patient has normal renal function, a diuretic such as furosemide (Lasix) can be administered. Calcium chloride or calcium gluconate (Kalcinate) can also be administered. Another option for treatment is to give sodium polystyrene sulfonate (Kayexalate), which acts at the bowel to capture potassium and excrete it via feces. Alternatively, if the patient is in renal failure, dialysis can reduce K^+ (see Box 7-4).

Calcium Imbalances

Calcium and phosphorus are the major mineral contents of bone. A small amount of these electrolytes, which are regulated by vitamin D and parathyroid hormone (PTH), is found in the circulation. The major function of vitamin D is to facilitate the absorption of calcium from the gastrointestinal tract into the bloodstream; once in the bloodstream, PTH controls calcium levels. When the plasma calcium level is low, PTH is stimulated; when the plasma calcium level is high, PTH is inhibited.

PTH acts on bone to mobilize calcium and raise blood levels. There is a reciprocal relationship between calcium and phosphate; when there is an increase in calcium in the blood, there is a decrease in phosphate—and vice versa. Calcitonin, a hormone produced by the thyroid, acts at the bone and kidneys to remove calcium from the circulation.

Calcium is an important element in the body because of its role in the formation and function of bones and teeth, normal clotting, and regulation of neuromuscular irritability. It is stored in the bone, bound to plasma proteins, and bound with organic ions such as citrate. A small amount of calcium also remains free. This free, or ionized, calcium interacts in normal physiologic functions. The ionized form participates in cellular activities such as enzymatic reactions; neuron excitability; muscle contraction; release of hormones, neurotransmitters, and other chemical messengers; blood vessel contractility; cardiac contractility and automaticity; and blood clotting. Calcium is found in both ECF and ICF.

Because calcium is highly protein bound, interpretation of calcium levels is based on serum albumin levels. About half of the calcium in the body is bound to albumin. Hypoalbuminemia can cause the appearance of low calcium levels called pseudohypocalcemia. In pseudohypocalcemia, there is a normal level of body calcium with more in the ionized state than in the bound state because there is a diminished amount of albumin able to carry calcium.

Hypocalcemia

Hypocalcemia consists of a blood calcium level of less than 8.7 mg/dL in adults. Acute hypocalcemia is manifested by neuromuscular excitability, which is demonstrated in individuals as a subjective experience of paresthesias around the mouth, hands, and feet; muscle spasms of the face, hands, and feet; laryngeal spasm; seizures; and death. Cardiovascular effects of

---

BOX 7-4. Causes of Hypokalemia and Hyperkalemia

Causes of Hypokalemia	Causes of Hyperkalemia
• Alkalosis	• Addison's disease
• Diuretic therapy	• Burns (can redistribute K^+ into ECF from ICF)
• Elevated glucocorticoids	• Digitalis toxicity
• Excessive gastrointestinal, renal, or skin losses	• Excessive administration of K^+ sparing diuretics (Spironolactone)
• Hyperaldosteronism	• Extreme exercise
• Inadequate intake	• Hemolysis of red blood cells
• Laxative abuse	• Hypoaldosteronism
• Nasogastric suction	• Medications: antibiotics such as Bactrim, ACE inhibitors, chemotherapeutic agents, and immunosuppressive agents such as cyclosporine
• Redistribution of potassium (K^+) between the intracellular and extracellular spaces	• Metabolic acidosis
	• Na^+ depletion
	• Renal failure
	• Trauma (can redistribute K^+ into ECF from ICF)

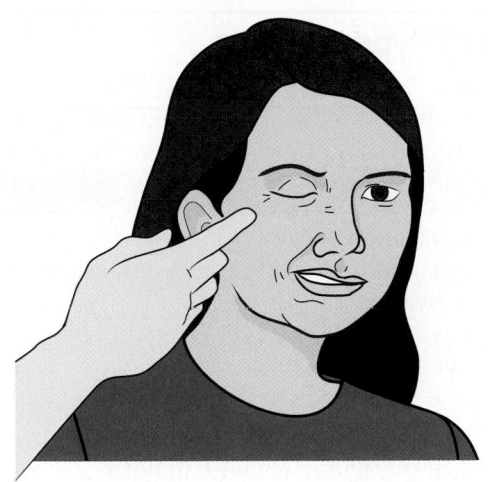

FIGURE 7-14. Chvostek's sign. (From Williams, L., & Hopper, P. (2011), *Understanding medical-surgical nursing.* 4th ed. Philadelphia, PA: F.A. Davis Company, with permission.)

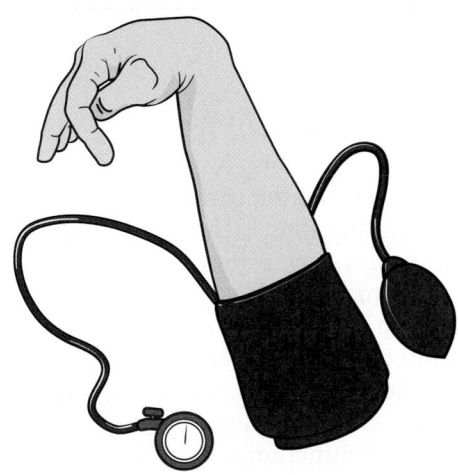

FIGURE 7-15. Trousseau's sign. (From Williams, L., & Hopper, P. (2011), *Understanding medical-surgical nursing.* 4th ed. Philadelphia, PA: F.A. Davis Company, with permission.)

hypocalcemia include hypotension, arrhythmias (particularly heart block and ventricular fibrillation), and failure to respond to cardioactive drugs. Chronic hypocalcemia causes bone pain and fragility, dry skin and hair, cataracts, depression, and dementia. Chvostek's sign and Trousseau's sign are examples of neuromuscular irritability caused by chronically low calcium levels (see Fig. 7-14 and Fig. 7-15).

Treatment of hypocalcemia requires calcium replacement. Oral calcium supplements with vitamin D are often used, as vitamin D is needed for calcium absorption from the intestine.

Hypercalcemia

Hypercalcemia is a calcium level greater than 10 mg/dL. Hypercalcemia will occur when the amount of calcium entering the ECF exceeds calcium excretion by the kidneys. The two common causes are hyperparathyroidism and cancer. In hyperparathyroidism, the PTH is overproduced, and the hormone pulls excessive amounts of calcium out of the bones and into the bloodstream. Cancer-related hypercalcemia is caused by malignant cells invading the bone, causing bone destruction. Cancer also releases a parathyroid-like hormone, causing an increase in serum calcium levels.

The signs and symptoms of hypercalcemia involve decreased neuromuscular excitability. Muscle flaccidity, proximal muscle weakness of the lower extremities, bone tenderness, and decreased neuromuscular activity of the bowel causing constipation are the main effects. High calcium concentrations in the urine increase susceptibility to renal calculi. The heart responds to hypercalcemia with increased contractility and ventricular arrhythmias. Other nonspecific effects include dulled consciousness, depression, anorexia, nausea, vomiting, and ulcers. Hyperreflexia and tongue fasciculations may also occur.

Treatment involves enhancement of urinary excretion of calcium and inhibition of bone breakdown. Increased fluids and loop diuretics enhance calcium excretion. Bisphosphonates, such as alendronate, and calcitonin are used to inhibit bone breakdown. Dialysis can be used in patients with kidney or heart failure (see Box 7-5).

Phosphorus Imbalances

Phosphorus is an essential component of bone, red blood cells, enzymatic processes, formation of adenosine triphosphate (ATP), acid-base balance, and cellular building blocks. Phosphorus is found in bone and circulates in the blood as phosphate (PO_4-). They are incorporated into nucleic acids of DNA and RNA and the phospholipids of the cell membrane. The kidneys excrete phosphate, and the parathyroid glands regulate the phosphate level in the blood. Phosphate has a reciprocal relationship with calcium in the blood, meaning that when calcium is low in the bloodstream, phosphate is high and vice versa.

Hypophosphatemia

Hypophosphatemia consists of a blood level of phosphate lower than 2.5 mg/dL There are three main causes of hypophosphatemia: decreased intestinal absorption of phosphorus, increased excretion of phosphorus by the kidneys, and an intracellular shift of phosphate. Low phosphate causes red blood cell, white blood cell, and platelet dysfunction, as well as neural dysfunction and disturbed musculoskeletal function. Lack of sufficient phosphate can cause tremors, paresthesias, hyporeflexia, anorexia, dysphagia, muscle weakness, joint stiffness, bone pain, and osteomalacia. Treatment of hypophosphatemia is replacement therapy.

Hyperphosphatemia

Hyperphosphatemia is a PO_4- level of 4.5 mg/dL or greater in the blood. The most common cause of hyperphosphatemia is kidney failure, where the kidneys are

BOX 7-5. Causes of Hypocalcemia and Hypercalcemia

Causes of Hypocalcemia	Causes of Hypercalcemia
• Alcohol abuse	• Decreased elimination of calcium
• Drugs: loop diuretics, anticonvulsants, calcitonin, gentamycin, phosphates	• Drugs: diuretics, chemotherapy, androgens, estrogen, lithium, theophylline
• Hyperphosphatemia	• Excess vitamin D
• Hypoalbuminemia	• Hyperparathyroidism
• Hypomagnesemia	• Increased bone resorption of calcium
• Hypoparathyroidism	• Increased intestinal absorption of calcium
• Inadequate dietary intake or inadequate vitamin D	• Malignancy such as bone, multiple myeloma, blood, breast, and lung cancer
• Malabsorption	• Prolonged immobility
• Pancreatitis	• Renal insufficiency
• Sepsis	

unable to excrete excessive phosphorus. Hyperphosphatemia is usually accompanied by hypocalcemia, and many of its symptoms are related to low calcium levels. Treatment is directed at correcting the cause of the disorder. Calcium-based phosphate binders, such as sevelamer and lanthanum carbonate, inhibit gastrointestinal absorption of phosphate. Dialysis can also reduce hyperphosphatemia (see Box 7-6).

BOX 7-6. Causes of Hypophosphatemia and Hyperphosphatemia

Causes of Hypophosphatemia	Causes of Hyperphosphatemia
Alcohol withdrawal	Chemotherapy
Antacid abuse	Excessive vitamin D
Burns	Hyperthyroidism
Decreased intestinal absorption of PO_4-	Hypoparathyroidism
Diabetic ketoacidosis	Laxative/enema excess
Hyperalimentation (nutrient-rich intravenous solution)	Massive cellular injury
	Renal failure
	Sarcoidosis
Hypercalcemia	Tuberculosis
Hyperparathyroidism	
Increased renal loss of PO_4-	
Lack of vitamin D	
Respiratory alkalosis	

Magnesium Imbalances

Magnesium (Mg^{++}) is largely stored in bone and, like calcium, is protein-bound within the bloodstream. It is the most abundant cation in the intracellular fluid. About 60% of the body's magnesium is found in the bones. It is required for many cellular metabolic processes, such as functioning of nerve conduction, replication and transcription of DNA, translation of RNA, intracellular enzyme reactions, and all processes that require ATP. The cardiovascular system requires magnesium for vasodilation and normal functioning. Magnesium also affects sodium and potassium levels both inside and outside the cell membrane. Magnesium can also compete with and exert effects on calcium-mediated processes, because of its effect on the parathyroid gland.

Magnesium is ingested from the diet in meats, seafood, green vegetables, and some sources of ground water. It is absorbed from the intestine, reabsorbed in the loop of Henle, and then excreted by the kidney. It is inhibited by high plasma calcium levels and high PTH levels. Magnesium also assists in release of PTH. There is an interdependent relationship between Mg^{++} and K^+: when K^+ decreases, so does Mg^{++} and vice versa.

Hypomagnesemia

Hypomagnesemia is a magnesium blood level of less than 1.5 mEq/L. In this disorder, Mg^{++} ions are released from bone in exchange for increased uptake of calcium. It usually occurs in conjunction with hypocalcemia and hypokalemia. Causes of hypomagnesemia are prolonged diarrhea, laxative abuse, increased renal excretion of magnesium, sepsis, burns, and serious wounds requiring debridement. Signs and symptoms of low Mg^{++} are similar to those of low Ca^{++} and K^+ levels. These include neuromuscular manifestations such as tetany, Chvostek's sign, Trousseau's sign, and cardiac arrhythmias. There may be ECG changes similar to those of hypokalemia. More serious manifestations may be respiratory muscle paralysis, complete heart block, and coma. Treatment of hypomagnesemia is replacement therapy, commonly with magnesium sulfate.

Hypermagnesemia

Hypermagnesemia is a magnesium blood level of greater than 2.5 mEq/L. Magnesium is often used to treat cardiac disorders and pregnancy-related eclampsia, and levels must be carefully monitored. The most common cause of hypermagnesemia is renal dysfunction. High Mg^{++} inhibits acetylcholine release and can cause diminished neuromuscular function, demonstrated by hyporeflexia and muscle weakness. Magnesium also blocks calcium channels and can cause cardiovascular effects such as hypotension and arrhythmias. Severely high Mg^{++} levels (greater than 10 mEq/L) can cause cardiac arrest. To counteract hypermagnesemia, intravenous calcium or dialysis can be used (see Box 7-7).

BOX 7-7. Causes of Hypomagnesemia and Hypermagnesemia

Causes of Hypomagnesemia	Causes of Hypermagnesemia
• Alcoholism	• Alcohol withdrawal
• Citrated blood	• Antacid abuse
• Diarrhea	• Burns
• Drugs such as diuretics, aminoglycoside antibiotics, amphotericin, cyclosporine	• Decreased intestinal absorption of PO_4-
• Liver failure	• Diabetic ketoacidosis
• Malabsorption	• Hyperalimentation (nutrient-rich intravenous solution)
• Malnutrition	• Hypercalcemia
• Renal failure	• Hyperparathyroidism
	• Increased renal loss of PO_4-
	• Lack of vitamin D
	• Respiratory alkalosis

Chapter Summary

- The human body is 60% water and it is contained in three different compartments: intracellular, interstitial, and extracellular.

- The extracellular compartment is within the bloodstream, intracellular is within each cell, and interstitial is in the tissue between the cells and bloodstream.

- Hypovolemia stimulates the RAAS.

- Blocking angiotensin converting enzyme (ACE) inhibits the conversion of angiotensin I to angiotensin II in the RAAS.

- Angiotensin II is a potent vasoconstrictor and stimulates the adrenal gland to secrete aldosterone.

- Aldosterone increases sodium and water reabsorption into the bloodstream and excretes potassium into the urine.

- The posterior pituitary secretes ADH, which causes water reabsorption into the bloodstream.

- SIADH causes excess secretion of ADH and excess water reabsorption, which results in hypervolemia and dilutional hyponatremia.

- Electrolytes Na^+, K^+, Ca^{++}, Mg^{++}, and PO_4- are the main ionic solutes in the blood.

- Sodium has a major influence on hydration status.

- Starling's Law of Capillary Forces explains that there are two major forces at every capillary-cell interface in the body: hydrostatic and osmotic pressure. Hydrostatic pressure forces fluid out of the capillary pores into the tissues and osmotic pressure pulls water from the tissues into the bloodstream.

- There are three types of intravenous solution: isotonic, hypotonic, and hypertonic. The loss of body water, whether acute or chronic, can cause a range of problems from mild lightheadedness to convulsions and coma. Conversely, the administration of excess water can be lethal to the patient.

Making the Connections

Pathophysiology	Signs and Symptoms	Physical Assessment Findings	Diagnostic Testing	Treatment
Dehydration | Lack of body water in intracellular and extracellular fluid.				
	Thirst. Dry mucous membranes. Weakness.	Low urine output. Dark urine. Poor skin turgor. Dry mucous membranes. Hypotension. In infants, depressed fontanelle.	High blood urea nitrogen (BUN). Oliguria. Hypernatremia caused by low water in blood.	Oral fluids. IV 0.45% NaCl.
Overhydration | Excess of body water in ICF and ECF.				
	Edema. Weight gain.	Dyspnea caused by pulmonary fluid accumulation. Crackles in lungs. Edema, either ankle or sacral. Weight gain. Ascites.	Dilutional hyponatremia.	Diuretic.
Hyponatremia | Serum sodium lower than 135 mEq/L. Commonly caused by heart failure, diuretic therapy, cirrhosis, nephrosis, excess water intake, SIADH.				
	Muscle cramps. Weakness. Headache. Depression. Anxiety. Lethargy. Confusion. Anorexia Nausea. Vomiting.	Weakness. Depression. Anxiety. Lethargy. Confusion. Vomiting.	Serum sodium less than 135 mEq/L.	Depends on cause of low sodium. Slow replacement of sodium if true hyponatremia. Tolvaptan if true hyponatremia. Restriction of water intake if caused by dilutional hyponatremia.
Hypernatremia | Serum sodium greater than 145 mEq/L. Commonly caused by loss of water, fluid restriction, hypertonic IV fluids, diaphoresis with more water loss than sodium, tube feedings without adequate free water, Cushing's syndrome, diabetes insipidus.				
	Decreased salivation. Thirst. Headache. Agitation. Seizures.	Decreased skin turgor if low water volume. Decreased reflexes. Tachycardia. Weak, thready pulse. Hypertension or hypotension depending on water volume.	Serum sodium greater than 145.	If caused by inadequate water: Replace with IV fluid 0.45% NaCl.

Continued

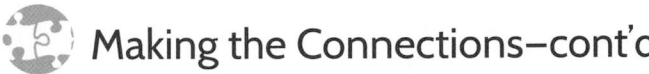

Making the Connections—cont'd

Pathophysiology	Signs and Symptoms	Physical Assessment Findings	Diagnostic Testing	Treatment
Hypokalemia | Serum potassium level less than 3.5 mEq/L. Commonly caused by dietary deficiency, diuretics, vomiting, diarrhea, NG suction, hyperaldosteronism, salt wasting kidney disease, GI surgery, alkalosis, laxative abuse.				
	Anorexia, nausea, vomiting. Muscle weakness. Muscle cramps. Paresthesias. Confusion.	Postural hypotension. Increased sensitivity to digitalis toxicity. Muscle weakness.	Serum potassium level less than 3.5 mEq/L. ECG dysrhythmias ECG: U wave.	Oral or parenteral K^+.
Hyperkalemia | Serum potassium level greater than 5.2 mEq/L. Commonly caused by excessive intake, aldosterone deficiency, Na^+ depletion, acidosis, tissue trauma, burns, extreme exercise, renal failure, Addison's disease (lack of cortisol), hemolysis, potassium-sparing diuretics, ACE inhibitors.				
	Nausea, vomiting. Intestinal cramping. Diarrhea. Paresthesias. Muscle weakness. Muscle cramping. Dizziness.	Muscle weakness. Dizziness.	Serum potassium level greater than 5.2 mEq/L. ECG changes, including peaked T wave. Risk of cardiac arrest with severe K^+ excess.	An infusion of 50% dextrose, 10 units of regular insulin, and 75 mEq of sodium bicarbonate. Lasix. Calcium chloride or Calcium gluconate (Kalcinate). Sodium polystyrene sulfonate (Kayexalate®).
Hypocalcemia | Serum calcium level less than 8.5 mg/dL. Commonly caused by hypoparathyroidism, malabsorption syndrome, hypomagnesemia, hyperphosphatemia, renal failure, insufficient vitamin D, hypoalbuminemia, diuretic therapy, diarrhea, acute pancreatitis, gastric surgery, massive blood transfusion.				
	Body-wide muscle cramps (tetany). Laryngeal spasm Paresthesias. Bone pain, deformities, fracture. Dry skin, hair. Confusion. Seizure.	Increased neuromuscular excitability (tetany). Hyperactive reflexes. Positive Chvostek's and Trousseau's sign. Hypotension. Seizure. Dementia possible.	Serum calcium level less than 8.5 mg/dL. Arrhythmias. Heart block. Ventricular fibrillation.	Administration of Ca^{++} and vitamin D.
Hypercalcemia | Serum calcium level greater than 10.5 mg/dL. Commonly caused by excessive calcium in diet, excessive vitamin D, immobility, hyperparathyroidism, hypophosphatemia, diuretics, ACE inhibitors, lithium therapy, prolonged immobility, malignancy of bone or blood.				
	Anorexia. Nausea, vomiting. Constipation. Muscle weakness. Bone fracture possible.	Decreased neuromuscular excitability. Ataxia. Loss of muscle tone. Hypertension.	Serum calcium level greater than 10.5 mg/dL. Urine hematuria/calcium. Kidney stone possible. Low bone density (osteopenia, osteoporosis). Hypertension. Heart block.	Increased fluids and loop diuretics enhance calcium excretion. Bisphosphonates and calcitonin are used to inhibit bone breakdown. Dialysis may be necessary.

Continued

Making the Connections—cont'd

Pathophysiology	Signs and Symptoms	Physical Assessment Findings	Diagnostic Testing	Treatment

Hypophosphatemia | Serum phosphorus level less than 2.5 mg/dL. Can be caused by ingestion of excess antacids (aluminum and calcium), severe diarrhea, lack of vitamin D, hypercalcemia, alkalosis, hyperparathyroidism, diabetic ketoacidosis, alcoholism.

| | Tremor. Lack of coordination. Paresthesias. Confusion. Seizures. Muscle weakness. Joint stiffness. Bone pain. | Tremor. Ataxia. Muscle weakness. Decreased reflexes. | Serum phosphorus level less than 2.5 mg/dL. Complete blood count; low hemoglobin, hematocrit, hemolytic anemia. Platelet dysfunction; bruising. White blood cell dysfunction; infections. Low bone density Osteomalacia. | Replacement of PO_4-. |

Hyperphosphatemia | Serum phosphorus level greater than 4.5 mg/dL. Can be caused by laxatives, enemas containing phosphate, massive trauma, heat stroke, rhabdomyolysis, tumor lysis syndrome, potassium deficiency, hypocalcemia, kidney failure, hypoparathyroidism.

| | Paresthesias. Muscle cramps. | Tetany. Hypotension. | Cardiac arrhythmias. | Calcium-based phosphate binders and dialysis reduce hyperphosphatemia. |

Hypomagnesemia | Serum magnesium level less than 1.5 mg/dL. Can be caused by malnutrition/malabsorption Excessive loss of GI fluids. Alcoholism/cirrhosis, diuretic therapy, hyperparathyroidism, hyperaldosteronism, diabetic ketoacidosis, thyroid malfunction, pancreatitis, NG suction, fistulas.

| | Muscle cramps. Personality change. Uncontrollable movements. | Positive Chvostek's and Trousseau's sign. Nystagmus. Positive Babinski sign. Hypertension. | Serum magnesium level less than 1.5 mg/dL. ECG: tachycardia, arrhythmias. | Replacement Mg^{++} therapy. |

Hypermagnesemia | Serum magnesium level greater than 2.5 mg/dL. Can be caused by excessive use of Mg containing antacids and laxatives, untreated diabetic ketoacidosis, excessive Mg infusion, renal failure.

| | Lethargy. Confusion. Weakness. | Decreased reflexes (hyporeflexia). Hypotension. Weak muscles. | Serum magnesium level greater than 2.5 mg/dL. ECG: Arrythmias. Cardiac arrest possible. | IV calcium or dialysis. |

Bibliography

Albert, N. M. (2012). Fluid management strategies in heart failure. *Crit Care Nurs.* 32(2), 20–32.

Arora, S. K. (2011). Hypernatremic disorders in the intensive care unit. *J Int Care Med,* May 16. Epub ahead of print.

Bergwitz, C., Collins, M. T., Kamath, R. S., & Rosenberg, A. E. (2011). Case records of the Massachusetts General Hospital. Case 33-2011. A 56-year-old man with hypophosphatemia. *N Engl J Med,* 365(17), 1625–1635.

Chawla, A., Sterns, R. H., Nigwekar, S. U., & Cappuccio, J. D. (2011). Mortality and serum sodium: do patients die from or with hyponatremia? *Clin J Am Soc Nephr,* 6(5), 960–965.

Friedewald, V. E., Emmett, M., Gheorghiade, M., & Roberts, W. C. (2011). The editor's roundtable: pathophysiology and management of hyponatremia and the role of vasopressin antagonists. *Am J Card,* 107(9), 1357–1364.

Guevara, M., & Ginès, P. (2010). Hyponatremia in liver cirrhosis: pathogenesis and treatment. *End Nutr,* 57 Suppl 2, 15–21.

Kim, E., Barrett, K. E., Barman, S. M., Boitano, S., & Brooks, H. (2012). *Ganong's review of medical physiology.* 24th ed. New York: McGraw-Hill/Lange Medical Books.

Lee, J. W. (2010). Fluid and electrolyte disturbances in critically ill patients. *Electro Blood Pres,* 8(2), 72–81.

Lehrich, R. W., & Greenberg, A. (2011). Hyponatremia and the use of vasopressin receptor antagonists in critically ill patients. *J Int Care Med,* May 13. Epub ahead of print.

Marco Martínez, J. (2010). Hyponatremia: classification and differential diagnosis. *Endo Nutr,* 57 Suppl 2, 2–9.

Simmons, S. (2010). Acute dehydration. *Nurs,* 40(1), 72.

Strunden, M. S., Heckel, K., Goetz, A. E., & Reuter, D. A. (2011). Perioperative fluid and volume management: physiologic basis, tools and strategies. *Ann Int Care,* 1(1), 2.

Thanavaro, J. L. (2011). Diagnosis and management of primary aldosteronism. *Nurse Pract,* 36(4), 12–21.

Vaidya, C., Ho, W., & Freda, B. J. (2010). Management of hyponatremia: providing treatment and avoiding harm. *Cleveland Clin J Med,* 77(10), 715–726.

Verbalis, J. G. (2010). Managing hyponatremia in patients with syndrome of inappropriate antidiuretic hormone secretion. *Endo Nutrition,* 57 Suppl 2, 30–40.

Veronese, N., Bolzetta, F., Mosele, M., Manzato, E., & Sergi, G. (2011). A case of hypocalcemia. *Intl Emer Med,* Mar 3. Epub ahead of print.

Wakil, A., Ng, J. M., & Atkin, S. L. (2011). Investigating hyponatraemia. *Brit Med J,* 342(10), 1118–1136.

Wunderlich, R. (2013). Principles in the selection of intravenous solutions replacement: sodium and water balance. *J Infus Nurs,* 36(2), 126–130. doi: 10.1097/NAN.0b013e318283440d.

Acid-Base Imbalances

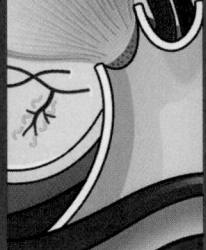

Key Terms

Acid

Acidic

Acidosis

Alkaline

Alkalosis

Anion gap (AG)

Arterial blood gas (ABG)

Base

Buffer

Metabolic acidosis

Metabolic alkalosis

Oxygen (SaO$_2$) saturation of blood

Partial pressure of carbon dioxide (Pco$_2$)

Partial pressure of oxygen (Po$_2$)

pH

Pulse oximetry

Respiratory acidosis

Respiratory alkalosis

Every second, a multitude of physiologic biochemical reactions occur within the body. Just as cells require sufficient oxygen and nutrients, cellular function requires an acid-base balance within the cell environment. Cellular proteins contain many acidic and basic groups within their structure; a change in the pH of the cellular environment can alter their structure and function. Cellular mechanisms constantly change the acidity or alkalinity of the bloodstream, making neutralization continuously necessary. To prevent the cellular environment from becoming too acidic or basic, buffer systems exist and are important to homeostasis. The buffer system created within the blood stream by carbonic acid (H$_2$CO$_3$) is discussed in this chapter.

Basic Concepts of Acid-Base Balance

Understanding the physiology of acid-base balance is key to understanding respiratory and metabolic disorders. The starting point for this knowledge is the basic chemistry of acids, bases, and buffers.

Acids, Bases, and Buffers

An **acid** is defined as any compound that donates hydrogen ions (H$^+$) in solution. A **base** is a compound that accepts an H$^+$ ion in solution. When H$^+$ ions predominate in a solution, the solution is **acidic.** When basic ions predominate in a solution, the solution is **alkaline.**

In body fluids, the concentration of H$^+$ ions is extremely low compared with other ions; however, the H$^+$ ion is a very strong acid, so it must be kept within a very precise range in the bloodstream. Because the hydrogen ion concentration is so small, it is expressed in terms of **pH,** which is the negative logarithm (p) of the H$^+$ ion concentration in mEq/L. For example, a pH value of 4 indicates that the H$^+$ concentration of a solution is 10^{-4} (0.00001 mEq/L). The pH value is inversely related to the H$^+$ ion concentration; a low pH indicates a high concentration of H$^+$ ions and a high pH, a low concentration of H$^+$ ions.

Physiologic pH is maintained through the interaction of acids, bases, and buffers. A **buffer** is a neutralizer that attempts to balance the pH. The carbonic acid (H$_2$CO$_3$) buffer system balances the pH of the bloodstream. When H$_2$CO$_3$ dissociates, it yields a hydrogen ion (H$^+$) and a bicarbonate ion (HCO$_3$$^-$). The chemical reaction of H$_2$CO$_3$ formation and dissociation (CO$_2$ + H$_2$O $\leftrightarrow$ H$_2$CO$_3$ $\leftrightarrow$ H$^+$ + HCO$_3$$^-$) is constantly occurring within the bloodstream to maintain physiologic pH for cellular homeostasis. The carbonic acid buffer system can absorb or release hydrogen ions in response to pH changes in the body.

Metabolic Processes

Cellular metabolism produces large quantities of carbon dioxide (CO$_2$) and acid. For example, the metabolism of fats and carbohydrates leads to the formation of large amounts of CO$_2$. The CO$_2$ combines with water (H$_2$O) in the bloodstream to form H$_2$CO$_3$. Acids are also produced during hypoxic states when pyruvate, a product of anaerobic metabolism, is converted to lactic acid. Other acids are produced during the metabolism of positively charged amino acids and hydrolysis of phosphate.

Most bases come from metabolism of negatively charged amino acids and from oxidation and consumption of organic anions such as lactate and citrate, which produce HCO$_3$$^-$. Deviations of pH of the bloodstream outside the normal range of 7.35 to 7.45 can have profound effects on cellular function and can be potentially life-threatening. Cellular enzymes can only function well within a narrow range of blood pH, and any deviation from this can result in disturbances in a wide range of body systems. Because there are numerous cellular processes that can change the pH environment, the carbonic acid buffer system is necessary.

Balancing Acidity and Alkalinity of the Bloodstream

Whenever blood pH changes, the body attempts to maintain acid-base balance via the lungs and the kidneys (see Fig. 8-1). The lungs attempt to reestablish homeostasis by regulating CO_2, whereas the kidneys attempt to compensate by excreting or reabsorbing H^+ or HCO_3^- as necessary. In this way, both the lungs and the kidneys regulate acid-base balance in the body.

The lungs can increase or decrease ventilation as needed to correct pH within the bloodstream. When the lungs increase respiratory rate, they eliminate CO_2. This shifts the buffer equation to the left and decreases H^+ like so: $CO_2 + H_2O \Leftarrow H_2CO_3 \Leftarrow H^+$ and HCO_3^-. The lungs can pull H^+ out of the bloodstream via increased breathing, or hyperventilation. When the lungs decrease the rate of ventilation they cause retention of CO_2, which increases the amount of acid. This is a shift of the buffer equation to the right like so: $CO_2 + H_2O \Rightarrow H_2CO_3 = \rightarrow H^+$ and HCO_3^-. The lungs can create more acid in the bloodstream via slowed breathing, or hypoventilation.

> ### CLINICAL CONCEPT
> The lungs and kidneys maintain acid-base balance; Therefore, if ventilation is suboptimal or if renal dysfunction occurs, acid-base imbalance can result.

Respiratory Regulation of Blood pH
The pressure of CO_2 in the bloodstream must be maintained at a level that ensures H^+ concentrations remain in the narrow limits required for optimal protein function.

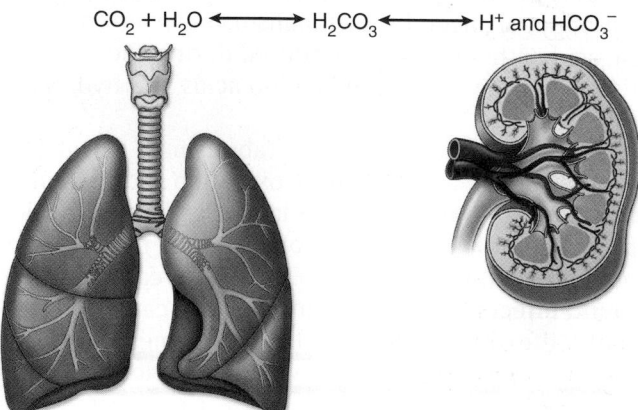

$$CO_2 + H_2O \longleftrightarrow H_2CO_3 \longleftrightarrow H^+ \text{ and } HCO_3^-$$

Figure 8-1. Acid-base balance via the lungs and kidneys.

Partial pressure of carbon dioxide (Pco$_2$) is normally maintained in the range of 35 to 45 mm Hg. Chemoreceptors in the brain and in the carotid bodies sense H^+ concentrations and influence ventilation to adjust the PCO_2, **partial pressure of oxygen (Po$_2$)**, and pH. This is a feedback system that keeps PCO_2 within its narrow normal range.

Arterial chemoreceptors sense increases in PCO_2 and, in turn, stimulate the respiratory center in the medulla to raise respiratory rate. The increased respiratory rate attempts to blow off excess CO_2. Two important premises to understand are: (1) hyperventilation blows off CO_2 and (2) hypoventilation causes retention of CO_2. When CO_2 is exhaled, H^+ ion diminishes and blood pH increases. For every change in the pressure of arterial CO_2, there is an inversely proportional change in the pH. In this way, the lungs attempt to correct disturbances in acid-base balance. The compensation by the lungs begins immediately and is usually only mildly effective. Therefore, medical interventions are commonly necessary to facilitate balancing the bloodstream's pH.

Renal Regulation of Blood pH
The kidneys control pH by adjusting the amount of HCO_3^- that is reabsorbed into the bloodstream or excreted into the urine. The kidney also can regulate reabsorption of H^+ into the bloodstream, as well as H^+ that is excreted. Metabolic compensation by the kidney increases or decreases H^+ and HCO_3^- absorption as needed to correct the pH balance. The kidney's compensation is slow and may take days to reach maximal effectiveness. Therefore, medical interventions are commonly necessary to facilitate balancing the bloodstream's pH.

> ### CLINICAL CONCEPT
> Hyperventilation of the lungs decreases CO_2 in the blood, thereby reducing acid in the blood and increasing blood pH.
>
> Hypoventilation of the lungs increases CO_2 in the blood, thereby increasing acid in the blood and decreasing blood pH.
>
> The kidneys are able to conserve or excrete H^+ or HCO_3^- as needed by the body.

Arterial Blood Gases

An **arterial blood gas (ABG)** is a laboratory study that measures the values involved in the oxygenation, acidity, and alkalinity of the arterial blood. Blood pH, Po_2, Pco_2, and HCO_3 are the values indicated by an ABG. In addition, a procedure called **pulse oximetry** can measure the **saturation of hemoglobin with oxygen (SaO$_2$)**. A pulse oximeter is a noninvasive sensor placed on the patient's finger.

Analysis of ABGs can determine if there is an acid-base imbalance within the bloodstream and whether or not the imbalance is caused by a respiratory or metabolic problem. The clinician has to compare the patient's ABGs to normal and interpret the results. Normal ABG values are the following:

- **Blood pH:** 7.35 to 7.45
- **Pco$_2$:** 35 to 45 mm Hg
- **Po$_2$:** 90 to 100 mm Hg
- **HCO$_3^-$** 22 to 26 mEq/L
- **SaO$_2$:** 95% to 100%.

Such information is vital when caring for patients with a critical illness. A clinician commonly uses the radial or femoral artery to obtain the blood sample. Alternatively, an indwelling arterial catheter is sometimes used for patients who require frequent ABG measurement.

 CLINICAL CONCEPT

When measuring ABGs, it's important to remember that low Po$_2$ is classified as hypoxia or hypoxemia, elevated Pco$_2$ is termed hypercapnea, and diminished Pco$_2$ is termed hypocapnea.

Analysis of Arterial Blood Gases

The ability to interpret ABGs affords an understanding of the etiology behind acid-base disorders. If blood pH is lower than 7.35, the bloodstream is acidic and the condition is termed **acidosis** (also called acidemia). If the blood pH is greater than 7.45, the bloodstream is basic and the condition is **alkalosis** (also called alkalemia). When interpreting ABGs, the clinician needs to determine if the patient is enduring an acid-base imbalance and, if so, the source of the imbalance. The sources of acidic or alkalotic blood can be respiratory or metabolic in nature. Disorders of the lungs can cause respiratory acid-base imbalances. Common respiratory disorders that affect blood pH are chronic obstructive pulmonary disease (COPD), infection, foreign body obstruction, and asthma. Metabolic acid-base imbalances can be caused by many different conditions, including drug toxicity, diabetes, renal failure, toxic ingestion, and excessive gastrointestinal losses. Interpretation of ABGs can decipher if the acid-base imbalance is of respiratory or metabolic etiology. The clinician needs to interpret ABG values in relation to the whole clinical picture, not just the laboratory values. The patient's vital signs, history, and physical examination are integral to the diagnosis of acid-base imbalances. It is also important to understand that the body will attempt to compensate and reverse acid-base imbalances in the body. The kidney, if healthy, is commonly the organ that compensates. It does so by excreting or reabsorbing H$^+$ or HCO$_3^-$ according to the body's needs. The lungs can also attempt to compensate, if healthy, by slowing or increasing rate of breathing. When analyzing ABG results in conjunction with all other indicators, use questions in a step-by-step process (see Box 8-1). Remember to evaluate the whole clinical picture, including Po$_2$ and SaO$_2$.

BOX 8-1. Steps for Interpretation of Basic Arterial Blood Gas Disturbances

Step 1. Begin by asking if the blood pH shows an acidic, basic, or normally balanced bloodstream. If blood pH is less than 7.35, the condition is acidosis. If the blood pH is greater than 7.45, the condition is alkalosis. If the pH is between 7.35 and 7.45, it is normal.

Step 2. Determine if the blood pH is caused by a respiratory or a metabolic problem. What is the Pco$_2$? If the Pco$_2$ is greater than 45 mm Hg, the lungs are hypoventilating and adding H$^+$ (acid) to the blood. If the Pco$_2$ is lower than 35 mm Hg, the lungs are hyperventilating, and pulling H$^+$ out of the blood. If the Pco$_2$ is normal, the lungs are not the origin of the problem.

Step 3. Compare the Pco$_2$ and blood pH. Is the acid-base imbalance caused by a respiratory or metabolic source? Can the pH be caused by the patient's Pco$_2$? If the Pco$_2$ is high, the body is retaining CO$_2$. If the Pco$_2$ is low, the body is blowing off CO$_2$. A high Pco$_2$ is usually caused by a respiratory disorder. Also, an abnormal Po$_2$ or SaO$_2$ is evidence of a respiratory problem.

Step 4. Determine if the condition is a compensated or uncompensated condition. If the pH is normal, this is a compensated condition. If pH is abnormal, it is an uncompensated condition. Analyze the HCO$_3^-$ and Pco$_2$ to evaluate the method of compensation by the body. The kidneys compensate for respiratory disorders and the lungs and kidneys can compensate for metabolic disorders.

CASE STUDY 1

Patient A is enduring an asthma attack and brought into the ED. The patient's vital signs are Temp: 98.4°F, Pulse: 110 beats/min, Resp rate: 24 shallow breaths/min, BP 136/86 mm Hg.

ABGs are:

- Blood pH: 7.30
- Pco$_2$: 58 mm Hg
- Po$_2$: 88 mm Hg
- HCO$_3^-$: 28 mEq/L
- SaO$_2$: 88%.

Continued

BOX 8-1. Steps for Interpretation of Basic Arterial Blood Gas Disturbances—cont'd

Step 1. Does the blood pH show an acidotic, alkalotic, or normal bloodstream?

In this problem, the blood is acidic at pH 7.30 which is less than 7.35; therefore, the condition is acidosis.

Step 2. What is the P_{CO_2}?

There is an elevated P_{CO_2} of 58 mm Hg, which indicates the lungs are hypoventilating.

A high P_{CO_2} shifts the equation to the right. This is evident in the chemical equation:

$CO_2 + H_2O \rightarrow H_2CO_3 \rightarrow H^+$ and HCO_3^-. Excess H^+ is created by a high Pa_{CO_2}.

Step 3. Is the acid-base imbalance caused by a respiratory or metabolic source?

The high P_{CO_2} indicates a ventilation problem and the P_{O_2} and Sa_{O_2} are also low, further confirming a lung problem.

Step 4. Is this a compensated or uncompensated problem?

The pH is abnormal; therefore, the condition is un-compensated. The way the body is attempting to compensate is reabsorption of HCO_3^- at the kidney.

Result

Because of the low blood pH and high P_{CO_2}, this is uncompensated respiratory acidosis. The kidney is attempting to compensate through the reabsorption of HCO_3^-.

CASE STUDY 2

Patient B is unconscious and brought into the ED because of suspected drug toxicity. Vital signs include Temp: 97.8°F, Pulse: 90 beats/min, Resp rate: 12 breaths/min, BP 100/70 mm Hg.

The patient's ABGs are:

- Blood pH: 7.29
- P_{CO_2}: 32 mm Hg
- P_{O_2}: 95 mm Hg
- HCO_3^-: 13 mEq/L
- Sa_{O_2}: 98%.

Using the previous step-by-step process:

Step 1. Does the blood pH show an acidotic, alkalotic, or normal bloodstream?

In this problem, the blood is acidic at 7.29 because the pH is less than 7.35; therefore, the condition is acidosis.

Step 2. What is the P_{CO_2}?

The P_{CO_2} is 32 mm Hg, which is low. This indicates the lungs are eliminating CO_2 excessively.

Step 3. Is the acid-base imbalance caused by a respiratory or metabolic source?

The lungs cannot be the cause of the acidic pH because P_{CO_2} is low. Also, because the P_{O_2} and Sa_{O_2} are normal, the lungs are functioning well. The acidotic ABG is probably caused by a metabolic cause.

Step 4. Is this a compensated or uncompensated problem?

The pH is abnormal, so the condition is uncompensated. The lungs in this case are trying to compensate for the high H^+ in the bloodstream by blowing off CO_2, but it is not completely neutralizing the acids.

Result

Because of the low blood pH and low P_{CO_2}, the condition is uncompensated metabolic acidosis. The lungs are attempting to compensate by blowing off CO_2 shown by a low CO_2 of 32 mm Hg. You can calculate anion gap by $(Na^+ + K^+) - (Cl^- + HCO_3^-)$. This can narrow down your list of possible causes of metabolic acidosis.

CASE STUDY 3

Patient C is having an anxiety attack and comes to the ED. Vital signs; Temp 98.1°F, Pulse 121 beats/min, Resp rate 28 breaths/min, and BP 138/88 mm Hg.

The patient's ABGs are:

- Blood pH: 7.58 mm Hg
- P_{CO_2}: 28 mm Hg
- P_{O_2}: 93 mm Hg
- HCO_3^-: 26 mEq/L
- Sa_{O_2}: 92%.

Step 1. Does the blood pH show an acidotic, alkalotic, or normal bloodstream?

In this problem, the blood is basic because the pH is greater than 7.45; therefore, the condition is alkalosis.

Step 2. What is the P_{CO_2}?

The P_{CO_2} is 28 mm Hg, which means that the lungs are hyperventilating, blowing off CO_2.

The lungs are pulling H^+ out of the blood, so the chemical equation moves to the left. $CO_2 + H_2O \leftarrow H_2CO_3 \leftarrow H^+$ and HCO_3^-

Step 3. Is the acid-base imbalance caused by a respiratory or metabolic source?

As indicated by the low P_{CO_2}, the alkalosis is caused by the respiratory problem of hyperventilation, so this is respiratory alkalosis. The P_{O_2} and Sa_{O_2} are on the low side, additionally indicating a pulmonary problem.

Step 4. Is this a compensated or uncompensated problem?

The pH is abnormal; therefore, this is uncompensated. The kidneys are attempting to compensate by excreting HCO_3^-.

Result

Because of the high blood pH, low P_{CO_2}, and low HCO_3^-, this is uncompensated respiratory alkalosis.

CASE STUDY 4

Patient D has endured 3 days of nausea and vomiting caused by a virus. Vital signs: Temp 101.1°F, Pulse: 98 beats/min, Resp rate 12 breaths/min, BP 90/60 mm Hg.

The patient's ABGs are:

- Blood pH: 7.61 mm Hg
- P_{CO_2}: 49 mm Hg

BOX 8-1. Steps for Interpretation of Basic Arterial Blood Gas Disturbances—cont'd

- Po_2: 99 mm Hg
- HCO_3^-: 49 mEq/L
- SaO_2: 99%.

Step 1. Does the blood pH show an acidotic, alkalotic, or normal bloodstream?

In this problem, the blood is basic because at 7.61, it is greater than 7.45; therefore, alkalosis is present.

Step 2. What is the Pco_2?

The Pco_2 is 49 mm Hg, which is high at greater than 45 mm Hg. If the blood is alkalotic, it cannot be caused by the high Pco_2. Also, the Po_2 and SaO_2 are normal, indicating normal lung function. Therefore, the lungs are not causing the alkalosis.

Step 3. Is the acid-base imbalance caused by a respiratory or metabolic source?

Alkalosis cannot be caused by the lungs if Pco_2 is 49 mm Hg. This is a metabolic problem, so this is metabolic alkalosis. The chemistry is: $CO_2 + H_2O \leftarrow H_2CO_3 \leftarrow H^+$ and HCO_3^-.

Step 4. Is this a compensated or uncompensated problem?

The pH is abnormal, so this is uncompensated. The body is attempting to retain acids in the bloodstream by slow respirations (which increases CO_2) and reabsorption of H^+ and excretion of HCO_3^- at the kidney.

Result

Because of a high blood pH and high Pco_2, this is an uncompensated metabolic alkalosis. The lungs are attempting to compensate by breathing slowly but cannot accomplish full compensation. The kidneys are attempting to eliminate HCO_3^-.

CASE STUDY 5

Patient E presents to the ED in a coma with no history. The ABGs are:

- Blood pH: 7.37
- Pco_2: 47 mm Hg
- Po_2: 85 mm Hg
- HCO_3^-: 26 mEq/L
- SaO_2: 87%.

Step 1. Does the blood pH show an acidotic, alkalotic, or normal bloodstream?

In this problem, the blood pH is between 7.35 and 7.45, which is within the normal range.

Step 2. What is the Pco_2?

The Pco_2 is 47 mm Hg. This is a high Pco_2, which means the lungs are hypoventilating. Hypoventilation causes retention of CO_2, which yields H^+ (acidosis). It is also apparent that there is low Po_2 and SaO_2, so a pulmonary problem exists.

Step 3. Is the acid-base imbalance caused by a respiratory or metabolic source?

The HCO_3^- is normal, so we are not dealing with a metabolic problem. There is a respiratory problem indicated by the high Pco_2. The chemistry is: $CO_2 + H_2O \rightarrow H_2CO_3 \rightarrow H^+$ and HCO_3^-.

Step 4. Is this a compensated or uncompensated problem?

This is a compensated respiratory problem because the blood pH is normal. The kidneys are trying to reabsorb enough HCO_3^- to neutralize the H^+ caused by high Pco_2.

Result

Because of the normal pH, high Pco_2, and normal HCO_3^-, this is compensated respiratory acidosis.

Anion Gap

The bloodstream contains positively charged ions (cations) and negatively charged ions (anions). Clinical laboratory reports measure the most numerous cations; [Na^+] and [K^+] and anions; [Cl^-] and [HCO_3^-] in the bloodstream. Under normal conditions, the bloodstream contains a small amount of unmeasured anions and unmeasured cations. The term **anion gap (AG)** represents the concentration of the unmeasured anions in the bloodstream. An anion gap exists in disorders of **metabolic acidosis** where there are a large number of unmeasured, pathological acids in the bloodstream (e.g., diabetic ketoacidosis). The ions that exist within the bloodstream can be represented as follows:

$$[Na^+] + [K^+] + \text{unmeasured cations} = [Cl^-] + [HCO_3^-] + \text{unmeasured anions.}$$

To maintain electrochemical balance, the body's total number of cations should equal the total number of anions. The anion gap is defined as the quantity of anions not balanced by cations in the bloodstream. Normally, there are a small number of unbound, free anions not balanced by cations in the bloodstream; this is referred to as a normal anion gap (see Fig. 8-2). The major unmeasured anions include negatively charged plasma proteins (albumin), sulphates, and phosphates.

In metabolic acidosis a large amount of pathological, unmeasured acids can be in the bloodstream. When a large amount of unmeasured acids is in the bloodstream, HCO_3^- binds to the acids. This causes a decrease in HCO_3^- within the bloodstream. The decrease in HCO_3^- increases the anion gap (see Fig. 8-2).

The anion gap can be measured by: $[Na^+ + K^+] - [Cl^- + HCO_3^-]$. The formula assumes that the patient has a normal albumin level. Low serum albumin reduces the accuracy of the anion gap calculation.

The normal range for the anion gap is 8 to 16 mEq/L, although laboratories may slightly differ in their reference range. The anion gap can be high, normal, or low.

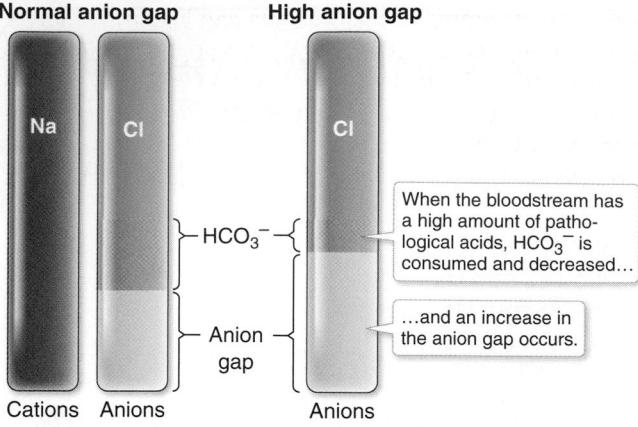

Figure 8-2. The normal anion gap versus high anion gap within the bloodstream. The bloodstream normally has a certain level of unbound anions, called the normal anion gap. When the bloodstream has an increased amount of acids, as in diabetic ketoacidosis, the anion gap is increased.

A normal anion gap has a small number of unmeasured anions in the bloodstream (see Fig. 8-2). A high anion gap has a value between 16 and 20 mEq/L, which indicates a high number of pathological acids in the bloodstream such as lactic acid or ketoacids (e.g., diabetic ketoacidosis). Bicarbonate ions bind to these pathological acids in the bloodstream and diminish the [HCO$_3^-$], which raises the anion gap. A low anion gap is uncommon, but can be caused by decreased unmeasured anions (usually low protein, especially hypoalbuminemia), increased unmeasured cations, or laboratory error.

CLINICAL CONCEPT

An anion gap, a lack of anions in the bloodstream, exists in metabolic acidosis. Calculating the anion gap is clinically useful, as it helps to differentiate types of metabolic acidosis disease states.

Metabolic acidosis with an elevated anion gap is found in the following conditions:

- lactic acidosis
- ketoacidosis
- renal failure
- overdose of acetylsalicylic acid (ASA), also known as aspirin
- ingestion of methanol or ethylene glycol.

Metabolic acidosis with a normal anion gap is found in the following conditions:

- GI loss of HCO$_3^-$
- increased renal HCO$_3^-$ loss
- hypoaldosteronism
- ingestion of ammonium chloride
- hyperalimentation.

The Relationship of K$^+$ and H$^+$

The transcompartmental exchange of K$^+$ and H$^+$ is important in the regulation of acid-base balance. Both K$^+$ and H$^+$ ions are positively charged and both ions move freely between the intracellular (ICF) and extracellular fluid compartments (ECF). When excess H$^+$ is present in the bloodstream (ECF), it moves into the body cells (ICF) in exchange for K$^+$. This shift causes an increase of K$^+$ ions in the bloodstream. Likewise, when excess K$^+$ is present in the bloodstream (ECF), it moves into the body cells (ICF) in exchange for H$^+$. This shift causes an increase of H$^+$ ions in the bloodstream. Therefore, alterations in K$^+$ levels in the body affect acid-base balance. Potassium shifts are more pronounced in acidosis than alkalosis and are greater in metabolic acidosis than respiratory acidosis.

An important aspect of the K$^+$ and H$^+$ exchange is its effect on the resting membrane potential of neurons. In acidosis, H$^+$ moves into the cell and K$^+$ moves out of the cell into the bloodstream. Increased levels of blood K$^+$ cause resting membrane potential of neurons to become less negative, which leads to hyperexcitability. In alkalosis, decreased levels of H$^+$ are available to move into the cell, so K$^+$ moves into the cell. A decreased level of K$^+$ in the blood causes resting membrane potential of neurons to become more negative and less excitable. Changes in neural excitability are also influenced by changes in ionized calcium (Ca^{++}). Some calcium circulates in the bloodstream attached to albumin and some calcium is in free, ionized form. In acidosis, albumin has less affinity for calcium. Therefore, in acidosis, the free ionized Ca^{++} is increased, which makes neurons less excitable. In alkalosis, albumin binds tightly to calcium; therefore, the amount of free ionized Ca^{++} is reduced, making neurons more excitable.

Pathophysiologic Concepts Regarding Acid-Base Imbalances

There are four states of acid-base imbalance in the bloodstream:

1. Respiratory acidosis
2. Respiratory alkalosis
3. Metabolic acidosis
4. Metabolic alkalosis.

Each has a different etiology, clinical presentation, compensatory mechanism, and treatment.

Respiratory Acidosis

Respiratory acidosis occurs when the body accumulates too much CO$_2$ or cannot exhale sufficient CO$_2$ (hypercapnea), which shifts the carbonic acid buffer equation to the right, thereby producing more H$^+$ and HCO$_3^-$. CO$_2$ + H$_2$O $\Rightarrow$ H$_2$CO$_3^-$ $\Rightarrow$ H$^+$ and HCO$_3^-$.

BOX 8-2. Causes of Respiratory Acidosis

PULMONARY

- Chronic obstructive lung disease, such as asthma, emphysema, and bronchiectasis
- Pulmonary edema
- Pneumonia
- Airway obstruction, such as laryngospasm, bronchospasm, and aspiration
- Underventilation by mechanical ventilation
- Hypoventilation secondary to obesity, postoperative pain, abdominal distention, or use of abdominal binders
- Excessive fatigue or weakness of rib cage muscles
- Cystic fibrosis

NONPULMONARY

- Overdosage of anesthetic, sedatives, and narcotics
- Neuromuscular disorders, such as Guillain Barré, myasthenia gravis, and advanced multiple sclerosis
- Severe spinal deformities
- Central nervous system depression related to cerebral infarct, meningitis, or trauma
- Cardiopulmonary arrest

Because H+ is such a strong acid, this makes the blood acidic. This can occur rapidly or over an extended period of time. In this situation, the P_{CO_2} will rise above 45 mm Hg and the pH will drop below 7.35. Respiratory acidosis is an indicator of hypoventilation from inadequate oxygen and carbon dioxide exchange within the lungs.

Epidemiology

The incidence of respiratory acidosis is different for its varied etiologies.

Etiology

Common causes of respiratory acidosis are listed in Box 8-2.

Pathophysiology

The lungs normally excrete CO_2 through ventilation, which pulls acid out of the blood. This is shown through the leftward shift of the chemical reaction: $CO_2 + H_2O \leftarrow H_2CO_3 \leftarrow H^+$ and HCO_3^-. Any alteration in ventilation that affects elimination of carbon dioxide can cause a respiratory acid-base disorder.

The Pa_{CO_2} is normally maintained within the range of 35 to 45 mm Hg. In disorders that raise P_{CO_2} greater than 45 mm Hg (hypercapnea), respiratory acidosis occurs. In acute respiratory acidosis, the respiratory center in the medulla is stimulated to breathe faster to rid the body of CO_2. Also, the kidneys attempt to compensate by excreting acids and reabsorbing HCO_3^-.

However, with chronic respiratory acidosis, as in long-term chronic obstructive pulmonary disease (COPD), the respiratory center in the medulla can become insensitive to high CO_2 levels. The body can adjust to high P_{CO_2} levels, and patients with hypercapnea live with precariously balanced blood pH values. The kidneys compensate for the high CO_2 by excreting H+ ions; with this compensation, blood pH can remain normal or near normal.

 CLINICAL CONCEPT

Patients with long-term COPD retain CO_2, which increases susceptibility to respiratory acidosis.

Clinical Presentation

Patients in respiratory acidosis complain of anxiety, restlessness, headache, lethargy, fatigue, shortness of breath, rapid breathing, and cough. Advanced respiratory acidosis leads to confusion, somnolence, and possible coma. The effects of excess CO_2 are commonly referred to as carbon dioxide narcosis.

Physical Examination Findings

The thoracic examination of patients with respiratory acidosis usually reveals obstructive lung disease. The signs include diffuse wheezing; hyperinflation of lungs; barrel-shaped chest in emphysema; decreased breath sounds; hyperresonance on percussion; and prolonged expiration. Rhonchi may also be heard. Cyanosis and clubbing may indicate the presence of chronic hypoxia. Confusion, disorientation, somnolence, or stupor can be present with high levels of P_{CO_2}.

ALERT! Respiratory acidosis can occur in severe asthma despite the patient being tachypneic. The breathing rate is increased, but the breaths are very shallow and do not eliminate CO_2. CO_2 accumulates, causing increased production of acids in the bloodstream.

Compensatory Mechanisms

In acute respiratory acidosis, the kidneys attempt to compensate by reabsorbing HCO_3^- and excreting H+, which brings blood pH to normal. Persons who have chronically high P_{CO_2} levels develop insensitivity to the P_{CO_2} levels and maintain normal blood pH. However, they are in delicate acid-base balance and can easily suffer respiratory acidosis with minor increases in P_{CO_2}.

Treatment

Treatment of respiratory acidosis is directed at improving ventilation. Oxygen is administered to improve ventilation. Bronchodilation is attempted via oral and parenteral adrenergic agents. Pulmonary infection requires treatment. If these do not improve ventilation, endotracheal intubation with mechanical ventilation is necessary.

Respiratory Alkalosis

Respiratory alkalosis occurs when the levels of CO_2 in the blood are low. When the P_{CO_2} falls, the pH of the bloodstream rises. When the lungs blow off an excess of CO_2, a deficit in H_2CO_3 occurs. The carbonic buffer equation shifts to the left, pulling off H^+ ions. Lack of sufficient H^+ in the bloodstream makes the blood alkalotic: $CO_2 + H_2O \Leftarrow H_2CO_3^- \Leftarrow H^+$ and HCO_3^-.

Epidemiology
Respiratory alkalosis is the most common acid-base abnormality observed in patients who are critically ill. It is associated with numerous illnesses and is a common finding in patients on mechanical ventilation.

Etiology
Common causes of respiratory alkalosis are listed in Box 8-3.

Pathophysiology
Respiratory alkalosis is most commonly caused by hyperventilation, which refers to a high rate of ventilation. The patient is breathing at a rate greater than normal, more than 20 breaths per minute. Hyperventilation causes excessive elimination of CO_2 from the lungs. In the carbonic buffer system, excess CO_2 elimination pulls the chemical equation toward the left; $CO_2 + H_2O \leftarrow H_2CO_3 \leftarrow H^+$ and HCO_3^-. The elimination of CO_2 leads to less acid in the bloodstream, causing the blood to become alkaline. Hyperventilation may or may not be associated with dyspnea.

BOX 8-3. Causes of Respiratory Alkalosis

PULMONARY
- Pneumonia
- Pulmonary edema
- Pulmonary embolus
- Asthma
- Lung disease with shortness of breath (asthma, pneumonia, ARDS, fibrosis, pulmonary embolism)
- Hypoxia with hyperventilation
- Overventilation by mechanical ventilation

NONPULMONARY
- Anxiety
- Pain
- Liver disease
- Fever/infection/sepsis
- Central nervous system disorders (tumors, cerebrovascular accidents)
- Salicylate intoxication
- Alcohol intoxication

Acute hypocapnea causes lack of H^+ and HCO_3^-. Decreased H^+ ion and HCO_3^- upsets the ionic balance of other ions in the bloodstream. An intracellular shift of K^+ and PO_4^- occurs, which reduces the blood level of these ions. There is also enhanced binding of ionized calcium to albumin, which reduces Ca^{++} levels in the bloodstream. Many of the symptoms present in persons with respiratory alkalosis are related to the hypocalcemia and hypokalemia that occurs in association with hypocapnea. Changes in potassium and calcium levels affect the resting membrane potentials of neuromuscular tissue and cardiac tissue. Therefore, many of the effects of respiratory alkalosis are within the central nervous system, peripheral nervous system, muscles, and cardiac tissue.

Clinical Presentation
In respiratory alkalosis, the central and peripheral nervous systems are stimulated, which causes tingling of extremities (paresthesias), muscle cramps, tetany, dizziness and/or syncope, confusion, anxiety, seizures, and coma. Cardiac symptoms include palpitations, dysrhythmias, and hypotension.

Physical Assessment Findings
Many patients enduring hyperventilation appear anxious and are frequently tachycardic. In acute hyperventilation, there is obvious chest wall movement and use of intercostal muscles to breathe. In patients with chronic hyperventilation, these physical findings may not be obvious. Muscle spasms, as well as Chvostek's and Trousseau's signs may be elicited because of hypocalcemia. Patients may have pulmonary disease and have signs such as crackles and rhonchi. Cyanosis may be present if the patient is hypoxic. The patient may have focal neurological signs or a depressed level of consciousness. Cardiac rhythm disturbances often occur.

Compensatory Mechanisms
The kidneys attempt to compensate in respiratory alkalosis by reabsorbing H^+ into the bloodstream and excreting HCO_3^-. This can take hours to days to accomplish, so the need for medical intervention is apparent. In compensated respiratory alkalosis, blood pH can be normal or near normal and P_{CO_2} will be low.

Treatment
Treatment of respiratory alkalosis lies in identifying the underlying trigger that has produced hyperventilation. Pain management or sedation may be required to slow and control the respiratory rate. One common treatment for respiratory alkalosis is to have the patient breathe into a paper bag. This allows for rebreathing of exhaled CO_2 to bring CO_2 levels back up to a normal range. A CO_2 rebreather is a type of breathing apparatus that recycles the exhaled gas and adds O_2 to compensate for the oxygen consumed by the user.

Metabolic Acidosis

An excess of acid or a loss of HCO_3^- in the blood causes metabolic acidosis. In metabolic acidosis, HCO_3^- will be lower than 22 mEq/L and the pH will be lower than 7.35. An accumulation of acid occurs whenever the rate of cellular metabolism increases. Also, accumulation of acid occurs in the absence of insulin, as in diabetes mellitus. In uncontrolled diabetes mellitus, ketoacids accumulate in the bloodstream. Diabetic ketoacidosis is one of the most common causes of metabolic acidosis. Metabolic acidosis also occurs in widespread ischemia when anaerobic metabolism occurs and yields lactic acid. A large amount of cellular ischemia, as occurs in severe hypotension, can cause lactic acidosis, which is another type of metabolic acidosis. Toxic ingestion or medication overdose commonly cause states of metabolic acidosis. Excessive vomiting with GI loss of pancreatic HCO_3^- is also known to cause metabolic acidosis.

Epidemiology
Morbidity and mortality in metabolic acidosis are dependent on the underlying condition.

Etiology
Common causes of metabolic acidosis are listed in Box 8-4.

BOX 8-4. Causes of Metabolic Acidosis

INCREASED NONCARBONIC ACIDS
- Diabetic ketoacidosis
- Lactic acidosis
- Alcoholic ketoacidosis
- Uremic acidosis
- Ingestion of toxic substances (antifreeze, aspirin)
- Intestinal, biliary, or pancreatic fistulas
- Hypocalcemia, hypokalemia, or hypomagnesemia

BICARBONATE LOSS
- Prolonged diarrhea
- Renal tubular acidosis
- Interstitial renal disease
- Ureterosigmoid loop
- Ingestion of acetazolamide or ammonium chloride

Pathophysiology
Metabolic acidosis is a condition characterized by an arterial pH of lower than 7.35 in the absence of an elevated P_{CO_2}. It is caused by one of three mechanisms:

1. increased production of acids
2. decreased excretion of acids
3. loss of base.

In metabolic acidosis there is an excess of H^+ and the body attempts to compensate. With excess H^+ in the bloodstream, chemoreceptors sense high H^+ and stimulate the respiratory center to increase respiratory rate. The resulting hyperventilation decreases the P_{CO_2} in an attempt to remedy the acidosis and increase the pH back toward normal. In compensating for metabolic acidosis, hyperventilation causes loss of CO_2 and the carbonic acid buffer reaction pulls to the left; $CO_2 + H_2O \leftarrow H_2CO_3 \leftarrow H^+$ and HCO_3^-; thereby removing H^+.

There are changes in potassium in metabolic acidosis. Excess hydrogen ions in the bloodstream move into the intracellular compartment (ICF) and replace intracellular potassium. Potassium moves out of the cell into the bloodstream. For every decrease in the serum pH by 0.1, a concomitant increase in the potassium blood level by 0.5 mEq occurs. As a result, hyperkalemia can occur, which has cardiac effects such as arrhythmias, peaked T waves, QRS widening, and ventricular fibrillation. Other effects of excessive acid in the bloodstream include insulin resistance, increased protein degradation, and reduced adenosine triphosphate (ATP) synthesis. Also, in acidosis, hemoglobin has less affinity for oxygen.

Tachycardia is the most common cardiovascular effect seen with a mild metabolic acidosis. As the serum pH falls below 7.2, myocardial depression occurs because hydrogen ions diminish the heart's contractility. Hypotension can also occur because acid stimulates peripheral vasodilation.

Metabolic acidosis is mainly divided into processes that are associated with a normal anion gap (8 to 16 mEq/L) or an elevated anion gap (greater than 16 mEq/L) (see section on Anion Gap).

Clinical Presentation
The symptoms of metabolic acidosis are widespread and manifested by changes in neurological, respiratory, gastrointestinal, and cardiovascular function. The patient complains of respiratory distress. Neurological symptoms include headache, drowsiness, confusion, seizures, neuromuscular fatigue, twitching, and coma. Gastrointestinal symptoms such as nausea, vomiting, and anorexia are common. Cardiovascular symptoms present as hypotension, dysrhythmias, decreased cardiac contractility, hyperkalemia, and diminished response to catecholamines.

Physical Assessment Findings
The patient is tachypneic and in respiratory distress. Cardiovascular signs may include weak pulses, tachycardia, hypotension, and arrhythmia. The patient may

have gastrointestinal pain and vomiting. Excessive vomiting can lead to dehydration. Signs of dehydration may include tachycardia, dry mucous membranes, and delayed capillary refill. Patients with diabetic ketoacidosis may present with fruity odor to their breath. Metabolic acidosis can also cause confusion, lethargy, and possibly coma or seizures.

Compensatory Mechanisms

In metabolic acidosis, if the kidneys are healthy, they will reabsorb HCO_3^- into the bloodstream and excrete H^+. The lungs attempt to reduce H^+ by deep, rapid breathing to blow off CO_2. Elimination of CO_2 will pull H^+ out of the bloodstream. This type of deep, rapid breathing is often referred to as Kussmaul's breathing. Kussmaul's breathing is particularly common in metabolic acidosis caused by diabetic ketoacidosis. Compensatory mechanisms require hours to days to completely remedy the condition. Therefore, medical intervention is needed.

Treatment

Treatment is directed at identifying and correcting the underlying disorder and restoring electrolyte and fluid balance. Intravenous sodium bicarbonate may be utilized in severe cases of metabolic acidosis where the pH is lower than 7.20. Caution needs to be taken as excessive use of sodium bicarbonate may produce a rebound metabolic alkalosis. In **metabolic alkalosis,** K^+ enters the cell and there is a rapid decrease in serum potassium (hypokalemia). In addition, excessive sodium bicarbonate can cause an increase in serum sodium (hypernatremia) and fluid overload. All types of metabolic acidosis require treating the etiology. For example, if the etiology is diabetic ketoacidosis, insulin is needed to remedy the acidosis. If the metabolic acidosis is caused by kidney failure; hemodialysis is required.

Metabolic Alkalosis

Metabolic alkalosis is caused by excessive loss of acids, shift of H^+ ions into the intracellular space, or increase in bicarbonate in the bloodstream. The blood pH will be greater than 7.45 and there is an elevated bicarbonate concentration greater than 26 mEq/L.

Epidemiology

Metabolic alkalosis is the most common acid-base disturbance that occurs in hospitalized patients. It accounts for approximately 50% of all acid-base disorders. Mortality rates have been reported as 45% in patients with an arterial blood pH of 7.55 and 80% when the pH was greater than 7.65.

Etiology

For the causes of metabolic alkalosis see Box 8-5.

Pathophysiology

Depletion of H^+ ions is the most common cause of metabolic alkalosis. The organ systems involved in

---

> ### BOX 8-5. Causes of Metabolic Alkalosis
>
> - Bicarbonate ingestion
> - Excess IV sodium bicarbonate
> - Potassium wasting diuretics
> - Loss of gastric fluids from vomiting, gastric suctioning, diarrhea, or binge-purge syndrome
> - Cushing's syndrome
> - Primary hyperaldosteronism
> - Secondary hyperaldosteronism

metabolic alkalosis are mainly the kidneys and GI tract because H^+ ions are easily lost via these two excretory systems. Gastric secretions contain large amount of hydrochloric acid (HCl) and any process that depletes gastric fluid can cause metabolic alkalosis such as severe vomiting or gastrointestinal tract suctioning.

Metabolic alkalosis can also occur in hypokalemia. In the presence of hypokalemia, there is a shift of hydrogen ions into the intracellular space to replace the lack of K^+. This depletes the amount of H^+ in the bloodstream, causing alkalosis. Diuretic treatment commonly causes hypokalemia, which in turn can lead to metabolic alkalosis. Hyperaldosteronism of Cushing's syndrome is also a cause of hypokalemia because aldosterone causes excretion of K^+. With excess loss of K^+, H^+ ions enter the cells from the bloodstream and deplete the blood of H^+. Therefore, metabolic alkalosis can occur in hypokalemia of hyperaldosteronism.

Another cause of metabolic alkalosis commonly occurs in cardiac resuscitation. Administration of large amounts of sodium bicarbonate are needed to neutralize the lactic acidosis that occurs in cardiac arrest. The excessive amount of sodium bicarbonate in the bloodstream often exceeds the capacity of the kidneys to excrete it. Excess bicarbonate remains in the bloodstream, thereby causing metabolic alkalosis.

Clinical Presentation

The symptoms of metabolic alkalosis are widespread, affecting the neurological, cardiovascular, gastrointestinal, and musculoskeletal systems. These patients present with various symptoms such as confusion, dizziness, agitation, weakness, vomiting, diarrhea, and possibly seizures.

Physical Assessment Findings

The physical signs of metabolic alkalosis are nonspecific and multisystemic. Metabolic alkalosis can cause changes in K^+ and Ca^{++} electrolyte levels. In alkalosis, the lack of H^+ causes increased amounts of K^+ to enter the cells, leaving less K^+ in the bloodstream. Hypokalemia can cause muscular weakness, myalgia, muscle spasms, and cardiac arrhythmias. Also in metabolic alkalosis, albumin affinity for Ca^{++} is enhanced, causing more Ca^{++} ions to be bound in the bloodstream. This decreases the free, ionized calcium concentration in the bloodstream and causes hypocalcemia. Therefore, signs of hypocalcemia such as tetany, Chvostek's sign, and Trousseau's sign may be present. Fluid volume status can also change in metabolic alkalosis. Assessment includes evaluation of orthostatic changes in blood pressure and heart rate, mucous membranes, presence or absence of edema, skin turgor, weight change, and urine output.

Patients with bulimia self-induce vomiting, which often depletes their gastric HCl and causes metabolic alkalosis. Patients with bulimia often have erosions of teeth enamel and dental caries because of repeatedly exposing their teeth to gastric acid.

Compensatory Mechanisms

In metabolic alkalosis, the kidneys attempt to compensate by reabsorbing H^+ into the bloodstream and excreting HCO_3^-. This can take days to occur to the point of adequate compensation; therefore, medical intervention is necessary. The lungs attempt to compensate by slowing breathing rate to retain CO_2, which synthesizes acid. However, this may cause hypoxemia, especially in patients with respiratory problems.

Treatment

Treatment of metabolic alkalosis includes electrolyte and fluid replacement. Potassium-sparing diuretics may be administered if the source of alkalosis is from diuretic use. Acetazolamide is a carbonic anhydrase inhibitor used to treat conditions of moderate to severe metabolic or respiratory alkalosis. It does this by interfering with bicarbonate (HCO_3^-) reabsorption in the kidneys.

Chapter Summary

- An acid is defined as any compound that donates hydrogen ions (H^+) in solution.

- A base is a compound that accepts an H^+ ion in solution.

- When H^+ ions predominate in a solution, the solution is acidic. When basic ions predominate in a solution, the solution is alkaline.

- The lungs and the kidneys regulate the body's acid-base balance.

- Blood pH, pressure of oxygen (P_{O_2}), pressure of carbon dioxide (P_{CO_2}), and bicarbonate ion concentration (HCO_3^-) are the values indicated by an arterial blood gas (ABG).

- The pH of blood is 7.35 to 7.45. If the bloodstream has a pH of lower than 7.35, this is acidosis; if greater than 7.45, it is alkalosis.

- The chemical buffering system that consistently maintains the acid-base equilibrium is $CO_2 + H_2O \leftrightarrow H_2CO_3 \leftrightarrow H^+$ and HCO_3^-.

- During hypoventilation the lungs retain CO_2; during hyperventilation, the lungs blow off CO_2.

- The greater the CO_2 in the body, the greater the formation of H^+.

- There are four possible acid-base disturbances: respiratory acidosis, respiratory alkalosis, metabolic acidosis, and metabolic alkalosis.

- If the P_{CO_2} is high, the lungs are hypoventilating. If the P_{CO_2} is low, the lungs are hyperventilating.

- Hypoventilation, which causes P_{CO_2} greater than 45 mm Hg, results in respiratory acidosis; hyperventilation, which causes P_{CO_2} less than 35 mm Hg, results in respiratory alkalosis.

- An excess of acid or a loss of HCO_3^- in the blood causes metabolic acidosis. In metabolic acidosis, HCO_3 will be lower than 22 mEq/L and the pH will be lower than 7.35.

- Metabolic alkalosis is caused by excessive loss of acids, shift of H^+ ions into the intracellular space, or increase in bicarbonate in the bloodstream. The blood pH will be greater than 7.45 and the bicarbonate concentration greater than 35 mEq/L.

- Metabolic acid-base imbalances affect levels of serum electrolytes. Metabolic acidosis causes H^+ to enter cells, replacing K^+. Potassium increases in blood, causing hyperkalemia. Albumin has increased affinity for Ca^{++} in metabolic alkalosis. Less free Ca^{++} is left in the bloodstream, causing hypocalcemia.

Making the Connections

Disorder and Pathophysiology	Signs and Symptoms	Physical Assessment Findings	Diagnostic Testing	Treatment

Respiratory Acidosis | Lungs are not ventilating; retaining too much CO_2 which creates too much H^+. The chemistry of the bloodstream: Excess $CO_2 + H_2O \rightarrow H_2CO_3 \rightarrow H^+$ and HCO_3^-.

| | Dyspnea. Respiratory distress. Patient may be lethargic, stuporous, or comatose. | Diminished respiratory rate. Cyanosis. Clubbing if chronic hypoxia. | Blood ph less than 7.35. P_{CO_2} greater than 45 mm Hg. P_{O_2}: low. Urine: acidic. | Treat the lung disorder for better ventilation. Bronchodilation. Antibiotics if pneumonia. Intubation and mechanical ventilation if needed. |

Respiratory Alkalosis | Lungs are hyperventilating; losing too much CO_2 which creates too little H^+ in the blood. The chemistry of the bloodstream: $CO_2 + H_2O \leftarrow H_2CO_3 \leftarrow H^+$ and HCO_3^-.

| | Hyperventilation. Anxiety. Palpitations. Paresthesias. Patient may have pain. | High respiratory rate Tachycardia. | Blood ph greater than 7.45. P_{CO_2} less than 35 mm Hg. Urine: basic. | Slow the breathing rate; CO_2 rebreather. Patient may need sedative. |

Metabolic Acidosis | Excessive acid in the bloodstream (e.g., ketoacids or lactic acid) or excessive loss of HCO_3^- (e.g., pancreatic dysfunction). With excess H^+, the chemical equation shifts to the left, creating more CO_2 that leaves via the lungs:

$$CO_2 + H_2O \leftarrow H_2CO_3 \leftarrow H^+ \text{ and } HCO_3^-.$$

| | Symptoms according to etiology of disorder: respiratory distress, headache, drowsiness, confusion, seizures, fatigue. GI symptoms of nausea, vomiting, and anorexia are common. | Tachycardia. Hypotension, weak pulses. Dehydration signs may be present: dry mucous membranes, poor skin turgor, and delayed capillary refill. Patients with diabetic ketoacidosis may present with fruity odor to their breath. Metabolic acidosis can also cause confusion, lethargy, and possibly coma or seizures. | Blood ph less than 7.35. P_{CO_2} normal or slightly low. Serum K^+: high. Urine: acidic. ECG changes caused by hyperkalemia: arrhythmias, peaked T waves, QRS widening, and ventricular fibrillation possible. | Sodium bicarbonate IV. Treat etiologic disorder (for example, if diabetic ketoacidosis, treat diabetes). |

Continued

Making the Connections—cont'd

Disorder and Pathophysiology	Signs and Symptoms	Physical Assessment Findings	Diagnostic Testing	Treatment
Metabolic Alkalosis | Excessive base in the bloodstream (such as toxic ingestion) or lack of sufficient acid in the bloodstream caused by high loss of H^+ (such as loss of HCl with excessive vomiting). Excess base shifts chemistry to the left: $$CO_2 + H_2O \leftarrow H_2CO_3 \leftarrow H^+ \text{ and } HCO_3^-.$$	Symptoms according to etiology of disorder; often related to decreased calcium ionization resulting from low H^+ level. Low Ca^{++} levels cause: tetany, irritability, disorientation, and seizures. Prolonged vomiting may be the cause.	Chvostek's sign. Trousseau's sign. Hypotension or hypertension may be present. Patients with bulimia often have erosions of teeth enamel and dental caries.	Blood ph greater than 7.45. P_{CO_2} normal or slightly high. Urine: basic. Serum ionized Ca^{++} low. ECG may show dysrhythmias.	IV Acetazolamide.

Bibliography

American Society of Nutrition. (2008). Acid-base symposium. *J Nutr.* 138, 413S–414S.

Barrett, K. E., Barman, S. M., Boitano, S., & Brooks, H. L. (2012). *Ganong's review of medical physiology.* 24th ed. New York: McGraw-Hill.

Hall, J. (2011). *Guyton and Hall textbook of medical physiology.* 12th ed. New York: Saunders.

Harwani, S., Baumhover, N., Berry, C., Denison, D., Langraff, T., & Mathis, D. (2009). *CCRN certification for adult, pediatric and neonatal critical care nurses.* New York: Kaplan Publishing Co.

Jones, M. B. (2010). Basic interpretation of metabolic acidosis. *Crit Care Nurse,* 30(5), 63–69.

Lawes, R. (2009). Body out of balance: understanding metabolic acidosis and alkalosis. *Nursing,* 39(11), 50–54.

McPhee, S. J., & Papdakis, M. A. (2012). *Current medical diagnosis and treatment.* New York: Lange/McGraw-Hill.

Myall, K., Sidney, J., & Marsh, A. (2011). Mind the gap! An unusual metabolic acidosis. *Lancet,* 377(9764), 526.

Woodrow, P. (2010). Essential principles: blood gas analysis. *Nurs Crit Care,* 15(3), 152–156.

UNIT 4
INFECTION AND INFLAMMATION

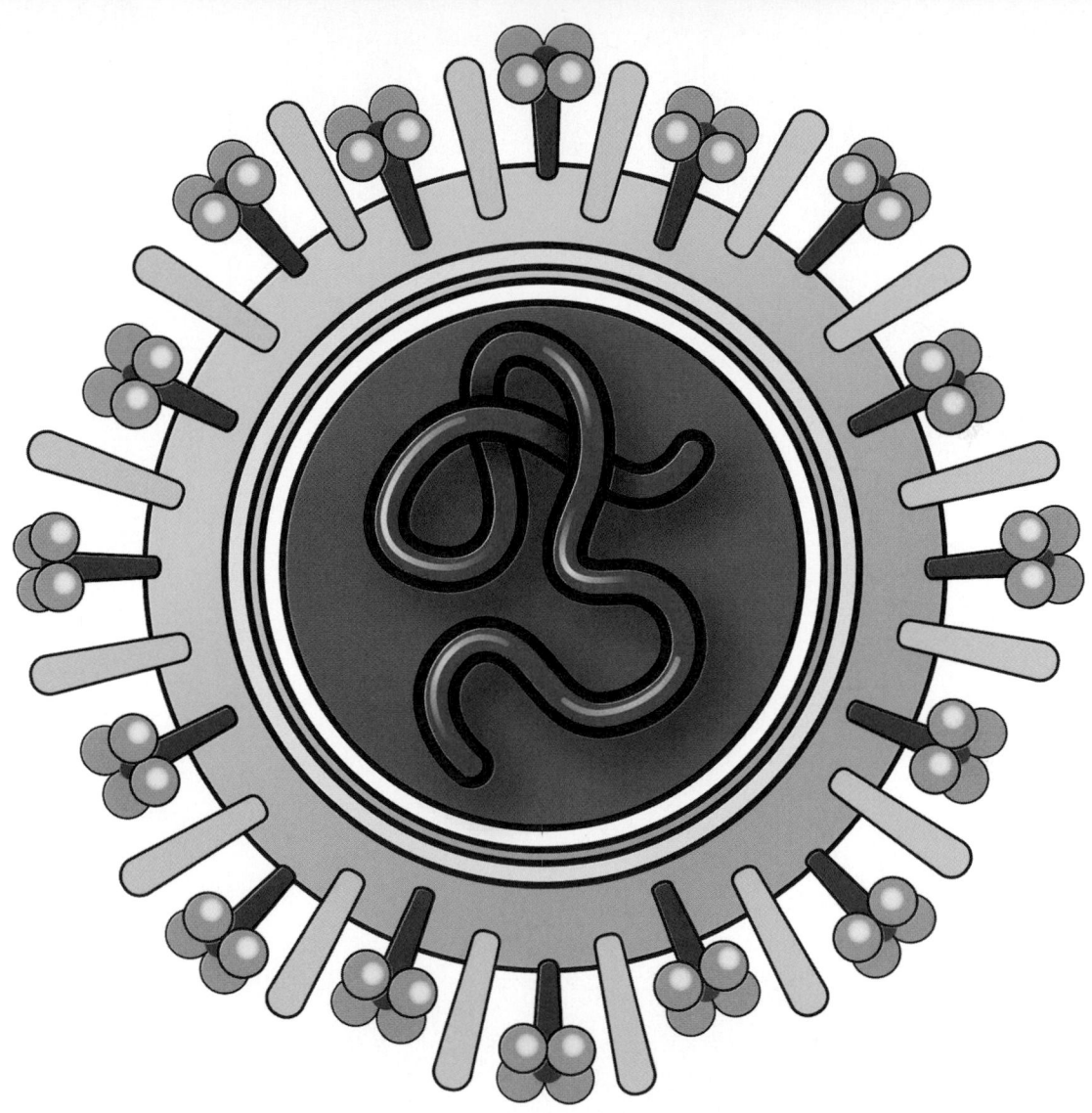

Chapters

Inflammation and Dysfunctional Wound Healing

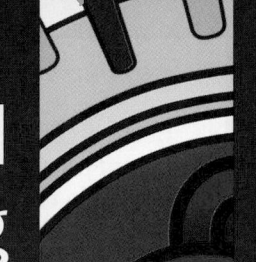

Key Terms

Chemotaxis

Contracture

C-reactive protein (CRP)

Cytokines

Erythrocyte sedimentation rate (ESR)

Granuloma

Histamine

Inflammation

Interleukins (ILs)

Leukocytosis

Leukopenia

Lymph node

Lymphocytes

Phagocytosis

Primary intention

Prostaglandins (PGs)

Purulent exudate

Pyrogens

Secondary intention

Stricture

Tertiary intention

Transudate

White blood cell (WBC) differential

Wound dehiscence

Wound evisceration

Inflammation is a protective, coordinated response of the body to an injurious agent. It involves many cell types and inflammatory mediators that initiate, modulate, amplify, and terminate this response. There are characteristic cellular products, tissue changes, and systemic responses associated with inflammation. The intensity of the inflammatory reaction is usually proportional to the extent of the tissue injury. The major aims of inflammation are to wall-off the area of injury, prevent spread of the injurious agent, and bring the body's defenses to the region under attack.

Inflammation and the Inflammatory Response

The inflammatory response is a multistaged process that involves vascular and cellular changes, but may also include systemic changes. White blood cells (WBCs) are brought to the damaged area, and they secrete substances that control the process from initial injury to resolution or long-term inflammation. The inflammatory response is most efficient when it rids the body of injury, enhances healing processes, and resolves. In some disorders, such as rheumatoid arthritis, tuberculosis (TB), and atherosclerosis, inflammation can persist and ultimately cause unremitting damaging effects on the body; these are considered chronic inflammatory conditions. See Box 9-1 for examples of inflammatory conditions.

Inflammatory conditions can cause discomfort, organ dysfunction, and diminished quality of life. Cell biologists continue to uncover micromolecular-level mediators of inflammation and precise targets for drugs. Our

---

> ### BOX 9-1. Inflammatory Conditions
>
> In most cases, the terminology that indicates inflammation of tissue or an organ uses the suffix *-itis*. For example, the term *acute pharyngitis* means inflammation of the pharynx; it is commonly known as sore throat.
>   Other inflammatory conditions include:
>
> - **Appendicitis:** inflammation of the appendix
> - **Hepatitis:** inflammation of the hepatocytes or liver
> - **Colitis:** inflammation of the colon
> - **Arthritis:** inflammation of arthrus tissue or joints.

current knowledge base regarding inflammation is less than complete, but research continues to enhance our understanding of this complex physiologic response.

Types of Inflammation

There are two types of inflammation: acute and chronic. Acute inflammation occurs rapidly in reaction to cell injury, rids the body of the offending agent, enhances healing, and terminates after a short period, either hours or a few days. Chronic inflammation occurs when the inflammatory reaction persists, inhibits healing, and causes continual cellular damage and organ dysfunction.

Acute Inflammation

Acute inflammation can be triggered by various injurious stimuli, such as infections, microbial toxins, physical injury, surgery, cancer, chemical agents, tissue necrosis, foreign bodies, and immune reactions. Regardless of etiology, all acute inflammatory reactions cause the same characteristic vascular, cellular, and systemic changes. These reactions are orchestrated by responses to various inflammatory mediators. The acute inflammatory reaction involves three main stages:

1. vascular permeability
2. cellular chemotaxis
3. systemic responses.

Vascular Permeability. During the vascular phase at a site of inflammation, inflammatory mediators such as histamine and bradykinin enable the blood vessels to dilate and become more permeable. This permits fluids, WBCs, and platelets to travel out to the site of injury or infection. Vasodilation of the arterioles is followed by enhanced capillary permeability, allowing fluid to flow out of the blood vessels to the injured tissues (Fig. 9-1). The increased fluid in the tissues dilutes the toxin and lowers the pH of the surrounding fluids so they are not conducive to microbial growth.

The inflamed area immediately starts to become congested, warm, red, and swollen from the vasodilation and fluid extravasation into the tissues from the capillaries. These effects can occur internally within an organ or externally on the surface of the body, depending on where the cell injury and inflammation is occurring.

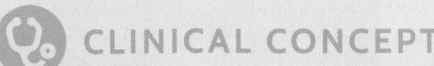

CLINICAL CONCEPT

The classic external signs of inflammation are known as the five cardinal signs: rubor (redness), tumor (swelling), calor (heat), dolor (pain), and loss of function.

The fluid that leaves the capillaries is a protein-rich filtrate of blood that contains WBCs. The WBCs surround and consume the foreign material in a process called **phagocytosis.** As the WBCs perform defensive activities, the fluid increases within the tissue spaces and causes edema, or swelling. If the fluid is rich in protein from WBCs, microbial organisms, and cellular debris, it is called **purulent exudate,** or pus. In contrast, fluid that contains little protein and is mainly a watery filtrate of blood is called **transudate.**

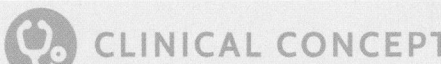

CLINICAL CONCEPT

An example of purulent exudate is the whitish-green drainage emitted from an infected wound. An example of a transudate is the clear fluid contained within a noninfected blister. Both are types of fluid that result from inflammation.

Cellular Chemotaxis. During the cellular phase of inflammation, a chemical signal from microbial agents, endothelial cells, and WBCs attracts platelets and other WBCs to the site of injury. This is referred to as **chemotaxis.** Once the WBCs arrive at the site of inflammation, they line up along the endothelium in the area of inflammation in a process called margination. They then release many different inflammatory mediators that act in various ways. Some mediators amplify the inflammatory process, some attract more WBCs to the area of injury, and others attempt to stop the inflammatory process. Each will be discussed in the following text.

Cytokines and Acute Phase Proteins. Some of the inflammatory mediators released by WBCs are referred to as **cytokines;** these include tumor necrosis factor (TNF-alpha) and **interleukins (ILs).** Cytokines modulate the inflammatory reaction by amplifying or deactivating the process. Simultaneously, they cause localized and systemic effects. One of the systemic effects of cytokines is stimulation of the liver to release substances called acute phase proteins. Acute phase proteins include **C-reactive protein (CRP),** fibrinogen, serum amyloid A, and many other substances. These proteins influence the inflammatory process by stimulating, modulating, and deactivating the reaction. The acute phase proteins, just as cytokines, initiate, amplify, or sustain the inflammatory process, and some exert negative, dampening effects.

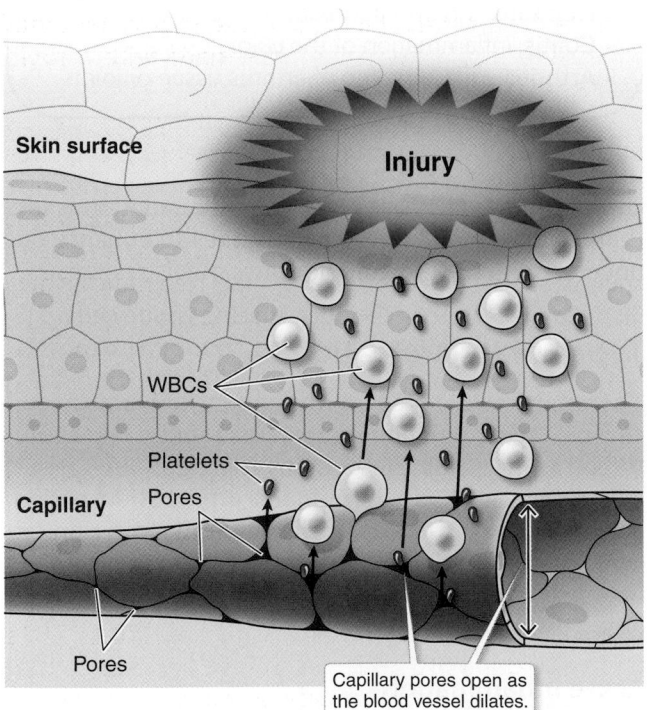

Figure 9-1. The vascular permeability phase of inflammation. Inflammation stimulates dilation of blood vessels and the opening of capillary pores. The capillary pores allow fluid and cells, such as WBCs and platelets, out to the area of injury.

CRP is a key acute phase protein secreted by the liver that is both pro-inflammatory and anti-inflammatory in action. It is integral to identifying foreign material for the immune system, activates the complement system, stimulates other inflammatory cytokines, and prevents WBC adhesion to endothelium.

 CLINICAL CONCEPT

An elevated-level CRP in the bloodstream indicates active inflammation. Another laboratory test that is used to diagnose inflammation is **erythrocyte sedimentation rate (ESR),** which is a measure of the rate at which red blood cells (RBCs) precipitate out of the plasma; it is influenced by fibrinogen levels in the blood. Because fibrinogen levels in the blood can now be measured directly, ESR is considered an imprecise indicator of inflammation. However, ESR is still commonly used for monitoring the activity of many inflammatory diseases.

Leukocytosis. In the cellular phase of inflammation, there is an increase in the number of WBCs released from the bone marrow into the bloodstream. WBCs are also known as leukocytes, and an elevated number of WBCs in the bloodstream is known as **leukocytosis.** During inflammation, the WBC count in the blood commonly increases from a normal baseline of 4,000 to 10,000 cells/mL to 15,000 to 20,000 cells/mL. The term *leukemoid reaction* is used to describe an extreme, extraordinary elevation in number of WBCs. Leukemoid reactions can raise the WBC count to 50,000 cells/microliter or more. These reactions can occur in conditions such as leukemia.

 CLINICAL CONCEPT

Leukopenia is a term used to indicate too few WBCs.

Types of White Blood Cells. There are five basic types of WBCs:

1. neutrophils
2. lymphocytes
3. eosinophils
4. basophils
5. monocytes (see Fig. 9-2).

 CLINICAL CONCEPT

Neutrophils are also referred to as polymorphonuclear leukocytes (PMNs); in their immature form, they are called bands or stabs.

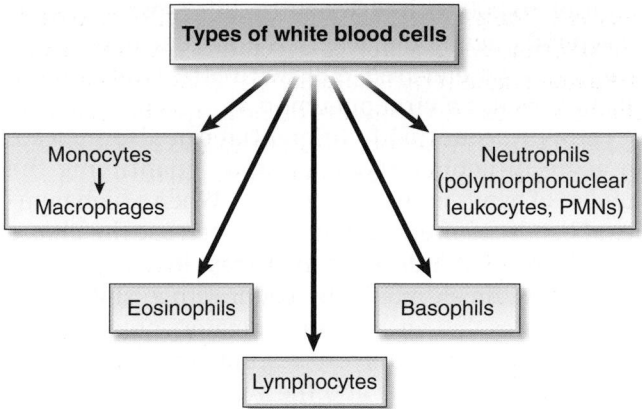

Figure 9-2. Types of WBCs.

Neutrophils, basophils, and eosinophils are referred to as granulocytes because they contain obvious cytoplasmic granules when examined under the microscope. These cytoplasmic granules contain important enzymes and inflammatory mediators to support the inflammatory process and fight infection. Mature neutrophils also have multisegmented nuclei and are sometimes known as segmented neutrophils (segs).

A large inflammatory response creates an urgent need for WBCs at the site. Neutrophils, which are the first responders, rush to the site within the first 24 to 48 hours. They begin the process of phagocytosis of the foreign matter immediately. However, they have a short life span of approximately 10 hours to a few days. As mature neutrophils die off and the supply becomes exhausted, the bone marrow responds with a rapid release of immature neutrophils.

During this phase of the inflammatory response, as the neutrophils are involved in phagocytosis of microbial organisms and cellular debris, there is a respiratory burst from the mitochondria. This burst releases free radicals that disrupt microbial membranes, leading to their destruction. Unfortunately, the free radicals may also damage some of the surrounding tissue cells.

After the initial 24 to 48 hours, monocytes are activated, congregate at the site, and become efficient macrophages that use phagocytosis to rid the body of foreign material and cellular debris. Monocytes have a long life span of weeks to months and become the predominant cell at the injury site.

A laboratory test called a **white blood cell (WBC) differential** is used in the diagnosis of infection and inflammation. This test is part of a complete blood count (CBC) with differential, which quantifies RBCs and WBCs. A WBC with differential measures total number of WBCs and calculates the percentages of specific types of WBCs within the total. The result of the laboratory test shows the predominate type of WBC responding to the infectious agent and can be used to indicate the etiology of inflammation. For example, a patient with pneumonia who has an elevated total WBC count of 16,000 with 90% neutrophils most likely has a bacterial pneumonia, whereas a patient with pneumonia and an elevated WBC with 90% lymphocytes most likely has a viral pneumonia.

The WBC count with differential can also indicate an acute inflammatory reaction by quantifying the number of bands in the bloodstream. When a high number of bands are present, clinicians often use the phrase "shift to the left," indicating an increase in newly formed neutrophils. An elevated WBC count with a "shift to the left" indicates that an acute inflammatory process is occurring. As inflammation resolves, immature neutrophils become less numerous and the WBC count returns to normal.

Systemic Response. Persons enduring acute inflammation experience symptoms throughout the whole body, known as systemic responses, such as fever, pain, lymphadenopathy (swollen lymph nodes), anorexia, sleepiness, lethargy, anemia, and weight loss. Chemical mediators produced during the inflammation reaction are responsible for many of these systemic effects. Prostaglandins (PGs), leukotrienes, TNF-alpha, and ILs are inflammatory mediators released from WBCs. Investigations continue to reveal increasing information about the role of these mediators in modulating inflammation. They are also under intense scrutiny in pharmacological research for development of specific anti-inflammatory drugs. Researchers are studying the micromolecules involved in inflammation in order to find specific targets for anti-inflammatory drugs. There are many drugs that target TNF-alpha, such as etanercept (Enbrel®) and infliximab (Remicade®).

Fever. Fever, an increase in body temperature, is a common manifestation of inflammation and infection. Microbial organisms, bacterial products, and cytokines all act as **pyrogens,** which are substances that cause fever. Pyrogens activate PGs to reset the hypothalamic temperature-regulating center in the brain to a higher level. A higher body temperature is theorized to increase the efficiency of WBCs in their defense of the body against foreign invaders (see Fig. 9-3).

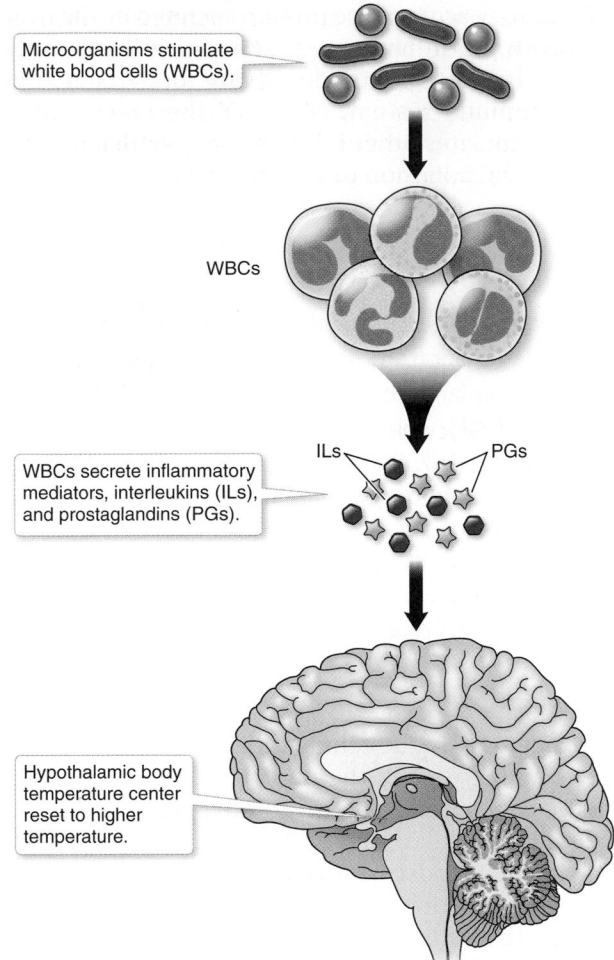

Figure 9-3. The fever response. Microorganisms enter the body and stimulate WBCs. Pyrogens are inflammatory mediators that are released by WBCs. Pyrogens reset the hypothalamic temperature center in the brain to create fever. Fever assists the WBCs in performing their activities in infection.

ALERT! Never give children or adolescents aspirin or any salicylate-containing products to control a fever. Research has demonstrated a link between salicylate use and Reye's syndrome in children and adolescents who have viral infections. Reye's syndrome is a life-threatening disorder in which mitochondrial failure leads to liver failure and encephalopathy.

The sensation of chills often accompanies fever. When the set-point of the hypothalamic temperature-control center is suddenly changed from normal (98.6°F) to a higher temperature, it takes some time before the body reaches the new higher set-point. Initially, the blood temperature is less than the new higher set-point and the person has a sensation of being cold. The blood vessels constrict and the body attempts to conserve and generate heat. To reach the

CLINICAL CONCEPT

Fever, although advantageous to the immune system, can reach levels high enough to cause seizures and brain damage. Therefore, it is recommended to keep fever below 102°F through the use of antipyretic medications such as aspirin, ibuprofen, or acetaminophen. These medications inhibit prostaglandin formation and, thus, reduce fever.

new hypothalamic temperature set-point, the muscles shiver to generate body heat. The sensation of cold and muscle shivering are experienced as chills, which continue until the body reaches the higher hypothalamic temperature set-point. When the stimulus for the fever resolves, pyrogens stop stimulating PGs, and the hypothalamic temperature returns to normal levels. The feverish body must adapt to the new, lower hypothalamic set-point. In response, vasodilation and intense sweating (diaphoresis) occur to dissipate the body heat. As body temperature declines, the patient appears flushed and diaphoretic because of widespread vasodilation.

Histamine Release. **Histamine** is an inflammatory mediator released from basophils, platelets, and mast cells, and it has many systemic effects. It causes arteriolar vasodilation, large artery vasoconstriction, and increased permeability of venules.

Mast cells, located in tissues adjacent to blood vessels, are the richest source of histamine. Physical injury, immune reactions, cytokines, and other inflammatory mediators stimulate histamine release. Commonly, sneezing, rhinorrhea (runny nose), eye tearing, sinus inflammation, and pharyngeal irritation are consequences of histamine released in the upper respiratory tract.

Effects of Prostaglandins, Leukotrienes, and Their Enzymatic Pathways. **Prostaglandins (PGs)** are released from WBCs and other cell membranes through a series of reactions. During inflammation, an enzyme called phospholipase is stimulated and acts on phospholipids, constituents of the WBC cell membrane. Phospholipids are broken down into arachidonic acid, which undergoes further enzymatic action by cyclooxygenase and lipooxygenase. The cyclooxygenase pathways produce PGs and the lipooxygenase pathway produces leukotrienes. Some PGs perpetuate negative effects of inflammation, and other PGs are needed for protective bodily functions. Leukotrienes provoke bronchiole inflammation in asthma.

There are two different enzymes involved in the formation of PGs from arachidonic acid: cyclooxygenase-1 (cox-1) and cyclooxygenase-2 (cox-2). Each pathway yields a different type of PG. The cox-1 pathway enzymatically breaks down arachidonic acid into helpful PGs and the cox-2 pathway yields harmful PGs. The PGs formed from the cox-1 pathway stimulate gastric mucous production, enhance renal perfusion, and assist platelets to aggregate and form clots. The PGs formed by the cox-2 pathway perpetuate inflammation; cause pain, fever, swelling, and muscle contractions; and potentiate effects of other inflammatory mediators (see Fig. 9-4).

Systemic Effects of TNF-Alpha and ILs. TNF-alpha, IL-1, and IL-6 are major cytokines produced by macrophages in the inflammation reaction and have been shown to induce fever, loss of appetite, and lethargy. TNF-alpha also promotes lipid and protein mobilization, which causes weight loss and cachexia, the wasting of

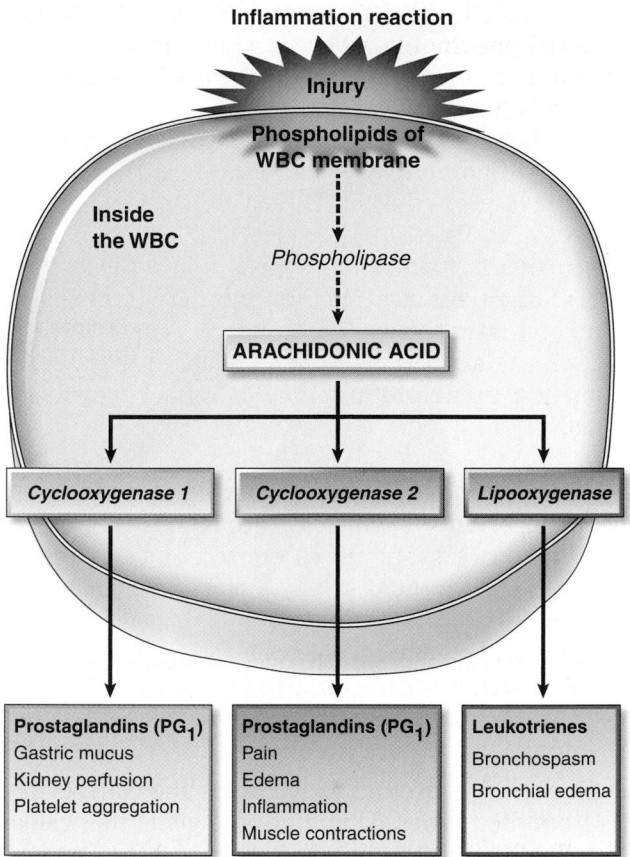

Figure 9-4. Prostaglandin and leukotriene synthesis pathways within the WBC. Injury stimulates inflammation, which attracts WBCs to the area of injury. Within the WBC, phospholipase acts upon phospholipids to yield arachidonic acid, which is then converted to PGs via the cyclooxygenase 1 or cyclooxygenase 2 pathway or to leukotrienes via the lipooxygenase pathway. The PGs created by the cyclooxygenase 1 pathway are needed to secrete gastric mucus and enhance renal perfusion and thrombus formation. The PGs created by the cyclooxygenase 2 pathway cause uncomfortable symptoms of inflammation, such as fever, edema, and pain. Leukotrienes cause bronchospasm and bronchiole edema.

lean body mass. TNF-alpha can enhance release of WBCs into the bloodstream and facilitate the release of pituitary corticotropin and adrenal corticosteroids in the body. In an infected bloodstream, which is a condition known as sepsis, TNF-alpha provokes hypotension, widespread vasodilation, increased heart rate, and decreased blood pH.

Lymphadenopathy. Lymphadenopathy, or lymphadenitis, is a term used to describe the enlargement of lymph nodes because of inflammatory processes. **Lymph nodes** are small bean-sized masses of tissue located in various regions of the body, including the neck, axillary regions, central thoracic region, inguinal areas, and gastrointestinal tract. **Lymphocytes** mature within a lymph node, and during an inflammatory process, lymph nodes become enlarged (Fig. 9-5). Because of the active proliferation of lymphocytes, lymph nodes enlarge and become tender. Lymphatic fluid or

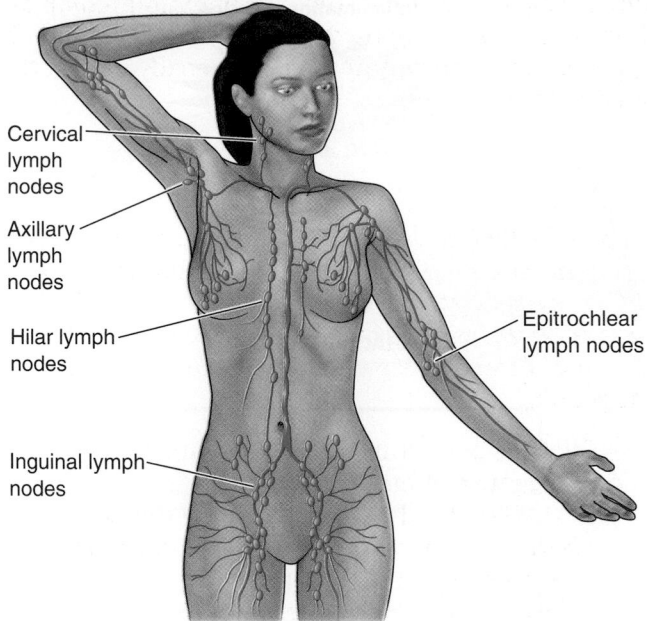

Cervical lymph nodes

Axillary lymph nodes

Hilar lymph nodes

Epitrochlear lymph nodes

Inguinal lymph nodes

Figure 9-5. Regions of the lymph nodes in the body.

lymph circulates around body tissues and collects debris from the tissues. The injurious agents that cause the inflammation can invade lymph, and then spread to other lymph nodes.

Outcomes of Acute Inflammation. Acute inflammation will result in one of three outcomes:

1. complete resolution
2. healing by connective tissue
3. chronic, persistent inflammation that does not recede.

Ideally, acute inflammation is a short-lived reaction that eliminates an injurious agent, allows little tissue destruction, and terminates by facilitating the regeneration of normal tissue. Resolution involves normalization of vascular permeability, deactivation of chemical mediators, elimination of cellular debris and edema, and apoptosis of WBCs.

At times, severe tissue injury and a large acute inflammatory reaction preclude the regeneration of normal cells. This happens when inflammation involves tissues incapable of regenerating cells or when inflammatory exudates and cellular debris cannot be adequately cleared at the conclusion of the inflammatory reaction. At these times, resolution and healing occur through the proliferation of connective tissue. Cellular debris and exudates are reabsorbed and fibrous scar tissue, rather than regenerated cells, replace damaged cells. Finally, there are times when acute inflammation cannot be resolved because of persistence of the injurious agent or other interference with healing. In these cases, inflammation becomes a chronic, persistent condition with failure to resolve and extensive tissue damage.

Chronic Inflammation

An inflammatory reaction that persists for a prolonged time, from weeks to months, without resolution or healing is considered a chronic inflammatory disorder. There are specific etiologic agents known to cause chronic inflammation, but a persistent, unremitting inflammatory reaction can also occur for unknown reasons. Certain microorganisms such as *mycobacteria tuberculi*, the etiologic agent of TB, and *treponema pallidum*, the cause of syphilis, cause chronic inflammation. Viruses, parasites, fungi, and bacteria can also cause chronic inflammatory disorders, as can prolonged exposure to toxic agents. Examples include long-term exposure to coal dust inhaled by coal miners, which results in anthracosis (black lung disease), a chronic pulmonary disease. Alternatively, occupational exposure to carbon tetrachloride can cause chronic liver inflammation.

Autoimmune diseases, such as rheumatoid arthritis and systemic lupus erythematosus, are chronic inflammatory disorders. In autoimmune disease, an unknown offending agent, also called an antigen, incites an inflammatory reaction that initiates production of antibodies that attack the body's own tissues. The antibodies produce a persistent inflammatory reaction that causes chronic tissue damage.

In contrast to acute inflammation, which is manifested by vascular permeability and neutrophil proliferation, chronic inflammation is characterized by the predominance of monocytes, lymphocytes, and macrophages. In acute inflammation, the products of activated macrophages eliminate injurious agents such as microbes and initiate the process of healing. In chronic inflammation, however, these same products, when constantly secreted by macrophages, cause tissue damage. The destructive macrophage products include free radicals, proteases, cytokines, angiogenesis growth factors, and fibroblast activators. Tissue is repeatedly damaged, healing is delayed, and connective tissue replaces injured cells. As tissue damage causes cell death, necrotic tissue stimulates an inflammatory reaction. As a result, tissues undergoing chronic inflammation can have regions demonstrating acute inflammation as well.

Chronic inflammation often causes a distinctive histological pattern of granulomatous changes. A **granuloma** is an area where macrophages have aggregated and are transformed into epithelial-like or epithelioid cells. The epithelioid cells are surrounded by lymphocytes, fibroblasts, and connective tissue. Frequently, the epithelioid cells fuse to form giant cells within the granuloma. TB is the prototypical granulomatous chronic inflammatory disease. On histological examination of the lungs, a TB granuloma is characterized by an aggregate of macrophages surrounding mycobacteria tuberculi bacterial organisms. After acute infection, neutrophils and monocytes surround but cannot kill TB bacteria. The WBCs attracted to the area of infection can only wall off the bacteria. Eventually this region,

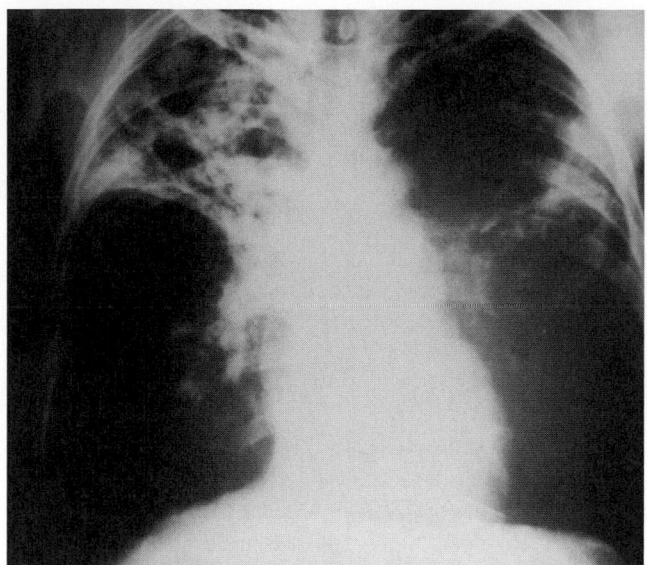

Figure 9-6. Chest x-ray showing TB. *(Courtesy of CDC.)*

infiltrated with macrophages, becomes a chronic inflammatory granuloma called a tubercle. The tubercle can be identified on histological examination and x-ray of the lungs (see Fig. 9-6).

Cellular Regeneration, Tissue Repair, and Healing

Tissue healing and regeneration are the desirable outcomes of cell injury and inflammation. Optimal regenerative healing occurs when injured cells are replaced by cells of the same type, leaving no trace of residual injury. Certain tissue injuries, such as those involving loss of tissue because of gouging injuries, cannot heal by cellular replacement. In situations such as this, cells are replaced by connective tissue, which leaves a scar. Cellular regeneration is controlled by signals from the environment that either stimulate or inhibit proliferation. Tissues are composed of different populations of quiescent, actively dividing, and terminally differentiated cells.

The Cell Cycle

Tissue healing depends on the type of cells that have been injured. There are three types of body cells that differ according to their ability to regenerate: labile, stable, or permanent cells. Each of these cell types are in a different stage within the cell cycle. These stages are:

- G0: Cells are resting or quiescent and not undergoing mitotic division.
- G1: Cells enter the cell cycle during this stage, where they make preparations for mitosis and then continue on to the S phase.
- G2: Cells continue to undergo necessary activities before mitosis.
- S: Cells undergo chromosomal duplication in preparation for mitotic division.
- M: Cell completes mitosis and divides to regenerate itself.

See Figure 9-7 for the stages of the cell cycle.

Labile Cells

Cells that continuously proceed through the cell cycle are called labile cells. Labile cells continually divide and replicate throughout life, replacing cells that are constantly eliminated. For example, skin, oral mucosal cells, gastrointestinal mucosal lining cells, and genitourinary mucous membrane cells are continuously sloughed and require replacement. The bone marrow is continuously active as it synthesizes blood cells. Cancer cells are considered labile cells because they are constantly dividing.

Figure 9-7. The cell cycle. Almost all cells divide into two daughter cells via mitosis. The cell goes through the stages shown and repeats. G0 – G1 – S – G2 – M. The time between mitosis phases, which includes G1, S, and G2, is called interphase. (From Thompson, G. S. (2013). *Understanding anatomy and physiology.* Philadelphia, PA: F.A. Davis Company, with permission.)

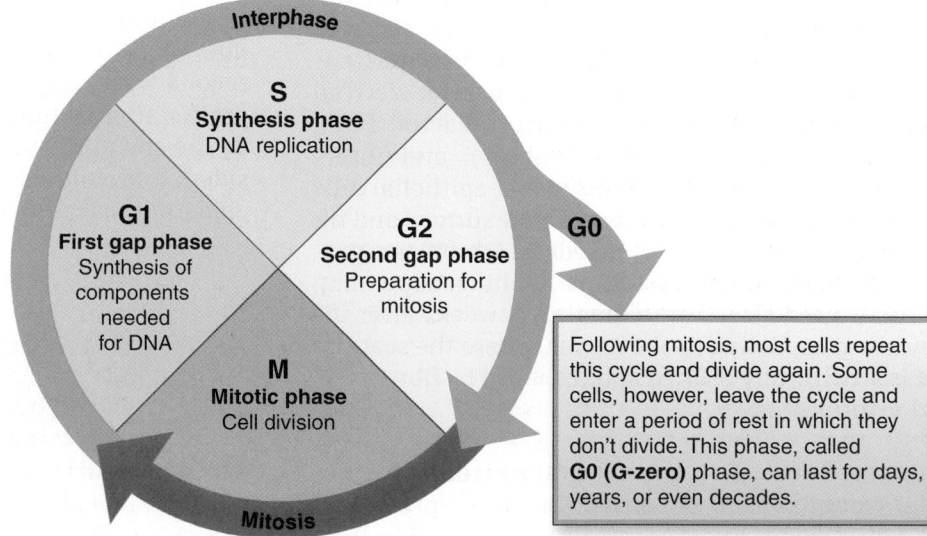

Stable Cells

Stable cells are cells that are in a resting stage until stimulated, when they then enter the cell cycle. Examples of stable cells are bone cells and hepatocytes. Both of these kinds of cells require major stimuli to enter the cell cycle, undergo mitosis, and regenerate. After fracture, bone cells enter the cell cycle to regenerate and repair bone tissue. Hepatocytes undergo mitosis and regenerate the liver after surgical, traumatic, or chemical injury.

Permanent Cells

Permanent cells cannot regenerate and therefore do not enter the cell cycle. Neurons and cardiac myocytes are considered permanent cells that do not undergo mitosis and have lost the ability to proliferate. For example, brain cells involved in stroke and myocardial cells involved in infarction are considered dead and unable to function. However, researchers are investigating the regenerative potential of neurons and cardiac cells. Studies are showing that adult stem cells in areas previously thought to consist of solely permanent cells, such as the heart, can be coaxed into regeneration and mitosis.

Normal Wound Healing

Wound healing is divided into three phases:

1. inflammation
2. proliferation, granulation tissue formation, and epithelialization
3. wound contraction and remodeling.

Inflammation occurs in the acute phase immediately after injury, and has been described previously. In the subsequent proliferation phase, granulation tissue forms. The fibroblast, a connective tissue cell that synthesizes collagen and provides the extracellular matrix in wound healing, is the key cell involved in this process. As early as 24 to 48 hours after injury, fibroblasts and vascular endothelial cells form the granulation tissue that serves as the foundation of scar tissue. The granulation tissue then secretes growth factors and cytokines such as vascular endothelial growth factor (VEGF), platelet-derived growth factor (PDGF), fibroblast growth factor (FGF), tissue growth factor-beta (TGF-beta), and interleukin-1 (IL-1). Also during this phase, epithelial cells migrate and proliferate to form a new surface and fill in the gap between the wound edges. Fibroblasts produce collagen for days, weeks, or months, depending on the wound size. Approximately 3 weeks after injury, the remodeling phase begins, where the scar tissue is structurally refined and reshaped by fibroblasts and myofibroblasts.

Primary, Secondary, and Tertiary Intention

Skin wounds heal by either of three processes: primary, secondary, or tertiary intention (see Fig. 9-8).

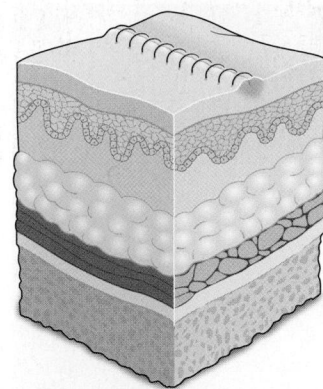
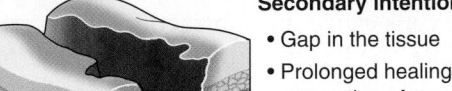
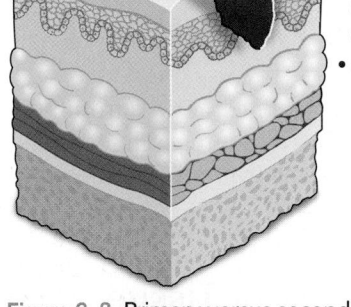

Primary intention
- No gap in the tissue
- Simple reapproximation of edges of wound
- Simple reepithelialization
- Surgical incision type of healing

Secondary intention
- Gap in the tissue
- Prolonged healing involving generation of granulation tissue and more complex tissue
- Scar tissue formation

Figure 9-8. Primary versus secondary intention healing.

The nature of the wound determines the process the body uses. Healing by **primary intention,** also called primary union, is the least complicated type of wound repair. The edges of the wound are clearly demarcated, cleanly lacerated, easily brought together, and there is no missing tissue within the injured area. A surgical wound is the best example of this type of injury, which usually undergoes a simple, rapid healing process. Within 24 hours, WBCs congregate and a fibrin clot develops at the site. After 24 to 48 hours, simple epithelialization predominates as the major process that closes the wound. By day 5, granulation tissue progressively fills in the incision space and new blood vessel growth is maximal. During the second week, there is accumulation of collagen and proliferation of fibroblasts within the incisional scar. By the end of the first month, inflammation has subsided, and connective tissue covered by an intact epidermis makes up the wound site.

> ## 🩺 CLINICAL CONCEPT
>
> Primary intention is best exemplified by healing of a clean, surgical laceration. It requires predominately surface reepithelialization and reestablishment of tissue integrity of the approximated edges.

When there is extensive loss of tissue within a wound, the repair process is more complex; in this case, **secondary intention,** also called secondary union, healing begins (see Fig. 9-8). Regeneration of the same cells to replace lost tissue is not possible. Abundant granulation and fibrous tissue is necessary to fill the defect and restore the original structure of tissue. The inflammation process within this type of wound is more intense and longer in duration. The formation of granulation tissue requires extensive time and support for the healing process.

The phase that differentiates primary from secondary intention is wound contraction. Wound contraction occurs because of myofibroblasts, which are connective tissue cells with smooth muscle characteristics. These specialized cells cause the contraction of the wound's edges to close the tissue gap. Substantial scar formation and thinning of the epidermis occurs. Wounds of this type are highly susceptible to infection, complications, and deformity.

In **tertiary intention,** also called tertiary union, the wound is missing a large amount of deep tissue and is contaminated. It is cleaned and left open for 4 to 5 days before closure. The wound may require temporary packing with sterile gauze and have extensive drainage. By the fifth day, WBC phagocytosis of contaminated tissues occurs and the processes of epithelialization, collagen deposition, and maturation take place. Foreign materials are walled off by macrophages and other types of leukocytes to form granulomas. There is prominent scarring with healing. Commonly this type of wound requires a skin graft.

 CLINICAL CONCEPT

Pressure ulcers and severe burns are examples of wounds that require secondary and tertiary intention healing. These wounds have large areas of missing skin, dermis, and deeper tissue, which are replaced by scar tissue.

Primary, secondary, and tertiary intention wounds do not regain full tensile strength of unwounded skin after healing is completed. Clinicians and patients need to be aware of the weakened integrity of the skin and underlying tissues. Careful support of the area to facilitate healing is necessary during the first few weeks after surgery. After sutures are removed, usually 1 to 2 weeks later, wounded skin is again in a vulnerable, weakened state. The healed wound builds to a maximal tensile strength of 70% to 80% after 3 months.

Factors That Affect Wound Healing

Wound healing is a complex phenomenon, and many body systems are involved in supporting the process. Healing requires a sufficient supply of nutrients and oxygen, as well as efficient removal of tissue debris and invading microorganisms. Box 9-2 summarizes the positive and negative factors involved in wound healing; each is discussed in detail in the following text.

Nutrition

Successful wound healing depends on adequate protein, carbohydrates, fats, vitamins, and minerals obtained from optimal nutrition. Protein is particularly necessary for cellular regeneration and synthesis of connective tissue. For wounds to heal, a patient must be in a state of positive nitrogen balance. Nitrogen balance is defined as the difference between nitrogen intake and nitrogen excretion. Protein is the best source of nitrogen in the diet. When a patient's nitrogen intake exceeds nitrogen excretion, the resultant positive nitrogen balance suggests the availability of protein for wound repair.

Carbohydrates can be used for energy in order to spare protein sources for tissue healing. Fats are essential components of cell membranes that are synthesized during the healing process.

Most vitamins are essential cofactors for the body's metabolic activities. They are particularly important in wound healing. The role of vitamins and other trace elements in successful wound healing is listed in Table 9-1.

BOX 9-2. Factors Involved in Wound Healing

- **Nutrition:** Lack of adequate nutrients, particularly protein, decreases cellular regeneration and metabolic function.
- **Oxygenation:** Oxygen is needed for neutrophil phagocytosis and collagen synthesis.
- **Circulation:** Lack of adequate circulation predisposes the individual to ischemia, infarction, and consequent infection of necrotic tissue, also known as gangrene.
- **Immune strength:** Diabetes, corticosteroid use, cancer, human immunodeficiency virus, and immunosuppressant agents diminish WBC activity, delay wound healing, and predispose to infection.
- **Contamination:** Foreign bodies present in a wound diminish healing ability and predispose to infection. Sutures that remain too long can act as foreign bodies and inhibit healing. Surgically inserted devices such as pacemakers, heart valves, and orthopedic or prosthetic implants can become sources of infection and predispose the patient to septicemia.
- **Obesity:** Adipose tissue does not heal efficiently and approximated edges cannot be sutured together easily.
- **Age:** The regeneration process of infants and young children is superior to that of adults. Studies show that fetal wounds heal without fibrosis or scarring. Elderly adults have the slowest healing process.

TABLE 9-1. Vitamins, Minerals, and Wound Healing

Substance	Function in Wound Healing
Vitamins A and C	• Build proteins • Fortify epithelial mucous membranes • Increase collagen strength
Vitamin B_{12}	• Enable cell replication • Support growth of RBCs • Maintain nervous system • Enable synthesis of nucleic acids
Vitamin D	• Foster absorption of calcium from gastro-intestinal tract
Vitamin K	• Enable synthesis of coagulation factors
Folate	• With vitamin B_{12}, enables synthesis of nucleic acids
Calcium, Phosphorus	• Support bone growth
Iron	• Essential for synthesis of hemoglobin and RBCs • Required for mitochondrial functioning
Zinc, Copper, Manganese	• Needed for cellular metabolism

Obesity tends to impair wound healing because adipose tissue is less vascular and, in turn, deficient in oxygen. Oxygen is needed for neutrophil phagocytosis and collagen synthesis, two activities integral to efficient wound healing. Surgical procedures on obese patients require more time and cause more tissue trauma. In addition, surgical wound closure is more difficult in obese patients because of the tension on the sutures. These factors increase the risk of wound infection.

Blood Flow and Oxygen Delivery

Arterial and venous circulation should be optimal in the region that requires healing, as healing tissue needs a rich supply of nutrients and oxygen delivered via arterial blood flow as well as adequate waste removal provided by efficient venous flow. Bacteria, cellular debris, necrotic tissue, and local toxins need to be eliminated as tissue regenerates. Wounds that attempt to heal under ischemic conditions require lengthier time periods and are susceptible to infection. Ischemia fosters the growth of anaerobic bacteria such as *Clostridium perfringens*, the microorganism that causes gangrene.

Brisk arterial blood flow is needed to deliver maximal oxygen to the area. Oxygen facilitates collagen synthesis and WBC function. Without oxygen, WBCs cannot kill phagocytosed microorganisms and collagen growth is deficient. Hyperbaric oxygen, which is 100% oxygen delivered at two times normal atmospheric pressure, facilitates collagen synthesis, angiogenesis, neutrophil phagocytic activity, and fibroblast proliferation.

Immune Strength

A strong immune system that is capable of eliminating dead tissue, walling off foreign matter, and killing microorganisms is required for optimal wound healing. A brisk inflammatory response is needed in the initial stages of tissue injury, followed by efficient phagocytic WBC function and strong acquired immune reactions. The infant who is naïve immunologically and the elderly patient who is naturally immunosuppressed are vulnerable to suboptimal wound healing because of susceptibility to infection. However, in general, immunocompetent children have more efficient healing processes than adults. Studies show that fetal wounds heal without fibrosis or scarring. Compared with adult wounds, fetal wounds are richer in hyaluronic acid, a component thought to facilitate cellular regeneration and collagen synthesis. Elderly patients heal less efficiently because of aged skin, thinned dermal layer, reduced collagen and fibroblast synthesis, and greater potential for secondary conditions that reduce blood flow to the area.

Conditions that cause immunosuppression, such as cancer, human immunodeficiency virus, diabetes mellitus, and corticosteroid use, may delay healing of the body. Diabetes mellitus decreases the phagocytic ability of neutrophils and macrophages, which hinders the inflammation response in wound healing. Diabetes mellitus also injures small arterial blood vessels, diminishing peripheral circulation. Decreased peripheral circulation diminishes the arteriolar blood flow to peripheral nerves which, in turn, decreases sensation. Individuals with diabetes mellitus gradually develop increasing sensory deficit of the lower extremities, particularly of the feet. Lack of sensation and circulation in the feet predispose the individual to wound formation. For example, a person with diabetes mellitus who wears an ill-fitting shoe can develop a blister that goes unrecognized because of lack of pain sensation in the feet. This simple blister can quickly become an infected foot wound because of the diabetic patient's lack of sensation, diminished circulation, and decreased WBC function.

Corticosteroids, potent anti-inflammatory agents, suppress the inflammation phase of wound healing. These drugs also inhibit collagen synthesis, which is integral to the proliferative and remodeling phases of wound healing. Therefore, patients on corticosteroids can become immunosuppressed and experience poor wound healing.

Infection is the single most important cause of delayed healing. The wound's susceptibility to infection is influenced by the patient's immune strength, the type of wound present, and conditions of injury. The presence of infection perpetuates the inflammation phase and delays the formation of granulation tissue and collagen synthesis. Foreign bodies present within the wound are major impediments to the healing process and increase risk of infection. Vigorous irrigation, cleansing, and removal of necrotic tissue and foreign matter are necessary to facilitate optimal wound healing. Sutures can act as foreign bodies if they are not removed in a timely manner from the healing wound site. Surgically inserted devices such as pacemakers, heart valves, and orthopedic or prosthetic implants can become sources of infection and predispose the patient to septicemia.

Dysfunctional Wound Healing

Wounds can fail to heal properly if the factors needed to support healing are lacking. Individuals who are poorly nourished or immunocompromised are at risk for suboptimal wound outcomes. In addition, the healing wound must be protected if it is to close properly. Finally, the processes involved in functional wound healing may become overly aggressive and lead to complications (see Box 9-3).

Wound Rupture

Most wounds require structural support and immobility for the initial healing period. Undue tension on the wound can inhibit the approximation of edges and epithelialization of the surface. There is particularly high tension on edges of abdominal wall wounds because of the mechanical stresses of coughing, vomiting, and the Valsalva maneuver. When previously closed wound edges open and rupture, the condition is called **wound dehiscence.** In rare cases, internal tissues and organs can extrude from the open wound, a condition called **wound evisceration.** Abdominal wounds are most susceptible to these conditions.

> **ALERT!** Wound dehiscence and evisceration require immediate wound protection with sterile, saline-moistened dressings and prompt surgical evaluation.

Keloid Formation

Wound healing can be complicated by hyperplastic epithelialization and collagen formation. The excessive accumulation of epithelium and collagen can form a hypertrophic scar, also called a keloid. The etiology of keloid formation is unknown; however, it is more common in persons of African descent. Keloids can be reduced by cosmetic surgery.

Contractures

Wound contraction, the last step in second intention healing, can become exaggerated and result in a deformity called a **contracture,** which is an inflexible shrinkage of wound tissue that pulls the edges toward the center of the wound. Contractures often occur in burn wounds and limit mobility when they occur across a joint surface. A related type of wound complication is a **stricture,** which is a complication of wound healing that causes narrowing or closure of an open area of the body. A duct, canal, or tube may develop a stricture caused by scar tissue. For example, if the esophagus is injured, a stricture would reduce the diameter and narrow or completely close off the tubular open area for passage of food.

Fistula

A fistula is an abnormal connection between two different areas of tissue or organs. A fistula can form with abnormal wound healing and cause complications. An example is a tracheoesophageal fistula, which is a connection between trachea and esophagus. Aspiration of contents from the esophagus can obstruct the trachea.

Adhesions

Adhesions are abnormal bands of internal scar tissue that can form following invasive surgical procedures. These bands of scar tissue can limit mobility if they form within a joint as in adhesive capsulitis of the shoulder (frozen shoulder). Alternatively, adhesions can form around internal organs, cause pain or obstruction, and require surgical excision.

BOX 9-3. Possible Complications of Wound Healing

- **Keloid:** hyperplasia of scar tissue
- **Contractures:** inflexible shrinkage of wound tissue that pulls the edges toward the center of the wound
- **Dehiscence:** opening of a wound's suture line
- **Evisceration:** opening of wound with extrusion of tissue and organs
- **Stricture:** an abnormal narrowing of a tubular body passage from the formation of scar tissue (e.g., esophageal stricture)
- **Fistula:** an abnormal connection between two epithelium-lined organs or vessels that normally do not connect (e.g., Tracheoesophageal fistula)
- **Adhesions:** internal scar tissue between tissues or organs

Chapter Summary

- Inflammation is an essential process for protecting the body during injury or infection.
- In the initial phase, WBCs are attracted to the site of the injury in a process called chemotaxis.
- Blood vessel walls become more permeable so fluid and WBCs can move out of the bloodstream to the site of injury.
- Types of WBCs include neutrophils, eosinophils, basophils, lymphocytes, and monocytes, which turn into macrophages.
- The five cardinal signs of inflammation are rubor (redness), tumor (swelling), calor (heat), dolor (pain), and loss of function.

- C-reactive protein and erythrocyte sedimentation rates increase in acute inflammation.
- Inflammation can undergo healing and resolution or persist as chronic inflammation.
- Healing involves one of three processes: primary, secondary, or tertiary intention.
- Nutrition status, oxygen supply, steroid use, diabetes, and immunosuppression affect the process of healing.
- There are many possible complications of wound healing including keloid formation, contracture, stricture and fistula formation, wound dehiscence, and evisceration.

Bibliography

Arias, C. A., & Murray, B. E. (2009). Antibiotic-resistant bugs in the 21st century—a clinical super-challenge. *N Engl J Med,* 360(5), 439–443. doi: 10.1056/NEJMp0804651.

Barrett, K. E., Barman, S. M., Boitano, S., & Brooks, H. L. (2012). *Ganong's review of medical physiology.* 24th ed. New York: McGraw-Hill.

Centers for Disease Control and Prevention (CDC). (2013). Measles—United States, January 1–August 24, 2013. *MMWR Morb Mortal Wkly Rep,* 62(36), 741–743. Erratum in: *MMWR Morb Mortal Wkly Rep.* 2013 Sep 20;62(37):774.

Cowman, S., Gethin, G., Clarke, E., et al. (2012). An international eDelphi study identifying the research and education priorities in wound management and tissue repair. *J Clin Nurs,* 21(3-4), 344–353. doi: 10.1111/j.1365-2702.2011.03950.x. Epub 2011 Dec 9.

Defay, F., De Serres, G., Skowronski, D. M., et al. (2013). Measles in children vaccinated with 2 doses of MMR. *Ped,* 132(5), e1126–e1133. doi: 10.1542/peds.2012-3975.

Eltzschig, H. K., & Carmeliet, P. (2011). Hypoxia and inflammation. *N Engl J Med,* 364(7), 656–665.

Gethin, G. (2012, March 12). Understanding the inflammatory process in wound healing. *Brit J Comm Nurs,* Suppl, S17–S18, S20, S22.

Hall, J. (2011). *Guyton and Hall textbook of medical physiology.* 12th ed. New York: Saunders.

Huskins, W. C., Huckabee, C. M., O'Grady, N. P., et al. (2011). Intervention to reduce transmission of resistant bacteria in intensive care. *N Engl J Med,* 364(15), 1407–1418. doi: 10.1056/NEJMoa1000373.

Kang, J., Sickbert-Bennett, E. E., Brown, V. M., Weber, D. J., & Rutala, W. A. (2014, April 25). Changes in the incidence of health care-associated pathogens at a university hospital from 2005 to 2011. *Am J Infect Control,* pii: S0196-6553(14)00213-2. doi: 10.1016/j.ajic.2014.03.019.

Knol, M., Urbanus, A., Swart, E., et al. (2013, Sep 5). Large ongoing measles outbreak in a religious community in the Netherlands since May 2013. *Euro Surveill,* 18(36), pii=20580.

Kumar, V., Abbas, A. K., Fausto, N., & Aster, J. (2010). *Robbins and Cotran pathologic basis of disease.* 8th ed. Philadelphia, PA: Elsevier Saunders.

Longo, D., Fauci, A., Kasper, D., et al. (2011). *Harrison's principles of internal medicine.* 18th ed. New York: McGraw-Hill.

Lowy, F. D. (2013). Methicillin-resistant *Staphylococcus aureus:* where is it coming from and where is it going? *JAMA Intern Med,* 173(21), 1978–1979. doi: 10.1001/jamainternmed.2013.8277.

McPhee, S. J., & Papdakis, M. A. (2012). *Current medical diagnosis and treatment.* New York: Lange / McGraw-Hill.

Nicks, B., Ayello, E., Woo, K., Nitzki-George, D., & Sibbald, R. G. (2010). Acute wound management: revisiting the approach to assessment, irrigation, and closure considerations. *Int J Emerg Med,* 3(4), 399–407. Published online 2010 August 27. doi: 10.1007/s12245-010-0217-5.

Porter, M., & Kelly, J. (2014). Pressure ulcer treatment in a patient with spina bifida. *Nurs Stand,* 28(35), 60–69. doi: 10.7748/ns2014.04.28.35.60.e7943.

Reuter, S., Ellington, M. J., Cartwright, E. J., et al. (2013). Rapid bacterial whole-genome sequencing to enhance diagnostic and public health microbiology. *JAMA Intern Med,* 173(15), 1397–1404. doi: 10.1001/jamainternmed.2013.7734.

Sane, J., Gouma, S., Koopmans, M., et al. (2014, April). Epidemic of mumps among vaccinated persons, the Netherlands, 2009–2012. *Emerg Infect Dis,* 20(4), 643–648. doi: 10.3201/eid2004.131681.

Sepkowitz, K. A. (2013). Clostridium difficile leaves the hospital—what's next? *JAMA Intern Med,* 173(14), 1367–1368. doi: 10.1001/jamainternmed.2013.7940.

Swindon, Wiltshire, Bath, and North East Somerset Wound Group. (2011). Identification, diagnosis and treatment of wound infection. *Nurs Stand,* 26(11), 4–8.

Tredget, E. E., & Ding, J. (2009). Wound healing: from embryos to adults and back again. *Lancet,* 373(9671), 1226–1228.

Infectious Diseases

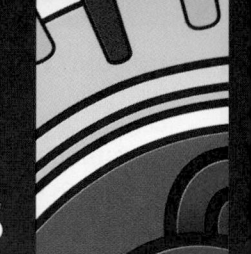

Key Terms

Antibody titer

Congenital

Dermatophytes

Epidemiology

Exanthem

Gram negative

Gram positive

Group A beta hemolytic streptococcus (GABHS)

Immunocompetence

Incidence

Infection

Inoculum

Methicillin-resistant *Staphylococcus aureus* (MRSA)

Nosocomial infection

Opportunistic infection

Portal of entry

Prevalence

Reservoir

Septicemia

Vancomycin-resistant *Staphylococcus aureus* (VRSA)

Vector

Virulence

Infectious diseases are found among people of all ages, races, and geographic locations. They can be difficult to manage because of human susceptibilities, environmental factors, and their ability to evolve and develop resistance to antibiotics. Across the world infectious disease is a significant cause of morbidity, disability, and death.

Many infectious diseases of viral origin, such as measles, mumps, and rubella, were once the bane of childhood, but the advent of mandatory immunizations has helped to lessen their impact. Parasitic infections, such as malaria, are present in developing countries but are uncommon in industrialized regions; with the increase in international travel, however, diseases previously endemic to specific regions have the potential to spread across the globe.

Clinical settings contain different populations of bacteria, viruses, fungi, and parasites; many of them are resistant to drugs. All patients, particularly those who are immunosuppressed, are susceptible to microbial invasions developing into nosocomial infections. Therefore, all clinicians, regardless of setting, need to be aware of prevention, pathophysiology, diagnosis, and treatment of infectious disease.

Basic Concepts of Infection

Humans are constantly exposed to microorganisms. Pathogens, specific microorganisms that are capable of causing infectious disease, are categorized as viruses, bacteria, fungi, and parasites. These pathogens are capable of invading, colonizing, and stimulating an inflammatory reaction in host tissues. *Host* is the term used to describe the human or animal invaded and colonized by a pathogen, whereas **infection** describes the invasion, colonization, and multiplication of pathogens within the host. Colonization indicates that a pathogen is living within the host, but does not mean infection exists. Infection is diagnosed when there is isolation of a pathogen or evidence of its presence and pathogen-related host symptoms.

Different pathogens have varying disease-producing potential, which is called **virulence.** There are various virulence factors that enhance the pathogen's ability to infect the host; examples of virulence factors include pathogenic toxins that destroy host cells, adhesion factors that enhance attachment of the pathogen to the host cells, and evasive factors that shield or hide the pathogen from the host's immune system. The severity of infection depends on the pathogen's virulence and the strength of the host's defenses at the time of infection.

A reservoir and a vector may also be involved in an infectious process. A **reservoir** is a source of a pathogenic organism that may or may not be suffering from the disease caused by the pathogen. A child suffering from chickenpox would be considered a reservoir because he or she harbors the transmissible microorganism. Environmental objects, also called fomites, can also act as reservoirs of microorganisms. An unsanitary bathroom surface is an example of a fomite.

A **vector** is a living being that can carry the pathogenic organism from the reservoir to the host. Commonly a vector is an insect, such as a mosquito, tick, or housefly. A vector is not considered infected with the organism but is needed to transmit the pathogen to the host.

The study of infectious disease requires an understanding of pathogens at the population, individual, cellular, and molecular levels. For example, the human immunodeficiency virus (HIV) has infected so many people across the world that it has decreased the immune strength of the population as a whole. At the individual level, HIV causes immunosuppression and consequent susceptibility to opportunistic infections, which can be transmitted from individual to individual. At the cellular level, HIV attacks CD4 cells (also known as T helper cells) and macrophages, which are integral to the immune response. Loss of CD4 cells and macrophages causes dysfunction of other body systems. Finally, at the molecular level, there is a gene that confers resistance to HIV in certain individuals. Study of this gene may lead to the development of a vaccine that could prevent HIV infection.

Epidemiology, the study of disease distributions in human populations, uses specific terms. Epidemiological data include **incidence,** which is the number of new cases of infection within a population, and **prevalence,** which is the number of active ongoing cases of infection at any given time. A disease is considered endemic if the incidence and prevalence are relatively stable; an epidemic is an abrupt increase in the incidence of disease within a geographic region. A pandemic is a term used for global spread of a specific disease.

Normal Microbial Flora Versus Pathogens

The human body contains numerous species of bacteria that are considered normal flora. Normal microbial flora are organisms that perform advantageous functions for the life of the host and reside in a specific niche in the human body. Staphylococci live on skin surfaces; lactobacilli, *Escherichia coli* (*E. coli*), and bacteroides reside within the gastrointestinal tract; and streptococci are normal inhabitants of the vagina. Microorganisms that serve as normal flora secrete needed nutrients, perform necessary metabolic activities, and help defend the body against other microorganisms. Normal flora do not cause infection when they remain within the strict boundaries of their anatomic niche in the body. However, if normal flora bacteria invade noncolonized areas of the body, they can cause infection.

> ### CLINICAL CONCEPT
>
> Clinicians must be careful to not allow normal flora to invade sterile areas of the body when performing invasive procedures. For example, if an intravenous catheter is inserted without properly disinfecting the skin, staphylococci from the skin can be transferred into the bloodstream. Infection of the bloodstream is termed **septicemia.**

In general, all humans harbor the same normal flora. However, some individuals carry specific microbes that do not cause disease for them but can cause infection in others. These individuals, who can carry certain bacteria and transmit infection to susceptible individuals, are known as carriers.

>
> ### CLINICAL CONCEPT
>
> Mary Mallon was a cook for a number of families in New York in the early 1900s. Although healthy herself, Mary was a carrier of the bacteria that causes typhoid fever. Many members of the families she worked for became ill with typhoid, and several died. Each time, Mary moved onto another job, and the cycle repeated itself. Because of this, history remembers her as Typhoid Mary.

Individuals are exposed to many common microorganisms within the environment on a daily basis. The term **immunocompetence** refers to an individual's ability to protect oneself from infectious agents because of a strong immune system. Immunosuppression indicates that there is a defective immune system that is placing a person at risk for infections. From a young age, an immunocompetent person builds immune defenses and swiftly eliminates many microorganisms as threats of infection. However, if the individual becomes immunosuppressed, common microorganisms can overwhelm the weakened immune defenses and multiply within the body to cause an **opportunistic infection,** which is an infection caused by a microorganism that flourishes because of a host's deficient immune system.

Hospitalized patients are in a precarious situation with respect to pathogenic microorganisms. The hospital environment exposes bacteria to a wide variety of antibiotics. Bacteria can adapt to many antibiotics, resulting in a high number of bacteria within the hospital environment that are antibiotic resistant. Hospitalized patients are vulnerable to infection because of illness, surgery, and other invasive procedures. A patient infection caused by microorganisms inherent to the healthcare facility environment is called a **nosocomial infection.** Nosocomial infections may be difficult to treat because they are often caused by antibiotic-resistant bacteria.

> **ALERT!** Hospital personnel often inadvertently spread microbes from one patient to another because of lack of proper hand washing and poor sterile technique. Careful hand washing is critical to the patients' health.

Types of Microorganisms

There are many types of pathogenic microorganisms capable of causing infectious disease. Each microorganism has unique characteristics, mechanisms of disease, and methods of elimination. The clinician needs a broad understanding of the agents of infectious disease, diagnostic methods, and the antibiotics that can be used to eliminate them.

Bacteria

Bacteria are ubiquitous, free-living microorganisms within the environment that can be either advantageous or harmful to humans. The human body is colonized with bacteria as normal flora on the skin and within the oropharynx, gastrointestinal tract, and vaginal canal. Bacteria are categorized according to their shape, aerobic or anaerobic respiratory capability, and the laboratory staining of their cell wall structure.

The common shapes of bacterial microorganisms are round, called cocci, and rod-shaped, called bacilli. A small number of bacteria, called spirochetes, are spiral-shaped (Fig. 10-1). Chlamydiae, rickettsiae, and mycoplasma are unique types of bacteria that have distinctive features and cannot be categorized according to their shape.

Cocci bacteria can be found living unattached to each other in the environment in clusters. Alternatively, they can be found in chains, called streptococci, or in duos, called diplococci.

Gram staining is a laboratory procedure used to identify and highlight bacterial organisms within infected tissue. Bacteria stain differently according to the composition of their cell wall. The cell wall of bacterial organisms is made up of different percentages of peptidoglycan, an amino acid and sugar complex. **Gram-positive** bacteria have a thick, peptidoglycan-rich cell wall that takes on a characteristic purple color when subjected to the staining procedure in the laboratory. **Gram-negative** bacteria have a thin cell wall that contains fewer peptidoglycan and takes on a pink-colored stain.

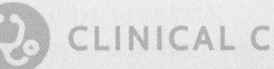

CLINICAL CONCEPT

Bacteria that take on Gram stain in the same manner share other features, such as antibiotic susceptibility. There are specific antibiotics for gram-positive and gram-negative bacteria.

A broad spectrum antibiotic can be used against both types of bacteria.

There are certain bacteria that cause common infectious diseases. Clinicians should be familiar with names and characteristic features associated with these bacteria (Table 10-1). Bacteria are usually referred to by the genus to which they belong, followed by the species, or name of the specific bacteria. For example, the bacteria that causes gonorrhea is called *Neisseria gonorrhoeae*, meaning it belongs to the genus *Neisseria* and the species *gonorrhoeae*. It is common to abbreviate the names of bacteria by using the capitalized initial of the genus, followed by the species name, such as *N. gonorrhoeae*. Both genus and species terms are italicized.

Viruses

Viruses are microorganisms that depend on a host cell's metabolic processes for their life cycle. They consist of a deoxyribonucleic acid (DNA) or ribonucleic acid (RNA) genome surrounded by a protein coat (see Fig. 10-2). In general, a virus enters a human cell and reprograms the infected cell to synthesize viral particles. This viral replication continues for the virus's life cycle, a time frame that varies for different types of viruses. Most viruses, such as influenza and rhinovirus, cause transient, acute illnesses. However, certain viruses such as

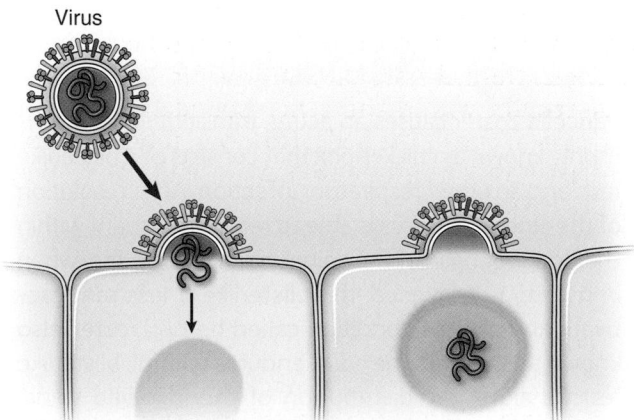

FIGURE 10-2. A typical virus has an outer envelope with specific surface structures designed to attach to a host cell surface. A protein coat lies beneath the envelope and the viral genome in the form of DNA or RNA are in the center. The goal of the virus is to inject its DNA or RNA into a host cell. The viral DNA or RNA can then direct the activities of the host cell and manufacture more viral particles.

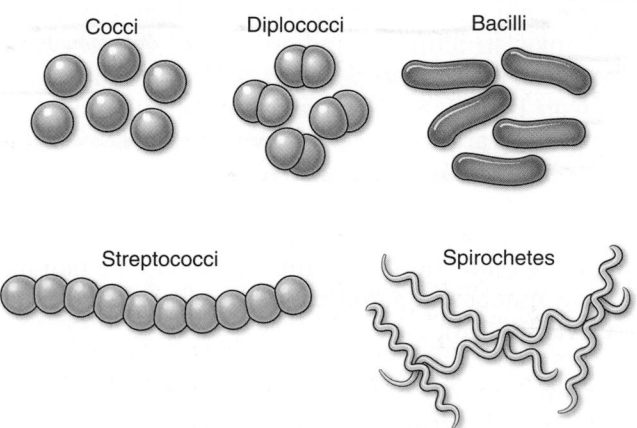

FIGURE 10-1. Categories of bacteria according to shape.

TABLE 10-1. Common Disease-Causing Bacteria

Species Name	Common Disease Presentation
Staphylococcus aureus	Skin and wound infections, impetigo, pneumonia, septicemia
Streptococcus pyogenes or group A beta-hemolytic streptococcus (GABHS)	Pharyngitis, impetigo, upper respiratory tract infection, rheumatic fever, scarlet fever, glomerulonephritis
Streptococcus pneumoniae (pneumococcus)	Community–acquired pneumonia
Escherichia coli	Urinary tract infection, wound infection, pneumonia, septicemia
Klebsiella pneumoniae	
Enterobacter aerogenes	
Pseudomonas aeruginosa	
Haemophilus influenzae	Meningitis, upper and lower respiratory tract infection
Legionella pneumophila	Legionnaire's disease
Bordetella pertussis	Whooping cough
Shigella	
Vibrio cholerae	Gastroenterocolitis
Campylobacter jejuni	
Enteropathogenic E. coli	
Salmonella	
Clostridium tetani	Tetanus
Clostridium botulinum	Botulism
Clostridium perfringens	Gas gangrene, necrotizing cellulites
Clostridium difficile	Pseudomembranous colitis
Mycobacterium tuberculosis	Tuberculosis
Bacillus anthracis	Anthrax
Borrelia burgdorferi	Lyme disease
Treponema pallidum	Syphilis
Neisseria meningitidis (meningococcus)	Meningitis
Neisseria gonorrhoeae	Gonorrhea

hepatitis B can persist and cause chronic infection, which damages tissues. Other viruses can cause acute illness; enter a dormant, nonreplicating stage; and then reactivate at a later time. The most common example of this type of viral infection involves herpes viruses.

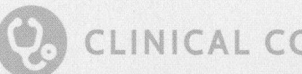

CLINICAL CONCEPT

Varicella zoster causes an acute, transient illness commonly known as chickenpox that consists of a blisterlike rash and an upper respiratory infection. After resolution of the illness, the virus is able to remain dormant within the dorsal ganglia of the spinal cord. Later in life, when immunity is weakened, this blisterlike illness can reactivate and cause a condition called herpes zoster, also known as shingles. The adult endures painful, blisterlike lesions along the distribution of the involved spinal nerve.

In addition to causing infections, some viruses can initiate cancer cell growth in host cells. An example of this type of virus is human papilloma virus, which can cause cervical cancer.

At present, antibiotic medications are able to kill various kinds of bacteria, but not viruses. Some antiviral drugs are available that can inhibit certain metabolic actions of viruses within host cells. There are a number of viruses that commonly cause human illness, and clinicians should be familiar with the names of these organisms (see Table 10-2).

Fungi

Fungi are moldlike organisms that can live on human tissue and cause infectious disease. They are diagnosed by the characteristic appearance of filamentous, or stringlike, structures found on culture. Fungal infections, also called mycoses, are classified as superficial or deep infections. **Dermatophytes,** such as tinea (ringworm), are fungi that cause superficial infections involving the skin, hair, or nails. Invasive, systemic mycoses, such as *C. albicans*, occur most often in an immunocompromised host and can cause fatal disseminated infection. The clinician should be familiar with a number of significant disease-causing fungi (see Table 10-3).

Parasites

Protozoa, helminths, and insects are parasites capable of causing infection in humans. Protozoa are single-celled

TABLE 10-2. Common Viruses That Cause Disease

Viral Pathogen	Common Disease Presentation
Adenovirus	Upper respiratory tract infection
Rhinovirus	
Coronavirus	
Influenza virus	Influenza
Respiratory syncytial virus (RSV)	Bronchiolitis, pneumonia
Mumps virus	Mumps, pancreatitis, orchitis
Norovirus virus	Gastroenteritis
Hepatitis A, B, C, D, and E virus	Acute or chronic hepatitis
Measles virus	Rubeola
Rubella virus	Rubella
Varicella zoster virus	Chickenpox, shingles
Herpes simplex virus 1	Cold sore
Herpes simplex virus 2	Genital herpes
Parvovirus	Erythema infectiosum
Coxsackie virus	Hand-foot-mouth disease, herpangina, Severe acute respiratory syndrome (SARS)
Epstein Barr virus	Infectious mononucleosis
Human papilloma virus	Condyloma accuminata
Human immunodeficiency virus (HIV1 and HIV2)	HIV infection and acquired immune deficiency syndrome (AIDS)
Regional hemorrhagic fever virus	Ebola, Marburg disease
Arboviral encephalitis viruses	Eastern equine encephalitis, Western equine encephalitis, Venezuelan equine encephalitis, St. Louis encephalitis

TABLE 10-3. Common Fungi That Cause Disease

Fungus	Common Disease Presentation
Candida	Candidiasis
Trichophyton	Tinea
Histoplasma	Histoplasmosis
Pneumocystis jirovecii	Pneumonia
Aspergillus	Aspergillosis
Coccidioides	Cocciodiomycosis

TABLE 10-4. Common Parasites That Cause Disease

Protozoan Parasites	Common Disease Presentation
Entamoeba histolytica	Amebic dysentery, liver abscess
Giardia lamblia	Giardiasis diarrheal illness
Trichomonas vaginalis	Vaginitis
Cryptosporidium	Enterocolitis
Toxoplasma gondii	Toxoplasmosis
Plasmodium	Malaria
HELMINTH PARASITES	
Taenia saginata	Tapeworm infection
Trichinella spiralis	Trichinosis
Schistosoma	Schistosomiasis
Trichuris trichuria	Whipworm
Enterobius vermicularis	Pinworms

organisms present within the environment that can infect the body through the skin and genitourinary and gastrointestinal tracts. Contaminated water, food, or disease-carrying insects can transmit protozoa. Mosquitoes that carry the plasmodium protozoan organism transmit malaria by injecting plasmodium into the human bloodstream. Other common clinical examples of protozoan infections are amebiasis and giardiasis, which are both acquired from contaminated water. Helminths are worms that can invade the body via the skin or gastrointestinal tract; examples include pinworms, tapeworms, and roundworms.

Insects can be the direct cause of disease or be a vector of disease. An insect that acts as a vector harbors a pathogen and transmits the pathogen to humans via its sting or bite. The deer tick acts as a vector, harboring the *Borrelia burgdorferi* (*B. burgdorferi*) bacterium that causes Lyme disease in humans. A few of the many significant disease-producing parasites are listed in Table 10-4.

Prions

Prions are unique proteinaceous infectious agents capable of causing brain diseases in animals and humans.

They are resistant to human proteases and have the ability to confer this resistance to other proteins in human cells. It is believed that prions enter neurons in the brain and convert existing proteins into prion-type protein. These abnormal proteins accumulate within large areas of brain tissue, causing distinctive histological changes within brain tissue and a condition called spongiform encephalopathy, literally meaning sponge-like damage to the brain. Prions cause animal diseases such as mad cow disease and scrapie, the latter being a disease among sheep. Among humans, prions cause Creutzfeldt-Jakob disease, which is an encephalopathy transmitted through infected beef.

All the spongiform encephalopathies are untreatable and fatal. Some forms of prion disease are inherited because of a defective gene that allows normal brain cell proteins to transform into abnormal prion-type proteins. Currently, prion-induced diseases are not fully understood.

Mechanisms of Infection

To gain entry and infect the host, pathogenic organisms must penetrate or overwhelm the host's defensive barriers. The human body has two primary levels of defenses:

1. innate immunity
2. adaptive immunity.

The innate defensive barriers include the skin, mucous membranes, phagocytic cells, ciliated cells, and mediators of the inflammatory reaction. Innate immunity is a nonspecific mechanism that defends the body against all types of pathogens immediately. Sensitized T lymphocytes and B lymphocytes, which have memory for specific antigens, comprise the defenses known as adaptive immunity. Adaptive immunity is developed with exposure to antigens and targets precise pathogens.

Portals of Entry

Pathogens can infect the body by skin contact, inhalation, ingestion, sexual transmission, insect or animal bites, or injection. The **portal of entry** for microorganisms can be the skin, respiratory, gastrointestinal, or urogenital tracts.

Skin. Skin is naturally resistant to infection because of its thick, dense composition and low pH (5.5). The health and integrity of skin is influenced by nutrition, hormones, physical activity, environmental exposures, and systemic disorders. External trauma, burns, insect bites, and other conditions, such as acute and chronic dermatoses, can cause breaks in skin integrity. Urticaria, eczema, acne, and psoriasis are examples of conditions that can cause breaches in intact skin.

The skin surface is inhabited by resident normal flora that include *Staphylococcus epidermidis* (*S. epidermidis*), *Staphylococcus aureus* (*S. aureus*), corynebacterium, and *Candida albicans* (*C. albicans*). The skin is most vulnerable to infection when there is a break in the integrity of the surface. Keeping the skin intact, dry, and clean can prevent most skin infections.

Persons with limited mobility should not put pressure on one area of the skin surface for a prolonged period. Pressure on areas of the skin that lie over bony prominences can cause an individual to develop pressure sores, also called decubitus ulcers, which are breaks in the skin that can evolve into wounds.

Dermatophytes, which cause fungal infections of the hair, nails, and skin, often occur without a breach in the integrity of the skin surface. Dermatophytes, like all fungi, thrive in moist, dark areas; spread from person to person; and are difficult to eliminate once established. A common dermatophyte is tinea or ringworm. There are many types of tinea infection, including *Tinea cruris*, which affects the groin region; *Tinea versicolor*, which affects the whole body; *Tinea capitus*, which affects the scalp; and *Tinea pedis*, commonly called "athlete's foot."

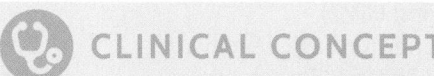

CLINICAL CONCEPT

Lack of position changes can lead to skin breakdown and decubitus ulcers, which are vulnerable to infection.

Respiratory Tract. Thousands of different microorganisms are inhaled into the respiratory tract every day. Many of these pathogens are transmitted by droplet infection. Droplets of fluid emitted from sneezes and coughs of infected individuals contain large inoculums of pathogens; when emitted into the air, these droplets are inhaled by individuals who then can become infected and transmit the pathogens to others.

There are several defense mechanisms that protect the respiratory portal of entry. After inhalation, large microorganisms are trapped by the mucous membranes and mucous secretions and swept away by the ciliated respiratory tract cells. These mechanisms are referred to as mucociliary defenses. Sneezing and coughing are reflexive defensive actions that attempt to expel infectious agents in response to irritation of the respiratory tract. Alveolar macrophages are present to phagocytose small microorganisms that penetrate beyond the mucociliary defenses. The respiratory epithelial cells also secrete interferon, which is the body's natural antiviral cytokine. Immunoglobulin A (IgA) is found in large amounts in the B lymphocytes of the respiratory tract and defend the body against inhaled antigens. Numerous cervical lymph nodes located within the oropharyngeal region store WBCs to defend against inhaled infectious agents.

Certain microorganisms are capable of evading the first line of defense of the respiratory tract. There are a variety of mechanisms that these microorganisms use to accomplish this. The influenza virus, *Haemophilus influenza* (*H. influenza*), *Bordetella pertussis* (*B. pertussis*), *Pseudomonas aeruginosa* (*P. aeruginosa*), and *Mycoplasma pneumoniae* (*M. pneumoniae*) are able to bypass the mucociliary defenses. *Streptococcus pneumoniae* (*S. pneumoniae*) and *S. aureus* often invade a host after a viral infection has impaired the mucociliary defenses. They then enter the alveoli and cause pneumonia. Pneumonia consists of widespread inflammation and infiltration of exudative fluid in the alveolar regions of the lungs. This infiltration is often referred to as a consolidation. *Mycobacterium tuberculosis* is unique because it can evade the phagocytic and killing effects of respiratory tract macrophages in the alveolar regions. Rhinoviruses, which cause the common cold, are able to thrive within the nasal passages and upper respiratory tract, despite the defense mechanisms. Inhaled fungi, such as *Pneumocystis carinii* (also called *Pneumocystis jirovecii*) and *C. albicans*, can become infectious agents when persons are immunosuppressed.

Gastrointestinal Tract. Most gastrointestinal pathogens are transmitted by food or drink contaminated with infectious agents. The fecal-oral route is often described as the method of transmission of gastrointestinal pathogens, which indicates ingested material was contaminated by fecal matter. Fecal matter contains a large **inoculum** of *E. coli* and *Enterococcus faecalis* (*E. faecalis*) and may harbor hepatitis A, many bacteria in the *Shigella* and *Salmonella* geni, *Vibrio cholerae*, or any number of other bacteria, viruses, or parasites. Fecal contamination of drinking water reservoirs may occur because of problems in sewage systems. This contamination may lead to significant levels of bacteria in drinking water, and it is necessary to perform frequent analysis of bacteria counts. Transmission of disease by the fecal-oral route may also be the result of food preparation by persons with poor hygiene or lack of sanitary food preparation methods.

The acidic conditions and mucous lining of the stomach and intestine protect the body from invasion of many pathogens. Pancreatic enzymes, bile, mucosal antimicrobial peptides, normal bacterial flora, and lymphoid tissue secretions of IgA antibodies also serve to defend the body against ingested pathogens. Infections via the gastrointestinal tract usually occur when defenses are weakened. Some microorganisms are relatively resistant to the body's protective mechanisms and may cause infection in an otherwise healthy host. *Helicobactor pylori* (*H. pylori*), *Shigella*, and *Giardia* cysts, for example, can resist the acidic environment of the stomach. Viruses such as rotavirus, hepatitis A, and Norwalk virus (also called Norovirus) can resist bile and pancreatic enzymes. Staphylococcus can grow on foods and secrete an enterotoxin, a toxic secretion that targets the gastrointestinal mucosa. The staphylococcal enterotoxin causes a diarrheal illness commonly called food poisoning. *Salmonella typhi*

(*S. typhi*), a bacteria found on some foods, can be absorbed from the GI tract, enter the lymphatic system and bloodstream, and cause a systemic infection. *Entamoeba histolytica* (*E. histolytica*), found in contaminated water, erodes the intestinal mucosa and causes a hemorrhagic, diarrheal illness called dysentery. Intestinal parasites can live in the intestine and absorb the host's nutrients.

Genitourinary Tract. Urogenital infections most commonly originate from entry of pathogens into the urethra. Urine outflow through the urethra serves as a protective mechanism that constantly flushes microorganisms out of the body. Certain organisms such as gonococcus and *E. coli* are capable of adhering to bladder mucosa epithelium and thus evade the protective mechanisms afforded by urine outflow.

Female anatomy predisposes to urinary tract infection (UTI) because of the close proximity of the rectal mucosa and urethra. The bowel is the natural habitat for *E. coli*, and urethral invasion into the bladder is common. Urinary tract infections can spread retrograde from the urethra and bladder and into the ureter and kidney. Pyelonephritis is an upper UTI that can occur in this manner.

Lactobacilli are colonized in the vaginal canal as normal flora. They break down glycogen stores and keep the vaginal pH low. The low pH is a defensive mechanism that wards off other microbial invaders. The vaginal pH can be altered if the normal flora are eradicated, which can occur as a side effect of antibiotic use. The vaginal canal then becomes susceptible to infection. Vaginal candidiasis is a common side effect of long-term antibiotic use.

Male semen and female vaginal fluids can also transmit microorganisms. Unsafe sexual practices allow for the spread of these microorganisms and the passage of sexually transmitted diseases, which are commonly viral and bacterial infections, between individuals.

Blood–Blood Transmission. Blood transfusion is the most common method of transmission of bloodborne infections, although blood donations are vigilantly screened to prevent transfusion of infected blood. Exposure to bloodborne pathogens can also occur through a needlestick or lacerating injury with a sharp instrument contaminated with infected blood. Intravenous drug users can contract infection from unsterile needles. Bloodborne pathogens can also enter the body via the eye, naso-oral mucous membranes, and skin. For this reason, universal precautions exist for handling patient body fluids and biohazardous material.

Following exposure to bloodborne pathogens, risk of infection depends on the type of exposure, amount of infected blood transferred to the recipient, and the number of pathogens contained in the infected blood. The most commonly transmitted bloodborne pathogens are hepatitis B, hepatitis C virus, and HIV.

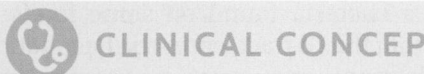

Maternal-Fetal Transmission. Some pathogens that cause infection in a pregnant woman can be transmitted to the developing fetus in two ways:

1. Pathogens that invade the maternal bloodstream and placenta can pass into the fetal circulation.
2. Maternal infection can be transferred during childbirth when infected vaginal secretions and membranes come in contact with the newborn.

When an infectious disease is passed from mother to newborn, it is called a **congenital** infection. Certain microorganisms are common causes of congenital infection, including cytomegalovirus (CMV), *Toxoplasma gondii* (*T. gondii*), *Treponema pallidum* (syphilis), rubella, herpes simplex virus, varicella zoster, parvovirus B19, group B streptococci, and HIV.

Stages of Infection

After a pathogen enters a host, there are five distinct stages of infection:

1. incubation period
2. prodromal stage
3. acute stage
4. convalescent stage
5. resolution phase.

Different pathogens have distinctive time periods for each stage.

The incubation period is the phase when the microorganism begins active replication without producing identifiable symptoms in the host. The duration of the incubation may be short, as in the case of rhinovirus, which causes the common cold and lasts about 24 hours, or prolonged, as in hepatitis B infection, which can last between 1 and 3 months. Some infections are highly contagious during this phase, and the host is usually unaware of the developing illness.

The prodromal stage occurs when the initial appearance of symptoms are apparent in the host. During this time, the host may have only a vague sense of illness with general malaise, myalgias, headache, or fatigue. It is also a time when the host is highly contagious to others.

The acute stage is the time period during which the host experiences the full infectious disease with rapid proliferation of the pathogen. The host's defenses are in full force and the inflammation reaction is fully engaged. The host's symptoms are heightened and more specific than in the prodromal stage. The patient remains contagious during this stage.

The convalescent stage is characterized by the body's attempt to contain the infection and progressively eliminate the pathogen. Resolution of symptoms begins to occur and may stretch over days, weeks, or months, depending on the pathogen.

The resolution phase is the time when there is total elimination of the pathogen from the body without residual signs or symptoms.

Immune Responses to Infection

Infection stimulates the body's immune system to defend against an invading pathogen. There are two major types of immunity: innate and adaptive. Innate immunity consists of nonspecific, cellular reactions that protect an individual who is exposed to a pathogen. Adaptive immunity consists of specific cellular responses that are stimulated when the body recognizes a pathogen it has encountered in the past. Adaptive immunity most effectively defends the body upon reexposure to a pathogen, whereas innate immunity defends the body in a general manner regardless of history of exposure to the pathogen.

Importantly, the function of the adaptive immune system is dependent on an intact innate immune system. Toll-like receptors (TLRs) on the surface of many cells of the innate immune system play a critical role in stimulating the adaptive immune response. TLRs are proteins on cell surfaces that detect specific pathogens. When a TLR detects a pathogen, it relays a signal to the cell's nucleus. The signal switches on specific genes that code for release of substances that perpetuate the innate immune response and stimulate the adaptive immune response.

The innate system is the first level of defense against invasion by pathogens. It consists of anatomical barriers, antipathogenic chemicals, and cellular reactions. The anatomical barriers of the innate immune system include the intact epithelial surfaces of the skin, as well as the respiratory, gastrointestinal, and genitourinary tracts. The skin and mucous membranes provide a mechanical and chemical barrier to pathogens. Skin and mucous membranes are protective coverings that secrete certain peptides and enzymes that have antibacterial, antifungal, and antiviral properties. The low pH of sweat also acts as a chemical antipathogenic barrier. In the nose and lungs, cilia act as anatomical barriers to sweep away debris and keep the airways clear. Tears, secreted by the lacrimal glands around the eyes, contain enzymes that help flush pathogens away. The acidic pH of gastric secretions acts as an antipathogenic barrier. In the lower gastrointestinal and genitourinary tract, mucus traps any ingested pathogens and expels them in the stool or urine.

An acute inflammatory reaction is triggered when the innate immune system is stimulated. The components of the inflammatory reaction act as cellular barriers in the innate immune system. These include white blood cells (WBCs), the complement system, coagulation system, and cytokines, which are active during the chemotaxis phase of an acute inflammatory reaction.

The complement system also responds to pathogens in the innate and adaptive immune systems. It is composed of enzymes, proteins, and chemical mediators that target and attack pathogens. The complement system acts to mediate antigen-antibody reactions in the adaptive immune responses and enhances the inflammatory reaction.

The adaptive immune system is the second line of defense against the invasion of pathogens. It requires more time to respond than the innate system of defense. The adaptive immune system is antigen-specific, reacts to a pathogen that it recognizes, and has memory for the pathogen. The main cells within this system are the lymphocytes, also called B and T cells. T cells are produced primarily in the thymus, and B cells arise primarily from the bone marrow. There are different types of T cells that take part in the adaptive immune response. These include cytotoxic and helper T cells. Cytotoxic T cells, also called CD8 cells, directly attack the pathogen, whereas helper T cells, also called CD4 cells, assist CD8 cells and stimulate the proliferation of B cells. B cells produce specialized glycoproteins known as immunoglobulins (Igs) that attack antigens. Igs may be undifferentiated and provide general defense against infection by binding to microbes. These nonspecific Igs, also called immunoglobulin D (IgD), are found on the surface of B cells. Once the invading antigens have been bound by the IgD, the B cells produce specific Igs that recognize and bind to particular foreign antigens.

Immunoglobulin M (IgM) is the earliest specific immunoglobulin to appear in response to exposure to antigen in the bloodstream. It is responsible for initiating further immune reactions. Immunoglobulin G (IgG) develops later in the course of infection and predominates for many years after exposure, conferring some long-lasting immunity against the specific antigen. Secretory IgA is an immunoglobulin found on mucosal surfaces and the bloodstream, and immunoglobulin E (IgE) is produced in response to allergies and parasitic infections. Table 10-5 summarizes these immunoglobulin functions.

Diagnosis of Infection

There are distinctive signs and symptoms exhibited by the host during specific infectious processes. Most infections present with nonspecific symptoms, such as fever, myalgias, lethargy, and anorexia. However, the specific symptoms experienced by the patient often reflect the specific system that is infected. For example, hepatitis presents with jaundice, a sign of liver dysfunction. *Salmonella* infection presents with intestinal symptoms such as nausea, vomiting, and diarrhea. Diagnosis of infection is based on the history, clinical symptoms, physical examination findings, and laboratory testing.

Laboratory Studies

Specimens of infectious material can be subjected to microscopic staining and culture procedures. Bacteria can be classified according to how their cell membrane absorbs a dye such as a Gram stain or acid-fast stain. A culture of the infected tissues or body fluids involves growing the microbes on a specific medium, such as agar, so they can be studied and identified. The extent of infection may be inferred from the number of microorganisms seen per microscopic high power field, or in a specific volume of substrate such as 1 milliliter.

TABLE 10-5. Immunoglobulins and Their Functions

Immunoglobulin	Functions	Most Active Phase of Infection
IgA	Protect mucous membranes of genitourinary, gastrointestinal, and pulmonary systems; found in breast milk and tears	Activity not related to infection; has a protective and preventive role
IgD	Attached to surface of B cells, binds antigens to the B cell	Early stage, when antigen has first entered the body
IgE	Found on mast cells in pulmonary and gastrointestinal tracts, active in allergic reactions	Not related to infection, found in persons with allergies Binds to mast cells and basophils to release histamine and leukotrienes
IgG	Confers long-term immunity, active against viruses, bacteria, antitoxins; moves across maternal-fetal barrier Most prevalent	Late disease, recovery, and long after Activates complement to release inflammatory and bactericidal mediators
IgM	Controls ABO blood reactions, initiates complement activity and further immune responses	Early disease

A culture can also be used to yield information about the organism's antibiotic susceptibility. Culture media can be infused with different antibiotics and growth or suppression of microbes can be observed.

At times, infection is difficult to diagnose and a biopsy of tissue may be needed for histological study. In histological study of tissue, the cells within a biopsy are examined under a microscope for signs of inflammation and infection. The tissue is scrutinized for evidence of the pathogenic organism or characteristic cell changes associated with the pathogen.

Infection can also be confirmed through serological testing that studies the blood serum for the existence of antibodies to the microorganism in the bloodstream. A sample of blood is withdrawn from the patient and tested for the presence of specific antibodies. For example, a person infected with syphilis would develop antibodies to *T. pallidum*, which can be confirmed in a serological study. The level of antibody within the bloodstream is called an **antibody titer,** and usually the titer corresponds to the level of exposure to the microbe. Serological testing can also assist in the staging of infection because levels of IgG and IgM can be measured. IgM is the first immunoglobulin to rise in response to infection; IgG rises later.

Direct antigen identification is another method that combines culture and microscopic procedures. The infectious agent is fused with artificially synthesized antibodies that are fluorescent. When the artificial antibody attaches to the antigen, the antigen-antibody complex fluoresces under the microscope, making them easier to identify and quantify.

Yet another technique for identifying an infectious agent is the polymerase chain reaction (PCR) technique that detects a microorganism's genetic material (DNA or RNA). A specimen containing the infectious agent is mixed with a reagent that targets the pathogen's DNA or RNA. The method can accurately detect extremely low levels of pathogen within a specimen. For example, the HIV RNA assay is a type of PCR diagnostic technique that can determine the number of human immunodeficiency viral particles present in the bloodstream.

Treatment and Eradication of Infection

Most infections are self-limiting and will resolve if allowed to progress through the stages of infection. However, when the infectious disease manifestations are prolonged or cause undue risk for the patient or those in contact with the patient, medical therapy is recommended. The treatment may involve antimicrobial agents, immunological boosting agents, or surgical removal of infected tissues.

Antimicrobial agents consist of a wide array of antibacterial, antiviral, antifungal, antiprotozoan, and antihelminthic medications. The most numerous among the antimicrobial agents are antibiotics or antibacterial medications. Bacteria are highly adaptable and commonly develop resistance to available antibiotics when exposed for a prolonged period of time. This resistance creates continual need for development of new antibiotic agents.

Prevention of Infection Through Immunization

Prevention of infectious disease through administration of vaccines is the most efficient method of controlling contagious disease within a population. Some infectious diseases, such as smallpox, have been virtually eliminated through the use of vaccines. Although vaccines offer long-term immunity, few confer lifelong immunity, and must be readministered at intervals to maintain protection. Recommended immunizations vary by age, health status, and exposure risk of the individual, but are based on protecting public health by decreasing the number of susceptible persons in a population.

Emerging Infectious Diseases

Emerging infectious diseases are defined as diseases that have newly appeared in the population and those that are rapidly increasing in incidence or geographic range. Emergence may be caused by the spread of a new agent, to the recognition of an infection that has been present in the population but has gone undetected, or to the realization that an established disease has an infectious origin. Emergence may also be used to describe the reappearance of a known infection after a decline in incidence.

Emergence Versus Reemergence

With the modern ability to travel anywhere in the world within 36 or fewer hours, unique infections are able to be easily and unknowingly transmitted to areas where they previously had not been found. Governments have regulations that bar individuals with certain infectious diseases from traveling, but it is nearly impossible to adequately screen every passenger. Furthermore, some diseases are contagious during the incubation and prodromal phases, whereas there are no obvious signs of sickness. In addition, some microbes can survive on inanimate objects, such as doorknobs, keyboards, and telephones, and are transported in this manner. Many emerging diseases arise when infectious agents in animals are passed to humans; these transmitted diseases are called zoonoses. As the human population expands into new geographical regions, the possibility that humans will come into close contact with animal species that are potential hosts of an infectious agent increases. When that factor is combined with increases in human density and mobility, it is easy to see that this combination poses a serious threat to human health.

Another factor that is especially important in the reemergence of disease is the acquired resistance of pathogens to antimicrobial medications such as antibiotics. Over time, bacteria and viruses can change and develop a resistance to antimicrobial medications, resulting in the forced disuse of treatments that were once effective in controlling disease. A wide variety of antibiotic-resistant bacteria that are currently challenging clinicians include **methicillin-resistant *Staphylococcus aureus* (MRSA), vancomycin-resistant *Staphylococcus aureus* (VRSA),** vancomycin-resistant enterococcus (VRE), and drug-resistant *Streptococcus pneumoniae* (DRSP).

Reappearance may also occur because of breakdowns in public health measures that had previously controlled a particular infection.

Infectious Agents and Bioterrorism

The world has become highly vigilant of the threat of bioterrorism in recent years. There are infectious agents that can be used as weapons and harm large segments of the population. Biological agents with the potential to be used as weapons can be classified based on ease of dissemination or transmission, potential for major public health impact, and requirements for public health preparedness. Agents of high concern include:

- *Bacillus anthracis* (anthrax)
- *Yersinia pestis* (plague)
- *Variola major* (smallpox)
- *Clostridium botulinum* toxin (botulism)
- *Francisella tularensis* (tularemia)
- filoviruses (Ebola hemorrhagic fever, Marburg hemorrhagic fever).

Many governments are engaged in research on how to protect their populations from this particular form of warfare.

Selected Bacterial Infections

Staphylococcus and streptococcus are two kinds of bacteria that are normal flora of the human body as well as instigators of infectious disease. In recent years these bacteria have become major challenges to clinicians because of antibiotic resistance. *Neisseria meningitidis*, also known as meningococcus, resides within the nasopharynx and can cause a serious bloodstream infection as well as meningitis. It is important to keep a high index of suspicion for meningococcal infection when examining schoolchildren, college students, and military recruits with flulike illness who live in close quarters such as dormitories.

Staphylococcal Infections

Staphylococci are hardy, gram-positive round microorganisms that form clusters. They are capable of surviving for prolonged periods on inanimate surfaces in variable conditions. One of the most important and ubiquitous strains is *S. aureus*, which colonizes the skin, vagina, nares, and oropharynx as normal flora. *S. aureus* can change from normal flora to an infectious agent and has become the leading cause of nosocomial infection and surgical wound infection. In the community, *S. aureus* is a major cause of skin and soft-tissue infections, respiratory infections, and, among intravenous drug abusers, endocarditis. *S. aureus* has developed resistance to many antibiotics, and strains such as MRSA and VRSA are commonly encountered in clinical settings. Because of an ability to produce three types of toxins, *S. aureus* can cause life-threatening illness such as septicemia. *S. aureus* can also cause a wide range of infections affecting almost every body system.

S. epidermidis, also a constituent of normal flora, and *Staphylococcus saprophyticus,* are other staph organisms that normally colonize the skin and can cause infection. However, *S. aureus* is a most virulent strain because it secretes proteases, produces hemolytic toxins that degrade host cells, and has the genetic ability to develop antibiotic resistance.

Antibiotic-Resistant *S. Aureus*

The introduction of the antibiotic penicillin in the 1940s dramatically reduced the morbidity and mortality associated with bacterial infections. Penicillin seemed to be a panacea until strains of penicillin-resistant organisms were found. Some strains of *S. aureus* could develop genetic changes that enabled the organism to secrete penicillinase. Penicillinase, also called *beta lactamase,* is an enzyme that destroys penicillin and allows the organism to resist the antibiotic. Penicillin-resistant *S. aureus* created a need for the development of new antibiotics that could resist beta lactamase. Methicillin has been the most commonly used drug for that purpose. However, within 1 year after the introduction of methicillin, methicillin-resistant strains of *S. aureus* were found. Despite a steady slow increase in the number of methicillin-resistant strains of *S. aureus*, methicillin and its derivatives, oxacillin, nafcillin, cloxacillin, and dicloxacillin were effective against *S. aureus* for many years. A dramatic rise in methicillin-resistant strains of *S. aureus* occurred in the 1990s.

Approximately 40% to 50% of *S. aureus* strains found in hospitals are resistant to methicillin, as well as to many other antibiotics. As resistant strains increased, vancomycin became the sole antibiotic effective against MRSA. However, with time and exposure to vancomycin, some strains of *S. aureus* have become resistant to vancomycin and its derivatives. Identifying an antibiotic to kill VRSA became the challenge for pharmacologists.

MRSA infection is especially problematic in hospitals and other congregate settings. Strict isolation procedures and universal precautions by health-care providers are necessary to prevent transmission of the infection. Scrupulous hand washing practices among health-care personnel is a key prevention strategy. Health-care providers should be vigilant about disinfecting diagnostic equipment such as stethoscopes when using them for multiple patients in the hospital environment. Patients with antibiotic-resistant infections should have dedicated equipment that is not used for any other patients.

Community-acquired MRSA infections are becoming a treatment challenge. The widespread use of broad spectrum antibiotics in health care and the addition of antibiotics in livestock feed exposes bacteria to our arsenal of antibiotics. This exposure allows bacteria to develop genetic changes leading to resistance.

Presently, *S. aureus*, enterococcus, and *S. pneumoniae* are the bacterial organisms most resistant to available antibiotics. It is a constant challenge for researchers to develop newer and more effective antibiotics in this era of continuing bacterial resistance.

Streptococcal Infections

There are a number of streptococcal organisms that cause human disease. **Group A beta hemolytic streptococcus (GABHS),** also called *Streptococcus pyogenes*, is a bacterium that causes many different infections. These bacteria have capsules that resist WBC phagocytosis and secrete substances that degrade tissue membranes. Streptococci can also release an exotoxin that can cause fever and rash.

Streptococci are gram-positive spherical organisms in chains that produce zones of hemolysis when cultured on blood agar, referred to as beta hemolysis. GABHS secretes large numbers of extracellular products that enhance its toxicity in the spread of infection through tissues. These products include streptolysins S and O, streptokinase, DNAases, protease, and exotoxins. GABHS can infect almost every body system; before the advent of antibiotics, it commonly caused serious complications. Rheumatic fever, streptococcal pharyngitis (strep throat), scarlet fever, glomerulonephritis, skin infections, pneumonia, necrotizing fasciitis, and toxic shock syndrome are among the many possible diseases caused by GABHS (see Fig. 10-3).

Other streptococcal bacteria can also cause a number of significant diseases. *S. pneumoniae* is the major cause of community-acquired pneumonia and can cause meningitis. *Streptococcus faecalis*, also called

E. faecalis, is a major cause of UTIs, nosocomial bacteremia, and endocarditis. *Streptococcus viridans* can also cause infective endocarditis.

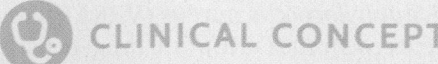

CLINICAL CONCEPT

In persons suffering from sore throat, a throat culture is the only method that can accurately diagnose or rule out GABHS pharyngitis. In some individuals, GABHS can cause rheumatic fever and rheumatic heart disease (RHD), a condition involving the development of a heart murmur. In RHD, an immune reaction occurs; antibodies developed against GABHS mistakenly attack heart valve tissue and cause valvular deformities.

Bacterial Pneumonias

Bacteria are hardy microorganisms that commonly invade the respiratory tract via the nasopharynx. Bacteria can invade lower respiratory tract tissues, stimulate inflammation, and create an exudative fluid that hinders oxygen exchange at the alveoli. Exudative fluid in and around the alveoli is referred to as a consolidation on chest x-ray, but is most commonly known as pneumonia.

Streptococcus Pneumoniae

S. pneumoniae (Pneumococcus) is the most common cause of community-acquired pneumonia. This is a gram-positive diplococcal bacterium that colonizes the nasopharynx. After colonization, organisms may gain access to areas of the upper and lower respiratory tracts by direct extension. Under normal conditions in a healthy host, anatomic and ciliary clearance mechanisms prevent clinical infection. However, clearance may be inhibited by chronic factors such as smoking, allergies, and bronchitis, as well as acute factors such as viral infection and allergies, both of which can lead to infection. Influenza is a common precursor of streptococcal pneumonia. Alternatively, pneumococci may reach normally sterile areas, such as the blood, peritoneum, cerebrospinal fluid, or joint fluid, by hematogenous spread after mucosal invasion. The most vulnerable individuals are children younger than 2 years old and adults aged 60 years and older. Pneumococcal pneumonia affects approximately 100 per 100,000 adults each year and has a mortality rate of 20% annually.

Classically, pneumonia is preceded by a viral illness that is followed by an acute onset of high fever—often with rigors, productive cough, pleuritic chest pain, dyspnea, tachypnea, tachycardia, sweats, malaise, and fatigue. The patient may report blood-tinged sputum. Patients typically appear ill and may have an anxious appearance. On physical examination, crackles can be heard in the lung region affected by the pneumonia.

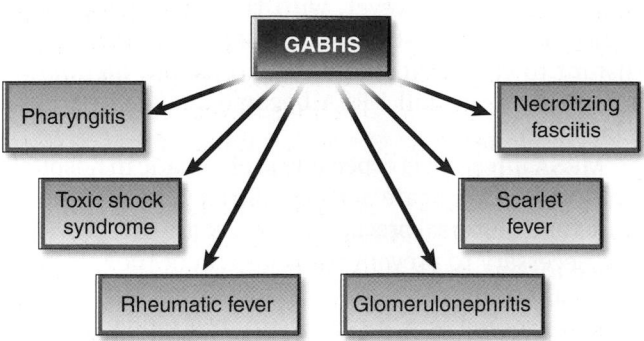

FIGURE 10-3. Diseases caused by GABHS.

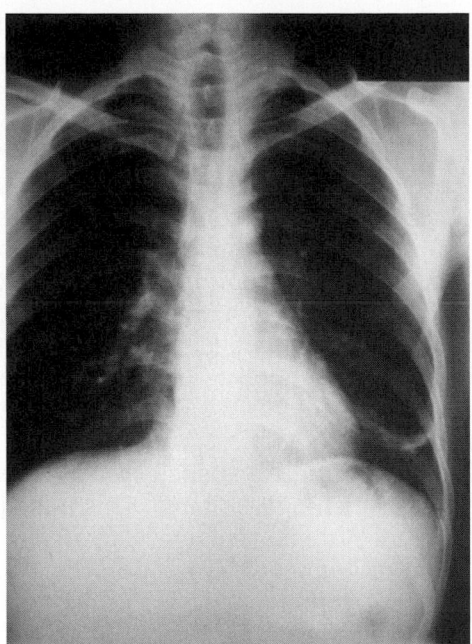

FIGURE 10-4. Chest x-ray showing lobar pneumonia. *(Courtesy of CDC/Dr. Thomas Hooten.)*

About half of all patients exhibit dullness to percussion over the involved lung region. Diagnostic tests include chest x-ray and sputum culture. Chest x-ray shows consolidation in the region of pneumonia (see Fig. 10-4). Antibiotic susceptibilities should be obtained routinely on all cultures with growth of *S. pneumoniae*. Antibiotic resistance is commonly encountered with this bacteria.

Pneumococcal vaccine every 5 to 10 years has been recommended for older adults and has greatly reduced infections. Routine childhood pneumococcal conjugate vaccine, introduced in 2000, has decreased rates of invasive pneumococcal infections by greater than 90%.

Mycoplasma Pneumoniae

Mycoplasma pneumonia is an infection of the lungs from the bacteria *M. pneumoniae,* a very small bacterium without a cell wall. It causes an atypical pneumonia that commonly affects people younger than 40 years. This type of pneumonia is often referred to as "walking pneumonia" because the affected individual does not appear very ill. Various studies suggest that it makes up 15% to 50% of all pneumonia cases in adults and even more in school-aged children. People at highest risk for mycoplasma pneumonia include those living or working in crowded areas such as schools and homeless shelters, although many people who contract mycoplasma pneumonia have no identifiable risk factor. It is spread by droplet infection. The symptoms are generally mild and appear over a period of 1 to 3 weeks. Common symptoms include fever, sore throat, chills, cough, myalgias, headache, and earache. In this type of pneumonia, headache and earache are unique symptoms. A complete physical examination and a chest x-ray are necessary. Sputum culture may

be necessary. Treatment includes specific antibiotics that affect bacteria without a cell wall, such as tetracyclines, and supportive measures.

Legionnaire's Disease

Legionnaire's disease is an acute respiratory infection caused by a gram-negative bacteria called *Legionella pneumophila* bacteria. The bacteria was named in 1976 when people who attended a Philadelphia convention of the American Legion suffered an outbreak of this disease. These bacteria are found most often in the warm, moist air conditioning systems of large buildings, though they have also been found in water delivery systems. The microbe is transmitted via aerosolized mist in the air. Person-to-person transmission has not been shown. Most infections occur in middle-aged or older people, although they also have been reported in children. Risk factors include alcoholism; cigarette smoking; diseases such as kidney failure or diabetes; diseases or medications that weaken the immune system, including cancer and steroids; long-term (chronic) lung disease such as chronic obstructive pulmonary disease (COPD); and use of a ventilator. Symptoms include dyspnea, chest pain, nonproductive cough, chills, hemoptysis, fever, nausea, vomiting, diarrhea, headache, arthralgias, and possible ataxia. These symptoms tend to get worse during the first 4 to 6 days and typically improve in another 4 to 5 days. Diagnostic tests include chest x-ray, sputum culture, and urine antigen test. Antibiotics are the major treatment measure.

Pseudomonas Infection

Pseudomonas is a gram-negative rod that is widespread in nature, inhabiting soil, water, plants, and animals, including humans. *P. aeruginosa* has become an important cause of infection, especially in patients with compromised host defense mechanisms. It is the most common pathogen isolated from patients who have been hospitalized longer than 1 week. It is a frequent cause of nosocomial infections such as pneumonia, UTIs, and bacteremia. Pseudomonal infections are complicated and can be life threatening.

P. aeruginosa is also the fourth most commonly isolated nosocomial pathogen, accounting for 10% of all hospital-acquired infections. It is found on the skin of some healthy persons and has been isolated from the throat and stool of 5% and 3% of nonhospitalized patients, respectively. The gastrointestinal carriage rates among hospitalized patients increases to 20% within 72 hours of admission. Predisposing conditions include placement of intravenous lines, severe burns, urinary tract catheterization, surgery, trauma, and premature birth (infants).

In pseudomonas pneumonia, patients have crackles, rhonchi, fever, cyanosis, retractions, and hypoxia. Shock may develop in patients with bacteremic pneumonia. Pseudomonal bacteremia occurs in association with malignancy, chemotherapy, acquired immunodeficiency disease (AIDS), burn wounds, and diabetes.

Diagnostic procedures depend on the site of pseudomonas infection. In pneumonia, sputum culture, chest x-ray, and blood cultures are necessary. Double antibiotic therapy is needed for treatment.

Bacterial Meningitis Infection

Meningitis is a potentially fatal infectious disease caused by inflammation of the meningeal layers that surround and protect the brain and spinal cord. Meningitis is most commonly caused by viruses or strains of bacteria. *S. pneumoniae* (pneumococcus), *Neisseria meningitides* (meningococcus), and *H. influenzae* are bacterial causes of meningitis. Bacterial meningitis is a very serious illness, whereas viral meningitis, also called aseptic meningitis, is usually a milder disorder.

The key signs of meningitis are fever, nuchal rigidity (stiff neck), and headache. Certain kinds of meningitis can present with an accompanying rash. Kernig's and Brudzinski signs are commonly exhibited by the patient during physical examination (see Fig. 10-5). The diagnosis of meningitis requires a lumbar puncture, a test that allows sampling and culturing of the cerebrospinal fluid. High dose antibiotic therapy is necessary for bacterial meningitis. Viral meningitis usually resolves by itself and requires supportive treatment. Complications of meningitis include seizures, brain damage, ischemia of extremities, and visual or hearing losses. Bacterial meningitis can be prevented by immunization with *Haemophilus influenzae* b (Hib), meningococcal, and pneumococcal vaccines.

Neisseria Meningitidis

Meningitis is commonly caused by the bacterium *N. meningitidis,* which is also known as meningococcus,

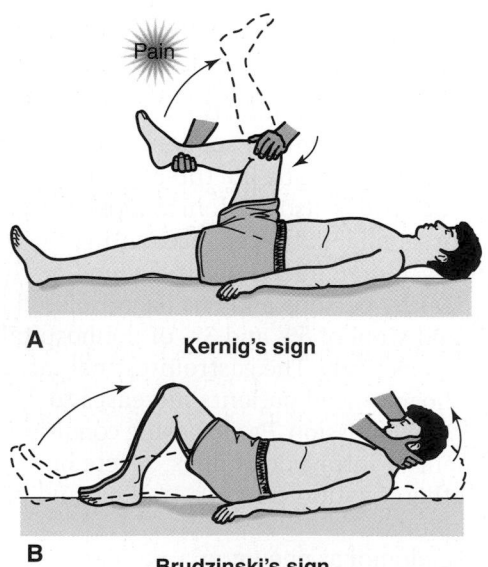

FIGURE 10-5. (A) In Kernig's sign, attempt to extend the leg at the knee. The patient feels pain in the neck and leg. (B) In Brudzinski's sign, the patient flexes knees and hips when you flex the neck. (From Williams, L. & Hopper, P. (2011), *Understanding medical-surgical nursing.* 4th ed. Philadelphia. PA: F.A. Davis Company.)

a gram-negative diplococcus bacteria. The human nasopharynx is a known reservoir for *N. meningitidis.* Meningococci spread from person to person by droplet infection. The prevalence is approximately 1 to 2 cases per 100,000 population, but outbreaks of meningococcal disease have occurred in some specific populations. Outbreaks often involve persons living in close quarters such as those who are incarcerated, college students living in dormitories, and military recruit populations. Although not common, school-age children have spread meningococcal infection to each other. Exposure of school-age children to meningococcus commonly requires prophylactic antibiotic treatment.

Meningococcal infection usually first occurs in the bloodstream as meningococcemia. This infection can range in severity from a transient bacteremia that is benign to an overwhelming infection that is rapidly fatal. Meningitis commonly occurs during the course of meningococcemia. At first, meningitis may seem like an upper respiratory illness with pharyngitis, fever, and chills. However, the disorder rapidly deteriorates into more severe symptoms such as high fever, malaise, weakness, myalgias, headache, nausea, vomiting, and arthralgias. Nuchal rigidity (stiff neck), photophobia, and headache are signs of meningitis. Nuchal rigidity can be confirmed on physical assessment by Kernig's and Brudzinski signs. Lethargy, drowsiness, or coma, which is an ominous sign, can occur. Alternatively, apprehension, restlessness, and, frequently, delirium can occur. Encephalopathy refers to mental status changes that can occur such as disorientation, confusion, and memory loss. A skin rash accompanies meningococcemia as a characteristic manifestation. The skin rash may advance from a few ill-defined petechial lesions to widespread purpura and ecchymotic areas within a few hours. Disseminated intravascular coagulation, vascular collapse, and ischemic necrosis of extremities can develop. Gangrene of extremities requires amputation.

Rapid diagnosis and treatment initiation is critical in meningitis because it is potentially fatal. Lumbar puncture is a necessary diagnostic procedure for analysis of the cerebrospinal fluid (CSF) in meningitis. Protein and WBCs will be elevated in the CSF because of the microbes. Glucose will be diminished in CSF because it is being utilized by the microbes. Bacteria can be cultured from the CSF. Magnetic resonance imaging (MRI) or computed tomography (CT) scan of the head can evaluate complications.

Treatment involves high doses of intravenous antibiotics, antiemetics, analgesics, corticosteroids, hydration, and antipyretics. The patient should be placed in isolation. Seizure precautions are necessary. Surgical amputation of gangrenous extremities may be required. Meningitis can leave a patient with complications of cognitive problems, as well as vision and hearing loss. Rifampin is advised for all those who have come in close contact with the person suffering from meningococcal infection. Meningococcal vaccine is recommended for adolescents and young adults, particularly those entering college who live in dormitories.

> **ALERT!** Nuchal rigidity, headache, photophobia, and high fever are key signs of meningitis.

CLINICAL CONCEPT

Patients with meningitis may exhibit opisthotonus—spasm of the whole body that causes legs, head, and neck to hyperextend and body to arch backwards.

Haemophilus Influenzae

H. influenzae is a small, gram-negative coccobacillus-shaped bacterium. The most virulent strain is Hib, which has a characteristic outer capsule. It accounts for more than 95% of *H. influenzae* invasive diseases in children and half of invasive diseases in adults. It can be manifested as bacteremia, meningitis, cellulitis, epiglottitis, septic arthritis, or pneumonia. Hib conjugate vaccine has led to dramatic declines in incidence and prevalence of these diseases. The most vulnerable populations include children and elders. Because of successful immunization during childhood, *H. influenzae* accounts for 5% to 10% cases of adult meningitis. Transmission is by direct contact or by inhalation of respiratory tract droplets. The incubation period is not known. The presence of a concomitant viral infection can potentiate the infection. The colonizing bacteria invade the mucosa and enter the bloodstream.

Meningitis is the most serious manifestation of Hib infection. Symptoms of upper respiratory infection before *H. influenzae* meningitis are common. Headache, nuchal rigidity, photophobia, altered mental status, and fever are the most common presenting features. Infants demonstrate irritability, fever, lethargy, poor feeding, and vomiting. As with other types of bacterial meningitis, diagnosis requires lumbar puncture and treatment involves high dose antibiotics. Complications include brain damage, as well as vision and hearing losses.

Gastrointestinal Bacterial Infections

Salmonella, *Shigella*, *Escherichia coli*, and Campylobacter are leading bacterial causes of gastroenteritis worldwide. They cause severe diarrheal illness and can be serious in infants and elderly adults. *E. coli* is also the cause of UTI commonly affecting women.

Salmonella

Salmonella is a rod-shaped, gram-negative, nonspore-forming, motile enterobacteria with flagella. *Salmonella* can be transmitted between animals and humans, but most infections are caused by ingestion of contaminated food. There are two main types of organism: *Salmonella enterica*, which causes gastroenteritis, and *Salmonella typhi (S. typhi)*, which causes typhoid fever. Both types secrete endotoxins that affect the gastrointestinal tract. The organism enters through the digestive tract and must be ingested in large numbers to cause disease in healthy adults. After a short incubation period of a few hours to 1 day, the organism multiplies in the intestinal lumen, causing fever, vomiting, and intestinal inflammation with diarrhea that is often mucopurulent and bloody. In infants and elderly adults, severe dehydration can occur. *Salmonella* can be found in uncooked foods, contaminated water, contaminated kitchen utensils, and in some animals such as reptiles. Animal fecal matter that contaminates eggs or vegetation can cause disease. It can also be caused by unsanitary food preparation by carriers of the organism.

S. typhi is particularly spread by human carriers. There is an estimated 16 to 33 million cases of typhoid fever annually, resulting in 216,000 deaths in endemic areas of Africa, Asia, and South America. Typhoid fever is a potentially fatal disease that causes high fever, cough, abdominal pain, watery diarrhea, and cardiac problems that include bradycardia and endocarditis. Liver involvement and intestinal perforation are common. Neuropsychiatric symptoms such as delirium also can occur. A distinctive rash called rose spots may occur on the lower chest and abdomen. Diagnosis is made by blood or stool culture and serological antibodies.

Salmonella can survive for weeks outside the body. It is not destroyed by freezing; however, heat can kill the organism after at least 10 minutes at 167°F.

According to the Centers for Disease Control and Prevention, approximately 5% of people who contract typhoid continue to carry the disease after they recover. These persons can transmit the infection to others. There are two vaccines available to prevent the disease. The organism is resistant to several different antibiotics but is sensitive to azithromycin.

Shigella

Shigella is a gram-negative, nonspore forming, nonmotile, rod-shaped bacteria related to *E. coli* and *Salmonella*. *Shigella* infection, called shigellosis, is an intestinal disease that causes severe diarrhea that is often bloody, a condition referred to as dysentery. *Shigella* causes approximately 90 million cases of severe dysentery, with at least 100,000 of these resulting in death each year, mostly among children in the developing world.

There are several different types of *Shigella* bacteria. Some secrete toxins; these can cause hemolytic uremic syndrome, a disorder of acute renal failure. The most common symptoms are diarrhea, fever, nausea, vomiting, stomach cramps, and flatulence. The stool may contain blood, mucus, or pus. In rare cases, young children may have seizures. Symptoms often begin 2 to 4 days after ingestion of contaminated food or water and last for weeks. A common cause of *Shigella* is direct contact of the bacteria in stool with diaper changes in a child care setting. Treatment consists of antibiotic therapy with agents such as ampicillin or fluoroquinolones.

Escherichia coli

E. coli are gram-negative, rod-shaped bacteria that inhabit the human intestine. There are multiple different strains. Although most strains of *E. coli* are harmless, the organisms can cause cholecystitis, bacteremia, cholangitis, UTI, traveler's diarrhea, neonatal meningitis, and pneumonia.

Several types are known to produce toxins that can cause severe gastroenteritis, diarrhea, and renal failure. A specific strain called *E. coli* 0157:H7 causes severe gastroenteritis and can cause hemolytic-uremic syndrome. This specific bacteria is one of the enterohemorrhagic *Escherichia coli* (EHEC). The EHEC bacteria are acquired by the fecal-oral route, usually in food or contaminated water. The bacteria live in the intestines of healthy cattle, and contamination of the meat can occur in the slaughtering process. Eating infected meat that is rare or undercooked is the most common way of acquiring the infection. Infection can also occur after consuming fecal-contaminated vegetation or unpasteurized milk, juice, or cider. Person-to-person transmission can also occur. Infants and elderly adults are most susceptible to illness caused by *E. coli* 0157:H7.

Infected persons can develop mild to severe diarrhea with abdominal cramps and blood in the stool. Usually little or no fever is present. In some people, particularly children younger than 5 years of age, the infection can cause a serious complication called hemolytic uremic syndrome (HUS). The patient has high amounts of RBC breakdown and renal failure. Diagnosis is made by stool culture or PCR. Transfusions of blood or blood clotting factors as well as kidney dialysis may be necessary. Hospitalization is usually required and most patients recover completely.

E. coli UTIs are caused by uropathogenic strains of *E. coli*. Uncomplicated lower UTIs, also called cystitis, occur primarily in females who are sexually active and are colonized by a uropathogenic strain of *E. coli*. The periurethral region is colonized from contamination with colonic bacteria, and the organism reaches the bladder during sexual intercourse. Males can endure UTI when urine stasis develops in the bladder, commonly caused by benign prostatic hyperplasia. The prostate obstructs urine outflow, and static urine serves as a perfect medium for bacterial growth. The most prominent symptoms are dysuria (burning on urination), frequency, and urgency. Fever is not an aspect of lower UTI. If fever is present, pyelonephritis should be ruled out.

An *E. coli* UTI can be treated with antibiotics and usually causes no complications. However, in elderly adults, UTI can become a serious bloodstream infection called urosepsis. Patients can develop acute illness with fever and severe hypotension. Intravenous antibiotics are required for urosepsis.

Campylobacter Jejuni

Campylobacter jejuni is a gram-negative, helical-shaped bacteria found in animal feces, particularly that of birds. It is one of the most common causes of gastroenteritis in the world, and usually produces diarrheal illness, and is self-limited. Contaminated food, particularly poultry, is a common source, though cattle infection can lead to infected beef. Improper meat or poultry preparation is the usual cause of infection. The illness can spread person to person. Homosexual males and immunosuppressed patients are at increased risk. The disorder causes abdominal pain, fever, and diarrhea, often containing blood. It can last 24 hours to a week. Specific culture media is required to diagnose the illness. Antibiotic treatment with erythromycin or ciprofloxacin is usually sufficient. Guillain-Barré syndrome has been noted as a complication that can develop 2 to 3 weeks after the gastroenteritis.

Cholera

Cholera is an infection of the small intestine caused by the bacterium *Vibrio cholerae*, a toxin-producing, flagellated bacterium. Cholera affects an estimated 3 to 5 million people worldwide, and causes 100,000 to 130,000 deaths a year. It is endemic in Africa and parts of Asia. The organism lives in nature, but can reach high levels in fecal-contaminated water. For unclear reasons, persons with O blood type are more susceptible than others. The main symptoms are profuse, watery diarrhea and vomiting. Transmission occurs primarily by drinking water or eating food that has been contaminated by the feces of an infected person. The severity of the diarrhea and vomiting can lead to rapid dehydration, electrolyte imbalance, and, in some cases, death. The diarrhea is extremely watery and has been referred to as "rice water" diarrhea. Some patients can lose 10 to 20 liters of fluid per day, so rehydration is continually needed.

There is a dipstick test available for diagnosis of cholera, and a positive test should be confirmed with stool culture. A number of safe vaccines are available. Water sanitation is the most effective means of prevention. Fluids, electrolytes, and doxycycline have been effective treatments.

Other Bacterial Infections

Bacteria such as diphtheria, tetanus, and pertussis are less common bacterial causes of infection mainly because of decades of successful immunization policies. However, because of a recent movement against vaccination, these microorganisms and their infections are reemerging. *Clostridium botulinum* and *Clostridium tetani* are neurotoxic bacteria that rarely cause disease. A tetanus booster every 10 years virtually eradicates the threat of *C. tetani*. *Clostridium difficile*, however, has become a dreaded source of nosocomial infection.

Diptheria, Pertussis, and Tetanus

Diptheria, pertussis, and tetanus are uncommon diseases in industrialized countries because of the success of routine immunization of children. Epidemics, however, can occur when immunization rates decline, as happened in Russia in the 1990s. A massive diptheria epidemic occurred and caused more than 5,000 deaths.

Corynebacterium diptheriae (*C. diptheriae*) is a toxin-producing bacteria that infects mucous membranes in the respiratory tract. It causes a distinctive gray-colored pseudomembrane consisting of sloughed epithelium, necrotic debris, white blood cells, and bacteria that line the respiratory tract. It presents with a sore throat, fever, and tonsillar exudate. Obstruction of the respiratory tract can occur, caused by the extensive pseudomembrane formation. Diphtheria antitoxin is administered to those who are infected. A combination of antibiotics, such as penicillin and erythromycin, are also administered. Other treatments may include IV fluids and oxygen; heart monitoring and intubation may be needed in severe cases. Individuals who come into contact with persons infected with *C. diptheriae* should receive an immunization or booster shot against diphtheria. Protective immunity lasts only 10 years from the time of vaccination, so it is important for adults to get a booster of tetanus-diphtheria (Td) vaccine every 10 years.

Pertussis, also called whooping cough, is an infection of the respiratory tract caused by *Bordetella pertussis* (*B. pertussis*). Bordetella is a toxin-producing bacteria that allows the binding of bacteria to respiratory ciliated cells. Other toxins produced by *B. pertussis* cause tissue necrosis and impairment of the immune responses mounted by the body. The infected individual has episodes of spasmodic forceful coughing with an audible whoop. The cough may be so forceful that it causes vomiting, subconjunctival hemorrhages, bulging eyes, and neck vein distention. Infants need hospitalization and have the highest mortality rate. Early treatment with antibiotics, IV fluids, and oxygen are necessary. Cough elixirs and expectorants are contraindicated. Diptheria-tetanus-pertussis (DTaP) vaccine is administered in 5 doses to infants at 2 months, 4 months, 6 months, 15 to 18 months, and children at age 6 years. A booster vaccine should be administered to children at age 10 to 12 years and every 10 years thereafter. In a pertussis outbreak, children younger than age 7 years should be kept away from those suspected of disease. Complications include pneumonia, convulsions, cerebral hemorrhage, and apnea.

Tetanus is a neurological disorder characterized by intense muscle spasms caused by *Clostridium tetani* (*C. tetani*), a toxin-producing, spore-forming anaerobic bacteria. *C. tetani* is a common organism found in soil and its spores can survive for many years under harsh conditions. Tetanus infection can occur after a penetrating injury such as a puncture wound or laceration. *C. tetani* toxin is released in the wound, binds to peripheral motor neurons, and is then transported to the spinal cord. The toxin blocks inhibitory neurotransmitters, causing hyperactivity of neurons. Infected persons may first notice increased muscle tone, particularly in the masseter muscles and jaw. For this reason, the term *lockjaw* has been used to describe the initial sign of tetanus infection. Generalized muscle spasms with the uncontrollable, rigid arching of the back may occur. Respiratory arrest, hypertension or hypotension, tachycardia or bradycardia, profuse sweating, and hyperpyrexia may result. Antibiotics are of little value in the treatment of tetanus; antitoxin is administered along with supportive treatments.

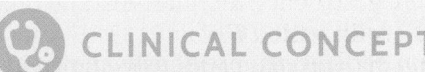

CLINICAL CONCEPT

Adults should receive Tdap vaccination every 10 years because it offers the best prevention against pertussis, tetanus, and diphtheria. Tdap stands for tetanus and diphtheria toxoids with acellular pertussis.

Botulism

Clostridium botulinum (*C. botulinum*) is a spore-producing, toxin-secreting bacteria found in soil. The toxin can be ingested or inhaled, or it can invade the body through breaches in the skin. In industrialized countries, most cases are food-borne and result from improper storage and packaging of canned foods. However, contaminated water, fish, cured ham, honey, and corn syrup have been sources. The botulinum toxin affects neurons and causes a descending paralysis, affecting the cranial nerves initially. Weakness progresses rapidly from the head down into the neck, arms, trunk, and legs. Nausea, vomiting, and abdominal pain may occur, as may dizziness, blurred vision, dry mouth, and a change in mental status. Pupillary reflexes may be absent in some patients. Approximately 100 cases occur per year in the United States with the majority in infants.

Botulism is a reportable disease and clinicians should contact the Centers for Disease Control and Prevention to obtain appropriate directions for treatment with antitoxin. Because botulinum toxin can be widely dispersed as an aerosol or food contaminant, it has the potential as a weapon in bioterrorism and biological warfare. Botulinum toxin is also used therapeutically to relieve muscle spasm and cosmetically for reduction of facial wrinkles. The toxin used for cosmetic purposes is known as onabotulinumtoxin A (Botox).

Clostridium Difficile

C. difficile is a spore-forming, toxin-secreting anaerobic bacteria. Spores of *C. difficile* are ingested and germinate in the small and large intestine. The organisms emit toxins that disrupt the intestinal mucosa, erode the intestinal epithelial cells, and form pseudomembranes that contain necrotic tissue, white blood cells, and mucus.

The most common predisposing factor is long-term antibiotic use because of consequent alteration of the normal flora in the gut. However, prolonged use of proton pump inhibitors can cause the condition, and contagion between patients is possible. Recently, the bacterium has become a source of nosocomial infection.

Prolonged frequent diarrhea, fever, and abdominal pain are the most common presenting symptoms. Stool culture to identify the presence of *C. difficile* is diagnostic of the condition. Discontinuation of the antibiotic in use is necessary, and supportive treatments, such as rehydration, may be initiated. Metronidazole may be used to control the diarrhea.

Clostridial Gas Gangrene

Clostridium perfringens, previously known as *Clostridium welchii,* is the most common cause of clostridial gas gangrene (80% to 90% of cases). Clostridial organisms can be found in soil and isolated from normal human colonic flora, skin, and the vagina. *C. perfringens* is a highly lethal organism that causes myonecrosis, a rapidly spreading necrotizing infection of skeletal muscle and surrounding tissue. The destruction of tissue is caused by toxins that are secreted by the organism. The toxin causes direct vascular injury, cellular necrosis, hemolysis, leukocyte degeneration, and polymorphonuclear cell damage. The process of myonecrosis can spread as fast as 2 cm per hour. Spreading infection often results in systemic toxicity and shock that can be fatal within 12 hours. If properly treated, the overall mortality rate is 20% to 30%. If untreated, the process is 100% fatal.

Clostridial infection usually occurs in a wound after trauma or surgery. The symptom that should alert the clinician to clostridial infection is severe, sudden pain that is out of proportion to physical findings at the wound site (see Box 10-1). On physical examination, the involved body part commonly demonstrates the following characteristics:

- edema
- erythema with purplish black discoloration
- extreme tenderness
- brownish skin discoloration (bronzing, brawny) with bullae
- profuse, "dish-watery," serous drainage from ruptured bullae
- discharge that may have a peculiar, "mousy," sweet odor
- crepitant tissue that may extend well beyond any skin discoloration or edema.

X-rays reveal fine gas bubbles within the soft tissues, dissecting into the intramuscular fascial planes and muscles. The wound discharge should be collected for culture and sensitivity. Penicillin is the preferred drug for clostridial infections. Patients allergic to penicillin may be treated with clindamycin or chloramphenicol. Surgical consultation is necessary and may result in amputation of the involved area.

BOX 10-1. Risk Factors for Clostridial Infection

Clostridia is a bacterial organism that can cause gangrene in ischemic tissue. The following risk factors make one susceptible to clostridia infection.

- Diabetes mellitus
- Peripheral vascular disease
- Alcoholism
- Drug abuse
- Advanced age
- Chronic debilitating disease(s)
- Immunocompromised state caused by:
  - steroid use
  - malnutrition
  - malignancy
  - acquired immunodeficiency syndrome (AIDS).

Tick-Borne Bacterial Disease

Lyme disease and Rocky Mountain spotted fever (RMSF) are the most common tick-borne illnesses in the United States. Both diseases are caused by bacterial parasites that are harbored by forest animals, such as deer. A tick feeds off the animal and then carries the bacterial parasite. Humans come in contact with the pin-sized ticks in forested regions and are commonly bit without awareness. Lyme disease and RMSF tick bites cause debilitating symptoms. Despite its name, RMSF can occur throughout the United States. Lyme disease is mainly found in the northeastern United States.

Lyme Disease. Lyme disease is caused by a bacterial spirochete called *Borrelia burgdorferi* a microorganism found in forest animals such as squirrels, rodents, and the white-tailed deer. A tick that feeds off one of these animals can harbor the microorganism. Neither the reservoir (deer) nor vector (tick) becomes ill because of the microorganism. However, the tick can bite a human, who can become infected with the microorganism and develop illness. Deer ticks are tiny, no larger than the point of a pencil, and the infected individual frequently cannot remember being bitten. After a lengthy incubation period of 3 to 32 days, a rash known as *Erythema migrans* begins as a painless red macule that expands slowly to form a targetlike lesion (see Fig. 10-6). Within a few days, the center of the lesion can become extremely erythematous, vesicular, and ulcerated. The legs, thighs, groin, and axilla are common sites of the lesion. Almost 20% of infected persons do not exhibit the characteristic skin lesion.

Skin involvement is usually followed by headache, mild stiffness of the neck, fever, chills, migratory musculoskeletal pain, arthralgias, and extreme fatigue. Early symptoms usually wane within several weeks. Cranial neuritis of the facial nerve can develop in some patients. In cranial neuritis, inflammation of the facial

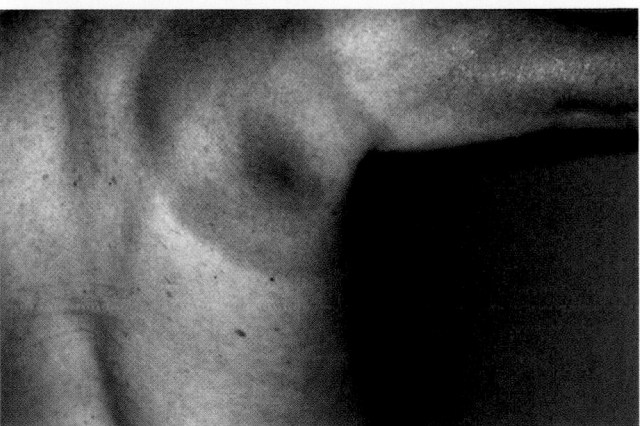

FIGURE 10-6. Erythema migrans. *(Courtesy of CDC.)*

nerve causes one side of the face to be paralyzed—a condition called Bell's palsy. The patient exhibits a one-sided facial droop when smiling and is unable to close the eye on the affected side. Months after the onset of *Borrelia* infection, approximately 60% of patients develop arthritis, usually of the large joints, particularly the knees.

Diagnosis of Lyme disease is difficult because positive cultures are only obtained early in the disease when most infected persons are unaware of the infection. Biopsy samples of the *Erythema migrans* lesion or involved joint fluid may reveal evidence of the *B. burgdorferi* organism. Lyme disease, however, is usually diagnosed by the characteristic history and clinical presentation of the patient, in addition to serological testing for the antibody to *B. burgdorferi*. The test for the antibody may be negative in the initial period of the disease, but after several weeks, most patients develop a positive antibody titer. Serological tests cannot distinguish between active and inactive infection. Patients can remain seropositive for many years after initial infection, even after antibiotic treatment.

Lyme disease is best treated early in the disease with oral and intravenous antibiotics. Oral antibiotic regimens may require treatment for 30 to 60 days, whereas intravenous regimens may be needed for only 14 to 28 days.

Rickettsia. Rickettsia comprise a specific type of bacteria known as obligate intracellular parasites because they must be within a living cell in order to reproduce. They can only be transmitted via vectors, usually fleas, ticks, or mites. As a class, rickettsia are responsible for a number of significant human diseases, including RMSF, typhus, and Q fever.

CLINICAL CONCEPT

Typhus and typhoid fever are not the same disease. Typhus is caused by any one of a number of *Rickettsia* bacteria, whereas typhoid fever is caused by *Salmonella typhi*.

Rocky Mountain Spotted Fever. The bacteria *Rickettsia rickettsii* (*R. ricketsii*) is a small gram-negative bacillus that may be harbored in a dog tick or a wood tick. *R. rickettsii* enters the skin through a tick bite and spreads along the lymphatic system. Initially, the classic triad of symptoms is fever, rash, and history of a tick bite. However, as with Lyme disease, most individuals do not recall being bitten by a tick. After entry into the lymphatic system, *R. rickettsii* rapidly infects the endothelial cells and causes increased vascular permeability, with resulting edema. Vascular permeability causes hypoalbuminemia, hypovolemia, hypotension, and reduced serum oncotic pressure. An inflammatory reaction follows, including activation of platelets and the fibrinolytic system. Various organ systems may be involved, including the pulmonary, cardiac, nervous, renal, hematopoietic, and hepatic systems.

Initial symptoms may include nonspecific systemic signs such as fever, nausea, vomiting, severe headache, muscle pain, and lack of appetite. Later signs and symptoms include rash, abdominal pain, joint pain, and diarrhea. The characteristic red, spotted (petechial) rash of RMSF is usually not seen until the sixth day or later after onset of symptoms. The rash involves the palms of the hands or soles of the feet, but 10% of patients may never develop it.

Serological or antibody testing is the most frequently used method for confirming cases of RMSF. The indirect immunofluorescence assay is a type of serology test that is generally considered the reference standard in RMSF.

Patients with RMSF are critically ill and require immediate intensive care and antibiotic treatment. Cardiac monitoring, hemodialysis, blood transfusion, and endotracheal intubation with ventilatory support may be required. Long-term health problems after acute infection may follow.

Selected Viral Infections

Viruses are ubiquitous and have the ability to mutate, which confounds treatment. They spread most often from human to human by droplet infection or via contact, and they require the cellular machinery of a living organism in order to reproduce. The common cold is a typical viral disorder.

Common Cold Viruses

Acute upper respiratory illnesses are the most common of human diseases. On average, adults suffer three to four upper respiratory illnesses per person per year. It is estimated that two-thirds to three-fourths of acute respiratory illnesses are caused by viruses. Rhinovirus, coronavirus, and adenovirus are the major causes of the common cold and all present in a similar manner. These viruses spread through direct contact or droplet infection. Frequently, the virus is transmitted from hands that have been in contact with respiratory secretions. They can survive for 1 to 3 hours on environmental surfaces, such as keyboards.

The incubation period for rhinovirus is 1 to 2 days and symptoms usually begin with rhinorrhea and sneezing. Illness generally lasts 4 to 9 days, and resolves spontaneously. Rhinovirus infection can lead to otitis media and sinusitis, or stimulate asthma in those who are susceptible to these conditions. Diagnosis is usually made on clinical presentation alone. Treatment is supportive, consisting of antihistamines and decongestants. Thorough hand washing and environmental disinfection can help prevent spread of the infection to others.

Influenza Virus

The three major types of influenza virus, A, B and C, are among the most common causes of upper and lower respiratory tract infection affecting all age groups. Influenza virus has been responsible for many pandemics and epidemics across the world. Some epidemics have been notable, such as the "Spanish flu" of 1918 that took many lives.

Outbreaks of influenza occur annually, and are particularly worrisome for the very young, elders, and those with chronic disease. These viruses possess surface antigens known as hemagglutinin and neuraminidase, proteins that facilitate entry into respiratory cells and enhance release of viral particles. The most extensive and severe outbreaks are caused by influenza A viruses because of their ability to undergo mutation. From year to year, the hemagglutinin and neuraminidase antigens of influenza A change because of genetic mutations. Influenza B virus causes outbreaks that are associated with less severe disease because genetic mutation causing variation in their hemagglutinin and neuraminidase antigens is less common. The periodic genetic mutations that occur in influenza viruses require new vaccine development each year.

Transmission of influenza occurs through droplet infection and aerosols generated by coughs and sneezes of individuals. Fomites and hand-to-hand contact also can spread the virus. Initially the virus enters the upper respiratory tract and then invades the lower respiratory tract mucous gland cells, alveolar cells, and macrophages. The infection usually presents as abrupt onset of fever, chills, headache, myalgias, arthralgias, cough, and sore throat. Uncomplicated influenza generally resolves over a 1-week period, although cough may persist for 2 weeks or longer. In elderly patients, postinfluenza weakness and fatigue can persist for several weeks. Influenza in elderly adults also increases susceptibility to pneumonia.

Influenza virus can be isolated from throat culture, nasopharyngeal secretions, or sputum. Treatment consists of antipyretic medications, hydration, and rest. Amantadine, rimantadine, zanamivir, and oseltamivir are antiviral medications that can be used to shorten the disease's course. Influenza vaccine is recommended annually for all persons older than age 6 months, but it is particularly important for elderly adults and the chronically ill. The influenza vaccine may not prevent an individual from developing active disease, but it is highly effective at preventing severe disease and complications. Health-care workers need to get annual immunization, because unimmunized persons can transmit the virus even if they do not become symptomatic themselves.

Epstein Barr Virus

Epstein Barr virus (EBV) is the cause of infectious mononucleosis, a common infection of adolescents and young adults. By adulthood, more than 90% of individuals have been infected with EBV and have developed antibodies to the virus.

EBV is spread by oral secretions because the virus infects the epithelium of the oropharynx and salivary glands. The virus is frequently spread from asymptomatic adults to children by transfer of saliva. Among adolescents and young adults, the virus is most often spread by kissing and so infectious mononucleosis has the nickname "the kissing disease." The virus initially binds to and infects the cells of the oropharynx. After the virus enters the oropharynx, it invades the bloodstream and has a predilection for B lymphocytes. The virus incites an immune response that causes proliferation of B lymphocytes within lymphoid tissue, resulting in lymphadenopathy. The cervical lymph nodes, which are most commonly involved, are tender and symmetrically enlarged. Pharyngitis, fatigue, headache, fever, chills, abdominal pain, nausea, and vomiting are usually presenting symptoms. Pharyngitis is often the most prominent sign with tonsillar enlargement and exudate. Some individuals develop periorbital edema and a papular rash on the trunk and arms. Administration of ampicillin during infection with EBV can provoke development of an erythematous maculopapular rash. Enlargement of the liver and spleen can also occur. Hepatomegaly can cause elevated liver enzymes and jaundice, whereas splenomegaly can predispose the patient to splenic rupture. Symptoms of infectious mononucleosis are self-limited and usually resolve within 4 weeks, although some individuals may require up to 6 months for full recovery.

White blood cell counts with examination of the cells show a lymphocytosis with atypical lymphocytes. These atypical cells are larger than normal lymphocytes, and contain large vacuoles in their cytoplasm. The heterophile antibody test is a specialized diagnostic test that can detect antibodies in acute EBV infection. Repeated testing may be necessary because antibodies develop throughout the illness and are most easily detected during the third week of infection. Heterophile tests usually remain positive for 3 months, although antibodies can persist for up to a year. A rapid monospot test is often used clinically, but it is not as accurate as the heterophile test.

After recovery from infectious mononucleosis, the virus is shed from the oropharynx for as long as 18 months after acute infection and may continue to be shed intermittently for many years in healthy EBV-positive individuals. As long as the virus is shedding, it may be transmitted to another individual. Furthermore, EBV has a unique ability to remain dormant within the body after recovery from acute infection. EBV remains in a dormant form within lymphoid tissue for life and reactivation is possible.

Treatment is supportive, which includes adequate hydration, nutrition, and rest. Splenomegaly increases the chance of splenic rupture and internal bleeding. Aspirin should be avoided to decrease the chance of bleeding. Other antipyretic medications such as acetaminophen are recommended for fever and sore throat. Corticosteroids may be necessary if there is severe tonsillar enlargement with impending airway obstruction. Antiviral medications have not shown to be effective in infectious mononucleosis.

Although rare, EBV is associated with nasopharyngeal cancer. It has also been implicated in chronic fatigue syndrome.

> **ALERT!** The individual with EBV infection and splenomegaly should not participate in strenuous activities or contact sports for at least 3 weeks or until the spleen returns to normal size.

Cytomegalovirus

Cytomegalovirus (CMV) is capable of causing a wide range of disorders in all age groups. It can cause an asymptomatic infection, birth defects in the fetus, mononucleosis-type syndrome in adults, and severe disseminated infection in immunosuppressed individuals. Initially, the virus infects the salivary epithelial cells and is shed in the saliva. CMV also commonly infects the genitourinary tract, shedding in the urine. In immunocompetent persons, CMV infection may be asymptomatic or present as a mild flulike illness or a mononucleosislike illness. The most common symptoms are extreme fatigue, fever, pharyngitis, lymphadenopathy, and, in some cases, splenomegaly.

In comparison to EBV mononucleosis, CMV mononucleosis has a lower incidence of cervical lymphadenopathy and negative heterophile test. CMV can cause pneumonia and hepatitis, which is usually self-limited and resolves without complication in immunocompetent individuals. However, CMV can cause more serious disseminated bloodstream infection of the immunosuppressed patient. Once in the bloodstream, the virus can be found in breast milk, saliva, feces, urine, cervical secretions, and semen. Transmission of the virus from person to person is facilitated by close living conditions and poor personal hygiene. It can be transmitted sexually, through blood transfusion, and by transplantation. In the immunocompromised individual, CMV can cause life-threatening pneumonitis, gastrointestinal disease, retinitis, hepatitis, encephalitis, and myeloradiculitis.

CMV antibodies are found in the bloodstream 4 to 7 weeks after infection and may persist for as long as 20 weeks. CMV antigen can also be isolated from tissue culture or from the bloodstream.

CMV is the most common congenitally acquired infection in infants. During pregnancy, women without immunity are susceptible to disseminated infection, which affects the placenta and is transferred to the fetus. Cervical excretion of the virus is common during pregnancy and can be transferred to the infant during delivery. CMV may also be transmitted to the infant through breast milk. Most children infected in utero appear healthy but may demonstrate symptoms of disease later in development. Ten percent are born with cytomegalic inclusion disease. The symptoms of cytomegalic inclusion disease include jaundice, splenomegaly, thrombocytopenia, intrauterine growth retardation, microcephaly, and retinitis. Children born with cytomegalic inclusion disease commonly develop neurological or cognitive impairment.

CMV is within the herpes family of viruses; like all herpes viruses, it has the potential to remain dormant in the body after the acute infection subsides.

Cell-mediated immunity is the most important defense mechanism against CMV. Patients with AIDS and immunosuppressed transplant recipients are most vulnerable.

At present there are no sufficiently effective antiviral medications to combat CMV infection.

Measles, Mumps, and Rubella

Measles, mumps, and rubella (MMR) were common childhood illnesses fewer than 50 years ago, but are now rare because of routine vaccination. Rubella and measles (also called rubeola) are referred to as viral **exanthems,** a term indicating rash. The clinical significance of MMR now lies mainly in their public health implications. As immunization has become mandatory in many economically developed countries, public knowledge and concern about these serious diseases has decreased dramatically. In some instances, a false sense of security has occurred, and people have become lax in adhering to recommendations for immunization. Some parents are refusing vaccination of their children because of fear of dangerous side effects, which is increasing the incidence of MMR. Health-care providers have an important role in educating the public about diseases that have become uncommon because of immunization programs. Additionally, people need accurate, easily understood information on the actual risks and benefits of vaccination.

Measles

The measles virus is an RNA virus of the genus *Morbillivirus* within the family *Paramyxoviridae*. Humans are hosts and infection is transmitted via respiratory droplets, which can remain active and contagious, either airborne or on surfaces, for up to 2 hours. The measles virus, once acquired, establishes a localized infection at the respiratory epithelium, after which the virus infects regional lymph nodes and endothelial cells, and then disseminates to distant organs. In immunocompetent individuals, measles virus infection induces an effective immune response, which clears the virus and results in lifelong immunity.

The CDC reports the childhood mortality rate from measles infection in the United States to be 0.1% to 0.2%. Globally, however, measles remains one of the leading causes of death in young children. According to the CDC, an estimated 10 million cases and 197,000 deaths caused by measles occur in children worldwide each year.

Measles has an incubation period of 7 to 14 days and a prodromal stage of 4 to 7 days. High fever, cough, upper respiratory illness, conjunctivitis with periorbital edema, and photophobia are major symptoms. There are unique white areas in the oral buccal mucosa called Koplik spots that appear in the prodromal stage. Koplik spots are considered pathognomonic for measles. After the appearance of Koplik spots, the characteristic tiny maculopapular, mildly pruritic rash appears on the body (see Fig. 10-7). The rash develops from head to toe and then fades after 5 to 7 days.

Diagnosis is usually made by clinical history and physical exam, and specific measles IgM and IgG immunoglobulins can be found in the blood. Rest, hydration, antipyretics, and other supportive therapy are required for treatment. Vitamin A supplements are also recommended because they have been found to decrease mortality and complications by 50%. Complications, which are more likely to occur in persons younger than 5 years or older than 20 years, include bacterial pneumonia, eye damage, and blindness.

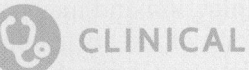

CLINICAL CONCEPT

All individuals should receive the MMR vaccine at 15 months, and a booster is recommended at age 18.

Rubella

Rubella, also known as German measles, is an RNA virus classified as a Rubivirus in the *Togaviridae* family. Before the rubella vaccine, epidemics of the disease were seen in young children, adolescents, and young adults in winter and early spring. Since development of the rubella vaccine, the number of rubella cases has decreased significantly. One major focus of infection is now unvaccinated adults.

The disease is spread by droplet infection from cough or sneeze and infects the respiratory epithelium. It has an incubation period of 14 to 19 days, with onset of a rash usually on the 15th day. The disease can be spread from a few days before rash to 5 to 7 days after the appearance of the rash. Patients are most contagious when the rash is erupting and are noncontagious after 7 days of rash.

The rash may be the first manifestation, followed by fever, sore throat, and rhinitis. The rash begins as discrete, red macules on the face that spread to the neck, trunk, and extremities. The macules may coalesce on the trunk. Appearance of the rash corresponds with the appearance of the rubella-specific antibody. The rash lasts 1 to 3 days, first leaving the face. Forchheimer spots, which are pinpoint red macules and petechiae over the soft palate and the uvula, can be seen just before or with the rash.

The hallmark of rubella is generalized, tender lymphadenopathy that involves all nodes, but particularly the suboccipital, postauricular, and anterior and posterior cervical nodes. Although less common in children, polyarthralgia and even polyarthritis may occur in adults and rarely may persist longer than 2 weeks.

The major complication of rubella is its teratogenic effects when pregnant women contract the disease, especially in the early weeks of gestation. The virus can be transmitted to the fetus through the placenta and can cause serious congenital defects, spontaneous abortions, and stillbirths. Serological studies show a rise in IgM antibodies in the beginning of the disease and IgG later in the disease. IgG remains and confers long-term immunity.

Treatment for rubella involves supportive therapy with antipyretics, hydration, and oatmeal baths, which can be used to soothe the pruritic rash. Vaccination with the MMR vaccine is usually administered to infants at 15 months and a booster is usually necessary at approximately age 18 years.

FIGURE 10-7. Measles rash. *(Courtesy of CDC/Dr. Heinz F. Eichenwald.)*

Mumps

Mumps is a paromyxovirus transmitted by droplet infection of a cough or sneeze. It has an incubation period of 14 to 25 days, after which time prodromal symptoms occur and last anywhere from 3 to 5 days. The most common presentation is parotitis, or swollen parotid salivary glands, which occur in 30% to 40% of patients. Other reported sites of infection are the testes, pancreas, eyes, ovaries, central nervous system, joints, and kidneys. A patient is considered infectious from about 3 days before the onset to up to 4 days after the start of active parotitis. Infections can be asymptomatic in up to 20% of persons.

The most common symptoms are parotitis, submaxillary/submandibular gland swelling, fever, and sore throat. The average length of illness is 5 days. Complications, including encephalitis and orchitis, are reported in 5% of patients. In the male, orchitis can result in sterility. Diagnosis is based on clinical examination, and mumps-specific IgG can be detected in the bloodstream. Testicular ultrasonography is needed to diagnose orchitis, whereas lumbar puncture is necessary for symptomatic meningitis or encephalitis. Treatment is supportive, including anti-inflammatory agents, intravenous hydration, and use of ice packs to decrease parotid or scrotal swelling. Prevention with the MMR vaccine is recommended for all children at age 15 months.

Varicella Zoster

The varicella zoster virus (VZV) causes the clinical syndrome varicella, which is more widely known as chickenpox. Varicella is largely a childhood disease, with more than 90% of cases occurring in children younger than 10 years old. As with MMR, varicella is becoming a less common disease because of immunization programs. The disease is benign in the healthy child, whereas increased morbidity is seen in adults and in patients who are immunocompromised. The adult who has not developed varicella as a child is susceptible to varicella pneumonia, which is a serious illness with prolonged recovery and potential complications.

Varicella is usually acquired by the inhalation of airborne respiratory droplets from an infected host. A history of exposure to an infected contact within the incubation period of 10 to 21 days is an important clue in the diagnosis. It is a highly contagious virus and is usually diagnosed on the basis of the characteristic rash and successive crops of lesions. The typical patient is infectious for 1 to 2 days before the development of rash and until the last vesicles have crusted over. The triad of rash, malaise, and low-grade fever are typical signs. The characteristic chickenpox vesicle, surrounded by an erythematous halo, is described as a "dewdrop on a rose petal" (see Fig. 10-8). Small, erythematous macules often first appear on the scalp, face, trunk, and proximal limbs, with rapid sequential

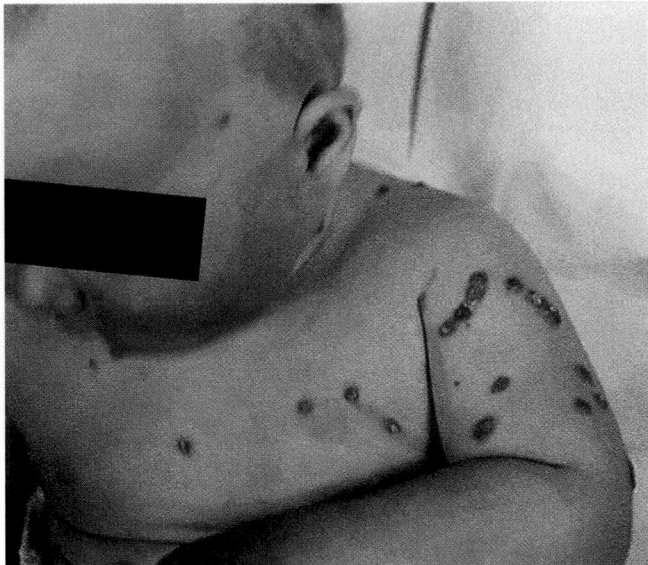

FIGURE 10-8. Varicella. *(Courtesy of CDC/Susan Lindsley.)*

progression over 12 to 14 hours to papules, clear vesicles, and pustules, with subsequent central umbilication and crust formation. Vesicles may appear on the palms and soles and on the mucous membranes, with painful, shallow, oropharyngeal, or urogenital ulcers. Intense pruritus commonly accompanies the vesicular stage of the rash. Diagnosis is most commonly based on history and physical exam. Treatment consists mainly of supportive measures such as antipyretics, hydration, oatmeal bath, and antihistamines for the pruritic rash. Oral acyclovir is used for persons at increased risk of severe varicella infections, most notably people older than 12 years. To prevent the disease, VZV is recommended in childhood.

Herpes zoster infection, also known as *shingles,* is a reactivation of varicella zoster. Following resolution of varicella, the varicella virus lies dormant in the dorsal root ganglia of the spinal nerves. In adulthood, during times of extreme stress or immunosuppression, the virus can become reactivated and cause herpes zoster infection. Upon reactivation, the virus migrates down the sensory nerve to the skin, causing a characteristic line of vesicular lesions, usually along a single dermatome. It may be followed by painful neuralgias for up to a year after reactivation. The incidence of herpes zoster increases with age, with older adults being disproportionately affected. Therefore, immunization with herpes zoster vaccine is advised for persons age 65 and older. Antiviral agents such as acyclovir can be prescribed to lessen the severity of the disorder.

Erythema Infectiosum (Fifth Disease)

Erythema infectiosum (E. infectiosum; Fifth disease) is a common childhood viral exanthem caused by human parvovirus B19. Acute infection involves an adaptive immune response, with the production of specific IgM antibodies and subsequent formation of immune

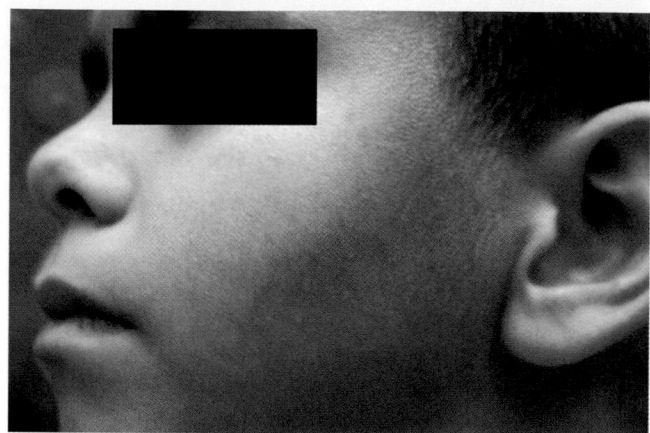

FIGURE 10-9. Erythema infectiosum. *(Courtesy of CDC.)*

complexes that deposit in skin and joints. The infection tends to occur in the late winter or early spring.

E. infectiosum typically has an incubation period of 4 to 14 days and is spread primarily via droplet infection during this period. The prodromal phase may include headache, low-grade fever, pharyngitis, and malaise. Classic skin rash follows within 3 to 7 days. The facial skin develops a classic slapped-cheek appearance that may appear like a sunburn and typically fades over 2 to 4 days (see Fig. 10-9). It is occasionally edematous.

Within 1 to 4 days of the rash appearing on the cheeks, the second stage skin rash develops. It is an erythematous macular-to-morbilliform rash over the extremity extensor surfaces that can involve the palms and soles.

After several days, most of the second stage skin rash fades into a lacy pattern, with particular emphasis on the proximal extremities. After starting to fade, the rash may recur over several weeks following physical stimuli such as exercise, sun exposure, friction, bathing in hot water, or stress.

Diagnosis is most commonly made by history and physical examination. It is a self-limited disorder. Treatment involves mainly supportive measures such as antipyretics, antihistamines, and hydration.

Herpes Simplex Virus

There are two herpes simplex viruses (HSV), HSV-1 and HSV-2. The two viruses cause disease in the same manner but are distinctly categorized because they usually infect different parts of the body. HSV-1 is the common cold sore virus, whereas HSV-2 is the cause of genital herpes infection.

Both HSV-1 and HSV-2 cause acute and latent infection. Acute infection is characterized by abrupt onset of vesicular lesions within the epidermis and mucous membranes. The fluid-filled vesicles contain active viral particles; transmission of the virus to others during this phase is common. After a few weeks, the acute phase ceases and is followed by a period of dormancy when there are no apparent lesions and the virus is inactive. During the latent period, the herpes viral DNA remains dormant within the nucleus of the affected individual's neurons and evades immune destruction. Reactivation of HSV frequently occurs during periods of stress, illness, or immunosuppression.

In active HSV-2, the lesions occur in the genital region and perineal area. During sexual activity or close skin contact, the virus can spread from these lesions to partners. At times, the affected individual may not have apparent symptoms of active lesions and can unknowingly spread the virus. (See Chapter 28: Sexually Transmitted Diseases for more on HSV-2.)

The characteristic cytological changes induced by HSV can be demonstrated in a specialized culture called a Tzanck smear. Alternatively, HSV DNA can be extracted from lesions by PCR. Supportive measures are used for treatment. Acyclovir is an antiviral medication often used to lessen the severity of the outbreak of HSV infection.

Poliomyelitis

Poliomyelitis is a disease that is caused by the polio virus. Historically, polio caused epidemics resulting in high death rates and disability. Currently, the disease is preventable through routine immunizations.

Polio enters the body through the fecal-oral route, usually from contaminated eating utensils, water sources, or through hand contamination from the stool of an infected person. The virus lives in the throat and intestinal tract of the infected person for approximately 1 week to 6 weeks. Upon initial infection with the poliovirus, 90% of individuals will have no symptoms for the first 2 weeks. Others will have short-term symptoms of headache, tiredness, fever, stiff neck and back, and generalized muscle pain. Unfortunately, the infected person is most contagious before the symptoms are manifested.

Polio causes damage to the motor neurons of the central nervous system. There are three related syndromes for polio. Abortive poliomyelitis is a nonspecific disease with a fever for 2 to 3 days. There is no central nervous system (CNS) involvement, and the patient may not even seek medical attention. The second syndrome is aseptic meningitis. Again, there is fever, but recovery is rapid and complete, without any complications. The third syndrome is paralytic poliomyelitis, which is the classic presentation. At one time the disease was called infantile paralysis. There is asymmetrical flaccid paralysis, deep tendon reflexes are decreased or absent, and sensation remains intact. Complications of poliomyelitis mostly affect the legs, although paralysis of the diaphragm muscle and swallowing mechanisms may be seen in cases called bulbar paralytic poliomyelitis.

There is no treatment for polio. Therapy is supportive and consists of mobility, support of the work of breathing, and prevention of complications such as aspiration. There is, however, a vaccine available. Jonas Salk developed the first polio vaccine in 1955; since then, the disease has been eradicated in areas where immunization is routine and widespread. There are two types of vaccines. The inactivated polio vaccine is an injectable vaccine that can be given at 2 months and 4 months of age. The other vaccine is the oral polio vaccine, which is administered early in infancy and again at 4 to 6 years. Boosters are recommended for world travelers.

Hantavirus

Hantaviruses, which belong to the *Bunyaviridae* family of viruses, were first recognized in the 1950s during the Korean War. There are five different viruses within the *Bunyaviridae* family; each is made up of a single-stranded RNA virus. They are rodent-borne viruses transmitted via inhalation. Humans breathe in the aerosolized virus from infected rodents' urine, droppings, or saliva.

The incidence of hantavirus infection varies depending on geography. In the countries of China and Russia, there are 20,000 to 100,000 cases reported annually. In the United States, there are approximately 400 reported cases per year, mostly in the states of New Mexico, California, Washington, and Texas.

Hantavirus can cause two separate syndromes: hemorrhagic fever with renal syndrome (HFRS) and hantavirus cardiopulmonary syndrome (HCPS). They have different symptoms.

HFRS has five phases, which occur after the incubation period of 2 to 4 weeks:

1. **Febrile phase:** characterized by fever and flulike symptoms lasting 3 to 7 days.
2. **Hypotensive phase:** characterized by decreasing platelets, tachycardia, and hypotension. This phase lasts for approximately 2 days.
3. **Oliguric phase:** features the onset of acute renal failure and proteinuria and lasts 3 to 7 days.
4. **Diuretic phase:** characterized by urine output of 3 to 6 liters/day, and may last for a few days or several weeks.
5. **Convalescent phase:** characterized by recovery of renal and respiratory function. This phase may last for a couple of weeks.

HCPS is the more fatal form of the hantavirus. If contracted, the symptoms are similar to the HFRS, but the cardiovascular shock is potentially fatal.

Serological testing is the method for a definitive diagnosis. IgG and specific kinds of IgM antibodies will be present upon testing. Treatment is based on symptomatology. Support of the respiratory system with early mechanical ventilation and administration of antiviral medications may be helpful. The earlier the disease is recognized and treated, the better outcome for the patient. Environmental rodent control is the principal strategy for preventing the virus.

West Nile Virus

West Nile virus (WNV) was first diagnosed in 1937 in Uganda, Africa, but did not appear in the United States until 1999. WNV is within the family of flaviviridae, part of the Japanese encephalitis antigenic complex of viruses. The virus is spread when a mosquito bites an infected bird, ingests its blood, and then bites a person. Mosquitoes carry the highest amount of viral load in the early fall. The risk of disease decreases in cold weather.

People who are infected with WNV may have one of three different syndromes, which range from an asymptomatic infection, to a mild febrile syndrome, to the virus entering the brain. In this last case, WNV may be deadly, causing encephalitis or meningitis. The highest risk groups are elderly individuals, those with compromised immune systems, and women who are pregnant.

Diagnosis of WNV is by complete blood count, which will indicate an elevated leukocyte count; lumbar puncture with CSF testing, which will show a predominance of lymphocytes as well as elevated protein levels; head CT scan and head MRI, which usually return negative findings; electroencephalogram (EEG), which may show generalized slowing in the frontal or temporal regions; and serology, checking for antibodies against the virus. The IgM antibody assay is most often used for diagnosis. WNV should be suspected if the patient presents with an acute febrile episode and symptoms suggestive of meningitis or flaccid paralysis during mosquito season.

There are no vaccines or treatments for WNV, but antiviral medications may be used. Complications are rare, but in severe cases permanent brain damage, muscle weakness, and death can occur.

The principal method of control is to avoid mosquitoes by using insect repellent and eradicating the mosquito breeding sites.

Hemorrhagic Viruses

Ebola and Marburg virus belong to the family of viruses known as the filoviruses. They are responsible for severe hemorrhagic fever. Both the Ebola and the Marburg viruses are classified as Category A bioterrorism agents because of their virulence, stability, and high infectivity as small-particle aerosols.

Ebola Virus

Ebola virus is extremely lethal and rapid in onset. It was first isolated in the Congo region of Africa and is called a hemorrhagic fever. It is hypothesized that the virus is a zoonosis, appearing first in animals, then spread to humans by contact. Transmission is by direct contact with the virus through blood and body fluids. Humans spread it to each other when in close contact or commonly in unsterile clinic conditions. The incubation period is from 2 to 21 days. The mechanism of entry into the body is unknown. The virus is activated, and then begins to release its own genetic material, causing the host to produce proteins for viral replication. It then rapidly spreads to other cells and continues to spread until all the cells have the virus. Death ensues within 7 to 14 days.

Diagnosis is through PCR and ELISA testing. Immediate isolation of the affected patient is necessary. Ebola hemorrhagic fever symptoms range from vomiting, diarrhea, and general body malaise to internal bleeding from organs and fever. Mortality rates are high, up to 90%. The cause of death has been attributed to shock and organ dysfunction. There is no standard treatment other than supportive. Health-care providers should isolate the affected patient and use mask, gloves, gown, and goggles when caring for patients. It is also important to prevent close contact with bodies of the deceased.

Marburg Virus

Marburg virus causes Marburg hemorrhagic fever. Similar to Ebola virus, it begins with infection of animals, such as nonhuman primates. The African fruit bat is a known reservoir of the virus.

The disease is transmitted via contact with infected bodily fluids. The disease occurs in sporadic outbreaks within Africa. It has also occurred in laboratory workers in Europe working with primate blood samples. The incubation period is 3 to 9 days. Early symptoms are fever, headache, and general malaise. After 5 days, a rash is noted on the trunk. Symptoms of late-stage Marburg hemorrhagic fever include jaundice, pancreatitis, weight loss, delirium, neuropsychiatric symptoms, and hemorrhage. Diagnosis is made using PCR. The mortality rate has been reported as high as 90%. There is no standard treatment. Health-care providers need to use full body protection precautions.

Selected Fungal Infections

Fungi are plantlike organisms that live in air, soil, plants, water, and even the human body. Fungi reproduce through tiny spores in the air. Fungal infections often affect those with a weakened immune system and those who are on prolonged antibiotics. They can affect the skin and nails, or they can infect the lungs, gastrointestinal tract, genitourinary tract, or vaginal tract. Some fungal infections are difficult to eradicate. Some common fungal infections include tinea (also called ringworm) infections, yeast infections, and skin and nail infections.

Candida

Candida is a common fungus in our environment and part of the normal flora. *C. albicans,* normally found in the gastrointestinal and vaginal tracts, is the most common type of Candida infection. Candida becomes pathogenic when an overgrowth of the Candida fungus occurs, commonly causing superficial diseases. The host immune response is one of the most important determinants of the type of infection that will be caused by Candida. An immunocompromised host can develop widespread dissemination of candida within the body, which can then progress to overwhelming sepsis. A bloodstream infection with candida is known as systemic candidiasis.

Oropharyngeal candidiasis, or thrush, is commonly seen in infants, denture wearers, and those individuals who are immunosuppressed, either because of chemotherapy or because of a primary immunocompromising disease such as AIDS. The common symptoms of thrush are dry mouth, the presence of fluffy white lesions on the tongue and buccal surfaces, and loss of taste. In more severe cases, patients may have difficulty eating and swallowing. Scraping the lesions and conducting microscopic examination can confirm the diagnosis; however, the presence of the characteristically white plaque lesions is usually diagnostic. Treatment consists of oral agents, such as a swish and swallow of an antifungal agent or an antifungal lozenge.

A more severe type of oral candidiasis is Esophageal candidiasis, which is found in patients who are immunocompromised and patients who have hematologic malignancies. The major symptom is painful swallowing, known as odynophagia. Endoscopic examination of the esophagus is the definitive diagnosis, but most times the diagnosis is made by history and clinical signs and symptoms.

Vulvovaginal candidiasis is yeast infection of the female outer genitalia and vaginal canal. It is commonly seen in women with increased estrogen levels, such as those taking oral contraceptives, estrogen therapy, and those who are pregnant. Other risk factors for vulvovaginitis include medications such as antibiotics and steroids, and comorbid conditions of diabetes and HIV infection. Women who use intrauterine devices and diaphragms are also at higher risk for vulvovaginitis. Clinical manifestations include itching and discharge, dyspareunia, dysuria, and vaginal irritation. Physical examination shows a classic white, curdlike watery discharge. Vulvular erythema and swelling may also be present.

Balanitis is a candida infection of the penis that is associated with severe burning and itching. The infection can also be found on the thighs, gluteal folds, buttocks, and scrotum.

Treatment for all the local Candida infections is antifungal medication, either orally or topically.

Aspergillus

Aspergillus is a fungus that grows on carbon sources, such as plants and starchy foods like bread and potatoes. The most common species of Aspergillus that may cause invasive disease are *A. fumigatus* and *A.*

flavus. Aspergillosis is the term used for a group of fungal diseases caused by aspergillus. Mainly a disease of the pulmonary system, it is characterized by a flulike illness, fever, cough, chest pain, dyspnea, and infiltrates on chest x-ray. It is an infection that occurs in immunocompromised, critically ill patients. Patients suffering from hematologic malignancies are particularly vulnerable to invasive fungal infections of the aspergillus type. The major forms of the disease are allergic bronchopulmonary aspergillosis, acute invasive aspergillosis, and disseminated invasive aspergillosis. Exposure to aspergillus can also cause a syndrome termed hypersensitivity pneumonitis, a pulmonary infection that is difficult to diagnose. Aspergillosis is treated with antifungals such as amphotericin B or itraconazole.

Cryptococcus

Cryptococcus is encapsulated yeast that causes meningitis or disseminated disease. There are 19 species in the genus *Cryptococcus*, but only *C. neoformans* is associated with disease in humans. Cryptococcosis is an invasive fungal infection seen in patients who are immunocompromised.

Disseminated cryptococcosis begins with infection of the lungs via inhalation. The infection moves from the lungs into the bloodstream, allowing dissemination to the brain and CNS. Cryptococcus is capable of secreting potent enzymes that allow for its penetration through the bloodbrain barrier. The organism's thick polysaccharide capsule protects it from phagocytosis by macrophages. Cryptococcal infection of the brain is rare, but has arisen in patients with AIDS. Diagnosis is by culture confirmation. Infection requires aggressive treatment with antifungal medications, surgical intervention, and supportive treatments.

Histoplasmosis

Histoplasmosis, also known as Darling's disease, is a fungal disease caused by *Histoplasma capsulatum*, which is a dimorphic fungus that is found in the soil of areas inhabited by bats and birds. It is the most prevalent endemic mycosis in the United States. Most cases of histoplasmosis are self-limiting, but some may develop into systemic infection, especially in patients who are immunocompromised. There are approximately 2,000 cases of acute infections per year in the United States.

Histoplasmosis gains entry into the body through inhalation into the respiratory tract. It then is germinated into yeast. Neutrophils, macrophages, lymphocytes, and natural killer cells are attracted to the site of infection. These defense mechanisms are usually adequate to control the infections, except in immunosuppressed individuals, who usually have a more severe disease course. However, the macrophage infiltration leads to the translocation of the fungus via the lymphatics to other areas. At autopsy, patients with disseminated histoplasmosis have involvement of the liver, spleen, bone marrow, adrenal glands, and the GI tract. Lesions have also been noted in the CNS.

Risk factors for severe disease include patients who are immunocompromised by disease or via treatment with immunosuppressive medications, such as corticosteroids, methotrexate, and tumor necrosis factor-alpha inhibitor therapies.

Pneumocystis Jirovecii

Pneumocystis jirovecii, previously known as *pneumocystis carinii,* is the organism responsible for *Pneumocystis* pneumonia, the most common opportunistic infection in patients infected with HIV. The organism has been recently renamed *Pneumocystis jirovecii* for the researcher, Otto Jirovec, who discovered the microbe as a cause of human infection. The organism, mistaken as a protozoan in the past, is categorized as a fungus.

Pneumocystis infection occurs most often in patients who are immunocompromised by AIDS, chemotherapy, or immunosuppressive agents for solid organ transplant recipients. The fungal organism is a normal inhabitant of the respiratory tract, and in healthy individuals does not cause disease. Severe immunosuppression allows proliferation, and macrophages cannot eradicate the organism. The fungal organism produces hardy spores. When the organism proliferates in the lungs, patients exhibit signs and symptoms of pneumonia that include fever, dyspnea, cough, crackles, hemoptysis, and pulmonary infiltrates on chest x-ray.

Diagnosis of PCP requires sputum analysis obtained by bronchoalveolar lavage, staining procedures that highlight pneumocystis cysts found in sputum samples, and lactic dehydrogenase levels, which indicate degree of lung involvement. Treatment requires antibiotic medication.

Coccidiomycosis

Coccidioides immitis is a fungal organism that resides in the soil of the western United States, Mexico, Central America, and South America. Coccidiomycosis is a fungal infection that is also known as Valley Fever. The fungus is usually dormant but develops long filaments that break off into airborne spores in rainy season. The spores disperse into the air with any disruption of the soil, such as during construction. Infection is caused by inhalation of the particles. It affects humans and animals; however, the disease is not transmitted from person to person. Immunosuppressed persons are more susceptible than others.

Initially the infection begins similar to the flu with coughing, fever, muscle aches, and headache. A macular skin rash can occur. It is usually self-limited in most persons; however, some can develop pneumonia, meningitis, bone and joint infection, or bloodstream infection. Chest x-ray, CT scan, serology, and blood culture are often done to diagnose the disease. Tissue biopsy may be required. Treatment consists of antifungal medications such as fluconazole.

Selected Parasitic Infections

Parasitic infections are uncommon in the United States but frequently affect individuals in underdeveloped countries. Diagnosis is a challenge for the clinician; however, antiparasitic agents are widely available and effective. Some parasitic infections, such as malaria, are endemic to certain areas of the world. With worldwide travel, persons of these areas often bring parasitic diseases to distant regions.

Malaria

There are four protozoan organisms that can infect humans and cause malaria:

1. *Plasmodium falciparum*
2. *Plasmodium vivax*
3. *Plasmodium ovale*
4. *Plasmodium malariae.*

All of these parasites are transmitted to humans via the Anopheles mosquito. Through widespread pesticide utilization in the 1950s, mosquito control has led to malaria eradication in North America, Russia, and Europe; however, it remains a problem in Africa, South and Central America, and parts of Asia.

Malaria most commonly occurs when the female Anopheles mosquito bites a human and injects the microscopic plasmodium parasites into the bloodstream. However, malaria can be transmitted to individuals from blood products, contaminated needlesticks, or organ transplantation. From the bloodstream, the parasites invade the liver and multiply within the hepatocytes, which then burst and release the organisms into the blood. The organisms enter red blood cells (RBCs), where they multiply vigorously and degrade the blood cell constituents, particularly hemoglobin. In *Fulminant parasitemia*, RBCs become deformed, obstruct small blood vessels, die, and accumulate within the spleen. This destruction of RBCs causes accumulation of bilirubin from hemoglobin breakdown, resulting in jaundice. Hemoglobinuria can also cause renal damage. The sequelae of malaria may also include hemolytic anemia, hepatomegaly, splenomegaly, and eventual splenic rupture.

The release of plasmodium organisms from dead RBCs induces an immune response within the host that includes a characteristic pattern of fever and chills that occurs every 2 to 3 days. Headache, myalgia, nausea, vomiting, and orthostatic hypotension are common. In many individuals, a strong immune response can suppress the disease so that the individual has asymptomatic periods in life.

Diagnosis of malaria is based on demonstration of the parasite within RBCs on a peripheral blood smear. Repeat blood smears are necessary to obtain a sample with proof of the organism. In general, patients with greater than 10^5 parasites per microliter are considered to have a poor prognosis. Serological testing that demonstrates the specific antibody against plasmodium is also used to diagnose malaria.

Chloroquine is the major medication used to treat malaria; however, resistant strains are widespread. Other medication regimens such as sulfadoxine plus pyrimethamine or quinine plus tetracycline are used for resistant organisms. Mefloquine is a prophylactic medication that is recommended for those who travel to areas where malaria remains a transmissible disease. Travelers are advised to consult the Centers for Disease Control and Prevention for up-to-date recommendations about malaria prophylaxis.

Toxoplasmosis

Toxoplasmosis is a disease caused by the parasite protozoan *Toxoplasma gondii*. It infects warm-blooded animals, including humans, but the primary host is the cat. Pregnant women and immunosuppressed individuals are at high risk for toxoplasmosis infection. In the pregnant woman, the infection may cause congenital disease in the fetus. The newborn can experience complications that range from vision impairment to significant learning disabilities or death. Most infants born with toxoplasmosis are asymptomatic at birth, though some have fever, maculopapular rash, hepatosplenomegaly, microcephaly, seizures, jaundice, thrombocytopenia, and rarely generalized lymphadenopathy. The symptoms of chorioretinitis, hydrocephalus, and intracranial calcifications have been considered the classic triad.

In the immunosuppressed adult, toxoplasmosis infection symptoms are similar to those of a mild flulike illness. The parasite can cause encephalitis and progressive neurological diseases that can also extend to the heart, liver, and eyes. Transmission can occur through the ingestion of raw or partly cooked meat, specifically pork, lamb, and venison. Oocysts (eggs of the organism) may be found on hands of people who handle the meat or on contaminated cooking utensils. Contamination can also occur by ingestion of toxoplasmosis-contaminated cat feces. For this reason, pregnant women and immunosuppressed individuals are cautioned against handling cat litter boxes. The infection can also be contracted from contaminated drinking water and infected organ transplant or blood transfusion.

Amebiasis and Giardiasis

Amebiasis and giardiasis are both water-borne protozoan infections. Amebiasis is caused by the protozoan parasite *Entamoeba histolytica*. Giardiasis is caused by *Giardia lamblia (G. lamblia)*. Amebiasis and giardiasis are contracted by consuming contaminated food or water containing the cyst stage of the parasite. The cyst stage is a hardy form of the organism that is resistant to gastric acid. After ingestion, the cysts can develop into the motile organism referred to as the trophozoite form. Trophozoites adhere to and lyse the epithelial cells of the gastrointestinal tract and cause necrosis. Organisms are commonly transmitted via contaminated water or the fecal-oral route. Anal-oral sexual activity can also transmit the organisms.

Individuals can carry the parasite for weeks to years, often without symptoms. The majority of cases of amebiasis and giardiasis are asymptomatic; however, significant morbidity and mortality are associated with the dysentery form of illness. The trophozoite form of the protozoan (motile organism) is responsible for the clinical syndrome referred to as dysentery. This syndrome is associated with nausea, vomiting, intense abdominal pain, tenderness, and copious diarrhea of watery stool, sometimes with blood. Microscopic identification of *E. histolytica* or *G. lamblia* in stool culture is the basis for diagnosis. Amebic dysentery is treated with metronidazole, amebicides, and supportive measures. Giardiasis is treated with metronidazole.

Leshmaniasis

Leshmaniasis is a disease caused by a protozoan of the genus *Leshmania* that infects mammalian reservoir hosts, and in particular rodents. The prevalence among soldiers returning from the Persian Gulf is higher than in the general population because sandflies that bite the infected rodents act as vectors by then biting humans. The protozoan invades the bloodstream and can then invade body organs. Asymptomatic infection is common, though the protozoan can cause fever, splenomegaly, lymphadenopathy, hepatomegaly, cachexia, and gray discoloration of the skin. Diagnosis is made by demonstration of the organism from microscopic staining, histological tissue sampling, or culture. Serological testing for specific *Leshmania*-specific cell-mediated immunity is also used. Vector control with pesticides, protective garments, and insect repellents are the best methods to prevent infection. Different types of antibiotic agents have been moderately effective for treatment.

Helminth Infections

Parasitic helminths, commonly known as worms, cause infectious disease in animals and humans. The parasite's life cycle, which ranges from egg to larva to adult stages, influences the clinical course and manifestations of the infection. Some of these infections can be transmitted directly from infected to uninfected persons; in others, eggs must mature outside the human host before the larva gains entry into the host. Alternatively, some parasitic worms mature from egg to adult and spend a part of their life cycle in the soil before becoming infective to humans.

In general, repeated or intense exposure to a multitude of helminths in the infective stage is required for infection to be established and disease to arise. Significant helminthic diseases include enterobiasis (pinworms), trichuriasis, ascariasis (roundworm), hookworm, strongyloides, trichinosis, filariasis, schistosomiasis, and tapeworm infection.

Many helminth infections are more prevalent in tropical areas with warm, moist climates. Trichuriasis, an infection with the helminth *Trichuris trichuria,* is one of the most prevalent worldwide; infection rates of up to 75% have been found in young schoolchildren in Puerto Rico. Ascariasis, hookworm infection, and strongyloidiasis are common infections in tropical countries with poor sanitation.

Enterobiasis is caused by pinworms and is a highly prevalent disease throughout the world, particularly in children. Unsanitary hygiene measures that spread the helminth via the fecal-oral route perpetuate the infection. Typically, children are infected by unknowingly touching pinworm eggs and putting their fingers in their mouths. The eggs are swallowed and hatch in the small intestine before maturing in the colon. Female worms then move to the child's anal area, especially at night, and deposit eggs. This usually causes intense itching. When the child scratches the perineal area, the eggs can get under the child's fingernails. These eggs can be transferred to other children, family members, and items in the house. A tape test can be done where a piece of cellophane tape is pressed against the skin around the anus, and removed. This should be done in the morning before bathing or using the toilet, because bathing and wiping may remove eggs. The tape is then placed on a slide to review with a microscope to look for eggs. The antihelminthic medication mebendazole is used to eradicate the infection.

Helminths can also be transmitted in undercooked food. Trichinosis is a disease caused by the *Trichinella* worm that is harbored within carnivorous animals. Contraction of the infection occurs by ingestion of the helminth within uncooked meat. When a person eats meat from an infected animal, *Trichinella* cysts break open in the intestines and grow into adult roundworms. The infection can move through the gastrointestinal wall and into the bloodstream. These organisms tend to invade muscle tissues, including the heart and diaphragm. They can also affect the lungs and brain. Intense abdominal pain, diarrhea, fever, and muscle pain occur. A muscle biopsy is needed to confirm diagnosis. The antihelminthic medication mebendazole is used for treatment. Avoiding raw meat and cooking meat well enough (to greater than 160°F) will prevent infection.

Taenia saginata, commonly known as the tapeworm, causes infection of humans mainly by ingestion of taenia eggs contained in undercooked beef or contaminated vegetation. After ingestion, the tapeworm attaches to the intestinal wall. The worm then depletes the patient of nutrients to support its own growth.

Tapeworms can grow to as long as 8 meters within the digestive tract and can live for years. Clinical signs and symptoms include abdominal pain, nausea, anorexia, weight loss, and passage of eggs in the stool. Segments of the worm can be passed in stool. If pork tapeworm larvae move out of the intestine, they can cause local growths and damage tissues such as the brain, eye, or heart. This condition is called cysticercosis. Infection of the brain can cause seizures and other nervous system problems. Avoiding raw meat and cooking meat well enough (to greater than 160°F) will prevent tapeworm infection. Freezing meats to −4°F for 24 hours also kills tapeworm eggs. Antihelminthic medications praziquantel and niclosamide are used for treatment.

Prion Infectious Disease

Prions are infectious agents composed of abnormal proteins. Similar to viruses, prions require a host, where it can use the host cell machinery to replicate itself. How a prion is formed is not completely understood. However, it is known that when a prion enters a healthy organism, it induces existing, properly formed proteins to convert into the disease-associated, prion forms. Newly synthesized prions then go on to convert more proteins into prions. Prion agents cause several diseases, and the diseases share a common symptom: progressive neurological deterioration of the brain.

Creutzfeldt-Jakob Disease

Creutzfeldt-Jakob disease (CJD) is a rare but fatal degenerative neurological disease caused by a prion. CJD causes progressive death of the brain's nerve cells; brain tissue pathology demonstrates a spongiform appearance of the brain tissue. It affects people between the ages of 45 and 75 years. The duration of the disease varies, but it is fatal within months or even weeks. In more than 85% of the cases, the duration of CJD is less than 1 year after onset of symptoms.

The first symptom of CJD is rapidly progressive dementia, with memory loss, personality changes, and hallucinations. This is accompanied by speech impairment,

myoclonus (involuntary jerky muscle movements), ataxia, and seizures. The diagnostic tests for the diagnosis of CJD are electroencephalography (triphasic spikes seen), CSF analysis for 14-3-3 proteins, and brain MRI, which shows high signal intensity bilaterally in the caudate nucleus and putamen. The only definitive diagnostic test, however, is biopsy of the brain. There is no treatment or cure for CJD.

Variant Creutzfeldt-Jakob Disease

Variant Creutzfeldt-Jakob disease is a new form of CJD that has been noted mostly in the United Kingdom and France. It is different from CJD in that it affects younger people, with the average age of onset at 33 years. It is believed to be caused by the same infectious agent that causes bovine spongiform encephalopathy (BSE), also called "mad cow disease." The symptoms begin with psychiatric problems or problems with hearing, seeing, or smelling. The first symptoms are noted for weeks or months, and then progress to poor muscle coordination, muscle spasms, and mental confusion. Death occurs an average of 13 months after the first symptoms are noted.

Bovine Spongiform Encephalopathy

Bovine spongiform encephalopathy, also known as mad cow disease, is a progressive neurological disorder of cattle; the infectious agent is unknown. The most accepted theory is that the agent is a prion.

The vast majority of cases of BSE have been reported from the United Kingdom, but other cases have been reported throughout Europe—and both Canada and the United States have reported at least one case.

The disease is spread via meat-and-bone meal fed to cattle. The mechanism of disease is unknown; however, the natural diet of cows is not meat, and this type of feed may be causative. In response to a BSE outbreak, the United Kingdom placed many restrictions on the meat industry, from the slaughter of cattle to the restriction of feed and how the meat is cooked. In the United States, the U.S. Department of Agriculture has placed a prohibition on the importation of livestock from countries where BSE is known to exist.

Chapter Summary

- The body's normal flora are organisms that colonize the body but do not normally cause infection.
- The body has an innate and adaptive immune system for defending against invading pathogens.
- An antibody titer is the level of antibodies against the pathogen in the bloodstream.
- When these defense mechanisms fail, the body is susceptible to colonization and infection by bacteria, viruses, prions, fungi, or parasites.

- In infectious disease, the host is the infected being, the reservoir is the source of pathogens, and the vector is the organism that can transmit the pathogen.
- The microorganism gains entry via a portal such as skin; the respiratory, gastrointestinal, or genitourinary tracts; or is transmitted via blood or maternal-fetal pathways.
- Bacteria are categorized as cocci, streptococci, bacillus, and spirochetes.

- Bacteria are categorized as gram negative or gram positive according to how their membranes take up Gram stain. Specific antibiotics are effective against each.

- The five distinct phases of infection are incubation, prodrome, infection, convalescence, and resolution.

- Culture and sensitivity is the common method of diagnosis in bacterial disease.

- Viral exanthems are specific rash-inducing infections that occur in childhood and include measles, rubella, and varicella.

- An opportunistic infection occurs in an immunosuppressed patient.

- A nosocomial infection is contracted from the clinical setting.

- MRSA, VRSA, VRE, and DRSP are known as antibiotic-resistant bacteria.

- In the United States, there are a wide number of antibiotic medications available to treat infectious diseases. There are also a great number of immunizations in the arsenal against infections.

- Many infectious diseases have been virtually eradicated in the United States because of successful vaccination campaigns.

- Microorganisms are constantly mutating and developing resistance to the available antibiotics. In addition, some individuals choose to not get immunized. These factors increase the susceptibility of the population to infectious disease.

- Certain highly virulent pathogens are considered possible bioterrorist weapons.

Bibliography

Arias, C. A., & Murray, B. E. (2009). Antibiotic-resistant bugs in the 21st century—a clinical super-challenge. *N Engl J Med*, 360(5), 439–443.

Biesbroeck, L., & Sidbury, R. (2013). Viral exanthems: an update. *Dermatol Ther*, 26(6), 433–438. doi: 10.1111/dth.12107.

Cayley, W. E., Jr. (2010). Neuraminidase inhibitors for influenza treatment and prevention in healthy adults. *Am Fam Phys*, 82(3), 242–244.

Centers for Disease Control & Prevention. (2011, February 4). Recommended adult immunization schedule—United States 2011. *MMWR*, 60(4).

Choby, B. A. (2009). Diagnosis and treatment of streptococcal pharyngitis. *Am Fam Phys*, 79 (5), 383–390.

Diep, B. A. (2013). Use of whole-genome sequencing for outbreak investigations. *Lancet Infect Disease,* 13(2), 99–101. doi: 10.1016/S1473-3099(12)70276-1. Epub 2012 Nov 14.

Edson, R. S., Bundrick, J. B., & Litin, S. C. (2011). Clinical pearls in infectious diseases. *Mayo Clin Proceed*. 86(3), 245–248.

Fauci, A. S., & Morens, D. M. (2012). The perpetual challenge of infectious diseases. *N Engl J Med*, 366(5), 454–461.

Feldmann, H., & Geisbert, T. W. (2011). Ebola haemorrhagic fever. *Lancet*, 377(9768), 849–862.

Hitzeman, N., & Dyer, A. (2010). Influenza vaccination of health care personnel working with older patients. *Am Fam Phys*, 82(7), 763–764.

Ilgenfritz, S., Dowlatshahi, C., & Salkind, A. (2013, October). Acute rheumatic fever: case report and review for emergency physicians. *J Emerg Med,* 45(4), e103–e106. doi: 0.1016/j.jemermed.2013.04.037. Epub 2013 Aug 2.

Kappagoda, S., Singh, U., & Blackburn, B. G. (2011). Antiparasitic therapy. *Mayo Clin Proceed*, 86(6), 561–583.

Kumar, V., Abbas, A. K., Fausto, N., & Aster, J. (2010). *Robbins & Cotran pathologic basis of disease.* 8th ed. Philadelphia, PA: WB Saunders.

Lambert, M. (2011). IDSA guidelines on the treatment of MRSA infections in adults and children. *Am Fam Phys*, 84(4), 455–463.

Leekha, S., Terrell, C., & Edson, R. (2011). General principles of antimicrobial therapy. *Mayo Clin Proceed*, 86(2), 156–167.

Lin, J. N., Chang, L. L., Lai, C. H., Lin, H. H., & Chen, Y. H. (2013). Group A streptococcal necrotizing fasciitis in the emergency department. *J Emerg Med*, 45(5), 781–788. doi: 10.1016/j.jemermed.2013.05.046.

Longo, D., Fauci, A., Braunwald, E., et al. (2012). *Harrison's principles of internal medicine.* 18th ed. New York: McGraw-Hill.

Lowy, F. D. (2013). Methicillin-resistant *Staphylococcus aureus*: where is it coming from and where is it going? *JAMA Intern Med*, 173(21), 1978–1979. doi: 10.1001/jamainternmed .2013.8277.

Lu, P. J., Euler, G. L., & Harpaz, R. (2011). Herpes zoster vaccination among adults aged 60 years and older, in the U.S. *Am J Prev Med*, 40(2), 1–6.

Luzuriaga, K., & Sullivan, J. L. (2010). Infectious mononucleosis. *N Engl J Med*, 362(21), 1993–2000.

Moss, W. J., & Griffin, D. E. (2012). Measles. *Lancet*, 379(9811), 153–164. Epub 2011 Aug 17.

Mulholland, E. K., Griffiths, U. K., & Biellik, R. (2012, May 10). Measles in the 21st century. *N Engl J Med,* 366(19), 1755–1757. doi: 10.1056/NEJMp1202396.

Parker Fiebelkorn, A., Redd, S. B., Gallagher, K., et al. (2010). Measles in the United States during the postelimination era. *J Infect Dis*, 202(10), 1520–1528.

Poland, G. A., & Jacobson, R. M. (2011). The age-old struggle against the antivaccinationists. *N Engl J Med,* 364(2), 97–99. doi: 10.1056/NEJMp1010594.

Post-polio syndrome: unraveling the mystery. (2011). *Nursing*, 41(2), 29–30.

Rivera, A. M., & Boucher, H. W. (2011). Current concepts in antimicrobial therapy against select gram-positive organisms: methicillin-resistant *Staphylococcus aureus*, penicillin-resistant pneumococci, and vancomycin-resistant enterococci. *Mayo Clin Proceed*, 86(12), 1230–1243.

Rossi, F., Diaz, L., Wollam, A., et al. (2014). Transferable vancomycin resistance in a community-associated MRSA lineage. *N Engl J Med,* 370(16), 1524–1531. doi: 10.1056/ NEJMoa1303359.

Salles, J. M., Salles, M. J., Moraes, L. A., & Silva, M. C. (2007). Invasive amebiasis: an update on diagnosis and management. *Exp Rev Anti-Infect Ther*, 5(5), 893–901.

Sandora, T. J., & Goldmann, D. A. (2012). Preventing lethal hospital outbreaks of antibiotic-resistant bacteria. *N Engl J Med*, 367(23), 2168–2170. doi: 10.1056/NEJMp1212370.

Sepkowitz, K. A. (2009). Forever unprepared—the predictable unpredictability of pathogens. *N Engl J Med*, 361(2), 120–121.

Shetty, P. (2010). Experts concerned about vaccination backlash. *Lancet*, 375(9719), 970–971.

Tan, L. K., Carlone, G. M., & Borrow, R. (2010). Advances in the development of vaccines against *Neisseria meningitidis*. *N Engl J Med*, 362(16), 1511–1520.

Temte, J. L. (2009). Basic rules of influenza: how to combat the H1N1 influenza (swine flu) virus. *Am Fam Phys*, 79(11), 938–939.

Thera, M. A., Doumbo, O. K., Coulibaly, D., et al. (2011). A field trial to assess a blood-stage malaria vaccine. *N Engl J Med*, 365(11), 1004–1013.

Thigpen, M. C., Whitney, C. G., Messonnier, N. E., et al. (2011). Bacterial meningitis in the United States, 1998–2007. *N Engl J Med*, 364(21), 2016–2025.

Usatine, R. P., & Tinitigan, R. (2010). Nongenital herpes simplex virus. *Am Fam Phys*, 82(9), 1075–1082.

Uyeki, T. M. (2010). 2009 H1N1 virus transmission and outbreaks. *N Engl J Med*, 362(23), 2221–2223.

Watkins, R. R., & Lemonovich, T. L. (2011). Diagnosis and management of community-acquired pneumonia in adults. *Am Fam Phys*, 83(11), 1299–1306.

Wright, W. F., Riedel, D. J., Talwani, R., & Gilliam, B. L. (2012). Diagnosis and management of Lyme disease. *Am Fam Phys*, 85(11), 1086–1093.

Disorders of the Immune System

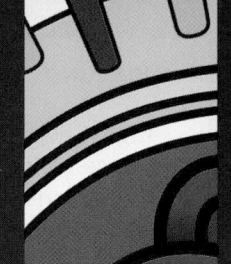

Key Terms

Acquired immune deficiency syndrome (AIDS)

Active acquired adaptive immunity

Adaptive immunity

AIDS

Amnestic response

Anergy panel

Antibody titer

Antigen

Autoimmune disease

Autoimmunity

B lymphocyte

Booster

CD4 cell

Cell-mediated immunity

Dendritic cell

HIV RNA assay

Human immunodeficiency virus (HIV)

Hypersensitivity

Immunodeficiency

Immunoglobulins (Igs)

Innate immunity

Major histocompatibility complexes (MHCs)

Molecular mimicry

Passive acquired adaptive immunity

Raynaud's phenomenon

Systemic anaphylaxis

T lymphocyte

Toxoid

Vaccine

The immune system is a complex defense mechanism that protects humans from a constant barrage of injurious agents in the environment, including microbes such as viruses, bacteria, fungi, and parasites. In addition, many foreign substances that are ingested, inhaled, and absorbed are potentially damaging agents. The immune system can decipher which substances are "self" versus "non-self." Non-self substances, also called **antigens,** are the targets of the immune system. A vital immune system, in conjunction with the inflammatory reaction of the body, rapidly identifies an antigen and subjects it to barriers and protective cellular forces that destroy the threat.

There are two basic parts of the immune system:

1. **innate immunity**
2. **adaptive immunity.**

The innate immune mechanism comes to the body's defense first and immediately. It is composed of the body's natural anatomic barriers, normal flora, white blood cells (WBCs), and protective enzymes and chemicals. Natural anatomic barriers include skin and mucous membranes, whereas normal flora includes bacteria that live on the skin and within the gastrointestinal (GI) tract. The WBCs are macrophages that phagocytose foreign debris and antigens. Interferon, cytokines, and hydrochloric acid are some of the protective enzymes and chemicals that protect the body from bacteria and viruses.

The adaptive immune system comes to the body's defense after the innate system. A more specific form of protection, the adaptive immune line of defense, is developed after exposure to antigens. However, after exposure, the adaptive immune mechanisms act rapidly, specifically, destructively, and with memory for every individual antigen it has encountered.

In a type of immune dysfunction called **immunodeficiency,** the immune system can weaken to the extent that it cannot destroy foreign invaders, and antigens can overwhelm the body. Alternatively, in a type of immune dysfunction called **autoimmunity,** the immune system can no longer distinguish between self and non-self. In autoimmune disorders, the immune system attacks non-self and self antigens indiscriminately. Lastly, in **hypersensitivity** disorders, which can take the form of a simple case of hives to life-threatening transplant rejection, the immune system can become overreactive against foreign invaders.

Basic Concepts of Immunity

Immunity is the way the body defends itself against injurious agents in the environment. To understand the mechanism of immunity, basic concepts of immunology need to be introduced first.

Innate Immunity

Innate immunity refers to natural mechanisms that ward off invaders as a first line of defense. The major component of innate immunity consists of anatomic barriers that block entry of environmental antigens, such as the nasal epithelium, which consists of mucus-producing cells and hairs that trap inhaled substances before they enter the respiratory tract. Innate immunity also consists of phagocytic cells that engulf and ingest microorganisms and other noxious substances. These cells, known as macrophages, provide constant surveillance in different organ systems; they are recruited to sites of infection and stimulate the inflammation reaction. Examples include alveolar macrophages in the lungs, Kupffer cells in the liver, and microglial cells in the brain. Innate barriers also include natural killer (NK) cells, which are a specific kind of T lymphocyte that directly attacks antigens, and the complement system of the inflammation reaction, which is a legion of proteins that bind to antigens in the innate system and to antibodies in the adaptive system. Lastly, innate immunity includes natural enzymes, bactericidal and antiviral substances, and acidic secretions that make the skin and mucous membranes inhospitable to pathogens.

If a foreign invader attempts to enter the body, it must deal with the innate immune system first. For example, when an individual inhales infectious bacteria, mucus and ciliated epithelium trap the pathogen in the respiratory tract, which allows the cough reflex to expel the microbe.

Other innate mechanisms of defense include processes within the GI tract. Within the initial section of the GI tract, pathogens are weakened by enzymes and antibacterial substances in the saliva. Further along in the GI tract, gastric mucus traps pathogens and destroys them with hydrochloric acid. Should the pathogen survive these innate defenses and make its way into the intestine and bowel, the body defends itself with normal flora—natural bacterial colonies that live in symbiosis with the body. Other innate barriers include tears, which flush pathogens out of the eyes; urine, which eliminates antigens from the genitourinary tract; and sweat, which acts as an antibacterial barrier on skin.

Once the innate line of defense is compromised, the inflammatory reaction begins within seconds and has the potential to last minutes or even days. If the innate defense mechanisms prove inadequate to deal with a foreign invader, the second line of defense, the adaptive immune system, is activated.

Monocyte–Macrophages

Macrophages arise from WBCs called monocytes. Monocytes leave the peripheral circulation and migrate to the tissues. Common locations where tissue macrophages are found include the lymph nodes, spleen, bone marrow, perivascular connective tissue, skin, lungs, liver, bone, central nervous system (CNS), synovial membranes, and serous cavities such as the peritoneal and pleural spaces. Macrophages mediate innate immune functions, such as destruction of bacteria and tumor cells. The macrophages ingest bacteria or viruses and then undergo apoptosis, or self-degeneration. Macrophages that are infected and apoptotic are phagocytosed by dendritic antigen-presenting cells (APCs). The destruction of pathogens by phagocytosis is largely mediated by cytokines.

Macrophage secretory products, which are more diverse than those of any other cells, have the ability to break down various types of antigens. Secretory products include hydrolytic enzymes, oxidative metabolites, TNF-alpha, interleukins (ILs), and other cytokines.

Cytokines

Cytokines are inflammatory mediators produced by WBCs, mainly macrophages and lymphocytes. These inflammatory mediators promote leukocyte recruitment and acute inflammation reactions; regulate lymphocyte growth, activation, and differentiation; activate macrophages; and stimulate growth and production of new blood cells.

Natural Killer Cells

NK cells are lymphocytes that contain cytoplasmic granules, which is why they are also called granular lymphocytes. They are part of the innate immune response and act as a first-line defense. NK cells can destroy tumor cells and virus-infected cells without previous exposure.

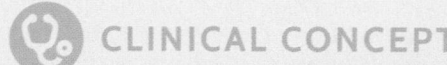

CLINICAL CONCEPT

Cytokines, which act as inflammatory mediators, include tumor necrosis factor-alpha (TNF-alpha), prostaglandins, and ILs. Many anti-inflammatory drugs are designed to counteract these mediators.

Adaptive Immunity

The adaptive immune system allows the body to recognize an antigen, target the specific antigen, limit its response to that antigen, and develop memory for the antigen for future reference. The adaptive immune system's ability to recognize and remember specific antigens is called specificity. The ability to respond again and again to specific antigens is caused by a memory response, which develops after a second exposure to an antigen.

The ability to distinguish self from non-self is another vital function of the adaptive immune system. Every human cell has surface antigens called **major histocompatibility complexes (MHCs),** also called human leukocyte antigens (HLAs). The adaptive immune system allows the body to distinguish between antigens that belong to the host versus antigens that are from an invader.

B Lymphocytes and T Lymphocytes

There are two major categories of adaptive immunity:

1. B lymphocyte immunity, also known as humoral immunity
2. T lymphocyte immunity, also known as **cell-mediated immunity**.

In both categories of adaptive immunity, the lymphocyte is the primary cell. Lymphocytes originate in the bone marrow in immature form and cannot initiate immunity until mature, which occurs as they pass through lymphoid tissues such as the thymus, spleen, and lymph nodes. **T lymphocytes,** also called T cells, mature within the thymus gland, which is a small gland located in midchest that degenerates with age. After maturation in the thymus, mature T cells are found in the bloodstream and T cell zones of lymph nodes. **B lymphocytes,** also called B cells, mature within the bone marrow, spleen, and lymph nodes.

CD4 and CD8 Cells

During the maturation process in the thymus, T cells begin developing surface antigens that differentiate them from one another. These are called cluster of differentiation (CD) antigens. The most common T cells that take part in cell-mediated immunity are called CD4 cells, also called T helper cells, and CD8 cells, also called cytotoxic T cells. CD4 cells and CD8 cells perform distinct but overlapping functions. The **CD4 cell** influences all other cells of the immune system, including other T cells, B lymphocytes, macrophages, and NK cells. The CD4 cells are involved in cell-mediated immunity and also assist in antibody-mediated adaptive immunity. The CD8 cell directly attacks an antigen. Human immunodeficiency virus (HIV) targets CD4 cells. By targeting CD4 cells, HIV defeats both cell-mediated and antibody-mediated immune responses, the human body's strongest two defense mechanisms.

Antigen-Presenting Cells

T cells cannot be activated by antigen alone; antigen-presenting cells (APCs) process the antigen first and induce cell-mediated immunity (see Fig. 11-1). APCs capture and attach to antigen and process it before the antigen is attacked. APCs include dendritic cells and macrophages. **Dendritic cells,** which are named for their numerous fine dendritic cytoplasmic projections, attach to the broadest range of antigens. They are located within epidermis and mucous membranes where antigens enter the body. When dendritic cells come in contact with bacteria or viruses, they release cytokines that stimulate cells of the innate and adaptive immune systems to respond.

Plasma Cells

B lymphocytes, also called B cells, are naïve or immature until they encounter antigens. After exposure to an antigen, B cells are stimulated to further mature into plasma cells. As plasma cells, they have the ability to produce specific proteins called immunoglobulins (Igs), also called antibodies, which attack the antigen. The process of B cell maturation into plasma cells and Ig production comprises antibody-mediated immunity, also called humoral immunity (see Fig. 11-2). Antibody-mediated immunity confers long-term immunity, though full initiation of this immune response takes time.

Upon first exposure to the antigen, the process of B cell maturation into plasma cells that synthesize

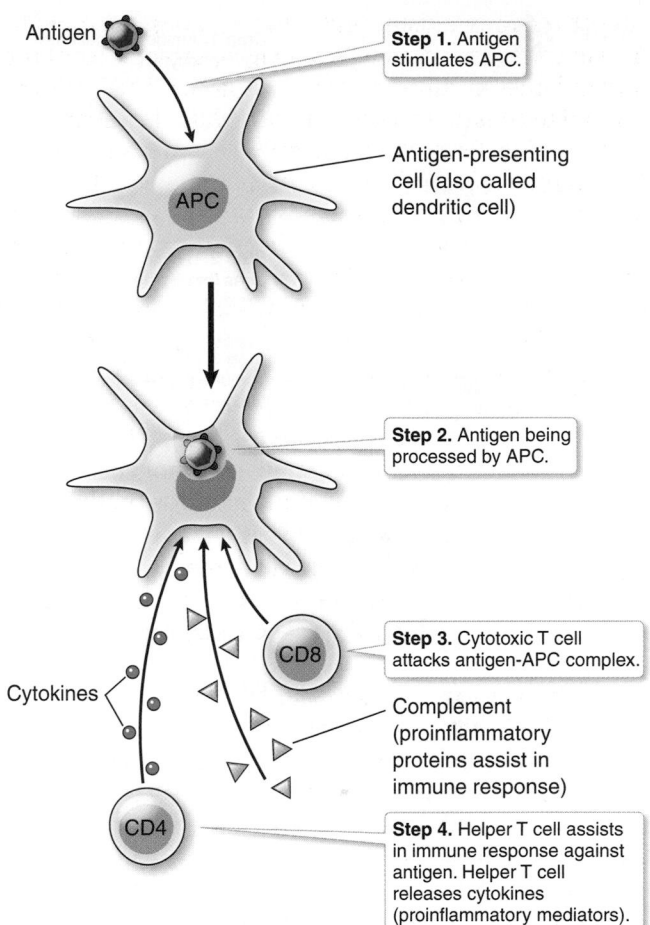

Figure 11-1. Cell-mediated immunity is an immune response that involves the activation of cytotoxic T lymphocytes, called CD8 cells. Step 1. An antigen provokes an antigen-presenting cell (APC). Step 2. The APC processes the antigen. Step 3. CD8 cells attack the antigen processed by the APC. Concurrently, a helper T cell assists the CD8 cell in the attack and yields cytokines that promote an inflammatory reaction. Proteins called complement also take part in the proinflammatory process.

immunoglobulins takes days to initiate. Problems can occur when pathogens overwhelm the body before full initiation of the antibody-mediated immune response. The components of the T cell-mediated immune response become activated more quickly than the antibody-mediated immune response. During the lag time of B cell maturation, CD4 cells attack antigens to blunt the pathogen effect on the body. In this manner, CD4 cells are integral to the antibody-mediated immune response.

Immunoglobulins

The terms antibody and immunoglobulin are interchangeable. An **immunoglobulin (Ig)** is a product of a plasma cell that is derived from a B lymphocyte. An antigen stimulates a B lymphocyte to mature into a plasma cell which, in turn, develops the ability to synthesize Igs. Antibody-mediated immunity involves five subtypes of Igs: IgM, IgG, IgA, IgE, and IgD. These Igs are categorized by structural and functional differences. They are continually circulating

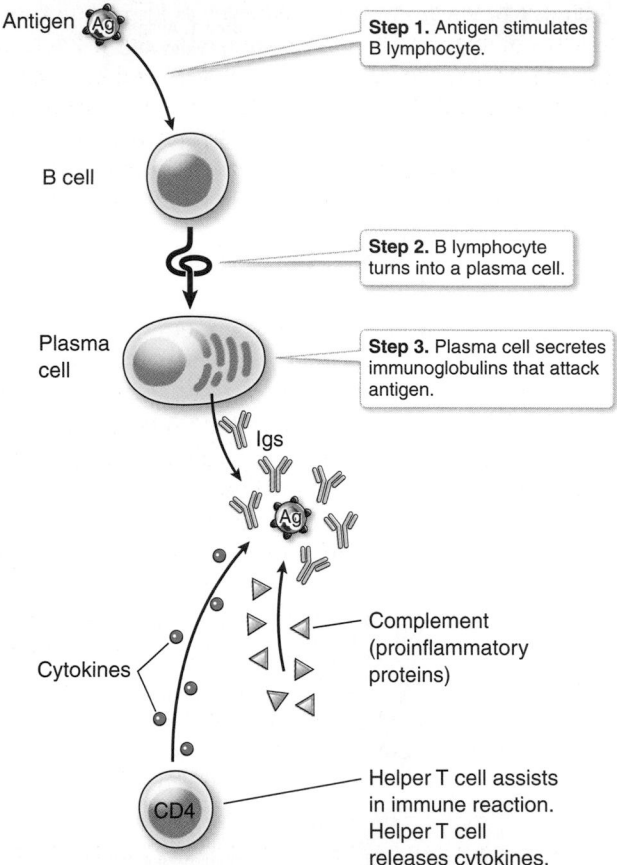

Figure 11-2. Antibody-mediated immunity is an immune response that involves the activation of B lymphocytes and Igs. Step 1. The antigen stimulates a B lymphocyte. Step 2. The B lymphocyte transforms into a plasma cell. Step 3. The plasma cell secretes Igs. Concurrently, a helper T cell assists in the attack and yields cytokines that promote an inflammatory reaction. Proteins called complement also take part in the proinflammatory process.

through the lymph system, bone marrow, and other lymphoid organs. As a group, Igs are responsible for neutralizing bacterial toxins, attacking viruses, promoting phagocytosis of bacteria, and activating and reactivating the immune response.

Igs circulate within the bloodstream and body fluids and float suspended and inactive. Once an antigen is presented and recognized, Igs directly attack the antigen. The initiation of the response begins with the binding of the immunoglobulin to antigen. Physically, once bound, the antigen is no longer able to bind to another cell, and therefore cannot infect any other cell nor reproduce its antigenic parts. Chemically, the antigen is targeted for phagocytosis, and proliferation of B cells begins with development of plasma cells ready to destroy the antigenic invader.

The body's antibody-mediated response to an antigen consists of two phases: primary and secondary. The primary phase occurs when the host cell is exposed to an antigenic invader and there is a lag time between recognition and proliferation of Igs to neutralize the invader. There can be a lag time of 5 to 7 days before

an increase in IgM, the primary immunoglobulin responder, can be detected. The increase in IgM marks the primary response. Once the pathogen is eradicated, the existing Igs degrade and immunoglobulin levels return to normal.

A second exposure to the same antigen initiates a secondary immune response, known as an **amnestic response,** that stimulates a quick increase in levels of Igs. During this time an increase in IgG occurs, comprising approximately 75% to 85% of total serum Igs. IgG is the predominant immunoglobulin made after the host's reexposure to antigen. IgA comprises 7% to 15% of total serum Igs, but it is mainly found within secretions, such as tears, saliva, nasal and respiratory secretions, GI fluid, and breast milk. IgE is usually present in very low concentrations in the blood but it rises to high levels in allergic reactions. IgD, which binds to basophils and mast cells in hypersensitivity reactions, comprises only 1% of Igs.

CLINICAL CONCEPT

IgM Igs are large antibodies that increase in the bloodstream after the first exposure to an antigen. During a pregnancy in which the mother and fetus have incompatible blood types, IgM antibodies are developed by the mother against the fetus's blood cells. However, because of their large size, they cannot cross the placenta and the fetus is protected.

Active Acquired Versus Passive Acquired Immunity

Adaptive immunity can be categorized as actively acquired or passively acquired. **Active acquired adaptive immunity** is obtained through exposure to an antigen or through immunization; it is developed after an individual experiences an illness or has exposure to a pathogen. For example, after a child contracts measles infection (rubeola), the child develops active acquired adaptive immunity: The child's body has to process the antigen and develop B cells and plasma cells that secrete Igs while enduring the disease. The child develops all the symptoms of disease but at the same time develops significant Igs for life. The Igs are specific for measles and are remembered by the B cells. Because the child's body actively developed immunity, future exposure to measles will be dealt with by the preformed Igs.

Alternatively, a child can receive a measles immunization to develop active acquired adaptive immunity. An immunization or **vaccine** is a specific formulation that contains a weakened, nondisease producing pathogen. It cannot cause actual disease but it can stimulate the adaptive immune system. The vaccine is "seen" by the adaptive immune system as an actual antigen, despite its nondisease producing attributes. The body recognizes the vaccine as an antigen and develops an immune response and memory of the antigen without direct disease contraction. Also, any future exposure to the antigen will be dealt with by the preformed Igs.

In both forms of active acquired immunity, the body recognizes an antigen, develops immune cells specifically against the antigen, attacks and neutralizes the antigen, remembers the antigen, and develops long-lasting immunity. The body has to perform the activities needed to develop immunity in both forms of active acquired adaptive immunity.

The other type of adaptive immunity is called **passive acquired adaptive immunity.** To gain this form of immunity, an individual is given premade, fully formed antibodies against an antigen. The patient is a passive recipient of the antibodies and his or her body does not have to perform the actions needed to develop immunity. It is immediate immunity, but it is also short-term immunity, not long lasting. An example involves hepatitis B immunoglobulin (called HBIg). If a member of a family develops hepatitis B infection, the other family members need immediate immunity, which can be conferred though administration of HBIg. The family members receive an injection of preformed IgG against hepatitis B for instant, short-term immunity. The family members can then be protected during their exposure to the infected individual.

 CLINICAL CONCEPT

An example of passive acquired adaptive immunity occurs when an infant is breastfed and receives fully formed maternally produced antibodies in breast milk.

Active acquired adaptive immunity is longer lasting than passive acquired adaptive immunity.

Vaccines

A vaccine or immunization can consist of either viral or bacterial components. Most viral vaccines consist of a live virus that has been inactivated. The inactivated viruses exhibit antigenic properties and stimulate an immune response but will not transfer disease to the host. Live virus vaccines, however, should only be used in individuals with strong immune responses and not in immunosuppressed individuals, as they can sometimes infect the recipient and even those in close contact with the recipient. These vaccines are given to young children with robust immune reactivity. It is important to recognize that some vaccine immunity administered to children can wear off by adulthood. Often adults require another dose of vaccine to stimulate the immune system's antigen memory; this is known as a **"booster"** vaccination.

Bacterial vaccines are derivatives of killed microorganisms or extracts of antigens or toxins. Some bacteria damage a host through injurious secreted exotoxins rather than cellular invasion. The vaccines produced against these toxin-producing bacteria are called **toxoids.** The toxoid type of vaccine is a modified form of the bacterial toxin that has no disease-producing effects. An example of a toxoid type of vaccine is the tetanus toxoid, which should be administered every 10 years.

In general, vaccines allow the body to recognize exposure and develop a response and memory of the antigen without direct disease contraction. Primary immune responses stimulated by vaccines are long lasting. However, some first responses are inadequate and boosters are required to obtain full immunity. Boosters restimulate the body to initiate immune responses and confer long lasting active immunity. Vaccines are often given to children in a series to accomplish this long-term resistance (see Chapter 10: Infectious Diseases). Hepatitis B vaccine and human papilloma virus (HPV) vaccine are examples of vaccines that require a series of doses for full immunity. Certain immunizations, such as tetanus toxoid, require routine boosters.

Anergy Panel
An **anergy panel** is a test of immunocompetence; it consists of common antigens that individuals are exposed to, such as mumps, candida, or trichophyton. These antigens are injected intradermally, just under the skin. The clinician inspects the patient's reaction to these antigens after a set time period. Individuals should have a positive skin reaction to one or more of these antigens, indicating general immunocompetence. No reaction to the skin test indicates a lack of immune responsiveness and immunodeficiency.

Antibody Screening and Titer
Antibody screening tests, referred to as **antibody titers,** are laboratory tests used to confirm adequate immune protection against a particular antigen by measuring IgM and IgG Igs. Because IgM is the immunoglobulin that responds first in infection, elevated IgM levels indicate a recent or current infection. IgG is a secondary responder, which means that levels rise after a second exposure to an antigen. IgG levels indicate previous exposure and immune competence to a particular antigen. The antibody screening test identifies the presence of the immunoglobulin, and the titer provides a measurement of the amount of immunoglobulin.

It is common to screen for rubella virus immunity. Women planning on becoming pregnant are given a rubella titer laboratory test for IgM to determine their immunity to rubella infection, as rubella infection can cause multiple birth defects in a developing fetus. If the woman is IgM negative, this indicates that she has not been exposed to rubella, never developed an infection to it, and also never developed immunity, which requires her to receive the rubella vaccine.

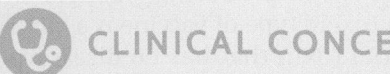

CLINICAL CONCEPT

Health-care providers, particularly those engaged in maternal-child health care, should have a rubella titer to ensure their own immunity to rubella. Without immunity, the health-care provider can transmit rubella to patients.

Allergy Testing

Allergy testing includes skin tests and serology blood tests. Skin tests measure the body's IgE reaction to an allergen by scratching or injecting a small amount of the allergen into the skin. Allergen preparations such as pollen, grass, or peanut extracts are used. The testing is considered positive for the allergen if the skin becomes red, swollen, and itchy.

Serology testing measures the presence of IgE, which is associated with allergic or hypersensitivity reactions. These serology tests are called the enzyme-linked immunosorbant assay (ELISA), radioallergosorbant test (RAST), and ImmunoCAP IgE test; they can evaluate the severity of allergy by measuring how much IgE reacts with allergen.

Hypersensitivity

The development of immunity can come with unintended consequences. Immune responses to environmental antigens lead to induction of protective defense mechanisms, but they can also lead to reactions that can be injurious to tissues. Injurious immune reactions can range from a mild allergic rash to life-threatening autoimmune diseases. The various damaging immune reactions are called hypersensitivity reactions and they involve either cell-mediated or antibody-mediated immune mechanisms. There are four types of hypersensitivity reactions:

1. type I immediate hypersensitivity
2. type II cytotoxic hypersensitivity
3. type III immune complex disorders
4. type IV delayed hypersensitivity.

Type I Immediate Hypersensitivity

Type I immediate hypersensitivity is a rapidly developed immune reaction that occurs after IgE Igs bind to mast cells and combine with antigen. This type of reaction, also called an allergy or atopic disorder, occurs in individuals previously exposed to an antigen.

Mast cells are key components in type I immediate hypersensitivity. These are cells that are widely distributed in the tissues—particularly the respiratory, nasal, and conjunctival epithelium. Mast cells have cytoplasmic granules that contain histamine, a potent vasodilator of arterioles and venules.

Immediate hypersensitivity reactions can present as local or systemic disorders. The nature of the local reaction depends on the portal of entry of an allergen. Common localized reactions include hives, which is a skin rash also called urticaria; nasal and conjunctival discharge; bronchial asthma; or allergic gastroenteritis. Common allergens include pollen, animal dander, dust, shellfish, peanuts, chocolate, and medications such as penicillin.

The mechanism of type I immediate hypersensitivity reactions involve CD4 cells, IgE antibodies, eosinophils, and mast cells (see Fig. 11-3). The first step in the synthesis of IgE is the presentation of the antigen to CD4 cells by dendritic antigen-presenting cells. The CD4 cells produce cytokines, which stimulate IgE-producing B lymphocytes and attract eosinophils to the area. Mast cells bind with the IgE antibodies and, in turn, the IgE antibodies bind to the allergen. This stimulates the release of histamine from mast cells. Other inflammatory mediators such as proteases, heparin, leukotrienes, prostaglandins, and platelet-activating factor (PAF) also are involved in the reaction. Within minutes, symptoms of allergy result, including urticaria, allergic rhinitis, conjunctivitis, and bronchospasm.

Allergic Rhinitis

Exposure to allergens such as mold, animal dander, or pollen leads to the development of allergic rhinitis, a type I immediate hypersensitivity response. The incidence of allergic rhinitis is increasing, and it is now one of the most common medical disorders. Approximately 50% of people in the United States have a positive skin test to one of the 10 most common allergens that lead to the development of allergic rhinitis. Allergic rhinitis is also associated with the development of asthma, sinusitis, and respiratory infections.

Exposure to the allergen triggers the production of IgE and the release of inflammatory mediators. These mediators include histamine, prostaglandins, and leukotrienes. The result is vasodilation, smooth muscle constriction of the bronchioles, and mucous hypersecretion. The most common symptoms include watery eyes, sneezing, and rhinorrhea. The secretions are white or clear in an allergic response. Symptoms may progress to coughing and bronchospasm. Nasal polyps may develop in chronic cases of allergic rhinitis.

It is important to ask if there is a personal or family history of asthma or other allergic illnesses. Nasal secretions demonstrate the presence of eosinophils. Diagnostic testing can determine the presence of IgE antibodies to common allergens. Treatment involves the use of antihistamines, intranasal corticosteroids, and decongestants.

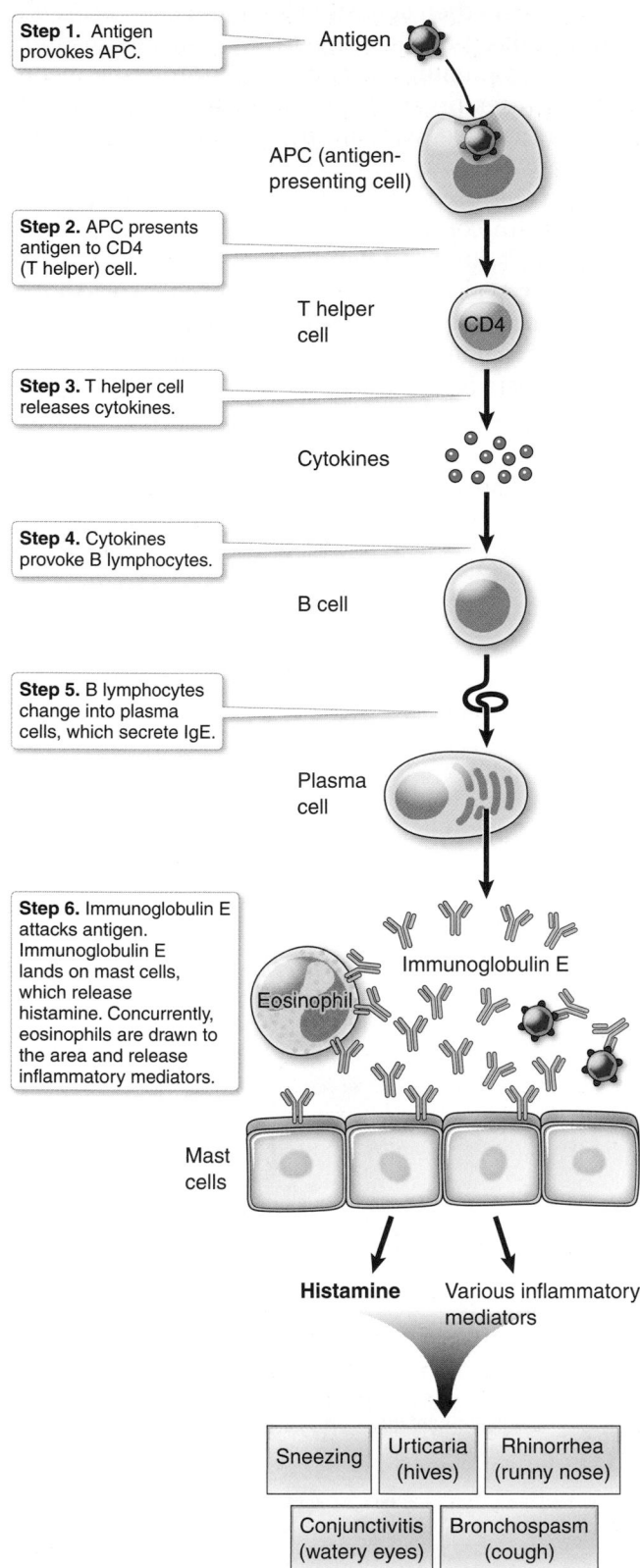

Step 1. Antigen provokes APC.

Antigen

APC (antigen-presenting cell)

Step 2. APC presents antigen to CD4 (T helper) cell.

T helper cell

CD4

Step 3. T helper cell releases cytokines.

Cytokines

Step 4. Cytokines provoke B lymphocytes.

B cell

Step 5. B lymphocytes change into plasma cells, which secrete IgE.

Plasma cell

Step 6. Immunoglobulin E attacks antigen. Immunoglobulin E lands on mast cells, which release histamine. Concurrently, eosinophils are drawn to the area and release inflammatory mediators.

Immunoglobulin E

Eosinophil

Mast cells

Histamine   Various inflammatory mediators

| Sneezing | Urticaria (hives) | Rhinorrhea (runny nose) |

| Conjunctivitis (watery eyes) | Bronchospasm (cough) |

Figure 11-3. Immediate hypersensitivity reaction. Step 1. Antigen provokes an antigen-presenting cell. Step 2. Antigen is presented to CD4 cell. Step 3. CD4 cell releases cytokines. Step 4. Cytokines provoke a B lymphocyte. Step 5. B lymphocyte turns into a plasma cell that secretes immunoglobulin E. Step 6. Igs attack antigen. Igs land on mast cells and provoke release of histamine. Eosinophils are attracted to the area and release other inflammatory mediators. Within minutes, symptoms of allergy result, including sneezing, urticaria, rhinorrhea, conjunctivitis, pharyngitis, and cough.

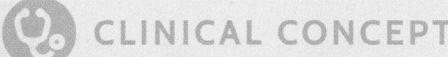

CLINICAL CONCEPT

During a physical examination, the nasal mucosa appears pale because of the swelling from an allergic response. The mucosa is erythematous if the symptoms are caused by an infection.

Systemic Anaphylaxis

Systemic anaphylaxis is a severe, life-threatening type I immediate hypersensitivity reaction. Extremely small doses of an allergen can trigger this overwhelming allergic reaction within minutes after exposure. Although patients at risk can generally be identified by a previous history of allergy, any individual can endure an anaphylactic reaction at any time in life.

Within minutes after exposure, itching, urticaria, and skin erythema appear, followed by bronchoconstriction. Laryngeal edema, tongue swelling, and angioedema can occur. Because of widespread vasodilation, blood pressure drops and can induce vascular shock, at which point the disorder is anaphylactic shock. The patient may lose consciousness and require cardiac monitoring. This is a medical emergency and requires rapid response from emergency medical personnel. IV or IM antihistamines, glucocorticoids and epinephrine are immediately required. The patient needs cardiac monitoring and periodic blood pressure measurement until recovery. Patients should be aware of the allergen that triggered the reaction and wear a medic-alert bracelet or necklace. Also for prophylaxis, the patient should carry an EpiPen (predrawn syringe of epinephrine) at all times.

ALERT! Patients with allergic urticaria should be carefully observed for signs of anaphylaxis. Anaphylaxis is a medical emergency that requires vigilant monitoring of the patient's vital signs, respiratory status, and electrocardiogram. Immediate injection of epinephrine is required.

Type II Cytotoxic Hypersensitivity

Type II cytotoxic hypersensitivity is mediated by Igs directed toward antigens present on cell surfaces. The antigens may be intrinsic to the cell membrane or they may take the form of an exogenous antigen, such as a drug metabolite, that is attached to a cell surface. In simpler terms, Igs target cells coated with antigen in type II cytotoxic hypersensitivity. Antibody-mediated cell destruction and phagocytosis occur in these reactions (see Fig. 11-4).

The classic type II hypersensitivity reaction is a transfusion reaction in which cells from an incompatible

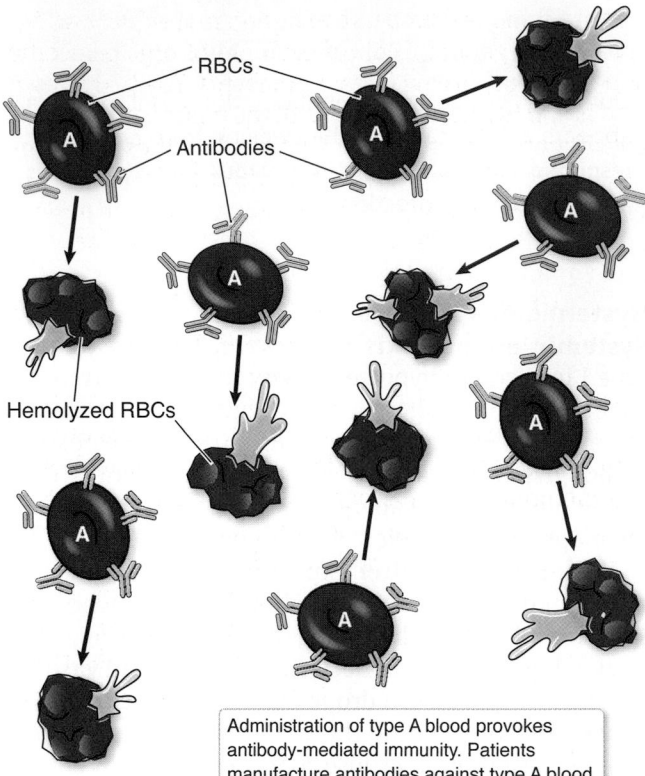

Administration of type A blood provokes antibody-mediated immunity. Patients manufacture antibodies against type A blood.

Figure 11–4. Type II cytotoxic hypersensitivity reaction. A patient has type B blood and is mistakenly administered a transfusion with type A blood. The donor RBCs stimulate antibody formation by the patient against the transfused blood. Patient anti-A antibodies attack the transfused type A red blood cells, causing hemolysis.

donor react with host Igs. For example, if type A blood from a donor is administered to a type B recipient, the anti-A Igs of the recipient will attack and destroy the type A red blood cells, causing a massive hemolytic reaction. Another example includes certain drug reactions in which Igs are produced that react with a drug that has coated host cells. The Igs attack and destroy the drug-coated cells.

CLINICAL CONCEPT

Health-care providers need to be vigilant when administering blood products. The donor and recipient blood type must match to avoid a transfusion reaction or type II cytotoxic hypersensitivity reaction. At least two different clinicians should confirm that the patient's blood type and the blood to be infused are the same.

Type III Immune Complex Hypersensitivity

Type III hypersensitivity reactions occur when antigen combines with Ig within circulation and these

complexes are then deposited in tissues (see Fig. 11-5). The deposition of the antigen-Ig complexes, also referred to as immune complexes, within tissue membranes causes organ dysfunction. Immune-complex disorders can be systemwide, where immune complexes are deposited in many different organs. An example of this occurs in systemic lupus erythematosus (SLE), where complexes are deposited in the kidney, blood vessels, lung, and skin. Immune complex-mediated disorders can also be localized to specific tissues in the body, such as the joints in rheumatoid arthritis (RA). The antigen of an immune-complex disease may not be identifiable. There is an unidentifiable antigen that triggers the type III hypersensitivity reactions in SLE and RA.

Type IV Delayed Hypersensitivity

Type IV delayed hypersensitivity is initiated by T lymphocytes that have had previous exposure to an antigen.

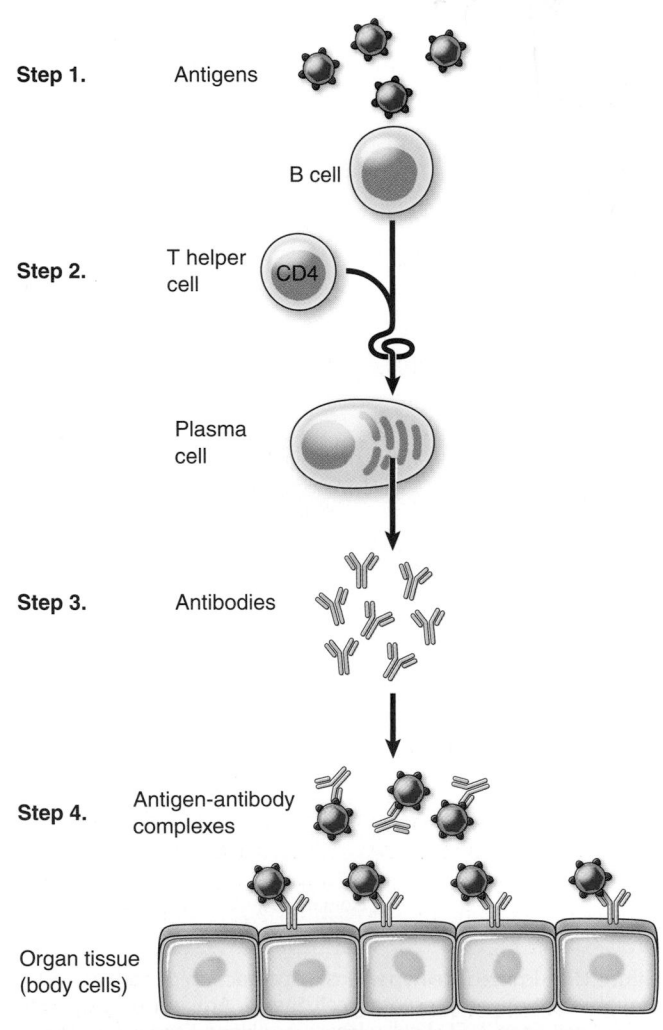

Figure 11–5. Type III hypersensitivity reactions involve the antigenic stimulation of Igs that combine with the antigen to form immune complexes. Step 1. Antigen provokes B cells. Step 2. The B cells transform into plasma cells with the assistance of CD4 cells. Step 3. Plasma cells secrete Igs. Step 4. Antigen combines with Igs within circulation and these complexes are then deposited in tissues. The deposition of the antigen-Ig complexes within tissue membranes causes organ dysfunction.

The T lymphocytes that are sensitized to the antigen do not attack the antigen until days after initial exposure. The inflammatory reaction that occurs in delayed hypersensitivity is referred to as contact dermatitis.

Because the inflammation reaction occurs days after exposure to the antigen, it is sometimes difficult to diagnose the source of the antigen. A classic example of this type of delayed hypersensitivity reaction occurs with exposure to poison ivy, a plant that usually grows wild in grassy fields and gardens in the United States. The person's exposure to poison ivy occurs days before the appearance of a vesicular, erythematous rash on the hands or other part of the body. At times, the patient may not be able to recall exposure to the antigen in a type IV hypersensitivity reaction.

Another important example of type IV delayed hypersensitivity occurs in transplant rejection. Donor tissue has major histocompatibility complexes (MHCs) on its cells that differ from a recipient's MHCs. The donor tissue cells are antigenic to the recipient and the recipient's T cells target the donor tissue. The T cells destroy the donor's foreign MHC-bearing transplant cells and cause rejection of the transplant. This usually takes a few days to become apparent.

 CLINICAL CONCEPT

The Mantoux test is a tuberculosis (TB) screening test that demonstrates type IV delayed hypersensitivity. The patient receives a subcutaneous injection of tuberculin, which is a protein component of the myobacteria tuberculi, on his or her forearm and then waits 48 hours for a result. If there is a reaction of erythema and induration of 10 mm or greater, active TB disease is probable. If the reaction is 5 mm or fewer, there has probably been exposure to TB in the past. If there is no erythema, there has been no exposure to TB or infection.

Pathophysiology of Selected Autoimmune Disorders

Autoimmune disease encompasses immune reactions against self antigens that result from the loss of self-tolerance. Under normal conditions, the immune system is vigilant in its surveillance and recognition of non-self antigens. The immune system can precisely distinguish self from non-self, and its purpose is to preserve and protect the body from injurious non-self invaders. In autoimmune disease, T cells or Igs cannot make a distinction between non-antigenic cell surface markers and antigenic foreign cell surface markers. The body's own immune system becomes intolerant to its own cells, attacks its own tissues, and renders organs dysfunctional. The body develops Igs against its own tissues, known as autoantibodies.

Autoimmune disorders can be organ-specific or widespread and generalized. An example of organ-specific autoimmunity occurs in type 1 diabetes. The body's own T cells and Igs attack beta cells of the pancreas and cause an inflammatory response that renders these insulin-producing cells nonfunctional. The patient incurs an unrecoverable insulin deficiency and contracts a permanent condition of diabetes. In multiple sclerosis, another autoimmune disease, the body's T cells attack myelin, the white matter of the CNS. Individuals suffer neuropathy of motor and sensory neurons that result in gait disturbance and loss of sensation.

An example of a generalized autoimmune disease is systemic lupus erythematosus (SLE). In SLE, Igs are developed against the body's deoxyribonucleic acid (DNA), cell membranes, and blood cells. Individuals with SLE endure a classic facial skin rash, kidney dysfunction, joint inflammation, or cardiac and lung dysfunction.

The underlying etiologic mechanisms of autoimmune diseases remain unclear. However, some autoimmune disorders are associated with infectious disease. It is theorized that a mechanism called **molecular mimicry** is involved in some autoimmune disorders. In molecular mimicry, an infectious agent is composed of antigens that have the same amino acid sequences as some self antigens. Immune responses are mounted against the foreign microbial antigens and the immune cells mistake the body's own tissues for foreign antigens. Although the immune cells attack antigen, they also attack the normal tissue with the similar composition.

An example of molecular mimicry occurs in rheumatic fever (see Fig. 11-6). In this disease, Group A beta hemolytic streptococcus (GABHS) infects the throat, causing a disorder called streptococcal pharyngitis, which is commonly known as strep throat. The body reacts by developing Igs against the streptococcal proteins and destroys the strep organisms. In a small percent of individuals, the body's antistreptococcal Igs not only attack the strep organisms, they also attack myocardial proteins, specifically cardiac valvular tissue. The anti-strep Igs are subjected to molecular mimicry as the myocardial proteins are mistakenly attacked along with the strep organisms. There is a molecular similarity of the myocardial cell protein structure and strep organism cell structure. The result is antistrep Igs attack the microbes but also attack heart tissue which, in turn, results in myocarditis with irreversible valvular deformity, also known as rheumatic heart disease.

Systemic Lupus Erythematosus

SLE, commonly called lupus, is a multisystem autoimmune disease characterized by autoantibodies, particularly antinuclear antibodies (ANAs). SLE is a chronic disease that can have an acute or insidious onset. It is characterized by remissions and exacerbations with fever, skin rash, joint inflammation, and damage to the kidney and serosal membranes.

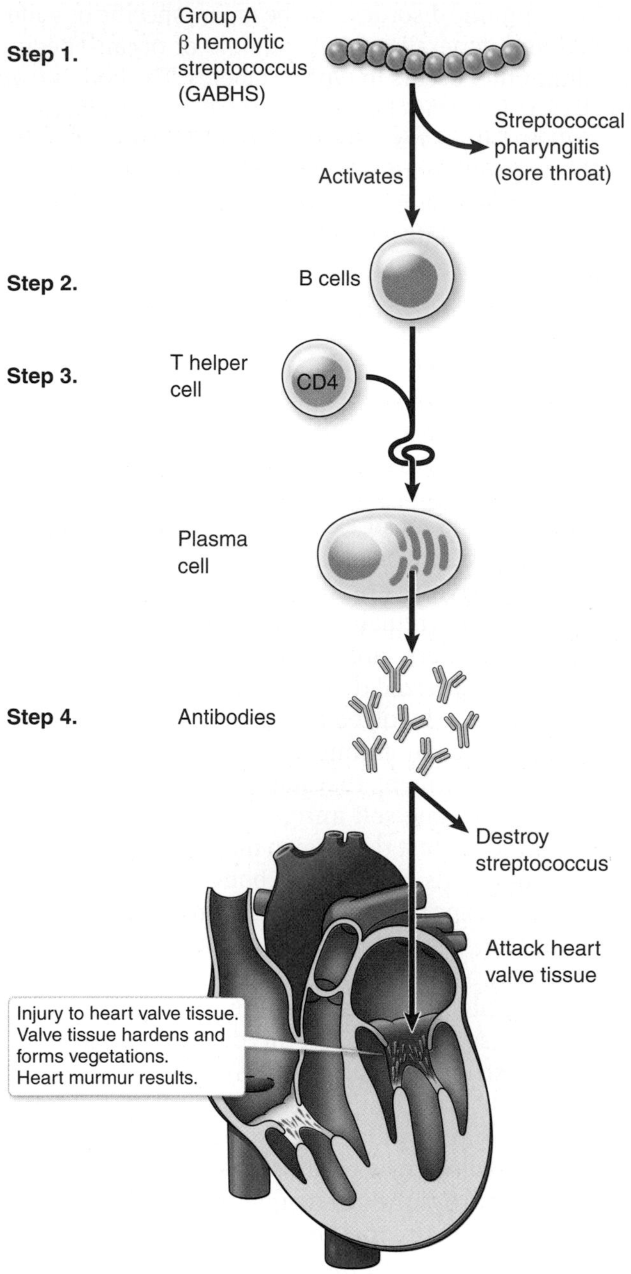

Step 1. Group A
β hemolytic
streptococcus
(GABHS)

→ Streptococcal
pharyngitis
(sore throat)

Activates

Step 2. B cells

Step 3. T helper
cell   CD4

Plasma
cell

Step 4. Antibodies

→ Destroy
streptococcus

Attack heart
valve tissue

Injury to heart valve tissue.
Valve tissue hardens and
forms vegetations.
Heart murmur results.

Figure 11–6. The process of rheumatic heart disease: molecular mimicry. An example of molecular mimicry occurs in rheumatic fever. Step 1. In this disease, GABHS infects the throat. Step 2. Streptococcus activates B cells. Step 3. The B cells transform into plasma cells that secrete antibodies. CD4 cells assist in this reaction. Step 4. The antibodies destroy the streptococcus organisms. In a small percent of individuals, the body's anti-streptococcal antibodies not only attack the strep organisms, they also attack myocardial proteins, specifically cardiac valvular tissue, resulting in heart murmur.

Epidemiology

The incidence of SLE is 2 to 5 cases per 100,000 population annually. It is mainly a disease of women, as women are 8 to 10 times more likely to develop SLE than men. Women of child-bearing age account for 65% of all SLE cases. African American women are 2 to 3 times more likely to develop SLE than Caucasians; those of Asian and Hispanic descent are also diagnosed more frequently than Caucasians.

Etiology/Risk Factors

The cause of SLE is unknown. Risk factors include genetic predisposition and environmental, hormonal, and immunological elements. In the majority of individuals, multiple genetic alterations are most likely responsible. At least eight chromosomal regions are linked to SLE, with chromosomes 1 and 6 having the most commonly documented linkage.

There are some environmental and hormonal factors that can trigger SLE. The presence of Epstein Barr virus (EBV) antibodies significantly increases the risk of SLE. The risk is noted to be more intense in African Americans, as EBV increases risk five- to six-fold in this racial group. Drugs such as hydralazine, procainamide, quinidine, phenytoin, isoniazid, and penicillamine can also induce SLE-like reactions. Exposure to ultraviolet light exacerbates the disease. The hormone most often linked to SLE is estrogen, with exacerbations of disease often occurring in women during menses or pregnancy.

Pathophysiology

The pathological process of SLE involves formation of autoantibodies, particularly antinuclear antibodies. Specific types of autoantibodies include anti-double stranded DNA antibodies (anti-dsDNA) and anti-Smith (anti-Sm) antibodies. Antibodies form immune complexes that are deposited in organs and tissues such as the skin, synovium, glomeruli, and lungs. The deposition of immune complexes triggers an inflammation reaction that damages organ membranes. There is also destruction of the microvasculature within the affected organ.

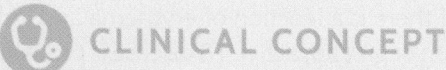

CLINICAL CONCEPT

The kidney is commonly affected in SLE, as deposition of immune complexes leads to glomerular damage.

Clinical Presentation

The symptoms of SLE can vary depending on the organ that is affected. General symptoms include fever, fatigue, myalgias, and arthralgias, but these symptoms are vague and often lead to misdiagnosis. There is a classic butterfly rash across the bridge of the nose and cheeks that is pathognomonic for SLE. Joint inflammation and musculoskeletal symptoms occur in 90% of patients. Other signs include splenic enlargement, pleural effusion, vasculitis, pericarditis, anemia, and thrombocytopenia.

The kidney is notably the worst affected organ in SLE. Nephrotic syndrome with hypertension and hematuria are common manifestations. Nephrotic syndrome often causes edema; periorbital or peripheral edema are common. Raynaud's phenomenon, which is episodic vasospasm of the arteries supplying the fingers, is common; it is observed as a tricolor change in the fingers from cyanosis to pallor to rubor (see Fig. 11-7).

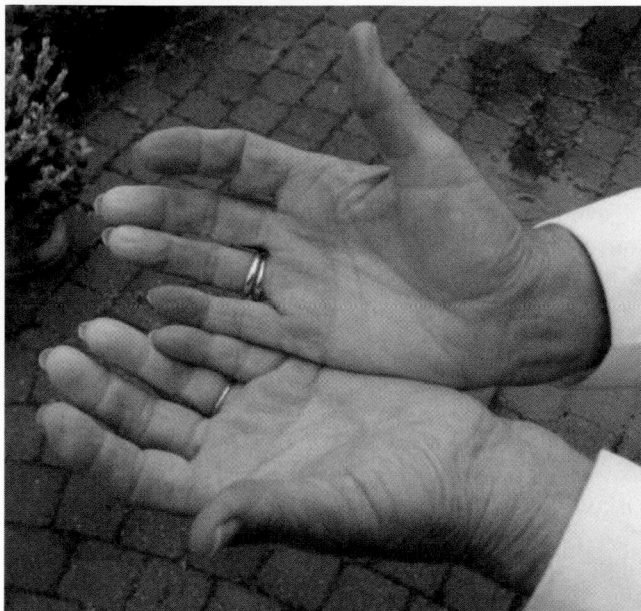

Figure 11–7. Raynaud's phenomenon. *(Wikipedia: Courtesy of Jamclaassen.)*

Accelerated ischemic coronary artery disease can also develop in patients with SLE. This may present as atypical chest pain and needs to be distinguished from pulmonary symptoms of SLE. Pleuritis and pleural effusion are also frequently endured by patients with SLE. Headache, which has similar features to a migraine, is a common complaint. Mood disorders are also common. Leukopenia, anemia, and thrombocytopenia can develop in SLE because of antibody targeting of blood cells. Leukopenia predisposes the patient to infection and thrombocytopenia increases risk of bleeding.

Diagnosis

The diagnosis of SLE is based on a detailed patient history, physical examination, and laboratory tests. The American College of Rheumatology has developed 11 criteria that are specific for accurate diagnosis of SLE (see Box 11-1). The health-care provider can make a diagnosis of SLE if four or more criteria are present.

No single laboratory test can diagnose SLE, but several laboratory tests may support the diagnosis. The immunofluorescent ANA test is most commonly performed in making a diagnosis of SLE. More than 95% of individuals with SLE have high ANA levels, though ANA is not specific to SLE alone. Other autoimmune diseases, cancers, inflammatory disorders, and chronic renal and liver disease can also cause elevated ANA.

The ANA test should be followed by anti-dsDNA and anti-Sm antibody levels, which are more specific to patients with SLE. Other antibodies are also frequently present in SLE, including antiribosomal, antineuronal, anti-Ro, and anti-La antibodies. Complement levels C3 and C4 are often diminished in SLE because they are consumed by immune complexes formed in the disease.

Erythrocyte sedimentation rate (ESR) and C-reactive protein (CRP) are elevated in SLE. A CBC with differential often reveals anemia, leukopenia, and thrombocytopenia. Urinalysis may show proteinuria, hematuria, casts, or pyuria. Serum creatinine level is needed to monitor renal involvement of SLE. Liver enzymes may be elevated in acute SLE or in response to medications. Creatinine phosphokinase levels may be elevated in cases of SLE-induced myositis.

X-rays may show joint and soft-tissue swelling and osteopenia. Chest x-ray is necessary to rule out pneumonitis. Magnetic resonance imaging of the brain may show changes consistent with SLE of the CNS. Skin biopsy of the butterfly rash can also help diagnose SLE.

Treatment

The course of SLE is unpredictable, with remissions and exacerbations occurring over many years. Treatment includes nonsteroidal anti-inflammatory drugs (NSAIDs), antimalarial drugs, corticosteroids, Methotrexate (MTX), and immunosuppressive drugs. Combination therapy with NSAIDs and the antimalarial drug hydroxychloroquine provides additive anti-inflammatory effects. The goal is to reduce the amount of time of exacerbations of disease. Improvement in signs and symptoms often occurs after 8 weeks of therapy.

Because SLE causes severe inflammation, corticosteroids such as prednisone are often used for short-term treatment. MTX can be used as an alternative to antimalarial drugs. Weekly MTX treatment can control joint and skin symptoms, but liver toxicity can occur with MTX, so liver enzymes must be monitored.

For those patients with severe disease, the immunosuppressant cyclophosphamide also may be included in the treatment regimen.

ALERT! Those treated with immunosuppressant drugs for inflammatory disorders are at increased risk for developing infections.

Rheumatoid Arthritis

Rheumatoid arthritis (RA) is a chronic autoimmune, inflammatory disorder that affects the joints and may have systemic effects. There are specific criteria for diagnosis of this disorder.

Epidemiology

The prevalence of RA in the adult population is fairly constant at 0.5% to 1%. Prevalence increases with age, and the disorder is 2 to 3 times more common in females than in males.

Etiology

The cause of RA is unknown. Autoimmune mechanisms are notable in RA; however, what instigates the immune reaction is unclear. Genetic, environmental, hormonal, immunological, and infectious factors may play significant roles. Genetic factors account for 50% of the risk for developing RA. There are several genes being studied. Genes that program for MHCs are involved along with the presence of resistance and susceptibility genes referred to as *PTPN22* and *TRAF5*.

Numerous infectious agents have been under study as potential causes of RA, including *Mycoplasma* organisms, EBV, and rubella virus. Synovial fluid of RA patients has been found to contain high levels of anaerobic bacterial antibodies; therefore, a bacterial cause is possible. Females are largely affected by RA, so sex hormones may also play a role. Studies show RA regresses during pregnancy and it recurs in the postpartum period. Also, there is a decreased incidence of RA in women using oral contraceptives.

Pathophysiology

In RA, the body's immune system attacks its own synovial tissues, stimulating an inflammatory process that results in destruction of cartilage, bone, tendons, and ligaments. An unknown, initial antigenic stimulus provokes an antigen-presenting cell (APC) to begin the sequence of events in the RA inflammation cascade. Antigen-presenting cells (APCs) activate T cells (T lymphocytes), which play a key role in the destruction of joint components. Following activation, T cells secrete cytokines, which recruit other WBCs to the synovial regions, escalating the inflammatory process. Once set in motion, the inflammation becomes persistently fueled by reactivated T cells and cytokines that constantly attract other WBCs into the joint space.

Among the other WBCs recruited are B cells (B lymphocytes), which secrete Igs. B cells secrete an autoantibody commonly referred to as rheumatoid factor (RF), which can be found in large quantities in the synovial fluid, although in up to 30% of patients, serum RF is negative.

Concurrently, WBCs such as macrophages and monocytes produce proinflammatory cytokines such as TNF-alpha, ILs, and matrix metalloproteases. Together with the cellular components involved in RA, these cytokines incite the inflammation, causing a chronic, persistent destructive, autoimmune process.

Continual inflammation of the synovial membrane causes hypertrophy; this region of the joint becomes known as the pannus in RA (see Fig. 11-8).

Clinical Presentation

Classic symptoms of RA include symmetrical, tender, swollen joints, most commonly of the fingers, wrists, knees, hips, and feet. In addition, patients often experience fatigue, fever, and general malaise. Patients commonly report painful, stiff joints lasting approximately 30 minutes to an hour in the morning or after a period of prolonged rest. The chronic joint inflammation experienced by RA patients results in permanent damage of the surfaces of joints. As the disease progresses, RA patients become increasingly limited in their mobility.

Diagnosis

The diagnosis of RA is based on several clinical criteria and laboratory tests. Clinical criteria include the presence of morning stiffness in the joints; polyarthritis, which includes the hand joints; symmetrical arthritis; and subcutaneous rheumatoid nodules for a minimum of 6 weeks. The diagnosis of RA should not be confused with osteoarthritis, as there are key differences (see Table 11-1). The diagnosis of RA is made according to a set of specific criteria developed by the American College of Rheumatology (see Box 11-2).

In the hands, characteristic involvement includes the metacarpal and proximal interphalangeal joints, with sparing of the distal interphalangeal joints in the fingers. There are two classic rheumatoid deformities in the fingers: Swan neck deformity and Boutonniere

Major diagnostic evidence includes elevated serum RF, ESR, and CRP. Anti-citrullinated protein antibodies (ACPAs) are also present in up to 70% of patients. ACPAs are biomarkers similar to RF that indicate erosion of the synovial membrane of joints. Serum RF may be negative in up to 30% of patients, making early diagnosis difficult. Periodic monitoring of indicators of inflammation in RA is necessary to assess the disease's progress.

Treatment

Treatment of RA involves anti-inflammatory agents such as NSAIDs, specific agents known as disease-modifying antirheumatic drugs (DMARDs), and immunosuppressive drugs such as MTX. Biological agents made up of monoclonal antibodies are proving to be very effective. There are a number of anti-TNF alpha biological agents, including etanercept and infliximab. These drugs block the action of TNF-alpha, a destructive cytokine.

Sarcoidosis

Sarcoidosis is a chronic, autoimmune multisystem disorder of unknown origin characterized by an accumulation of T lymphocytes, macrophages, and epithelioid granulomas in various organs. Any organ can be involved, though the most frequently affected is the lung. Other organs that can be involved include the skin, eye, liver, and lymph nodes. The disease can be episodic with relapses and remissions over many years.

Epidemiology

Sarcoidosis affects females more commonly than males with a prevalence of 10 to 40 per 100,000 in the United States. African American females are more commonly affected than Caucasian females. Most individuals with sarcoidosis present with signs of the disease between the ages of 20 and 40 years.

Pathophysiology

There is an accumulation of macrophages, T cells, and inflammatory mediators in affected organs. The acute inflammatory process is followed by chronic inflammation. In chronic inflammation there is formation of granulomas, which are aggregates of macrophages, epithelial-like cells, and other inflammatory mediators surrounded by T cells. Characteristic giant cells are found within the granulomas. The granulomas and inflammatory changes cause architectural distortions within organs and may cause organ dysfunction, particularly of lungs, liver, and lymph nodes.

Clinical Presentation

Sarcoidosis can range from an asymptomatic disorder to a disease with extensive dysfunction of organs. It is unclear why some patients are mildly affected and some are severely affected. Symptoms include fever, fatigue, malaise, anorexia, and weight loss. Some patients may develop arthritis at the ankles, wrists,

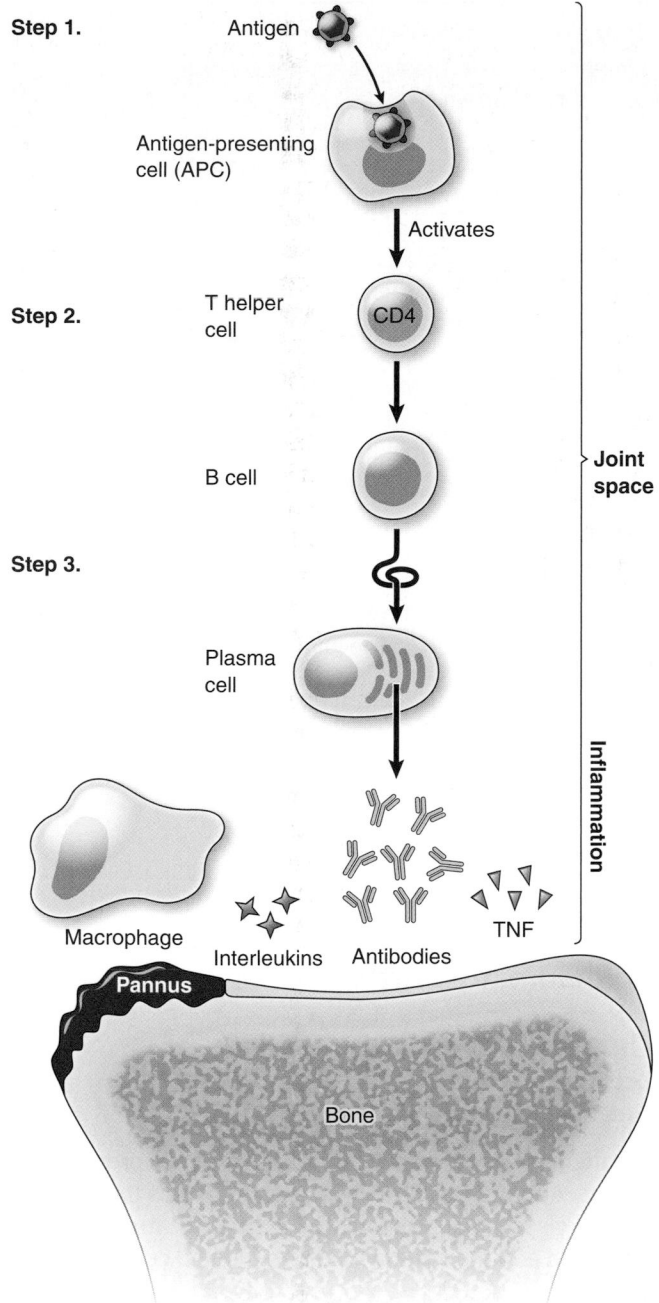

Figure 11-8. The inflammatory process in rheumatoid arthritis. Step 1. Within the joint space, an unknown antigenic stimulus provokes antigen-presenting cells (APCs). Step 2. The APCs process T cells and other WBCs, including B cells and macrophages, which are attracted to the joint space. Step 3. B cells transform into plasma cells, which secrete destructive antibodies, and macrophages secrete proinflammatory, damaging cytokines, including tumor necrosis factor (TNF), ILs, and metalloproteases (MPs), which persistently fuel the inflammatory process.

deformity. With severe hand deformity there is a distinctive ulnar deviation of the metacarpal bones (see Fig. 11-9). Also, a cystic nodule in the popliteal region called a Baker's cyst is common. Nodular fibrotic tissue accumulation in the lungs, termed rheumatoid nodules, may be found.

TABLE 11-1. Rheumatoid Arthritis Versus Osteoarthritis

	Rheumatoid Arthritis	Osteoarthritis
Etiology	Autoimmune disease	Wear and tear or overuse of joints caused by excessive weight bearing. Traumatic injury can predispose to osteoarthritis
Age	20 to 40 years old	Older than age 50
Population affected	Women are predominately affected	Both women and men affected
Pain	Stiffness in morning but better with use of joint	Stiffness in morning and worse with use of joint Rest decreases pain
Movement	Movement of joint decreases pain	Movement of joint increases pain
Joints	Symmetrical involvement of joints; hands most commonly affected initially	Symmetrical or asymmetrical involvement of small and large joints
Diagnosis	Specific rheumatological association criteria and x-ray	X-ray
Time frame	Gradual with exacerbations and remissions	Gradual over years and steady decline of health of joints
Associated symptoms	Systemic disease; feeling of being ill, fever, elevated WBC count	Limited to the joint pain
Key characteristics	Swan neck and Boutonniere deformity of fingers with ulnar deviation of metacarpal bones Rheumatoid nodule in lung; Baker's cyst in popliteal space	Herbeden's and Bouchard's nodes of fingers

BOX 11-2. Diagnostic Criteria for Rheumatoid Arthritis

The following American College of Rheumatology (ACR) criteria are used to diagnose rheumatoid arthritis. A score of ≥ 6/10 is needed for classification of a patient as having definite RA.

JOINT INVOLVEMENT

1 large joint	0
2 to 10 large joints	1
1 to 3 small joints (with or without involvement of large joints)	2
4 to 10 small joints (with or without involvement of large joints)	3
Greater than 10 joints (at least 1 small joint)**	5

SEROLOGY (AT LEAST 1 TEST RESULT IS NEEDED FOR CLASSIFICATION)

Negative RF and negative ACPA	0
Low-positive RF or low-positive ACPA	2
High-positive RF or high-positive ACPA	3

ACUTE-PHASE REACTANTS (AT LEAST 1 TEST RESULT IS NEEDED FOR CLASSIFICATION)

Normal CRP and normal ESR	0
Abnormal CRP or abnormal ESR	1

DURATION OF SYMPTOMS

Less than 6 weeks	0
Greater than or equal to 6 weeks	1

The criteria are aimed at classification of newly presenting patients. Although patients with a score of less than 6/10 are not classifiable as having RA, their status can be reassessed and the criteria might be fulfilled cumulatively over time.

Joint involvement refers to any swollen *or* tender joint on examination, which may be confirmed by imaging evidence of synovitis. Distal interphalangeal joints, first carpometacarpal joints, and first metatarsophalangeal joints are excluded from assessment. Large joints refers to shoulders, elbows, hips, knees, and ankles. Small joints refer to the metacarpophalangeal joints, proximal interphalangeal joints, second through fifth metatarsophalangeal joints, thumb interphalangeal joints, and wrists.

**In this category, at least 1 of the involved joints must be a small joint; the other joints can include any combination of large and additional small joints, as well as other joints not specifically listed elsewhere.

Abbreviation key: ACPA: anti-citrullinated protein antibody. CRP: C-reactive protein. ESR: erythrocyte sedimentation rate. RF: Rheumatoid factor.

Adapted from Aletaha, D., Neogi, T., & Silman, A. J. (2010). 2010 Rheumatoid arthritis classification criteria: An American College of Rheumatology/European League Against Rheumatism collaborative initiative. *Arthr Rheum, 62,* 2569–2581

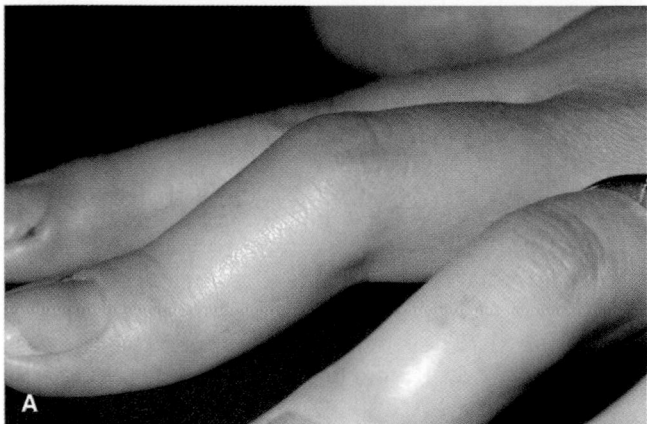

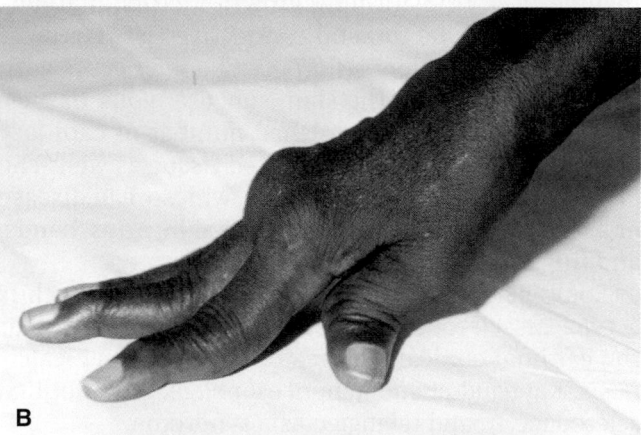

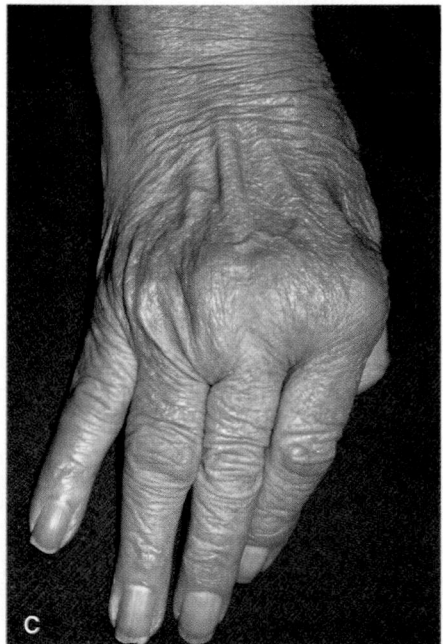

Figure 11–9. Classic rheumatoid deformities in the fingers: A. Boutonniere deformity. *(From Dr. P. Marazzi/Science Source.)* B. Swan neck deformity. *(From Sue Ford/Science Source.)* C. Ulnar deviation of the fingers on the hand. *(From SPL/Science Source.)*

on the face around eyes and nose, on the back, and on the extremities. Parotid gland and lymph node enlargement are commonly found in patients with sarcoidosis. Respiratory tract abnormalities, which mainly consist of interstitial lung disease, cause most of the morbidity and mortality in sarcoidosis.

Diagnosis

Diagnosis involves a chest x-ray, which shows a typical pattern of bilateral hilar lymphadenopathy, a hallmark of the disease. No blood tests are diagnostic of sarcoidosis, though most affected individuals have elevated levels of angiotensin-converting enzyme. A biopsy of a sarcoid lesion in a lymph node or in cells recovered from bronchoalveolar lavage is mandatory to make a definitive diagnosis.

Treatment

The prognosis for those affected is good. Disease clears spontaneously in 50% of patients, though approximately half of all patients have some permanent mild organ dysfunction. Treatment involves use of glucocorticoids, chemotherapy, and immunosuppressive drug regimens.

Sjögren's Syndrome

Sjögren's syndrome is a chronic, autoimmune disease characterized by dry eyes, also called keratoconjunctivitis sicca, and dry mouth, also called xerostomia. These major symptoms occur because of immunologically mediated destruction of lacrimal and salivary glands. It can present as an isolated disorder or in combination with other autoimmune diseases.

Epidemiology

Sjögren's syndrome occurs most commonly in women between ages 50 and 60 years. Approximately 60% of individuals with Sjögren's disease also suffer from RA.

Pathophysiology

In Sjögren's syndrome there is a lymphocytic infiltration of many of the body's exocrine glands. The infiltrate consists mainly of T cells, B cells, plasma cells, and inflammatory mediators.

There is excess proliferation of lymphocytes, which interferes with glandular function. The main targets are salivary and lacrimal glands; however, respiratory and GI involvement are also seen. The infiltrate mainly surrounds ducts and vessels within glandular tissue. Ductal epithelial cells show hyperplasia, which eventually protrude into the lumen of the ducts. The hyperplastic cells obstruct the lumen of the ducts, preventing secretions such as tears and saliva from release. Regions of lymphocytic infiltration in glands eventually undergo fibrosis and atrophy. The lack of secretions from affected glands can cause complications. Lack of tears causes drying of the cornea and lack of saliva causes dryness and breakdown of the oral mucosa.

knees, and elbows. Many patients have cough, dyspnea, and chest discomfort if the respiratory system is affected. Patients often develop a characteristic skin rash called erythema nodosum, which manifests as tender erythematous nodules on the anterior surface of the legs. A nonspecific maculopapular rash can develop

Clinical Presentation

Symptoms include blurred vision, burning and itching of the eyes, and thickened secretions that can block tear ducts. Dry mouth makes swallowing difficult and renders the patient with a decreased ability to taste. Oral mucous membranes become cracked and fissured. Manifestations of extraglandular involvement, such as synovitis, pulmonary fibrosis, and peripheral neuropathy, are seen in a third of patients. Parotid gland enlargement can sometimes be evident.

Diagnosis

Autoantibodies are a key characteristic of Sjögren's syndrome. ANAs and antibodies against cellular components are found. Antibodies referred to as SS-A (Ro) and SS-B (La) are diagnostic of the syndrome and are detected in up to 90% of those affected. Diagnosis requires a biopsy of the lip tissue to examine minor salivary glands. The lymph nodes are commonly enlarged and infiltrated with dysplastic B cells. Because of lymphocytic proliferation, persons with Sjögren's syndrome have a 40-fold increased risk of developing lymphoid malignancies.

Treatment

Treatment is aimed at symptomatic relief and limitation of damaging effects of xerostomia and keratoconjunctivitis sicca. Ophthalmic solutions to replace tears and medications that stimulate salivary gland function are used, as are glucocorticoids and immunosuppressive agents.

Scleroderma

Scleroderma, also known as systemic sclerosis, is a chronic, autoimmune disease of unknown origin characterized by abnormal accumulation of fibrous tissue in the skin and various organs. The skin is most noticeably affected, but the GI tract, kidneys, muscles, and lungs are frequently involved as well.

Epidemiology

An estimated 40,000 to 165,000 persons in the United States are affected by scleroderma. Women between 30 and 50 years old are most commonly affected, and the disorder occurs more often in African American women than Caucasian women.

Etiology

The cause of scleroderma is unclear; however, there are numerous gene mutations associated with scleroderma. Genetic mutations that produce abnormal B cells, T cell components, and cytokines have been implicated. Among the many genes under scrutiny are BANK1, a gene located at 4q24, BLK, located at 8p23, and CD247, located at 1q22. A gene mutation on the X chromosome, called *IRAK1*, which codes for a protein integral to both innate and adaptive immune system pathways may be the cause of the female predominance in this disease. Exposure to toxic substances has also been associated with scleroderma. These include silica, organic solvents, hydrocarbons, epoxy resins, and pesticides.

Pathophysiology

In scleroderma, there is an inflammatory reaction with injury to the endothelial lining of blood vessels. The endothelial reaction leads to a cascade of changes that involve fibroblasts, T lymphocytes, macrophages, and mast cells. These activated cells infiltrate the vasculature, skin, and some organs. Inflammatory mediators that play an important part in the reaction include IL-4, transforming growth factors, platelet-derived growth factor, and connective tissue growth factor. Extensive deposition of collagen occurs with resulting fibrosis in the skin, subcutaneous tissues, and deep tissues. A diminished number of capillary branches are noted in the affected tissue as well. The disorder may present as a diffuse, widespread disease or a localized disease limited to the skin, arms, hands, and fingers.

Some persons develop CREST syndrome, which is a type of scleroderma. Its name is an acronym for the cardinal clinical features of the syndrome: calcinosis, Raynaud phenomenon, esophageal dysmotility, sclerodactyly, and telangiectasia syndrome.

In CREST syndrome there is a loss of esophageal motility; sclerodactyly, which is the contracture of fingers caused by the tightening of the skin covering the hands; and **Raynaud's phenomenon,** which is a vasoconstrictive disorder of the extremities that causes fingers and toes to become ischemic.

Clinical Presentation

Initial complaints are vague at times because of scleroderma's widespread involvement of the body. The disorder can present as an inflammatory musculoskeletal problem. The patient commonly complains of muscle aches, joint pain, and swelling with limited range of motion. The most noticeable sign is the skin involvement, which renders skin shiny, smooth, and stretched in appearance, particularly on the face and hands. There is a facial masklike appearance with loss of normal wrinkles and nasolabial folds. The skin on the hands can become so stiff as to cause contractures of the fingers.

As the disorder continues, dysphagia is common because of esophageal dysmotility. Abdominal pain, intestinal obstruction, and malabsorption with weight loss and anemia can occur, as can cardiac dysfunction and malignant hypertension.

Diagnosis

Diagnosis of scleroderma is based on patient symptoms and physical examination findings. There is commonly an elevation in ANAs. Antibodies called antitopoisomerase-1 and anti-sci-70 appear in the blood of 40% of patients. Other diagnostic tests include pulmonary spirometry, chest x-ray, electrocardiogram, echocardiogram, and 24-hour holter monitoring when scleroderma is widespread. Computed tomography of the lungs demonstrates a "ground glass" or "honeycomb" appearance because of development of pulmonary fibrosis. Esophageal manometry, which measures pressure and motility, shows esophageal involvement in 90% of patients.

Treatment

Currently there is no specific treatment for scleroderma. Medications used to control symptoms include NSAIDs, corticosteroids, and immunosuppressant agents. Fibrosis of body organs, such as the lungs and myocardium, can lead to death.

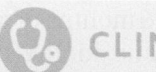

CLINICAL CONCEPT

Upon exposure to cold, many persons with an autoimmune disorder exhibit Raynaud's phenomenon of the fingers, a tricolor change of blue (cyanosis) to red (erythema) to white (pallor).

Polyarteritis Nodosa

Polyarteritis nodosa is a disease characterized by necrotizing inflammation of blood vessel walls. The vascular lesions resemble those found in type III hypersensitivity reactions, which are caused by immune complex deposition. The trigger or etiologic agent is unknown, but any type of blood vessel can be involved: arteries, arterioles, veins, or venules. Tissue ischemia can occur distal to the inflamed blood vessel.

Polyarteritis nodosa typically involves renal and visceral blood supply. Diagnosis is confirmed by the presence of anti-neutrophil cytoplasmic antibodies in the bloodstream. Typically a disease of young adults, it can be episodic and remitting with long symptom-free intervals. Clinical manifestations include fever, myalgias, arthralgias, hypertension, abdominal pain, peripheral neuritis, and malaise. Renal involvement is often severe and the cause for death. Treatment involves the use of corticosteroids and immunosuppressant agents.

Pathophysiology of Selected Immunodeficiency Disorders

Immunodeficiencies can be divided into primary, or congenital, and secondary, or acquired, disorders. Most primary immunodeficiency diseases are genetic and most manifest during infancy, between the ages of 6 months and 2 years. These patients may show deficiencies of innate or adaptive immunity. Many of the primary immunodeficiency disorders are X-linked, which is why they mostly manifest in males.

The major acquired immunodeficiency disorders develop after birth because of disorders with immunosuppressive effects, such as lymphoma, leukemia, or HIV infection.

Severe Combined Immunodeficiency Disease

Severe combined immunodeficiency disease (SCID) is a constellation of genetically distinct syndromes all having defects of both antibody-mediated and cell-mediated immune responses. The incidence is 1 case per 50,000 to 75,000 births. The most common form is X-linked, which is why the disease presents most frequently in males.

The syndrome is associated with a diverse number of genetic defects that result in malfunction of the T cell and B cell immune systems. Infants usually present with many different kinds of infection during early weeks of life and are diagnosed by age 3 months. Affected infants present with diarrheal illness, pneumonia, skin infections, thrush, extensive diaper rashes, and failure to thrive. Patients are susceptible to recurrent severe infections by a wide array of pathogens. Live vaccines must not be administered because these can cause life-threatening illness in immunosuppressed individuals. Diagnosis must be made before severe life-threatening infections occur so that the immunity can be restored with bone marrow transplant, which can lead to long-term survival. With bone marrow and other stem cell reconstitution techniques, many patients with SCID can develop normal immunocompetence. Without treatment, death from infection usually occurs within the first 2 years of life.

IgA Deficiency

IgA deficiency is one of the most common primary immune deficiencies. It occurs in 1 in 500 to 700 Caucasian persons per year in the United States. It is less common in African Americans, with an incidence of 1 in 6,000 persons. It is usually diagnosed through routine screening of family members of individuals with another primary immune deficiency.

In most cases, individuals affected with IgA deficiency are asymptomatic but are at higher risk for atopic diseases and autoimmune diseases. In many instances, IgA deficiency is caused by a genetic defect, though the deficiency can be acquired as well. Medications that can cause IgA deficiency include D-penicillamine, sulfasalazine, fenclofenac, gold, captopril, chloroquine, phenytoin, and valproic acid. In addition, some infections can increase susceptiblity to IgA deficiency, including rubella, cytomegaloviruses, toxoplasma gondii, and Epstein Barr virus. Benzene exposure has also been associated with IgA deficiency.

Those older than 6 months who have recurrent upper and lower respiratory tract infections with encapsulated bacteria (e.g., *Haemophilus influenzae, Streptococcus pneumoniae*) should be evaluated for IgA deficiency.

Persons with absent secretory IgA have an increased incidence of severe respiratory infections, GI infections, and cancer. Lack of secretory IgA has been hypothesized to compromise the defense against infection with *Helicobacter pylori*, which is thought to be a cause of stomach cancer. RA and SLE are the most common autoimmune disorders associated with deficiencies of IgA. Other conditions, such as ulcerative colitis, inflammatory bowel disease, Crohn's disease, and pernicious anemia, have been described in IgA-deficient individuals. Individuals with chronic obstructive pulmonary disease are also often found to have IgA deficiency.

Persons with absent IgA can present with recurrent respiratory tract infections, including swelling, pain, or tenderness upon palpation over the maxillary and frontal sinuses; chronic otorrhea, scarred or perforated tympanic membranes, and decreased auditory acuity or even deafness; chronic nasal discharge; fever; nonproductive or productive cough; and dyspnea. GI findings may include abdominal distention, cramps after eating, diffuse pain, and increased peristalsis.

Normal levels of IgM and IgG and indetectable levels of serum IgA are diagnostic of the disorder. Pulmonary function tests may show an obstructive pattern in patients with IgA deficiency, and jejunal biopsy specimens of patients with IgA deficiency who have chronic diarrhea and malabsorption may show blunting of the villi.

If patients are symptomatic with increased infections, monthly injections of Igs are the treatment of choice. Sinus surgery can frequently help relieve chronic obstruction and promote drainage. Tympanostomy tubes may also be helpful in reducing the risk of decreased hearing and secondary defective speech development in children with chronic otitis.

Chronic Mucocutaneous Candidiasis

Chronic mucocutaneous candidiasis (CMC) is caused by the inability of the T lymphocyte to respond to challenges of the fungus *Candida albicans*. Without this ability, individuals experience recurrent and severe candidiasis infections of mucous membranes and skin. *Candida albicans* is a fungal organism that is part of the normal flora of the skin, GI tract, and vaginal canal.

Eighty percent of CMC cases present in children younger than 3 years old. Children often present with persistent oral candidiasis (thrush) and candida dermatitis. Potassium hydroxide (KOH) preparation is used to diagnose candida infection. Scrapings from the infected site are suspended in 10% to 20% KOH and microscopically examined. The presence of yeast cells and pseudohyphae confirms the diagnosis.

Iron deficiency is common in patients with CMC, as are endocrine disorders such as thyroid disease. Thymoma and myasthenia gravis are also associated with CMC. Systemic antifungal therapy is the mainstay of CMC therapy. It may be used alone or in combination with an immunomodulatory agent. Topical agents alone are usually ineffective.

Hypogammaglobulinemia

Hypogammaglobulinemia is a condition of decreased number of Igs related to a defect in B cell development and maturation. With this decreased production, the immune system cannot respond to and initiate the immune/inflammatory response. The disorder can be caused by genetic defects or can be acquired. Acquired hypogammaglobulinemia can be caused by immunosuppressant medications, renal loss of Igs, GI immunoglobulin loss, B cell-related malignancies, and severe burns. Renal loss of Igs occurs in nephrotic syndrome, in which IgG loss is usually accompanied by albumin loss. GI loss occurs in protein-losing enteropathies and intestinal lymphangiectasia.

Patients with hypogammaglobulinemia experience an increased incidence of infections starting at an early age. Symptoms typically begin at 6 months of age when maternal antibodies start to wane in the newborn. Severe candidiasis and *Pneumocystis jiroveci* pneumonia are common before 2 years of age. Encapsulated bacteria such as *Streptococcus pneumoniae*, *Streptococcus pyogenes*, *Haemophilus influenzae*, and *Staphylococcus aureus* are pathogens that commonly cause respiratory infections. Diarrhea with malabsorption syndrome is reported in more than 50% of patients. Gastritis with achlorhydria and pernicious anemia may occur. *Giardia lamblia* and *Campylobacter* species are the pathogens involved in the GI manifestations in many of these patients.

The diagnosis of hypogammaglobulinemia is made after a child is 2 years of age. Before age 2, low immunoglobulin levels in the blood can be caused by a normal delay of B-cell maturation. Although no pathognomonic physical examination finding is typical, lymphadenopathy, splenomegaly, and hepatomegaly can all be present. Failure to thrive is a common diagnosis. Abnormal lung examination indicating bronchiectasis caused by frequent respiratory infections is common. A patient could also have a positive fecal occult blood test secondary to invasive bacterial infection.

Hallmarks of the disease are a lack of Igs and an impaired antibody response to vaccination. IgG levels persistently below the 5th percentile for age are usually present in this disorder. Decreased levels of IgA are also common in this group, and low IgM levels may be seen, but less frequently. Most infants have normal lymphocyte counts for age.

Treatment consists of bone marrow transplantation, immunoglobulin transfusions, and prophylactic antibiotics. Live vaccines should not be administered to the patient or family members.

Wiskott-Aldrich Syndrome

Wiskott-Aldrich syndrome (WAS) is an X-linked recessive disease characterized by eczema, thrombocytopenia, and vulnerability to infectious disease. The syndrome is caused by a genetic defect that affects development of T cells, platelets, and Igs. In WAS, T cells and IgM are usually deficient and thrombocytopenia is common. The genetic defect is found at Xp11.22; because it is X-linked, it is found almost exclusively in boys. It is an uncommon disorder with an incidence of 4 in 1 million live male births.

Because of a lack of platelets, WAS usually present with bleeding; in male infants, prolonged bleeding from circumcision is commonly one of the first symptoms. Purpura or unusual bruising and blood in the stool can occur early. Because of IgM deficiency, infections caused by encapsulated organisms can cause life-threatening complications, including pneumonia, meningitis, and sepsis. *Pneumocystis jiroveci* and viral infections are also seen. Eczema develops in 81% of patients. Patients frequently become anergic (completely immuno-incompetent) and are vulnerable to overwhelming infections and sepsis.

To diagnose the condition, antibody-mediated immune function is tested by measuring the patient's ability to develop antibody responses to standard vaccines such as pneumococcal vaccine and tetanus toxoid. Cell-mediated immune function is evaluated by examining lymphocyte responses to antigens and the patient's ability to react to an anergy panel, which consists of candidal, mumps, trichophyton, and tetanus toxoid antigens.

Treatment consists of bone marrow transplantation, immunoglobulin transfusions, and prophylactic antibiotics. Live vaccines should not be administered to the patient or family members. Bone marrow transplant can be curative. Without treatment, the average survival is 8 to 11 years.

DiGeorge Syndrome

DiGeorge syndrome is an isolated T cell deficiency that results from maldevelopment of the thymus gland. The disease is caused by a genetic deletion at 22q11. The infant born with this genetic mutation has organ defects that include congenital cardiac abnormalities, parathyroid gland maldevelopment with hypocalcemic tetany, and absence of the thymus gland. Facial abnormalities characteristic of the disease include micrognathia (underdeveloped jaw), hypertelorism (eyes that are wide apart), and a shortened philtrum (top lip disfigurement). Incidence is 1 per 2,000 to 4,000 in the general population. It is a frequent cause of cleft palate and congenital heart defects.

Eighty percent of affected infants have congenital heart defects, complications of which are usually the first life-threatening effects of the disease. Tetralogy of Fallot and ventricular septal defects are common. Recurrent infections usually present in patients older than 3 to 6 months. The facial features of this syndrome are often subtle and go unnoticed until later in childhood. The overall incidence of immune dysfunction is 77% and recurrent infections are usually observed. Autoimmune diseases such as juvenile RA often occur with the disease. Hypocalcemia can cause seizures early

in development. Developmental delay and learning difficulties are observed in 70% to 90% of patients.

To diagnose the syndrome, a karyotype can reveal the characteristic gene deletion at 22q11. Lymphocyte counts and serum calcium will be abnormal. Cardiac catheterization can demonstrate the cardiac defects.

Multidisciplinary coordinated health care with use of multiple specialists is necessary to ensure that these patients receive optimal medical care. The patient needs consultations from a cardiac surgeon, immunologist, endocrinologist, developmental psychologist, and craniofacial surgical specialist. Cardiac defects were previously a common cause of death; however, with proper surgical care, there is only a 4% mortality rate. The patient's immunoglobulin levels are normal; however, because of the deficiency of CD4 T cells, immune responses are impaired. Treatment involves transplanted thymus gland, preventive antibiotics, and immunoglobulin infusions.

Human Immunodeficiency Virus Infection

Human immunodeficiency virus (HIV) infection is a disease that causes an acute infection syndrome usually followed by a lengthy asymptomatic period. If HIV infection progresses without treatment, it can advance to **acquired immune deficiency syndrome (AIDS).** HIV first came to the public's attention because of an unusual outbreak of disease among homosexual males in Los Angeles in 1981. At that time, there was no name for the disease, but it was known to be associated with severe immune deficiency, *Pneumocystis carinii* pneumonia, and Kaposi's sarcoma, which were highly unusual diseases contracted by healthy homosexual males. The Centers for Disease Control (CDC) took intense interest in examining the outbreaks, and by 1983 a new organism, HIV, was isolated. By 1984, HIV was confirmed as the causative agent of AIDS. The infection quickly became an epidemic and pandemic before it was known that sexual contact and blood products transmit the disease. Before treatments were discovered, many individuals died and HIV infection was thought to be fatal. Today, thanks to advances in diagnostic testing and treatment, many individuals who have HIV never see the disease progress to AIDS, allowing them to live a normal life with chronic HIV infection.

Epidemiology

In the United States, over 1.1 million people are infected with HIV annually—and of those persons, up to a quarter are unaware of their diagnosis. Globally, there are current epidemics of HIV infection in sub-Saharan Africa, Russia, Ukraine, and Southeast Asia. South Africa has the highest prevalence of HIV, with 1 in 5 persons carrying the infection. The CDC and World Health Organization have declared AIDS the most rapidly spreading epidemic in the world.

Etiology

HIV mainly infects CD4 cells, also known as helper T cells. The virus fuses with CD4 surface receptors and inserts its ribonucleic acid (RNA) into the cell. Through the use of a viral enzyme, reverse transcriptase, viral RNA is transformed into DNA and inserted into the CD4 cell's genome. The HIV genes code for synthesis and proliferation of more virus by the host CD4 cell. The active CD4 cell becomes a factory of HIV particles. However, if the CD4 cell is inactive, the virus can remain dormant within the CD4 cell until the cell begins to replicate. This period of dormancy is one of the reasons HIV is difficult to treat.

CD4 cells have a specific surface receptor that is targeted by the HIV virus. The CD4+ surface receptor is also found on macrophages and other cells within the CNS, which is why HIV also targets these cells. After HIV uses the CD4 cell for replication of itself, it destroys the cell and moves on. Viruses move from one CD4 cell to another, using them as factories and then destroying them. The infected CD4 cell can no longer function within cell-mediated immune responses nor assist antibody-mediated immune responses. By destroying the CD4 cell, HIV weakens the body's two categories of adaptive immunity. By destroying macrophages, HIV weakens the body's innate immunity as well (see Fig. 11-10).

Pathophysiology

After contraction of the virus, acute HIV infection presents as a flu-like viral syndrome. Many persons disregard the early symptoms as influenza or a mild viral syndrome and do not seek medical attention. The syndrome resolves and the patient becomes asymptomatic. During this initial phase there is no rise in antibodies or serological representation of disease; this is because of the length of time needed for the immune system to recognize the invader and begin making antibodies against the virus. For most individuals, the development of antibodies to HIV requires from 2 weeks to 6 months. Early in the disease, HIV is a silent, asymptomatic

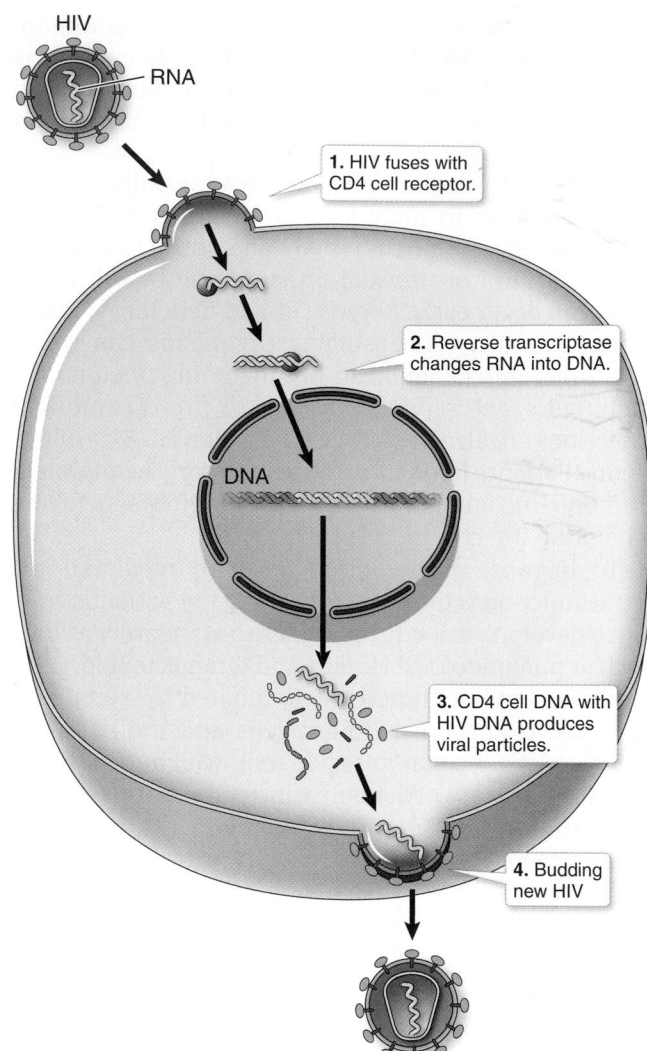

Figure 11–10. The life cycle of human immunodeficiency virus. Step 1. The virus fuses with CD4 cell surface receptor. Step 2. After fusion, HIV inserts its RNA into the cell. Through the use of a viral enzyme, reverse transcriptase, viral RNA is transformed into DNA. Step 3. The CD4 cell synthesizes HIV virus particles. Step 4. Viruses are assembled and new viruses are released.

infection. Although antibodies are not present early in the infection, viral particles can be detected in the bloodstream.

The asymptomatic period of HIV replication and CD4 cell destruction is called the latent period; this period can last from 6 months to 10 years, depending on the individual. During this time, the infected individual is able to transmit the disease. As the virus replicates, the CD4 cell count begins to show a steady decline caused by destruction by the virus. There is significant immunological impairment when the CD4 cell count goes below 500 and an affected individual starts to become susceptible to opportunistic infections. When the CD4 cell count diminishes to 200 and there is existence of an opportunistic infection, the diagnosis of AIDS is made. Without intervention, the strength of the immune system continues to decline, opportunistic infection overwhelms the body, and death is imminent (see Fig. 11-11).

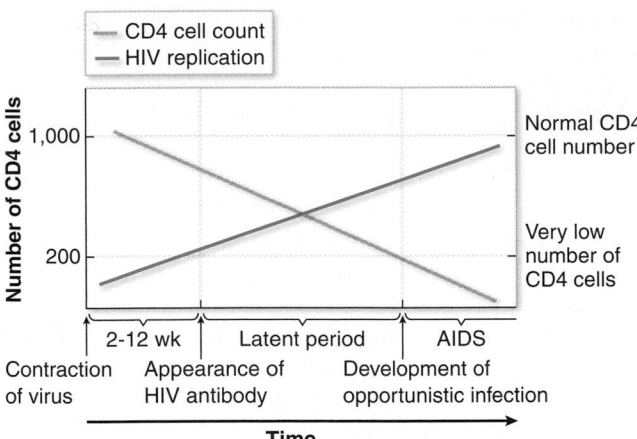

Figure 11–11. The clinical course of HIV infection. There is a 2 week to 6 month period from the time of contraction of the virus to the appearance of the HIV antibody. This is called the window period, when the blood does not demonstrate any HIV antibody. After the virus is contracted, the virus replicates by infecting an increasing number of CD4 cells. As time goes on, CD4 cell number decreases. The latent period is a span of time of increasing viremia when the patient is asymptomatic but the virus is gradually destroying CD4 cells. When there is a low number of CD4 cells, the patient is immunosuppressed and susceptible to opportunistic infection. When the patient has developed an opportunistic infection and has fewer than 200 CD4 cells, the HIV infection is then termed acquired immunodeficiency syndrome (AIDS).

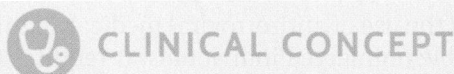 CLINICAL CONCEPT

Kaposi sarcoma is associated with HIV infection. It is a cancerous condition of the endothelium caused by the herpes virus, exhibited by red to purple papular lesions on the skin and mucous membranes.

Clinical Presentation

Early in the disease process the physical examination may be completely normal. Acute HIV infection presents as a mild flulike illness called acute retroviral syndrome. The patient may experience vague symptoms of fever, lymphadenopathy, arthralgias, headache, pharyngitis, fatigue, and GI symptoms that last for approximately 1 to 2 weeks. If the patient seeks health care at this time, a detailed patient history is most important. High-risk behaviors such as unprotected sexual activity, anal intercourse, and intravenous drug abuse should alert the health-care provider of the patient's susceptibility to HIV infection. At-risk populations include heterosexuals who engage in unprotected sexual activity, especially teens and young adults. Heterosexual females are at higher risk of HIV infection than heterosexual males. Homosexual males who engage in unprotected sexual activity are also at high risk. The activity of anal intercourse is particularly a high risk behavior. Persons with a history of sexually transmitted disease are at high risk, as are intravenous drug users who share needles and those who are exposed to bloodborne pathogens.

Despite the fact that donor blood and donor organs are screened for HIV, persons who require frequent transfusions such as hemophiliacs or those who have undergone transplantation are also at risk for HIV infection. Offspring of HIV-positive mothers can contract infection during pregnancy or through breastfeeding. Although not a common occurrence, HIV transmission is also possible through unsanitary tattooing, piercing, dental, and manicure instruments. Substance abusers who share instruments such as spoons or straws are also at risk. Saliva is not known to transmit infection, although an infected individual can pass the virus through saliva to another person with open mouth wounds

Diagnosis

To diagnose acute HIV infection, the **HIV RNA assay** is the earliest and most sensitive test. It is a measure of how much virus is in the bloodstream, also called viral load. If viral load measures fewer than 10,000 copies/mL, there is a low risk of the development of AIDS at the time of measurement. However, if viral load measures greater than 100,000 copies/mL, there is a high risk of the development of AIDS.

Inversion of the CD4 to CD8 ratio also occurs early in infection. This occurs because there is a decrease in number of CD4 cells and the CD8 cells remain unaffected. Normally, in an infection the CD4 to CD8 ratio is 2:1. This ratio reverses with HIV infection: The CD4 to CD8 ratio becomes 1:2.

HIV antibody develops slowly after contraction of the virus. There is a window period when the patient is antibody negative, also called serologically negative. Seroconversion occurs when antibody appears in the bloodstream. This can occur from 2 weeks to 6 months after contraction of the virus, though, in some individuals, this window period can be prolonged. It is during this time when there is no discernible antibody in the bloodstream that infected individuals often pass the virus to others unknowingly.

After seroconversion, HIV antibody can be tested by enzyme linked immunosorbent assay (ELISA). If the ELISA test is negative, the patient is negative for HIV. However, a positive test must be confirmed by the Western Blot test, which is highly sensitive for HIV antibody. There are some over-the-counter HIV tests available; some use saliva or cheek cells and some require a small blood sample. These commercial screening tests detect HIV antibody, but still require a confirmatory Western Blot test.

The number of CD4 cells decreases over the time of viral replication. The normal CD4 count is 700 to 1,200 cells per microliter. At a CD4 count of 500 cells, there is significant immune impairment. At 200 CD4 cells, opportunistic infections commonly overwhelm the body. When CD4 cells fall to low levels, the patient commonly experiences symptoms of persistent fever, night sweats, weight loss, and opportunistic infections. Kaposi's sarcoma often develops and leaves purple-blue blotches on the skin. Opportunistic infections associated with

HIV infection include recurring candida infection, *Pneumocysitis carinii* (also called *Pneumocystis jiroveci*) pneumonia, toxoplasmosis, cryptococcus, and TB. A CD4 count of 200, the presence of an opportunistic infection, and HIV antibody make the diagnosis of **AIDS**.

CLINICAL CONCEPT

A CD4 cell count of 200, an opportunistic infection and HIV antibody make the diagnosis of AIDS.

In those who are HIV positive, CD4 lymphocyte counts should be performed every 6 months. However, those patients with CD4 counts of fewer than or equal to 350 cells per microliter should have their counts performed every 3 months.

CLINICAL CONCEPT

Blood donations are screened for HIV using the p24 antigen test. The risk of contracting HIV infection from donor units of blood is between 1 in 1.4 million and 1 in 1.5 million units.

Treatment

Treatment of HIV and AIDS has posed a great deal of difficulty for the health-care community for a number of reasons. Because of the latency of the disease, an infected individual commonly does not seek treatment until symptomatic with an opportunistic disorder, when the immune system is already greatly compromised. HIV is highly mutatable and development of a vaccine or an effective antibody has proved impossible to date. Although the body produces antibodies to the disease, they are not effective combatants in the fight against the disease. Also, HIV can remain dormant in the body within non-replicating CD4 cells.

The only treatment that has been successful in long-term treatment of HIV infection is antiretroviral therapy (ART) (previously called HAART, highly active retroviral therapy). During this therapy, three different kinds of antiretroviral medications are used to decrease the viral load. These medications work to suppress viral replication within infected cells.

There are several types of antiretroviral medications and each has a different mechanism of action. Treatment attacks the virus at different stages in its development and counteracts HIV development of drug resistance. Reverse transcriptase inhibitors such as zidovudine (AZT) inhibit the reverse transcriptase enzyme. This blocks the transformation of the viral RNA into DNA so HIV cannot insert its directions into the CD4 cell genome. Protease inhibitors block HIV at a stage of protein building in its development within the CD4 cell. These drugs inhibit the synthesis of complete virus structures within the CD4 cell; examples include fosamprenavir and atazanavir.

Another agent used in the treatment of HIV is enfuvirtide (Fuzeon), which blocks the initial entry of HIV into CD4 cells. It has been shown to greatly reduce viral load. Although not a cure, the ART regimen along with prophylactic antibiotics to prevent opportunistic infection has been successful in the control of HIV infection. The T cell's CCR5 coreceptor for HIV is also a site of ART. Maraviroc, a CCR5 receptor antagonist, blocks HIV connection to the CD4 cell (see Box 11-3).

When HIV was first discovered in the 1980s, the life expectancy of patients with the disease was 2 years at most. Today, with ART treatment approaches and the prevention of opportunistic infections, patients with HIV can live a long life from their date of diagnosis. HIV is no longer a life-threatening illness; it is a chronic disease with effective treatment.

Preventive Treatment. HIV preexposure prophylaxis (PrEP) is the use of antiretroviral medications in highly susceptible uninfected individuals. It requires taking a single combination pill daily consisting of emtricitabine and tenofovir (called Truvada®). PrEP is a strategy being used in partners when one spouse is HIV positive and the other spouse is HIV negative. When taken consistently PrEP has been shown to reduce the risk of HIV infection in persons of high risk by 92%. It is currently being used with success in men who have sex with men and IV drug abusers.

BOX 11-3. Human Immunodeficiency Virus Resistors

C–C chemokine receptor type 5 (CCR5) is a protein that is encoded by the CCR5 gene. The CCR5 gene codes for a receptor on CD4 cells that binds with HIV. Certain populations, however, have inherited a mutation resulting in the deletion of the CCR5 gene; these individuals do not have a receptor for HIV on their CD4 cells. Homozygous carriers of this mutation are resistant to HIV-1 infection.

Chapter Summary

- The immune system is a complex defense mechanism that protects humans from a constant barrage of injurious agents in the environment.

- The immune system deciphers which substances are "self" versus "non-self." Non-self substances, also called antigens, are the targets of the immune system.

- The innate line of immunity is the nonspecific defenses that act against all antigens. Innate immunity includes defenses provided by skin, mucous membranes, enzymes, and macrophages.

- The adaptive immune line of defense is developed after exposure to antigens and has memory for antigens. Specific T cells and B cell antibodies are synthesized against specific antigens.

- Adaptive immunity has two categories: cell-mediated (T lymphocyte) and antibody-mediated (B lymphocyte). After exposure, the adaptive immune mechanisms act rapidly, specifically, destructively, and with memory for every individual antigen it has encountered.

- After exposure to antigen, T lymphocytes attack antigens themselves.

- After exposure to antigens, B lymphocytes are transformed into plasma cells that release antigen-attacking Igs.

- There are two types of adaptive immunity: active and passive. Active adaptive immunity occurs when an individual contracts a disease and builds Igs against the antigen or when an individual receives a vaccine. Passive adaptive immunity occurs when an individual receives fully formed antibodies to use against antigen.

- Although the immune system is designed for protection, dysfunction of the immune system can wreak havoc within the body. Immunodeficiency, immune hypersensitivity, and autoimmunity can occur when the immune system dysfunctions.

- There are four types of hypersensitivity reactions. Type I is immediate hypersensitivity, which is an allergic or atopic reaction. Type II is a cytotoxic reaction, such as a transfusion reaction. Type III occurs by immune complex deposition, as in rheumatoid arthritis. Type IV is delayed hypersensitivity, such as the body's delayed reaction to the Mantoux TB test, which develops after 48 hours.

- Autoimmune disease occurs when the body cannot decipher between self and non-self and antibodies attack the body's own tissues.

- HIV is able to undermine both the cell-mediated and antibody-mediated protective defenses of the body by attacking the CD4 cell.

- HIV can be transmitted via semen, vaginal secretions, breast milk, blood, and transplanted tissues.

- The HIV antibody requires 2 weeks to 6 months for development. The window period of HIV infection occurs from the time of contraction of the virus to antibody development.

- The HIV RNA assay is the earliest and most sensitive test of HIV. It measures viral particles or viral load.

- Opportunistic infection and a CD4 count of fewer than 200 are the diagnostic conditions for AIDS.

- Although there is no cure at present, millions are living with and managing their chronic HIV infection because of a triple drug regimen called ART.

- PrEP is a strategy to prevent HIV infection in uninfected but highly vulnerable persons. PrEP is showing efficacy in men who have sex with men and IV drug abusers.

 ## Making the Connections

Disorder and Pathophysiology	Signs and Symptoms	Physical Assessment Findings	Diagnostic Testing	Treatment
Allergic Rhinitis (Type 1 Immediate Hypersensitivity)	Exposure to allergen triggers B cells to produce plasma cells, which in turn secrete Igs. IgE, eosinophils, and mast cells interact to release inflammatory mediators such as histamine, leading to tissue edema.			
	Sneezing. Conjunctivitis. Rhinorrhea.	Copious clear secretions from nose. Pale nasal mucous membranes. Erythema of conjunctiva.	Nasal secretions containing eosinophils. Skin testing to identify specific allergens.	Antihistamines. Intranasal anti-inflammatory corticosteroid.

Continued

Making the Connections–cont'd

Disorder and Pathophysiology	Signs and Symptoms	Physical Assessment Findings	Diagnostic Testing	Treatment

Systemic Anaphylaxis (Severe Type I Immediate Hypersensitivity) | Anaphylaxis is an exaggerated allergic reaction that is a medical emergency. Exposure to allergen triggers B cells to produce plasma cells which, in turn, secrete Igs. IgE, eosinophils, and mast cells interact to release a persistent, high amount of inflammatory mediators such as histamine, leading to tissue edema.

	Pruritic urticaria (itchy hives). Coughing. Stridor. Asthma attack. Extreme anxiety. Fainting.	Urticaria. Edema of tongue. Bronchospasm. Laryngeal edema. Facial edema (angioedema). Hypotension.	Elevated IgE level. Eosinophils in nasal and bronchial secretions. Severe hypotension.	Medical emergency IV or IM antihistamines, corticosteroids and epinephrine required.

Rheumatoid Arthritis | Autoimmune disease mainly involving T cells and inflammatory mediators that attack joints and synovial membranes.

	Painful, tender joints, particularly of hands, wrists, fingers. Systemic symptoms may be present such as fever, malaise, fatigue, anorexia.	Joint swelling. Joint deformities, particularly of metacarpal joints and proximal interphalangeal joints of fingers. Swan's and Boutiniere's deformity. Ulnar deviation of hands.	Elevated ESR, CRP, leukocyte count. RF may be positive. X-ray of regions of joint destruction.	Anti-inflammatory meds: NSAIDs, MTX, DMARDs.

Systemic Lupus Erythematosus | Chronic autoimmune, inflammatory disease with unclear antigen that triggers innate and adaptive immune reactions. Affects skin, heart, lungs, kidneys, and blood cells. Patient can experience remissions and exacerbations.

	Classic butterfly rash across the bridge of nose and cheeks. Fever. Joint pain and swelling. Fatigue. Weight loss.	Rash. Fever. Weight loss. Joint inflammation. Splenic enlargement. Pleural effusion. Vasculitis. Pericarditis. Anemia. Thrombocytopenia. Cardiac valve deformities and renal dysfunction are common.	Antibodies to double-stranded DNA and the Smith (Sm) antigen.	Corticosteroids and immunosuppressive drugs.

Severe Combined Immunodeficiency | Genetically distinct syndromes all having defects of both humoral and cell-mediated immune responses.

	Chronic infection. Candidiasis. Severe diaper rash. Failure to thrive.	Chronic infections. Candidiasis. Severe diaper rash. Failure to thrive.	Immunoglobulin level.	Bone marrow transplant.

Continued

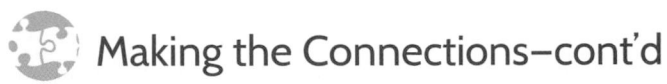

Making the Connections–cont'd

Disorder and Pathophysiology	Signs and Symptoms	Physical Assessment Findings	Diagnostic Testing	Treatment
DiGeorge Syndrome | Isolated T cell deficiency that results from maldevelopment of the thymus gland. Caused by a genetic mutation mapped to 22q11 and 10p.				
	Chronic infections.	Infant has facial abnormalities characteristic of the disease: micrognathia, hypertelorism, and a shortened philtrum.	Lack of T lymphocytes.	Thymus gland transplant. Ig infusions. Antibiotics.
Sarcoidosis | Chronic, autoimmune multisystem disorder of unknown origin characterized by an accumulation of T lymphocytes and macrophages and epithelioid granulomas in various organs.				
	Fever. Fatigue. Malaise. Anorexia. Weight loss. Some patients may develop arthritis at the ankles, wrists, knees, and elbows. Many patients have cough, dyspnea, and chest discomfort if the respiratory system is affected.	Characteristic skin rash called erythema nodosum. Tender erythematous nodules on the anterior surface of the legs. Nonspecific maculopapular rash can develop on the face, around eyes and nose, on the back, and on the extremities. Parotid gland and lymph node enlargement.	Histological examination of lymph nodes. Chest x-ray.	Anti-inflammatory and immunosuppressive agents.
Scleroderma | Autoimmune disease mainly involving collagen infiltration of skin and some organs.				
	Appearance of shiny, stretched skin, particularly of face and hands.	Appearance of shiny, stretched skin, particularly of face and hands. Finger contractures. Raynaud's phenomenon.	Histological examination of skin. Antinuclear antibodies.	Anti-inflammatory and immunosuppressive agents.
Human Immunodeficiency Virus (HIV)/Acquired Immunodeficiency Syndrome | HIV is contracted via blood, sexual activity, transplacental route, or breastfeeding. HIV replicates within the CD4 cells and kills the CD4 cell. As virus increases in the blood, CD4 cell count decreases, which diminishes both humoral and cell-mediated immunity, leaving the patient susceptible to opportunistic infections.				
	May be asymptomatic. Early symptoms may include a flulike syndrome. Late symptoms may include weight loss and symptoms of opportunistic infections.	Signs may be absent if early in disease. Late in disease, signs are those of the opportunistic infections such as lymphadenopathy, fever.	HIV RNA assay. HIV antibody: ELISA and Western Blot: CD4 cell count.	ART triple drug regimen.

Bibliography

American College of Rheumatology. (2012). Scleroderma (Systemic Sclerosis) fact sheet. Retrieved from http://www.rheumatology.org/Practice/Clinical/Patients/Diseases_And_Conditions/Scleroderma_(also_known_as_systemic_sclerosis)/

Anglemyer, A., Horvath, T., & Rutherford, G. (2013). Antiretroviral therapy for prevention of HIV transmission in HIV-discordant couples. JAMA, 310(15), 1619–1620. doi: 10.1001/jama.2013.278328.

Barrett, K., Barman, S., Boitano, S., & Brooks, H. (2012). Ganong's review of medical physiology. 24th. ed. New York: Lange Medical Books/McGraw-Hill Medical Publishing Division.

Boztug, K., Schmidt, M., Schwarzer, A., & Banerjee, P. P. (2010). Stem-cell gene therapy for the Wiskott-Aldrich syndrome. N Engl J Med, 363(20), 1918–1927.

Brown, S. R., & Kennelly, C. (2014). AAFP recommends universal screening for HIV infection beginning at age 18 years of age. Am Fam Phys, 89(8), 614–617.

Burgess, M. J., & Kasten, M. J. (2014). Human immunodeficiency virus: what primary care clinicians need to know. Mayo Clin Proceed, 88(12), 1468–1474. doi: 10.1016/j.mayocp.2013.07.010.

Celum, C., Wald, A., Lingappa, J. R., et al. (2010). Acyclovir and transmission of HIV-1 from persons infected with HIV-1 and HSV-2. N Engl J Med, 362(5), 427–439.

Centers for Disease Control and Prevention. (2014). Pre-exposure prophylaxis (PrEP). Retrieved from http://www.cdc.gov/hiv/prevention/research/prep/

Chang, H. J., Burke, A. E., & Glass, R. M. (2010). JAMA patient page. Sjögren syndrome. JAMA, 304(4), 486.

Chasela, C. S., Hudgens, M. G., Jamieson, D. J., et al. (2010). Maternal or infant antiretroviral drugs to reduce HIV-1 transmission. N Engl J Med, 362(24), 2271–2281.

Chu, C., & Selwyn, P. A. (2010). Diagnosis and initial management of acute HIV infection. Am Fam Phys, 81(10), 1239–1244.

Chu, C., & Selwyn, P. A. (2011). Complications of HIV infection: a systems-based approach. Am Fam Phys, 83(4), 395–406.

Cohen, M. S., Shaw, G. M., McMichael, A. J., & Haynes, B. F. (2011). Acute HIV-1 Infection. N Engl J Med, 364(20), 1943–1954. doi: 10.1056/NEJMra1011874.

Crowson, C. S., Matteson, E. L., Myasoedova, et al. (2011). The lifetime risk of adult-onset rheumatoid arthritis and other inflammatory autoimmune rheumatic diseases. Arthritis & Rheumatism, 63(3), 633–639.

Fauci, A. S., Marston, H. D., & Folkers, G. K. (2014). An HIV cure: feasibility, discovery, and implementation. JAMA, 312(4), 335–336. doi: 10.1001/jama.2014.4754. No abstract available. Erratum in: JAMA. 2014 Aug 13;312(6):652.

Furst, D. E., Tseng, C. H., Clements, P. J., et al. (2011). Adverse events during the Scleroderma Lung Study. Am J Med, 124(5), 459–467.

Gilliam, B. L., Riedel, D. J., & Redfield, R. R. (2011). Clinical use of CCR5 inhibitors in HIV and beyond. J Trans Med, 27 (9 Suppl), S1–S9.

Guatelli, J. (2010). How innate immunity can inhibit the release of HIV-1 from infected cells. N Engl J Med, 362(6), 553–554.

Günthard, H. F., Aberg, J. A., Eron, J. J., et al. (2014). Antiretroviral treatment of adult HIV infection: 2014 recommendations of the International Antiviral Society-USA Panel. JAMA, 312(4), 410–425. doi: 10.1001/jama.2014.8722.

Hampton, T. (2010). HIV study shines spotlight on women. JAMA, 304(3), 257–258.

Jones, C. E., Naidoo, S., De Beer, C., et al. (2011). Maternal HIV infection and antibody responses against vaccine-preventable diseases in uninfected infants. JAMA, 305(6), 576–584.

Kuehn, B. M. (2014). Physicians focus on primary care for patients with HIV. JAMA, 311(1), 17–18. doi: 10.1001/jama.2013.284509.

Kumar, V, Abbas, A. K., Fausto, N., & Aster, J. (2010). Robbins & Cotran pathologic basis of disease. 8th ed. Philadelphia, PA: WB Saunders.

Lallemant, M., & Jourdain, G. (2010). Preventing mother-to-child transmission of HIV—protecting this generation and the next. N Engl J Med, 363(16), 1570–1572.

Latinovic, O., Kuruppu, J., Davis, C., Le, N., & Heredia, A. (2009). Pharmacotherapy of HIV-1 infection: focus on CCR5 antagonist maraviroc. Clin Med Ther, 1, 1487–1510.

Lee, K. C. (2014). Screening for HIV. Am Fam Phys, 89(8), 665–666.

Longo, D., Fauci, A., Kasper, D. L., et al. (2012). Harrison's principles of internal medicine. 18th ed. New York: McGraw-Hill.

Mandell, B. F. (2010). HIV: just another chronic disease. Cleveland Clin J Medicine, 77(8), 489.

Marrazzo, J. M., del Rio, C., Holtgrave, D. R., et al. (2014). HIV prevention in clinical care settings: 2014 recommendations of the International Antiviral Society-USA Panel. JAMA, 312(4), 390–409. doi: 10.1001/jama.2014.7999. Erratum in: JAMA. 2014 Aug 13;312(6):652. JAMA. 2014 Jul 23-30;312(4):403.

Mathers, B. M., & Cooper, D. A. (2014). Integrating HIV prevention into practice. JAMA, 312(4), 349–350. doi: 10.1001/jama.2014.8606.

Mays, M. (2012). The genetics of scleroderma: looking into the post-genomic era. Curr Opin Rheum, 24(6), 677–684. doi: 10.1097/BOR.0b013e328358575b.

McInnes, I. B., & Schett, G. (2011). The pathogenesis of rheumatoid arthritis. N Engl J Med, 365(23), 2205–2219.

Metsch, L. R., Feaster, D. J., Gooden, L., et al. (2013). Effect of risk-reduction counseling with rapid HIV testing on risk of acquiring sexually transmitted infections: the AWARE randomized clinical trial. JAMA, 310(16), 1701–1710. doi: 10.1001/jama.2013.280034.

Mills, E. J., Bärnighausen, T., & Negin, J. (2012). HIV and aging—preparing for the challenges ahead. N Engl J Med, 366(14), 1270–1273.

Mitka, M. (2011). Treatment for lupus, first in 50 years, offers modest benefits, hope to patients. JAMA, 305(17), 1754–1755.

Mofenson, L. M. (2010). Protecting the next generation—eliminating perinatal HIV-1 infection. N Engl J Med, 362(24), 2316–2318.

Robinson, M., Cook, S. S., & Currie, L. M. (2011). Systemic lupus erythematosus: a genetic review for advanced practice nurses. J Am Acad Nurs Pract, 23(12), 629–637.

Saguil, A. (2013). Antiretroviral preexposure prophylaxis for preventing HIV infection in high-risk individuals. Am Fam Phys, 88(3), 172–173.

Segerstrom, S., & Miller, G. (2004). Psychological stress and the human immune system: a meta-analytic study of 30 years of inquiry. Am Psych Assoc, 130(4), 601–630.

Sherin, K., Klekamp, B. G., Beal, J., & Martin, N. (2014). What is new in HIV infection? *Am Fam Phys*, 89(4), 265–272.

Smith, D. K., Koenig, L., Martin, M., et al. (2014). *Preexposure prophylaxis for the prevention of HIV infection–2014: a clinical practice guideline.* United States Public Health Service; Centers for Disease Control and Prevention (U.S.); National Center for HIV/AIDS, Viral Hepatitis, STD, and TB Prevention (U.S.).

Steinbrook, R. (2012). Preexposure prophylaxis for HIV infection. *JAMA*, 308(9), 865–866. doi: 10.1001/jama.2012.9885.

Stephenson, J. (2010). Scientists explore use of anti-HIV drugs as a means to slow HIV transmission. *JAMA*, 303(18), 1798–1799.

Stevens, L. M., Lynm, C., & Glass, R. M. (2010). JAMA patient page. HIV infection: the basics. *JAMA*, 304(3), 364.

Taege, A. (2011). Seek and treat: HIV update 2011. *Cleveland Clin J Med*, 78(2), 95–100.

The 2010 ACR-EULAR classification criteria for rheumatoid arthritis. Retrieved from http://www.rheumatology.org/practice/clinical/classification/ra/ra_2010.asp

Thompson, M. A., Aberg, J. A., Cahn, P., et al. (2010). Antiretroviral treatment of adult HIV infection: 2010 recommendations of the International AIDS Society–USA panel. *JAMA*, 304(3), 321–323.

Torpy, J. M., Perazza, G. D., & Golub, R. M. (2011). JAMA patient page. Rheumatoid arthritis. *JAMA*, 305(17), 1824.

Tsokos, G. C. (2011). Systemic lupus erythematosus. *N Engl J Med*, (22), 2110–2121.

van Lunzen, J., Fehse, B., & Hauber, J. (2011). Gene therapy strategies: can we eradicate HIV? *Current HIV/AIDS Reports.* Feb 18 Epub

Vaughn, J. A., & Miller, R. A. (2011). Update on immunizations in adults. *Am Fam Phys*, 84(9), 1015–1020.

Voelker, R. (2011). Stroke increase reported in HIV patients. *JAMA*, 305(6), 552.

Volkow, N. D., & Montaner, J. (2010). Enhanced HIV testing, treatment, and support for HIV-infected substance users. *JAMA*, 303(14), 1423–1424.

Wasserman, A. M. (2011). Diagnosis and management of rheumatoid arthritis. *Am Fam Phys*, 84(11), 1245–1252.

Weiner, L. M., & Lotze, M. T. (2012). Tumor-cell death, autophagy, and immunity. *N Engl J Med*, 366(12), 1156–1158. doi: 10.1056/NEJMcibr1114526.

Wheeler, T. (2010). Systemic lupus erythematosus: The basics of nursing care. *Brit J Nurs*, 19(4), 249–253.

Wood, E., Kerr, T., Rowell, G., et al. (2014). Does this adult patient have early HIV infection?: The Rational Clinical Examination systematic review. *JAMA*, 312(3), 278–285. doi: 10.1001/jama.2014.5954. Review.

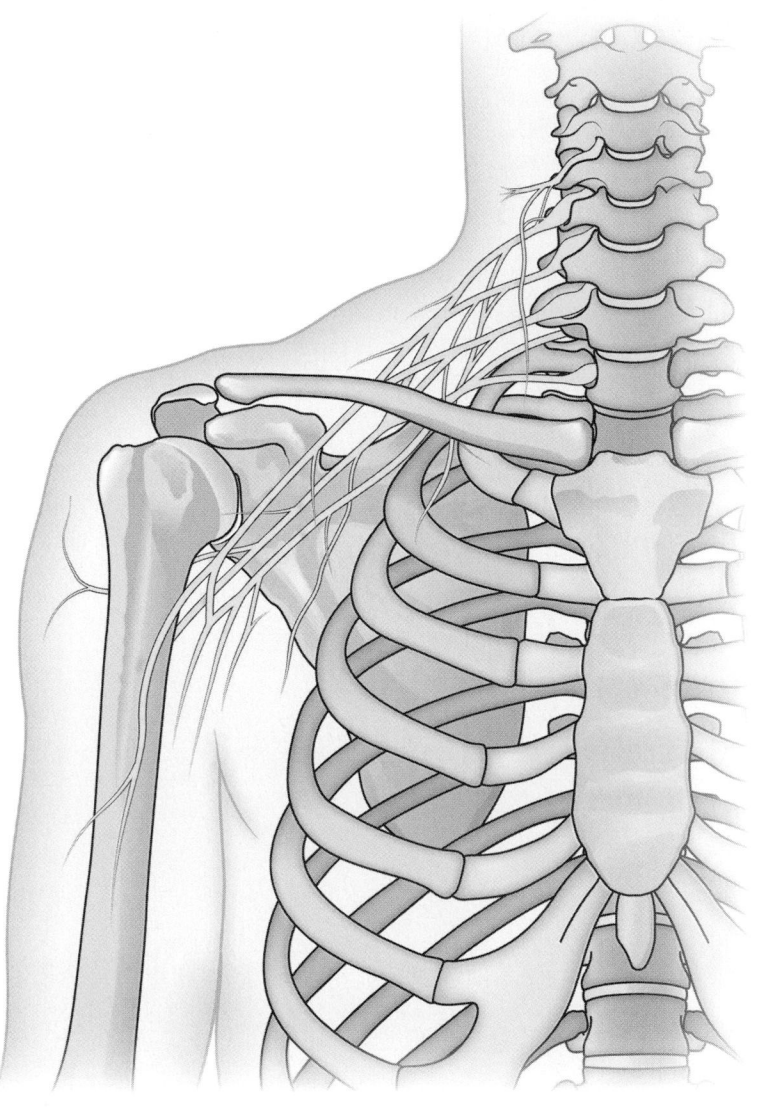

UNIT 5
HEMATOLOGIC DISORDERS

Chapters

CHAPTER 12 Disorders of White Blood Cells

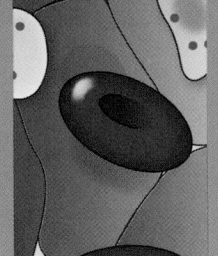

Key Terms

Allogeneic hematologic stem cell transplant

Autologous hematologic stem cell transplant

Bands

Blast cells

Leukemia

Leukemoid reaction

Leukocytosis

Lymphoma

Multiple myeloma (MM)

Myelodysplastic syndrome (MDS)

Neutropenia

Neutrophilia

Philadelphia chromosome (PhC)

Plasmacytoma

Pluripotent stem cells

Segs

Tumor lysis syndrome

Tyrosine kinase

White blood cells (WBCs), also called leukocytes, protect the body against infection. They function within the innate and adaptive divisions of the immune system. Those found in the innate division, known as macrophages, are the first line of defense against foreign invaders, also called antigens. In the adaptive division, specialized WBCs called B lymphocytes and T lymphocytes attack specific antigens while maintaining a memory of these antigens for future defensive action.

All WBCs are manufactured in the bone marrow and released. Lymphocytes mature further within lymphoid tissue, such as the lymph nodes, tonsils, adenoids, thymus gland, and spleen.

Infections, immune diseases, and hematologic neoplasms are the main disorders that affect WBCs. Hematologic neoplasms, the major disorder of WBCs reviewed in this chapter, include the leukemias and lymphomas. These cancerous disorders target WBCs, but they also have effects on red blood cells (RBCs) and platelets. Hematology, the study of the blood cells, and oncology, the study of cancers, are closely related fields, and specialist clinicians are usually skilled in both types of disease.

Epidemiology

Leukemias and **lymphomas** are the neoplastic disorders that affect WBCs. Lymphomas are solid tumors of lymphoid cells, and they affect approximately 3% of the U.S. population per year. Examples include Hodgkin's lymphoma, which affects people between 15 to 20 years of age and those aged 50 to 70 years. It is one of the most curable of the hematologic cancers, and affects 1 in 25,000 people annually. The disease accounts for slightly fewer than 1% of all cancers worldwide.

Leukemias cause proliferation of cancerous WBCs. Worldwide, leukemia affects approximately 350,000 people per year, with 90% of those cases being diagnosed in adults. It is, however, the third most common cancer in children.

Basic Concepts of WBC Function

WBCs are the major defenders of the body. The bone marrow produces them in response to inflammation or infection. Macrophages are WBCs of the innate immune system, which are always ready and waiting to defend. Lymphocytes, part of the adaptive immune system, act against specific antigens for which they have memory.

Categories of WBCs

The normal range of total WBCs in the body is between 4,100 and 10,900 cells per microliter (uL). They are divided into three major categories: monocytes (also known as macrophages), lymphocytes, and granulocytes. There are also three types of granulocytes: neutrophils, eosinophils, and basophils, with neutrophils comprising the majority of the granulocytes. WBCs without granules such as monocytes and lymphocytes are sometimes called agranulocytes. There are two types of lymphocytes: T cells and B cells. Each type of WBC has its own normal range (see Table 12-1).

Synthesis and Maturation of WBCs

All blood cells arise from a small number of undeveloped, precursor cells called **pluripotent stem cells** in the bone marrow during the process of hematopoiesis.

TABLE 12-1. WBC Differential	
WBC Count	**4.1-10.9 x10³/μL**
• Polymorphonuclear wbcs	• 35% to 80%
• Immature polys	• 0% to 10%
• Lymphocytes	• 20% to 50%
• Monocytes	• 2% to 12%
• Eosinophils	• 0% to 7%
• Basophils	• 0% to 2%

These precursor cells have the potential to become any type of blood cell. The bone marrow is stimulated to produce specific types of blood cells according to the body's needs. WBCs have a short life span and need constant replenishment by the bone marrow. To produce WBCs, the bone marrow begins with pluripotent stem cells called myeloid and lymphoid stem cells. Granulocyte and monocyte cells are derived from myeloid stem cells and lymphocytes from lymphoid stem cells. Immature precursor cells for each cell line are called **blast cells.** From the blast cell stage, each type of WBC begins to differentiate and mature along a committed cell line (see Fig. 12-1). Lymphocytes mature to a certain extent in the bone marrow, but then leave and complete the maturation process in lymphoid tissue (see Fig. 12-2). B lymphocytes mature to an extent in bone marrow and then develop into plasma cells, which are antibody-producing cells, within lymph nodes. T lymphocytes continue the maturation process mainly within the thymus gland, where they become T helper (CD4) and cytotoxic T cells (CD8) and then move into lymph nodes for proliferation.

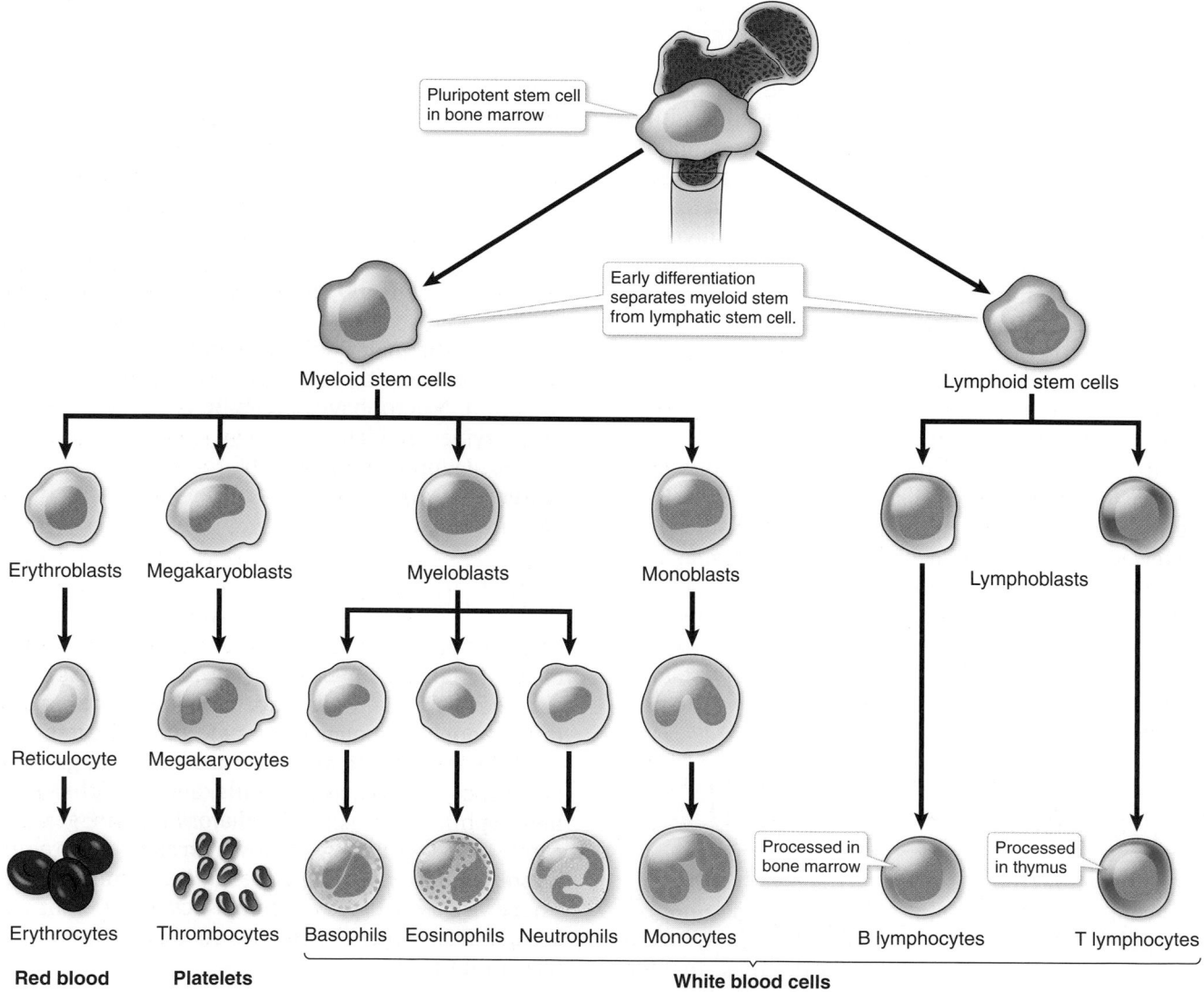

FIGURE 12-1. Hematopoiesis. All blood cells are derived from a pluripotent stem cell that has the ability to become any kind of blood cell. From the pluripotent stem cell, there is a differentiation into either a myeloid or a lymphoid line of stem cells. From the myeloid stem cell line, erythroblasts, myeloblasts, monoblasts, and megakaryocytes can be formed and developed into mature cells. Erythroblasts develop into RBCs. Myeloblasts and monoblasts develop into different types of WBCs. Megakaryocytes develop into platelets. From the lymphatic stem cell line, lymphoblasts can be formed and develop into mature lymphocytes.

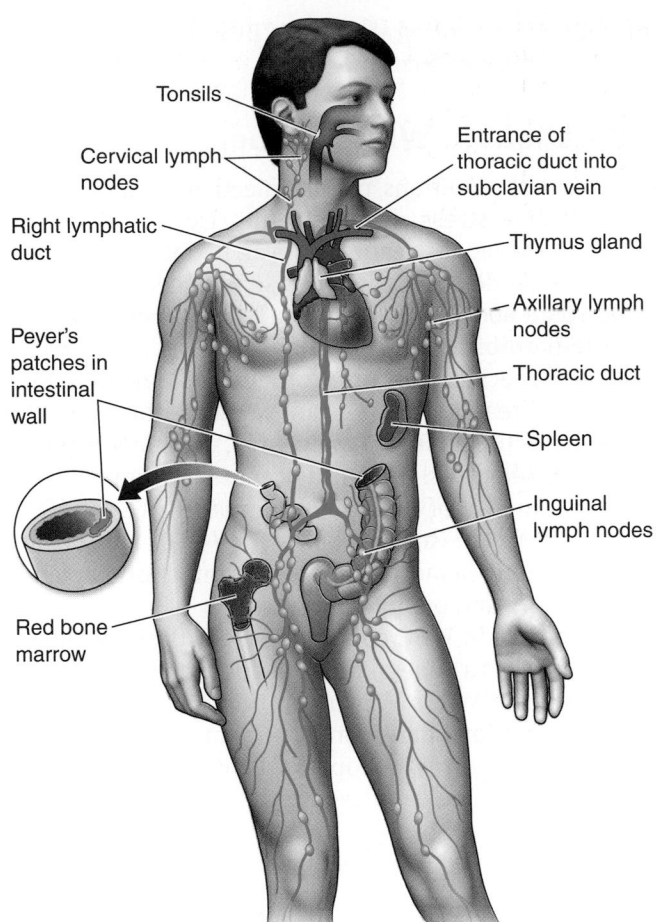

Tonsils

Cervical lymph nodes

Right lymphatic duct

Peyer's patches in intestinal wall

Red bone marrow

Entrance of thoracic duct into subclavian vein

Thymus gland

Axillary lymph nodes

Thoracic duct

Spleen

Inguinal lymph nodes

FIGURE 12-2. The lymphatic system.

Lymph nodes are located at various sites throughout the body. For example, the spleen is an organ rich in lymphoid tissue. In addition, the gastrointestinal, respiratory, and genitourinary tracts are guarded by zones of lymphoid tissue and high numbers of macrophages.

Monocytes

Monocytes make up 3% to 7% of circulating WBCs. When they leave the circulation and enter tissue, they mature into macrophages, which are found in large quantities in the spleen and other organs. They have the ability to exit and reenter circulation while maintaining their primary function, which is phagocytosis. In phagocytosis, the macrophage engulfs, ingests, and enzymatically destroys antigenic substances and cellular debris. Another important function of monocytes is their ability to synthesize and secrete cytokines, substances that enhance inflammation and stimulate function of other WBCs.

Lymphocytes

Lymphocytes make up 20% to 35% of circulating WBCs. There are two main types of lymphocytes: B lymphocytes (B cells) and T lymphocytes (T cells). Lymphocytes are part of the adaptive branch of the immune system. After exposure to an antigen, lymphocytes recognize, target, and have memory for specific antigens. They endow the body with long-term immunity (see Chapter 11: Disorders of the Immune System for more information).

Granulocytes

Granulocytes are WBCs with chemical-containing granules in their cytoplasm. Their granules contain powerful digestive enzymes capable of killing microorganisms and then catabolizing debris during phagocytosis. The three types of granulocytes—eosinophils, basophils, and neutrophils—are classified by the chemical makeup of their granules. Laboratory differentiation is possible because different granules stain differently when dye is applied.

Neutrophils. Neutrophils make up 60% to 70% of the WBCs in circulation. Like macrophages, they are the first responders to an infection, stressful event, or inflammatory reaction. Antigens, epinephrine, and corticosteroids stimulate generation and release of neutrophils in the bloodstream. Mature neutrophils, also called polymorphonuclear leukocytes, have a life span of 1 to 2 days, and new recruits from the bone marrow are necessary during infection or inflammation. Under the microscope, mature neutrophils have a segmented, multilobed nucleus as opposed to immature neutrophils, which have a bandlike nucleus. Because of the shape of their nucleus, mature neutrophils are referred to as **segs,** whereas immature neutrophils are called **bands.** The bone marrow releases immature neutrophils when the mature neutrophil supply in circulation is exhausted. Bands in circulation indicate that the bone marrow is working very hard to manufacture enough WBCs for the infection or inflammatory disorder in the body. In severe acute infection or inflammation, the bone marrow cannot keep up with the body's need for mature neutrophils, so it releases bands. If a laboratory test indicates a high number of bands in circulation, this is referred to as a "shift to the left."

At the first sign of cell injury, neutrophils leave circulation and enter the tissues, where they lyse (break down) bacteria by releasing lysosomal enzymes stored in their granules. When a neutrophil phagocytizes an invading organism or cellular debris, it releases a respiratory burst of free radicals called superoxides $[O_2^-]$ that contribute to injury of surrounding tissues (see Fig. 12-3).

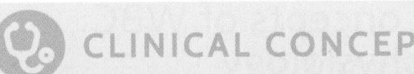

CLINICAL CONCEPT

Macrophages function within the innate immune system and are the first responders in defense against antigen.

CLINICAL CONCEPT

Purulent exudate, commonly called pus, is a whitish-green-colored discharge from a site of injury that contains dead neutrophils, infectious material, and cellular debris.

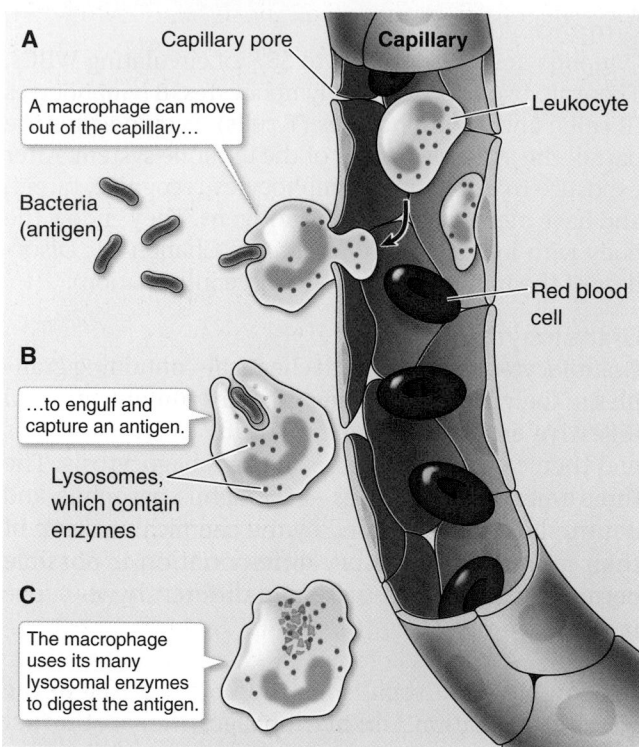

FIGURE 12-3. Phagocytosis of bacteria by a macrophage. A macrophage can move out of the capillary to engulf and capture an antigen. The macrophage uses its many lysosomal enzymes to digest the antigen.

Eosinophils. Eosinophils are WBCs that are generated by the bone marrow and mainly released during allergic reactions and parasitic infection. They include granules in the cytoplasm that contain chemical mediators and enzymes, such as histamine, eosinophil peroxidase, ribonuclease, deoxyribonuclease, lipase, and plasminogen. These mediators are released following activation of the eosinophil and are toxic to both parasites and host tissues. In healthy individuals, eosinophils make up about 1% to 6% of all WBCs, but their number rises during allergic reactions or parasitic infection.

Basophils. Basophils make up fewer than 1% of circulating WBCs but rise in response to infection. Their granules have chemical mediators, including histamine, prostaglandin, leukotrienes, and heparin. Basophils are generated and released by the bone marrow in response to many inflammatory reactions, particularly parasitic infection. The mediators histamine and heparin assist in the migration of neutrophils to an inflammatory site.

Basic Concepts of WBC Pathophysiology

WBCs can rise or become deficient in number, indicating a specific pathophysiologic condition and corresponding side effects. Additionally, there are conditions of neoplastic proliferation of WBCs that can disrupt normal immune function.

Alterations in WBC Number

Pathological conditions, mainly infection, inflammation, and extreme stress, stimulate the rise in number of WBCs in the bloodstream. However, neoplasms or bone marrow disorders can also increase WBC count. A rise in WBC count above 11,000/uL is called **leukocytosis.**

A **leukemoid reaction** is leukocytosis in excess of 50,000/μL because of causes other than leukemia. In a leukemoid reaction there is an excess of normal, early neutrophil precursors: myelocytes, metamyelocytes, and promyelocytes. In contrast, acute leukemia shows a predominance of cancerous, immature WBCs called blasts. There are various causes for a leukemoid reaction, including hemorrhage, specific infections, splenic dysfunction, and organ necrosis.

A decrease in WBC count below 4,000 /uL is leukopenia, which is a general term that describes a decrease in all types of WBCs. Any agent that diminishes bone marrow function or any condition that causes destruction of WBCs causes leukopenia. Leukopenia increases risk of infection, decreases signs of infection, and diminishes healing ability.

Neutrophils are the most common type of WBC affected in leukopenia. Filgrastim (Neupogen®) is a stimulant of the bone marrow that can increase leukocyte synthesis, specifically neutrophils.

Neutrophils

The most common type of WBC that rises in leukocytosis is the neutrophil. **Neutrophilia** is the term used for neutrophil predominance in the WBC count; it is defined as a neutrophil count above 7,700/uL in patients with a total WBC count of fewer than 11,000/uL. It is usually secondary to infection, inflammation, or malignancy, but it can also be caused by additional factors such as smoking, stress, and drugs. In fact, cigarette smoking has been estimated to raise the WBC count in smokers by about 25%, and the total WBC count may remain elevated for up to 5 years after cessation. The rise in neutrophil levels is theorized to occur as the result of smoking-related inflammation. Drugs that cause neutrophilia include glucocorticoids, lithium, and epinephrine.

 CLINICAL CONCEPT

WBC count is measured using a laboratory test called a complete blood count with differential (CBC with differential). It measures total RBCs, hemoglobin (Hgb), hematocrit (Hct), platelets, total WBCs, and the percentage of each type of WBC present. When the WBC count contains a large number of immature neutrophil bands, this is referred to as a "shift to the left."

BOX 12-1. Common Causes of Neutropenia

- Infections, more commonly viral infections, but also bacterial or parasitic infections
- Medications, including medications that may damage the bone marrow or neutrophils, including cancer chemotherapy, chloramphenicol, phenothiazines, allopurinol, carbamazepine, and phenylbutazone
- Vitamin deficiencies, including megaloblastic anemia caused by vitamin B_{12} or folate deficiency
- Diseases of the bone marrow, including leukemias, myelodysplastic syndrome, aplastic anemia, myelofibrosis, and any cause of bone marrow suppression
- Radiation therapy
- Hemodialysis machinery
- Heart-lung machinery used in cardiac bypass
- Congenital (inborn) disorders of bone marrow function or of neutrophil production, such as Kostmann syndrome
- Autoimmune destruction of neutrophils (either as a primary condition or associated with another disease such as Felty's syndrome) or from drugs stimulating the immune system to attack the cells
- Hypersplenism, which refers to the increased sequestration and/or destruction of blood cells by the spleen

Neutropenia, which is the lack of sufficient number of neutrophils, is the most frequent kind of leukopenia. It is diagnosed in patients with fewer than 1,500 neutrophils/uL. A decrease in neutrophil number can occur rapidly and may occur because of deficient marrow function, WBC destruction, or a shift of neutrophils into various tissues.

There are many causes of neutropenia (see Box 12-1). With moderate to severe neutropenia (less than 1,000/uL), the body's immune defenses are significantly impaired, though monocytes are still active and will cause a rise in body temperature. Neutropenia with fever is evidence of infection.

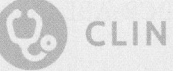 CLINICAL CONCEPT

Neutropenia increases susceptibility to infection and diminishes the external signs of inflammation.

Monocytes

Monocytic leukocytosis is defined as a total WBC count greater than 11,000/μL, primarily caused by a monocyte count above 800/μL. An elevated monocyte count in the presence of a normal total WBC count is called monocytosis. It is seen in the acute and chronic monocytic types of leukemia and can occur in acute bacterial infections and tuberculosis. Monocytopenia, an abnormally low number of monocytes, can be caused by high-dose steroids, but is usually a result of a malignancy.

Eosinophils

Eosinophilia is an abnormally high number of eosinophils in the blood. Normally, there are no more than a few hundred eosinophils among all WBCs. In eosinophilia, there are greater than 600 cells/uL in the bloodstream. Eosinophilia is usually a result of an allergy or parasitic infection. Leukemia, as well as certain medications, toxins, and autoimmune disease, can cause eosinophilia.

Basophils

Basophilic leukocytosis is a rare condition most often associated with basophilic or mast cell types of acute or chronic leukemia. Other causes include hypersensitivity or inflammatory reactions, parasitic infection, hypothyroidism, ulcerative colitis, and varicella virus. Basopenia, an abnormally low number of basophils, is usually the result of a malignant disorder.

Lymphocytes

Lymphocytosis is an increase in lymphocytes within the bloodstream. Because thymus-derived T cells decrease in number as a person ages, the definition of lymphocytosis also changes as a person ages:

- **Infant:** lymphocyte count greater than 9,000/uL
- **Children:** lymphocyte count greater than 7,000/uL
- **Adults:** lymphocyte count greater than 4,000/uL.

Lymphocytosis is a sign of infection, particularly in children. In elderly individuals, lymphoproliferative disorders, including chronic lymphocytic leukemia (CLL) and lymphomas, often present with lymphadenopathy and lymphocytosis.

Lymphocytopenia, a decrease in lymphocytes, is a result of a decreased production in the bone marrow because of an acquired or inherited immunodeficiency. Alternatively, it can occur because of lymphocyte destruction from radiation or chemotherapy. It, too, is diagnosed at different levels at different ages:

- **Children:** lymphocyte count lower than 3,000/uL
- **Adults:** lymphocyte level lower than 1,500/uL
- **Elderly:** lymphocyte count lower than 1,400/uL.

In some cases, lymphocytopenia can be further classified according to the kind of lymphocytes that are reduced. In T lymphocytopenia, there are too few T lymphocytes, but a normal number of other lymphocytes. This is usually caused by human immunodeficiency virus (HIV) infection, an inherited disorder, severe infection, radiation, or chemotherapy. In B lymphocytopenia, there are too few B lymphocytes, but normal numbers of other lymphocytes. This is usually caused by medications that suppress the immune system. In NK lymphocytopenia, a rare disorder, there are too few natural killer cells, but normal numbers of other lymphocytes.

Myelodysplastic Syndrome

A **myelodysplastic syndrome (MDS)** is a broad term used for disorders of the stem cells in the bone marrow. In this syndrome, all or part of bone marrow hematopoiesis is disorderly and ineffective and differentiation of all or one category of precursor stem cells into committed cell lines is impaired. The patient suffers deficient numbers of all blood cells or one type of blood cell: WBCs, RBCs, or platelets. The median age at diagnosis of a MDS is between 60 and 75 years; few patients are younger than age 50 and MDS diagnoses are rare in children. Males are slightly more commonly affected than females. Estimates of incidence are on the order of 10,000 to 20,000 new cases per year in the United States, with incidence increasing as the age of the population increases.

MDS is caused by environmental exposures such as radiation and benzene; other risk factors have been reported inconsistently. Secondary MDS occurs as a toxic effect of cancer treatment. Signs and symptoms are nonspecific and generally related to the diminished number of all blood cells. The clinical presentation is similar to that of hematologic neoplasms. Lack of RBCs causes anemia, lack of WBCs causes infections, and lack of platelets causes increased susceptibility to bleeding and bruising. MDS can lead to complete bone marrow failure or leukemia. Treatment involves transfusion of the deficient type of blood cells and chemotherapy.

Hematologic Neoplasms

The hematologic neoplasms are types of cancer that affect blood, bone marrow, and lymph nodes. They account for 9.5% of new cancer diagnoses in the United States. These cancers are classified by whether the malignancy is mainly located in the blood (leukemia) or in lymph nodes (lymphomas). Within the category of hematologic neoplasms, lymphomas are more common than leukemias.

Leukemias commonly develop in precursor stem cells of the bone marrow from a specific cell line. The abnormal cells appear similar to the immature forms of these cells, also called blasts. These blasts continue to proliferate and do not differentiate into mature cells.

Lymphomas are hematologic neoplasms that specifically arise from abnormal proliferation of B or T lymphocytes. The tumors typically begin in the lymph nodes but can develop from any lymphoid tissue.

Etiology

Hematologic cancers can develop from any agent that damages the deoxyribonucleic acid (DNA) of developing cells in the bone marrow. The damage turns on

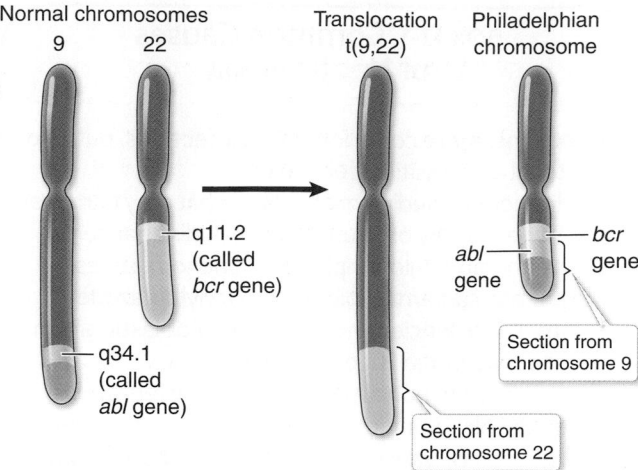

FIGURE 12-4. Formation of the Philadelphia chromosome. A section of the long arm of chromosome 9 breaks off and a section of the long arm of chromosome 22 breaks off. The broken sections from each chromosome switch positions. The section from chromosome 9 binds to chromosome 22, whereas the broken section from chromosome 22 binds to chromosome 9. The translocation of these chromosomes is involved in the etiology of chronic myelogenous leukemia.

oncogenes or turns off tumor suppressor genes in the individual's genome, causing abnormal blood cell development. These malignancies are sometimes associated with a single gene abnormality such as the **Philadelphia chromosome (PhC)** or changes to whole chromosomes such as trisomy (3 chromosomes instead of 2) or monosomy (1 chromosome instead of a pair).

The PhC is an abnormality that results from a translocation of a gene (see Fig. 12-4). The translocation is between chromosome 9 and chromosome 22; part of chromosomes 9 and 22 actually change places with each other. The translocation causes a fusion of the parts of the two genes. A gene called the break point cluster (BCR) gene on chromosome 22 fuses with the Abelson leukemia virus (ABL) gene on chromosome 9. This translocation is commonly referred to as the BCR-ABL oncogene. The protein formed by the directions of these genes is the enzyme **tyrosine kinase,** which causes leukemia in hematopoietic cells. Many new drugs used to treat leukemias are tyrosine kinase inhibitors that prevent BCR-ABL from inciting leukemic changes.

Risk Factors

Exposure to any agent that can damage DNA is a risk for a hematologic cancer. Exposure to intense radiation and contact with benzene are known predisposing factors for leukemia. Some viruses have been found to predispose to hematologic cancers, such as Epstein Barr virus (EBV), HIV, and human T-lymphotropic virus (HTLV). Chronic gastric infection with *Helicobacter pylori* is also associated with lymphoma.

Lymphomas have also been associated with congenital or acquired immunodeficiency disorders, including

BOX 12-2. Risk Factors of Hematologic Neoplasms

- Repeated exposure to the chemical benzene, which is found in cigarette smoke, the most common known cause of exposure to this toxin, and in certain industrial settings; strict regulation of its use has decreased exposure in the workplace
- Repeated exposure to herbicides and pesticides such as Agent Orange
- Certain genetic disorders such as Down syndrome, Fanconi anemia, Shwachman syndrome, and Diamond-Blackfan syndrome
- Past chemotherapy or radiation treatments for other cancers
- History of other blood cancers or disorders, such as polycythemia vera, idiopathic myelofibrosis, primary thrombocythemia, and myelodysplastic syndromes
- Viral causes, including EBV, HIV, and HTLV
- Bacteria, including *H. pylori*, related to mucosa-associated lymphoid tissue lymphoma

those resulting from immunosuppression treatment. See Box 12-2 for a list of common risk factors for hematologic malignancies.

Pathophysiology

Each specific type of leukemia or lymphoma has a specific pathophysiologic process. Leukemias are states of neoplastic proliferation involving WBCs other than lymphocytes. Lymphomas are neoplasms of lymphocytes and are commonly solid tumors found in lymphoid tissue. Regardless of the type of neoplasm, leukemias and lymphomas cause similar pathophysiologic conditions in the body. Nonfunctional, cancerous WBCs proliferate and overwhelm the bone marrow and other lymphoid tissue. The cancerous WBCs increase to excess numbers and they crowd and suppress development of the other blood cells in the bone marrow—healthy WBCs, RBCs, and platelets.

Clinical Presentation

As with any illness, assessment begins with a complete history and physical examination. A complete list of all medications, including over-the-counter medications and supplements, needs to be obtained. Many medications and supplements can alter the production and number of WBCs. Past history of toxic or occupational exposures should be assessed to investigate possible risk factors associated with hematologic disorders. For example, history of benzene exposure is related to leukemia. History of herbicide or insecticide exposure is associated with some types of lymphoma. Past medical and surgical disorders are important because some illnesses predispose

to leukemias or lymphomas. For example, persons with EBV are at risk for development of Burkitt's lymphoma.

Family history and psychosocial history are important because many hematologic disorders can be caused by genetic abnormalities or behavioral risk factors. For example, CLL is often found among family members. Unsafe sexual practices can predispose individuals to HIV infection, which is a risk factor for lymphoma.

Signs and Symptoms. Key symptoms seen in patients with leukemia or lymphoma are those related to bone marrow suppression. Bone marrow becomes overwhelmed by the proliferation of neoplastic blood cells that crowd out healthy blood cells. The symptoms are related to low RBC count (anemia), WBC count (leukopenia), or platelets (thrombocytopenia) (see Box 12-3 for symptoms of hematologic neoplasms).

Physical examination may reveal enlarged lymph nodes, splenomegaly, or both. An enlarged lymph node is the result of proliferative neoplastic cells and may be noticed by the patient or clinician on a physical exam. Splenomegaly may be present, the result of excessive infiltration of neoplastic blood cells or excessive hemolysis performed by an overactive spleen. In leukemia or lymphoma, splenomegaly is often the initial symptom.

Diagnosis

CBC with differential is usually the initial laboratory test with abnormal findings that begins the investigation into hematologic malignancy. Bone marrow biopsy and genome investigation of abnormal cells follows.

CBC With Differential. A CBC with differential is an important initial diagnostic test used to identify which specific type of WBC is causing the neoplastic disorder. The CBC identifies rbc number, Hgb, Hct, platelet number, and proportions of specific WBCs in the bloodstream. This is the basic diagnostic test that most often initiates further investigation into a hematologic neoplasm.

Bone Marrow Aspiration. Blood cells develop from their precursor cells in the bone marrow. It is through aspirating and examining this marrow that the etiology of the illness can be determined. Typical results of bone marrow aspiration, also known as bone marrow biopsy, would demonstrate an adequate amount of precursor cells with other cells in various stages of maturation. Changes in the cell types or increased presence of immature cells are often seen in hematologic disorders. Most aspiration procedures use the hip bone as the source of bone marrow.

Fluorescence In-Situ Hybridization. Fluorescence in-situ hybridization (FISH) is used to analyze cells for

---

BOX 12-3. Common Signs and Symptoms of Hematologic Neoplasms

Common signs and symptoms of hematologic neoplasms are caused by the excessive proliferation of neoplastic blood cells that overwhelm the bone marrow and crowd out and suppress development of healthy cells. Neoplastic cells also invade the lymph nodes, spleen, and liver.

- Anemia: caused by decreased red blood cells; chronic tiredness, shortness of breath, pallor, sometimes chest pain
- Neutropenia: decreased normal WBCs, which causes increased susceptibility to infections
- Thrombocytopenia: decreased platelets, which increases susceptibility to bleeding and ecchymosis (bruising), nosebleeds (epistaxis), gingival bleeding, or subcutaneous hemorrhaging resulting in purpura or petechiae
- Bone pain: caused by excessive proliferation of neoplastic cells inside the bone marrow of many different bones, most commonly the sternum, femur, and tibia
- Lymphadenopathy: excessive proliferation of abnormal lymphocytes
- Splenomegaly: excessive proliferation of abnormal lymphocytes
- Hepatomegaly: excessive proliferation of lymphocytes
- Abdominal feeling of fullness: caused by an enlarged spleen or liver putting pressure on stomach
- Unintentional weight loss: caused by decreased appetite
- Fever, chills: caused by hypermetabolic state resulting from constant neoplastic cell production

---

chromosome defects. It can be performed on tissue, peripheral blood, or bone marrow, where it detects and localizes the presence or absence of specific DNA sequences on chromosomes. This diagnostic test can be used to identify a specific chromosome, show translocations and deletions, or identify extra-chromosomal fragments of chromatin.

Flow Cytometry. Flow cytometry is a diagnostic technique frequently used in leukemia, as it aids in staging and prognosis. It is a technique for examining cells and analyzing DNA by suspending tissue in fluid and passing it through an electronic detection apparatus that uses laser light.

Treatment

The treatment regimen in hematologic neoplasms is based on the type of disorder. There are basic types of treatment commonly utilized: chemotherapy, monoclonal antibodies, radiation, stem cell transplants, and surgery.

Chemotherapy. Most chemotherapeutic agents target rapidly dividing cells, including cancer cells. However, chemotherapy causes ancillary effects on rapidly dividing healthy cells such as skin, gastric mucosa, and bone marrow. Hair loss, disruption of the gastric mucosa, and bone marrow suppression occur in chemotherapy. Neutropenia is a major complication of chemotherapy with its associated risk of life-threatening infection. This threat can be reduced by the administration of a neutrophil stimulant such as filgrastim (Neupogen) to increase the production of neutrophils.

Monoclonal Antibodies. Monoclonal antibodies are highly specific antibodies that can target a single antigen; in this case, specific types of cancer cells. In the laboratory, a tumor antigen is identified and introduced to myeloma cells, which are cells that continually synthesize antibodies. The myeloma cells are genetically reprogrammed so that they continually synthesize antibodies specifically against the tumor antigen. As a result, monoclonal antibodies are a supply of laboratory-produced antibodies against tumor antigen. These antibodies are administered to the cancer patient and they precisely target and destroy tumor cells.

Radiation. Radiation therapy is the use of high-dose x-rays to treat cancer cells, particularly cancer cells that are not totally removed by surgery. Radiation therapy is often used for the treatment of non-Hodgkin's lymphoma (NHL), Hodgkin's lymphoma (HL), and all types of leukemia. Radiation therapy may be used alone or in combination with chemotherapy. For lymphoma or leukemia, radiation therapy may be administered from a machine outside the body that directs radiation to the cancer (external radiation). Or it may be given inside the body (internal radiation) through radiation that is sealed inside of seeds, wires, or catheters. The way radiation is given depends on the type and stage of cancer being treated.

Stem Cell Transplants. Bone marrow stem cell transplantation has long been used as treatment for hematologic malignancies. Initially in this procedure, the patient's diseased bone marrow is completely ablated or partially ablated. Ablation destroys the patient's diseased bone marrow using intense chemotherapy, radiation, or both. During ablation, the patient is severely immunosuppressed and highly susceptible to infection. After ablation is achieved, healthy bone marrow stem cells are infused into the patient. Healthy bone marrow cells are harvested from a donor who has a matching tissue type to the recipient. These are called **allogeneic hematologic stem cell transplants.** The donor has a large bore needle inserted into the pelvis to obtain healthy bone marrow, and then cells are administered to the recipient. When successful, the donor's healthy bone marrow cells replace the recipient's cancerous bone marrow. However, bone marrow transplant rejection occurs frequently.

CLINICAL CONCEPT

Siblings are most often found to have matching types of tissue for bone marrow transplant.

An alternative procedure that is commonly used is **autologous hematologic stem cell transplant.** This kind of transplant involves initial extraction of healthy hematopoietic stem cells from the patient and storage of the harvested cells in a freezer. The patient is then treated with high-dose chemotherapy with or without radiation to destroy the patient's malignant cell population at the cost of partial or complete bone marrow ablation. In partial bone marrow ablation, the patient is not completely immunosuppressed. After complete or partial bone marrow ablation, the patient's own stored healthy stem cells are returned to his or her body, where they replace destroyed tissue and resume the patient's normal blood cell production. Autologous transplants have the advantage of lower risk of infection during the immunocompromised portion of the treatment because the recovery of immune function is rapid. Also, the incidence of patients experiencing rejection is very rare because the donor and recipient are the same individual.

Umbilical cord stem cells are also being used as stem cell transplants for hematologic cancers with varying rates of success. Cord blood has a higher concentration of hematologic stem cells than is normally found in adult blood. However, the small quantity of blood obtained from an umbilical cord (typically about 50 mL) makes it more suitable for transplantation into small children than into adults.

Complications

Serious complications of treatment are always a possibility regardless of what method is used. Aside from life-threatening infection and graft rejection, **tumor lysis syndrome** is a serious but infrequent complication. It results from rapid cell destruction of a large number of tumor cells all at once. The lysed cells release their intracellular contents into the surrounding tissues and circulation, causing hyperuricemia (from purine breakdown), hyperkalemia, and hyperphosphatemia with secondary hypocalcemia. The uric acid crystals can cause damage to the glomeruli and nephron tubules, causing renal failure.

CLINICAL CONCEPT

Tumor lysis syndrome is most often seen 48 to 72 hours after initiation of cancer treatment and can cause acute renal failure.

Pathophysiology of Selected WBC Disorders

Leukemia

Leukemia is a cancer of developing WBCs within the bone marrow. The cancerous WBCs are arrested at an early stage of development, proliferate uncontrollably, and do not function. As discussed previously, there are two basic categories of cells within the bone marrow: myeloid and lymphoid cells. Leukemias that affect the myeloid lineage are called myelocytic leukemias. Leukemias that affect the lymphoid lineage are called lymphocytic leukemias.

CLINICAL CONCEPT

Myelocytic leukemias are also called myelogenous, myeloblastic, or nonlymphocytic leukemias, whereas lymphocytic leukemias are also called lymphoblastic or lymphogenous leukemias.

Acute Lymphocytic Leukemia

Acute lymphocytic leukemia (ALL) is an aggressive cancer that is more common in children than adults. It represents 23% of cancer diagnoses in children younger than 15 years of age. Children younger than age 6 years comprise 75% of pediatric ALL cases. Survival rates are over 80% in children, but only 20% to 40% in adults. Approximately 20% to 30% of adults with ALL have the PhC, which is associated with chemotherapy-resistant disease.

Risk Factors There is no known cause of ALL, but previous chemotherapy or radiation therapy for other diseases increases the risk. In children, prenatal exposure to high doses of radiation is thought to be a common risk factor. In adults, risk factors include being male, white, older than 70 years, and having radiation exposure or genetic disorders such as Down syndrome.

Pathophysiology In ALL, the stem cell precursors for T or B lymphocytes in the bone marrow do not function and do not mature beyond the lymphoblast stage. As the lymphoblasts become more numerous, there is less room for healthy WBCs, RBCs, and platelets, leading to anemia, susceptibility to infection, and suppressed clotting. Lymph nodes also contain large numbers of lymphoblast cells, which crowd out healthy lymphocytes.

The central nervous system (CNS), kidneys, and testicles can be infiltrated with lymphoblast cells. Meningeal involvement is as high as 85%, especially with T-cell ALL.

Patients with T-cell ALL have a worse prognosis than those with B-cell ALL. There is a 5-year survival rate of 75% for those with T-cell ALL and an 84% survival rate for those with B-cell disease. Age at diagnosis is an important indicator of survival. Children aged 1 to 9 years have a higher disease-free survival rate than older children, adolescents, and infants. There is also a higher rate of treatment-related mortality in children with Down syndrome.

Clinical Presentation. It is important to gather a complete history and perform a comprehensive physical exam on the patient with signs of ALL. However, the patient's initial history may not prompt quick recognition of ALL by the clinician because symptoms can be vague and mistakenly attributed to other disorders. Frequently, the patient presents with a nonspecific array of symptoms that is erroneously attributed to a viral syndrome. The medical, surgical, and family history are frequently unremarkable. The psychosocial history may include occupational exposure to toxins such as benzene or radiation, which increase risk. However, many sufferers of ALL have no such history. Past use of chemotherapy agents for cancer can also increase risk. Habits such as smoking increase susceptibility to ALL.

Signs and Symptoms. Clinical signs and symptoms of ALL are related to the extent of replacement of the bone marrow with blast cells. Because cancerous lymphoblasts do not function and crowd out other WBCs in the bone marrow, patients may present to the clinician with frequent infection, ranging from infected tonsils, canker sores, and diarrhea to life-threatening pneumonia or opportunistic infections.

Also because of lymphoblast numbers overwhelming RBCs in the bone marrow, the patient may present with fatigue, dyspnea, and pallor related to anemia. Some patients experience other vague symptoms, such as fevers, chills, night sweats, and other flulike symptoms. Additionally, blast cells proliferate within lymph nodes and the spleen and liver, which increase the size of these organs. An enlarged lymph node or spleen is often the initial sign of ALL. Some patients experience nausea or a feeling of fullness caused by an enlarged liver and spleen; this can result in unintentional weight loss.

Blast cell proliferation within the marrow in the center of bones leads to persistent bone pain, which is most pronounced at the sternum, tibia, and femur.

Because of the crowding of platelets by blast cells, patients will have unexplained bruising, gingival bleeding, epistaxis (nosebleeds), and extremely heavy bleeding with menstrual periods. If the blast cells invade the CNS, neurological symptoms such as headaches can occur.

Diagnosis. It is difficult for the clinician to diagnose ALL based on history and physical assessment alone. A CBC with differential is necessary and may present the first diagnostic sign of ALL. The WBC count is markedly elevated. A bone marrow biopsy demonstrates hypercellularity with predominantly lymphoblasts. A bone marrow lymphoblast count of over 20% of total WBC is sufficient for a diagnosis of ALL.

Treatment. The aims of ALL treatment regimens are rapid restoration of bone marrow function, adequate prophylactic treatment of sanctuary sites (sites that may have concealed blast cells such as the CNS), and maintenance therapy to eliminate minimal or undetectable disease. The overall goal is to put the patient into remission, which is a period of undetectable or no disease. The faster the response to treatment, the better the prognosis for all types of ALL. Bone marrow transplantation from a tissue-matched sibling and chemotherapy are commonly used treatments in children and young adults. Older adults are mainly treated with chemotherapy agents.

Chemotherapy for ALL is a multidrug regimen. The overall duration of treatment is usually about 36 months. Patients with a good early response to initial chemotherapy have a 65% to 70% 5-year event-free survival rate.

Chronic Lymphocytic Leukemia

CLL is the most common type of leukemia in the United States and other Western countries, but it is rare in China and Japan. It is a B-cell lymphocyte malignancy with more than 17,000 people diagnosed yearly in the United States. The disease is found in elderly individuals, with a median age at diagnosis of 70 years. The male-to-female ratio is 2:1. As the population ages, the incidence of CLL is speculated to rise. One of the primary risk factors appears to be family history of CLL or any B-cell malignancy.

Risk Factors. Male gender, advanced age, Caucasian race, and family history of hematologic cancer are risk factors for CLL. Exposure to certain herbicides and insecticides, including Agent Orange used during the Vietnam War, have also been linked to an increased risk of CLL.

Etiology. Genetic changes are the fundamental cause of CLL. Exposure to any agent that can disrupt DNA is an etiologic agent. Over 80% of patients with CLL have some type of chromosomal abnormality, with trisomy 12 being the most common. Other chromosome anomalies are deletions in chromosome 6, 11, 13, 14, and 17.

Pathophysiology. Over 95% of CLL cases involve B cells that have failed to differentiate from precursor B cells into mature B cells in the bone marrow. In the peripheral blood, these cells resemble mature B cells, but they synthesize and release low levels of immunoglobulin (Ig), mutated Igs, or no Ig at all. They are referred to as B-CLL lymphocytes. B-CLL lymphocytes contain excess proto-oncogene bcl 2. This proto-oncogene bcl 2 is a suppressor of apoptosis (programmed cell death), resulting in long life for the B-CLL cells. There is constant proliferation of B-CLL precursor cells in the bone marrow. The accumulation of B-CLL cells results in crowding of the bone marrow and consequent decreased development of RBCs, WBCs, and platelets. The proliferation of B-CLL cells also occurs in the lymph nodes and spleen, causing lymphadenopathy and splenomegaly.

About 60% of cases of CLL have B-CLL cells that yield a mutated Ig. The B-CLL cells that produce this abnormal Ig have a specific antigen on their surface called CD38. Patients with greater than 20% CD38 type B-CLL cells have aggressive disease and an unfavorable prognosis. Patients with fewer than 20% CD38 B-CLL cells have a more favorable prognosis.

DNA analysis has also distinguished two major types of CLL with different prognoses. Zeta-chain-associated protein tyrosine kinase 70 (ZAP-70) is an enzyme produced by some B-CLL cells. Tyrosine kinases cause unregulated growth of the cell, which leads to development of cancer. Therefore, tyrosine kinase inhibitors, such as imatinib, are often effective cancer treatments. Patients with B-CLL cells that are positive for the marker ZAP-70 have poor prognosis with an average survival of 5 years. Patients with B-CLL cells that are negative for ZAP-70 have a good prognosis with an average survival rate of more than 25 years.

Clinical Presentation. Early in the disorder, patients commonly have an unremarkable history that does not include any diagnostic clues for CLL. Patients may present later in the disease with complaints of enlarged, but painless, lymph nodes; fatigue; fever; and pain in the upper left portion of the abdomen, which may be caused by an enlarged spleen, night sweats, weight loss, and frequent infections. Patients may report a family history of hematologic cancer. Occupational history is important because CLL is associated with exposure to certain herbicides and insecticides.

Signs and Symptoms. Most people do not have symptoms early in CLL, but a routine blood test returns a high WBC count and further investigation reveals the disorder. As the disease advances, the patient suffers lymphadenopathy, splenomegaly, hepatomegaly, and, eventually, anemia and infections. The patient typically suffers from symptoms similar to those of hematologic neoplasms.

Diagnosis. CLL is usually first suspected by the presence of a lymphocytosis on a CBC with differential test. This abnormality is frequently an incidental finding on a routine medical visit. The hallmark of CLL is lymphocytosis with a WBC count of greater than 20,000/uL. The bone marrow is infiltrated with characteristic small lymphocytes. The presence of lymphocytosis in an elderly individual should raise strong suspicion for CLL, and a confirmatory diagnostic test, in particular flow cytometry, should be performed.

Treatment. Treatment of CLL varies with the clinical stage and the presence or absence of symptoms. With the ability to identify cell mutations using flow cytometry and FISH, treatment is started even if no symptoms are present when the B-CLL cell mutation identifies an unfavorable prognosis.

Chemotherapy can be curative or palliative therapy. Early chemotherapy is considered for all patients with high-risk biological or genetic markers predicting a poor long-term prognosis. Monoclonal antibodies have been effective against B-CLL cells with specific identifying markers such as ZAP-70 or CD38.

Nonablative stem cell transplantation, which only partially suppresses the patient's immune system, reduces relapses for high-risk patients. This regimen is less intensive and does not cause as much damage to patients' normal tissues as a conventional fully ablative regimen. Treatment has resulted in complete remission rates of over 90% of patients without negative prognostic mutations and over 70% of patients with negative prognostic mutations.

Acute Myelogenous Leukemia

Acute myelogenous leukemia (AML) is caused by the proliferation of undifferentiated (blast) myeloid cells in the bone marrow. The bone marrow will have more than 20% blast cells. With the proliferation of blasts, the production of normal blood cells by the bone marrow is reduced. The result includes anemia from lack of RBCs, bleeding disorders from lack of platelets, and infections from neutropenia. The genetic mutations in the abnormal myeloid cells cause a change in the normal apoptosis. The proliferation of the blasts continues with infiltration beyond the bone marrow to the blood, tissues, spleen, and liver. AML can also invade the skin with the myeloid blasts causing a diffuse rash or raised nodules. If the blasts invade the lungs, there are symptoms similar to pneumonia.

Previous chemotherapy and radiation therapy for a variety of cancers including breast cancer and Hodgkin's lymphoma have been a cause of AML.

The increased incidence of AML following the 1986 Chernobyl nuclear disaster in Russia was directly proportional to the radiation exposure. There are numerous cell mutations that occur in AML, and treatment is devised according to these.

Chronic Myelogenous Leukemia

Chronic myelogenous leukemia (CML) is a disorder characterized by an overproduction of mature myeloid cells in the bone marrow. Similar to CLL, it arises from a BCR-ABL oncogene mutation in a single pluripotent hematopoietic stem cell. The median age at diagnosis is 50 years. CML accounts for about 15% to 20% of leukemia in adults, with slightly more males than females diagnosed. Like other leukemias, exposure to ionizing radiation is a known risk. Ninety-five percent of adults with CML have the PhC.

The clinical course is divided into three phases:

1. chronic phase, where neutrophils begin to lose their differentiation
2. accelerated phase, where neutrophils are more undifferentiated and unable to function
3. blast crisis phase, where myeloid blast cells do not differentiate at all.

During the chronic phase, the bone marrow is about 10% myeloid blast cells. This leads to a gradual increase in blasts within the peripheral blood, causing leukocytosis. The accelerated phase has 10% to 20% blast cells in the bone marrow and the peripheral blood. The blast crisis phase has over 20% blast cells in the peripheral blood and the bone marrow.

Symptoms of a blast crisis include all the usual symptoms of leukemia. There is crowding of the bone marrow with blast cells that causes a decreased number of normal WBCs, RBCs, and platelets. Symptoms caused by frequent infection, anemia, and thrombocytopenia are common such as fever, fatigue, weakness, and bleeding. Bone pain also occurs, caused by the excessive proliferation of blasts that stretch the bone marrow. Symptoms that may mean a poor prognosis include splenomegaly, older age, genetic mutations in addition to PhC, basophilia, and eosinophilia.

Fatigue is a common complaint of patients with CML. Other symptoms include abdominal fullness from hepatomegaly and splenomegaly, night sweats, and a low grade fever. The fever is caused by the hypermetabolic state related to the overproduction of WBCs, which can rise to greater than 100,000 cells. As the WBC count increases, patients may have respiratory distress because of pulmonary accumulation of WBCs. The WBC count may be as high as 150,000/uL at diagnosis.

CML is both treatable and curable. Because tyrosine kinase activity is needed for the action of PhC, drugs that inhibit this enzyme are used to treat CML. Tyrosine kinase inhibitors, such as imatinib (Gleevec[R]), can induce a complete remission in over 90% of all patients treated. Allogenic bone marrow transplantation is also indicated for some patients with CML before imatinib.

Lymphomas

Lymphoma is the most common type of blood cancer in the United States. Lymphoma falls into one of two major categories:

1. Hodgkin's lymphoma (HL, previously called Hodgkin's disease)
2. Non-Hodgkin's lymphoma (NHL).

NHLs account for 83% of lymphoma cases, with HL accounting for the other 17%. In the United States, about 66,000 of new cases of NHL and 8,500 new cases of HL occur per year. Lymphoma can occur at any age, including childhood. HL is most common in two age groups: adults 15 to 20 years of age and people 50 years of age and older. NHL is more likely to occur in older people.

NHL and HL may be associated with the same symptoms, and often have similar appearance on physical examination. However, they are readily distinguishable via microscopic examination. HL develops from a specific abnormal B lymphocyte line, whereas NHL may derive from either abnormal B or T cells and are distinguished by unique genetic markers.

There are five subtypes of HL and about 30 subtypes of NHL. The different subtypes and the classification are based on microscopic appearance as well as genetic and molecular markers. Many of the NHL subtypes look similar, but they are functionally different and respond to different therapies with different probabilities of cure. HL subtypes are microscopically distinct, and typing is based upon the microscopic differences as well as extent of disease. The risk factors, signs, and symptoms are similar for all lymphomas (see Box 12-4 and Box 12-5).

Staging of Lymphoma

Lymphomas are evaluated and classified according to size, spread, microscopic appearance, and genetic and

---

BOX 12-4. Risk Factors of Lymphomas

- Age older than 60 years
- HIV and other autoimmune disorders
- EBV
- *H. pylori*
- Hepatitis C
- Immunosuppressive therapy
- Exposure to toxic chemicals
- Occupational exposure to toxic chemicals, such as pesticides, herbicides, benzene, and other solvents
- Hair dye usage, especially before 1980
- Family history of lymphoma

BOX 12-5. Signs and Symptoms of Lymphoma

The first sign of lymphoma is often a painless enlarged lymph node in the neck, under an arm, or in the groin. The enlarged lymph node sometimes causes other symptoms by pressing against a vein or lymphatic vessel (swelling of an arm or leg), nerve (pain, numbness, or tingling), or the stomach (early feeling of fullness). Other signs and symptoms of lymphoma include:

- Splenomegaly
- Hepatomegaly
- Enlargement of the spleen or liver, causing abdominal pain or discomfort
- Fevers
- Chills
- Unexplained weight loss
- Night sweats
- Lack of energy
- Itching, most commonly in the lower extremity, but can occur anywhere, be local, or spread over the whole body.

molecular markers, and then assigned a stage and grade. Staging of lymphoma is based on its size and the extent of spread in the body. Also, lymphoma is often described as "bulky" or "nonbulky." Nonbulky indicates the tumor is small; bulky means the tumor is large. Nonbulky disease has a better prognosis than bulky disease. Lymphomas have a complex classification system (see Box 12-6).

Non-Hodgkin's Lymphoma

NHLs can be caused by cancerous T cells, B cells, or NK cells and are classified according to cell type and aggressiveness. They usually develop among middle age and older adults and are 50% more frequent in men than women. Children and young adults are occasionally diagnosed with NHL; in these patients, the lymphomas are more aggressive.

Etiology. Chromosomal translocations are the genetic hallmark of lymphomas. A common translocation in NHL is the translocation of genes at 14q32 and 18q21 present in 85% of follicular lymphomas. Why the translocations occur is unknown, although there is evidence that oncogenic pathogens may be involved.

BOX 12-6. Grades, Stages, and Letter Classifications of Lymphoma

The grade of a lymphoma is based on the rate of growth, stage is based on regions involved, and letter classification further describes the tumor symptoms and spread.

GRADE
- **Low grade**: These are slow-growing lymphomas. Low-grade lymphomas are often widespread when discovered, but because they grow slowly, they usually do not require immediate treatment unless organ function is compromised. They are rarely cured and can transform over time to more aggressive types.
- **Intermediate grade**: These are rapidly growing, aggressive lymphomas that usually require immediate treatment; they are often curable.
- **High grade**: These are very rapidly growing, aggressive lymphomas that require immediate, intensive treatment and are much less often curable intermediate grade lymphomas.

STAGE
- **Stage I (early disease):** Lymphoma is located in a single lymph node region or in one area or organ outside the lymph node.
- **Stage II (locally advanced disease):** Lymphoma is located in two or more lymph node regions, all located on the same side of the diaphragm or in one lymph node region and a nearby tissue or organ.
- **Stage III (advanced disease):** Lymphoma affects two or more lymph node regions, or one lymph node region and one organ, on opposite sides of the diaphragm.
- **Stage IV (widespread or disseminated disease):** Lymphoma is outside the lymph nodes and spleen and has spread to another area or organ such as the bone marrow, bone, or central nervous system.

LETTER CLASSIFICATION
Both HL and NHL are further classified with letters:

- An "A" or "B" designation indicates whether the person with lymphoma had symptoms such as fevers or weight loss at the time of diagnosis. "A" indicates no such symptoms, and "B" indicates symptoms.
- An "E" designation indicates that the tumor spread directly from a lymph node into an organ or that a single organ outside the lymphatic system is affected with no apparent lymphatic involvement.
- If the spleen is involved, an "S" designation is added.

Some pathogens that have been associated with the development of NHL include HIV, EBV, *Helicobacter pylori*, HTLV-I, hepatitis C, and human herpesvirus-8.

The viral pathogens introduce their genes into affected lymphocytes, causing mutations in the genome of the affected cells. The mutations involve either stimulation of oncogenes or inhibition of tumor suppressor genes, either of which causes uncontrolled proliferation of the affected lymphocytes. HIV specifically causes lymphoma of the brain, which causes focal neurological signs and mental status changes. It is a late complication of HIV infection. Hepatitis C increases the risk of B-cell NHL by 30%. Chronic infection with *Helicobacter pylori* in the stomach is associated with gastric mucosa-associated lymphocytic tumor.

Risk Factors. The risk factors for NHL are similar to those for all lymphomas (see Box 12-4).

Pathophysiology. NHLs consist of over 20 different lymphomas, which all have a distinct microscopic appearance. About 85% of NHLs form in lymph tissue from mutated B cells, 15% develop from T-cell mutations, and fewer than 1% arise from NK cells. Lymphomas are also grouped by certain properties, such as size, shape, and appearance of cells within a lymph node. The appearance within a lymph node is described as follicular (round clusters of abnormal cells) or diffuse (abnormal cells spread throughout the node).

Tumors are characterized by the level of differentiation, the size of the cell of origin, the origin cell's rate of proliferation, and the histological pattern of growth. For many of the B-cell NHL subtypes, the pattern of growth and cell size may be important determinants of tumor aggressiveness. Tumors that grow in a nodular or follicular pattern are generally less aggressive than lymphomas that proliferate in a diffuse pattern. Lymphomas of small lymphocytes generally have a milder course than those of large lymphocytes, which may have intermediate-grade or high-grade aggressiveness.

Clinical Presentation. The patient with NHL may come to the attention of the health-care provider because of a variety of different symptoms (see Box 12-5). The patient should be questioned about past medical history, particularly infection with EBV, HIV, hepatitis C, or gastric ulcer (caused by *H. pylori*). Immunosuppressive treatments can also predispose individuals to NHL. Occupational exposures and family and psychosocial history are also important. Toxic exposure to herbicides, pesticides, benzene, and radiation are known risk factors. Unsafe sex practices or intravenous drug abuse can predispose individuals to HIV, another risk factor.

Signs and Symptoms. In patients with NHL, the patient or clinician often notices an enlarged, painless lymph node, which initiates further investigation. Other signs and symptoms for NHL are listed in Box 12-5.

Diagnosis. Although a variety of laboratory and imaging studies are used in the evaluation and staging of suspected NHL, a lymph node biopsy is the mainstay of diagnosis. The diagnostic studies commonly performed for a patient with suspected NHL include blood studies, bone marrow aspiration, abdominal computed tomography scan, and nuclear medicine studies.

Treatment. For early stage disease, radiation is the key treatment. However, a combination of chemotherapy and radiation is commonly needed. Prognosis for lymphoma-free survival is based on specific factors (see Box 12-7).

Hodgkin's Lymphoma

HL, a malignancy of B lymphocytes, is the most common lymphoma in young adults and children older than 10 years. It is one of the few pediatric malignancies that is similar to the adult form.

HL has a worldwide incidence of 62,000 cases per year. Compared with North America and Europe, HL is relatively rare in Japan and China. Overall, HL is somewhat more common in males than in females. The observed male predominance is particularly evident in children, in whom 85% of the cases are in males. Age-specific incidence rates of HL peak in young adults (aged 15 to 34 years old) and older individuals (greater than 55 years old).

Etiology. The cause of HL is unknown, but EBV has been found in malignant B lymphocytes. Exposure to

---

BOX 12-7. Prognostic Factors for Non-Hodgkin's Lymphoma

The International Prognostic Index for NHL includes five risk factors:

1. Age older than 60 years
2. Stage III or IV disease
3. High lactic dehydrogenase (present with large amount of tumor breakdown products)
4. More than one extranodal site
5. Poor performance status, as a measure of general health; from these factors, the following risk groups were identified:
   - **Low risk:** one risk factor, 5-year lymphoma-free survival (LFS) of 70%
   - **Intermediate risk:** two to three risk factors, 5-year LFS of 49% to 50%
   - **Poor risk:** four to five risk factors, 5-year LFS of 26%.

The prognostic models were developed to evaluate groups of patients and are useful in developing therapeutic strategies.

Adapted from A predictive model for aggressive non-Hodgkin's lymphoma. (1993). The International Non-Hodgkin's Lymphoma Prognostic Factors Project. *N Engl J Med* 329(14), 987–994.

carcinogens, viruses, and genetic and immune mechanisms have been proposed, but none have been proven.

Pathophysiology. Classic HL is commonly diagnosed by the presence of Reed-Sternberg (RS) cells in the lymphoid tissue. The RS cell is a large malignant B cell with two nuclei that give the cell the appearance of owl's eyes. About 50% of patients have EBV in their RS cells.

The malignancy is thought to start in one area, such as a lymph node, and then spread throughout the lymphatic system. The cervical lymph nodes, mediastinal nodes, and spleen are commonly involved in most cases. There are various types of HL, each with different growth patterns and required treatments.

Clinical Presentation. The patient with HL usually has no dramatic symptoms. The patient or clinician may discover a painless, enlarged lymph node. Alternatively, the patient can experience symptoms of sore throat, fever, trouble swallowing, shortness of breath, abdominal pain, or other various symptoms associated with the enlargement of lymphoid tissue in the body. As with all cancer patients, a complete history and physical is necessary.

Signs and Symptoms. Patients with HL present with solid tumors of lymphoid tissue. Enlargement of lymphoid tissue at lymph nodes or extra nodal sites such as the thymus gland, spleen, liver, or tonsils usually occurs. Symptoms depend on the affected site. Waldeyer's ring, a circular arrangement of lymphoid tissue in the pharynx, which includes the palatine, pharyngeal, and lingual tonsils, is a common site of involvement.

CLINICAL CONCEPT

A lymphoma in the thymus gland may produce chest pain or pressure from an enlarging tumor. A lymphoma can also place pressure on the trachea, possibly causing shortness of breath or coughing. If a lymphoma is placing pressure on the superior vena cava SVC, it may provide SVC syndrome with edema of the head and arms. If a lymphoma involves lymphatic tissue below the diaphragm, there may be abdominal distention with splenomegaly.

Diagnosis. Diagnosis is made after biopsy of nodal and extranodal sites. Flow cytometry and DNA analysis identify chromosomal translocations and molecular rearrangements. Bone marrow biopsy is done in the presence of anemia, leukopenia, or thrombocytopenia to rule out leukemia. Predictors for poor survival include advanced age at onset, multiple extranodal sites, and the presence of significant symptoms such as weight loss. Clinical staging is done after history and physical

---

BOX 12-8. Prognostic Factors for Hodgkin's Lymphoma

Several risk factors have been extensively evaluated and shown to play a role in treatment outcomes for HL. For HL, the International Prognostic Index includes the following seven risk factors:

1. Male sex
2. Age 45 years or older
3. Stage IV disease
4. Albumin lower than 4.0 g/dL
5. Hgb lower than 10.5 g/dL
6. Elevated WBC count of 15,000/mL
7. Low lymphocyte count lower than 600/mL or lower than 8% of total WBC.

The absence of any of the above risk factors is associated with an 84% rate of control of Hodgkin's disease, whereas the presence of a risk factor is associated with a 77% rate of disease control. The presence of five or more risk factors is associated with a disease control rate of only 42%.

Adapted from Hasenclever, D., Diehl, V. (1998). A prognostic score for advanced Hodgkin's disease. International Prognostic Factors Project on Advanced Hodgkin's Disease. *N Engl J Med, 339*, 1506–1514.

---

exam, lab studies, and thoracic, pelvic, and abdominal CT scans. PET scans are used to evaluate response to treatment.

Treatment. HL has a potential cure rate of 70% using treatment methods. Staging of the disease involves risk factors, lymph nodes involved, and dissemination of disease. The more localized the disease, the more favorable the diagnosis.

Localized disease is usually treated with radiation. Chemotherapy for HL involves two or more drugs, usually given intravenously in cycles. More than 75% of newly diagnosed patients with HL can be cured with combination chemotherapy or radiation. The 5-year survival rate is 85% for patients 65 years and younger. The survival rate for patients older than age 65 years drops to 50%, probably because of more advanced disease, a higher number of risk factors, and comorbidities. Prognosis for lymphoma-free survival is based on specific factors (see Box 12-8).

Multiple Myeloma

Multiple myeloma (MM) is a hematologic neoplasm that arises in B lymphocytes, causing proliferation of abnormal plasma cells in the bone marrow and consequent synthesis of abnormal Igs or Ig fragments. It is an incurable B-cell malignancy that affects approximately 55,000 people in the United States yearly. MM accounts for 1.1% of all malignancies and is the second most common hematologic neoplasm in the

United States. It has a higher incidence in men than women (2:1) and African Americans than Caucasians (2:1). The current 5-year survival rate in newly diagnosed MM is 33% according to the American Cancer Society.

Etiology

The cause of MM is unknown, although genetic and chromosomal changes are found in affected patients. It has a wide spectrum of presentations with three main forms of the disorder. It ranges from a benign disorder called monoclonal gammopathy of undetermined significance (MGUS) to smoldering MM to active, highly destructive MM. The transformation from MGUS or smoldering myeloma to active MM is a result of critical chromosomal translocations in the DNA of affected plasma cells.

As the disease progresses, additional genetic events occur that affect prognosis. Deletions of p53 are seen in some B cells that go on to become neoplastic plasma cells. There may be loss of chromosome 13 and activation of oncogenes. The deletion of chromosome 13 is associated with a very poor prognosis. The genetic mutation results in a complete dysregulation of the cell cycle, allowing the proliferation of neoplastic plasma cells. Translocations of chromosome 4 and 14, or loss of the short arm of chromosome 17 also have poor outcomes. Translocations at chromosome 11 and 14 have a favorable prognosis. Patients are placed into risk categories based on genetic or chromosomal changes.

Risk Factors

The cause of MM is unknown, but there is a possible association with exposure to chemicals, including Agent Orange and exposure to radiation. Genetic factors are involved and there is evidence of MM in families.

Pathophysiology

MM is characterized by neoplastic plasma cells (derived from abnormal B cells) that proliferate within the bone marrow. In the bloodstream these aberrant plasma cells synthesize abnormal Ig proteins that precipitate out of the blood into organs and become filtered into the urine. It is a generalized disorder that leads to bone destruction, bone marrow failure, renal failure, neurological complications, and amyloidosis. The pathology of myeloma depends on the neoplastic plasma cell identified on bone marrow biopsy. Normally, each type of plasma cell produces only one type of Ig. Healthy Ig proteins are composed of two identical heavy chains and two identical light chains (see Fig. 12-5).

When one particular type of plasma cell proliferates abnormally, it causes an excess of its synthesized abnormal Ig and Ig fragments. The abnormal Ig and fragments are referred to as monoclonal proteins or M-proteins. Some myelomas secrete only whole Igs and some overly secrete Ig fragments. Bence Jones myeloma, identified in 1848 by Dr. Henry Bence Jones, is a myeloma in which only the light chains of Ig structure are produced; these light chains were formerly called Bence Jones proteins.

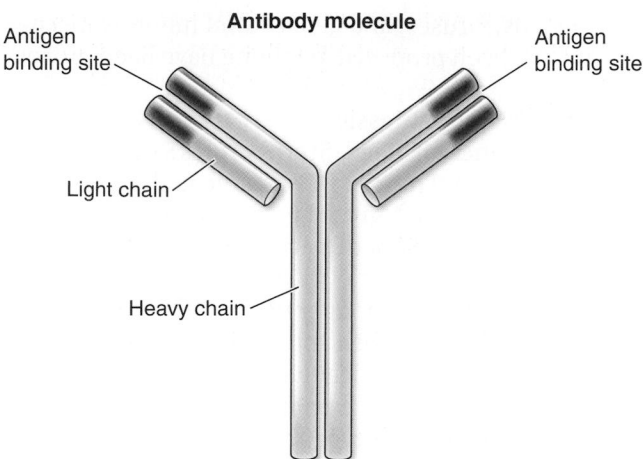

Antibody molecule

Antigen binding site

Antigen binding site

Light chain

Heavy chain

FIGURE 12-5. Antibody structure. Antibodies, also called immunoglobulins (Igs), are proteins synthesized by plasma cells. Plasma cells are formed from B cells. Each antibody consists of four polypeptides—two heavy chains and two light chains joined to form a Y-shaped molecule. The polypeptide tips of the Y vary among different antibodies and give the antibody its specificity for antigen.

MGUS is a result of the overproduction of a specific plasma cell in the bone marrow that causes an increase in a specific Ig. This disorder is similar to MM but is benign. It is defined by three criteria:

1. The presence of a serum monoclonal protein (M-protein) whether IgA, IgG, or IgM, at a concentration of 3 g/dL or lower (more would indicate MM or another disorder)
2. Fewer than 10% plasma cells in the bone marrow (higher than 10% is considered smoldering myeloma)
3. The absence of lytic bone lesions, anemia, hypercalcemia, and renal insufficiency related to the plasma cell proliferative process (no symptoms of MM).

MGUS is present in 3.2% of the general population older than age 50 years and in 5.3% of people older than 70 years. The highest rate of 8.9% is in men older than age 85. Patients with MGUS are at risk for progression to MM, with the risk of progression to MM based on the proportion of neoplastic plasma cells in the bone marrow and the M-protein level in the bloodstream. The overall risk of progression to MM is 10% yearly for those with smoldering myeloma, but only 1% yearly for persons with MGUS.

In active MM, there is an increase in osteoclast activity that causes bone resorption at an accelerated rate. The cytokines in the myeloma cells stimulate osteoclastic activity and inhibit osteoblastic activity, causing bone destruction and preventing bone formation. As proliferation in bone marrow occurs, it causes lytic bone disease, leading to bone destruction, marrow and renal failure, extraosseous involvement, and neurological complications. Vertebral bones are commonly involved. There may be a reduction in height because of vertebral collapse. The bone destruction also causes serum hypercalcemia. Radiculopathy is a frequent neurological occurrence from compression of a nerve by a paravertebral plasmacytoma (neoplastic plasma cell tumor) in the lumbosacral area.

> **ALERT!** Patients with MM can suffer vertebral lesions that cause spinal cord compression. Severe back pain, paresthesias of the lower extremities, and bladder or bowel incontinence may indicate cord compression that can result in permanent spinal cord damage. This is a medical emergency that requires immediate treatment.

The most common MM proliferative Igs are IgG and IgA. Proliferation of IgG accounts for about 60% to 70% of all myeloma and IgA accounts for about 20%. IgD and IgE are rarely the product in MM. IgM can be proliferative in MM, but high amounts of IgM are usually related to another disease called Waldenstrom's macroglobulinemia. With high amounts of circulating Igs, hyperviscosity of the blood can occur. Because Igs are of differing size, with IgM being very large, it causes the greatest increase in viscosity. IgG and IgE are smaller and cause less of a problem.

Clinical Presentation

Clinical symptoms are the result of the disease progression. Bone pain, especially in the back, is a common complaint at diagnosis. It is a result of lytic destruction and the formation of plasmacytomas. Lytic lesions are rounded, punched-out areas of bone found most commonly in vertebra, the skull, ribs, humerus, and femur. Bone scans may not reflect the lytic destruction seen on x-ray. Osteopenia is seen on bone density study.

Weakness, pallor, and fatigue associated with anemia occur. The anemia is a normocytic, normochromic anemia. There may be a decreased vitamin B_{12} level and Rouleaux formation of RBCs. Rouleaux formation is a phenomenon when RBCs collect in clumps and appear as stacks of coins. It is found in patients with elevated serum protein levels.

There is frequently an infection because of the deficiency in antibody-mediated immunity. The myeloma cells outnumber and crowd out normal plasma cells, which causes low levels of normal Igs. The risk of infection is greatest at the time of diagnosis and will decrease as the disease responds to treatment. Most deaths from infection occur early during treatment when the body has little natural immunity available.

Renal disease is present in one-half of patients at the time of diagnosis and contributes to a poor prognosis. The two major causes of renal insufficiency are hypercalcemia and myeloma cast nephropathy. Hypercalcemia occurs because of bone breakdown, and calcium can precipitate in the kidney, causing kidney stones. Myeloma cast nephropathy is characterized by the presence of large, waxy, laminated casts or deposits in the distal and collecting tubules of the kidneys. They are formed from precipitated abnormal light chains that have collected in the tubules. Proximal tubules are also damaged by the large protein load. Hypercalciuria as well as hyperuricemia contribute to kidney damage.

Diagnosis

MM is diagnosed as having 10% or more plasma cells in the bone marrow, the presence of M-proteins in blood and urine, and organ or tissue damage as a result of the proliferation of the plasma cells. **Plasmacytomas,** or tumors of plasma origin, may be found on tissue biopsy.

Treatment

Treatment of MM in asymptomatic patients is usually deferred. Tumor growth is slow in the beginning of the disorder. Thus, there may be no early treatment but periodic monitoring. MGUS requires yearly observation, whereas smoldering myeloma requires observation every 2 to 3 months.

Treatment is chemotherapy followed by autologous stem cell transplantation. Initially, if a single lesion called an isolated plasmacytoma is found in the bone, it is treated with radiation and followed up with chemotherapy to reduce spread. Bisphosphonate therapy is administered to reduce bone disease, fractures, and skeletal complications, improving survival.

Chapter Summary

- WBCs are an integral part of the body's defense against antigens.
- WBCs are born in the bone marrow and released in response to the body's needs. After bone marrow synthesis, lymphocytes, also called B cell and T cells, need to mature within lymphoid tissue that includes the lymph nodes, tonsils, adenoids, thymus gland, and spleen.
- All WBC synthesis is stimulated by infections, inflammatory reactions, extreme stress, and neoplasms.
- Bacterial infections particularly stimulate neutrophil synthesis, whereas allergic reactions and parasitic infections provoke eosinophil and basophil production.
- Lymphocytes classically respond to viral infection.

- Leukocytosis greater than 11,000/uL is most commonly indicative of infection; however, neoplastic disease of the WBCs also causes a rise in number of WBCs.
- In leukemia, there is a neoplastic proliferation of WBCs that are arrested in early development within the bone marrow.
- Cancerous WBCs are nonfunctioning and crowd out normal WBCs, RBCs, and platelets. Infection, anemia, and thrombocytopenia are the effects of leukemia.
- Lymphoma is a cancerous proliferation of lymphoid tissue, often first presenting as an enlarged lymph node.

- There are different types of leukemia and lymphoma, but all cause the same basic condition: immunosuppression.
- Susceptibility to infection is often the first sign of a WBC hematologic neoplasm.
- Similar treatments are used to combat leukemias and lymphomas: chemotherapy, radiation, and bone marrow transplantation.
- MM is a unique kind of neoplastic condition that involves overproliferation of Ig fragments. It can present as vertebral lumbosacral pain.

 Making the Connections

Pathophysiology	Signs and Symptoms	Physical Assessment Findings	Diagnosis	Treatment
Myelodysplastic Syndrome | Disorder of one or more stem cell lines in the bone marrow; RBCs, WBCs, or platelets; can lead to complete bone marrow suppression.				
	Deficient number of healthy WBCs causes infection and lack of signs of inflammation. Deficient healthy RBCs cause fatigue, weakness, pallor. Deficient healthy platelets cause bruising and bleeding, such as nosebleeds.	Infection, fever, or lack of signs of inflammation. Bruises or nosebleeds caused by thrombocytopenia. Pallor, tachycardia caused by anemia.	CBC with differential shows excess WBCs. Bone marrow aspiration demonstrates abnormal WBCs in bone marrow and lack of RBCs and platelets.	Transfusion of specific deficient blood cells.
Acute Lymphocytic Leukemia | Stem cell precursors of B cells or T cells do not function and do not mature beyond lymphoblast stage.				
	Frequent infection, fatigue, dyspnea, fever, chills, night sweats, other flulike symptoms. Bone pain caused by overproliferation of lymphoblasts in bone marrow.	Infection and fever caused by inadequate healthy WBCs. Blast cell proliferation in spleen and liver causes hepatomegaly and splenomegaly. Deficient platelets cause signs of bruising and nosebleeds.	CBC with differential and bone marrow aspiration show immature lymphoblast count greater than 20%.	Chemotherapy. Bone marrow transplantation.
Chronic Lymphocytic Leukemia | Immature B cell proliferation in bone marrow; B cells do not synthesize Igs.				
	Frequent infection caused by deficient healthy WBCs, fatigue, dyspnea caused by anemia, fever, chills, night sweats, and other	Infections. Pallor. Bruises. Nosebleeds. Lymphadenopathy, splenomegaly, and hepatomegaly.	CBC with differential; lymphocytosis greater than 20,000 cells/uL. Excessive number of lymphocytes.	Chemotherapy. Monoclonal antibodies. Bone marrow transplantation.

Continued

Making the Connections—cont'd

Pathophysiology	Signs and Symptoms	Physical Assessment Findings	Diagnosis	Treatment
	flulike symptoms caused by deficient WBCs. Spontaneous bruising caused by lack of platelets. Bone pain caused by overproliferation of lymphoblasts in bone marrow, lymphadenopathy, splenomegaly, hepatomegaly.			

Acute Myelogenous Leukemia | Proliferation of myeloid blast cells in bone marrow. Overproliferation of lymphoblasts in organs such as lymph nodes, spleen, and liver.

Pathophysiology	Signs and Symptoms	Physical Assessment Findings	Diagnosis	Treatment
	Frequent infection caused by deficient healthy WBCs. Fatigue and dyspnea caused by anemia. Spontaneous bruising caused by lack of platelets. Bone pain caused by overproliferation of lymphoblasts in bone marrow. Lymphadenopathy, infiltration of skin, lungs, and other organs with lymphoblast cells.	Infections. Pallor. Bruises. Nosebleeds. Lymphadenopathy, splenomegaly, and hepatomegaly.	CBC with differential; bone marrow aspiration with lymphocytosis greater than 20%.	Chemotherapy. Monoclonal antibodies. Bone marrow transplantation.

Chronic Myelogenous Leukemia | Overproliferation of mature myeloid cells in bone marrow. Overproliferation of myeloid cells in organs such as lymph nodes, spleen, and liver; lymphadenopathy, splenomegaly, and hepatomegaly.

Pathophysiology	Signs and Symptoms	Physical Assessment Findings	Diagnosis	Treatment
	Frequent infection caused by deficient healthy WBCs. Fatigue and dyspnea caused by anemia. Spontaneous bruising caused by lack of platelets. Bone pain caused by overproliferation of myeloid cells in bone marrow. Abdominal fullness caused by liver and spleen pressure on stomach, causing decreased appetite.	Infections. Pallor. Bruises. Nosebleeds. Lymphadenopathy, splenomegaly, and hepatomegaly.	CBC with differential, bone marrow aspiration shows excessive WBCs.	Tyrosine kinase inhibitor. Bone marrow transplantation.

Continued

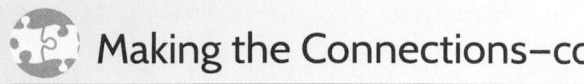

Making the Connections—cont'd

Pathophysiology	Signs and Symptoms	Physical Assessment Findings	Diagnosis	Treatment
Non-Hodgkin's Lymphoma (NHL) | Proliferation of abnormal B cells, T cells, or natural kill cells.				
	Fever, chills, night sweats, weight loss, fatigue. Lymphatic blockage causing lymphedema or nerve impingement, which causes numbness and tingling caused by enlarged lymph node.	Painless enlarged lymph node, splenomegaly, hepatomegaly. Lymphedema. Nerve impingement can cause weakness and sensory loss in an extremity.	CBC with differential, HIV serology, serum chemistry, chest x-ray, lymph node biopsy, bone marrow aspirate. Excessive WBCs in CBC and bone marrow. HIV positive often associated with NHL.	Chemotherapy. Bone marrow transplantation. Radiation. Monoclonal antibodies.
Hodgkin's Lymphoma | Enlarged, malignant B cells called RS cells that contain EBV.				
	Sore throat, fever, trouble swallowing, shortness of breath, abdominal pain.	Pharyngeal edema and erythema. Painless enlarged lymph node, signs of infection, splenomegaly, enlarged thymus.	Pharyngeal CBC with differential; biopsy of lymph node; flow cytometry; bone marrow aspirate; computed tomography of abdomen, thorax, or pelvis; positron emission tomography scan; CBC and bone marrow shows excessive WBCs. Biopsy shows RS cells.	Chemotherapy. Radiation.
Multiple Myeloma | Neoplastic plasma cells that synthesize abnormal Igs and Ig fragments.				
	Bone pain. Nerve pain, numbness, and tingling can occur if spinal nerve impingement occurs.	Tenderness over involved bone; commonly vertebrae in lumbosacral area. Vertebral bone fracture common. Nerve impingement can cause weakness and sensory loss in an extremity.	CBC shows excessive WBCs. Bone marrow shows excessive WBCs. Urine shows fragmented Igs called M-proteins.	Chemotherapy. Bone marrow transplantation. Bisphosphonates.

Bibliography

Adès, L., Itzykson, R., & Fenaux, P. (2014). Myelodysplastic syndromes. *Lancet*, Mar 20. pii: S0140-6736(13)61901-7.

Amsberg, G. K., & Schafhausen, P. (2013). Bosutinib in the management of chronic myelogenous leukemia. *Biol*, 7, 115–122.

Armitage, J. O. (2010). Early-stage Hodgkin's lymphoma. *N Engl J Med*, 363(7), 653–662.

Armitage, J. O. (2012). My treatment approach to patients with diffuse large B-cell lymphoma. *Mayo Clin Proceed*, 87(2), 161–171.

Barrett, K. E., Barman, S. M., Boitano, S., & Brooks, H. L. (2010). *Ganong's review of medical physiology*. 23rd ed. New York: McGraw-Hill/Lange Medical Series. 11.

Brown, J. R. (2014). A new era of treatment for chronic lymphocytic leukaemia? *Lancet Oncol*. 15(1), 3–5. doi: 10.1016/S1470-2045(13)70558-8. Epub 2013 Dec 10.

Canellos, G. P., Niedzwiecki, D., & Johnson, J. L. (2009). Long-term follow-up of survival in Hodgkin's lymphoma. *N Engl J Med*, 361(24), 2390–2391.

Cheson, B. D., & Leonard, J. P. (2008). Monoclonal antibody therapy for B-cell non-Hodgkin's lymphoma. *N Engl J Med*, 359(6), 613–626.

Cortes, J. E., Kantarjian, H., Shah, N. P., et al. (2012). Ponatinib in refractory Philadelphia chromosome-positive leukemias. *N Engl J Med*, 367(22), 2075–2088.

Cortes, J. E., Talpaz, M., & Kantarjian, H. (2014, February 6). Ponatinib in Philadelphia chromosome-positive leukemias. *N Engl J Med*, 370(6), 577. doi: 10.1056/NEJMc1315234.

Davies, J. (2011). First-line therapy for CML: nilotinib comes of age. *Lancet Oncol*, 12(9), 826–827.

Davis, A. S., Viera, A. J., & Mead, M. D. (2014). Leukemia: an overview for primary care. *Am Fam Phys*, 89(9), 731–738.

DeVita, V. T., & Costa, J. (2010). Toward a personalized treatment of Hodgkin's disease. *N Engl J Med*, 362(10), 942–943.

Ferrara, F. (2010). Treatment of older patients with acute myeloid leukaemia. *Lancet,* 376(9757), 1967–1968.

Ferrara, F., & Schiffer, C. A. (2013). Acute myeloid leukaemia in adults. *Lancet*, 381(9865), 484–495.

Georgopoulos, K. (2009). Acute lymphoblastic leukemia—on the wings of IKAROS. *N Engl J Med,* 360(5), 524–526. Epub 2009 Jan 8.

Godley, L. A. (2012). Profiles in leukemia. *N Engl J Med,* 366(12), 1152–1153. doi: 10.1056/NEJMe1200409. Epub 2012 Mar 14.

Hillmen, P. (2010). Chronic lymphocytic leukaemia—moving towards cure? *Lancet*, 376(9747), 1122–1124.

Howard, S. C., Jones, D. P., & Pui, C. H. (2011). The tumor lysis syndrome. *N Engl J Med*, 364(19): 1844–1854. doi: 10.1056/NEJMra0904569.

Inaba, H., Greaves, M., & Mullighan, C. G. (2013). Acute lymphoblastic leukaemia. *Lancet*, 381(9881), 1943–1955.

Jabbour, E., & Kantarjian, H. (2012). Chronic myeloid leukemia: 2012 update on diagnosis, monitoring, and management. *Am J Hem*, 87(11), 1037–1045.

Klemm, J., & Mehr, S. R. (2012). Chronic myelogenous leukemia. *Am J Man Care,* 18(3 Spec No.), SP105–SP107.

Korde, N., Kristinsson, S. Y., & Landgren, O. (2011). Monoclonal gammopathy of undetermined significance (MGUS) and smoldering multiple myeloma (SMM): novel biological insights and development of early treatment strategies. *Blood*, 117(21), 5573–5581.

Kumar, S. K., Mikhael, J. R., Buadi, F. K., et al. (2009). Management of newly diagnosed symptomatic multiple myeloma: updated Mayo Stratification of Myeloma and Risk-Adapted Therapy (mSMART) consensus guidelines. *Mayo Clin Proceed,* 84(12), 1095–1110.

Kyle, R. A. (2011). Role of maintenance therapy after autologous stem cell transplant for multiple myeloma: lessons for cancer therapy. *Mayo Clin Proceed*, 86(5), 419–420.

Landgren, O., & Waxman, A. J. (2010). *Multiple myeloma precursor disease. JAMA,* 304(21), 2397–2404.

Lenz, G., & Staudt, L. M. (2010). Aggressive lymphomas. *N Engl J Med,* 362(15), 1417–1429.

Linker, C. A. (2010). Blood disorders. In S. J. McPhee & M. A. Papadakis, *Current medical diagnosis & treatment.* New York: McGraw-Hill/Lange Medical Series.

Longo, D., Fauci, A. S., Kasper, D. L., et al. (2011). *Harrison's principles of internal medicine.* 18th ed. New York: McGraw-Hill.

Lowry, L., Hoskin, P., & Linch, D. (2010). Developments in the management of Hodgkin's lymphoma. *Lancet*, 375(9717), 786–788.

Lyons, R. M. (2012). Myelodysplastic syndromes: therapy and outlook. *Am J Med,* 125(7 Suppl), S18–S23.

McPhee, S. J., & Hammer, G. D. (2009). *Pathophysiology of disease: an introduction to clinical medicine.* 6th ed. New York: Lange Medical Books.

Milpied, N. (2013). Myeloablation for lymphoma—question answered? *N Engl J Med*, 369(18), 1750–1751. doi: 10.1056/NEJMe1309182.

Mohundro, M. M., & Mohundro, B. L. (2012). On the horizon for multiple myeloma. *Am J Man Care,* 18(3 Spec No.), SP140–SP143.

Palumbo, A., & Anderson, K. (2011). Multiple myeloma. *N Engl J Med*, 364(11), 1046–1060.

Pang, W. W., Pluvinage, J. V., Price, E. A., et al. (2013). Hematopoietic stem cell and progenitor cell mechanisms in myelodysplastic syndromes. *Proc Natl Acad Sci U S A.*, 110(8), 3011–3016.

Radich, J. (2013). Genetically informed therapy in leukemia. *N Engl J Med,* 368(19), 1838–1839. doi: 10.1056/NEJMe1302363.

Rai, K. R., & Barrientos, J. C. (2014). Movement toward optimization of CLL therapy. *N Engl J Med,* 370(12), 1160–1162. doi: 10.1056/NEJMe1400599.

Rajkumar, S. V., Larson, D., & Kyle, R. A. (2011). Diagnosis of smoldering multiple myeloma. *N Engl J Med.* 2011 Aug 4;365(5):, 474–475. doi: 10.1056/NEJMc1106428.

Rowley, J. D. (2013). Genetics. A story of swapped ends. *Science*, 340(6139), 1412–1413.

Russell, N. H. (2012). Improving outcomes for elderly patients with AML. *Lancet Oncol*, 13(11), 1065–1066.

Saglio, G., Kim, D. W., Issaragrisil, S., et al. (2010). Nilotinib versus imatinib for newly diagnosed chronic myeloid leukemia. *N Engl J Med*, 362(24), 2251–2259. Epub 2010 Jun 5.

Schmitz, N., Ziepert, M., Vitolo, U., & German High-Grade Non-Hodgkin's Lymphoma Study Group; Fondazione Italiana Linfomi. (2014). The role of myeloablation for lymphoma. *N Engl J Medicine,* 370(6), 574–575. doi: 10.1056/NEJMc1314757#SA1.

Sharma, S. P. (2013, August). Targeting the B-cell signalling pathway in CLL and MCL. *Lancet Oncol.* 14(9), e343.

Steidl, C., Lee, T., Shah, S. P., et al. (2010). Tumor-associated macrophages and survival in classic Hodgkin's lymphoma. *N Engl J Med*, 362(10), 875–885.

Tefferi, A. (2010). Myelodysplastic syndromes—many new drugs, little therapeutic progress. *Mayo Clin Proceed*, 85(11), 1042–1045. doi: 10.4065/mcp.2010.0502.

Tefferi, A., Lasho, T. L., Jimma, T., et al. (2012). One thousand patients with primary myelofibrosis: The Mayo Clinic experience. *Mayo Clinic Proceedings*, 87(1), 25–33. doi: 10.1016/j.mayocp.2011.11.001.

Townsend, W., & Linch, D. (2012). Hodgkin's lymphoma in adults. *Lancet*, 380(9844), 836–847.

Valent, P. (2010). Exploring the curative potential of BCR-ABL1-targeting drugs for chronic myeloid leukaemia. *Lancet Oncol*, 11(11), 1010–1011.

Wilcox, R. A. (2010). Cancer-associated myeloproliferation: old association, new therapeutic target. *Mayo Clin Proceed*, 85(7), 656–663.

Zhang, F. H., Ling, Y. W., Zhai, X., et al. (2013). The effect of imatinib therapy on the outcome of allogeneic stem cell transplantation in adults with Philadelphia chromosome-positive acute lymphoblastic leukemia. *Hematology,* 18(3), 151–157.

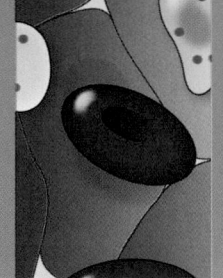

CHAPTER 13

Disorders of Red Blood Cells

Key Terms

Agglutinogens

Alloimmune hemolysis

Anemia

Aplastic anemia

Cold agglutinin syndrome

Erythropoiesis

Hemoglobinopathy

Hemolysis

Hyperbilirubinemia

Intrinsic factor (IF)

Oxyhemoglobin dissociation curve

Pernicious anemia

Pica

Polycythemia

Reticulocyte

Subacute combined degeneration

Vaso-occlusive crisis

Warm agglutinin syndrome

The main function of the red blood cell (RBC), also called an erythrocyte or corpuscle, is to deliver oxygen to the body's tissues. It is solely designed to carry oxygen on its large hemoglobin (Hgb) molecule. The major pathophysiologic condition involving RBCs is **anemia,** a condition in which there is insufficient delivery of oxygen to the tissues caused by inadequate number of mature, healthy RBCs in the blood. Insufficient oxygen delivery to the tissues produces signs and symptoms related to cellular hypoxia and lack of cell energy.

Anemia has various causes, including blood loss, nutritional deficiencies, defective Hgb, bone marrow failure, and chronic disease. It is a common disorder that affects more than 3 million people in the United States across all age, ethnic, and racial groups. Although anemia occurs in both men and women, women of childbearing age are at higher risk than men. Older adults, especially those with chronic medical problems, are also at increased risk.

Another less common disorder of RBCs is **polycythemia,** which is a disorder characterized by overproliferation of all blood cells in the bone marrow.

Epidemiology

Anemia is the most common problem associated with RBCs. In the United States, approximately 6.6% of men and 12.4% of women have anemia. The prevalence of the disorder increases with age and is prevalent in 44.4% of men 85 years and older. In undeveloped countries, prevalence of anemia is estimated to be 2 to 5 times greater than in the United States. Growing children commonly suffer from anemia in undeveloped countries.

Certain races and ethnic groups have an increased prevalence of genetic factors associated with particular anemias. For example, sickle cell anemia (SCA) is common in Africa, the Middle East, and the Mediterranean

region. In areas of poor socioeconomic conditions, deficient diet leads to an increased prevalence of anemia. For instance, iron deficiency anemia is much more prevalent in countries where there is little meat in the diet. Anemia of chronic disease (ACD) is commonplace in populations with a high incidence of chronic infectious disease, such as malaria, tuberculosis, and acquired immune deficiency syndrome (AIDS). Although most prominent in elderly individuals, anemia also occurs during infancy and adolescence. Growth spurts in adolescence predispose to anemia. Infants weaned from breast milk to cow's milk also are at risk for anemia.

Basic Concepts of RBC Physiology

Hematopoiesis is the process by which all blood cells are formed in the bone marrow. The bone marrow is constantly in a state of synthesis of RBCs, white blood cells (WBCs), and platelets. RBCs, the only cells that carry oxygen, have a life span of 120 days. The body is in a state of constant renewal of the RBC supply.

Synthesis of Erythrocytes

Erythropoiesis is the specific series of steps in the bone marrow that leads to the synthesis of mature RBCs. All RBCs begin as pluripotent stem cells in the bone marrow that are stimulated to become erythroid precursor cells. Each precursor goes through a series of changes until it becomes a mature erythrocyte released by the bone marrow (see Fig. 13-1). The nucleus of the RBC is expelled in one of the last stages of erythropoiesis, which is why the RBC has no genetic material in its mature state.

The last stage of erythropoiesis involves formation of the **reticulocyte,** an immature RBC. Reticulocytes usually remain in the bone marrow until fully matured

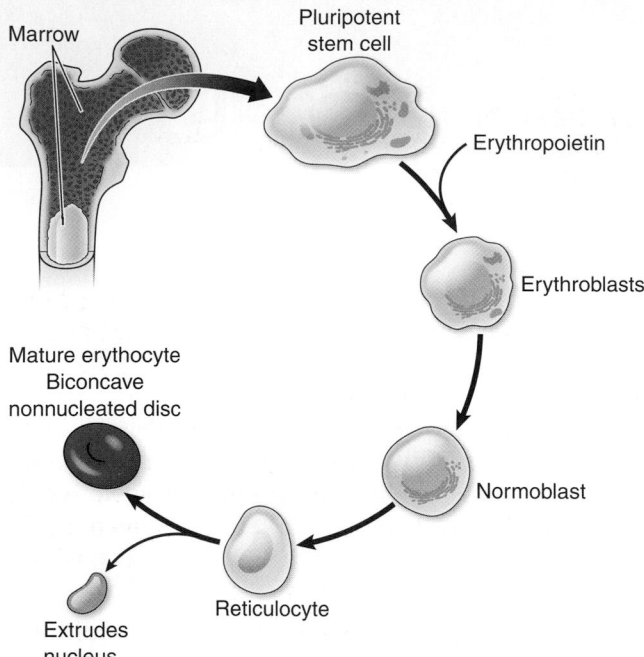

FIGURE 13-1. Erythropoiesis is the process of maturation of a pluripotent stem cell into mature erythrocytes in the bone marrow. Under the influence of EPO, the pluripotent stem cell in the bone marrow develops into a nucleated erythroblast and then into a normoblast. The normoblast extrudes its nucleus to become a reticulocyte and then fully matures into a nonnucleated erythrocyte. In times of acute hemorrhage, rapid blood loss creates a situation where the bone marrow cannot synthesize a sufficient number of mature erythrocytes. In acute hemorrhage, reticulocytes are allowed out of the bone marrow and circulate within the bloodstream. A high reticulocyte count indicates that the bone marrow is working hard to replace lost erythrocytes.

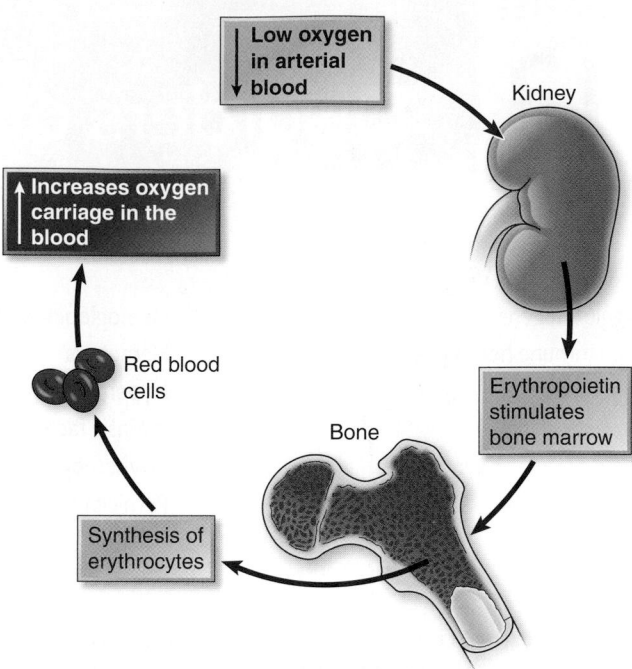

FIGURE 13-2. Synthesis of erythrocytes. The kidney releases the hormone acronym erythropoetin (EPO) in response to hypoxia sensed in the bloodstream. EPO activates the bone marrow to synthesize erythrocytes. The extra erythrocytes raise the blood's oxygen-carrying ability; this is sensed by the kidney, which in turn shuts down EPO synthesis.

as an RBC. However, when the bone marrow cannot synthesize enough RBCs to keep up with their loss, as in blood loss or hemolysis, reticulocytes are released into the circulation. Normally, the reticulocyte count in the bloodstream is approximately 1%, reflecting the daily replacement of approximately 1% of the RBC population. However, when there is a large loss of mature RBCs, there is a markedly higher percentage of reticulocytes in the bloodstream; this is called reticulocytosis. High numbers of reticulocytes in the bloodstream commonly indicates bleeding or brisk RBC destruction. Conversely, abnormally low numbers of reticulocytes occur in conditions of bone marrow suppression or other causes of poor RBC production.

Hypoxia is the major stimulus for erythropoiesis. The kidney senses hypoxia in the bloodstream and releases the hormone erythropoietin, which stimulates the bone marrow. When stimulated by erythropoietin, the bone marrow synthesizes RBCs from stem cell erythroid precursors. The resulting increase in the number of RBCs reverses the hypoxia (see Fig. 13-2).

Substances needed for adequate synthesis of healthy RBCs include protein, iron, vitamin B_{12}, and folic acid. Iron is the main nutritional element needed for Hgb synthesis. Hgb is composed of a heme and globin compound. Heme is composed of iron ($Fe+2$) and a protein called porphyrin. Porphyrin is metabolized into a protein called biliverdin, a green-colored compound that colorizes bile, feces, and ecchymoses. Biliverdin is further broken down into bilirubin, a yellow-colored compound that is a constituent of bile. In conditions where there is a high amount of breakdown of RBCs, bilirubin accumulates in the bloodstream, a condition called **hyperbilirubinemia** (see Fig. 13-3). Bilirubin adheres to elastin, a component of connective tissue contained in the skin and sclera of the eye. The skin and sclera take on an obvious yellow stain, resulting in a condition called jaundice (also called icterus) (see Fig. 13-4). Jaundice is often a sign of a high amount of RBC breakdown but can also occur in liver disorders.

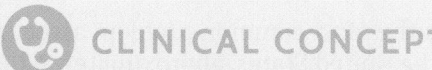
CLINICAL CONCEPT

The number of reticulocytes is a good indicator of bone marrow activity, because it represents recent production of RBCs. A high reticulocyte count indicates that the bone marrow is working hard to keep up with RBC loss.

The Erythrocyte

The unique design of the erythrocyte produces efficient transport of oxygen. It does not have a nucleus,

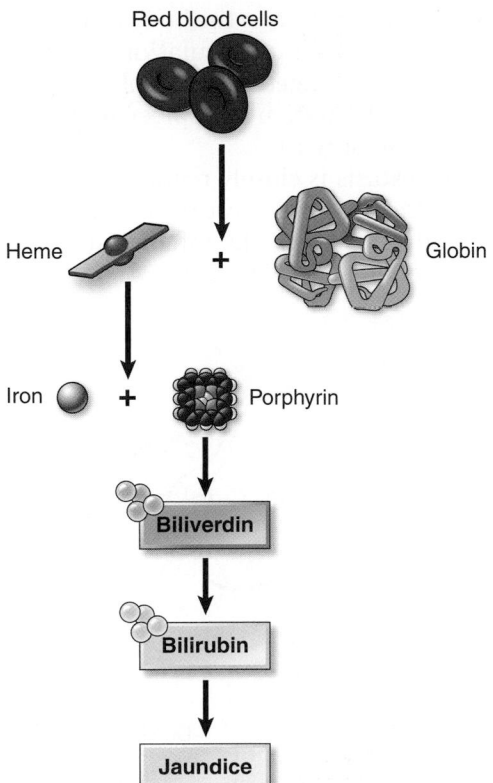

Red blood cells

Heme + Globin

Iron + Porphyrin

Biliverdin

Bilirubin

Jaundice

FIGURE 13-3. Hgb breakdown from erythrocytes. Hemoglobin breaks down into heme + globin. Heme further breaks down into iron (Fe++) and porphyrin. Porphyrin breaks down into biliverdin, which is transformed into a yellow substance called bilirubin. High bilirubin levels in the bloodstream cause jaundice, which is a yellowish color obvious in the skin and sclera of the eyes. Therefore, a large amount of RBC breakdown (hemolysis) causes jaundice.

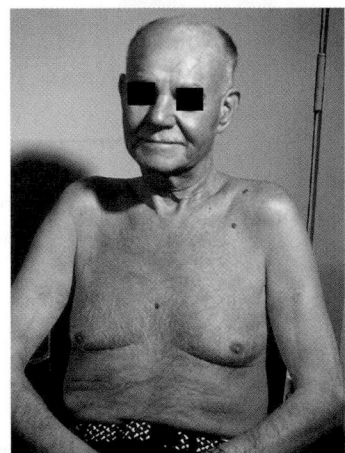

FIGURE 13-4. Person with jaundice. (From Dillon, P. (2007). *Nursing health assessment.* 2nd ed. Philadelphia, PA: F.A. Davis Company, with permission.)

allowing more room for Hgb, which fills the erythrocyte and produces its red color. Erythrocytes are biconcave discs, providing a large surface area for diffusion (see Fig. 13-5).

Approximately 95% of oxygen travels in the circulation attached to Hgb, whereas only 5% is directly

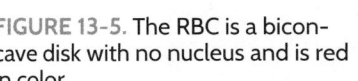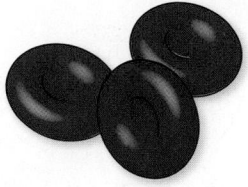

FIGURE 13-5. The RBC is a biconcave disk with no nucleus and is red in color.

dissolved in the plasma. Hgb also carries carbon dioxide away from tissues, but most carbon dioxide travels in the form of soluble bicarbonate (HCO_3^-) in the plasma. Erythrocytes are very flexible and easily change shape in order to pass through small capillaries. They have a limited life expectancy, generally lasting about 120 days. The spleen removes aged, lysed, and dead RBCs from circulation. In the spleen, RBCs are broken down into their component parts, which are recycled to make new red blood cells.

CLINICAL CONCEPT

The spleen, a highly vascular organ, is the "graveyard of RBCs" and an organ of immunity. It sequesters abnormally shaped and hemolyzed RBCs and destroys them. Splenomegaly occurs when there is a large amount of RBC breakdown occurring in the body.

Hemoglobin

The RBC carries oxygen because of the affinity of Hgb for oxygen. Oxygen attaches to Hgb at the pulmonary capillaries and from there it is delivered to tissues. Hgb carries oxygen to cells and carries carbon dioxide away from cells and back to pulmonary circulation. In adults, the Hgb molecule is composed of four polypeptide chains referred to as alpha 1, alpha 2, beta 1, and beta 2. Each chain has an atom of iron that can carry an oxygen atom, allowing for each Hgb to carry four oxygen atoms (see Fig. 13-6). The synthesis of Hgb is greatly dependent on the availability of iron. A lack of iron results in small amounts of Hgb in each RBC and a resulting low amount of oxygen carriage in the blood. Normal Hgb is called Hgb A.

In the fetus until early infancy there is a specific kind of Hgb called Hgb F. This Hgb has four alpha chains and a very high affinity for oxygen. It can facilitate transfer of oxygen across the placenta. Hgb F is replaced by Hgb A by 6 months of age. The formation of the four polypeptide chains that make up Hgb is directed by genes within the deoxyribonucleic acid (DNA) of the early RBC. In disorders called hemoglobinopathies, there is an abnormal structure of Hgb because of a genetic mutation. For example, in sickle cell anemia (SCA), there is a mutation in one of the genes that directs the synthesis of the beta polypeptide chains. Within one of the beta chains there is an abnormal

Hemoglobin

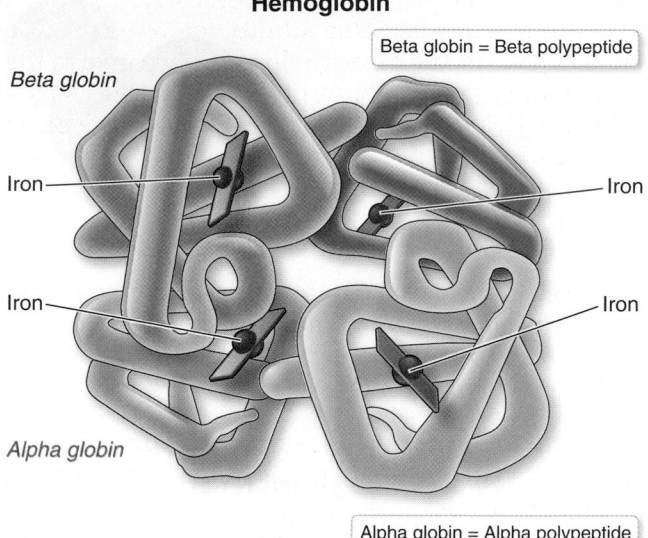

FIGURE 13-6. Structure of Hgb. The Hgb molecule consists of two beta polypeptide chains and two alpha polypeptide chains. There are four iron atoms that bind to oxygen.

substitution of the amino acid valine for glutamic acid. Because of this mutation, persons with SCA have a different Hgb called Hgb S.

Iron Metabolism

Iron is needed in the diet to synthesize Hgb in RBCs and myoglobin, a component of muscle cells. Cellular enzymes, which are used in various metabolic processes, also require iron for optimal function. Iron is mainly absorbed in the duodenum and upper jejunum. Some iron is sequestered within the intestinal cells and some is released into the bloodstream. The epithelial intestinal cells are constantly sloughed and excreted, and with loss of the cells, there is loss of iron. When absorbed into the bloodstream from the GI system, iron is transported by a protein called transferrin. Iron that is bound to transferrin and other sites in the body is represented within the measurement called total iron binding capacity (TIBC).

Transferrin carries iron to the bone marrow for erythropoiesis. Membrane receptors on erythroid precursors in the bone marrow avidly bind transferrin. About 10% to 20% of absorbed iron goes into a storage pool in cells of the reticuloendothelial system, which is made up of the macrophages throughout the body. The storage of iron occurs in ferritin complexes that are present in all cells, but most commonly found in the bone marrow, liver, and spleen. The liver's stores of ferritin are the primary physiologic source of reserve iron in the body.

The composition of the diet influences iron absorption. Citrate and vitamin C can form complexes with iron that increase absorption, whereas tannates in tea can decrease absorption of iron. The iron in heme found in meat is the most readily absorbed kind of iron. Only a small fraction of the body's iron is gained or lost

each day. Most of the iron in the body is recycled when old RBCs are taken out of circulation and destroyed. The RBC iron is scavenged by macrophages within the reticuloendothelial system and spleen and returned to the storage pool for reuse.

Iron homeostasis is closely regulated via intestinal absorption. Increased absorption is signaled by decreasing iron stores, hypoxia, inflammation, and erythropoietic activity (see Fig. 13-7).

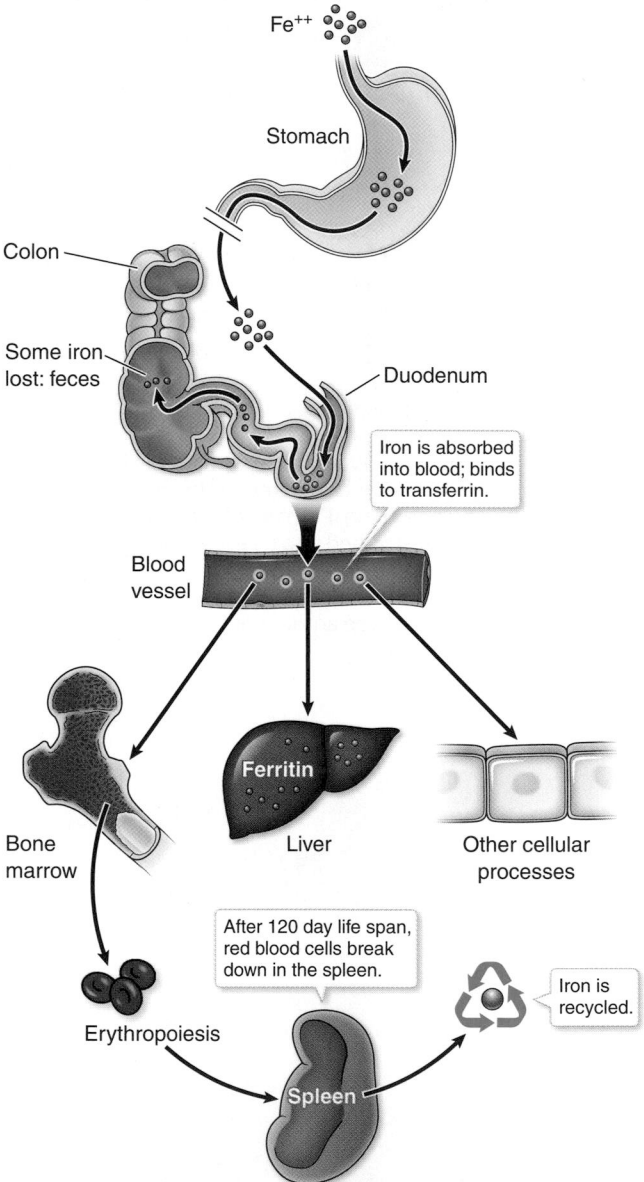

FIGURE 13-7. Normal iron absorption and metabolism. Iron is absorbed from the diet in the duodenum and jejunum. Only 10% of iron in the diet is absorbed, and it is in the intestinal epithelium until absorption into the bloodstream. Some of the intestinal epithelium is sloughed daily, and so some iron is lost in the feces daily. After absorption into the bloodstream, iron is carried by a protein called transferrin, which carries iron in the bloodstream to the bone marrow. In the bone marrow, iron is used for the synthesis of red blood cells. Iron is also delivered to the liver for storage as ferritin. Some iron is also used in cellular processes. As RBCs die, they are transported to the spleen for breakdown; the iron is absorbed back into the bloodstream and recycled in the body.

Oxyhemoglobin Dissociation

The sole purpose of the RBC is to transport oxygen from the pulmonary capillaries to the cells and carbon dioxide away from the cells back to the lungs. At high levels of arterial oxygen pressure (PO_2), Hgb has a strong affinity for oxygen and it is fully saturated. However, as PO_2 diminishes, Hgb sites for oxygen go unfilled, and Hgb becomes less attracted to oxygen. Hgb starts to drop all its oxygen as PO_2 falls below 60 mm Hg.

The **oxyhemoglobin dissociation curve** is an important tool for understanding how blood carries and releases oxygen (see Fig. 13-8). The oxyhemoglobin dissociation curve represents the relationship between PO_2 and the affinity of Hgb to oxygen. When PO_2 is 100 mm Hg, Hgb is totally saturated with oxygen atoms. This is the ideal and highest level of oxygen-hemoglobin affinity. However, at PO_2 of approximately 60 mm Hg, Hgb affinity for oxygen dramatically falls and oxygen is given up to the tissues.

There are some conditions that decrease or increase affinity of Hgb for oxygen. An increase of carbon dioxide in the blood, fever, increased 2,3 diphosphoglycerate (2,3 DPG), and a decrease in pH (acidosis) results in a reduction of the affinity of Hgb for oxygen. These conditions shift the sigmoid-shaped oxy-Hgb dissociation curve to the right, showing less affinity of Hgb for oxygen. Because Hgb has less affinity, it gives up oxygen to the tissues easily. Conversely, an increase of

pH in the blood (alkalosis), decreased 2,3 DPG, and hypothermia increase Hgb affinity for oxygen. These conditions shift the oxy-Hgb dissociation curve to the left, showing greater affinity of Hgb for oxygen. Oxygen is held by Hgb tighter than normal and less is given up to the tissues.

The effect of pH on the Hgb's ability to bind oxygen is called the Bohr effect. When pH is low (acidosis), Hgb binds oxygen less strongly, and when pH is high (alkalosis), Hgb binds more tightly to oxygen. Because of the Bohr effect, Hgb gives up oxygen to tissue easily during low pH. Alternatively, the Haldane effect occurs when oxygen is high in concentration in the bloodstream and it saturates Hgb sites. Hgb binds oxygen tightly and O_2 displaces carbon dioxide from Hgb. In deoxygenated blood, Hgb has free sites for binding to carbon dioxide.

2, 3 DPG is an organic phosphate bound to Hgb in RBCs. It is a by-product of the breakdown of glycogen to glucose. It reduces the affinity of Hgb for oxygen, shifting the oxygen dissociation curve to the right and thereby assisting the unloading of oxygen to tissues.

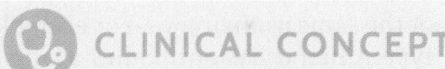

CLINICAL CONCEPT

Oxygen delivery to tissues is affected by both oxy-Hgb saturation and the amount of Hgb in the blood. If the oxygen saturation is 100% and Hgb level is normal, oxygen delivery to the tissues is ideal. However, if oxygen saturation of blood is 100% and Hgb is low (as in anemia), oxygen delivery will be inadequate and cellular hypoxia will result.

ALERT! Hgb has greater affinity for carbon monoxide (CO) compared with oxygen. If there are high levels of CO in the environment, oxygen will be displaced off Hgb sites and saturated with CO. This deoxygenated state is often fatal.

Blood Types

There are surface antigens on all body cells, including RBCs. Specific types of antigens on the surface of RBCs are called **agglutinogens.** There are two different types of agglutinogens, type A and type B. The ABO blood type classification system categorizes blood into four types according to these agglutinogens: type A, B, AB, and O.

Another antigen on the surface of RBCs is Rh factor, also called D antigen. If the RBC surface has the Rh factor, it is categorized as positive (Rh+); if it does not have the Rh factor, it is called negative (Rh-). All blood types are either Rh+ or Rh-. Individuals inherit their blood type from their parents. The A and B antigens

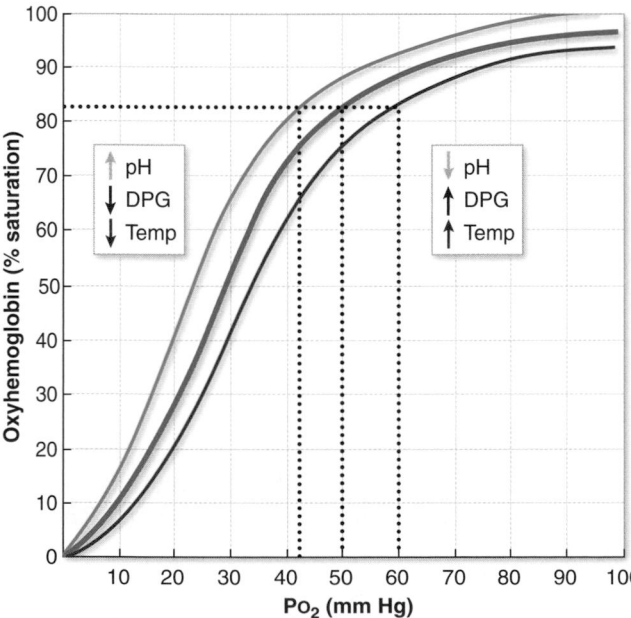

FIGURE 13-8. Oxygen-hemoglobin dissociation curve. The normal binding of Hgb to oxygen (O_2) is depicted in blue. Normally, when the partial pressure of oxygen (PO_2) in blood is 100 mm Hg, there is great affinity of Hgb for oxygen and great saturation. At approximately PO_2 60 mm Hg there is a dramatic drop in affinity of Hgb for oxygen (blue). In fever, high carbon dioxide, acidosis, and high DPG, there is less affinity of Hgb for O_2 and less saturation (red). In alkalosis, hypothermia, and low DPG, there is greater affinity of Hgb for O_2 and greater saturation (green).

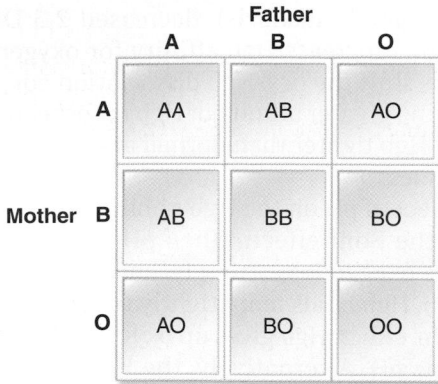

FIGURE 13-9. Punnett square for inheritance of blood types.

are encoded by different alleles, one from the mother and the other from the father. A gene called the O allele codes for a nonfunctional protein that does not produce surface molecules. The person with O blood has no antigens on his or her RBCs. The possible combinations of alleles that can yield the blood type of offspring can be configured with a Punnett square (see Fig. 13-9).

Individuals develop antibodies to blood antigens that are not the same as their own. For example, a person with type A blood has antibodies against type B blood called anti-B antibodies. A person with type O blood has no antigens on the surface of his or her RBCs; however, they have both anti-A and anti-B antibodies (see Table 13-1).

The ABO system is the blood-group system used in human-blood transfusion. If a person receives a different type of blood than his or her own from a donor, antibodies attack the infused RBCs and cause a transfusion reaction that involves hemolysis. For example, if a person with type A blood receives a type B blood transfusion, the anti-B antibodies of the recipient will attack the type B RBCs of the donor blood. The person with type O negative blood can donate blood to persons with any type of blood because they have no surface antigens on their RBCs. Individuals with type AB + blood can accept any kind of foreign blood because they do not have antibodies.

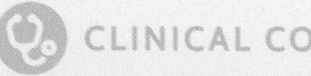 CLINICAL CONCEPT

A person with type O negative blood is known as a universal donor, whereas a person with AB positive blood is known as a universal recipient.

Basic Concepts of RBC Pathophysiology

Anemia is the most common disorder that affects RBCs. There is inadequate oxygen delivery to the

TABLE 13-1. Blood Types and Antibodies

Type A, B, or AB blood has antigens on the RBC surface and specific antibodies in the plasma. Type O blood has no antigens on the RBC surface and stimulates no antibody formation in the recipient. However persons with Type O blood have anti-A antibodies and anti-B antibodies. Therefore type O persons cannot receive A or B type blood.

Type AB blood has both A and B antigens on the surface of the RBCs and will not stimulate any antibodies in the recipient.

A transfusion will work if a person who is going to receive blood has a blood group that doesn't have any antibodies against the donor blood's antigens. If a person who is going to receive blood has antibodies matching the donor blood's antigens, the red blood cells in the donated blood will agglutinate.

Example 1: Type O blood can be given to all persons because the recipient will not build antibodies against any antigen. However, only type O blood can be given to type O recipients because O persons have anti-A and anti-B antibodies..

Example 2: Type A blood individuals cannot give blood to type B recipients because the recipient has anti-A antibodies. Type B blood individuals cannot give blood to type A recipients because the recipient has anti-B antibodies.

Blood Type	Antibody
A	Anti-B antibody
B	Anti-A antibody
AB (both surface antigens) Universal recipient	No antibodies
O (no surface antigens) Universal donor	Anti-A antibody Anti-B antibody Anti-Rh antibody
Rh-negative Rh-positive (D antigen)	No antibodies

tissues either because of deficient Hgb, abnormal Hgb, or low number of RBCs. Polycythemia, the opposite kind of disorder, causes too many RBCs in circulation.

Anemia

Anemia is the major pathophysiologic condition affecting RBCs. It can be defined as a decreased RBC mass that becomes clinically apparent when levels of Hgb and hematocrit (Hct) are less than normal. A complete blood count (CBC) measures all RBCs and RBC characteristics. Different types of anemia produce different CBC results.

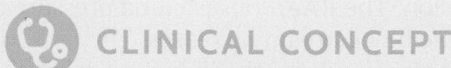

Complete Blood Count

The CBC is one of the basic diagnostic procedures used when investigating any disorder in the body. It can be ordered as a CBC with differential when the measure of WBCs is also needed. The CBC includes Hgb, Hct, a number of RBCs, mean corpuscular volume (MCV), mean corpuscular hemoglobin (MCH), and MCH concentration (MCHC) (see Table 13-2).

Hemoglobin

Hgb is a direct measure of the amount of Hgb in a given volume of blood. Normal values differ for men and women. The normal range for men is 13 to 18 gm/dL, whereas the normal range for women is 12 to 16 gm/dL. Females and African American males are usually 1 to 2 gms lower than white males. Women have lower Hgb and Hct than men because of monthly menstrual blood loss. Persons who live at high altitudes normally have higher Hgb and Hct because their environment naturally has lower oxygen concentration. The low oxygen in their bloodstream constantly stimulates renal erythropoietin (EPO) which, in turn, stimulates the bone marrow to synthesize RBCs. A high number of RBCs is called secondary polycythemia or erythrocytosis.

Hematocrit

Hct is the percentage of blood that consists of RBCs. The normal range for men is 45% to 52%, whereas the normal range for women is 37% to 48%.

Total RBC Count

Total RBC count is a measure of the number of RBCs in a given volume of blood. This value is usually between 4.5 and 5.5 x 10^6 cells per cubic millimeter for males and 4.0 to 4.9 x 10^6 cells per cubic millimeter for females.

Mean Corpuscular Volume

MCV is the volume of one RBC. This value reflects red cell size as seen under the microscope. It is used to classify the anemia as either microcytic, megaloblastic (also called macrocytic), or normocytic. The normal value of MCV is 80 to 100 femoliters.

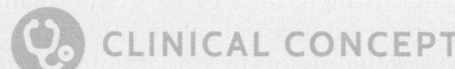

MCH and MCHC

MCH is the average amount of Hgb in an average RBC. Normal MCH is 27 to 32 picograms. MCHC is the average concentration of Hgb in a given volume of RBCs. The normal range is 32% to 36%.

TABLE 13-2. CBC Normal Values*

To understand how to interpret a CBC, the following are the parameters, their definition, and the normal levels.

Parameter	Definition	Normal Levels
Total red blood cells x 10^6	Number of RBCs per liter	Males: 4.5 to 5.5 Females: 4.0 to 4.9
Hgb	Amount of Hgb in blood g/dL	Males: 13 to 18 Females: 12 to 16
Hct	Packed RBC volume; fraction of the whole blood that consists of RBC	45% to 52 % males 37% to 48% females
MCV	Size of the RBC	80 to 100
MCH	Mass of the RBC	27 to 32
MCHC	Concentration of Hgb (color)	32% to 36 %
RBC distribution width	Measures the variation in RBC size and shape	11 to 15
Platelets	Cells that assist clotting	90,000 to 450,000
Reticulocytes	Immature RBCs	1%

*Different labs have minor differences in normal values.

> ### CLINICAL CONCEPT
>
> MCH and MCHC can be used to indicate the color of the RBCs. A low value for either indicates that cells are pale or hypochromic.

In anemia, when MCV is normal and MCHC is normal, size and color of the RBCs are normal. This is characterized as a normocytic normochromic (NCNC) anemia. The most common cause of NCNC anemia is blood loss, as the lack of RBC mass and low Hgb and Hct occurs because there is a deficient number of RBCs.

When MCV and MCHC are both decreased, the size and color of the RBCs are abnormal. A low MCV indicates small size of RBCs, and a low MCHC indicates pale color of RBCs. This is categorized as microcytic hypochromic (MCHC) anemia. This most commonly occurs in iron deficiency.

When MCV is high, the RBCs are abnormally large; this is also referred to as megaloblastic or macrocytic. This most commonly occurs in vitamin B_{12} and folic acid deficiency.

RBC Distribution

RBC distribution width (RDW) measures the variation in RBC size and width.

Platelets

Platelets are the blood cells that cause clotting of the blood. If the total amount of platelets is too low, bleeding or bruising can occur; if it's too high, clotting can occur. The normal value is 90,000 to 450,000 platelets in the blood.

Reticulocyte Count

Reticulocyte count measures the number of new RBCs in the blood and helps to determine whether the bone marrow is producing new red cells at an appropriate rate. Increased reticulocyte numbers associated with anemia suggest accelerated destruction or loss of RBCs. Normal reticulocyte count is approximately 1% of total RBCs.

Basic Pathophysiologic Concepts Related to Anemia

There are various possible etiologies for anemia. The physiologic response to anemia varies according to the etiology and rate of onset. With anemia caused by acute blood loss, a sudden reduction in oxygen-carrying capacity occurs along with a rapid decrease in intravascular volume, with resultant hypoxia and hypovolemia. Hypovolemia will trigger baroreceptors and the activity of the sympathetic nervous system. The heart will beat faster in an attempt to accomplish greater blood oxygenation. Also, the renin-angiotensin-aldosterone system (RAAS) is provoked to remedy the hypovolemia and hypotension. The RAAS raises blood pressure and volume of the bloodstream increases. The hypoxia in the bloodstream stimulates the kidney to release erythropoietin, which stimulates the bone marrow to synthesize more RBCs. Acute blood loss incites emergency remedies by the body.

In chronic blood loss, the body slowly loses RBCs over a long period of time. The blood volume lost may not be perceptible by the patient, and the small blood volume lost is not the main problem as the body can replace it. However, the body is unable to synthesize healthy RBCs, which requires iron, vitamin B_{12}, and folic acid. The stores of these nutrients slowly become exhausted because of loss of the blood's nutrients. In other words, the RBCS are slowly, constantly lost, with the iron, vitamin B_{12}, and folic acid that they contain. Normally, after the RBC's death, the RBC components are recycled in the spleen. In chronic blood loss, however, there is no recycling; the RBCs produced by the bone marrow become deficient in these nutrients. The RBCs become particularly iron deficient because iron stores become exhausted quicker than stores of vitamin B_{12} and folic acid. Iron-poor RBCs cannot carry oxygen required by the tissue. Tissue hypoxia results, which can cause ischemia of the heart muscle and weakening of peripheral musculature. Cerebral hypoxia occurs and organs become dysfunctional because of the lack of tissue oxygenation. A similar process of dysfunctional erythropoiesis occurs when anemia is caused by vitamin B_{12} or folic acid deficiency.

With hemolytic anemias, the RBCs become prematurely destroyed and dead RBCs accumulate in the spleen, causing splenomegaly. The circulation contains fewer RBCs and less oxygen delivery occurs, resulting in diminished tissue oxygenation.

Clinical Manifestations of Anemia

A thorough history and physical examination is needed to diagnose anemia. Commonly, anemia causes subtle symptoms and the patient may be unaware of the disorder. In addition, physical findings can be understated. Incidental findings on a laboratory test are often the way individuals discover that they have anemia.

History

Asymptomatic anemia is common, as it usually occurs gradually over a long period of time without an obvious initiating event. Patients may complain of fatigue and being generally run down. The patient's medication list should be reviewed because some drugs can cause hemolytic anemia, folic acid deficiency, or bone marrow suppression. It is important to ask about diet and nutritional intake, especially in elderly patients, where lack of adequate diet and impaired absorption play a role in the development of anemia.

The gastrointestinal tract is a common site for slow blood loss, and it is important to ask about the appearance of the stool, especially the color, and any history of stomach or intestinal disorders, such as gastric ulcers or inflammatory bowel disease, which can produce bleeding. Black tarry stools, also called melena, contain blood from gastrointestinal bleeding.

In women of childbearing age, it is important to ask about menstrual periods and any history of uterine problems. Menorrhagia, which is excess menstrual blood loss, often goes unreported and is a common cause of iron deficiency anemia. Last menstrual period is important because ectopic pregnancy or spontaneous abortion can cause acute blood loss.

Past medical history is important as certain diseases such as kidney problems or chronic disorders can cause anemia. Some infections predispose to anemia, such as infectious mononucleosis, mycoplasma, and malaria. Family history is important, as certain anemias such as sickle cell anemia, hereditary spherocytosis, and thalassemia are inherited disorders. Social habits should be investigated, as lifestyle choices such as alcohol abuse can lead to anemia.

Signs and Symptoms

The appearance and severity of symptoms depend on whether the anemia developed rapidly or slowly. Symptoms of anemia are frequently overlooked by the patient and attributed to tiredness. For a list of the common symptoms associated with all anemias, see Box 13-1.

Physical Examination

The vital signs in anemia may reveal tachypnea and tachycardia. The patient's complexion may be pale, as may be the conjunctiva of the eye, nail beds, creases in the palm of the hand, and the buccal mucosa. Persons with hemolytic anemia may exhibit jaundice. Splenomegaly is a sign that the spleen is hyperactive, which would occur in hemolytic anemia.

> ### BOX 13-1. Common Signs and Symptoms of Anemia
>
> Different types of anemia have distinctive symptoms. However, the common signs and symptoms of all types of anemia include:
>
> - Pallor of skin, conjunctiva, nailbeds, and buccal mucosa
> - Excessive fatigue
> - Weakness
> - Shortness of breath, especially with activity
> - Exercise intolerance
> - Palpitations (tachycardia)
> - Chest pain
> - Dizziness or feeling faint
> - Headache
> - Nutritional anemias can cause glossitis, cheilitis, koilonychia, or pica.

Some types of chronic anemia cause hair loss, koilonychia, cheilitis, and glossitis. Koilonychia is an abnormal spoon shape of the nails. Cheilitis are sores on the corners of the mouth, and glossitis is a smooth, swollen red tongue.

Diagnosis

The diagnostic tests used in the investigation of all anemias are the CBC, discussed earlier in the chapter, and the peripheral blood smear, which allows microscopic visualization of blood cells, including their size, shape, color, coating, and any abnormal fragments or cellular material. If anemia is difficult to diagnose, a bone marrow aspiration or biopsy is performed. The bone marrow is usually taken from the hip bone and examined for abnormalities such as signs of neoplastic disease.

A cardiovascular examination is needed with anemia. Echocardiogram and electrocardiogram (ECG) are needed to assess cardiovascular health. Additional diagnostic tests are indicated based on type of anemia. For more specific diagnostic studies, see each type of anemia.

Treatment

There are many different treatments because there are a wide range of causes of anemia. In anemia caused by blood loss, transfusion may be the only treatment. For treatment of specific anemias, see their respective sections.

Pathophysiology of Selected RBC Disorders

Different types of anemia can be categorized according to etiology. Anemia caused by decreased RBC mass includes acute and chronic blood loss and RBC loss caused by hemolysis. Anemia can also be caused by lack of sufficient RBC synthesis. Iron, vitamin B_{12}, and folic acid deficiency cause insufficient synthesis of RBCs. Hemoglobinopathies cause anemia because of abnormal Hgb structure, which causes deficient oxygen carriage. Hemolysis can be caused by hemoglobinopathy, medication side effects, transfusion reaction, and autoimmune reactions against RBCs.

Anemias Caused by Decrease in RBC Mass

A decrease in RBC mass can occur mainly through acute blood loss, chronic blood loss, or hemolysis. The adult has a total blood volume of approximately 5 liters and can usually lose 500 mL of blood without serious or lasting effects. However, if the loss reaches 1,000 mL or more, serious adverse effects such as hypovolemic shock and cerebral hypoperfusion can occur. Blood loss can be acute or chronic and hemolysis can be mild or severe.

Anemia of Acute Blood Loss

Anemia of acute blood loss is a precipitous drop in the RBC population caused by hemorrhage. Trauma is the most common cause of acute hemorrhage. Acute anemia can also result from significant acute internal blood loss into the thoracic and abdominal cavities caused by rupture of an artery or an organ. Elderly adults and children are at highest risk of death with acute external blood loss because of less resilience. There are many different traumatic causes of anemia caused by blood loss; incidence depends on the etiology.

Risk Factors. Recent trauma is the major risk factor for acute blood loss, and the blood loss can be either overt or occult. Abdominal trauma predisposes to rupture of the spleen, a highly vascular organ. Head trauma can predispose to epidural or subdural hematoma, which is blood loss between the layers of meninges in the cranium. History of aortic aneurysm can predispose to rupture of the aorta. Anticoagulants increase the risk of blood loss because of the prolonged clotting time of the blood. History of hematologic neoplasms increases the risk of bleeding because of lack of platelets. A family history of hereditary blood disorders that cause bleeding such as von Willebrand disease or hemophilia increases risk. Alcohol abuse can cause formation of esophageal varices, which are fragile and cause acute blood loss. In females, acute blood loss can occur during pregnancy, particularly early when the patient may not be aware of the pregnancy. Ectopic pregnancy or spontaneous abortion, also called miscarriage, are common causes of acute blood loss.

Etiology. Acute blood loss is a rapid loss of blood as in hemorrhage caused by trauma, childbirth, rupture of a major blood vessel, or organ. Severe gastrointestinal bleeding can occur in disorders such as esophageal varices or penetrating peptic ulcer.

Pathophysiology. In acute blood loss, all blood cells and plasma volume are lost. It is a rapid development of a NCNC anemia because cells are normal in size and color but deficient in number. The lack of sufficient number of RBCs to carry oxygen causes tissue hypoxia. The severity of the signs and symptoms of NCNC anemia depend on the amount of blood loss. When Hgb falls below 12 g/L, erythropoiesis is activated and the bone marrow starts to synthesize RBCs. In acute hemorrhage, the loss of RBCs can be too fast for the bone marrow to replace them with mature RBCs, so reticulocytes are released into the bloodstream. Reticulocytosis and other compensatory mechanisms are activated in acute hemorrhage. Because of the fluid lost from the bloodstream there is compensatory stimulation of the sympathetic nervous system, systemic arterial vasoconstriction, fluid shifts from tissues into the capillaries, stimulation of the RAAS, and antidiuretic hormone (ADH) release. These mechanisms attempt to diminish the effect of the lost blood volume, and they all act to increase fluid volume in the bloodstream. The increase in fluid volume within the bloodstream can result in hemodilution. Hemodilution of the circulating blood is exhibited by a decrease in Hct.

Clinical Presentation. A thorough history and physical examination are needed in acute blood loss. If trauma is the etiology, the patient often is not able to give the history. Clinicians must use physical assessment skills to assess bleeding source and volume lost. If the patient is able to give a history, there are specific questions to ask in regard to possible causes of acute blood loss.

History. If there is obvious trauma, the patient should be asked about the incidents that led to the trauma. This can give the clinician specific guidance for the physical examination. In acute blood loss, time is of the essence and finding the source of bleeding is a priority. The manner in which the trauma occurred can give clues as to the presence of internal bleeding.

If the patient is not in an acute state of traumatic blood loss, more detailed questions can be asked. The patient should be asked about current medications. Often the medication list can give the clinician clues as to what is causing the acute blood loss. It is important to ask about use of aspirin, nonsteroidal anti-inflammatory drugs (NSAIDs), or corticosteroids. When used long term, these drugs are common causes of gastrointestinal bleeding. Past medical history can give information about risk factors for bleeding. For example, does the patient have a history of hematologic malignancy or clotting disorder? Is the patient on anticoagulant medications? Social habits are also important as these can cause increased risk of bleeding. For example, alcohol abuse can lead to bleeding from esophageal varices.

Signs and Symptoms. Signs and symptoms seen with acute blood loss depend on the volume lost:

- Loss of less than 15% of total blood volume causes orthostatic hypotension and anxiety.
- Loss of 15% to 30% of total blood volume results in the activation of compensatory mechanisms designed to increase blood volume and oxygen delivery to vital organs. Baroreceptors in the arteries sense a drop in BP and stimulate the sympathetic nervous system to increase heart rate and vasoconstrict arteries. The kidney senses low volume of blood and releases renin, which kicks off the RAAS. Water is conserved by ADH, which decreases urine output to fewer than 30 mL/hr. Restlessness and changes in level of consciousness occur as perfusion of the brain is decreased.
- Loss of 30% to 40% of total volume results in worsening of the previous signs, with tachycardia above 120 beats per minute; weak, rapid pulse associated with the loss of Hgb and plasma volume;

cool, pale skin; hypotension; and urine output of 5 to 15 mL/hr.

- Loss greater than 40% of total volume causes profound shock (severe hypotension) with confusion and decreased level of consciousness, heart rate above 140 beats per minute, scant or no urine output, and profound hypotension. Shock can reach an irreversible stage when compensatory mechanisms become exhausted.

Vital signs in acute blood loss include hypotension, tachycardia, and tachypnea. Pallor, cool clammy skin, and loss of consciousness develop as bleeding worsens. If bleeding is apparent, then a complete examination of the region of trauma is needed. If bleeding is occult, a complete physical exam is necessary to rule out internal bleeding. The left upper quadrant of the abdomen should be palpated to assess the spleen, as splenic rupture is often the source of bleeding caused by abdominal trauma. In head trauma, the clinician should rule out epidural and subdural hematoma, as these are sources of occult bleeding. Patients with severe gastrointestinal bleeding will vomit blood or excrete blood in the stool. Patients with blood loss require a thorough chest, abdomen, and pelvic examination. Digital rectal exam with fecal occult blood test (FOBT) can detect signs of gastrointestinal bleeding.

ALERT! When rapid bleeding is overt or suspected, danger signs include hypotension, heart rate above 110 bpm, complaints of thirst, and urine output of fewer than 30 mL/hr.

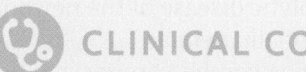 **CLINICAL CONCEPT**

Patients bleeding because of esophageal varices often exhibit a large loss of blood via vomiting, which is referred to as hematemesis. Blood mixed with stomach acid and mucus in vomitus is referred to as "coffee ground" emesis. Patients losing large amounts of blood via the rectum exhibit hematochezia, which is bright red blood in the stool.

Diagnosis. Hemorrhage that is overt or occult will cause a rapid NCNC anemia with reticulocytosis on a CBC. Platelet count should be reviewed on the CBC to assess clotting ability. Blood pressure may be in the hypotensive range of less than 100 mm Hg systolic. In cases where acute blood loss is occult, reticulocytosis is an important diagnostic sign indicating the bone marrow is rapidly generating RBCs to replace those lost. Blood chemistry studies, serum creatinine, and arterial blood gases (ABGs) are important because acute blood loss can cause irregularities in these values. The

patient should have an FOBT to investigate the possibility of bleeding from the gastrointestinal tract. A pregnancy test should be performed on women of childbearing age. The patient should have lab testing for blood type and crossmatching in case of the need for transfusion. A computed tomography (CT) scan of the abdomen and pelvis can assist with recognition of occult internal bleeding. If the patient has head trauma or is unconscious, a CT scan of the head is important.

Treatment. Immediate treatment includes establishing hemostasis, restoring blood volume, and treating shock. An intravenous normal saline solution should be infused until a matching blood product can be infused. Transfusion is currently the only reliable way to restore blood volume and oxygen-carrying capacity. If blood is not immediately available, plasma is the most suitable substitute. If the amount of blood lost is not large, erythropoiesis will restore normal volume and Hgb over time. After the patient is stabilized, endoscopy and colonoscopy should be done to investigate gastrointestinal bleeding.

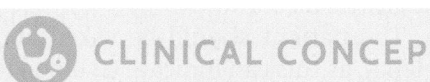 **CLINICAL CONCEPT**

Reticulocytosis indicates that the bone marrow is synthesizing a large amount of RBCs, usually because of blood loss.

Anemia of Chronic Blood Loss

In anemia of chronic blood loss, the patient is enduring a slow, gradual blood loss via the gastrointestinal tract or excessive monthly menstrual loss. Alternatively, there may be hemolysis of blood cells, which slowly diminishes blood cell mass. Chronic blood loss is usually subtle and asymptomatic.

The incidence of anemia caused by chronic blood loss depends on the underlying cause. Approximately 100,000 patients are admitted to U.S. hospitals annually for upper gastrointestinal bleeding, of which peptic ulcer is a common cause. Lower gastrointestinal bleeding accounts for approximately 20% to 33% of episodes of gastrointestinal bleeding, with an annual incidence of about 20 to 27 cases per 100,000 population in Western countries. Colon cancer is a common cause of lower GI bleeding.

Excessive monthly menstrual blood loss, known as menorrhagia, is another common cause of chronic blood loss. Menorrhagia affects nearly 2 million women each year in the United States. Heavy menstrual bleeding has been reported in approximately 10% to 15% of all women at some point during their life. Among these women, as many as 20% will go on to develop anemia.

Risk Factors. In chronic blood loss, risk factors include gastrointestinal disorders such as gastric ulceration, inflammatory bowel disease, and colon cancer. The chronic use of aspirin or NSAIDs can predispose individuals to gastric ulceration and slow bleeding. In females, chronic blood loss commonly occurs because of menorrhagia; large losses of menstrual blood monthly can lead to anemia.

Pathophysiology. The major problem that arises with chronic blood loss is iron deficiency anemia. The RBCs are the largest iron depot in the body. When RBCs are lost, iron is lost and not recycled in the body. Slow loss of RBCs gradually depletes the body's iron stores.

Clinical Presentation. In chronic blood loss, patients may not complain of symptoms, which then requires investigation into possible unrecognized problems. It is important to obtain a list of medications. The patient may not be aware of overuse of aspirin and NSAIDs that can lead to gastric ulceration. The patient may report use of over-the-counter antacids, proton pump inhibitors such as lansoprazole (Prilosec®), or acid suppressants such as ranitidine (Zantac®). Frequent use of these medications can indicate the patient is attempting to treat gastric ulceration.

History. The patient should be asked about dark stools (melena), as this can indicate GI blood loss. Past medical and surgical history is important, especially regarding GI problems. Women may report episodes of excessive menstrual bleeding. The patient should also be questioned about her last menstrual period to investigate the possibility of pregnancy. Social habits such as smoking, caffeine, and alcohol use are important because these are risk factors for development of gastric ulcer.

Signs and Symptoms. Signs and symptoms of anemia such as pallor, weakness, exercise intolerance, and fatigue may not develop in an obvious manner. The patient is usually not aware of the slow decrease in Hgb and Hct. Also, physical signs and symptoms are not as dramatic as in acute blood loss. Gastrointestinal symptoms may be present, such as those of esophagitis and gastric ulceration. Gastric ulcer symptoms include epigastric burning and a gnawing pain that occurs between meals. The patient may have melena. Women may not have apparent signs of excessive menstrual blood loss and should be questioned about this. Soaking through one menstrual pad or one tampon per hour is usually indicative of menorrhagia. Alternatively, a menstrual period that lasts greater than 1 week can be indicative of menorrhagia.

CLINICAL CONCEPT

In chronic, slow blood loss, the physical examination is often unremarkable. Alternatively, the patient may show general signs of anemia such as pallor, tachycardia, and tachypnea.

Diagnosis. In chronic blood loss, the CBC commonly demonstrates MCHC anemia. The slow bleeding gradually depletes Hgb, Hct, and iron stores. Therefore, blood tests should include serum Fe++, serum ferritin, total iron binding capacity (TIBC), and serum transferrin. Blood chemistry, serum creatinine, and liver function tests should be done. An endoscopy can view disorders in the upper gastrointestinal tract such as bleeding ulcer. A colonoscopy can examine any disorders of the lower gastrointestinal tract such as inflammatory bowel disease, polyps, or colon cancer. An FOBT is important to investigate gastrointestinal bleeding that is exhibited in the stool. In women of childbearing age, a pregnancy test is necessary. Women may require an abdominal or pelvic image study, as well.

Treatment. For chronic blood loss, treatment consists of remedying the source of bleeding. The patient may need gastric ulcer medications or inflammatory bowel treatment. If the patient has a severe gastrointestinal ulceration, polyp, or colon cancer, a gastroenterologist and surgeon should be consulted. For women with probable excessive menstrual blood loss, a gynecologist should be consulted. Commonly, the patient needs iron replacement treatment; usually oral Ferrous sulfate or intramuscular iron administration is sufficient to rebuild the Hgb and Hct. In rare cases, the person with chronic blood loss requires blood transfusion. When Hgb falls below 7 g/dL, transfusion is considered.

Hemolytic Anemia

Hemolysis, another cause of decreased RBC mass, can occur because of various disorders, including hemoglobinopathies, medication side effects, autoimmune disorders, hereditary spherocytosis, blood transfusion reactions, and hemolytic disease of the newborn (HDN). They represent 5% of all anemias.

Hemolytic anemias can be categorized as acute or chronic and intravascular or extravascular. Intravascular hemolytic anemia occurs within the circulating blood. Extravascular hemolytic anemia occurs because of splenic destruction of the RBCs, RBC lysis in the reticuloendothelial system, or mechanical destruction as in prosthetic valve damage of RBCs.

CLINICAL CONCEPT

Drugs that are known to trigger hemolytic anemia include cephalosporins, quinidine, penicillins, levodopa, methyldopa, and NSAIDs.

Hemolytic anemia occurs when erythrocyte destruction outpaces RBC synthesis by the bone marrow. When RBC destruction occurs in autoimmune disorders, the body's immune system acts as though the RBCs are antigens and produces antibodies against them. This most often occurs in systemic autoimmune problems such as systemic lupus erythematosus or vasculitis. If the antibody causing the destruction of the RBCs is of the IgG class, the hemolysis will occur at any temperature, which is called **warm agglutinin syndrome.** If the antibody against the RBCs is of the IgM class, this is called **cold agglutinin syndrome,** in which hemolysis occurs at low temperatures. There are also drugs that are known to produce hemolytic anemia, which disappears when the drug is withdrawn.

Alloimmune hemolysis occurs when antibodies are formed against antigens on the RBC surface. This occurs in transfusion reactions and hemolytic disease of the newborn (HDN). In HDN, the mother forms antibodies that attack the RBCs of the fetus. This is most commonly associated with Rh incompatibility, but may also occur in ABO incompatibility. The same mechanism occurs in the hemolysis that occurs with the transfusion of incompatible blood.

Signs and Symptoms. Signs and symptoms include the general signs of anemia: fatigue, pallor, shortness of breath, and tachycardia. Additional signs and symptoms related to the hemolysis include chills, jaundice (caused by increased bilirubin levels produced by the breakdown of the rbcs cells), dark urine (caused by increased urobilinogen), and an enlarged spleen, which occurs as a result of the spleen's efforts to remove the increased numbers of damaged and broken RBCs from the circulation.

Diagnosis. Diagnosis involves assessing the CBC and bone marrow response, through evaluation of the reticulocyte count. Reticulocyte count is elevated when the bone marrow cannot keep up with RBC destruction. It is also important to measure the products of erythrocyte destruction such as methemoglobin and bilirubin. The peripheral smear in hemolytic anemia will show anisocytosis, poikilocytosis, and spherocytosis. These are terms that indicate misshapen and damaged RBCs, which is the appearance of lysed RBCs. Once the presence of hemolysis has been established, a variety of tests are performed to determine the exact cause. These include Hgb electrophoresis, bone marrow examination, and tests for the presence of autoantibodies.

Treatment. Treatment depends on the type and cause of the hemolytic anemia and may include folic acid and iron replacement, corticosteroids, and, in some emergent situations, transfusions. In cases of autoimmunity, treatments may include immunosuppressive drugs and splenectomy.

Specific Types of Hemolytic Anemias

Hemoglobinopathies, hereditary spherocytosis, HDN, and transfusion reactions are all causes of hemolytic anemia. Certain hemoglobinopathies are prevalent among people of different cultures. HDN commonly occurs, but to a mild extent.

Hemoglobinopathy. A **hemoglobinopathy** is an inherited disorder of the structure of the Hgb molecule that can lead to destruction of the RBC. The abnormal Hgb cannot carry oxygen efficiently and the blood undergoes frequent hemolysis. SCA and thalassemia are common hemoglobinopathies.

Sickle Cell Anemia. SCA is one of the most common inherited hemoglobinopathies. It is a disease found mainly in those of African, Middle Eastern, and Mediterranean ancestry. In the United States, the SCA gene is present in approximately 8% of African Americans. More than 2 million people in the United States, nearly all of them of African American ancestry, carry the sickle cell gene. Individuals with a sickle cell gene carry the trait, but do not endure full blown sickle cell disease. Individuals with two sickle cell genes, one from the mother and one from the father, experience the full severity of the disease. SCA occurs in 1 in every 500 African Americans.

For centuries it has been known that individuals with SCA are resistant to malaria. In the past, malaria was a major cause of death in the regions where SCA is prominent—Africa and the Middle East. Even today, malaria infects more than 300 million persons every year. Malaria organisms live within RBCs but cannot thrive in RBCs carrying the Hgb defect of SCA. Over the years, SCA carriers living in malaria-ridden locales have had a survival benefit compared with noncarriers, allowing them to live longer and have more children. This benefit is what evolutionary biologists call heterozygote advantage, and it explains why the sickle cell trait has persisted in areas where malaria is common.

SCA is caused by an abnormal kind of Hgb called Hgb S that distorts the RBC's shape upon exposure to hypoxia or severe stress. These RBCs are less able to deliver oxygen to tissues and are fragile when they change into a characteristic sickle shape. Some sickled RBCs are destroyed by the immune system, causing hemolysis. These sickled RBCs can also occlude capillaries and cause ischemia in various organs throughout the body.

Individuals can be heterogeneous for the SCA genetic mutation, where they only carry the trait. Carriers have different amounts of Hgb S in their circulation, which causes a spectrum of clinical disease presentations. Some carriers do not have enough Hgb S to suffer any symptoms; however, some carriers do have enough Hgb S to exhibit symptoms of disease. Some persons who only carry the trait can manifest all the complications of SCA when exposed to high stress, hypoxia, dehydration, or infection. More than 30,000 patients have homozygous Hgb S disease, which indicates that both alleles have the genetic mutation; these patients have the most severe form of the disease. Males and females are affected equally.

Although hematologic changes indicative of the disorder are evident as early as the age of 10 weeks, clinical signs of SCA usually do not appear until the first year of life. This is because fetal Hgb levels decline at approximately 6 months of age and then Hgb S starts to control oxygen transport. SCA persists for the entire life span, and those with the full spectrum of clinical disease have a shortened life span. After the individual is 10 years old, rates of complications increase. Renal disease is one of the major complication of SCA. The average survival time after the diagnosis of renal disease is about 4 years, and the median age of death is 27 years, despite dialysis treatment.

Etiology. SCA occurs because of a gene mutation that directs abnormal synthesis of the Hgb molecule. Normally, the Hgb molecule is composed of four polypeptide chains, a pair of alpha and a pair of beta chains. The SCA gene mutation causes one of the beta polypeptide chains to be abnormal as one of the amino acids in the chain, valine, is substituted for glutamic acid. This changes the Hgb molecule into Hgb S, the major type of Hgb in SCA. This mutation causes structural fragility of the SCA RBCs, where upon exposure to hypoxia or stress, the RBC contorts into a sickle shape.

SCA is transmitted by a recessive trait. Some individuals are homozygous (two traits for Hgb S) and endure severe disease, and some are heterozygous (one trait for Hgb S and one trait for normal Hgb A) and only carry the trait. Chances for offspring to be born with SCA can be configured on a Punnett square (see Fig. 13-10).

Persons with SCA have both Hgb S and normal Hgb A in their bloodstream. There is a spectrum of the degree of severity of disease according to the amount of Hgb S that exists in circulation. Those who are homozygous for the disorder have the majority of their RBCs in the form of Hgb S. Persons with sickle cell trait can possess up to 40% Hgb S in their circulation. These individuals tend to suffer mild anemia but upon exposure to extreme stress can develop symptoms of severe SCA.

Pathophysiology. The genetic mutation in SCA causes synthesis of Hgb that is more fragile and inefficient at carrying oxygen. Under conditions of hypoxia, severe stress, infection, or dehydration, the SCA Hgb tends to polymerize and become distorted in shape which, in turn, causes the RBC to change into a crescent

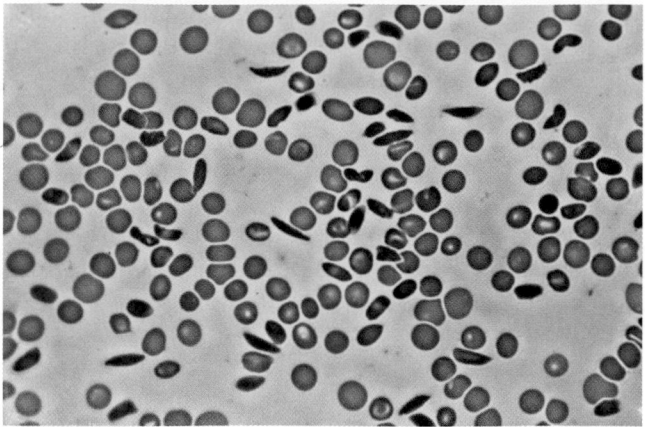

FIGURE 13-11. Peripheral smear with sickled cells. (*From Biology Pics/Science Source.*)

or sickle-shaped cell (see Fig. 13-11). The RBCs can reoxygenate and resume normal condition, but with frequent episodes of sickling they remain distorted. These abnormal RBCs have a severely shortened life span of only 10 to 20 days, as they are broken down by the spleen at a rate much faster than the bone marrow can replace them, resulting in severe hemolytic anemia.

The misshapen RBCs also cannot pass easily through capillaries. They become trapped, blocking blood flow and creating obstructions to distal tissues and organs. The occlusion in these vessels causes ischemia and consequent tissue hypoxia, which leads to organ damage and possible infarction. The episodes of ischemia, called **vaso-occlusive crises,** can occur in various organs of the body. Common sites obstructed by sickled RBCs are the chest, abdomen, long bones, and joints. Multiple sites are often involved simultaneously.

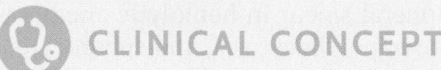

CLINICAL CONCEPT

Vaso-occlusive episodes are extremely painful for the patient. Ischemia and infarction cause chronic damage of the liver, spleen, heart, kidneys, and retina.

The spleen can become ischemic and dysfunction can begin early in childhood because of the high amount of lysed RBCs that must be processed. This diminishes the spleen's immune function, which increases the risk of infection in the patient with SCA. Children are particularly vulnerable to severe bacterial infections and sepsis.

Clinical Presentation. The common signs of anemia are present, particularly the fatigue and exercise intolerance. The frequent hemolysis of RBCs causes a high amount of heme breakdown in circulation with concomitant hyperbilirubinemia. High bilirubin in the bloodstream causes jaundice and bile concentration in the gallbladder, often leading to gallstones.

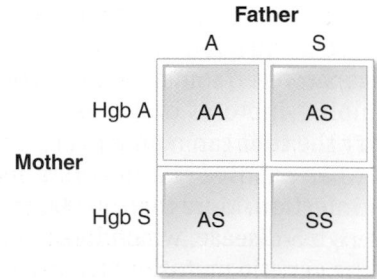

FIGURE 13-10. Punnett square for offspring of parents who are carriers of the SCA trait. Hgb AA represents normal Hgb. Hgb AS represents SCA trait. Hgb SS is SCA disease. When the Punnett square is configured for two parents with sickle cell trait, the following are the risks for having an affected offspring: 25% chance of having a child with full SCA disease, 50% chance of having a child with the SCA trait, and 25% chance of having a child with normal Hgb.

Episodes of vaso-occlusion cause severe pain, fever, tachycardia, and anxiety. Vaso-occlusive crises can be triggered by different stressors, including exposure to cold, hypoxia, infection, dehydration, acidosis, emotional stress, high exertion, and pregnancy. The pain's location will vary with the area of the circulation affected. Multiple sites of pain occurring simultaneously is common. Repeated crises can require three to four hospitalizations a year.

Chest pain can occur with tachypnea, fever, cough, and low arterial saturation. The chest pain can mimic myocardial infarction, pulmonary embolism, or pneumonia. Commonly experienced by sufferers of SCA, this is called acute chest syndrome and leads to pulmonary infarction and possible respiratory failure.

Children are particularly susceptible to severe infections, growth retardation, osteomyelitis, and stroke. Children commonly suffer repeated strokes due to cerebral infarction with resulting neurological sequela such as paralysis.

Hand-foot syndrome is a complication that occurs because of painful ischemia and infarctions in the hands and fingers. The formation of ischemic ulcerations of the lower extremities is common. A painful disorder of male patients called priapism can occur because of blockage of veins in the penis. Renal necrosis can also occur with all the signs and symptoms of renal failure. Retinal ischemia and hemorrhages can lead to retinal detachment with its symptoms of partial blindness.

Diagnosis. A blood sample is screened for the presence of Hgb S as part of the routine screening of newborns, but it can also be done on patients of any age. Early identification of these infants associated with improved treatments have more than doubled the life expectancy of these patients. Hgb electrophoresis can differentiate which patients with Hgb S are homozygous and which are heterozygous. A CBC can assess for anemia and a peripheral blood smear can show the typical sickle-shaped cells. Reticulocytosis indicates a high amount of hemolysis is occurring. Genetic counseling of parents who are carriers or sufferers of SCA is necessary to discuss the chance of passing the gene to offspring.

Treatment. The combination of oxygen, hydration, pain medications, and prophylactic antibiotics are used to treat vaso-occlusive crises and complications. A high amount of fluid is administered intravenously in an effort to flush out occlusive areas of cells. Pain medications, such as opiates, are commonly needed, but these are problematic as they can lead to dependence.

Hydroxyurea, an antitumor drug, has proven effective in decreasing vaso-occlusive episodes. It increases the level of fetal Hgb in erythrocytes; this treatment does not cure the disease but helps decrease the disorder's severity and the occurrence of occlusive episodes.

Much of the treatment for SCA is directed at preventing and managing the disease's complications. Prophylactic antibiotics are used to prevent infection.

All required immunizations are administered. Patients take folic acid supplements to prevent aplastic crisis in the bone marrow. Patients are also educated to avoid the triggers that cause crises. Splenic sequestration crisis is a disorder of ischemia and occlusion of vessels in the spleen. This usually requires splenectomy which, in turn, increases risk of infection.

Bone marrow transplant allows replacement of defective bone marrow with healthy marrow. Blood transfusions can increase the number of normal RBCs and help to reduce the anemia. However, because blood transfusions contain iron, chronic use of transfusions can lead to iron overload, which is toxic to the body and requires the use of iron-chelating agents.

Other experimental treatments include gene therapy to replace the defective gene with a corrected copy to promote the production of normal Hgb by the bone marrow. Researchers are also exploring ways to suppress the defective gene and to reactivate the gene responsible for producing fetal Hgb. Nitric acid, which helps keep blood vessels open and reduces the adhesiveness of RBCs, is low in persons with SCA and replacement may help decrease the formation of the sickle cells.

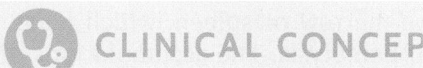

CLINICAL CONCEPT

Splenectomy causes immunodeficiency and increased risk of infection with encapsulated bacteria such as *Streptococcus pneumoniae*, *Haemophilus influenza* type B, Klebsiella, and Salmonella.

Thalassemia. Thalassemia resembles SCA in that it is a genetic disorder that causes defects in Hgb synthesis. The similarity of the two diseases extends to the cultural background of affected individuals. Thalassemia mainly affects persons of Mediterranean, African, and Southeast Asian descent. It affects 200 million persons worldwide and is one of the most common genetic disorders in the world. Approximately 15% of African Americans are carriers of the trait. The minor form of disease occurs in 3% of African Americans, whereas the major form of disease occurs in fewer than 1%.

Etiology. Thalassemia is a condition caused by a genetic defect. Thalassemia minor occurs if one defective gene is inherited from one parent. Persons with this form of the disorder are carriers of the disease and usually do not have symptoms. Risk factors for thalassemia include:

• Asian, Chinese, Mediterranean, or African American ethnicity
• Family history of the disorder.

In thalassemia, the genes that code for Hgb formation are missing or variant; consequently, some proteins needed for Hgb synthesis are abnormal or absent. It affects the alpha and beta polypeptide chains of the Hgb molecule. Alpha and beta thalassemia are the two main types of the disease. In alpha thalassemia, an alpha chain is missing and in beta thalassemia, a beta chain is absent. Sometimes the disease is called alpha thalassemia or beta thalassemia, depending on the specific Hgb component affected.

Thalassemia has an autosomal recessive inheritance pattern similar to that seen in sickle cell disease. A child who inherits defective genes from both parents is homozygous for the abnormal Hgb and exhibits moderate to severe disease. Homozygotes have a form of the disease called thalassemia major. Those who are heterozygous for the defective Hgb are carriers; they can have a mild form of the disease called thalassemia minor. Beta thalassemia major, also called Cooley's anemia, is the most severe form of the disease.

Pathophysiology. In both thalassemia major and minor, one of the polypeptide chains of the Hgb structure is deficient, leading to reduced Hgb synthesis and decreased RBCs. However, within the RBC, the unaffected polypeptide chains continue to be synthesized and accumulate. The accumulation of polypeptide chains interferes with normal maturation of the RBC. The affected RBCs become defective and destroyed in the bone marrow or spleen, which leads to large amounts of hemolysis. The accumulations of normal polypeptide chains within the RBCs develop into pathological fragments called Heinz bodies, which are pathognomonic for thalassemia.

The bone marrow also attempts to compensate for the loss of RBCs with an exaggerated rate of erythropoiesis in the bone marrow. Osteopenia of bone marrow occurs because of the large space taken by maturing erythrocytes.

Clinical Presentation. The signs and symptoms of thalassemia include the expected signs of anemia: fatigue, weakness, pallor, and exercise intolerance. Those with the trait usually have no overt symptoms and endure a mild anemia. In the more severe forms of disease, the signs and symptoms appear in early childhood and require frequent transfusions.

Because of the high amount of erythropoiesis needed to replace lysed RBCs, the bone marrow expands inside all the bones, causing pain. The bones become weak, enlarged, and distorted, particularly the cranial bones. Children often develop a characteristic chipmunk appearance because of hyperplasia of the marrow in the cheek bones. The skull develops tiny bone deformities that resemble "hair on end" in an x-ray (see Fig. 13-12).

The spleen and liver become filled with dead RBCs and enlarged because of the high amount of RBC destruction. The hepatomegaly and splenomegaly cause a protuberant abdomen. The large amount of hemolysis and required transfusions cause iron overload, also called hemochromatosis. The myocardium, liver, kidney, and pancreas can be affected by iron overload. Also, the great amount of hemolysis in the bloodstream

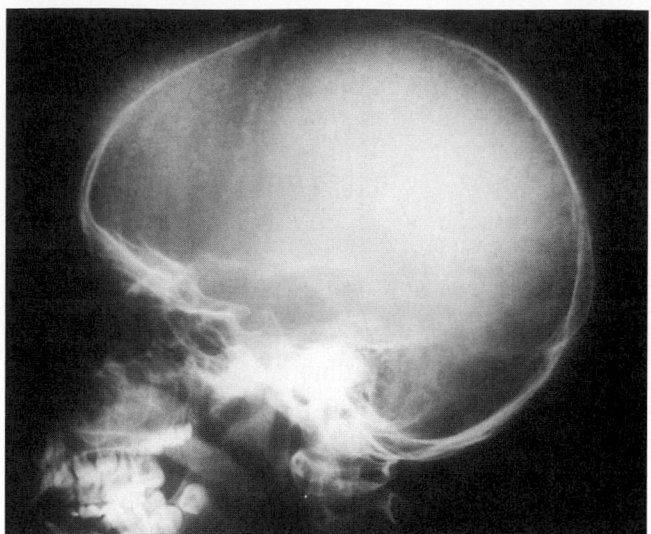

FIGURE 13-12. Hair-on-end appearance of skull bone formation in thalassemia. (*From Biophoto Associates/Science Source.*)

causes hyperbilirubinemia with resulting jaundice and dark urine. Concentrated bile in the gallbladder can form gallstones with right upper quadrant abdominal pain and tenderness.

Diagnosis. Diagnostic studies include a CBC, which reveals an MCHC anemia. Hgb electrophoresis provides additional information about the types of Hgb present in the RBCs. The abnormal Hgb found in beta thalassemia is termed Hgb A 2. It is important to distinguish alpha thalassemias from iron deficiency anemia to avoid inappropriate treatment with iron, so tests of iron levels in the blood and iron stores need to be included.

Radiographically, the skeletal response to marrow proliferation consists of thinning of cortical bone and resorption of cancellous bone, which results in a generalized loss of bone density.

Treatment. Treatment depends on the severity of the disease. Those persons who have the trait and are asymptomatic require no treatment. Genetic counseling is necessary so individuals understand the chance of passing the trait on to offspring. The mainstays of treatment for those with the more severe forms of the disease are transfusions and prevention of infection. All immunizations should be administered as required. If splenomegaly occurs, splenectomy becomes necessary and this increases the risk of infection. As with SCA, the regular transfusions lead to iron buildup in the body and necessitate iron chelation treatments to avoid the toxic effects of the iron. Folic acid supplementation helps the body build normal red cells. As with SCA, enhancement of fetal Hgb levels lessens the disease's severity. Gene therapy in which the abnormal gene or genes are replaced with normal genes is being studied as a way to cure the disease. Bone marrow or stem cell transplants have cured thalassemias in some children but are still considered experimental.

Hereditary Spherocytosis. Hereditary spherocytosis is a familial hemolytic disorder that is caused by a lack of membrane proteins in RBCs. The lack of membrane integrity causes fragility and gives RBCs a characteristic spherical shape. In the United States, the disorder's incidence is approximately 1 case in 5,000 people. It is most common among people of Northern European descent.

Hereditary spherocytosis is an autosomal dominant disorder. Only heterozygous individuals are identified in the population, suggesting that the homozygous state is incompatible with life. The major problem in this disorder involves the spleen and fragile RBCs. Spherocytic RBCs are sequestered and destroyed, after which they accumulate in the spleen. There are variations in the disease's expression in individuals. Some of those affected have no symptoms, whereas others can have anemia, splenomegaly, jaundice, and bilirubin gallstones.

The major complications are aplastic anemia crisis, megaloblastic anemia, hemolytic anemia, cholecystitis and cholelithiasis, and severe neonatal hemolysis. Aplastic anemia crisis occurs when Hgb levels fall rapidly and severely because of ongoing destruction of spherocytes that is not balanced with new RBC production. Blood transfusions and splenectomy are required treatment. Megaloblastic anemia crisis can also occur where there is inadequate folic acid for erythropoiesis. Patients with hereditary spherocytosis are instructed to take supplementary folic acid (1 mg/dL) for life in order to prevent a megaloblastic crisis. Severe neonatal hemolysis requires transfusion and phototherapy to rid the body of bilirubin.

Blood Transfusion Reactions. Hemolytic transfusion reactions are the result of antibodies in the recipient's blood directed against antigens on the donor's erythrocytes. This results in rapid intravascular hemolysis of the donor RBCs. ABO incompatibility caused by clerical error is the most frequent cause. In hemolytic transfusion reactions, symptoms usually occur after a small amount of blood has been transfused and almost always before the unit is transfused completely (see Box 13-2). Hemolytic transfusion reactions occur in 1 per 40,000 transfused units of packed RBCs.

Nonhemolytic febrile reactions and minor allergic reactions are the most common transfusion reactions, each occurring in 3% to 4% of all transfusions. Nonhemolytic febrile reactions and extravascular hemolysis are observed more commonly in patients who have developed antibodies from prior transfusions. Proteins in the donor plasma can also cause minor allergic reactions.

Nonhemolytic febrile reactions are thought to stem from the formation of cytokines during the storage of the blood. This anaphylactoid nonhemolytic reaction is observed more frequently with components containing large amounts of plasma, such as whole blood, pooled platelets, and fresh frozen plasma. Minor allergic reactions are associated with urticaria.

Nonhemolytic febrile reactions do not occur as rapidly as acute hemolytic reactions. They occur between

---

BOX 13-2. Signs and Symptoms of Hemolytic Transfusion Reaction

Hemolytic transfusion reactions occur when the wrong blood type is administered to a patient. The wrong type of donor blood will stimulate the recipient's development of antibodies against the donor blood cells. The following are symptoms of this hemolytic reaction:

- Fever
- Chills
- Flushing
- Nausea
- Burning at intravenous line
- Chest tightness
- Restlessness
- Apprehension
- Joint pain
- Back pain
- Tachycardia
- Tachypnea.

In severe cases of hemolytic transfusion reaction, hypotension, oozing from the IV site, diffuse bleeding, hemoglobinuria, oliguria, shock, and renal failure can occur.

---

1 and 6 hours after transfusions and are associated with the nonspecific symptoms of fever, chills, and malaise. Some patients may complain of dyspnea. These nonspecific symptoms also occur with a hemolytic transfusion reaction. These reactions seldom proceed to hypotension or respiratory distress.

Anaphylactic reactions occur in 1 per 20,000 transfused units. Risk of transfusion-related hepatitis B is approximately 1 per 350,000 units transfused. Risk for hepatitis C is 1 per 2 million units transfused. Risk of transfusion-related HIV infection is 1 per 2 million units transfused.

Anaphylactic reactions most often are observed in those patients with a hereditary immunoglobulin A (IgA) deficiency. Some of these patients have developed complement-binding anti-IgA antibodies that cause anaphylaxis when exposed to donor IgA. In anaphylactic reactions, symptoms usually occur with fewer than 10 mL of blood transfused and only rarely occur more insidiously. Anaphylactic reactions to blood transfusion are associated with rapid development of dyspnea, flushing, urticaria, abdominal pain, bronchospasm, hypotension, facial swelling, and edema of the tongue.

In hemolytic transfusion reactions, pharmacological treatment is aimed at increasing renal blood flow and preserving urinary output. The transfusion should be stopped immediately with suspicion of a reaction. A normal saline intravenous drip should be substituted for the blood. Acetaminophen is used for fever. Diuretics such as furosemide, antihistamines such as diphenhydramine, and steroids such as Solu-Medrol can be used. In anaphylaxis, the goals of therapy are to maintain airway and hemodynamic stability and reverse the underlying process. Commonly required medications include epinephrine, corticosteroids, antihistamines, and vasopressors such as dobutamine.

CLINICAL CONCEPT

It is mandatory for two clinicians to double check the patient blood type and donor blood type before administration of a transfusion. All patients receiving blood products should be placed on continuous cardiac monitoring and pulse oximetry.

Hemolytic Disease of the Newborn. HDN involves an antigen-antibody reaction between a mother's antibodies and her newborn infant's RBCs at the time of birth. The mechanism of HDN involves maternal synthesis of antibodies against the surface A, B, or Rh antigens, also called D antigens, on fetal or neonatal RBCs. Antibodies that react against ABO blood antigens are

of the IgM class, which are large in size and cannot pass through the placenta during pregnancy. Therefore, a mother with a different blood type than the fetus can carry the pregnancy without problems. It is only during delivery, when maternal and infant blood may mix, that ABO incompatibility can occur between mother and infant. Some of the infant's RBCs can enter the maternal circulation and stimulate an antibody reaction in the mother. The mother's antibodies, in turn, can enter the infant's circulation and attack infant RBCs. In these cases, the infant may experience a mild hemolysis because of ABO incompatibility. The infant endures a mild hyperbilirubinemia caused by RBC breakdown and exhibits mild jaundice, but it is usually short-lived. Exposure to sunlight or phototherapy is used to break down the bilirubin in the infant. A severe hemolytic reaction called erythroblastosis fetalis can occur if a fetus is Rh-positive and the mother is Rh-negative (see Box 13-3).

RBC Maturation Defects

Necessary nutrients used to synthesize RBCs include iron, vitamin B_{12}, and folic acid. Iron is an essential element of Hgb synthesis and multiple metabolic

---

BOX 13-3. Erythroblastosis Fetalis

Erythroblastosis fetalis can occur if a fetus is Rh-positive and the mother is Rh-negative. It is a severe hemolytic reaction in the Rh-positive fetus caused by anti-Rh antibodies from the mother. This usually occurs in cases where the mother has had prior exposure to the Rh antigen and has formed Rh antibodies.

The mother was most likely sensitized to Rh-positive blood during a previous pregnancy at delivery, when mixing of maternal and infant blood occur. Other ways in which the mother could have been exposed to the Rh-positive antigen include fetal-maternal hemorrhage caused by trauma, abortion, childbirth, ruptures in the placenta during pregnancy, or medical procedures carried out during pregnancy that breach the uterine wall. Once the Rh antibodies

are formed in the mother, they cross the placenta into the fetal circulation and attack the fetal (RBCs), causing a high amount of hemolysis. The fetus suffers hemolytic anemia, which can be severe. Severe hemolytic anemia of the fetus can cause heart failure with hepatomegaly, splenomegaly, hyperbilirubinemia, and possible death. The infant can be stillborn. However, if the fetus can survive the hemolysis, hyperbilirubinemia occurs because of the large amount of RBC lysis. The neonate exhibits high bilirubin at birth, which can lead to kernicterus. At delivery, Rhogam, a medication that coats Rh-positive RBCs, is administered to mothers to prevent the mother from developing Rh antibodies. This prevents erythroblastosis fetalis from occurring in following pregnancies.

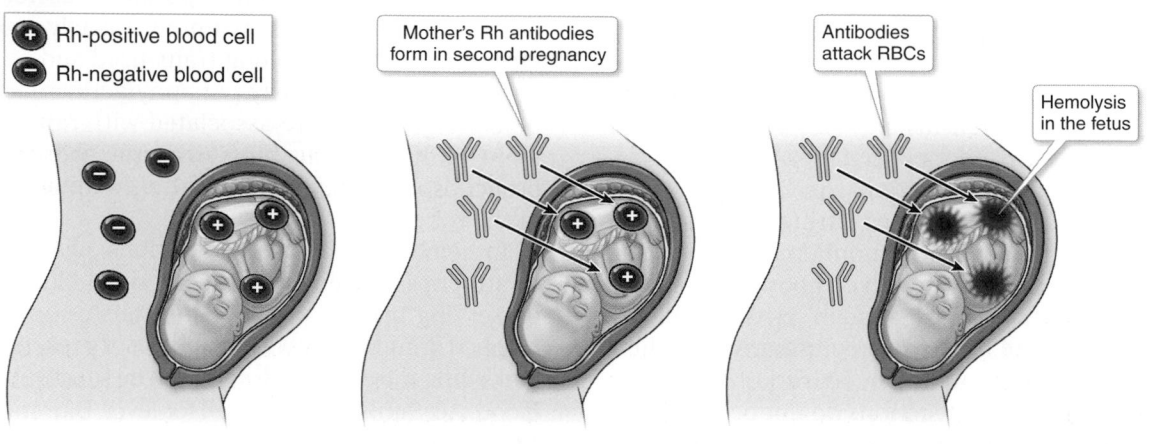

processes, and vitamin B$_{12}$ and folic acid are necessary components of DNA synthesis. Any deficiency of these components can lead to decreased erythropoiesis in the bone marrow which, in turn, leads to anemia. The bone marrow is constantly generating new blood cells: RBCs, WBCs, and platelets. Disturbance of bone marrow function can lead to anemia, leukopenia, and thrombocytopenia. Complete disruption of bone marrow function inhibits manufacture of all blood cells, a condition called **aplastic anemia.** Aplastic anemia is a life-threatening disorder that can be caused by cancer, sepsis, or radiation exposure.

Iron Deficiency Anemia

Iron deficiency is the most common cause of anemia worldwide. Its prevalence is approximately 50% in underdeveloped countries and 10% in developed countries. In countries where little meat is in the diet, iron deficiency anemia is 6 to 8 times more prevalent than in North America and Europe. The highest prevalence of iron deficiency occurs in women of childbearing age and elderly adults. Approximately 15% of women between ages 20 and 45 years are iron deficient. Prevalence of anemia in the older adult ranges from 8% to 44%, with the highest prevalence in men aged 85 years and older.

Gastrointestinal bleeding can cause chronic blood loss, which is a cause of iron deficiency. A recent study showed that 60% of individuals with colon cancer have iron deficiency.

The following groups of people have an increased risk of iron deficiency anemia:

- Women of childbearing age: Because women lose blood during menstruation, women in general are at greater risk of iron deficiency anemia. Pregnancy, delivery, and breastfeeding use a great deal of iron.
- Infants and children: Infants who are weaned from formula to cow's milk may need extra iron because of the low iron in cow's milk. Children and adolescents need extra iron during growth spurts.
- Vegetarians: Individuals who don't eat meat may have a greater risk of iron deficiency anemia if they don't supplement their diet with iron-rich foods.
- Elderly adults: Poor diet and lack of stomach acid can cause iron deficiency.
- Individuals with gastrointestinal bleeding: Persons with peptic ulcer, esophageal varices, or cancer of the gastrointestinal tract can lose blood in the stool.

Etiology. The most common causes of iron deficiency are inadequate intake, excessive menstrual blood loss, and gastrointestinal blood loss. Meats contain the most absorbable kind of iron compared with plants, so vegetarians have to be vigilant about eating iron sources such as green leafy vegetables, beans, mushrooms, and soy.

The adult male absorbs and loses about 1 mg of iron from an average diet containing 10 to 20 mg daily. During childbearing years, an adult female loses an average of 2 mg of iron daily and must absorb a similar quantity of iron in order to maintain equilibrium. With each pregnancy, a woman loses about 500 mg of iron. In menstruating women, menstrual blood loss is highly variable, ranging from 4 to 100 mg of iron lost per period.

Healthy newborn infants have a total body iron of 250 mg, which is obtained from maternal sources transplacentally. Breastfeeding mothers need considerably more iron in the diet because the growing infant draws from the maternal storage. For the infant, breast milk and formula have adequate iron, but when the child is weaned, iron deficiency often occurs because cow's milk is iron deficient.

Iron deficiency is also the most common type of anemia seen in teenagers, as it is related to increased demand for RBCs during growth spurts, which occur during these years. Adolescents also suffer iron deficiency because of poor diet; girls are particularly at risk.

Elderly individuals frequently suffer from poor iron nutrition caused by lack of meat in the diet. Also, elderly individuals commonly have achlorhydria, or a lack of hydrochloric acid (HCl), of the stomach, which is a natural physiologic change of aging that decreases iron absorption in the stomach. Persons who frequently use antacids such as histamine-2 antagonists or proton pump inhibitors are also at risk for iron deficiency caused by lack of gastric HCl. For men, loss of blood from the GI tract is the most common cause for iron deficiency anemia. GI problems that can cause bleeding include gastritis, ulcerations, esophageal varices, and carcinomas. In both men and postmenopausal women, colon cancer frequently presents with iron deficiency anemia caused by undetected chronic blood loss from the GI tract. In certain geographic areas, intestinal parasites, particularly hookworm, cause iron deficiency because of blood loss from the GI tract.

> ## CLINICAL CONCEPT
>
> The majority of patients with a new diagnosis of colorectal cancer are iron deficient at presentation.

ALERT! The appearance of iron deficiency in an adult male means gastrointestinal blood loss until proven otherwise.

Physiology. Iron is needed in the diet to synthesize Hgb. The heme portion of Hgb contains iron that carries oxygen atoms. Lack of sufficient iron leads to poor oxygen transport by iron-deficient Hgb molecules. Iron is absorbed from the gastrointestinal tract and some is stored in the intestinal cells before crossing into the bloodstream. Every day, intestinal epithelial cells are constantly sloughed and excreted, so some ingested iron is lost. Approximately 0.5 to 1.5 mg of iron is ingested and 1 mg is lost in the feces daily. In the bloodstream, iron is carried to storage sites by transferrin. Blood loss in excess of 20 mL per day is greater than the amount of iron that can be absorbed from the GI tract. Under these conditions, the body must use stored iron from ferritin complexes in the reticuloendothelial cells (mainly macrophages from various sites), bone marrow, liver, and spleen. When iron stores become depleted, serum ferritin complexes and transferrin become depleted. Once the circulating transferrin becomes depleted of iron, Hgb synthesis is impaired and iron-deficient erythropoiesis starts to occur. As Hgb synthesis decreases, RBC numbers diminish. The RBCs that are synthesized are abnormally small (microcytic) and pale (hypochromic). When iron deficiency is severe, the process of erythropoiesis in the bone marrow is affected and fewer RBCs are produced.

Clinical Presentation. A thorough history and physical examination are important in a patient suspected of iron deficiency anemia. History questions of particular importance include age; current medications, including over-the-counter drugs; current history of GI symptoms; current menstrual history in women; history of past health disorders; and social habits. Current medications can indicate current health disorders endured by the patient. For example, frequent use of NSAIDs and aspirin can cause gastric ulceration with slow, gradual gastrointestinal blood loss. It is important to know the frequency of alcohol use and if the patient smokes. These activities predispose to GI bleeding as well. Menstruating women should be asked about the duration and volume of menstrual blood loss. All patients should be asked about dark stool, which can indicate melena (blood in stool).

Signs and Symptoms. The signs and symptoms of iron deficiency anemia are those of anemia in general; fatigue, weakness, and exercise intolerance. If iron deficiency is caused by GI blood loss, the patient may have melena. Women of childbearing age may have menorrhagia.

Iron deficiency also has some specific signs, including hair loss; cheilitis; glossitis; nail changes called koilonychias, which are spoon-shaped nails; and pica. **Pica,** a unique sign of iron deficiency, is a craving for nonfood substances such as ice, clay, starch, chalk, dirt, or other material. At times, an individual craves specific food items to excess, such as carbohydrates. Cold intolerance and feeling of tingling or numbness in the fingers occurs in many who are iron deficient.

Physical Examination. The physical examination is commonly unremarkable except for pallor of the conjunctiva, nailbeds, and palms. In severe cases of anemia, splenomegaly may be found on the abdominal exam.

Diagnosis. Iron deficiency anemia is primarily a laboratory diagnosis. Useful tests include a CBC, peripheral smear, serum iron, TIBC, and serum ferritin (see Box 13-4). Serum iron and ferritin are decreased, but TIBC is high because there are many free iron-binding sites in the body. A peripheral blood smear will often show signs of iron deficiency before the CBC exhibits abnormalities. Because GI blood loss is often the reason for iron deficiency anemia, a FOBT should be done along with other diagnostic tests. A colonoscopy or endoscopy are indicated if the FOBT is positive.

When iron and folate deficiency occur, the peripheral smear reveals a population of macrocytes mixed among the MCHC cells. This combination of microcytes and macrocytes can erroneously normalize the MCV. Chronic lead poisoning may produce a CBC with mild microcytosis. The incidence of lead poisoning is greater in individuals who are iron deficient than in healthy subjects because increased absorption of lead occurs in individuals who are iron deficient. Paint in old houses has been a source of lead poisoning in children and painters.

Treatment. In most patients, the iron deficiency should be treated with oral iron therapy (ferrous sulfate), and the underlying etiology should be corrected to avoid recurrence of anemia. Vitamin C enhances absorption of iron. Oral iron can cause gastritis and constipation. Parenteral iron therapy, either intramuscular or intravenous, is an option, but anaphylaxis is a risk factor. The patient can be advised to use iron cookware, as iron can naturally seep into foods prepared in this way.

BOX 13-4. Diagnosis of Iron Deficiency Anemia

Iron deficiency anemia has specific count; complete blood count (CBC) indicative of the disorder. There are also some additional specific laboratory tests needed for the diagnosis:

- Hgb: low
- Hct: low
- MCV: low (microcytic)
- MCH: low
- MCHC: low (hypochromic)
- Serum Fe++: low
- Serum ferritin: low
- Total iron-binding capacity: high
- Peripheral blood smear: shows small, pale blood cells.
- FOBT should be done.

Vitamin B$_{12}$ Deficiency

Vitamin B$_{12}$, also called cyanocobalamin or cobalamin, is a cofactor for two important processes: synthesis of DNA in RBCs and normal myelin synthesis of neurons. Lack of vitamin B$_{12}$ results in an inability of the body to make enough mature RBCs and allows breakdown of the myelin sheath of some of the body's sensory and motor nerves.

The exact prevalence of vitamin B$_{12}$ deficiency is unknown, but it is known that **pernicious anemia,** which results from vitamin B$_{12}$ deficiency, is a common cause of anemia throughout the world, especially in persons of European or African descent. Dietary deficiency of vitamin B$_{12}$ is also a common cause, particularly in vegetarians. Globally, according to various studies, low vitamin B$_{12}$ is prevalent in 25% to 70% of persons in undeveloped countries. It is a severe problem in India, Mexico, Central and South America, and selected areas in Africa.

According to the U.S. Framingham Offspring study, up to 39% of adults are vitamin B$_{12}$ deficient, particularly elderly individuals. Prevalence is greater than 20% in the elderly population, commonly caused by intestinal malabsorption. Malabsorption caused by gastric bypass surgery is also an increasingly common cause of vitamin B$_{12}$ deficiency. The gastric bypass procedure is becoming increasingly performed for treatment of obesity.

Etiology. In persons who lack meat in the diet, vitamin B$_{12}$ deficiency is common. The most absorbable sources of vitamin B$_{12}$ are in animal products such as meat and dairy foods. Those who follow a strict vegetarian diet are at risk for this problem, as are those with poor diets related to aging, alcoholism, and economic factors.

Vitamin B$_{12}$ stores in the liver can last for years. An average diet contains between 5 to 30 micrograms per day, with the daily requirement being 1 to 3 micrograms per day. Body stores of vitamin B$_{12}$ are approximately 2 to 3 mg, sufficient for 3 to 4 years if supply is cut off.

In elderly patients, vitamin B$_{12}$ deficiency is caused primarily by food-cobalamin malabsorption or pernicious anemia. Food-cobalamin malabsorption syndrome is characterized by the inability to release vitamin B$_{12}$ from food or from intestinal transport proteins. This syndrome is defined by vitamin B$_{12}$ deficiency in the presence of sufficient food and B$_{12}$ intake.

Pernicious anemia, another disorder common in elderly individuals, occurs as a result of a lack of **intrinsic factor (IF),** an essential carrier protein of vitamin B$_{12}$ in the stomach. Without IF, vitamin B$_{12}$ is not absorbed into the bloodstream (see Fig. 13-13). Achlorhydria can also be responsible for vitamin B$_{12}$ deficiency. Frequent use of proton pump inhibitors such as omeprazole (Prilosec), which can cause achlorhydria, also have been found to be a cause of vitamin B$_{12}$ deficiency.

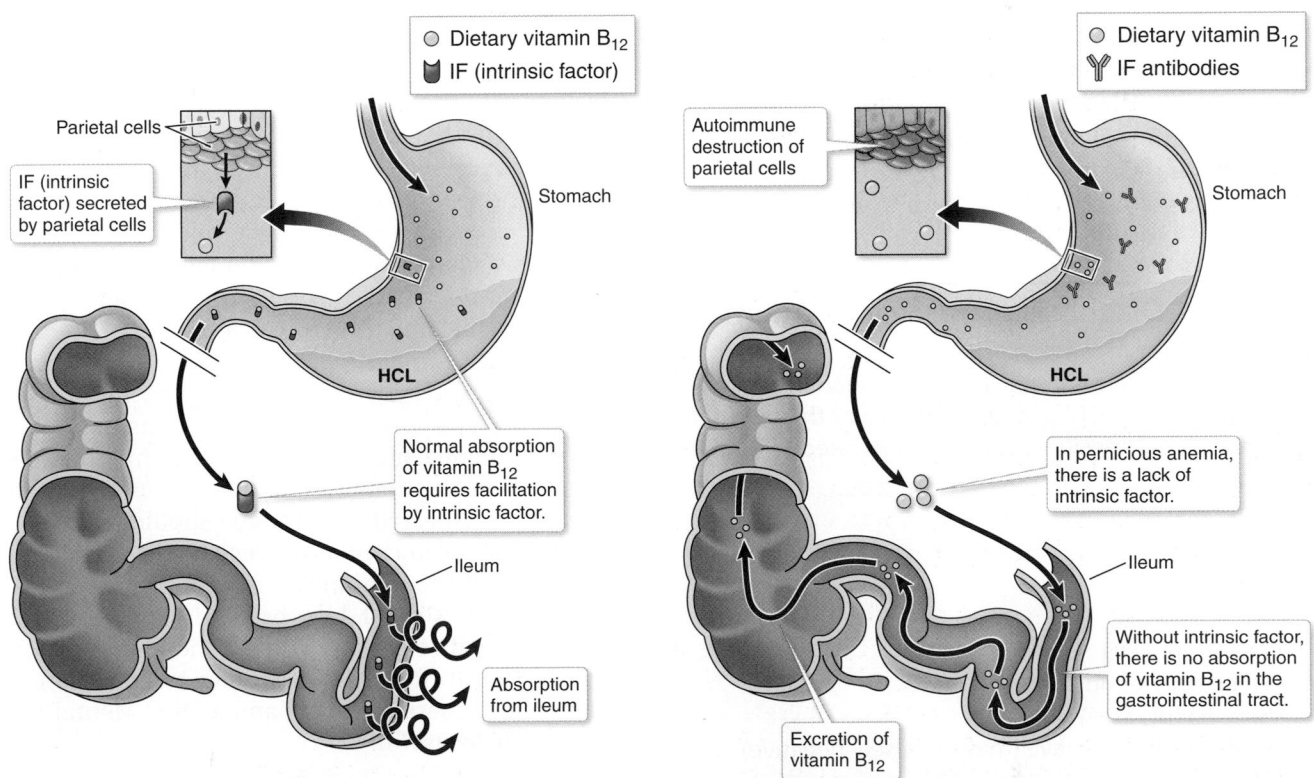

FIGURE 13-13. In pernicious anemia, there is autoimmune destruction of IF in the stomach. IF is necessary for absorption of vitamin B$_{12}$ in the gastrointestinal tract; without IF, vitamin B$_{12}$ is not absorbed.

Pathophysiology. Food-cobalamin malabsorption syndrome and pernicious anemia are important disorders to understand when it comes to vitamin B_{12} deficiency—and both affect older adults.

Food-cobalamin malabsorption is caused primarily by gastric atrophy. Over 40% of patients older than 80 years have gastric atrophy and achlorhydria. Normally, the absorption of vitamin B_{12} from the stomach into the bloodstream requires adequate gastric HCl and IF. Gastric mucosal atrophy, common in elders, diminishes the cells that secrete HCl and IF.

In pernicious anemia, for unclear reasons, the body develops antibodies to IF. The antibodies destroy the IF and consequently vitamin B_{12} cannot be absorbed into the bloodstream. This autoimmune destruction of IF is most commonly seen in the elderly.

Other factors that contribute to malabsorption of vitamin B_{12} in elderly individuals include chronic carriage of *Helicobacter pylori*. The proliferation of the bacteria *H. pylori* in the stomach, a common cause of gastric ulceration, can interfere with vitamin B_{12} absorption into the bloodstream.

Other causes of vitamin B_{12} malabsorption include long-term ingestion of biguanides (metformin) and antacids, including H_2-receptor antagonists and proton pump inhibitors, drugs that are commonly prescribed to the elderly. Chronic alcoholism, gastric bypass surgery for obesity, pancreatic exocrine failure, celiac disease, Crohn's disease, and Sjögren's syndrome are other causes of cobalamin malabsorption (see Box 13-5).

Vitamin B_{12} Deficiency: Effects on the Body. Both vitamin B_{12} and folic acid are necessary for DNA synthesis. The rapidly dividing blood cell precursors of the bone marrow are constantly synthesizing DNA, which means that deficiency of either vitamin B_{12} or folic acid negatively affects hematopoiesis. Vitamin B_{12} is a vital factor in folic acid metabolism. During the many transformations of folate from one form to another, some of the folate is accidentally converted to an inactive metabolite. This is called the folate trap, and the only way for the active form to be regenerated involves a reaction in which a form of vitamin B_{12} acts as a cofactor. Lack of vitamin B_{12} results in more folate being trapped in this inactive form, resulting in a failure to synthesize adequate DNA for new cells. Red blood cells with inadequate vitamin B_{12} develop into megaloblastic cells and have difficulty exiting the bone marrow.

Vitamin B_{12} deficiency also has an effect on the neurological system, but the mechanism is not well understood. Central nervous system demyelination occurs, but how vitamin B_{12} deficiency exactly leads to demyelination remains unclear. Myelin defects and abnormal neural conduction occur mainly in the dorsal horns and corticospinal tract of the spinal cord. The disorder is referred to as **subacute combined degeneration**, which is manifested as numbness and weakness in the extremities and gait disturbance. In addition, synthesis of serotonin, norepinephrine, and dopamine are affected by lack of vitamin B_{12}. This suggests that vitamin B_{12} deficiency affects neurotransmitter synthesis and may be relevant to mental status changes, such as depression and memory loss.

Clinical Presentation. The history and physical examination may or may not lead the clinician to suspect vitamin B_{12} deficiency. This is often not readily apparent to the patient through symptoms or to the clinician via physical assessment findings. Those patients at highest risk include vegetarians and elderly individuals.

Signs and Symptoms. Signs and symptoms of vitamin B_{12} deficiency anemia include those of other anemias: fatigue, exercise intolerance, dyspnea, weakness, and tachycardia. The patient may also have glossitis. Symptoms usually develop slowly over time, with nervous system changes such as numbness and tingling in the hands and feet, unsteady gait, balance problems, and mental changes possibly being noticed first. Mental changes such as depression and memory impairment that mimic dementia can occur. Optic atrophy and consequent visual impairment can also occur.

Physical Examination. The physical examination of the patient with vitamin B_{12} deficiency may be unremarkable. The exam should involve assessment for signs of anemia such as pallor and tachycardia. Signs of pallor in the conjunctiva and palms of the hand should be inspected. The tongue should be inspected for glossitis. The cranial nerves should be examined. Sensation of the extremities should be assessed. Gait and balance should be observed. Romberg's sign, imbalance with eyes closed in a standing position, may be positive. If the patient exhibits mental changes, a depression assessment tool and a Mini-Mental Status Exam may be useful.

Diagnosis. Diagnosis begins with establishing that anemia is present, based on the CBC. Additional tests should be done to assess vitamin B_{12} levels, as well as

---

BOX 13-5. Diagnosis of Pernicious Anemia

Pernicious anemia is a specific type of vitamin B_{12} deficiency. There are CBC results indicative of the disorder and additional specific laboratory tests needed for the diagnosis.

- Hgb: low
- Hct: low
- MCV: high
- MCH: normal
- MCHC: normal
- Reticulocytes: low
- Vitamin B_{12} assay: low
- IF antibodies: positive (may be falsely negative)
- Parietal cell antibodies: positive
- Gastrin: high
- *H. pylori* antibodies: may be positive

folate, homocysteine (tHCy), and methylmalonic acid (MMA) levels. The concentration of total tHCy in serum and plasma is elevated in both folate and cobalamin deficiencies, whereas MMA in serum, plasma, or urine is a specific marker of cobalamin function. In the CBC, there is decreased Hgb, decreased Hct, and increased MCV, which indicate megaloblastic anemia. There is also a deficiency of reticulocytes, as the bone marrow is weakly producing RBCs. Peripheral blood smear demonstrates enlarged oval RBCs, referred to as macrocytosis, and some misshapen RBCs, a condition referred to as anisocytosis and poikilocytosis. Leukopenia may be present. Neutrophils have nuclei that are characteristically hypersegmented and multilobed. A serum B_{12} assay is done that indicates the amount of vitamin B_{12} in the bloodstream. Other blood tests include bilirubin levels and presence of IF antibodies and parietal cell antibodies, though these antibodies are not always exhibited in a blood test. Bilirubin may be elevated because of death of immature RBCs in the bone marrow.

Treatment. The main goal of treatment is correction of the anemia, which is accomplished by first remedying the underlying cause, such as poor nutrition. If the cause is not readily remedied, then the patient needs administration of vitamin B_{12} intramuscularly. Insufficient dietary intake is corrected by recommending a diet rich in sources of vitamin B_{12} and through the use of oral supplements. Replenishment of body stores can be accomplished with six 1,000 microgram intramuscular injections of hydroxocobalamin given at 3- to 7-day intervals. For maintenance therapy, 1,000 micrograms of vitamin B_{12} intramuscularly every 3 months is sufficient. If an intramuscular regimen is not possible, the patient can take large daily oral doses (1,000 to 2,000 micrograms) of vitamin B_{12}. Before administering vitamin B_{12} replacement, it is important to assess folic acid level to assess for the need of folate. Synthesis of folate is mediated by vitamin B_{12}; therefore, the lack of vitamin B_{12} will cause diminished folate (also called folic acid).

Folic Acid Deficiency

A deficiency of folic acid, also called folate, results in a megaloblastic anemia similar to that seen with vitamin B_{12} deficiency. Folic acid is a form of B vitamin found in a variety of foods, including whole grains, beans, and green leafy vegetables such as spinach. In the United States and developed countries, foods are fortified with folic acid, so in these countries folic acid deficiency is uncommon; however, underdeveloped countries that do not have fortified food have higher rates of folic acid deficiency. In the United States, patients at risk for folic acid deficiency include:

- Pregnant and lactating women
- Alcohol abusers
- Patients taking certain drugs, such as phenytoin, sulfonamides, oral contraceptives, anticonvulsants, or methotrexate

- Elderly adults because of malnutrition and co-morbid medical conditions
- Individuals with celiac disease or inflammatory bowel disease
- Patients with chronic inflammatory disorders such as rheumatoid arthritis, tuberculosis, psoriasis, bacterial endocarditis, and systemic infections.

Etiology. A healthy individual has about 500 to 20,000 mcg of folate in body stores and needs 50 to 100 mcg of folic acid per day in order to replenish the daily degradation and loss through urine and bile. Although folic acid deficiency from malnutrition can occur, malabsorption of folic acid from the GI tract is a much more common cause. Folic acid deficiency occurs in gluten-induced intestinal disorders, intestinal resection surgery, Crohn's disease, and celiac disease. It is also seen in patients taking certain drugs, such as methotrexate, triamterene, trimethoprim, anticonvulsants, certain antibiotics, and oral contraceptives.

Increased demand for folic acid, which plays a vital role in neural development in the fetus, occurs with pregnancy as well as during lactation. During pregnancy, up to 400 mcg of folic acid is needed daily; prenatal vitamins are a good source. Newborn infants have a demand for folic acid that is 10 times that of an adult. The B vitamins such as thiamine and folic acid are often deficient in alcohol abusers.

Because folic acid is loosely bound to plasma proteins, dialysis can remove folic acid, causing deficiency. Chronic intake of alcohol other than beer causes folic acid depletion, though the mechanism is unknown. Hematologic disorders such as chronic hemolytic anemia, particularly SCA, can also cause folic acid deficiency. Chronic inflammatory disorders such as rheumatoid arthritis, tuberculosis, psoriasis, bacterial endocarditis, and systemic infections increase the demand for folic acid.

Pathophysiology. In order to understand folic acid deficiency, it is necessary to comprehend the synthesis of activated folic acid, as well as the effects of folic acid deficiency on DNA synthesis.

Folic Acid and DNA Synthesis. The common feature of all megaloblastic anemias is a defect in DNA synthesis that affects rapidly dividing cells in the bone marrow. Folic acid is needed in reactions that lead to DNA synthesis. Within the plasma, folate is present, mostly in the 5-methyltetrahydrofolate (5-methyl THFA) form, and is loosely associated with plasma proteins in circulation. The 5-methyl THFA enters the cell via a diverse range of folate transporters with differing affinities and mechanisms. Once inside, 5-methyl THFA must be demethylated to THFA, the active form participating in folate-dependent enzymatic reactions. Vitamin B_{12} is required in this conversion, and in its absence, folate is trapped as 5-methyl THFA. This is referred to as folate trapping. Without vitamin B_{12}, folic acid cannot become active to participate in DNA synthesis.

Folic Acid and Prevention of Fetal Neural Tube Defects. Spina bifida, also called myelomeningocele, is a disorder of the spinal cord that can develop in the fetus during the first month of gestation. In spina bifida, some vertebrae overlying the spinal cord are underdeveloped and do not fuse around the spinal cord. This can allow a portion of the spinal cord to protrude outside of the vertebrae. Other neural tube defects include anencephaly and encephalocele, conditions in which a portion of the cerebral neural tube protrudes through the skull. Anencephaly is not compatible with life.

If not severe, spina bifida can be surgically repaired after birth, but this usually does not restore complete normal function to the affected part of the spinal cord. Intrauterine surgery for spina bifida has also been performed. The incidence of spina bifida can be decreased by up to 70% when daily folic acid supplements are taken before conception. The mechanism by which folic acid prevents spinal cord deformities is unclear.

Folic Acid and Prevention of Cardiovascular Disease. Homocysteine (tHCy) is an amino acid that requires folic acid for its breakdown. Without sufficient folic acid, tHCy levels accumulate and can cause injury to the endothelial lining of arteries. Some studies have linked elevated blood levels of tHCy to increased risk of premature coronary artery disease, stroke, and venous blood clots. These studies have led to speculations that high tHCy levels could contribute to atherosclerosis, which is why some clinicians are prescribing folic acid to prevent cardiac disease and atherosclerosis.

Clinical Presentation. A thorough history and physical examination is necessary if folic acid deficiency is suspected. However, the deficiency does not cause overt symptomatology nor does it cause obvious physical assessment findings. In alcohol abusers and those who are malnourished, folic acid deficiency is probable.

Signs and Symptoms. Folic acid anemia usually progresses over several months, and the patient typically does not exhibit symptoms until the Hct level reaches very low levels, lower than 20%. At that point, symptoms such as weakness, fatigue, difficulty concentrating, irritability, headache, palpitations, and shortness of breath can occur. Heart failure can develop in light of high-output cardiac compensation for the decreased tissue oxygenation. Angina pectoris may occur in predisposed individuals because of increased cardiac work demand. Tachycardia, postural hypotension, and lactic acidosis are other common findings.

Physical Examination. The physical examination of the patient with folic acid deficiency may be unremarkable. Signs of anemia such as pallor, tachycardia, and cheilitis may be present. In pregnant women, folic acid supplementation should begin as soon as pregnancy is discovered. Infants also should have vitamins containing folic acid.

Diagnosis. Blood and bone marrow findings exhibit megaloblastic anemia that is indistinguishable from

---

> ### BOX 13-6. Diagnosis of Folic Acid Deficiency
>
> Folic acid and vitamin B_{12} deficiency cause a megaloblastic anemia, but it is important to differentiate them with specific laboratory tests.
>
> - Hgb: low
> - Hct: low
> - MCV: high
> - MCH: normal
> - MCHC: normal
> - Folic acid level: low
> - tHCy: high
> - MMA level: normal

vitamin B_{12} deficiency. It is important to decipher folic acid from vitamin B_{12} deficiency (see Box 13-6). Because vitamin B_{12} is necessary for activation of folic acid, simply supplementing the diet with folic acid alone can bypass the need for vitamin B_{12}. Administering folic acid can mask the vitamin B_{12} deficiency. However, vitamin B_{12} is necessary for neurological health and it needs to be replaced as well.

A vitamin B_{12} assay and folic acid level should be done together. However, blood folic acid levels have false positive and false negative results. The best test for folic acid deficiency as the cause of megaloblastic anemia is a comparison of serum tHCy level and a level of its metabolite, methylmalonic acid (MMA). A normal MMA level with an elevated tHCy level indicates that folic acid is not assisting in the metabolism of homocysteine, which is diagnostic for folate deficiency.

Treatment. Commonly, treatment consists of oral replacement of folic acid at the dose of 1 mg/day. This will restore tissue levels. Oral doses of 5 to 15 mg of folic acid can be absorbed in those with malabsorption. Long-term therapy is needed when the underlying cause cannot be corrected. It is important to measure vitamin B_{12} levels to investigate if treatment with B_{12} is also needed.

> **ALERT!** Before treating a patient with folic acid in megaloblastic anemia, it is important to exclude vitamin B_{12} deficiency. Treating the patient with only folic acid would correct the anemia but not prevent the neurological damage associated with vitamin B_{12} deficiency.

Lack of Bone Marrow Production of RBCs

The lack of bone marrow synthesis of RBCs is a possible cause of anemia. Although, uncommon, when this type of anemia occurs, it often involves WBCs and platelets as well. Therefore, infection and lack of clotting are accompanying symptoms.

Lack of Erythropoietin

Lack of EPO causes anemia, as there is a lack of stimulation of the bone marrow to synthesize RBC. The anemia will be NCNC because, although the RBCs that are synthesized are normal, there is a scarcity of them. There is also a lack of reticulocytes in the peripheral blood and bone marrow because the progenitor cells and immature forms of RBCs are deficient.

The most common cause of EPO deficiency is renal failure. However, hypometabolic states such as hypothyroidism and hypopituitarism, as well as protein deficiency, also decrease production of EPO. In renal failure, the degree of anemia depends on the severity of the renal dysfunction.

Therapy is directed at the underlying cause. In cases like chronic renal disease where normal function cannot be reestablished, recombinant EPO can be administered to stimulate production of a normal level of RBCs. Transfusion is usually not required.

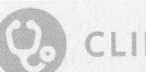

CLINICAL CONCEPT

In renal failure, EPO is currently used to stimulate RBC production and correct the anemia.

Aplastic Anemia

In aplastic anemia, the bone marrow fails, resulting in hypocellular bone marrow and pancytopenia, which is a deficiency of all blood cells. Approximately 80% of the time, the problem is acquired because of infections such as hepatitis, human immunodeficiency virus, or Epstein-Barr virus; exposure to toxic levels of radiation or chemicals such as benzene; certain drugs; or immune disease.

Aplastic anemia is rare, but can occur at any age. There is an increase in cases in people older than 60 years of age. It occurs in 2 persons per million in the United States. The major causes of death among this population are infection caused by lack of WBCs and bleeding caused by lack of platelets.

In bone marrow failure, early forms of hematopoietic cells are greatly diminished; the stem cell pool is reduced to fewer than 1%. The bone marrow often contains fat instead of blood cells.

In drug-induced or chemical damage of the bone marrow, direct tissue injury occurs because of toxic metabolites. High doses of radiation also cause direct cell injury. However, in cases caused by other agents, the disorder may be immune-mediated. Activated cytotoxic T cells are present in patients with aplastic anemia and these diminish with immunosuppressive therapy. However, the sustained autoimmune response is not well understood.

Signs and symptoms can develop abruptly or gradually. Symptoms caused by thrombocytopenia are petechiae, bleeding gums, easy bruising, nosebleeds, and heavy menstrual bleeding. The lack of RBCs will produce the typical symptoms of anemia, including fatigue, pallor, tachycardia, and tachypnea. Lack of white cells increases the risk for infections. Patients commonly do not appear sick despite the lack of blood cells. The physical examination may be unremarkable.

Diagnosis begins with the CBC, which will reveal pancytopenia. Some small amounts of enlarged RBCs may be found, making for a mild megaloblastic anemia. The reticulocyte, WBC, and platelet count will be low. Bone marrow examination reveals severe hypocellularity with lack of hematopoietic cells and a predominance of fat cells. Additional tests are needed to identify the cause. Aplastic anemia can be mild, moderate, or severe. The severe form is life-threatening with extremely low blood cell counts and requires immediate hospitalization.

Blood transfusions will be required until the diagnosis is confirmed and specific treatment is started. However, the goal of treatment is to achieve independence from transfusions. The use of transfusions should be limited where possible to decrease the occurrence of sensitization, which would increase the risk of rejection in candidates for bone marrow transplantation. Infections are the major cause of mortality, so preventive use of broad spectrum antibiotic therapy is recommended, particularly for those patients with indwelling catheters. Early use of antifungal agents should be considered for those with persistent fever.

Bone marrow transplantation from an HLA-matched sibling donor is the preferred treatment. The risk of rejection, also called graft versus host disease (GVHD), increases with the patient's age. The use of antithymocyte globulin induces recovery in 50% of patients. The addition of the drug cyclosporine increases recovery in 70% of patients. Prophylactic antibiotics and platelet, RBC, and WBC transfusions are necessary. Bone marrow stimulants such as filgrastim (Neupogen®) and epoetin-alfa (Epogen®) can be used to stimulate the marrow to make more cells and provide symptom relief.

Immunosuppressive therapy is preferred if the patient is older than 60 years or if no matched sibling donor is available. The response to therapy in aplastic anemia, unlike other autoimmune diseases, is slow and can take anywhere from 4 to 12 weeks for initial improvement to as long as 6 months for resolution. Most patients improve enough to become transfusion independent and demonstrate clinical improvement. Follow-up is important with this therapy as relapse is common.

In cases of aplastic anemia caused by radiation or chemotherapy, the marrow usually recovers once the treatment is stopped. Bone marrow-stimulating drugs (Epogen® and Neupogen®) are used to relieve the symptoms until the marrow recovers.

Anemia of Chronic Disease

Anemia of chronic disease (ACD) develops as a result of chronic disorders such as infection, inflammation, cancer, heart failure, diabetes, and stroke. It is a side effect of a long-term disorder that weakens the body. The long-term disorder is a disease such as rheumatoid arthritis or other autoimmune disease, tuberculosis or other chronic infection, or inflammatory bowel disease, chronic heart failure, or kidney failure. It is particularly common among elderly patients, as they often have one or more chronic diseases and take multiple medications that may contribute to their anemia. The mechanisms of ACD include a decrease in RBC survival time, blunted erythropoietic response in the bone marrow, and impaired iron metabolism in the cell, resulting in an inefficient recycling of iron from old RBCs. Therefore, there is a lack of available iron for erythropoiesis. The clinician will need to distinguish this anemia from iron deficiency anemia, though this can be difficult as ACD and iron deficiency anemia frequently coexist in elderly individuals. The serum ferritin and transferrin levels are recommended to evaluate iron.

Signs and symptoms are usually those of the underlying disease accompanied by signs and symptoms of anemia, principally fatigue, pallor, and tachycardia. The anemia is usually NCNC but may become microcytic over time. Iron stores are usually normal.

Treatment should focus on the underlying disease. Transfusions are not recommended but the use of recombinant EPO has been effective. Because of the blunted response to EPO, higher than usual doses are needed to be effective.

Polycythemia

Polycythemia can be described as the opposite of anemia. Instead of a deficit of RBCs, there is an overabundance of RBCs in polycythemia. In primary polycythemia, there is hyperproliferation of all blood cells. Secondary polycythemia is more common, and it is a hyperproliferation of the RBCs. Secondary polycythemia occurs in response to chronic blood hypoxia.

Primary Polycythemia. In primary polycythemia, also called polycythemia vera, there is an excess of all blood cell types—RBCs, WBCs, and platelets—in the bone marrow. The excess RBCs make the blood viscous and it flows slowly, especially through small vessels. The slow blood flow and thrombocytosis result in the formation of clots, which can incite a number of serious problems, including heart attack and stroke. The etiology of primary polycythemia is unknown, but chromosomal abnormalities are associated with 30% of cases. These include a mutation at 20q, trisomy 8, and mutation at 9p. A mutation of the gene at 9p activates the enzyme tyrosine kinase, which appears to be involved in the cause of the disorder.

Primary polycythemia is rare, more often seen in adults older than age 60 years and rarely in persons younger than age 20 years. It occurs more often in men than women. Primary polycythemia is usually diagnosed by an incidental finding on a CBC. Hgb can be as high as 20 g/dL and Hct greater than 60%. Symptoms are usually related to hyperviscosity of the blood. Systolic hypertension and deep venous thrombosis may be presenting signs. Neurological symptoms related to cerebral blood flow, such as vertigo, tinnitus, headache, visual disturbances, and transient ischemia attacks, are experienced by patients. Ischemia of organs, easy bruising, nosebleeds, or gastrointestinal bleeding may occur because of vascular stasis. A complication called erythromelalgia causes ischemia and infarction in the lower extremities. The patient experiences pain, numbness, erythema, and digital necrosis. Body-wide pruritus is a chronic problem without relief from antihistamines. Splenomegaly can occur because of the constant breakdown of blood cells. Because the patient has an excess of blood cells, a large amount of cellular breakdown occurs daily. The large amount of cellular DNA further breaks down into purines, which become uric acids. The patient often develops hyperuricemia and gout.

The most useful diagnostic test in primary polycythemia is EPO level. A normal level of EPO is an indication that the polycythemia is occurring without any stimulus from EPO. For treatment, patients require periodic phlebotomy. Aspirin or anticoagulants are given to prevent clots. Allopurinol is a medication to keep uric acid low. Splenectomy may be required. Myelosuppressive agents may be ordered to reduce the overproduction of cells by the bone marrow. Hydroxyurea is the most commonly used myelosuppressive agent. Bone marrow transplantation may be curative in young patients. Most persons with primary polycythemia can live long lives without functional impairment with the described treatments.

Secondary Polycythemia. Secondary polycythemia, also called erythrocytosis, is a more common disorder than primary polycythemia. It is caused by prolonged hypoxia as a compensatory effort by the body to improve oxygen delivery. Hypoxia constantly stimulates EPO, which in turn provokes the bone marrow to produce RBCs. Persons with chronic hypoxia such as those who suffer from COPD, spend long periods at high altitudes, or have severe heart or lung disease are most likely to have secondary polycythemia.

The signs and symptoms develop slowly, and the patient can be asymptomatic for years. The various symptoms include headache; dizziness; weakness; shortness of breath, especially when lying down (called orthopnea); feelings of fullness on the left side of the abdomen caused by splenic enlargement; vision changes; redness and itching of the skin; and unexplained bleeding. The person may also experience angina and abdominal pain.

Secondary polycythemia is often an incidental finding on a CBC. Hgb levels usually do not become greater than 17 or 18 g/dL. It should be suspected when the person has an abnormally high Hgb or Hct level and a high EPO level. Secondary polycythemia may be reversed depending on whether the underlying cause of hypoxia can be eliminated.

Chapter Summary

- RBCs are synthesized in the bone marrow in response to EPO secretion by the kidneys.
- RBCs are nonnucleated cells that carry oxygen on an Hgb molecule. Iron is necessary to form Hgb.
- The reticulocyte is an immature RBC that is produced in high numbers by active bone marrow.
- A breakdown product of RBC is bilirubin. Jaundice occurs when there is a high amount of bilirubin in the bloodstream.
- The spleen is the graveyard of RBCs. Splenomegaly and splenic dysfunction can occur if a constant amount of RBCs need to be processed by the spleen.
- Anemias are disorders in which there is a lack of mature, healthy RBCs, leading to impaired oxygen delivery to cells and tissues.
- Causes of anemia include blood loss, accelerated destruction of erythrocytes, and failure of erythrocyte production.
- Common symptoms of anemia include fatigue, dyspnea, exercise intolerance, pallor, and tachycardia.
- Diagnosis of anemia begins with a CBC, which establishes the presence of the disorder. The indices MCV, MCH, and MCHC provide information about possible causes.

- Anemias can be categorized according to how they appear on a peripheral blood smear. The various descriptive categories include normocytic, normochromic, microcytic, hypochromic, or megaloblastic.
- Iron deficiency is the most common cause of anemia. Menorrhagia and GI bleeding are the most common causes of iron deficiency anemia.
- Vitamin B_{12} deficiency causes megaloblastic anemia and neurologic dysfunction of the spinal nerves.
- Pernicious anemia is vitamin B_{12} deficiency caused by autoimmune destruction.
- SCA and thalassemia are the most common disorders of Hgb structure.
- Vaso-occlusive crises can occur when individuals with SCA endure hypoxia, stress, or infection.
- Transfusion, a mainstay of treatment in anemia, is commonly used when Hgb is 7 g/dL.
- Type O blood is the universal donor; type AB is the universal recipient.
- Secondary polycythemia is stimulated by chronic hypoxia of the bloodstream.
- Bone marrow transplantation requires a donor with matching tissue type of the recipient.

 Making the Connections

Pathophysiology	Signs and Symptoms	Physical Assessment Findings	Diagnosis	Treatment
Anemia | Lack of adequate numbers of mature, healthy RBCs results in insufficient oxygen delivery to tissues. The cells are unable to meet the demand for oxygen, causing an oxygen deficit. Because oxygen demand is higher with activity, the deficit is worse with increased activity or stress.				
	Unusual fatigue. Decreased ability to carry out activities of daily living. Shortness of breath that worsens with activity. Dizziness. Cold intolerance. Headache possible. Chest pain possible.	Pallor. Tachypnea. Tachycardia. Cold extremities.	Decreased Hgb and Hct levels. Decreased RBC count. Reticulocyte count is increased if there is a normal bone marrow response.	Depends on the cause of the anemia: Standard treatment is blood transfusion. Avoidance of stress and increased activity. Oxygen. Dietary modifications to increase iron sources.
Anemia Caused by Hemorrhage, Rapid Blood Loss | Trauma or severe GI bleeding causes the body to lose large amounts of blood. Sympathetic nervous system response causes increased heart rate and peripheral vasoconstriction.				

Continued

Making the Connections—cont'd

Pathophysiology	Signs and Symptoms	Physical Assessment Findings	Diagnosis	Treatment
Activation of the renin-angiotensin system results in retention of water by the kidney, which increases blood volume and blood pressure.				
	Depends on volume of blood loss. • Less than 15% loss: anxiety and orthostatic hypotension. • 15% to 30% loss: restlessness, changes in level of consciousness (LOC). • 30% to 40% loss: further decrease in LOC. Faint, dizziness, apprehension. Feels cold. • Greater than 40% loss: profound shock. Patient may report hematemesis if blood loss is from esophageal varices. Melena and hematochezia if blood loss from lower GI tract.	Postural blood pressure drops. Changes in LOC. Narrowed pulse pressure. Urine output lower than 30 mL/hr. Tachycardia greater than 120. Weak pulse, hypotension, cool, pale. Heart rate greater than 140. Scant or no urine output. Profound hypotension.	Low Hgb and Hct. Low RBC count. Normochromic, normocytic anemia. High reticulocyte count. FOBT may be positive if GI bleed.	Identify the bleeding site and restore hemostasis. Transfusion to restore RBCs and blood volume. Avoid inotropic drugs in the setting of low blood volume. Oxygen. Elevate feet.
Anemia Caused by Chronic Blood Loss | Gradual, slow blood loss from GI tract or caused by heavy menses. Colon cancer is a common cause of chronic blood loss via the GI tract. Slow loss of blood depletes the body of iron.				
	Fatigue, weakness, or no symptoms. Some shortness of breath with activity. Dark stool possible (melena). If excessive menstrual blood loss, the patient has excessive use of pads or tampons per day.	Mild tachycardia. Pallor. Melena: FOBT positive stools if GI bleed. Unusually heavy menses if caused by menorrhagia.	Low Hgb and Hct. Low RBC count. Low serum iron and ferritin levels caused by loss of iron stores and inability to recycle iron.	Identify the site of the blood loss and establish hemostasis. If blood loss has been severe, transfusions are required. Iron replacement therapy is needed for hemopoiesis.
Hemolytic Anemia | Accelerated RBC destruction exceeds erythrocyte production. Causes: mechanical turbulence caused by prosthetic cardiac valves; autoimmune response leading to destruction of RBCs by antibodies. Can be an adverse effect of medication. The spleen enlarges because it is working hard to remove damaged RBCs.				
	Fatigue, pallor, shortness of breath. Chills, jaundice possible.	Tachycardia as compensatory response to anemia. Pallor. Jaundice caused by excess breakdown on RBCs, which releases bilirubin into blood. Dark urine caused by bilirubin in urine. Enlarged spleen caused by high activity.	Decrease in Hgb and Hct. Increased reticulocyte count. Increased bilirubin, methemoglobin, and urobilinogen levels, which are breakdown products of RBCs. Tests for autoantibodies: IgM class is called cold agglutinins; IgG class is called warm agglutinins.	If medication suspected as etiology, stop medication. Folic acid and iron replacement. Corticosteroids. Autoimmune diagnosis may require immunosuppressive drugs and splenectomy.

Continued

Making the Connections—cont'd

Pathophysiology	Signs and Symptoms	Physical Assessment Findings	Diagnosis	Treatment

Pernicious Anemia | A specific type of vitamin B_{12} anemia caused by a lack of IF. Lack of IF results in impaired absorption of vitamin B_{12} from stomach. Autoimmune destruction of IF by antibodies is the cause of IF deficiency. Nerve and blood cells need vitamin B_{12} to function properly, so neurological functions are impaired. RBCs cannot be properly synthesized and neurons in the dorsal columns of the spinal cord show loss of myelination.

| | Usual symptoms of anemia: pallor, shortness of breath with activity, fatigue. Vitamin B_{12} deficiency. Neurological symptoms, including numbness and tingling of hands and feet, gait disturbances, and lack of coordination. Depression and dementia also may be caused by vitamin B_{12} deficit. | Unsteady gait. Positive Babinski reflex. Loss of deep tendon reflexes. Personality changes; dementialike symptoms and depression. Neurological changes are often seen before the anemia is diagnosed. Red, smooth tongue; glossitis. Sore mouth; chelitis. | Enlarged oval-shaped RBCs. Hgb and Hct may be low or normal. Megaloblastic, macrocytic anemia. Low serum levels of vitamin B_{12} and folic acid. High levels of tHCy in blood. | Treatment with vitamin B_{12} Replacement of vitamin B_{12}; intramuscular injection every 3 months. Nasal spray available. Diet rich in meat, eggs, milk, and dairy products. |

Folic Acid Deficiency Anemia | Lack of sufficient folic acid in diet results in a megaloblastic anemia very similar to vitamin B_{12} deficiency.

| | Usual signs and symptoms of anemia: pallor, fatigue, shortness of breath with activity, possible dizziness. | Patient is usually asymptomatic except for anemia signs; pallor, cold extremities may be present. Fetal adverse effects; lack of full spinal cord development; open neural tube defect. Infant often born with spina bifida, which causes paraplegia. | Folic acid levels lower than 4 ng/mL. Low Hgb and Hct levels. MCV high. Elevated tHCy levels. | Oral replacement of 1 mg folate/day. Diet rich in breads, pasta, asparagus, green leafy vegetables such as spinach, and beans. |

Iron Deficiency Anemia | Most common cause of anemia in general. Iron is essential for the formation of heme, the part of Hgb responsible for attaching oxygen for transport. Normal erythropoiesis cannot occur.

| | Usual signs and symptoms of anemia: pallor, fatigue, shortness of breath, dizziness. Pica. | Pallor. Tachycardia. Red, swollen tongue; glossitis. Sores of mouth; cheilitis. Enlarged spleen. | Microcytic anemia. Hypochromic anemia. Decreased Hgb and Hct. Low serum iron and serum ferritin levels. Increased total iron binding capacity. Absence of iron in the bone marrow. | Oral supplements such as ferrous sulfate. If iron malabsorption is present, imferon IM or IV. Vitamin C helps the body absorb more iron. |

Aplastic Anemia | Deficiency of all cells produced by the bone marrow including RBCs, WBCs, and platelets. Radiation, severe infection, or cancer can cause this deficiency of bone marrow.

| | Severe signs and symptoms of anemia: high output heart failure can occur. Increased susceptibility to infections caused by WBC deficiency. | Severe pallor. Easy bruising, petechiae, and easy bleeding that is hard to stop, such as nosebleeds. Severe infections. | CBC reveals pancytopenia; no synthesis of any type of blood cell. Low reticulocyte count indicates failure of marrow response. | Transfusions. Leuko-poor blood transfusions preferred because fewer WBCs will allow for less chance of hypersensitivity. |

Continued

Making the Connections—cont'd

Pathophysiology	Signs and Symptoms	Physical Assessment Findings	Diagnosis	Treatment
	Increased bleeding risk caused by platelet deficiency.		Bone marrow exam reveals hypocellularity with lack of hematopoietic cells and predominance of fat cells.	Bone marrow stimulants such as Filgrastim and Epoetin. Bone marrow transplant. Prophylactic broad spectrum antibiotic.

Anemia of Chronic Disease | Results from a chronic disorder that leads to decreased RBC survival time, blunted erythropoietic response in the bone marrow, impaired cellular iron metabolism, and inefficient recycling of iron from old RBCs. The chronic disease, which is often an autoimmune disorder, chronic infection, or chronic cause of inflammation, causes a weakening of the bone marrow.

Pathophysiology	Signs and Symptoms	Physical Assessment Findings	Diagnosis	Treatment
	Signs and symptoms of the underlying disease along with the symptoms of anemia.	Pallor. Fatigue. Tachycardia. Shortness of breath with activity. Signs of the chronic disease, which is the etiology.	Normocytic, normochromic (NCNC) anemia. Iron stores are normal, unlike those in a patient with iron deficiency anemia. Serum transferrin levels and transferrin receptor levels are normal.	Treatment focuses on the underlying disease. Recombinant EPO has been successful.

Sickle Cell Anemia | Most common hemoglobinopathy, which is a genetic disorder that causes production of flawed Hgb structure: Hgb S is produced instead of normal Hgb. Flawed Hgb provokes a hemolytic reaction by the body and poor oxygen carriage by the abnormal RBCs. Autosomal recessive inheritance pattern. RBCs polymerize or clump under certain conditions such as hypoxia or dehydration. Distorted RBCs block blood flow in the microcirculation, leading to ischemia and damage to tissues and organs. These RBCs also have a shortened life span, leading to a secondary anemia.

Pathophysiology	Signs and Symptoms	Physical Assessment Findings	Diagnosis	Treatment
	Usual signs and symptoms of anemia, particularly fatigue and reduced activity tolerance. During vaso-occlusive episodes, severe pain. Long bones often affected. Pain can be in any area of body. Stroke and myocardial infarction can occur early in childhood.	Weakness caused by anemia. Shortness of breath with activity. Stunted growth. Jaundice caused by accelerated breakdown of abnormal cells. Increased infections caused by splenic dysfunction. Enlargement of the spleen.	CBC to assess for anemia: low Hgb and Hct. Commonly an NCNC or microcytic hypochromic. Peripheral blood smear shows crescent-shaped RBCs. Screen blood sample for presence of Hgb S, the altered sickle cell Hgb. Part of routine screening of newborns. RBC breakdown causes hyperbilirubinemia. Infections with encapsulated bacterial organisms is common because of splenic dysfunction.	Prevention and management of pain; opiates commonly needed. Prophylactic antibiotics to reduce infections. Educate patients to avoid triggers that cause crises. Bone marrow transplant if suitable donor available. Transfusions to increase numbers of normal cells. IV hydration during crisis. Hydroxyurea given during crisis.

Continued

Making the Connections—cont'd

Pathophysiology	Signs and Symptoms	Physical Assessment Findings	Diagnosis	Treatment

Thalassemia | A common hemoglobinopathy Abnormal Hgb structure; two types of disease: alpha or beta Genetic disorder with autosomal recessive inheritance Hemolysis of abnormal RBCs occurs and large amounts of erythropoiesis in the bone marrow leads to deformities and weak ening of bones. Spleen enlarges because of hyperactivity.

| | Usual signs of anemia; can be severe depending on Hgb and Hct deficiency. Can have heart failure if severe anemia. Weakness. Pallor. Shortness of breath with activity. Tachycardia. Palpitations. Hemolysis causes high bilirubin levels, which leads to jaundice. | Stunted growth. Enlarged spleen and liver. Jaundice. Dark urine. Characteristic bone abnormalities: chipmunk cheeks and hair on end skull deformities. | CBC; low Hgb and Hct. MCHC anemia. Electrophoresis to determine type of Hgb present. Splenomegaly. X-ray shows osteopenia, characteristic bone deformity. | Genetic counseling. Transfusions. Bone marrow transplant. Prophylactic antibiotics to reduce infections. |

Polycythemia | An excess of RBCs causes blood to be more viscous and increases peripheral vascular resistance. Blood flow slows, especially in smaller vessels, leading to increased clotting. **Primary polycythemia** results from a gene mutation that occurs after conception. High numbers of RBCs, WBCs, and platelets cause high viscosity of blood. **Secondary polycythemia** is a compensatory response to chronic hypoxia associated with smoking, living at high altitudes, and chronic diseases of the lungs and heart.

| | Headache. Dizziness. Weakness. Shortness of breath, especially when lying down. Feeling of fullness on the left side of the abdomen. May have angina and abdominal pain. | Enlarged spleen and liver. Redness and itching of the skin, especially after a warm bath. Unexplained bleeding or clotting. Flushed face caused by excessive numbers of RBCs. | CBC reveals abnormally high Hgb and Hct, with high WBC and platelet counts. Increased vitamin B_{12} and uric acid levels. Serum EPO is very low in primary polycythemia vera but high in secondary polycythemia. | Periodic phlebotomy. Myelosuppressive agents such as hydroxyurea. Low-dose aspirin to reduce clotting. Antihistamines for itching. In secondary polycythemia, control or elimination of cause. |

Bibliography

Akinsheye, I., Alsultan, A., Solovieff, N., et al. (2011, April 13). Fetal hemoglobin in sickle cell anemia. *Blood*. Epub ahead of print.

Balarajan, Y., Ramakrishnan, U., Ozaltin, E., Shankar, A. H., & Subramanian, S. V. (2011). Anaemia in low-income and middle-income countries. *Lancet*, 378(9809), 2123–2135. Epub 2011 Aug 1.

Bross, M. H., Soch, K., & Smith-Knuppel, T. (2010). Anemia in older persons. *Am Fam Phys*, 82(5), 480–487.

Bull-Henry, K., & Al-Kawas, F. H. (2013). Evaluation of occult gastrointestinal bleeding. *Am Fam Phys*, 87(6), 430–436.

Chiche, L., Mancini, J., Arlet, J. B., & BDOSE study investigators. (2013, May 24). Indications for cobalamin level assessment in departments of internal medicine: a prospective practice survey. *Post Med J*. Epub ahead of print.

Drüeke, T. B. (2013). Anemia treatment in patients with chronic kidney disease. *N Engl J Med*, 368(4), 387–389.

Fishbane, S. (2010). The role of erythropoiesis-stimulating agents in the treatment of anemia. *Am J Man Care*, 16 Suppl Issues, S67–S73.

Friedrich, M. J. (2011). Advances reshaping sickle cell therapy. *JAMA*, 305(3), 239–240, 242.

Geller, A. K., & O'Connor, M. K. (2008). The sickle cell crisis: a dilemma in pain relief. *Mayo Clin Proceed*, 83(3), 320–323.

Hannemann, A., Weiss, E., Rees, D. C., Dalibalta, S., Ellory, J. C., & Gibson, J. S. (2011). The properties of red blood cells from patients heterozygous for HbS and HbC (HbSC Genotype). *Anemia*. Epub 2010 Oct 13.

Higgs, D. R., Engel, J. D., & Stamatoyannopoulos, G. (2012). Thalassaemia. *Lancet*, 379(9813), 373–383. Epub 2011 Sep 9. Review.

Johnson, M. A., Dwyer, J. T., Jensen, G. L., et al. (2011). Challenges and new opportunities for clinical nutrition interventions in the aged. *J Nutr*, 141(3), 535–541.

Kessenich, C. R., & Cronin, K. (2013). Fecal occult blood testing in older adult patients with anemia. *Nurse Practitioner*, 38(1), 6–8.

Kumar, A. (2009). Perioperative management of anemia: limits of blood transfusion and alternatives to it. *Cleveland Clin J Med*, 76 Suppl 4, S112–S118.

Landgren, O., & Waxman, A. J. (2010). Multiple myeloma precursor disease. *JAMA*, 304(21), 2397–2404.

Langan, R. C., & Zawistoski, K. J. (2011). Update on vitamin B_{12} deficiency. *Am Fam Phys*, 83(12), 1425–1430.

Lawrence, C. (2011). Blood. *Lancet*, 377(9773), 1231.

Lin, K. W. (2009). Screening for sickle cell disease in newborns. *Am Fam Phys*, 79(6), 507–508.

Longo, D., Fauci, A. S., Kasper, D. L., Hauser, S. L., Jameson, J. L. & LoScalzo, J. (2011). *Harrison's principles of internal medicine.* 18th ed. New York: McGraw-Hill.

Lopez-Contreras, M. J., Zamora-Portero, S., Lopez, M. A., Marin, J. F., Zamora, S., & Perez-Llamas, F. (2010). Dietary intake and iron status of institutionalized elderly people: relationship with different factors. *J Nutr, Health Aging*, 14(10), 816–821.

McGann, P. T., & Ware, R. E. (2011). Hydroxyurea for sickle cell anemia: what have we learned and what questions still remain? *Curr Opin Hem*, 18(3), 158–165.

Mehari, A., Gladwin, M. T., Tian, X., Machado, R. F., & Kato, G. J. (2012). Mortality in adults with sickle cell disease and pulmonary hypertension. *JAMA*, 307(12), 1254–1256.

Milman, N. (2011). Anemia—still a major health problem in many parts of the world! *Ann Hem*, 90(4), 369–377.

Muncie, H. L., Jr., & Campbell, J. (2009). Alpha and beta thalassemia. *Am Fam Phys*, 80(4), 339–344.

Quinn, C. T., McKinstry, R. C., Dowling, M. M., et al. (2013). Acute silent cerebral ischemic events in children with sickle cell anemia. *JAMA Neurol*, 70(1), 58–65.

Rees, D. C., Williams, T. N., & Gladwin, M. T. (2010). Sickle-cell disease. *Lancet*, 376(9757), 2018–2031. Epub 2010 Dec 3.

Roy, R. R., & Thomas, M. R. (2010). 25-year-old woman with anemia. *Mayo Clin Proceed*, 85(3), e9–e12.

Schnuelle, P., Mueller, A., & Schmitt, W. H. (2013). A case of pica-like, nutrient-induced, severe iron-deficiency anemia. *Am J Med*, 126(12), e1–e2. doi: 10.1016/j.amjmed.2013.07.032.

Sharma, S., Sharma, P., & Tyler, L. N. (2011). Transfusion of blood and blood products: indications and complications. *Am Fam Phys*, 83(6), 719–724.

Short, M. W., & Domagalski, J. E. (2013). Iron deficiency anemia: evaluation and management. *Am Fam Phys*, 87(2), 98–104.

Stabler, S. P. (2013). Clinical practice. Vitamin B_{12} deficiency. *N Engl J Med*, 368(2), 149–160.

Taylor, C., Kavanagh, P., & Zuckerman, B. (2014). Sickle cell trait—neglected opportunities in the era of genomic medicine. *JAMA*, 311(15), 1495–1496. doi: 10.1001/jama.2014.2157.

Thum, T., Kalantar-Zadeh, K., & Anker, S. D. (2011). Erythropoietin in kidney disease and type 2 diabetes. *N Engl J Med*, 364(4), 384–386.

Tolich, D. J., Blackmur, S., Stahorsky, K., & Wabeke, D. (2013). Blood management: best-practice transfusion strategies. *Nursing*, 43(1), 40–47.

Torpy, J. M., Lynm, C., & Golub, R. M. (2012). JAMA patient page. Blood transfusion. *JAMA*, 307(22), 2448.

Van Vranken, M. (2010). Evaluation of microcytosis. *Am Fam Phys*, 82(9), 1117–1122.

Weatherall, D. J. (2011a). Hydroxycarbamide for sickle-cell anaemia in infancy. *Lancet*, 377(9778), 1628–1630.

Weatherall, D. J. (2011b). Systems biology and red cells. *N Engl J Med*, 364(4), 376–377.

Yang, D. T., & Cook, R. J. (2012). Spurious elevations of vitamin B_{12} with pernicious anemia. *N Engl J Med*, 366(18), 1742–1743.

Disorders of Platelets, Hemostasis, and Coagulation

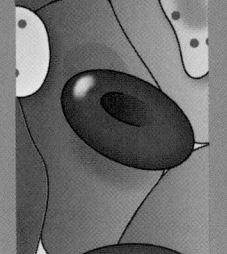

Key Terms

Activated partial thromboplastin time (aPTT)

Antiphospholipid syndrome

Coagulation factors

Disseminated intravascular coagulation (DIC)

Extrinsic pathway

Fibrinolysis

Glycoprotein (GP) IIb/IIIa receptor

Hemostasis

Heparin

Immune thrombocytopenic purpura (ITP)

Intrinsic pathway

Low molecular weight heparin (LMWH)

Plasmin

Prothrombin time (PT)

Thrombocytopenia

Thrombocytosis

Thrombopoietin

Thrombosis

Thrombotic thrombocytopenic purpura (TTP)

Thrombus

Tissue plasminogen activator

Platelets and coagulation factors are the major elements involved in blood clotting, and an abnormality in either can cause either excessive bleeding or excessive clotting. The normal range of platelets is 150,000 to 400,000 cells/uL. **Thrombocytopenia** is the term for a low number of platelets, less than 100,000/uL which can cause bleeding. **Thrombocytosis** is the term for an excessive number of platelets, greater than 750,000/uL, which can cause excessive clotting. A wide number of medications can trigger an antibody reaction to platelets, causing lysis of platelets and thrombocytopenia. A viral or bacterial infection can also stimulate antibody destruction of platelets for unknown reasons. In disorders such as polycythemia, a hyperactive disorder of the bone marrow, too many platelets can lead to development of thrombi (clots); as a result, occlusion of blood vessels can occur, and this can give rise to stroke, myocardial infarction, deep venous thrombosis, pulmonary emboli, and peripheral arterial disease.

Epidemiology

Platelet or coagulation disorders are uncommon in clinical practice. Thrombocytopenia most often accompanies hematologic cancers such as leukemia, which inhibits development of all blood cells in the bone marrow. **Immune thrombocytopenic purpura (ITP),** a disorder that specifically targets platelets, can be triggered by a wide variety of medications and has an incidence of 66 cases per million persons per year. Because coagulation factors are synthesized by the liver, cirrhosis caused by alcoholism is probably the most common cause of deficient coagulation. Up to 20% of heavy drinkers develop cirrhosis and consequent risk of bleeding.

Disseminated intravascular coagulation (DIC) is the most commonly acquired disorder of coagulation. Often triggered by sepsis, it occurs in 1% of all hospitalized patients. The most common genetic disease of coagulation, hemophilia A, affects 1 out of 5,000 male newborns per year. Hemophilia B, also called Christmas disease, is less common and affects 1 out of 30,000 male babies per year.

Basic Concepts of Bleeding and Clotting Physiology

The process of clotting involves the process of hemostasis, the function of platelets, and the activated coagulation cascade. An understanding of all these concepts is necessary in order to comprehend pathological conditions of clotting and bleeding.

Hemostasis

Hemostasis is a protective mechanism whereby the formation of a thrombus prevents excessive blood loss from the body. It has three major steps:

1. vasoconstriction
2. development of a platelet plug
3. blood coagulation.

Platelets, also called thrombocytes, are the cells in the body that make up clots and assist in hemostasis. Hemostasis is divided into two stages: primary hemostasis and secondary hemostasis. In primary hemostasis, platelets form a fundamental platelet plug. In secondary hemostasis, coagulation factors undergo a process known as the coagulation cascade, which leads to fibrin formation and, eventually, a finished fibrin clot. A clot, also known as a **thrombus,** is a collection of aggregated platelets reinforced by fibrin. Platelets and coagulation factors are activated to form a thrombus when the body is injured, a blood vessel wall is damaged, or blood flow is sluggish or stagnant. The coagulation system's formation of fibrin is counterbalanced by a system of fibrinolytic (clot dissolving) mechanisms that ensure that the hemostatic effect is regulated and does not extend inappropriately.

In pathological states, hemostatic events can escape normal control mechanisms because of either inherited or acquired defects, resulting in **thrombosis,** which is the generation of an occlusive thrombus (clot) that obstructs blood flow in an artery or vein. Coronary, cerebrovascular, and venous thrombosis are some of the consequences.

Platelets

Platelets begin as immature cells called megakaryocytes in the bone marrow. Megakaryocytes have no nucleus, deoxyribonucleic acid, or ribosomes, and they cannot synthesize proteins. However, they mature into platelets that have powerful granules, which contain procoagulant substances.

Platelet formation is stimulated by the hormone **thrombopoietin,** which is synthesized by the liver. A reduction in platelet number in the bone marrow stimulates this hormone. The normal platelet has a life span of 7 to 10 days. Almost one-third of all platelets reside in the spleen, but when enlarged and hyperactive, the spleen can sequester up to 80% of platelets.

Under normal conditions, the endothelial lining of blood vessels is a smooth, antithrombotic surface. However, when injured, inflammatory mediators and prothrombotic substances released by the endothelium draw platelets to the area. Exposed collagen and von Willebrand factor (vWF) released by the endothelium activate platelets which, in turn, stimulate coagulation factors and draw additional platelets to the site. Platelet adhesion results in the activation of the **glycoprotein (GP) IIb/IIIa receptor,** which binds to fibrinogen from the coagulation cascade and enhances further platelet aggregation. Activated platelets release adhesive proteins, growth factors, and thromboxane A2 that promote platelet aggregation, draw more platelets to the site, and facilitate blood clot formation. This leads to formation of an occlusive platelet thrombus that is stabilized by fibrin.

CLINICAL CONCEPT

Some antiplatelet agents work as GPIIb/IIIa receptor blockers to diminish platelet and fibrinogen linkage and inhibit clot formation. Abciximab (Reopro®) is an example of a GPIIb/IIIa inhibitor.

The Coagulation Factors

Secondary hemostasis requires a stepwise activation of proteins in the blood called **coagulation factors** that take part in a complex cascade. The cascade ultimately forms fibrin strands, which strengthen the platelet plug formed in primary hemostasis. The coagulation cascade has two pathways: the **intrinsic pathway,** also known as the contact activation pathway, and the **extrinsic pathway,** also known as the tissue factor (TF) pathway. The pathways are triggered by different events but ultimately end in the same final pathway that synthesizes fibrin. The two pathways both terminate in the same steps: the activation of factor X, which converts prothrombin to thrombin and, in turn, converts fibrinogen to fibrin. The coagulation cascade is best understood by reviewing the various step-by-step reactions portrayed in Figure 14-1.

Extrinsic Pathway

The extrinsic pathway is stimulated by trauma to a blood vessel that occurs because of an external injury such as a laceration. Factor VII is activated and comes into contact with TF located on injured membrane components such as fibroblasts and leukocytes. The two components form an activated complex called TF-factor VII. TF-factor VII activates factor IX and factor X. The activation of factor X by TF-factor VII is almost immediately impeded by an extrinsic pathway inhibitor. Factor X and its cofactor, factor V, form a complex that activates prothrombin to thrombin. Both the extrinsic and intrinsic pathways arrive at this significant step, which leads to the ultimate conversion of fibrinogen into fibrin (see Fig. 14-1). The clotting time of the extrinsic pathway can be measured by the **prothrombin time (PT)** diagnostic test.

Intrinsic Pathway

The intrinsic pathway is stimulated by tissue damage incurred by injury to the endothelial lining of a blood vessel as in inflammation or atherosclerosis. The pathway can also be triggered by stasis of blood as occurs in atrial fibrillation. The pathway begins with activation of factor XII; from there, activation of a number of factors occurs until factor X is reached (see Fig. 14-1). Factor X activates the conversion of prothrombin to thrombin, which leads to the ultimate conversion of fibrinogen into fibrin. The blood clotting time of the intrinsic pathway can be measured by the **activated partial thromboplastin time (aPTT)** diagnostic test.

Final Pathway in the Coagulation Cascade

Both intrinsic and extrinsic pathways go through an array of complex step-by-step reactions to arrive at a common final pathway: conversion of prothrombin into thrombin. Thrombin has many functions, mainly the conversion of fibrinogen to fibrin, the major building block of a clot. Calcium and vitamin K are required for the proper functioning of the coagulation cascade.

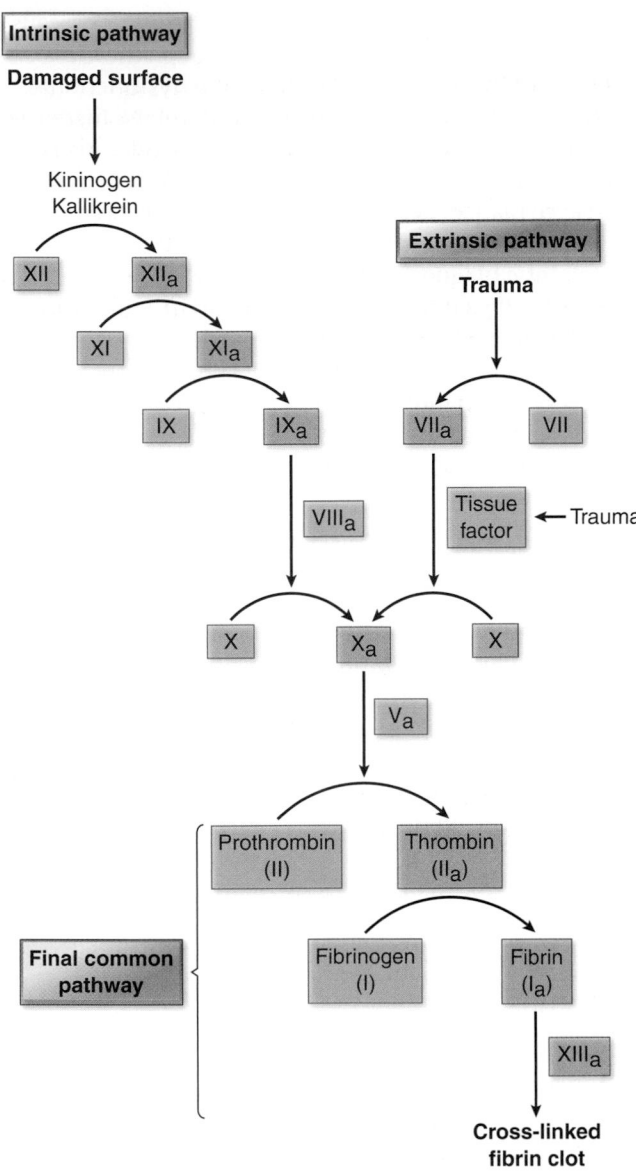

FIGURE 14-1. The coagulation cascade is a sequence of coagulation factors, synthesized by the liver, that form a clot. There are two different pathways that can activate the coagulation cascade: the intrinsic and extrinsic pathways, both of which end in a final common pathway that stimulates prothrombin to form thrombin and fibrinogen to form fibrin. The intrinsic pathway is stimulated by any damage to the endothelial surface of a blood vessel, as in arteriosclerosis, or any turbulence in blood flow, as in atrial fibrillation. The extrinsic pathway is stimulated by external trauma to a blood vessel, as happens in a laceration.

These can be obtained from the diet through consumption of dairy foods and green leafy vegetables. Vitamin K is fat-soluble, meaning it is stored in fatty tissue. Any disorder that decreases absorption of fat will decrease absorption of vitamin K.

Clot Dissolution
There are three substances that act to decrease clot formation and dissolve clots:

1. plasmin
2. plasminogen
3. tissue plasminogen activator (tPA).

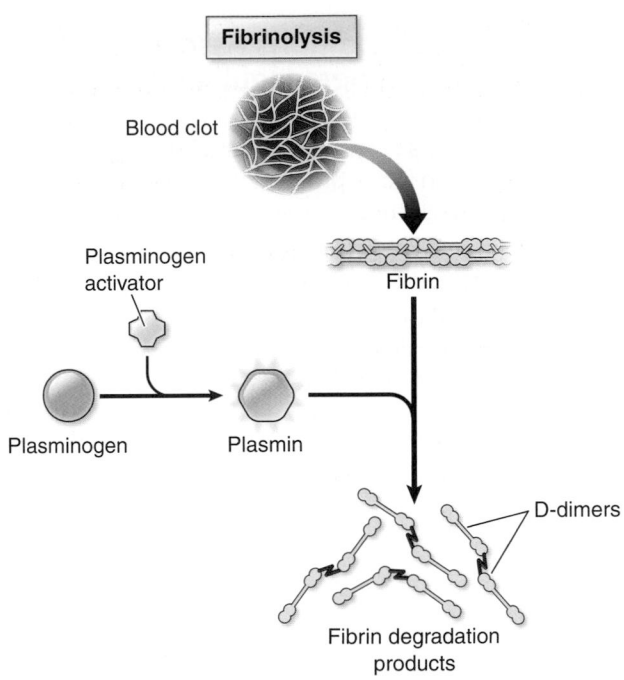

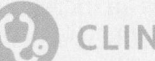

FIGURE 14-2. Fibrinolysis. After a clot is formed, the body can dissolve it using plasmin. Plasminogen activator catalyzes the transformation of plasminogen into plasmin. Plasmin then catalyzes the breakdown of fibrin into fibrin degradation products, also called D-dimer.

These substances are involved in limiting the size of the clot and act to eventually dissolve it. Blood clots are dissolved by a process termed **fibrinolysis.** The main enzyme responsible for this process is **plasmin,** which is regulated by various activators and inhibitors. Plasmin activates **tissue plasminogen activator,** which dissolves clots. After the clot is dissolved, blood flow can be reestablished and tissue healing can take place (see Fig. 14-2).

> ### CLINICAL CONCEPT
>
> Arterial thrombi are referred to as white thrombi because they are rich in platelets but scarce in RBCs. Venous thrombi are referred to as red thrombi because they have a large number of RBCs and small number of platelets.

Basic Concepts of Bleeding and Clotting Pathophysiology

Pathophysiologic problems of clotting can develop because of inadequate or excessive platelet number, platelet dysfunction, inadequate coagulation factors, or defective coagulation cascade activity. Inadequate platelet number, missing coagulation factors, and decreased coagulation activity can lead to bleeding problems, whereas excessive platelet number and enhanced coagulation activity can lead to hypercoagulability and complications of excessive thrombus formation (see Box 14-1).

Clotting Disorders

A susceptibility to clot formation occurs with thrombocytosis, enhanced platelet activity, or increased activation of coagulation factors. Enhanced platelet activity can occur with disturbances in blood flow and endothelial damage. Increased activation of coagulation factors occurs with stasis of blood flow, increase in procoagulation factors, or decrease in anticoagulation factors.

Increased Platelet Number and Activity

Thrombocytosis, which describes an increased number of platelets in excess of 750,000/uL, is a disorder that can occur after splenectomy, because the spleen sequesters and lyses dead platelets; without the spleen, the body is unable to eliminate platelets. Platelet excess also occurs in myeloproliferative disorders, such as polycythemia or leukemia where the bone marrow is hyperactive.

There are two types of thrombocytosis: primary and secondary. Primary thrombocytosis, also known as essential thrombocytosis, occurs in the bone marrow. The cause is unknown, but the increased number of platelets enhance the risk of clot formation. Secondary thrombocytosis, also called reactive thrombocytosis, is an elevated platelet count caused by another primary condition, such as iron deficiency anemia, cancer, inflammation, infection, surgery, or myeloproliferative disorders. In secondary thrombocytosis, the exact mechanism for development of thrombocytosis is unclear, but the excessive number of platelets does not cause excessive clotting. In fact, in myeloproliferative disorders such as polycythemia vera, elevated platelet count leads to

bleeding. Platelet counts can rise into the millions, causing a paradoxical risk of bleeding. Although there are excessive numbers of platelets, many are dysfunctional.

Aside from an excess number of platelets, increased platelet activity can lead to enhanced platelet aggregation and increased susceptibility to blood clot formation. Increased platelet activation most commonly occurs with disturbances in blood flow and endothelial damage. Atherosclerotic plaques disrupt smooth blood flow through arteries, and plaque rupture exposes an irregular surface that attracts platelets and promotes clot formation. Smoking, elevated lipids and cholesterol, hypertension, diabetes, and immune reactions can cause vessel injury that draws platelets to the site and predisposes to platelet aggregation and thrombus formation.

Increased Coagulation Activity

Increased activation of the coagulation system is caused by stasis of blood flow, increase in procoagulation factors, or decrease in anticoagulation factors. Sluggish or stagnant blood flow is a common cause of venous thrombus formation, which often occurs in the lower extremities of immobile, sedentary, or postoperative patients. A deep vein thrombosis (DVT) in the femoral vein can travel into the inferior vena cava and flow into the right atrium and ventricle, and then into the pulmonary artery, causing a pulmonary embolism (see Fig. 14-3). Heart failure, which causes weakened pumping of blood, can also lead to venous stasis in the

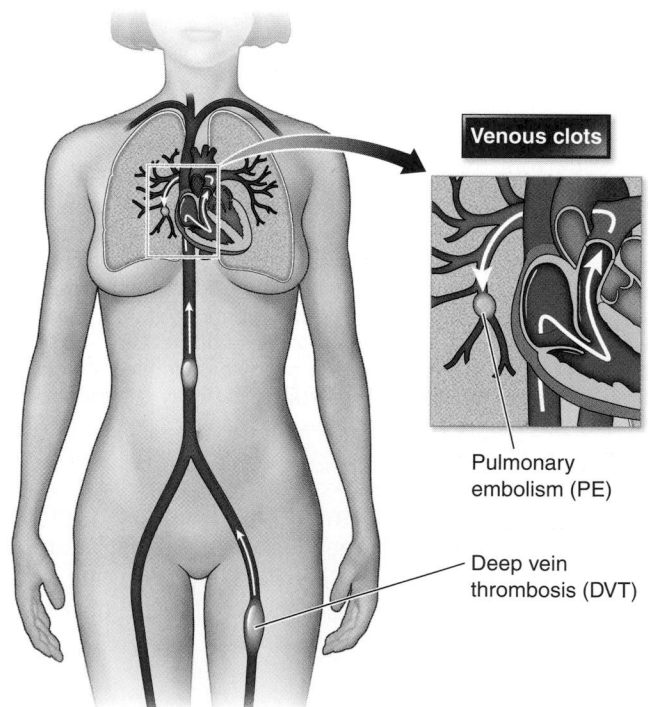

Venous clots

Pulmonary embolism (PE)

Deep vein thrombosis (DVT)

FIGURE 14-3. A femoral DVT can break away from the leg vein, ascend into the interior vena cava, and then enter the heart's right atrium. From the right atrium, the thrombus enters the right ventricle, then flows into the pulmonary artery and into the lung's arterial system. It lodges in a pulmonary arterial vessel and blocks the circulation from becoming oxygenated.

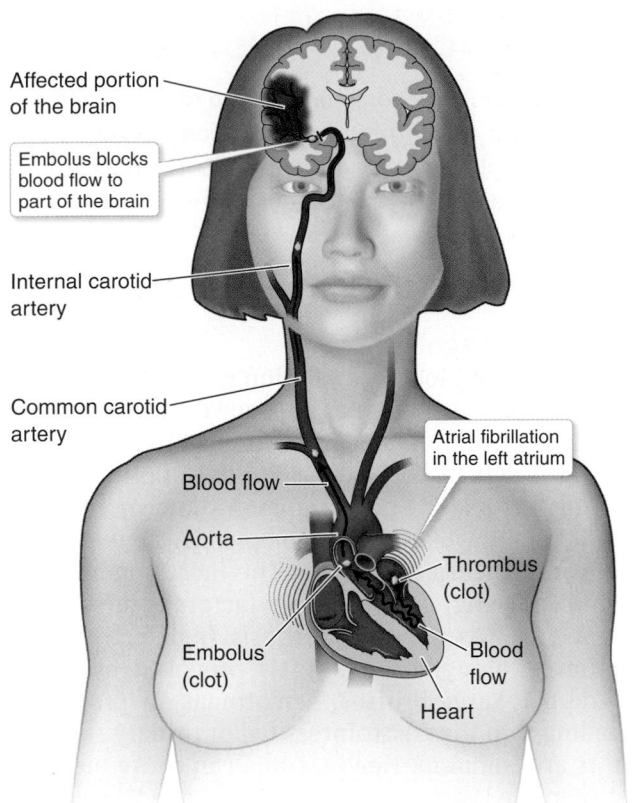

Affected portion of the brain

Embolus blocks blood flow to part of the brain

Internal carotid artery

Common carotid artery

Atrial fibrillation in the left atrium

Blood flow

Aorta

Thrombus (clot)

Embolus (clot)

Blood flow

Heart

FIGURE 14-4. How atrial fibrillation leads to cerebral embolism that causes ischemic stroke. The fibrillating left atrium is not contracting and stasis of blood in the atrium leads to clot formation. The clot travels from the left atrium to the left ventricle and into the aorta before moving up the brachiocephalic artery to the common carotid artery; at this point, it is referred to as an embolism. The common carotid artery divides into the internal and external carotid artery. The clot travels up the internal carotid artery and then lodges in a section of the middle cerebral artery, causing ischemic stroke.

lower extremities, which predisposes to thrombus formation. Atrial fibrillation, which causes a noncontracting atrium, leads to stagnation of arterial blood in the left atrium. Stagnant blood tends to form arterial thrombi that then travel to the left ventricle, then to the aorta, and into any systemic artery. Commonly, an arterial thrombus from the left atrium travels up to the carotid arteries and into the brain, causing ischemic stroke (see Fig. 14-4).

High estrogen levels increase hepatic synthesis of coagulation factors and decreased antithrombotic factors, which is why oral contraceptives, the high estrogen levels of pregnancy, and the postpartum period are risk factors for the formation of a venous thrombus.

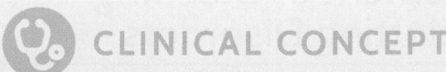

CLINICAL CONCEPT

The incidence of stroke, thromboemboli, and myocardial infarction is greater in women who use oral contraceptives, particularly those women aged 35 years and older and in those who smoke.

A hypercoagulability state is also common in cancer because tumor cells secrete prothrombotic substances. A reduction in the body's natural anticoagulants, antithrombin (AT) and protein C, predisposes to arterial and venous thromboses. Deficiencies of AT or protein C occur as genetic disorders. Elevated homocysteine levels, which occur along with a vitamin B deficiency, have also been associated with increased venous and arterial thrombi.

A condition called **antiphospholipid syndrome** is associated with formation of multiple clots. The cause of this disorder is unknown, but there is a high prevalence in persons with autoimmune disease. Antiphospholipid antibodies are found in the bloodstream, but it is unclear how the antibodies lead to formation of clots. In this syndrome, thrombosis can be precipitated by trauma, surgical procedures, use of drugs such as oral contraceptives, and abrupt withdrawal of anticoagulant drugs. Increased predisposition to formation of clots increases incidence of stroke, myocardial infarction, ischemia, and gangrene of the lower extremities. Glomerular and renal arterial clots often lead to renal failure. Women with antiphospholipid syndrome often have a history of recurrent pregnancy loss because of clotting of the placenta. In catastrophic antiphospholipid syndrome, multiple thrombotic events with resulting vascular occlusions occur simultaneously in the body over a period of days. Multiple organ infarctions can also occur—and are often fatal

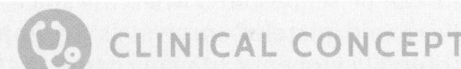

CLINICAL CONCEPT

Women with antiphospholipid syndrome tend to endure repeated miscarriages.

Bleeding Disorders

Bleeding disorders and impairment of blood clotting occur because of decreased platelet number, defects associated with platelets, coagulation factors, and vascular integrity (see Box 14-2). The normal number of platelets (150,000 to 450,000 cells/uL) must be severely depleted to levels between 10,000 and 20,000/uL before hemorrhagic problems or spontaneous bleeding arise.

Decreased Platelet Number and Activity

Thrombocytopenia can result from decreased platelet synthesis in the bone marrow, increased sequestering of platelets in the spleen, or decreased platelet life span. Dilutional thrombocytopenia can occur from multiple transfusions because blood stored for more than 24 hours has little or no platelets.

Decreased platelet production can result from suppression of bone marrow, as occurs in aplastic anemia, or from replacement of bone marrow by cancer cells, as in leukemia. Reduced synthesis of platelets can also occur

BOX 14-2. Conditions Associated With Increased Susceptibility to Bleeding

Conditions that decrease platelet number, diminish platelet activity, or cause defective coagulation can increase the blood's susceptibility to bleeding.

DECREASED PLATELET NUMBER OR ACTIVITY
- Aplastic anemia
- Cancer in the bone marrow
- Extracorporeal circulation
- Folate deficiency
- Hypersplenism
- Infections in the bone marrow (very rare)
- Myelodysplasia
- Renal failure
- Vitamin B_{12} deficiency
- Various medications

DEFECTIVE COAGULATION
- Cirrhosis (chronic liver disease)
- Hemophilia
- Vitamin K deficiency
- Von Willebrand disease

with human immunodeficiency virus (HIV) infection, exposure to radiation, or use of antineoplastic drugs.

There may be normal production of platelets with excessive pooling of platelets in the spleen. A majority of platelets can be sequestered when the spleen is enlarged. Decreased platelet survival is an important cause of thrombocytopenia. In many cases, premature destruction of platelets is caused by antiplatelet antibodies. Antibody-mediated platelet destruction occurs in idiopathic thrombocytopenic purpura (ITP). Decreased platelet survival may also occur as the result of mechanical injury associated with prosthetic heart valves or cardiopulmonary bypass surgery.

Impaired Platelet Activity

Acquired platelet dysfunction is common and usually caused by antiplatelet therapy agents or as a side effect of other drugs. Use of aspirin and other nonsteroidal anti-inflammatory drugs (NSAIDs) is the most common cause of impaired platelet function. Aspirin (acetylsalicylic acid) produces irreversible acetylation of platelet cyclooxygenase, the enzyme required for synthesis of the procoagulant, thromboxane A2, in inflammation. The antiplatelet effects of aspirin last for the life of the platelet, usually 7 to 10 days. The antiplatelet effects of other NSAIDs are reversible and last only for the duration of the drug action.

Acquired platelet dysfunction commonly occurs in renal failure. The high nitrogenous waste products in the bloodstream cause decreased platelet adhesion and lysis of the cells. Impaired platelet function may also result from inherited disorders of adhesion or acquired defects caused by drugs, disease, or extracorporeal circulation.

 CLINICAL CONCEPT

Aspirin prolongs bleeding time for up to 7 days and so it should be avoided for a week before surgery. Low doses of aspirin are recommended for the prevention of heart attack and stroke because they inhibit platelet aggregation.

Defective Coagulation

Impairment of blood coagulation can result from deficiencies of one or more of the known clotting factors. Deficiencies can arise because of defective synthesis, inherited defects, or increased consumption of the clotting factors. The most commonly known inherited disorders of coagulation are hemophilia A, hemophilia B, and von Willebrand disease. The most common acquired deficiency of coagulation factors occurs in liver disease, such as alcoholic cirrhosis. In defective coagulation, prolonged bleeding is provoked by injury or trauma. Large bruises, hematomas, or prolonged bleeding into the gastrointestinal or urinary tracts or joints are common. Head trauma can cause bleeding between the layers of the meninges, called a subdural hematoma.

Impaired Synthesis of Coagulation Factors. The coagulation factors are synthesized in the liver; therefore, clotting of blood depends on a healthy liver. In liver disease, such as cirrhosis, coagulation factors are not manufactured and bleeding often results. Some coagulation factors require vitamin K for normal function, which is why vitamin K deficiency can cause the liver to produce dysfunctional clotting factors. Vitamin K is a fat-soluble vitamin produced by intestinal bacteria. When the intestinal flora is disrupted as in broad spectrum antibiotic treatment, vitamin K is not produced and coagulation can be impaired. Impaired fat absorption caused by liver or gallbladder disease also leads to vitamin K deficiency and possible clotting dysfunction.

 CLINICAL CONCEPT

Vitamin K is administered to newborns because they have undeveloped intestinal flora to synthesize the vitamin.

Assessment of Bleeding and Clotting Disorders

The patient with a suspected bleeding or clotting disorder should have a complete history and physical examination. The clinician needs to ask specific questions regarding occurrences of nosebleeds, spontaneous bruising, or prolonged bleeding with trauma. The patient's body should be examined for any clues to bleeding susceptibility such as bruises. Clotting disorders are more difficult to assess because the effects of hypercoagulability are coronary, cerebrovascular, venous and peripheral arterial thromboses, or organ infarction.

History

Patient history can reveal risk factors of bleeding and clotting disorders. Patient medications should be reviewed because a multitude of drugs can cause thrombocytopenia (see Box 14-3). Vitamin K deficiency can diminish clotting ability. Oral contraceptives and estrogen can increase clotting risk.

Past medical history is important because cancer and other disorders can lead to clotting problems. Malignant tumors often secrete coagulation substances, leading to thrombi. Deep venous thrombi are common in patients with cancer. Venous stasis, peripheral arterial disease, atherosclerosis, and atrial fibrillation all increase susceptibility to clot formation. On the other hand, hematologic cancers of the bone marrow, such as leukemia, can inhibit the synthesis of platelets in the bone marrow and lead to bleeding. A recent viral or bacterial infection can be a catalyst for thrombocytopenia. Spleen, kidney, and autoimmune disease commonly cause platelet destruction. Liver disease can cause coagulation factor deficiency. Cushing's disease, Marfan's syndrome, Ehlers-Danlos disorder, and connective tissue diseases can all cause a tendency for bleeding that initially appears with bruising.

Women should be questioned about menorrhagia, excessive loss of blood at menses, as it is an initial symptom of von Willebrand disease. Pregnancy and the postpartum period are associated with hypercoagulability, and the formation of deep venous thromboses is common. Repeat miscarriages can indicate antiphospholipid syndrome, a disorder that causes multiple clots. Social habits such as smoking and alcohol abuse can contribute to coagulation disorders. Smoking increases coagulability, whereas alcohol abuse can lead to cirrhosis of the liver, resulting in decreased coagulation factors. Family history is important in assessment because many bleeding disorders have an inheritance pattern, including the X-linked recessive hemophilias.

Signs and Symptoms

During the physical examination, the clinician should look for signs of bleeding. Ecchymoses or large bruises may be the first symptom of platelet deficiency. Less remarkable bleeding such as petechiae or purpura may also be apparent (see Fig. 14-5). Spontaneous bleeding such as nosebleeds (epistaxis), bleeding from the gums, and abnormal vaginal bleeding can occur when platelet count decreases to fewer than 20,000 cells/uL. Other signs of bleeding to look for include excessive bleeding with trauma and occult bleeding from the gastrointestinal tract. In addition to signs of bleeding, the spleen may be enlarged because of increased activity.

BOX 14-3. Drugs Associated With Thrombocytopenia

There are a wide variety of drugs that can destroy platelets and decrease platelet number, including:

- Antidepressants
- Antiepileptic drugs
- Antihistamines
- Anti-inflammatory drugs
- Antimicrobials
- Antineoplastic drugs
- Benzodiazepines
- Cardiac medications and diuretics
- Gold salts
- Heparin
- Histamine-2 antagonists
- Illicit drugs, including cocaine and heroin
- Iodinated contrast agents
- Quinine/Quinidine group
- Retinoids
- Sulfonylurea drugs
- Miscellaneous drugs, including
  - Actinomycin-D
  - Aminoglutethimide
  - Danazol
  - Desferrioxamine
  - Levamisole
  - Lidocaine
  - Morphine
  - Papaverine
  - Tamoxifen
  - Ticlopidine.

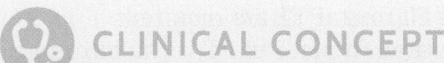

CLINICAL CONCEPT

Petechiae, pinpoint red-purple areas of bleeding that resemble a rash, can be the first sign of thrombocytopenia.

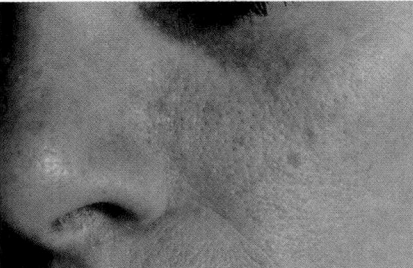

FIGURE 14-5. **Petechiae.** (From Dillon, P. (2007). *Nursing health assessment*. 2nd ed. Philadelphia, PA: F.A. Davis Company, with permission.)

Clotting disorders are more difficult to diagnose based on physical examination. Coronary and cerebrovascular thromboses, stroke, myocardial infarction, deep venous thrombosis, pulmonary embolism, and arterial thrombi of the extremities are the most common disorders associated with increased formation of clots. All of these disorders have a wide variety of symptoms and physical assessment findings.

Diagnosis

Complete blood count (CBC) with platelet count, peripheral blood smear, PT, and aPTT are all key components in the evaluation of the patient with a bleeding or clotting disorder. PT reflects the activity of coagulation factors I, II, V, VII, and X, which measures the integrity of the extrinsic pathway of coagulation. It also measures the clotting time from the activation of factor VII through the formation of the fibrin clot. The aPTT measures the function of factor XII through the fibrin clot in the intrinsic pathway.

Both PT and aPTT are measured in terms of seconds—the time it takes for the blood to clot. Both the PT and aPTT are based on normal values established by the laboratory. For PT, the normal range is 10 to 14 seconds. For the aPTT, the normal range is 30 to 40 seconds. The greater the patient's PT or aPTT compared with normal values, the longer it takes for the patient's blood to clot. Anticoagulants prolong the time it takes for blood to clot, and thereby hinder formation of clots. To acquire an anticoagulant therapeutic effect on the blood, the clinician aims for the PT and aPTT to be prolonged. For example, a clinician can administer an anticoagulant with the aim of prolonging clotting time to 2 times normal. Because normal PT is 10 to 14 seconds, the clinician would want to see the PT at 20 to 28 seconds to assure the therapeutic effect of the anticoagulant. It is important to recognize that a prolonged clotting time can lead to the undesired complication of bleeding. Therefore, when administering anticoagulants, frequent monitoring of PT and aPTT are required.

A test used in place of PT is the international normalized ratio (INR), which is a method of standardizing the measurement of clotting. The INR is calculated from the PT while avoiding the wide difference in normal ranges for PT. If a blood sample has an INR of 1, this indicates the blood has a normal clotting time. The greater the INR, the longer it takes for the blood to clot. For example, an INR of 3 indicates that the blood is taking 3 times the normal time to clot. A common target range for INR in anticoagulant use (e.g., warfarin) is 2 to 3. In some cases, if more intense anticoagulation is required, the target range may be as high as 3 to 4. Prothrombin time, aPTT, or INR laboratory tests are most commonly monitored when a patient is on anticoagulation medications. There are other specific laboratory tests that assist in diagnosis of clotting and bleeding disorders (see Table 14-1).

Treatment

There are various types of anticoagulants commonly used in clinical practice. Some agents inhibit platelet aggregation, whereas others block the activity of vitamin K. A few different agents work by impeding the steps of the coagulation cascade. Thrombolytic agents are used in emergency situations to travel directly to a clot and dissolve it.

Antiplatelet, Anticoagulation, and Thrombolytic Therapy

Antithrombotic drugs that decrease the body's ability to form clots include antiplatelet, anticoagulant, and thrombolytic agents. Thrombolytic agents are also called fibrinolytic agents or "clot-busters." Arterial and venous clots are major causes of morbidity and mortality. Arterial clots lead to obstruction of arterial blood supply, thereby causing ischemia and infarction of major organs. Stroke, myocardial infarction, and limb ischemia are the result of clots that form in arterial vessels. Deep venous thrombosis, a clot that forms in the deep veins of the lower extremity, can lead to pulmonary embolism, which is often fatal. Platelets, coagulation factors, and the endothelium of blood vessels interact to generate clots. Arterial clots are rich in platelets, whereas venous clots are predominately composed of fibrin and trapped red blood cells (RBCs). Thrombolytic agents are used to directly dissolve arterial or venous clots, such as obstructive coronary artery clots that cause myocardial infarction, cerebral clots that cause ischemic stroke, and venous clots that form pulmonary emboli.

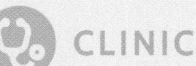 CLINICAL CONCEPT

Antiplatelet agents are the main agents used to prevent arterial clots, whereas anticoagulants are more effective to prevent venous clots. Thrombolytic agents are used to dissolve arterial or venous clots.

Antiplatelet Drugs

Platelets adhere to the exposed collagen surface of the injured endothelial lining of arterial vessels. They synthesize and release adenosine diphosphate (ADP) and thromboxane A2, which activate other circulating platelets and recruits them to the site of injury. Disruption of the endothelial lining also exposes tissue factor (TF), which initiates the coagulation cascade. Activated platelets bind to the coagulation factors for assembly of a thrombus that attracts more platelets, enhancing clot formation. When platelets are activated, the GPIIb/IIIa receptor on the platelet surface binds to fibrinogen and acts as a bridge between adjacent platelets, increasing the size of the clot. Antiplatelet drugs, which target different steps

TABLE 14-1. Common Laboratory Tests for Platelets, Coagulation Activity, and Bleeding Disorders

Lab Test	What Does It Measure?	Meaning of Abnormal Results
CBC	Counts and evaluates size and shape of platelets. RBCs, and white blood cells (WBCs). Proportions of the different types of WBCs in circulation. Measures hemoglobin (Hgb), hematocrit (Hct), and size and color of RBCs.	Decreased Hgb/Hct indicates anemia. Increased WBCs indicates inflammation or infection. Decreased platelet number indicates increased bleeding tendency.
D-dimer	Measures fibrin degradation products.	If elevated, indicates recent clotting activity may be caused by acute or chronic condition, such as a thromboembolism or DIC or pulmonary embolism.
Fibrin degradation products	Reflects clotting activity.	If increased, indicates recent blood clot formation and breakdown.
Fibrinogen	Reflects clotting ability and activity.	If low, may indicate decreased production or increased use of fibrinogen; may be elevated with infection and inflammation.
aPTT	Measures time to clot; evaluates the intrinsic pathway of coagulation cascade.	Prolonged aPTT suggests need for further tests. May indicate: • Coagulation factor deficiency • Inhibition of factor VIII • Nonspecific inhibitor, such as lupus anticoagulant • Patient on heparin.
Platelet aggregation	Evaluates platelet's ability to adhere and form clumps.	If abnormal, there is an increased risk of excessive bleeding; may indicate presence of one of several disorders such as von Willebrand disease.
PT	Measures time to clot; evaluates the extrinsic pathway of coagulation cascade.	Most common use is monitoring warfarin anticoagulant therapy. Prolonged PT may suggest need for further tests. May be elevated in inherited or acquired coagulation disorders.

in the process of platelet aggregation, include aspirin, clopidrogrel (Plavix®), dipyridamole (Aggrenox®), and GPIIb/IIIa receptor antagonists (Abciximab [Reopro®]). Aspirin is the most commonly used antiplatelet medication; it is recommended in small doses of 70 to 150 mg daily to prevent myocardial infarction.

In cases where there are an excessive number of platelets, such as essential thrombocytosis, medications such as hydroxyurea are used to suppress platelet production by the bone marrow. In cases of severe life-threatening thrombocytosis, a procedure called platelet pheresis is performed to immediately lower the platelet count to safer levels. In this procedure, blood is removed from the patient, platelets are removed, and blood is returned to the patient.

Anticoagulant Drugs
There are parenteral and oral forms of anticoagulants. Parenteral agents include standard heparin, **low molecular weight heparin (LMWH),** and fondaparinux (Arixtra®). The oral anticoagulants include warfarin (Coumadin®), dabigatran (Pradaxa®), and rivaroxaban (XareltoR).

Heparin. **Heparin** acts as an anticoagulant by activating anti-thrombin (AT), the body's natural clot dissolving substance. It acts to limit the extension of a clot, though it does not prevent clot formation. It can be administered intravenously or subcutaneously.

Heparin binds to plasma proteins in circulation, which causes reduced anticoagulant activity. Because levels of plasma proteins vary from person to person, heparin has an unpredictable anticoagulant response. The blood level of heparin has to be individually titrated for each patient and careful coagulation monitoring is essential. Subtherapeutic levels predispose the patient to additional clot formation, whereas excessive levels subject the patient to bleeding episodes.

The aPTT lab test monitors heparin activity. Antifactor X levels can also be used to monitor heparin therapy.

For prophylaxis of clot formation, heparin is usually given in small fixed doses subcutaneously 2 to 3 times a day. In contrast, when a clot already exists, much higher therapeutic doses are administered intravenously. Heparin takes time to rise to a therapeutic level, and frequent monitoring of its level in the bloodstream is required. Therapeutic heparin dose is based on a control aPTT (approximately 30 to 40 seconds), and the aim is to keep heparin at a level that maintains aPTT 2 to 3 times the control value.

There are some drawbacks to using heparin. It has an unpredictable anticoagulant response, it requires constant monitoring, and it takes time to reach therapeutic levels in the blood. Also, side effects include thrombocytopenia, osteoporosis, elevated liver enzymes, and bleeding. However, a positive feature is that protamine sulfate can be used to neutralize heparin if bleeding occurs.

Low Molecular Weight Heparin. LMWH, which consists of small fragments of heparin, exerts its anticoagulant effect by activating AT. It binds to plasma proteins, but not as strongly as standard heparin; this allows LMWH to have a more predictable anticoagulant response. It can be administered, usually subcutaneously, once or twice a day without coagulation monitoring.

There are fixed dosages recommended for venous versus arterial clots. LMWH has a shorter half-life and fewer side effects than standard heparin.

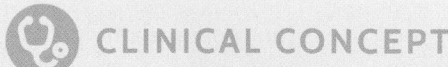

CLINICAL CONCEPT

If bleeding occurs in a patient on standard heparin, the antidote, protamine sulfate, is necessary. To counteract bleeding in a patient on low molecular weight heparin, simply stopping the drug is all that is necessary.

Fondaparinux. Fondaparinux (Arixtra®) causes factor Xa inhibition, which inhibits prothrombin from forming thrombin. It is a subcutaneous agent given once daily and is used most commonly for thromboprophylaxis in general surgical and high-risk orthopedic patients. It produces a predictable anticoagulant effect after administration in fixed doses because it does not bind to plasma protein. It has few side effects.

Dabigatran (Pradaxa^R) is a direct thrombin (also called factor IIa) inhibitor that is given orally. It is used to prevent stroke in patients with atrial fibrillation that is not caused by a heart valve disorder. Venous thrombi are also inhibited by dabigatran and perioperative administration is common. Its effects last 24 hours and it does not require monitoring of INR, PT, or PTT. However, a drawback of this category of drug is that its effect is not easily reversed.

Rivaroxaban (Xarelto®) is an oral factor Xa inhibitor that is well absorbed from the gastrointestinal tract and peaks approximately 4 hours after a dose. It is recommended for nonvalvular atrial fibrillation and can prevent arterial and venous clots. The effects of rivaroxaban can last up to 24 hours and once daily dosing is recommended. It does not require monitoring of INR, PT, or PTT. A drawback of this category of drug is that its effects cannot be easily reversed as warfarin.

Vitamin K Antagonists. Warfarin (Coumadin®) is a vitamin K antagonist that interferes with the synthesis of the vitamin K-dependent clotting factors prothrombin, factor VII, IX, and X. Warfarin is almost completely absorbed by the gastrointestinal tract, and levels peak in the blood about 90 minutes after drug administration.

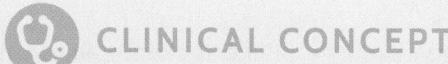

CLINICAL CONCEPT

Oral anticoagulants, such as warfarin, require frequent monitoring of PT or INR. Genetic factors that involve liver metabolism may make some individuals require smaller doses of warfarin. Fluctuations in dietary vitamin K intake can also affect warfarin level.

A wide variety of drugs and various disease states can modify the anticoagulant effect of warfarin, so close monitoring of warfarin level is necessary. PT has been the lab test used to monitor warfarin levels in the past, but the INR is preferable. When using the PT test, the normal value is approximately 10 to 14 seconds, and for adequate anticoagulation, the aim is to keep the PT between 1.5 to 2 times the normal value. For example, if a patient's normal PT is 12 seconds and warfarin is administered to inhibit clotting, a PT value of 18 to 24 seconds would be considered in therapeutic range. When using the INR laboratory test, the aim is to keep the therapeutic level between 2 and 3 times the normal value of 1 for adequate coagulation. An INR of 2 or 3 would be therapeutic.

Warfarin is usually started at a dose of 5 to 10 mg; when at the therapeutic level, monitoring is advised every 2 to 3 weeks. The major side effect is bleeding, and it is contraindicated in pregnancy. A rare complication is skin necrosis of the body's fatty areas. Bleeding can be reversed by administering vitamin K.

Thrombolytic Agents

Thrombolytic agents can be used to dissolve thrombi. They can be administered systemically or be delivered via catheters directly into the thrombus. Systemic delivery is used in acute myocardial infarction, acute ischemic stroke, and pulmonary emboli. The goal is to dissolve the clot and reestablish blood flow.

Commonly used thrombolytic agents include streptokinase, urokinase, and recombinant tissue-type plasminogen activator, also known as alteplase. All of these agents convert plasminogen to plasmin, and plasmin then degrades the fibrin matrix of a thrombus. With ischemic stroke, ideally, the goal is to treat the patient in less than 3 to 4 hours from the time of the acute event. Thrombolytic therapy is indicated in patients with evidence of ST segment elevation myocardial infarction (STEMI) or new left bundle branch block presenting within 12 hours of the onset of symptoms if there are no contraindications to fibrinolysis.

Pathophysiology of Selected Coagulation Disorders

There are some important disorders that cause bleeding because of thrombocytopenia. These include drug-induced thrombocytopenia, heparin-induced thrombocytopenia (HIT), immune thrombocytopenic purpura (ITP), and **thrombotic thrombocytopenic purpura (TTP).** Hemophilia and von Willebrand disease (vWD) also cause bleeding, but in these disorders the bleeding is caused by coagulation factor problems. Disseminated intravascular coagulation (DIC) is severe malfunction of the coagulation system, which causes unpredictable episodes of both bleeding and clotting.

Drug-Induced Thrombocytopenia

Drug-induced thrombocytopenia has been associated with more than 1,500 medications, with heparin, antimalarial drugs, and sulfonamides being some of the most common causes of the disorder. Because there are so many drugs associated with thrombocytopenia, all drugs should be suspect in a patient without another apparent cause of thrombocytopenia. Herbal and over-the-counter medications are included as possible causes.

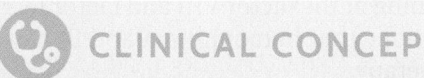

> ### CLINICAL CONCEPT
>
> Often drug-induced thrombocytopenia is misdiagnosed as autoimmune disease because the drugs induce antigen-antibody reactions.

Typically, a patient will have taken the offending drug for about 1 week or intermittently over a longer period before presenting with petechial hemorrhages and purpura that are indicative of thrombocytopenia. Occasionally, symptoms develop within 1 or 2 days after the first exposure to a drug. Platelet count can decrease to levels of 20,000 or lower. Systemic symptoms such as lightheadedness, chills, fever, nausea, and vomiting often precede bleeding symptoms. Severely affected patients have epistaxis or bleeding from the gums, gastrointestinal tract, or urinary tract. If the causative medication is stopped, symptoms usually resolve within 2 days, and the platelet count returns to normal in less than a week.

Heparin-Induced Thrombocytopenia

HIT is different from thrombocytopenia induced by other drugs because it is not associated with bleeding, but it is paradoxically associated with increased risk of thrombosis. The disorder results from the development of an antibody to heparin. Some individuals who develop the antibody do develop low platelet count, but the majority develop clots. HIT can occur with standard heparin or LMWH and develops after approximately 5 to 10 days after exposure. Thrombi can develop in the arterial or venous vessels. Direct thrombin inhibitors are used as treatment of HIT.

Immune Thrombocytopenic Purpura

Immune thrombocytopenic purpura, also called ITP, is one of the most common autoimmune disorders. It is caused by autoantibodies that develop against platelets. The antigenic target in most patients appears to be the platelet GPIIb/IIIa complex. The complex is attacked by IgG antibodies, and these platelet-antibody complexes are phagocytosed by macrophages and destroyed by the spleen.

Acute ITP is more common in children and usually follows a viral infection. It is characterized by sudden onset of petechiae and purpura and is a self-limited disorder with no treatment. In contrast, a chronic form of the disorder is usually seen in adults, with a peak incidence between ages 20 and 50 years; it is usually seen twice as often in women as it is in men. It may be associated with other immune disorders such as acquired immune deficiency syndrome or systemic lupus erythematosus.

ITP is a diagnosis of exclusion; all other possible diagnoses should be investigated, particularly drug-induced thrombocytopenia. The condition presents with signs of bleeding, such as petechiae, purpura, bleeding from gums, epistaxis, and abnormal menstrual bleeding. Because the spleen is the site of platelet destruction, splenic enlargement may occur. Hemorrhage represents the most serious complication; intracranial hemorrhage is the most lethal. Diagnosis usually is based on severe thrombocytopenia (fewer than 20,000 cells/mL) and exclusion of other causes. Treatment includes use of corticosteroid drugs, IV immunoglobulin (IVIg), platelet transfusion, and the use of immunosuppressive drugs. Splenectomy may be necessary.

Thrombotic Thrombocytopenic Purpura

TTP is a combination of thrombocytopenia, hemolytic anemia, thrombotic vascular occlusions, fever, and neurological abnormalities. In TTP there is a deficiency of metalloproteases that act on vWF. The persistence of unmodified vWF causes platelet adhesion and aggregation. The exact etiology of TTP is unclear. For unknown reasons, TTP is common in persons with HIV infection, as well as pregnant women.

The onset is abrupt and the outcome can be fatal. Widespread vascular occlusions consist of clots in arterioles and capillaries of many organs, including the heart, brain, and kidneys. Erythrocytes become fragmented as they circulate through the partly occluded vessels and cause hemolytic anemia. The clinical manifestations include purpura, petechiae, and neurological symptoms ranging from headache to seizures and altered consciousness.

Although the etiology of TTP is unknown, the initiating event seems to be widespread endothelial damage and activation of intravascular thrombosis. Toxins produced by certain strains of *E. coli* (*E. coli* O157:H7) are a trigger for endothelial damage and an associated condition called hemolytic-uremic syndrome (HUS) that is characterized by acute renal failure, hemolytic anemia, and thrombocytopenia.

Treatment for TTP includes plasmapheresis, a procedure that involves removal of the blood's plasma portion and replacement with fresh frozen plasma; this treatment is continued until remission occurs. With plasmapheresis, there is a complete recovery in 80% to 90% of cases.

Hemophilia

There are two forms of hemophilia based on the deficiency of a specific coagulation factor. Hemophilia A is caused by deficiency of factor VIII, whereas hemophilia B is caused by lack of factor IX. Both are X-linked, recessive disorders that primarily affect males. Women carry the trait for either disease but do not suffer the bleeding problems. Hemophilia A is the more common form, comprising 80% of hemophilia cases. Both diseases have similar pathophysiologic mechanisms and symptoms because of a deficient or dysfunctional coagulation factor.

Hemophilia A is mainly a hereditary disorder, but there is no familial history of the disorder in approximately 30% of newly diagnosed cases. Approximately 90% of persons with hemophilia A produce insufficient quantities of factor VIII, with the remaining 10% producing a defective form of factor VIII. There is a wide spectrum of the severity of disease, with up to 50% affected by mild hemophilia.

In mild or moderate forms of the disease, bleeding usually does not occur unless trauma provokes it. The mild disorder may not be detected in childhood. In severe hemophilia, bleeding can be spontaneous. Characteristically, bleeding occurs in soft tissue, the gastrointestinal tract, and the hip, knee, elbow, and ankle joints. Bleeding into muscle tissue can compress arteries and veins and cause compartment syndrome. Joint bleeding usually begins when a child begins to walk. After a joint is affected, the joint is commonly subjected to repeated bleeding, causing inflammation of the synovium with acute pain and swelling. Without proper treatment, chronic bleeding and inflammation can cause joint fibrosis and contractures, resulting in major disability. Bleeding into the oropharyngeal spaces, central nervous system, or retroperitoneum can be fatal and requires immediate treatment.

When hemophilia is a known familial disorder, carrier detection and prenatal diagnosis should be done. Diagnosis of the disease involves complete blood cell (CBC) count, coagulation studies, a factor VIII assay for hemophilia A, and a factor IX assay for hemophilia B. The hemoglobin/hematocrit are usually normal or low values. Platelet counts are normal. On coagulation studies, the PT, which assesses the extrinsic coagulation pathway, is normal, whereas the aPTT, which assesses the intrinsic coagulation pathway, is prolonged.

Factor VIII replacement therapy is initiated when bleeding occurs or as prophylaxis in hemophilia A. Factor IX is the replacement treatment for persons with hemophilia B. Recombinant factor VIII and recombinant factor IX are synthetic forms of the coagulation factors, and these are the preferred treatments to reduce the risk of transmitting HIV or other viruses from donor pools of coagulation factors. Although donor pools of coagulation factors are screened, there is a slight risk of contamination with HIV or hepatitis infection. For this reason, individuals with hemophilia should receive the hepatitis B vaccine.

Desmopressin acetate (DDAVP), which is a synthetic analog of vasopressin, may be used to prevent bleeding in persons with mild hemophilia A. This synthetic vasopressin stimulates the release of vWF, a carrier of factor VIII, from the endothelium, thus increasing factor VIII levels 2-fold to 3-fold for several hours.

The cloning of the factor VIII and factor IX genes has led to the hope that hemophilia A and B may be cured by gene therapy.

Essential Thrombocytosis

Essential thrombocytosis (ET; also called primary thrombocythemia) is a rare, chronic disorder of the bone marrow. It is a disorder of megakaryocyte proliferation that increases the number of circulating platelets. The excess of platelets increases susceptibility to clot formation. However, many of the excessive platelets do not function; consequently, there can be an increased susceptibility to bleeding. The disorder causes a platelet count greater than 600,000/µL, splenomegaly, and a tendency for coagulation or bleeding episodes.

Epidemiology

There is an incidence of approximately 6,000 cases of ET each year in the United States. ET is more frequent in older patients with a median age at diagnosis of 60 years. Both sexes are affected equally. Death commonly occurs from clotting episodes that lead to myocardial infarction or stroke. For unclear reasons, some patients with ET develop the complication of acute myelogenous leukemia (AML).

Etiology/Pathophysiology

There is no known etiology of ET. The presence of a gene mutation called *JAK2* on chromosome 9p is present in 50% of patients with ET. The significance of this gene mutation is unclear but it is found in syndromes that cause hyperproliferation of blood cells. In ET there is an excessive number of platelets; some show less ability to aggregate, which leads to susceptibility to bleeding. Other platelets show hyperaggregation tendencies, which leads to clot formation.

Clinical Presentation

Approximately 25% to 33% of patients with ET are asymptomatic at diagnosis. Most symptomatic patients present with clots in small or large blood vessels. However, some patients may present with bleeding because of dysfunctional platelets. There are neurological symptoms that include headache and paresthesias of the fingers and toes. Some patients suffer ischemia of the fingers and toes that causes burning and erythema, a condition called erythromelalgia. Patients often report symptoms associated with transient ischemic attacks caused by clots that lodge in a cerebral artery. Symptoms of TIAs include unsteadiness, vertigo, dizziness, syncope, seizures, and dysarthria.

Clots in the large veins and arteries are common and may result in occlusion of the leg, coronary, and renal arteries. Clots can also develop in the splenic, hepatic, leg, and pelvic veins. Pulmonary hypertension can result because of clotting in the pulmonary vasculature. In contrast, the gastrointestinal tract, gums, urinary tract, joints, and brain are susceptible to bleeding. Patients also report fever, diaphoresis, and pruritus. ET is also known to cause complications during pregnancy such as an increase in spontaneous abortions, ischemia of the placenta, intrauterine growth retardation, and fetal death.

Diagnosis

A CBC count is necessary for the diagnosis of ET. An unexplained, excessive number of platelets is noted on the CBC. There may also be an excessive number of WBCs and RBCs. On bone marrow biopsy, megakaryocytic hyperplasia is common. The PT and aPTT studies are usually within reference ranges. The bleeding time may or may not be prolonged. Blood chemistry studies reveal elevated uric acid (UA) levels in 25% of patients at diagnosis. CT scan or ultrasound of the spleen may reveal splenomegaly.

Treatment

Medications that inhibit megakaryocyte maturation into platelets are used in ET. Some medications include hydroxyurea, anagrelide, interferon alfa, and phosphorous-32 (^{32} P). Low-dose aspirin may be useful in treating patients with symptoms of microvascular clotting. In emergencies, plateletpheresis, a procedure that removes excess platelets from the bloodstream, may be useful if there is severe thrombocytosis. Lifestyle modifications are also recommended such as weight loss for obese patients and smoking cessation for smokers.

von Willebrand Disease

vWD is a genetic disorder transmitted as an autosomal trait that causes a deficiency of or defect of vWF. vWF is a protein that connects platelets to the endothelial lining of blood vessels and binds to factor VIII of the coagulation cascade. vWF deficiency causes decreased platelet adhesion and reduced levels of active factor VIII, which result in defective clot formation.

Epidemiology

vWD has an incidence of approximately 125 persons per million. Males and females are equally affected; however, females have a more evident course of disease because vWD causes severe menstrual bleeding. vWD presents as a spectrum from mild to severe forms of the disorder.

Etiology/Pathophysiology

The etiology of vWD is a gene mutation on the short arm of chromosome 12. The gene is expressed in megakaryocytes and endothelial cells. vWF functions to enhance platelet aggregation and platelet adhesion to endothelium, and stops the degradation of factor VIII. Consequently, without vWF there is defective hemostasis and lack of factor VIII, which increases the patient's susceptibility to bleeding and hemorrhage.

Clinical Presentation

Symptoms of vWD include easy bruising, excessive menstrual blood loss, and bleeding from the nose, mouth, and gastrointestinal tract. Many persons are unaware of the disorder until a surgical or dental procedure results in abnormally prolonged bleeding.

Diagnosis

In order to diagnose vWD, laboratory tests need to demonstrate a deficiency of vWF. This may be difficult to obtain as many conditions can stimulate production of vWF. Stress, estrogen, growth hormone, and vasopressin can stimulate vWF and increase amounts in the blood. The patient's amount of vWF can fluctuate, so obtaining an accurate result can be difficult. Laboratory tests include PT, aPTT, factor VIII activity, and concentration of vWF antigen in the bloodstream (vWF:Ag). The aPTT is usually prolonged because of low levels of factor VIII.

Treatment

Most cases of vWD are mild and do not require treatment. In severe cases, factor VIII products that contain vWF are infused to replace the deficient clotting factors. The disorder is also treated with Desmopressin (DDAVP), a synthetic form of vasopressin, which stimulates the endothelial cells to release vWF and plasminogen activator.

Hemolytic-Uremic Syndrome

HUS is a disorder that causes progressive renal failure, hemolytic anemia, and thrombocytopenia. HUS is the most common cause of acute renal failure in children and is increasingly occurring in adults. There are two forms of the disorder: shiga-toxin-producing HUS (Stx-HUS) and non-shiga-toxin-producing HUS (non-Stx-HUS).

Epidemiology

Stx-HUS is the more common form of the disease, with an incidence of 0.5 to 2.1 cases per 100,000 persons per year. However, in children younger than 5 years, the incidence is 6.1 cases per 100,000 persons per year. Non-Stx-HUS accounts for 5% to 10% of all cases of HUS, and the incidence in children is about one-tenth that of Stx-HUS.

Etiology

In North America and Western Europe, 70% of cases of Stx-HUS are caused by *Escherichia coli* serotype O157:H7. In Asia and Africa, HUS is often caused by Stx-producing *Shigella dysenteriae* serotype 1. *Streptococcus pneumoniae* infection accounts for 40% of all cases of non-Stx-HUS in the United States. Other causes of non-Stx-HUS include other strains of bacteria, viruses, fungi, drugs, malignancies, vaccinations, transplantation, pregnancy, and other underlying medical conditions such as antiphospholipid syndrome and systemic lupus erythematosus (see Box 14-4).

Pathophysiology

E. coli O157:H7 is one of many strains of the rod-shaped bacterium *E. coli*. Although most strains are harmless and live in the intestines of healthy humans and animals, *E. coli* O157:H7 produces a powerful toxin (called Stx) and is considered an enterohemorrhagic strain of *E. coli*. *E. coli* O157:H7 is found in the environment and in animal intestines, particularly cattle. Most illness is caused by ingestion of contaminated produce, water, or undercooked meat. Other sources include unpasteurized milk and juice and contact with infected live animals. Waterborne transmission can occur by swimming in contaminated lakes or pools, or drinking inadequately treated water. Flies have been shown to carry *E. coli* O157:H7 as well. The organism is easily transmitted from person to person via the fecal-oral route and has caused epidemics in child day-care centers.

Once ingested the *E. coli* O157: H7 bacterium closely adheres to the mucosal lining of the human intestine. It irritates the intestinal mucosa and causes a bloody, diarrheal illness. When in the bloodstream, the *E. coli*

BOX 14-4. Etiologies of Hemolytic Uremic Syndrome

Causes of Stx-HUS include bacterial infections, viral infections, and vaccinations.

BACTERIAL INFECTIONS
- *Campylobacter jejuni*
- *E. coli* O157:H7
- *Legionella pneumophila*
- *Mycoplasma* species
- *Neisseria meningitidis*
- *S. dysenteriae*
- *S. pneumoniae*
- *Salmonella typhi*
- *Yersinia pseudotuberculosis*

VIRAL INFECTIONS
- Coxsackievirus
- Echovirus
- Epstein-Barr virus
- Herpes simplex virus
- HIV
- Influenza virus

VACCINATIONS
- Influenza triple-antigen vaccine
- Polio vaccine
- Typhoid-paratyphoid A and B (TAB) vaccine

Causes of non-Stx-HUS syndrome include conditions, disorders, and medications. No cause is identified in about 50% of all cases of sporadic non-Stx-HUS.

CONDITIONS AND DISORDERS
- Allogenic hematopoietic cell transplantation
- Cancers, chiefly mucin-producing adenocarcinomas
- Collagen-vascular disorders, such as systemic lupus erythematosus and antiphospholipid antibody syndrome
- Malignant hypertension
- Pregnancy and postpartum period
- Primary glomerulopathies
- Transplantation

MEDICATIONS
- Anticancer agents, including mitomycin, cisplatin, bleomycin, and gemcitabine
- Antiplatelet agents, including ticlopidine and clopidogrel
- Chemotherapeutic agents, including mitomycin-C, cisplatin, bleomycin, gemcitabine, carmustine, oxaliplatin, pentostatin, bevacizumab, and sunitinib
- Immunotherapeutic agents, including cyclosporine and tacrolimus
- Oral contraceptives
- Quinine

O157:H7 toxin directly damages endothelial cells and binds to WBCs. The toxin causes the lysis of RBCs and formation of arteriolar and capillary microthrombi. The route by which the toxin is transported from the intestine to the kidney is unclear.

Clinical Presentation

The patient usually reports gastroenteritis, fever, and bloody diarrhea for 2 to 7 days. Patients should be questioned about recent foods eaten and sources of the food. The patient needs to recall ingestion of any raw foods, untreated water, or recent association with sick individuals. The source of the gastroenteritis is not always clear. The disorder causes abdominal pain, dehydration, fatigue, and a very low urine output. Acute renal failure is diagnosed soon after infection. The physical findings commonly include hypertension, edema, lethargy, and pallor.

Diagnostic Tests

In the diagnosis of HUS, a urinalysis will reveal mild proteinuria and hematuria. Blood urea nitrogen and serum creatinine may be high, which indicate renal insufficiency. On the peripheral blood smear, fragmented RBCs are seen, as well as thrombocytopenia. Bilirubin levels may be elevated because of a large amount of hemoglobin breakdown. Stool culture should be done to check for *E. coli* O157:H7 and *Shigella* bacteria.

Study of kidney tissue will reveal the characteristic findings of HUS: obstructive microthrombi of the capillaries and arterioles in the kidney. These are small clots that cause ischemia and infarctions of renal tissue.

Treatment

Supportive therapy, the major form of treatment, includes maintenance of fluid and electrolyte balance, blood-pressure control, and dietary protein restriction. If diarrhea is severe, parenteral nutrition may be necessary. Between 20% and 40% of patients develop seizures, so prophylactic treatment with phenytoin (Dilantin®) may be necessary.

Antibiotics are used if the patient is septic, in which case azithromycin may be effective. If end-stage renal disease (ESRD) develops, hemodialysis and renal transplantation are recommended.

Treatment of non-Stx-HUS requires plasma exchange (also called plasmapheresis) early in the course of the disease. In plasma exchange, the patient's plasma component of blood is removed and replaced with donor plasma. Plasma exchange treatment should be started within the first 24 hours of the patient's illness and then continued once or twice a day for at least 2 days after complete recovery. Aspirin to inhibit platelet aggregation is used in combination with plasma exchange.

In *S. pneumoniae* non-Stx-HUS plasma treatment is contraindicated. Renal transplantation is not an option for non-Stx-HUS because there is a 50% recurrence rate in the transplanted kidney and 90% chance of transplant failure.

Disseminated Intravascular Coagulation

DIC is a disorder of both clot formation and bleeding episodes in critically ill patients. There is active formation of fibrin clots with simultaneous depletion of coagulation factors and platelets. In addition, there is suppression of fibrinolysis. The resultant clinical condition is characterized by episodes of both coagulation and hemorrhage. The patient unpredictably begins to form clots, which can lead to ischemia of organs. The patient also undergoes random periods of spontaneous bleeding.

Epidemiology

DIC occurs in 30% to 50% of patients with sepsis. It can occur in all races and affects males and females equally. The presence of DIC can double the risk of death in sepsis. In cases of major trauma, the occurrence of DIC doubles the mortality rate.

Etiology

DIC occurs in critically ill patients and is a complication of a wide number of conditions (see Box 14-5). It is most commonly observed in patients with sepsis and septic

---

BOX 14-5. Conditions Associated With DIC

There are many types of conditions that can trigger DIC. These include obstetric disorders, cancers, infections, shock, transfusion reactions, trauma, or surgery.

CANCER
- Leukemia
- Metastatic cancer

HEMATOLOGIC CONDITIONS
- Blood transfusion reactions

INFECTIONS
- Acute bacterial infections such as meningococcal meningitis
- Acute viral infections
- Rickettsial infection such as Rocky Mountain spotted fever
- Parasitic infection such as malaria

OBSTETRIC CONDITIONS
- Abruptio placenta
- Dead fetus syndrome
- Pre-eclampsia or eclampsia
- Amniotic fluid embolism

SHOCK
- Septic shock
- Severe hypovolemic shock

TRAUMA OR SURGERY
- Burns
- Massive trauma
- Surgery involving extracorporeal circulation
- Snake bite
- Heatstroke

shock. Sepsis, caused by both gram-positive and gram-negative organisms, is commonly associated with DIC; however, other organisms—including viruses, fungi, and parasites—may cause DIC as well. In infections caused by gram-negative bacteria, endotoxins released from the bacteria activate both the intrinsic and extrinsic pathway of coagulation. In addition, endotoxins inhibit the anticoagulant activity of protein C. In obstetrical conditions, particularly those involving shock, hypoxia, acidosis, and fetal death can provoke DIC. Other clinical conditions that can trigger DIC include massive trauma, burns, shock, meningococcemia, and malignant disease.

Pathophysiology

The main mechanisms of DIC are uncontrolled synthesis of thrombin, suppression of anticoagulant mechanisms, and abnormal fibrinolysis. Together, these abnormalities lead to excessive fibrin deposition in small and mid-sized blood vessels. The fibrin deposition in blood vessels obstructs the blood supply to organs, particularly the lungs, kidneys, and brain, with consequent organ failure. Persistent activation of coagulation results in the depletion of clotting factors and platelets, which, in turn, leads to bleeding. Further aggravation of bleeding occurs because of increased fibrinolysis. The coagulation system is severely dysfunctional in DIC, swinging from extreme clotting activity to severe anticoagulant activity.

Clinical Presentation

Although coagulation and formation of microemboli may characterize DIC in the initial phase, its most harmful effects are more directly related to the bleeding problems that occur. The bleeding may be present as petechiae, purpura, oozing from puncture sites, severe hemorrhage, or uncontrolled postpartum bleeding. Cardiovascular shock is a common complication. Microthrombi may obstruct blood vessels and cause ischemia and infarction of the kidneys, heart, lungs, and brain. As a result, renal, circulatory, or respiratory failure can occur.

Diagnosis

Platelet counts are moderately to severely reduced in DIC. Hemolytic anemia can develop as RBCs become damaged when passing through vessels obstructed by thrombi. The peripheral blood smear can demonstrate evidence of abnormally shaped RBCs caused by hemolysis. Fibrinolysis is also an important feature of DIC, and fibrin breakdown is demonstrated by elevations in the D-dimer lab test, the most sensitive lab test for DIC. Clotting times (both aPTT and PT) are elevated. AT levels as well as individual coagulation factors are diminished in DIC.

Treatment

To treat DIC, it is necessary to control the primary disease, replace clotting factors, and prevent further activation of clotting mechanisms. Transfusions of fresh frozen plasma, platelets, or fibrinogen-containing cryoprecipitate may correct the clotting factor deficiency. Heparin may be given to decrease blood coagulation, thereby interrupting the clotting process. The use of antifibrinolytic agents may reduce bleeding episodes, and protein C concentrates can be effective.

Chapter Summary

- Platelet formation is stimulated by the hormone thrombopoietin, which is synthesized by the liver.
- The normal platelet count is 150,000 to 450,000 cells/uL, and their life span is 7 to 10 days.
- Almost one-third of all platelets reside in the spleen; when enlarged and hyperactive, the spleen can sequester up to 80% of platelets.
- Numerous GP receptors (GPIIb/IIIa) on the surface of a platelet assist in clot formation. Some antiplatelet agents work as GPIIb/IIIa receptor blockers to diminish platelet aggregation.
- The activated platelet surface provides the major physiologic site for coagulation factor activation.
- Coagulation factors are produced in the liver and require vitamin K.
- Clots formed because of stasis of blood or endothelial injury are created via the intrinsic pathway.
- Clots formed because of external trauma to a blood vessel are created via the extrinsic pathway.

- Acquired deficiencies of coagulation are the most frequently encountered disorders in the clinical area. Causes include liver disease, vitamin K deficiency, and DIC.
- The most common hereditary bleeding disorder is hemophilia. In these disorders, blood coagulation is hindered. Bleeding can be occult, as in gastrointestinal blood loss, or apparent, as in traumatic hemorrhage.
- Many different drugs can cause thrombocytopenia.
- In platelet dysfunction or deficiency, lesions such as petechiae may be seen on physical examination. Spontaneous bleeding can occur as bruises, nosebleeds, bleeding from the gums, or vaginal bleeding.
- Hypercoagulability of the blood causes susceptibility to clotting. Clots can occlude blood vessels and cause tissue ischemia, infarction, or gangrene. Stroke, myocardial infarction, peripheral arterial disease, deep venous thrombosis, and pulmonary embolism are all caused by blood clots.

- The INR is a standard measurement of clotting. If a blood sample has an INR of 1, this indicates normal clotting. The greater the INR, the longer it takes for the blood to clot.
- For adequate anticoagulation, an INR should be maintained between 2 and 3.
- The greater the patient's PT or aPTT compared with normal values, the longer it takes for the patient's blood to clot, which can increase risk for bleeding.
- Aspirin is commonly used to decrease platelet aggregation.

- Protamine sulfate is a heparin antagonist.
- Vitamin K antagonizes warfarin.
- Patients on anticoagulants should avoid eating green leafy vegetables.
- Disseminated intravascular coagulation, where the coagulation system dysfunctions and causes both clotting and bleeding, can occur in critically ill patients, particularly those who are septic.

 Making the Connections

Pathophysiology	Signs and Symptoms	Physical Assessment Findings	Diagnostic Tests	Treatment
Immune Thrombocytopenic Purpura (ITP) | Antibody destruction of platelets triggered by an antigen because of an unknown cause. The antigenic target appears to be the platelet GPIIb/IIIa complex. The complex is attacked by IgG antibodies.				
	Purpura. Petechiae. Mucosal bleeding. Ecchymoses. GI bleeding. Heavy menstrual blood loss.	Mucocutaneous bleeding, ecchymoses, gastrointestinal or excessive menstrual bleeding. Retinal hemorrhages possible.	Decreased platelet count. Peripheral smear may show enlarged platelets. Iron deficiency may be present. Serum protein electrophoresis and immunoglobulin levels to detect possible hypogammaglobulinemia, and a direct antiglobulin test (also called Coomb's test).	Corticosteroid, IV immunoglobulin, immunosuppressive agents.
Thrombotic Thrombocytopenic Purpura (TTP) | Deficiency of or antibodies to metalloproteases that cleave vWF. The persistence of vWF causes platelet adhesion and aggregation.				
	Petechiae and purpura of lower extremities. Fever. Anemia. Renal injury or failure. Neurological dysfunction such as confusion or coma.	Petechiae and purpura of lower extremities. Fever.	Decreased platelet count caused by platelet adhesion. Hemolysis. Microvascular thrombosis. Increased bilirubin caused by breakdown of RBCs. Increased reticulocyte count caused by increased bone marrow activity to replace lysed RBCs Negative direct antiglobulin test. Peripheral smear has schistocytes, which are odd-shaped RBCs caused by hemolysis.	Plasma exchange, immunomodulatory medications, splenectomy, glucocorticoids.

Continued

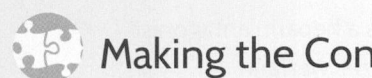 Making the Connections–cont'd

Pathophysiology	Signs and Symptoms	Physical Assessment Findings	Diagnostic Tests	Treatment
Drug-Induced Thrombocytopenia | Antibody attack on platelets in presence of certain drugs.				
	Petechiae. Purpura.	Petechiae. Purpura.	Decreased platelet count and antibodies to drug metabolites.	Stop medications.
Hemolytic-Uremic Syndrome (HUS) | Renal failure, hemolytic anemia, thrombocytopenia commonly preceded by *E. coli* O157:H7 infection.				
	Fever, abdominal pain, pale skin, fatigue and irritability, bruising or bleeding of nose and mouth, reduced urination, edema.	Hx of diarrheal illness caused by *E. coli* O157:H7; may have blood in urine because of large amount of hemolysis; bloody diarrhea.	Decreased platelet count, normal aPTT, and normal PT; low RBC caused by hemolysis; high bilirubin caused by RBC breakdown. Stool culture for *E. coli* O157:H7. Increased serum creatinine caused by renal insufficiency and renal failure.	Supportive treatment with dialysis, plasma exchange may be used.
Essential Thrombocytosis | High platelet number because of an unknown cause.				
Secondary Thrombocytosis is almost always caused by iron deficiency; inflammation, cancer, or infection; or underlying myelodysplastic disorder. The patient may have had a splenectomy.				
	May have no symptoms. When symptoms do appear, they can be caused by abnormal blood clotting and cause stroke, heart attack, or deep venous thrombosis.	May have no physical assessment abnormalities. Possible signs include stroke, heart attack, or deep venous thrombosis.	Increased platelet count. May have low iron, low serum ferritin, or high total iron-binding capacity indicating iron deficiency anemia. Erythrocyte sedimentation rate and C-reactive protein may be elevated because of inflammation. Bone marrow shows excessive platelets. Splenectomy may be evident through imaging studies.	Aspirin or antiplatelet drugs. Plateletpheresis.
von Willebrand Disease | A major adhesion molecule that ties platelets to exposed endothelial tissue. Hereditary and involves diminished vWF protein, decreased function of vWF, and decreased factor VIII levels.				
	Excessive bleeding caused by trauma, surgical procedures, or at menses.	Excessive bruising or bleeding with minor trauma, spontaneous nosebleeds, bleeding from gums, or menorrhagia.	CBC, decreased platelet count, aPTT, and PT show prolonged bleeding time. Diminished vWF.	Desmopressin acetate, which releases vWF and factor VIII from endothelial stores. vWF replacement. Antifibrinolytic agents.

Continued

Making the Connections–cont'd

Pathophysiology	Signs and Symptoms	Physical Assessment Findings	Diagnostic Tests	Treatment
Disseminated Intravascular Coagulation (DIC) | Secondary to another disease. Overactivation of the clotting mechanism. Commonly caused by sepsis.				
	Petechiae. Purpura. Hematomas. Shortness of breath. Severe pain in back, chest, and muscles Vomiting.	Clotting and bleeding occur at the same time. Severe hypotension.	Increased PT, increased aPTT, CBC. Increased fibrin-split products. Decreased fibrinogen. D-dimer level increased.	Fresh frozen plasma transfusion for bleeding (has most amount of coagulation factors), heparin, fibrinolytic drugs for excessive clotting, and treatment underlying disease.
Hemophilia A | Genetic disorder; lack of factor VIII causes decreased clotting ability.				
	Bruises. Nosebleeds. Gum bleeds. Hemarthrosis.	Bleeding, pain, skin, and oral mucosa; history of bleeding, infections, or controlling bleeding.	Normal PT. Increased PTT. Normal platelet count. Decreased factor VIII levels.	Factor VIII transfusion until bleeding stops; genetic counseling.
Hemophilia B | Genetic disorder; lack of factor IX causes decreased clotting ability.				
	Bruises. Nosebleeds. Gum bleeds. Hemarthroses.	Bleeding, pain, skin, and oral mucosa; history of bleeding, infections, or controlling bleeding.	Normal PT. Increased PTT. Normal platelet count. Decreased factor VIII levels.	Factor IX transfusion until bleeding stops; genetic counseling.

Bibliography

Achterbergh, R., Vermeer, H. J., Curtis, B. R., et al. (2012). Thrombocytopenia in a nutshell. *Lancet, 379*(9817), 776.

Alpert, J. S. (2012). New directions in anticoagulation. *Am J Med*, 125(3), 217–218. doi: 10.1016/j.amjmed.2011.11.002.

Argulian, E. (2013). Atrial fibrillation and acute myocardial infarction: antithrombotic therapy and outcomes. *Am J Med*, 126(5), e19. doi: 10.1016/j.amjmed.2012.09.017.

Baruch, L. (2013). Laboratory monitoring of anticoagulant medications: focus on novel oral anticoagulants. *Postgrad Med*, 125(2), 135–145. doi: 10.3810/pgm.2013.03.2647.

Berntorp, E., & Shapiro, A. D. (2012). Modern haemophilia care. *Lancet*, 379(9824), 1447–1456.

Binder, W. D., Traum, A. Z., Makar, R. S., & Colvin, R. B. (2010). Case records of the Massachusetts General Hospital. Case 37-2010. A 16-year-old girl with confusion, anemia, and thrombocytopenia. *N Engl J Med*, 363(24), 2352–2361.

Carrier, M., Khorana, A. A., Moretto, P., et al. (2014). Lack of evidence to support thromboprophylaxis in hospitalized medical patients with cancer. *Am J Med*, 127(1), 82–86.e1. doi: 10.1016/j.amjmed.2013.09.015. Epub 2013 Oct 5.

Connolly, S. J., Eikelboom, J., Joyner, C., et al. (2011). Apixaban in patients with atrial fibrillation. *N Engl J Med*, 364(9), 806–817.

Connolly, S. J., Ezekowitz, M. D., Yusuf, S., et al. (2009). Dabigatran versus warfarin in patients with atrial fibrillation. *N Engl J Med, 361*(12), 1139–1151.

Crownover, B. K., Sleuwen, L., Carls, C., & Ketterman, B. (2010). Diagnosing von Willebrand disease. *Am Fam Phys*, 81(12), 1415–1418.

CURRENT-OASIS 7 Investigators, Mehta, S. R., Bassand, J. P., Chrolavicius, S., et al. (2010). Dose comparisons of clopidogrel and aspirin in acute coronary syndromes. *N Engl J Med*, 363(10), 930–942.

Decousus, H., Prandoni, P., Mismetti, P., et al. (2010). Fondaparinux for the treatment of superficial-vein thrombosis in the legs. *N Engl J Med, 363*(13), 1222–1232.

Deedwania, P. C. (2013). New oral anticoagulants in elderly patients with atrial fibrillation. *Am J Med*, 126(4), 289–296.

EINSTEIN Investigators, Bauersachs, R., Berkowitz, S. D., Brenner, B., et al. (2010). Oral rivaroxaban for symptomatic venous thromboembolism. *N Engl J Med*, 363(26), 2499–2510.

Gafter-Gvili, A., Mansur, N., Bivas, A., Zemer-Wassercug, N., Bishara, J., Leibovici, L., & Paul, M. (2011). Thrombocytopenia in *Staphylococcus aureus* bacteremia: risk factors and prognostic importance. *Mayo Clin Proceed*, 86(5), 389–396.

Gauer, R. L., & Braun, M. M. (2012). Thrombocytopenia. *Am Fam Phys*, 85(6), 612–622.

George, J. N. (2010). Management of immune thrombocytopenia—something old, something new. *N Eng J Med*, 363(20), 1959–1961.

Hemmelgarn, B. R., Moist, L. M., Lok, C. E., et al. (2011). Prevention of dialysis catheter malfunction with recombinant tissue plasminogen activator. *N Engl J Med*, 364(4), 303–312.

Hunt, B. J. (2014). Bleeding and coagulopathies in critical care. *N Engl J Med*, 370(9), 847–859. doi: 10.1056/NEJMra1208626.

Hylek, E. M. (2010). Therapeutic potential of oral factor Xa inhibitors. *N Engl J Med*, 363(26), 2559–2561.

Imbach, P., & Crowther, M. (2011). Thrombopoietin-receptor agonists for primary immune thrombocytopenia. *N Engl J Med*, 365(8), 734–741.

Kaandorp, S. P., Goddijn, M., van der Post, J. A., et al. (2010). Aspirin plus heparin or aspirin alone in women with recurrent miscarriage. *N Engl J Med*, 362(17), 1586–1596.

Kallistratos, M. S., Poulimenos, L. E., & Manolis, A. J. (2014). New oral anticoagulants and the risk for intracranial hemorrhage. *JAMA Neurol*, 71(3), 370–371. doi: 10.1001/jamaneurol.2013.5963.

Kar, A. (2012). Making hemophilia a global priority. *Lancet*, 380(9838), 216–217.

Kimmel, S. E., French, B., Kasner, S. E., et al. (2013). A pharmacogenetic versus a clinical algorithm for warfarin dosing. *N Engl J Med*, 369(24), 2283–2293. doi: 10.1056/NEJMoa1310669. Epub 2013 Nov 19.

Komócsi, A., Vorobcsuk, A., & Aradi, D. (2013). New oral anticoagulants in acute coronary syndromes: what does a meta-analysis tell us?—Reply. *JAMA Intern Med*, 173(9), 835. doi: 10.1001/jamainternmed.2013.424.

Kuter, D. J., Rummel, M., Boccia, R., et al. (2010). Romiplostim or standard of care in patients with immune thrombocytopenia. *N Engl J Med*, 363(20), 1889–1899.

Lassen, M. R., Gallus, A., Raskob, et al. (2010). Apixaban versus enoxaparin for thromboprophylaxis after hip replacement. *N Engl J Med*, 363(26), 2487–2498.

Lip, G. Y., Laroche, C., Dan, G. A., et al. (2014). 'Real-world' antithrombotic treatment in atrial fibrillation: the EURObservational Research Programme Atrial Fibrillation General Pilot survey. *Am J Med*, Jan 28. pii: S0002-9343(14)00069-2. doi: 10.1016/j.amjmed.2013.12.022. Epub ahead of print.

Maag, R. L., & Chuang, C. H. (2013). Uncommon complications of heparin-induced thrombocytopenia. *Am J Med*, 126(11), e5–e6. doi: 10.1016/j.amjmed.2013.06.032.

McCrae, K. (2011). Immune thrombocytopenia: no longer 'idiopathic'. *Cleveland Clin J Med*, 78(6), 358–373.

Mitka, M. (2012). New anticoagulants offer options beyond warfarin to reduce stroke risk. *JAMA*, 308(17), 1727–1728. doi: 10.1001/jama.2012.14623.

Mitka, M. (2014). Another novel oral anticoagulant matches warfarin. *JAMA*, 311(3), 233–234. doi: 10.1001/jama. 2013.284833.

New oral anticoagulants for acute venous thromboembolism. *JAMA*, 311(7), 731–732. doi: 10.1001/jama.2014.202.

Nurden, A. T. (2011). Sustaining platelet counts in chronic ITP. *Lancet*, 377(9763), 358–360.

Olah, Z., Bereczky, Z., Szarvas, M., & Boda, Z. (2011). Coagulation: cascade! *Lancet*, 378(9792), 740.

Padrini, R., & Pengo, V. (2010). Dosing of clopidogrel and aspirin in acute coronary syndromes. *N Engl J Med*, 363(25), 2465–2466.

Prophylaxis versus episodic treatment to prevent joint disease in boys with severe hemophilia. Manco-Johnson M. J., Abshire, T. C., Shapiro, A. D., Riske, B., Hacker, M. R., Kilcoyne, R., Ingram, J. D., Manco-Johnson, M. L., Funk, S., Jacobson, L., Valentino, L. A., Hoots, W. K., Buchanan, G. R., DiMichele, D., Recht, M., Brown, D., Leissinger, C., Bleak, S., Cohen, A., Mathew, P., Matsunaga, A., Medeiros, D., Nugent, D., Thomas, G. A., Thompson, A. A., McRedmond, K., Soucie, J. M., Austin, H., Evatt, B. *N Engl J Med*. 2007 Aug 9;357(6): 535–44.

PROTECT Investigators for the Canadian Critical Care Trials Group and the Australian and New Zealand Intensive Care Society Clinical Trials Group, Cook, D., Meade, M., Guyatt, G., et al. (2011). Dalteparin versus unfractionated heparin in critically ill patients. *N Engl J Med*, 364(14), 1305–1314. Epub 2011 Mar 22.

Provan, D., & Newland, A. C. (2011). Guidelines for immune thrombocytopenia. *N Engl J Med*, 364(6), 580–581.

Punnoose, A. R., Lynm, C., & Golub, R. M. (2012). *JAMA* patient page. Hemolytic uremic syndrome. *JAMA*, 307(10), 1098.

Reiffel, J. A. (2014). Novel oral anticoagulants. *Am J Med*, 127(4), e16–e17. doi: 10.1016/j.amjmed.2013.06.004.

Ruiz-Irastorza, G., Crowther, M., Branch, W., & Khamashta, M. A. (2010). Antiphospholipid syndrome. *Lancet*, 376(9751), 1498–1509.

Sarosiek, S., Crowther, M., & Sloan, J. M. (2013). Indications, complications, and management of inferior vena cava filters: the experience in 952 patients at an academic hospital with a level I trauma center. *JAMA Intern Med*, 73(7), 513–517. doi: 10.1001/jamainternmed.2013.343.

Siasos, G., Tousoulis, D., & Stefanadis, C. (2011). CYP2C19 genotype and outcomes of clopidogrel treatment. *N Engl J Med*, 364(5), 481–482.

Slichter, S. J., Kaufman, R. M., Assmann, S. F., et al. (2010). Dose of prophylactic platelet transfusions and prevention of hemorrhage. *N Engl J Med*, 362(7), 600–613, 637.

Teachey, D. T. (2010). Dabigatran versus warfarin for venous thromboembolism. *N Engl J Med*, 362(11), 1050–1051.

Thachil, J., Fitzmaurice, D. A., & Toh, C. H. (2010). Appropriate use of D-dimer in hospital patients. *Am J Med*, 123(1), 17–19. doi: 10.1016/j.amjmed.2009.09.011.

Toth, P. P. (2013). Stroke prevention in patients with atrial fibrillation: focus on new oral anticoagulants. *Postgrad Med*, 125(3), 155–161. doi: 10.3810/pgm.2013.05.2670.

Visser, J., Cohen, D., & Bloemenkamp, K. W. (2010). Antithrombotic medications and recurrent miscarriage. *N Engl J Med*, 363(9), 887–888.

Wanat, M. A. (2013). Novel oral anticoagulants: a review of new agents. *Postgrad Med*, 125(4), 103–114. doi: 10.3810/pgm.2013.07.2683.

Wechsler, L. R. (2011). Intravenous thrombolytic therapy for acute ischemic stroke. *N Engl J Med*, 364(22), 2138–2146.

Wells, P. S., Forgie, M. A., & Rodger, M. A. (2014). Treatment of venous thromboembolism. *JAMA*, 311(7), 717–728. doi: 10.1001/jama.2014.65.

Winkelmayer, W. C. (2011). Tackling the Achilles' heel of hemodialysis. *N Engl J Med*, 364(4), 372–374.

Yawn, B., Nichols, W. L., & Rick, M. E. (2009). Diagnosis and management of von Willebrand disease: guidelines for primary care. *Am Fam Phys*, 80(11), 1261–1268.

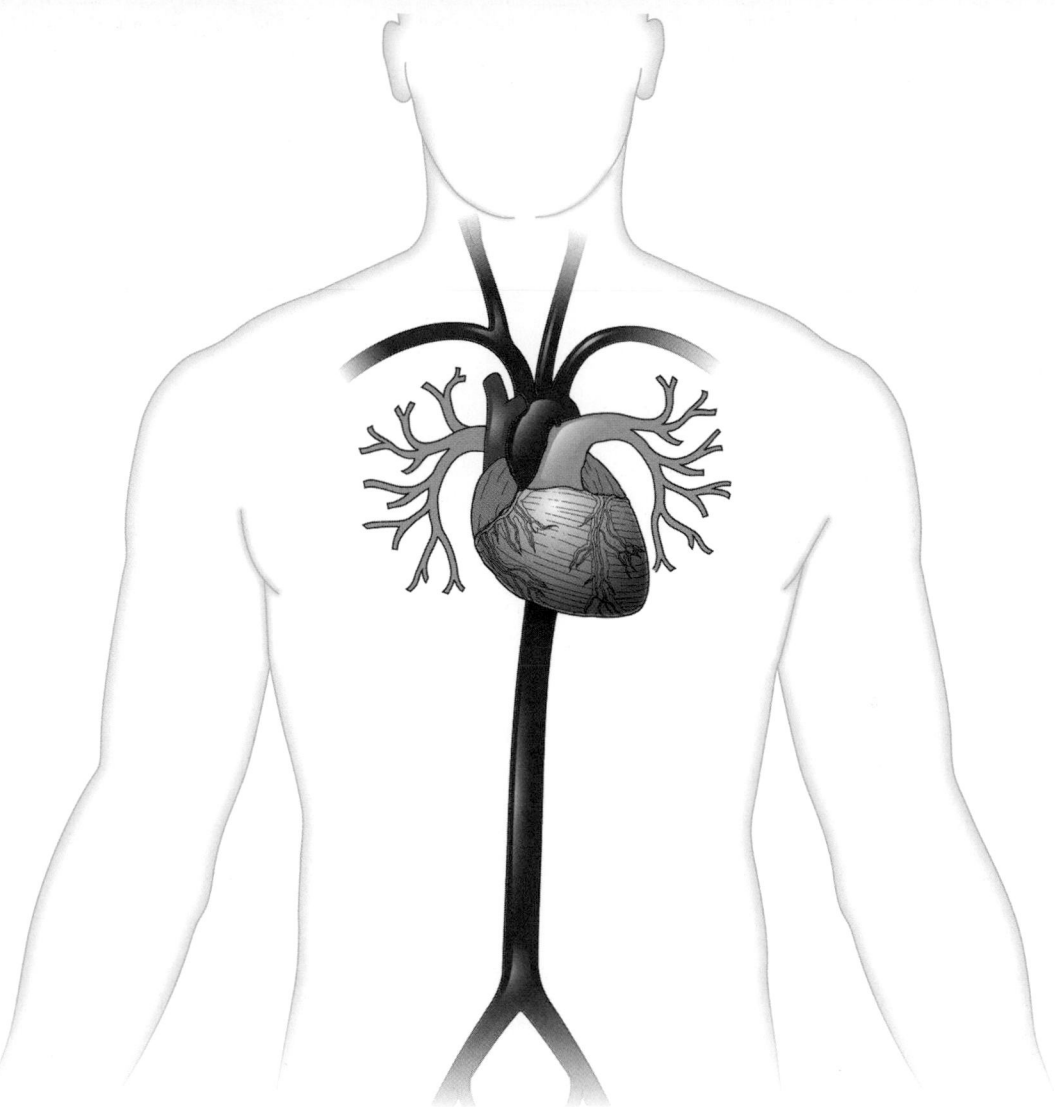

UNIT 6
DISORDERS OF CARDIOVASCULAR FUNCTION

Chapters

Arterial Disorders

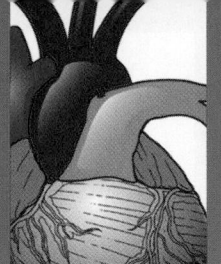

Key Terms

Aneurysm

Ankle-brachial index (ABI)

Artery

Atherosclerosis

Baroreceptor

Cardiac output (CO)

Cholesterol

Diastole

Endothelium

High-density lipoprotein (HDL)

Hyperlipidemia

Hypertension (HTN)

Intermittent claudication

Low-density lipoprotein (LDL)

Natriuresis

Peripheral arterial disease (PAD)

Pulse pressure

Renin

Renin-angiotensin-aldosterone system (RAAS)

Stroke volume (SV)

Systole

Triglyceride

The arterial system is composed of large- and medium-sized arteries and arterioles. **Arteries** are muscular-walled blood vessels with large amounts of elastic fibers. The elasticity of the arteries allows them to contract and dilate according to the body's needs. The heart's pumping action is reflected in the arteries—there is a large volume of blood pumped through the arteries with the heart's contraction; when the heart relaxes, the volume within the arteries rests. Arteries direct blood out of the heart to the tissues of the rest of the body, thereby supplying the tissues with oxygenated blood and nutrients. A key concept to understand is that the greater the pressure of blood within the arteries and arterioles, the higher the resistance against the heart pump. The main artery that arises from the heart is the aorta, the body's largest and most muscular arterial vessel.

Basic Physiologic Concepts of Arterial Structure and Function

Cardiovascular health depends mainly on the heart and the arteries. The arteries are muscular blood vessels that maintain blood pressure (BP) throughout the body. Their composition is significant because their inner lining, called **endothelium,** undergoes key changes that predispose individuals to **atherosclerosis.** The muscular walls of the arteries respond to autonomic impulses that signal blood flow needs. Pulsations in the arteries are reflective of the heart's contractile function. To assess heart function, the pulses of the radial, carotid, and brachial arteries are most commonly used. Blood flow and BP are largely regulated by sensors in the arterial walls. Blood constituents such as lipids, glucose, nicotine, and others can affect the artery's reactivity and

undermine the health of the endothelium. Understanding the artery's structure and function is fundamental to full comprehension of the workings of the cardiovascular system.

The Composition of the Arterial Wall

Artery walls are composed of three layers (see Fig. 15-1):

1. **Tunica intima:** The innermost layer of the artery wall. It is composed of a thin layer of endothelial cells that lie adjacent to each other and have contact with the blood. The endothelium is a smooth, contiguous surface of cells that blankets all the inner linings of the arteries. The endothelium is a metabolically active tissue that releases substances, reacts to chemical mediators, and responds to blood contents.
2. **Tunica media:** The middle layer of the artery wall. It is composed of smooth muscle that can constrict and dilate to change the artery's diameter. The smooth muscle is innervated by autonomic nerves, which are the sympathetic, also called adrenergic, and parasympathetic, also called cholinergic, nerve fibers. There are alpha-adrenergic and beta-adrenergic nerves. Alpha-adrenergic nerve fibers are excitatory and cause vasoconstriction, whereas beta-adrenergic fibers are inhibitory and cause vasodilation. The vascular smooth muscle relies on extracellular calcium for depolarization. Calcium enters membrane channels to evoke contraction and vasoconstriction.
3. **Tunica externa:** The outermost covering of the artery wall; it is also called the tunica adventitia. It is largely composed of connective tissue that provides support for the artery.

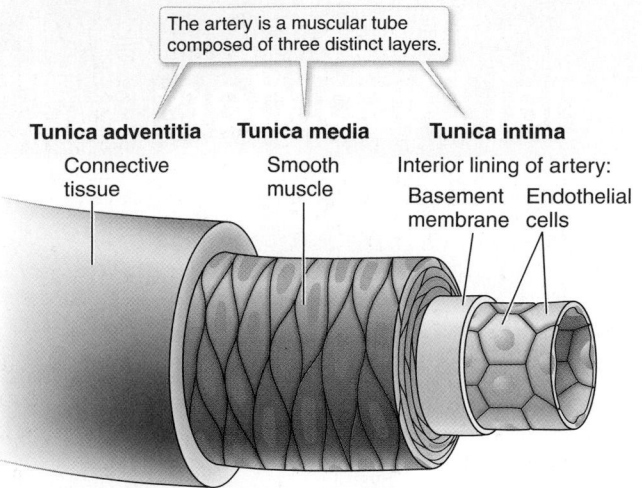

The artery is a muscular tube composed of three distinct layers.

Tunica adventitia
Connective tissue

Tunica media
Smooth muscle

Tunica intima
Interior lining of artery:
Basement membrane
Endothelial cells

FIGURE 15-1. The three layers of arteries: tunica intima (endothelium), tunica media (smooth muscle), and tunica adventitia (outer connective tissue).

CLINICAL CONCEPT

Calcium channel blocker (CCB) medications block vasoconstriction of arteries.

The Endothelium as Active Tissue

The endothelium is composed of a blanket of endothelial cells, which are specialized squamous epithelial cells. These cells line the interior surface of arteries, from the heart to the smallest arterioles and capillaries. The endothelium forms an interface between the blood and the artery walls. The endothelium of the interior surfaces of the heart chambers is called the endocardium.

Endothelial cells have distinct metabolic functions, including fluid filtration, maintenance of blood vessel tone, hemostasis, angiogenesis (the formation of new blood vessel growth), neutrophil chemotaxis, and hormone secretion. The endothelium acts as a semipermeable barrier between the vessel lumen and surrounding tissue, controlling the passage of biochemical substances and the transit of white blood cells (WBCs) into and out of the bloodstream. Endothelial cells also produce nitric oxide (NO), which stimulates dilation of blood vessels, and endothelin, which provokes constriction of vessels.

To stimulate angiogenesis, endothelial cells produce vascular endothelial growth factor (VEGF). Collateral branches of arterioles form in response to VEGF. When blood volume is excessive, endothelial cells produce C-type natriuretic peptide to diurese the body and allow excretion of excess water. Substances that oppose each other are produced by the endothelium. Prostacyclin (PG12), which breaks down clots, and thromboxane A2 (TXA2), which enhances clot formation, are also secreted by the endothelial cells. In some organs, there are highly differentiated endothelial cells that perform

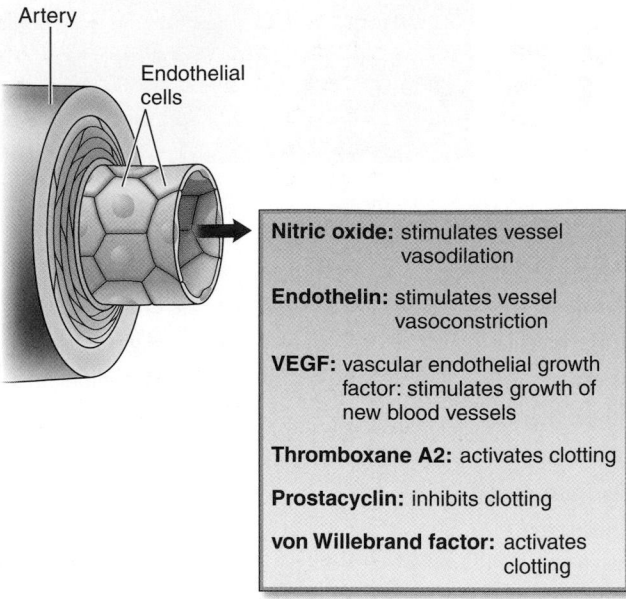

Artery

Endothelial cells

Nitric oxide: stimulates vessel vasodilation

Endothelin: stimulates vessel vasoconstriction

VEGF: vascular endothelial growth factor: stimulates growth of new blood vessels

Thromboxane A2: activates clotting

Prostacyclin: inhibits clotting

von Willebrand factor: activates clotting

FIGURE 15-2. The endothelium is a metabolically active tissue. It can secrete chemical mediators that activate vasodilation, vasoconstriction, clotting, and new growth of blood vessels. It can also secrete factors that inhibit clotting.

filtering functions. Examples of such unique endothelial structures include the renal glomerulus and the blood-brain barrier.

Endothelial injury causes endothelial dysfunction, which is the key early event in the development of atherosclerosis. Endothelial injury incites the inflammation reaction, which brings WBCs to the site of damage. The WBCs engulf and phagocytose lipids in the region and form lipid-laden macrophages called foam cells. There is also lack of release of nitric oxide, which decreases blood vessel vasodilation capability. Simultaneously, there is release of excessive quantities of von Willebrand factor, which promotes platelet aggregation and adhesion to the endothelial surface. These reactions together provide the elements for vascular dysfunction and atherosclerotic plaque construction (see Fig. 15-2).

CLINICAL CONCEPT

Dysfunctional endothelium is seen in patients with coronary artery disease (CAD), diabetes mellitus, hypertension, and hypercholesterolemia, as well as in smokers.

Blood Flow Regulation

In the cardiovascular system, the arteries are the most influential structures in control of blood flow. The arteries are vessels of high volume, high pressure, and high or low resistance, depending on their state of vasoconstriction or vasodilation. The elements of volume, pressure, and resistance regulate the blood flow through the arteries. Optimal circulatory function requires volume that fills the blood vessel and pressure to move the blood into all areas of body tissues. Pressure of blood flow is determined by the difference between the two ends of a vessel. In the arterial system, large areas of artery diameter gradually feed into smaller areas of artery diameter. Blood flow is inversely related to the diameter of the blood vessel. When blood flows from a larger area of vessel diameter to a smaller area of vessel diameter, pressure increases in the vessel. Resistance is the amount of obstruction to blood flow caused by vessel diameter, vessel length, and blood viscosity, which is the thickness of the fluid caused by the particles in solution. In the bloodstream, this is fairly constant. The relation of pressure, resistance, and blood flow is expressed in the equation:

Blood flow = Pressure of blood/
Resistance of blood

In the circulatory system, blood flow is analogous to **cardiac output (CO),** which is the amount of blood that flows from the heart's left ventricle per minute. The pressure of blood is the arterial BP, which measures the force against the walls of arteries as the heart pumps blood through the body. The resistance is the total peripheral vascular resistance (PVR) caused by the blood vessels within the circulatory system. The mathematical calculation of blood flow is:

CO = BP /PVR

Varying mathematical relationships can be inferred from this equation:

CO = BP /PVR can also be expressed
as CO × PVR = BP

How BP changes in relation to CO and PVR can be seen using mathematical relationships. If BP is constant and PVR increases, then CO decreases. If blood vessel diameter decreases, PVR increases. If PVR is increased, BP increases. If PVR is constant and BP increases, then CO increases. If CO is constant and PVR increases, then BP increases.

Blood flow normally is laminar, which means that the flow is smooth and parallel to the horizonal lines of the vessels. This allows a smooth, low friction flow of blood where blood cells and constituents flow in a streamlined central axis through the vessel. In areas where the endothelium is not smooth, injured, or inflamed, blood flow tends to become turbulent. Turbulent blood flow causes areas of blood to move perpendicular to vessel walls and predisposes to small areas of stagnant blood (see Fig. 15-3). The nonstreamlined and stagnant movement of blood causes blood constituents, such as RBCs, WBCs, platelets, and coagulation factors, to come in contact with the arterial endothelial lining. The stasis of blood and stimulation of endothelium predisposes to thrombus (clot) formation. Areas of turbulence often occur in damaged and arteriosclerotic sections of artery walls; therefore, these areas are predisposed to thrombus formation.

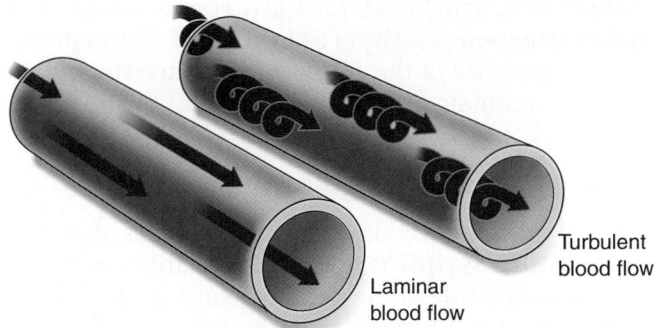

FIGURE 15-3. Laminar versus turbulent blood flow in a blood vessel.

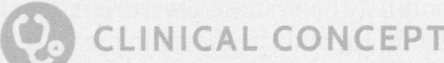

CLINICAL CONCEPT

Turbulent blood flow often produces whooshing sounds called bruits that can be heard through the stethoscope.

Arterial Wall Tension

In a blood vessel, wall tension is the force in the vessel wall that opposes the distending pressure inside the vessel. The internal pressure expands the vessel until it is inhibited by the tension in the vessel wall. The smaller the vessel's radius, the greater the pressure needed to overcome wall tension. Laplace's law is used to express the effect of the radius on wall tension:

Intraluminal pressure = Tension/Radius
or tension = Pressure × radius

or

P = T / r or T = P × r

Wall tension is also inversely related to wall thickness: The thicker the vessel wall, the lower the tension, and vice versa. This can be expressed as the following mathematical equation:

Tension = Pressure × radius / wall thickness

or

T = P × r / wall thickness

In **hypertension (HTN),** arterial vessel walls hypertrophy and become thicker, thereby reducing the tension and minimizing the wall stress. Laplace's law can be applied to the pressure required to maintain the patency of small blood vessels. When the thickness of the vessel wall remains constant, it takes more pressure to overcome wall tension and keep the vessel open as its radius decreases in size. There is a critical pressure where the vessels collapse and blood can no longer flow through them.

Distention and Compliance

Compliance is defined as the total quantity of blood that can be accommodated by a given part of the circulatory system for each millimeter rise in pressure. Compliance is the distention capacity of a blood vessel. The high distention capacity of the aorta and large arteries allows them to accommodate the high output of the heart.

Blood Pressure Regulation

Arterial BP is a reflection of the cardiac cycles of systole and diastole. **Systole** is the period of cardiac contraction, and **diastole** is the period of cardiac relaxation. In the arteries, BP rises when the left ventricle contracts in systole and ejects blood from the chamber. This is followed by the decline of blood pressure, and the left ventricle ends its contraction in diastole. In healthy adults, the systolic pressure is ideally lower than 120 mm Hg and the diastolic pressure is ideally lower than 80 mm Hg. Numerous research investigations such as The Framingham Heart Study have demonstrated that when systolic and diastolic pressure are maintained at these values, there is a diminished risk of cardiovascular disease (CVD) (see Box 15-1). The difference between the systolic and diastolic arterial BP is called the **pulse pressure,** which ideally is approximately 40 mm Hg.

In a healthy adult, approximately 70% of blood is ejected from the left ventricle during systole; this volume ejected per contraction is called the **stroke volume (SV).** Within the left ventricle, there is approximately 100 mL of blood and 70% of this volume is ejected; therefore, SV is approximately 70 mL.

The average heart rate (HR) is 70 beats per minute. Mathematically, one can multiply SV by HR to obtain the volume of blood per minute ejected from the left ventricle. The volume of blood ejected by the left ventricle per minute is the cardiac output. Therefore, SV multiplied by HR is equal to CO (SV × HR = CO). In the healthy adult, 70 mL of SV × 70 heart beats /minute = 4,900 mL blood/minute (approximately 5 liters).

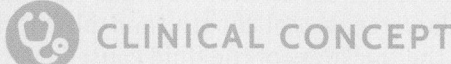

CLINICAL CONCEPT

Normal CO is approximately 5 liters blood/minute.

The systolic and diastolic components of BP are determined by CO and PVR. This is mathematically expressed as BP = CO x PVR. The PVR is mainly influenced by the diameter of the arterial blood vessel. The diameter is regulated by the autonomic nervous system innervation of the smooth muscle wall of the artery and arteriole. Arteries and arterioles are frequently referred to as resistance vessels because they constrict or relax to control the outflow of blood into the capillaries. Mathematical relationships of blood pressure, cardiac output, and PVR can be expressed as:

$$CO \times PVR = BP$$

or

$$CO/BP = PVR$$

or

$$CO = BP/PVR$$

CO is determined by BP and PVR. The body has to adjust PVR and BP inversely to maintain cardiac output. For example, to maintain CO when BP decreases, the body has to raise total peripheral resistance by arterial vasoconstriction.

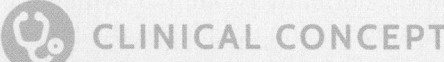

CLINICAL CONCEPT

As PVR increases, BP and CO increase. As PVR decreases, BP and CO decrease.

Baroreceptor: Neural Mechanisms of Blood Pressure Regulation

Short-term regulation of BP is aimed at correcting temporary imbalances that occur when the body changes position or endures exercise. The cardiovascular regulation center in the brain is in the lower pons and medulla, where modulation of the autonomic nervous system occurs. The center transmits sympathetic and parasympathetic signals to the heart and blood vessels. The parasympathetic impulses are transmitted via the vagus nerve to the heart and blood

---

BOX 15-1. The Framingham Heart Study

In 1948, the Framingham Heart Study under the direction of the National Institutes of Health began as a novel research project. At the time, little was known about the causes of heart disease and stroke, but the death rates for CVD had been increasing steadily since the beginning of the century and had become an American epidemic. The objective of the study was to identify the common factors that contribute to CVD by following a group of 5,209 men and women between the ages of 30 and 62 from the town of Framingham, Massachusetts. These participants were the first to undergo extensive physical examinations and interviews about factors related to CVD development. Since 1948, the subjects have continued to return to the study every 2 years for a detailed medical history, physical examination, and laboratory tests; in 1971, the study enrolled a second generation—5,124 of the original participants' adult children and their spouses—to participate in similar examinations. A wealth of information has been revealed about CVD risk factors from this study. In 2002, the study entered a new phase, the enrollment of a third generation of participants, the grandchildren of the original participants. The study continues today.

vessels. The sympathetic impulses travel to the heart and blood vessels via the spinal cord and peripheral nerves. The vagus nerve slows down HR and the sympathetic stimulation increases the HR and contractility. The sympathetic simulation also causes vasoconstriction of the arteries.

Within the walls of arteries, particularly the carotid artery and aortic arch, are BP sensors known as **baroreceptors.** When baroreceptors detect a drop in BP, they respond rapidly by stimulating the sympathetic nervous system (SNS). The SNS stimulates an increase in HR and contractility and stimulates contraction of vascular smooth muscle in the arteries. The increase in heart rate, contractility, and vasoconstriction cause BP to quickly increase in response to the drop in blood pressure. This baroreceptor reflex is commonly exhibited when an individual goes from a lying position to a sitting and standing position. The change in position from lying to sitting or standing causes a brief drop in BP that is sensed by the baroreceptors, which in turn stimulate the SNS to enact a reflexive increase in HR and vasoconstriction. The sensitivity of baroreceptors are key to the maintenance of BP. As individuals age, baroreceptor sensitivity decreases.

> **CLINICAL CONCEPT**
>
> Orthostatic hypotension is a drop in BP that occurs when changing position from lying to standing. The drop in BP causes decreased cerebral perfusion, which leads to dizziness. This is often experienced by elderly adults and individuals on antihypertensive medications.

The Renin-Angiotensin-Aldosterone System

The **renin-angiotensin–aldosterone system (RAAS)** is a key part of BP regulation. This multistep reaction raises BP in response to diminished circulation in the body. When the BP or blood volume in the body is diminished, the kidney is sensitive to the drop in blood pressure. **Renin** is an enzyme that is released by the juxtaglomerular apparatus of the nephrons in response to decreased perfusion. When the circulation to the kidney is diminished, renin is released into the bloodstream and stimulates the liver to release a large protein called angiotensinogen. In the lungs, angiotensinogen is transformed into angiotensin I; angiotensin-converting enzyme (ACE) changes angiotensin I into angiotensin II. Angiotensin II is a potent arterial vasoconstrictor and stimulates the adrenal gland to release the hormone aldosterone. The arterial vasoconstriction raises blood pressure. Aldosterone works at the nephron to increase sodium and water reabsorption into the bloodstream and secrete potassium into the nephron tubules. The sodium and water increase the volume of the bloodstream and blood pressure, whereas potassium is excreted in the urine (see Fig. 15-4).

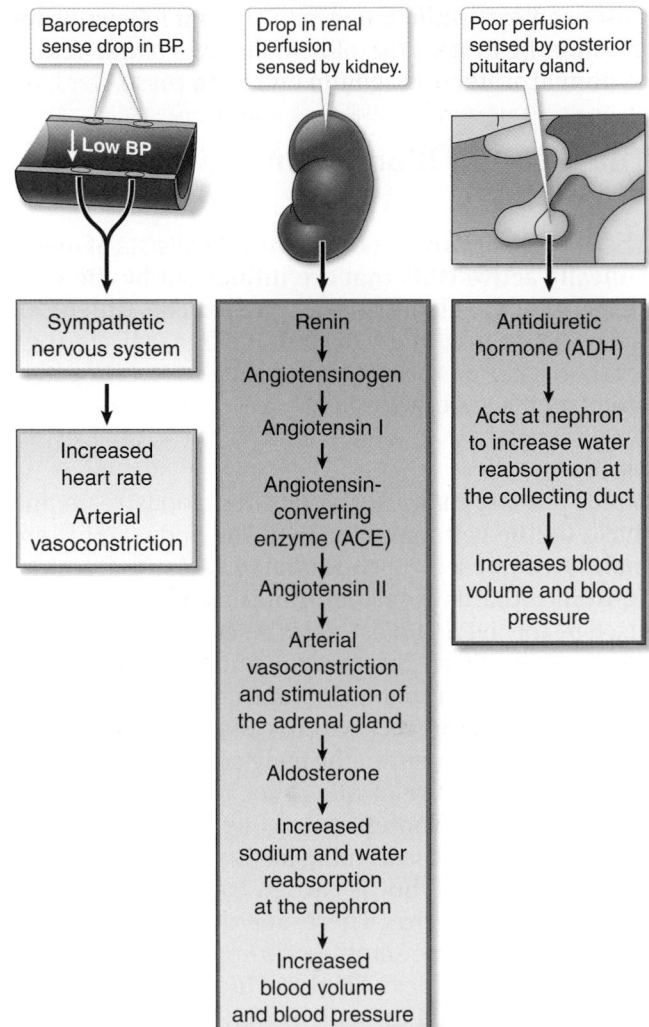

FIGURE 15-4. Body mechanisms that maintain blood pressure. 1. Baroreceptors located in the arterial wall sense decreases in BP and stimulate the SNS. The SNS stimulates the heart to increase rate and activates arterial vasoconstriction. 2. The RAAS is activated when the kidneys sense low blood pressure. The effect of the RAAS is increased blood volume and vasoconstriction. 3. The posterior pituitary gland senses low perfusion and secretes ADH, which acts at the nephron to increase water reabsorption; this raises blood volume and blood pressure.

The Posterior Pituitary–Antidiuretic Hormone Mechanism

Another important hormone that is secreted in response to diminished BP is antidiuretic hormone (ADH), which is also called vasopressin. The posterior pituitary secretes ADH when it senses a drop in blood volume or BP or an increase in blood osmolarity. ADH acts at the nephron to increase water reabsorption into the bloodstream, thereby raising blood volume and BP.

Natriuresis

Natriuresis is natural diuresis promoted by the heart and brain. The heart releases atrial natriuretic peptide (ANP) and the brain releases brain natriuretic peptide (BNP) in response to excess water in the bloodstream. The natriuretic peptides act at the nephrons to release excess water into the urine. Natriuresis decreases the water content in the blood, and sodium follows water out into the urine. When BP and blood volume return to normal, water and sodium excretion cease.

The Effect of Blood Composition on Arteries

The endothelial lining of the arteries consists of metabolically active cells that are influenced by the constituents of the bloodstream. Common constituents of the blood include lipids, glucose, and free radicals. High levels of any of these components have a negative effect on the endothelium.

Lipids

Lipids are fats that circulate in the bloodstream and make up the cell membranes in the body. Lipids are mainly composed of **cholesterol,** a fatty steroidal substance that is ingested from the diet and synthesized by the liver. Cholesterol is an essential structural component of cell membranes and it assists in the maintenance of proper membrane permeability. In addition to its importance within cells, cholesterol is an important component in the body's hormonal systems for the manufacture of bile acids, steroid hormones, and vitamin D. Cholesterol is ingested via animal products such as meat, milk, butter, and cheese; it is insoluble in blood but is carried by proteins to form soluble lipoproteins. There are different types of lipoproteins: Some contain cholesterol and others contain triglycerides. **Triglycerides** are large lipid molecules acquired through diet and stored as fat tissue. Lipoproteins are classified by size and lipid content: There are **low-density lipoproteins (LDLs)** and **high-density lipoproteins (HDLs).** HDL is excreted from the body, which is why it is considered good cholesterol, whereas LDL is deposited on artery walls, which is why it is considered bad cholesterol. The deposition occurs at areas of endothelial injury where inflammation is occurring. WBCs phagocytose the LDL and form lipid-laden macrophages called foam cells; the foam cell is the preliminary change in the endothelium that leads to larger collections of fat, inflammatory mediators, and platelets called atherosclerotic plaque (see section on Hyperlipidemia).

Glucose

Chronically high circulating levels of glucose in the bloodstream cause harm to the endothelial lining of arteries. Glucose reacts with the cell membranes of endothelial cells in a process called glycosylation (also called glycation). The glucose reacts with vessel wall proteins and forms advanced glycosylation end products (AGEs), which injure the smooth endothelial surface. This type of endothelial injury is a precursor to endothelial inflammation and formation of atherosclerotic plaque. In addition, the stimulation by AGEs causes endothelium to secrete endothelin, a hormone that causes potent vasoconstriction. Continuous high

glucose levels, like those that occur in uncontrolled diabetes, predispose to arteriosclerosis and vasoconstricted arteries. These changes occur throughout the body, which is the reason diabetes is a risk factor for severe atherosclerosis and acute cardiovascular events such as stroke and myocardial infarction (MI).

Free Radicals

Free radicals, also called reactive oxidative species, are molecules with a single unpaired electron in its shell. They have a strong affinity for cell membranes and cause damage to the artery endothelial lining. These molecules have an oxidative effect and set up areas of inflammation in the artery. The areas of inflammation become the preliminary change that set up formation of atherosclerotic plaque.

Nicotine

Nicotine, a common ingredient in cigarettes, is a potent vasoconstrictor of arteries, particularly the coronary arteries. Nicotine is known to immediately increase blood pressure, and significant remnants of nicotine remain in the body for 6 to 8 hours after smoking a cigarette. It also activates the SNS, acting via splanchnic nerves to the adrenal medulla, and stimulates the release of epinephrine, which increases HR and causes central nervous system stimulation.

Homocysteine

Homocysteine is an amino acid that is integrally involved in the metabolism of folic acid and B vitamins. Deficiencies of folic acid and B vitamins cause decreased breakdown of homocysteine. Elevated levels of homocysteine in the bloodstream lead to damage of the endothelial lining of the arteries. High homocysteine levels are linked to thrombosis formation and CVD.

Pathophysiology of Arterial Disorders

CVD begins in the body's arteries. Atherosclerosis is the fundamental change in the body that initiates widespread CVD. There are many agents that can injure the endothelial lining of arteries, and this damage is the inciting event for atherosclerosis. One of the major predisposing conditions for atherosclerosis is hyperlipidemia. The risk factors and etiology of this condition have been clearly investigated. Essential HTN, another inciting condition for widespread CVD, is common within the population. However, its etiology is still unclear.

Hyperlipidemia

Hyperlipidemia refers to elevated levels of lipids in the bloodstream, mainly cholesterol and triglycerides. In more precise terms, hypercholesterolemia refers to elevated cholesterol levels, whereas hypertriglyceridemia refers to elevated triglyceride levels. Hyperlipidemia is one of the major conditions that lead to atherosclerosis, the basic disorder of all forms of CVD. The specific type of cholesterol that contributes to atherosclerosis is LDL. Elevated levels of LDL are often accompanied by decreased levels of HDL cholesterol. High levels of LDL cholesterol and low levels of HDL cholesterol predispose to CVD.

Approximately 20% of adults older than age 20 years are estimated to have hyperlipidemia, although this is thought to be a low estimate because many adults have not been tested for LDL levels and many of those diagnosed are undertreated. In adults, risk of hypercholesterolemia increases with advancing age.

Etiology

Cholesterol is a necessary lipid component of body structures. It is a major component of all cell membranes, is needed to maintain cell stability, and is also a basic constituent of steroid hormones and bile acids, two components involved in many physiologic functions. All cells are capable of synthesizing cholesterol, but the liver is most effective at its production, metabolism, and excretion. Cholesterol is largely acquired by the body via diet and liver production.

Liver Synthesis of Cholesterol. The liver synthesizes cholesterol and releases it as very low density lipoprotein, which is altered to become intermediate density lipoproteins. These, in turn, are broken down into LDL. LDL transports cholesterol to the tissues, where it is deposited within artery walls. Reverse cholesterol transport occurs when HDL takes cholesterol from the bloodstream and returns it to the liver for excretion. HDLs maintain low levels of tissue and plasma cholesterol, so high levels of HDL keep cholesterol levels in check. HDL also enhances excretion of cholesterol. However, with low levels of HDL, the body cannot initiate sufficient reverse cholesterol transport. Low HDL allows cholesterol-rich atherosclerotic plaques to accumulate on arterial walls. High levels of HDL have a protective effect against atherosclerosis.

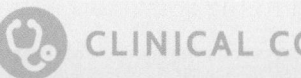

CLINICAL CONCEPT

HDL cholesterol is cardioprotective because it carries cholesterol away from artery walls to be excreted.

Dietary Sources of Lipids. Dietary sources of lipids include saturated and unsaturated fats as well as trans-fatty acids. A saturated fat is a fatty acid with a single carbon chain and every available bonding site filled or bonded with hydrogen ions. Saturated fats are usually solid forms of animal fat. The most apparent example is the fat contained in meats. Other sources of saturated fats are animal products such as eggs, butter, cheese, and dairy products. An unsaturated fatty acid is chemically a carbon chain with one or more unsaturated

double bonds. Unsaturated double bonds are easily broken down compared with saturated bonds. Commonly, unsaturated fats are liquid forms of fat. If there is only one unsaturated double bond, it is called a monounsaturated fatty acid; if there is more than one double bond, it is a polyunsaturated fat. Dietary sources of monounsaturated fats include olive oil, peanut oil, and canola oil. Vegetable oils such as sesame, corn, and safflower oils; fish; and margarine represent polyunsaturated fats.

Trans-fatty acids are manufactured and used to extend the life of polyunsaturated fats in processed foods. This is done by taking the polyunsaturated double-bonded carbon chain and forcing the double bond to break so that hydrogen ions can be introduced at these sites, thereby "transforming" the polyunsaturated fats into trans-fats via the hydrogenation process. Trans-fats have been linked to increased levels of LDL and the formation of plaque in the arterial vessels, as well as decreased levels of HDL.

Risk Factors

Several conditions can increase lipid levels in the bloodstream. The genetic disorder familial hypercholesterolemia (FH) is a disorder of elevated levels of cholesterol in the bloodstream. One in 500 persons is affected by familial hypercholesterolemia. In FH, a gene mutation on the short arm of chromosome 19 causes a deficiency of LDL receptors in the body. Without LDL receptors, the liver cannot efficiently metabolize LDL cholesterol, so high levels of LDL cholesterol accumulate in the bloodstream. Extremely high cholesterol levels and premature CVD occur in affected persons. Polygenic hypercholesterolemia is the more common form of hyperlipidemia prevalent in the population. The condition is the result of a number of different gene mutations and is influenced by diet. Individuals develop excess levels of cholesterol in the bloodstream but not as high as in familial hypercholesterolemia.

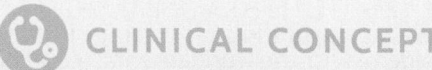

CLINICAL CONCEPT

Persons with FH develop severely elevated blood cholesterol levels, atherosclerosis, and MI (heart attack) at an early age.

Diabetes mellitus, both type 1 and type 2, are associated with elevated lipid levels. In diabetes mellitus, there is decreased hepatic removal of LDL from the circulation as well as increased levels of free fatty acids (FFA). The increased FFAs are the result of enhanced lipolysis, an action that enables fat stores to be used as the cells' alternative energy source. Elevated levels of blood glucose cause glycosylation of endothelial cells, which has a damaging effect on the arterial lining. The damaged areas attract WBCs and platelets and facilitate lipid deposition in vessel walls. Atherosclerotic plaque develops on artery walls throughout the body. Diabetes mellitus accelerates widespread development of atherosclerosis.

Obesity is a condition that causes excess cutaneous body fat, visceral fat accumulation, and elevated blood lipid levels. Hypercholesterolemia and hypertriglyceridemia are common in obese individuals. Elevated blood lipid levels enhance development of atherosclerosis.

Hypothyroidism is associated with decreased LDL receptors in the liver. Fewer liver receptors for LDL cause less LDL metabolism and excretion. This, in turn, leads to elevated LDL levels, which enhances development of atherosclerosis. Increased synthesis of lipids also occurs with the kidney disorder called nephrotic syndrome. Therefore, it is important to identify and treat disorders that lead to elevated lipid levels.

Low physical activity or sedentary lifestyle predisposes to hyperlipidemia. LDL cholesterol increases and HDL levels decrease with lack of physical activity.

A diet that is high in cholesterol, saturated fats, and trans-fats will increase LDL levels. In addition, certain medications increase lipid levels in the bloodstream. These drugs include progestins, anabolic steroids, corticosteroids, diuretics, and beta adrenergic blockers.

Pathophysiology

The finding of LDL cholesterol and triglyceride-rich lipoproteins in atherosclerotic plaque has provided substantial evidence for their direct role in atherosclerosis, which begins with injury of the endothelium. Endothelial inflammation occurs and macrophages rush to the area along with platelets. The prelude to atherosclerosis occurs as macrophages engulf and ingest LDL. As LDL accumulates within the WBCs, they develop a foamy appearance and are referred to as foam cells. Foam cells deposited along the vessel wall accumulate and form fatty streaks; this is a preliminary stage in the development of atherosclerotic plaque.

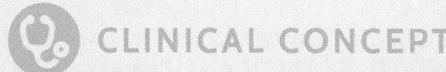

CLINICAL CONCEPT

Hyperlipidemia is the fundamental condition that causes atherosclerosis.

Clinical Presentation

Clinicians seeking diagnostic signs of hyperlipidemia should interview the patient about the existence of other cardiovascular problems such as HTN, angina, or MI. Thorough descriptions of diet and activity level are also key elements in the patient history. Commonly, individuals with hyperlipidemia report a diet high in fat. In addition, patients often describe a sedentary lifestyle and lack of exercise in the daily routine.

A family history of CVD is also frequently reported. Parents, siblings, or other relatives commonly have HTN, high cholesterol, MI, angina, or stroke. A family history of premature MI, which occurs in persons under age 40, is particularly indicative of familial hypercholesterolemia. The patient should also be questioned about current medications and the existence of predisposing disorders, such as hypothyroidism, diabetes, or kidney disease.

Signs and Symptoms. Patients do not usually report any symptoms associated with hyperlipidemia because it is largely a silent disorder. Persons may report symptoms related to angina or MI.

Physical Examination. Physical examination findings often include xanthoma and xanthelasma, yellowish cholesterol deposits under the skin and around the eyes (see Fig. 15-5). Arcus senilis may be noted in the ophthalmological exam. This is a yellow-white ring around the cornea of the eye that consists of cholesterol deposits. The patient may also exhibit signs and symptoms of metabolic syndrome, which is a constellation of disorders that include central obesity, glucose intolerance, hyperinsulinemia, HTN, and hyperlipidemia.

Diagnosis

To reduce atherosclerotic CVD risk in adults, the 2013 American College of Cardiology (ACC) and American Heart Association (AHA) have established specific categories for evaluating blood lipid levels (Table 15-1). These guidelines are recommended for diagnosis and treatment of lipid disorders.

In addition to a history and physical examination, blood samples for lipoproteins, cholesterol, and triglycerides should be obtained. Testing must also rule out possible causes of elevated lipid levels, such as hypothyroidism, diabetes mellitus, obstructive liver disease, and kidney disease. Therefore, blood glucose, thyroid-stimulating hormone, blood urea nitrogen (BUN), serum creatinine, and liver enzymes should be checked. Because cholesterol levels are affected by food, a complete lipoprotein analysis must be drawn following a 9- to 12-hour fast.

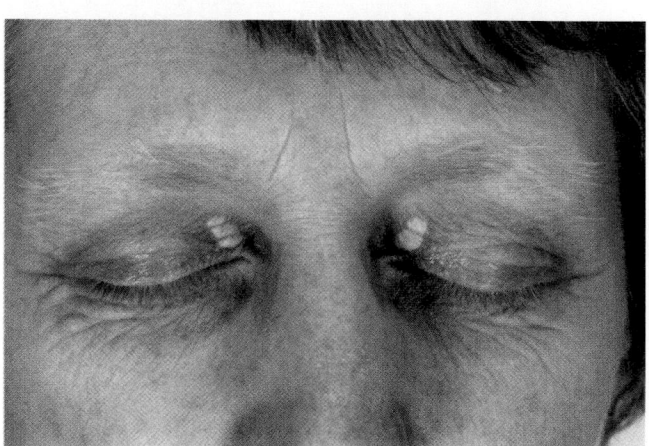

FIGURE 15-5. Xanthoma/Xanthelasma. *(From Biophoto Associates/ Science Source.)*

TABLE 15-1. AHA/ACA Classification of Cholesterol Categories

Total Cholesterol	Category
Less than 200 mg/dL	Desirable
200 to 239 mg/dL	Borderline high
240 mg/dL and above	High

LDL Cholesterol	Category
Less than 100 mg/dL	Optimal * (if patient is very high risk with CHD goal of 70 mg/dL or lower)
100 to 129 mg/dL	Near optimal/above optimal
130 to 159 mg/dL	Borderline high
160 to 189 mg/dL	High
190 mg/dL and above	Very high

HDL Cholesterol	Category
Less than 40 mg/dL	Poor: Major risk factor for heart disease
40 to 59 mg/dL	Good
60 mg/dL and above	Ideal: Considered cardioprotective

Triglycerides	Category
Less than 150 mg/dL	Ideal
150 to 199 mg/dL	Borderline high
200 to 499 mg/dL	High
500 mg/dL or above	Very high

*In those with very high-risk who have established CHD and multiple risk factors, including diabetes, metabolic syndrome, or severe or poorly controlled risk factors, the guidelines offer a new therapeutic option of aggressively treating LDL levels to lower than 70 mg/dL. In very high-risk patients with LDL levels less than 100 mg/dL, AHA/ ACA 2013 guidelines support using drug therapy to bring LDL cholesterol down to below 70 mg/dL.
Adapted from Stone, N. J., Robinson, J., Lichtenstein, A. H., et al. (2013). 2013 ACC/AHA guideline on the treatment of blood cholesterol to reduce atherosclerotic cardiovascular risk in adults. *J Am College of Card.* doi:10.1016/j.jacc.2013.11.002. Volume 63 issue 25 Pt B pp. 2889–2934.

Treatment

Lifestyle changes are a fundamental part of hyperlipidemia treatment. A low-fat diet that is particularly low in cholesterol is necessary. The patient should aim to keep dietary cholesterol lower than 300 mg per day. Fats should be limited to fewer than 30% of total dietary calories. Saturated fat must be strictly limited. Monounsaturated fats such as olive oil and polyunsaturated fats such as vegetable oil are preferable. Physical activity should be included in the daily routine; usually 30 minutes of vigorous walking is sufficient. Also, the individual should refrain from smoking and limit alcohol use. A glass of red wine daily has been shown to reduce CVD risk in some individuals. Fish oils, also known as omega-3 fatty acids, have been shown to reduce triglycerides. Fish oil can be taken as a supplement or obtained through fish such as mackerel, tuna, salmon, bluefish, anchovy, sardines, herring, and trout. High fiber is also a recommended component of the diet to reduce hyperlipidemia.

Medications called statins or HMG-CoA reductase inhibitors, such as atorvastatin (Lipitor®), rosuvastatin (Crestor®), and simvastatin (Zocor®), are first-line agents that are recommended if diet and exercise do not lower bloodstream lipids to desired levels. These agents block the liver enzyme that assists in the manufacture of cholesterol. Statins diminish cholesterol synthesis and can reverse atherosclerotic plaque formation. Pre-existent atherosclerotic plaque has been shown to diminish with statin treatment. The 2013 American Cardiology Association (ACA) and AHA guidelines recommend statin therapy for the following groups:

- People without CVD who are 40 to 75 years old and have a 7.5% or higher risk for having a heart attack or stroke within 10 years.
- People with a history of a cardiovascular event (heart attack, stroke, stable or unstable angina, peripheral artery disease, transient ischemic attack (TIA), or coronary or other arterial revascularization).
- People 21 and older who have a very high level of LDL cholesterol (190 mg/dL or higher).
- People with type 1 or type 2 diabetes who are 40 to 75 years old.

Bile acid sequestrants such as cholestyramine (Questran®) are second-line agents for the treatment of elevated LDL cholesterol. These block bile acid absorption in the gastrointestinal tract. The main component of bile acids is cholesterol; therefore, these agents prevent cholesterol absorption from the intestine into the bloodstream. Fibrates such as gemfibrozil (Lopid®) and fenofibrate (Tricor®) are used as first-line treatment for elevated triglyceride concentrations and may be prescribed in combination with the other drug classes. These medications decrease triglyceride secretion by the liver. Nicotinic acid (niacin) is an optional medication for all lipid disorders. Niacin blocks breakdown of fats, lowers LDL levels, and raises HDL levels. Niacin is often combined with statins, but is also effective as a single agent. Ezetimibe (Zetia®), another type of medication, decreases intestinal absorption of fat, and is often used as a second-line therapy because of its effectiveness, safety, and lack of side effects.

Hypertension

HTN is the elevation of BP to values that are correlated with cardiovascular damage. It is called the silent killer because it has no symptoms and can lead to fatal CVD. The American Heart Association (AHA) and American College of Cardiology (ACC) has established that HTN exists when two or more diastolic BP measurement on at least two or more clinical visits is 80 mmHg or greater, or when the systolic BP readings on two or more clinical visits is consistently 130 mmHg or greater. According to the AHA and ACC there are five different categories of BP according to numerical values: normal blood pressure,

Blood Pressure (BP) Classification	Systolic BP (mmHg)	Diastolic BP (mmHg)
Normal	Less than 120	and less than 80
Elevated	120 to 129	and less than 80
Stage 1 Hypertension	130 to 139	or 80 to 89
Stage 2 Hypertension	140 or greater	or 90 or greater
Hypertensive crisis*	Greater than 180	and/or greater than 120

TABLE 15-2. Blood Pressure Classification

*Immediate hospitalization required if there are signs of organ damage.
Data from 2017 ACC/AHA/AAPA/ABC/ACPM/AGS/APhA/ASH/ASPC/NMA/
PCNA Guideline for the Prevention, Detection, Evaluation, and Management
of High Blood Pressure in Adults: A Report of the American College of
Cardiology/American Heart Association Task Force on Clinical Practice
Guidelines. J Am Coll Cardiol 2017; Nov 13.

elevated blood pressure, stage 1 HTN, stage 2 HTN and hypertensive crisis (see Table 15-2).

Controversy currently exists between the recommended BP goals of the AHA, ACA, and Joint National Committee on Prevention, Detection, Evaluation, and Treatment of Hypertension eighth report (JNC-8). In 2014, the JNC-8 made the following recommendations for the management of hypertension in certain groups of adults: age 60 and older with high BP, optimal BP is less than 150/90; age 30 to 59 with high BP, optimal BP is less than 140/90; and adults with diabetes or chronic kidney disease, optimal BP is less than 140/90. However, these recommendations differ from the BP goals recommended by the AHA and ACC. The JNC-8 expert panel also recommended how to achieve optimal BP measurements. It recommended that persons with high BP adopt healthy lifestyle changes. These include weight loss, limitation of salt intake, diet rich in fruits and vegetables and whole grains; and at least 30 minutes of physical activity daily. The JNC-8 also recommends specific drug therapy for African Americans and all persons with diabetes. For Caucasian persons, an ACE inhibitor, angiotensin-receptor blocker (ARB), calcium channel blocker (CCB), or thiazide-type diuretic are the best medications for control of HTN. For African Americans, a CCB or thiazide-type diuretic is the best initial medication for HTN. Among individuals with declining kidney function or diabetes, a low dose of an ACE inhibitor or ARB are preferred treatment for HTN. ACE inhibitors and ARB medications protect the kidneys from further damage.

The strong association between HTN and CAD has been well established by epidemiological studies. HTN is a major independent risk factor for CAD, stroke, and renal failure. The diagnosis and consequent treatment of HTN over the last 50 years has resulted in major reductions in cardiovascular morbidity and mortality. There are two main categories of HTN: primary HTN, also called essential HTN, and secondary HTN. Primary HTN is the most common type, but its etiology is unknown. Secondary HTN affects a much smaller percentage of the population and is the result of some pathology in another system or organ.

Epidemiology

HTN is one of the most common worldwide diseases. Because of the associated morbidity and mortality and the cost to society, it is an important public health challenge. Approximately 78 million people in the United States are affected by HTN. Overall, approximately 20% of the world's adults are estimated to have HTN. Substantial improvements have been made with regard to improving awareness and treatment of the disorder, but approximately 30% of adults are still unaware of their HTN; up to 40% of people with HTN are not receiving treatment and, of those treated, up to 67% do not have their BP controlled to lower than 140/90 mm Hg. In many countries, 50% of the population older than 60 years has HTN. Many more people are at risk for developing the disease, falling into a category known as prehypertension.

Etiology

Primary HTN accounts for 90% to 95% of adult cases; a small percentage of patients have a secondary cause. Primary HTN has no known cause. Secondary HTN is clearly a side effect of another systemic disorder such as Cushing's disease, pheochromocytoma, kidney disease, or hyperaldosteronism (see Box 15-2). Treating the systemic disorder will lower BP in secondary HTN.

Risk Factors

There are many risk factors for HTN, including:

- age
- African American ethnicity
- family history
- obesity
- diabetes mellitus
- sedentary behavior
- tobacco use
- excess sodium in diet
- insufficient potassium in diet
- insufficient vitamin D in diet
- excess alcohol
- stress.

Pathophysiology

HTN has two major negative effects on the cardiovascular system. It exerts high damaging forces against all the endothelial linings of the arteries. It also causes high resistance against the heart's left ventricle. BP in the aorta is elevated when there is HTN in the systemic arteries. High aortic pressure places an excessive workload on the heart's left ventricle, raising the intramyocardial wall tension in the ventricular muscle. Over time, this results in left ventricular hypertrophy (LVH) as the muscle works harder to eject blood into the aorta (see Fig. 15-6). The

---

BOX 15-2. **Causes of Secondary Hypertension**

Secondary HTN occurs when a disorder causes elevated BP as a side effect.

RENAL CAUSES
- Chronic kidney disease
- Liddle syndrome
- Polycystic kidney disease
- Renin-producing tumor
- Urinary tract obstruction

CARDIOVASCULAR CAUSES
- Coarctation of aorta
- Collagen-vascular disease
- Vasculitis

ENDOCRINE CAUSES
- Acromegaly
- Congenital adrenal hyperplasia
- Cushing syndrome
- Hyperaldosteronism, primary
- Pheochromocytoma
- Hyperparathyroidism
- Hyperthyroidism and hypothyroidism

NEUROGENIC CAUSES
- Brain tumor
- Bulbar poliomyelitis
- Intracranial HTN

DRUGS AND TOXINS
- Adrenergic medications
- Alcohol
- Cocaine
- Cyclosporine, tacrolimus
- Decongestants containing ephedrine
- Erythropoietin
- Herbal remedies containing licorice or ephedrine
- Nonsteroidal anti-inflammatory medications
- Oral contraceptives

OTHER CAUSES
- Hypercalcemia
- Obstructive sleep apnea
- Pregnancy-induced HTN

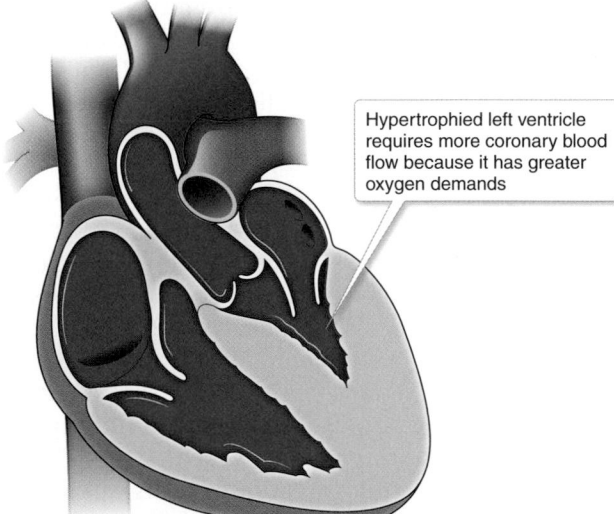

Hypertrophied left ventricle requires more coronary blood flow because it has greater oxygen demands

FIGURE 15-6. Long-term HTN leads to left ventricular hypertrophy. The left ventricle hypertrophies because of the excessive resistance in the aorta in HTN. The enlarged muscle of the left ventricle then requires extra coronary artery blood flow because of the increased energy needs of the large muscle. However, extra supply of coronary artery blood flow is unavailable and so the left ventricle is susceptible to ischemia and infarction.

enlarged left ventricle develops into a prominent muscle that requires increased circulation and oxygen. However, the coronary blood flow available is inadequate for the enlarged ventricular muscle. The enlarged left ventricle, which hypertrophied because of HTN, becomes susceptible to ischemia, infarction, and heart failure.

HTN predisposes all the systemic arteries to injury. It creates a high shearing force against all arterial

vessel walls, which causes weakening and injury of the endothelium. Arteries particularly damaged by HTN include those of the retina, kidneys, brain, and lower extremities. Damaged retinal arteries can lead to blindness, injured renal arteries can lead to renal failure, and damaged cerebral arteries can lead to hemorrhagic stroke.

The RAAS plays a role in the regulation of BP and its elevation. In certain circumstances, hypersensitivity to angiotensin II with its resulting arterial vasoconstriction and increased blood volume is believed to contribute to primary HTN. Research has also shown that stress can cause persistently elevated levels of angiotensin II. Chronic stress stimulates renin and sets off the RAAS, which increases total blood volume and causes widespread arterial vasoconstriction. The result of chronic stimulation of the RAAS is HTN.

Other studies have examined renin activity in the body. Some individuals are known to be high renin secretors. High renin activity results in the same outcomes as discussed with angiotensin II sensitivity, such as chronic cycling of the RAAS. This cycling causes widespread arterial vasoconstriction, increases circulating blood volume, and elevates blood pressure.

 CLINICAL CONCEPT

In population studies, African American individuals on average have higher BP measurements compared with Caucasians. Many African American individuals have been identified as having high sensitivity to sodium. The AHA

Continued

recommends daily dietary sodium intake of 1,500 mg. However, the average daily American diet consists of more than double this amount, mainly because of processed foods. In the body, excess sodium increases water content of the blood, which results in high blood volume and elevated blood pressure. In persons with high sensitivity to sodium, any excess sodium in the diet intensely increases blood volume and blood pressure.

Clinical Manifestations

HTN is a silent, gradual process that most commonly has no symptoms until it causes organ dysfunction. In reviewing the patient's history, it is important to determine if any disorders are present that can predispose to HTN such as Cushing's disease, pheochromocytoma, diabetes, kidney disease, or hyperaldosteronism. The patient's list of medications should be checked for possible medication-induced HTN. Such medications include steroids, sympathetic stimulants, or MAO inhibitor antidepressants.

The clinician should ask the patient about symptoms correlated with target organ damage of HTN. The target organs of HTN are the heart, brain, extremities, retina, and kidney. Symptoms such as chest pain, dyspnea on exertion, palpitations, headache, vision disturbances, dizziness, weakness in an extremity, leg pain, or edema can be indications of target organ damage. Additionally, if the patient indicates that these symptoms are present, it is necessary to determine the quality, character, duration, and associated symptoms. The patient should also be asked about diet, physical activity, and smoking. Foods that are high in saturated fat and salt such as fast food and processed food raise blood pressure. Sedentary activity and excessive alcohol use are also associated with HTN.

Signs and Symptoms. Primary HTN commonly has no signs or symptoms. The disease may be quite advanced before it is detected or diagnosed, and may have already caused target organ damage. Rarely, persons with HTN complain of headache, nosebleeds, blurred vision, or palpitations.

Physical Examination. A complete physical examination of the patient should be completed with focus on the cardiovascular system. Accurate measurement of both the systolic and diastolic BP is needed to identify those at risk and to monitor the success of therapy. The individual should be comfortably seated for at least 5 minutes. No caffeine, exercise, or smoking should have taken place 30 minutes before taking the measurement. The arm should be supported and the cuff large enough for the bladder to cover 80% of the upper arm. The accurate calibration of the sphygmomanometer is critical. At least two measurements should be taken and the average recorded. To diagnose HTN, there should be at least two separate measurements of high BP on two different days.

Fundoscopic examination is a procedure that uses an ophthalmoscope to assess the retina and optic nerve. There are characteristic changes in the retinal vessels caused by HTN. This is the only place the clinician can gather information about the health of the body's arteries using physical examination techniques.

There should be an examination of the chest for indications of HTN. The clinician should palpate the chest for the point of maximal impulse (PMI). In long-term untreated HTN, the left ventricle hypertrophies. This causes the PMI to be palpable further left in the chest, at the 5th intercostal space toward the axillary line. There also may be a visible left ventricular lift of the chest. When listening to the heart, the clinician may hear an S_4 sound, which occurs before S_1 because of a less compliant left ventricle in LVH.

The health of the peripheral arteries is essential when assessing a patient for HTN. The clinician should use the stethoscope to listen for bruits over the aorta, carotid, and renal arteries. Bruits are indicative of turbulent blood flow caused by aneurysm or arterial stenosis (narrowing).

Examination of the peripheral arteries of the lower extremities is also important in patients with HTN. Inspect and palpate the lower extremities for signs of peripheral arterial obstruction. The clinician should focus on the color, temperature, sensation, and pulses in the lower legs and feet. Pallor, coolness, decreased sensation, and weak pulses are indications of peripheral arterial obstruction.

Diagnosis

Diagnostic evaluation of HTN should rule out any potential causes of an elevated BP and determine if there is any target organ damage. Testing includes a 12-lead ECG, urinalysis, complete blood count (CBC), blood glucose, serum potassium, serum creatinine, and serum calcium. An electrocardiogram (ECG) can provide information about hypertensive cardiac effects such as LVH. The urinalysis, BUN, and serum creatinine levels can identify early indications of hypertensive injury to the kidneys. The presence of protein in the urine, a condition known as proteinuria, in conjunction with elevated BUN and serum creatinine level, is indicative of renal damage.

Diagnostic testing should rule out such disorders as hyperthyroidism, kidney disease, diabetes, pheochromocytoma, and Cushing's disease, which cause secondary HTN.

Treatment

Treatment focuses initially on lifestyle modifications such as diet, stress reduction, physical activity, and smoking cessation, as these have been shown to have a significant effect to lower blood pressure.

Diet. The National Heart, Lung, and Blood Institute (NHLBI) advocates the DASH diet, which stands for

Dietary Approaches to Stop Hypertension. The DASH diet includes low sodium (1,500 mg), low-fat foods—mainly fruits, vegetables, whole grains, poultry, fish, and low-fat dairy products. The benefits of reducing saturated and trans-fats from the diet and reducing sodium have repeatedly been proven to be effective. Also beneficial is a diet rich in folic acid, as folic acid has been shown to reduce homocysteine, which at high levels causes endothelial injury.

Stress Reduction and Physical Activity. Stress has been proven to play a significant role in the development of HTN. Complementary medicine or healing modalities have long established the powerful connection between the mind and body. Biofeedback, relaxation techniques, and yoga are all methods of stress reduction. Sedentary lifestyle has been shown to predispose individuals to HTN. Physical activity is also advocated as a way to deal with stress. Endorphins are released with physical activity and these help to reduce stress.

Smoking Cessation

Smoking cessation is recommended for cardiovascular health. Nicotine is an arterial vasoconstrictor that raises BP and increases resistance to blood flow. The left ventricle must contract with greater force, thereby causing it to hypertrophy when there is arterial vasoconstriction. The left ventricle can become exhausted by the high resistance it must pump against in the aorta; eventually, heart failure occurs. In addition, free radicals contained in cigarette smoke are known to damage the endothelial linings of the arteries. The endothelial damage initiates the development of arteriosclerosis. By stopping smoking, the nicotine stimulus for vasoconstriction and the free radical damage leading to arteriosclerosis can be eliminated. Also, the arterial resistance against the left ventricle can be relieved.

Treatment

It is important to note that lifestyle modifications and pharmacological agents are both needed in the management plan when diet and exercise are not enough to lower blood pressure. Pharmacological agents such as diuretics, ACE inhibitors, angiotensin receptor blockers (ARBs) or beta-adrenergic blockers may need to be added to the regimen. Diuretics decrease the water content of the bloodstream. ACE inhibitors block ACE that changes angiotensin I into angiotensin II in the RAAS. Angiotensin II receptor blockers diminish angiotensin II activity. Beta blockers diminish the effects of the SNS on the heart and arteries, thereby decreasing HR and blocking vasoconstriction.

Complications

HTN is responsible for damage to target organs, which include the heart, retina, kidney, brain, and peripheral arteries. When it is not well controlled, it contributes to the development of hypertensive heart disease, heart failure, and renal failure. Additionally, it is the major contributing factor to fatal intracerebral hemorrhage.

Hypertensive heart disease is a compensatory response to increased afterload, or the force the heart must pump against in order to eject blood. LVH develops when the left ventricle must pump blood against excess arterial resistance for a prolonged period of time. The enlarged left ventricle muscle wall has an increased need for circulation and oxygen. However, there is an inadequate coronary artery blood supply for the enlarged muscle; as a result, this region becomes susceptible to ischemia and infarction. Long-term HTN often leads to left ventricular myocardial ischemia and infarction. Also, as the left ventricle hypertrophies, the enlarged muscle protrudes into the left ventricular chamber, reducing the chamber's capacity. As a result, reduced volume of blood fills the left ventricle, which reduces the volume of blood ejected with each contraction or stroke volume (SV). At the same time, when the left ventricular wall hypertrophies, the interventricular septum also enlarges and diminishes the right ventricle's filling capacity. Both left and right ventricle SV decrease; as a result, there is an overall reduction in cardiac output. If this does not resolve with treatment, the heart fails to supply adequate circulation to the body. HTN is the most common predisposing factor of heart failure.

All arteries are subjected to the effect of hypertensive damage. HTN weakens the walls of arteries, increasing susceptibility to development of bulges in arterial walls called **aneurysms.** Aneurysms cause turbulent blood flow and are susceptible to rupture. The most common areas for aneurysm development are the aorta and cerebral arteries (see Fig. 15-7).

There are multiple hypertensive effects on the brain. HTN places excess pressure on cerebral arteries and arterioles. The major concern is cerebral hemorrhage from hypertensive damage to small vessels within the brain. Acute elevations in BP can cause the rupture of cerebral blood vessels or hemorrhagic stroke. Although hemorrhagic stroke accounts for about 10% of all strokes, the mortality is very high. Also, because HTN accelerates formation of atherosclerosis, there is an increased risk of plaque formation in the cerebral arteries, which leads to thrombotic or embolic obstruction within the brain. This can be manifested by a TIA or ischemic stroke.

Altered blood flow from HTN contributes to the development of hypertensive encephalopathy, which is described as a cerebral edema from arteriolar spasm. A patient who presents with this condition may display confusion, changing level of consciousness, and seizures.

HTN also contributes to retinal changes called hypertensive retinopathy (see Fig. 15-8). In response to HTN, the retinal vessels become thickened with a narrowing of the vessel lumen. Higher pressures make the vessels kinked and tortuous. This gives an appearance of arteriovenous (AV) nicking at points where arteries and veins cross. Increased pressure leads to microhemorrhages within the retina. Cholesterol deposits in

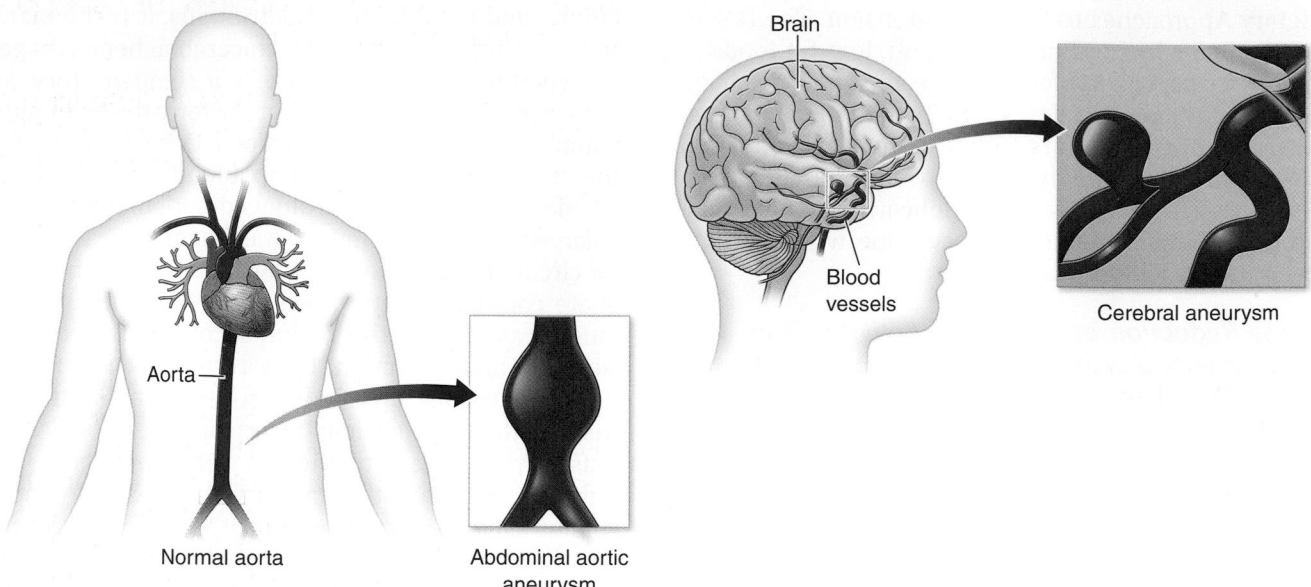

FIGURE 15-7. An aneurysm is a weakening in the wall of an artery. It is susceptible to rupture. 1. Abdominal aortic aneurysm. 2. Cerebral aneurysm.

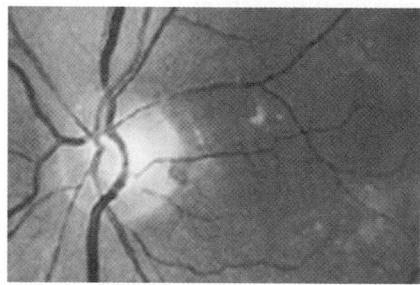

FIGURE 15-8. Hypertensive retinopathy. (From Dillon, P. (2007). *Nursing health assessment.* 2nd ed. Philadelphia, PA: F.A. Davis Company, with permission.)

arterioles give the vessels an appearance like copper-silver wiring. Small vessel infarcts in the retina give an appearance of cotton wool spots.

Renal disease is a common occurrence because of HTN. Because HTN is associated with an accelerated atherosclerosis, the afferent and efferent arterioles of the nephrons become obstructed by plaque. Also, the fragile capillaries of the glomeruli are damaged by the high blood pressure. These detrimental changes of HTN decrease the glomerular filtration rate, which causes waste products to accumulate in the blood. Consequently, serum creatinine rises and BUN increases. Glomerular injury increases glomerular permeability and loss of proteins into the urine, called proteinuria or microalbuminuria. As hypertensive disease continues, renal failure and end-stage renal disease can result.

Atherosclerosis

The basic physiologic change that causes CVD is atherosclerosis, which is the gradual process by which atherosclerotic plaque builds on the body's arterial walls. The terms *atherosclerosis* and *arteriosclerosis* are interchangeable. Atherosclerosis is a chronic, progressive disease with a long asymptomatic phase. It is a pathological series of changes that take place in the tunica intima, media, and adventitia of the artery, but primarily in the tunica intima, the innermost layer of the arterial wall. Spanning the whole arterial system, the endothelium sustains insults from many different agents and releases factors involved in atherogenesis.

Epidemiology

Clinical manifestations of atherosclerosis, including CAD, cerebrovascular disease, and peripheral arterial disease, will occur in two of three men and one in two women after age 40 years. Almost 60% of deaths are caused by CVD; this same death rate applies to atherosclerosis.

Etiology

The endothelial cells are exposed to all the constituents of the bloodstream, some of which can be injurious. Endothelial injury is the fundamental change that serves as the precursor of atherosclerosis. Agents that commonly harm the endothelium include oxidizing free radicals, the shearing force of high blood pressure, high circulating glucose levels, and elevated levels of LDL. Their injurious influence is widespread, encompassing the extensive endothelial lining throughout the body. Endothelial injury, as with any injury in the body, stimulates the inflammatory reaction, a chain of events that involves WBCs, platelets, clotting factors, cytokines, and various other inflammatory mediators. Atherogenesis, the development of arteriosclerotic plaque, is an inflammatory process that includes LDL—an added constituent to the other inflammatory mediators affecting the endothelium.

Risk Factors

The risk factors associated with atherosclerosis are categorized as modifiable or nonmodifiable (see Table 15-3). It is important to distinguish between the two because

TABLE 15-3. Risk Factors of Cardiovascular Disease

Nonmodifiable	Modifiable
AGE	**DIET**
Males greater than 45 years Females greater than 55 years (post-menopause)	Excess saturated fat and cholesterol Excess salt Lack of sufficient potassium Lack of folic acid
GENDER	**PHYSICAL ACTIVITY**
Males greater than females Postmenopausal females have same risk as males	Lack of exercise
RACE/ETHNICITY	**OBESITY**
African Americans greater than Caucasian Americans	Body mass index greater than 30 Triglycerides greater than 150 mg/dL Central adiposity
FAMILY HISTORY	**LIFESTYLE FACTORS**
Familial hypercholesterolemia Polygenic hypercholesterolemia Genetic disposition to DM, HTN, MI, or stroke	Tobacco use Excessive alcohol use High stress
	OTHER DISORDERS THAT ACCELERATE CVD
	HTN BP greater than 140/90 mm Hg Diabetes mellitus

the treatment of women with CVD is often less aggressive than that received by men.

Age. The physiologic changes associated with age contribute to the development of atherosclerosis and CVD. As people age, the blood vessels become less elastic and walls become fibrotic. In addition, arteries are more likely to develop atherosclerotic plaque formation with age.

Diabetes Mellitus. Diabetes mellitus accelerates the development of atherosclerosis. Patients with type 1 or type 2 diabetes mellitus often have significantly elevated triglycerides and LDL cholesterol levels, along with a lower level of HDL cholesterol. Therefore, patients with diabetes mellitus are at greater risk for developing atherosclerosis and cardiac pathology. Diabetes mellitus causes microvascular and macrovascular changes that compromise circulation to the myocardium as well as other organs. Also, as blood glucose levels rise in poorly controlled diabetes mellitus, endothelial cells decrease their production of the vasodilator nitric oxide. The endothelium also increases production of thromboxane A2 (TXA2), a clot enhancer. In addition, thrombolysis is diminished because of decreased plasminogen activator function. These conditions enhance clot formation, which could obstruct blood flow through arterial vessels. Finally, glucose interacts with the endothelium of the arterial wall through a process called glycosylation. Glycosylation stimulates endothelial cell secretion of endothelin, a potent vasoconstrictor. Therefore, diabetes promotes atherosclerosis, clot formation, and constriction of arteries. When the conditions of atherosclerosis, clot enhancement, and vasoconstriction occur in the coronary arteries or arteries of the extremities, there is an increased risk of heart attack and peripheral arterial occlusive disease.

Family History. Having a family history of CVD increases the patient's risk. There are multiple genes that are known to increase susceptibility to atherosclerosis and hyperlipidemia. However, the risk is not solely caused by genetics. Cultural and family influences on diet and lifestyle contribute to this risk factor as well.

treatment can be implemented to counteract modifiable factors.

Gender. Gender is an important issue in the development of atherosclerosis. Men have a greater risk and incur MI earlier in life than women. Atherosclerosis and CVD develop in men by age 45 years and in women by age 55 years. The reason for the difference in risk is that premenopausal women's estrogen activity is considered cardioprotective. Premenopausal estrogen levels in the female raise HDL. However, after menopause, women are more likely to die from MI than men. In fact, CVD kills more women than breast cancer annually. A possible explanation for this is that women often present with different symptoms from men. Additionally,

Tobacco Use. Tobacco use has been identified as a risk factor for atherosclerosis. Cigarette smoke contains oxidizing free radicals that cause endothelial injury. Also, smoking decreases levels of HDL, which allows cholesterol to deposit on arterial walls and facilitate the formation of atherosclerotic plaque. The nicotine found in cigarettes causes vasoconstriction, which contributes to occlusion of arterial blood vessels. Lastly, cigarette smoking is also associated with increased coagulability via stimulation of platelet activity and elevation of fibrinogen and factor VII levels.

Hypertension. HTN is an elevated arterial BP that causes direct and indirect cardiovascular damage. Increased pressure from within the arterial vessel causes endothelial injury, which initiates atherosclerosis. Also, within the damaged area of the endothelium there is decreased release of nitric oxide, the chemical of vasodilation, and increased release of endothelin, a potent vasoconstrictor. The net result is arterial vasoconstriction and initiation of atherosclerosis in the area subjected to high blood pressure.

Once atherosclerotic plaque is fully developed, elevated pressure within the blood vessel increases the stress on the area of plaque and commonly causes plaque rupture. A piece of plaque travels to a more distal, narrower branch of the artery and creates an obstruction at this site. Ischemia of tissue is the end result. When this occurs in a coronary artery, it causes myocardial ischemia, also called angina pectoris.

Obesity. Obesity is a global epidemic in both children and adults. It is associated with numerous disorders such as atherosclerosis, diabetes, HTN, osteoarthritis, certain cancers, and sleep apnea. Obesity is an independent risk factor for CVD and is associated with an increased risk of morbidity and mortality. Excess adipose tissue places extra demands on the heart, as the heart has to pump high amounts of blood to supply the excess body tissue. Excess adipose tissue is also known to be insulin resistant, which increases the risk of diabetes. In addition, obesity increases coagulation factors, thereby increasing the risk for thrombosis. Commonly, persons with obesity have metabolic syndrome, which is a syndrome consisting of HTN, glucose intolerance, and hyperlipidemia.

The body mass index (BMI) calculation has been devised to evaluate an individual's body weight in relation to cardiovascular risk. A BMI greater than 30 is considered a cardiovascular health risk. (See Chapter 5: Obesity and Nutritional Imbalances for more information on BMI.)

Lifestyle. A high-fat diet, high stress levels, and a sedentary lifestyle contribute to the development of atherosclerosis. A diet high in saturated fat, cholesterol, and trans-fatty acids brings more fat into the body for the manufacture of LDL cholesterol. LDL becomes the major component in atherosclerotic plaque, which eventually narrows and vasoconstricts the arteries.

Excessive stress elevates levels of hormones that initiate the fight-or-flight response. With acute stress, stimulation of the endocrine system and SNS occurs, which raises HR and vasoconstricts blood vessels. These conditions increase BP and pulse, which are detrimental if prolonged. Also, long-term stress causes overactivation of the RAAS, which results in high BP. High BP damages the endothelium, and endothelial injury is the initial step in atherosclerosis.

Sedentary lifestyle and lack of exercise also increase the risk of atherosclerosis. Obesity and lower levels of HDL cholesterol are associated with sedentary behavior. Lower levels of HDL also decrease cholesterol excretion. Accumulation of cholesterol in the bloodstream enhances development of atherosclerotic plaque.

Pathophysiology

After endothelial injury, the development of arteriosclerotic plaque begins in a sequential pattern. Endothelial inflammation draws WBCs and platelets to the site of injury. One of the first changes in the endothelium involves WBCs that engulf and ingest LDL cholesterol. These lipid-rich WBCs form the foundation for arteriosclerotic plaque.

Formation of Foam Cells. Injured endothelial cells produce molecules that have adhesive properties called vascular cell adhesion molecule 1 (VCAM-1) and chemoattractant protein-1 (MCP-1). These adhesive molecules attract and bind circulating WBCs to the endothelium of arterial vessels. The adhered WBCs on the intima are then incorporated into the layer beneath the endothelium, the tunica media, where smooth muscle is located. The WBCs differentiate into macrophages that engulf and ingest LDL. At this point in atherogenesis, there is visible cholesterol within the cytoplasm of macrophages. These LDL-laden macrophages become known as foam cells. Foam cells can accumulate LDL and create atherosclerotic plaque. However, foam cells can also transmit the cholesterol back to the bloodstream where the circulating HDL could bind with it and transport it to the liver for excretion, a process called reverse cholesterol transport. If the level of LDL remains significantly elevated in the bloodstream, the stimulus for atherosclerosis remains and the foam cells do not participate in reverse cholesterol transport.

Foam cells store cholesterol until they undergo apoptosis and release the stored lipid into the tunica media layer of the arterial wall. Macrophages release inflammatory cytokines that cause attraction of fibroblasts and increase the number of endothelial cell LDL receptors. This amplifies the binding of LDL to macrophages and creates more foam cells, which in turn leads to increased lipid deposits and fibrotic changes within the arterial wall.

Fibroblast activity is enhanced by inflammatory mediators: metalloproteinases, cytokines, growth factors, and plasmin. The arterial wall becomes less elastic because fibroblasts invade the vascular smooth muscle layer. Continual formation of foam cells and fibrosis within the vessel wall increases its thickness and promotes growth of foam cells that become fatty streaks. The fibrosis also diminishes the artery's vasodilation ability.

Formation of Fatty Streaks and Atherosclerotic Plaque. Lipid-rich, fibrotic changes of foam cells begin to form fatty streaks that are obvious on microscopic examination of the artery. As the lipid-rich fatty streak enlarges, it becomes an atherosclerotic plaque that protrudes into the vessel lumen, reducing the artery's diameter. Early in this process there may be no patient symptoms. However, with time, the plaque enlarges and becomes calcified and covered with a fibrous platelet cap. When this occurs, it is referred to as an atheroma. The vessel's elastic quality stretches to its limit to accommodate the expanding plaque and the vessel becomes stiff or hardened. For this reason, atherosclerosis is referred to as hardening of the arteries. Some obstruction of the arterial lumen occurs, vasodilatory capacity of the artery is diminished, and the patient may begin to have symptoms, particularly during exertion. Exertion brings on symptoms because extra blood supply is needed and vasodilation is required during exercise; the stiff, atherosclerotic wall is less able to accommodate these needs. Over time plaque calcifies, making it more fragile and susceptible to rupturing into pieces (see Fig. 15-9).

Plaque Rupture. There is an inflammatory sequence of events that can lead to plaque rupture. This is a complex process involving many mediators. Activated vascular endothelial cells and inflammatory WBCs secrete mediators that promote atheroma formation. Additionally, smooth muscle cells and platelets are a source of inflammatory mediators and clotting factors. The release of these mediators inhibits normal substances such as nitric oxide (NO) that should ordinarily prevent clot formation and vessel spasm. The plaque is constantly being remodeled, which increases the risk that plaque rupture will occur. The plaques that are most likely to rupture are those with large areas of extracellular lipids, foam cells, inflammatory cells, calcification, and those with a thin fibrous platelet cap. Although the actual trigger for plaque rupture is not clearly defined, once it occurs there is bleeding into the atheroma. This is followed by the release of substances that draw platelets to the site and promote platelet aggregation. This is when a piece of plaque or clot generated by the plaque can break loose and travel to an arterial site where it can obstruct blood flow. The vessel's subsequent occlusion leads to the signs and symptoms of ischemia and infarction.

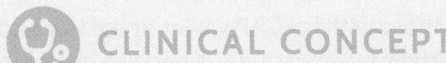

CLINICAL CONCEPT

C-reactive protein (CRP), which is a protein released with inflammation, is associated with increased risk of plaque rupture in atherosclerosis. This is measured as the high sensitivity CRP (hs-CRP) blood level.

Clinical Manifestations

Atherosclerosis is a gradual process that has no symptoms until it causes organ dysfunction. In reviewing the patient's history, it is important to determine if any disorders are present because of atherosclerosis. The clinician should ask the patient about episodes of chest pain, shortness of breath, palpitations, leg pain, or dependent edema. These questions are aimed at detecting atherosclerosis of the coronary arteries and peripheral arteries of the extremities. Additionally, if the patient indicates that these symptoms are present, it is necessary to

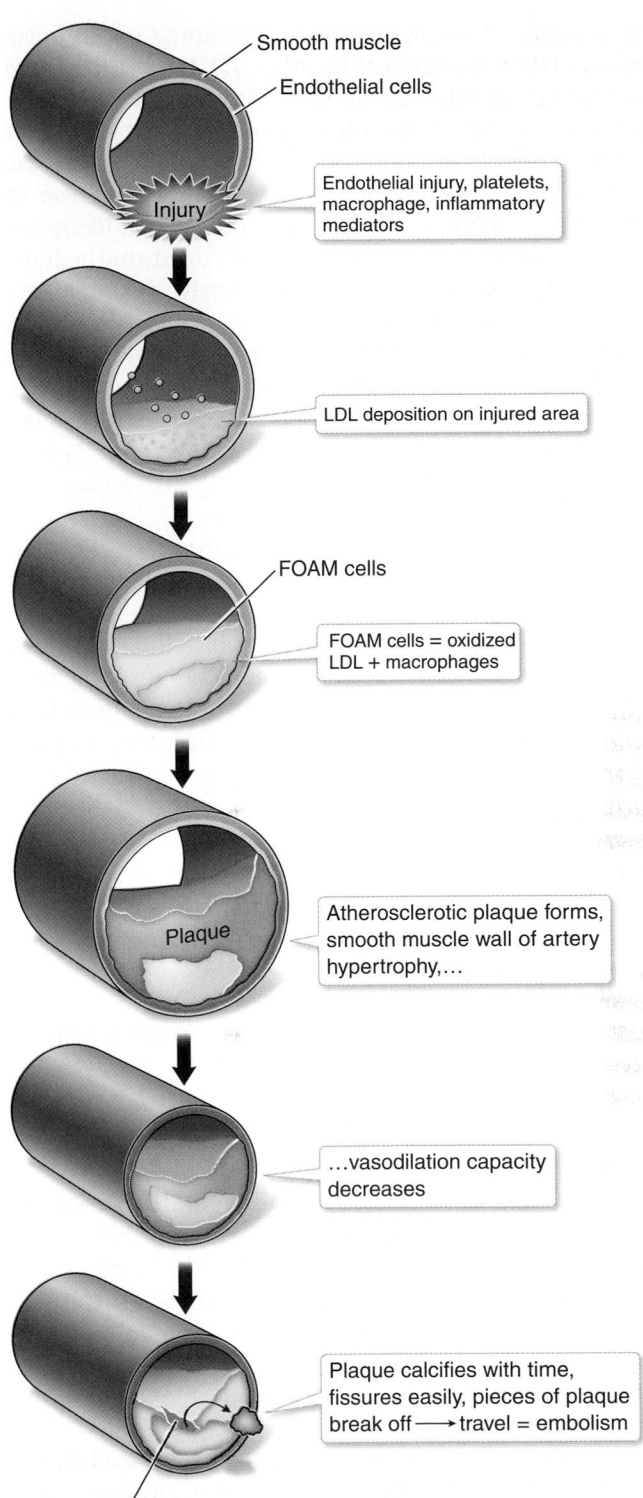

Smooth muscle
Endothelial cells
Endothelial injury, platelets, macrophage, inflammatory mediators
Injury

LDL deposition on injured area

FOAM cells
FOAM cells = oxidized LDL + macrophages

Plaque
Atherosclerotic plaque forms, smooth muscle wall of artery hypertrophy,...

...vasodilation capacity decreases

Plaque calcifies with time, fissures easily, pieces of plaque break off ⟶ travel = embolism

Fissure

FIGURE 15-9. The development of atherosclerotic plaque.

determine the quality, character, duration, and associated symptoms. The patient should be asked about smoking, diet, and exercise in daily activity.

Signs and Symptoms. During physical examination, the clinician should look for clues of atherosclerosis and CVD. Examining a patient at rest can provide information about CVD status. Is the individual obese? Is the individual short of breath at rest? Are there changes in skin color indicating pallor or cyanosis? Are pulses weak in the lower extremities? Is BP elevated? Is the pulse rapid? Does the patient have an S_4? Are bruits heard over the carotid arteries or aorta? Does the patient have apparent xanthoma or xanthelasma or arcus senilis? Is the PMI further left of the midclavicular line toward the axilla? Do you hear a heart murmur? If the answer to any of these questions is yes, then the patient likely has altered cardiovascular function. If on exertion the individual experiences chest pain or excessive dyspnea, cardiovascular function is probably compromised. A patient with chest pain may be pale and diaphoretic. Dependent edema could be indicative of heart failure. Cyanosis is indicative of decreased oxygen delivery to the tissues, another indication of heart failure.

Physical Examination

There are few outward physical symptoms associated with atherosclerosis. However, physical examination should include assessment of blood pressure. Additionally, a retina examination with an ophthalmoscope may reveal arteriosclerotic retinal artery changes indicative of atherosclerosis. In the body, turbulent blood flow through narrow areas of arteriosclerotic arteries causes a unique sound called a bruit. Bruits may be heard with a stethoscope over the carotid arteries, abdominal aorta, and renal arteries. Arterial areas narrowed by arteriosclerosis are called areas of stenosis.

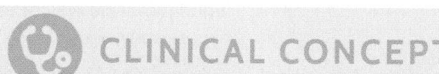

CLINICAL CONCEPT

Arterial bruits and regions of arterial stenosis are signs of severe atherosclerosis.

Diagnosis

To diagnose CVD there are various laboratory tests and procedures. The constituents of the blood, endothelial function, and inflammatory mediators can be measured to provide information about risk of CVD. Cardiac catheterization is a widely used technique to diagnose coronary arteriosclerosis. CT calcium scan and ultrasound are also used in the investigation of CVD.

Lipid Profile. Atherosclerosis begins with elevated lipids circulating in the bloodstream. Therefore, diagnostic tests for atherosclerosis include those for hyperlipidemia: total cholesterol, LDL, HDL, and triglycerides. If hyperlipidemia is present, additional tests are needed for diabetes mellitus, hypothyroidism, and liver disease. Body mass index should be calculated because obesity is commonly present with hyperlipidemia and atherosclerosis.

Endothelial Function. The endothelium plays a key role in the development of atherosclerosis; endothelial injury and resultant dysfunction is often the catalyst for atherogenesis. Endothelium-dependent vasodilation can be assessed in the coronary and peripheral circulations, both invasively and noninvasively. Endothelial function of the coronary arteries can be assessed using intracoronary Doppler techniques to measure coronary blood flow in response to stimulation with acetylcholine. This can be accomplished during cardiac catheterization. In patients with healthy endothelial function, infusion of acetylcholine incites vasodilation. In patients with atherosclerosis, endothelial dysfunction becomes apparent by vasoconstriction or blunted responses to acetylcholine.

An ultrasound of the arm's brachial artery is also a noninvasive measure of endothelial cell function. A BP cuff is placed around the upper arm, which is then inflated and occludes blood flow to the forearm for 5 minutes. When the pressure is released, reactive hyperemia of the forearm should occur because of brisk vasodilation. If the forearm has delayed return of circulation, this is indicative of suboptimal arterial elasticity and endothelial injury. This technique has the advantage of being noninvasive and can readily identify populations with reduced endothelial function.

C-Reactive Protein. C-reactive protein (CRP) is an acute phase protein produced by the liver in response to inflammation in the body. CRP is produced in response to atherosclerosis, which is basically an inflammatory process. Studies have associated elevated CRP with high rates of cardiac events. According to the American Heart Association (AHA), high sensitivity CRP (hs-CRP) is a blood test that can help predict a cardiovascular event or stroke and help direct evaluation and therapy. People with elevated hs-CRP values have the highest risk of CVD; those with lower values have less of a risk.

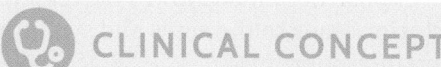

CLINICAL CONCEPT

Individuals who have hs-CRP results in the high end of the normal range have 1.5 to 4 times the risk of having an MI as those with hs-CRP values at the low end of the normal range.

Homocysteine Level. Homocysteine is an amino acid that can be measured in the blood. The body uses folic acid to metabolize and break down homocysteine into usable amino acid components. Lack of sufficient folic acid causes accumulation of homocysteine in the bloodstream, called hyperhomocysteinemia. Hyperhomocysteinemia, in turn, causes endothelial injury. Lack of sources of folic acid in the diet can predispose individuals to this risk of endothelial injury.

Calcium Computed Tomography Scan. Calcification is part of the progression of atherosclerotic plaque lesions. Calcium is obvious on x-ray and its deposition in vessels can be detected via a computed tomography (CT) scan. These CT images may be just one sign of

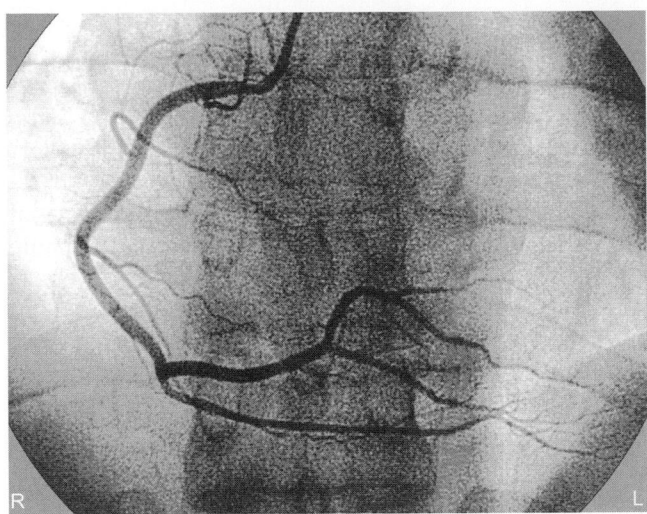

FIGURE 15-10. Coronary angiography. *(From BSIP/Science Source.)*

atherosclerosis, and clinicians need to review these scans along with patient symptoms and risk factors. Cardiac artery calcium CT scans are increasingly utilized to screen patients for potential cardiac episodes. There are studies being conducted to examine the relationship between the calcium scan value and its predictive worth in identifying patients who need to undergo cardiac catheterization or other invasive interventions.

Cardiac Angiography. Angiography is a radioopaque dye study using the cardiac catheterization procedure with x-rays to view blocked vessels (see Fig. 15-10). Sometimes referred to as cardiac catheterization, this test is the gold standard for diagnosing CAD, but it has risks because it is invasive and requires the introduction of a catheter into the body, as well as a contrast medium.

Angiography can show the outline of a blood vessel, as well as how much an atherosclerotic lesion extends into the vessel's lumen. The health-care provider is given an outline but nothing more in terms of the constituents of the lesion; sometimes, the lesion may be missed. Results from cardiac angiography help determine whether treatment with coronary artery bypass graft (CABG) surgery or percutaneous coronary intervention (PCI), such as angioplasty, may be effective.

Intravascular Ultrasonography. Intravascular ultrasonography allows for detailed assessment of the coronary arteries. Intracoronary ultrasound, via small catheters, provides a cross-sectional image of the coronary arteries, thereby providing visualization and quantization of plaque. This technology can be used to determine if a patient is a candidate for PCI. The calcium within the atherosclerotic plaque is echogenic, which allows it to be imaged on ultrasound.

Treatment
The medical treatment for atherosclerosis is the same as that for hyperlipidemia. There are surgical treatments

for atherosclerosis of the coronary arteries and obstructed arteries of the extremities. CABG surgery and PCI are commonly implemented to reperfuse ischemic areas of the heart caused by obstructed coronary arteries. Angioplasty with stent placement is a common type of PCI. CABG surgery utilizes vessel grafts that are placed to circumvent areas of obstruction caused by coronary arteriosclerosis.

Peripheral Arterial Disease

Peripheral arterial disease (PAD) (also called peripheral arterial occlusive disease; PAOD) is a disorder that involves arteriosclerosis of an extremity's peripheral arteries. This peripheral arterial occlusive disease is caused by arteriosclerotic plaque that obstructs blood flow to an area of a lower extremity. Occlusive disorders may be acute or more gradual in nature. In an acute occlusion, sudden disruption in blood flow leads to ischemia which, if untreated, could result in infarction and necrosis of tissue. More often, PAD is a chronic disorder that can be silent for years. The most common site for an occlusion is the femoral artery located above the knee, though obstruction can occur in the iliac, popliteal, or tibial arterial vessels.

Epidemiology
Peripheral artery disease affects up to 20% of individuals aged 65 years and older. Before age 65, PAD is more common in men; after age 65, both sexes are affected equally. With advanced age, the incidence of PAD continues to rise, such that at age 85 years and older, 50% to 65% of the population is affected by the disorder. PAD is probably more prevalent than studies show because as PAD is developing, it is a silent disease.

In general, African Americans have a higher incidence of PAD than Caucasians. Among persons who have a history of smoking and diabetes, the prevalence of PAD is as high as 50%.

Approximately 40% to 60% of persons with PAD also have CAD and cerebral artery disease, and patients who have PAD are 3 to 4 times more likely to suffer a stroke than the general population.

Etiology
Arteriosclerosis is the most common cause of PAD. Similar to CAD, arteriosclerotic plaque can accumulate in the peripheral arteries of the extremities. Diabetes mellitus accelerates development of PAD. The uncontrolled glucose levels in the bloodstream cause endothelial injury, which initiates arteriosclerosis throughout the body. Blood vessel injury is particularly apparent in the lower extremities in diabetes.

Risk Factors
The risk factors for PAD are the same as those for arteriosclerosis, including age older than 45 years for men and older than 55 years for women, HTN, high-fat diet, sedentary lifestyle, obesity, family history, and hyperlipidemia. Diabetes mellitus and smoking independently

increase the risk of PAD by 3 to 4 times. Chronic kidney disease, cancer, hypercoagulable states, and obesity are other risks associated with increased incidence of PAD.

Pathophysiology

In PAD, there is a reduction in arterial blood flow to the body's peripheral arteries. Arteries such as the carotid artery in the neck and femoral arteries in the legs are commonly affected. PAD typically develops gradually over time in persons with atherosclerosis. PAD of the lower extremities causes characteristic symptoms. Reduced arterial blood flow leads to tissue ischemia, which presents as **intermittent claudication**, a cramping leg pain that occurs with exertion and is usually relieved by rest. Persons with PAD can often predict how much exercise of the leg will trigger pain.

The location of pain experienced with PAD varies depending on the vessels affected. In aortoiliac disease, the pain is often in the low back or across the buttocks, whereas in femoral or popliteal arterial disease, the pain or discomfort is usually in the calf.

Intermittent claudication is a classic symptom of PAD that occurs because of ischemia of muscle tissue. In arterial obstruction, lack of circulation causes an imbalance between tissue demand for oxygen and blood supply. During exertion, muscle tissue requires increased oxygenated blood. An obstructed artery cannot furnish the needed oxygenated blood. Therefore, muscle tissue undergoes anaerobic metabolism, which yields 2 ATP and lactic acid. The 2 ATP are an inadequate amount of energy and the lactic acid is noxious to muscle tissue and causes pain. If the demand for oxygen is reduced, then the pain will subside. The patient can stop exercising to rest the muscle in order to reduce its oxygen demand and relieve the pain. Intermittent claudication is similar to angina, an episodic pain that occurs because of ischemia. However, the pain in PAD is caused by episodes of ischemia in the leg rather than the chest.

The pathophysiology of intermittent claudication is not limited to an imbalance between oxygen supply and demand. Metabolic changes in skeletal muscle that occur with ischemic episodes contribute to the pain. Injury to endothelial cells, nerve cells, and muscle tissue may occur as a result of ischemia, followed by reperfusion of the tissue. During reperfusion, free radicals are produced, causing oxidative stress. Oxidative stress, in turn, results in injury to the vascular bed and alterations in muscle metabolism, which contribute to claudication.

Clinical Presentation

When assessing the patient who is suspected of having PAD, clinicians should focus on the signs of arteriosclerosis. Patients with signs of arteriosclerosis in the coronary arteries or cerebral arteries are likely to have arteriosclerosis of the extremities as well. Patient history of HTN, hyperlipidemia, diabetes mellitus, CAD, or MI are significant predisposing factors to PAD. The patient should be questioned about specific symptoms related to ischemia of the limbs, such as pain, numbness and tingling, and coolness of the extremities. It is important to ask if the patient has leg pain or numbness upon exertion. The pain or numbness associated with PAD in the lower extremities is intermittent, associated with exertion, and relieved by rest.

Clinical manifestations seen with peripheral arterial disorders include diminished or absent pulses, palpable coolness, paresthesias, pallor, and pain of the lower extremity on exertion. The symptoms commonly worsen with elevation of the limb. Sensory assessments from distal to proximal should be carried out, including light touch, pain and temperature sensation, tactile discrimination, vibratory sensation, proprioception, and deep tendon reflexes. Loss of sensation in the feet is common in PAD; however, the patient may not be aware of this deficit.

In PAD, one limb's pulses may be weakened or absent compared with the other limb's pulses, so peripheral pulses of the lower extremities should be compared. Lower extremity peripheral pulses include the femoral, popliteal, dorsalis pedis, and posterior tibial.

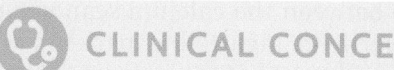

CLINICAL CONCEPT

Symptoms of PAD are not usually present until approximately 70% of the arterial lumen is occluded, so it is important to remember that PAD may be present without apparent symptoms.

Diagnosis

In addition to peripheral pulse assessment, the **ankle-brachial index (ABI)** should be assessed to determine the severity of PAD. The ABI is a comparison of upper and lower extremity systolic BP whereby the ankle pressure is divided by the brachial pressure. When done properly, this noninvasive, inexpensive, simple test has become the diagnostic test of choice for detecting PAD. ABI measures are assessed when the patient has been supine for at least 5 minutes. To assess ABI, a Doppler sphygmomanometer device measures the systolic BP in the brachial artery of each arm and in the ankles. The ABI is calculated by first assessing the systolic BP in both upper extremities by auscultating the brachial artery with a Doppler. Next, the ankle systolic pressure is measured using a Doppler over the posterior tibial artery or the dorsalis pedis artery with the cuff firmly wrapped around the ankle above the malleolus. The ABI is calculated by dividing each ankle systolic pressure by the corresponding systolic brachial pressure. This will provide an ABI for both extremities.

Generally, the ABI in a healthy person is approximately 1 or slightly greater than 1, because the ankle pressure is the same or slightly higher than the brachial systolic pressure. An ABI of lower than 1 indicates that the ankle pressure is lower than the arm systolic pressure (see Table 15-4 for significance of ABI readings).

TABLE 15-4. Ankle-Brachial Index

The ABI is the ratio of the BP in the lower legs to the BP in the arms. Normally, there is slightly higher BP in the legs compared with the arms. The ABI is calculated by dividing the systolic BP at the ankle by the systolic BP in the arm. An ABI that is greater than or equal to 1 is normal. An ABI that is lower than 1 indicates PAD. A Doppler ultrasound blood flow detector and a sphygmomanometer are usually needed to calculate ABI.

Category	ABI Calculation
Normal	1 or greater
Minimal PAD	0.8 to 0.95
Moderate PAD	0.4 to 0.8
Severe PAD	0.4 or lower

Right arm systolic pressure

Left arm systolic pressure

Right ankle systolic pressure

Left ankle systolic pressure

An ABI lower than 1 indicates PAD. A pulse volume recording detects the volume of blood flow through the limb. This test is particularly beneficial when the ABI cannot be calculated or is questionable because of calcified arteries.

Serum laboratory tests that should be assessed include complete blood count (CBC), hemoglobin, hematocrit, platelet count, lipid profile, and nonspecific tests of inflammation such as erythrocyte sedimentation rate (ESR) and CRP. Other useful diagnostic tests include impedance arterial plethysmography, pulse oximetry, ultrasonography, magnetic resonance angiography (MRA), conventional angiography, computerized tomography, and duplex ultrasonography. Plethysmography is a noninvasive diagnostic test to measure changes in the size of blood vessels by determining blood volume. Impedance plethysmography diagnoses arterio-occlusive disease of the extremities through application of a series of BP cuffs that measure the amplitude of each pulse wave. An angiogram is an examination where dye is injected into the circulation and radiographic images are taken to determine the integrity of blood vessels. The arteriogram is invasive and carries some risk to the patient with compromised circulation. Consequently, better angiographic studies utilize computerized tomography (CT) or magnetic resonance imaging (MRI) to provide cross-sectional three-dimensional views of the vessel with or without use of contrast.

ALERT! In patients with suspected or confirmed PAD, a pulse that is not palpable may indicate a critical lack of blood flow.

CLINICAL CONCEPT

Peripheral circulation can be assessed by checking capillary refill. Normal capillary refill time is less than 3 seconds.

Treatment

As in many disease processes, the initial focus of patient care in PAD should be on prevention and health promotion. Prudent lifestyle choices can prevent many of the vascular changes that occur over time. Regular exercise, weight control, abstention from smoking, maintenance of normal blood sugar levels in the presence of diabetes, and healthy cholesterol and lipoprotein levels reduce the risk of injury to the arteries that precedes disease. Exercise stimulates growth of collateral vessels, which improves blood flow. Walking regimens of 30 minutes per day at least 3 times per week have been shown to provide significant benefits.

Pharmacological treatment generally includes medications to reduce blood cholesterol, control blood pressure, inhibit platelet aggregation, and dilate peripheral vessels. The phosphodiesterase type-3 inhibitor cilostazol (Pletal®) significantly increases walking distances. Another drug, pentoxifylline (Trental®), a blood viscosity reducing agent, has shown mixed results in the treatment of claudication. Thrombolytic agents known as clot busters are also used in PAD. Best results occur when catheter-directed thrombolytic therapy takes place within 2 weeks of the onset of symptoms.

Surgery for PAD includes revascularization procedures such as bypass grafts and the placement of stents. A common procedure is femoral popliteal bypass grafting. Revascularization usually involves grafting synthetic vessels to bypass the areas of occlusion.

Aneurysm

An aneurysm is a weakening in an artery wall that causes a localized area of bulging or dilation. The weakened segment of the artery creates an outpouching that is susceptible to rupture. The disrupted wall can cause turbulent blood flow within the artery. The brain and the aorta are the typical sites for aneurysms to occur. Of the two sites, an abdominal aortic aneurysm (AAA) is the most common type of aneurysm.

Epidemiology

An AAA, the most common type of aneurysm, is found in 5% to 7% of persons older than age 60 years. As the population ages, the incidence of AAA is expected to increase. Rupture of AAA causes 15,000 deaths each year. Compared with females, males have a 3- to 8-fold higher risk of AAA formation.

Abdominal aortic aneurysms are twice as prevalent in Caucasians compared with African Americans. Elderly white males older than age 80 years with risk factors for heart disease have the highest incidence of AAA. Aortic aneurysm is often an incidental finding on examination when the patient presents to health care for another reason.

Cerebral aneurysms occur in about 1% to 5% of the U.S. population. Clinical manifestations increase with age, reaching a peak in people aged 55 to 60 years. Most patients with cerebral aneurysm are asymptomatic until the aneurysm ruptures, which results in a subarachnoid hemorrhage (SAH). About 65% of individuals with SAH from a cerebral aneurysm die suddenly before reaching health care; 25% die within a day of suffering SAH. Cerebral aneurysms are more common in African Americans than Caucasians. Approximately 15% of strokes are caused by ruptured cerebral aneurysms.

Etiology

Aneurysms are usually the result of damage to the artery lining from atherosclerosis, but may also be caused by degenerative vascular disease, infection, collagen vascular disease, or trauma. There is a probable genetic predisposition to the development of intracerebral aneurysms; the existence in some families runs as high as 10%, approximately 10 times higher than that found in the general population. Genetic mutations found on chromosomes 9, 8, and 4 are associated with cerebral aneurysm and are currently under investigation.

Risk Factors

Atherosclerosis, smoking, and HTN are major risk factors for the formation and rupture of aneurysms. Genetic factors are likely involved as there is a high incidence of aneurysm within families. Arteriosclerotic plaque invades the wall of the artery and undermines its strength; in addition, blood flow rushing by this area of arteriosclerosis contributes to the reduced strength of the wall. HTN is a constant force against arterial walls that also weakens the integrity of blood vessels. Connective tissue disorders such as Marfan or Ehlers-Danlos syndrome increase the risk of aortic aneurysm.

Pathophysiology

In an aneurysm, a region of arterial wall bulges and contains an uneven interior surface. The wall becomes weaker as blood flows against it and blood can collect within it. The dreaded sequel of an aneurysm is rupture, leading to internal hemorrhage. However, during the formation of an aneurysm, blood can enter the bulging pouch in the wall and become stagnant or turbulent. The stagnant blood inside the aneurysm can give rise to platelet aggregation, resulting in thrombus development. If thrombi embolize to other organs, they can lodge in small arterial vessels and cause ischemia, necrosis, or gangrene of distant organs.

Aneurysms are classified by their size, shape, and location. Size and location may influence treatment and prognosis. Aneurysms may also be classified as true aneurysms or false aneurysms. A true aneurysm involves all three layers of the vessel wall, whereas a false aneurysm is a hematoma where the clot is actually outside the arterial wall. Aneurysm shapes include fusiform and saccular. A fusiform aneurysm occurs when all the layers of the blood vessel's wall dilate equally, whereas a saccular aneurysm occurs when there is a weakness on only one side of the vessel with a pouchlike bulge.

Cerebral aneurysms, sometimes called berry aneurysms, are commonly small berrylike outpouchings off the circle of Willis within the subarachnoid space.

Clinical Presentation

Clinical presentation of an aneurysm depends on its size, location, and integrity. Aortic aneurysms tend to develop gradually, with 75% being undetected until they rupture. Rupture may be the first sign of an AAA. Before rupture, symptoms of an AAA include abdominal, flank, or back pain. If the aneurysm is large it can put pressure on adjacent organs. Nausea, vomiting, bowel, or ureteral compression symptoms can occur. An abrupt onset of severe constant back, flank, or abdominal pain occurs with rupture of AAA.

Cerebral aneurysms are usually silent. However, if the cerebral aneurysm is large it can put pressure on adjacent tissues such as cranial nerves. Headache and cranial nerve dysfunction can be signs of a cerebral aneurysm. Rupture of a cerebral aneurysm causes a SAH, and the classic symptom is a very severe headache; the patient usually complains of the worst headache he or she has ever experienced. Most SAHs are fatal.

During assessment of arteries, normally no sound should be heard over the smooth blood flow of an artery. However, the turbulent blood flow through a large aneurysm may be heard with a stethoscope as a bruit.

An AAA may be detected by inspection and palpation of the abdomen in a thin patient. A pulsatile mass may be evident in someone with a scaphoid abdomen. With rupture of an AAA, circulation to the lower extremities will be diminished, resulting in cool pale extremities with diminished or absent pulses. When an AAA ruptures, the patient will feel acute pain and go into shock. Manifestations of shock include cold clammy skin, decreased blood pressure, increased heart rate, and changes in the patient's level of consciousness.

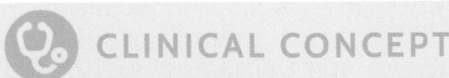
CLINICAL CONCEPT

Auscultation of a bruit over the abdominal aorta suggests presence of an aneurysm.

> **ALERT!** If a pulsatile mass is evident in the abdomen during inspection or light palpation, deep palpation should not be performed until the possibility of AAA is ruled out.

Diagnosis

Most often, aneurysms are found incidentally because they are usually silent until they rupture. Ultrasonography is the diagnostic test of choice for detection and follow up of AAAs because of its lack of invasiveness, lack of a need for contrast, and its sensitivity between 95% and 100%.

X-rays can only show a large calcified aortic silhouette and do not indicate the size of the AAA. Ultrasound can indicate the size, location, and progression of the AAA. Contrast CT scan provides detailed information on the size and location of an aneurysm. Magnetic resonance angiography (MRA), which can indicate the size and location of AAAs, does not require contrast, but it is less accurate than a CT or ultrasound. MRI can also indicate the size and location of AAAs.

Treatment

Preventive medical treatment for an aneurysm includes smoking cessation and reductions in BP and blood volume. After initial identification of an AAA, periodic follow up is needed to assess progression and susceptibility to rupture. Because of the significant risks associated with surgery, AAAs are not usually operated on until the aortic diameter exceeds 4.5 cm.

Surgical treatment usually involves endovascular repair with graft or stent placement. Endovascular repair is performed by removing the aneurysm and replacing the section of aorta with a synthetic graft or stent. For cerebral aneurysms, microsurgical and endovascular procedures aim to impede the blood flow from the cerebral circulation into the aneurysm. This is accomplished by inserting a clip, coil, or band around the neck of the aneurysm.

Aortic Dissection

Aortic dissection is a potentially lethal disorder of the aorta that involves a tear in the arterial lining between the tunica media and intima. Blood flows within the tear and commonly forms a hematoma within the wall.

Epidemiology

Aortic dissection is 2 to 3 times more common than rupture of the abdominal aorta. When left untreated, about 33% of patients die within the first 24 hours, and 50% die within 48 hours. The 2-week mortality rate approaches 75% in patients with undiagnosed ascending aortic dissection. African Americans are affected more than Caucasians. Males are affected more than females. Affected persons are commonly in the 50- to 65-year-old age range. Approximately 2,000 cases are reported in the United States annually.

Etiology

Aortic dissection is caused by genetic predisposition, HTN, and arteriosclerosis. Aortic dissection is more common in patients with connective tissue disorders, congenital aortic stenosis, or a bicuspid aortic valve. Individuals with Marfan syndrome are particularly at risk for the disorder. More than 70% of patients with aortic dissection have HTN. It is also common in those with a family history of aortic dissection.

Pathophysiology

The wall of the aorta is composed of collagen, elastin, and smooth muscle. With aging, collagen breakdown and atherosclerotic changes weaken the wall of the aorta. Because the aorta is under constant pulsatile stress, it is prone to injury and disease. If an aneurysm is present, the aorta is particularly susceptible to rupture because of high wall tension.

In aortic dissection, the aortic wall undergoes a splitting of the layers between the inner lining and middle muscular wall. Blood starts to flow between the layers, which traumatizes the region and causes more of a gap between the wall layers. Eventually, a hematoma develops in the region that protrudes into the lumen. The dissection of the aortic wall forms a false lumen in the aorta, which ends in a blind pouch that collects blood and can reduce blood flow to the major arteries arising from the aorta. Aortic dissection occurs most commonly in the first few centimeters of the aortic arch, with 90% occurring within 10 cm of the aortic valve (see Fig. 15-11).

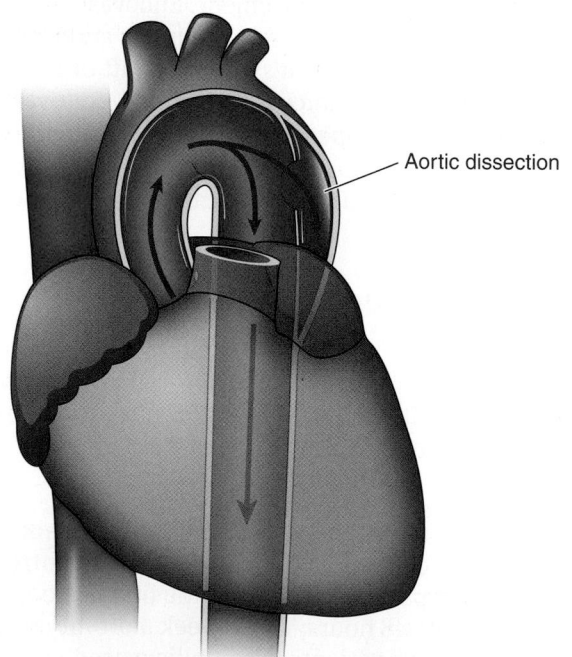

— Aortic dissection

FIGURE 15-11. Aortic dissection occurs when there is a tear in the inner wall of the aorta, which causes blood to flow between the layers of the wall of the aorta, forcing the layers apart. The separation of the layers of the aorta creates another lumen where blood flows and widens the tear in the layers. Aortic dissection increases risk of aortic rupture and is a medical emergency.

Clinical Presentation

With aortic dissection, onset of symptoms is usually sudden. The patient may complain of severe pain in the chest or back associated with a ripping or tearing sound. Pallor, tachycardia, and diaphoresis may be present. BP elevation or difference from one side to the other may be evident. The pain of aortic dissection is similar to MI.

HTN may result from the patient's anxious state or underlying essential HTN. However, with severe aortic dissection, HTN is usually present. There may be a difference in BP in the right and left arm; a difference of greater than 20 mm Hg should increase the suspicion of aortic dissection.

Signs of aortic regurgitation caused by dysfunction of the aortic valve may be present, including bounding pulses, wide pulse pressure, and diastolic murmur. Acute, severe aortic regurgitation may result in heart failure. Signs of heart failure include dyspnea, orthopnea, bibasilar crackles, or elevated jugular venous pressure.

Other cardiovascular manifestations include findings suggestive of cardiac tamponade, which is a condition caused by pressure around the heart, limiting its pumping action. Signs include muffled heart sounds, hypotension, and jugular venous distention. The superior vena cava can be compressed from the abnormally shaped aorta. The signs of this include wide pulse pressure and pulse deficit or asymmetry of peripheral pulses.

Neurological deficits occur in up to 20% of cases. The most common neurological deficits are syncope (fainting, losing consciousness) and decreased level of consciousness. Syncope may be the result of increased stimulation of the vagus nerve, hypovolemia, or dysrhythmia. Other causes of syncope or altered mental status include stroke from compromised blood flow to the brain or spinal cord.

Diagnosis

Patients require an ECG and chest x-ray. CT and MRI of the chest are also usually performed to reveal aortic dissection. Some studies have shown use of transesophageal echocardiogram (TEE) is best because it can best visualize the aortic arch. Intravascular ultrasound and angiography are also sometimes used to guide surgical repair.

Treatment

Aortic dissection is treated by surgery to repair the tear in the aorta with a graft. Aortic stenting is also done when the dissection is in the thoracic aorta. Medical management includes pain relief, usually with opiates, and beta blockers and nitrates to decrease BP, if necessary.

Vasculitis

Vasculitis, the inflammation of arterial vessels, most often occurs as a result of an autoimmune disorder.

Many of the vasculitis disorders are considered to be immune complex-mediated diseases where antigens and antibodies are formed. An excess amount of antigens is deposited in the vessel walls, leading to inflammation. With some disorders, the antigen has not been clearly identified. Vasculitis disorders are categorized according to their involvement of either large, medium, or small-size arterial vessels.

Large-sized vessel vasculitis includes temporal arteritis (TA), also called giant cell arteritis, and Takayasu arteritis. TA generally affects the branches of the aorta that supply the head. Takayasu arteritis typically involves the aorta and its main branches. Vasculitis affecting medium-sized blood vessels include the disorders known as polyarteritis nodosa (PAN) and Kawasaki disease. PAN is an inflammatory condition of arteries and arterioles that can occur in any organ of the body. Kawasaki disease is mainly a disease that affects children and causes problems in the heart. The most common types of vasculitis of small-sized arterioles include Raynaud's disease and thromboangiitis obliterans (TAO) (see Table 15-5).

Temporal Arteritis

TA is a common type of vasculitis affecting patients older than 50 years. The disorder mainly involves inflammation of the superficial temporal arteries; however, the aorta, carotid, subclavian, vertebral, and iliac arteries are often affected as well.

Epidemiology. TA typically occurs in Caucasian, older adult patients. Women are affected by TA 2 to 3 times more frequently than men. The average age of onset is 72 years, rarely affecting individuals under age 50. Incidence increases with age and can range from 1 in 10,000 to 5 in 10,000 annually in the United States. The most serious complication of TA is blindness. Studies show bilateral visual loss occurs in up to 33% of patients.

Etiology. The exact etiology of TA is unknown. The inflammation cascade is involved, although the event that triggers the cascade remains uncertain. It may be an autoimmune disease because, on biopsy, there is a preponderance of T cells that attack the arterial wall. Many infectious pathogens have been suggested as triggers, such as parvovirus B19 and Chlamydia species, but the involvement of microbial pathogens is still unclear.

Risk Factors. The etiology of TA involves both genetic and environmental influences. There is some evidence that persons with human leukocyte surface antigens HLA-DR4 and HLA-DRB104 are more susceptible than others.

Pathophysiology. TA is a chronic, systemic vasculitis, primarily affecting the walls of medium- and large-sized arteries. Inflammation is apparent across all layers of the wall of an artery with infiltration by lymphocytes, macrophages, and multinucleated giant cells. The arterial walls become thickened and arterial lumens become narrowed, which causes distal ischemia of tissues.

The temporal artery is affected, often resulting in headache in the region of the artery. Other commonly affected vessels include the ophthalmic artery and the central retinal artery, which causes visual impairment.

The inflammatory changes seen in TA are also seen in polymyalgia rheumatica (PMR). PMR and TA may have the same underlying disease process. The symptoms of PMR include pain and stiffness in the shoulder and pelvic musculature, as well as systemic signs of fever, malaise, and weight loss. Approximately half of patients initially presenting with TA also develop PMR.

Clinical Presentation. Headache is the most common symptom reported and occurs in over two-thirds of

TABLE 15-5. **Other Vasculitides**	
Vasculitide	**Description**
Wegener's granulomatosis	Vasculitis of small arterioles and venules. It can affect many organs of the body, but it usually involves the kidneys, the lungs, and the upper respiratory tract. Certain antibodies such as antineutrophil cytoplasmic antibodies are associated with Wegener's disease and may be detected in the blood in these patients.
Henoch-Schonlein purpura	A small-vessel vasculitis that also affects many different organs. This vasculitis is seen in infants, children, and adults, but it is more common in children between ages 4 and 7 years.
Hypersensitivity vasculitis	A small-vessel vasculitis that may be related to an allergic insult to blood vessels. The main areas of involvement are cutaneous, as they damage the small vessels of the skin; therefore, they may also be called predominantly cutaneous vasculitis or cutaneous leukocytoclastic vasculitis.
Essential cryoglobulinemia vasculitis	A small-vessel vasculitis related to cryoglobulins, which are small protein complexes that can precipitate in cold temperatures. They may cause vascular inflammation by depositing in the vessel walls.

patients with temporal arteritis. The headache tends to be sudden in onset and localized to the temporal region. The headache pain of TA is unique and unlike past headaches according to the patient. Therefore, TA should be considered as a diagnosis in any new type of headache in patients older than 50 years old.

TA tends to affect the branches of the carotid artery, and symptoms vary depending on the region of the ischemic artery. Superficial temporal artery involvement can cause severe scalp tenderness. Patients may also present with apparent areas of scalp ischemia and necrosis. Pain in the jaw often occurs in patients with involvement of the maxillary artery.

Sudden loss of vision may also be an initial symptom. Initial visual symptoms are usually episodic, occurring as unilateral visual loss or diplopia. If left untreated, permanent blindness can result.

Systemic symptoms caused by widespread inflammation are common. Fever, malaise, memory impairment, anorexia, weight loss, fatigue, and depression are often reported. The pain and stiffness of PMR is an initial symptom in about half of all cases of temporal arteritis.

Diagnosis. Elevated ESR and CRP are signs of inflammation in temporal arteritis. However, up to 20% of patients with TA do not present with these inflammatory indices. CBC may show leukocytosis, anemia, or thrombocytosis. Elevated liver enzymes, particularly alkaline phosphatase, are present in about one-half of patients with temporal arteritis. Color duplex ultrasound of the temporal arteries show a "halo" sign around the temporal artery. A definitive diagnosis is based on a temporal artery biopsy.

Treatment. Steroid treatment is the most common therapy used in temporal arteritis. Low-dose aspirin use is recommended as well. The patient may require oral steroids for 1 to 2 years, which can lead to complications that mandate treatment. Long-term steroids can cause glucose intolerance, osteoporosis, gastric ulceration, and immune deficiency. Some rheumatologists recommend including methotrexate and azathioprine in the treatment regimen to decrease the amount of steroids needed.

Takayasu Arteritis

Takayasu arteritis is a rare, systemic, large-vessel vasculitis of unknown cause that most commonly affects women under 50 years old. It is defined as granulomatous inflammation of the aorta and its major branches. Arteries throughout the body can be involved with multiorgan effects.

Epidemiology. Takayasu arteritis affects approximately 2.6 persons per million per year worldwide. It is observed more frequently in patients of Asian or Indian descent. Approximately 80% of patients with Takayasu arteritis are women of an average age of approximately 30 years old.

Etiology. The etiology of Takayasu arteritis is unclear; however, it is an autoimmune, inflammatory disorder.

Microorganisms proposed as etiologic agents that may trigger the disease include spirochetes, Mycobacterium tuberculosis, and streptococcal organisms. Genetic factors may play a role in the pathogenesis. Individuals with the human leukocyte surface antigen HLA-Bw52 are particularly affected.

Pathophysiology. Takayasu arteritis is an inflammatory disease of large- and medium-sized arteries that particularly affects the aorta and its branches. The inflammatory process affects the wall of the aorta, causing narrowing, obstruction, or aneurysms. Vascular complications include HTN, most often caused by renal artery stenosis, aortic insufficiency, pulmonary HTN, and aortic aneurysm.

Clinical Presentation. There are three stages of disease. During the first stage, the patient suffers a flulike illness that includes fever, general malaise, and fatigue. This stage occurs before the inflammatory changes of the arteries.

The second stage involves inflammatory changes of the arteries that cause stenosis, aneurysms, and ischemia of tissue. The patient has various complaints including pain in extremities and joints, dyspnea, palpitations, headaches, rash, hemoptysis, and weight loss. The patient can also suffer various symptoms of arterial insufficiency and ischemia, including arm numbness, claudication in the legs, visual impairment, stroke, TIA, seizures, and paralysis of extremities.

The third stage of Takayasu arteritis is referred to as the burned-out stage, when fibrosis develops in the arteries and symptoms subside. However, this stage does not occur in all patients, and does not indicate full recovery. Patients in remission can suffer a relapse of severe illness.

Diagnosis. Laboratory tests indicative of inflammation, such as ESR and CRP, are elevated. Leukocyte count may be normal or slightly elevated. Normochromic, normocytic anemia may be present. Antiendothelial antibodies may be present in the blood. Angiography is the standard test for diagnosis and evaluation of the disease. CT scan, ultrasound, and MRA are used in the diagnosis.

Treatment. Treatment in Takayasu arteritis involves controlling the inflammatory process and controlling HTN. Corticosteroids are the mainstay of therapy for active disease. Use of cytotoxic agents methotrexate, azathioprine, and cyclophosphamide may allow tapering of chronic corticosteroid treatment. Antitumor necrosis factor (anti-TNF) agents such as etanercept and infliximab are sometimes effective.

Bypass graft surgery and percutaneous balloon angioplasty are used. Angioplasty and stenting are effective to treat recurrent stenosis. Other procedures include aneurysm clipping and revascularization.

HTN is treated with antihypertensive agents, and low-dose aspirin may have a therapeutic effect in large vessel vasculitis. Antiplatelet agents, heparin, and warfarin can be used to prevent ischemic stroke.

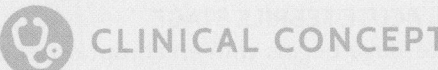

CLINICAL CONCEPT

Pregnancy can exacerbate HTN and cardiovascular complications in Takayasu arteritis, leading to high rates of morbidity and mortality.

Polyarteritis Nodosa

PAN is a rare, systemic necrotizing inflammation of the small- and medium-sized arteries that can occur anywhere in the body. The vascular inflammation leads to aneurysms, thrombosis, ischemia, and infarction in the body's organs.

Epidemiology. PAN has an incidence of about 3 to 4.5 cases per 100,000 persons annually. PAN occurs in men more often than women and predominately affects individuals aged 45 to 65 years of age.

Etiology. The etiology of PAN is unknown. However, viral infections, including human immunodeficiency virus (HIV) infection, hepatitis C virus (HCV) infection, and particularly hepatitis B virus (HBV) infection, have been associated with PAN. HBV was once the cause of up to 30% of PAN cases. However, with the advent of hepatitis B vaccine, the incidence of HBV-PAN has significantly decreased to fewer than 8% of all PAN cases. Other infectious organisms that are associated with PAN include tuberculosis, varicella-zoster virus, parvovirus B19, cytomegalovirus, human T-cell leukemia virus, streptococcal species, *Klebsiella* species, *Pseudomonas* species, *Yersinia* species, *Toxoplasma gondii*, *Rickettsiae*, trichinosis, and sarcosporidiosis. It is unclear how these microorganisms may cause PAN. Malignancies, rheumatoid arthritis (RA) and Sjögren's syndrome have also been associated with PAN. Because of effective treatments of RA, PAN has become less common in RA.

Pathophysiology. PAN is an inflammatory disorder found in arteries, mainly at bifurcation points where arteries branch off from each other. Inflammation starts in the interior lining of the artery but eventually involves the entire arterial wall. The inflammation destroys the entire wall of the artery and leads to necrosis. The weakened arteries develop aneurysms that rupture and hemorrhage. Thrombi often develop at the sites of the inflammation. With progression of the disease, the arterial wall thickens and can protrude into the lumen to cause obstruction of the artery. Arterial obstruction can lead to tissue ischemia or infarction in organs.

Clinical Presentation. PAN is a spectrum of disease ranging from single-organ involvement to widespread multiorgan failure. The patient first presents with vague, flulike symptoms of fever, malaise, fatigue, anorexia, myalgia, and arthralgias. With progression of the disorder, patients often complain of symptoms related to TIAs, particularly monocular blindness. Arteritis of the cerebral arteries can lead to cerebral hemorrhages, encephalopathy, and seizures.

Inflammation of the peripheral nerves develops in as many as 60% of patients. The neuropathy can involve motor or sensory nerves and is often asymmetrical, affecting one limb more than the other. Skin involvement that causes rash, cutaneous ischemia and infarction, gangrene, and Raynaud's phenomenon are common in PAN. Gastrointestinal involvement can present as abdominal pain, nausea, and vomiting, with or without obvious GI bleeding. Bowel ischemia and infarctions can occur.

Many patients with PAN suffer renal involvement. Renal ischemia causes flank pain and HTN. Renal failure develops in a small percentage of patients and may require dialysis. PAN can also affect the coronary arteries, leading to myocardial ischemia and infarction. Ophthalmic artery involvement presents as blurred vision. Infarction of genitourinary organs such as the testicle and ovary can occur.

Diagnosis. Angiography, CT, and MRI scans are used to examine the body for characteristic lesions. Aneurysms are often seen in the liver, kidney, and mesenteric arteries. When possible, a biopsy of involved tissue is collected to aid in the diagnosis. Biopsy reveals a necrotizing inflammation of the artery walls. Electromyography (EMG) studies may reveal neurological and muscle involvement. Nerve biopsy characteristically reveals axonal degeneration and fiber loss.

Treatment. Currently, corticosteroids are the standard treatment. The cytotoxic drug cyclophosphamide is added to the regimen when steroids do not yield results or when PAN includes major organ involvement. For patients with PAN associated with hepatitis B virus, antiviral medications, steroids, and plasmapheresis are used.

Kawasaki Disease

Kawasaki disease, or Kawasaki syndrome, is a type of vasculitis that affects children. The disorder has also been called mucocutaneous lymph node syndrome and infantile periarteritis nodosa.

Epidemiology. Epidemics of Kawasaki disease primarily occur in the late winter and spring. In the United States, approximately 3,000 children are hospitalized annually for Kawasaki disease. The disorder occurs most commonly in Asian children, especially those of Japanese descent, and is slightly more common in males than in females. Approximately 90% to 95% of cases occur in children younger than 10 years old. In the United States, the incidence peaks in children aged 18 to 24 months.

Etiology. The etiology of Kawasaki disease is unknown, but most evidence points to an infectious causative agent. Possible infectious causes include parvovirus B19, meningococcus, Mycoplasma pneumoniae, Klebsiella pneumoniae bacteremia, adenovirus, cytomegalovirus, parainfluenza type 3 virus, Rotavirus infection, measles, Epstein-Barr virus, mite-associated bacteria, and tick-borne diseases. Some studies theorize that Kawasaki disease is caused by an RNA virus that enters through the respiratory route and causes disease in genetically predisposed individuals.

Studies also show that autoimmunity and genetic predisposition may be involved in the etiology. A genetic predisposition is based on the fact that siblings of affected children have a 10 to 20 times higher probability of developing Kawasaki disease than the general population. A genetic mutation at 19q13.2 is significantly associated with an increased susceptibility to developing Kawasaki disease.

Pathophysiology. Kawasaki disease is a vascular inflammatory disease that occurs most prominently in the coronary arteries but also occurs in veins, capillaries, small arterioles, and larger arteries. Early in the disease, the arterial endothelium and muscle wall become edematous. WBCs rush to the area followed by CD8 lymphocytes and immunoglobulin A-producing plasma cells. The WBCs secrete various cytokines, including tumor necrosis factor, VEGF, interleukins (IL)-1, IL-4, and IL-6; and metalloproteinases that target the endothelium of arteries and cause vascular damage.

In severely affected vessels, there is necrosis of smooth muscle cells in the walls. The artery walls weaken and layers can separate and split, leading to aneurysms. With time, the active inflammatory cells are replaced by fibroblasts and monocytes. Fibrous tissue begins to form within the vessel wall and the inner lining thickens. The arterial vessel eventually becomes narrowed and obstructed by a thrombus. Commonly death occurs from an MI secondary to thrombosis of a coronary aneurysm or from rupture of a large coronary aneurysm.

Clinical Presentation. Most children with Kawasaki disease present with fever. Affected children are usually treated with antibiotics but fever persists. Fever can be accompanied by vomiting, decreased oral intake, cough, diarrhea, rhinorrhea, abdominal pain, and joint pain. There are four stages: acute, subacute, convalescent, and chronic phase (see Box 15-3).

Diagnosis

No specific laboratory test is used to diagnose Kawasaki disease; however, ESR, CRP, and alpha 1-antitrypsin levels are elevated at first. They usually return to normal 6 to 10 weeks after the onset of the illness. On CBC, mild-to-moderate normocytic, normochromic anemia

---

BOX 15-3. The Four Stages of Kawasaki Disease

STAGE 1: ACUTE FEBRILE STAGE

The acute stage begins with an abrupt onset of fever and lasts approximately 7 to 14 days. The fever is typically high-spiking and remittent, with peak temperatures ranging from 102°F to 104°F (39°C to 40°C) or higher. This fever is not responsive to antibiotics or antipyretics and can persist for up to 3 to 4 weeks if untreated. With appropriate therapy, high-dose aspirin, and intravenous immunoglobulin, the fever typically remits within 48 hours.

In addition to fever, signs and symptoms may include bilateral conjunctivitis (90%), anterior uveitis (70%), perianal erythema (70%), erythema and edema on the hands and feet, strawberry tongue, and lip fissures. Hepatic, renal, and gastrointestinal dysfunction can occur. Myocarditis, pericarditis, and lymphadenopathy (75%) occur. Commonly there is a single, enlarged, cervical lymph node measuring approximately 1.5 cm.

STAGE 2: SUBACUTE STAGE

The subacute stage begins when the fevers have abated, and it continues until week 4 to 6. The hallmarks of this stage are desquamation of the digits, thrombocytosis (the platelet count may exceed 1 million/μL), and the development of coronary aneurysms. The risk for sudden death is highest at this stage.

Other characteristics of the subacute stage are by persistent irritability, anorexia, and conjunctival injection. Persistence of fever beyond 2 to 3 weeks may be an indication of recrudescent Kawasaki disease. If fever persists, the outcome is less favorable because of a greater risk of cardiac complications.

STAGE 3: CONVALESCENT PHASE

The convalescent phase is marked by complete resolution of clinical signs of the illness, usually within 3 months of presentation. During this stage, most of the clinical findings resolve; however, deep transverse grooves across the nails (Beau lines) may become apparent 1 to 2 months after the onset of fever.

During the convalescent stage, cardiac abnormalities may still be apparent. Smaller coronary artery aneurysms tend to resolve on their own (60% of cases), but larger aneurysms may expand, and MI may occur. In patients whose echocardiograms were previously normal, however, detection of new aneurysms is unusual after week 8 of the illness.

STAGE 4: CHRONIC PHASE

This stage is of clinical importance only in patients who have developed cardiac complications. Its duration is of lifetime significance because an aneurysm formed in childhood may rupture in adulthood. In some cases of aneurysms rupturing in adult life, careful reviews of past medical histories have revealed febrile childhood illnesses of unknown etiology.

is observed in the acute stage. The WBC is moderate to high, with 50% of patients having a WBC count greater than 15,000/μL. The CBC shows a left shift, which indicates immature WBCs are rising within the bloodstream in an acute infection.

During the subacute stage, platelet count increases in the second and third week. Platelet counts average 700,000/μL, but levels as high as 2 million have been observed.

In the convalescent stage, the levels of platelets and other inflammatory mediators begin to return to normal values. Laboratory values may require 6 to 8 weeks to normalize.

Levels of antineutrophil cytoplasmic antibodies, antiendothelial cell antibodies, antinuclear antibody, and rheumatoid factor are all within the reference range. Culture results are negative as are tests for adenovirus. Urinalysis may show mild-to-moderate numbers of WBCs and proteinuria. Two urine biomarkers—proteins called meprin and filamin—may be present.

Echocardiography is the main diagnostic study used to evaluate for coronary artery aneurysms. Echocardiograms should be obtained at the time of Kawasaki disease diagnosis, at 2 weeks, and at 6 to 8 weeks after the onset of the illness. These may need to be performed more frequently in high-risk patients.

Magnetic resonance imaging, MRA, and CT scanning are other noninvasive tests that can be used to evaluate coronary artery abnormalities.

On electrocardiography (ECG), tachycardia, prolonged PR interval, ST-T wave changes, and decreased R waves may indicate myocarditis. Q waves or ST-T wave changes may indicate MI. Cardiac enzyme and troponin levels are elevated if MI is present.

Some patients may require cardiac catheterization and angiography. Coronary CT angiography and MRA may also be used to evaluate the coronary arteries.

Liver enzyme tests may show elevated serum transaminase values in 40% of affected patients. Elevated alanine aminotransferase (ALT) levels can indicate serious disease. Bilirubin values are elevated in 10% of affected patients.

A chest x-ray should be done to evaluate for cardiomegaly or pneumonitis, or confirm existence of heart failure.

If the patient has joint involvement, an arthrocentesis may be indicated to analyze synovial fluid. Synovial fluid analysis in patients usually shows numerous WBCs, ranging from 125,000 to 300,000/μL, with normal glucose levels and negative culture results.

Lumbar puncture may be indicated in patients with signs of meningitis; 50% of children with Kawasaki disease show evidence of aseptic meningitis on lumbar puncture.

Some children present with many of the clinical signs of Kawasaki disease, but do not have all the required diagnostic criteria. These children are diagnosed with "incomplete" Kawasaki disease.

Treatment

The aim of treatment for Kawasaki disease is to prevent CAD and to relieve symptoms. Intravenous immunoglobulin (IVIg), the major treatment, has been shown to decrease autoantibodies and diminish the proliferation of inflammatory mediators. If there is no success with IVIg, corticosteroids and the anti-TNF agent, infliximab (Remicade®), are used. Cyclophosphamide and methotrexate have also been used with some success in IVIg-resistant disease. Aspirin is used to decrease platelet aggregation. Antiplatelets and anticoagulants may be needed to prevent thromboses.

Raynaud's Disease

Raynaud's disease causes vasospasm of the arterioles of the hands and sometimes the feet. It is a primary disorder, whereas Raynaud's phenomenon is secondary to other diseases, such as scleroderma, and other autoimmune disorders. Raynaud's phenomenon can also occur because of exposure to cold or vibration.

Epidemiology. Raynaud's disease occurs in 11% of women and 8% of men and does not usually cause serious complications. However, in rare cases, it can cause ischemia of an affected body part. Raynaud's phenomenon is commonly a sign of autoimmune disease, including scleroderma (progressive systemic sclerosis), systemic lupus erythematosus, and hyperviscosity syndromes. Raynaud's disease usually occurs in the second or third decade of life.

Etiology. The disease affects primarily young women and is often precipitated by cold temperature or stress. There may also be a genetic predisposition to the disorder.

Pathophysiology. The pathophysiology is unclear in Raynaud's disease, but it is theorized to be an exaggerated reflex sympathetic stimulus that causes vasoconstriction. There is endothelial dysfunction, deficiency of the vasodilatory mediator NO, and high levels of endothelin-1, a potent vasoconstrictor. High levels of circulating angiotensin are also present, which have vasoconstrictive effects. Research indicates that patients with Raynaud's disease or phenomenon repeatedly undergo cutaneous vasoconstriction in response to many stressful stimuli.

An important neuropeptide, calcitonin gene-related peptide, is a potent vasodilator secreted by nerves that supply blood vessels. In patients with Raynaud's disease, there is a diminished number of calcitonin gene-related peptide-releasing neurons in skin biopsy samples. Neuropeptide Y, a potent vasoconstrictor, is increased in Raynaud's phenomenon secondary to scleroderma.

In Raynaud's disease, there is increased platelet activation and aggregation. In addition, an increased production of platelet thromboxane A2, a potent vasoconstrictor, has been found in patients. There is also an impaired fibrolytic system that contributes to vascular obstruction.

Clinical Presentation. Signs of disease occur bilaterally and include pain, blanching of the skin, and numbness and coolness of the fingers and toes. Lack of oxygen to the tissue can cause cyanosis. When vasospasm subsides, blood flow returns to the extremity, causing rubor, paresthesia, and throbbing pain.

Diagnosis/Treatment. Diagnosis involves a wide variety of laboratory tests to rule out autoimmune disease. Treatment is aimed at prevention of vasospasm by avoidance of precipitating factors. Smoking cigarettes and exposure to cold should be avoided. Stress-reduction practices such as yoga or meditation are recommended. Medications that reduce vasospasm or increase blood flow in this disorder include calcium channel blockers, angiotensin II receptor antagonists, and vasodilators. A surgical treatment called sympathectomy may be required if the disorder is severe.

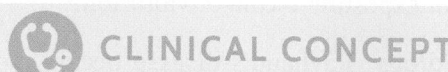

CLINICAL CONCEPT

In both Raynaud's disease and phenomenon, there is a classic tricolor change of white (pallor), blue (cyanosis), and red (rubor) in the fingers.

Thromboangiitis Obliterans

TAO, also known as Buerger's disease, is an inflammatory disorder of unknown etiology where the small- and medium-sized arteries and veins of the hands and feet are affected by inflammation, vasospasm, and thrombus formation. Thrombus formation most likely occurs as a result of reduced blood flow through the spasmodic, inflamed vessels. There may also be an autoimmune component to this disorder.

Epidemiology. TAO is mostly found in young adult males between ages 20 and 45 years who smoke. Its prevalence has been estimated at 12.6 to 20 cases per 100,000 population. Incidence has been decreasing because of the overall trend of smoking cessation in the United States; 43% of patients with the disease who continue to smoke develop ischemia, necrosis, and gangrene of the fingers, which then require amputation.

Etiology. The etiology of TAO is unknown; however, cigarette smoking is known to initiate the disease. Increased prevalence occurs in individuals with cellular types HLA-A9, HLA-A54, and HLA-B5, which suggests a genetic component to the disease.

Pathophysiology. The disease mechanism underlying TAO is unknown. It is theorized that smoking is a trigger of an immunological reaction that leads to vasospasms and inflammatory thrombi of the fingers. Patients demonstrate hypersensitivity to tobacco, elevated antiendothelial cell antibody titers, and impaired peripheral vasodilation.

Clinical Presentation. Symptoms include a deep red skin color caused by increased capillary blood flow. Dusky or cyanotic skin color also occurs as deoxygenated blood collects in the tissues. Thin, shiny skin is a result of chronic nutrient deficiency to the tissues. There is palpable coolness of the extremities and pain. Raynaud's phenomenon, which is a tricolor change in skin of fingers and toes, is often seen with the disorder. Patients may also complain of claudication of the hands, feet, forearm, and calves. Other signs include severe ischemia of fingertips, trophic nail changes, painful ulcerations, and susceptibility to gangrene.

Diagnosis. No specific laboratory tests confirm or exclude the diagnosis of TAO. The primary goal of the laboratory tests is to exclude other disease processes. Tests for antinuclear antibody, rheumatoid factor, anticentromere antibody, and antiphospholipid antibodies are done.

Angiogram is the best diagnostic test in TAO because it demonstrates the occlusive lesions of the small- and medium-sized vessels. Angiogram can show that arteriosclerosis is not the primary disease causing the vascular occlusion. There are characteristic branches of blood vessels around areas of occlusion in TAO known as "corkscrew" collaterals.

Treatment. Treatment for TAO includes smoking cessation, vasodilators to reduce vasospasm, and exercises to promote blood flow. Necrosis and gangrene of the fingers or toes requires amputation.

Arterial Ulcers

Arterial ulcers are ischemic skin wounds that develop gradually because of lack of blood flow to the extremity. Obstructive atherosclerosis causes lack of oxygen and blood delivered to the lower extremity. The extremity is pale and pulses may be absent or diminished. Toenails are thickened and yellowed and capillary refill is delayed. The leg is often painful and elevation worsens pain. Dangling the leg brings circulation into the leg and improves pain and circulation. Arterial ulcers are usually located distally at the tips of the toes, the heel, or the lateral malleolus. Diagnosis is usually made by clinical examination in a patient with known peripheral arterial disease. Patients often have diabetes and require strict glucose control. Treatments for arterial ulcers vary, depending on the severity of the arterial disease. Antibiotics may be needed to prevent infection. Endovascular therapy or bypass surgery to restore circulation to the affected leg may be required. It is important to protect the skin from further injury and breakdown. The patient should avoid pressure and weight-bearing on the affected leg. Surgical debridement, which is the removal of necrotic tissue from wounds, is commonly done to accelerate healing. Frequently, special shoes or orthotic devices are required.

Chapter Summary

- The artery wall is composed of three distinct layers: tunica intima, tunica media, and tunica externa.
- The tunica intima is composed of endothelial cells that are metabolically active and exposed to blood constituents that are potentially damaging.
- High blood pressure, high lipids, high glucose levels, free radicals, and high homocysteine levels in the blood can cause endothelial injury, which is the inciting event that starts the process of atherogenesis.
- Low-density lipoprotein (LDL) is the type of cholesterol that is deposited on artery walls.
- High-density lipoprotein (HDL) is the type of cholesterol that is excreted.
- Hyperlipidemia, which consists of high total cholesterol, high LDL, and elevated triglycerides, predisposes individuals to atherosclerosis.
- HTN is defined as either a systolic BP of 140 mm Hg or greater or a diastolic BP of 90 mm Hg or greater, which is found during at least two different clinical visits.
- The target organs of HTN include the retina, kidney, heart, brain, and peripheral arteries of the extremities.
- HTN causes arterial damage throughout the body, left ventricular hypertrophy, hemorrhagic stroke, retinopathy, and glomerular injury.

- Artery walls can become weakened and form aneurysms. Turbulent blood flow within an aneurysm can be heard as a bruit through the stethoscope.
- An abdominal aortic aneurysm, the most common type of aneurysm, is usually asymptomatic until time of rupture.
- Aortic dissection is a disorder where the layers of the wall of the aorta tear and split apart. Blood then collects in between the walls of the aorta.
- PAD, peripheral arterial disease of a lower extremity, is common in hyperlipidemia, HTN, and diabetes.
- The symptoms of PAD in a lower extremity include pulselessness intermittent claudication (pain), pallor, paresthesias, paresis (weakness), and palpable coolness.
- An ABI of lower than 1 indicates PAD.
- Vasculitis is inflammation of the arterial vessels that is often caused by autoimmune disease.
- Raynaud's phenomenon is a tricolor change in the fingertips from white (pallor), blue (cyanosis), to red (erythema) when exposed to cold or stress.
- Thrombangitis obliterans (TAO) is a vasculitis that is exacerbated by cigarette smoking.

 ## Making the Connections

Disorder and Pathophysiology	Signs and Symptoms	Physical Assessment Findings	Diagnostic Testing	Treatment
Hyperlipidemia | Elevated total cholesterol in bloodstream caused by excess ingestion of fatty foods or liver synthesis of cholesterol. Specifically, elevated LDL and elevated triglycerides in the bloodstream is harmful to cardiovascular health. LDL is deposited on arterial walls, leading to formation of atherosclerotic plaque. Low HDL in the bloodstream is also harmful because HDL normally carries cholesterol away to be excreted. All these conditions predispose individuals to atherosclerosis and cardiovascular disease.				
	None.	Xanthoma. Xanthelasma. Retinal blood vessel changes in some affected persons— copper-silver wiring, cotton wool spots. Arcus senilis	Total cholesterol greater than 200 mg/dL. LDL greater than 100 mg/dL. HDL less than 40 mg/dL. Triglycerides greater than 150 mg/dL.	Diet low in fat to reduce cholesterol ingested. Exercise daily to raise HDL. Antilipidemia agents such as statin medications that reduce liver synthesis of cholesterol.

Continued

Making the Connections—cont'd

Disorder and Pathophysiology	Signs and Symptoms	Physical Assessment Findings	Diagnostic Testing	Treatment
Hypertension | Elevated BP, which causes endothelial injury and increases susceptibility to atherosclerosis. HTN directly targets the small arteries of the retina, glomerulus, and brain, as well as peripheral arteries throughout the body. High pressure in cerebral arteries can cause stroke. It targets the heart by causing high aortic resistance against the left ventricle, which causes left ventricular hypertrophy. LVH is a risk factor for MI.				
	None.	Headache in some affected persons. BP greater than 140/90 mm Hg. S_4 heart sound. Retinal blood vessel changes in some affected persons– arteriovenous nicking, flame hemorrhages caused by retinal artery rupture.	Increased renin levels in some affected persons, which in turn will cause constant cycling of the renin-angiotensin-aldosterone system. ECG shows LVH in some affected persons.	Low-salt, low-fat diet. Exercise daily will lower BP over the long term. Antihypertensive agents such as beta blockers decrease HR and inhibit. vasoconstriction. Diuretics decrease the water content of blood. Calcium antagonists inhibit vasoconstriction. ACE inhibitors or angiotensin II receptor blockers are used.
Atherosclerosis | Widespread arterial wall plaque composed of lipid, platelets, fibroblasts, and WBCs, which protrudes into arterial lumen. The arteriosclerotic plaque hardens over time and calcifies. It then can rupture into pieces that travel as emboli and can lodge in smaller diameter arteries to cause ischemia in tissue.				
	None.	Retinal blood vessel changes in some affected persons– opper-silver wiring, cotton wool spots. Carotid, aortic, or renal artery bruits are found in some affected persons.	Elevated hs-CRP. Total cholesterol greater than 200 mg/dL. LDL greater than 130 mg/dL in most affected persons. HDL less than 40 mg/dL in most affected persons. Elevated blood homocysteine level.	Diet low in fat, low in salt to diminish formation of cholesterol and decrease BP. Antilipidemic medications. Folic acid to lower homocysteine. Anticoagulant such as aspirin. Keep BP low. Exercise daily.
Peripheral Arterial Disease | Arteriosclerosis within the lower extremities that obstructs blood flow to the legs.				
	Pain: Intermittent claudication, especially with muscle activity. Pallor of leg. Paresthesia. Palpable coolness of leg.	Pallor. Palpable coolness. Pulselessness. Paresis or paralysis. Pain with activity and on elevation.	Elevated hs-CRP. Total cholesterol greater than 200 mg/dL. LDL greater than 130 mg/dL in most affected persons. HDL less than 40 mg/dL in most affected persons. Elevated blood homocysteine level. ABI less than 1.	Diet low in fat, low in salt to diminish formation of cholesterol and decrease BP. Antilipidemic medications. Folic acid to lower homocysteine. Anticoagulant such as aspirin. Keep BP low. Exercise daily to build collateral branches of leg arteries. Vasodilator medications.

Continued

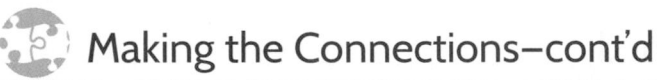

Making the Connections–cont'd

Disorder and Pathophysiology	Signs and Symptoms	Physical Assessment Findings	Diagnostic Testing	Treatment
Aneurysm | Weakening of an arterial wall with a localized area of dilatation. Blood flow is turbulent in these areas, thrombosis is more common in these areas, and rupture of the aneurysm can be fatal.				
	Cerebral aneurysm most commonly has no symptoms. Headache, seizure, or abrupt loss of consciousness occurs with rupture. If aneurysm places pressure on cranial nerve, then there will be cranial nerve dysfunction. AAA: nausea; vomiting; bowel or bladder disturbances; back, flank, or abdominal pain. May have sudden severe pain and symptoms of shock with rupture.	Cerebral aneurysm: Presentation may include headache or cranial nerve dysfunction. May have seizure activity or abrupt loss of consciousness with rupture. In AAA, pulsatile mass may be palpated or visible.	Bruit may be heard over an aortic aneurysm. Chest x-ray can often show thoracic aortic aneurysm. Computed tomography scan can show aortic aneurysm. MRA can show cerebral arterial aneurysm.	Keep BP low. Use surgical intervention to clip off cerebral aneurysm or place stent or graft within aorta to repair aneurysm.
Aortic Dissection | A disorder that causes splitting of layers of the wall of the aorta. The wall develops a gap that fills with blood.				
	Sudden chest pain that radiates to the back. Possible loss of consciousness.	Sudden hypotension, loss of consciousness. Pallor. Tachycardia. Difference of 20 mm Hg BP over brachial arteries of 2 arms.	Chest x-ray. TEE. Angiography. MRI.	Regulate BP. Pain medication. Immediate surgery to repair aortic wall.
Raynaud's Disease | Vasospastic disorder of the arterioles and arteries of the hands and feet. Often vasospasms occur because of autoimmune disease; antigen-antibody complexes are deposited in tissues.				
	Pain, numbness, and coolness of the extremity, beginning distally.	Tricolor changes, blanching, and cyanosis followed by rubor with return of blood flow when vasospasm abates.	Diagnostic studies should investigate if an autoimmune disorder is present: CBC with differential, liver function tests, renal function tests, serum glucose (fasting), erythrocyte sedimentation rate, CRP, antinuclear antibody, rheumatoid factor, anticentromere antibody, and antiphospholipid antibodies. Angiogram: best diagnostic imaging test.	Smoking cigarettes and exposure to cold should be avoided. Calcium channel blockers, and other vasodilators are used. Sympathectomy may be carried out if noninvasive medical measures are unsuccessful.

Continued

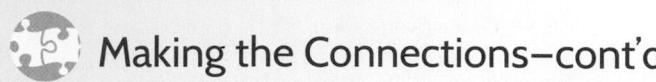
Making the Connections–cont'd

Disorder and Pathophysiology	Signs and Symptoms	Physical Assessment Findings	Diagnostic Testing	Treatment
Vasculitis | Inflammation and vasospastic condition of small- and medium-sized arteries, which can be caused by bacteria, virus, or autoimmune disease. The walls of the arteries become degraded, necrotic, and develop thrombi and aneurysms. Examples of vasculitis include PAN, Kawasaki disease, and Thromboangiitis obliterans.				
	Depending on the location of vasculitis, symptoms usually include systemic manifestations such as fever and symptoms localized to the artery involved.	Signs and symptoms depend on the specific arteries involved. Coronary artery vasculitis can cause MI. Vasculitis of a cerebral artery can cause stroke and seizures. Vasculitis of the renal artery can cause renal failure. Vasculitis of the fingers and toes can cause ischemia and gangrene.	Angiography. MRI. Computed tomography scan. EMG. Biopsy of vessel.	

Bibliography

Allen, N. B., Siddique, J., Wilkins, J. T., et al. (2014). Blood pressure trajectories in early adulthood and subclinical atherosclerosis in middle age. *JAMA*, 311(5), 490–497.

Alpert, J. S. (2012). A few unpleasant facts about atherosclerotic arterial disease in the United States and the world. *Am J Med*, 125(9), 839–840.

Bauchner, H., Fontanarosa, P. B., & Golub, R. M. (2014). Updated guidelines for management of high blood pressure: recommendations, review, and responsibility. *JAMA*, 311(5), 477–478. doi: 10.1001/jama.2013.284432.

Bhattacharya, V. (2011). Peripheral artery disease in primary care. *Clin Ad*, March 2011, 73–76.

Bonow, R. O., Maurer, G., Lee, K. L., et al. (2011). Myocardial viability and survival in ischemic left ventricular dysfunction. *N Engl J Med*, 364(17), 1617–1625. doi: 10.1056/NEJMoa1100358. Epub 2011 Apr 4.

Braverman, A. C. (2011). Aortic dissection: prompt diagnosis and emergency treatment are critical. *Cleveland Clin J Med*, 78(10), 685–696.

Criqui, M. H., Denenberg, J. O., Ix, J. H., et al. (2014). Calcium density of coronary artery plaque and risk of incident cardiovascular events. *JAMA*, 311(3), 271–278. doi: 10.1001/jama.2013.282535.

Dawber, T. R., & Kannel, W. B. (1966). The Framingham Study: an epidemiological approach to coronary heart disease. *Circ*, 34, 553–555. Retrieved from http://circ.ahajournals.org

Drozda, J., Jr., Messer, J. V., Spertus, J., et al. (2011). ACCF/AHA/AMA-PCPI 2011 performance measures for adults with coronary artery disease and hypertension: a report of the American College of Cardiology Foundation/American Heart Association Task Force on Performance Measures and the American Medical Association-Physician Consortium for Performance Improvement. *J Am Coll Cardiol*, 58(3), 316–336. doi: 10.1016/j.jacc.2011.05.002. Epub 2011 Jun 14.

Eckel, R. H., Jakicic, J. M., Ard, J. D., et al. (2013). 2013 AHA/ACC guideline on lifestyle management to reduce cardiovascular risk: a report of the American College of Cardiology/American Heart Association Task Force on Practice Guidelines. *J Am Coll Cardiol*, Nov 7. pii: S0735-1097(13)06029-4. doi: 10.1016/j.jacc.2013.11.003. Epub ahead of print.

Ghaffari, S., & Pourafkari, L. (2010). Images in clinical medicine. Aortic dissection during diagnostic aortography. *N Engl J Med*, 363(13), e18.

Grayburn, P. A. (2012). Interpreting the coronary-artery calcium score. *N Engl J Med*, 366(4), 294–296. doi: 10.1056/NEJMp1110647.

Grotta, J. C. (2013). Clinical practice. Carotid stenosis. *N Engl J Med*, 369(12), 1143–1150. doi: 10.1056/NEJMcp1214999.

Hauk, L. (2012). ACCF/AHA update peripheral artery disease management guideline. *Am Fam Phys*, 85(10), 1000–1001.

Hennion, D. R., & Siano, K. A. (2013). Diagnosis and treatment of peripheral arterial disease. *Am Fam Phys*, 88(5), 306–310.

Hoffman, G. S. (2010). Therapeutic interventions for systemic vasculitis., *Journal of American Medical Association (JAMA)*. 304(21), 2413–2414.

James, P. A., Oparil, S., Carter, B. L., et al. (2014). 2014 evidence-based guideline for the management of high blood pressure in adults: report from the panel members appointed to the Eighth Joint National Committee (JNC 8). *JAMA*, 311(5), 507–520. doi: 10.1001/jama.2013.284427.

Katz, M. H. (2014). Evolving treatment options in coronary artery disease. *JAMA Intern Med*, 174(2), 231. doi: 10.1001/jamainternmed.2013.7492.

Keaney, J. F., Jr., Curfman, G. D., & Jarcho, J. A. (2014). A pragmatic view of the new cholesterol treatment guidelines. *N Engl J Med*, 370(3), 275–278. doi: 10.1056/NEJMms 1314569. Epub 2013 Nov 27.

Keller, D. L. (2011). Giant cell arteritis. *Cleveland Clin J Med*, 78(8), 512. doi: 10.3949/ccjm.78c.08001.

Kelly, R. B. (2010). Diet and exercise in the management of hyperlipidemia. *Am Fam Phys*, 81(9), 1097–1102.

Khera, A. V., Cuchel, M., de la Llera-Moya, M., et al. (2011). Cholesterol efflux capacity, high-density lipoprotein function, and atherosclerosis. *N Engl J Med,* 364(2), 127–135. doi: 10.1056/NEJMoa1001689.

Krumholz, H. M. (2014). The new cholesterol and blood pressure guidelines: perspective on the path forward. *JAMA*, 311(14), 1403–1405. doi: 10.1001/jama.2014.2634.

LaBoon, A., & Mastracci, T. M. (2013). A 67-year old man with an abdominal aortic aneurysm. *Cleveland Clin J Med*, 80(3), 161–167.

Linsel-Nitschke, P., Samani, N. J., & Schunkert, H. (2010). Sorting out cholesterol and coronary artery disease. *N Engl J Med*, 363(25), 2462–2463.

Longo, D., Fauci, A., Kasper, D. L., et al. (Eds.). (2011). *Harrison's principles of internal medicine.* 18th ed. New York: McGraw-Hill.

Magid, D. J., & Green, B. B. (2013). Home blood pressure monitoring: take it to the bank. *JAMA*, 310(1), 40–41.

McConaghy, J. R., & Oza, R. S. (2013). Outpatient diagnosis of acute chest pain in adults. *Am Fam Phys,* 87(3), 177–182.

McDermott, M. M., Reed, G., Greenland, P., et al. (2011). Activating peripheral arterial disease patients to reduce cholesterol: a randomized trial. *Am J Med*, 124(6), 557–565.

Medicines for lowering cholesterol. (2011). *Am Fam Phys*, 84(5), 561–562.

Minder, C. M., Blaha, M. J., Horne, A., et al. (2012). Evidence-based use of statins for primary prevention of cardiovascular disease. *Am J Med,* 125(5), 440–446.

Mitka, M. (2012). AHA statement calls attention to risk of peripheral artery disease in women. *JAMA*, 307(14), 1474–1475.

Murrow, J. R. (2010). The role of non-statin therapy in managing hyperlipidemia. *Am Fam Phys,* 82(9), 1056–1057.

National Heart Lung and Blood Institute. The Dietary Approaches to Stop Hypertension—Sodium Study (DASH-Sodium). Retrieved from https://biolincc.nhlbi.nih.gov/studies/dashsodium/

National Institute of Health. National Heart, Lung, and Blood Institute (NHLBI). The seventh report of the Joint National Committee on Prevention, Detection, Evaluation, and Treatment of High Blood Pressure. Washington, DC. Retrieved from www.nhlbi.nih.gov

Navar-Boggan, A. M., Pencina, M. J., Williams, K., Sniderman, A. D., & Peterson, E. D. (2014). Proportion of US adults potentially affected by the 2014 hypertension guideline. *JAMA*, 311(14), 1424–1429. doi: 10.1001/jama.2014.2531.

Nicholls, S. J., Ballantyne, C. M., Barter, P. J., et al. (2011). Effect of two intensive statin regimens on progression of coronary disease. *N Engl J Med*, 365(22), 2078–2087. doi: 10.1056/NEJMoa1110874. Epub 2011 Nov 15.

Olin, J. W., & Sealove, B. A. (2010). Peripheral artery disease: current insight into the disease and its diagnosis and management. *Mayo Clin Proceed*, 85(7), 678–692.

Peterson, E. D., Gaziano, J. M., & Greenland, P. (2014). Recommendations for treating hypertension: what are the right goals and purposes? *JAMA*, 311(5), 474–476. doi: 10.1001/jama.2013.284430.

Pflieger, M., Winslow, B. T., Mills, K., & Dauber, I. M. (2011). Medical management of stable coronary artery disease. *Am Fam Phys*, 83(7), 819–826.

Polonsky, T. S., McClelland, R. L., Jorgensen, N. W., et al. (2010). Coronary artery calcium score and risk classification for coronary heart disease prediction. *JAMA*, 303(16), 1610–1616.

Psaty, B. M., & Weiss, N. S. (2014). 2013 ACC/AHA guideline on the treatment of blood cholesterol: a fresh interpretation of old evidence. *JAMA*, 311(5), 461–462. doi: 10.1001/jama.2013.284203.

Rudisill, H. M., Kelsberg, G., & Safranek, S. (2011). FPIN's clinical inquiries. Effective therapies for intermittent claudication. *Am Fam Phys*, 84(6), 699, 703–704.

Sarafidis, P. A., & Bakris, G. L. (2014). Early patterns of blood pressure change and future coronary atherosclerosis. *JAMA*, 311(5), 471–472. doi: 10.1001/jama.2013.285123.

Sharma, P., Sharma, S., Baltaro, R., & Hurley, J. (2011). Systemic vasculitis. *Am Fam Phys*, 83(5), 556–565.

Sipahi, I., Akay, M. H., Dagdelen, S., Blitz, A., & Alhan, C. (2014). Coronary artery bypass grafting vs percutaneous coronary intervention and long-term mortality and morbidity in multivessel disease: meta-analysis of randomized clinical trials of the arterial grafting and stenting era. *JAMA Intern Med*, 174(2), 223–230. doi: 10.1001/jamainternmed.2013.12844.

Stone, G. W., Maehara, A., Lansky, A. J., et al. (2011). A prospective natural-history study of coronary atherosclerosis. *N Engl J Med*, 364(3), 226–235. doi: 10.1056/NEJMoa1002358. Erratum in: *N Engl J Med*. 2011 Nov 24;365(21):2040.

Stone, N. J., Robinson, J., Lichtenstein, A. H., et al. (2013). 2013 ACC/AHA guideline on the treatment of blood cholesterol to reduce atherosclerotic cardiovascular risk in adults: a report of the American College of Cardiology/American Heart Association Task Force on Practice Guidelines. In *J Am College Card. 63* (25 Pt. B), 2889-2934. doi: 10.1016/j.jacc.2013.11.002.

Tripolt, N. J., & Sourij, H. (2014). New American College of Cardiology and American Heart Association cholesterol treatment guidelines: subjects with type 2 diabetes are under treated with high-intensity statins. *Diabet Med*, Feb 25. doi: 10.1111/dme.12420. Epub ahead of print.

Usman, M. H., Qamar, A., Gadi, R., et al. (2012). Extended-release niacin acutely suppresses postprandial triglyceridemia. *Am J Med,* 125(10), 1026–1035.

Villa-Forte, A. (2011). Giant cell arteritis: suspect it, treat it promptly. *Cleveland Clin J Med*, 78(4), 265–270.

Vijan, S. (2013). Diabetes: treating hypertension. *Am Fam Phys*, 87(8), 574–575.

Wireman Cook, H. (2014). Chronic arterial hypertension. *JAMA*, 311(14), 1451. doi: 10.1001/jama.2013.279439.

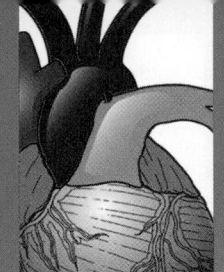

Ischemic Heart Disease and Conduction Disorders

Key Terms

Action potential

Acute coronary syndrome (ACS)

Angina pectoris

Cardiac tamponade

Cardiac troponin I (cTnI)

Coronary artery bypass graft (CABG)

Coronary artery disease

Depolarization

Dressler's syndrome

Dysrhythmias

Electrocardiogram (ECG)

Endocardium

Epicardium

Myocardial infarction (MI)

Myocardium

Non-ST elevation myocardial infarction (NSTEMI)

Percutaneous transluminal coronary angioplasty (PCTA)

Pericardial effusion

Pulsus paradoxus

Septic emboli

Stable angina

ST segment elevation myocardial infarction (STEMI)

Unstable angina

The heart is a muscular pump approximately the size of a fist that sits left of the midline in the chest, within the mediastinum of the thoracic cavity, a space between the lungs and beneath the sternum. The broadest part of the heart, called the base, is at the upper right, where the great vessels enter and leave the heart, including the aortic arch and pulmonary arteries. The pointed end of the heart, called the apex, is at the lower left.

Off the aortic arch are the coronary arteries, which perfuse the myocardium and supply the heart muscle with blood. Arteriosclerosis commonly affects these arteries and can obstruct vital blood to the heart muscle. Obstruction of a coronary artery can lead to **acute coronary syndrome (ACS),** which is a disorder caused by myocardial ischemia. If myocardial ischemia is prolonged, **myocardial infarction (MI)** occurs, which can cause death.

Researchers have been investigating coronary arteriosclerosis, myocardial ischemia, and MI for more than 50 years, and in that time there have been many technological advances in diagnosis and medical and surgical treatment of cardiovascular disease. In fact, many persons survive their first or second MI. However, despite the advances in medical technology, arteriosclerosis remains the number-one killer of much of the world's population. Heart disease is the cause of death in 25% of the U.S. population, and **coronary artery disease** is the most common form of heart disease. In 2010, coronary artery disease alone cost the United States $108.9 billion.

Structure and Function of the Heart

The heart is an organ composed of unique muscle tissue that is innervated by specialized neurons and perfused by coronary arteries. These neurons and arteries are not only vital to the heart's muscle tissue, they are vital for the individual's life. It is essential to understand the structure and function of the cardiovascular system in order to comprehend the consequences of heart disease.

Heart anatomy is sometimes difficult to understand because the aorta and pulmonary artery sit upon the base in a twisted fashion. To understand the heart's anatomy, it is useful to look at an image of the heart with the great vessels untangled (see Fig. 16-1).

The Heart Wall

The heart is composed of three layers of tissue: the epicardium, myocardium, and endocardium. The **epicardium** is the outermost layer that covers the entire heart and great vessels and then folds over to form the parietal layer that lines the fibrous membrane called the pericardium (see Fig. 16-2). Between the visceral layer and parietal layer of pericardial membrane is the pericardial cavity. This space contains approximately 30 to 50 mL of serous fluid, which acts as a lubricant to minimize friction as the heart contracts and relaxes. When the chest is opened, the heart lies beneath the sternum, covered by the pericardium. The coronary arteries are interwoven within the heart's muscular layer and are vaguely apparent as they are covered by the translucent pericardial membrane.

The **myocardium** is the heart's muscular layer that contracts; it is controlled by the autonomic nervous system. This thick wall of cardiac muscle is different from smooth or skeletal muscle. Cardiac muscle cells are densely packed together and separated by gap junctions that are low resistance pathways from one cardiac cell to another. When electrically stimulated, the myocardium

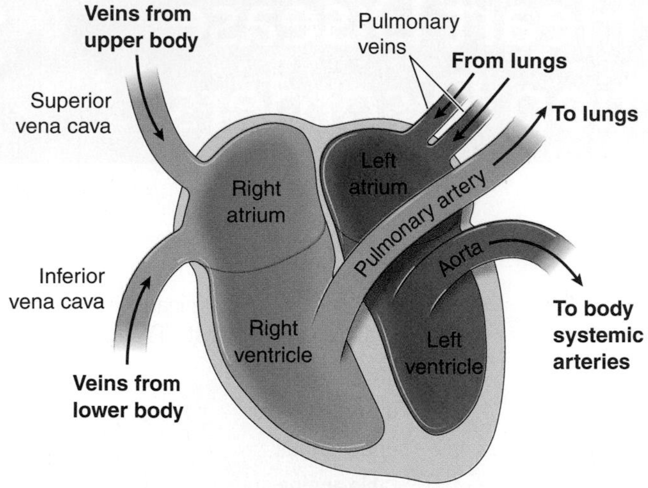

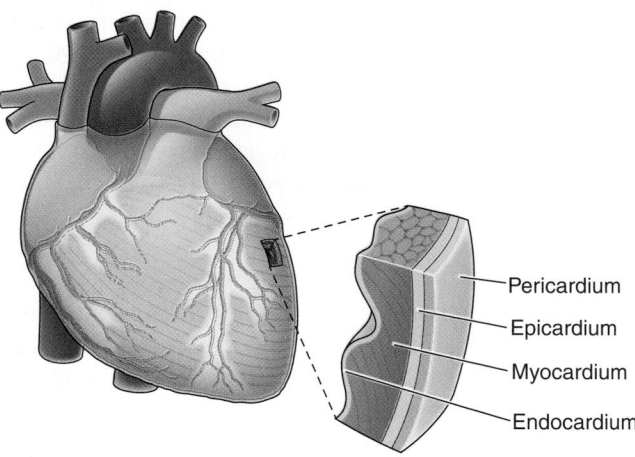

FIGURE 16-1. The SVC and IVC bring venous blood up from the body into the right atrium. The right atrium moves blood into the right ventricle, which pumps blood into the pulmonary artery, which then delivers it to the lungs for oxygenation. After oxygenation, the blood returns via the pulmonary veins into the left atrium, where it then moves into the left ventricle before being pumped into the aorta to the rest of the body. The arteries gradually become arterioles, which supply the capillary beds of all tissues; the veins then bring blood out of the tissues back up to the heart.

FIGURE 16-2. Dissection of the heart wall: pericardium, epicardium, myocardium, and endocardium.

behaves as a single unit rather than a group of isolated cells. An impulse travels rapidly so that the heart muscle contracts as one unit. Compared with other kinds of muscle, cardiac muscle can store very little calcium. It relies heavily on an influx of extracellular calcium ions for contraction.

The **endocardium** is a very thin, three-layered membrane that lines the interior heart and covers the valves. The innermost layer consists of endothelial cells supported by a thin layer of fibrous tissue, similar to the inner lining of an artery. The middle layer consists of dense fibrous tissue with elastin. The outer layer is denser connective tissue that contains blood vessels and nerves continuous with the myocardium. The four heart valves are part of the endothelium, which include the mitral, aortic, tricuspid, and pulmonic valves.

Coronary Circulation

When the chest is opened and one can look straight down onto the heart, the coronary arteries are obvious as they pierce through the myocardium. There are two major coronary arteries: the right and the left main coronary artery. These arteries arise from the aortic arch just as the aorta arises from the left ventricle of the heart. The left main coronary artery branches off into the left anterior descending (LAD) artery, which travels down the heart's vertical axis along the left ventricle, and the circumflex artery, which travels toward the back of the heart. The LAD artery supplies the left ventricle and is most commonly involved in myocardial infarction. As the major arteries pass through the myocardium, they give rise to smaller branches that supply different areas of the muscle.

The right coronary artery arises from the aortic arch and travels down over the right atrium. It then moves down along the right ventricle and branches off into the posterior descending artery, which travels around to the back and supplies the posterior portion of the heart (see Fig. 16-3).

Coronary artery anatomy is similar in most individuals. Athletic persons tend to have more branches off the left and right coronary artery, as exercise stimulates the construction of collateral vessels. These extra branches benefit the heart because the collaterals provide more avenues of circulation to the heart muscle. In arteriosclerosis, where there is possible obstruction of coronary blood vessels, the additional paths of circulation are of benefit (see Fig. 16-4).

The Chambers of the Heart

The heart contains four chambers:

1. right atrium
2. left atrium

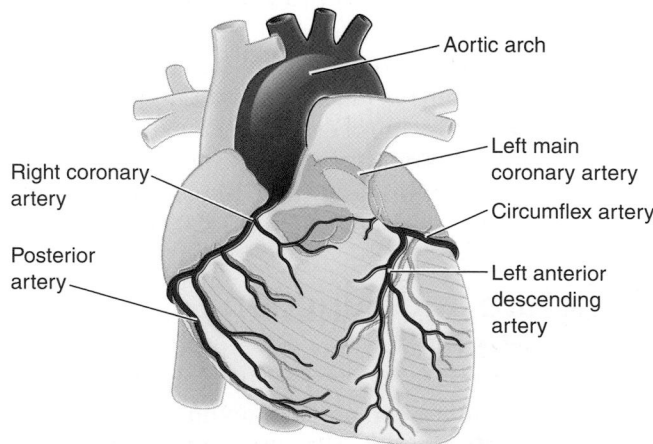

FIGURE 16-3. How the coronary arteries originate from the aorta.

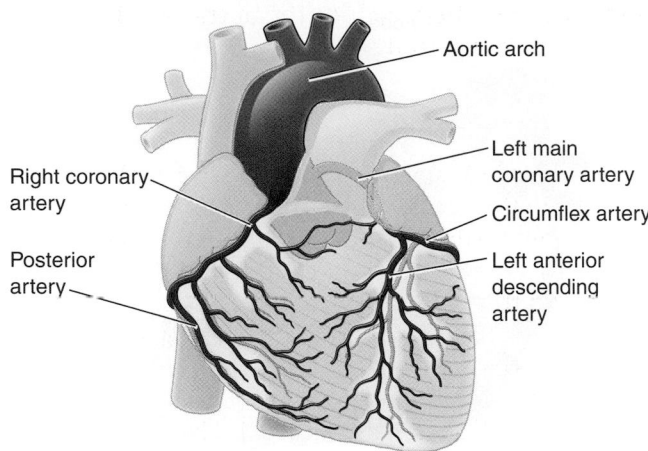

FIGURE 16-4. The physically fit heart has many collateral branches off the major coronary arteries.

3. right ventricle
4. left ventricle.

Atria are thin-layered chambers that contract and relax. These chambers sit on top of the stronger walled ventricles that also contract and relax. The right atrium collects blood from the superior vena cava (SVC) and inferior vena cava (IVC), the major veins of the body. The right atrium empties its blood into the right ventricle, which ejects its contents into the pulmonary artery. The left atrium empties its blood into the left ventricle, which ejects its contents into the aorta. The pulmonary artery is the entrance into the pulmonary circulatory system and the aorta is the entry into the systemic circulatory system (see Fig. 16-5).

Pulmonary and Systemic Circulation

The circulatory system can be divided into two parts: the pulmonary circulation and systemic circulation. The pulmonary system moves blood from the pulmonary artery into the lungs and allows oxygenation and gas exchange at the capillary bed. It then moves blood into the pulmonary vein, which empties into the left atrium. This is the only area in the body where an artery carries deoxygenated blood and a vein carries oxygenated blood (see Fig. 16-6).

The systemic circulation begins at the aorta where blood obtained from the left ventricle is moved into the tissues for oxygenation. The cells absorb the oxygen and deoxygenated blood is carried back to the heart via the veins. The veins from the lower section of the body drain into the IVC and the veins from the upper section of the body drain into the SVC. Both the SVC and IVC empty into the right atrium.

The pulmonary circulatory system functions as a low pressure system. The low pressure allows the blood to move through the lungs slowly, which is important for gas exchange. The systemic circulation is a high pressure system. Its pulsations reflect the contractions of the left ventricle; it must work against gravity to move blood into the body's tissues.

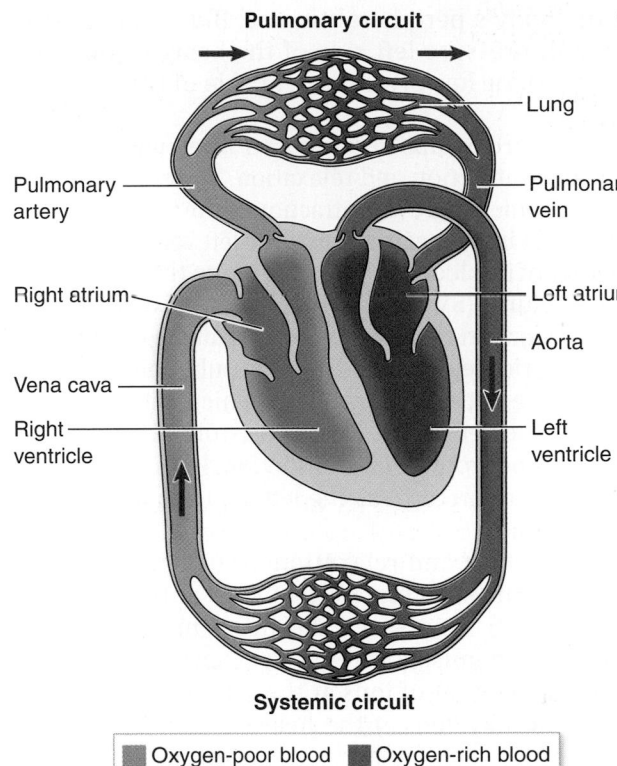

FIGURE 16-5. The heart showing the right ventricle pushing blood into the pulmonary arterial circulation and into the lungs. The pulmonary venous circulation brings blood back to the left atrium. The pulmonary artery carries blood to the lungs for oxygenation. The pulmonary veins carry oxygenated blood back to the heart from the lungs.

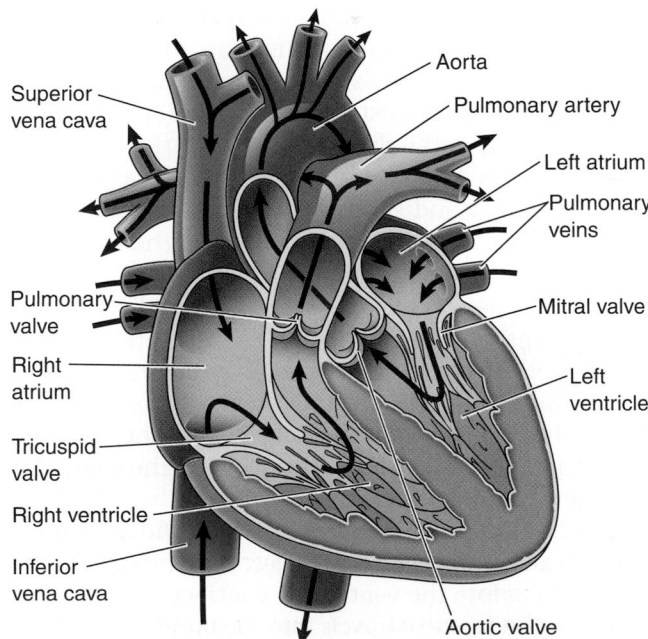

Figure 16-6. The heart with pulmonary and arterial circulation.

Systolic and Diastolic Function

The heart is composed of two pumps: the right ventricle and the left ventricle. The right ventricle must push blood through the pulmonary circulation and the left ventricle pushes blood through the aorta to all the body's peripheral tissues. Blood moves from the high pressure left side of the heart through the tissues to the low pressure right side of the heart and lungs.

The heart pumps according to a regular, rhythmic cycle of contraction and relaxation. Systole is the time frame in which there is contraction of the ventricles. During systole in the healthy adult, the left ventricle ejects a majority of its blood (70% into the aorta; this is called the stroke volume (SV), which is also known as the left ventricular ejection fraction (LVEF). Also during systole, the right ventricle ejects blood into the pulmonary artery.

Diastole is the time frame in which there is relaxation of the ventricles. During diastole, the ventricles accept blood from atrial contraction. In the left ventricle, this is referred to as the left ventricular end diastolic volume.

Contraction and relaxation occur because of the heart's neuromuscular system. The autonomic nervous system innervates the heart muscle. Within each cardiac muscle cell, neural control is governed by the movement of ions at the cell membranes. The conduction system of the heart is constructed in a precise manner. The nerve tracts direct impulses in a specific direction from the atria down into the ventricles.

The Conduction System

Heart muscle is capable of generating and conducting its own nerve impulses. There is a specialized pathway of conductive tissue that maintains an orderly impulse sequence for the heart's contraction and relaxation. The specialized conductive tissue includes the sinoatrial (SA) node in the right atrium; the atrioventricular (AV) node, which is located centrally in the heart in between the atria and ventricles; and the bundle of His, which travels down the septum between the ventricles and Purkinje fibers in the walls of both ventricles (see Fig. 16-7). The conduction system can be divided into two systems, one that stimulates the atria and one that stimulates the ventricles. The impulse begins in the SA node within the right atrium, called the heart's pacemaker. It travels to the AV node, which provides one-way conduction of the impulse down into the ventricles through the bundle of His.

The transmission is slightly delayed at the AV node so that the atria can contract and eject their blood into the ventricles before the ventricular contraction. From the AV node, the impulse travels into the bundle of His and then into the Purkinje fibers. The Purkinje fibers divide into right and left bundles that fire rapidly to allow for simultaneous excitation of the right and left ventricles.

Action Potential

A nerve impulse that occurs in cardiac tissue is called an **action potential.** Action potentials are electrical

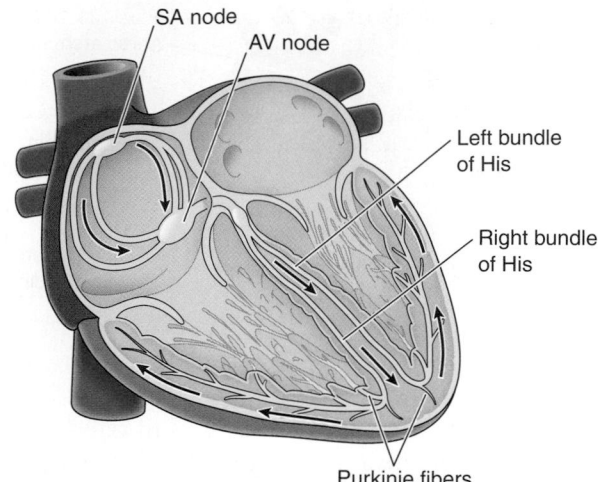

FIGURE 16-7. Conduction system through the heart. Impulses begin in the SA node of the right atrium and continue down into the AV node. The impulses then run down the right and left bundle of His to the Purkinje fibers.

currents caused by the movement of positive and negative ions in and out of the cardiac cell membrane. When stimulated, the cardiac muscle generates a five-phase action potential. Initially, the action potential rises in voltage in the stage called **depolarization,** also referred to as phase 0. It reaches a maximal point and then slightly decreases in voltage, also called phase 1. After phase 1, there is a long plateau called phase 2. Phase 3 features rapid repolarization until, in phase 4, it returns to baseline at the resting membrane potential (see Fig. 16-8).

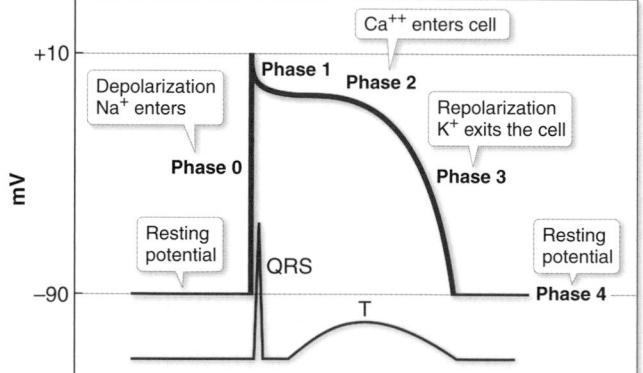

FIGURE 16-8. The cardiac action potential has five phases: During phase 0, membrane permeability to sodium ions increases, producing depolarization. During phase 1, there is partial repolarization because of a decrease in sodium permeability. Phase 2 is the plateau phase of the cardiac action potential. Membrane permeability to calcium increases during this phase, maintaining depolarization and prolonging the action potential. Membrane permeability to calcium decreases somewhat toward the end of phase 2. In phase 3, repolarization occurs, caused by the exit of potassium ions. At phase 4, there is a resting membrane potential.

The membrane of cardiac muscle has three types of ion channels that allow the voltage changes during the phases of the action potential. These are fast sodium channels, slow calcium-sodium channels, and potassium channels. At rest, the cardiac membrane is at −90 mV. In phase 0 the opening of fast sodium channels causes the initial upstroke of the action potential called depolarization. The entry of sodium ions into the cell causes a shift of electrical potential from −90 mV to +20 mV. Phase 1 occurs at the peak of the action potential; there is then an abrupt decrease in sodium permeability of the cardiac cell membrane. Phase 2 is the plateau of the action potential caused by slow opening of sodium-calcium channels. Calcium ions enter the muscle cell and are integral to the contractile action of the cardiac muscle fibers. Phase 3 is the rapid repolarization that causes a decrease of the action potential down toward resting potential. During phase 3, the influx of calcium ceases and there is a sharp rise in potassium permeability of the cardiac cell membrane. Potassium ions move out of the cell and the resting cell membrane potential is reestablished. In phase 4, the sodium-potassium pump is activated, moving sodium out of the cell and bringing potassium into the cell.

Absolute Refractory Period

The heart pump contracts and relaxes because of the ion channel movements of the action potential. There is a period in the action potential during which no stimuli can generate another action potential. This period is known as the absolute refractory period, and it includes phases 0, 1, 2, and part of phase 3. During this time, the cells cannot depolarize again under any circumstances. In other words, a second contraction cannot be stimulated until the first contraction's action potential phases are competed. The absolute refractory period maintains alternating periods of the heart's contraction and relaxation. This protects the heart from fatal dysrhythmias. When a second impulse interferes with the phases of a first action potential in progress, rhythm disturbances, called dysrhythmias, occur.

Dysrhythmias

Dysrhythmias, also called arrhythmias, are disorders of cardiac rhythm. There are two categories of cardiac dysrhythmias: supraventricular and ventricular. The supraventricular dysrhythmias include those generated at the SA node, atria, and AV node. The ventricular dysrhythmias include those generated in the ventricular conduction system; bundle of His, Purkinje fibers, and ventricular muscle.

(**ALERT!** Ventricular dysrhythmias are potentially fatal.)

The heart can beat excessively fast in tachyarrhythmias or excessively slow in bradyarrhythmias. Heart block occurs when impulses of the conduction system are blocked, most commonly at the AV node. In complete heart block, the atria and ventricles beat independently of each other.

An ectopic pacemaker is an excitable area outside the normal conduction pathway. A premature ventricular contraction (PVC) occurs when an ectopic pacemaker initiates a contraction. Several PVCs in a row lead to ventricular tachycardia, where the ventricle is beating independently without waiting for the completion of each action potential. This can lead to ventricular fibrillation, where the heart is beating so rapidly that the ventricle is actually quivering and not ejecting any blood.

Electrocardiogram

An **electrocardiogram (ECG)** is a recording of the electrical activity of the heart that can be measured from certain points on the body. Electrodes can be placed on the skin and electrical current will project a pattern on a graph depicting the phases of resting potential, depolarization, plateau, and repolarization of the heart. There are points designated as P, Q, R, S, and T that represent different points within the phases of action potentials generated by cardiac muscle.

The P wave represents the SA node and atrial depolarization, the QRS complex represents ventricular depolarization, and the T wave represents ventricular repolarization (see Fig. 16-9). The horizontal axis of an ECG measures time in seconds, whereas the vertical axis measures amplitude of the impulse in millivolts (mV) (see Fig. 16-10). The ECG records the potential difference in charge between two electrodes as the depolarization and repolarization waves move through the heart. The shape of the tracing is determined by the direction in which the impulse spreads through the heart in relation to the electrode placement. A depolarization wave that moves toward the electrode registers positive or upward deflection. Conversely, a depolarization wave that moves away from the electrode registers negative or downward deflection. Conventionally, 12 leads are recorded for a diagnostic ECG, each providing a view of the heart's electrical forces from a different position on the body (see Fig. 16-11).

Selected Pathophysiologic Disorders of the Heart

The most common cardiac disorders cause ischemia of the heart muscle; ACS is a term used for ischemic disorders of the heart that occur suddenly and require immediate treatment. Other disorders of the heart

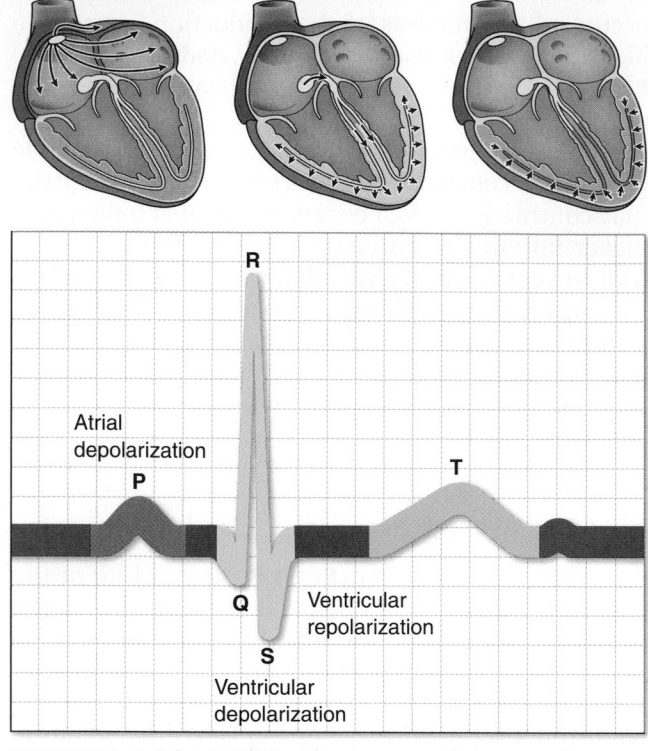

Activation of the atria   Activation of the ventricles   Resting of heart

FIGURE 16-9. A basic ECG with corresponding parts of the heart activated during points on the ECG. The P wave on the ECG represents atrial depolarization. The QRS complex represents ventricular depolarization. The T wave represents the phase of repolarization or resting of the ventricles.

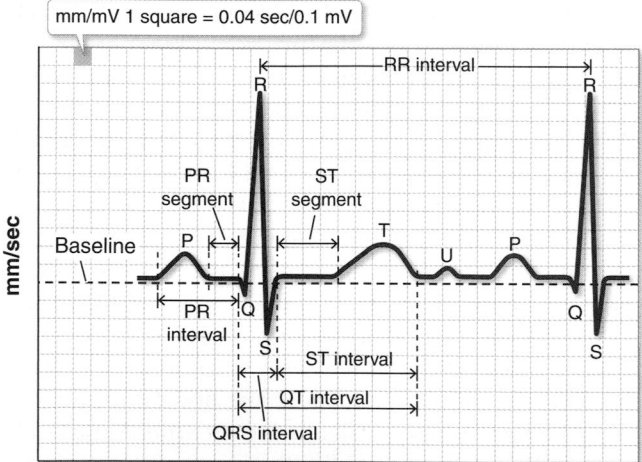

FIGURE 16-10. A detailed description of an ECG waveform. P wave = activation (depolarization) of atria. PR interval = time interval between onset of atrial depolarization and onset of ventricular depolarization. QRS complex = depolarization of ventricles, consisting of the Q, R, and S waves. QT interval = time interval between onset of ventricular depolarization and end of ventricular repolarization. R-R interval = time interval between two QRS complexes. T wave = ventricular repolarization. ST segment plus T wave (ST-T) = ventricular repolarization. U wave = time probably after depolarization (relaxation) of ventricles. The ST segment should be on the baseline in normal ECG but, above or below baseline in MI or myocardial ischemia.

include infection and inflammatory conditions. Although these are less common, they can have similar damaging effects on the heart.

Ischemic Heart Disease

Ischemic heart disease is a disorder caused by the deprivation of blood to the myocardium of the heart. When coronary blood flow is interrupted or obstructed, the result is a lack of tissue circulation, which is termed ischemia. Myocardial ischemia can be temporary, where perfusion of the myocardium is reestablished. Alternatively, it can be prolonged and lead to myocardial infarction, the death of heart muscle tissue. Arteriosclerosis of the coronary arteries can be exhibited suddenly, as in ACS, or it can be a known chronic disease called stable angina.

Acute Coronary Syndrome
ACS can take either of two forms: unstable angina (UA) or MI. There are two main types of MI: **ST segment elevation myocardial infarction (STEMI)** and **non-ST elevation myocardial infarction (NSTEMI).**

Unstable Angina. The term *angina pectoris* is derived from the Latin words *angere,* which means to choke, and *pectus,* which translates to chest. These two words aptly describe the sensations that many patients use when explaining cardiac chest pain. **Angina pectoris** is the squeezing pain in the chest that occurs when there is lack of blood flow to the myocardium (termed myocardial ischemia). Angina can be described as stable or unstable. **Stable angina** is chronic chest pain that the patient has experienced in the past and feels similar to past episodes. The patient has a prescribed medication for episodes of stable angina and self-medicates for treatment. **Unstable angina** is chest pain that is occurring for the first time by a patient, a sudden pain in the chest that is caused by myocardial ischemia.

ALERT! UA is an emergency situation requiring immediate medical attention.

UA is also the term used for chest pain that is more severe than usually experienced by the patient with chronic angina. The change in pain pattern often indicates that new regions of the heart are undergoing myocardial ischemia. This is also an emergency situation.

Epidemiology. Approximately 9 million persons suffer from angina in the United States, with 500,000 new cases diagnosed annually. The prevalence of angina rises with increasing age, with a mean age of onset of

12 leads

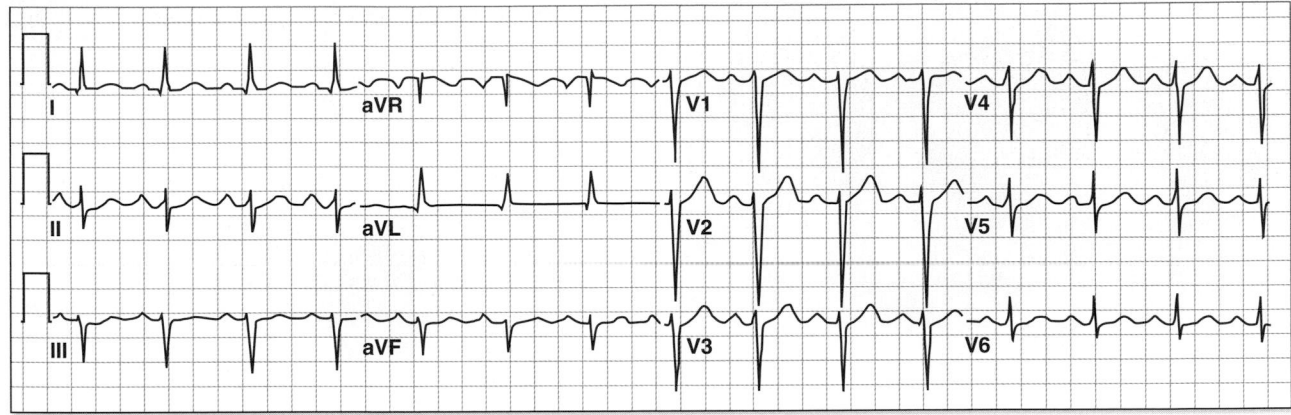

Rhythm strips lead II

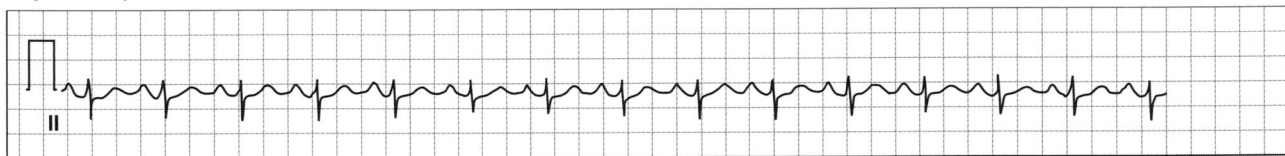

FIGURE 16-11. A 12-lead ECG will show a short segment of the recording of each of 12 leads placed on the patient's body. The ECG is arranged in a grid of four columns by three rows, the first columns being the limb leads (I, II, and III), the second column the augmented limb leads (aVR, aVL, and aVF), and the last two columns being the chest leads (V1 to V6). Each column will usually record the same moment in time for the three leads; the recording will then switch to the next column, which will record the heart beats after that point. Each of these segments is short, perhaps one to three heart beats only, depending on the heart rate, and it can be difficult to analyze any heart rhythm that shows changes between heart beats. To help with the analysis, it is common to print one or two rhythm strips as well. This will usually be lead II, which shows the electrical signal from the atria, and the P wave, which shows the rhythm for the whole time the ECG was recorded, usually 5 to 6 seconds.

62 years. There is a slightly greater prevalence of angina in women than men. Women often suffer angina equivalents, which are signs of myocardial ischemia that differ from the classic chest pain. Women also often delay obtaining medical attention for angina, which can lead to a worse outcome. Studies also show that there is less aggressive treatment for women with angina, compared with men. In general, we know less about coronary artery disorders in women compared with men. This is because women have been underrepresented in research studies regarding cardiovascular disease.

Etiology. The etiology of angina pectoris is myocardial ischemia, which results from coronary artery atherosclerosis. Atherosclerotic plaque accumulates in the coronary arteries when hyperlipidemia and endothelial injury affect the arterial lining. Angina is most often experienced in relation to exertion when the heart muscle needs more circulation to supply the cells with more oxygen. During exercise, the plaque-filled, obstructed coronary arteries cannot supply oxygenated blood to the cardiac muscle. Ischemia causes cellular hypoxia, and so the myocardial cells undergo anaerobic metabolism, which yields two adenosine triphosphate (ATP) and lactic acid. Studies have shown that adenosine may be the main chemical mediator of anginal pain. Lactic acid is also noxious to muscle cells. During

ischemia, lactic acid and adenosine (from breakdown of ATP) are both diffused into the extracellular space, causing pain.

Pathophysiology. There are several pathophysiologic processes by which cardiac muscle cells suffer ischemia and lack of sufficient oxygen. A coronary artery can be blocked by a thrombus (blood clot) that obstructs blood flow to the heart muscle. This is called a coronary thrombosis and is a common cause of myocardial ischemia. A coronary thrombosis is a consequence of endothelial injury and platelet aggregation. If the coronary artery diameter is blocked by 50% to 70%, an inadequate amount of blood flows past the blockage, resulting in ischemia. Another more common cause of myocardial ischemia is accumulation of hardened atherosclerotic plaque in a coronary artery. As arteriosclerotic plaque ages, it calcifies and becomes fragile. A piece of calcified plaque often breaks off, embolizes (travels) downstream, and lodges in a small diameter arteriole. After lodging in the arteriole, the piece of plaque obstructs blood flow to the distal myocardial tissue (see Fig. 16-12). A third and less common way that myocardial ischemia can occur is by coronary artery vasospasm. Prinzmetal or variant angina is caused by a coronary artery spasm. The vascular spasm obstructs blood flow through the coronary artery, creating ischemia in the surrounding myocardial

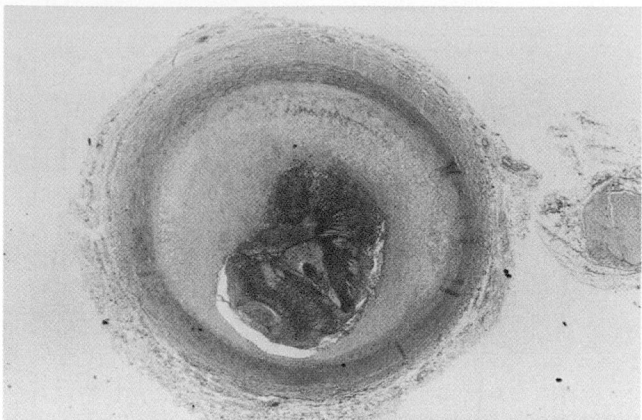

FIGURE 16-12. Coronary atherosclerosis. *(From Biophoto Associates/ Science Source.)*

tissue. When the artery relaxes, circulation is returned to the myocardium.

The least common pathophysiologic process that can cause angina is related to anemia. In anemia, the respiratory and circulatory systems are working properly, but there are not enough red blood cells (RBCs) or hemoglobin to carry the oxygen. The blood itself has a deficit of oxygen. In anemia, when exertion occurs, the lack of oxygen-carrying ability of the RBCs becomes most apparent. Exertion requires an increased amount of oxygen delivery to myocardial cells. However, in anemia there is an inadequate supply of oxygen in the blood to meet the metabolic demands of the cardiac muscle. Cardiac muscle cells enter anaerobic metabolism, resulting in angina pectoris.

Clinical Presentation. The patient with angina commonly has a history of chest pain brought on by exertion or stress. Patients report retrosternal chest discomfort and use terms such as pressure, choking, squeezing, or heaviness on the chest to describe the sensation. Classic cardiac chest pain is a crushing sensation felt on the left side of the chest, radiating into the left shoulder down the left arm. Alternatively, cardiac pain can radiate to the jaw, back, neck, right arm, or epigastric region. A significant characteristic of angina is that it is precipitated by exertion or stress and the pain lasts approximately 1 to 5 minutes. It can be relieved by rest and the use of medications called nitrates, if prescribed. Significantly, the intensity of pain does not change with respirations, cough, or change in position. Additional stressors that can bring on angina include exposure to cold, eating a large meal, and emotional stress.

Symptoms referred to as anginal equivalents may occur instead of classic angina symptoms. Anginal equivalents often occur in women and include symptoms such as episodic dyspnea, dizziness, lightheadedness, or pain of the jaw, epigastric region, or back in response to exertion or stress (see Fig. 16-13). Patients

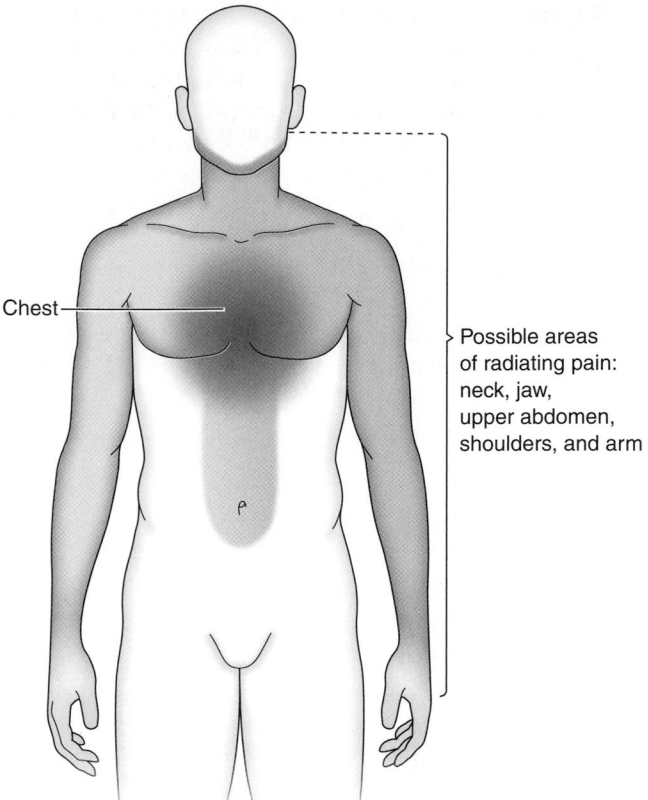

Chest

Possible areas of radiating pain: neck, jaw, upper abdomen, shoulders, and arm

FIGURE 16-13. Pain distribution of angina pectoris and myocardial infarction. The classic pain associated with ischemic heart disease is retrosternal, crushing chest pain that radiates down the left arm. Some patients describe a pressurelike pain, as if something is sitting on the chest. Pain can also radiate into the epigastric region, jaw, right arm, or back. Dyspnea, diaphoresis, pallor, and weakness are commonly associated with the pain.

with angina commonly suffer from hyperlipidemia or hypertension and have a family history of cardiovascular disease. Diabetes is also a common disorder in the patient history.

Physical Examination. There are some physical examination findings that can be noted when observing patients with angina. Commonly, individuals will clench their fist over their sternum when experiencing the pain of angina. This is known as a positive Levine's sign and is consistent with angina pectoris and MI. The individual may become pale, dyspneic, and diaphoretic. The pulses may be weak and there may be signs of hyperlipidemia such as xanthomas or xanthelasmas. Heart rate may be normal, bradycardic, or tachycardic, and there may be extra beats or irregular rhythm.

ALERT! If the patient with angina takes 3 nitroglycerin (NTG) tablets within a 10-minute period without relief of chest pain, assume the patient is enduring an MI.

Diagnosis. Diagnostic tests for angina are similar to those of arteriosclerosis (see Chapter 15: Arterial Disorders). Blood pressure measurement, total blood cholesterol, low-density lipoprotein (LDL), high-density lipoprotein (HDL), and triglycerides are measured. Additional tests include ECG, serum electrolytes, high sensitivity C-reactive protein (hs-CRP), homocysteine, cardiac enzymes, cardiac troponins (cTn), chest x-ray, calcium computed tomography (CT) scan, cardiac angiogram, cardiac catheterization, and intravascular ultrasonography. In angina pectoris, the ECG can show ST depressions or ST elevations. However, ST elevation is more commonly associated with acute MI. It is important to recognize that an ECG is not a confirmatory test of MI.

CLINICAL CONCEPT

The ECG can appear similar in angina pectoris and myocardial infarction, so cardiac troponin (cTn) is the laboratory test that is used to confirm diagnosis of MI.

A diagnostic test specifically for angina is a thallium stress test, which is a nuclear scan used to show myocardial perfusion during exercise. The patient exercises to maximal level on a treadmill or stationary bicycle while a radioactive substance called thallium is injected into the bloodstream. The thallium highlights the coronary artery blood flow to the heart stressed by exercise. This test is useful in patients who are suspected of having angina pectoris and can show the extent of coronary artery obstruction and perfusion defects in the heart. If the patient has had an MI, this scan will demonstrate the affected region of the heart.

Treatment. The goals of treatment of UA are to relieve symptoms, slow the progression of the ischemic disease, and reduce future occurrences. Ultimately, the goal is to prevent an MI and premature death. Patients mainly need education and assistance to reduce modifiable risk factors such as smoking, stress, diet, and weight. Contributing pathology such as hypertension, diabetes mellitus (DM), and hyperlipidemia must be addressed with patients to develop approaches that will reduce these risk factors.

Oxygen should be administered to the patient suffering from angina pectoris if SaO$_2$ is lower than 95%. Major medications that are used to treat angina pectoris include nitrates and aspirin. Nitrates are available as a sublingual tablet, nasal spray, paste, patch, or intravenous (IV) preparation. Nitroglycerin (NTG) sublingual tablets are classically used. Nitrates are potent vasodilators that widen the coronary arteries to deliver optimal circulation to the myocardial muscle. Aspirin can diminish platelet aggregation to decrease clot formation. Other drugs such as anticoagulants, beta blockers, and calcium channel blockers are also used to control anginal symptoms and reduce myocardial ischemia.

ALERT! NTG and other nitrate preparations can cause severe hypotension. NTG should not be administered with sildenafil (Viagra®) because of the risk of severe hypotension.

Surgery is an option, as percutaneous coronary interventions (PCI) are often used to treat angina pectoris and MI. These procedures aim to ensure perfusion in the areas of the myocardium denied of circulation because of coronary artery disease. **Percutaneous transluminal coronary angioplasty (PCTA)** is a procedure that utilizes a catheter with a balloon at the tip (see Fig. 16-14). The catheter is inserted using a peripheral artery such as the femoral artery in the leg or radial artery of the wrist. The catheter is inserted and threaded up the aorta into the obstructed coronary artery. At the point of obstruction, the balloon is inflated and pushes the plaque content against the walls of the artery, a procedure referred to as angioplasty. Alternatively, the plaque can be reduced using a specialized blade or laser tip on the catheter in a procedure referred to as an atherectomy. Often a catheter is inserted with a stent at the end. A stent is a surgical steel, meshlike, tubular structure

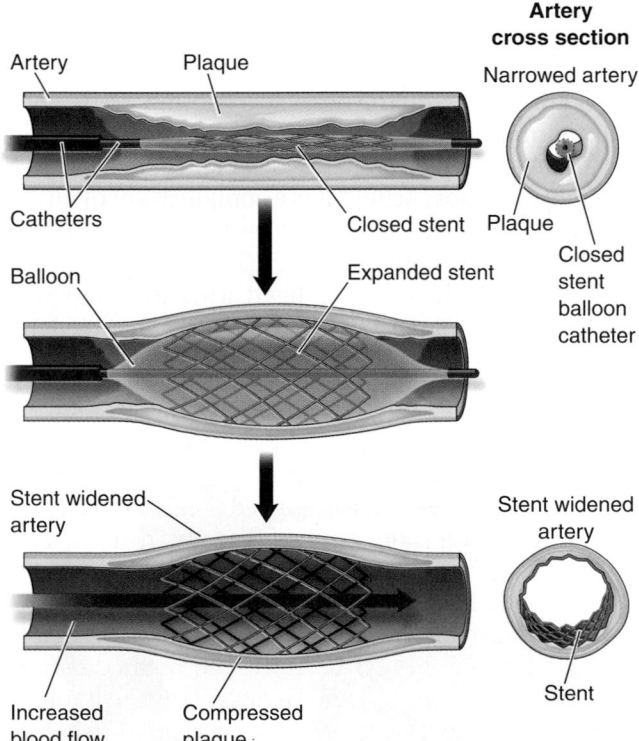

FIGURE 16-14. Percutaneous coronary transluminal angioplasty (PCTA) is the technique of mechanically widening narrowed or obstructed arteries that result from atherosclerosis. An empty and collapsed balloon on a guide wire, known as a balloon catheter, is passed into the narrowed coronary arteries and then inflated. The balloon causes compression of plaque against the internal wall of the artery. The result is an opened blood vessel for improved flow; the balloon is then deflated and withdrawn. A stent may or may not be inserted at the time of the ballooning to ensure the vessel remains open.

that is inserted at the area of obstruction. The stent structurally reinforces the wall of the coronary artery, maintains an open vessel, and prevents reblockage with plaque. Drug-eluting stents can be used that release anticoagulants along with the stent.

Coronary artery bypass graft (CABG) surgery creates new routes around narrowed and blocked arteries, allowing sufficient blood flow to deliver oxygen and nutrients to the heart muscle. Traditionally, an incision is made down the middle of the chest through the sternum (sternotomy) for access to the heart. Alternatively, minimally invasive direct CABG (MIDCABG) procedures are performed via very small incisions in the chest.

The most commonly used vessel for the bypass is the saphenous vein from the leg. Bypass grafting involves sewing the graft vessels to the coronary arteries beyond the narrowing or blockage. The other end of this vein is attached to the aorta or left internal mammary artery. Depending on the extent of obstructions in the coronary arteries, triple, quadruple, or quintuple bypasses can be performed. These types of revascularization procedures have increased survival for many individuals with CAD.

Traditionally, CABG is performed using a cardiopulmonary heart pump. The heart is stopped and the heart pump keeps the blood oxygenated until surgery is completed. Alternatively, another procedure allows CABG without using cardiopulmonary heart pump (referred to as "off pump"), with the heart still beating. This significantly minimizes the side effects and complications that may be seen after CABG (see Fig. 16-15).

Complications. Acute MI is a complication of angina pectoris and it usually occurs in the same area of ST segment change as noted by the ECG. The greater the involvements of the patient's heart with atherosclerosis and coronary vessel stenosis, the greater the incidence of MI for patients who have angina.

Coronary artery bypass

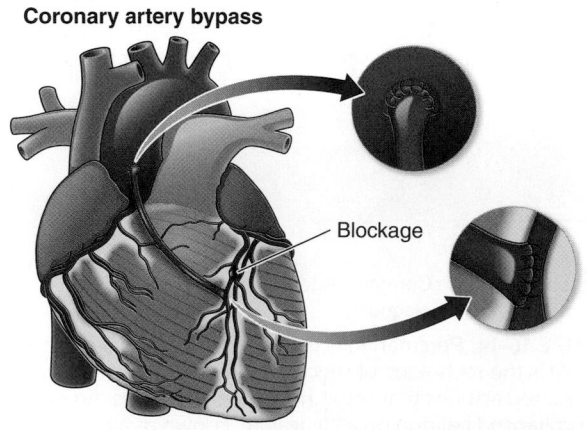

FIGURE 16-15. CABG is a surgical treatment for ischemic heart disease. During CABG, a healthy artery or vein from the body is connected, or grafted, to a blocked coronary artery. The grafted artery or vein goes around the blocked portion of the coronary artery. This creates a new path for oxygen-rich blood to flow to the heart muscle. Surgeons can bypass multiple coronary arteries during one surgery.

Myocardial infarction

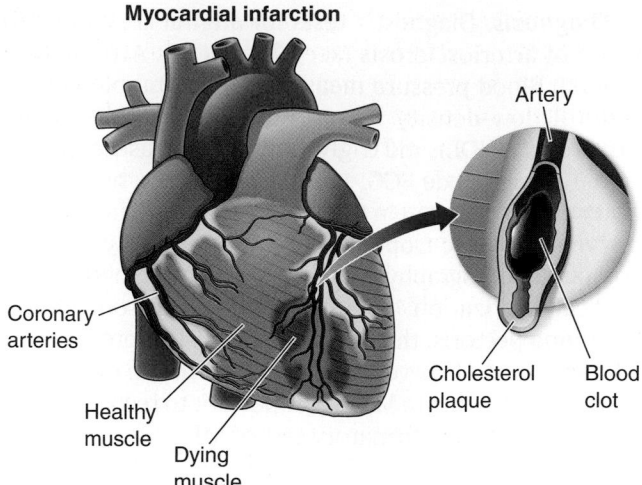

FIGURE 16-16. Prolonged ischemia leads to MI.

Acute Myocardial Infarction. Acute MI is an ACS that occurs when the heart tissue endures prolonged ischemia without recovery (see Fig. 16-16). Myocardial cells suffer irreversible damage because of hypoxia and die in a process referred to as ischemic necrosis. MIs are classified according to findings on an ECG such as STEMI or NSTEMI.

Frequently, acute MI occurs because a coronary artery is completely obstructed by atherosclerotic plaque or clot and blood flow carrying oxygen to the myocardium is blocked. More commonly, a ruptured piece of atherosclerotic plaque breaks off and travels distally within a coronary artery to an area where it obstructs blood flow. Another common scenario of acute MI occurs when an atherosclerotic plaque ruptures and the exposed plaque area attracts platelets and forms a thrombus over the region. The thrombus then breaks off and travels within the bloodstream distally to a narrow area of a coronary artery and causes obstruction. Regardless of how it occurs, MI is a dead area of the cardiac muscle that is not perfused with coronary artery blood flow.

Acute MI can also result if the coronary artery supply remains constant but the myocardial metabolic demands increase, as in the case of severe hypertension, left ventricular hypertrophy, or severe aortic valve stenosis. In all these cases, the left ventricle must pump against a great deal of resistance, which increases its need for extra coronary artery blood flow that is not available. The ventricle muscle endures ischemia; if ischemia is prolonged, infarction develops.

MI occurs because of a disparity between the oxygen needs of the myocardium and the oxygen available to the myocardium. The influences on the heart that increase myocardial oxygen demand include the following:

- changes in heart rate
- increased muscle mass
- increased systemic blood pressure.

However, MI can occur in different ways and can be classified according to how the injury occurred.

Epidemiology. Acute MI is the leading cause of death in the United States and in other industrialized nations throughout the world. Each year approximately 1.5 million Americans suffer an MI and 500,000 die from the event. Despite the public health service campaigns to educate the public about the signs and symptoms of MI and the importance of calling for medical assistance when experiencing the earliest symptoms, 250,000 individuals die of MI before arrival at a hospital each year. Hesitation and delayed request for emergency care are major causes of death resulting from MI. Once patients are at the hospital and treated, survival rates for patients with acute MI are 90% to 95% in the United States. Approximately 50% of individuals who suffer an MI are younger than 65 years old. Persons older than age 65 often suffer silent, asymptomatic MI.

Etiology. The etiology of MI is coronary artery atherosclerosis. MI begins with coronary artery obstruction, which causes ischemia (see angina pectoris).

Pathophysiology. MI occurs because of prolonged ischemia of the cardiac tissue. Damage to myocardial cells occurs when needed oxygen is either not arriving at the cells or is inadequate in amount. The extent of damage caused by an MI is influenced by three factors:

1. location or level of occlusion in the coronary artery
2. length of time that the coronary artery has been occluded
3. heart's availability of collateral circulation.

These three factors play a significant role in determining if the heart muscle will be able to survive an acute MI episode. The longer the period of coronary artery occlusion and the greater the area of myocardial ischemia, the more extensive the death of heart muscle. If, however, oxygen-enriched blood flow can be restored to the at-risk tissue, the heart muscle can be saved from necrosis and the extent of damage to the myocardium can be reduced.

Prolonged ischemia of longer than 30 minutes usually causes irreversible cellular damage and necrosis, leading to decreased contractile force and alteration of conduction in the myocardium. The necrotic cells are inactive electrically and their cell membranes rupture, releasing their cellular contents into the interstitial spaces. These cellular contents can be measured and serve as diagnostic markers of myocardial injury. For example, creatinine phosphokinase (CPK) and cardiac troponin (cTn) are released by these necrotic cells.

Ischemic myocardial cells undergo changes associated with insufficient oxygen supply and anaerobic metabolism. Failure of the sodium-potassium ATPase pump occurs because of lack of energy. Potassium concentration increases in the extracellular space and sodium remains inside the cell. There is also an increase in lactic acid from anaerobic metabolism, which leads to an increase in the hydrogen ion concentration surrounding the cell. Both of these changes contribute to changes in the myocardial cellular membrane potential. This is seen on an ECG as ST segment changes.

MI tissue changes are evident within 12 to 24 hours. The myocardium becomes pale, progressing to a mottled appearance over the next 3 to 5 days. As phagocytic cells remove necrotic debris, the myocardial wall becomes soft and relatively thin. There is interstitial edema and evidence of microscopic hemorrhage. After 5 days, the fibroblasts begin collagen deposition and scar formation. Scar formation begins at the periphery of the infarcted tissue and gradually moves inward. The scar is well established at about 2 weeks. However, it can take as long as 2 months for completion of scar formation.

The area of infarct is surrounded by an area of injury and an ischemic zone. Some of the cells in the injured area will recover. The ischemic zone has relatively viable, salvageable tissue (see Fig. 16-17). The area of infarct and ischemic zone boundaries can change postinfarction depending on the success of measures to restore blood supply such as angioplasty and thrombolytic therapy.

The ultimate size of the infarct is dependent upon the ischemic zone. Reversal of ischemia will decrease the amount of necrosis. The ischemic zone can be reduced by decreasing myocardial oxygen consumption and by increasing oxygen delivery to the tissues.

The location of the infarcted myocardium is important in terms of recovery and potential complications. For instance, inferior wall infarctions usually occur from right coronary artery occlusions and can be associated with variable degrees of heart block. The AV node usually receives its blood supply from the same vessel that nourishes the inferior wall. Thus, alterations in AV nodal conduction would be seen in an inferior wall acute MI.

Reperfusion Injury. Early treatment of the acute MI involves measures to restore myocardial blood flow. However, rapid restoration of blood flow to the myocardium also contributes to injury because ischemic myocardial tissue is less able to respond to normalized levels of oxygen and nutrients, a situation known as myocardial stunning. Reperfusion injury is most likely caused by oxidized free radicals generated by white blood cells and the cellular response to restored blood

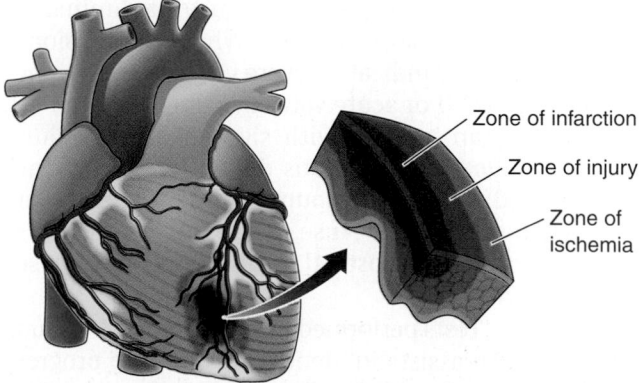

Zone of infarction

Zone of injury

Zone of ischemia

FIGURE 16-17. In acute MI, the infarcted region of the heart is surrounded by a zone of injury and a zone of ischemia. Zones surrounding the infarction are salvageable tissue that can be treated with reperfusion procedures.

flow. Blood flow through damaged microvessels gives the tissue a hemorrhagic appearance. Clinically, reperfusion injury is characterized by arrhythmias and reduced contractile function.

Clinical Presentation. The patient suffering an MI commonly has risk factors in his or her history congruent with atherosclerosis and angina pectoris. Elevated blood cholesterol levels, in particular LDL, are associated with atherosclerosis and the occurrence of an MI. They also contribute to the development of angina pectoris, which can lead to MI. DM, both type 1 and type 2, causes an acceleration of atherosclerosis and hyperlipidemia. Patients with DM are at high risk for developing cardiac pathology and MI. They also have microvascular and macrovascular changes that compromise circulation of cardiac tissue. Hypertension is also consistently associated with a higher risk of MI. This risk can be reduced if patients maintain a regimen of medication and lifestyle modifications to lower BP.

Smoking or the use of tobacco has been identified as a cardiac risk factor for many years. The free radicals contained in the smoke cause endothelial injury, which kicks off the chain of events that lead to atherosclerosis. Nicotine in cigarettes causes arterial vasoconstriction. The combination of atherosclerosis and vasoconstriction of coronary arteries leads to myocardial ischemia; if ischemia is prolonged, the result is MI.

Another important risk factor is family history. Having a family history of coronary disease increases the patient's risk for MI. However, family history is not solely caused by genetic influences; lifestyle choices are influenced by family also. Diet, food preferences, food preparation, and exercise regimen are all part of family influence.

Signs and Symptoms. MI can present with very specific signs and symptoms, or no symptoms at all. Although each patient may experience unique symptoms, there are some that are characteristic (see Box 16-1). When there are no signs or symptoms, it is referred to as a silent MI (see Box 16-2).

Physical Examination. During MI, if chest pain is ongoing, the patient may appear anxious, diaphoretic, and pale. They often demonstrate Levine's sign and respiratory distress. Peripheral pulses may be diminished and hypertension may be present. When hypotension is present, it usually indicates severe ventricular dysfunction caused by MI or acute valve dysfunction. After MI, the patient can present with signs of heart failure, which include jugular venous distention, pulmonary crackles, and a third heart sound (S_3). A new heart murmur may be present because of papillary muscle dysfunction, a common post-MI complication that causes valve dysfunction.

Diagnosis. Tests performed to diagnose an MI include an ECG, which assists in identifying an MI in progress or documenting an MI that has already occurred. The finding of ST elevation or ST depression on the ECG is indicative of ACS, but ECG alone cannot confirm MI. The clinician needs to rely on blood tests to diagnose MI.

BOX 16-1. Signs and Symptoms of Myocardial Infarction

- Diaphoresis
- Dyspnea
- Extreme anxiety
- Levine's sign (fist to chest)
- Pallor
- Retrosternal crushing chest pain that radiates to shoulder, arm, jaw, or back
- Weak pulses

BOX 16-2. Silent Myocardial Infarction

Silent MI has been shown to occur far more frequently than anginal episodes in patients with coronary artery disease. Both an increase in myocardial oxygen demand and abnormalities of coronary vasomotor tone appear to play a significant role in the genesis of silent ischemia. Recent data show that in excess of 40% of patients with stable angina have frequent episodes of silent ischemia. Silent MI and asymptomatic MI affect the elderly and those with diabetes more than any other population of patients with cardiovascular disease risk. Most silent ischemic episodes occur during minimal or no physical exertion. Exercise testing appears to be the most suitable laboratory diagnostic test to document silent MI in asymptomatic individuals. An ECG will reveal a deep Q wave when performed on a person with a prior MI.

When heart cells die, their membranes are disrupted and intracellular contents slowly spill into the bloodstream. To confirm if the patient is suffering from acute MI, blood is examined for specific cardiac enzymes and cardiac proteins, particularly CPK-MB fraction, a cardiac enzyme, and troponin I (cTnI), a cardiac protein. CPK-MB levels begin to rise within 4 hours after MI, peak between 18 and 24 hours, and subside over 3 to 4 days. The cardiac proteins are cardiac cardiac troponin I (cTnI) and troponin T (TnT). **Cardiac troponin I (cTnI)** is highly specific for cardiac muscle necrosis. Serum levels rise 4 to 8 hours after onset of chest pains, peak at 12 to 16 hours, and return to baseline within 5 to 9 days.

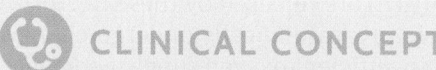 CLINICAL CONCEPT

cTnI is considered the preferred biomarker for diagnosing MI.

It is a cardiac-specific contractile protein that is not normally found in serum and is released only when myocardial cell death has occurred. For early detection of

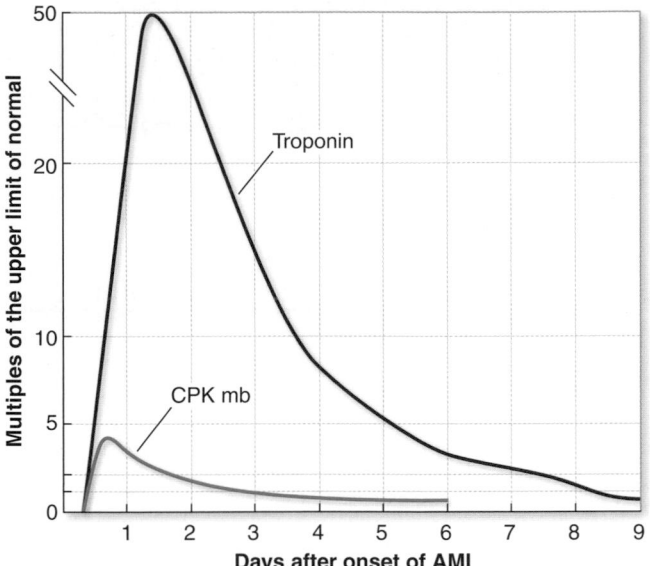

FIGURE 16-18. A graph of cardiac biomarkers that indicate MI. The most sensitive indicator of MI is CTn. The cardiac enzyme CPK-MB is also elevated.

myocardial necrosis, sensitivity of troponin is superior to that of the cardiac enzymes.

When MI is suspected, clinicians usually order serial cardiac CPK and cTnI every 8 to 12 hours for 1 to 2 days to follow the progression of MI. The rise and fall of these biomarkers provides an indication of the extent of myocardial cell death (see Fig. 16-18).

The information from an echocardiogram is limited because it cannot differentiate an acute MI from an old MI. Therefore, an echocardiogram alone cannot diagnose acute MI.

CLINICAL CONCEPT

After confirming the presence of cardiac biomarkers indicative of MI, an MI can be categorized as STEMI or NSTEMI according to the ECG. An MI that is classified as STEMI indicates that the infarction is completely through the heart wall, whereas NSTEMI indicates that the MI is subendocardial and not completely through the heart wall.

An echocardiogram may also be done to identify what portion of the heart is affected by the MI. When the heart muscle has been injured by the restriction of its oxygenated blood supply, the immediate response of the heart cells is to cease muscle contraction in the region of infarction. Contractile dysfunction occurs at the area of vessel occlusion in the cardiac muscle and the echocardiogram can identify abnormal wall motion within the infarcted portion of the heart.

Radionuclide myocardial perfusion imaging has excellent sensitivity to detect early acute MI. Perfusion imaging can be used to determine the extent and measurement of infarction. A radionuclide dye is injected into the bloodstream and it highlights areas of the heart that lack perfusion.

Treatment. In acute MI, the main focus of treatment is to reestablish the flow of blood to the heart muscle to minimize damage. It is essential that patients seek medical assistance as soon as possible for reperfusion to be achieved.

An antiplatelet agent such as aspirin can be taken as soon as the patient experiences chest pain. Oxygen should be administered if the O_2 saturation is less than 95%. Nitrates are administered, but male patients must be asked if they are taking medications for erectile dysfunction, because adding nitrates would result in severe hypotension or shock. Morphine sulfate is usually administered to relieve pain, improve gas exchange, and relieve anxiety.

Depending on the time between the onset of pain and the presentation in the emergency department, a thrombolytic agent may be given. Ideally, thrombolytic agents are used within 4 hours of the beginning of the MI. Because of the risk for uncontrolled bleeding, there are strict criteria regarding administration of thrombolytic agents. Other pharmacotherapeutic agents are given such as beta blockers and unfractionated or low molecular weight heparin. Glycoprotein IIb/IIa antagonists and angiotensin-converting enzyme (ACE) inhibitors are also prescribed later in the course of recovery.

A PCTA can be performed in the course of early MI. CABG surgery may also be an option. Later in the course of recovery after the acute MI, cardiac stress testing and cardiac rehabilitation are essential.

Complications. There are some potential complications that can occur after a patient sustains an MI. Common complications include dysrhythmia, papillary muscle rupture, thromboembolism, ventricular rupture, pericarditis, heart failure, and cardiogenic shock.

Postmyocardial Infarction Dysrhythmias. The incidence of arrhythmias after MI is greatest early after the onset of MI symptoms. Within the first 24 hours of STEMI, ventricular tachycardia (VT) and ventricular fibrillation (VF) can occur without any preceding rhythm disturbance. The mechanisms responsible for infarction-related arrhythmias include autonomic nervous system imbalance, electrolyte disturbances, and ischemia of conductile cardiac tissue. Almost all post-MI arrhythmias are the result of a phenomenon known as reentry. Normally, an electrical impulse is conducted through the heart in an orderly sequential manner beginning at the SA node to AV node through the bundle of His and finally through the Purkinje fibers. The normal ECG demonstrates a P wave, representing atrial contraction; a QRS complex, representing ventricular contraction; and a T wave, which represents the heart's repolarization or refractory period. Normally, the electrical impulse dies out after the sequence is completed and the refractory period takes place. However, ischemic and infarcted cardiac tissue do not conduct impulses; therefore, impulses are slowed or blocked at these areas. The slowing or blocking of impulses causes some impulses

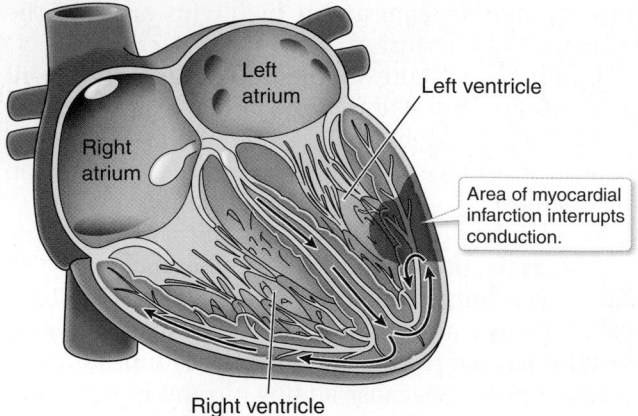

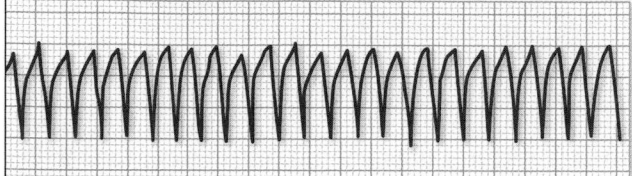

Ventricular tachycardia

FIGURE 16-19. Conduction disturbances are common complications of acute myocardial infarction. They are induced by ischemia and necrosis of the conduction system.

to change direction and travel antegrade or retrograde (see Fig. 16-19). This causes some depolarized areas to receive an extra impulse without refractory time, creating disrupted conduction and causing some of the cardiac conductile tissue to fire inappropriately. The heart develops excitable areas that begin to act as ectopic pacemakers outside the normally functioning nodes.

Atrioventricular Block. AV block is associated with anterior and inferior wall MI. In anterior wall infarction, heart block is related to ischemic malfunction of the conduction system, commonly caused by extensive myocardial damage. AV block occurs when the SA atrial impulse fails to be conducted to the ventricles, usually causing bradycardia. The ECG shows a prolonged PR interval with slowed heart rate of fewer than 60 beats per minute (see Fig. 16-20). Temporary electrical pacing provides an effective means of raising heart rate in patients with bradycardia caused by AV block.

Atrial Fibrillation. Atrial fibrillation (AF) is the most commonly encountered arrhythmia in the clinical setting, with the highest prevalence within the elderly population. AF is present in almost 30% of those aged 80 to 89 years and complicates MI in 5% to 10% of cases. It is defined as the absence of coordinated, rhythmic atrial contractions. There are multiple, irregular fibrillatory P waves on the ECG that represent multiple, rapid reentrant impulses moving around in the atrial chamber. The multiple irregular P waves may or may not stimulate a concomitant irregular, rapid ventricular response (see Fig. 16-21).

When ventricular rate increases to tachycardic levels, AF can cause decompensation of the ventricle in the form of myocardial ischemia or heart failure. AF can also

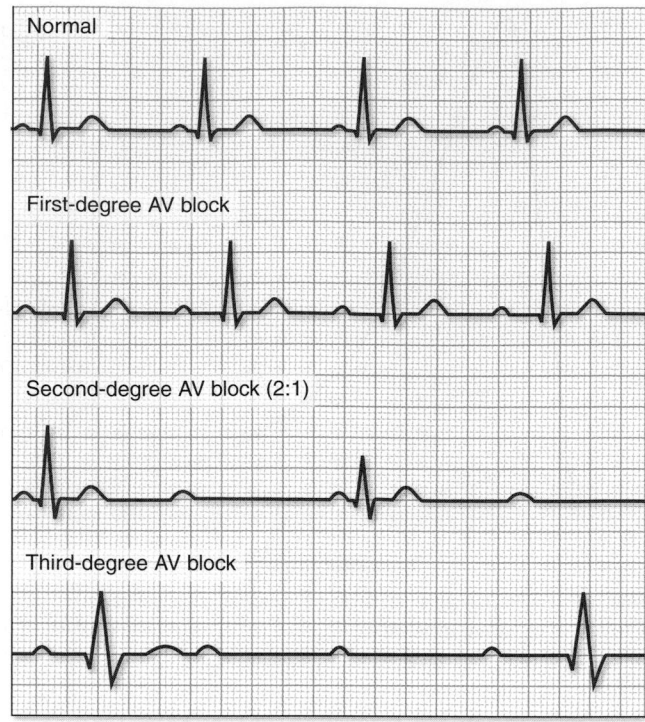

FIGURE 16-20. AV block rhythm disturbances. There is a pause after the P wave and a dropped beat in the AV block.

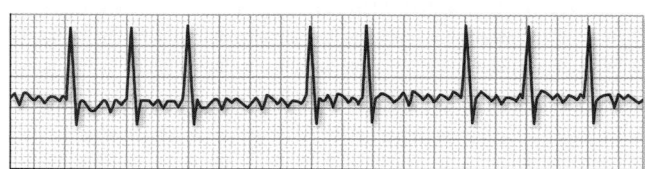

FIGURE 16-21. In atrial fibrillation, the atria are quivering and not effectively contracting. The rhythm is irregular and the ECG shows multiple P waves.

increase the risk of embolic stroke. The noncontracting, quivering atria in AF allow for stasis of blood and subsequent clot formation. A clot can form in the left atrium, travel into the left ventricle, then move into the aorta and up the subclavian artery to the internal carotid and middle cerebral artery of the brain. The rate of ischemic stroke in the presence of AF is 2 to 7 times the rate of stroke in patients without AF.

ALERT! AF can cause thrombus formation and embolism to the brain. It is a frequent cause of ischemic stroke.

Premature Ventricular Contractions. Sporadic PVCs are the most common arrhythmia occurring with MI. During PVCs, the ventricle beats independently without waiting for the sequential conduction initiated by the SA or AV nodes. PVCs do not have a P wave or T wave and are characterized by a wide, bizarre QRS (see Fig. 16-22). Their form on the ECG indicates that they do not follow an atrial contraction and do not allow

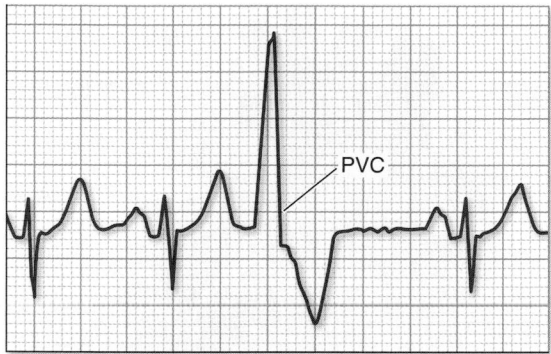

FIGURE 16-22. Premature ventricular contractions (PVCs) are beats that begin in the ventricle without waiting for a signal from the SA or AV node. A PVC has no P wave preceding it and no T wave after it. This ineffective contraction of the ventricle can lead to ventricular tachycardia. A PVC can occur singularly or in sequences. Three PVCs in a row constitutes ventricular tachycardia.

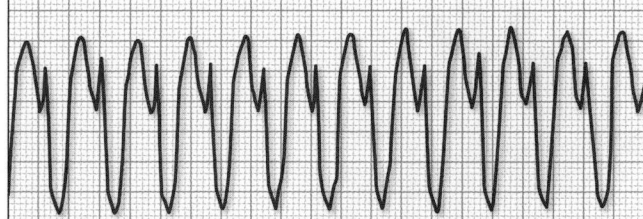

FIGURE 16-23. VT is a beat that begins in the ventricle without waiting for a signal from the SA or AV node. It is an erratic rhythm with few efficient contractions. The impulses have no P wave preceding them and no T wave after them. This rhythm heralds ventricular fibrillation.

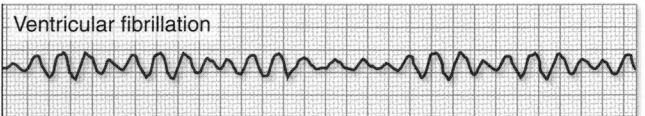

FIGURE 16-24. VF is an erratic rhythm with no effective contractions. The ventricle is quivering rather than contracting. This is considered cardiac arrest and requires defibrillation.

for a refractory period. PVCs may occur singularly or in patterns of bigeminy, trigeminy, quadrigeminy, or other sequential patterns. In bigeminy, a PVC occurs every other beat. In trigeminy, a PVC occurs after every two normal beats. Two sequential PVCs are termed couplets and require vigilance because three PVCs in a row constitutes ventricular tachycardia, a dangerous cardiac rhythm. Sporadic, infrequent PVCs do not require treatment.

PVCs that are frequent, in that there are more than 10 per hour, or complex, such as those occurring in couplets, are associated with increased mortality. Cardiac mortality occurs in association with significantly impaired ventricular function. Patients may experience palpitations with PVCs. If frequent, PVCs can diminish cardiac output and cause fatigue, dizziness, and more severe arrhythmia. Three or more PVCs in a row constitutes VT.

Ventricular Tachycardia. Sustained VT is defined as VT that persists for greater than 30 seconds or VT associated with hemodynamic compromise. The ECG demonstrates a series of widened QRS waves without preceding P waves or any T waves that follow (see Fig. 16-23). With VT, the rate of the QRS waves, which represent rapid, ineffective ventricular contractions, is greater than 100 beats per minute. Also, the ventricular contractions do not allow for effective pumping of blood, severely diminishing cardiac output. Patients are aware of a sudden onset of rapid heart rate and may experience dyspnea, palpitations, and lightheadedness.

VT is often treated with antiarrhythmic drugs, but when VT causes significant hemodynamic compromise, cardioversion is necessary. When treating a patient with VT, the clinician should have the defibrillator ready for use because rapid VT commonly initiates VF.

Ventricular Fibrillation. VF is often precipitated by a single, early PVC falling on the T wave of a previous impulse. The T wave indicates repolarization or the

refractory period for the ventricle. The lack of a refractory period is dangerous; often, the rhythm degenerates into a rapid, repetitive sequence of VT that deteriorates into VF. The word *fibrillation* means quivering; in VF; the ventricle is quivering and not contracting effectively to pump blood out of the chamber. The ECG shows bizarre waves with no discernible P, QRS, or T waves (see Fig. 16-24).

Onset of VF is rapidly followed by loss of consciousness and, if untreated, death. Most patients who have successfully treated VF within the first 48 hours of the onset of acute MI have a good long-term prognosis with a low rate of recurrence or cardiac death. Cardiac pulmonary resuscitation and defibrillation are the treatments for VF. Patients can also have cardioverters/defibrillators surgically implanted, which promptly recognize and terminate life-threatening ventricular arrhythmias.

Papillary Muscle Rupture. When the heart sustains an MI in the left ventricle, the injury often involves a papillary muscle. These small muscular projections are tethered to the heart valve leaflets via stringlike structures called chordae tendineae (see Fig. 16-25). In the left ventricle, papillary muscle rupture causes the mitral valve to be unable to close. In papillary muscle rupture, with each contraction of the left ventricle, blood flows upward through the loose mitral valve into the left atrium. This causes a mitral valve regurgitant murmur, also called mitral insufficiency. As a consequence, mitral regurgitation often causes backup of blood into the left atrium, pulmonary veins, and pulmonary capillaries, causing pulmonary edema. Patient signs and symptoms include dyspnea, cough, pulmonary crackles, and heart murmur heard at the 5th intercostal space left midclavicular line. Treatment includes surgical valve repair and diuretic agents.

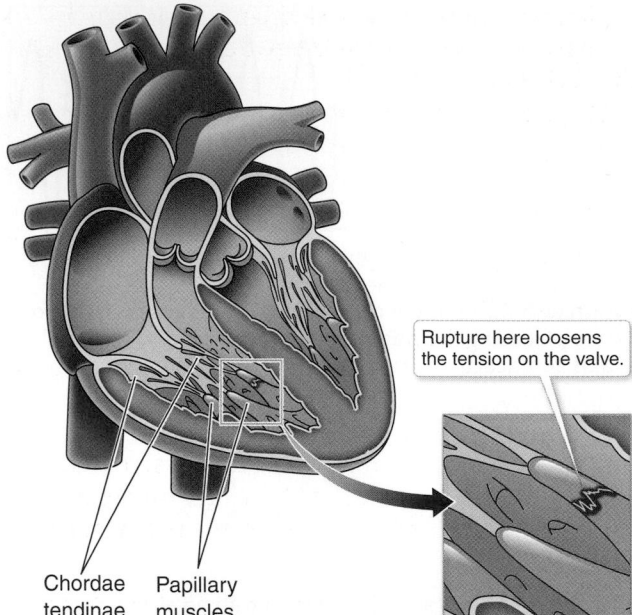

FIGURE 16-25. Papillary muscle rupture. A papillary muscle is attached to membranous strings called chordae tendineae, which are attached to the mitral and tricuspid valve leaflets. With MI, papillary muscle rupture can occur and the fixation of the valve leaflets comes loose. Blood then flows upward through the floppy valve with contraction of the ventricle, and this causes a regurgitant heart murmur.

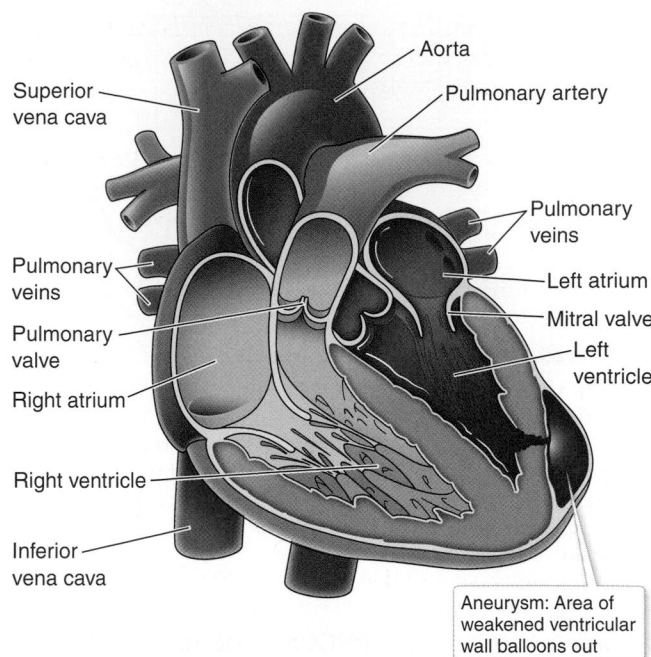

FIGURE 16-26. A ventricular aneurysm is a weakening in the ventricular wall that often occurs after myocardial infarction. This floppy area of dilated wall has turbulent blood flow within it. Thrombi often develop within the aneurysm.

Thromboembolism. After MI, the atrial and ventricular muscles are not contracting fully. The areas of infarction consist of dead tissue, which is noncontractile. In this noncontractile chamber, stagnant blood collects and is susceptible to clotting. A clot then can travel out of the heart into the pulmonary or aortic artery and become a thromboembolism, which can potentially obstruct blood flow through pulmonary or systemic arteries. Anticoagulant and thrombolytic therapies may be needed to break up the clot.

Ventricular Aneurysm and Rupture. After MI, a portion of the heart wall is infarcted and damaged so that it is noncontractile, necrotic, and scarred. The tensile strength of necrotic tissue is much less compared with normal myocardium. The weakened area is constantly exposed to the shearing force of blood and the pressure of adjacent contractile tissue. These conditions can contribute to the formation of a weakened bulging of the wall (see Fig. 16-26). When this occurs in the ventricle, the weakened area is a ventricular aneurysm with potential for rupture. Ventricular rupture causes a sudden drop in blood pressure and inadequate peripheral tissue perfusion. The patient loses consciousness and shows signs of shock. Surgical intervention to repair the rupture is needed immediately.

Pericarditis. Pericarditis is the inflammation of the pericardial membrane that surrounds the heart. It usually appears on the second or third day after MI. The patient experiences sharp, stabbing pain that is aggravated with deep inspiration and positional changes. The classic sound heard through the stethoscope is called a pericardial friction rub, which may or may not

be present. Pericarditis can occur as a component of **Dressler's syndrome,** which is a hypersensitivity reaction to the tissue necrosis of MI. Dressler's syndrome includes pericarditis, pleuritis, and pneumonitis and is treated with anti-inflammatory agents.

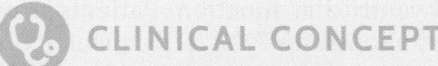

CLINICAL CONCEPT

The murmur of pericarditis, called pericardial friction rub, is a scratchy, rough sound.

Heart Failure. Heart failure, weakening of the ventricles of the heart, is a common complication of MI. The heart's pumping action becomes impaired, blood volume accumulates in the chambers, and hydrostatic pressure builds backward in the cardiovascular system. Hydrostatic pressure builds within the left ventricle, left atrium, pulmonary veins, and in the pulmonary capillaries. Pulmonary edema, a severe symptom of heart failure, develops. Symptoms include dyspnea, cough, pulmonary crackles, and peripheral edema. If the heart is severely damaged from an extensive MI, heart failure can worsen into cardiogenic shock. In cardiogenic shock, the ventricles are unable to pump sufficient blood to the rest of the body, causing blood pressure to drop abruptly (see Chapter 17: Heart Failure).

Prinzmetal Angina. Prinzmetal angina, also known as variant angina, was originally described by Prinzmetal in 1959 and is significantly different from classic angina because patients with Prinzmetal angina have chest pain at rest. This type of angina is caused by coronary artery vasospasm. It can also be associated with MI, life-threatening ventricular arrhythmias, and sudden death.

Epidemiology. Prinzmetal angina affects approximately 4 out of 100,000 people per year in the United States. About 2% of patients with angina have coronary artery spasm. For unknown reasons, the prevalence of coronary spasm is higher in Japan and Korea than in the Western countries.

Etiology. The etiology of coronary artery spasm is unclear, but there are several theories concerning this condition. Within the myocardium, there may be reduced amounts of the vasodilatory substance nitric oxide (NO). Elevated LDL cholesterol causes decreased production and inactivation of NO. Lack of NO is associated with coronary artery muscle thickening and enhanced sensitivity to vasoconstrictors. Also, the region of coronary artery spasm in Prinzmetal angina typically occurs at or adjacent to atherosclerotic plaque. Because of this, endothelial dysfunction is hypothesized to be the cause of the spasm. As an alternative theory, abnormal magnesium metabolism, which results in hypercontraction of smooth muscle cells in coronary artery walls, may be the cause of variant angina. Lastly, it is also proposed that hyperinsulinemia and insulin resistance are related to etiology of variant angina, although the exact mechanisms of these associations have not been defined.

Pathophysiology. In Prinzmetal angina there is a localized area of vasospastic muscle wall in one or more coronary arteries for reasons that are unclear. Coronary artery vasospasm in Prinzmetal angina obstructs blood flow to the myocardium and the area undergoes temporary ischemia. Ischemia initiates anaerobic metabolism, which yields 2 ATP and lactic acid, an irritant to cardiac muscle cells. Vasospasm can occur at rest, last a few minutes, and cause the same squeezing chest pain as typical angina. Vasospasm can be mild with hardly any constriction apparent in the vessel wall or severe with tight spasm causing complete arterial obstruction. The vasospasm eventually subsides and the patient's symptoms are relieved.

Clinical Presentation. Patients with Prinzmetal angina commonly do not have many cardiovascular risk factors. History of episodes of squeezing chest pain may be all that the patient reports. However, the patient should be asked about cardiovascular risk factors such as hypertension, hyperlipidemia, fat and salt in the diet, sedentary lifestyle, and family history. The patient should be specifically asked about cigarette smoking because this is common in those with Prinzmetal angina.

Another commonality in a small percentage of patients is the concurrent conditions of migraine headaches and Raynaud's phenomenon. As in Prinzmetal angina, these two conditions are caused by an abnormality in the vasomotor tone of vessels.

The pain pattern for variant angina is unlike classic angina. Unlike the exercise intolerance observed with patients with typical angina, patients with variant angina have normal exercise tolerance. Most episodes of chest pain occur when the patient is at rest and in the early morning hours.

Diagnosis. Patients with Prinzmetal angina are usually admitted to the hospital for observation, evaluation, and initiation of therapy. Diagnosis includes cardiac monitoring for 24 to 48 hours, coronary angiography, and serial cardiac enzyme assays. During angiography, coronary artery spasm is often provoked by chemical means, using ergonovine maleate, a vasoconstrictor. The coronary vasoconstriction of Prinzmetal angina can be visualized by the angiographic demonstration of spontaneous or induced coronary vessel spasm that causes chest pain in patients at rest. The ECG may include ST-segment elevation or depression. Patients with Prinzmetal angina often have atherosclerosis of a major coronary artery; however, the vasospasm occurs in a different coronary artery.

If the patient is experiencing a prolonged period of chest pain, an ECG may show bradycardia, tachycardia, and an elevated ST-segment. The transient elevated ST-segment and complaint of chest pain at rest provide the rationale for diagnosis of variant angina. An ECG is necessary to document an elevated ST-segment during the period of chest pain. An ambulatory ECG Holter monitor can demonstrate the cardiac irregularities of the patient during a 24- to 48-hour period.

Treatment. Initially IV or sublingual NTG may be given, as well as a calcium blocker antagonist. Long-acting nitrates are commonly ordered to prevent recurrent episodes.

Complications. Acute MI is a complication of Prinzmetal angina and is usually in the same area of ST segment change as noted by the ECG during the prior anginal attack. The greater the involvement of the patient's heart with atherosclerosis and coronary vasospasm, the greater the incidence of MI for patients who have Prinzmetal angina. Patients can also have rhythm disturbances caused by the vasospasms and resulting ischemia of contractile tissue.

Chronic Coronary Artery Disease. Chronic coronary artery disease, also called stable angina, is characterized by recurring episodes of chest pain caused by transient myocardial ischemia. The prevalence of stable angina is unclear. In the United Kingdom, a study revealed almost 1 in 3 patients with stable angina have anginal pain at least once a week. The etiology and risk factors for stable angina are the same as those for unstable angina. The patient has coronary artery disease, usually with at least one artery that is 70% obstructed. Patients with stable angina either cannot withstand surgical intervention for their CAD or have had surgical interventions that have not been successful to relieve their chest pain. They have chronic episodes of angina for which they self-medicate. The chest pain of stable angina usually occurs during exertion or any conditions that increase the heart's work demands. Stable angina has a predictable pattern that has been experienced by the patient. The patient is usually on a daily medication that aims to prevent angina episodes such as long-acting nitrates, calcium antagonists, beta blockers, or antiplatelet medications. The patient also has sublingual or nasal spray NTG that can act immediately for "breakthrough" episodes of angina pain. The pain usually recedes with rest and NTG medication. Worsening of angina pain, sudden-onset angina at rest, or angina lasting more than 15 minutes are symptoms of unstable angina. Diagnostic studies and treatment is then similar to that of unstable angina.

Cardiac Inflammation and Infection

A few cardiac disorders are caused by inflammation and infection. Infective endocarditis (IE) is the most common type of cardiac infection. Heart valve disease occurs as a result of IE. Myocarditis is often caused by viruses that attack the cardiac muscle tissue. Pericarditis, which affects the outer layer around the heart, commonly occurs after MI.

Infective Endocarditis

IE is a noncontagious infection of the cardiac endothelium that most commonly affects the heart valves. It is mainly caused by bacteria, although fungi can also be the infection's etiologic agent. Normally, the cardiac endothelium is a smooth membrane that helps regulate vascular tone, inflammation, thrombosis, and vascular remodeling. Damaged valves and turbulent blood flow within the heart create areas of impact that wear away at the smooth endothelial surface. These rough areas of the heart's membranous surface are prone to infection and provoke aggregation of platelets to form a thrombus. Intracardiac devices such as prosthetic valves can incite the same conditions.

Epidemiology. The incidence of IE in the general population is estimated to be between 3 to 9 cases per 100,000, but incidence is greater among patients with underlying valvular heart disease and those who inject illicit IV drugs. Women are affected by IE twice as much as men. More than one-third of cases of IE are caused by hospital-acquired infections. There is an increased incidence in persons older than age 65 with the highest incidence in those aged 74 to 79 years. The incidence of IE is rising because of longer survival of patients with degenerative heart diseases, increased implantation of prosthetic heart valves, and aging of the population.

 CLINICAL CONCEPT

Pacemaker-associated endocarditis can develop in patients with implantation of these devices caused by nosocomial infection or because of erosion of pacemaker components.

IE is difficult to diagnose and is associated with a death rate of up to 35%. Bacterial antibiotic resistance has become a significant obstacle in the treatment of this disease.

Etiology

A select group of bacteria are the major etiologic agents that cause IE. The leading causative organisms are *Streptococcus viridans (S. viridans)* and *Staphylococcus aureus (S. aureus),* which account for 80% of all cases. Prosthetic valve endocarditis is an increasingly common cause of IE, possibly because of the increasing numbers of valvular replacement surgeries within the growing elderly population. Prosthetic valve endocarditis is caused by *S. aureus* and *Staphylococcus epidermidis (S. epidermidis)* and is frequently a result of contamination during surgery. These are often methicillin-resistant *S. aureus* (MRSA) infections. Other microorganisms that cause IE include enterococci and a group of organisms known by the acronym *HACEK:* **H**aemophilus, **A**ctinobacillus, **C**ardiobacterium, **E**ikenella, and **K**ingella.

Pathophysiology. Bacterial endocarditis is the most common form of IE. Microorganisms that cause IE enter the bloodstream from mucosal surfaces or sites of localized infection. A common port of entry for *S. aureus* is the skin in IV drug use. When microbes infect the bloodstream, bacteremia develops and allows microorganisms to travel into the heart, where they adhere to damaged endothelial tissue or attach to thrombi within the heart. Once adherent, the microorganisms multiply and attract white blood cells and platelets, which release cytokines and coagulation factors. Stimulation of the coagulation cascade results in fibrin deposition and, eventually, development of a vegetation. A vegetation is a tiny mass that contains microorganisms, a meshwork of fibrin, and cellular components that are similar to thrombi. Microorganisms continually proliferate, are shed into the bloodstream, and stimulate development of additional vegetations. Cytokines attracted to the area provoke a persistent cycle of inflammation, which damages intracardiac structures, particularly heart valves. Vegetations are most commonly found on valve leaflets and fragments of vegetations can embolize into the circulation. Carried by the bloodstream, these fragments, called **septic emboli,** can initiate infection or ischemia in remote tissues.

Fungal endocarditis can occur in immunosuppressed patients and those who require prolonged use of indwelling central vascular catheters. The most common fungal species is *Candida albicans.*

In approximately 10% of all cases of endocarditis, an infectious agent cannot be found. This can occur because of prior antibiotic treatment, difficulty isolating the microbial agent, or deeply lodged microbes within vegetations that are not released into the bloodstream. There is also a type of endocarditis characterized by sterile thrombi that do not contain microorganisms.

Nonbacterial, thrombotic endocarditis (NBTE) occurs in severely debilitated patients, such as those suffering cancer, extensive burns, or sepsis. Indwelling vascular catheters, systemic lupus erythematosus (SLE), and carcinoid syndrome also predispose to NBTE. SLE is associated with Libman-Sacks endocarditis, which occurs because of an immune-mediated attack on the endocardium. In carcinoid syndrome, a tumor that usually originates in the gastrointestinal tract releases large amounts of serotonin and other vasoactive substances that stimulate fibrotic changes in the endocardium and valvular tissue.

IE can occur as an acute or subacute infection. Acute IE develops suddenly, and the patient becomes critically ill and in need of medical attention. Subacute IE develops more gradually and symptoms may be subtle initially. Individuals with subacute infection may be unaware of the severity of the illness and delay obtaining medical attention.

Clinical Presentation

Individuals with IE usually present with nonspecific symptoms, including fever, chills, anorexia, weight loss, myalgias, and arthralgias. Fever may be low or absent in elderly or severely debilitated persons. The development of a new heart murmur or worsening of a pre-existent murmur are important diagnostic signs. With severe valvular dysfunction, signs of heart failure such as edema may be present.

Signs of ischemia or infarction of the extremities, spleen, kidney, bowel, or brain may be the initial clinical manifestations of IE. Signs consistent with the damage caused by septic emboli may also be present; in the brain, septic emboli can lodge in a cerebral artery or arteriole and cause an ischemic stroke. Neurological symptoms from embolic stroke occur in up to 40% of patients with IE. Patients may also present with meningitis, seizures, encephalopathy, or abscesses of the brain. The kidney can also be damaged by septic emboli or immune-mediated glomerulonephritis. Septic emboli can lodge in the lungs, particularly in IV drug abusers. In IV drug abusers, the veins are the portal of entry; *S. aureus*, the flora of the skin, most commonly causes bacteremia. Septic emboli from *S. aureus* travel from the peripheral vein into the IVC and into the right side of the heart. As a result, the tricuspid valve is most often affected in IV drug users, and tricuspid murmurs are common. From the tricuspid valve, septic emboli travel easily into the right ventricle, then the pulmonary artery (see Fig. 16-27). The patient demonstrates cough, pleuritic chest pain, and a distinctive pneumonia on x-ray consisting of nodular infiltrates.

Classic clinical manifestations of IE caused by septic emboli include petechiae, splinter hemorrhages, Janeway lesions, Osler's nodes, and Roth spots. Splinter hemorrhages appear as red, linear streaks in the nailbeds. Janeway lesions are erythematous, nontender lesions on the palms and soles. Osler's nodes are subcutaneous nodules in the pulp of the fingertips that

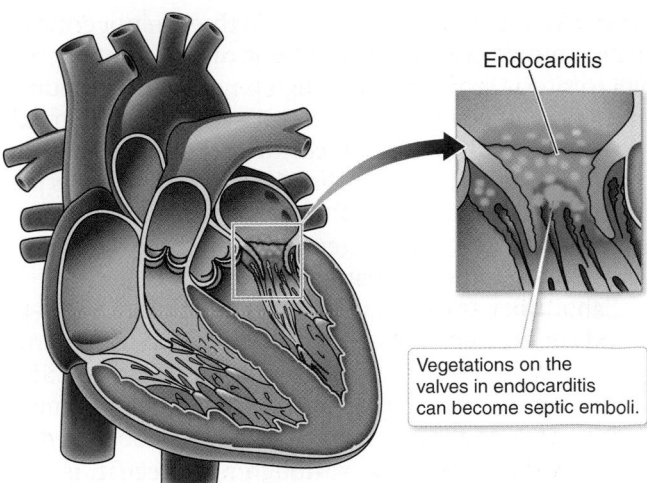
Endocarditis

Vegetations on the valves in endocarditis can become septic emboli.

FIGURE 16-27. In infectious endocarditis, lesions called vegetations form on the heart valves. Vegetations on the valvular leaflets can become septic emboli.

persist for hours or days. Roth spots are oval retinal hemorrhages with pale centers. These signs are pathognomonic for IE and they are seen in persons who suffer prolonged illness without treatment.

Diagnosis. A definitive diagnosis of IE is based on a set of specific clinical signs, as well as laboratory and echocardiographic findings, called the Duke criteria (see Box 16-3). To diagnose IE, a patient must exhibit

---

BOX 16-3. The Duke Criteria of Infective Endocarditis

Clinical criteria for IE requires that two major criteria are met, one major and three minor criteria are met, or that five minor criteria are met.

MAJOR CRITERIA
- Positive blood cultures from at least two separate cultures drawn 12 hours apart
- Evidence of IE on echocardiogram, such as a vegetation, abscesses, or valve perforation
- New regurgitant murmur

MINOR CRITERIA
- Predisposing heart condition such as mitral valve prolapse, rheumatic or congenital heart disease, or IV drug abuse
- Temperature greater than 100.4°F (38°C)
- Presence of embolic disease or hemorrhage
- Presence of immunological phenomena, such as glomerulonephritis, Osler's nodes, Roth spots, or rheumatoid factor
- Positive blood culture but major criteria not met
- Positive echocardiogram but major criteria not met

Adapted from Li, J. S., Sexton, D. J., Mick, N., et al. (2000). Proposed modifications to the Duke criteria for the diagnosis of infective endocarditis. *Clin Infect Dis*, 30(4), 633–638.

two major criteria, or one major and three minor criteria, or five minor criteria. Assessment of a patient for the Duke criteria requires a thorough physical examination, multiple blood cultures, laboratory tests, and echocardiography. Multiple blood cultures are necessary because in IE there are fewer than 100 microorganisms per mL of blood and it is difficult to obtain a sample of blood containing the etiologic agent. At least three blood cultures drawn 12 hours apart is the preferred method.

Laboratory tests are necessary, including complete blood count, electrolytes, creatinine, blood urea nitrogen, glucose, erythrocyte sedimentation rate (ESR), coagulation panel, and urinalysis. Anemia is common in subacute endocarditis. Leukocytosis is observed in acute endocarditis. ESR, although not specific, is elevated in more than 90% of cases. Glomerulonephritis, which causes proteinuria and microscopic hematuria, is present in approximately 50% of cases. Decreased complement and the presence of rheumatoid factor are evident in subacute endocarditis.

A transthoracic echocardiogram can demonstrate new onset valvular dysfunction, vegetations, abscess, or prosthetic-valve dysfunction. New onset of regurgitant valvular dysfunction is particularly indicative of IE. Transesophageal echocardiography is significantly more accurate than transthoracic echocardiogram and is the preferred diagnostic procedure.

Treatment

Treatment of IE consists mainly of IV antibiotics for 6 weeks or a more prolonged course. The antibiotic should be precisely bactericidal for the cultured microorganism. Microbes within vegetations on infected valves are difficult to penetrate, necessitating high serum levels of IV antibiotics. After appropriate treatment is initiated, recovery should occur within 2 weeks. Blood cultures should be repeated daily until sterile. Persistent fever despite antibiotic therapy often indicates paravalvular or extracardiac abscesses. Laboratory indicators of inflammation such as elevated ESR resolve slowly and do not reflect response to treatment. Vegetations may not change in size with treatment. Surgical intervention may be necessary in patients who do not respond to antibiotic therapy, those with heart failure, or those with persistent septic emboli. As many as 40% of patients with prosthetic valve IE require surgical intervention.

After recovery from IE, the patient needs to be vigilant about prevention of recurrence. Prophylactic antibiotics are necessary in recovered patients anytime there is a risk for bacteremia, as in surgical procedures, certain invasive dental treatments, bronchoscopy, endoscopy, cystoscopy, or localized infections.

Complications

Regurgitant heart valve defects, intracardiac abscesses, and heart failure are the major cardiac complications of IE. Heart murmurs occur in 85% of affected individuals. Heart failure is usually the result of abnormal blood flow dynamics caused by valvular dysfunction, but it can also result from inflammation of the myocardium. Abscesses can form within the heart and erode through the endocardium or pericardium, causing pericarditis. Infection of the endocardium can also interrupt the cardiac conduction system and provoke dysrhythmias.

Extracardiac complications are most often caused by the septic valvular vegetations, which tend to break apart and embolize. Septic arterial emboli, which occur in 50% of patients, can lodge in remote tissues and form abscesses, particularly in the lungs, spleen, brain, and meninges. Septic emboli can also weaken the walls of arterial vessels and create mycotic aneurysms. Mycotic cerebral aneurysms form in 2% to 15% of patients, causing headaches, focal neurological signs, and cerebral artery rupture, leading to intracerebral hemorrhage. Septic emboli can also obstruct the circulation of extracardiac tissues and cause ischemia or infarction. This often occurs in the extremities, brain, lung, bowel, kidneys, and spleen. Ischemic stroke occurs in up to 40% of patients. The emboli can also lodge in the kidney and cause renal infarction and stimulate immune-mediated glomerulonephritis. When formed on the structures of the right side of the heart, septic emboli can cause pulmonary embolism.

Myocarditis

Myocarditis, also called inflammatory cardiomyopathy, is an inflammatory disease of the myocardium that can range from a mild disorder to a lethal condition. The myocardium undergoes inflammation with degeneration and necrosis of cardiac myocytes. It does not involve myocardial ischemia; however, conduction disruption is common.

Epidemiology. The incidence of myocarditis is estimated at 1 to 10 cases per 100,000 persons. As many as 1% to 5% of patients with acute viral infections may have involvement of the myocardium. The incidence of myocarditis is similar between males and females, although young males are particularly susceptible. Susceptible populations include immunocompromised individuals, pregnant women, and infants.

Etiology. Viruses are the most common causes of myocarditis in the United States and Europe. Coxsackieviruses A and B account for a large proportion of the cases. Many different bacteria, fungi, and parasites can cause myocarditis, as well as drugs and toxins. Other causes include radiation, hypersensitivity reactions, or exposure to toxic substances such as cocaine. Risk factors of myocarditis include viral infections; systemic infections caused by bacteria, fungi, or parasites; autoimmune disease; and a multitude of toxins, drugs, and chemotherapeutic agents. Myocarditis is the cause of cardiac transplant rejection.

Pathophysiology. Myocarditis is inflammation of the muscle layer of the heart's wall. It can occur by direct invasion of a pathogen or a toxin that is liberated by a pathogen. It can also occur as an immunological mechanism initiated by an infectious agent. Cardiac myocytes undergo destruction with large infiltration of T cells and WBCs that liberate tissue-damaging cytokines. Often the etiologic organism is not found. It is believed that an organism often begins the process of cellular destruction; however, continued inflammation is then caused by an autoimmune mechanism.

Clinical Presentation. Patients with myocarditis can demonstrate varying clinical presentations from no symptoms to severe chest pain, chills, fever, and dyspnea. Patients may report a flulike syndrome of fever, myalgia, arthralgia, pharyngitis, tonsillitis, and upper respiratory infection. Symptoms of palpitations or syncope can occur. Sudden cardiac death can develop because of ventricular arrhythmias or AV block. Adults can develop heart failure years after an episode of myocarditis.

On physical examination, cardiac auscultation may reveal an S_3 gallop rhythm, which is an extra beat heard after S_2. A pericardial friction rub is also possible. Depending on the etiology, there may be various other signs such as lymphadenopathy, rash, or those of the Jones criteria seen in rheumatic fever.

Diagnosis. Laboratory studies involved in the diagnosis include a CBC that demonstrates leukocytosis, elevated ESR, and CRP, which indicates inflammation. The cTn and cardiac enzymes are elevated, indicating cardiac muscle damage. The blood is analyzed for various viral antibody titers such as coxsackievirus, influenza, Epstein-Barr virus, hepatitis, human immunodeficiency virus (HIV), and cytomegalovirus. Presence of a viral genome within a biopsy of myocardium confirms a viral etiology. An echocardiogram can reveal heart dysfunction and degree of heart failure if present. A diagnostic test called antimyosin scintigraphy can identify myocardial inflammation. Gallium scanning is used to investigate myocardial cellular infiltration. Positron emission tomography scanning has been used to assess the degree and location of inflammation.

Treatment. Treatment focuses on symptom management and decreasing myocardial workload. Activity is restricted during a recovery period of 6 months or more. Treatment measures for heart failure such as diuretics, nitrates, and beta blockers are often necessary. Antiarrhythmic agents, corticosteroids, and immunosuppressant medications are commonly used. Pacemaker insertion may be needed. In severe cases of heart failure, cardiac transplantation is considered.

Pericarditis

Pericarditis is inflammation of the pericardium and epicardium, the folds of serous membrane that surround the heart's exterior. The pericardium is a tough, outer membrane that secures the heart in position and is attached to the sternum and thoracic structures. The inner layer is the epicardium, which is directly attached to the heart's surface. In between these layers is the pericardial space that contains 30 to 50 mL of serous fluid that acts as lubricant.

When the pericardium undergoes inflammation, fluid accumulates in the pericardial space. The fluid is called a **pericardial effusion** and it surrounds the heart. If the fluid accumulates to high levels of 200 mL or greater, it can compress the heart, causing a condition called **cardiac tamponade.** In cardiac tamponade, the heart chambers are restricted by the surrounding pericardial fluid so they cannot stretch and fill with blood (see Box 16-4).

Epidemiology. Studies indicate that a diagnosis of acute pericarditis occurs in approximately 1 per 1,000 hospital admissions. This is thought to be a low estimate because many persons do not have symptoms with pericarditis. Acute pericarditis and MI present in a similar manner; chest pain and ST elevation on ECG. However, pericarditis occurs in only 1% of patients with acute chest pain and ST elevation. In general, males are affected by pericarditis more frequently than females. Pericarditis occurs in 6% to 20% of patients with advanced renal failure. Pericardial effusion occurs in 21% of cancer patients and up to 43% of acquired immune deficiency syndrome (AIDS) patients. After MI, Dressler's syndrome, a disorder that includes pericarditis, occurs in 5% to 6% of patients. Pericardial effusions, some of which go undetected, are estimated to occur in 28% of MI patients.

Etiology. Viral infection is a common cause of pericarditis. Viruses such as coxsackievirus, influenza, Epstein-Barr virus, varicella, hepatitis, mumps, and HIV cause pericarditis. Rheumatic fever, autoimmune disease, renal failure, tuberculosis, metabolic disorders, and high doses of radiation can also cause pericarditis. Pericarditis commonly occurs after myocardial infarction, a condition called Dressler's syndrome. Malignancies of the lung, breast, and skin, as well as leukemia and lymphoma, are associated with pericarditis.

Pathophysiology. Inflammation of the pericardium can occur because of a direct effect of a pathogen, such as a pathogen's toxin, or autoimmune reaction. Pericarditis often occurs along with myocarditis in viral or bacterial infection or autoimmune inflammatory disorders such as SLE, Sjögren's syndrome, or rheumatoid arthritis. In pericarditis, the capillaries that supply the pericardial membrane become highly permeable. The capillary pores allow plasma proteins and fibrinogen to leave the bloodstream and enter the pericardial cavity. This creates a fibrin-rich, exudative edema that envelops the heart; as it heals, it forms scar tissue. Commonly, adhesions form between the layers of the pericardium, which can restrict optimal filling of the ventricles.

BOX 16-4. Pericardial Effusion

Pericardial effusion is the presence of fluid in the pericardial cavity. Normally, the pericardial cavity contains approximately 40 mL of clear filtrate of blood. A small amount of pericardial fluid around the heart may not cause any symptoms. However, a large amount of fluid, such as 200 mL or more, causes compression against the heart, inhibiting filling of the chambers. Like pericarditis, pericardial effusions can be caused by such disorders as infection, autoimmune reactions, or systemic inflammatory conditions. To diagnose pericardial effusion, an echocardiogram is done. The echocardiogram will show the excess fluid surrounding the heart and can demonstrate the decrease in left ventricular ejection volume. Treatment is aimed at removal of the pericardial fluid in a procedure called pericardiocentesis. Pericardial fluid analysis can assist in the determination of etiology. Treatment depends on the etiology of the effusion.

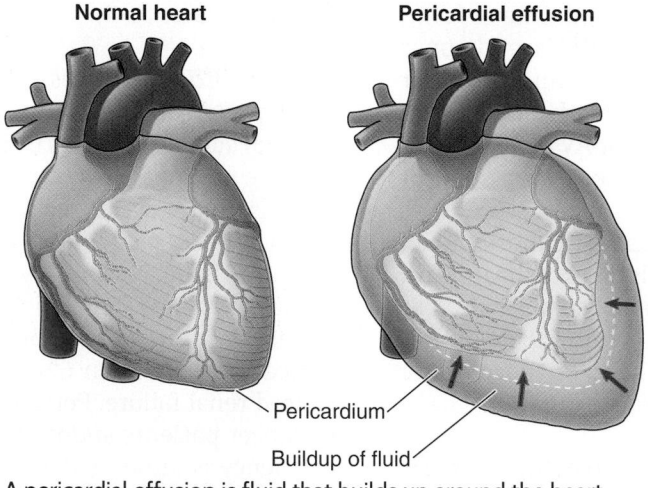

Normal heart   **Pericardial effusion**

Pericardium

Buildup of fluid

A pericardial effusion is fluid that builds up around the heart within the pericardial cavity.

Dressler's syndrome is a specific type of pericarditis that develops in some persons post-MI. This autoimmune reaction follows an MI after 2 to 3 weeks. Cardiac proteins released during an MI stimulate immunoglobulins that combine with the proteins to form immune complexes. The immune complexes are deposited in the pericardium, causing inflammation and fluid collection in the pericardial sac.

Clinical Presentation. The signs of acute pericarditis include chest pain, fever, dyspnea, pericardial friction rub, and specific ECG findings. The chest pain of pericarditis is described as sharp and sudden, and it worsens with deep breathing, swallowing, and coughing. The pain can radiate into the neck, jaw, abdomen, or back. A pericardial friction rub, which is a scratching sound, can be heard through the stethoscope. Symptoms of cardiac tamponade, called the Beck triad, can be present; they include hypotension, jugular vein distention, and muffled heart sounds. A finding called pulsus paradoxus occurs in 70% to 80% of patients with cardiac tamponade. **Pulsus paradoxus** is exhibited by a decrease in systolic blood pressure of 10 mm Hg or more with inspiration. In pulsus paradoxus, the thorax, which is full of air in inspiration, places pressure on the heart and diminishes the volume ejected from the left ventricle into the aorta.

Diagnosis. The ECG in pericarditis shows ST segment elevations in multiple leads, which can appear as ECG changes of MI. Increased blood urea nitrogen and increased serum creatinine occur in pericarditis of renal failure. Otherwise, laboratory values can be normal, but if there is a concurrent MI or a great degree of cardiac stress, there may be elevated levels of cardiac markers such as cTn and CPK-MB.

Treatment. Treatment depends on the etiology of pericarditis. If infection is present, antibiotics are administered. Anti-inflammatory agents such as aspirin, NSAIDs, or corticosteroids are also given. Surgical drainage of the pericardial space may be needed.

Chapter Summary

- Three layers compose the wall of the heart: endocardium, myocardium, and epicardium.
- The two coronary arteries, the right and left main coronary arteries, are branches off the arch of the aorta.
- The LAD artery, which supplies the left ventricle with coronary blood flow, is most commonly affected by arteriosclerosis.
- Risk factors of coronary artery disease and MI include male gender, age greater than 45 years for males, age greater than 55 years for females, hyperlipidemia, hypertension, smoking, diabetes, and family history of cardiovascular disease.
- ACS can take either of two forms: UA or MI.
- There are two main types of myocardial infarction: STEMI or NSTEMI.
- Cardiac chest pain is a crushing type of pain that usually radiates down the left arm and is accompanied by dyspnea, diaphoresis, and pallor.
- Elevated cTn is the best indicator of MI.
- STEMI commonly indicates a transmural MI.
- Prinzmetal or variant angina is caused by vasospasm of a coronary artery.

- Common complications of MI include dysrhythmias, heart failure, pericarditis, ventricular aneurysm, ventricular thrombosis, thromboembolism, and papillary muscle rupture.
- The most common rhythm disturbance post-MI is the PVC; three or more PVCs is called ventricular tachycardia.
- VT predisposes to ventricular fibrillation, which is considered cardiac arrest and requires defibrillation.
- The leading causes of IE are *S. viridans* and *S. aureus*.
- Clinical manifestations of IE are heart murmur, petechiae, splinter hemorrhages, Janeway lesions, Osler's nodes, and Roth spots.
- Myocarditis is most often caused by a viral infection.
- Pericarditis can be accompanied by a pericardial effusion that can cause cardiac tamponade.
- Cardiac tamponade is the compression of the heart by surrounding pericardial fluid that inhibits the heart chambers from completely filling with blood.

 Making the Connections

Disorder and Pathophysiology	Signs and Symptoms	Physical Assessment Findings	Diagnostic Testing	Treatment
Unstable Angina Pectoris | UA pectoris, chest pain caused by myocardial ischemia, is part of ACS. There is inadequate coronary artery blood flow to the heart muscle. Ischemia develops, which causes myocardial cell hypoxia, triggering anaerobic metabolism. Anaerobic metabolism yields 2 ATP and lactic acid. Lactic acid is noxious to muscle cells, and 2 ATP is inadequate energy for the needs of the myocardial tissue. Other types of angina include: • Stable angina: episodes of myocardial ischemia that are predictable and have the same pain pattern. Patient self-medicates with NTG. • Prinzmetal angina: caused by vasospasm of the coronary artery.				
	An episode of retrosternal crushing, squeezing chest pain with radiation to the left arm, jaw, epigastric area, or back with a duration of 1 to 15 minutes. Chest pain most commonly occurs with exertion and is accompanied by dyspnea, diaphoresis, and pallor.	Vital signs show increased respiratory rate, slowed heart rate, and low blood pressure. Patient often brings fist to chest (Levine's sign), indicating the crushing feeling on the chest. Pallor, dyspnea, and diaphoresis are apparent. Pulses are weak.	ECG shows ST depression or ST elevation or T-wave inversions. Cardiac catheterization with coronary angiogram will show areas of coronary artery occlusion caused by arteriosclerosis. Cardiac enzymes are used to rule out MI. The cTn is used to rule out MI.	Low-fat diet. Daily exercise. Oxygen. Nitrates (NTG sublingual or nasal spray). 1 Aspirin/day. Anticoagulants. Possible procedures include PCTA, stent placement in the affected coronary artery, and CABG.

Continued

Making the Connections–cont'd

Disorder and Pathophysiology	Signs and Symptoms	Physical Assessment Findings	Diagnostic Testing	Treatment

Myocardial Infarction | Acute MI is an ACS that occurs when myocardial ischemia is prolonged and death of tissue (infarction) occurs. Can be a STEMI if it is a transmural MI or an NSTEMI if it is a subendocardial MI.

	Signs and Symptoms	Physical Assessment Findings	Diagnostic Testing	Treatment
	Steady retrosternal crushing, squeezing chest pain with radiation to the left arm, jaw, back, or epigastric region. Accompanied by pallor, dyspnea, and diaphoresis. Commonly occurs with exertion. Patient may lose consciousness.	Vital signs show increased respiratory rate, slowed heart rate, and low blood pressure. Levine's sign. Decreased level of consciousness (LOC) possible. Pallor. Diaphoresis. Respiratory distress. Diminished peripheral pulses.	Elevated troponin I. Elevated CPK-MB fraction. ECG shows ST elevation or ST depression, as well as inverted T waves. Cardiac catheterization with angiography shows coronary artery obstruction. Radionuclide angiogram. CT scan. Calcium CT scan.	IV nitrates. Morphine. Aspirin. Oxygen. Heparin. Thrombolytic agent to dissolve the clot for some eligible persons. Possible PTCA with stent placement or coronary artery bypass graft. Cardiac rehabilitation.

Endocarditis | A noncontagious infection of the cardiac endothelium that most commonly affects the heart valves. It is mainly caused by bacteria; *S. viridans* or *S. aureus*. Damaged valves are prone to infection and provoke aggregation of platelets to form a thrombus. Intracardiac devices such as prosthetic valves can incite the same conditions.

	Signs and Symptoms	Physical Assessment Findings	Diagnostic Testing	Treatment
	Nonspecific symptoms, including fever, chills, anorexia, weight loss, myalgias, and arthralgias. Fever may be blunted or absent in elderly or severely debilitated persons.	Fever may be present. New heart murmur or changed preexistent heart murmur. Septic emboli form and can be manifested as infarction in organs such as the brain, which causes signs of stroke-neurological deficits. Clinical signs caused by septic emboli include petechiae, splinter hemorrhages, Janeway lesions, Osler's nodes, and Roth spots.	At least three blood cultures are performed at three different times of the day. Transthoracic echocardiogram or trans-esophageal echocardiogram is used to visualize heart valves. Laboratory tests are necessary, including CBC, electrolytes, serum creatinine, blood urea nitrogen, blood glucose, ESR, CRP, coagulation panel, and urinalysis. Anemia is common in subacute endocarditis. Leukocytosis is observed in acute endocarditis. ESR, although not specific, is elevated in more than 90% of cases. Glomerulonephritis, which elevates serum creatinine and causes proteinuria and microscopic hematuria, is present in approximately 50% of cases.	Treatment consists mainly of parenteral antibiotics for 6 weeks or a more prolonged course. Surgical removal of prosthetic device may be necessary.

Continued

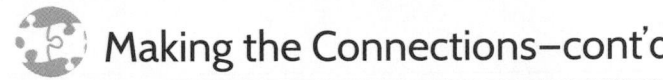

Disorder and Pathophysiology	Signs and Symptoms	Physical Assessment Findings	Diagnostic Testing	Treatment

Myocarditis | Myocarditis is inflammation of the muscle layer of the heart's wall. It can occur by direct invasion of a pathogen or a toxin that is liberated by a pathogen. It can also occur as an immunological mechanism initiated by an infectious agent.

	Signs and Symptoms	Physical Assessment Findings	Diagnostic Testing	Treatment
	Chest pain, chills, fever, and dyspnea. Patients may report a flulike syndrome of fever, myalgia, arthralgia, pharyngitis, tonsillitis, and upper respiratory infection. Symptoms of palpitations or syncope can occur. Sudden cardiac death can develop because of ventricular arrhythmias or AV block. Adults can develop heart failure signs and symptoms, including ankle edema, ascites, and dyspnea with exertion. Patient's may be asymptomatic.	On physical examination, cardiac auscultation may reveal an S_3 gallop rhythm indicative of heart failure. A pericardial friction rub and other signs such as lymphadenopathy and rash can be present, depending on etiology.	CBC, which demonstrates leukocytosis; elevated ESR and CRP, which indicate inflammation; and cTn and cardiac enzymes, which are elevated with myocardial injury. Various viral antibody titers are drawn. Presence of a viral genome within a biopsy of endomyocardium is confirmatory. Echocardiogram can reveal heart function and degree of heart failure, if present. Antimyosin scintigraphy can identify myocardial inflammation. Gallium scanning is used to investigate myocardial cellular infiltration. Positron emission tomography has been used to assess the degree and location of inflammation.	Decrease myocardial workload, including activity restrictions. Treatment measures for heart failure such as diuretics, nitrates, and beta blockers are often necessary. Antiarrhythmic agents, corticosteroids, and immunosuppressant medications are commonly used. Pacemaker insertion may be needed. In severe cases of heart failure, cardiac transplantation is considered.

Pericarditis | Inflammation of the serous membrane that surrounds the heart. Fluid can collect within the layers of pericardium and cause pericardial effusion.

	Signs and Symptoms	Physical Assessment Findings	Diagnostic Testing	Treatment
	Retrosternal sharp chest pain that worsens with inspiration and coughing. Fever can accompany dyspnea. The pain can radiate into the neck, jaw, abdomen, or back.	A pericardial friction rub may be heard through the stethoscope. Signs of cardiac tamponade, called the Beck triad, are hypotension, jugular vein distention, and muffled heart sounds. Pulsus paradoxus may be exhibited by a decrease in systolic blood pressure of 10 mm Hg or more with inspiration.	The ECG shows ST segment elevations in multiple leads, which can appear as ECG changes of MI. Other diagnostic studies can show increased blood urea nitrogen, or increased blood creatinine in cases of uremic pericarditis. If there is MI or a great degree of cardiac stress, there may be increased cardiac markers like cTn and CPK-MB. Echocardiogram can show pericardial effusion.	Antibiotic treatment and pericardiocentesis. Nonsteroidal anti-inflammatory drugs or other anti-inflammatory agents. Treatment aimed at etiology.

Bibliography

Alexander, J. H., Lopes, R. D., James, S., et al. (2011). Apixaban with antiplatelet therapy after acute coronary syndrome. *N Engl J Med*, 365(8), 699–708. Epub 2011 Jul 24.

Alpert, J. S., Thygesen, K. A., White, H. D., & Jaffe, A. S. (2014). Diagnostic and therapeutic implications of type 2 myocardial infarction: review and commentary. *Am J Med*, 127(2), 105–108. doi: 10.1016/j.amjmed.2013.09.031. Epub 2013 Oct 16.

Anavekar, N. S., Schultz, J. C., De Sa, D. D., et al. (2011). Modifiers of symptomatic embolic risk in infective endocarditis. *Mayo Clin Proceed*, 86(11), 1068–1074.

Bates, E. R., & Jacobs, A. K. (2013). Time to treatment in patients with STEMI. *N Engl J Med*, 369(10), 889–892. doi: 10.1056/NEJMp1308772.

Bayturan, O., Tuzcu, E. M., Lavoie, A., et al. (2010). The metabolic syndrome, its component risk factors, and progression of coronary atherosclerosis. *Arch Int Med*, 170(5), 478–484.

Berry, J. D., Dyer, A., Cai, X., et al. (2012). Lifetime risks of cardiovascular disease. *N Engl J Med*, 366(4), 321–329. doi: 10.1056/NEJMoa1012848.

Bhatt, D. L. (2010). Controversies in non-ST-elevation acute coronary syndromes and percutaneous coronary interventions. *Cleveland Clin J Med*, 77(2), 101–109.

Bock, C. T., Klingel, K., & Kandolf, R. (2010). Human parvovirus B19-associated myocarditis. *N Engl J Med*, 362(13), 1248–1249.

Christiansen, E. H., & Jensen, L. O. (2013). Sex and percutaneous coronary intervention. *Lancet*, 382(9908), 1864–1865. doi: 10.1016/S0140-6736(13)62030-9.

Dalen, J. E., & Devries, S. (2014). Diets to prevent coronary heart disease 1957–2013: what have we learned? *Am J Med*, 127(5), 364–369. doi: 10.1016/j.amjmed.2013.12.014. Epub 2013 Dec 30.

Davidson, L., Wilcox, J., Kim, D., et al. (2014). Clinical features of precocious acute coronary syndrome. *Am J Med*, 127(2), 140–144. doi: 10.1016/j.amjmed.2013.09.025. Epub 2013 Oct 15.

Dawber, T. R., & Kannel, W. B. (1966). The Framingham Study: an epidemiological approach to coronary heart disease. *Circulation*, 34, 553–555. Retrieved from http://circ.ahajournals.org

Drozda, J., Jr., Messer, J. V., Spertus, J., et al. (2011, July 12). ACCF/AHA/AMA-PCPI 2011 performance measures for adults with coronary artery disease and hypertension: a report of the American College of Cardiology Foundation/American Heart Association Task Force on Performance Measures and the American Medical Association-Physician Consortium for Performance Improvement. *J Am Coll Cardiol*, 58(3), 316–336. doi: 10.1016/j.jacc.2011.05.002. Epub 2011 Jun 14.

Fan, T., & Smallman, D. P. (2014). Screening for coronary heart disease with electrocardiography. *Am Fam Phys*, 89(2), 79–80.

Ferreyra, M. C., Chavarría, E. R., Ponieman, D. A., & Olavegogeascoechea, P. A. (2013). Silent brain abscess in patients with infective endocarditis. *Mayo Clin Proceed*, 88(4), 422–423.

Fuster, V. (2010). Fine-tuning therapy for acute coronary syndromes. *N Engl J Med*, 363(10), 976–977.

Graber, M. A., Darby-Stewart, A., & Dachs, R. (2010). Can ECG rule out ACS if performed while the patient is having chest pain? *Am Fam Phys*, 82(10), 1185.

Hall, S. L., & Lorenc, T. (2010). Secondary prevention of coronary artery disease. *Am Fam Phys*, 81(3), 289–296.

Hoen, B., & Duval, X. (2013). Infective endocarditis. *N Engl J Med*, 368, 1425–1433.

Hoffmann, U., Truong, Q. A., & Schoenfeld, D. A. (2012). Coronary CT angiography versus standard evaluation in acute chest pain. *N Engl J Med*, 367(4), 299–308.

Htwe, T. H., & Khardori, N. M. (2012). Cardiac emergencies: infective endocarditis, pericarditis, and myocarditis. *Med Clin N Am*, 96(6), 1149–1169.

Johnston, S. S., Bell, K., Gdovin, J., Jing, Y., & Graham, J. (2012). Coronary artery bypass graft surgery in acute coronary syndrome: incidence, cost impact, and acute clopidogrel interruption. *Hosp Prac*, 40(1), 15–23.

Jolly, S. S., Yusuf, S., Cairns, J., et al. (2011). Radial versus femoral access for coronary angiography and intervention in patients with acute coronary syndromes (RIVAL): a randomised, parallel group, multicentre trial. *Lancet*, 377(9775), 1409–1420. Epub 2011 Apr 4.

Joshi, N. V., Vesey, A. T., Williams, M. C., et al. (2014). 18F-fluoride positron emission tomography for identification of ruptured and high-risk coronary atherosclerotic plaques: a prospective clinical trial. *Lancet*, 383(9918), 705–713. doi: 10.1016/S0140-6736(13)61754.

Kaiser, C., Galatius, S., Erne, P., et al. (2010). Drug-eluting versus bare-metal stents in large coronary arteries. *N Engl J Med*, 363(24), 2310–2319.

Khandaker, M. H., Espinosa, R. E., Nishimura, R. A., et al. (2010). Pericardial disease: diagnosis and management. *Mayo Clin Proceed*, 85(6), 572–593.

Kolte, D., Khera, S., Palaniswamy, C., et al. (2013). Early invasive versus initial conservative treatment strategies in octogenarians with UA/NSTEMI. *Am J Med*, 126(12), 1076–1083.e1. doi: 10.1016/j.amjmed.2013.07.024.

Kumar, V., Abbas, A. K., Fausto, N., & Aster, J. (2010). *Robbins and Cotran pathologic basis of disease*. 8th ed. Philadelphia, PA: Saunders Elsevier.

Kwong, J. S., & Yu, C. M. (2013). New oral anticoagulants in acute coronary syndromes: what does a meta-analysis tell us? *JAMA Int Med*, 173(9), 834–835.

Last, A. R., Ference, J. D., & Falleroni, J. (2011). Pharmacologic treatment of hyperlipidemia. *Am Fam Phys*, 84(5), 551–558.

Lefebvre, C. W., & Hoekstra, J. (2010). Approach to non-ST segment elevation acute coronary syndrome in the emergency department: risk stratification and treatment strategies. *Hosp Prac*, 38(2), 40–49.

Li, J. S., Sexton, D. J., Mick, N., et al. (2000). Proposed modifications to the Duke criteria for the diagnosis of infective endocarditis. *Clin Infect Dis*, 30(4), 633–638. Epub 2000 Apr 3.

Libby, P. (2013). Mechanisms of acute coronary syndromes and their implications for therapy. *N Engl J Med*, 368(21), 2004–2013.

Linsel-Nitschke, P., Samani, N. J., & Schunkert, H. (2010). Sorting out cholesterol and coronary artery disease. *N Engl J Med*, 363(25), 2462–2463.

Litt, H. I., Gatsonis, C., Snyder, B., et al. (2012). CT angiography for safe discharge of patients with possible acute coronary syndromes. *N Engl J Med*, 366(15), 1393–1403.

Longo, D., Fauci, A. S., Kasper, D. L., et al. (2011). *Harrison's principles of internal medicine*. 18th ed. New York: McGraw-Hill.

May, A. E. (2013). Antiplatelet therapy after coronary stenting: for how long? *Lancet*, 382(9906), 1684–1685. doi: 10.1016/S0140-6736(13)61756-0. Epub 2013 Sep 1.

McConaghy, J. R., & Oza, R. S. (2013). Outpatient diagnosis of acute chest pain in adults. *Am Fam Phys*, 87(3), 177–182.

McManus, D. D., Huang, W., Domakonda, K. V., et al. (2012). Trends in atrial fibrillation in patients hospitalized with an acute coronary syndrome. *Am J Med*, 125(11), 1076–1084.

McMullin, N., Lindsell, C. J., Lei, L., et al. (2011). Outcomes associated with small changes in normal-range cardiac markers. *Am J Emerg Med*, 29(2), 162–167.

McPhee, S. J., & Ganong, W. F. (2009). *Pathophysiology of disease: An introduction to clinical medicine.* Lange Medical Books/McGraw-Hill Publishing.

Merella, P., Casu, G., & Meloni, I. (2010). Dosing of clopidogrel and aspirin in acute coronary syndromes. *N Engl J Med*, 363(25), 2466–2468.

Meune, C., Balmelli, C., Twerenbold, R., et al. (2011). Patients with acute coronary syndrome and normal high-sensitivity troponin. *Am J Med*, 124(12), 1151–1157.

Nabel, E. G., & Braunwald, E. (2012). A tale of coronary artery disease and myocardial infarction. *N Engl J Med*, 366(1), 54–63. doi: 10.1056/NEJMra1112570. No abstract available. Erratum in: *N Engl J Med*. 2012 Mar 8;366 (10):970.

Nicholls, S. J., Ballantyne, C. M., Barter, P. J., et al. (2011). Effect of two intensive statin regimens on progression of coronary disease. *N Engl J Med*, 365(22), 2078–2087. doi: 10.1056/NEJMoa1110874. Epub 2011 Nov 15.

Nielsen, N., Wetterslev, J., Cronberg, T., et al. (2013). Targeted temperature management at 33°C versus 36°C after cardiac arrest. *N Engl J Med*, 369(23), 2197–2206. doi: 10.1056/NEJMoa1310519. Epub 2013 Nov 17.

Park, S. J., Kim, Y. H., Park, D. W., et al. (2011). Randomized trial of stents versus bypass surgery for left main coronary artery disease. *N Engl J Med*. 2011 Apr 4. Epub ahead of print.

Pflieger, M., Winslow, B. T., Mills, K., & Dauber, I. M. (2011). Medical management of stable coronary artery disease. *Am Fam Phys*, 83(7), 819–826.

Pierce, D., Calkins, B. C., & Thornton, K. (2012). Infectious endocarditis: diagnosis and treatment. *Am Fam Phys*, 85(10), 981–986.

Pinto, D. S. (2010). A 43-year-old man with angina, elevated troponin, and lateral ST depression: management of acute coronary syndromes. *JAMA*, 303(1), 54–63.

Redberg, R. F. (2012). Coronary CT angiography for acute chest pain. *N Engl J Med*, 367(4), 375–376.

Roe, M. T., & Ohman, E. M. (2012). A new era in secondary prevention after acute coronary syndrome. *N Engl J Med*, 366(1), 85–87. Epub 2011 Nov 13.

Saffitz, J. (2009). The heart. In E. Rubin & H. M. Reisner, *Essentials of Rubin's pathology.* 5th ed. Philadelphia, PA: Lippincott, Williams, & Wilkins.

Sagar, S., Liu, P. P., & Cooper, L. T., Jr. (2012). Myocarditis. *Lancet*, 379(9817), 738–747.

Seehusen, D. A. (2011). Statins for primary cardiovascular prevention. *Am Fam Phys*, 84(7), 767–768.

Stone, G. W., Maehara, A., Lansky, A. J., et al. (2011). A prospective natural-history study of coronary atherosclerosis. *N Engl J Med,* 364(3), 226–235.

Torpy, J. M., Burke, A. E., & Glass, R. M. (2010). *JAMA* patient page. Acute coronary syndromes. *JAMA*, 303(1), 90.

Tricoci, P., Huang, Z., Held, C., et al. (2012). Thrombin-receptor antagonist vorapaxar in acute coronary syndromes. *N Engl J Med*, 366(1), 20–33. Epub 2011 Nov 13.

Viera, A. J., & Sheridan, S. L. (2010). Global risk of coronary heart disease: assessment and application. *Am Fam Phys*, 82(3), 265–274.

Wald, D. S., Morris, J. K., Wald, N. J., et al. (2013). Randomized trial of preventive angioplasty in myocardial infarction. *N Engl J Med*, 369(12), 1115–1123. doi: 10.1056/NEJMoa1305520.

Wald, D. S., Morris, J. K., Wald, N. J., & PRAMI Investigators. (2014, January 16). Preventive angioplasty in myocardial infarction. *N Engl J Med,* 370(3), 283. doi: 10.1056/NEJMc1314696.

Weintraub, W. S., Grau-Sepulveda, M. V., Weiss, J. M., et al. (2012). Comparative effectiveness of revascularization strategies. *N Engl J Med*, 366(16), 1467–1476. doi: 10.1056/NEJMoa1110717. Epub 2012 Mar 27.

Heart Failure

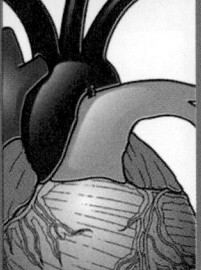

Key Terms

Afterload

Angiotensin-converting enzyme (ACE)

Ascites

Cardiac contractility

Cardiomyopathy

Central venous pressure (CVP)

Chronotropic function

Diastolic dysfunction

Heart failure

Hydrostatic pressure

Inotropic function

Jugular vein distension (JVD)

Left ventricular ejection fraction (LVEF)

Orthopnea

Paroxysmal nocturnal dyspnea (PND)

Preload

Pulmonary capillary wedge
  pressure (PCWP)

Pulmonary hypertension

Starling's capillary forces

Systolic dysfunction

Heart failure is a clinical condition commonly resulting from a weakened ventricular muscle that is unable to sufficiently pump blood into the arterial circulation to meet the needs of the tissues. Less commonly, heart failure can be caused by the ventricle's inability to expand and fill with sufficient blood volume. With an inability to fill, the ventricle cannot pump blood into the peripheral or pulmonary circulatory system. When it is accompanied by fluid retention, it is sometimes called congestive heart failure.

Heart failure should not be confused with cardiac arrest, which is the cessation of all heart activity. A failing heart has a weakened ventricle but continues to pump blood to supply the body with circulation. However, a weakened ventricle cannot adequately eject its blood volume; this creates pressure changes within the heart's chambers. The consequent pressure changes within the heart's chambers and great vessels cause major systemic effects.

Heart failure is a disease of epidemic proportions within the United States, with more than 550,000 patients diagnosed with it each year. It affects 5 million Americans and causes 300,000 deaths annually. It also is the most common cause of hospitalization. Regardless of age, the lifetime risk of developing heart failure is approximately 20% for all patients older than 40 years, and its incidence in persons age 65 and older is 10 per 1,000—numbers that are only expected to increase as the aged segment of the population grows. As the treatment for other cardiovascular diseases has improved, more persons are surviving into old age with chronic cardiovascular conditions. Mortality rates from ischemic heart disease, myocardial infarction (MI), and dysrhythmias have been significantly reduced over the last few decades, and prevalence of cardiovascular morbidity has increased among survivors. Ironically, this has increased the prevalence of heart failure within the population. Persons with cardiovascular disease are surviving acute cardiac events and living longer with chronic cardiac disorders.

Hypertension (HTN) is the greatest risk factor for the development of heart failure, as more than 75% of patients with heart failure are treated for HTN before developing it. About 22% of men and 46% of women will develop heart failure within 6 months following an acute MI. Other causes of heart failure include coronary artery disease and metabolic syndrome; a history of diabetes mellitus also increases the risk of developing the disorder. Women are often diagnosed with heart failure at an older age than men because natural estrogen is cardioprotective. After menopause, the risk of cardiovascular disease for men and women are equal. Within the U.S. population, there is a greater prevalence of heart failure among African Americans compared with Caucasian Americans. Many researchers are investigating the causes for this disparity (see Box 17-1).

Basic Physiologic Concepts of Heart Function

The heart's failure as a pump creates widespread consequences throughout the body and activates specific compensatory mechanisms. It is essential to understand the following key concepts related to the heart's physiology before understanding the pathophysiology of heart failure.

Cardiac Output

Cardiac output is the amount of blood that the heart pumps out of the left ventricle each minute. In general, cardiac output is diminished in heart failure, because the left ventricle is weakened and cannot adequately

BOX 17-1. Prevalence of Heart Failure Among African Americans

Mortality from heart failure is 2.5 times greater among African Americans compared with Caucasians younger than 65 years of age. African Americans develop heart failure at an earlier age and the hospitalization rates are substantially higher than those among Caucasians. Between the ages of 45 and 64, African American males have a 70% higher risk for heart failure than Caucasian males. African American females between the ages of 45 and 54 have a 50% greater risk for developing heart failure than Caucasian females. The reason for the increased morbidity and mortality in African American heart failure patients is unclear. Past research demonstrates that HTN is the specific cause for heart failure among a majority of African Americans, and conventional forms of antihypertensive medication are ineffective for this population. Current research focuses on specific pharmacological treatments that target the distinctive pathological mechanisms of heart failure and HTN in African Americans. The field of pharmacogenomics is in its infancy but can increase efficacy of drugs by matching specific medications to specific patients.

pump blood out of the chamber. It is based on heart rate (HR), the rate at which the heart beats, and stroke volume (SV), the volume of blood pumped out of the ventricle with each contraction. In mathematical terms, cardiac output = HR × SV (see Box 17-2).

Because cardiac output varies by body size, a hemodynamic measurement termed cardiac index can be calculated to give a more accurate assessment of each individual's cardiac output. Cardiac output divided by an individual's body surface area yields the cardiac index.

HR is controlled by the sympathetic (adrenergic) and parasympathetic (cholinergic) nervous systems. Adrenergic stimulation raises HR and cholinergic stimulation

BOX 17-2. Normal Cardiac Output

Cardiac output = SV × HR
SV = milliliters of blood ejected per ventricular contraction
HR = number of ventricular contractions per minute

In a healthy heart, SV equals approximately 70 mL of blood ejected per ventricular contraction. The average HR is 70 beats per minute or 70 contractions/minute. Therefore, cardiac output equals 70 mL/contraction x 70 contractions/minute or a blood volume of 4,900 mL/minute (approximately 5,000 mL or 5 liters/minute).

slows heart rate. SV is influenced by preload, afterload, and cardiac contractility.

Preload

Preload can be defined as the volume of blood in the heart at the end of diastole. Essentially, preload factors are those that affect cardiac output but occur before contraction. Most commonly, in clinical settings, preload refers to the volume of blood that enters the right atrium from the venous system (see Fig. 17-1).

As blood flows into the right atrium, it empties into the right ventricle during diastole. The preload volume of blood that originates from the venous system and ultimately empties into the right ventricle can also be called the ventricular end diastolic volume. Preload causes stretch and increased pressure within the ventricular chamber, which increases SV. With increased venous return, preload increases, and SV is enhanced. If venous return is diminished, preload decreases, and SV is reduced. However, excessive venous return can overload a weakened ventricle, resulting in decreased cardiac output leading to heart failure. This relationship is described in the Frank-Starling law (see Box 17-3).

Afterload

Afterload can be described as the amount of resistance that the ventricle must overcome in order to pump

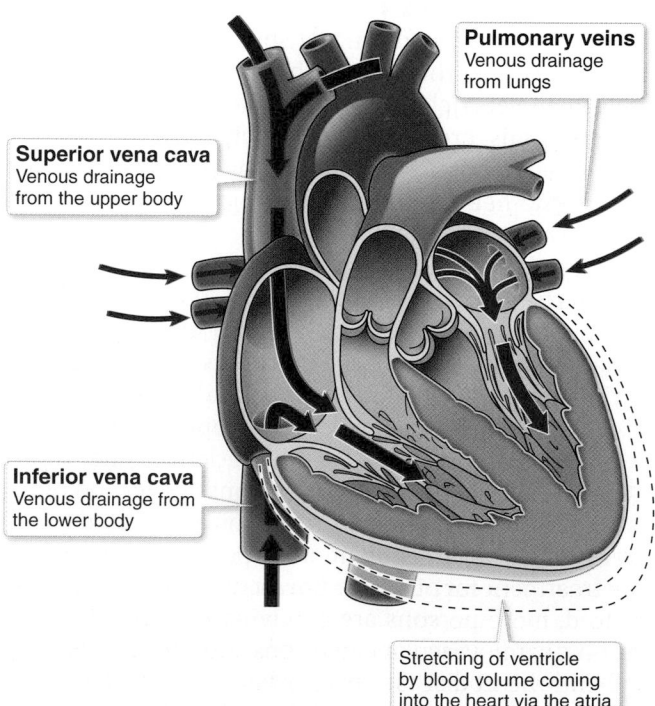

Pulmonary veins
Venous drainage from lungs

Superior vena cava
Venous drainage from the upper body

Inferior vena cava
Venous drainage from the lower body

Stretching of ventricle by blood volume coming into the heart via the atria

FIGURE 17-1. Cardiac preload. Preload is a volume of blood that stretches the right or left ventricle of the heart. It can be referred to as the ventricular end-diastolic volume that is achieved by the passive filling of the ventricle from the atria. In the clinical setting, the volume of blood entering the right atrium is most often referred to as preload.

BOX 17-3. The Frank-Starling Law

The relationship between cardiac contractility, preload, afterload, SV, and cardiac output of the heart is called the Frank-Starling law. This mechanism describes how the ventricle can adjust its pumping force to accommodate various levels of preload and afterload. An increase in left ventricular end-diastolic volume (preload) will increase the blood volume in the ventricle, which in turn produces an increase in cardiac output. The force of contraction of the healthy heart is directly related to the blood volume that fills the ventricle in diastole (preload). The maximum force of contraction of the ventricle occurs when an increase in preload stretches muscle fibers to 2½ times their resting length.

Evaluating the heart's effectiveness as a pump is based on the relationship between preload and its SV. SV varies directly with preload and inversely with afterload. In the healthy heart, an increased volume of blood filling the ventricle stretches ventricular myocardial fibers and consequently increases cardiac contractility and SV. Cardiac output is enhanced by preload (see Fig. 17-1) and can be reduced by afterload (see Fig. 17-2).

The strength of the heart's cardiac contractility has a major effect on SV. As the heart pump fails, cardiac contractile strength diminishes and the ventricle ejects a progressively decreased amount of SV from preload (see Fig. 17-3). Decreased SV, in turn, diminishes cardiac output. Cardiac contractile strength can be weakened by such conditions as direct injury of the myocardium, excessive afterload, or extremely low preload.

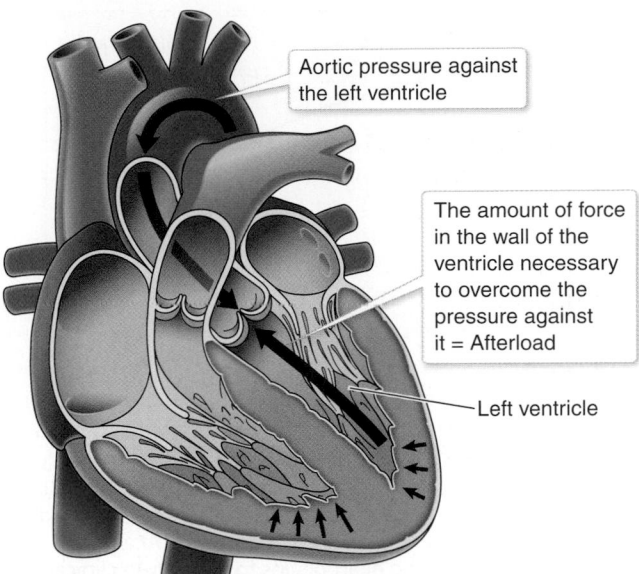

FIGURE 17-2. Cardiac afterload. Afterload is the force that the ventricle must overcome in order to eject its contents. It is the tension or stress developed in the wall of the ventricle during ejection. In the clinical setting, afterload is most commonly measured as the aortic pressure against the left ventricle. Aortic pressure reflects the systemic arterial pressure. Therefore, if there is high systemic arterial pressure (also referred to as HTN), this is considered high afterload.

blood out of the heart. The greater the pulmonary vascular resistance, the greater the afterload against the right ventricle. Pulmonary HTN, which is high pressure within the pulmonary arteries, creates high afterload for the right ventricle.

The greater the systemic arterial vascular resistance, the greater the afterload against the left ventricle. Most commonly, afterload describes the workload of the left ventricle or resistance exerted by the pressure within the aorta against the left ventricle (see Fig. 17-2). Pressure within the aorta is a reflection of systemic arterial blood pressure; therefore, systemic HTN creates high afterload for the left ventricle.

Cardiac Contractility

Cardiac contractility refers to the myocardium's ability to stretch and contract in response to the filling of the heart with blood. As blood fills the ventricle during diastole, tension in the heart muscle wall steadily increases, and stretching of the chamber occurs. Actin and myosin filaments of the myocardial muscle wall interact to create a force of contraction. The muscle filaments can change the force of contraction with varying amounts of stretch caused by blood volume or preload. SV is the amount of blood within the ventricle that is

ejected with each contraction. Therefore as preload increases, SV increases and the actin-myosin filaments in the heart wall stretch to accommodate the increased volume. These conditions enhance contractility in a healthy heart (see Fig. 17-3).

Contractility can also be influenced by afterload. As afterload increases, the heart's workload increases, which can negatively affect contractility. If the afterload becomes excessive, the ventricle's ability to eject blood is lessened; consequently, SV is diminished. Also,

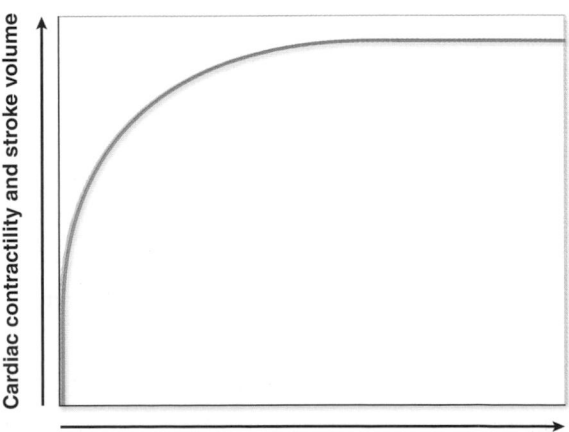

FIGURE 17-3. How changes in preload affect the contractility and SV of the healthy heart. As ventricular end diastolic volume (preload) increases, myocardial contractility and SV increase until a maximal level is reached. In the healthy heart, cardiac contractility and SV increase until the stretch of myocardial muscle fibers is 2 1/2 times their resting length.

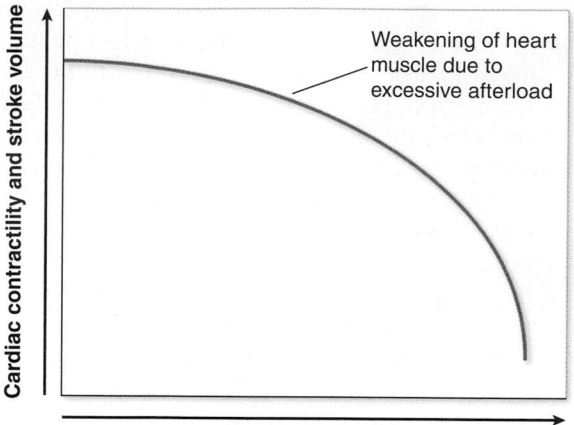

FIGURE 17-4. How changes in the afterload affect contractility and the heart's SV. As peripheral arterial resistance (afterload) increases, cardiac contractility and SV decrease. At a level of maximal afterload, the heart begins to weaken. In clinical settings, afterload is most commonly defined as the systemic arterial blood pressure or aortic pressure force exerted against the left ventricle.

the heart muscle is burdened with resistance and contractility decreases (see Fig. 17-4).

In the failing heart, an increase in preload causes high blood volume filling the ventricle; however, the weakened ventricular muscle may not have the strength to pump the excessive volume out. SV decreases when the weakened ventricle cannot optimally eject its blood. Also, the ventricular muscle's fibers can become overly taxed by the burden of the excessive filling of blood in the chamber and contractile force diminishes. Therefore, in a failing heart, with increased preload filling the weakened ventricle, contractility and SV can decrease (see Fig. 17-5).

Contractility is also influenced by the autonomic nervous system, acid-base balance, and electrolytes. Strong sympathetic nervous system (SNS) activity provides enhanced contractility because of stimulation of

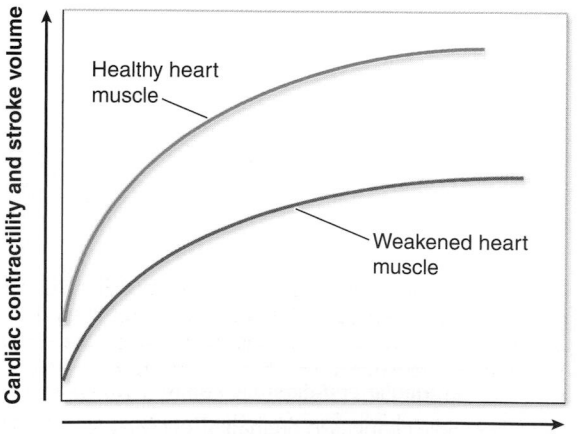

FIGURE 17-5. How increasing preload influences contractility and SV in the failing heart. As ventricular end-diastolic volume (preload) increases, a weakened heart muscle develops decreased cardiac contractility and SV.

beta-1 adrenergic receptors in the heart. Activation of the parasympathetic nervous system stimulates the vagal or cholinergic receptors in the heart, which decreases the force of contraction. Also, impaired calcium activity within cardiac ventricular muscle can negatively affect contractility.

Inotropic Versus Chronotropic Function of the Heart. The **inotropic function** of the heart refers to the force of contraction of the cardiac muscle. The heart's contractility can be influenced by the amount of calcium available for interaction between the actin and myosin filaments of the cardiac muscle fibers. Sympathetic stimulation can increase force of contraction, which is referred to as a positive inotropic effect.

Chronotropic function refers to HR. When digitalis is administered, it decreases HR by slowing conduction of impulses through the atrioventricular (AV) node; therefore, it has a negative chronotropic effect. Beta-adrenergic blocking agents antagonize the SNS effect on the heart by slowing impulses at the sinoatrial (SA) node, also a negative chronotropic effect. Conversely, epinephrine, an adrenergic or sympathetic stimulant, has positive inotropic and positive chronotropic effects on the heart. Under the influence of epinephrine, the heart has a greater force of contraction and increased heart rate.

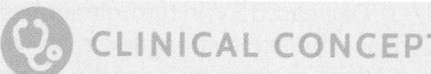

CLINICAL CONCEPT

The cardiac glycoside drug digitalis is a positive inotropic agent and a negative chronotropic agent because it increases force of ventricular contraction of the heart and decreases the heart rate.

High Capillary Hydrostatic Pressure and Edema. There are two major opposing pressure forces at every capillary bed in the body: hydrostatic pressure and oncotic (osmotic) pressure. Together, these opposing pressure forces are known as **Starling's capillary forces.** At every capillary–cell interface, there are three fluid compartments: intracellular, extracellular, and interstitial. Intracellular fluid is found inside the cells, interstitial fluid surrounds the cells, and extracellular fluid is located inside the capillary.

Capillary membranes are semipermeable, which means they allow diffusion of fluid out of the blood through the capillary pores into the interstitial and intracellular spaces. Fluid within the blood exerts **hydrostatic pressure,** a force that attempts to push fluid out of the capillary pores into the interstitial and intracellular spaces. Particles within the blood, such as albumin, sodium, and glucose, exert oncotic or osmotic pressure.

Oncotic (osmotic) pressure is a force that attempts to pull fluid from the interstitial and intracellular spaces into the capillary. Oncotic pressure forces and hydrostatic pressure forces oppose each other at every

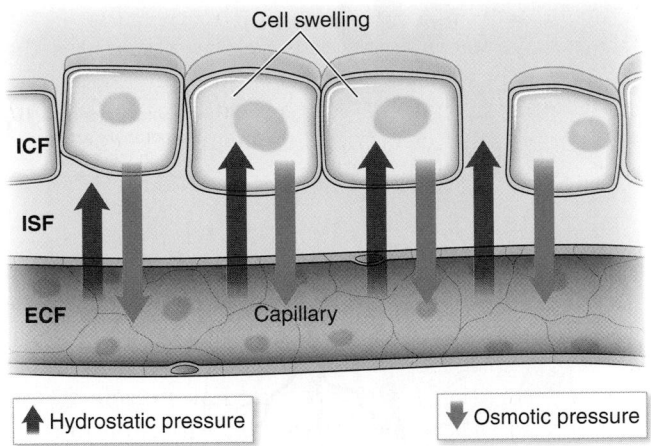

Cell swelling

ICF

ISF

ECF   Capillary

⬆ Hydrostatic pressure   ⬇ Osmotic pressure

FIGURE 17-6. Edema fluid in interstitial fluid space and intracellular fluid space caused by high hydrostatic pressure. Edema occurs because of high hydrostatic pressure in capillary blood into interstitial spaces and intracellular spaces. Fluid accumulation in and around the cells is edema, which causes swelling.

capillary membrane. Under normal conditions, these forces balance each other out, creating an equilibrium that exists at the capillary beds.

When hydrostatic pressure increases within the capillary, the forces become unbalanced. A high hydrostatic pressure force can overcome the opposing balancing effect of the oncotic pressure. High capillary hydrostatic pressure causes fluid to diffuse out of the capillary pores into the interstitial and intracellular spaces. This collection of fluid, which traverses into the interstitial and intracellular spaces, is called edema (see Fig. 17-6).

Hemodynamic Monitoring. A hemodynamic monitor measures pressures within the chambers and vessels of the right and left sides of the heart. Hemodynamic monitoring is accomplished by right heart cardiac catheterization or placement of a Swan-Ganz catheter. These are distinct invasive procedures that employ a specialized cardiac catheter device to diagnose heart disease and monitor treatment in heart failure.

A cardiac catheter is capable of measuring pressure and flow within the heart chambers. It is connected to a transducer that converts the pressure waves into a digital read that can be seen on a monitor screen. The catheter is inserted into a large vein for right heart hemodynamic assessment and the femoral artery for left heart hemodynamic assessment.

To directly measure right heart pressures, a Swan-Ganz catheter is threaded into the subclavian vein and advanced into the inferior vena cava (IVC) and right atrium. Pressure measurement within the IVC is referred to as **central venous pressure (CVP).** The catheter can measure CVP, which is the same as right atrial pressure at this location. The catheter can be further advanced into the right ventricle and pulmonary artery and then wedged into a pulmonary capillary (see Fig. 17-7). Pressures within the right ventricle, pulmonary artery, and pulmonary capillary bed can be

measured by the catheter at points along its path. When the catheter remains in place, it can provide a continuous measure of pulmonary capillary pressure. Upon inflation of the balloon on the tip of the Swan-Ganz catheter, the pressure reading is referred to as **pulmonary capillary wedge pressure (PCWP).**

To directly measure left heart pressures, a catheter is inserted into the femoral or radial artery and advanced against the flow of blood into the aorta; it is then further advanced into the left ventricle (see Fig. 17-8). Measurements can be taken of aortic pressure and systolic and diastolic pressures of the left ventricle from the catheter tip. **Left ventricular ejection fraction (LVEF),** the volume of blood pumped with each ventricular contraction, can be approximated from the systolic and diastolic pressure measurements. In healthy individuals, approximately 60% to 70% of blood volume in the left ventricle is pumped out with each contraction. A LVEF lower than 40% is indicative of heart failure.

The cardiac catheter inserted into a peripheral artery and into the aorta can be threaded into the coronary arteries. Radiopaque dye can be injected to illuminate the lumens of the coronary arteries and visualize the blood flow. Obstruction to blood flow,

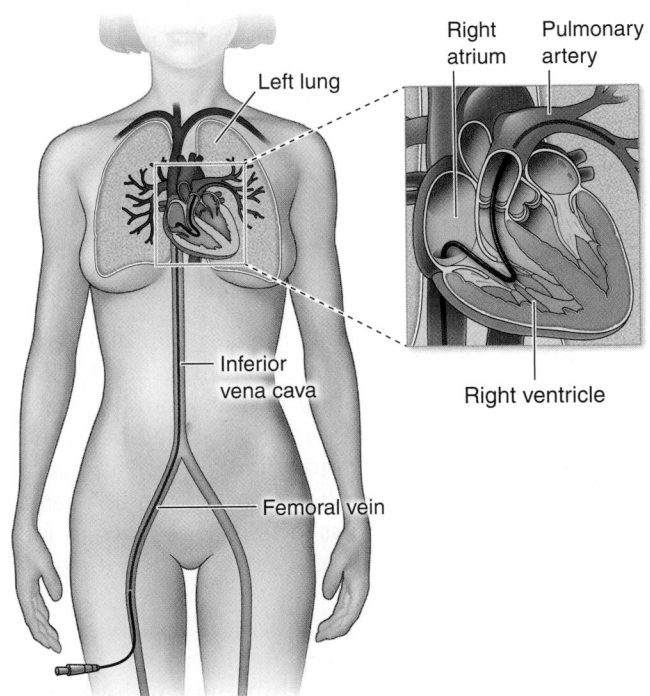

FIGURE 17-7. Cardiac catheterization. Cardiac catheterization can be done via the venous system or the arterial system, depending on the goal of the procedure. In this diagram, right-sided cardiac catheterization is shown. The goal of right-sided cardiac catheterization is to obtain the pulmonary capillary pressure (also called PCWP). The catheter is inserted via a peripheral vein, commonly the femoral vein. It is then threaded into the inferior vena cava, right atrium, right ventricle, and into the pulmonary artery. Finally it is wedged in a pulmonary capillary. The PCWP is used to assess the severity of left ventricular failure.

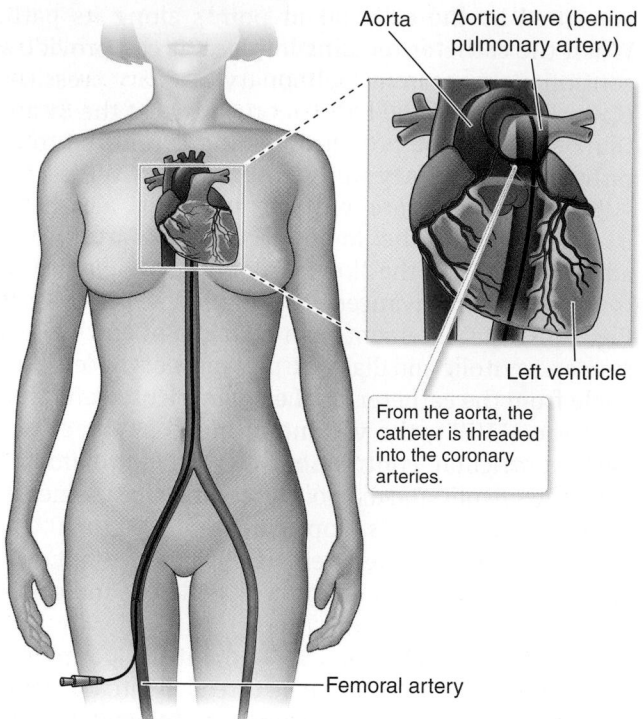

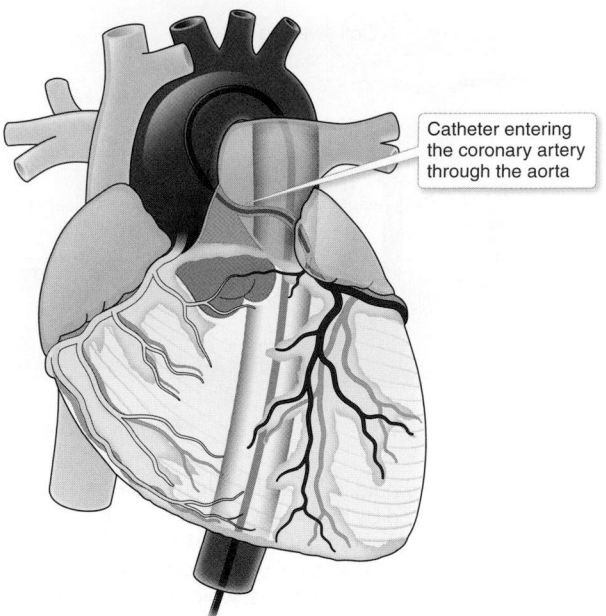

FIGURE 17-9. In left-sided cardiac catheterization, a catheter is inserted into a peripheral artery and then into the aorta. From the aorta, the catheter is threaded into the coronary arteries. At that point, an opaque dye is infused to outline the interior of the coronary arteries. A specialized x-ray called a coronary angiogram is then completed.

FIGURE 17-8. Cardiac catheterization. Cardiac catheterization can be done via the venous system or the arterial system, depending on the goal of the procedure. In this diagram, left-sided cardiac catheterization is shown. The goal is visualization of the coronary arteries. The catheter is inserted via a peripheral artery, commonly the femoral artery. It is then threaded into the aorta and into the coronary arteries. An opaque dye is infused into the coronary arteries in order to highlight them in a specialized x-ray called a coronary angiogram. The interior structure of the coronary arteries can then be examined.

thrombi, arteriosclerotic plaque, aneurysm, or other malformations of the arteries can be visualized through this procedure (see Fig. 17-9).

The healthy heart exhibits ranges of normal hemodynamic measurements. In the failing heart, these measurements become abnormal and can be used to differentiate right-sided versus left-sided heart dysfunction. Abnormal hemodynamic measurements obtained from cardiac catheterization can be used to diagnose right-sided versus left-sided ventricular failure. Cardiac catheterization is also used to diagnose coronary artery disease.

Cardiovascular Regulatory Mechanisms

There are major sensors within the cardiovascular system that respond to decreased blood pressure and blood volume. The major mechanisms include the renin-angiotensin-aldosterone system (RAAS), which is triggered by the kidney. The autonomic nervous system senses low circulation via baroreceptors that are embedded within the arteries. The posterior pituitary releases antidiuretic hormone (ADH) in response to decreased blood volume or blood pressure. In addition, there are substances in the body that regulate circulation to the tissues and cardiovascular

changes: endothelin, nitric oxide, natriuretic peptides and TNF.

Renin-Angiotensin-Aldosterone System. The RAAS is a major mechanism in the regulation of arterial blood pressure. It is a compensatory mechanism that raises blood pressure and increases blood volume in response to decreased renal perfusion (see Fig. 17-10).

Renin is an enzyme that is released from the juxtaglomerular apparatus of the kidney in response to decreased renal perfusion. When blood pressure drops, renal perfusion diminishes, which, in turn, provokes renin release. After release, renin circulates and reacts with angiotensinogen, a protein synthesized by the liver. Angiotensinogen is then cleaved into a smaller protein, angiotensin I. Angiotensin I circulates, and in the lungs it is transformed into angiotensin II by **angiotensin-converting enzyme (ACE).**

Angiotensin II is a potent arterial vasoconstrictor that raises blood pressure within the systemic arterial system. It is also a trigger for myocardial changes referred to as ventricular remodeling. Frequent stimulation of angiotensin II will activate genetic changes in the cardiac myocyte that lead to hypertrophy, apoptosis, and myocardial fibrosis. As some cardiac myocytes hypertrophy, the ventricular muscle enlarges. Other cardiac myocytes degenerate, causing ventricular muscle weakness. As the myocardium degenerates it becomes infiltrated with collagenous fibrous tissue, which is noncontractile and nonconductive.

In addition, angiotensin II stimulates the adrenal gland to release aldosterone. Aldosterone is a hormone that acts at the nephron to increase sodium and water

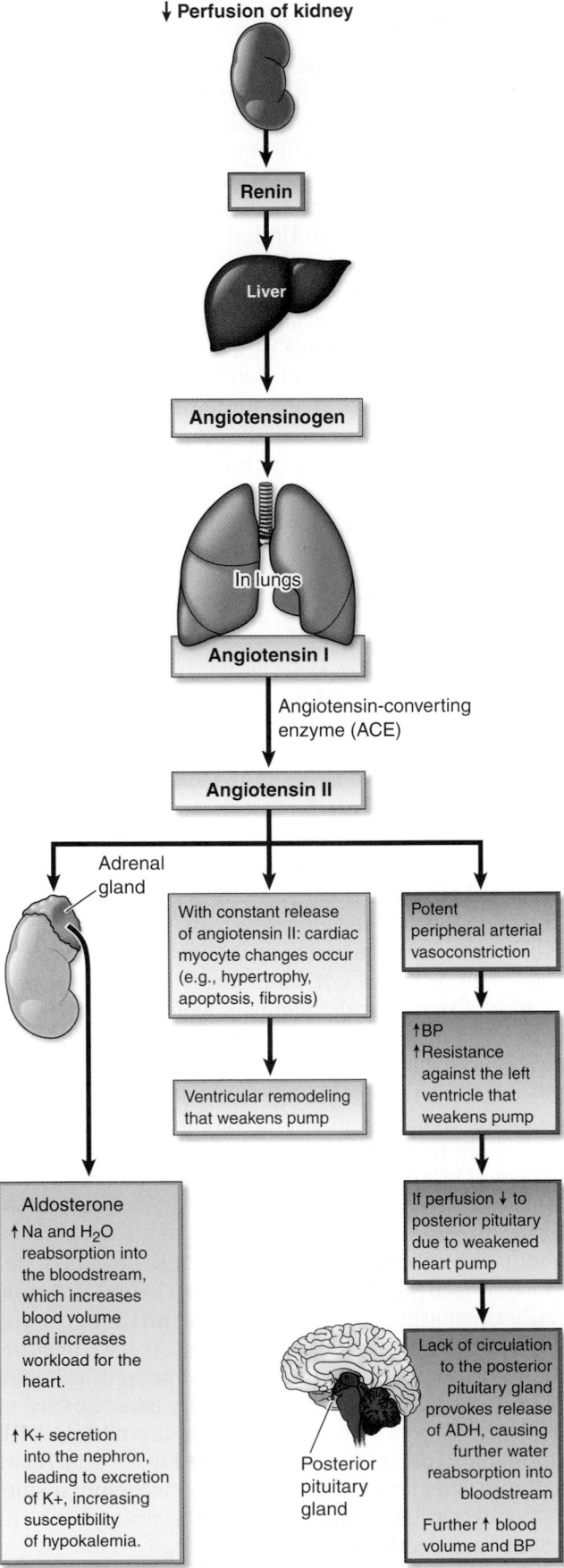

↓ Perfusion of kidney

Renin

Liver

Angiotensinogen

In lungs

Angiotensin I

Angiotensin-converting
enzyme (ACE)

Angiotensin II

Adrenal
gland

With constant release
of angiotensin II: cardiac
myocyte changes occur
(e.g., hypertrophy,
apoptosis, fibrosis)

Potent
peripheral arterial
vasoconstriction

↑BP
↑Resistance
against the left
ventricle that
weakens pump

Ventricular remodeling
that weakens pump

If perfusion ↓ to
posterior pituitary
due to weakened
heart pump

Aldosterone

↑ Na and H₂O
reabsorption into
the bloodstream,
which increases
blood volume
and increases
workload for the
heart.

↑ K+ secretion
into the nephron,
leading to excretion
of K+, increasing
susceptibility
of hypokalemia.

Posterior
pituitary
gland

Lack of circulation
to the posterior
pituitary gland
provokes release
of ADH, causing
further water
reabsorption into
bloodstream

Further ↑ blood
volume and BP

FIGURE 17-10. The RAAS. In heart failure, the RAAS continuously cycles and increases weakening of the heart. The net effect of the RAAS is increased blood volume, increased resistance against the heart, increased workload on the heart, and ventricular remodeling that weakens the heart.

reabsorption from the distal tubule into the bloodstream. It also increases secretion of potassium into the nephron tubule, resulting in potassium excretion. The sodium and water retention caused by aldosterone increases total blood volume and raises blood pressure.

Although the RAAS is a vital compensatory mechanism and major regulator of blood pressure, it has detrimental effects in heart failure. The net effects of the RAAS are elevated blood pressure and blood volume, which increase workload for the left ventricle. In left ventricular failure (LVF), this extra blood volume and high blood pressure further weakens the heart pump. Because this can be a vicious cycle, it can be said that heart failure begets heart failure. This mechanism is explained in more detail within the neurohormonal forward failure effects of LVF.

Natriuretic Peptides. Within the circulatory system, increased water and sodium retention raises blood volume. High blood volume entering the heart stretches the heart's atrial chambers, which activates the release of natriuretic peptides from the atrial myocytes. Atrial natriuretic peptide (ANP) is a protein molecule that induces a process of natriuresis, which is increased excretion of sodium and water by the nephron. Release of ANP stimulates the glomerulus to increase filtration of the blood, inhibits reabsorption of sodium at the proximal tubule, blocks release of renin and aldosterone, and opposes the vasoconstrictive effects of angiotensin II. All these actions enhance the excretion of water from the body and decrease blood volume.

Similarly, when increased blood volume causes increased ventricular volume and stretch, the ventricular myocytes release B-type natriuretic peptide (BNP). BNP exerts the same effects as ANP, inducing the process of natural diuresis. In heart failure, both these natriuretic peptides are released because of the increased blood volume and edema.

CLINICAL CONCEPT

An elevated level of BNP is commonly used as a diagnostic indicator in heart failure. Synthetic BNP is also administered as a therapeutic pharmacological agent in heart failure to induce diuresis.

Endothelin. Endothelin is a peptide that is secreted by the heart's endothelium and vasculature in heart failure. It is often elevated in heart failure following an acute MI. It stimulates vasoconstriction of the arterial blood vessels, which increases resistance against the left ventricle. Increased resistance causes high workload for the left ventricle. If resistance becomes excessive, the workload strains the heart. Endothelin also provokes fibrotic changes within the myocardium, which is part of the heart's ventricular remodeling, which occurs in heart failure.

Tumor Necrosis Factor-Alpha. In heart failure, elevated levels of tumor necrosis factor-alpha (TNF-alpha) are present in the bloodstream and cardiac muscle. TNF-alpha is an inflammatory cytokine that stimulates hypertrophy, fibrotic changes, and cell death, or apoptosis of the myocardium. It also negatively affects the heart's inotropic function. This leads to dilation of the ventricle with decreasing cardiac output. Myocardial apoptosis, degeneration of heart muscle, puts further strain on the functional myocytes. The net effect is diminished strength of ventricular contraction, worsening heart failure, and detrimental remodeling of the heart.

Nitric Oxide. Nitric oxide (NO) is a potent vasodilator produced by vascular endothelial cells. Through its vasodilator action, it is a local regulator of blood flow to the tissues.

Antidiuretic Hormone. Another physiologic response to decreased tissue perfusion is the release of ADH from the posterior pituitary gland. This hormone promotes water reabsorption into the bloodstream at the nephron in the kidneys and also has vasoconstrictor effects.

Autonomic Nervous System Regulation. Cardiovascular homeostasis is promoted by the activity of the autonomic nervous system. The heart is richly innervated by both the sympathetic and parasympathetic neurons. The parasympathetic nervous system stimulates cholinergic receptors to slow the HR and decrease the force of contraction. Conversely, sympathetic stimulation of beta-1 adrenergic receptors results in an increase in HR and a strengthening of the force of contraction, which results in increased SV and cardiac output. However, sympathetic stimulation also leads to activation of alpha-adrenergic receptors within arterial vessel walls, which results in vasoconstriction.

Basic Pathophysiologic Concepts of Heart Failure

There are four major pathological changes that can lead to the development of heart failure:

1. increased fluid volume or volume overload
2. impaired ventricular filling
3. degeneration of ventricular muscle
4. decreased ventricular contractile function.

Any one of these can lead to a reduction in cardiac output and compensatory mechanisms associated with heart failure. Heart failure is initiated by a precipitating event, and the four pathological changes occur over time.

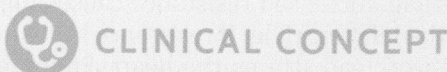
CLINICAL CONCEPT

It is important to identify the most likely cause of heart failure, because it will guide treatment.

Epidemiology

Heart failure is the fastest-growing clinical cardiac disease entity in the United States, affecting approximately 2% of the population. It is the most frequent cause of hospitalization in individuals older than age 65 years. The American Heart Association (AHA) estimates that there are approximately 5.8 million people with heart failure in the United States and 23 million people with the disorder worldwide. The prevalence of heart failure and left ventricular dysfunction increases steeply with age. As an example, the Framingham Heart Study found a prevalence of heart failure in men of 8 per 1,000 at age 50 to 59 years, increasing to 66 per 1,000 at ages 80 to 89 years; similar values were noted in women. Women, however, develop the disorder later than men and live longer with the chronic condition. The prevalence of heart failure in African Americans is reported to be 25% higher than in whites.

Etiology

There are many causes of heart failure; however, the most common cause is ischemic heart disease. Repeated episodes of coronary insufficiency denies the heart muscle of needed oxygen and nutrients. Many persons are surviving more than one MI, and many different areas of infarcted ventricular muscle cause a diminished contractile force. Chronic HTN is another major cause of heart failure because the left ventricle must overcome the high resistance of aortic pressure. Eventually the ventricular muscle becomes exhausted. Chronic obstructive pulmonary disease (COPD) can cause right ventricular changes that lead to a type of heart failure called cor pulmonale. Obstructive pulmonary disease causes hypoxia, which constricts the pulmonary arterial vessels in the lungs. This pulmonary HTN eventually causes exhaustion of the right ventricle. RVF eventually affects the left ventricle and heart failure develops. There are other less common causes of heart failure, but they all have the same effect; weakening of the left ventricle—the body's main pump.

Ischemic Heart Disease
About 75% of patients with heart failure develop it because of ischemic heart disease, also called ischemic cardiomyopathy. Coronary artery insufficiency is the primary cause of ischemic heart disease. Lack of sufficient coronary circulation causes repeated ischemia or infarction of the myocardium. The consequence of repeated MI is a scarred, fibrotic heart muscle with diminished contractile strength (see Fig. 17-11). Heart failure occurs as a result of repeated ischemic insults to the myocardium, which weakens the strength of ventricular contractions.

Chronic Hypertension
Chronic HTN is the leading cause of LVF. Long-term high systemic arterial blood pressure causes high aortic pressure, which creates a high workload or increased

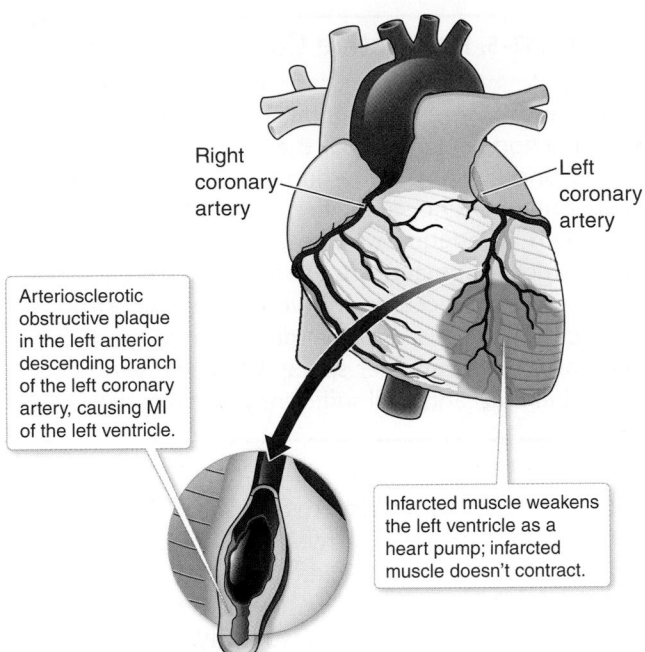

Right coronary artery

Left coronary artery

Arteriosclerotic obstructive plaque in the left anterior descending branch of the left coronary artery, causing MI of the left ventricle.

Infarcted muscle weakens the left ventricle as a heart pump; infarcted muscle doesn't contract.

FIGURE 17-11. Repeated episodes of ischemic heart disease (ischemic cardiomyopathy) leads to a weakened heart muscle or heart failure. Ischemic cardiomyopathy or repeated episodes of ischemic heart disease is a leading cause of heart failure. Repeated ischemic insults to the myocardial muscle weakens the heart muscle and creates a suboptimal heart pump. One of the most common areas of arteriosclerosis is in the left coronary artery, a major arterial supply of the left ventricle. The LV is the most common site of ischemia and MI. Infarcted heart muscle doesn't contract or conduct impulses. Repeated myocardial infarcts are extremely harmful to the strength of the ventricular muscle, which predisposes the individual to heart failure.

resistance for the left ventricle. In response to the resistance caused by the high arterial pressure, the left ventricle hypertrophies. As the ventricular muscle increases in size, it requires increased circulation from the existing coronary artery supply. Eventually, the coronary artery supply cannot sufficiently perfuse the enlarged left ventricle. This condition predisposes the hypertrophied left ventricle to ischemic injury because of inadequate coronary arterial perfusion. A hypertrophied left ventricle is more apt to sustain ischemia and MI, which results in weakening of the muscle. Therefore, the hypertrophied left ventricle is detrimental to the heart's health.

In addition, the enlarged cardiac muscle wall encroaches on the left ventricular chamber. As the muscle wall enlarges, it leaves less filling space within the chamber, which results in a condition termed restrictive cardiomyopathy. Over time, the hypertrophied left ventricle impedes optimal ventricular filling and becomes increasingly predisposed to ischemia. These conditions lead to severely impaired left ventricular contractile function (see Box 17-4).

Chronic Pulmonary Disease

Chronic pulmonary disease is the leading cause of RVF. When pulmonary disease is the etiology of RVF, the condition is referred to as cor pulmonale. In cor

BOX 17-4. How Chronic HTN Leads to Left Ventricular Failure

- High systemic arterial blood pressure is reflected in the aorta as high aortic pressure.
- High aortic pressure creates increased resistance against the left ventricle, which causes left ventricular hypertrophy.
- The hypertrophied left ventricle requires increased coronary circulation, and demand eventually exceeds coronary artery supply.
- The hypertrophied left ventricle becomes predisposed to ischemia and systolic dysfunction.
- The hypertrophied left ventricle impedes optimal ventricular filling, causing restrictive cardiomyopathy and diastolic dysfunction type of heart failure.

pulmonale, the initiating event of heart failure is a lung disease that causes chronic hypoxia. The heart starts out in good health until a lung disease exerts detrimental effects on the right ventricle.

To understand cor pulmonale, the basic premise to comprehend is that chronic hypoxia stimulates vasoconstriction of the pulmonary arterial circulation. In turn, vasoconstriction of the pulmonary arterial circulation creates high pulmonary artery pressure or **pulmonary hypertension.** In pulmonary HTN, the right ventricle, which must pump its contents into the pulmonary artery, is confronted with increased resistance. This increased workload on the right ventricle eventually causes right ventricular hypertrophy. As the right ventricle muscle wall enlarges, it requires increased coronary circulation. Demand for coronary blood flow eventually exceeds supply and the right ventricle sustains ischemia. Ischemic insults to the right ventricle consequently weaken the muscle, leading to RVF (see Fig. 17-12).

 CLINICAL CONCEPT

Long-standing pulmonary disease that causes chronic hypoxia can lead to cor pulmonale; one of the most common lung conditions that leads to cor pulmonale is COPD.

Cardiomyopathies

The term **cardiomyopathy** is most commonly used to describe a disease that targets the heart muscle itself. Cardiomyopathy generally infers that the myocardium has been directly injured by an agent or damaged as a side effect of another disease process. Infections that cause myocarditis, autoimmune disorders such as sarcoidosis, neuromuscular diseases such as muscular dystrophy, and alcoholic toxicity are examples of conditions that can directly injure the myocardium.

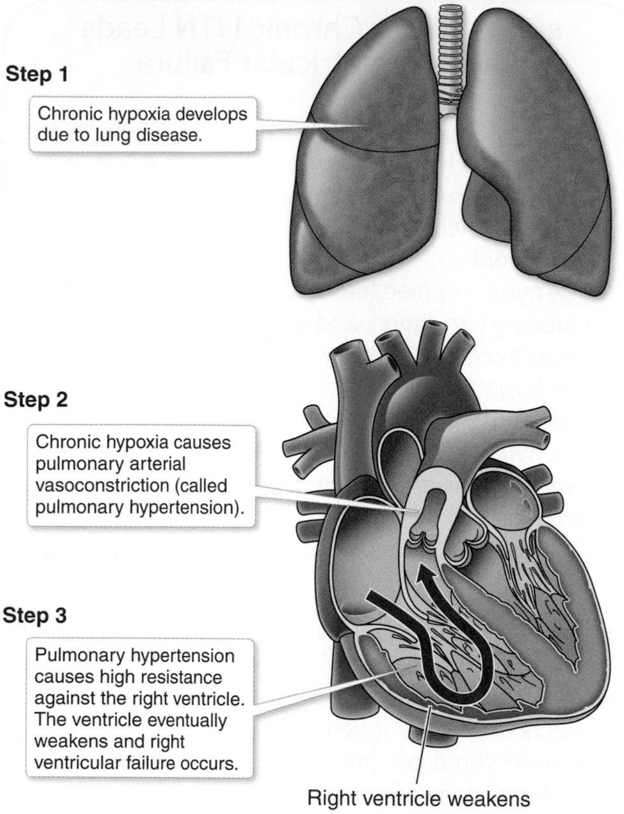

Step 1

Chronic hypoxia develops due to lung disease.

Step 2

Chronic hypoxia causes pulmonary arterial vasoconstriction (called pulmonary hypertension).

Step 3

Pulmonary hypertension causes high resistance against the right ventricle. The ventricle eventually weakens and right ventricular failure occurs.

Right ventricle weakens

FIGURE 17-12. Cor pulmonale. Cor pulmonale is right-sided heart failure that develops because of lung disease. The heart starts out healthy but, because of chronic lung disease, the right side of the heart weakens. The events occur as follows: Step 1: The lung is diseased and causes chronic hypoxia. Step 2: Chronic hypoxia causes pulmonary arterial vasoconstriction. Step 3: The pulmonary vasoconstriction causes high resistance against the right ventricle and eventually weakens the right ventricle.

Ischemic cardiomyopathy is a term used to describe the diffuse myocardial fibrosis and scarring of the heart muscle caused by coronary artery insufficiency and MI. Dilated cardiomyopathy is another term used to describe enlargement and hypertrophy of the left or right ventricles in response to chronic injury. The distended ventricle loses contractile ability and exhibits poor systolic function. The enlarged ventricle becomes prone to dysrhythmias, stasis of blood, and consequent formation of emboli.

Cardiomyopathies are also described as restrictive or hypertrophic. In restrictive cardiomyopathy, the ventricle is impeded from filling to full capacity (see Box 17-5). Fibrotic changes of the myocardium, pericardial effusion, and pericarditis are disorders that restrict the ventricle's ability to fully expand. In hypertrophic cardiomyopathy, the left ventricular muscle is enlarged, usually on the side of the interventricular septum. The asymmetric hypertrophy of the left ventricle causes muscle wall stiffness and can obstruct the ejection of blood into the aorta during systole. Primary hypertrophic cardiomyopathy is commonly caused by a genetic predisposition for the muscular enlargement of the interventricular septal wall of the left ventricle.

BOX 17-5. Restrictive Cardiomyopathy

A minority of cases of heart failure result from diastolic dysfunction, an inability of the ventricle to relax, expand, and fill sufficiently during diastole. Restrictive cardiomyopathy occurs when the ventricle is unable to attain an adequate volume of blood because of a constrictive structural problem. This ventricular filling deficiency can occur in left ventricular hypertrophy, myocardial fibrosis, or pericarditis. Each of these conditions create a smaller space within the ventricular chamber that cannot fill sufficiently with blood volume.

Chronic HTN is referred to as a secondary cause of hypertrophic cardiomyopathy. HTN usually causes more diffuse enlargement of the left ventricle, not limited to the interventricular septal wall region, than is seen in primary hypertrophic cardiomyopathy.

Dysrhythmias

Dysrhythmias, also known as irregular heart rhythms, are common precipitating causes of heart failure. Tachydysrhythmias, rapid irregular rhythms of the ventricle, reduce the time available for ventricular filling, which can precipitate heart failure. Bradydysrhythmias, which are slow irregular rhythms of the ventricle, can slow the HR excessively, minimize cardiac output, and precipitate heart failure. Atrial dysrhythmias can diminish the atrial "kick" volume emptied into the ventricle, which in turn decreases SV. Decreased SV lessens the blood pumped out of the ventricle to meet the needs of the tissues.

Heart Valve Abnormalities and Cardiac Infections

Various heart valve disorders such as mitral regurgitation, which is insufficient closure of the mitral valve, and aortic stenosis, which is the narrowing of the aortic valve, cause pressure changes within the heart chambers, which can lead to heart failure.

Mitral Regurgitation. Mitral regurgitation, also known as mitral insufficiency, occurs when the mitral valve does not close completely during systole. As the left ventricle contracts, blood from the ventricle refluxes back into the left atrium. This increased blood volume in the left atrium increases backward pressure within the pulmonary veins. Pulmonary capillary hydrostatic pressure increases as a result, and fluid diffuses out of the capillaries into the pulmonary interstitium.

Mitral regurgitation commonly occurs after transmural MI of the left ventricle. The infarction commonly injures the papillary muscles, which are muscular projections that extend from the internal left ventricular wall. These small muscular projections are attached to the chorda tendineae, which are membranous, stringlike cords that hold the heart valve leaflets in place. Chordae tendineae and papillary muscles assist in valve function. When rupture of a papillary muscle occurs because of MI of the left ventricle, the mitral valve becomes incompetent (see Fig. 17-13). The mitral valve leaflets become loose and do not come together to close off blood flow from the left atrium to the left ventricle. This dysfunction of the valve causes a classic, holosystolic murmur heard loudest at the heart's apex. As the left ventricle contracts during systole, blood refluxes upward into the left atrium through the incompletely closed mitral valve. Consequently, backward pressure builds into left atrium pulmonary veins and pulmonary interstitium.

Aortic Stenosis. Aortic stenosis is often caused by calcification of the aortic valve with aging, a process called aortic sclerosis. This produces a narrowing of the aortic valve that impedes the ejection of blood flow from the left ventricle into the aorta during systole (see Fig. 17-14). Aortic stenosis causes increased resistance against the left ventricle, which eventually causes left ventricular hypertrophy (LVH). As discussed previously, LVH is a precursor of events that lead to left ventricular failure.

Other Abnormalities. Aortic stenosis and mitral regurgitation are common heart valve disorders that lead to heart failure, but other disruptions of heart valve function can also lead to pressure changes within the heart chambers and eventual right or left ventricular failure.

Endocarditis and myocarditis, infections of the heart muscle, can cause detrimental biochemical and structural changes within the myocardium. These changes can lead to rapid deterioration of the contractile strength of the ventricular muscle. Rheumatic fever, a streptococcal infection, can lead to rheumatic heart disease, a cause of valve deformities.

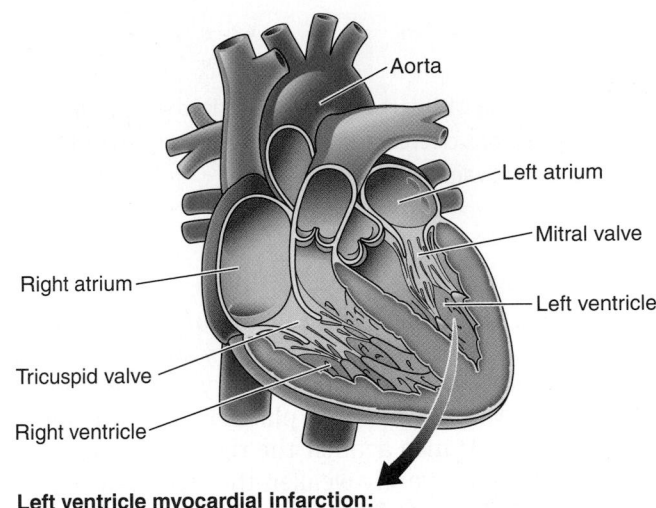

Left ventricle myocardial infarction:

FIGURE 17-13. Papillary muscle rupture after MI with resulting mitral regurgitation. The event occurs as follows: Step 1: Papillary muscles are attached to the mitral valve leaflets by stringlike cords called chordae tendineae. Step 2: MI ruptures papillary muscles of left ventricle. Step 3: The mitral valve leaflets become unattached to the ruptured papillary muscles, causing dysfunction of the mitral valve and regurgitation of blood up through the mitral valve into the left atrium.

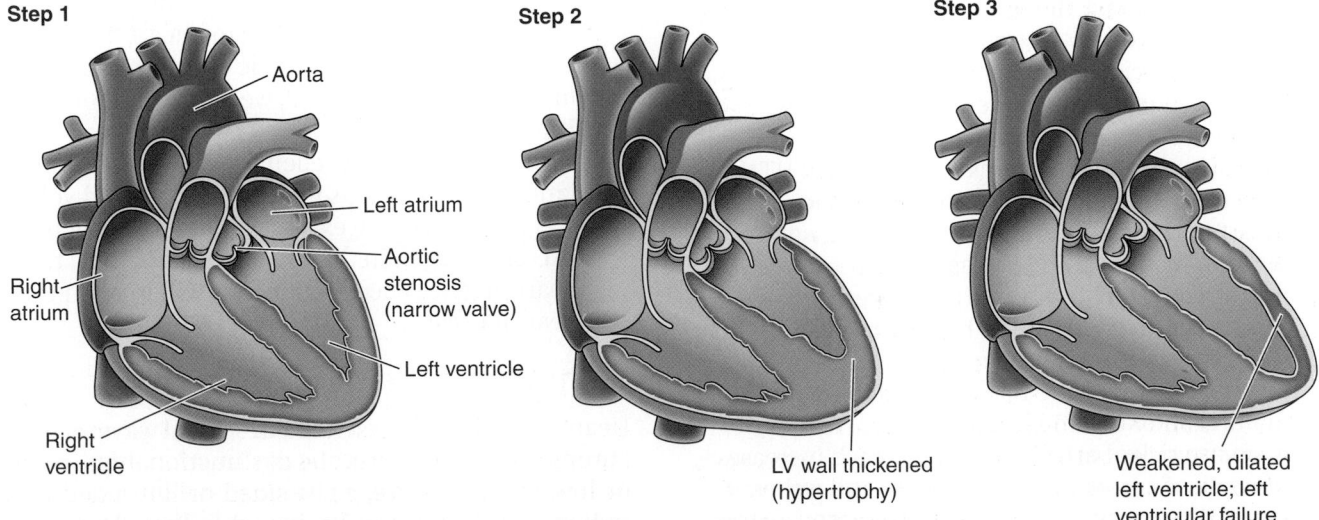

FIGURE 17-14. Development of LVH and LVF caused by aortic stenosis. Aortic stenosis is the narrowing of the aortic valve. A narrowed aortic valve creates excessive resistance against the left ventricle. It is difficult for the left ventricle to pump its blood forward into the aorta. Step 1 shows aortic stenosis. Step 2 shows how the left ventricle hypertrophies because of the increased resistance. Step 3 shows how eventually the left ventricle fails when exhausted from excessive workload because of the narrowed aortic valve.

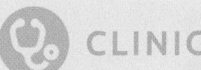

CLINICAL CONCEPT

A major cause of heart valve disease in the past, rheumatic fever, has decreased in prevalence because of the widespread availability of antibiotics.

Pulmonary Embolism

A pulmonary embolism can cause acute RVF. An embolus lodged in the pulmonary artery suddenly raises pressure within the pulmonary artery. This acute rise in pulmonary artery pressure places an overwhelming amount of resistance against the right ventricle. This can rapidly and severely weaken the right ventricular muscle, causing acute RVF.

Risk Factors

There are a number of risk factors for heart failure, including the following:

- **Age:** Heart failure risk increases with advancing age. Heart failure is the most common reason for hospitalization in people age 65 years and older.
- **Ethnicity:** Heart failure occurs more often in African Americans than Caucasians. African Americans more often develop heart failure before age 50 years and die from the condition compared with Caucasians.
- **Family history and genetics:** People with a family history of cardiomyopathies are at increased risk of developing heart failure. Cardiomyopathies are diseases of the heart that cause hypertrophy, dilation, or rigidity of myocardium. Currently, there are investigations into the genetic basis of these diseases.
- **Diabetes:** Diabetes increases risk of arteriosclerosis throughout the body, including the coronary arteries. Coronary arteriosclerosis leads to coronary insufficiency, myocardial ischemia, and MI. These syndromes of ischemic heart disease weaken the heart muscle.
- **Obesity:** Obesity is associated with both HTN and type 2 diabetes, conditions that place the heart at risk for arteriosclerosis. HTN also causes development of LVH with associated coronary insufficiency. These conditions together cause decreased strength of the heart muscle.
- **Lifestyle factors:** Smoking and sedentary lifestyle increase the risk for developing heart failure. Smoking and lack of physical activity increase risk of arteriosclerosis, which increases the risk of coronary artery disease and ischemic heart disease. Smoking also causes vasoconstriction of arterial blood vessels. These problems lead to high workload and decreased coronary blood supply of the heart muscle.
- **Medications:** Long-term use of anabolic steroids, which are male hormones used to build muscle mass, increases the risk for heart failure. The drug itraconazole (Sporanox), used to treat skin, nail, or other fungal infections, has occasionally been linked to heart failure. The cancer drug imatinib (Gleevec) has been associated with heart failure cases, and other chemotherapy drugs, such as doxorubicin, can increase the risk for later developing heart failure years after cancer treatment. Cancer radiation therapy to the chest can also damage the heart muscle.
- **Sleep apnea:** Sleep apnea can cause hypoxia and increases risk of rhythm disturbances. Chronic hypoxia can lead to pulmonary artery vasoconstriction, which leads to pulmonary HTN. Pulmonary HTN increases risk of RVF. Rhythm disturbances can weaken the heart muscle contractility.
- **Congenital heart defects:** Structural heart defects that occur in gestation and become apparent during the newborn period are called congenital heart defects. These defects may involve valvular abnormalities, imperfections in the heart wall, or anatomical problems with the aorta or pulmonary artery. These conditions cause changes in pressures within the heart chambers that can lead to excess workload for the heart and weakening of the heart muscle.
- **Viruses:** Although uncommon, certain viral infections can cause myocarditis, which weakens the heart muscle.
- **Alcohol abuse:** Excess long-term alcohol use can cause alcoholic cardiomyopathy and lead to heart failure. Patients who consume more than 2 drinks per day have a 1.5- to 2-fold increase in HTN compared with persons who do not drink alcohol, and this effect is most prominent when the daily intake of alcohol exceeds 5 drinks. Long-term HTN causes increased resistance against the left ventricle, eventually causing heart failure. Alcohol itself also has a toxic effect on the heart muscle, causing a dilated, weak myocardium.
- **Kidney conditions:** Kidney conditions can cause excess blood volume, edema, HTN, and accumulation of nitrogenous waste. Excess blood volume and HTN can cause excess workload for the heart. Excess nitrogen in the bloodstream is toxic to the heart muscle. These conditions will weaken the heart muscle.

Pathophysiology

Heart failure can be described in several ways: acute or chronic, systolic or diastolic dysfunction, high-output or low-output failure, right-sided or left-sided heart failure, and forward or backward failure. These contrasting descriptions are academic distinctions that explain the disorder's various mechanisms. However, these distinctions are often pertinent only early in the disease. Late in the course of heart failure, the distinctions become blurred.

The heart is a singular muscular organ that depends on the efficiency, rhythmicity, and strength of all its chambers. The biochemical and pressure changes that affect the myocardium in heart failure eventually affect both ventricles. A defect or weakness of one side of the heart will gradually lead to effects on the other side, causing a mixed clinical presentation of signs and symptoms late in the disease. Patients encountered in the clinical setting are often in the late stages of heart failure when theoretical distinctions become less applicable. Clinically, most patients in heart failure present with a combination of right-sided and left-sided ventricular failure, systolic and diastolic dysfunction, and both backward and forward failure effects. However, in order to better understand the complexities of this disorder, it is best to describe these mechanisms in terms of the previous distinctions for academic purposes.

Acute Versus Chronic Heart Failure

Acute heart failure describes the rapid, sudden development of heart failure that is often caused by substantial ventricular muscle injury as in massive MI. Sudden severe shock is often referred to as cardiogenic shock; it occurs when there is a significant loss of the ventricle's ability to pump blood adequately to maintain optimal blood pressure within the body. It often occurs because of extensive acute MI.

Chronic heart failure is a more common disorder, where the heart gradually suffers weakening over a long period of time.

Systolic Versus Diastolic Dysfunction

A weakened heart may exhibit dysfunction during systole, diastole, or both. In **systolic dysfunction,** also known as systolic heart failure, the weakened ventricle has difficulty ejecting blood out of the chamber. The ventricle is a poor forward pump which, in turn, causes inadequate ventricular emptying. SV and cardiac output, both functions of forward heart pumping action, are diminished. Blood accumulates in the weakened ventricle, elevating pressure within the chamber; this causes a backup of hydrostatic pressure into the atrium above it.

In **diastolic dysfunction,** also known as diastolic heart failure, the ventricle has difficulty relaxing, is less elastic, and cannot expand fully. The stiff ventricle cannot fill with blood adequately and therefore pumps out insufficient blood volume. SV and cardiac output are diminished because there is low blood volume in the ventricle (see Fig. 17-15).

High-Output Versus Low-Output Failure

High-output failure and low-output failure are less common mechanisms of heart failure. In high-output failure, the heart cannot pump sufficient amounts of blood to meet the high circulatory needs of the tissues. The heart is driven to high rates and contractile force to facilitate the delivery of blood to tissues demanding a greater amount of circulation. Under the strain of this effort, the heart can weaken and the ventricle can fail. High-output heart failure can be caused by systemic conditions that require increased arterial circulation caused by high metabolic demands, but this is a relatively uncommon occurrence. However, it is associated with thyrotoxicosis, AV shunting, severe anemia, Paget's disease of the bone, and thiamine deficiency.

In contrast, low-output failure occurs when the heart is unable to fill with adequate amounts of blood to pump out to the tissues. This is not a common cause of heart failure, but it can occur in conditions of impaired venous return to the heart. With less than adequate venous return, there is a lack of sufficient blood to recirculate through the heart and into the pulmonary and systemic arterial circulation. Consequently, in low output failure, insufficient blood volume is pumped into the circulation, causing a lack of delivery of adequate oxygen to the tissues. For example, low output failure can occur in traumatic injuries that block venous return from the legs up to the heart.

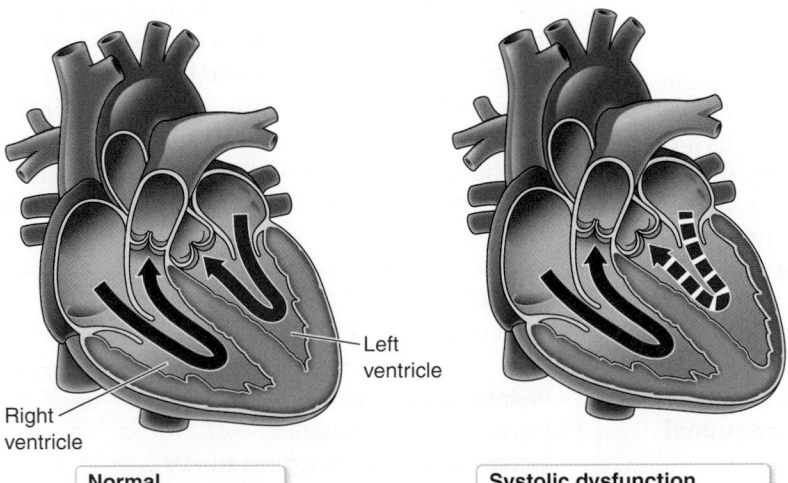
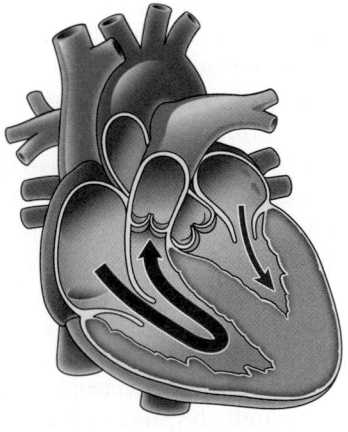

Left ventricle

Right ventricle

Normal
The ventricles fill normally with blood.

Systolic dysfunction
Weak distended left ventricle cannot pump blood forward.

Diastolic dysfunction
Stiff nonelastic left ventricle with less filling of blood.

FIGURE 17-15. Normal heart function versus systolic function versus diastolic function.

LVF Versus RVF

The simplest way to understand heart failure is by studying the process in terms of left ventricular failure (LVF) and right ventricular failure (RVF). Failure of each side of the heart has distinctive consequences and can be simplified by visualizing each side of the weakened heart as having backward failure and forward failure effects (see Fig. 17-16 and Fig. 17-17). Essentially, backward effects are the result of a backup of hydrostatic pressure. Forward effects occur from decreased perfusion of the brain, kidney, and other vital organs. The heart is one organ; what happens to the right side will have consequences on the left side. Although heart failure usually involves both right and left ventricles, LVF and RVF will be explained individually for academic purposes in the following discussion.

Left Ventricular Failure. LVF can be explained in terms of systolic and diastolic dysfunction. Left ventricular diastolic dysfunction occurs from reduced relaxation or increased stiffness of the ventricular muscle. The increased afterload of HTN is commonly the cause for the development of these changes in the left ventricle. HTN causes increased resistance against the left ventricle, and the left ventricular muscle hypertrophies to compensate for the increased workload. LVH creates a noncompliant, enlarged, stiff-walled ventricular chamber. The thickened, muscular ventricular wall encroaches into the left ventricular chamber and diminishes the size of the left ventricle's interior. This leads to decreased left ventricular filling, as well as reduced SV and cardiac output. Because the ventricular filling or diastolic phase of heart function is most affected, this condition is often termed diastolic dysfunction.

Alternatively, left ventricular systolic dysfunction occurs when there is reduced forward pumping strength of the ventricular muscle. The left ventricle is weak and cannot eject its blood volume into the aorta, thereby decreasing SV and cardiac output. Systolic dysfunction of the left ventricle has two major consequences: backward effects and forward effects of failure. The backward effect of a failing left ventricle creates a buildup of hydrostatic pressure in the left atrium, pulmonary veins, and pulmonary capillaries. The forward failure effects cause decreased perfusion of the brain, kidneys, and other organs.

The backward effects consist of a buildup of hydrostatic pressure backward up into the left atrium and pulmonary vasculature, which causes fluid extravasation into the pulmonary interstitial and intracellular spaces. The opening and closing of alveoli against this fluid is heard as crackles through a stethoscope and is exhibited as cough, dyspnea, orthopnea, and **paroxysmal nocturnal dyspnea (PND)** by the patient.

The forward effects of the weak left ventricle cause inadequate ejection of blood into the aorta and diminished perfusion throughout the whole arterial circulatory system. The decreased perfusion of vital tissues

activates a neurohormonal response that includes stimulation of the RAAS, ADH, and SNS.

When the kidney senses decreased perfusion, it releases renin from the nephron juxtaglomerular apparatus and initiates cycling of the RAAS. Simultaneously, with decreased forward pumping of blood, the aorta and peripheral arteries experience diminished blood flow, which initiates other compensatory mechanisms. The baroreceptors within the artery walls sense a drop in blood pressure and this activates the SNS. The SNS stimulates adrenergic receptors in the heart and blood vessels to create further effects. Adrenergic stimulation of the heart increases HR and adrenergic stimulation of the vasculature causes vasoconstriction.

Also, in response to diminished perfusion, the posterior pituitary gland releases ADH, which acts at the nephrons to increase water reabsorption into the bloodstream and, in turn, leads to increased blood volume.

> **ALERT!** Diminished perfusion of the kidney is particularly significant in LVF; it stimulates the secretion of renin from the juxtaglomerular apparatus of the nephron, which initiates cycling of the RAAS.

Cycling of the RAAS. The RAAS plays a major role in the neurohormonal effects of heart failure. After release, renin circulates and reacts with angiotensinogen, a protein synthesized by the liver. Angiotensinogen is cleaved into a smaller protein; angiotensin I. Angiotensin I circulates, and in the lungs it is transformed into angiotensin II by angiotensin converting enzyme (ACE). Angiotensin II has significant widespread systemic effects that worsen heart failure (see Box 17-6). Also, as mentioned previously, angiotensin II promotes the development of ventricular hypertrophy.

Angiotensin II is a potent arterial vasoconstrictor and exerts this effect on the systemic arterial system. This widespread vasoconstriction raises peripheral arterial resistance, which increases afterload for the weakened heart. The failing left ventricle, which is already weakened, is further challenged by the increased peripheral resistance against it. In addition, angiotensin II stimulates the adrenal gland to release aldosterone.

Aldosterone causes sodium and water retention and potassium excretion from the bloodstream. The sodium

---

BOX 17-6. Effects of Angiotensin II in Heart Failure

- Peripheral arterial vasoconstriction
- Increased blood pressure
- Increased resistance against the LV
- Cardiac myocyte hypertrophy
- Detrimental ventricular remodeling
- Stimulation of adrenal aldosterone

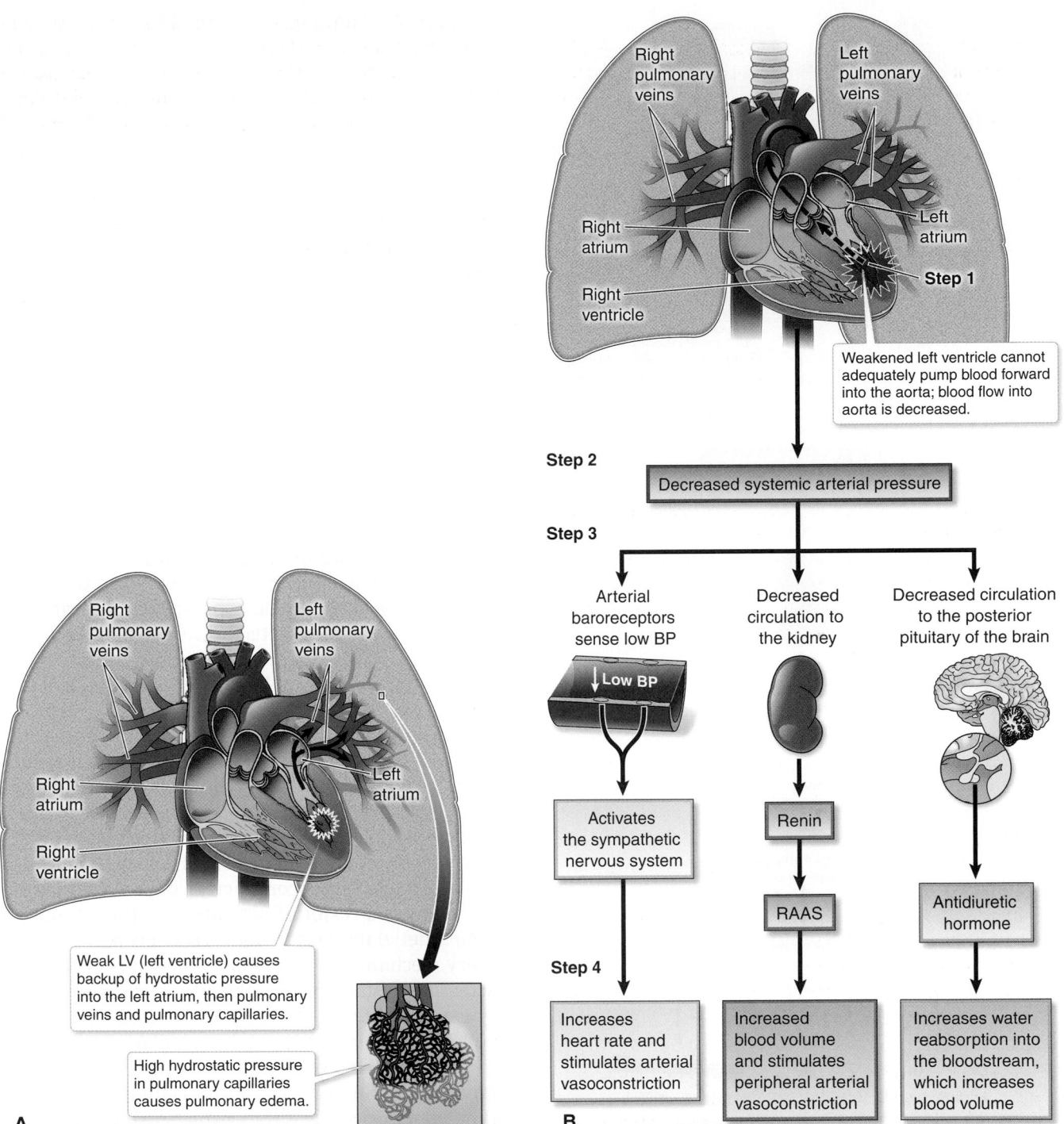

FIGURE 17-16. LVF. LVF can be studied by looking at the backward effects versus the forward effects of LVF. **(A)** Backward effects of left ventricular failure. A weakened left ventricle cannot pump all its blood forward into the aorta and consequently causes buildup of hydrostatic pressure in the left ventricle that is transmitted to the left atrium. The elevated hydrostatic pressure is further transmitted backward into the pulmonary veins and then pulmonary capillaries. High hydrostatic pressure within the pulmonary capillaries causes pulmonary edema. **(B)** Forward effects of left ventricular failure. Step 1: The failing left ventricle cannot adequately pump blood forward into the aorta. Step 2: Aortic pressure falls and systemic arterial pressure drops. Step 3a: Baroreceptors in the arteries sense a drop in BP and stimulate SNS, which increases HR and stimulates peripheral arterial vasoconstriction. The increased HR further weakens the left ventricle. The increased arterial vasoconstriction increases resistance against the ventricle. Step 3b: As decreased blood flows into the systemic circulation and the kidney, the kidney secretes renin. Step 4: This stimulates the RAAS, which increases blood volume and blood pressure. This further increases the left ventricle's workload and weakens the ventricle more. Step 3c: Decreased circulation to the posterior pituitary gland of the brain causes secretion of ADH. ADH causes reabsorption of water into the bloodstream.

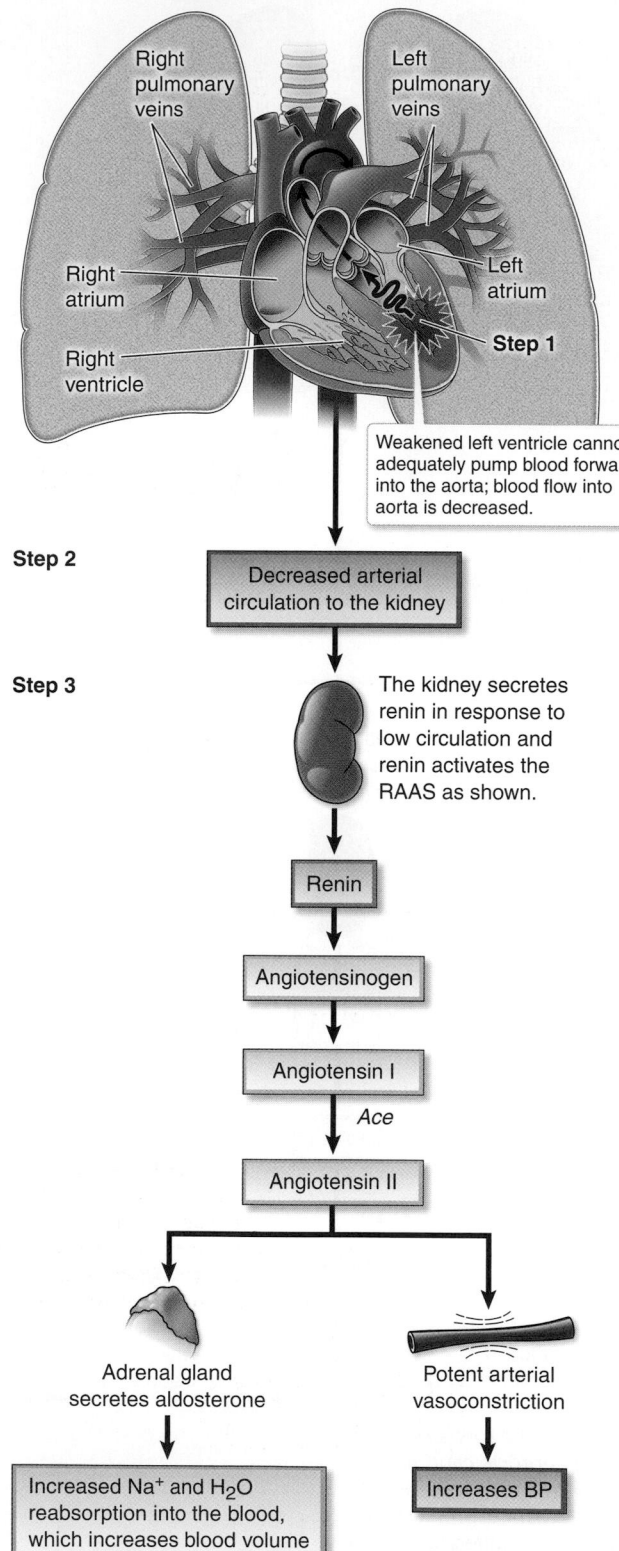

Step 1

Weakened left ventricle cannot adequately pump blood forward into the aorta; blood flow into aorta is decreased.

Step 2

Decreased arterial circulation to the kidney

Step 3

The kidney secretes renin in response to low circulation and renin activates the RAAS as shown.

Renin

Angiotensinogen

Angiotensin I

Ace

Angiotensin II

Adrenal gland secretes aldosterone

Potent arterial vasoconstriction

Increased Na⁺ and H₂O reabsorption into the blood, which increases blood volume

Increases BP

FIGURE 17-17. Forward failure effects of LVF stimulate the kidney to secrete renin and activate RAAS. Step 1: The failing left ventricle cannot adequately pump blood forward into the aorta. Step 2: Aortic pressure falls and systemic arterial pressure drops. Decreased blood flow to the kidney causes renin secretion. Step 3: This stimulates the RAAS, which increases blood volume and blood pressure. This further increases the workload of the left ventricle and weakens the ventricle more.

and water retention increases total blood volume and raises blood pressure. Therefore, the stimulation of aldosterone by angiotensin II further challenges the weakened left ventricle. The net effects of angiotensin II and aldosterone include an increased blood pressure and blood volume as well as increased resistance against the left ventricle. These conditions require the failing ventricle to pump out a greater volume of blood against high resistance within the arterial circulation. As a result, the effects of angiotensin II and aldosterone further strain the weakened left ventricle, resulting in diminished forward pumping of blood into the aorta, which further diminishes arterial circulation and organ perfusion (see Fig. 17-18).

ALERT! Hypokalemia, which increases risk of cardiac dysrhythmias, can occur in heart failure caused by the constant stimulation of aldosterone.

An increasingly weakened left ventricle further diminishes renal perfusion, which stimulates renin and provokes persistent cycling of the RAAS. As the RAAS cycles, the weakened heart continually deteriorates. Excess blood volume created by the constant cycling of the RAAS increases workload for the left ventricle, worsening heart failure. Without treatment, left ventricular heart failure leads to worsening LVF.

Adrenergic Stimulation. SNS activation occurs early in heart failure. Initially in LVF, there is a drop in arterial blood pressure caused by the inadequate forward pumping of blood into the aorta. The decline in blood pressure stimulates baroreceptors within arterial walls, which sense pressure changes. Baroreceptors, in turn, activate the SNS. Vasoconstriction of peripheral arteries occurs as a result of activation of the adrenergic (sympathetic) nervous system. This acts as a compensatory mechanism to raise blood pressure, but it also increases resistance within the arterial circulation. The increased resistance acts as increased afterload against the left ventricle, which further challenges the heart. Simultaneously, adrenergic stimulation increases HR by activating the SA node. The already failing heart is then stimulated to increase its rate, which further strains the ventricle (see Fig. 17-19).

Progressive Ventricular Remodeling. A weakened heart muscle activates the secretion of certain molecules that cause detrimental cellular changes within the myocardium. Molecular substances such as angiotensin II, aldosterone, endothelin, TNF-alpha, catecholamines, insulinlike growth factor, and growth hormone provoke genetic changes, apoptosis, and hypertrophy of cardiac myocytes, as well as collagen deposits and myocardial fibrosis (see Fig. 17-20). During the course of heart failure, these molecules cause changes in the heart that lead to enlargement and dilation of the left ventricle.

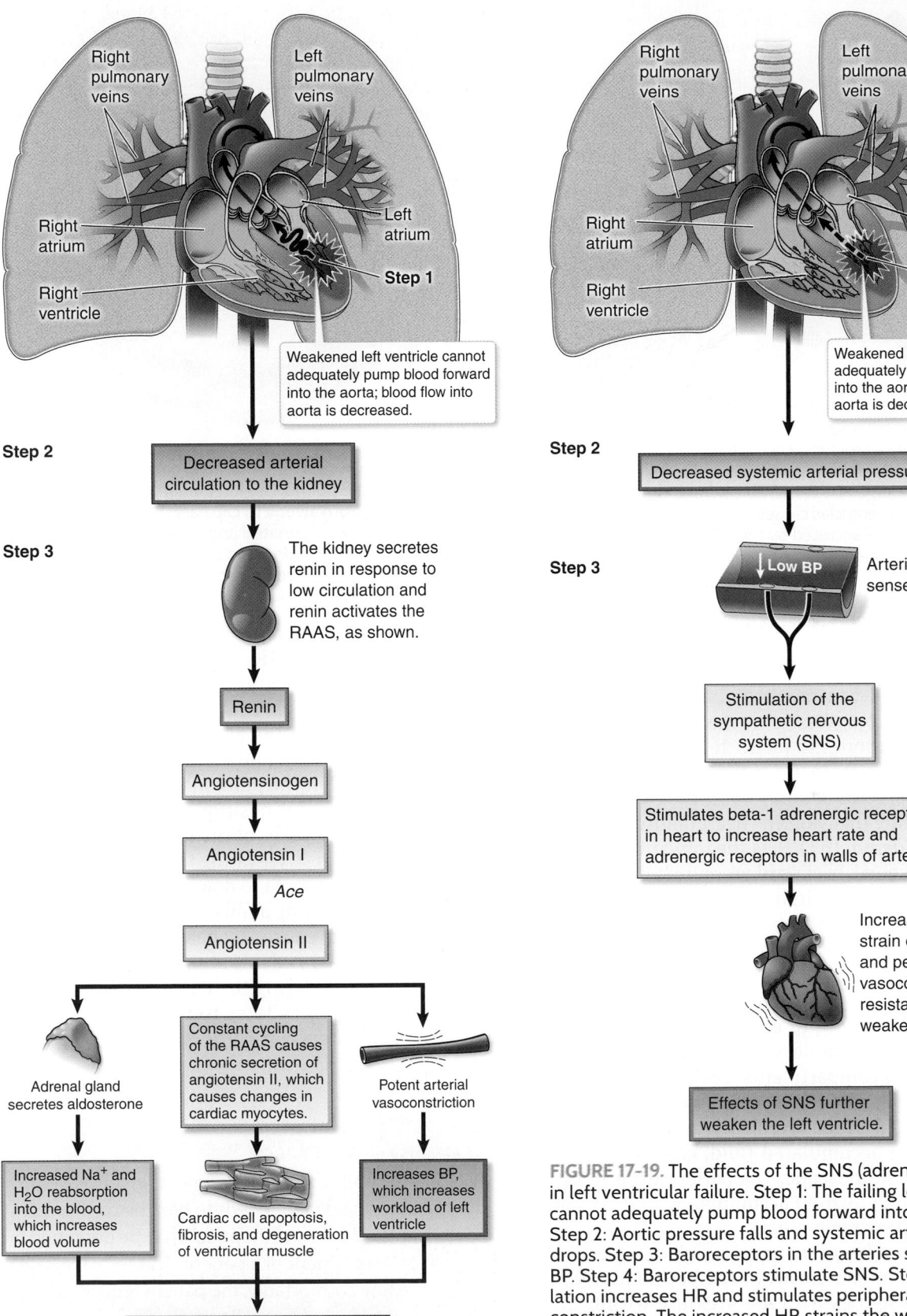

Right pulmonary veins

Left pulmonary veins

Right atrium

Left atrium

Right ventricle

Step 1

Weakened left ventricle cannot adequately pump blood forward into the aorta; blood flow into aorta is decreased.

Step 2

Decreased arterial circulation to the kidney

Step 3

The kidney secretes renin in response to low circulation and renin activates the RAAS, as shown.

Renin

Angiotensinogen

Angiotensin I

Ace

Angiotensin II

Adrenal gland secretes aldosterone

Constant cycling of the RAAS causes chronic secretion of angiotensin II, which causes changes in cardiac myocytes.

Potent arterial vasoconstriction

Increased Na⁺ and H₂O reabsorption into the blood, which increases blood volume

Cardiac cell apoptosis, fibrosis, and degeneration of ventricular muscle

Increases BP, which increases workload of left ventricle

These effects are detrimental to left ventricular function and LVF worsens.

FIGURE 17-18. There are many detrimental effects of activation of the RAAS in left ventricular failure.

Right pulmonary veins

Left pulmonary veins

Right atrium

Left atrium

Right ventricle

Step 1

Weakened left ventricle cannot adequately pump blood forward into the aorta; blood flow into aorta is decreased.

Step 2

Decreased systemic arterial pressure

Step 3

↓ Low BP

Arterial baroreceptors sense low BP.

Stimulation of the sympathetic nervous system (SNS)

Stimulates beta-1 adrenergic receptors in heart to increase heart rate and adrenergic receptors in walls of arteries

Increased heart rate puts strain on the failing heart and peripheral artery; vasoconstriction increases resistance against the weakened left ventricle.

Effects of SNS further weaken the left ventricle.

FIGURE 17-19. The effects of the SNS (adrenergic) stimulation in left ventricular failure. Step 1: The failing left ventricle cannot adequately pump blood forward into the aorta. Step 2: Aortic pressure falls and systemic arterial pressure drops. Step 3: Baroreceptors in the arteries sense a drop in BP. Step 4: Baroreceptors stimulate SNS. Step 5: SNS stimulation increases HR and stimulates peripheral arterial vasoconstriction. The increased HR strains the weakened left ventricle. The increased arterial vasoconstriction increases resistance against the ventricle, weakening the left ventricle further.

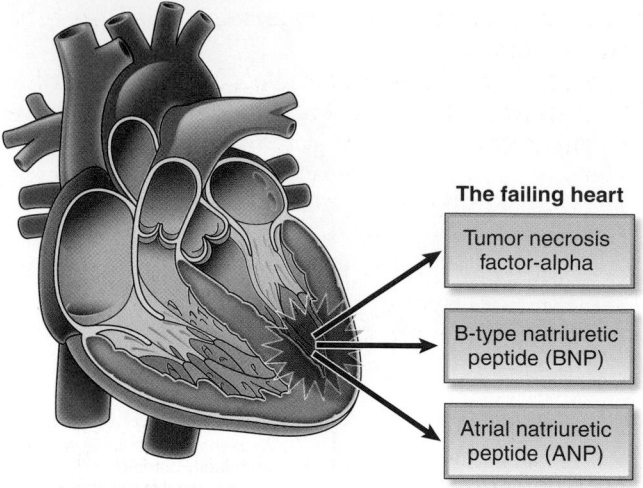

FIGURE 17-20. Molecular substances activated during heart failure. During heart failure, molecular substances are secreted. TNF-alpha, insulinlike growth factor, growth hormone, and endothelin cause detrimental ventricular remodeling. The ventricular cells undergo apoptosis, fibrosis, and degeneration. BNP secreted by the ventricles causes water loss from the body (called natriuresis). ANP secreted by the atria enhances water loss from the body (called natriuresis).

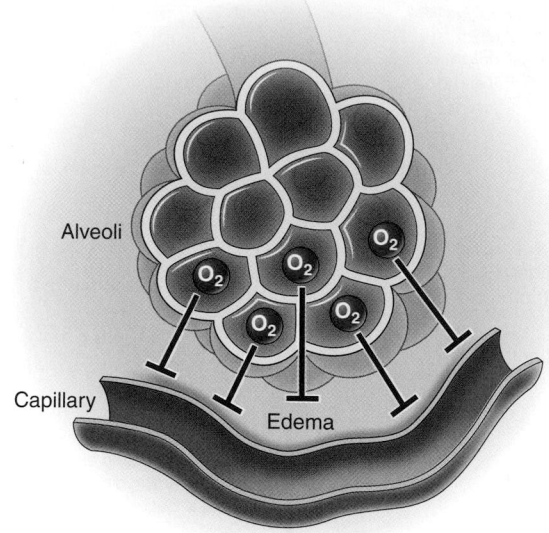

FIGURE 17-21. Pulmonary edema. Pulmonary edema is a fluid accumulation in the pulmonary interstitial spaces that hinders oxygen diffusion from alveoli to capillary. The blood cannot become sufficiently oxygenated and hypoxemia develops. The patient suffers severe dyspnea, cough, and pink frothy sputum. Pulmonary edema can occur in left ventricular failure.

As these cellular changes occur, the ventricular myocardium progressively weakens. Additionally, there is impaired calcium utilization in the ventricular myocytes, leading to reduced contractile force. This triggers a vicious cycle with progressive weakening of the heart muscle, which continues to incite detrimental cellular changes. This cycle within the myocardium contributes to a continuous process of unfavorable progressive ventricular remodeling that worsens heart failure.

Pulmonary Edema. In LVF, as the forward ventricular pump is weakened, backward pressure builds within the left atrium, resulting in high hydrostatic pressure in the pulmonary veins. This high hydrostatic pressure is transmitted further backward into the pulmonary capillary bed. At the pulmonary capillaries, high hydrostatic pressure causes fluid extravasation into the interstitial spaces, leading to edema. Edematous fluid builds within the pulmonary interstitial spaces and intracellular fluid compartments and hinders oxygen diffusion from the alveoli into the pulmonary capillaries (see Fig. 17-21). As the alveoli attempt to open and close against the accumulated fluid, crackles can be heard through a stethoscope. The patient experiences dyspnea and cough as fluid accumulates between the alveoli and capillary membranes.

Changes caused by pulmonary vascular congestion appear as vessel engorgement in the perihilar region on chest x-ray. High hydrostatic pressure within the pulmonary veins can also cause pleural effusion, which is edema accumulation in the pleural cavity. Pleural effusion can be identified on chest x-ray as a fluid level within the pleural cavity.

Clinical Presentation. Orthopnea. As fluid accumulates in the pulmonary interstitial spaces, the patient may experience **orthopnea,** which is a sensation of dyspnea

when lying flat. When a patient is in the supine position, the fluid accumulation in the lungs becomes distributed throughout the lung fields. The supine position disperses the fluid within the lungs, which worsens the oxygen diffusion from the alveoli into the pulmonary capillaries. The standing position allows gravitational forces to pull fluid in the pulmonary interstitial spaces downward. While in this position, any fluid in the lungs is pulled toward the bases of the lungs. When a patient is supine or on bedrest, elevating the patient's head will redistribute pulmonary fluid downward toward the lung bases and ease breathing ability (see Fig. 17-22). For this reason, excess fluid caused by heart failure may be noticeable as pulmonary edema at night when the patient is supine. However, during the day when the patient is standing and fluid gravitates to the lung bases, there may be no respiratory difficulty.

🩺 CLINICAL CONCEPT

Clinically, orthopnea can be described in terms of how many pillows the patient needs to breathe comfortably. For example, "2 pillow orthopnea" may be described in the clinical assessment of a patient. This term indicates that to breathe comfortably, the patient requires a head elevation at a level of two pillows.

Paroxysmal Nocturnal Dyspnea. PND is a unique symptom experienced by the patient who is experiencing the backward effects of LVF. PND is sudden shortness of breath that occurs in the middle of the night, disrupting a patient's sleep.

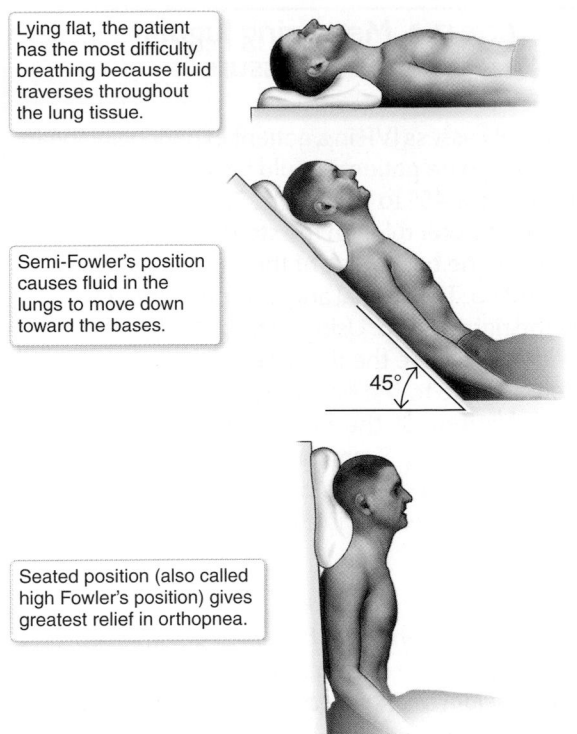

Lying flat, the patient has the most difficulty breathing because fluid traverses throughout the lung tissue.

Semi-Fowler's position causes fluid in the lungs to move down toward the bases.

45°

Seated position (also called high Fowler's position) gives greatest relief in orthopnea.

FIGURE 17-22. Orthopnea. Orthopnea is the feeling of shortness of breath when in a flat, supine position. Orthopnea most often occurs in LVF when fluid builds in the lungs. In the flat, supine position, the patient's pulmonary fluid traverses throughout the lung tissue. The person has the most difficulty breathing in this position. As the head of the bed is raised, orthopnea can be relieved because the fluid in the lungs is pulled downward to the bases of the lungs. Semi-Fowler's position (head at a 45° angle) can ease breathing and the seated position can bring more relief because fluid is in the bases of the lungs. With fluid only in the bases of lungs, the patient can breathe easier.

This symptom occurs because of the fluid accumulation in the lungs caused by backward effects of LVF. When the patient is in the supine position while asleep, any fluid in the pulmonary interstitium widely disperses over the lung fields. The fluid within the interstitial spaces hinders oxygen transfer from the alveoli into the capillaries and the patient experiences hypoxia. When the patient is in the standing position, this same fluid accumulation in the lungs is less noticeable because gravitational forces pull it downward into the lung bases.

 CLINICAL CONCEPT

Patients often describe PND as nightmares or night terrors that awaken them from sleep. Commonly, a patient is not able to accurately describe PND as shortness of breath because it occurs during sleep.

Cerebral Symptoms. With diminished strength of the left ventricle to pump blood into the arterial circulation, perfusion of the brain decreases. The patient may manifest decreased cerebral perfusion as confusion, headache, memory loss, insomnia, anxiety, or disorientation.

Constitutional Symptoms. Because of the diminished strength of the left ventricle, the organs receive less blood flow. Decreased gastrointestinal perfusion may cause anorexia, nausea, and abdominal discomfort. Reduced skeletal muscle perfusion can cause weakness and exercise intolerance. Poor urinary output and suboptimal filtration of blood can occur because of diminished renal perfusion. Diminished peripheral circulation results in decreased pulses bilaterally, as well as cold, pale extremities.

Right Ventricular Failure. In right-sided heart failure, the backward failure effects are most significant. In backward failure, the right ventricle is weak and has difficulty pumping all of its blood forward into the pulmonary artery. The ventricle's inability to pump its contents forward causes a backup of blood, raising hydrostatic pressure within the right heart chambers. Unejected blood accumulates in the right ventricle, increasing pressure within the ventricle, which in turn causes increased backward pressure in the right atrium. From the right atrium, backward hydrostatic pressure builds in the superior and inferior vena cava and consequently builds within the systemic venous system. Increased pressure within the venous system, also called central venous pressure, raises pressure in all the veins, which is transmitted as increased hydrostatic pressure in all peripheral capillary beds, causing edema. Continued backup of fluid contributes to organomegaly, or enlargement of the liver and spleen, and ascites, or fluid accumulation in the peritoneal cavity (see Fig. 17-23).

With weakening of the right ventricle, forward contractile force into the pulmonary artery is diminished. This decreases pulmonary arterial blood flow, which results in suboptimal alveolar-oxygen diffusion into the capillaries and, in turn, causes hypoxemia. The patient also may experience hypoxia and cyanosis. Compared with the backward failure effects of venous congestion and peripheral edema in RVF, forward failure effects are less dramatic.

Clinical Presentation.
Jugular Venous Distension. As the right ventricle weakens, pressure builds within the right atrium, superior vena cava (SVC), and IVC. Demonstrable congestion within the SVC is exhibited in the jugular veins of the neck. **Jugular venous distension (JVD),** or bilateral bulging blue neck veins, becomes the clinical sign of backward pressure within the SVC.

Elevated jugular venous pressure (JVP) is a classic sign of the backward effects of RVF (see Box 17-7). Pressure in the jugular veins is a reflection of right atrial pressure and CVP, which are important clinical indicators of right ventricular function. As the right ventricle fails, right atrial pressure increases, which in turn increases CVP and JVP. Hence, RVF raises JVP.

Under normal conditions, jugular veins are collapsed and not visible in the seated or standing patient. Neck veins may be slightly distended under normal conditions

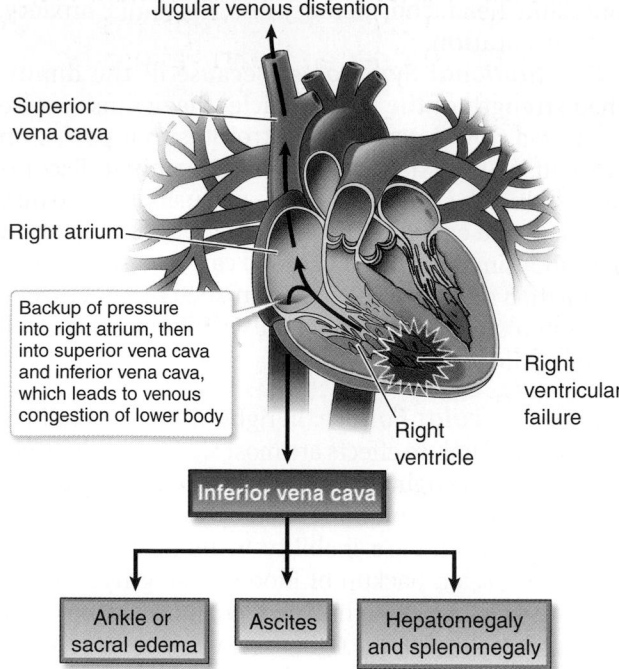

FIGURE 17-23. Right ventricular failure. The backward effects of RVF cause high hydrostatic failure in the right ventricle, which backs up into the right atrium and superior and inferior vena cava. From the vena cava, hydrostatic pressure builds throughout the body, causing widespread venous congestion. Venous congestion in the SVC is exhibited as JVD. Venous congestion in the gastrointestinal system is exhibited as peritoneal edema, which is called ascites. Venous congestion in the liver and spleen are exhibited as hepatomegaly and splenomegaly. Accumulation of hydrostatic pressure in the veins of the legs is exhibited as ankle edema. If the patient is in the supine position, sacral edema can occur.

BOX 17-7. Backward Effects of Right Ventricular Failure

- Jugular vein distension: result of high SVC pressure
- Elevated jugular venous pressure
- Elevated central venous pressure: high SVC and IVC pressure
- Ascites: backup of hydrostatic pressure in peritoneum
- Hepatomegaly: venous congestion/swelling of liver
- Splenomegaly: venous congestion/swelling of spleen
- Ankle or sacral edema

---

when the patient is supine. However, in RVF, jugular veins are distended even when the patient is upright (see Box 17-8).

Venous Congestion of Gastrointestinal Tract. As the right ventricle fails, hydrostatic pressure builds backward into the right atrium and throughout the venous system. As venous pressure rises, venous congestion in the GI tract occurs. Venous drainage diminishes within the gastrointestinal tract. Anorexia, nausea, early satiety, postprandial fullness, indigestion, and

---

BOX 17-8. Measuring Jugular Venous Pressure

To accurately assess JVP in a patient experiencing heart failure, the supine patient should have the head of the bed raised to a 45° to 60° angle. The clinician should place a centimeter ruler on the sternal angle of the patient's chest, the bony ridge of the sternum adjacent to the second rib. The sternal angle is approximately 5 cm above the right atrium. Using a straight edge, the clinician should measure the distance in centimeters from the sternal angle to the horizontal level of the highest visible pulsations of the distended neck veins. This measurement plus 5 cm provides an approximate measure of jugular venous pressure. The following is an example of how JVP is clinically noted in patient assessment:

Neck:
+ JVD: jugular veins 9 cm from right atrium at 45°
alternatively
+ JVD: jugular veins 4 cm above sternal angle at 45°

This assessment indicates that the clinician observed a level of jugular vein distension at 9 cm above the right atrium or 4 cm above the sternal angle, which is considered elevated JVP.

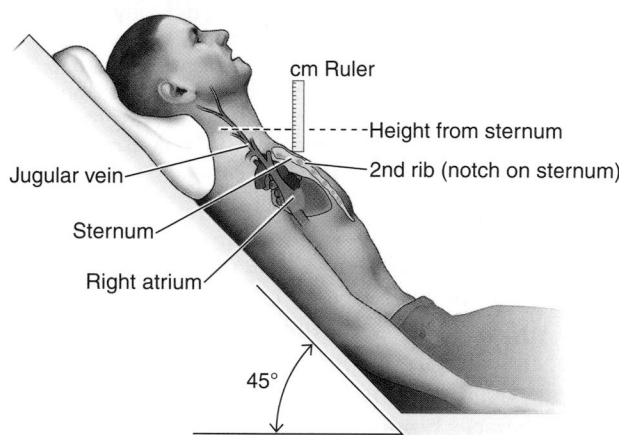

To assess JVP, the supine patient should have the head of the bed raised to a 45° to 60° angle. The clinician should place a centimeter ruler on the sternal angle of the patient's chest, the bony ridge of the sternum adjacent to the second rib. The sternal angle is approximately 5 cm above the right atrium. Using a straight edge, the clinician should measure the distance in centimeters from the sternal angle to the horizontal level of the highest visible pulsations of the distended neck veins.

---

impaired intestinal absorption are conditions associated with poor gastrointestinal venous drainage. The liver and spleen endure venous congestion, which leads to engorgement within both organs.

Aside from organ dysfunction, venous engorgement leads to hepatomegaly and splenomegaly. Jaundice, coagulation problems, impaired drug metabolism, and elevated liver enzymes can develop because of the severe venous congestion of the liver. The liver's portal vein develops high pressure, which is referred to as high portal venous pressure. To confirm hepatic congestion caused by RVF, the clinician can elicit positive hepatojugular reflux.

CLINICAL CONCEPT

In order to elicit hepatojugular reflux, the patient is supine and the clinician presses on the liver. Pressure on the liver increases portal venous pressure and in turn raises jugular venous pressure, producing visible JVD.

Increased hydrostatic pressure within all the gastrointestinal veins is transmitted to the capillary beds, which creates edema within the peritoneal cavity, called **ascites.** In ascites, the patient develops a fluid-filled, distended abdomen. The abdominal distension of ascites can restrict full thoracic excursion during inspiration, impairing respiratory function.

Peripheral Edema. Venous congestion within the lower body causes high hydrostatic pressure within all the capillary beds of the extremities and leads to edema. Edematous fluid accumulation is influenced by gravitational forces. If the patient is supine or on bedrest, edema tends to accumulate around the sacral region. If the patient is in the supine position for prolonged periods, sacral edema increases the skin's fragility and can lead to skin breakdown. Erythema of the skin and edema in the sacral area is the first sign of pressure in this area. Sacral edema predisposes the patient to formation of sacral decubitus ulcers. Because of the gravitational forces, dependent ankle edema develops in the standing or ambulatory patient. The feet and lower legs may also develop edema in RVF.

ALERT! If RVF is severe, peripheral edema can be massive and gradually affect most of the tissues in the body, a condition called anasarca.

Biventricular Heart Failure. The heart is a single muscular organ that requires efficient functioning of all its chambers in a rhythmic, coordinated, and resilient manner. Dysfunction of any one chamber causes compensatory changes within the other chambers. If dysfunction of one heart chamber persists, compensatory mechanisms become exhausted, begin to diminish, and decompensation of the whole organ occurs. Failure of one side of the heart ultimately results in detriment of the other side of the heart.

In the clinical setting, a patient most often presents in biventricular failure, which is combined left- and

---

BOX 17-9. Signs and Symptoms of Biventricular Heart Failure

LEFT VENTRICULAR FAILURE
- Dyspnea
- Cough
- Orthopnea
- PND
- Weak peripheral pulses
- Decreased cerebral perfusion; confusion, disorientation

RIGHT VENTRICULAR FAILURE
- JVD
- Ascites
- Gastrointestinal disturbances caused by venous congestion
- Hepato-jugular reflux
- Hepatomegaly
- Splenomegaly
- Peripheral edema; ankle or sacral edema; fingers, feet

---

right-sided heart failure. Depending on the extent of the disease, the patient commonly presents with a combination of the signs and symptoms of left and right ventricular failure. LVF produces pulmonary symptoms such as cough, dyspnea, and orthopnea, whereas RVF produces such systemic edema signs as JVD, ascites, hepatomegaly, and ankle edema. A patient in biventricular heart failure will exhibit a constellation of these signs and symptoms (see Box 17-9).

Clinical Presentation of Heart Failure

The diagnosis of heart failure is established by observable clinical manifestations, patient history, and laboratory findings. Patients commonly present to the clinician when combined RVF and LVF exists.

History

In mild to moderate heart failure, the patient may appear in no distress and clinical manifestations may be minimal at rest. However, the patient may report dyspnea upon exertion, dyspnea when lying flat for more than a few minutes, or a nocturnal cough. These are early signs of pulmonary interstitial fluid accumulation caused by failure of the left ventricle. Confusion, difficulty concentrating, and headache can occur with decreased cerebral perfusion. Cold, pale legs and feet may be noticeable to the patient caused by diminished circulation in the extremities.

The patient may notice swelling in the ankles or fingers, which is indicative of increased venous pressure. Patients may report tight rings or shoes because of fluid retention. Abdominal swelling and gastrointestinal symptoms, such as anorexia or a feeling of fullness, may be patient complaints associated with RVF. The patient may have increased frequency of urination and nocturia caused by excess fluid accumulation. Weight gain of 2 lb. or more per day is often indicative of fluid retention.

Signs and Symptoms

Pulmonary crackles may not be audible in early LVF. With more moderate heart failure, as pulmonary capillary pressure rises, bilateral pulmonary crackles can be heard further and further up from the bases of the lungs.

In early stages of RVF, the jugular veins may not be visibly distended at rest. However, elevated venous pressure may become observable by positive hepatojugular reflux when the abdomen is deeply palpated over the liver. Ascites, hepatomegaly, and splenomegaly may not be present or minimally apparent in mild heart failure.

The diagnosis of mild to moderate heart failure is most often inferred by the patient history of risk factors, dyspnea on exertion, orthopnea, and PND episodes. PND is often described in terms of night terrors, nightmares, or a choking feeling that awakens one from sleep. Clinical manifestations may not be overtly apparent in the resting patient early in heart failure, so the patient history must be carefully evaluated.

In moderate to severe heart failure, the pulses are usually diminished and cyanosis of the lips and nailbeds may be observed. Distended jugular neck veins are best observed with the patient in Fowler's position at a 45° angle.

Cardiomegaly or left ventricular enlargement may be demonstrated by shifted point of maximal impulse or apical pulse. When the left ventricle is enlarged, the apical pulse, normally located at the left fifth intercostal space midclavicular line, can be palpated further into the left axillary region.

Upon auscultation of the heart, a third and fourth heart sound may be heard through the stethoscope. The third heart sound (S_3) is a low-pitched sound heard after S_2, during rapid filling of the ventricle in the early part of diastole. In children and young adults, an S_3 may be normal. In adults older than age 40 years, the presence of an S_3 is abnormal and indicative of heart failure. High ventricular end diastolic volume and increased pressure within the chambers consequent to heart failure are responsible for a third heart sound.

A fourth heart sound (S_4) is heard when the atrium contracts against a noncompliant, stiff ventricle. Normally, when the atrium contracts, there is no sound. An S_4 is a low-pitched sound heard at the end of diastole, before S_1. An S_4 commonly occurs in chronic HTN, caused by the structural changes that occur in the left ventricle as a result of high blood pressure. In HTN, high aortic pressure creates high resistance and hypertrophy of the left ventricle. The hypertrophic left ventricle is less elastic and distensible. Atrial contraction against this stiff left ventricle causes an audible S_4 during diastole.

Upon palpation of pulse, resting tachycardia is often present in moderate or severe heart failure. Moist, inspiratory crackles may be heard over the lung bases bilaterally. Pulmonary edema is exhibited by coarse, bilateral crackles widely dispersed over the lung fields. A bilateral pleural effusion may develop as a result of high pulmonary venous pressure, causing diffusion of fluid into the pleural cavity.

Ascites occurs as a consequence of hepatic venous congestion, which causes diffusion of fluid into the peritoneal cavity. Fluid within the peritoneal cavity can be demonstrated by the finding of 'shifting dullness' on physical examination. Turning patients on their side allows the clinician to percuss dullness over the dependent portion of the abdomen where peritoneal fluid has shifted. Tympany can be percussed at the superior aspect of the patient's abdomen, where there is no peritoneal fluid. A palpable, enlarged liver and spleen may be evident on examination of the abdomen. Pressure on the liver will transmit elevated venous pressure into the jugular veins as hepatojugular reflux.

Symmetric, dependent edema is often apparent in the ankles in the ambulatory patient and may be most observable in the evening. In bedridden patients, dependent edema accumulates over the sacral region. Patients sense edema when fingers or feet swell to cause rings or shoes to fit tightly. Edema can be exhibited as facial puffiness or periorbital swelling. Weight gain can occur when several liters of edematous fluid accumulates in interstitial spaces of the body.

Daily weight measurement is recommended in the clinical assessment of patients in heart failure. Weight fluctuation of 2 lb. or more from day to day is often caused by fluid retention or edema. The skin over the extremities may be cool and pale because of decreased perfusion. The pulses of the extremities, particularly the dorsalis pedis pulses, are symmetrically diminished.

Diagnosis

To establish a diagnosis of heart failure, at least one of the major criteria and two of the minor criteria should be present from the Framingham Criteria for Diagnosis of Congestive Heart Failure (see Table 17-1).

Laboratory and Diagnostic Studies

There are a number of laboratory and diagnostic studies when it comes to diagnosing heart failure.

Brain Natriuretic Peptide. In heart failure, as the ventricle stretches in response to increased blood volume, the myocardium secretes BNP, a natural diuretic substance. This peptide, which is secreted by the heart, enhances the body's ability to allow water loss from the kidneys which, in turn, decreases blood volume. BNP is elevated in the bloodstream in heart failure as well as other conditions, particularly pulmonary disease.

TABLE 17-1. Framingham Criteria for Diagnosis of Congestive Heart Failure

Major Criteria	Minor Criteria	Major or Minor Criteria
Paroxysmal nocturnal dyspnea	Bilateral extremity edema	Weight loss of 4.5 kg or more over 5 days of treatment for heart failure
Jugular vein distension	Night time cough	
Pulmonary crackles	Dyspnea on exertion	
Cardiomegaly	Hepatomegaly	
Auscultation of S_3 heart sound	Pleural effusion	
Increased CVP (greater than 16 cm H_2O)	Reduced pulmonary vital capacity by one-third from normal	
Positive hepatojugular reflux	Tachycardia (120 beats/min or greater)	

To establish a diagnosis of heart failure, at least one of the major criteria and two of the minor criteria should be present from the Framingham Criteria for Diagnosis of Heart Failure.

Adapted from Ho, K. K. L., et al. (1993). *Circ*, 88, 107, 1993; taken from *Harrison's Principles of Internal Medicine*, 2005, p. 1371.

ALERT! Levels of BNP greater than 500 are considered indicative of heart failure.

Serum Electrolytes. In heart failure, blood volume increases because of excess water within the bloodstream. This excess water commonly dilutes the serum electrolytes, sodium and potassium, causing dilutional hyponatremia and hypokalemia. In addition, with the constant cycling of the RAAS in heart failure, aldosterone causes potassium excretion from the kidneys. The repeated simulation of the RAAS increases the risk of hypokalemia. Imbalances in serum electrolytes, particularly potassium, can have adverse effects on myocardial function. Hypokalemia predisposes the heart to dysrhythmias. In heart failure, serum electrolytes require periodic monitoring and correction if abnormal.

Chest X-Ray. A chest x-ray delineates the cardiac shadow and pulmonary fields. In heart failure, cardiomegaly, or enlargement of the heart, is commonly seen. Often the left ventricle is enlarged to a greater extent than the right ventricle. Cardiomegaly is often caused by LVH or dilatation of the ventricles. The pulmonary fields may show vasculature congestion as increased opacity in the vessels.

Kerley A lines and Kerley B lines are specific pulmonary x-ray findings indicating the vasculature congestion of heart failure. These findings, interpreted by the radiologist, appear as opaque linear shadows representing the engorged blood vessels of the lungs. The chest x-ray of pulmonary edema shows dense opaque vessel shadows in the perihilar regions of the lung fields called either "bat wing density" or "butterfly pattern" (see Fig. 17-24).

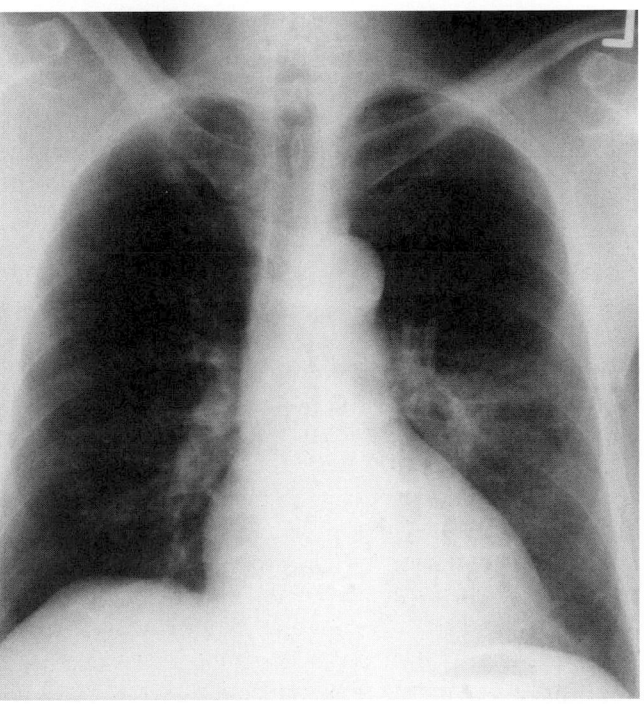

Figure 17-24. Chest x-ray showing heart failure. The heart is enlarged (cardiomegaly), and blood vessels are prominent in the hilar lung fields, which represents pulmonary venous congestion. Kerley lines are horizontal lines in the base of the lungs close to the chest wall. They are the result of interstitial edema in the lungs. *(From Southern Illinois University/Science Source.)*

Electrocardiogram. The electrocardiogram (ECG) may demonstrate various abnormalities in heart failure. LVH or enlargement is exhibited by the wave forms derived from the chest leads. Other changes of the ST segment, T wave, or QRS complex may be apparent. There are no specific ECG signs of heart failure.

Echocardiogram. An echocardiogram is a type of non-invasive sonogram that can demonstrate the activity and structures of the heart. It is commonly used to evaluate the size and function of the ventricles, valve structure, and function. Left ventricular ejection fraction (LVEF) can be estimated using this diagnostic modality.

Multiple-Gated Acquisition Scan. A multiple-gated acquisition scan, also known as radionuclide ventriculography, is a nuclear medicine procedure that involves injecting a small amount of radioactive dye into a peripheral vein. The radiopaque dye illuminates the heart on x-ray as it contracts. Similar to an echocardiogram, this procedure demonstrates the volume of blood pumped out of the ventricle with each contraction. The LVEF can be determined using this nuclear diagnostic procedure.

Cardiac Catheterization and Angiography. A specialized cardiac catheter can be used to perform hemodynamic monitoring within the heart or study the coronary arteries. A cardiac catheter can be inserted via the femoral vein, femoral artery, or subclavian vein depending on its intended purpose. If the goal is to measure hemodynamic pressures and volumes within the right side of the heart, a catheter can be inserted into the femoral vein, threaded into the IVC and then moved into the right atrium and right ventricle. If the goal is to measure pressures and volumes within the left side of the heart, a catheter can be inserted into the femoral artery, then into the aorta and left ventricle.

A cardiac catheter can also be used to study the health of the coronary circulation. Commonly, a cardiac catheter is first inserted into the femoral artery in the leg and threaded into the aorta against the flow of blood, and then into the openings of the coronary arteries.

The cardiac catheter can enter either the right or left coronary artery via the aorta. Radiopaque dye is injected via the catheter, which illuminates the coronary artery under study. The dye allows visibility of the artery structure on an x-ray called an angiogram or arteriogram. Angiography can be used to illuminate any artery in the body that is accessible via catheter.

Basic Hemodynamic Measurements of LVF Versus RVF

In the failing heart, pressure changes within the heart chambers and great vessels cause abnormal hemodynamic measurements. Specific hemodynamic pressure changes occur that characterize right versus left heart failure. These values can be used to differentiate RVF from LVF or monitor the efficacy of heart failure treatment. These values are monitored in an intensive care setting (see Table 17-2).

TABLE 17-2. Basic Hemodynamic Measurement Changes in Heart Failure

Hemodynamic Measure	Normal Value Range	Description	Hemodynamic Changes Occurring in Heart Failure
Central venous pressure (CVP)	1 to 5 mm Hg	Volume of blood returning to the right atrium from the venous circulation (e.g., can be referred to as preload)	In right ventricular failure, backward buildup of hydrostatic pressure increases right atrial pressure and CVP
Pulmonary artery pressure	17 to 32/4 to 13 mm Hg	Pressure within the pulmonary artery which acts as resistance against the right ventricle	
Cardiac output (CO)	4 to 8 liters/min	Total volume of blood pumped out by the heart per minute	Decreases as ventricles fail
Systemic arterial blood pressure	90 to 140/60 to 80 mm Hg	Blood pressure within the arteries	Blood pressure decreases with left ventricular failure
Pulmonary capillary wedge pressure (PCWP)	12 to 15 mm Hg	Pressure within the pulmonary capillary bed	In LVF, backward failure effects cause backup of hydrostatic pressure in the pulmonary capillaries, which increases PCWP
Left ventricular ejection fraction (LVEF)	50% to 70% of blood in ventricle Lower than 40% indicative of LVF	The volume of blood ejected with each contraction of the left ventricle (can be referred to as stroke volume [SV])	In LVF, LVEF is decreased

Classification Systems of Heart Failure

There are two major classification systems that describe the stages of heart failure according to the patient's symptoms: The New York Heart Association (NYHA) Classification and the American Cardiology Association/American Heart Association (ACC/AHA) Classification. Each classification system aims to help clinicians evaluate the severity of heart failure in their patients (see Table 17-3 and Table 17-4).

Treatment

Different types of interventions are available for heart failure. Lifestyle modification such as changing to a low-fat diet, smoking cessation, and increasing physical activity are basic health promotion strategies. Pharmacological agents, such as beta blockers and ACE inhibitors, are the cornerstone of treatment. Finally there are intracardiac interventions, such as pacemakers, that can greatly improve the life of a patient with heart failure.

Lifestyle Modifications

The patient with heart failure should limit fluid, salt, cholesterol, and alcohol consumption. A low-salt diet consisting of no more than 1.5 grams of sodium per day is commonly recommended. If the patient is ambulatory, a daily walking regimen is also recommended.

TABLE 17-3. The New York Association (NYHA) Classification of Heart Failure

Class	Patient Symptoms
CLASS I–MILD HEART FAILURE	No limitation of physical activity. Ordinary physical activity does not cause undue fatigue, palpitations, or dyspnea.
CLASS II–MILD HEART FAILURE	Slight limitation of physical activity. Comfortable at rest, but ordinary physical activity results in fatigue, palpitations, or dyspnea.
CLASS III–MODERATE HEART FAILURE	Marked limitation of physical activity. Comfortable at rest, but less than ordinary physical activity causes fatigue, palpitations, or dyspnea.
CLASS IV–SEVERE HEART FAILURE	Unable to carry out any physical activity without discomfort. Symptoms of cardiac insufficiency at rest. If any physical activity is undertaken, discomfort is increased.

TABLE 17-4. American College of Cardiology/American Heart Association (ACC/AHA) Classification of Heart Failure

Stage	Description	Examples
Stage A	Patients susceptible to heart failure because of the presence of conditions placing them at high risk. Patients have no identifiable structural or functional abnormalities of the myocardium, pericardium, or cardiac valves, and have not shown heart failure signs or symptoms.	Systemic HTN, coronary artery disease, diabetes mellitus, history of cardiotoxic drugs, alcohol abuse, rheumatic fever, or family history of cardiomyopathy.
Stage B	Patients who have developed structural heart disease strongly associated with heart failure development but who have not shown heart failure signs or symptoms.	LVH or fibrosis, left ventricular dilatation or hypocontractility, asymptomatic valvular heart disease, or previous MI.
Stage C	Patients who have current or prior symptoms of heart failure associated with underlying structural heart disease.	Dyspnea or fatigue caused by systolic dysfunction or asymptomatic patients undergoing treatment for prior symptoms of heart failure.
Stage D	Patients with advanced structural heart disease and marked symptoms of heart failure at rest despite maximal medical therapy and who require specialized interventions.	Patients who are frequently hospitalized for heart failure and cannot be safely discharged from the hospital, patients in the hospital awaiting heart transplant, patients at home receiving continuous intravenous support for symptom relief or being supported with a mechanical circulatory assist device, or patients in a hospice setting for the management of heart failure.

If obese, the patient should begin a weight loss program that includes daily weight measurement.

Following a daily medication schedule, periodic physical examinations, and laboratory tests are essential, as is smoking cessation if the patient smokes. Yearly flu vaccination and periodic pneumococcal vaccine are needed.

Pharmacological Therapies

Pharmacological therapies to treat patients with heart failure include diuretics, ACE inhibitors, beta-adrenergic blockers, inotropics, synthetic natriuretic peptides, nitrates, and arterial vasodilators.

Diuretics. Diuretics enhance water loss from the body by decreasing blood volume and sodium retention, also called diuresis. This occurs through the induction of changes at the nephrons of the kidney, which decrease reabsorption of sodium and water into the bloodstream. The main effect of diuretics in heart failure is a reduction in pulmonary interstitial fluid and peripheral edema. Loop diuretics, such as furosemide, torasemide, and bumetanide, are commonly used and can have a dramatic initial effect when administered intravenously. Patients are often maintained on low doses of oral diuretics, such as thiazides, to manage heart failure.

CLINICAL CONCEPT

Electrolyte imbalances, particularly hypokalemia, are a common side effect of diuretic therapy. Hypokalemia can worsen heart function and increase risk of cardiac dysrhythmias. If hypokalemia becomes a problem, patients can be given potassium supplements or placed on potassium-sparing diuretics.

A specific potassium-sparing diuretic, spironolactone, is often recommended. Spironolactone is an aldosterone antagonist that inhibits sodium and water reabsorption at the nephron. Blocking aldosterone also causes decreased excretion of potassium at the nephron and potassium is conserved within the bloodstream; this means that a potential side effect of a potassium-sparing diuretic is hyperkalemia, which increases risk of cardiac arrest.

ALERT! With all diuretics, the clinician needs to periodically monitor the patient's serum electrolytes, particularly serum potassium.

Angiotensin-Converting Enzyme Inhibitors. Many experts consider ACE inhibitors, such as ramipril, captopril, and lisinopril, as the cornerstone of heart failure treatment. These drugs inhibit ACE, which in turn blocks the conversion of angiotensin I to angiotensin II in the RAAS. Blocking the formation of angiotensin II inhibits peripheral vasoconstriction and the stimulation of aldosterone.

ACE inhibitors decrease resistance against the left ventricle (afterload) and diminish sodium and water retention in the bloodstream. They also inhibit the detrimental effects of the RAAS in heart failure and decrease ventricular hypertrophy. These drugs lower blood volume and blood pressure to ease the heart's work.

ALERT! Adverse effects of ACE inhibitors include hyperkalemia, angioedema, and cough.

CLINICAL CONCEPT

Angiotensin receptor blockers (ARB) inhibit the action of angiotensin II. These drugs have a similar effect as ACE inhibitors, because they block the detrimental effects of angiotensin II and the RAAS in heart failure. ARBs are often used when patients cannot tolerate ACE inhibitors.

Beta-Adrenergic Blockers. Beta-adrenergic blockers, such as metoprolol, atenolol, and carvedilol, inhibit the effects of the SNS on the heart and vasculature. In heart failure, baroreceptors sense low arterial pressure caused by the heart's low contractile force and, in turn, stimulate the SNS. The SNS increases HR and stimulates peripheral vasoconstriction, both of which are detrimental to the failing heart. Stimulation of a weakened heart to pump faster further strains the heart.

Peripheral vasoconstriction increases resistance against the left ventricle (afterload). Beta-adrenergic blockers inhibit these processes, and therefore reduce strain on the weakened heart.

ALERT! Beta-adrenergic blockers are contraindicated in patients with bradycardia, AV block, and hypotension; they should be used with caution in patients with asthma and diabetes.

Inotropic Agents. Inotropic agents increase the contractile force of the heart muscle. Increasing the force of contraction of the heart muscle is called a positive inotropic effect. Additionally, inotropic agents often have chronotropic effects on the heart as well. Chronotropic effects are influences on the heart's rate or number of beats per minute. The most commonly used inotropic drugs are digitalis (digoxin), dobutamine, dopamine, and milrinone.

Digitalis exerts positive inotropic and negative chronotropic effects on the heart; it is a cardiac glycoside that increases the force of contraction of the ventricular muscle, thereby increasing the strength of the heart as a pump. Concurrently, digitalis slows conduction through the AV node, thereby slowing heart rate.

> **ALERT!** Before administering digitalis, the clinician should measure the apical pulse for one full minute. Digitalis can slow the HR excessively and is contraindicated in patients with bradycardia.

> **ALERT!** The clinician should carefully monitor the patient's serum potassium level because digitalis in conjunction with hypokalemia causes cardiac dysfunction and serious dysrhythmias.

Dopamine is a catecholamine that stimulates the heart's beta-1 receptors. It increases both the inotropic and chronotropic responses of the heart. In addition, dopamine stimulates alpha-adrenergic receptors of arteries, causing vasodilation. Dopamine preserves perfusion of the peripheral organs, particularly the kidneys, as it increases the contractile force and rate of the heart.

Dobutamine, a synthetic catecholamine, also acts on the heart's beta-1 receptors. It consequently increases contractility of the heart and heart rate.

Milrinone, a phosphodiesterase inhibitor, also increases contractility of the heart muscle through a different mechanism. This drug increases calcium availability to the cardiac myocytes, which increases the muscle's overall force of contraction.

> **ALERT!** All inotropic drugs may have negative side effects and require careful monitoring of the heart because they can induce dysrhythmias, tachycardia, and activate the RAAS.

Synthetic Natriuretics. BNP is a natural substance secreted by the endothelium in heart failure to induce diuresis of the body. It is also available as nesiritide, a form of medication that acts at the renal vasculature to induce diuresis. Nesiritide, which is able to act rapidly, can decrease both pulmonary congestion and edema in heart failure when administered intravenously.

> **ALERT!** Certain ancillary drugs, such as ACE inhibitors, antihypertensives, nitroglycerin, and some diuretics should not be used in conjunction with nesiritide. Severe hypotension can result from potent diuresis and vasodilator addictive effects of these drugs used together.

Nitrates. Nitrates are arterial and venous vasodilators that enhance coronary circulation and decrease the heart's workload. Commonly used nitrates for heart failure are nitroglycerin, isosorbide dinitrate, and nitroprusside. Through stimulation of NO, nitrates promote arterial dilation. These drugs significantly lower arterial blood pressure, thereby decreasing resistance against the heart. Through venous dilation, they also lower venous pressure, which decreases the volume of blood entering the heart. Nitrates also directly stimulate dilation of the coronary arteries, which enhances delivery of oxygenated blood to the heart muscle. Nitrates have been found to be more effective than other drugs for heart failure in African Americans.

> **ALERT!** Nitrates can exert a detrimental hypotensive effect if combined with sildenafil-type medications for erectile dysfunction.

Arterial Vasodilators. Dilation of the arterial circulation decreases aortic pressure and the resistance against the left ventricle. Arterial dilators significantly reduce workload for the weakened heart in heart failure and lower blood pressure. These medications facilitate the weakened heart's ability to pump more efficiently against reduced afterload.

Interventional Cardiology Procedures

There are a number of cardiac interventions that require catheterization or surgery. Specific kinds of pacemakers and intra-arterial pump devices are used to stave off the effects of heart failure. Finally, there is cardiac transplantation, which can be successfully accomplished if the patient is eligible and the right tissue match is found.

Cardiac Resynchronization Therapy

In heart failure, the right and left ventricles may differ in the timing of their contraction. This dyssynchronous ventricular wall motion can contribute to a weakened force of contraction of the heart. Cardiac resynchronization therapy (CRT), also known as biventricular pacing, is a technique that places a specialized pacemaker in a region that activates both the left ventricular wall and septum of the heart. CRT can optimize the pumping function of the heart by coordinating impulse conduction through the ventricles, thereby synchronizing the contraction of the ventricles. An implantable cardiac defibrillator (ICD) can also be used in conjunction with CRT to counteract life-threatening rhythm disturbances.

Intra-Aortic Balloon Pump. In patients with severe heart failure, an intra-aortic balloon pump may be used in conjunction with interventional cardiac procedures, such as percutaneous transluminal angioplasty (PCTA). PCTA uses a catheter to clear the lumens of obstructed coronary arteries. An intra-aortic balloon pump may be needed during PCTA in patients with inadequate ventricular function for such a procedure.

An intra-aortic balloon pump may also be used in patients with end-stage heart failure awaiting transplant. A balloon pump attached to a cardiac catheter is inserted via a peripheral site into the thoracic aorta. The balloon is inflated during diastole, thus increasing aortic pressure during diastole and increasing coronary blood flow. The balloon is deflated before and during early left ventricular ejection, thus reducing aortic pressure and afterload.

Cardiac Assist Devices. There are cardiac assist devices, such as extracorporeal heart pumps, that are used to assist those in end-stage heart failure until a heart transplant is available. Most devices take blood from the left ventricle via a cannula and propel it into the ascending aorta. They are surgically placed in the subcutaneous tissue of the abdominal region with an attachment to an external pumping mechanism.

Cardiac Transplantation. Patients who have developed end-stage or stage D heart failure may be candidates for cardiac transplantation. Eligibility for this surgical procedure involves the age of the patient and the existence of comorbidities, such as peripheral or cerebrovascular disease, obesity, diabetes, or cancer. The United Network of Organ Sharing is a private organization under contract with the federal government that matches donors with heart transplant recipients. Allocation of donor hearts is decided by the network according to a set of conditions and priorities. A match of blood and tissue type, compatibility of gross body size between donor and recipient, and therapeutic immunosuppression of the recipient are some of the prerequisite conditions for heart transplant.

The International Society for Heart and Heart-Lung Transplantation monitors the survival of heart transplant patients. Over 90% of patients in the registry return to normal and unrestricted function following transplantation. About 67% of patients survive longer than 3 years. The average post-transplant survival time has been 9.3 years.

Chapter Summary

- The lifetime risk of developing heart failure is approximately 20% for all patients older than 40 years.

- Many individuals are surviving episodes of acute ischemic heart disease; eventually the damage endured by these insults is demonstrated as chronic heart failure.

- Chronic heart failure is often the result of longstanding HTN, multiple MI, or long-term diabetes mellitus.

- LVF mainly causes pulmonary symptomatology: dyspnea on exertion, cough, orthopnea, paroxysmal nocturnal dyspnea, cyanosis, and crackles on auscultation.

- LVF can cause pulmonary edema, which can be exhibited by pink, frothy sputum and loud, coarse crackles.

- In LVF, the RAAS is constantly stimulated, which increases blood volume, blood pressure, and left ventricular resistance; these compensatory mechanisms place more strain on the weak heart.

- Sympathetic stimulation occurs in LVF, which causes increased HR and further strain on the weak heart.

- When there is a question as to whether dyspnea is caused by a pulmonary origin or cardiovascular origin, the BNP diagnostic test is used.

- In RVF, symptoms are mainly caused by venous congestion in the body.

- The classic signs of RVF are jugular venous distension, ascites, hepatomegaly, splenomegaly, and ankle or sacral edema.

- An S_3 gallop rhythm is common in heart failure.

- A Swan-Ganz catheter is used to monitor the patient's cardiovascular hemodynamic measurements in cases of severe heart failure.

- Preload is the volume of blood that is returning to the heart—the right atrial volume.

- Afterload is the amount of resistance against the ventricle—commonly the aortic pressure.

- In LVF, LVEF is decreased and PCWP is increased.

- A LVEF of lower than 40% constitutes heart failure.

- Management of heart failure requires lifestyle modification and pharmacological interventions. If heart failure is severe, interventional cardiovascular procedures are available.

- Some common agents used in heart failure include ACE inhibitors, beta blockers, diuretics, digitalis, and the aldosterone antagonist Spironolactone.

- ACE inhibitors and beta blockers are the cornerstone treatment in heart failure.

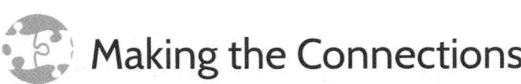

Making the Connections

Pathophysiology	Signs and Symptoms	Physical Assessment Findings	Diagnostic Testing	Treatment
LVF (backward effects)	Weak left ventricle causes a backup of hydrostatic pressure in the left atrium, pulmonary veins, and pulmonary capillaries. Hydrostatic pressure increases in lungs. Fluid builds in pulmonary interstitium, often to the point of pulmonary edema.			
	Cough (cough with pink frothy sputum equals pulmonary edema). Dyspnea. Orthopnea. PND.	Pulmonary bibasilar crackles (Widespread pulmonary coarse, loud crackles equals pulmonary edema). Cyanosis. S_3 or S_4 audible through stethoscope.	Pulmonary congestion on chest x-ray (Kerley A and B lines) caused by pulmonary interstitial fluid. Cardiomegaly on chest x-ray caused by enlarged, dilated ventricles. Elevated BNP caused by elevated water volume in bloodstream. Elevated PCWP caused by backup of hydrostatic pressure.	Fowler's position to ease breathing. Oxygen for hypoxia caused by pulmonary edema. Diuretics to rid body of excess water. Natriuretics (BNP) to rid body of excess water. Low-sodium diet to decrease water retention. Fluid restriction. Daily weight measurement to monitor water weight gain.
LVF (forward effects)	Weak left ventricle forward pumping of blood into the aorta, peripheral, and cerebral arteries. Kidneys sense low circulation caused by weak forward pump of heart. Kidneys release renin. RAAS is triggered. Blood volume increases, blood pressure increases. Peripheral vasoconstriction occurs. The SNS is triggered by baroreceptors in the arterial walls caused by decreased blood pressure. SNS causes increased HR and vasoconstriction of peripheral arteries. These compensatory mechanisms worsen LVF.			
	Cool, pale extremities. Confusion, disorientation. Edema. Nocturia.	Decreased peripheral pulses. Cool, pale extremities. Confusion, disorientation. S_3 or S_4 audible through stethoscope.	Decreased LVEF. HR may be high. Pulses weak.	Fowler's position. Oxygen. Diuretics. Low-sodium diet. Fluid restriction. Daily weight. ACE inhibitors (ACEi) or angiotensin receptor blockers (ARB). Nitrates. Inotropic agents. Beta-adrenergic blockers.
RVF (backward effects)	Weak right ventricle causes backup of hydrostatic pressure into the right atrium, superior vena cava, and jugular veins, then into inferior vena cava, causing venous congestion in gastrointestinal, peritoneal, hepatic, and splenic veins.			
	Jugular neck vein distension. Swelling (rings, shoes may feel tight). Anorexia, indigestion. Abdominal swelling.	JVD. Weight gain. Ascites. Hepatojugular reflux. Hepatomegaly. Splenomegaly. Ankle or sacral edema. Ascites; shifting dullness on abdominal exam. S_3 or S_4.	Elevated jugular venous pressure. Elevated central venous pressure. Dilutional hyponatremia. Hypokalemia.	Daily weight measurement. Low-sodium diet. Fluid restriction. Inotropic agents. Diuretics/Natriuretics. Nitrates. ACEi and ARBs.

Bibliography

American Academy of Family Physicians; American Academy of Hospice and Palliative Medicine; American Nurses Association; American Society of Health-System Pharmacists; Heart Rhythm Society; Society of Hospital Medicine, Bonow, R. O., Ganiats, T. G., Beam, C. T., et al. (2012). ACCF/AHA/AMA-PCPI 2011 performance measures for adults with heart failure: a report of the American College of Cardiology Foundation/American Heart Association Task Force on Performance Measures and the American Medical Association-Physician Consortium for Performance Improvement. *J Am Coll Card*, 59(20), 1812–1832. Epub 2012 Apr 23.

American College of Cardiology/American Heart Association (ACC/AHA). (2010). 2010 guidelines for assessment of cardiovascular risk in asymptomatic adults. Executive Summary. Retrieved from http://circ.ahajournals.org/cgi/reprint/CIR.0b013e3182051bab

American Heart Association. (2009). ACCF/AHA practice guideline: focused update: ACCF/AHA guidelines for the diagnosis and management of heart failure in adults. *Circ*, 119, 1977–2016.

American Heart Association. (2010). Acute heart failure syndromes: emergency department presentation, treatment, and disposition: current approaches and future aims. A scientific statement from the American Heart Association. *Circ*, 122, 1975–1996.

American Heart Association. (2011). Heart disease and stroke statistics—2011 update. *Circ*, 123, e18–e209. Retrieved from http://circ.ahajournals.org/cgi/content/full/123/4/e18

Anker, S. D., Koehler, F., & Abraham, W. T. (2011). Telemedicine and remote management of patients with heart failure. *Lancet*, 378(9792), 731–739.

Armstrong, P. W. (2011). Aldosterone antagonists—last man standing? *N Engl J Med*, 364(1), 79–80.

Barrett, K. E., Barman, S. M., Boitano, S., & Brooks, H. L. (2012). *Ganong's review of medical physiology*. 24th ed. New York: Lange McGraw-Hill.

Bibbins-Domingo, K., Pletcher, M. J., Lin, F., et al. (2009). Racial differences in incident heart failure among young adults. *N Engl J Med*, 360(12), 1179–1190.

Birnie, D. H., Sapp, J. L., Yee, R., Healey, J. S., & Rouleau, J. L. (2010). Cardiac-resynchronization therapy for mild-to-moderate heart failure. *N Engl J Med*, 363(25), 2385–2395.

Cheng, J. W., & Nayar, M. (2009). A review of heart failure management in the elderly population. *Am J Ger Pharm*, 7(5), 233–249.

Cullan, A., Grover, M., & Hitchcock, K. (2011). FPIN's clinical inquiries: brain natriuretic peptide for ruling out heart failure. *Am Fam Phys*, 83(11), 1333–1334.

Desai, A. S., & Stevenson, L. W. (2010). Connecting the circle from home to heart failure disease management. *N Engl J Med*, 363(24), 2364–2367.

Dunlay, S. M., Pereira, N. L., & Kushwaha, S. S. (2014). Contemporary strategies in the diagnosis and management of heart failure. *Mayo Clin Proc*, Mar 29. pii: S0025-6196(14)00053-6. doi: 10.1016/j.mayocp.2014.01.004. Epub ahead of print.

Francis, G. S. (2011). Neurohormonal control of heart failure. *Cleveland Clin J Med*, 78(Suppl 1), S75–S79.

Gersh, B. J., Simari, R. D., Behfar, A., Terzic, C. M., & Terzic, A. (2009). Cardiac cell repair therapy: a clinical perspective. *Mayo Clin Proceed*, 84(10), 876–892.

Goldenberg, I., Kutyifa, V., Klein, H. U., et al. (2014). Survival with cardiac-resynchronization therapy in mild heart failure. *N Engl J Med*, 370(18), 1694–1701. doi: 10.1056/NEJMoa1401426. Epub 2014 Mar 30.

Holzmeister, J., & Leclercq, C. (2011). Implantable cardioverter defibrillators and cardiac resynchronisation therapy. *Lancet*, 378(9792), 722–730.

Jessup, M., Abraham, W. T., Casey, D. E., et al. (2009). 2009 focused update: ACCF/AHA guidelines for the diagnosis and management of heart failure in adults: a report of the American College of Cardiology Foundation/American Heart Association Task Force on Practice Guidelines: developed in collaboration with the International Society for Heart and Lung Transplantation. *Circ*, 119(14), 1977–2016.

Kane, G. C., Karon, B. L., Mahoney, D. W., et al. (2011). Progression of left ventricular diastolic dysfunction and risk of heart failure. *JAMA*, 306(8), 856–863.

King, M., Kingery, J., & Casey, B. (2012). Diagnosis and evaluation of heart failure. *Am Fam Phys*, 85(12), 1161–1168.

Klapholz, M. (2009). Beta-blocker use for the stages of heart failure. *Mayo Clin Proceed*, 84(8), 718–729.

Krum, H., & Teerlink, J. R. (2011). Medical therapy for chronic heart failure. *Lancet*, 378(9792), 713–721.

Kumar, V., Abbas, A. K., Fausto, N., & Aster, J. (2010). *Robbins & Cotran pathologic basis of disease*. 8th ed. Philadelphia, PA: WB Saunders.

Lambert, M. (2012). NICE updates guidelines on management of chronic heart failure. *Am Fam Phys*, 85(8), 832–834.

Longo, D., Fauci, A., Kasper, D. L., et al. (Eds.). (2011). *Harrison's principles of internal medicine*. 18th ed. New York: McGraw-Hill.

Matlock, D. D. (2009). Defibrillators in heart failure and quality of life. *N Engl J Med*, 360(2), 187–188.

McMurray, J. J. (2010). Clinical practice. Systolic heart failure. *N Engl J Med*, 362(3), 228–238.

Moss, A. J. (2010). Preventing heart failure and improving survival. *N Engl J Med*, 363(25), 2456–2457.

Moss, A. J., Hall, W. J., Cannom, D. S., et al. (2009). Cardiac-resynchronization therapy for the prevention of heart-failure events. *N Engl J Med*, 361(14), 1329–1338.

Neubauer, S., & Redwood, C. (2014). New mechanisms and concepts for cardiac-resynchronization therapy. *N Engl J Med*, 370(12), 1164–1166. doi: 10.1056/NEJMcibr1315508.

New York Heart Association (NYHA). (2015). NYHA classification of heart failure. Retrieved from http://www.hfsa.org/hfsa-wp/wp/stages-of-heart-failure/

On the horizon in heart failure. (2011). *Lancet*, 378(9792), 637.

Piña, I. L., & O'Connor, C. (2009). BNP-guided therapy for heart failure. *JAMA*, 301(4), 432–434.

Pitt, B., Pfeffer, M. A., Assmann, S. F., et al. (2014, April 10). Spironolactone for heart failure with preserved ejection fraction. *N Engl J Med*, 370(15), 1383–1392. doi: 10.1056/NEJMoa1313731.

Ramani, G. V., Uber, P. A., & Mehra, M. R. (2010). Chronic heart failure: Contemporary diagnosis and management. *Mayo Clin Proceed*, 85(2), 180–195.

Resynchronization-Defibrillation for Ambulatory Heart Failure Trial Investigators: Tang, A. S., Wells, G. A., Talajic, M., et al. (2009). Advanced heart failure treated with continuous-flow left ventricular assist device. *N Engl J Med*, 361(23), 2241–2251.

Shah, A. M., & Mann, D. L. (2011). In search of new therapeutic targets and strategies for heart failure: recent advances in basic science. *Lancet*, 378(9792), 704–712.

Steffel, J., Holzmeister, J., & Abraham, W. T. (2011). Recent advances in cardiac resynchronization therapy. *Postgraduate Medicine*, 123(2), 18–26.

Taylor, A. L. (2005). The African American Heart Failure Trial: a clinical trial update. *Am J Card*, 96(7B), 44–48.

Torpy, J. M., Lynm, C., & Golub, R. M. (2011). *JAMA* patient page. Heart failure. *JAMA*, 306(19), 2175.

Weiss, B. D. (2014). Sodium restriction in heart failure: how low should you go? *Am Fam Phys*, 89(7), 508–510.

Wexler, R. K., Elton, T., Pleister, A., & Feldman, D. (2009). Cardiomyopathy: an overview. *Am Fam Phys*, 79(9), 778–784.

Yancy, C. W. (2005). Heart failure in African Americans. *Am J Card*, 96(7), 3–12.

Yancy, C. W. (2008). Race-based therapeutics. *Curr Hyper Rep*, 10, 276–285.

Zheng, H., Chen, Y., Chen, J., Kwong, J., & Xiong, W. (2011). Shengmai (a traditional Chinese herbal medicine) for heart failure. *Cochrane Database System Rev.* Feb 16; 2: CD005052.

Valvular Heart Disease

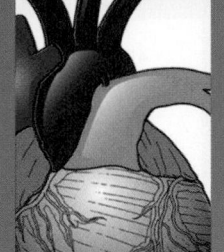

Key Terms

Bruit

Chordae tendineae

Echocardiography

Heart murmur

Hypertrophic cardiomyopathy (HCM)

Mitral valve prolapse (MVP)

Papillary muscles

Regurgitant

Rheumatic fever (RF)

Rheumatic heart disease (RHD)

S_3 gallop

Stenosis

Thrill

The heart valves are specialized cardiac tissue that direct the flow of blood through the heart's chambers. They consist of thin leaflets of endothelium-covered fibrous tissue that open and close in synchrony with the heart's contractions.

The heart valves can sustain injury that deforms their structure; this, in turn, can disrupt blood flow through the heart, alter chamber pressures, increase workload, incite thrombus formation or infection, and diminish the heart's pumping ability. Most valve disorders create turbulent blood flow that can be detected by auscultation as a heart murmur. Echocardiography is the gold standard for diagnosis of valve dysfunction.

Valvular heart disease can result from a number of disorders, including congenital defects, myocardial infarction (MI), trauma, infection, and inflammatory conditions. Valvular dysfunction can vary in degree from mild and asymptomatic to severe and rapidly fatal. Clinical consequences depend on the severity of valve impairment, rate of development of the dysfunction, and the heart's ability to compensate for the impairment. Heart failure is a common result of untreated valvular disease.

Regardless of etiology, valvular disorders can be surgically repaired or replaced with mechanical or tissue-derived prosthetic valves. Because valvular disorders can cause turbulent or stagnant blood flow within the heart, prevention of clot formation is a key treatment modality. Also, because deformed or prosthetic valves can act as a site for infection, patients require prophylactic antibiotics before any invasive procedure.

Epidemiology

One of the major causes of heart valve disorders in the past was **rheumatic fever (RF).** It would begin as an acute streptococcal throat infection and eventually lead to **rheumatic heart disease (RHD),** an inflammatory condition of the heart and heart valves. The heart's involvement was often silent in the acute phase of the disease, although heart valve deformities became obvious later in life. Commonly, there is a lengthy asymptomatic period of 30 to 40 years from onset of RF to the development of cardiac valve problems. With the widespread use of antibiotics, prevalence of RHD in the United States has declined and the incidence is 1 in 100,000 persons. However, the prevalence of RHD remains high in underdeveloped nations. In India, for example, the prevalence is approximately 100 to 150 cases per 100,000, and in Africa the prevalence is 35 cases per 100,000.

Most valvular disorders in the United States and in developed nations are caused by congenital heart disease, MI, arteriosclerosis, and aging. Valvular abnormalities caused by congenital heart disease can remain silent and asymptomatic until adulthood. Mitral insufficiency is a common valvular disorder caused by MI. Up to 20% of individuals who suffer MI also endure the complication of mitral insufficiency. Mitral valve prolapse (MVP), a type of mitral insufficiency, is diagnosed in 4% of the population, but has been found to be asymptomatic in as many as 20% of the population. With age, calcific changes occur in the mitral and aortic valves; heart murmurs involving these two valves are common in the elderly population.

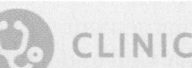
CLINICAL CONCEPT

Because of the expanding population of elderly adults, mitral and aortic stenosis are the most common valvular disorders encountered in the clinical area.

Basic Concepts of Cardiac Valve Function

The four chambers of the heart are separated from one another by atrioventricular valves. The tricuspid valve, located between the right atrium and right ventricle,

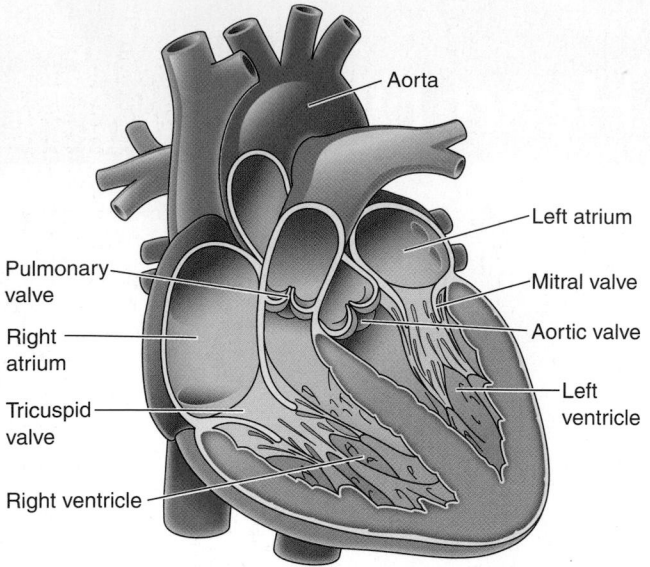

FIGURE 18-1. Heart anatomy showing the mitral, tricuspid, aortic, and pulmonic valves. In the diagram, the mitral and tricuspid valves are open. The aortic and pulmonic valves are closed.

is constructed of three valve leaflets. The mitral valve, between the left atrium and left ventricle, has two leaflets. The pulmonary artery and aorta each have a semilunar valve at their entry; the term semilunar describes their half-moon shape (see Fig. 18-1).

Anatomy and Function of Cardiac Valves

To understand valvular heart disease, a thorough knowledge of the anatomy and function of the heart's four valves is necessary. The mitral and tricuspid valves, located between the atria and ventricles, are attached to the myocardium via support structures called chordae tendineae and papillary muscles. **Chordae tendineae** are stringlike membranes that are tethered to the leaflets of the valve and anchored to tiny muscular projections of the myocardium, called **papillary muscles.** Damage to the chordae tendineae or papillary muscles can cause valvular instability.

During diastole, the ventricles fill with blood from the atria and pressure builds within the ventricular chamber. The increased pressure and enlargement of the ventricle cause tension in the ventricular wall and papillary muscles. As the tension builds in the ventricular wall, the chordae tendineae become taut and pull downward on the atrioventricular valve leaflets, keeping the valve closed. During systole, the mitral and tricuspid valves must remain closed despite the high pressure exerted by the contracting left and right ventricles as they push blood into the aorta and pulmonary artery (see Fig. 18-2).

The open aortic valve allows blood to flow from the left ventricle into the aorta during systole, whereas the open pulmonic valve allows blood flow from the right ventricle into the pulmonary artery during systole. During diastole, the ventricles receive blood from the atria, and the aortic and pulmonic valves must be closed for optimal ventricular chamber filling (see Fig. 18-3).

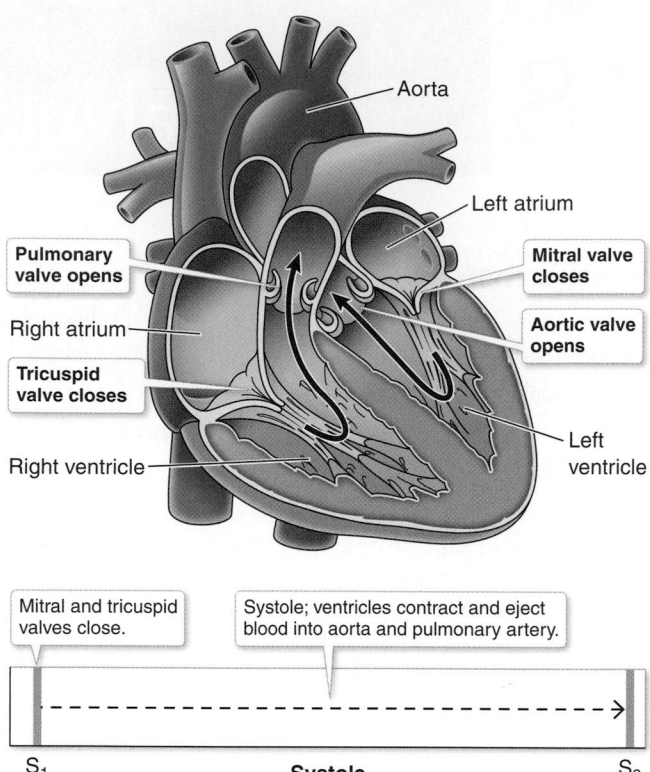

FIGURE 18-2. Normal valvular actions during systole when the ventricles contract. When the ventricles contract, the mitral and tricuspid valves close; this causes the first heart sound (S_1). Blood is then ejected from the ventricles into the open aortic and pulmonic valves.

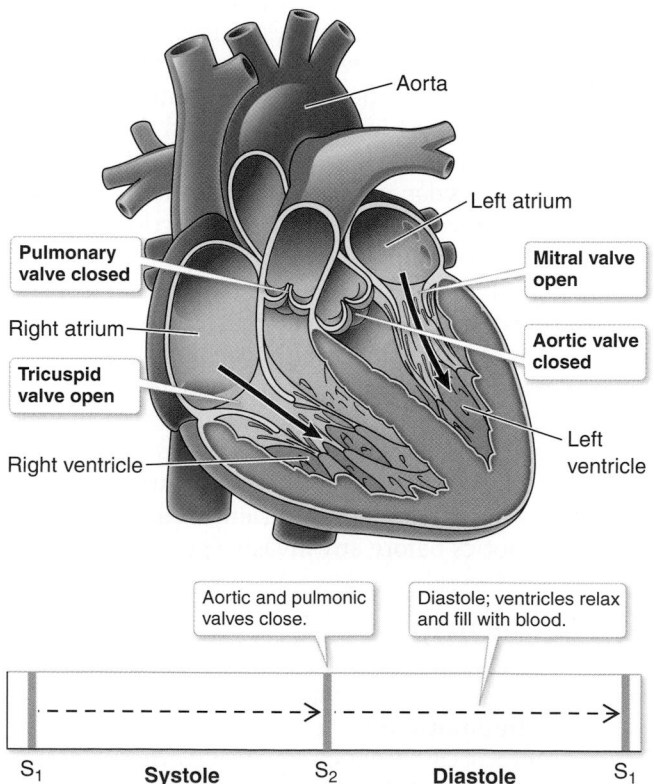

FIGURE 18-3. Normal valvular actions during diastole when the ventricles relax and fill with blood. When the ventricles relax, the aortic and pulmonic valves close; this causes the second heart sound (S_2). Blood can flow from atria to ventricles through open mitral and tricuspid valves.

First and Second Heart Sounds

The first heart sound (S_1) and the second heart sound (S_2) are vibrations transmitted through the chest wall that are caused by the closure of the heart valves. They are sometimes referred to as sounding audibly as "lub-dub." Closure of the mitral and tricuspid valves transmit S_1, whereas closure of the aortic and pulmonic valves transmit S_2.

During systole, as the ventricles contract, the mitral and tricuspid valves close, creating S_1. During systole, the aortic and pulmonic valves are open, allowing blood to flow into the respective vessels through their openings. When normal valves are open, the blood flow through them usually does not transmit a sound. Only valve closure should cause the heart sounds. During diastole, as the ventricles fill with blood from the atria, the aortic and pulmonic valves close, creating S_2.

Frequently, a split of the S_2 sound can be heard, created by the initial closure of the aortic valve and later closure of the pulmonic valve. This is a normal phenomenon often heard with deep inspiration and is referred to as an audible A_2 and P_2—a split S_2. A_2 refers to the aortic closure and P_2 refers to the pulmonic valve closure. The split of S_2 occurs because, with deep inspiration, there is thoracic cage expansion that allows widening of the pulmonary arterial vessels. The widened arterial diameters enhance the capacity of the pulmonary artery and an increased amount of blood can be accepted by the expanded vessel. The increased capacitance of the pulmonary artery allows more blood to enter from the right ventricle, and this prolongs the right ventricle's ejection time. Consequently, there is a slight delay in the pulmonic artery valve closure, causing the split of S_2, with the aorta closing first (A_2) and the pulmonary valve closing later (P_2).

Third Heart Sound

At times during diastole, as blood flows rapidly from the atria into the ventricles, the vibrations of the blood flow against the ventricular wall can be heard as a third heart sound (S_3) (see Fig. 18-4). This can be a normal sound in children and young adults, but in older adults it can indicate decreased ventricular muscle elasticity; in this age group, S_3 is often called an **S_3 gallop** and may be present in heart failure.

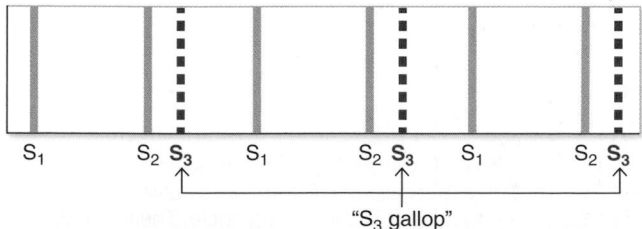

FIGURE 18-4. S_3 is a sound heard during diastole because of filling of the ventricle with a high amount of blood flow. This is commonly caused by heart failure. S_3 is heard after S_2 (closure of the aortic and pulmonic valves) and before S_1 (closure of the mitral and tricuspid valves). It is often referred to as an "S_3 gallop."

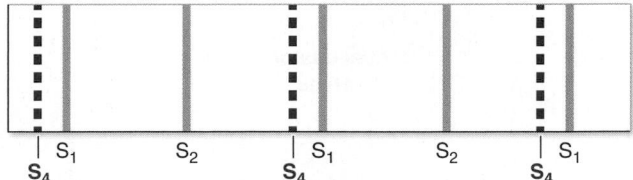

FIGURE 18-5. S_4 is an echo heard because of atrial contraction against a noncompliant, stiff left ventricle. This often occurs in LVH created by long-term hypertension. S_4 is heard just before S_1.

Fourth Heart Sound

Finally, although not usually heard in healthy individuals, atrial contraction may be auscultated as a fourth heart sound (S_4). At the end of diastole, the atria contract to eject an extra volume of blood into the ventricle; this is known as the atrial kick. This late diastolic phase immediately precedes systole and, therefore, occurs slightly before S_1.

An S_4 commonly occurs when the left atrium contracts against a noncompliant, stiff left ventricle. It is a low-pitched sound, best heard with the bell piece of the stethoscope. S_4 is associated with hypertension, because long-term hypertension causes left ventricular hypertrophy that creates a noncompliant, stiff left ventricle (see Fig. 18-5).

Cardiac Valve Auscultation

There are anatomical sites on the chest where auscultation of the sounds created by a specific valve can be heard best. The mitral valve is best heard at the apex of the heart at the fifth intercostal space, midclavicular line. The tricuspid valve is heard best at the left sternal border, fourth intercostal space. The pulmonic valve is best heard at the base of the heart, at the second intercostal space, left sternal border, and the aortic valve, at the second intercostal space, right sternal border (see Fig. 18-6).

Basic Pathophysiologic Concepts of Heart Valve Dysfunction

Heart murmurs are sounds transmitted through the chest wall heard with a stethoscope caused by turbulent blood flow through the heart or great vessels. Most commonly, they are caused by heart valve deformity, valve dysfunction, or defects in the heart wall.

Types of Heart Murmurs

There are two types of heart murmurs: pathologic and physiologic murmurs. Physiologic heart murmurs, sometimes called innocent or functional heart murmurs, may be heard in states of high blood flow within the heart. Anxiety, stress, fever, anemia, overactive thyroid, and pregnancy will cause physiologic murmurs. These heart

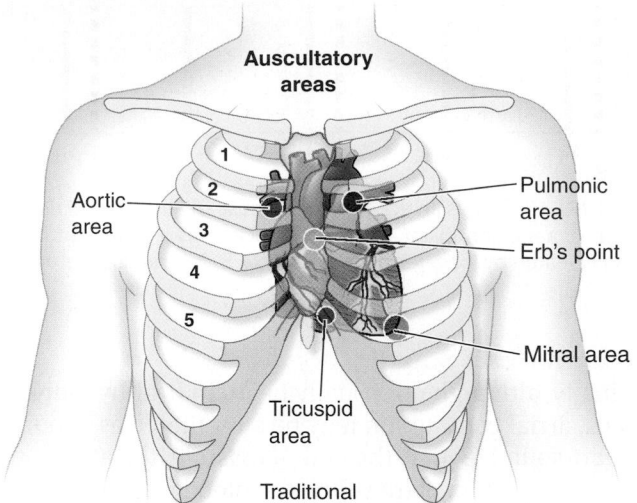

FIGURE 18-6. Cardiac auscultation sites where heart valves are heard best. Aortic valve: second intercostal space, right sternal border. Pulmonic valve: second intercostal space, left sternal border. Erb's point: third intercostal space, left sternal border. Tricuspid valve: fourth or fifth intercostal space, left sternal border. Mitral valve: fifth intercostal space, left midclavicular line.

murmurs are usually faint, intermittent, occur in a small area of the chest, and usually do not cause symptoms.

Pathologic heart murmurs are sounds caused by abnormalities of the heart that include valvular deformities, valvular dysfunction, and heart wall defects. Cardiac valve problems commonly cause deleterious hemodynamic consequences such as heart failure. They also cause symptoms such as shortness of breath, dizziness, chest pains, or palpitations. Pathologic heart murmurs usually require medical intervention to prevent complications, whereas physiologic murmurs do not.

Types of Valvular Dysfunction

There are two major types of valvular dysfunction that cause pathologic heart murmurs. A valve may be narrowed, in which case it does not allow blood to flow freely across it. This abnormality is called **stenosis,** which is caused by a narrow valve orifice or a valve that does not open completely. The other type of valvular deformity is a **regurgitant** or incompetent valve. In this valvular abnormality, the valve does not close properly, which allows leakage of blood across it, a condition referred to as a valvular insufficiency.

Hemodynamic Changes Caused by Valvular Dysfunction

Blood flow across a stenotic valve meets high resistance, which causes turbulent blood flow, less efficient movement of blood from one chamber to the other, and excess volume left behind. Blood is forced through a small space, which creates a heart murmur audible with the stethoscope. For example, in mitral stenosis, blood from the left atrium meets resistance when flowing

through the narrowed mitral valve into the left ventricle. Blood flow through the stenotic valve is turbulent and a diminished, limited volume moves from the left atrium into the left ventricle. As a result, the left ventricle has an inadequate volume of blood to eject forward and an excess volume of blood left behind. The volume left behind backs up and accumulates in the left atrium. The left atrium eventually is stretched and enlarged because of the greater amount of blood it can accommodate.

A stenotic valve can also cause excess workload for the heart muscle, as in the case of aortic stenosis. When the aortic valve is narrowed, the left ventricle must push against high resistance created by the narrow aortic orifice to eject its blood into the aorta. The high workload causes hypertrophy of the left ventricular muscle. Left ventricular hypertrophy eventually leads to other problems, such as inadequate coronary blood flow and ischemia (see Fig. 18-7).

When there is valvular insufficiency, a different kind of turbulent blood flow occurs. A valve that does not make a firm seal will allow leakage of blood from one chamber to another. This occurs in regurgitant valves. For example, in mitral insufficiency, after the mitral valve closes and the left ventricle contracts during systole, the mitral valve leaflets do not close tightly. As the pressure builds within the left ventricle during

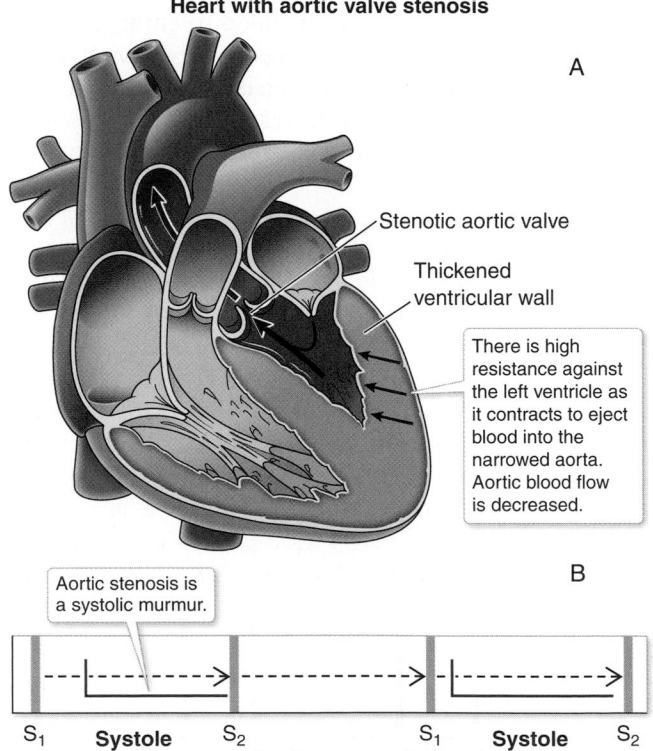

Heart with aortic valve stenosis

A

Stenotic aortic valve

Thickened ventricular wall

There is high resistance against the left ventricle as it contracts to eject blood into the narrowed aorta. Aortic blood flow is decreased.

B

Aortic stenosis is a systolic murmur.

S₁   **Systole**   S₂   S₁   **Systole**   S₂

FIGURE 18-7. Aortic stenosis. **(A)** Aortic stenosis is narrowing of the aortic valve. Because of the narrowed valve, there is increased resistance against the left ventricle. The result is left ventricular hypertrophy and decreased aortic blood flow. **(B)** When blood flows into the narrowed aorta, there is a turbulent sound (heart murmur) heard through the stethoscope that occurs after S₁ systole. The murmur can be early, mid, late, or holosystolic.

systolic contraction, the mitral leaflets are pushed apart and blood regurgitates upward into the left atrium. This causes pressure changes within the left atrium and ventricle. Because some blood flows up into the left atrium, the left ventricle has less blood volume to eject into the aorta. Also, because of the loose valve leaflets, the left atrium collects and accommodates extra accumulated blood volume. The extra blood volume causes dilatation and stretching of the left atrium, which leads to stasis of blood and thrombus formation. Also, decreased blood flow ejected into the aorta causes less filling of the coronary arteries, which eventually causes ischemia of the myocardium (see Fig. 18-8).

Common Pathologic Consequences of Valve Dysfunction

Heart valve deformities can lead to pressure changes within heart chambers, changes in blood fluidity, and disruption of cardiac function. Dysrhythmias, myocardial ischemia, stroke, and heart failure are consequences of valvular deformity. When valvular deformity causes distension and enlargement of a heart chamber, such as the right atrium, the conduction system is stretched and disrupted, causing dysrhythmia. Blood flow in the stretched atrium becomes nonlaminar, turbulent, and static—all conditions that predispose to thrombus formation. Thrombi travel in the bloodstream where they become emboli. Once a thromboembolism is formed, it can lodge within a small diameter vessel and cause obstruction and tissue ischemia anywhere in the body. A thromboembolism can lodge in the pulmonary arterial vasculature or cerebral arteries, both of which are potentially fatal conditions.

Valvular stenosis can lead to MI and heart failure because it often causes hypertrophy of the myocardium, which leads to ischemia and eventual infarction. An example of this disorder occurs in pulmonic stenosis, where the right ventricle has to push its blood volume through the resistance of the narrow pulmonic valve. With time right ventricular hypertrophy occurs, which eventually suffers inadequate coronary artery supply. This leads to ischemia, infarction, and right ventricular failure. Furthermore, there is backup of blood from the failing right ventricle into the right atrium and venous vessels; the venous congestion causes all the classic signs of right ventricular failure.

Assessment of Cardiac Valve Dysfunction

Valvular dysfunction often occurs in patients who are unaware of a heart problem. A clinician often detects a heart murmur as an incidental finding on a physical examination. Alternatively, patients may present to a health-care provider because of symptoms of dizziness, chest pain, syncope, or heart failure. It may be these symptoms that lead to the diagnosis.

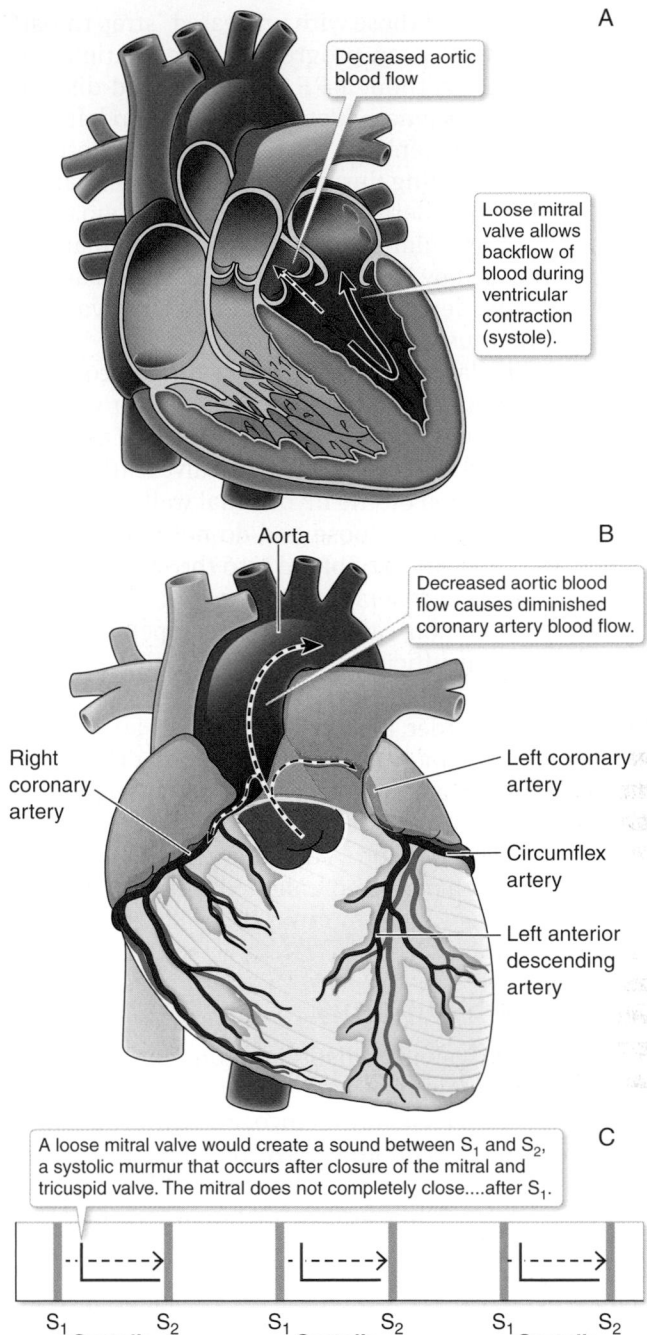

FIGURE 18-8. **(A)** Mitral insufficiency. In mitral insufficiency, the mitral valve leaflets are loose and allow blood to back up into the left atrium when the left ventricle contracts during systole. During systole, the blood flow into the aorta is decreased because some of the blood is flowing up into the left atrium. **(B)** Because the aorta has diminished blood flow, the coronary arteries, which come off the aorta, suffer lack of blood flow. **(C)** The murmur of mitral insufficiency occurs after S_2 during diastole when the ventricles are filling with blood. The sound you hear is that of backflow up through the loose mitral valve into the left atrium.

History

Rheumatic fever (RF) is a major risk factor for heart valve disorders. Acute RF can be a sequela of a previous group A beta hemolytic streptococcal (GABHS) infection of the upper respiratory tract called "strep throat."

A small minority of those with untreated "strep throat" develop RF, which can progress to Rheumatic Heart Disease (RHD). Although RF is a childhood disease, RHD does not become evident until adulthood. It usually becomes apparent as a heart murmur diagnosed as an incidental finding during a physical examination. Adults who are elderly and who had undiagnosed or untreated RF as children may be suffering valvular dysfunction caused by RHD. However, widespread antibiotic use has decreased the incidence of valvular dysfunction caused by RF.

MI, particularly of the inferior wall, is a common cause of valvular dysfunction. In an inferior wall MI, the papillary muscles and chordae tendineae are commonly ruptured, which detaches the valve leaflets from their fixed position on the myocardial wall. The mitral valve leaflets become loose and do not close tightly, which allows backflow of blood into the left atrium.

Myxomatous degeneration of the mitral valve leaflets is another common cause of an incompetent mitral valve. Mitral insufficiency and mitral valve prolapse (MVP) occur in this manner. There is a genetic component to this disorder, and most individuals affected are unaware of the murmur until adulthood. There is a female predominance of mitral valve prolapse.

Arteriosclerotic calcification of heart valves caused by aging is also common. A disorder called aortic sclerosis, caused by a narrowed, calcified aortic valve, often presents as a new heart murmur in an aged adult.

Signs and Symptoms

Patients with valvular disorders commonly become symptomatic upon physical exertion. Dyspnea, excessive fatigue, exercise intolerance, and syncope (fainting) are common symptoms. Severe valvular disorders can cause palpitations and symptoms of heart failure such as cough, edema, ascites, orthopnea, or paroxysmal nocturnal dyspnea.

Physical Assessment

Heart murmurs should be carefully assessed and fully described to assist in identifying the cause. The clinician should begin with careful inspection of the anterior chest to look for the apical impulse. Palpation of the anterior chest can confirm the characteristics of the apical impulse and detect cardiac thrills, which are vibrations transmitted through the chest wall from turbulent blood flow. Percussion is usually not performed on the chest wall to detect murmurs. Auscultation, however, is the most valuable clinical assessment technique. The clinician can auscultate from the base of the heart to the apex or vice versa.

Both the diaphragm and the bell of the stethoscope are useful when assessing heart murmurs. The diaphragm best detects high-pitched sounds, whereas the bell is more sensitive to low-pitched sounds. The clinician should listen to the heart with the patient in the supine position and inch the stethoscope carefully across the chest, listening for S_1, S_2, and any extra sound at every location. Throughout the examination the clinician should decipher systole and diastole according to S_1 and S_2.

Auscultation at the anatomic sites of the valves on the chest is most important. However, heart murmurs can cause echoes and may radiate toward different areas, and these anatomic sites may not reflect the actual valvular origin of the murmur. In addition, the anatomic valve sites on the chest wall are inaccurate in individuals with an enlarged heart, heart anomalies, or dextrocardia.

Clinical Description of a Heart Murmur

To fully assess a heart murmur, the clinician needs to describe the following characteristics:

- **Grade (based on volume):** A heart murmur is subjectively graded according to its volume by the examiner. A murmur can be Grade 1, where it is faintly audible with the stethoscope, to Grade 6, where it is so loud it can be heard with the stethoscope off the surface of the chest (see Box 18-1).
- **Timing:** To describe the timing, the clinician must ascertain where the murmur occurs in relation to S_1 and S_2 to determine whether the murmur occurs in systole or diastole. Systolic murmurs can be early, late, or holosystolic. A murmur that begins after S_1 fades and stops before a clear S_2 is heard may be early systolic or midsystolic in timing. A murmur that begins simultaneously with S_1 and ends on S_2 without a gap is described as pansystolic or holosystolic (see Fig. 18-9). A murmur that begins shortly before S_2 and ends at S_2 is late systolic in timing.

  Similarly, murmurs can be described in terms of diastole. A murmur that begins at S_2 and fades before S_1 is heard can be described as early diastolic in timing. A middiastolic murmur starts a short time after S_2 is heard and fades before S_1. A late diastolic murmur starts after S_2 is clearly heard and continues up to S_1.

BOX 18-1. Heart Murmur Grading

Heart murmurs are graded on a 6-point scale as follows:

- **Grade 1:** Very faint, heard only after listener has "tuned in"; may not be heard in all positions
- **Grade 2:** Quiet, but heard immediately after placing the stethoscope on the chest
- **Grade 3:** Moderately loud
- **Grade 4:** Loud with a palpable thrill
- **Grade 5:** Very loud, with thrill. May be heard when stethoscope is partly off the chest wall
- **Grade 6:** Very loud, with thrill. May be heard with stethoscope off the chest wall.

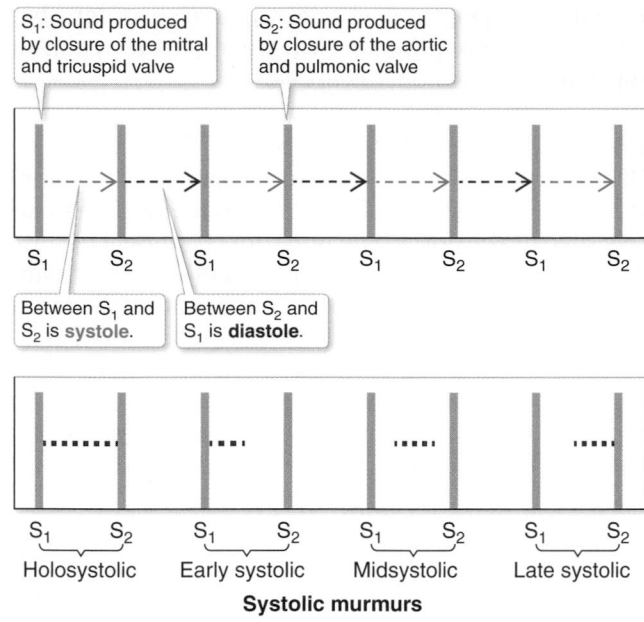

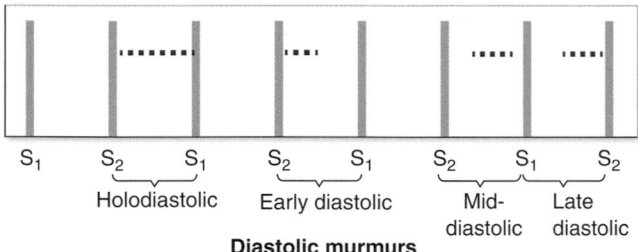

FIGURE 18-9. The timing of a heart murmur. A heart murmur can be heard during systole or diastole. The first heart sound (S_1) occurs when the mitral and tricuspid valves close. After S_1, systolic murmurs occur. The second heart sound (S_2) occurs when the aortic and pulmonic valves close. After S_2, diastolic murmurs occur. Heart murmurs can be described as early, mid, late, or holosystolic. Alternatively, heart murmurs can be described as early, mid, late, or holodiastolic.

- **Location of maximal intensity:** The clinician should listen to all areas of the chest with the stethoscope to determine the location of maximal intensity of the heart murmur.
- **Radiation:** The clinician should listen around the area of maximal intensity to determine if the murmur radiates to other regions, such as into the carotid arteries or into the axillary region.
- **Pitch:** The murmur's pitch should be described as high, medium, or low. A low-pitched sound is best heard with the bell piece of the stethoscope, whereas other sounds are heard well with the diaphragm.
- **Quality:** The quality of a murmur can be characterized as harsh, rough, blowing, rumbling, or musical.
- **Shape:** The shape of a murmur can be characterized as crescendo, which becomes louder in intensity over time; decrescendo, which becomes softer over time; or a steady plateau, which is unchanging in intensity (see Fig. 18-10).

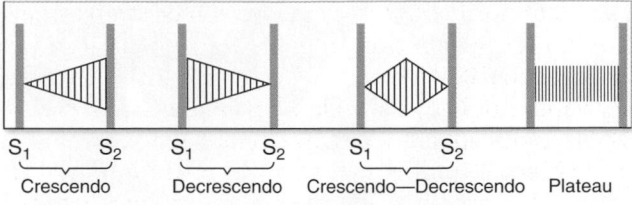

Shape of a murmur

FIGURE 18-10. Describing a heart murmur.

A murmur may be accompanied by a **thrill,** which is a humming vibration over an area of the heart that is palpable through the chest wall. At times a bruit may accompany a heart murmur. A **bruit** is a whooshing sound of turbulent blood flow heard through the stethoscope over an artery; a bruit may indicate an obstruction, aneurysm, or arterial malformation.

A fully described heart murmur may be documented as follows: "Grade 2/6, high pitched, harsh, decrescendo murmur heard best in the fifth intercostal space, left sternal border with radiation to the axilla."

> ### CLINICAL CONCEPT
> Throughout the heart's physical examination, the clinician should distinguish systole and diastole according to S_1 and S_2.

> ### CLINICAL CONCEPT
> Whenever a heart murmur is detected, the clinician should describe it thoroughly and document its presence during physical assessment. Echocardiography can determine the diagnosis.

Diagnosis

Echocardiography is the gold standard for the diagnosis of valvular heart disease. There are three types of echocardiographic techniques used for cardiac diagnostic study:

1. transthoracic echocardiography (TTE)
2. transesophageal echocardiography (TEE)
3. Doppler echocardiography.

TTE is a noninvasive technique that uses sound waves that reflect off cardiac structures to produce images of the heart. In TTE, an echocardiogram transducer is placed directly on the chest wall and moved to various locations on the chest surface to transmit images of the heart's interior structures.

Alternatively, in TEE, an ultrasound transducer is placed on an endoscope and inserted into the esophagus to obtain a closer image of the heart. In the sedated

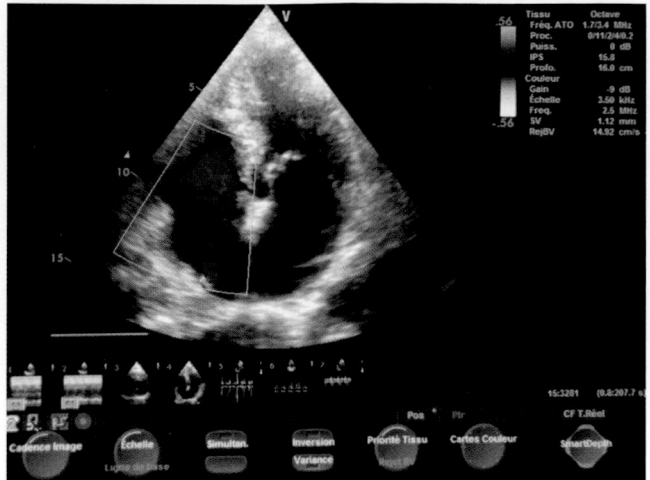

FIGURE 18-11. Example of an echocardiogram. *(From AJPhoto / Science Source.)*

patient, TEE can provide visualization of heart structures because of the close proximity of the esophagus to the heart. TEE is more sensitive than TTE and is the preferred method to visualize heart valves and small intracardiac lesions.

Doppler echocardiography uses sound waves to measure the velocity of blood flow across valves and within cardiac chambers. It can visualize abnormal blood flow patterns in color. Echocardiograms are usually performed with the patient in the resting state. Further information can be obtained by visualizing cardiac structures during exercise or pharmacological-induced stress.

Echocardiograms are instantaneous images that enable clinicians to immediately determine cardiac structure abnormalities (see Fig. 18-11). They can be used to determine the etiology and morphology of valve disorders, estimate severity, and quantify left ventricular ejection fraction. Regional wall abnormalities of the heart can also be detected, which often indicate myocardial ischemia. Patients with valvular disease often require echocardiograms annually, even in the absence of symptoms.

Cardiac catheterization and arteriography (angiography) are also used in patients with valvular disorders. A cardiac catheter can be threaded from a peripheral vein or artery into the right or left side of the heart to visualize the chambers and coronary arteries. Preoperatively, coronary angiography is advisable to determine left ventricular function and the health of the coronary arteries. Some patients may have coronary artery obstructions that can be surgically treated at the same time as valve repair or replacement.

Treatment

There are a number of medical and surgical treatments for heart valve disorders. Individuals can be treated symptomatically with various pharmacological agents and lifestyle modifications. Medical therapies can remedy the symptoms of mild valvular disorders, but most patients require surgical treatment to repair or replace a dysfunctional heart valve.

Medication

Heart valve disorders often cause changes of the pressures within the heart chambers and major blood vessels such as the aorta. The pressure changes can cause a change in shape or conductivity within heart chambers. Thrombosis and dysrhythmias are often the result of these heart valve effects. Long-term changes in pressures can cause complications such as heart failure, ischemic heart disease, and stroke. To prevent these complications and to normalize the pressures and conduction within the heart, many different medications can be used.

Nitrates and vasodilators can reduce venous return, peripheral resistance, and ischemic chest pain. Beta-adrenergic blockers can prevent tachydysrhythmias and lower peripheral arterial resistance. Digitalis, diuretics, and salt restriction can be used to treat heart failure associated with valve disorders. Exercise restrictions can limit strain on the heart. Anticoagulant therapy is commonly prescribed because deformed heart valves, stasis of blood, and turbulent blood flow can lead to thrombus formation. Atrial fibrillation, a common side effect of valvular dysfunction, particularly predisposes to thrombus formation. Thromboembolism can be prevented with anticoagulant therapy. Additionally, deformed or artificial valves can act as a site for bacterial growth if a patient develops bacteremia. Therefore, antibiotic therapy is recommended prophylactically whenever the patient undergoes dental treatment or other invasive procedures.

Surgery

Surgical treatment of valvular disorders can be lifesaving. However, surgical risk, morbidity, and mortality depend on the extent of the valvular disease, myocardial function, and general medical condition of the patient. When left ventricular function is impaired, surgical risk increases. Increased risk is also associated with advanced age, comorbidities such as diabetes or renal disease, and pulmonary hypertension.

Valvotomy, valvuloplasty, and valve replacement are the common surgical procedures used to restore normal heart valve function. Depending on the condition, the procedure may be performed as traditional open heart surgery or a minimally invasive percutaneous surgical procedure.

A percutaneous balloon valvuloplasty is a procedure used when a patient has stenosis of a valve but is too ill to endure surgery. A catheter is directed into the heart and threaded into the affected valvular region. Inflation of a balloon on the tip of the catheter pushes open a stenotic area for a temporary remedy.

Valvotomy is a more common surgical repair procedure that involves reshaping a heart valve by a commissurotomy, quadrangular resection, decalcification, annuloplasty, and leaflet patching. In a commissurotomy, narrowed valve leaflets are opened to allow for unrestricted blood flow through a valve. In a quadrangular resection, a floppy valve is stabilized to allow complete closure of the valve and limit regurgitation of blood flow. An annuloplasty reinforces a dilated valve ring, enhancing the heart valve's structural integrity.

Commonly, valvotomy is not a practical remedy, and a valve replacement is performed. A bioprosthetic valve or an artificial mechanical valve are options for valve replacement. A bioprosthetic valve is commonly made from porcine (pig), bovine (cow), or human cadaver tissue. Mechanical valves can last a lifetime for the patient; however, they act as a site for thrombus formation and predispose the patient to thromboembolism. Therefore, anticoagulation therapy is necessary for life with mechanical valves. Bioprosthetic valves are not associated with thrombus formation and, therefore, do not require anticoagulation therapy. However, bioprosthetic valves do not have the durability of mechanical valves. Studies show that 30% of patients need to replace their bioprosthetic heart valve after 10 years, and 50% need a replacement after 15 years.

> **ALERT!** Deformed or artificial valves can act as a site for bacterial growth.

CLINICAL CONCEPT

In patients with valvular disorders, antibiotics should be administered prophylactically before any invasive treatment such as dental work or insertion of an IV catheter.

Pathophysiology of Selected Heart Valve Disorders

The most common valvular disorders are mitral and aortic stenosis, which account for two-thirds of all valvular disease. Calcific aortic sclerosis, which occurs because of arteriosclerosis and aging, causes stenotic deformity of the aortic valve and is the most common valve disorder of all.

Mitral Valve Disorders

The mitral valve disorders include mitral stenosis, mitral insufficiency, and mitral valve prolapse (MVP). These are some of the most common heart murmurs heard in clinical practice.

Mitral Stenosis

Mitral stenosis is one of the most common heart valve disorders. It is a common sequel to rheumatic fever (RF) or a consequence of calcification of the mitral valve that occurs with aging.

Epidemiology. Patients with mitral stenosis commonly become symptomatic between age 30 and 40 years old and are predominately female. If the valvular stenosis is mild, patient survival is greater than 80% after 10 years. However, when mitral stenosis is severe, there is only a 15% survival if untreated.

Etiology. The most common risk factor for mitral stenosis is RF. In many individuals RF leads to RHD if untreated. Most cases of mitral stenosis caused by RHD occur 10 to 30 years after RF. The patient may not recall having childhood RF. The prevalence of RHD in developed nations is steadily declining with an estimated incidence of 1 in 100,000. However, in underdeveloped countries RF incidence remains high.

Pathophysiology. In mitral stenosis, the mitral valve is thickened, fibrotic, and narrowed. The stiff valve impedes blood flow from the left atrium into the left ventricle. The murmur of mitral stenosis is heard when blood attempts to squeeze through the narrow mitral valve during left ventricular filling or diastole. As the rigid mitral valve opens, often an opening snap can be heard followed by a diastolic murmur (see Fig. 18-12).

The best location to hear the murmur of mitral stenosis is at the apex of the heart during diastole, after S_2 and before S_1. Placing the patient in the left lateral decubitus position can accentuate the murmur.

In normal adults, the mitral valve opening is 4 to 6 cm in diameter. A valve is considered stenotic when it is less than 4 cm in diameter; it is regarded as severely stenotic when the opening is reduced to less than 2 cm. In severe mitral stenosis, there is a lack of blood flow from the left atrium into the left ventricle, which diminishes cardiac output. When the mitral valve opening is severely narrowed, the left atrium becomes overloaded with blood and high hydrostatic pressure builds in the pulmonary veins. This creates high pulmonary capillary pressure, congestion of the pulmonary vessels, and pulmonary edema.

In long-standing mitral stenosis, the left atrium becomes volume overloaded, overstretched, and dilated. A distended atrial wall can stretch cardiac conduction fibers, causing episodes of atrial fibrillation. Atrial fibrillation causes stasis of blood in the left atrium and predisposes to thrombus formation. A thrombus that forms in the left atrium can travel into the left ventricle, aorta, and systemic circulation. An embolic thrombus commonly travels from the left atrium, into the left ventricle, and into the aorta. From the aorta it can travel into the brachiocephalic artery, which leads to the common carotid and internal carotid artery. From the internal carotid artery it can then travel into a branch of the middle cerebral artery and cause an ischemic stroke.

Clinical Presentation. Dyspnea on exertion and cough are usually the initial symptoms associated with the pulmonary vascular congestion of mitral stenosis.

Mitral stenosis

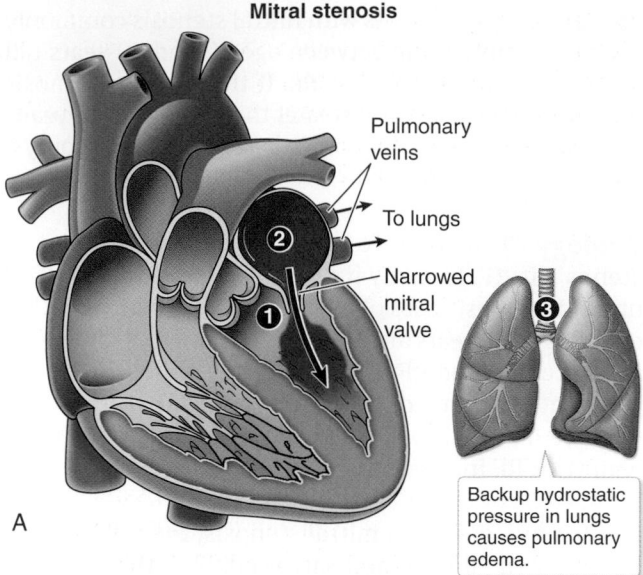

A

1. Narrow mitral valve hinders blood flow into the left ventricle.

2. Blood backs up in the left atrium, causing left atrial enlargement.

3. Hydrostatic pressure builds backward into the pulmonary veins. Congested pulmonary veins cause pulmonary edema.

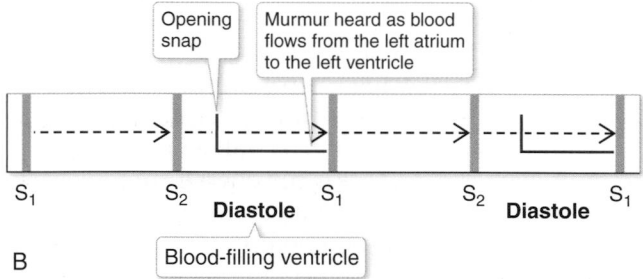

B

FIGURE 18-12. Mitral stenosis. **(A)** In mitral stenosis, the mitral valve is narrowed and blood flow from the left atrium to the left ventricle is hindered. As a result, blood backs up into the left atrium and stretches the chamber, creating an enlarged left atrium. Hydrostatic pressure builds backward from the left atrium into the pulmonary veins, causing increased venous congestion of the lungs and pulmonary edema. **(B)** The murmur of mitral stenosis occurs after S_2 during diastole as the blood flows from the left atrium to fill the left ventricle. Commonly, an opening snap is heard when the stiff mitral valve opens.

Pulmonary edema can occur if hydrostatic pressure rises to high levels within the pulmonary capillaries. In the supine position, the patient experiences orthopnea. When the patient lies flat during sleep, hypoxia, which presents as paroxysmal nocturnal dyspnea (PND), may be experienced. A patient may describe PND as awakening in the middle of the night because of a night terror.

In long-standing mitral stenosis, atrial fibrillation can occur, which causes an irregular pulse, possible tachycardia, and thrombus formation in the left atrium. The patient may complain of palpitations. Atrial fibrillation is a common predisposing condition to ischemic stroke, and symptoms of stroke can occur. Symptoms of stroke include hemiparesis (weakness over half the body), facial droop, or slurring of speech.

Diagnosis. The best diagnostic study for mitral stenosis is echocardiogram, which can be done via the transthoracic or transesophageal method. An electrocardiogram (ECG) and chest x-ray are necessary. Computed tomography (CT) scan and magnetic resonance imaging (MRI) scan of the brain should be done if atrial fibrillation is suspected.

Treatment. Anticoagulant therapy is prescribed to prevent atrial clot formation. Beta blockers, calcium blockers, or digitalis can be used to control atrial fibrillation. Surgery and prosthetic valve implantation will resolve the mitral valve problem. After implantation of a prosthetic valve, it is recommended that the patient receive preventive antibiotics before undergoing dental treatment or other invasive procedures.

Mitral Insufficiency

Mitral insufficiency is the most common valve problem caused by myocardial infarction (MI). Studies show that up to 59% of patients develop mitral insufficiency after MI. Mitral insufficiency after MI causes an increased risk of death and heart failure. The patient with mitral insufficiency is often clinically asymptomatic; therefore, after MI the heart should always be assessed using echocardiography. Echocardiograms show noncontractile areas of the ventricle, regurgitation of blood through the mitral valve, and estimates left ventricular ejection fraction.

Mitral insufficiency is also one of the most common valve problems caused by genetic disorders such as Marfan and Ehlers-Danlos syndromes. Both these disorders cause connective tissue abnormalities of the mitral valve. Mitral valve prolapse, often asymptomatic, is a condition of mild mitral insufficiency.

Epidemiology. The incidence of acute and chronic mitral insufficiency is approximately 5 in 10,000 people in the United States. In the past, RHD was the most common cause of mitral insufficiency. Antibiotic treatment has made RHD less common, and myxomatous degeneration of the mitral valve and MI are the leading causes of mitral insufficiency today. Mitral valve prolapse (MVP) has been estimated to affect as many as 20% of middle-aged and older adults, mostly women. Many have asymptomatic, undiagnosed MVP.

Etiology. The most common causes of mitral insufficiency include MVP, RHD, infective endocarditis, mitral annular calcification, cardiomyopathy, and ischemic heart disease. In underdeveloped regions of the world, RHD is the major cause of mitral insufficiency. Risk factors for mitral insufficiency include female sex, lower body mass index, advanced age, renal dysfunction, prior MI, prior mitral stenosis, and prior MVP.

Pathophysiology. In mitral insufficiency, the mitral valve fails to close completely, allowing blood to back up into the left atrium as the left ventricle contracts. In myocardial infarction (MI), rupture of a papillary muscle often causes mitral insufficiency. Infarction of the ventricle muscle wall often causes damage and rupture of the papillary muscle and chordae tendineae, thereby causing instability of one or more of the mitral valve leaflets.

Mitral insufficiency is commonly a holosystolic murmur heard best at the apex, often with radiation into the axilla. With each systolic contraction, the incompetent mitral valve allows backward flow of blood into the left atrium. Consequently, left atrial overload and distension are common. This is often a progressive disorder that causes buildup of blood volume in the left atrium and then into the left ventricle, which creates dilatation of both left heart chambers. With time, the increasing enlargement and stretch of the left-sided heart chambers cause tension on the mitral valve leaflets, which worsens the incompetence of the mitral valve.

Because of the backup of blood volume from the regurgitant mitral valve into the left atrium, hydrostatic pressure rises and the pulmonary veins become congested. With increased hydrostatic pressure in the pulmonary veins, pulmonary capillary pressure increases, and pulmonary edema can occur.

Clinical Presentation. Patients with mitral insufficiency may be asymptomatic until the mitral valve allows so much blood to back up into the left atrium that there is not enough forward output into the aorta from the left ventricle. The lack of blood pumped into the aorta may diminish the blood flow through the coronary arteries, at which point the patient can suffer chest pain, pallor, diaphoresis, and dyspnea of myocardial ischemia. With time, atrial fibrillation can develop in the overstretched, dilated left atrium. This can lead to thrombus formation. An S_3 is often heard, indicating excess blood volume flowing from the left atrium into the left ventricle.

Diagnosis. Echocardiogram is the best diagnostic test for mitral insufficiency. It can accurately estimate the diminished left ventricular ejection fraction present in mitral insufficiency. Chest x-ray may demonstrate cardiomegaly if there is left atrial dilatation. ECG should be performed to rule out MI.

Treatment. Treatment includes medications such as anticoagulants to decrease the risk of thrombus formation, beta blockers to control heart rate, and nitrates to dilate the coronary arteries. Diuretics may be necessary if pulmonary edema is present. Surgical repair is recommended rather than implantation of a prosthetic valve. Surgery is commonly performed through the percutaneous route. Prophylactic antibiotics are recommended before invasive procedures.

Mitral Annular Calcification

Calcium deposits can develop in the rim, also called the annulus, of the mitral valve. Usually, this occurs with age and causes no dysfunction. At times, however, the irregular, hard calcifications can cause narrowing and rigidity of the mitral valve, causing incomplete emptying of the left atrium. Alternatively, the calcium deposits can cause the rigid valve leaflets to remain partially open and allow regurgitation of blood into the left atrium during left ventricular contraction. The calcium deposits can also become areas that harbor bacteria and predispose individuals to infective endocarditis. Often, mitral annular calcification can be visualized on a chest x-ray as an opacity surrounding the mitral valve. Echocardiography, CT, and MRI scans of the heart are used in the diagnosis. Asymptomatic mitral annular calcification does not require specific medical therapy. However, blood can back up into the left atrium and pulmonary vasculature, causing pulmonary edema. Alternatively, the left atrium can become stretched out and susceptible to atrial fibrillation and thromboembolism formation. The possible consequence of pulmonary edema requires diuretics and the prevention of thromboembolism requires anticoagulants. Surgery is usually not performed unless the mitral valve is severely affected.

Mitral Valve Prolapse

Often referred to as Barlow's syndrome, floppy valve syndrome, or systolic-click syndrome, **mitral valve prolapse (MVP)** is a common cause of mitral insufficiency in the United States. It is a disorder that most commonly affects females, ages 14 through 30 years. It is a frequent finding in persons with genetic connective tissue disorders such as Marfan syndrome, osteogenesis imperfecta, and Ehlers-Danlos syndrome. It can arise from RF, ischemic heart disease, or cardiomyopathies, but in most cases the cause is unknown. It often goes undetected because the disorder is commonly asymptomatic. It is known to exist in 4% of the population, but it is estimated that up to 20% have asymptomatic MVP.

In MVP, one or both mitral valve leaflets are loose and floppy because of myxomatous degeneration of the valve tissue–an excess of mucopolysaccharide. The mitral valve leaflets are thickened and the attached chordae tendineae are thin and easily ruptured.

During left ventricular contraction, the loose mitral valve leaflets prolapse upward into the left atrium. The prolapse allows regurgitation of blood into the left atrium during systole. This causes a systolic murmur as blood flows out of an unsealed mitral valve. In some individuals, a midsystolic click may be heard, signaling the opening of the loose mitral valve leaflets. The tension in the wall of the contracting left ventricle pushes the incompetent mitral valve open into the left atrium. This turbulent, backward blood flow can create a midsystolic, holosystolic, or late systolic murmur, which is why the characteristic murmur heard in MVP is a midsystolic click followed by a systolic murmur (see Fig. 18-13).

Severe MVP can cause symptoms similar to angina. When MVP allows blood to flow backward into the left atrium, the blood volume within the left ventricle diminishes. This in turn decreases the blood volume into the aorta. With less aortic blood flow, there is diminished

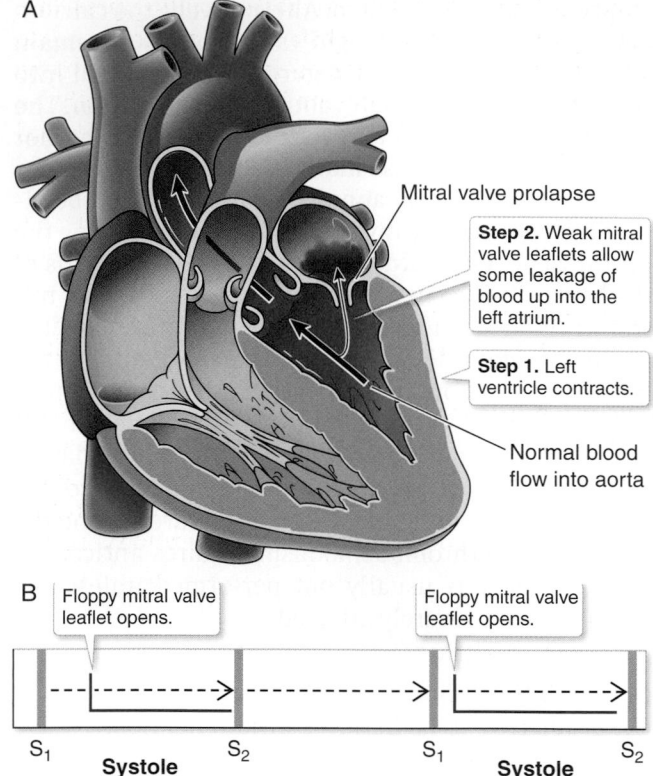

A

Mitral valve prolapse

Step 2. Weak mitral valve leaflets allow some leakage of blood up into the left atrium.

Step 1. Left ventricle contracts.

Normal blood flow into aorta

B

Floppy mitral valve leaflet opens.

Floppy mitral valve leaflet opens.

S₁ **Systole** S₂   S₁ **Systole** S₂

FIGURE 18-13. Mitral valve prolapse. (a) In mitral valve prolapse, there is a weak mitral valve. When the left ventricle contracts during systole, the mitral valve leaflets billow up and leak some blood backward into the left atrium. (b) The murmur of MVP occurs during systole.

coronary artery blood flow. The affected individual can experience coronary insufficiency, which causes myocardial ischemia. Chest pain, dyspnea, and fatigue are common symptoms.

Echocardiography is the diagnostic procedure used in MVP. The majority of persons affected by MVP have no untoward effects. Approximately 3% of those affected develop one of the following complications: infective endocarditis, mitral insufficiency, dysrhythmias, or leaflet thrombi that embolize into the arterial circulation. Patients should avoid caffeine, smoking, alcohol, and drugs that act as stimulants. For patients who are symptomatic, beta blockers are often given to decrease heart rate. Also, anticoagulants may be recommended. Oral contraceptives should not be used as these can increase the risk of thrombus formation. If mitral prolapse is severe, surgery is considered. Prophylactic antibiotics before dental treatment or invasive procedures are only recommended if prolapse is severe.

Aortic Valve Disorders

The aortic valve disorders include aortic stenosis and aortic insufficiency. Aortic stenosis is the most common valve disorder of elderly adults.

Aortic Stenosis

The most common cause of aortic stenosis is aortic sclerosis, which is the calcification of the aortic valve

orifice that occurs in the elderly. Also, a congenitally malformed bicuspid aortic valve is often responsible for aortic stenosis.

Epidemiology. Aortic sclerosis is the most common cause of aortic stenosis in the United States, and approximately 30% of persons older than age 65 years exhibit this disorder.

Etiology. The valve in aortic sclerosis becomes inflamed, calcified, and rigid, demonstrating changes seen in atherosclerosis. Hypercholesterolemia accelerates sclerosis of the aortic valve, and individuals with aortic sclerosis usually suffer from coronary atherosclerosis as well.

In middle-age adults, aortic stenosis is most commonly caused by a congenital bicuspid aortic valve which, with its two leaflets, creates a significantly narrower opening than the normal three leaflet aortic valve. This structural defect is present at birth in 1% to 2% of the population and can be a silent condition, or cause symptoms later in life. Symptoms often occur with aging when calcification and atherosclerotic plaque accumulate on the narrow bicuspid aortic valve, which further constricts the orifice.

Pathophysiology. Regardless of the etiology, in aortic stenosis the aortic valve is narrow and left ventricular outflow of blood is obstructed. The ejection of blood, which occurs during left ventricular contraction in systole, is hindered by the resistance of the distorted aortic valve.

As a compensatory mechanism to aortic stenosis, the left ventricle hypertrophies and the patient can remain asymptomatic for many years. Eventually the left ventricle muscle mass exceeds its coronary artery blood supply and myocardial ischemia can result. Therefore, left ventricular ischemia or angina pectoris is a common sequela of aortic stenosis.

Clinical Presentation. Aortic stenosis is a systolic murmur, occurring after S_1 and before or into S_2. The murmur characteristically is an ejection murmur heard after S_1, which is crescendo, low pitched, and rough ending before S_2. It is heard best at the second right intercostal space with the patient in the seated position and leaning forward, as it commonly radiates up into the carotid arteries.

An early systolic opening snap may be heard as the stiff aortic valve opens during systole. As the valve becomes increasingly rigid and calcified with time, this sound disappears. In severe aortic stenosis, the closure of the aortic valve may be later than that of the pulmonic valve, and a split S_2 may be heard.

Dyspnea, chest pain, and syncope are the three classic symptoms of severe aortic stenosis. Exertional dyspnea occurs because in aortic stenosis the left ventricle is unable to empty all its blood into the narrowed aorta. The blood volume backs up into the left ventricle and atrium, resulting in overload of the left heart chambers. The hydrostatic pressure in the left atrium increases backward pressure in the pulmonary veins and pulmonary capillaries. High hydrostatic pressure in the pulmonary capillaries causes pulmonary edema. Consequently, the patient is short of breath, especially when there is stress on the heart. Exertional angina or chest pain occurs because there is a diminished volume of blood entering the narrowed aortic valve and the aortic blood volume is less than optimal. Less blood volume in the aorta causes less blood flow into the coronary arteries, and the result is coronary insufficiency and ischemia of heart muscle.

Exertional syncope occurs because of the lack of sufficient blood volume entering the aorta and its branches. The blood volume in the brachiocephalic, common carotid, internal carotid, and cerebral arteries is diminished. Lack of sufficient cerebral artery blood flow causes syncope.

Diagnosis. Diagnostic studies include echocardiography, chest x-ray, and ECG. Cardiac catheterization and angiography are performed to evaluate the coronary arteries, as well as aortic and left ventricular pressure. Generally, the incidence of associated coronary artery disease has been reported to be 50% in patients with aortic stenosis who are older than 50 years. Exercise stress testing is contraindicated in symptomatic patients with severe aortic stenosis, but it may be considered in asymptomatic patients with aortic stenosis. Radionuclide ventriculography is performed to evaluate myocardial perfusion at rest and during exercise. A B-type natriuretic peptide (BNP) blood level is recommended because high or steadily rising BNP can be predictive of heart failure.

Treatment. Treatment for aortic stenosis is aortic valve replacement. For patients who cannot tolerate surgery, percutaneous aortic balloon valvuloplasty is performed. Medical treatment such as diuretic therapy in aortic stenosis may provide temporary symptom relief but is generally not effective long term.

Hypertrophic Cardiomyopathy

Hypertrophic cardiomyopathy (HCM) is another disorder that inhibits ejection of blood from the left ventricle. In HCM, the interventricular septum of the left ventricle is disproportionately enlarged because of a structural derangement of muscle fibers.

Etiology. HCM is a genetic disorder, affecting 1 in 500 adults in the United States. There are more than 150 different genetic mutations associated with the abnormal cardiac muscle proteins that cause this structural disorder of the interventricular septum. It is slightly more common in males than females and is the leading cause of sudden death in young athletes.

Pathophysiology. In HCM, the left ventricle is asymmetically hypertrophied, which is different from the concentric hypertrophic changes that occur because of hypertension. The left ventricle is also stiff and noncompliant, creating high diastolic filling pressure. Left ventricular outflow obstruction occurs because during systole the anterior mitral valve leaflet opens against the enlarged interventricular septum. Both the septum and the mitral leaflet obstruct outflow of blood from the left ventricle into the aorta (see Fig. 18-14).

Clinical Presentation. Many patients with HCM are asymptomatic, and there is no associated hypertension or aortic valve deformity. However, this disorder can cause sudden death in children, adolescents, and young adults, often during or after physical exertion. Ventricular dysrhythmias, which are associated with HCM, are commonly the cause of death. Trained athletes with HCM may have no symptoms before sudden cardiac arrest during strenuous exercise. In symptomatic patients, the most common complaints are similar to those in aortic stenosis: dyspnea, chest pain, fatigue, and syncope.

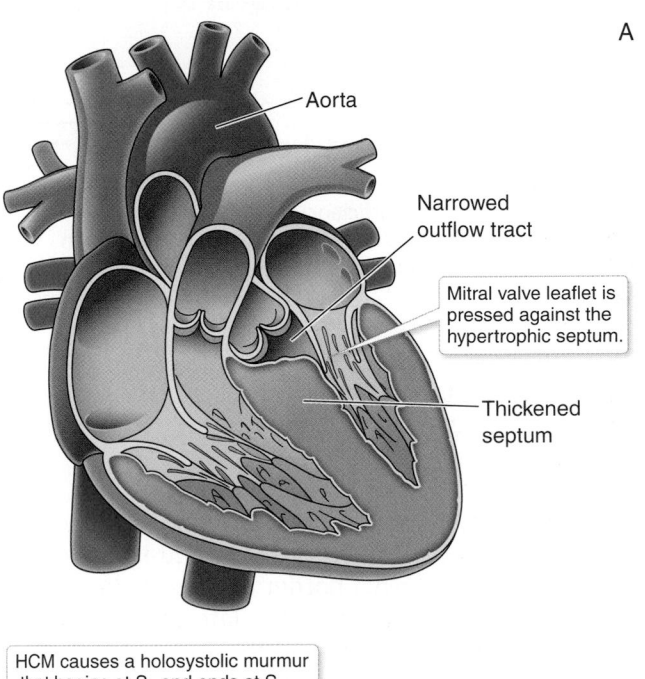

A

Aorta

Narrowed outflow tract

Mitral valve leaflet is pressed against the hypertrophic septum.

Thickened septum

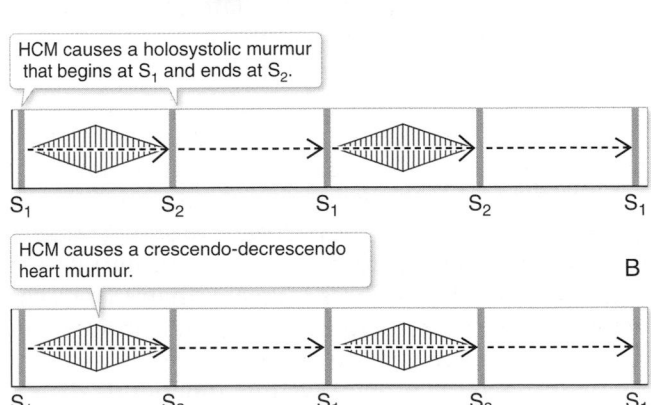

HCM causes a holosystolic murmur that begins at S_1 and ends at S_2.

S_1 S_2 S_1 S_2 S_1

HCM causes a crescendo-decrescendo heart murmur.

B

S_1 S_2 S_1 S_2 S_1

FIGURE 18-14. Hypertrophic cardiomyopathy. **(A)** In HCM, the interventricular septum is enlarged. When left ventricular contraction occurs, the enlarged septum obstructs blood flow into the aorta. As the left ventricle contracts, one of the leaflets of the mitral valve also obstructs blood flow into the aorta. With obstructed blood flow, the aorta receives decreased blood flow. **(B)** The heart murmur of HCM is a crescendo-decrescendo holosystolic murmur. It occurs after S_1 during left ventricular contraction as the blood from the ventricle squeezes through the obstruction into the aorta.

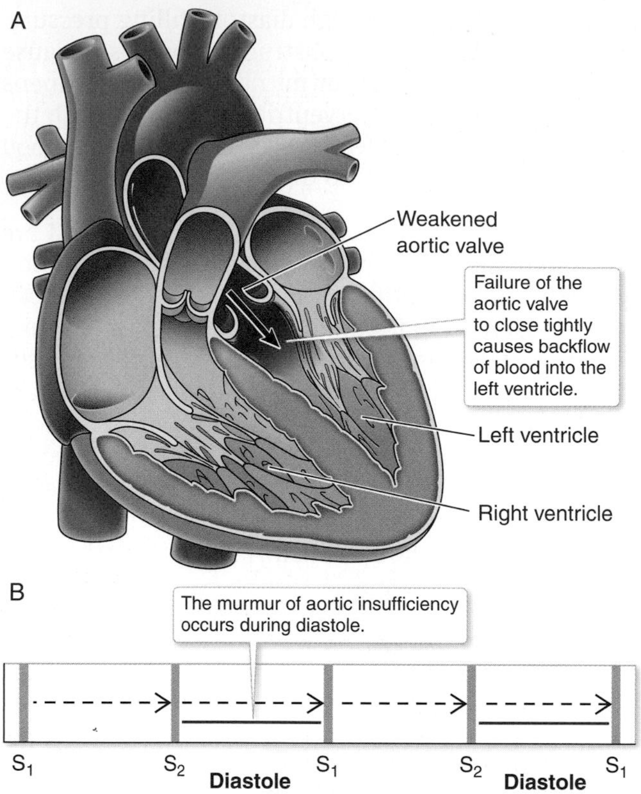

A

Weakened aortic valve

Failure of the aortic valve to close tightly causes backflow of blood into the left ventricle.

Left ventricle

Right ventricle

B

The murmur of aortic insufficiency occurs during diastole.

S_1 S_2 **Diastole** S_1 S_2 **Diastole** S_1

FIGURE 18-15. Aortic insufficiency. **(A)** In aortic insufficiency, the aortic valve is weak and does not close completely. In diastole, the aortic valve should be tightly closed. However, in diastole, as the left ventricle is filling with blood, the aorta leaks blood back into the ventricle. **(B)** The heart murmur of aortic insufficiency occurs after S_2 when the aortic valve should be closed. After S_2, there is a sound of the leakage of blood back into the left ventricle from the aorta.

Severe HCM causes a harsh, diamond-shaped systolic murmur, which begins after S_1 and is heard best at the lower left sternal border and apex. Ejection of blood flow is usually impeded in late systole, and the murmur occurs after a clear S_1 is heard (see Fig. 18-15). HCM may be accompanied by mitral insufficiency, which causes a holosystolic murmur.

Diagnosis. Echocardiography, color Doppler flow studies, CT, and MRI of the heart are performed to diagnose HCM. The hallmarks of the obstruction of HCM consist of systolic anterior motion of the anterior mitral valve leaflet, septal wall thickness of greater than 15 mm, and asymmetrical septal hypertrophy. Echocardiography also reveals diastolic dysfunction with decreased elasticity of the left ventricle. Systolic function is normal and the left ventricular ejection fraction may be high at the time of diagnosis. However, the left ventricular diameter is usually smaller than normal. A cardiac catheterization is useful to show the extent of outflow obstruction, hemodynamics within the atria and ventricles, the characteristics of the left ventricle, and coronary artery anatomy. ECG and Holter monitoring for 24 hours may be needed to study the electrical activity of the heart.

Treatment. Strenuous exercise is contraindicated in HCM. Medications usually include beta blockers and calcium channel blockers to decrease blood pressure and work of the heart. Digitalis is avoided as well as nitrates unless there is coronary artery disease. Sympathetic stimulants are avoided because of their effect of increasing heart rate. Cautious use of diuretics is recommended because they can reduce left ventricular outflow.

Surgical removal of excess septal muscle (left ventricular myomectomy) is performed if medical therapies are not effective. Replacement of the mitral valve may be necessary. Pacemaker insertion or an implantable cardioverter-defibrillator may be recommended because some patients are susceptible to ventricular arrhythmias.

An interesting procedure called transvenous catheter ablation may be performed in HCM. In this procedure, there is chemical destruction of the enlarged septal myocardial tissue. It is done by infusing 96% ethanol into the left anterior descending artery; this causes a therapeutic infarction of the excessive interventricular septal myocardium. This leads to a remodeling of the septum, which decreases the marked septal hypertrophy characteristic of HCM and results in a decrease of left ventricular obstruction.

Aortic Insufficiency

Rheumatic fever (RF) is the cause of aortic insufficiency in approximately two-thirds of patients. Other causes include congenital bicuspid aortic valve, infective endocarditis, Marfan syndrome, ankylosing spondylitis, long-term hypertension, syphilitic aortitis, and temporal and Takayasu arteritis.

Pathophysiology. In aortic insufficiency, the aortic valve is thickened and shortened, which prevents its proper closure. As a result, after the left ventricle pumps its blood volume into the aorta, there is backflow of blood into the left ventricle from the incompetent aortic valve. When aortic insufficiency is severe, the regurgitant backflow of blood can cause volume overload in the left ventricle. As left ventricular end-diastolic volume increases, the left ventricle becomes dilated and loses contractile ability. As a result, stroke volume and left ventricular ejection fraction can diminish and the patient will start to show signs of left ventricular failure.

In advanced stages, there is an overloaded left ventricle with backward buildup of hydrostatic pressure into the left atrium, pulmonary veins, and pulmonary capillaries. Pulmonary edema can occur in severe cases. Volume overload within the pulmonary vasculature occurs which, in turn, raises pressure within the pulmonary artery, leading to increased resistance against the right ventricle. The right ventricle then fails because of intense resistance.

Both left and right ventricular failure can occur in aortic insufficiency. In severe aortic insufficiency, the left ventricle can be stretched and dilated, causing the heart to become extremely large and overdistended. This enlarged myocardial muscle can eventually exceed coronary artery supply, causing myocardial ischemia. The patient then suffers angina pectoris and possibly MI.

Clinical Presentation. The murmur of aortic insufficiency is best heard in the third intercostal space along the left sternal border with the patient in the seated position, leaning forward. It is typically a high-pitched, blowing, decrescendo diastolic murmur. It is heard after the aortic valve closes at S_2.

During systole, S_1 is heard because of closure of the atrioventricular valves and the open aortic valve. During diastole, the ventricles are filling with blood and the aortic valve closes to produce an audible S_2. The regurgitant backflow from the aortic valve into the left ventricle is heard in diastole, after or coinciding with S_2. The backflow of blood can continue until S_1 or cease before S_1.

Another kind of sound, termed an Austin Flint murmur, can be heard in severe aortic insufficiency. This is a soft, low-pitched, rumbling middiastolic bruit produced by regurgitant blood flow from the aorta, which disrupts the anterior mitral valve leaflet. This occurs when there is a large amount of regurgitant blood flowing into the left ventricle when the aortic valve should be closed, but is incompletely sealed, during diastole.

In advanced stages of aortic insufficiency, there is both left and right ventricular failure with symptoms such as orthopnea, paroxysmal dyspnea, diaphoresis, hepatomegaly, ascites, and peripheral edema.

In aortic insufficiency, the left ventricular impulse can often be visible through the chest wall and is usually displaced laterally and inferiorly. A diastolic thrill is often palpable along the left sternal border and a systolic thrill may be palpable in the jugular notch of the sternum up toward the carotid arteries.

Diagnosis. Echocardiography is the major diagnostic test. ECG and laboratory studies that pertain to the etiology of the valvular disorder, such as blood cultures in infectious endocarditis, should also be done. An exercise treadmill test can evaluate coronary artery supply of the myocardium during exertion. Cardiac catheterization is useful to evaluate hemodynamic pressures in the heart chambers.

Treatment. Dobutamine is recommended to augment cardiac output and sodium nitroprusside to reduce afterload in hypertensive patients. Vasodilators may be used to enhance arterial circulation. Surgical implantation of a mechanical or bioprosthetic aortic valve is commonly performed. Mechanical valves are more durable but require long-term anticoagulation because of increased risk of thrombosis. Bioprosthetic valves are less durable and can deteriorate over time, but avoid the need for long-term anticoagulation.

Pulmonic Valve Disorders

The pulmonic valve is not a common site of pathology, but it is associated with disorders such as pulmonary stenosis and pulmonary insufficiency.

Pulmonic Stenosis

Pulmonic valve disorders can be caused by pulmonary hypertension, congenital rubella infection, or carcinoid syndrome. Pulmonic stenosis is a narrowing of the pulmonic valve, the entrance to the pulmonary artery from the right ventricle. Patients with mild pulmonic stenosis are usually asymptomatic and do not experience progression of the disease.

In severe pulmonic stenosis, blood must squeeze through the restrictive opening into the pulmonary artery during systole. Right ventricular ejection is prolonged and there is usually a delay in the closure of the pulmonic valve, causing a late P_2 component of S_2. The murmur is usually a harsh, systolic, crescendo-decrescendo sound heard best at the second intercostal space, left sternal border; this is commonly preceded by a systolic ejection sound. With right ventricular failure, the right atrium and ventricle enlarge and the patient experiences symptoms such as jugular venous distension, ascites, hepatomegaly, splenomegaly, and peripheral edema.

Diagnosis involves use of echocardiography, ECG, cardiac catheterization, and pulmonary angiogram. Medical treatment to diminish the effects of right ventricular failure includes diuretics and angiotensin-converting enzyme (ACE) inhibitors. Surgical valvotomy or percutaneous balloon valvuloplasty are the recommended treatment options.

Pulmonic Insufficiency

The most common disease affecting the pulmonic valve is regurgitation secondary to pulmonary hypertension, which is high blood pressure within the pulmonary arterial vasculature. Lung diseases that cause chronic hypoxia often cause pulmonary hypertension by stimulating vasoconstriction of pulmonary arterial vessels. Chronic obstructive pulmonary disease is an example of a disease that causes pulmonary hypertension.

In pulmonary hypertension, the valve of the pulmonary artery endures high pressure, becomes incompetent, and does not completely close during diastole. Incomplete closure of the pulmonic valve causes regurgitation of pulmonary artery blood back into the right ventricle during diastole. The murmur produced by this regurgitant flow is referred to as a Graham Steell murmur; it is a high pitched, decrescendo, blowing murmur heard best at the second intercostal space left sternal border, coinciding with or following S_2.

Diagnosis involves use of color Doppler echocardiography, cardiac catheterization, and pulmonary angiogram. Valve replacement and medical treatment for right-sided heart failure are recommended.

Tricuspid Valve Disorders

Tricuspid valve disorders include tricuspid stenosis and insufficiency. These are the least common valve disorders.

Tricuspid Stenosis

Tricuspid stenosis is mainly a sequela of RHD or infective endocarditis (IE). It is most commonly seen in intravenous drug abusers with IE. Staphylococcal organisms inhabit the skin and needle puncture allows the organisms to invade the venous bloodstream, which empties into the right side of the heart. The infection is then within the bloodstream (sepsis) and affects the tricuspid valve. Staphylococcal emboli can develop and gain entry into the lungs via the right ventricle and pulmonary artery.

In tricuspid stenosis, narrowing of the tricuspid valve hinders free flow of blood from the right atrium into the right ventricle during diastole. During diastole, the tricuspid valve should be open and allow filling of the right ventricle. With obstructed outflow into the right ventricle, hydrostatic pressure builds in the right atrium and backward into the venous system.

High hydrostatic pressure builds in the superior and inferior vena cava, evidenced by peritoneal, hepatic, and splenic congestion and peripheral edema. High pressure in the superior vena cava is demonstrated by jugular vein distension, which appears as bulging, blue enlarged veins in the neck. Peripheral edema is demonstrated by ascites, hepatomegaly, splenomegaly, and ankle or sacral edema.

On auscultation of tricuspid stenosis, the opening snap of the narrowed tricuspid valve may be heard early in diastole after S_2 over the left lower sternal border. The murmur is accentuated with inspiration because with chest expansion, there is distension and decreased resistance within the pulmonary arteries, which diminishes resistance against the right ventricle.

Echocardiography, cardiac catheterization, and blood cultures are used in diagnosis. Treatment mainly involves valve replacement, anticoagulants, and antibiotic medications. Treatment for right ventricular failure includes diuretics, digitalis, and ACE inhibitors. In infectious endocarditis, tricuspid valve removal is often performed. Most patients tolerate loss of the tricuspid valve well for years.

Tricuspid Insufficiency

Tricuspid regurgitation commonly occurs because of dilatation of the tricuspid valve annulus, which hinders complete closure of the valve leaflets. It can be caused by several disorders, including right ventricular infarction, rheumatic fever, infectious endocarditis, congenital heart disease, cardiomyopathy, pulmonary hypertension, and cor pulmonale.

Ebstein's anomaly is a congenital disorder that causes displacement of the tricuspid valve leaflets downward into the right ventricle. The tricuspid valve is placed low in the right ventricle, creating a small right ventricular chamber and large right atrium. Ebstein's anomaly commonly causes tricuspid insufficiency, atrial dysrhythmias, and right ventricular dysfunction.

Tricuspid insufficiency occurs because a loose tricuspid valve allows blood flow to back up from the right ventricle into the right atrium during systole. The S_1 sound is created by the closure of the tricuspid and mitral valves. However, with incomplete closure of loose tricuspid valve leaflets, a holosystolic murmur is heard that may make S_1 inaudible. The murmur is heard best along the left lower sternal border, and a right ventricular thrill may be palpable along the sternal border on the chest wall. As with tricuspid stenosis, the murmur of tricuspid insufficiency is accentuated with inspiration because expansion of the thoracic cage allows increased venous return.

The blood flow that backs up from the right ventricle into the right atrium causes distension and dilatation of the right atrium. With stretching of the right atrial wall, the SA node and conductive tissue are disrupted and atrial fibrillation can develop. With time, volume overload of the right atrium and right ventricle causes right ventricular failure and associated symptoms. In right ventricular failure, venous congestion causes jugular venous distension, ascites, hepatomegaly, splenomegaly, and ankle or sacral edema.

Echocardiography, cardiac catheterization, and blood cultures are used in diagnosis. Blood cultures are necessary because infectious endocarditis is common. A large number of patients with tricuspid insufficiency are intravenous drug abusers. Puncture of veins with unsterile needles frequently leads to blood infection (sepsis), which requires antibiotic therapy. Medications for right ventricular failure such as diuretics, digitalis and ACE inhibitors are also used. In Epstein's anomaly, valve replacement is usually necessary. However, in infective endocarditis, the tricuspid valve is usually removed. Most patients can still have normal heart function with loss of the tricuspid valve.

Chapter Summary

- Heart valves are structures composed of fibrous tissue covered by endothelial cardiac tissue.
- Heart valves direct the blood through the heart and great vessels.
- Heart valves can be damaged or deformed because of genetic disorders, infectious agents, myocardial infarction, the aging process, and atherosclerosis.
- A heart murmur is the classic auscultatory finding indicative of valvular heart disease; it is described according to its occurrence in the cardiac cycle, volume, pitch, and location of auscultation on the chest wall.
- There are classic landmarks on the chest wall where the sounds of specific heart valves can be heard best.

- Echocardiography is the method of choice to precisely diagnose valvular disease. Damaged valves can cause a variety of complications, including blood flow turbulence and stasis, heart chamber pressure changes, thrombi formation, heart failure, and sepsis.
- Stenotic valves are narrowed and restrict blood flow, whereas insufficient valves do not close completely, allowing regurgitant blood flow.
- Aortic stenosis, mitral stenosis, mitral valve prolapse, and mitral insufficiency are among the most common valvular disorders.

- Aortic sclerosis and mitral annular calcification are common causes of heart murmurs in elderly adults.
- HCM is the most common cause of sudden death of young athletes.
- Infectious endocarditis in intravenous drug abusers commonly causes tricuspid valvular dysfunction.
- Before any invasive procedure such as dental treatment or catheter placement, most patients with a valvular disorder should have antibiotics administered to prevent possible endocarditis and septicemia.

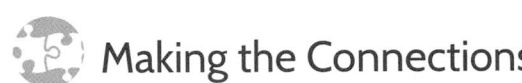 Making the Connections

Disorder and Pathophysiology	Signs and Symptoms	Physical Assessment Findings	Diagnostic Testing	Treatment
Mitral Stenosis | Narrowed mitral valve opening; blood flow hindered from left atrium into left ventricle during diastole. Left atrial pressure builds and backs up into pulmonary veins to pulmonary capillaries, causing pulmonary edema.				
	Dyspnea, cough, fatigue, orthopnea, PND.	Opening snap, diastolic murmur fifth intercostal space left sternal border after S_2 before S_1. If severe, bibasilar pulmonary crackles.	Echocardiogram showing narrowed mitral valve; may show left atrial enlargement from backflow of blood. ECG may show atrial fibrillation caused by enlarged left atrium.	Oxygen. Anticoagulation to prevent clot formation in enlarged, stretched left atrium. Heart failure medications such as diuretics, ACE inhibitors, digitalis, beta blockers. Surgical valve replacement.
Mitral Insufficiency | Incompetent mitral valve leaflets that cannot close; during systolic contraction of left ventricle, blood regurgitates up into the left atrium. Left ventricular ejection is decreased and backup of blood into the left atrium, pulmonary veins, and pulmonary capillaries occurs, which causes pulmonary edema. Aortic blood volume is diminished, as is blood volume entering coronary arteries. Myocardial ischemia results.				
	Dyspnea, cough, fatigue, orthopnea, PND. Chest pain (angina).	Holosystolic murmur, fifth intercostal space, left sternal border radiating into the axilla. S_3 may be heard. If severe, bibasilar pulmonary crackles heard. Pallor, diaphoresis, respiratory distress.	Echocardiogram showing regurgitant mitral valve leaflets; may show left atrial and ventricular enlargement. ECG may show atrial fibrillation.	Oxygen. Anticoagulation to prevent clot formation in the left atrium. Heart failure medications such as diuretics, ACE inhibitors, digitalis, and beta blockers. Coronary artery disease medications such as oxygen, morphine, and nitrates if myocardial ischemia. Surgical valve replacement.

Continued

Making the Connections–cont'd

Disorder and Pathophysiology	Signs and Symptoms	Physical Assessment Findings	Diagnostic Testing	Treatment

Mitral Valve Prolapse | A disorder caused by a myxomatous degeneration of one or both mitral valve leaflets that makes them floppy. One or both mitral valve leaflets occasionally prolapse into the left atrium during systolic contraction of the left ventricle, allowing for some regurgitation of blood flow up into the left atrium.

| | Asymptomatic in many affected persons; if severe, ischemic chest pain, dyspnea, and fatigue occur. | Midsystolic or late systolic murmur heard after a midsystolic click, at left lower sternal border. | Echocardiogram showing regurgitant mitral valve leaflet; may show left atrial and ventricular enlargement. | Commonly no treatment is necessary. If myocardial ischemia: oxygen, nitrates, beta blockers, morphine. |

Aortic Stenosis | Narrowed aortic valve opening; blood flow hindered from fully ejecting into aorta from left ventricle; coronary arteries suffer lack of sufficient blood flow. Aortic blood flow is low and may diminish blood flow to cerebral arteries. Left ventricle can also fail because of high resistance of aortic opening.

| | Chest pain (angina pectoris), fatigue, exertional dyspnea, exertional syncope (fainting caused by lack of cerebral blood flow). | Systolic ejection murmur, second intercostal space, right sternal border, opening snap, crescendo, low-pitched murmur after S_1 before S_2, split S_2 ($P_2 A_2$). | Echocardiogram showing narrowed aortic valve, left ventricular enlargement, left ventricular hypertrophy caused by excess resistance of aorta against left ventricle. Cardiac catheterization to measure hemodynamic pressures in heart chambers. | Treatment according to symptoms of angina or heart failure. Anticoagulation to prevent clot formation on valve deformity or left ventricular failure. Surgical valve replacement. |

Hypertrophic Cardiomyopathy | Interventricular septum is disproportionately enlarged, the left ventricle is eccentrically hypertrophied, and the anterior mitral leaflet opens against the enlarged septum, creating an obstructed outflow of blood from the left ventricle into the aorta.

| | Commonly asymptomatic. Sudden ventricular dysrhythmias can occur, causing sudden death. Few patients experience chest pain, dyspnea, and fatigue as warning signs. | Harsh, diamond-shaped systolic murmur; begins after S_1 at the lower left sternal border and apex. Ejection of blood flow is usually unimpeded until late in systole; therefore, the murmur occurs after a clear S_1. | Echocardiogram shows an enlarged interventricular septum, left ventricular hypertrophy. ECG needed to check for ventricular dysrhythmias. Cardiac catheterization to check hemodynamic pressure changes in heart chambers. | Surgical reduction of the interventricular septum (cardiac myomectomy). Implantable cardioverter-defibrillator. Medications for angina or for heart failure. depending on patient condition. |

Aortic Insufficiency | Incompetent aortic valve allows leakage of blood back into left ventricle and possibly left atrium, insufficient blood flow forward into aorta.

| | Chest pain (angina pectoris), fatigue, exertional dyspnea, exertional syncope (fainting), cough, dyspnea, PND, and orthopnea. | Diastolic murmur, third intercostal space, left sternal border, high-pitched, blowing, decrescendo. If severe, bibasilar pulmonary crackles. | Echocardiogram shows regurgitant aortic valve, left ventricular dilatation from excess regurgitant blood volume. Cardiac catheterization. | Anticoagulation to prevent clot formation. Angina or heart failure medications, depending on the patient presentation. Surgical valve replacement. |

Continued

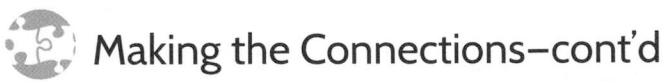

Making the Connections–cont'd

Disorder and Pathophysiology	Signs and Symptoms	Physical Assessment Findings	Diagnostic Testing	Treatment
Tricuspid Stenosis | Narrowed tricuspid valve hinders free flow of blood into the right ventricle during diastole; blood damming in the right atrium causes high hydrostatic pressure to build backward into the venous system.				
	Signs of increased venous pressure, jugular venous distension, ascites, hepatomegaly, splenomegaly, or ankle or sacral edema.	Opening snap after S_2, diastolic murmur over left lower sternal border, inspiration accentuates murmur.	Echocardiogram shows narrowed tricuspid valve, right atrial dilatation from obstructed blood flow, central veins congested. ECG may show atrial fibrillation. Blood cultures.	Anticoagulation to prevent clot formation. Heart failure medications. Surgical valve replacement or removal of valve. Antibiotics if infective endocarditis.
Tricuspid Insufficiency | Incompetent tricuspid valve does not close during right ventricular contraction, regurgitation of blood flow into the right atrium with each right ventricular contraction; increases backward pressure into the venous system.				
	Signs of increased venous pressure, jugular venous distension, ascites, hepatomegaly, splenomegaly, or ankle or sacral edema.	Blowing, holosystolic murmur at lower left sternal border that may obscure S_1, prominent right ventricular pulsation, accentuated murmur with inspiration.	Echocardiogram showing incompetent tricuspid valve, right atrial dilatation from regurgitant blood flow, central veins congested. ECG may show right atrial fibrillation. Blood cultures.	Anticoagulation to prevent clot formation. Heart failure medications. Surgical valve replacement. Antibiotics if infective endocarditis.
Pulmonic Stenosis | Narrowed pulmonic valve does not allow sufficient blood flow into the pulmonary artery; backup of blood into right ventricle, right ventricle hypertrophies against increased pulmonary artery resistance.				
	Fatigue, dyspnea, signs of right ventricular failure; jugular venous distension, ascites, hepatomegaly, splenomegaly, or ankle or sacral edema.	Harsh, systolic, crescendo-decrescendo murmur at the second intercostal space, left sternal, commonly preceded by a systolic ejection sound, split S_2 with delayed P_2.	Echocardiogram showing narrowed pulmonic valve, right ventricular hypertrophy, right ventricular and right atrial dilatation from built up blood, central veins congested. ECG may show atrial fibrillation.	Anticoagulation to prevent clot formation. Heart failure medications. Surgical valve replacement.
Pulmonic Insufficiency | Incompetent pulmonic valve allows regurgitant blood flow from pulmonary artery into right ventricle; dilatation of the right ventricle and right atrium possible with backup of hydrostatic pressure into the venous system.				
	Fatigue, dyspnea, signs of right ventricular failure; jugular venous distension, ascites, hepatomegaly, splenomegaly, or ankle or sacral edema.	Graham Steell murmur; a high-pitched, decrescendo, blowing murmur heard best at the second intercostal space, left sternal border coinciding with or following S_2.	Echocardiogram shows incompetent pulmonic valve, right ventricular and right atrial dilatation from built up blood, central vein congestion. ECG may show atrial fibrillation.	Anticoagulation to prevent clot formation. Heart failure medications. Surgical valve replacement.

Bibliography

Anilkumar, M. (2013). Patent ductus arteriosus. *Card Clin*, 31(3), 417–430. doi: 10.1016/j.ccl.2013.05.006.

Aronow, W. S. (2013). A review of the pathophysiology, diagnosis, and treatment of aortic valve stenosis in elderly patients. *Hosp Pract* (1995), 41(4), 66–77. doi: 10.3810/hp.2013.10.1082.

Barrett, K. E., Barman, S. M., Boitano, S., & Brooks, H. L. (2012). *Ganong's review of medical physiology*. 24th ed. New York: Lange/McGraw-Hill.

Bonow, R. O. (2013). Improving outlook for elderly patients with aortic stenosis. *JAMA*, 310(19), 2045–2047. doi: 10.1001/jama.2013.281825.

Bouzas-Mosquera, A., Alvarez-Garcia, N., & Peteiro, J. (2010). Repair of mitral-valve prolapse. *N Engl J Med*, 362(9), 857.

Brinkley, D. M., & Gelfand, E. V. (2013). Valvular heart disease: classic teaching and emerging paradigms. *Am J Med*, 126(12), 1035–1042. doi: 10.1016/j.amjmed.2013.05.022. Epub 2013 Oct 11.

Carabello, B. A., & Paulus, W. J. (2009). Aortic stenosis. *Lancet*, 373(9667), 956–966.

Chandrashekhar, Y., Westaby, S., & Narula, J. (2009). Mitral stenosis. *Lancet*, 374(9697), 1271–1283.

Chang, H. J., Lynm, C., & Glass, R. M. (2009). *JAMA* patient page. Hypertrophic cardiomyopathy. *JAMA*, 302(15), 1720.

Choby, B. A. (2009). Diagnosis and treatment of streptococcal pharyngitis. *Am Fam Phys*, 79(5), 383–390.

Desai, C. S., & Bonow, R. O. (2012). Transcatheter valve replacement for aortic stenosis: balancing benefits, risks, and expectations. *JAMA*, 308(6), 573–574. doi: 10.1001/jama.2012.9427.

Dorn, G. W., 2nd. (2013). Shared genetic risk for sclerosis of valves and vessels. *N Engl J Med*, 368(6), 569–570. doi: 10.1056/NEJMe1215152. No abstract available. Erratum in: *N Engl J Med*. 2013 Jun 20;368(25):2442.

Dunne, B., Marr, T., Kim, D., et al. (2014). Infective endocarditis. *Heart Lung Circ*, Mar 6. pii: S1443-9506(14)00081-X. doi: 10.1016/j.hlc.2014.02.010. Epub ahead of print.

Enriquez-Sarano, M., Akins, C. W., & Vahanian, A. (2009). Mitral regurgitation. *Lancet*, 373(9672), 1382–1394.

Erwin, J. P., & Otto, C. M. (2014). Infective endocarditis: old problem, new guidelines and still much to learn. *Heart*, May 3. doi: 10.1136/heartjnl-2014-305836. Epub ahead of print.

Feldman, T., Foster, E., Glower, D. D., et al. (2011). Percutaneous repair or surgery for mitral regurgitation. *N Engl J Med*, 364(15), 1395–1406.

Foster, E. (2010). Clinical practice. Mitral regurgitation due to degenerative mitral-valve disease. *N Engl J Med*, 363(2), 156–165.

Grimard, B. H., & Larson, J. M. (2008). Aortic stenosis: diagnosis and treatment. *Am Fam Phys*, 78(6), 717–724.

Hough, A., & Woods, D. (2014). Antithrombotic therapy after transcatheter aortic valve replacement. *JAMA*, 311(12), 1249–1250. doi: 10.1001/jama.2014.1180.

Jackson, G., Camargo, C., Ling, L. F., Kalahasti, V., & Rimmerman, C. M. (2013). The clinical picture: fever, dyspnea, and a new heart murmur. *Cleveland Clin J Med*, 80(9), 559–561. doi: 10.3949/ccjm.80a.12049.

Kodali, S. K., Williams, M. R., Smith, C. R., et al. (2012). Two-year outcomes after transcatheter or surgical aortic-valve replacement. *N Engl J Med*, 366(18), 1686–1695. Epub 2012 Mar 26.

Kumar, V., Abbas, A. K., Fausto, N., & Aster, J. C. (2010). *Robbins & Cotran pathologic basis of disease*. 8th ed. Philadelphia, PA: Saunders/Elsevier.

Lahaye, S., Lincoln, J., & Garg, V. (2014). Genetics of valvular heart disease. *Curr Cardiol Rep*, 16(6), 487. doi: 10.1007/s11886-014-0487-2.

Leon, M. B., Smith, C. R., Mack, M., et al. (2010). Transcatheter aortic-valve implantation for aortic stenosis in patients who cannot undergo surgery. *N Engl J Med*, 63(17), 1597–1607.

Longo, D. L., Fauci, A. S., Kasper, D. L., et al. (2011). *Harrison's principles of internal medicine*. 18th ed. New York: McGraw-Hill.

Ma, I., & Tierney, L. M. (2010). Name that murmur—eponyms for the astute auscultician. *N Engl J Med*, 363(22), 2164–2168. doi: 10.1056/NEJMon1006947.

Mack, M. J., Brennan, J. M., Brindis, R., et al. (2013). Outcomes following transcatheter aortic valve replacement in the United States. *JAMA*, 310(19), 2069–2077. doi: 10.1001/jama.2013.282043.

Maganti, K., Rigolin, V. H., Sarano, M. E., & Bonow, R. O. (2010). Valvular heart disease: diagnosis and management. *Mayo Clin Proceed*, 85(5), 483–500.

Manning, W. J. (2013). Asymptomatic aortic stenosis in the elderly: a clinical review. *JAMA*, 310(14), 1490–1497. doi: 10.1001/jama.2013.279194.

Marijon, E., Mirabel, M., Celermajer, D. S., & Jouven, X. (2012). Rheumatic heart disease. *Lancet*, 379(9819), 953–964.

Martínez-Sellés, M., Muñoz, P., Estevez, A., et al. (2008). Long-term outcome of infective endocarditis in non-intravenous drug users. *Mayo Clin Proceed*, 83(11), 1213–1217.

Maurice, J. (2013). Rheumatic heart disease back in the limelight. *Lancet*, 382(9898), 1085–1086.

McGee, S. (2010). Etiology and diagnosis of systolic murmurs in adults. *Am J Med*, 123(10), 913–921.e1. doi: 10.1016/j.amjmed.2010.04.027.

McPhee, S. J., & Papadakis, M. A. (2012). *Current medical diagnosis and treatment*. New York: Lange/McGraw-Hill.

Michelena, H. I., Topilsky, Y., Suri, R., & Enriquez-Sarano, M. (2011). Degenerative mitral valve regurgitation: understanding basic concepts and new developments. *Postgraduate Med*, 123(2), 56–69.

Nishimura, R. A., Carabello, B. A., Faxon, D. P., et al. (2008). ACC/AHA 2008 guideline update on valvular heart disease: focused update on infective endocarditis: a report of the American College of Cardiology/American Heart Association Task Force on Practice Guidelines endorsed by the Society of Cardiovascular Anesthesiologists, Society for Cardiovascular Angiography and Interventions, and Society of Thoracic Surgeons. *J Am Coll Card*, 52(8), 676–685. doi: 10.1016/j.jacc.2008.05.008.

Nishimura, R. A., & Otto, C. (2014). 2014 ACC/AHA valve guidelines: earlier intervention for chronic mitral regurgitation. *Heart*, Mar 31. doi: 10.1136/heartjnl-2014-305834. Epub ahead of print. No abstract available.

Nishimura, R. A., Otto, C. M., Bonow, R. O., et al. (2014a). 2014 AHA/ACC guideline for the management of patients with valvular heart disease: a report of the American College of Cardiology/American Heart Association Task Force on Practice Guidelines. *J Am Coll Cardiol*. 2014 Mar 3. pii: S0735-1097(14)01279-0. doi: 10.1016/j.jacc.2014.02.536. Epub ahead of print. No abstract available.

Nishimura, R. A., Otto, C. M., Bonow, R. O., et al. (2014b). 2014 AHA/ACC guideline for the management of patients with valvular heart disease: executive summary: a report of the American College of Cardiology/American Heart Association Task Force on Practice Guidelines. *J Am Coll Cardiol*, Mar 3. pii: S0735-1097(14)01280-7. doi: 10.1016/j.jacc.2014.02.537. Epub ahead of print. No abstract available.

Novaro, G. M., Houghtaling, P. L., Gillinov, A. M., Blackstone, E. H., & Asher, C. R. (2013). Prevalence of mitral valve prolapse and congenital bicuspid aortic valves in black and white patients undergoing cardiac valve operations. *Am J Card*, 111(6), 898–901. doi: 10.1016/j.amjcard.2012.11.051. Epub 2012 Dec 28.

Omer, S., Kar, B., Cornwell, L. D., et al. (2013). Early experience of a transcatheter aortic valve program at a Veterans Affairs facility. *JAMA Surg*, 148(12), 1087–1093. doi: 10.1001/jamasurg.2013.3743.

Otto, C. M. (2008). Calcific aortic stenosis—time to look more closely at the valve. *N Engl J Med*, 359(13), 1395–1398.

Otto, C. M., & Verrier, E. D. (2011). Mitral regurgitation—what is best for my patient? *N Engl J Med,* 364(15), 1462–1463.

Penny, D. J., & Vick, G. W. (2011). Ventricular septal defect. *Lancet,* 377(9771), 1103–1112.

Pierce, D., Calkins, B. C., & Thornton, K. (2012). Infectious endocarditis: diagnosis and treatment. *Am Fam Phys*, 85(10), 981–986.

Rahimtoola, S. H. (2014). The year in valvular heart disease: 2014. *J Am Coll Cardiol.* 2014 Jan 30. pii: S0735-1097(14)00337-4. doi: 10.1016/j.jacc.2014.01.024. Epub ahead of print. Review.

Schaff, H. V. (2011). Transcatheter aortic-valve implantation—at what price? *N Engl J Med*, 364(23), 2256–2258. Epub 2011 Jun 5.

Smith, C. R., Leon, M. B., Mack, M. J., et al. (2011). Transcatheter versus surgical aortic-valve replacement in high-risk patients. *N Engl J Med*, 364(23), 2187–2198. Epub 2011 Jun 5.

Tajouri, T. H., Kumar, G., & Klarich, K. W. (2010). 51-year-old man with heart murmur. *Mayo Clin Proceed,* 85(11), 1052–1055.

Taubert, K. A. (2008). Endocarditis prophylaxis: an evolution of change. *Am Fam Phys*, 77(4), 421–422.

Verma, S., & Mesana, T. G. (2009). Mitral-valve repair for mitral-valve prolapse. *N Engl J Med,* 361(23), 2261–2269.

Watkins, H., Ashrafian, H., & Redwood, C. (2011). Inherited cardiomyopathies. *N Engl J Med*, 364(17), 1643–1656.

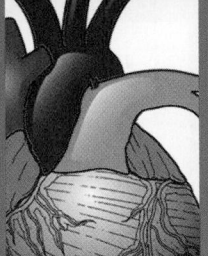

Disorders of the Venous System

Key Terms

D-dimer test

Deep venous thromboembolism (DVT)

Gradient compression stockings

Greenfield filter

Homan's sign

International normalized ratio (INR)

Pneumatic compression device

Pulmonary embolism

Sclerotherapy

Stasis dermatitis

Varicose veins

Venous ulcer

Ventilation-perfusion scan (V-Q scan)

Virchow's triad

Wells criteria

Chronic venous disorders of the lower limbs rank among the most common conditions affecting individuals. There is a wide spectrum of disease that varies from asymptomatic, minor **varicose veins** to disabling deep venous thrombosis. In contrast to many other chronic conditions, patients often accept venous disease as a slowly progressive condition related to aging and do not seek health care for these disorders. Although venous disease is most common in adults older than age 50, immobility at any age increases susceptibility to **deep venous thromboembolism (DVT)**—a potentially fatal disease.

Epidemiology

There are mainly three different types of venous disease: venous insufficiency, DVT, and varicose veins. Venous disease is a common disorder that is more prevalent in women, increases with age, and is a major cause of illness. Between 6% and 30% of all medical expenditures for cardiovascular disease are for venous disease. Chronic venous disease of the legs commonly occurs in the general population and is underreported. Studies estimate that the prevalence of varicose veins, the most common venous disorder, is as high as 56% in men and 60% in women. **Venous ulcers** are less common, affecting approximately 0.3% of the adult population. Deep venous thrombosis is one of the most underdiagnosed diseases, but studies estimate it affects 80 persons per 100,000 annually.

Basic Concepts of Venous Structure and Function

Veins are thin-walled, flexible blood vessels that return blood to the heart. Their walls are composed of three layers: tunica intima, which is an endothelial cell

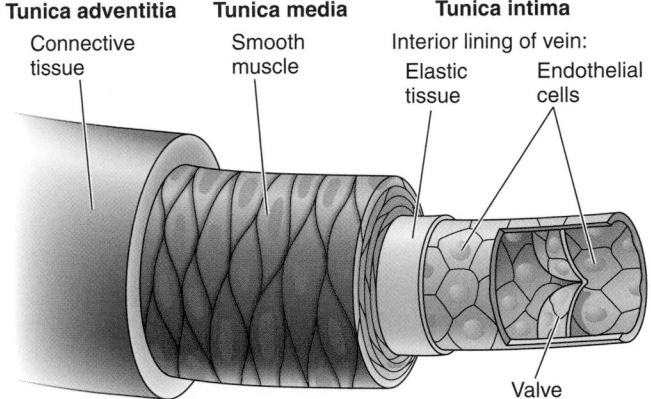

Tunica adventitia — Connective tissue

Tunica media — Smooth muscle

Tunica intima — Interior lining of vein: Elastic tissue, Endothelial cells

Valve

Figure 19-1. Anatomy of a vein. A vein is a collapsible, thin-walled vessel. Different from arteries, veins contain a thin wall of smooth muscle and valvular structures.

lining; tunica media, a thin layer of smooth muscle; and tunica adventitia, an exterior layer of connective tissue (see Fig. 19-1).

There are two systems of veins: (1) superficial, small diameter veins and (2) deep, large diameter veins. Perforating veins connect the two systems. Blood from the skin and subcutaneous tissue collects in the superficial veins, which empty into the perforating veins. From the perforating veins, blood travels into the deep veins, which empty into the body's major venous vessels, the inferior and superior vena cava, which empty into the right atrium.

The venous system and right side of the heart are low pressure regions. Veins do not pump blood as do arteries; instead, they direct blood toward the heart. In the extremities, veins rely on the supportive action of skeletal muscles that help pump the blood toward the heart. When an individual is walking, the gastrocnemius muscle in the calf provides pumping action for venous blood to return to the heart. Also, within the lumen of the veins are valves that prevent retrograde flow of venous blood (see Fig. 19-2).

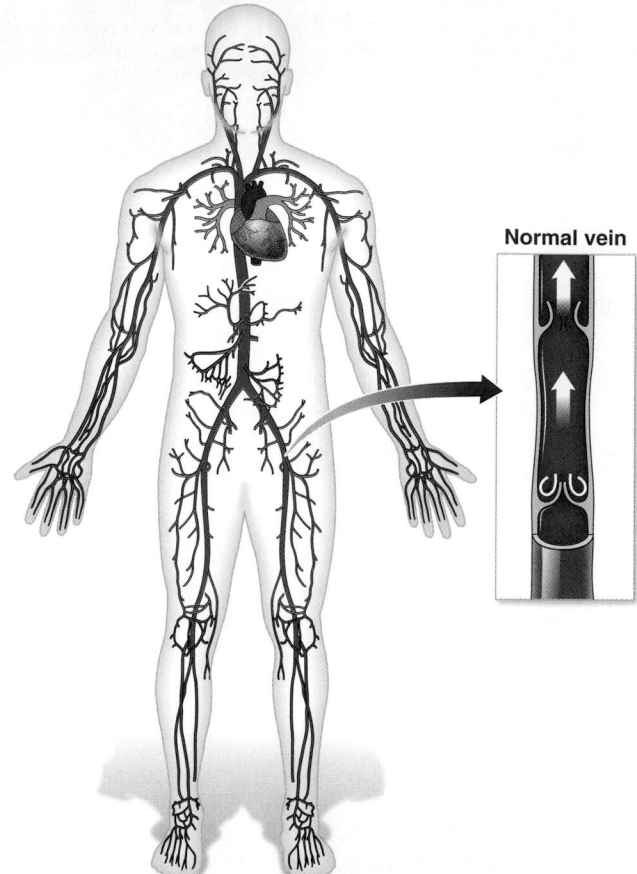

Figure 19-2. Valves of a deep vein. Valves keep the flow of venous blood up toward the heart.

Normal vein

Veins carry deoxygenated blood back to the right side of the heart and into the pulmonary artery, moving to the lungs for oxygenation. The exception to this rule occurs in the pulmonary veins and pulmonary artery. Pulmonary veins carry oxygenated blood from the lungs to the left atrium. The pulmonary artery carries the deoxygenated blood into the lungs from the right ventricle. The deoxygenated blood within the veins is a dark red color, which appears blue because of the light dispersion on the skin.

Veins are large capacity vessels that carry almost two-thirds of the body's blood volume. Their walls can expand to hold a large volume of blood, which renders the system susceptible to stasis of blood. The number of valves and anatomy and structural strength of veins differ among people. The hardiness of the veins is an inheritable quality, which explains familial predisposition to development of venous insufficiency.

Basic Pathophysiologic Concepts of Venous Dysfunction

The return of venous blood to the heart constantly opposes the downward pull of gravity. The unidirectional blood flow up to the heart is dependent on valvular competence and skeletal muscle contraction against the vessel walls. Prolonged standing or any obstruction to upward blood flow from the lower extremities places excess pressure on the valves of the veins. Obesity and pregnancy are the two main conditions that cause weakness of the valve leaflets with resultant retrograde flow of venous blood. Retrograde blood flow leads to stasis of venous blood and susceptibility to thrombus formation, the conditions known as venous insufficiency.

Venous insufficiency occurs in the superficial or deep venous system. Superficial venous incompetence is the most common form of venous disease. In superficial venous insufficiency, the deep veins are normal, but venous blood flows backward through distended superficial veins in which the valves have failed. The superficial veins that become distended and distorted under the high pressure are termed **varicose veins**.

Venous insufficiency in the deep veins can also occur as in the superficial veins because of valvular dysfunction. In deep venous insufficiency, after prolonged standing, the veins are completely filled, and all the venous valves are open. Venous congestion and high hydrostatic capillary pressure develop in the lower extremities, which causes edema in the interstitial tissues. Within the tissue there is poor clearance of waste products, cellular debris, carbon dioxide, and lactic acid. Wounds in this area are difficult to heal.

Unlike superficial vein insufficiency, deep venous insufficiency can lead to deep venous thrombosis, a potentially fatal condition. Thrombus formation can occur in a deep vein in the leg and then travel within the bloodstream, at which point it is called **deep venous thromboembolism (DVT)**.

Pathophysiology of Selected Venous Disorders

The major venous disorders include chronic venous insufficiency, DVT, varicose veins, and venous ulcers.

Deep Venous Thromboembolism

DVT is a term that is used to encompass both deep venous thrombosis and pulmonary embolism (PE). DVT occurs when a thrombus develops in a deep leg vein accompanied by inflammation. The thrombus can travel as an embolism within the venous system, then enter the lungs, where it becomes a PE, a potentially fatal consequence.

Epidemiology

The exact incidence of DVT is unknown because many episodes go undiagnosed; however, data indicate that DVT occurs in 80 patients per 100,000 annually. It is estimated that approximately 1 person in 20 will develop DVT over the course of his or her lifetime. Approximately 600,000 hospitalizations per year occur for DVT in the United States.

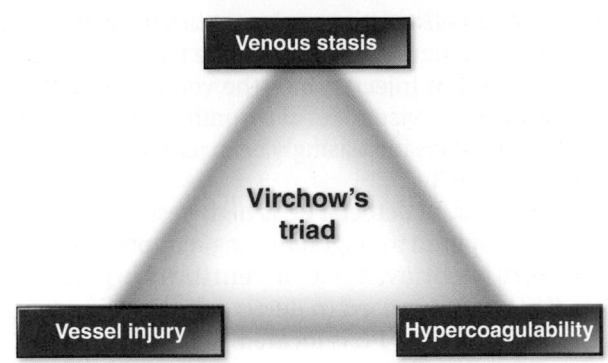

Figure 19-3. Virchow's triad. Virchow's triad describes the three risk factors that contribute to formation of a venous clot: hypercoagulability, venous stasis, and vascular damage.

Etiology

The predisposing factors to DVT are venous stasis, vascular damage, and hypercoagulability, a trio of risk factors that together are known as **Virchow's triad** (see Fig. 19-3). Venous stasis occurs because of poor venous return associated with sedentary behavior or valve dysfunction in the leg veins. Venous blood tends to pool in the lower extremities, and stagnant blood forms clots. Conditions that cause vascular damage such as surgery or trauma can also lead to DVT. Vein injury often leads to endothelial injury, inflammation, platelet aggregation, and stimulus of the coagulation cascade, which in turn causes formation of a clot. Any condition that causes hypercoagulability of blood can also lead to DVT. Cancers, which commonly secrete coagulation factors, and high estrogen states, which increase blood coagulability, increase risk of DVT as well. Other conditions that can contribute to formation of DVT are obesity and smoking, as both increase the risk of clot formation. Orthopedic surgery in particular causes a high risk of DVT because of vein injury during surgery and venous stasis, commonly associated with postoperative conditions.

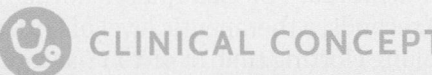

CLINICAL CONCEPT

DVT occurs in 50% of postoperative orthopedic surgery patients.

Pathophysiology

DVT occurs when a thrombus develops in a deep vein in the lower extremity. The thrombus forms at an area of inflammation in the vein. The sequel to DVT is **pulmonary embolism (PE).** A venous thrombus can travel from the leg vein into the inferior vena cava (IVC) and then continue upward into the right side of the heart and into the pulmonary arterial circulation. When the thrombus enters the pulmonary circulation, it becomes a PE, which is frequently fatal (see Fig. 19-4). Venous

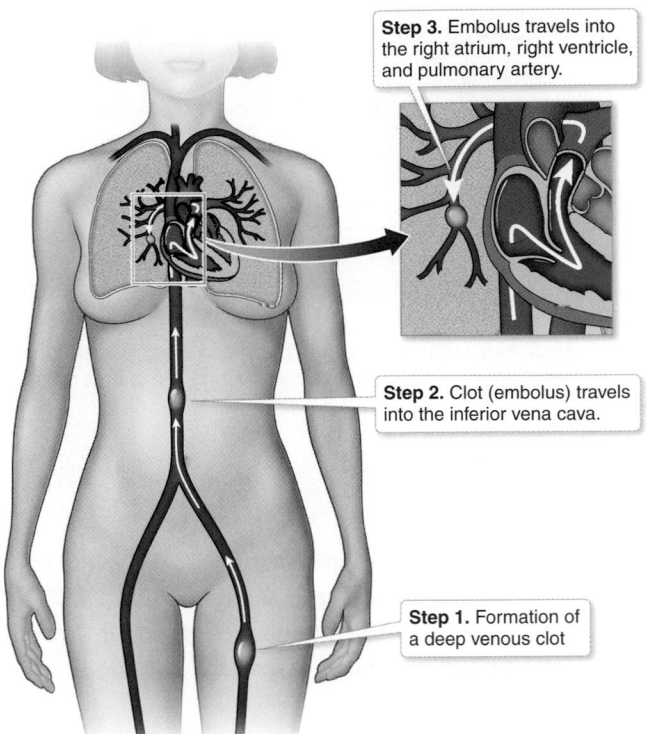

Step 3. Embolus travels into the right atrium, right ventricle, and pulmonary artery.

Step 2. Clot (embolus) travels into the inferior vena cava.

Step 1. Formation of a deep venous clot

Figure 19-4. Formation of a PE from a DVT. A clot (called a DVT) forms in the deep vein of a lower extremity and travels into the IVC. From the IVC, the clot travels into the right atrium of the heart, then right ventricle, and finally lodges in a pulmonary artery or arteriole. At the pulmonary arteriole, the PE can obstruct the diffusion of oxygen into the bloodstream.

thrombi often form silently and increase in size without producing manifestations. Deep venous thrombi can develop in the hips, knee, calf, or pelvic veins. Any condition that increases coagulation of the venous blood can cause DVT.

Clinical Presentation

The patient that develops DVT will commonly have a condition that causes either venous stasis, venous injury, or hypercoagulability. A patient may have venous stasis caused by immobility or sedentary behavior. The patient may have a history of venous injury such as trauma or recent surgery. The patient should be questioned about recent history of cancer, recent surgery, use of estrogen, and smoking, as these conditions increase the risk of DVT.

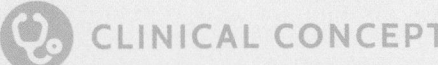

CLINICAL CONCEPT

Any surgical procedure can increase the risk for DVT, especially those of the lower extremity.

The physical examination findings associated with DVT include redness, ropiness, tenderness, or warmth over a vein; edema; and a positive **Homan's sign** (see Fig. 19-5).

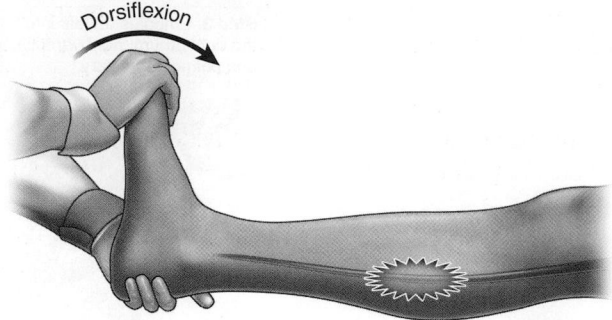

Figure 19-5. Homan's sign. Homan's sign can be an indication of a DVT. Dorsiflexion of the foot causes pain in the calf at the location of a DVT.

 CLINICAL CONCEPT

Homan's sign is pathognomonic for DVT. For Homan's sign, place the patient in the supine position with a straight knee and dorsiflex the patient's foot. If DVT is present, pain will be elicited in the calf.

Diagnosis

DVT is diagnosed through clinical examination in conjunction with the **D-dimer test,** which is a blood test that detects the presence of fibrin clot degradation products in the blood. The **Wells criteria** is used to evaluate clinical signs of DVT such as leg swelling and tenderness along a vein. The criterion summarizes the risk of DVT with a score between 0 and 3. D-dimer levels may be elevated in any medical condition where clots form, so the level is only used to rule out DVT, not to confirm a diagnosis of DVT. D-dimer levels remain elevated in DVT and PE for about 7 days. A negative D-dimer assay in combination with a Well's criteria score of fewer than 2 rules out the possibility of DVT. All patients with a positive D-dimer assay and a Wells criteria score of greater than or equal to 2 require duplex ultrasonography, which is a test that combines ultrasound images with Doppler blood flow studies. The absence of normal phasic Doppler signals arising from changes to venous flow in an extremity provides indirect evidence of venous occlusion.

Another diagnostic test, impedance plethysmography (IPG), is a noninvasive procedure that records changes in blood volume of an extremity. IPG can determine the

 CLINICAL CONCEPT

MRI is the diagnostic test of choice for suspected iliac vein or IVC thrombosis when CT venography is contraindicated or technically inadequate. In suspected calf vein thrombosis, MRI is more sensitive than any other noninvasive study.

existence of an obstruction such as a thrombus in venous outflow. CT venography is an invasive test that requires contrast medium injected into the venous system and CT scanning to visualize a thrombus in the lower extremity. MRI has increasingly been used for evaluation of suspected DVT.

The best test to detect a PE is high-resolution multidetector computed tomographic angiography (MDCTA). If this test is not available, a **ventilation-perfusion scan (V-Q scan)** is used to detect a lack of circulation in the lungs where a PE is located.

Treatment

Preventive strategies should be employed in all patients at increased risk for DVT. While a patient is immobile, sequential venous compression devices may be used to promote venous return. These devices are usually used with antiembolism stockings. They alternate inflation and deflation of chambers to provide sequential pressure over the lower extremity and promote venous return. When the patient is out of bed in a chair, his or her feet should be elevated to promote venous return. The patient should be taught not to stand for prolonged periods, to avoid constricting garments, to elevate legs periodically during the day, and to ambulate or do leg exercises that will promote blood flow and reduce venous stasis.

Patients are also treated prophylactically with drugs that interfere with clotting. Factor Xa inhibitors, direct thrombin inhibitors, low molecular weight heparin, unfractionated heparin, and warfarin are the medications used for DVT. To monitor the therapeutic effects of heparin and warfarin, prothrombin time (PT) and activated partial thromboplastin time (aPTT) lab tests have been used. Each of these tests measures the time it takes for the blood to clot; PT measures the extrinsic coagulation system and aPTT measures the intrinsic coagulation system. The actual blood clotting time is given in seconds and the normal blood clotting time is given for comparison. The goal is to prolong clotting time in DVT, so a clotting time that is 1.5 to 2.5 times normal is achieved. For example, if normal clotting time is 30 seconds, a therapeutic level of anticoagulant would prolong clotting time to 45 to 75 seconds. While the patient is on anticoagulants, the PT and aPTT have to be measured often. A simpler blood test called an **international normalized ratio (INR)** can also be used to monitor anticoagulant therapy. The INR indicates clotting time, which has to be kept in a specific range to avoid excessive anticoagulation. An INR result between 2 and 3 is commonly required for adequate anticoagulation.

Thrombolytic agents, also known as "clot busters," are effective in DVT; these agents directly dissolve an existing clot. Only patients with no risk of bleeding are eligible for treatment.

A **Greenfield filter,** also known as an IVC filter, is often inserted to block clots from traveling up from the lower extremity to the pulmonary circulation (see

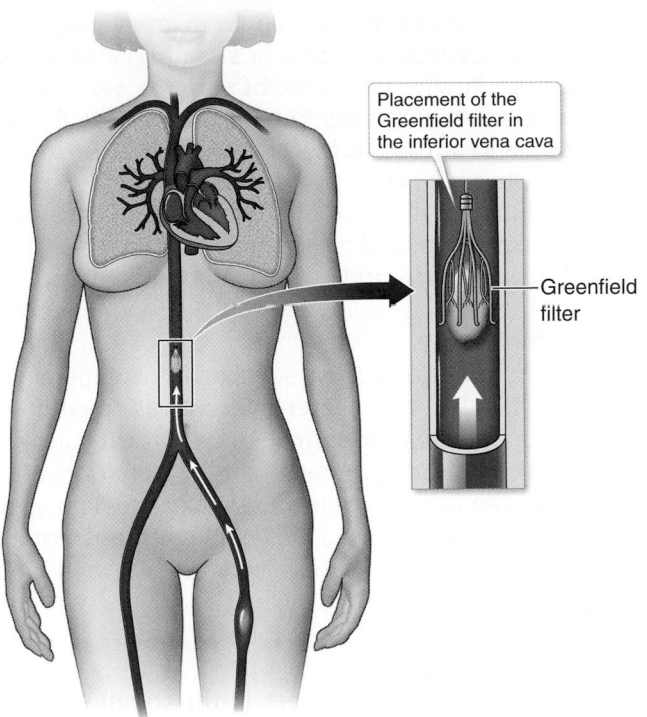

Figure 19-6. Greenfield filter. A Greenfield filter is an apparatus placed in the IVC that can trap a clot as it moves upward with venous flow. It can prevent a DVT from becoming a PE.

CLINICAL CONCEPT

When using warfarin, an effective INR is 2 to 3 for prophylaxis of DVT in most patients. Low molecular weight heparin, factor Xa inhibitors, and direct thrombin inhibitors do not require PT/aPTT or INR monitoring.

Fig. 19-6). These filters are inserted with the use of abdominal ultrasonography. Surgical removal of a thrombus, also called thrombectomy, may be used if other treatments prove ineffective.

Chronic Venous Insufficiency

Chronic venous insufficiency (CVI) occurs as a result of damage to valves in the deep veins of the legs. Valves may become incompetent as a result of impaired venous return caused by trauma, central obesity, pregnancy, or prolonged standing. Valve damage leads to impaired venous return and abnormally high venous pressure in the venous system, which in turn leads to pooling and stasis of blood in the lower extremities. Venous congestion will affect capillary filtration by inhibiting movement of fluid and waste products out of the interstitial spaces.

Clinical Presentation

Clinical presentation of venous insufficiency includes thin shiny skin, dusky discoloration, edema, poor healing,

and reduced or absent hair distribution. A circumferential dusky discoloration called **stasis dermatitis** is often noted around the ankle, instep, and lower leg (see Fig. 19-7). The discoloration is caused by the buildup of hemosiderin in the tissues. Hemosiderin is the iron-containing pigment found in hemoglobin that is liberated from disintegration of red blood cells. Chronic venous congestion will lead to edema, waste product accumulation, and impaired healing. Edema occurs because stasis of blood increases hydrostatic pressure, resulting in fluid movement out of the vascular compartment into the interstitial spaces.

Diagnosis

Key diagnostic tests for peripheral venous disorders include Doppler ultrasonography, photoplethysmography, and venography. Ultrasonography and photoplethysmography determine venous blood flow. Venography can be used to identify occlusions and patterns of collateral blood flow.

Treatment

Graduated compression is the main treatment of venous insufficiency. **Gradient compression stockings** are supportive hosiery that provide higher compression at the ankle than proximally up the leg. **Pneumatic compression devices** are also available that use inflatable compression sleeves on the legs to enhance venous blood flow. Graduated compression in combination with anticoagulant or antiplatelet medications are common medical treatments. Catheter-delivered thrombolytic agents may also be used.

Surgical therapy can be used to improve venous circulation by removing the major reflux pathways through venoablation methods. **Sclerotherapy,** radio frequency ablation (RFA), and endovenous laser therapy (EVLT) are

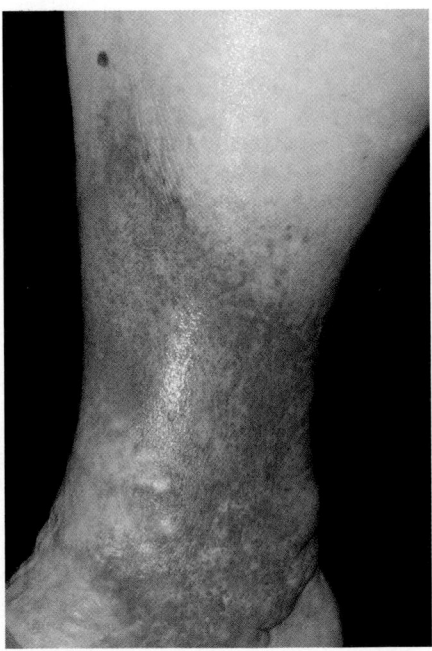

Figure 19-7. Stasis dermatitis. *(From Dr. P. Marazzi/Science Source.)*

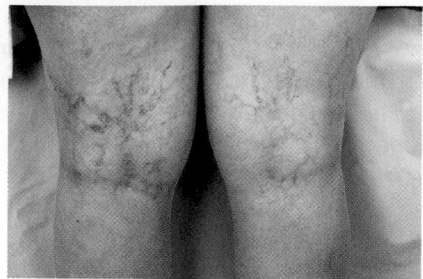

Figure 19-8. Varicose veins. (From Dillon, P. (2007). *Nursing health assessment.* 2nd ed. Philadelphia, PA: F.A. Davis Company, with permission.)

some venoablation procedures that aim to destroy the refluxing superficial veins by either injection of a sclerosing substance, passing a laser over the vein, or using thermal injury.

Varicose Veins

A varicose vein, also called a varicosity, is an abnormally dilated superficial vein (see Fig. 19-8). Leg veins are most commonly affected because they hold a large amount of blood. In the absence of disease, the action of muscles on the deep veins helps to promote venous return. The superficial veins have less supporting tissue than do deep veins; thus, varicosities are more likely in superficial veins.

Epidemiology

Investigators have found that prevalence rates of varicose veins are generally higher in industrialized countries and in more developed regions. The prevalence of visible varicose veins in the United States is 15% in men and 27.7% in women. Visible varicose veins are more prevalent in Hispanic individuals (26.3%) and less prevalent in Asian individuals (18.7%).

 CLINICAL CONCEPT

Prevalence of varicose veins increases with age. In one study, 40-year-old individuals had a prevalence of 22%, 50-year-olds a prevalence of 35%, and 60-year-olds a prevalence of 41%.

Etiology

The cause of varicose veins is high pressure within the superficial veins that weaken venous valves. High pressure is known to occur in prolonged standing, sitting, pregnancy, and obesity. The landmark Framingham Heart Study investigated the risk factors of varicose veins in more than 3,800 subjects. Findings indicate that the incidence of varicose veins is higher among women than men. The women with varicose veins were found to be obese, have lower levels of physical activity, and have higher systolic blood pressure. Women who

reported spending 8 or more hours in an average day in sedentary activities (sitting or standing) also had a significantly higher incidence of varicose veins than those who spent 4 or fewer hours a day in such activities. For men, varicose veins were associated with lower levels of physical activity and higher smoking rates. These results suggest that increased physical activity, smoking cessation, and weight control may help prevent varicose veins among adults at high risk.

Pathophysiology

Varicose veins occur because of valvular incompetence in the legs. Valve incompetence occurs as a result of pressure on the valves over time. Gravitational pull and prolonged standing promote blood stagnation and pooling in the lower extremities. Valves are damaged from chronic pressure, and become less competent at preventing backflow from one section of the vein into another.

Diagnosis

Clinical examination of the legs in the standing position reveals the regions of varicose veins. The duplex ultrasound, which highlights the major superficial vein in the leg, the great saphenous vein, has become the most useful tool for diagnosing varicose veins.

Treatment

Treatment for varicose veins aims to remove the superficial veins either through surgery, endovenous ablation, or sclerotherapy ablation. Sclerotherapy is the most commonly used treatment. Under ultrasound guidance, a sclerosing substance is injected into the collapsed varicose veins, destroys the vessel's endothelial layer, and causes fibrosis of the remainder of the vessel. The body eventually reabsorbs all dead vascular tissue layers. Elastic supportive stockings, which compress the superficial veins, are also recommended.

Venous Ulcers

Venous ulcers, also called venous stasis ulcers, occur in lower extremities affected by venous insufficiency. They are wounds caused by trauma or pressure on the lower limbs. Skin breakdown, tissue damage, and necrosis occur because of lack of venous circulation.

The prevalence of venous ulcers in the general population is not known. However, venous ulcers are seen in 2.5% of patients admitted to long-term care facilities. This rate is believed to be much higher than the overall population prevalence.

Pathophysiology

Sluggish circulation, poor tissue oxygenation, deprivation of cellular nutrition, and impaired waste product removal are the pathophysiologic changes found in venous stasis ulcers. Tissue that is attempting to heal has high metabolic demands that cannot be met because of venous insufficiency.

Clinical Presentation

A venous ulcer is dark red in color, has an uneven margin, is usually painful, and is accompanied by a large amount of edema and drainage (see Fig. 19-9). Most ulcers are located medially over the ankle just above the medial malleolus of the lower leg. Pulses are usually present and capillary refill time is normal.

Treatment

Lifestyle modifications will reduce the pressure on the valves and may reduce edema. These modifications include avoidance of prolonged standing, institution of a regular exercise program, avoidance of constrictive clothing, and the wearing of elasticized compression gradient stockings. Measures are aimed at promoting venous return and decreasing venous pooling. Susceptibility to infection is high with venous ulcers because poor circulation impairs the immune and inflammatory response. Specialized wound care measures are usually necessary such as antibiotic-impregnated semipermeable or occlusive dressings. Topical medications that contain epidermal,

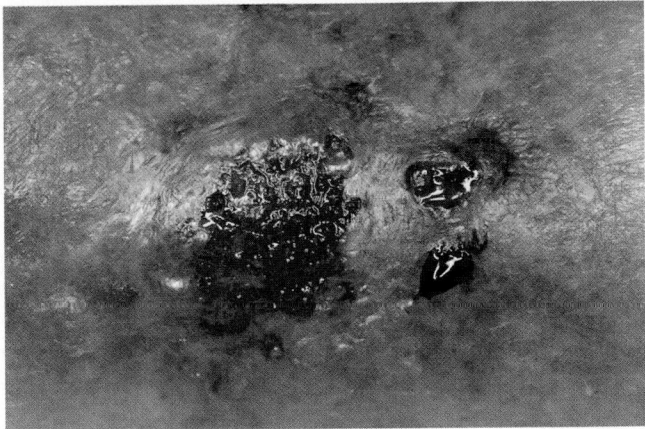

Figure 19-9. Venous ulcer. *(From Roberto A. Penne-Casanova/Science Source.)*

fibroblastic, and platelet-derived growth factors are used to assist chronic wounds with establishing healthy granulation tissue. Intermittent pneumatic compression has been shown to increase healing compared with no compression.

Chapter Summary

- Veins bring blood back to the heart. Major vessels are the inferior and superior vena cava, which empty into the right atrium.

- Veins are unique in that they have valves that prevent retrograde blood flow.

- Venous insufficiency can occur in the superficial veins or deep veins.

- Venous insufficiency occurs because of incompetent venous valves, which allow for retrograde blood flow and stagnation.

- Superficial venous insufficiency causes varicose veins, a mainly cosmetic problem with no serious consequences.

- The major superficial vein in the leg is the great saphenous vein.

- Prolonged standing, sitting, sedentary behavior, obesity, and pregnancy increase susceptibility to varicose veins.

- Deep venous insufficiency causes edema, heaviness of the leg, and dusky color of the lower leg; these result from incomplete clearance of waste products, as well as accumulation of hemosiderin, carbon dioxide, and lactic acid.

- The most serious consequence of deep venous insufficiency is DVT, which is a thrombus of a leg vein that travels via the leg veins into the IVC, then into the right side of the heart into the pulmonary artery.

- Virchow's triad of venous stasis, vascular damage, and hypercoagulability are risk factors for DVT.

- The signs of DVT include tenderness, redness, ropiness, warmth, and swelling over a vein in the leg.

- Dorsiflexion of the ankle that produces pain in the calf is called Homan's sign. Homan's sign is pathognomonic for DVT.

- DVT usually becomes a thromboembolism and can evolve into a PE.

- PE is often a cause of death in those who have an undiagnosed venous thrombus.

- Venous ulcers occur because of trauma in areas of venous insufficiency.

- A common area for venous ulcer is the ankle area above the medial malleolus.

Making the Connections

Disorder and Pathophysiology	Signs and Symptoms	Physical Assessment Findings	Diagnostic Testing	Treatment
Chronic Venous Insufficiency | Veins are unable to keep blood moving in unidirectional flow up to the heart. Incompetent veins allow venous stasis and risk for thrombus formation.				
	Heaviness of the legs. Sensation of fullness of the legs. Fatigue.	Edema and dusky, tan discoloration (hyperpigmentation) circumferentially with apparent distended veins.	Doppler ultrasonography demonstrates reduced blood flow in veins. Photoplethysmography and venography are used to identify location of clot.	Graduated compression over the lower legs via support hosiery or pneumatic compression device. Low molecular weight heparin. Educate patient on risk reduction and wearing of support hose. Teach patient not to stand for prolonged periods, to avoid constricting garments, to elevate legs periodically during the day, and to ambulate or perform leg exercises that will promote blood flow and reduce venous stasis.
Varicose Veins | Dilated, distended superficial veins that are incompetent and have retrograde blood flow.				
	Heaviness and sensation of fullness in legs. Aching, muscle cramps, itching, and increased fatigue in lower leg muscles.	Visible tortuous, dilated veins.	Duplex ultrasound highlights the anatomy of the major superficial vein in the leg, the great saphenous vein.	Sclerotherapy is commonly used to destroy the endothelial layer of the distended vein. The vein then fibroses and is reabsorbed by the body. Educate patient on risk reduction and wearing of support hose. Teach patient not to stand for prolonged periods, to avoid constricting garments, to elevate legs periodically during the day, and to ambulate or do leg exercises that will promote blood flow and reduce venous stasis.

Continued

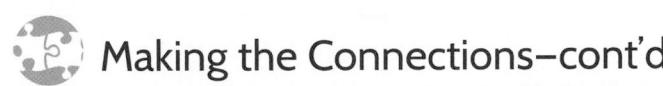

Making the Connections–cont'd

Disorder and Pathophysiology	Signs and Symptoms	Physical Assessment Findings	Diagnostic Testing	Treatment
Deep Vein thromboembolism | Inflammation and thrombus formation in the vein. Thrombus becomes an embolism that can travel up into the IVC and into the right side of the heart and pulmonary artery to cause a pulmonary embolism.				
	Tenderness, warmth, redness, swelling, and ropiness over a vein in the leg.	May have positive Homan's sign (only in 10% of cases). Unilateral leg edema, tenderness, ropiness, warmth, and erythema over a vein.	Duplex ultrasonongraphy demonstrates reduced venous flow. Radiopaque venography and impedance plethysmography identify the location of the clot. D-dimer blood test is positive (high amount of fibrinogen in blood). Follow clotting/bleeding time with either PT/aPTT or INR.	Antiplatelet drugs, low molecular weight heparin, or unfractionated heparin used, followed by warfarin. Monitor anticoagulant effects and levels. Monitor for signs of embolus—pulmonary, myocardial, or cerebral. Advise bedrest initially. Educate patient on risk reduction and wearing of support hose. Teach patient not to stand for prolonged periods, to avoid constricting garments, to elevate legs periodically during the day, and to ambulate or do leg exercises that will promote blood flow and reduce venous stasis.
Venous Ulcer | Venous ulcers are wounds caused by trauma or pressure on the lower limbs. Skin breakdown, tissue damage, and necrosis occur because of lack of venous circulation.				
	Dark red color, edema, and irregular margins of skin breakdown, often located around the medial ankle region.	Dark red color, edema, and irregular margins of skin breakdown, often located around the medial ankle region.	Apparent on physical examination.	Measures are aimed at promoting venous return and decreasing infection. Antibiotic-impregnated semipermeable or occlusive dressings are used. Topical medications that contain epidermal, fibroblastic, and platelet-derived growth factors are used to assist chronic wounds with establishing healthy granulation tissue. Intermittent pneumatic compression has been shown to increase healing compared with no compression.

Bibliography

Agnelli, G., & Becattini, C. (2010). Acute pulmonary embolism. *N Engl J Med,* 363(3), 266–274.

Bates, S. M., Jaeschke, R., Stevens, S. M., et al. (2012). Diagnosis of DVT: antithrombotic therapy and prevention of thrombosis, 9th ed: American College of Chest Physicians evidence-based clinical practice guidelines. *Chest,* 141(Suppl 2), e351S–e418S.

Büller, H. R., Ten Cate-Hoek, A. J., Hoes, A. W., et al. (2009). Safely ruling out deep venous thrombosis in primary care. *Ann Int Med,* 150(4), 229–235.

Decousus, H., Prandoni, P., Mismetti, P., et al. (2010). Fondaparinux for the treatment of superficial-vein thrombosis in the legs. *N Engl J Med,* 363(13), 1222–1232.

Douketis, J., Tosetto, A., Marcucci, M., et al. (2010). Patient-level meta-analysis: effect of measurement timing, threshold, and patient age on ability of D-dimer testing to assess recurrence risk after unprovoked venous thromboembolism. *Ann Int Med,* 153(8), 523–531.

EINSTEIN Investigators, Bauersachs, R., Berkowitz, S. D., Brenner, B., et al. (2010). Oral rivaroxaban for symptomatic venous thromboembolism. *N Engl J Med,* 363(26), 2499–2510.

Enden, T., Haig, Y., Kløw, N. E., et al. (2012). Long-term outcome after additional catheter-directed thrombolysis versus standard treatment for acute iliofemoral deep vein thrombosis (the CaVenT study): a randomised controlled trial. *Lancet,* 379(9810), 31–38.

Galioto, N. J., Danley, D. L., & Van Maanen, R. J. (2011). Recurrent thromboembolism. *Am Fam Phys,* 83(3), 293–300.

Goldhaber, S. Z., & Bounameaux, H. (2012). Pulmonary embolism and deep vein thrombosis. *Lancet,* 379(9828), 1835–1846.

Goldhaber, S. Z., Leizorovicz, A., Kakkar, A. K., et al. (2011). Apixaban versus enoxaparin for thromboprophylaxis in medically ill patients. *N Engl J Med,* 365(23), 2167–2177. doi: 10.1056/NEJMoa1110899. Epub 2011 Nov 13.

Hamdan, A. (2012). Management of varicose veins and venous insufficiency. *JAMA,* 308(24), 2612–2621. doi: 10.1001/jama.2012.111352.

Heit, J. A. (2012). Estimating the incidence of symptomatic postoperative venous thromboembolism: the importance of perspective. *JAMA,* 307(3), 306–307.

Howard, L., & Salooja, N. (2011). Outpatient management of pulmonary embolism. *Lancet,* 378(9785), 5–6.

Hull, R. D., Schellong, S. M., Tapson, V. F., et al. (2010). Extended-duration venous thromboembolism prophylaxis in acutely ill medical patients with recently reduced mobility: a randomized trial. *Ann Int Med,* 153(1), 8–18.

Jacobs, L. G., & Billett, H. H. (2009). Office management of deep venous thrombosis in the elderly. *Am J Med,* 122(10), 904–906.

Januel, J. M., Chen, G., Ruffieux, C., et al. (2012). Symptomatic in-hospital deep vein thrombosis and pulmonary embolism following hip and knee arthroplasty among patients receiving recommended prophylaxis: a systematic review. *JAMA,* 307(3), 294–303.

Kaatz, S., Qureshi, W., & Lavender, R. C. (2011). Venous thromboembolism: what to do after anticoagulation is started. *Cleveland Clin J Med,* 78(9), 609–618. doi: 10.3949/ccjm.78a.10175.

Kahn, S. R., Shapiro, S., Wells, P. S., et al. (2014, March 8). Compression stockings to prevent post-thrombotic syndrome: a randomised placebo-controlled trial. *Lancet,* 383(9920), 880–888. doi: 10.1016/S0140-6736(13)61902-9. Epub 2013 Dec 6.

Kumar, V., Abbas, A. K., Fausto, N., & Aster, J. (2009). *Robbins & Cotran pathologic basis of disease.* 8th ed. Philadelphia, PA: W.B. Saunders.

Kyrle, P. A., Rosendaal, F. R., & Eichinger, S. (2010). Risk assessment for recurrent venous thrombosis. *Lancet,* 376(9757), 2032–2039.

Longo, D. L., Fauci, A., Kasper, D. L., et al. (2011). *Harrison's principles of internal medicine.* 18th ed. New York: McGraw-Hill.

Lucassen, W., Geersing, G. J., Erkens, P. M., et al. (2011). Clinical decision rules for excluding pulmonary embolism: a meta-analysis. *Ann Int Med,* 155(7), 448–460.

Mumoli, N., & Giuntoli, S. (2011). Venous thromboembolism in progress. *Mayo Clin Proceed,* 86(6), 556.

Musani, M. H., Matta, F., Yaekoub, A. Y., et al. (2010). Venous compression for prevention of postthrombotic syndrome: a meta-analysis. *Am J Med,* 123(8), 735–740. doi: 10.1016/j.amjmed.2010.01.027.

Neumann, I., Rada, G., Claro, J. C., et al. (2012). Oral direct factor Xa inhibitors versus low-molecular-weight heparin to prevent venous thromboembolism in patients undergoing total hip or knee replacement: a systematic review and meta-analysis. *Ann Int Med,* 156(10), 710–719.

Raju, S., & Neglén, P. (2009). Clinical practice. Chronic venous insufficiency and varicose veins. *N Engl J Med,* 360(22), 2319–2327. doi: 10.1056/NEJMcp0802444.

Sareyyupoglu, B., Greason, K. L., Suri, R. M., et al. (2010). A more aggressive approach to emergency embolectomy for acute pulmonary embolism. *Mayo Clin Proceed,* 85(9), 785–790.

Shah, S. K., & Clair, D. G. (2013). Which lower-extremity DVTs should be removed early? *Cleveland Clin J Med,* 80(9), 546–547. doi: 10.3949/ccjm.80a.1214.

Sommers, B. D. (2010). Routine screening for silent pulmonary embolism is harmful and unnecessary. *Am J Med,* 123(12), e15. author reply e17. doi: 10.1016/j.amjmed.2010.05.033. Epub 2010 Oct 19.

Tafur, A. J., Kalsi, H., Wysokinski, W. E., et al. (2011). *The association of active cancer with venous thromboembolism location: a population-based study. Mayo Clin Proceed,* 86(1), 25–30.

Tapson, V. F. (2008). Acute pulmonary embolism. *N Engl J Med,* 358(10), 1037–1052.

ten Cate-Hoek, A. J. (2014, March 8). Elastic compression stockings—is there any benefit? *Lancet,* 383(9920), 851–853. doi: 10.1016/S0140-6736(13)62347-8. Epub 2013 Dec 6.

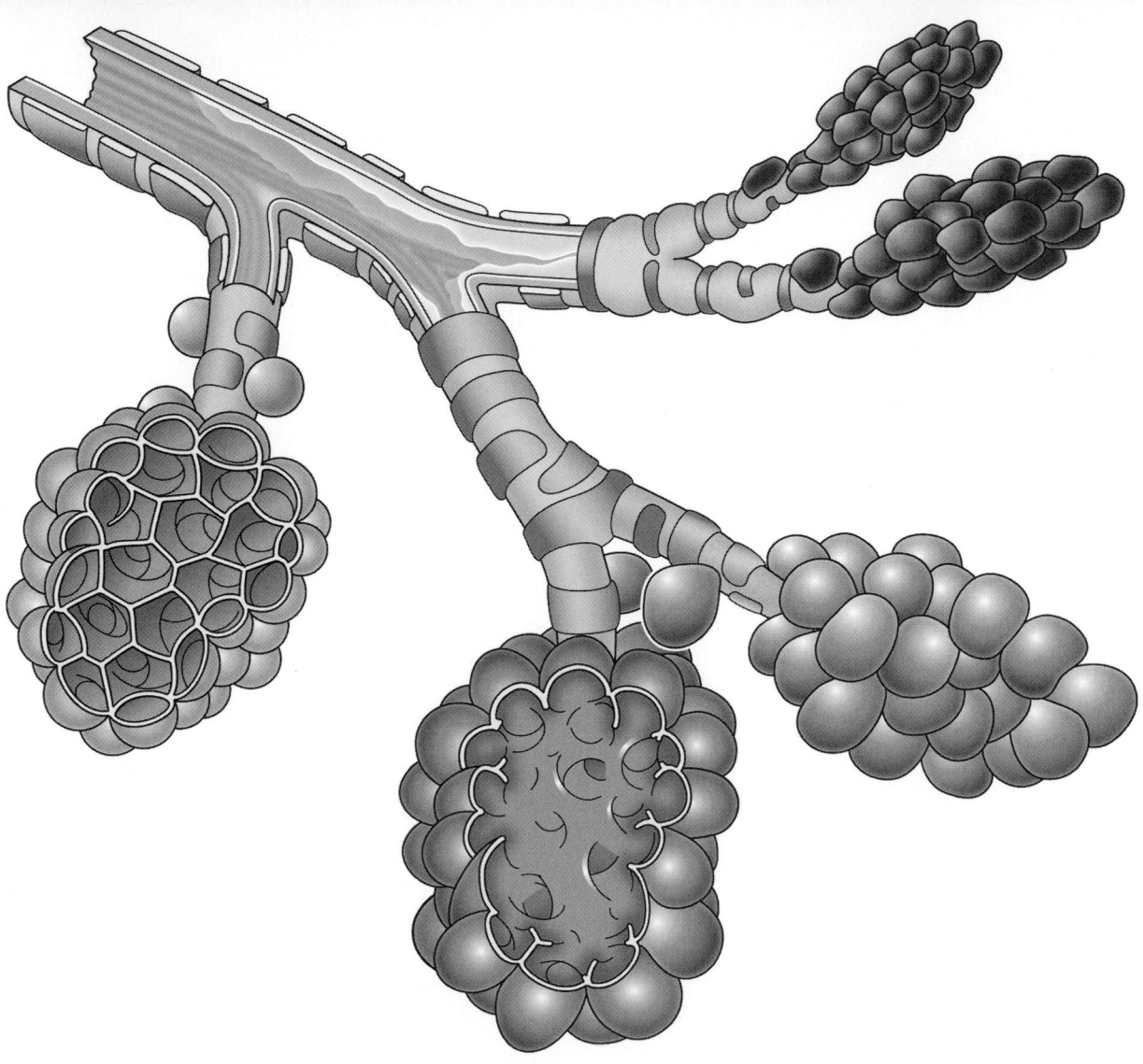

Chapters

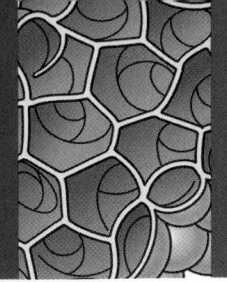

Respiratory Inflammation and Infection

Key Terms

Bradypnea	Hypercapnia	Pneumonia
Bronchitis	Hypoxia	Pulmonary aspiration
Diaphragm	Inspiration	Retractions
Epiglottitis	Mucociliary apparatus	Tachypnea
Expectoration	Oxyhemoglobin	Ventilation
Expiration	Perfusion	Ventilation-perfusion ratio (V-Q ratio)

Respiratory infections are common within the general population and range from the common cold to the life-threatening condition of tuberculosis (TB). Respiratory infections are highly contagious and often transmitted by casual contact. Infections are mainly caused by viruses and bacteria that are inhaled. The lungs are also at risk for exposure to inhalants such as smoke, allergens, and pollutants. Pneumonia and influenza virus have long been a cause of death for many persons, especially the elderly. However, immunizations such as pneumococcal and influenza vaccinations have reduced the frequency and severity of these respiratory infections. TB, a potentially fatal disease, remains a common respiratory infection worldwide. It has remained a scourge of the global population for centuries; over the years, it has developed resistance to many antibiotics.

Epidemiology

The most frequently acquired respiratory infection is the common cold. It can be caused by a variety of viruses found in the environment, such as rhinovirus, adenovirus, herpes simplex, and coronavirus.

 CLINICAL CONCEPT

Rhinoviruses, one of the major causes of the common cold, are found worldwide and account for about 40% of colds.

In the primary care setting, upper respiratory infection (URI) is one of the most frequent reasons for patients to seek care, with cough being one of the main symptoms. Cough is pathognomonic of acute bronchitis and pneumonia. Almost 5% of the general population in the United States develops acute bronchitis

annually, with the highest incidence during the fall and winter months. Pneumonia, a more serious infection, affects 5 out of 1,000 adults each year in the United States, with up to a 28% mortality rate. It is one of the most common diagnoses in elderly and immunosuppressed individuals.

TB is a unique respiratory infection caused by a resilient bacterial organism that can remain dormant in the body as latent TB. A potentially fatal disease, TB affects 2 billion persons worldwide. This infectious disease remains in the individual for a lifetime. Those who are immunosuppressed, such as individuals with human immunodeficiency virus (HIV), are highly susceptible to TB. The emergence of HIV infection in the 1980s stimulated a rise in TB as a global disease. It remains a challenging infection to treat because of its ability to mutate and develop resistance to antibiotics.

Basic Physiologic Concepts of Respiratory Function

The upper respiratory tract conducts air to the lower airways, protects the lungs from foreign matter, and warms, filters, and humidifies air as it enters the lungs. The lower respiratory tract participates in gas exchange by oxygenating blood and excreting carbon dioxide at the alveoli.

Lung Anatomy

The lungs sit in the center of the thoracic cage and receive air from the upper respiratory tract structures, which include the nose, oropharynx, larynx, trachea, and two main bronchi and bronchioles. There are two lobes of lung tissue on the left (the upper and lower lobes) and three lobes of lung tissue on the right (the upper, middle, and lower lobes).

The trachea divides into two main bronchi, which are shaped differently. The left bronchus is curved as it enters the lung tissue, whereas the right bronchus is vertical and wider, providing a straight path downward into the right lung (see Fig. 20-1). The shape of the right bronchus increases susceptibility of aspiration into the right middle and right lower lobes of the lung. **Pulmonary aspiration** occurs when material from the oropharynx enters the lower respiratory tract. Aspiration mainly occurs in patients who have trouble clearing their lungs, such as those with a diminished gag or cough reflex and patients with decreased level of consciousness. Consequences of pulmonary aspiration range from no injury at all to death within minutes from asphyxiation. Aspiration of small quantities of material is common, and healthy persons forcefully cough to remove the material from the trachea. However, people with significant underlying disease are at greater risk for developing aspiration pneumonia.

The two main bronchi branch into smaller bronchioles, which divide into respiratory bronchioles, alveolar ducts, and alveoli. At the alveoli, transfer of oxygen occurs into the capillaries and carbon dioxide transfers into the alveoli for exhalation.

Mucociliary Apparatus

During respiration, air enters the nasal passages and trachea and travels down to the lungs. Within the bronchioles, there is a specialized cellular mechanism called the **mucociliary apparatus,** which consists of ciliated pseudocolumnar epithelial cells and goblet cells that secrete mucus. The wavelike motion of the cilia enables the movement of mucus downward from the nasal passages to the throat. Inhaled particles such as dust, pollen, and pathogens are trapped by the mucus and removed from the air passages. Upward motion of the cilia moves the mucus from the bronchioles up to the throat, where it is swallowed.

Because the mouth, nose, and throat are exposed to the outside environment, they are colonized with bacteria that are normal flora, which are organisms that do not cause illness in a healthy person. The lower respiratory tract and alveoli do not have normal flora. They are kept free of microorganisms by the mucociliary apparatus that sweeps away and traps organisms in the upper respiratory tract. If the ciliated respiratory epithelium becomes damaged, however, there is an increased risk of lower respiratory infection.

Gas Exchange

Gas exchange of oxygen and carbon dioxide occurs within the respiratory bronchioles, alveolar ducts, and alveoli. Alveoli are thin-walled, balloonlike structures surrounded by pulmonary capillaries. This unique structure enables transfer of both oxygen and carbon dioxide. Air enters the alveolus and oxygen moves across the alveolar membrane to the red blood cells (RBCs). At the same time, carbon dioxide moves from the RBC into the alveolus to be excreted by exhalation (see Fig. 20-2).

Oxygen combines loosely with the heme portion of hemoglobin to form **oxyhemoglobin.** The most important function of hemoglobin is to combine with oxygen in the lungs and then release oxygen to the peripheral tissues. It then collects carbon dioxide from the tissues and carries it back to the lungs to be excreted. Each hemoglobin molecule can carry four oxygen molecules.

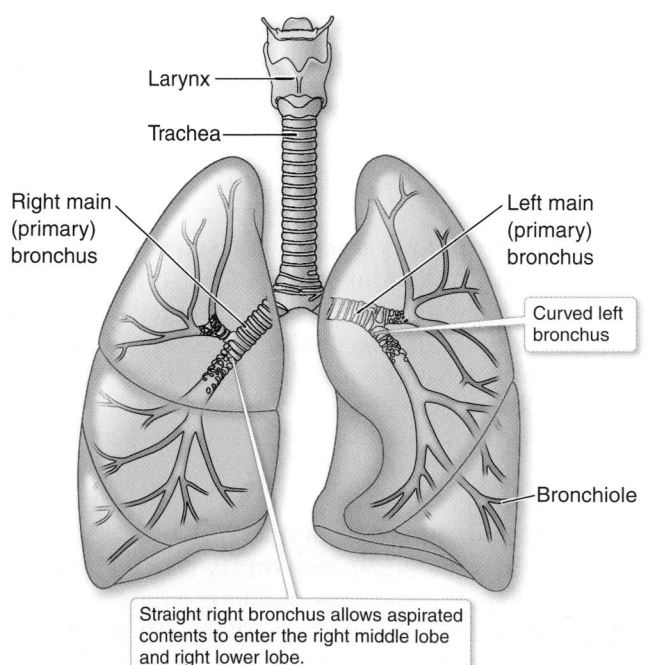

FIGURE 20-1. Shape of the bronchi. The left bronchus is curved and the right bronchus is more vertical. Because of the anatomy, aspiration often occurs into the right lung because of the straight route downward from the right bronchus.

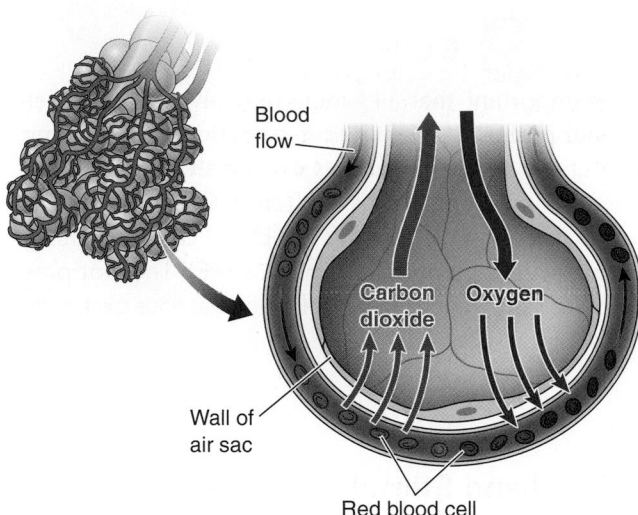

FIGURE 20-2. Oxygen and carbon dioxide gas exchange at alveoli.

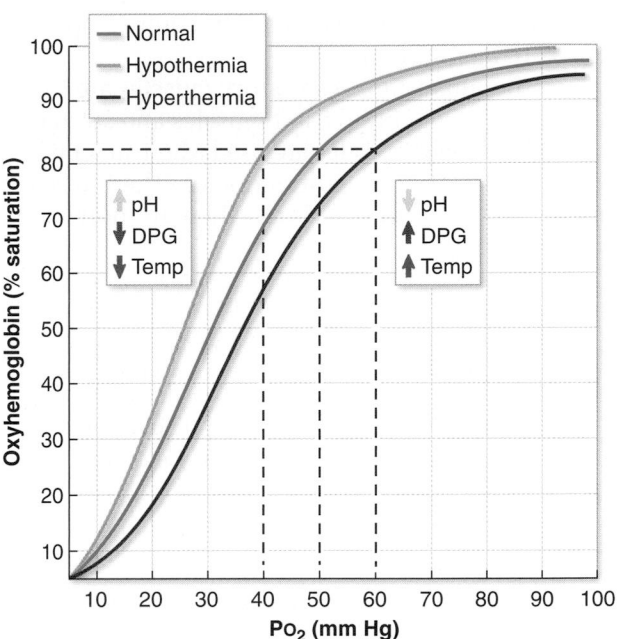

FIGURE 20-3. The oxyhemoglobin dissociation curve. The oxygen-hemoglobin dissociation curve demonstrates the proportion of hemoglobin that is saturated with oxygen on the vertical axis against the oxygen pressure in the bloodstream on the horizontal axis. Specifically, the oxyhemoglobin dissociation curve shows hemoglobin affinity for oxygen at different partial pressures of oxygen in the bloodstream (Po_2). (a) Under normal conditions, Hgb is fully saturated at 100 mm Hg; at approximately 50 mm Hg to 60 mm Hg Po_2 in the blood, hemoglobin affinity dramatically diminishes. (b) Under conditions of hyperthermia (fever), low pH (acidosis), high Pco_2, high CO (carbon monoxide), and increased 2,3-DPG*, there is less saturation of hemoglobin. Hgb affinity for oxygen is less than normal. (c) Under conditions of hypothermia, high pH (alkalosis), and low 2,3-DPG*, there is greater saturation of hemoglobin at an oxygen level of 50 mm Hg in the bloodstream. Hgb affinity for oxygen is greater than normal.

*2, 3-DPG is used in the metabolism of RBCs. It binds with greater affinity to deoxygenated hemoglobin than it does to oxygenated hemoglobin. It decreases Hgb affinity for oxygen, so it promotes the ability of RBCs to release oxygen near tissues.

CLINICAL CONCEPT

The percentage of hemoglobin saturated by oxygen can be measured using a pulse oximeter, a monitor usually placed on the finger.

The volume of oxygen dissolved in the plasma varies directly with the partial pressure of oxygen in the arteries. The relationship between the arterial pressure of oxygen and the percentage of saturation of oxygen in the blood is shown in the oxyhemoglobin dissociation curve (see Fig. 20-3).

If the pressure of oxygen in the arterial blood (Po_2) stays within the 90 to 100 mm Hg range, hemoglobin remains maximally saturated with oxygen and tissues remain oxygenated. When Po_2 falls below 60 mm Hg, hemoglobin drops all O_2 molecules off quickly. The desaturation of hemoglobin quickly leads to tissue hypoxia. It is important to keep hemoglobin fully saturated with Po_2 above 90 mm Hg to ensure optimal tissue oxygenation.

Erythropoietin, which is responsible for the stimulation of RBC production, is secreted by the kidneys in response to low oxygen levels in the bloodstream. Any condition that causes hypoxia, such as cardiac disease, lung disease, or change in atmospheric pressure, will stimulate erythropoietin. Erythropoietin then stimulates the bone marrow to produce more RBCs that can carry more oxygen to the tissues.

CLINICAL CONCEPT

In higher altitudes, there is a lower percentage of oxygen in the atmospheric air. This is why those who live at high altitudes have low Po_2, which constantly stimulates erythropoietin. This, in turn, increases production of RBCs and is why persons who live in mountainous areas have higher-than-normal hemoglobin and hematocrit levels.

Diaphragm and Respiratory Muscles

The **diaphragm** is a muscle that separates the abdomen from the thoracic cavity. During inhalation, the diaphragm moves downward or contracts at the same time the rib cage is being pulled up, resulting in lung expansion. The diaphragm is composed of both skeletal and smooth muscle; it is voluntarily and involuntarily controlled. During **inspiration,** the diaphragm allows expansion of the lungs by moving downward. When the diaphragm ascends, the rib cage moves down and the diaphragm compresses the lungs, promoting exhalation. The accompanying air movement with lung deflation is referred to as **expiration.**

The phrenic nerve, which originates as the fourth cervical spinal nerve (C4), innervates the diaphragm. It originates in the neck and traverses downward between the lung and heart to reach the diaphragm. When a spinal cord injury occurs at or above C4, motor and sensory conduction to the diaphragm is interrupted and respirations cease. The patient will require respiratory support to maintain life.

The other important respiratory muscles are the external and internal intercostal muscles and sternocleidomastoids. These muscles are used when an individual is short of breath. The contractions of the intercostal muscles are called **retractions** when an individual is using them to breathe.

> **ALERT!** It is critical to carefully assess all patients with spinal cord injuries for signs of respiratory distress. In spinal cord injuries affecting C4 or above, the patient needs rescue breathing or mechanical support.

Ventilation and Perfusion

Ventilation is the process of inspiration and expiration of air through the pulmonary airways. Physical factors affect the flow of air and oxygen content of the atmospheric air. At high altitudes there is low atmospheric pressure of air and diminished oxygen content. The decreased O_2 levels trigger an increase in the rate and depth of respiration.

Perfusion is the movement of blood through the pulmonary circulation, eventually providing oxygen to every part of the body. Oxygen and carbon dioxide are dissolved in the blood and transported throughout the body at the same time.

The **ventilation-perfusion ratio (V-Q ratio)** is defined as the ratio of the amount of air reaching the alveoli to the amount of blood reaching the alveoli; it is measured with a ventilation-perfusion (V-Q) scan. The ideal V-Q ratio occurs when ventilation and perfusion are equal or when there is ventilation and perfusion matching. When ventilation and perfusion are unequal, there is ventilation-perfusion mismatching. An area with no ventilation is termed a shunt. An area with no perfusion is termed dead space. The lungs have a built-in compensatory mechanism that attempts to match blood flow and ventilation: where there is little ventilation, pulmonary arterial vessels constrict. Pulmonary artery vasoconstriction leads to redistribution of blood flow to better-ventilated areas of the lung.

> 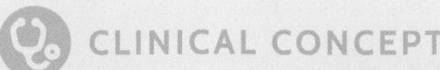 **CLINICAL CONCEPT**
>
> Hypoxia stimulates pulmonary arterial vasoconstriction. Patients with chronic hypoxia can develop chronic pulmonary vasoconstriction, referred to as pulmonary hypertension.

> **CLINICAL CONCEPT**
>
> It is important that all functioning alveoli have adequate perfusion. Ventilation-perfusion mismatching occurs when air cannot flow into an alveolus or blood flow around an alveolus is altered. One of the most common etiologies for this is a blood clot in the lung, also called a pulmonary embolus (PE). The clot prevents blood flow to the alveolus and gaseous exchange cannot take place.

Control and Stimulus of Breathing

Multiple different receptors control the process, rate, and depth of respirations during inspiration and expiration. Central chemoreceptors, located in the medulla, sense changes in carbon dioxide and blood pH and cause alterations in the rate and depth of respirations. An increase in CO_2 or a decrease in pH (acidosis) stimulates the central chemoreceptors, resulting in an increased rate of respirations. The end result is the return of the pH to normal.

Chemoreceptors in the medulla also sense the hydrogen (H+) concentration of the cerebral spinal fluid (CSF). An increase or decrease of pH in the arterial blood is reflected in a chemical change in the CSF. When CO_2 is retained, there is an increase in carbonic acid (H_2CO_3) in the blood. This increases the $PaCO_2$ level and lowers blood pH. In response to these changes, the respiratory center at the medulla stimulates respirations. High levels of CO_2, referred to as **hypercapnia,** stimulate the process of breathing.

Peripheral chemoreceptors, found in the aortic arch and bifurcation of the carotid artery (called carotid bodies), respond primarily to a decrease in arterial oxygen. A decreased level of oxygen in the blood is sensed by the peripheral chemoreceptors, which stimulate respirations; this is referred to as a hypoxic drive. A hypoxic drive takes over when CO_2 accumulation is not stimulating the medulla to control respiration, as in diseases such as emphysema.

The normal stimulus to breathe is hypercapnia, which is an increase of carbon dioxide in the blood. However, when central chemoreceptors are exposed to high levels of carbon dioxide for extended periods of time, they become less responsive. The blunted response to CO_2 allows the peripheral chemoreceptors of low O_2 to take over as the stimulus of respirations. The hypoxic drive becomes the main trigger for breathing. This response correlates with a PaO_2 level of about 60 mm Hg, the point at which oxygen fully dissociates from hemoglobin.

Baroreceptors, sensors of blood pressure, are also located in the aortic arch and carotid artery. Baroreceptors send signals to the autonomic nervous system, depending on blood pressure levels. When blood systolic pressure drops to 80 mm Hg or lower, the baroreceptors stimulate the sympathetic nervous system to increase heart and respiratory rate.

Proprioceptors, located in the muscles of movable joints, respond to body movement. When stimulated, respiratory rate and depth increases. The purpose of these receptors is to maintain adequate oxygen levels during periods of exercise.

The Hering-Breuer reflexes are stretch reflexes located in the bronchi and bronchioles. When the lungs inflate, neuronal impulses are sent up the vagus nerve to the medulla. The result is an inhibition of rate, rhythm, and duration of inspiration, which prevents the overdistention of the lungs.

Basic Pathophysiologic Concepts of Respiratory Function

There are several signs of lung pathophysiology. Dyspnea, or shortness of breath, is the most common sign of a pulmonary problem. At times it is difficult to decipher if dyspnea has a cardiac or pulmonary etiology. Cough, another common sign of pulmonary disease, usually develops because of an irritating stimulus in the bronchioles. However, heart failure can also be the cause of cough. Pulmonary symptoms have to be considered in the context of the whole patient—the compilation of the history, signs, symptoms, and laboratory studies together will lead to an accurate pulmonary or cardiac diagnosis.

Dyspnea

Dyspnea is the sensation of being short of breath; it is a common symptom of pulmonary or cardiovascular disease. If dyspnea is sudden, it can be caused by pulmonary embolism, acute coronary syndrome, pneumothorax, or aspiration. Orthopnea, the sensation of dyspnea when lying flat, is a common indication of heart failure. Nocturnal dyspnea is particularly associated with heart failure but can be caused by asthma. Acute episodes of dyspnea are most often caused by bronchospasm of asthma, whereas chronic, persistent dyspnea is commonly caused by chronic obstructive pulmonary disease.

Cough

A cough is an involuntary response to mechanical or chemical stimulation of the bronchial tree. It can occur as a result of a blockage in the airway caused by a foreign body, excess mucus, or aspirated fluids or foods. When this happens, coughing serves as a mechanism to eliminate the stimulant.

Coughing can be described as nonproductive or productive of mucus or sputum. The process of coughing up sputum is referred to as **expectoration.** Normal sputum is clear and thin in nature. In the presence of a bacterial infection, the production of sputum may become profuse and thick. The color may change to yellow or green. Pink-tinged, also called "rusty," sputum is often indicative of minor bleeding, as can occur when capillaries in the lungs rupture because of forceful coughing. Hemoptysis is the coughing up of a larger amount of blood, when the sputum clearly contains red blood. A cough with hemoptysis often is associated with TB or lung cancer. Grey-tinged sputum occurs from exposure to tobacco smoke.

Frequent, chronic coughing is a symptom that prompts individuals to see a health care provider. It can be a sign of infection, inflammation, gastroesophageal reflux, bronchospasm, heart failure, or neoplastic disease. In healthy individuals, cough frequently occurs as a result of a respiratory tract infection. Asthma can also present as a chronic cough. In elderly patients, chronic cough is frequently caused by heart failure or chronic obstructive pulmonary disease (COPD).

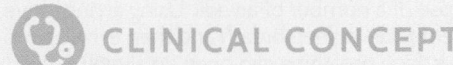

CLINICAL CONCEPT

Chronic cough is common in smokers. Exposure to secondhand smoke can trigger chronic coughing in children.

Hemoptysis

Hemoptysis is the production of sputum that contains blood. This is usually associated with serious illness such as infection, tumor, or TB. When assessing a patient complaining of hemoptysis, it is important to differentiate between blood in sputum versus blood from the gastrointestinal tract in vomitus. Blood from the gastrointestinal tract is referred to as hematemesis. Hematemesis usually consists of dark, coffee-colored blood, whereas hemoptysis contains bright red blood.

Atelectasis

Atelectasis is the collapse of a small number of alveoli resulting in reduced gas exchange. It can occur because of a compressive force on the alveoli, such as in that created by a mass. Alternatively, atelectasis can be caused by an obstruction of the bronchioles that inhibits the full inflation of alveoli. Atelectasis most commonly occurs postoperatively because of sedation. Under sedation, a patient's respiratory rate decreases and shallow breathing occurs. Some alveoli lack full inflation with shallow breathing, and atelectasis can occur. To treat atelectasis, the patient needs to cough and deep breathe to open all the alveoli (see Fig. 20-4). Atelectasis predisposes individuals to pneumonia.

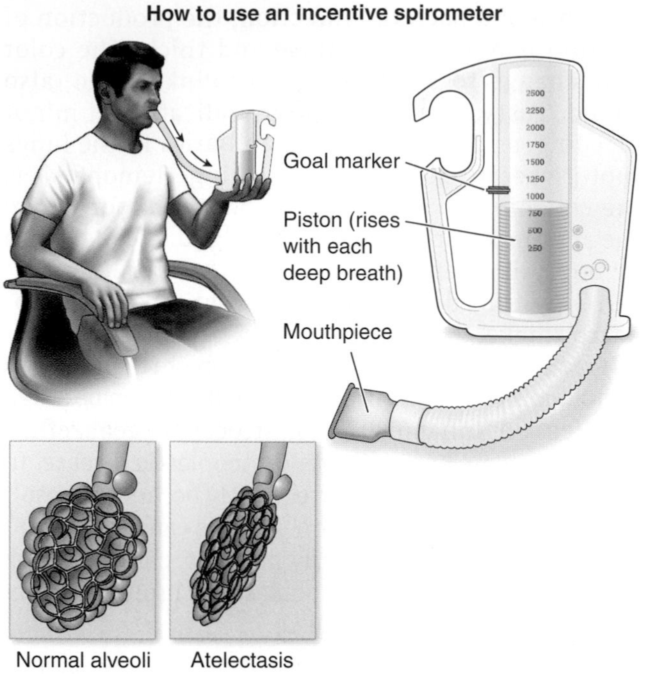

How to use an incentive spirometer

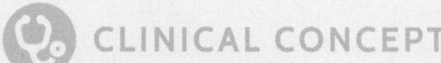

Goal marker

Piston (rises with each deep breath)

Mouthpiece

Normal alveoli   Atelectasis

FIGURE 20-4. Atelectasis and incentive spirometer. Atelectasis is the collapse of a number of alveoli. Using an incentive spirometer, a patient takes a deep breath and then exhales into the apparatus. The deep breathing can open up alveoli.

CLINICAL CONCEPT

Patients who undergo long surgical procedures often develop atelectasis. It is important to advise postoperative patients to cough, deep breathe, and use an incentive spirometer to reverse atelectasis.

Hypoxia

Hypoxia occurs when there are insufficient oxygen levels in the blood to meet the needs of tissue. It can be caused by any number of conditions that alter gas exchange across the alveolar membrane. Pulmonary edema, for example, creates a fluid barrier to oxygen transfer across the alveolar-capillary interface. The terms *hypoxia* and *hypoxemia* are used interchangeably. The term *hypoxemia* indicates lack of sufficient oxygen in the bloodstream, whereas the term *anoxia* indicates zero amount of oxygen in the blood.

The body's normal ventilatory stimulus is the accumulation of CO_2 in the bloodstream. As the CO_2 level rises, it stimulates the respiratory center in the medulla. However, with chronic CO_2 accumulation, the respiratory center becomes insensitive to high CO_2. Low O_2, or hypoxia, becomes the driving stimulus of respiration. Chemoreceptors in the aortic arch and carotid bodies sense low O_2 levels, which triggers the respiratory center. Hypoxia becomes the breathing stimulus in patients with chronic hypercapnia.

Chemical poisoning, such as that seen in carbon monoxide poisoning, can cause hypoxia. In this case, carbon monoxide binds to hemoglobin as carboxyhemoglobin, which has a much higher affinity for hemoglobin than oxygen and prevents oxygen from binding to the hemoglobin molecule. High levels of carbon monoxide in the bloodstream can be fatal.

Impending Respiratory Failure

Respiratory failure occurs when the pulmonary system fails to oxygenate the blood or fails to eliminate carbon dioxide sufficiently. It is classified as either hypoxemic or hypercapnic respiratory failure.

Hypoxemic respiratory failure occurs when the pressure of oxygen in arterial blood (PaO_2) is lower than 60 mm Hg with normal arterial carbon dioxide ($PaCO_2$). Many acute diseases of the lung can cause respiratory failure, including pulmonary edema, pulmonary embolism, pneumonia, or pneumothorax.

Hypercapnic respiratory failure occurs when carbon dioxide in arterial blood ($PaCO_2$) is greater than 50 mm Hg. Common causes of hypercapnia include COPD and asthma. Hypoxemia accompanies hypercapnic respiratory failure in persons who are breathing room air.

It is challenging to predict when a patient will cease independent breathing and incur respiratory failure. Serial arterial blood gases (ABGs) should be evaluated in all patients with respiratory problems. Usually there is a gradual increase in arterial carbon dioxide and decrease in arterial oxygen when a patient is developing respiratory failure (see Table 20-1). The patient typically appears distressed, may be using accessory respiratory muscles, and has difficulty maintaining a normal respiratory rate despite oxygen administration. Patients at risk of respiratory failure need intubation equipment ready at the bedside. The patient's whole clinical picture should be taken into account when deciding to intubate. After the patient's ventilatory status is corrected, the underlying pathophysiologic process that led to respiratory failure needs investigation.

Assessment

A complete history and physical examination is necessary to diagnose a pulmonary disorder. In the history, the patient should be asked about risk factors such as smoking or occupational toxins. Frequently, pulmonary and cardiac disorders present with the same symptoms.

History

A patient who presents with a pulmonary problem can have anything from a common cold to chronic heart failure. By asking specific questions in a thorough history, the clinician can try to categorize the symptoms as respiratory or cardiac in nature. It is important to ask the patient to completely describe the symptom and associated features. When and how

TABLE 20-1. Serial ABGs Demonstrating Trend Toward Respiratory Failure

This chart shows how a patient's ABGs decompensated over the course of an hour and a half, from 9 a.m. to 10:30 a.m. At 11:00 a.m., the patient stopped breathing and went into respiratory failure, needing intubation.

	9:00 a.m.	10:00 a.m.	10:30 a.m.	11:00 a.m.
BLOOD pH	7.36	7.35	7.32	7.30
P_{O_2}	90 mm Hg	80 mm Hg	66 mm Hg	60 mm Hg
P_{CO_2}	45 mm Hg	45 mm Hg	56 mm Hg	60 mm Hg
HCO_3-	21 mg/dL	21 mg/dL	17 mg/dL	12 mg/dL
INTERPRETATION OF ABGs	Normal	Hypoxia	Hypoxia and hypercapnia	Respiratory failure Patient intubated

did the symptom occur, suddenly or gradually? Has the symptom been present for a day, week, or month? The patient needs to be asked about symptoms of coronary artery disease to rule out dyspnea caused by cardiovascular disease. For example, does the patient suffer dizziness or chest pain when he or she has dyspnea? Usually dyspnea caused by cardiovascular disease worsens with exertion and is accompanied by diaphoresis and chest pain. The patient with dyspnea caused by heart failure commonly has edema. Ask the patient if lying flat causes difficulty with breathing, which is orthopnea, a classic symptom of heart failure. Nocturnal dyspnea is often a symptom of heart failure or asthma. If there is chest pain, the patient should fully describe it. Cardiac chest pain is crushing and a feeling of pressure. Pleuritic chest pain, caused by pleural membrane irritation, is sharp and worsens with deep breathing.

In respiratory infection, dyspnea and cough are often accompanied by fever and malaise. Sneezing, rhinorrhea, and a productive cough are classic features of upper respiratory infection (URI). A patient who has audible wheezing is usually exhibiting bronchospasm that may be caused by asthma. Ask the patient about current medications. Does the patient have any allergies? Rhinitis and sinusitis can be caused by allergy as well as infection. Acute bronchitis commonly occurs after an URI. Pneumonia is commonly a secondary infection after a viral infection such as influenza.

Signs and Symptoms

The patient's symptoms should be thoroughly described in terms of the mnemonic "OLDCART"—onset, location, duration, character, aggravating or relieving factors, and treatment. It is important to assess if dyspnea occurs with exertion or in the presence of edema. Exertional dyspnea commonly occurs with a cardiac condition. If ankle edema is present, this also often indicates a cardiac disorder. The signs of pulmonary edema of cardiac origin can present similarly to pneumonia. Both of these disorders cause crackles indicative of fluid in the lung tissue. However, if fever is present, the fluid is usually caused by an exudate in pneumonia. A chronic cough can be associated with asthma, heart failure, TB, lung cancer, or COPD. However, the patient usually demonstrates other symptoms that will narrow down the diagnosis. The chronic cough that is triggered by allergy is often asthma. A chronic cough that is accompanied by weight loss and hemoptysis is commonly caused by TB or lung cancer. A chronic cough in a smoker with cyanosis and a barrel-shaped chest is often indicative of COPD. The patient with cough, pallor, weak pulse, and ankle edema probably has heart failure. An astute assessment of the whole patient from head to toe is necessary to distinguish a pulmonary, cardiac, or infectious origin of a cough or dyspnea.

Physical Examination

After taking the patient's vital signs, the clinician should conduct a thorough physical examination. The pulmonary system requires use of all the physical assessment techniques: inspection, palpation, percussion, and auscultation.

Inspection

The patient should be seated with relaxed posture and arms resting comfortably at the side or in the lap. Observe the patient's breathing pattern and excursion of the chest wall with inhalation and exhalation. The patient's skin should be warm and without cyanosis or pallor. Extremities should be inspected for normal brachial and radial pulses and capillary refill in the fingernails should be less than 3 seconds. Clubbing of the fingertips can be a sign of chronic oxygen deprivation.

Assess the rate, rhythm, and depth of respirations by observing the rise and fall of the chest during respirations. The presence of retractions, visible indentation of the intercostal and supraclavicular spaces, is a sign of increased work of breathing and respiratory distress; they indicate that accessory muscles are necessary for inspiration. Normal respiratory rate is 12 to 20 breaths per minute. **Bradypnea** or hypoventilation is a respiratory rate less than 12 breaths per minute, whereas **tachypnea** or hyperventilation is a respiratory rate greater than 20 breaths per minute.

Palpation

Palpation involves examination of the chest wall with the fingers in order to identify areas of tenderness, changes in skin temperature, moisture, superficial lumps or masses, and skin lesions. Check symmetrical chest expansion by placing the hands on the posterior lateral chest wall with thumbs at the level of T9 or T10. Ask the patient to take a deep breath; the thumbs should move apart symmetrically.

Tactile fremitus is palpable vibration generated from the larynx and transmitted through the patient's bronchi to the chest wall. The examiner should place both hands on the patient's posterior chest and have the patient repeat the phrase "ninety nine." The examiner then moves down the posterior chest wall in a systematic manner as the patient repeats "ninety nine" (see Fig. 20-5). Vibration felt on the examiner's hands from both sides of the chest should be equal. An increased amount of vibration felt by one of the hands on the chest wall can indicate pneumonia in the region. A decreased amount of vibration can indicate pleural effusion.

Percussion

Percussion involves a specific technique of tapping tissues to elicit sounds. The examiner places a hand on the posterior chest wall between the patient's ribs. The examiner than takes his or her free hand and uses one or two fingers to strike the middle finger of the hand against the chest wall. The examiner does this down

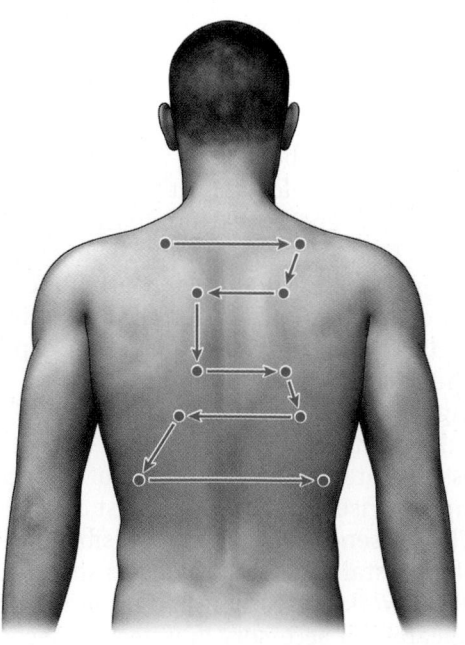

FIGURE 20-5. Palpation of the chest in systematic method.

the back of the patient. The changes in the specific tones are based on the density of the tissue. Tissues that contain air such as the lungs are described as resonant. Dull sounds indicate a solid mass or fluid consolidation. Hyperresonance indicates that the lungs are hyperinflated, which occurs in emphysema.

Auscultation

The flow of air through the bronchi, bronchioles, and into the alveoli can be assessed through auscultation of the lungs with a stethoscope. The presence of fluids or solid substances in the lung tissue can also be localized using auscultation. The characteristics of normal breath sounds vary according to the anatomical location within the lungs.

Over the trachea, breath sounds are very loud, tubular, and high-pitched. They are called bronchial breath sounds; expiratory sounds last longer than inspiratory sounds. Over the bronchi, bronchovesicular sounds are heard, which are equal in inspiration and expiration and have an intermediate intensity and pitch. They can be heard over the main bronchi located in the first and second interspaces anteriorly and between the scapulae posteriorly. Vesicular breath sounds are longer in inspiration than expiration, low pitched, and heard over the peripheral lung fields.

Abnormal Breath Sounds. Adventitious breath sounds are extra lung sounds superimposed over normal breath sounds present in various kinds of pulmonary dysfunction. Crackles, sometimes called rales, are noncontinuous sounds that occur when deflated alveoli open and close against fluid. They are commonly present in heart failure or pneumonia. Wheezes are high-pitched, whistling sounds related to the constricted diameter of the airways and may be inspiratory or expiratory in nature. Rhonchi are low-pitched, snorelike sounds present over inflamed bronchial airways. A friction rub is a grating, scratchy sound heard during inspiration and expiration with inflammation of the pleural surfaces.

Vocal resonance is the transmission of the sounds of speech through the lungs as heard when using the stethoscope. Vocal resonance is a physical assessment technique that can be used in the diagnosis of pneumonia. In the normal lungs, the sound of the patient's voice is muffled. To use vocal resonance in physical examination, the patient is asked to repeat a phrase such as "ninety nine" as the clinician listens with a stethoscope over different regions of the lungs. In bronchophony, the patient's words become clearer and louder over areas of pneumonia. In egophony, the patient is asked to repeat "e" as the clinician listens over different regions of the lungs. Over areas of pneumonia, the "e" will sound like "a." In whispered pectoriloquy, over normal lungs, whispered words are usually muffled. However when the clinician listens to areas of pneumonia, whispered sounds become clear and distinctive in whispered pectoriloquy.

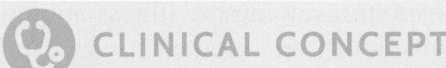

CLINICAL CONCEPT

When bronchial breath sounds are heard over the peripheral lung field, this commonly indicates pneumonia.

Diagnostic Testing

Diagnostic testing is an important component of respiratory assessment. ABGs provide information about gas exchange. Chest x-rays can visualize the structure of the chest and lungs. If an infection is suspected, culture and sensitivity testing is performed on sputum or swab of the throat. Computed tomography (CT) scanning and magnetic resonance imaging (MRI) can be useful when chest x-ray is inadequate. A V-Q scan is performed to investigate pulmonary embolus, if CT scan is inadequate.

Arterial Blood Gases. ABGs are serum blood values obtained through an arterial puncture. They enable identification of alterations in acid-base balance caused by respiratory diseases. ABG results include blood pH, partial pressure of O_2, CO_2, bicarbonate ion, and the saturation of Hgb (see Table 20-2). A pH of more than 7.45 indicates alkalosis and a pH of lower than 7.35 indicates acidosis (see Chapter 8: Acid-Base Imbalances).

The level of arterial oxygen (Pao_2) indicates the degree of oxygenation of the blood. The arterial carbon dioxide level ($Paco_2$) is an indicator of alveolar ventilation. The Pao_2 and $Paco_2$ values are useful in determining the ability of the lungs to provide oxygen and remove carbon dioxide. The pH of the blood is balanced by the lungs and the kidneys. The lungs regulate CO_2 and kidneys regulate conservation and excretion of acid (H+) and HCO_3^- (bicarbonate ion).

Culture and Sensitivity Testing. Culture and sensitivity of sputum samples can assist in the diagnosis of respiratory infection. Sputum that has been obtained by expectoration may be contaminated with normal flora from the mouth. Microscopic examination for the presence of epithelial cells from the oral mucosa can help determine if it is contaminated. Sputum cultures obtained by suctioning the respiratory tract or through bronchoscopy are less likely to be contaminated by normal flora. Acid-fast smears and cultures are the specific sputum test for TB. Cytology studies identify the presence of malignant cells.

Pulse Oximetry. Pulse oximetry can continuously monitor the oxygen saturation of hemoglobin (SaO_2). A small probe is attached to an extremity, usually the fingertip, although the forehead, earlobe, or toe may also be used. Infrared light passes over the extremity, reflects the blood pulsing through the tissue, and senses changes in oxygen saturation. Normal Sao_2 is 95% to 100%. A saturation level lower than 95% indicates that tissues are not receiving enough oxygen.

Chest X-Ray and Computed Tomography. Chest x-ray can identify adequate lung expansion or the presence of fluid in the lungs and can be used to evaluate the response to various treatments. A CT scan shows a more specific picture of the respiratory system and identifies different pathological conditions such as lung abscesses, tumors, TB, and pleural effusion.

Bronchoscopy. Bronchoscopy allows for direct visualization of the larynx, trachea, and bronchi, which can then allow for biopsy and removal of foreign objects. Secretions may also be removed using suctioning during the test.

Thoracocentesis. In thoracocentesis, a large bore needle is inserted through the chest wall into the pleural space and pleural fluid can be removed. Medication may also be inserted during the procedure. The procedure can be used to obtain specimens for culture and sensitivity or biopsy.

Treatment

Treatments of pulmonary disease include a variety of drugs and procedures. Bronchodilators reduce bronchospasm and antibiotics treat respiratory infections. Pulmonary embolism can be treated with thrombolytic and anticoagulant medications. Decongestant medications cause vasoconstriction that helps to reduce the inflammation and edema in the nasal passage and relieve nasal congestion. Antihistamine medications block the inflammatory effects of histamine in the airways. Antitussive medications can be used to control coughs. A warm saltwater gargle and mild analgesics can be used to treat pharyngitis (sore throat). Antiviral drugs, such as amantadine, are available to lessen the effects of viral infection in the respiratory tract.

TABLE 20-2. Normal Values of Arterial Blood Gases	
Value	Normal
pH	7.35 to 7.45
PCO_2	35 to 45 mm Hg
HCO_3^-	22 to 26 mEq/L
PO_2	90 to 95 mm Hg
% Hgb saturation with O_2	95% to 100%

ALERT! Coughing is important for ridding the airways of secretions, so clinicians do not want to inhibit coughing or oversedate the patient to a point that weakens the cough.

Pulmonary hygiene measures are used to clear the respiratory tract of mucus and purulent drainage. Methods used for pulmonary hygiene include suctioning of the airways, chest physiotherapy, incentive spirometry, and nasotracheal suction. Percussion over the chest loosens secretions and allows the cilia of the airways to remove material. Positioning is another method for promoting drainage of secretions. Intermittent positive pressure breathing physiotherapy is often used in nonintubated patients. Nebulizers can deliver humidified air with medication. Supplemental oxygen and mechanical ventilation are used when hypoxia or respiratory failure occur.

Pathophysiology of Selected Upper Respiratory Tract Disorders

Respiratory tract infections affect airway clearance and breathing patterns by changing the amount and character of secretions produced in the lungs. Risk factors for respiratory infection include stress and exposure to people infected with various microorganisms such as bacteria, viruses, and fungi. Any disease or condition that causes an immunocompromised state allows microorganisms to invade the body and proliferate rapidly, possibly resulting in infection.

More than 200 strains of virus cause upper respiratory tract infections. A common method of spreading viruses is the release of airborne droplet nuclei when the infected individual coughs, laughs, or sneezes. Pathogens are also commonly spread by hand-to-hand contact.

Acute Rhinitis

Acute rhinitis is a disorder that results in inflammation and irritation of the mucous membranes of the nose. Often called the common cold, rhinitis is caused by rhinovirus among other viruses and transmitted through airborne droplets. The incubation period is approximately 2 to 4 days. Rhinovirus is shed in large amounts and can occur a few days before cold symptoms are recognized by the patient. Viral shedding peaks on days 2 through 7 of the illness. A local inflammatory response to the virus in the respiratory tract leads to nasal discharge, nasal congestion, sneezing, and throat irritation. Slight fever may be present. Nasal mucociliary transport is markedly reduced during the illness and may be impaired for weeks. Diagnosis is mainly through physical examination and history. The nasal mucosa and nasal turbinates are red. The discharge from the nose is yellow to green in color. Pharyngeal erythema and earache may also be present.

Complete blood count (CBC) may show a high number of lymphocytes with viral infection and high number of neutrophils with bacterial infection. Both secretory immunoglobulin A and serum antibodies are involved in resolving the illness and protecting from reinfection.

Antihistamines, analgesics, and antipyretic medication such as acetaminophen are usually sufficient treatment. Corticosteroid nasal spray is often prescribed for allergic rhinitis.

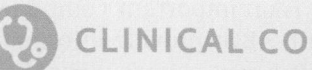

CLINICAL CONCEPT

Acute rhinitis can also be caused by allergies. In this case, it resembles the illness of the common cold; however, the interior nasal mucosa and turbinates are usually gray colored. Discharge from the nose is clear colored. The patient often has a crease at the tip of the nose from the constant maneuver of wiping upward from the nares, sometimes referred to as the "allergic salute." The patient's CBC usually shows a high number of eosinophils.

Acute Pharyngitis

Acute pharyngitis, an inflammation of the pharynx, is usually caused by a virus. If acute bacterial pharyngitis occurs, the cause is usually group A beta-hemolytic streptococcus (GABHS), also called *Streptococcus pyogenes*. The infection can spread from the pharynx to cause sinusitis and otitis media. In more severe cases, GABHS can cause bacteremia, pneumonia, meningitis, necrotizing fasciitis, rheumatic fever, rheumatic heart disease, scarlet fever, toxic shock syndrome, and glomerulonephritis.

In pharyngitis, assessment reveals red, swollen pharyngeal membranes and tonsils. The lymphoid follicles of the throat are swollen and often covered with white exudate; cervical lymph nodes are enlarged and tender. The patient may have a fever, malaise, and a sore throat, but typically has no cough.

Diagnosis is made with visual inspection and identification of the causative organism. A rapid screening test for streptococcal antigens and bacterial throat cultures are used to identify the organism causing the infection. To rule out Epstein-Barr virus (EBV), a heterophile blood test is necessary. Penicillin, erythromycin, or cephalosporins may be used to treat a bacterial infection. Saltwater gargle, as well as antipyretic and analgesic medications, are used to treat the fever and sore throat.

Acute Sinusitis

Sinusitis is an infection of the facial sinuses and membranes of the nose. The sinuses are mucus-lined cavities filled with air that drain into the nose. Sinusitis may be acute, subacute, or chronic. Acute sinusitis often accompanies a URI or an allergic reaction and may be caused by a virus, bacteria, or both.

Acute sinusitis caused by a virus usually lasts from 5 to 7 days. Bacterial sinusitis may last up to 4 weeks. Chronic sinusitis is an inflammation of the sinuses that persists for more than 12 weeks.

In sinusitis, the sinus cavity becomes obstructed because of accumulated fluid and edema caused by the inflammatory process. The fluid present in this area is an excellent medium for bacterial growth and infection. Symptoms include headache, facial pain or pressure over the sinus area, nasal obstruction, fatigue, purulent nasal discharge, fever, ear pain, dental pain, cough, decreased sense of smell, and sore throat. A sinus headache is usually made worse by the increased pressure that occurs when bending forward, coughing, or sneezing. Facial edema, nasal crusting, and purulent drainage in the nasal cavity may also be present.

Antimicrobial agents such as amoxicillin clavulanate (Augmentin), ampicillin (Ampicin) or third-generation cephalosporins may be used to treat the infection. Decongestant and antihistamine medications, saline sprays, and heated mist may help relieve symptoms. Mucolytic agents may decrease secretions.

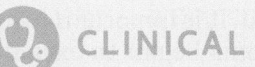

CLINICAL CONCEPT

In physical examination, a technique called transillumination of the sinuses using a penlight can be done to support a diagnosis of sinusitis.

Acute Tonsillitis

Acute tonsillitis is an acute infection of the tonsils and pharynx that is sometimes called pharyngotonsillitis. The most common causes of acute tonsillitis are GABHS or viruses such as EBV, adenovirus, herpes simplex virus, or cytomegalovirus. EBV is responsible for 19% of exudative tonsillitis in children; bacteria cause between 15% and 30% of the pharyngotonsillitis cases, and other cases are caused by other viruses. Sore throat, fever, and difficulty swallowing are the most common signs and symptoms. Cervical lymphadenopathy is a characteristic sign of EBV tonsillitis, also called infectious mononucleosis.

The physical examination demonstrates erythema and swelling of the tonsillar tissue and pharynx. Severe swelling of the tonsils with abscess, called quinsy, can cause swallowing difficulty. Throat culture is the best diagnostic test. To exclude EBV, a heterophile blood test is necessary. Some children are carriers of GABHS and do not develop pharyngotonsillitis but can transmit GABHS tonsillitis to others. These children can have a positive throat culture but do not have antibodies against GABHS. If there are recurrent infections or if severe tissue hypertrophy occurs, a tonsillectomy may be performed. If the infection is caused by GABHS, antibiotics are necessary.

Epiglottitis

Epiglottitis is the infection and inflammation of the epiglottis—the flap of tissue that sits atop the trachea to keep food from going into the trachea during swallowing. When inflamed, the epiglottis can obstruct the trachea. It may be caused by a respiratory infection, exposure to chemical substances in the environment, trauma, and various organisms, including bacteria, viruses, and fungi. Common organisms that cause epiglottitis include *Streptococcus pneumoniae*, *Haemophilus influenza*, Parainfluenza, varicella-zoster virus, herpes simplex virus type 1, and *Staphylococcus aureus*.

The disorder begins as inflammation and swelling between the base of the tongue and the epiglottis. The swelling pushes the epiglottis backward; as the process continues, complete blockage of the airway occurs, leading to suffocation and death.

X-rays and a laryngoscopic examination will show that the pharynx is inflamed, red, and stiff, and that the epiglottis is swollen. Blood tests will show signs of infection or inflammation, ABGs will confirm lack of gas exchange, and cultures may grow bacteria and indicate the causative organism. Neck x-ray shows a characteristic swelling of the pharyngeal tissues called "steeple" sign.

Immediate hospitalization is usually necessary, as there is a danger of sudden and unpredictable closing of the airway. Initial treatment includes making the person as comfortable as possible, humidified oxygen, and IV fluids. Antibiotics are given to control inflammation and stop the infection after the causative organism has been identified.

ALERT! Epiglottitis is a medical emergency. A laryngoscope and tracheostomy equipment should be available at the patient's bedside at all times because intubation may be needed.

Laryngitis and Tracheitis

Laryngitis is inflammation of the larynx, whereas tracheitis is inflammation of the trachea. The infection that causes both is usually viral in nature, although bacteria such as *Haemophilus influenza* can also cause the infection. Signs of acute laryngitis are hoarseness or complete loss of the voice. If the infection involves the larynx, trachea, and bronchi, then laryngotracheobronchitis, commonly called croup, occurs. Croup is mainly a children's disease.

In laryngitis, an irritating, high-pitched cough may be present. Tracheal involvement can produce a raspy cough or stridor, a high-pitched inhalation sound. Pleuritic chest pain may indicate pleural or other musculoskeletal involvement. The underlying cause of the cough is the irritation of the mucous membranes.

Eventually, sputum will be produced in response to the chronic irritation. Sputum is usually thin and may be yellow or green when bacteria are causing the infection. Thin mucoid sputum may indicate a viral or bacterial infection. Foul-smelling sputum may indicate a lung abscess. As airways narrow, the patient begins to wheeze mainly upon expiration.

There is no specific medical intervention for viral laryngitis other than resting the voice and managing the symptoms. If the infection has spread and proves to be bacterial, antibiotics may be administered. Bronchodilator medications are useful if the airway has narrowed and wheezing is present. Tracheitis can involve the epiglottis, in which case a medical emergency may occur.

Pathophysiology of Selected Lower Respiratory Tract Disorders

The lungs are constantly exposed to environmental pathogens and all types of pollutants, which increase susceptibility to infection. Aspiration of contents from the oropharynx can also increase the risk of respiratory infection. Infections of the lower respiratory tract hinder the exchange of oxygen and carbon dioxide, creating a vulnerability to hypoxia and hypercapnia.

Acute Bronchitis

Acute **bronchitis** is an inflammation of the bronchi and bronchioles caused by either bacterial or viral infection. Bronchitis can also be triggered by inhalation of toxic gases or chemicals.

Epidemiology
It is estimated that 44 out of 1,000 adults suffer acute bronchitis in the United States annually. This is likely a low estimate because not all individuals with acute bronchitis seek health care. Most episodes occur in fall or winter. Acute bronchitis occurs more frequently in populations with a low socioeconomic status and in people who live in urban and highly industrialized areas.

Etiology
Respiratory viruses are the most common causes of acute bronchitis. The most common viruses include influenza A and B, parainfluenza, respiratory syncytial virus, and coronavirus. Bacteria that cause acute bronchitis include *Mycoplasma* species, *Chlamydia pneumoniae*, *Streptococcus pneumoniae*, *Moraxella catarrhalis*, and *Haemophilus influenzae*. *Bordetella pertussis*, also called whooping cough, is a microorganism that can cause bronchitis. *B. pertussis* has had a recent resurgence in incidence in the United States after many years of successful eradication because of pertussis vaccine.

Cigarette smoking and exposure to pollutants or chemical irritants increase susceptibility to bronchitis.

Upper respiratory infections such as the common cold, sinusitis, and pharyngitis also increase susceptibility to acute bronchitis. Influenzae is commonly complicated by acute bronchitis.

Pathophysiology
In acute bronchitis, the bronchial tree undergoes an inflammatory response to a pathogen or irritant. The cells of the bronchial tissue are irritated and the mucous membrane becomes edematous, diminishing the bronchial mucociliary function. The air passages become obstructed by white blood cells (WBCs) and mucus. WBCs and inflamed respiratory epithelium secrete infectious exudate, cytokines, and proinflammatory mediators. There is a significant increase in the production of mucus, which causes a productive cough. Dysfunctional mucociliary movement and excess mucous secretion cause patients to frequently cough to clear the airway of secretions. Pleuritic chest pain with inhalation and exhalation, fever, and general malaise are also common.

Clinical Presentation
In the history, the patient may report that the illness began as a common cold. It is important to ask the patient when the symptoms began to exclude chronic bronchitis as the diagnosis. The clinician should ask about recent exposure of the patient to others who are ill, recent exposure to pollutants or occupational chemicals, and past medical history. It is important to know if the patient has a history of asthma because acute bronchitis sometimes presents with wheezing. The patient usually complains of sore throat, nasal discharge, muscle aches, and persistent cough. Fever and headache may occur in the beginning of infection. The initial days of infection can appear as the common cold. Cough becomes prominent as the disease progresses and can last from 10 to 20 days during the course of acute bronchitis. Sputum production is reported in most patients. Sputum may be clear, yellow, green, or even blood-tinged. Purulent sputum is reported in 50% of persons with acute bronchitis. Sputum color is not indicative of bacterial versus viral infection.

On physical examination, the patient may exhibit pharyngeal erythema, localized lymphadenopathy, and rhinorrhea. Rhonchi and wheezes can be heard across all lung fields. In severe cases, diffuse wheezes, high-pitched continuous sounds, and the use of accessory muscles can be observed. Coughing can clear some of the rhonchi and wheezes. Inspiratory stridor indicates that there may be mucous obstruction within the trachea.

Diagnosis
Diagnosis is mainly based on symptomatology, although a culture of respiratory secretions may be done. A CBC may be useful to distinguish bacterial infections

from nonbacterial infections. A chest x-ray is usually done to rule out pneumonia.

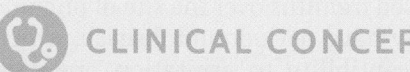

CLINICAL CONCEPT

Chronic bronchitis is diagnosed when a patient reports a history of bronchitis for 3 months out of the year for at least 2 years.

Treatment

Broad spectrum antibiotics are used to treat bacterial infections. Expectorant medications will assist the individual to cough up the exudate and mucus. Mucolytic agents can dissolve mucus. At times a bronchodilator is necessary if bronchospasm is present with cough. Cough suppressants may be needed at night to allow the individual to sleep.

Pneumonia

Pneumonia is inflammation of the lung tissue in which alveolar air spaces fill with purulent, inflammatory cells, and fibrin. Infection by bacteria or viruses is the most common cause, although inhalation of chemicals, aspiration of contents from the oropharynx or stomach, or infection by other infectious agents such as rickettsiae, fungi, and yeasts may occur.

Epidemiology

Pneumonia causes more disease and death in the United States than any other infection. There are various types of pneumonia depending on the setting in which it occurs: community acquired, nosocomial (hospital-acquired), and ventilator-associated. Etiologic pathogens vary widely, depending on the setting of the disease. More than 3 million cases occur annually in the United States. Pneumonia is more prevalent during the winter months and in colder climates. The incidence of pneumonia is greater in males than in females. Advanced age increases the incidence of, and the mortality from, pneumonia. Comorbidity and a diminished immune response and defense against aspiration increase the risk of bacterial pneumonia. Pneumonia is often the cause of death in chronically ill patients. For individuals aged 65 years and older, pneumonia and influenza are the sixth leading cause of death. In a 20-year study conducted in the United States, the average overall mortality rate in pneumococcal pneumonia with bacteremia was 20.3%; patients older than 80 years had the highest mortality rate, which was 37.7%. Up to 30% of nursing home patients die of pneumonia annually in the United States. Hospital-associated pneumonia (HAP) is a lung infection that is contracted after 48 hours of hospital admission. Among intubated and mechanically ventilated patients, the development of HAP is specifically called ventilator-associated pneumonia (VAP). Hospital-acquired pneumonia affects 5 to 10 per 1,000 patients annually in the United States and is a major cause of mortality. Approximately 60% of all deaths of patients with nosocomial infection are caused by HAP or VAP.

Etiologic and Risk Factors

Bacteria are the most common etiologic agents involved in pneumonia. Specific settings and conditions make certain types of pneumonia more common. Community-acquired pneumonia (CAP) is most often caused by *Streptococcus pneumoniae*. Other pathogens include *Haemophilus influenzae, Mycoplasma, Klebsiella, Staphylococcus,* and *Legionella* species and gram-negative organisms. Aspiration pneumonia is commonly caused by anaerobic bacteria swallowed from the oropharynx. Some pathogens, particularly *Staphylococcus* species, may be spread via the bloodstream to the lungs. Staphylococcus usually enters the bloodstream via an intravenous route from a central vein catheter or intravenous drug abuse. Staphylococcus is also the microorganism most commonly involved in hospital-associated pneumonia, specifically methicillin-resistant *Staphylococcus aureus* (MRSA). HAP is a major cause of mortality among critically ill patients. VAP is a specific type of HAP. In addition to MRSA, enterococcus is commonly involved in ventilator-associated pneumonia; specifically vancomycin-resistant enterococcus (VRE). Other microorganisms frequently involved in HAP and VAP are Pseudomonas, Klebsiella, and Acinetobacter. Legionella causes a unique kind of pneumonia, which is spread via water systems such as air conditioning, mists sprayed on produce in grocery stores, and hot tubs. Legionella pneumonia commonly affects small clusters of individuals living together in hotels, dormitories, or cruise ships. Mycoplasma is a small bacterialike organism that can cause a syndrome called walking pneumonia; in this mild pneumonia, the patient may not appear very ill but has persistent cough and, commonly, headache and earache.

One of the major risk factors for pneumonia is influenza infection. Viruses commonly alter the pulmonary immune defenses and make the lungs vulnerable to bacterial infection referred to as secondary pneumonia. Although influenza virus is the most common agent, other respiratory viruses, such as respiratory syncytial virus, parainfluenza viruses, adenovirus, and rhinoviruses, may also predispose individuals to pneumonia as a secondary bacterial infection.

Immunosuppression can predispose patients to pneumonia. In HIV infection and AIDs, pneumonia is commonly caused by *Pneumocystis jiroveci.* Pneumocystis is a yeastlike fungal organism formerly known as *Pneumocystis carinii.* Pneumocystis pneumonia is often referred to as PCP. Aspiration can also predispose the patient to pneumonia caused by accidental inhalation of substances refluxed from the stomach. Comatose patients and those with impaired gag reflex are at highest risk for aspiration pneumonia. Chronic gingivitis and periodontitis increase the risk of aspiration pneumonia and lung abscess. Other risk factors for pneumonia include lung cancer or tumors, COPD, and bronchiectasis. Smoking impairs resistance to infection. Alcohol or drug intoxication increases the risk of aspiration pneumonia with asphyxiation. Pneumonia is the second most common cause of nursing home-associated infection, after urinary tract infection. Postviral, aspiration, and bacterial pneumonias are major causes of death in nursing home residents.

Pathophysiology

Pneumonia is most commonly caused by inhalation of droplets containing bacteria or other pathogens. The droplets enter the upper airways and gain entry into the lung tissue. Pathogens adhere to respiratory epithelium and stimulate an inflammatory reaction. The acute inflammation spreads to the lower respiratory tract and alveoli. At the sites of inflammation, vasodilation occurs with attraction of neutrophils out of capillaries and into the air spaces. Neutrophils phagocytize microbes and kill them with reactive oxygen species, antimicrobial proteins, and degradative enzymes. There is an excessive stimulation of respiratory goblet cells that secrete mucus. Mucous and exudative edema accumulate between the alveoli and capillaries. The alveoli attempt to open and close against the purulent exudate; however, some cannot open. The sounds heard with the stethoscope over the alveoli opening against the exudative fluid are crackles. There is a layer of edema and infectious exudate at the capillary-alveoli interface that hinders optimal gas exchange. The patient can become hypoxic and hypercapnic, with obstructed exchange of O_2 and CO_2 at the pulmonary capillaries.

Clinical Presentation

When interviewing the patient, it is important to assess exposure to any other persons who are ill and evaluate if the patient has any aspiration risks or immunosuppression factors. The clinician should ask the patient about current medications, allergies, and past medical history. Conditions such as influenza, asthma, or COPD increase susceptibility to pneumonia. Social habits, such as smoking and use of alcohol or illicit drugs, are also factors that increase risk to pneumonia.

The clinical presentation of bacterial pneumonia usually starts with a sudden onset of symptoms. Cough, which may or may not be productive of sputum; fever; and chills are usually initial manifestations. Pleuritic chest pain, which is pain with deep breaths; dyspnea; hemoptysis; and decreased exercise tolerance develop as the disorder continues. Other nonspecific symptoms that may be seen with pneumonia include myalgias, headache, abdominal pain, nausea, and vomiting. Headache and earache, with less cough and fever, are the symptoms that occur with mycoplasma pneumonia.

On physical examination, the patient is likely to demonstrate fever, tachypnea, use of accessory muscles with breathing, tachycardia, and possibly cyanosis. Crackles are pathognomonic of pneumonia and the clinician can elicit egophony, bronchophony, and whispered pectoriloquy. There may be dullness to percussion and increased fremitus over the site of pneumonia. The patient may have periodontal disease, which can increase susceptibility to aspiration pneumonia with anaerobic infection. Poor cough and gag reflex increases the risk of aspiration pneumonia.

Otitis media or myringitis, which is inflammation of the tympanic membrane, typically occur in *Mycoplasma pneumoniae* infection.

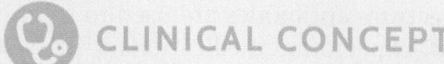

CLINICAL CONCEPT

Cough, crackles, and fever are the characteristic signs of pneumonia. In patients who are elderly, hypothermia may present instead of fever.

Diagnosis

A chest x-ray is the most important diagnostic study in pneumonia diagnosis (see Fig. 20-6). CBC with differential will suggest either a bacterial or viral infection. ABGs and pulse oximetry can demonstrate oxygenation. Sputum culture and sensitivity can exhibit the organism and antibiotic susceptibility. Ultrasound and thoracocentesis are useful if pleural effusion is suspected. Sputum, serum, and urinary antigen tests are available for *S. pneumoniae* and Legionella.

Treatment

Antibiotic therapy and oxygenation of the patient are key priorities in the treatment of pneumonia. Fowler's position and oxygen via nasal cannula or mask is recommended. The patient may require intravenous fluids if dehydrated. Analgesia, antipyretics, and bronchodilators

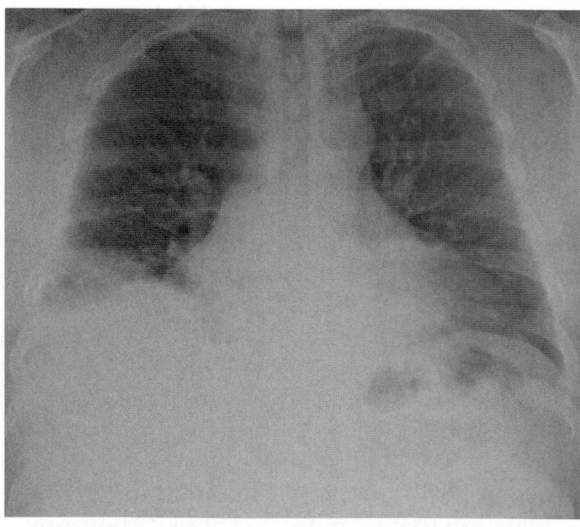

FIGURE 20-6. Chest x-ray showing pneumonia. (From Weber (2013). *Practical Radiology.* Philadelphia, PA: F.A. Davis Company, with permission.)

Patient characteristic*	Score
Nursing home resident	+10
Cancer	+30
Heart failure	+10
Stroke	+10
Kidney disease	+10
Altered level of consciousness	+20
Respiratory rate greater than 30/min	+20
Systolic BP lower than 90	+20
Fever	+15
Pulse greater than 125	+10
Blood ph lower than 7.35	+30
PO₂ lower than 60 mm Hg	+10
SaO₂ lower than 90%	+10
*Incomplete list **Risk score**	

0–90	**Low risk**
91–130	**Moderate risk**
Greater than 130	**High risk**

FIGURE 20-7. The pneumonia severity index. Some patients can recover from pneumonia with outpatient antibiotics. However, there are situations where pneumonia requires hospitalization. To decipher if the patient with pneumonia requires inpatient care, the PSI is often used. This can categorize the patient into classes according to risk. A score can be calculated using numerical values for different patient characteristics. Patients in Class I, II, and III are at low risk for death and can be treated as outpatients. Class IV and V require hospitalization. This table is a modified example of how the PSI is scored.

may be needed. To prevent pneumonia in the elderly, infants, and children with risk factors, pneumococcal vaccine is recommended.

 CLINICAL CONCEPT

In primary care, it is sometimes difficult to evaluate the need for hospitalization for the patient with pneumonia. The clinician can use the pneumonia severity index (PSI) as a guide for inpatient care and mortality risk (see Fig. 20-7).

Lung Abscess

A lung abscess is a localized area of purulent inflammation that results in tissue necrosis and a central area of liquefaction. A common cause of a lung abscess is the aspiration of oral contents containing anaerobic bacteria into the lungs.

Epidemiology

Lung abscess accounts for up to 4 to 5.5 per 10,000 hospital admissions each year in the United States. It occurs at any age, but most frequently from the sixth to eighth decades, and is predominantly seen in men. Immunosuppression is increasing the incidence of lung abscess in younger adults; however, specific statistics are unclear.

Etiology and Risk Factors

Lung abscess can develop as a complication of bacterial pneumonia. The exudate can form a walled-off, localized collection of infectious material. However, aspiration of anaerobic bacteria from the oral cavity is more often the etiology of lung abscess. Risk factors include advanced age, alcoholism, debilitation, malnutrition, HIV infection or other forms of immunosuppression, and malignancy. Intravenous drug abuse is a risk factor specifically for staphylococcal lung abscesses. Puncture of the skin allows entry of staphylococcal organisms into the bloodstream. Staphylococcal endocarditis usually occurs initially, followed by the development of septic emboli that travel into the lungs to form abscesses.

Pathophysiology

The oral cavity contains anaerobic bacteria as normal flora; aspiration of these bacteria often causes lung abscesses. Patients who aspirate anaerobic bacteria and develop a lung abscess are usually debilitated from other health problems or immunosuppressed. Septic emboli, which commonly develop from right-sided endocarditis, can also form lung abscesses. They are usually caused by tricuspid valve endocarditis with staphylococcal organisms. An abscess may also develop secondary to carcinoma of the bronchus; bronchial obstruction can cause an obstructive pneumonia, which may lead to abscess formation.

An abscess occurs after the alveoli have filled with fluid, purulent exudate, and microorganisms, causing the tissue to become necrotic. This process continues until the abscess ruptures and the contents empty into the bronchus, leaving a cavity filled with air and fluid. The purulent material released can obstruct bronchioles and the alveolar-capillary transfer of oxygen, which can eventually cause acute respiratory distress. Complications can occur if bacteria enter the bloodstream and cause sepsis. Bloodstream infection can lead to cerebral infection and meningitis.

Clinical Presentation

The major symptom of a lung abscess is copious amounts of foul-smelling sputum. Other symptoms include a productive cough, chills and fever, chest pain, malaise, and anorexia. Breath sounds are diminished, and crackles may be heard in the region of the abscess.

Diagnosis

A CBC may indicate leukocytosis, and a chest x-ray may show a thick solitary cavity with surrounding consolidation. The causative organism is usually identified by a sputum culture after the cavity has ruptured.

Treatment

Treatment for a lung abscess includes antibiotic therapy and surgical intervention. Bronchoscopy may be used to drain the abscess; if the pleural space is involved, a chest tube may be inserted. Postural drainage is often helpful in relieving the obstruction and promoting drainage.

Tuberculosis

TB is an infection caused by the bacillus *Mycobacterium tuberculosis*. Although TB is usually found in the lungs, it can be found in other parts of the body, such as the adrenal gland, vertebrae, and lymph nodes. It can spread within the bloodstream and cause multisystem disease.

Epidemiology

TB, the most common infectious disease in the world, is associated with the highest mortality rate of all infectious diseases. Globally, more than 1 in 3 individuals are infected with tubercle bacillus. There is a particularly high prevalence of TB in India and Asia. Two factors causing increased incidence of TB are an increased number of immunosuppressed individuals who easily contract the disease and the evolution of drug-resistant strains of the TB organism. Immunosuppressed persons include those with HIV infection, those on biological agents for autoimmune disease, and persons on cancer chemotherapy.

 CLINICAL CONCEPT

Persons with acquired immunodeficiency syndrome (AIDS) are 20 to 40 times more likely than persons who are immunocompetent to develop active TB. TB is the leading cause of mortality among persons infected with HIV.

TB is seven times more common in African Americans compared with non-Hispanic Caucasians. TB also has high incidence among immigrants in the United States. In 2011, more than 60% of cases of TB in the United States were reported to be among foreign-born persons. Approximately 54% of TB cases in 2011 were reported in persons from five countries: Mexico (21.3%), the Philippines (11.5%), Vietnam (8.2%), India (7.6%), and China (5.6%). An estimated 5 to 10 million people in the United States have latent TB infection. The World Health Organization (WHO) has estimated that 9.4 million persons are affected with TB annually. It is also estimated that 2 billion people have latent TB and that the disease killed 1.7 million people globally in 2009.

Etiology

TB is spread by the inhalation of airborne droplets containing *M. tuberculosis* bacilli. Persons at high risk

for contraction of TB are those who are immunosuppressed. Persons living in crowded environments are at risk when living with an infected person. Inhalation is the main route for transmission; approximately 20% of people in household contact with a TB patient develop infection. Populations at high risk for acquiring the infection include health-care personnel, urban residents, nursing home residents, and prisoners. Infection with HIV, intravenous drug abuse, alcoholism, silicosis, immunosuppressive therapy, cancer of the head and neck, hematologic malignancies, end-stage renal disease, intestinal bypass surgery or gastrectomy, chronic malabsorption syndromes, and low body weight also increase the risk for disease. Persons with diabetes have three times the risk of developing TB compared with individuals without diabetes. Travel to an area of the world where TB is endemic, such as China or India, is a risk factor.

CLINICAL CONCEPT

Biological agents used for the treatment of autoimmune disease will immunosuppress the patient and increase risk for TB.

Tumor necrosis factor-alpha (TNF-α) antagonists, used in the treatment of rheumatoid arthritis, psoriasis, and several other autoimmune disorders, have been associated with a significantly increased risk for TB. Patients taking a TNF-α antagonist should be screened for latent TB and counseled regarding the risk of TB. Patients on systemic or inhaled steroids are also at increased risk. Persons who regularly use inhaled steroids have 1½ times the risk. Smoking is a risk factor for relapse of TB in those who have inactive TB.

Pathophysiology

M. tuberculi is inhaled from another person's cough or sneeze and droplets pass down the airway, eventually settling in the bronchial tree. The TB organism is aerobic and prefers areas of lung tissue with high O_2 levels, such as the apex. Tissue inflammation occurs as the bacilli multiply and pulmonary macrophages and WBCs migrate to the infected area. Although WBCs cannot kill the organism, an immune response occurs that eventually walls off the infection. The lesion, called a tubercle, is a granulomatous accumulation of WBCs, bacilli, and fibrotic tissue. Eventually scar tissue grows around the tubercle, and the bacilli become inactive. Histologically, the lesion in TB is referred to as Ghon's focus; when calcified, it is called a Ranke complex.

The bacilli continue to multiply, and the macrophages degrade the bacteria. The macrophages continue to be stimulated, increase enzymes, and kill bacteria. The enzymes, however, also damage lung tissue. Necrotic lung tissue takes on a cheeselike appearance; histologically, it is called caseous necrosis. In this tissue, the bacilli remain dormant, though any impairment of the patient's immune response allows reactivation of TB infection. The bacilli reinfect the bronchial tree, allowing the patient to spread the disease.

Clinical Presentation

The signs and symptoms of pulmonary TB are chronic cough, which produces purulent sputum; hemoptysis; weight loss; anorexia; chest pain; and a low-grade fever with night sweats. Individuals who are elderly usually do not exhibit all the classic signs because they cannot mount a strong immune response.

Persons can present with TB of the bones, lymph nodes, meninges, or adrenal gland. Patients with tuberculous meningitis complain of headache that is either intermittent or persistent for 2 to 3 weeks. Fever may be low-grade or absent. Skeletal TB involves the vertebrae and is also called Pott's disease. Symptoms include back pain or stiffness, and lower-extremity paralysis occurs in up to half of the patients. TB can also involve the joints, causing swelling and stiffness. Scrofula is TB of the lymph nodes, which usually occurs in the neck. TB of the adrenal gland can cause decreased cortisol levels exhibited by severe hypotension and weakness.

On physical examination, pulmonary TB will be exhibited by crackles or bronchial sounds in the lungs over the area of involvement. Lymph nodes may be enlarged in the cervical, supraclavicular, or axillary areas. However, many persons exhibit no significant physical findings, so absence of physical signs does not exclude active TB. In patients who are immunosuppressed, classic symptoms are often absent. In fact, up to 20% of patients with active TB may not have any symptoms. Therefore, sputum testing is essential when chest x-ray is consistent with TB.

CLINICAL CONCEPT

Classic signs of TB are chronic cough, weight loss, night sweats, and hemoptysis.

Diagnosis

The Mantoux tuberculin skin test and sputum cultures for acid-fast bacilli confirm the diagnosis of TB. The Mantoux test can only indicate if an individual has had prior infection and sensitization to the organism *M. tuberculosis*. It does not differentiate inactive disease from active disease. A small amount of purified protein derivative (PPD), which is an extract of the tubercle bacillus, is injected intradermally into the forearm. After 48 hours, the site should be checked for a reaction of induration, which is indicated if the area is elevated and hardened. If there is no induration at the site, the test is negative and the individual is not infected. An induration of 5 to 15 mm may be positive depending on other patient conditions. A reaction greater than 15 mm of induration is interpreted as

positive in all persons. Patients suspected of positive reaction require a chest x-ray. In some countries of Europe, the Middle East, and Asia, individuals receive the Bacillus Calmette–Guérin (BCG) tuberculosis vaccine. If these individuals are given the Mantoux test, they will test positive, an indication of previous sensitization with PPD. The positive reaction does not necessarily mean that the individual is infected with TB, which is why most individuals who test positive are required to get a chest x-ray to check for active disease.

The interferon gamma release assay (IGRA) is a blood test used to diagnose TB. This test demonstrates if the immune system has been exposed to TB bacteria. A positive IGRA test requires further testing of the individual to decipher if there is latent TB or active TB. A chest x-ray or CT scan can rule out active TB. The IGRA result is not affected by previous BCG vaccine.

Sputum specimen for acid-fast staining of mycobacteria is the laboratory test necessary for diagnosis of TB. Serum testing for the TB organism can also be done. In infected tissue, polymerase chain reaction amplification techniques can be used to detect *M. tuberculosis*. Because sputum and blood testing are not always sensitive, particularly for the drug-resistant strains of TB, there have been investigations into the use of urine tests for TB. Although not used in clinical settings as yet, the urine test shows promise. Chest x-ray, as well as HIV testing, is important. If chest x-ray findings suggest TB and sputum smear is positive for acid-fast bacilli, then treatment is initiated.

The classic chest x-ray in TB exhibits a round granuloma, usually toward the apex of the lung (see Fig. 20-8). CT scan or MRI can also demonstrate the granulomatous mass in TB.

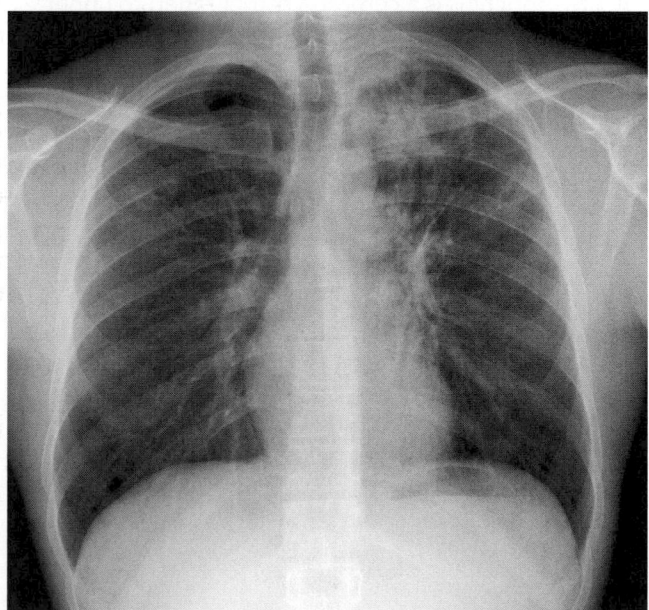

FIGURE 20-8. Chest x-ray showing TB. A round granuloma is highlighted by surrounding inflammatory tissue. Interior of lesion has tissue necrosis. *(From Du Cane Medical Imaging Ltd./Science Source.)*

Treatment

Antimicrobial medications, including isoniazid, rifampin, pyrazinamide, ethambutol, and streptomycin, are used in a combination therapy to treat patients with active TB and as prophylactic therapy for those who have had exposure and are at risk for developing active TB. The tubercle bacillus organism mutates rapidly and easily acquires resistance to any one drug. Multidrug therapy is required for a long period of time, usually 6 to 12 months, and may need to be longer in patients with an HIV infection or those with drug-resistant strains. Treatment protocols are based on the health of the patient and the type of TB strain.

Patients are placed in respiratory isolation until they are no longer considered contagious. Adequate hydration and nutrition are necessary to aid in recovery from the disease. TB is considered chronic in nature, as there is a potential for reactivation if a patient becomes immunosuppressed. Patient teaching is needed about the possibility of reoccurrence and spread of the disease. Because drug therapy extends over a prolonged period of time, the proper use of prescribed medicines needs to be reinforced.

Chapter Summary

- Upper respiratory infections are among the most common reasons that patients seek health care.
- Rhinitis is a common cold that is mainly caused by rhinovirus or adenovirus.
- GABHS is a common cause of pharyngitis; it can lead to rheumatic fever, rheumatic heart disease, glomerulonephritis, and other disorders.
- Epiglottitis, a condition that can occur as a complication of laryngitis and tracheitis, is a medical emergency that can cause asphyxiation.
- The right bronchus is vertical and wider than the left bronchus, making aspiration pneumonia more common in the right lung.
- Aspiration pneumonia can occur in debilitated persons, those with decreased level of consciousness, and persons with a weak gag or cough reflex.
- Acute bronchitis is a common complication to upper respiratory infection.
- Chronic bronchitis is diagnosed if the patient suffers bronchitis for 3 months out of the year for 2 years.
- Atelectasis commonly occurs in the postoperative period and predisposes individuals to pneumonia.

- Impending respiratory failure occurs when the patient's P_{O_2} decreases toward 60 mm Hg and PCO_2 increases toward 50 mm Hg.
- The most common cause of CAP is *S. pneumoniae*.
- Cough, fever, and crackles are classic signs of pneumonia.
- Septic emboli, which commonly develop from right-sided endocarditis, can form lung abscesses in IV drug abusers.
- Bronchial tumor obstruction of mucus and secretions can cause a lung abscess.
- Persistent cough, weight loss, night sweats, and hemoptysis are classic signs of TB.
- Immunosuppression caused by infection with HIV increases susceptibility to TB.
- The Mantoux tuberculin skin test is positive for active TB if the individual develops 15 mm or more of erythematous induration at the site of intradermal injection of PPD after 48 to 72 hours. Reactions of fewer than 15 mm need to be interpreted in terms of certain conditions.

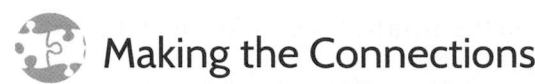

Making the Connections

Pathophysiology	Signs and Symptoms	Physical Assessment Findings	Diagnostic Testing	Treatment
Rhinitis | Inflammation of nasal mucosa and pharynx, commonly caused by viral infection.				
	Stuffed nose, nasal discharge, sneezing. Sore throat.	Nasal mucosa and turbinates red, nasal discharge, conjunctivitis possible. Pharyngeal erythema. Allergic rhinitis shows gray-colored nasal mucosa and turbinates.	CBC shows neutrophils in bacterial infection, lymphocytes in viral infection, and eosinophils in allergy.	Symptomatic treatment, antihistamines, and antipyretics. Acetaminophen. Corticosteroid anti-inflammatory nasal spray for allergic rhinitis.
Pharyngitis | Inflammation of pharynx, usually caused by a virus. It is important to test for GABHS as a bacterial cause of pharyngitis.				
	Malaise, fever, and sore throat.	Red, swollen pharyngeal membrane and tonsils. Lymphoid follicles swollen and covered with white exudate. Cervical lymph nodes tender.	Throat culture and sensitivity shows GABHS if present.	If throat culture is positive for GABHS, antibiotic such as penicillin, erythromycin, or cephalosporin. If viral pharyngitis, symptomatic relief, antipyretics, nonsteroidal anti-inflammatory drugs (NSAIDs), and antihistamines. Warm, saltwater gargle.
Sinusitis | Infection of facial maxillary and frontal sinuses, causing inflammation and the obstruction of the sinus cavity.				
	Headache, malaise, fever, stuffy, runny nose. Sore throat. Earache.	Facial pain or pressure over sinus area. Pain in sinuses that worsens with leaning forward, head-down position. Nasal obstruction and nasal discharge. Fever, headache, and ear pain. Decreased sense of smell. Sore throat.	Visual inspection and palpation of frontal and maxillary sinuses. No visualization of transmaxillary sinus light. Sinus x-rays.	Antibiotics if bacterial infection. Decongestants. Antihistamines. Saline sprays. Heated mist. Mucolytic agents. NSAIDs or acetaminophen.
Tonsillitis | Infection and inflammation of tonsils may be caused by GABHS.				
	Sore throat. Fever, malaise, anorexia, and pain with swallowing. May have earache with sore throat.	Red inflamed pharynx. Tonsillar tissues edematous and erythematous. White exudate over tonsillar tissue. Cervical lymphadenopathy.	Throat culture and sensitivity testing for GABHS.	Antibiotics if GABHS is etiology. Tonsillectomy if recurrent infections or severe tissue hypertrophy occurs.

Continued

Making the Connections–cont'd

Pathophysiology	Signs and Symptoms	Physical Assessment Findings	Diagnostic Testing	Treatment
Epiglottitis | Infection and inflammation of epiglottis caused by bacteria, viruses, or fungi (yeast). Swelling between the base of the tongue and epiglottis which, if untreated, may lead to airway blockage.				
	Severe sore throat with inability to speak and difficulty breathing Drooling of saliva caused by difficulty swallowing.	Red, swollen inflamed pharynx and tonsils. Swollen epiglottis.	Laryngoscopic exam. Neck x-rays. Increased WBC count. Arterial blood gas may show respiratory acidosis. Culture and sensitivity indicates causative organism.	Antibiotics. Humidified oxygen. IV fluids. Maintenance of the airway. Tracheostomy equipment at bedside.
Laryngitis and Tracheitis | Infection and inflammation of larynx or trachea; usually caused by a virus, but may be bacterial in nature.				
	Sore throat and difficulty speaking.	Hoarseness or complete loss of voice. Stridor may be heard. Irritating high pitch, brassy cough. Yellow, green, or mucoid sputum. Wheezing mainly upon exertion.	Arterial blood gas (respiratory acidosis). Throat culture and sensitivity.	Resting of the voice. Bronchodilators. Antibiotics. Treatment of symptoms. NSAIDs. Acetaminophen.
Acute Bronchitis | Infection and inflammation of the bronchi, caused by either bacteria or a virus. Loss of cilia from the respiratory cells lining the trachea and bronchi, resulting in impairment of mucociliary movement.				
	Cough, fever, sore throat, general malaise.	Fever possible. Cough. Mucus production. Rhonchi heard over lungs.	Chest x-ray to rule out pneumonia. CBC w/differential: High neutrophils usually indicate bacteria. Lymphocytes indicate virus. Sputum culture and sensitivity.	Expectorants. Cough suppressants. Antibiotics. Bronchodilator. Antipyretics. Acetaminophen.
Pneumonia | Infection and inflammation process in the lobes of the lungs caused by bacteria, viruses, fungi, parasites, mycoplasma, or chemicals. Exudates fill the alveolar air spaces, creating consolidation and impaired air exchange resulting in hypoxia.				
	Difficulty breathing. Fever, cough, chills, malaise, myalgias. Pleuritic chest pain. Sputum production.	Fever. Dyspnea. Diminished breath sounds. Increased tactile fremitus over pneumonia. Egophony, bronchophony, and whispered pectoriloquy elicited. Crackles. Increased sputum blood tinged to purulent. Tachycardia.	Chest x-ray. Sputum culture and sensitivity. Arterial blood gases. Pulse oximetry.	Antibiotics. Bronchodilators. Expectorants. Humidified oxygen. Antipyretics. Acetaminophen.

Continued

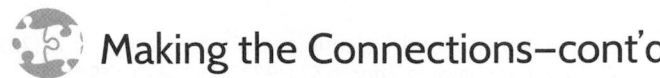 Making the Connections–cont'd

Pathophysiology	Signs and Symptoms	Physical Assessment Findings	Diagnostic Testing	Treatment
Lung Abscess | Localized area of infection and purulent inflammation, resulting in tissue necrosis. Usually caused by bacteria.				
	Fever, chills, productive cough. Pleuritic chest pain. Anorexia, cachexia.	Fever. Copious amounts of foul-smelling sputum. Productive cough. Decreased breath sounds in area of abscess.	Arterial blood gases. CBC (leukocytosis). Chest x-ray (solitary cavity with consolidation). Sputum culture.	Antibiotics. Surgical treatment. Bronchoscopy to drain abscess. Chest tube. Postural drainage. Humidified oxygen. Treatment of symptoms. Antipyretics.
Tuberculosis | Infection and inflammation of lung(s) caused by *M. tuberculosis*.				
	Chronic cough, weight loss, night sweats, and hemoptysis. Fever, malaise, dyspnea, pleuritic chest pain.	Cough with purulent sputum or hemoptysis. Weight loss. Fever.	Chest x-ray, positive Mantoux test showing greater than 10 mm, red, indurated area over intradermal injection site of PPD after 48 hours. Positive IGRA. Sputum culture; acid-fast bacilli.	Antimicrobial medications in combination therapy for long term. Adequate hydration and nutrition. Antipyretics.

Bibliography

Abubakar, I., Dara, M., Manissero, D., & Zumla, A. (2012). Tackling the spread of drug-resistant tuberculosis in Europe. *Lancet*, 379(9813), e21–e23. Epub 2011 Sep 14.

Albert, R. H. (2010). Diagnosis and treatment of acute bronchitis. *Am Fam Phys*, 82(11), 1345–1350.

Aring, A. M., & Chan. M. M. (2011). Acute rhinosinusitis in adults. *Am Fam Phys*, 83(9), 1057–1063.

Attridge, R. T., & Frei, C. R. (2011). Health care-associated pneumonia: an evidence-based review. *Am J Med*, 124(8), 689–697. doi: 10.1016/j.amjmed.2011.01.023. Epub 2011 Jun 12.

Barrett, K. E., Barman, S. M., Boitano, S., & Brooks, H. L. (2010). *Ganong's review of medical physiology.* 23rd ed. New York: McGraw-Hill/ Lange Medical Series.

Behr, M. A., Schwartzman, K., & Pai, M. (2013). Tuberculosis vaccine trials. *Lancet*, 381(9885), 2252–2253.

Bjornson, C. L., & Johnson, D. W. (2013). Croup in children. *Can Med Assoc J*, 185(15), 1317–1323. doi: 10.1503/cmaj.121645. Epub 2013 Aug 12.

Butt, S., & Swiatlo, E. (2011). Treatment of community-acquired pneumonia in an ambulatory setting. *Am J Med*, 124(4), 297–300. doi: 10.1016/j.amjmed.2010.06.027.

Cain, K. P., McCarthy, K. D., Heilig, C. M., et al. (2010). An algorithm for tuberculosis screening and diagnosis in people with HIV. *N Eng J Med*, 362(8), 707–716.

Chaisson, R. E., & Nuermberger, E. L. (2012). Confronting multidrug-resistant tuberculosis. *N Engl J Med*, 366(23), 2223–2224.

Chertow, D. S., & Memoli, M. J. (2013). Bacterial coinfection in influenza: a grand rounds review. *JAMA*, 309(3), 275–282. doi: 10.1001/jama.2012.194139.

Churchyard, G. J., Fielding, K. L., Lewis, J. J., et al. (2014). A trial of mass isoniazid preventive therapy for tuberculosis control. *N Engl J Med*, 370(4), 301–310. doi: 10.1056/NEJMoa1214289.

Czapran, A., Doherty, M., Haddon, A., & Labib, M. (2012). Recurrent aspiration and upper lobe cavitation. *Lancet,* 379(9810), 92. Epub 2011 Dec 21.

Dheda, K., Shean, K., Zumla, A., et al. (2010). Early treatment outcomes and HIV status of patients with extensively drug-resistant tuberculosis in South Africa: a retrospective cohort study. *Lancet*, 375(9728), 1798–1807.

Fourage, M., Bourguignat, C., Fermond, B., & Delobel, P. (2013). A recurrent tonsillitis. *Lancet,* 381(9862), 266.

Garbutt, J. M., Banister, C., Spitznagel, E., & Piccirillo, J. F. (2012). Amoxicillin for acute rhinosinusitis: a randomized controlled trial. *JAMA*, 307(7), 685–692.

Getahun, H., & Raviglione, M. (2013). Household tuberculosis interventions—how confident are we? *Lancet*, Jul 31. doi:pii: S0140-6736(13)61568-8. 10.1016/S0140-6736(13)61568-8. Epub ahead of print.

Gordin, F. M., & Masur, H. (2012). Current approaches to tuberculosis in the United States. *JAMA,* 308(3), 283–289.

Griffin, M. R., Zhu, Y., Moore, M. R., Whitney, C. G., & Grijalva, C. G. (2013). U.S. hospitalizations for pneumonia after a decade of pneumococcal vaccination. *N Engl J Med*, 369(2), 155–163.

Hoffner, S. E., & Jonsson, J. (2013). The need for improved tuberculosis control. *Lancet Infect Dis.* 13(9), 731–732.

Kahr, V., Barrett, N. A., Shankar-Hari, M., et al. (2010). A life-threatening sore throat masquerading as swine flu. *Lancet,* 375(9713), 524.

Keshavjee, S., Harrington, M., Gonsalves, G., Chesire, L., & Farmer, P. E. (2011). Time for zero deaths from tuberculosis. *Lancet,* 378(9801), 1449–1450.

Köser, C. U., Bryant, J. M., Becq, J., et al. (2013). Whole-genome sequencing for rapid susceptibility testing of *M. tuberculosis. N Engl J Med,* 369(3), 290–292.

Kranzer, K. (2011). Improving tuberculosis diagnostics and treatment. *Lancet,* 377(9776), 1467–1468. Epub 2011 Apr 18.

Laposata, M. (2010). *Laboratory medicine.* New York: McGraw-Hill/ Lange Medical Series.

Lawn, S. D., & Zumla, A. I. (2011). Tuberculosis. *Lancet,* 378(9785), 57–72.

Loeb, M. (2011). Community-acquired pneumonia. *Am Fam Phys,* 84(2), 218–219.

Longo, D. L., Fauci, A., Kasper, E., Hauser, S. L., & Jameson J. L. (2011). *Harrison's principles of internal medicine.* 18th ed. New York: McGraw-Hill.

Martin, A., Barrera, L., & Palomino, J. C. (2010). Biomarkers and diagnostics for tuberculosis. *Lancet,* 376(9752), 1539–1540.

McPhee, S. J., & Papadakis, M. A. (2010). *Current medical diagnosis & treatment 2010.* New York: McGraw-Hill/Lange Medical Series.

Moonan, P. K., Teeter, L. D., Salcedo, K., et al. (2013). Transmission of multidrug-resistant tuberculosis in the USA: a cross-sectional study. *Lancet Infect Dis,* 13(9), 777–784.

Randel, A., & Infectious Disease Society of America. (2013). IDSA updates guideline for managing group A streptococcal pharyngitis. *Am Fam Phys,* 88(5), 338–340.

Rangaka, M. X., & Wilkinson, R. J. (2013). Isoniazid prevention of HIV-associated tuberculosis. *Lancet Infect Dis.* 2013 Aug 14. doi: pii: S1473-3099(13)70218-4. 10.1016/S1473-3099(13)70218-4. Epub ahead of print.

Raviglione, M., Marais, B., Floyd, K., et al. (2012). Scaling up interventions to achieve global tuberculosis control: progress and new developments. *Lancet,* 379(9829), 1902–1913.

Ruuskanen, O., Lahti, E., Jennings, L. C., & Murdoch, D. R. (2011). Viral pneumonia. *Lancet,* 377(9773), 1264–1275.

Scherger, J. E. (2010). What is proper medication for patients with strep throat? *Am Fam Phys,* 81(11), 1318.

Small, P. M., & Pai, M. (2010). Tuberculosis diagnosis—time for a game change. *N Engl J Med,* 363(11), 1070–1071.

Török, M. E., & Farrar, J. J. (2011). When to start antiretroviral therapy in HIV-associated tuberculosis. *N Engl J Med,* 365(16), 1538–1540.

Torpy, J. M., Lynm, C., & Golub, R. M. (2011). *JAMA* patient page. Chronic sinusitis. *JAMA,* 306(18), 2048.

Undeland, D. K., Kowalski, T. J., Berth, W. L., & Gundrum, J. D. (2010). Appropriately prescribing antibiotics for patients with pharyngitis: a physician-based approach vs a nurse-only triage and treatment algorithm. *Mayo Clin Proceed,* 85(11), 1011–1015.

Wahls, S. A. (2012). Causes and evaluation of chronic dyspnea. *Am Fam Phys,* 86(2), 173–182.

Watkins, R. R., & Lemonovich, T. L. (2011). Diagnosis and management of community-acquired pneumonia in adults. *Am Fam Phys,* 83(11), 1299–1306.

Weber, R. (2014). Pharyngitis. *Prim Care,* 41(1), 91–98. doi: 10.1016/j.pop.2013.10.010. Epub 2013 Nov 21.

Wessels, M. R. (2011). Clinical practice. Streptococcal pharyngitis. *N Engl J Med,* 364(7), 648–655.

Wunderink, R. G., & Waterer, G. W. (2014). Clinical practice. Community-acquired pneumonia. *N Engl J Med,* 370(6), 543–551. doi: 10.1056/NEJMcp1214869.

Zoorob, R., Sidani, M. A., Fremont, R. D., & Kihlberg, C. (2012). Antibiotic use in acute upper respiratory tract infections. *Am Fam Phys,* 86(9), 817–822.

Zoorob, R., Sidani, M., & Murray, J. (2011). Croup: an overview. *Am Fam Phys,* 83(9), 1067–1073.

Zumla, A., Raviglione, M., Hafner, R., & von Reyn, C. F. (2013). Tuberculosis. *N Engl J Med,* 368(8), 745–755.

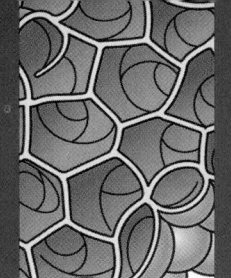

Restrictive and Obstructive Pulmonary Disorders

Key Terms

Asthma

Blue bloater

Bronchiectasis

Chronic obstructive pulmonary disease (COPD)

Compliance

Cor pulmonale

Emphysema

Forced expiratory volume (FEV)

Forced vital capacity (FVC)

Obstructive disease

Peak expiratory flow (PEF)

Pink puffer

Pleural effusion

Pleuritis (pleurisy)

Pneumothorax

Pulmonary function test (PFT)

Pulmonary hypertension

Restrictive disease

Total lung capacity (TLC)

Most lung disease can be clinically classified according to results on a **pulmonary function test (PFT).** Based on the results of these tests, pulmonary disorders can be categorized as obstructive or restrictive lung disease. **Obstructive disease** is characterized by an increase in resistance to airflow from the trachea and larger bronchi to the terminal and respiratory bronchioles. **Restrictive disease** is characterized by reduced expansion of lung tissue, with decreased total lung capacity. Lungs are stiff and noncompliant in restrictive disease.

Major obstructive lung diseases include emphysema, chronic bronchitis, bronchiectasis, and asthma. Major restrictive lung diseases include hypersensitivity pneumonitis, pulmonary fibrosis, pneumoconiosis, and thoracic cage deformities.

Epidemiology

More than 35 million Americans are living with chronic lung disease, such as asthma and chronic obstructive pulmonary disease (COPD). Long-term cigarette smoking is the primary cause of COPD, and great attention has been given to the effects of secondhand smoke. There is an increased prevalence of respiratory illness and reduced levels of pulmonary function in nonsmokers who reside with smokers. Nonsmokers exposed to secondhand smoke at home or work increase their risk of developing lung cancer by 20% to 30%.

Large numbers of individuals are also at risk for developing serious respiratory disorders as a result of occupational or environmental exposures. Approximately 2.4 million workers in the United States have been exposed to environmental causes of lung disease such as coal, silica, and asbestos. Radon gas, which is emitted from natural radium in earth materials and can be trapped indoors, is a risk factor for lung cancer. Levels of radon gas associated with lung cancer risk may be present in as many as 10% of households in the United States—and smokers who reside in households contaminated by radon have a potentially greater risk of lung cancer.

Respiratory illnesses have also been attributed to indoor chemical agents emitted from various kinds of synthetic fibers and building materials. Chemical agents such as formaldehyde, diisocyanates, and latex particles that circulate within the air of poorly ventilated buildings have been implicated as the cause of various respiratory complaints. Exact numbers are not available, but millions of workers inhale chemical agents and synthetic particles in unventilated workplaces daily.

Basic Concepts of Pulmonary Structure and Function

The lungs are spongelike organs that have the unique property of compliance, the flexibility to expand and contract. With inhalation, the lung tissue expands to bring in a large volume of oxygen for transfer into the bloodstream. With exhalation, the elastic lung tissue contracts to push out carbon dioxide. In addition, the bronchioles have the ability to dilate and constrict. Bronchodilation allows complete filling of the lungs with oxygen, whereas bronchoconstriction diminishes oxygenation.

Bronchodilation and Bronchoconstriction

The trachea divides into two main bronchi, which further divide into smaller diameter airways called the bronchioles. The bronchi and bronchioles are laced with smooth muscle controlled by the autonomic nervous system. The coordinated contraction and relaxation of the smooth muscle layer controls the diameter of these airways.

During inspiration, the smooth muscle of the airways relaxes, causing bronchodilation, which is the widening of the airways. Conversely, during exhalation, the smooth muscle of the airways contracts, stimulating bronchoconstriction, which is the narrowing of the airways.

Both types of autonomic nerves—sympathetic and parasympathetic nerves—innervate the bronchiole smooth muscle. Sympathetic nerves dilate the bronchioles, whereas the parasympathetic nerves constrict the bronchioles. The sympathetic nerves within the bronchioles specifically act on beta-2 adrenergic receptors within the walls of the airways. These receptors are similar to the beta-1 adrenergic receptors that are within heart tissue. Stimulation of beta-2 adrenergic receptors dilate the bronchioles and amplify the ventilatory capacity of the lungs. During times of high stress, the fight-or-flight response causes stimulation of the sympathetic nerves, which causes the bronchioles to dilate; this allows for maximal ventilation into the lungs. Stimulation of the sympathetic nervous system also causes blood vessel vasoconstriction and inhibition of bronchial secretions. Conversely, parasympathetic nervous system stimulation causes bronchoconstriction, blood vessel vasodilation, and an increase in bronchial secretions. Inflammatory mediators such as leukotrienes, which are secreted by white blood cells (WBCs), and histamine, which is released from mast cells, also stimulate bronchoconstriction.

Compliance

During the process of respiration, the lungs expand and contract. On inspiration, lungs expand and increase their total volume. On expiration, the lungs recoil based on their elasticity. The change in lung volume during this process is described as **compliance,** which is the flexibility of the lungs. Compliance is reduced by illness that makes the lungs stiffer, thereby increasing the work of breathing, as seen in bronchitis and pneumonia when the lungs are congested with fluid. Compliance is also reduced by inflammatory conditions such as pulmonary fibrosis and sarcoidosis.

The Pleural Membrane

The pleural membrane lines the thoracic cavity and envelopes the lungs. The outer layer lies on the chest wall and the inner layer adheres to the lung tissue. The inner and outer layers of the pleural membrane form a cavity known as the pleural space. A thin film of fluid called surfactant is contained within the pleural space to keep the membrane layers separated and lubricated. Other than surfactant, there is no air or fluid within the pleural space; it is a vacuum. Because it is a vacuum, the pleural space has negative intrathoracic pressure. When lung tissue fills with air during inspiration, the lung tissue develops positive intrathoracic pressure and expands into the vacuous pleural space. The lungs easily expand and retract during inhalation and exhalation within the empty pleural space. However, if air or fluid is contained within the pleural space, the positive pressure of the air or fluid pushes against the lung tissue and prevents its full expansion. Therefore, it is critical that the pleural space be completely devoid of air or fluid.

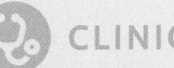

CLINICAL CONCEPT

The lungs are composed of spongy, compressible tissue, which is why they easily collapse when pressure is placed against them by pleural fluid, as in a pleural effusion, or air, as in a pneumothorax.

Basic Pathophysiologic Concepts of Pulmonary Disorders

There are two pathological conditions that can occur in lung disease: hypoxia and hypercapnia. Hypoxia occurs when the lungs cannot fully ventilate or acquire maximal oxygenation. Hypercapnia develops when the lungs cannot fully expel carbon dioxide. Hypoxia and hypercapnia often occur together because of suboptimal pulmonary ventilation.

Chronic Hypercapnia

When partial pressure of carbon dioxide (PCO_2) exceeds the upper limit of normal in the bloodstream (greater than 45 mm Hg), the condition is known as hypercapnia. Hypercapnia can develop because of bradypnea, which is an abnormally slow breathing rate. Slowed breathing allows accumulation of carbon dioxide (CO_2) in the bloodstream. The accumulation of blood CO_2 causes stimulation of the brain's respiratory center, found in the medulla, to increase breathing rate. CO_2 accumulation in the bloodstream stimulates the medulla and drives normal breathing.

Inadequate ventilation or any cause of obstructed gas exchange can cause hypercapnia; causes include asphyxiation, aspiration, pneumonia, pulmonary edema, thoracic muscle paralysis, and opiate toxicity. Some of the clinical features of acute hypercapnia include headache, drowsiness, intellectual impairment, and disorientation, all of which may progress to stupor and coma.

Hypercapnia and hypoxia are commonly simultaneous conditions. Chronic hypercapnia is a common finding in patients with progressive hypoxic lung disease. When chronic hypercapnia develops over a number of years, eventually the central chemoreceptors in the medulla become insensitive to CO_2 levels. The stimulus for breathing shifts to the chemoreceptors in the carotid and aortic bodies, which are triggered by low oxygen in the bloodstream. Patients with chronic hypercapnia incur a distinct change in their stimulus to breathe. Instead of

CO_2 accumulation being the stimulus to breathe, hypoxia becomes the impetus for the patient to take another breath. This is a significant change in physiologic response, which commonly occurs in severe COPD.

Chronic Hypoxia

Chronic hypoxia is a chronic lack of oxygen that occurs in respiratory dysfunction. The term is often used interchangeably with hypoxemia, which refers to diminished oxygen (O_2) levels in the blood. Body tissues vary in their vulnerability to hypoxia; some, such as bone, can withstand episodes of hypoxia for much longer time periods than others, such as the heart and brain.

If partial pressure of oxygen (PO_2) of tissues falls below a critical level, cellular aerobic metabolism ceases and anaerobic metabolism takes over with formation of lactic acid. Mild hypoxemia causes few symptoms because hemoglobin (Hgb) saturation remains high, at approximately 90%, with PO_2 levels as low as 70 mm Hg. However, there is a dramatic drop in Hgb's affinity for oxygen at PO_2 of 60 mm Hg. At a PO_2 of 60 mm Hg, Hgb starts to release all its oxygen molecules, placing the patient in a state of severe hypoxemia. Severe hypoxemia causes behavioral changes, restlessness, uncoordinated movements, impaired judgment, delirium, and eventually stupor and coma.

The body compensates for hypoxia by increasing ventilation, stimulating pulmonary vasoconstriction, and having the kidney release erythropoietin (see Fig. 21-1). Chronic hypoxia stimulates erythropoietin secretion by the kidney. Erythropoietin stimulates the bone marrow to synthesize red blood cells (RBCs). Chronic hypoxia causes constant synthesis of RBCs, a condition called erythropoiesis. Chronic hypoxia also causes pulmonary arterial vasoconstriction; this leads to pulmonary hypertension, a condition of high blood pressure within the pulmonary arterial system.

> **ALERT!** At a PO_2 of approximately 60 mm Hg, oxygen saturation of Hgb dramatically falls.

CLINICAL CONCEPT

Patients with chronic hypoxia develop pulmonary vasoconstriction, called pulmonary hypertension, which causes an increased workload for the right ventricle and can lead to right ventricular failure, a condition known as cor pulmonale.

Assessment

To thoroughly assess the patient with pulmonary disease, a detailed history and physical examination should

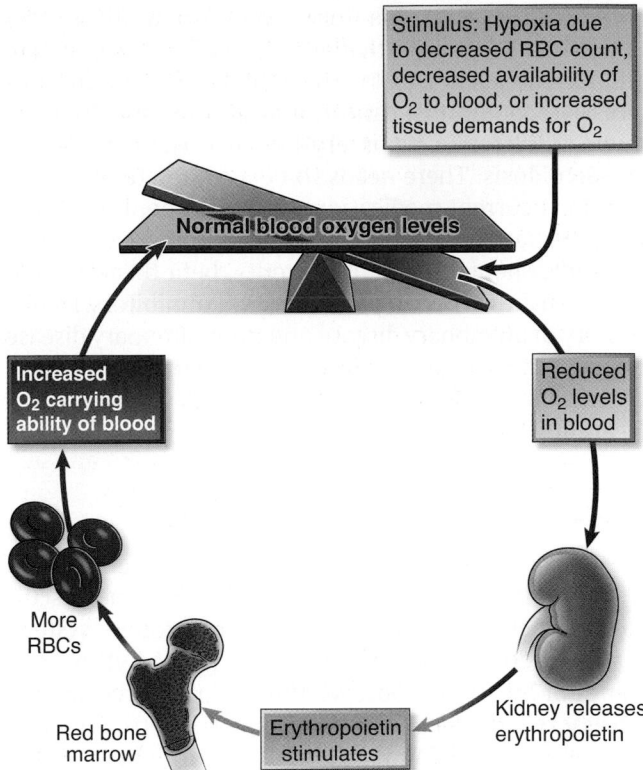

FIGURE 21-1. Erythropoiesis. When the blood develops hypoxia, the kidney secretes erythropoietin. Erythropoietin then stimulates bone marrow to synthesize RBCs.

be completed. The clinician should review all the risk factors for lung disease when taking a history. Smoking and occupational exposure are key risk factors to explore. All the components of physical examination—inspection, palpation, percussion, and auscultation—are used during pulmonary assessment.

Risk Factors

A history of current and past smoking habits should be sought from all patients. If the patient has smoked, the clinician should ask the patient the number of years he or she has smoked and multiply that number by the number of packs of cigarettes smoked per day; this yields a smoking history in pack-years. For example, a 76-year-old patient who has smoked two packs per day since age 16 years has a 120 pack-year smoking history (2 packs per day x 60 years). If the patient has no smoking history, the clinician should ask about exposure to secondhand smoke.

Occupational exposure to toxic agents should be investigated. Important agents include inorganic dusts such as asbestos and silica. Ask the patient about exposure to animals, pet dander, molds, pollen, ragweed, household dust, and cockroaches. Illicit drug use, particularly marijuana, cocaine, and intravenous drugs, needs to be discussed. Ask the patient about possible contact with individuals with respiratory infections and exposure to infectious agents such as tuberculosis.

A history of any respiratory or nonrespiratory disorder should be sought, particularly cardiac disease, human immunodeficiency virus (HIV) infection, immunosuppressive conditions, cancer, and autoimmune disease such as systemic lupus erythematosus, scleroderma, or sarcoidosis. There needs to be a complete list of the patient's current medications and treatments, particularly radiation therapy, immunosuppressive agents, steroids, chemotherapeutic agents, beta blockers, and angiotensin-converting enzyme (ACE) inhibitors. Family history of pulmonary disease and nonpulmonary disease should be investigated, particularly tuberculosis, asthma, cystic fibrosis, alpha-1 antitrypsin (AAT) deficiency, and heart disease.

Signs and Symptoms

The clinician should use the physical examination techniques of inspection, palpation, percussion, and auscultation when assessing the patient's pulmonary system. On inspection, note the patient's rate, rhythm, and depth of breathing. Observe the use of intercostal and accessory muscles, symmetrical or asymmetrical expansion of the chest, and structural abnormalities of the thoracic cage and spine. Observe the patient for dyspnea, which is breathing difficulty, and orthopnea, which is difficulty breathing when lying flat. The patient may cough while being examined. A cough is described as productive if sputum is expectorated with the cough; if blood is expectorated with the cough, this is called hemoptysis. Check the patient's hands for clubbing of the fingers, as this is a finding consistent with chronic hypoxia. Cyanosis, a bluish discoloration of the skin and mucous membranes, occurs with hypoxia; this is caused by the excessive concentration of deoxygenated Hgb in the small blood vessels.

Patients with chronic obstructive disease often have a characteristic barrel-shaped chest where the anterior and lateral diameter of the thoracic cage are equal. Normally, the lateral diameter is half the size of the anterior diameter.

Palpate the bony structures of the thoracic cage, such as the clavicles and ribs, for tenderness or fracture. Palpate the lymph nodes for tenderness or enlargement. Focus on the cervical, supraclavicular, infraclavicular, and axillary nodes. Inspect and palpate the oral cavity for lesions.

The clinician can use a unique palpation technique when assessing the lungs. Tactile fremitus is a palpation technique to assess the vibration in the lungs caused by vocalization. The patient is asked to repeat the words "ninety-nine" as the examiner palpates the vibrations transmitted though the posterior chest. Transmissions of vibrations increases over areas of pulmonary consolidation, such as pneumonia or neoplasm. Transmission of vibrations are decreased or absent over areas of pleural fluid.

The clinician can use percussion in physical examination of the chest. The normal sound percussed over lung tissue is called resonance. Percussion is performed with the index and middle finger of one hand tapping on the middle finger of the other hand over the posterior chest. Percussion of dull sounds is heard over consolidated areas of lung tissue or pleural fluid. Hyperresonance, a low, drumlike sound, is percussed over areas of emphysema or air in the pleural cavity.

On auscultation, the examiner should listen to the quality of breath sounds and for any adventitious sounds. Ask the patient to breathe in through the nose and out through the mouth slowly. Breath sounds are diminished by bronchial obstruction or by air or fluid in the pleural cavity. Tubular breath sounds, also called bronchial sounds, are heard over consolidated areas of the lung, as in pneumonia. Sound transmission can also be assessed by listening with the stethoscope to the vocal sounds of the patient transmitted through the lung and chest wall. The clinician may be able to elicit sounds referred to as bronchophony, egophony, and whispered pectoriloquy (see Chapter 20). The possible adventitious sounds heard with the stethoscope over the lungs are crackles, also called rales; wheezes; and rhonchi. Crackles are commonly heard in pneumonia and pulmonary edema.

Diagnosis

Chest x-ray is commonly the initial diagnostic study performed to evaluate patients with pulmonary signs and symptoms by assessing heart size, diaphragm borders, pulmonary tissue and vascularity, mediastinal lymph nodes, and pleural membranes (see Fig. 21-2). Anterior-posterior and lateral views of the lungs on chest x-ray are usually indicated. Increased opacity on chest x-ray usually indicates a solid mass or fluid. Increased radiolucency usually indicates air-filled or cystic conditions.

Further information about pulmonary health can be obtained from computed tomography (CT) scans, magnetic resonance imaging (MRI), ultrasonography, bronchoscopy, angiography, thoracocentesis, positron emission tomographic (PET) scans, arterial blood

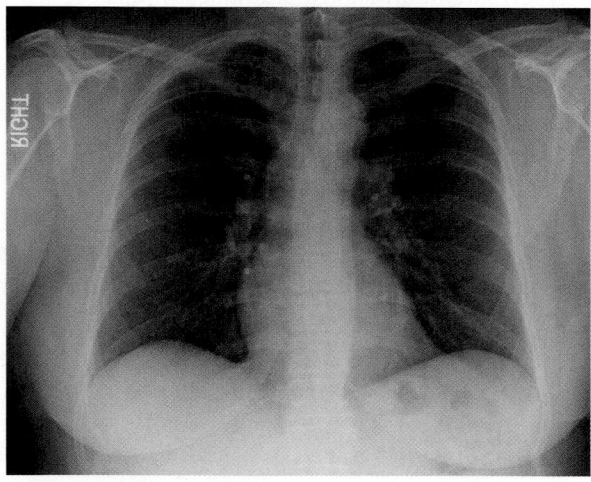

FIGURE 21-2. Normal chest x-ray. (From Weber, E.C. (2013). *Practical radiology*. Philadelphia, PA: F.A. Davis Company, with permission.)

BOX 21-1. (a) and (b). Lung Volumes Measured by a Pulmonary Function Test

(A)

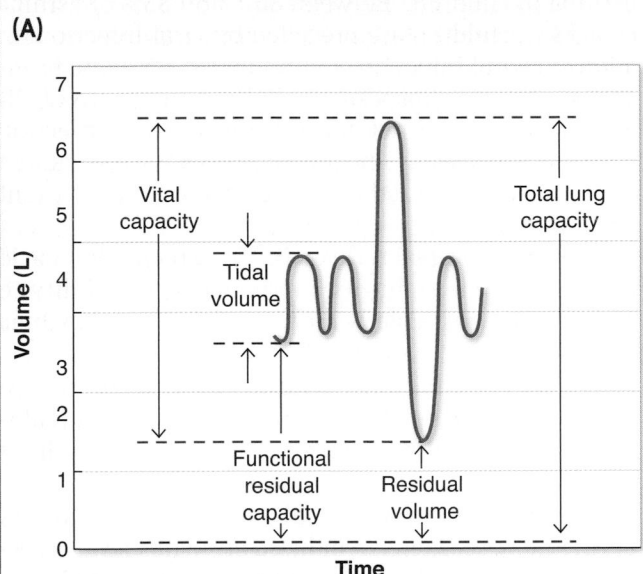

The more common lung function values measured with spirometry are:

- **Forced vital capacity (FVC):** This measures the amount of air an individual can exhale with force after inhaling as deeply as possible.
- **Forced expiratory volume (FEV):** This measures the amount of air an individual can exhale with force in one breath. The amount of air exhaled may be measured at 1 second (FEV1), 2 seconds (FEV2), or 3 seconds (FEV3). FEV1 divided by FVC can also be determined.
- **Forced expiratory flow 25% to 75% (FEV$_{25\%-75\%}$):** This measures the airflow halfway through an exhale.
- **Peak expiratory flow (PEF):** This measures how quickly an individual can exhale. It is usually measured at the same time as your FVC.

- **Total lung capacity (TLC):** This measures the amount of air in an individual's lungs after inhaling as deeply as possible.
- **Functional residual capacity (FRC):** This measures the amount of air in an individual's lungs at the end of a normal exhaled breath.
- **Residual volume (RV):** This measures the amount of air in an individual's lungs after a complete exhalation. It can be done by breathing in helium or nitrogen gas and seeing how much is exhaled.
- **Tidal volume (TV):** This shows an individual's usual relaxed breathing volumes in inhalation and exhalation.

(B) NORMAL FORCED EXPIRATORY VOLUME IN FIRST SECOND (FEV1) OF EXHALATION.

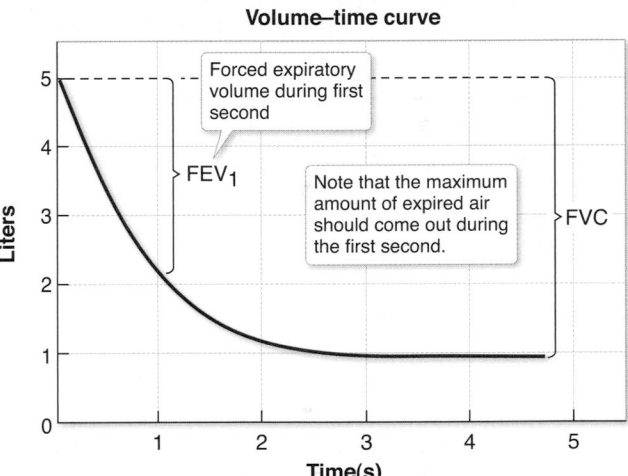

The FEV1 is the amount of air exhaled in the first second of expiration. Normally, approximately 80% of air in the lungs should be exhaled in the first second.

---

gas (ABG) analysis, pulse oximetry, and ventilation-perfusion (V-Q) scans.

Pulmonary disease can be categorized as obstructive or restrictive using PFTs, which measure different lung volumes as the patient exhales into a pulmonary spirometry device (see Box 21-1).

Treatment

Bronchodilators are commonly used in obstructive lung diseases to counteract bronchoconstriction. They are available as inhaler adrenergic agonists and inhaler anticholinergic agents. They come in the form of long-acting medication for maintenance therapy and short-acting, rescue medication for acute attacks of bronchoconstriction. Albuterol is a commonly used adrenergic rescue bronchodilator. Metaproteronol is a commonly used maintenance medication. Anti-inflammatory agents are available as inhaler corticosteroids, oral corticosteroids,

and oral leukotriene antagonists. Some inhalers contain a mixture of a long-acting bronchodilator and a corticosteroid as maintenance medication. Leukotriene antagonists are oral medications that counteract bronchial inflammation, and they need to be taken daily for maintenance. At times, patients require a short term of a low-dose oral corticosteroid such as prednisone when exacerbations of obstructive disease occur. Many patients with asthma and allergies carry a prefilled syringe of epinephrine for emergencies.

Patients may require a nebulizer for better absorption of medication. Nebulized adrenergic agonists deliver the medication in an easily absorbed mist that can get into the lower bronchial airways. Theophylline and aminophylline are phosphodiesterase inhibitors that can be used to enhance bronchodilation. Cromolyn sodium is a medication specifically used for exercise-induced asthma, whereas antibiotics are commonly used in obstructive diseases to counteract respiratory infections. Pleural disorders such as pleural effusion or pneumothorax require chest tube insertion and suction or thoracotomy. Surgical procedures are often needed to remove masses. A specific type of surgical procedure termed lung volume reduction surgery (LVRS) is used in emphysema. In LVRS, the most damaged alveoli are excised from the lung. Endotracheal intubation and mechanical ventilation are used in cases of respiratory failure.

Pathophysiology of Selected Obstructive Disorders

Obstructive disease is characterized by an increase in resistance to airflow from the trachea and larger bronchi to the terminal and respiratory bronchioles. The major obstructive lung diseases are asthma, COPD, and bronchiectasis.

Asthma

Asthma, also called hyperreactive airway disease, is a chronic inflammatory disorder that causes reversible airway constriction because of bronchial hyperreactivity. With each acute attack, permanent inflammatory changes develop in the bronchioles, so the aim of treatment is to prevent acute asthma attacks.

Epidemiology

Asthma is a common disease. Among adults in the United States, 106 per 1,000 are diagnosed with asthma per year, with an annual mortality rate of 2 per 100,000 persons. Poor clinical control of the disorder among patients is the major cause of nearly 2 million emergency department visits, 500,000 hospitalizations, and 5,000 deaths per year. The mortality rate is nearly 3 times higher in African American males than in Caucasian males and 2½ times greater in African American females than in Caucasian females.

Etiology

Asthma has many different etiologies and is considered a multifactorial genetic disorder caused by a combination of gene mutations and environmental factors.

Allergy is the most common etiology of asthma. There are a wide number of different allergens in the environment. Allergens include exhaust fumes, perfumes, pollen, grasses, flowers, dust, cigarette smoke, animal dander, molds, and spores. Tobacco smoke is particularly known for triggering bronchospasm.

Occupational exposure to chemical agents can also trigger asthma. More than 300 agents are known to stimulate bronchoconstriction. Employment settings with the highest risk of these chemical triggers include farming, painting, construction, landscaping, and janitorial work. Occupation-associated asthma can occur immediately after exposure to the chemical agent or as an immune-mediated disorder that occurs months to years after exposure.

Viral infections, such as those caused by rhinovirus and respiratory syncytial virus, are common triggers for asthma in children. Between 80% and 85% of asthma attacks in children are preceded by viral infection. In addition, viral infection commonly causes acute bronchitis with bronchospasm in adults. Adults with COPD are particularly at risk for viral respiratory infection with bronchospasm. Sinusitis is also a known stimulant of asthma; 50% of asthma patients have a concurrent sinus infection.

Gastroesophageal reflux (GERD), which allows acid to irritate the esophagus, increases susceptibility to asthma. It is particularly a cause of nocturnal asthma attacks.

A triad of conditions—asthma, aspirin sensitivity, and nasal polyps—are found in 5% to 10% of individuals with asthma. Nonsteroidal anti-inflammatory drugs (NSAIDs) have also been known to trigger asthma.

Asthma can be silent in individuals and only present during exercise. Exercise-induced bronchospasm occurs during vigorous physical activity in some individuals with airway hyperreactivity. Exposure to cold air often worsens exercise-induced asthma.

Pathophysiology

Asthma is a chronic inflammatory disease that causes episodes of spastic reactivity in the bronchioles. With each bout of acute bronchospasm in asthma, deleterious bronchial remodeling occurs. Prevention of asthma attacks is critical to avert bronchial airway alterations.

Allergy is a common stimulus of asthma. Allergens trigger the immune system, causing bronchial constriction, inflammation, and an increase in the size and number of goblet cells that secrete mucus. There is bronchoconstriction, bronchial edema, viscous mucus, and thickening of the bronchial basement membrane.

T lymphocytes are particularly involved in the pathophysiology of asthma. It is theorized that two types of helper T lymphocytes, Th1 and Th2, are active during asthma. Th1 cells are stimulated by microbes or allergens and assist B cells transform into plasma cells that produce immunoglobulin E (IgE). Th2 cells attract mast cells, eosinophils, and basophils, which promote inflammation. IgE binds to mast cells and provokes their degranulation, which releases mediators such as histamine and leukotrienes. Leukotrienes are responsible for the development of bronchoconstriction, bronchial hyperreactivity, edema, and eosinophilia. Histamine contributes to bronchospasm and inflammation. T cells release cytokines called interleukins that maintain the damaging effects of the asthma attack. Eosinophils migrate to the reactive airway, compounding cell damage and airway edema. A cholinergic effect maintains the bronchoconstriction, increased mucus production, and vasodilation.

Asthma is also commonly triggered by viral respiratory infections that stimulate the production of IgE directed toward the viral antigens. Viral and bacterial upper respiratory infections commonly cause bronchospasm and copious mucus production.

Exercise can induce asthma by provoking loss of heat and water from the tracheobronchial tree; it is particularly exaggerated by cold air.

Inhaled chemicals such as those contained in strong exhaust fumes induce bronchospasm by irritating receptors that stimulate a vagal reflex. Chemicals that trigger asthma include sulfur dioxide, nitrogen dioxide, ozone, toluene, epoxy resins, and formaldehyde commonly found in the workplace, as well as sulfites used in food processing.

Multiple episodes of asthma promote the process of airway remodeling, which involves proliferation of respiratory epithelium and hypertrophy of respiratory smooth muscle; it can also lead to a relatively fixed airway obstruction. Additionally, epithelial cell injury exposes the airway to triggers for hyperreactivity, resulting in more frequent episodes of bronchospasms.

There is a small group of persons with a clinical syndrome that includes asthma, nasal polyps with chronic sinusitis, and aspirin or NSAID sensitivity. The mechanism of this reaction is not well understood but is likely caused by some abnormality in the cyclooxygenase pathway of inflammation.

Also, those persons who suffer from GERD can experience asthma when gastric secretions reflux into the bronchi and act as a bronchospastic trigger. GERD is a common trigger of nocturnal asthma attacks that awaken patients from sleep.

Nocturnal asthma may also be caused by sleep-related circadian rhythm changes; these cause respiratory function to decrease during early morning hours. Concurrently, during the early morning hours, cortisol level, a natural anti-inflammatory substance, is low and eosinophil activity is increased.

Clinical Presentation

The clinician should assess the severity of the patient's asthma through a variety of important questions. A history of childhood asthma and family history are important. Questions to ask include:

- Are you experiencing dyspnea, wheeze, or cough?
- Are symptoms worse at night or after exercise?
- How often do you experience symptoms?
- Does exposure to certain environmental allergens such as dust or pet dander provoke symptoms? How about episodes of respiratory infection or GERD?
- What is your occupation? What kind of materials do you handle?

Signs and Symptoms. Asthma is characterized by wheezing, cough, dyspnea, and chest tightness. The severity of the symptoms depends on the degree of bronchial hyperresponsiveness and reversibility of the bronchial obstruction (see Fig. 21-3). Prolonged exhalations are commonly an early sign of airway obstruction. Severe attacks are accompanied by use of accessory muscles, distant breath sounds, and diaphoresis. The patient may only be able to speak one or two words

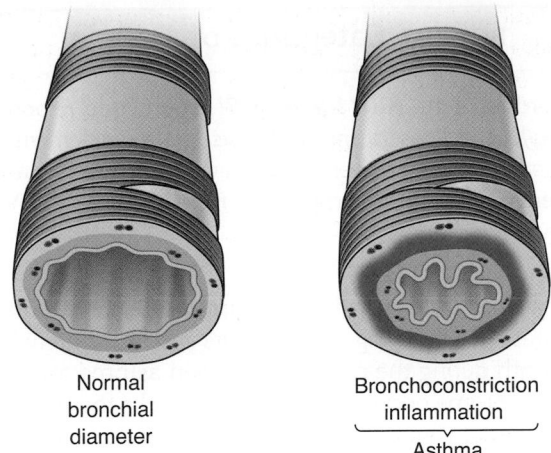

Normal bronchial diameter **Bronchoconstriction inflammation** **Asthma**

FIGURE 21-3. Bronchoconstriction in asthma.

before taking a breath. Patients going into respiratory failure caused by marked airway constriction have inaudible breath sounds and a repetitive, hacking cough. Rhonchi may be present if larger bronchial airways are involved. If the asthma is related to allergies, signs of chronic rhinitis may be present, including nasal edema, nasal polyps, rhinorrhea, and oropharyngeal erythema. Eczema, which indicates allergy, may be present on the patient's skin, particularly the neck and the antecubital or popliteal spaces.

Diagnosis

The diagnosis of asthma is based on a thorough history and physical examination, laboratory findings, and PFTs. The PFT measures of forced expiratory volume at 1 second (FEV1) and forced vital capacity (FVC) are used to diagnose and evaluate the severity of an asthma attack. During an acute asthma attack, FEV1 decreases, which diminishes the overall FEV1/FVC ratio. This ratio should then be reassessed after a bronchodilator is administered to diagnose and evaluate severity of asthma. The diagnosis of asthma should be considered if there is an increase of 12% or greater and 200 mL in FEV1 after inhaling a short-acting bronchodilator.

Categories of Asthma. Asthma is categorized according to the frequency of episodes, nocturnal symptoms, and PFT findings (see Box 21-2).

Treatment

Treatment guidelines have been developed by the National Asthma Education and Prevention Program. The guidelines utilize a stepwise approach to patient care based on the severity and frequency of symptoms as well as FEV1/FVC. Each step of treatment includes patient education, environmental control, and management of comorbidities, as well as medication. If a current treatment plan is not controlling the asthma, then treatment moves up a step to more aggressive therapy. The goal of treatment is to control asthma and prevent acute episodic exacerbations of bronchospasm.

BOX 21-2. Categories of Asthma

According to the *2007 NIH/NHLBI Expert Panel Report 3 (EPR3): Guidelines for the Diagnosis and Management of Asthma,* asthma categories are based on frequency and severity of asthma symptoms, FEV1, and FEV1/FVC measurements.

MILD INTERMITTENT

In mild intermittent asthma, symptoms occur less than 2 times a week during waking hours and less than twice a month during the night. In between asthma attacks, no symptoms occur at all, and the attacks themselves are generally brief, though their intensity can vary. The FEV1 is greater than 80% of normal during asthma attacks. The FEV1/FVC ratio is normal.

MILD PERSISTENT

In mild persistent asthma, symptoms are occurring more than twice a week, but not as often as daily. They may occasionally wake the patient up at night, but that happens less than 2 times a month. Asthma attacks may interfere with activity temporarily. The FEV1 is greater than or equal to 80% of normal during asthma attacks. The FEV1/FVC ratio is normal.

MODERATE PERSISTENT

In moderate persistent asthma, the disorder is starting to interfere more with daily living. Symptoms are cropping up every single day, and the patient needs to use a quick-relief inhaler daily. Asthma attacks are occurring at least twice a week, often interfere with activity, and may last for days at a time. The patient is probably also waking up 1 or more times a week with symptoms. FEV1 is between 60% and 80% of normal. The FEV1 / FVC ratio is reduced by 5%.

SEVERE PERSISTENT

In severe persistent asthma, the most severe form of the disorder, symptoms are basically continuous. Activity is severely limited and asthma attacks and night symptoms are frequent. The FEV1 is lower than 60% of normal. The FEV1/FVC ratio is reduced by more than 5%.

National Asthma Education and Prevention Program Expert Panel Report 3: Guidelines for the Diagnosis and Management of Asthma, 2007 U.S. Department of Health and Human Services, National Institutes of Health (NIH), National Heart, Lung, and Blood Institute (NHLBI).

Medications for asthma fall into two general classes: maintenance medication for daily use and rescue medication for acute episodes. Maintenance medications are long-acting bronchodilators and anti-inflammatory corticosteroids, usually in the form of inhaler medication. A common long-acting maintenance medication is a combination of adrenergic beta-2 agonist and corticosteroid. Alternatively, an anticholinergic inhaler can be administered if an adrenergic agonist is not effective. If additional maintenance control is needed, an oral leukotriene antagonist is usually added to the daily regimen. In addition, a phosphodiesterase inhibitor, theophylline or aminophylline, can be used to enhance bronchodilation.

Short-acting bronchodilators known as rescue medications are used for acute asthma attacks. These rescue medications are rapid-acting, adrenergic beta-2 agonists administered via an inhaler. If this is not sufficient to treat the acute attack, an oral corticosteroid is added to the regimen. An injection of epinephrine can also be administered if the acute exacerbation is severe.

Other asthma medications include cromolyn sodium, which stabilizes mast cells and can be used as preventive treatment before exercise or unavoidable exposure to known allergens. For allergic individuals, immunomodulator type medications may be helpful. Immunomodulators are monoclonal antibody medications that prevent binding of IgE to basophils and mast cells.

Studies show that a procedure called bronchial thermoplasty, performed using a bronchoscope, has decreased patients' need for rescue medications and lessens all symptoms. A catheter tip with a wire probe is used to deliver heat to the airway wall to decrease the mass of smooth muscle that constricts the airway.

Limitation of exposure to allergens in the patient environment is critical in asthma. Allergen immunotherapy, although controversial, can be tried if there is a definite association between asthma and unavoidable allergen triggers. Patients are slowly desensitized using incremental small amounts of the allergen.

Complications

Status asthmaticus is defined as persistent bronchoconstriction that endures despite attempts to treat the attack with medications. In this severe asthma attack, pulmonary gas exchange is diminished by the uneven distribution of ventilation resulting from generalized bronchoconstriction. The major physiologic abnormality is a grossly uneven V-Q distribution, leading to a dramatic fall in arterial oxygenation. If bronchoconstriction is not relieved, and the patient becomes exhausted and dehydrated, total alveolar ventilation fails, leading to cyanosis and carbon dioxide retention. Status asthmaticus can be fatal.

Chronic Obstructive Pulmonary Disease

Chronic obstructive pulmonary disorder (COPD) is a combination of chronic bronchitis, emphysema, and hyperreactive airway disease. It is characterized by the features of these three disorders.

Epidemiology

COPD is the third leading cause of death in the United States and a leading cause of disability. It is estimated that there are 12.7 million persons with COPD; most are over age 45. However, the prevalence is believed to be up to twice that number because of underreporting of individuals who do not seek health care. In the past, COPD had a higher prevalence in men, but from 1980 to 2000 the mortality rate from COPD increased dramatically in women; today, there are more women dying of COPD than men. In the United States, the economic burden of this disease, estimated at 24 billion dollars annually, is caused by the cost of medical care and days lost from work.

Etiology

Smoking is the major cause of COPD, as 90% of patients with COPD are smokers, but occupational and environmental exposures to chemicals, dusts, and secondhand smoke are also causes. COPD is caused by a combination of genetic susceptibility and environmental factors. One such genetic predisposition to COPD is caused by alpha-antitrypsin (AAT) deficiency. This rare genetic variant accounts for fewer than 1% of all COPD cases. AAT, a serum protein normally found in the lungs, inhibits elastase, a proteolytic enzyme released by WBCs. AAT deficiency allows elastase to destroy lung tissue unchecked. The genetic mutation causing AAT deficiency is found on chromosome 14. AAT deficiency leads to premature development of emphysema in young adults, often with chronic bronchitis and bronchiectasis.

Intravenous drug abuse has been associated with emphysema. This is caused by some of the components of the illicit drug that are injected into the bloodstream. Components such as talc enter the venous system and can travel to the right side of the heart and then into the pulmonary circulation and lung tissue.

Pneumocystis jiroveci infection in individuals with AIDS is associated with emphysematous changes in the lungs. Bullous cysts called pneumoceles are commonly found within lung tissue in AIDS sufferers.

Connective tissue diseases, which include Marfan syndrome and Ehlers-Danlos syndrome, also predispose individuals to emphysema. Connective tissue changes in the walls of the alveoli cause decreased elasticity and recoil of lung tissue.

Pathophysiology

COPD is characterized by poorly reversible airflow limitation caused by a combination of chronic bronchitis, emphysema, and hyperreactive airway disease. The characteristic features of chronic bronchitis are hypersecretion of mucus in the large and small airways, hypoxia, and cyanosis. Excessive mucus creates obstruction to inspiratory airflow that inhibits optimal oxygenation. To be diagnosed with chronic bronchitis, the individual has to have had a cough for 3 months out of the year for 2 consecutive years.

In **emphysema,** the characteristic finding is overdistention of alveoli with trapped air, which creates obstruction to expiratory airflow, loss of elastic recoil of the alveoli, and high residual volume of carbon dioxide in the lung. The airways are also hyperreactive to irritants, and episodes of bronchoconstriction are common in COPD.

The pathological changes leading to airflow limitation in COPD include narrowing, excessive mucus and fibrosis in the bronchioles, loss of alveolar elastic recoil, and smooth muscle hypertrophy. Inflammatory changes of chronic bronchitis cause permanent

remodeling of the pulmonary structure. The remodeled bronchioles demonstrate chronic inflammatory changes, thickening of the walls, and constriction of the lumens. Inflammation causes stimulation of macrophages followed by accumulation of neutrophils, T lymphocytes, and cytokines. Leukotrienes, interleukins, and tumor necrosis factor are among the inflammatory mediators that act in a proteolytic manner, chronically damaging lung structures. There is a proteolytic-antiproteolytic enzyme imbalance in the lungs of patients with COPD that leads to changes consistent with emphysema. Neutrophils and macrophages secrete proteases, elastases, and metalloproteinases, which are all proteolytic enzymes. Smoking activates proteolytic enzymes, which are released from neutrophils and macrophages. Cigarette smoke also contains free radicals that damage respiratory cell membranes and arterial endothelial cells. Concurrently, smoking inactivates the body's natural antioxidants and antiproteolytic enzymes (see Fig. 21-4).

In severe COPD, particularly in those areas demonstrating changes consistent with chronic bronchitis, there is poor ventilation and hypoxia. In areas of poor ventilation, hypoxia stimulates pulmonary arterial vasoconstriction. Pulmonary arterial vasoconstriction, which is called **pulmonary hypertension,** causes increased resistance in the main pulmonary artery and, in turn, increased resistance against the right ventricle. Chronic pulmonary hypertension causes right ventricular hypertrophy and eventual right ventricular failure. Right ventricular failure caused by pulmonary disease

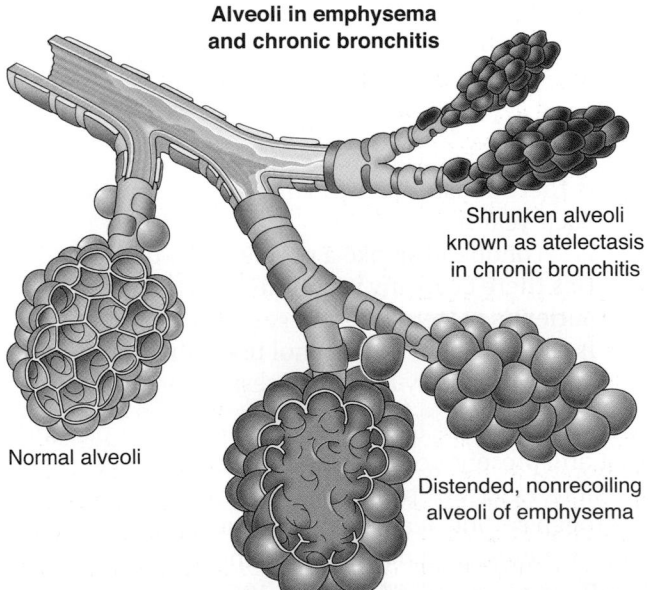

Alveoli in emphysema and chronic bronchitis

Shrunken alveoli known as atelectasis in chronic bronchitis

Normal alveoli

Distended, nonrecoiling alveoli of emphysema

FIGURE 21-4. The bronchioles and alveoli in COPD. COPD is a combination of chronic bronchitis and emphysema. In chronic bronchitis, there is inflammation, edema, and excess mucus production within the airways. In emphysema, there is an excess of air in the alveoli. The alveolar walls are weakened, distended, and cannot recoil. Some alveoli shown here are also atelectatic from lack of ventilation caused by chronic bronchitis.

is called **cor pulmonale.** In cor pulmonale, the patient suffers all the signs and symptoms consistent with right ventricular failure, including jugular venous distension, ascites, hepatomegaly, splenomegaly, and ankle or sacral edema.

In severe COPD, increased levels of CO_2 become chronic and the arterial chemoreceptors and respiratory center in the medulla become insensitive to high CO_2 levels. The normal respiratory drive stimulus changes from PCO_2 accumulation to low levels of PO_2. In severe COPD, hypoxia becomes the stimulus for breathing. In other words, the patient needs to be hypoxic to stimulate independent breathing. Administering high doses of oxygen can depress the patient's independent drive to breath and cause respiratory arrest. Careful, slow upward titration of oxygen is necessary when the patient requires oxygen therapy. Any agents that depress respiratory drive, such as tranquilizers, sedatives, and opiates, should be used with caution.

Clinical Presentation

Patient age and smoking history are important features in establishing a pattern of obstructive disease. Asthma occurs in all age groups; however, in general, COPD is a disease of older persons. The mean age of patients with emphysema is 65 years old. Patients with COPD caused by AAT deficiency are usually younger adults aged 40 to 50 years. Commonly, the patient with COPD complains of dyspnea and cough. It is important to ask what precipitates the dyspnea, such as climbing a flight of stairs, lifting heavy objects, walking several blocks, or the performance of activities of daily living such as bathing and dressing. This gives the examiner an idea of the severity of airflow limitation. Other questions to ask include:

- What is the frequency and quality of the cough? Is it productive of sputum? Is hemoptysis present? If so, how much?
- Has there been any wheezing?
- Is there a history of smoking? If so, what is the pack-year history?
- Is secondhand smoke a problem at work or home?
- Has there been any weight loss? What is the patient's pattern of exercise?
- Is there a history of alcohol use? Illicit drugs?
- Is there a family history of respiratory illness?

Along with these questions, ask about the patient's past and present occupations, particularly focusing on possible exposure to toxins such as asbestos, silica, hydrogen sulfide, lead, mercury, coal, cotton dust, and diisocyanates. Also make sure to include the patient's complete list of current medications, including herbal and over-the-counter medications, as well as allergies.

Signs and Symptoms. Signs and symptoms of COPD include those of chronic bronchitis, emphysema, and asthma. Dyspnea is usually the first symptom, initially occurring with heavy exertion. As the disease

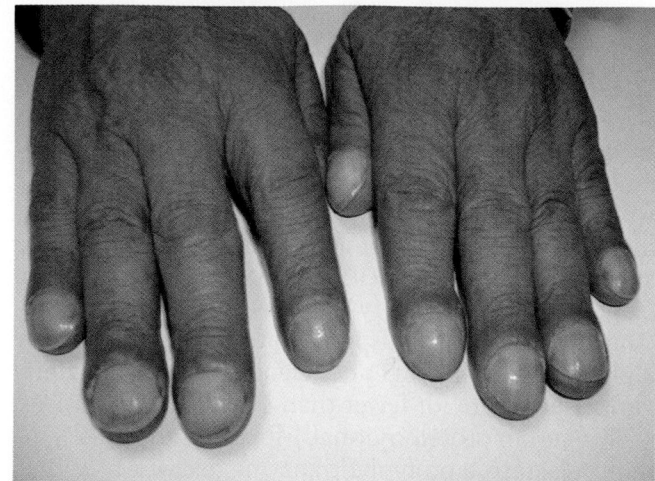

FIGURE 21-5. Clubbing of fingers occurs in chronic hypoxia. *(Courtesy of Desherinka.)*

progresses, dyspnea becomes increasingly worse with less and less vigorous exertion. Cough or wheezing may be a chief complaint. The cough may be productive and sputum should be expectorated for culture. Productive cough, hypoxia, and cyanosis are classic signs of chronic bronchitis. The hypoxia of chronic bronchitis stimulates pulmonary arterial vasoconstriction. Over time, because of the high resistance against the right ventricle, right ventricular failure occurs. The signs and symptoms of right-sided heart failure, such as jugular venous distension, ascites, hepatosplenomegaly, and ankle edema, develop after long-term chronic bronchitis.

Observe the patient for signs of respiratory distress, use of intercostal muscles or accessory muscles with breathing, and clubbing of the fingers (see Fig. 21-5).

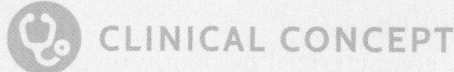

CLINICAL CONCEPT

Clubbing of fingers indicates chronic hypoxia.

Examine the thoracic cage structure. A barrel-shaped chest or increased anterior-posterior diameter is commonly present in patients with emphysema. Look at the patient's complexion. Cyanosis, commonly visible around the lips, indicates hypoxia. In those with a lengthy smoking history, the teeth or fingertips may be tobacco stained. Examine the jugular veins, abdomen, and ankles. Distended jugular veins, ascites, and ankle edema indicate cor pulmonale.

With regard to vital signs, particularly focus on respiratory rate, rhythm, and depth. Patients with COPD often have prolonged exhalation and purse the lips when exhaling. The examiner can palpate the posterior lung fields bilaterally for tactile fremitus. Vibrations over lung fields should be equal as the patient vocalizes "ninety-nine." The posterior lung fields can also be percussed bilaterally for resonance. In severe emphysema, hyperresonance may be percussed because of the extra air retained in the lungs. Auscultate the heart and note any abnormal sounds. Commonly wheezing is heard over the lung fields in COPD. Diminished breath sounds may suggest severe disease. Identify the location of any adventitious sounds.

 CLINICAL CONCEPT

Individuals with chronic bronchitis are known as **blue bloaters**—blue because of hypoxia and cyanosis and bloater because of the edema that occurs as a result of right ventricular failure. Individuals with emphysema are known as **pink puffers**—pink because they remain well-oxygenated until late in their disease, and puffer because they have a characteristic manner of exhalation using pursed lip breathing.

Diagnosis

Pulmonary function tests (PFTs) (also called spirometry) are a key part of the diagnosis of COPD. Airflow limitation of COPD is identified by a FEV1/FVC ratio of lower than 70%. FEV1 significantly diminishes in COPD because the patient's exhalation phase is slow and prolonged (see Fig. 21-6).

A complete blood count (CBC), blood chemistry panel, chest x-ray, electrocardiogram (ECG), and ABGs should be analyzed. In those individuals with mild to moderate disease, all laboratory data should be normal except for the PFTs. In severe COPD, the chest x-ray may have characteristics consistent with emphysema: flattened, low diaphragm borders and hyperinflation of both lung fields caused by retained air. The ECG commonly demonstrates a right axis deviation caused by right ventricular hypertrophy. Also in severe COPD, an enlarged heart may be visible on chest x-ray because of right ventricular failure. The pulmonary vasculature may be enlarged on chest x-ray if pulmonary hypertension exists because of chronic bronchitis. In those with severe hypoxia, the CBC will indicate erythrocytosis (high number of erythrocytes) caused by the constant secretion of erythropoietin from the kidney. Eosinophilia will be present if allergy exists.

 CLINICAL CONCEPT

Expiratory airflow limitation, demonstrated by a low FEV1, is the hallmark of COPD.

Treatment

Treatment of COPD involves a stepwise approach that begins with short-acting bronchodilator agents for patients with mild disease and incorporates long-acting

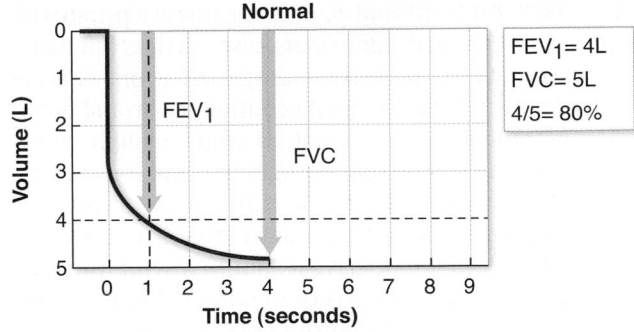

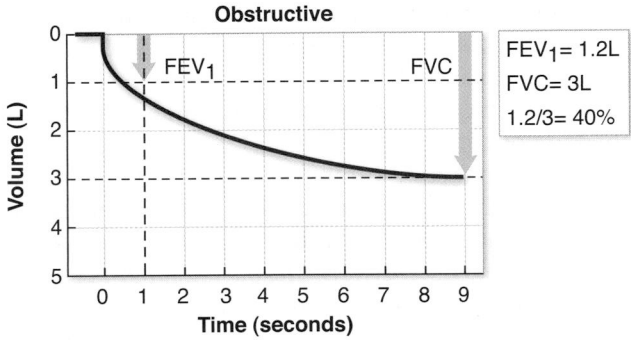

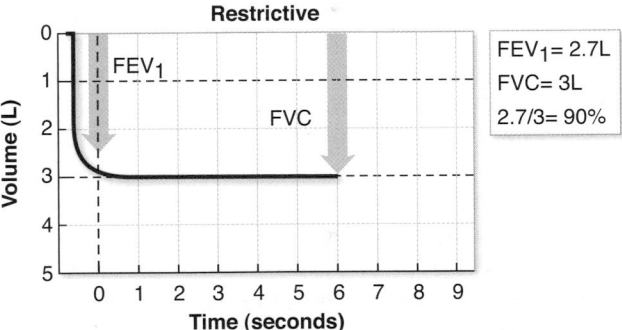

FIGURE 21-6. Spirometry measures in obstructive versus restrictive pulmonary disease. Forced expiration over 1 second (FEV1) is a simple PFT. A person inhales to total lung capacity and then exhales as completely as possible into a spirometer. The spirometer then prints out a curve on a graph. The graph will show total FVC and the amount of exhaled air in the first second of expiration. The FEV1 is compared with the FVC to diagnose an obstructive versus a restrictive pulmonary disease. (a) In a normal forced expiration curve, the total FEV that the healthy subject can expire in 1 second (FEV1) is about 80% of the total FVC. The FVC is approximately 5 liters. In a healthy subject, almost all of the air can be exhaled within the first second. (b) In an obstructive pulmonary condition, such as asthma, bronchitis, or emphysema, the FVC is reduced and the rate of expiratory flow is also reduced. The subject takes a prolonged time to exhale all the air from the lungs. Thus, an individual with an obstructive defect might have an FVC of only 3.0 liters, and in the first second of forced expiration, exhale only 1.2 liters, giving an FEV1/FVC ratio of 40%. (c) With a restrictive disease, such as interstitial pulmonary fibrosis, FVC is also reduced. However, because of the stiffness of the lung, there is a high recoil and the FEV1/FVC ratio may be normal or even greater than normal. For example, a patient with a restrictive condition might have a FVC of 3.0 liters, but the FEV1 might be as high as 2.7 liters, giving a FEV1/FVC ratio of 90%. The patient exhales the air rapidly in the first second.

agents into the treatment plan as the disease progresses in severity. Beta-2 adrenergic agonist inhalers stimulate bronchiole smooth muscle, leading to dilation, whereas anticholinergic inhaler agents counteract bronchoconstriction. Inhaled bronchodilators, which include short-acting and long-acting beta-2 agonists and long-acting anticholinergic agents, are the cornerstone of therapy. Inhaled bronchodilators are the treatment of choice in patients with COPD who have respiratory symptoms and an FEV1 that is lower than 60% of normal. Monotherapy with a long-acting beta-2 adrenergic agonist or an anticholinergic bronchodilator is recommended as first-line treatment. If monotherapy with a bronchodilator is insufficient, inhaled corticosteroids can be added to the regimen. Many inhaler preparations contain both a long-acting bronchodilator and corticosteroid agent combined in one canister.

Phosphodiesterase inhibitors, such as theophylline, can be added to the regimen when the patient is not responding adequately to bronchodilators. Oral corticosteroids are used when the patient has an acute exacerbation and is not responding adequately to bronchodilators. The patient needs to use oral corticosteroids in low doses for a short time and be weaned off them slowly.

Leukotriene antagonists are another type of agent used in asthma to counteract bronchoconstriction and inflammation in the bronchioles. These drugs block the lipoxygenase pathway of inflammation that yields leukotrienes.

Nonpharmacological interventions include smoking cessation, pneumococcal and influenza vaccine, pulmonary rehabilitation, and oxygen therapy. Pulmonary rehabilitation involves a slowly progressive program of aerobic exercise and endurance training with supervision. There is ventilatory muscle training in patients with decreased respiratory muscle strength and debilitating breathlessness. Pulmonary rehabilitation should be used for symptomatic patients who demonstrate an FEV1 lower than 50% of normal on PFTs.

Continuous oxygen therapy is indicated when arterial PO_2 is lower than or equal to 55 mm Hg or the saturation of oxygen in the blood is lower than or equal to 88%. Oxygen is also indicated if there is evidence of pulmonary hypertension, cor pulmonale, cognitive impairment caused by hypoxia, or polycythemia and a PO_2 of 56 to 59 mm Hg. Oxygen needs to be used in the lowest doses that can enhance the patient's oxygenation. Oxygen therapy requires slow upward titration to the level that assists the patient's oxygenation and still maintains the patient's independent respiratory drive.

ALERT! When administered to a patient with severe COPD, oxygen administration higher than 2 liters per minute will decrease or interrupt the stimulus for breathing and can result in respiratory arrest.

ALERT! Tranquilizers, sedatives, and opiates can depress respiratory drive and cause respiratory failure in patients with severe COPD.

Mechanical ventilator support via an endotracheal tube is indicated for patients with severe respiratory distress unrelieved by other therapies, life-threatening hypoxemia, severe hypercapnia, respiratory acidosis, or respiratory arrest. There is a 17% to 30% mortality rate for patients requiring mechanical ventilatory support. For patients older than 65 years who require critical care for COPD, mortality rate doubles to 60% regardless of the need for mechanical ventilation.

Lung volume reduction surgery (LVRS) is indicated in severe emphysema when nonsurgical therapies have proven to be limited in effectiveness. The goals of LVRS are to remove the most severely diseased areas of emphysematous lung and to decrease the degree of lung hyperinflation. The procedure removes the severely damaged alveoli that act as dead spaces that do not allow diffusion of oxygen into the circulation.

Bronchiectasis

Bronchiectasis is an uncommon disease, most often caused by untreated infections that lead to chronic inflammation and dilatation of bronchi. Infections that lead to bronchiectasis are frequently caused by *Pseudomonas aeruginosa*, *Haemophilus influenzae*, *Staphylococcus aureus*, tuberculosis, *Mycobacterium avium*, and klebsiella. Adenovirus and influenza virus are the main viruses that cause bronchiectasis. Aspergillus organisms that cause allergic bronchopulmonary aspergillosis can also lead to the disorder.

In bronchiectasis, the structural components of the bronchiole wall, including cartilage, muscle, and elastic tissue, are destroyed and replaced by fibrous tissue. Because of multiple infections over time, the bronchioles become irreversibly dilated. The permanently dilated airways commonly contain static, thick purulent secretions, and the peripheral airways are often obstructed or obliterated by secretions and replaced by fibrous tissue.

Patients typically present with persistent or recurrent cough and purulent sputum production. Hemoptysis caused by bleeding from inflamed airway mucosa occurs in 50% to 70% of patients. Dyspnea or wheezing indicates widespread bronchiectasis or underlying COPD. Chest x-ray may not reveal significant changes in order to diagnose bronchiectasis. Bronchography, which involves coating the airways with a radiopaque dye through a bronchoscope, can provide visualization of the dilated airways. CT scan can also provide a view of the dilated airways. Examination of sputum reveals a high amount of neutrophils and the infectious agent. Bronchoscopy may be necessary to investigate endobronchial obstruction and rule out neoplasm. PFTs demonstrate airflow obstruction similar to COPD and hyperreactive airways. A slow, prolonged FEV1 and decreased FEV1/FVC ratio are common findings.

Treatment involves elimination of the underlying problem such as infection. Mucolytic agents and aerosolized medications can decrease the viscosity of sputum. Bronchodilators to improve obstruction and clearance of secretions are useful in patients with hyperreactive airways. Antibiotics are also needed to clear the infection. Surgical excision of the involved region of lung may be considered. In patients with extensive disease, chronic hypoxemia may indicate long-term oxygen therapy. For select disabled patients, lung transplantation is a therapeutic option.

Obstructive Sleep Apnea

Obstructive sleep apnea (OSA), also called hypoventilation syndrome, is an intermittent cessation of airflow from the nose and mouth during sleep. It is characterized by recurrent episodes of sleep apnea of 2 to 3 minutes in duration.

In OSA, the upper airway closes repeatedly during sleep. Symptoms of OSA include loud snoring, choking or gasping during sleep, unrestful sleep, and daytime sleepiness. Basic factors, such as airway anatomy (e.g., large tonsils), nasal blockage, presence and distribution of body fat, and muscle tone, contribute to the severity of this disorder. Obesity is the most common risk factor. A specific form of OSA, Pickwickian syndrome, is caused by a short, thick neck circumference. OSA is worsened by the use of alcohol and sedative-hypnotic medications.

Diagnosis of OSA requires a sleep study, also called polysomnography. Patients are clinically observed overnight in a sleep laboratory and have various body functions measured.

Treatment includes behavioral changes such as abstinence from alcohol, smoking cessation, avoidance of the use of sedatives, weight loss, and continuous positive airway pressure (CPAP). Nasal CPAP prevents the airways from closing by delivering air through a mask that forces the air through the nasal passages. CPAP should be used for the entire sleep duration every night. A similar treatment, called BiPAP, also delivers positive air pressure. Alternatively, oral appliances that pull the tongue forward can be used in patients with mild OSA during sleep. Central nervous system stimulants may be recommended for those with daytime sleepiness. Surgery may be done to increase the size of the pharyngeal opening and upper airway.

Pathophysiology of Selected Restrictive Disorders

Diseases that prevent complete ventilation, diminish total lung capacity, and impede the opening of all the alveoli are referred to as restrictive pulmonary diseases. Pneumothorax and pleural effusion are the most common causes of restrictive respiratory diseases. Lung diseases that damage the lung tissue directly, such as pulmonary fibrosis and environmental lung disorders, can also cause restrictive disease, as can musculoskeletal disorders that cause structural alterations of the thoracic cage. Vertebral abnormalities such as kyphosis and scoliosis can restrict pulmonary function. Immunological-mediated disorders, such as sarcoidosis, cause restrictive lung disease. Neurological disorders such as muscular dystrophy, myasthenia gravis, and Guillan-Barré syndrome, all of which can impair full thoracic cage expansion, can also cause a restrictive pulmonary disorder.

Pneumothorax

A **pneumothorax,** also known as a collapsed lung, is the presence of air in the pleural cavity that causes collapse of a large section or whole lobe of lung tissue. Air can enter the pleural cavity because of chest trauma or rupture of alveoli (see Fig. 21-7). There are five types of pneumothorax:

1. primary spontaneous pneumothorax (PSP)
2. secondary spontaneous pneumothorax (SSP)

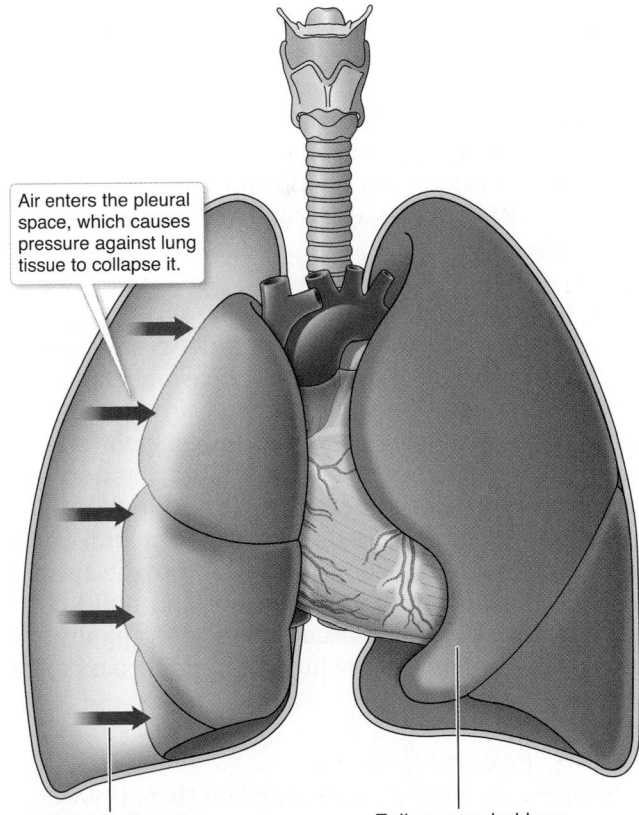

Air enters the pleural space, which causes pressure against lung tissue to collapse it.

Pneumothorax   Fully expanded lung

FIGURE 21-7. Pneumothorax. Pneumothorax is a collection of air in the pleural space that causes part or all of a lung to collapse. Normally, the pleural space is a vacuum with no air or fluid. The pressure in the lungs is greater than the pressure in the pleural space. However, if air enters the pleural space, the air presses against the lung tissue, causing the lung to collapse partially or completely. Pneumothorax can be either spontaneous or caused by trauma.

3. traumatic pneumothorax
4. tension pneumothorax
5. iatrogenic pneumothorax.

Primary Spontaneous Pneumothorax

PSP occurs in people without underlying lung disease and in the absence of an inciting event. Air is present in the intrapleural space without preceding trauma and without underlying clinical or radiological evidence of lung disease. This condition is commonly seen in tall, young men between the ages of 10 and 30 years old; it is rarely seen in people older than 40 years. The etiology is unclear, but ruptured alveoli are theorized to be the cause. The incidence of PSP is 7.4 to 18 cases per 100,000 persons per year for men and 1.2 to 6 cases per 100,000 persons per year for women. Some individuals who suffer PSP have a genetic predisposition. For example, PSP frequently occurs in persons with the genetic disorder Marfan syndrome. Cigarette smokers also have an increased risk of PSP.

Secondary Spontaneous Pneumothorax

SSP occurs in people with a wide variety of lung diseases. In SSP, an underlying pathological process occurs in the lung. Air enters the pleural space via ruptured blebs, which are overly distended and damaged alveoli. Patients with long-term emphysema often suffer SSP caused by ruptured alveoli. Other diseases that may be present when SSPs occur include tuberculosis, sarcoidosis, cystic fibrosis, malignancy, and idiopathic pulmonary fibrosis (IPF). *Pneumocystis jiroveci* pneumonia is a common cause of SSP in patients with acquired immune deficiency syndrome (AIDS).

Traumatic Pneumothorax

A traumatic pneumothorax is commonly caused by a penetrating wound of the thoracic cage and underlying pleural membrane. Commonly, a thoracic wound causes a rib fracture that punctures the pleural membrane. The punctured thoracic cage and pleural membrane create an opening between the pleural cavity and outside atmosphere. The open wound allows the pleural cavity, which is normally a vacuum, to pull air into the opening of the wound from the atmosphere and build up in the pleural space. The accumulated intrapleural air eventually compresses the lung tissue and causes lung collapse.

Tension Pneumothorax

A tension pneumothorax occurs when there is an escalating buildup of air within the pleural cavity that compresses the lung, bronchioles, cardiac structures, and vena cava. A tension pneumothorax occurs because there is a closed, penetrating wound that allows air into the pleural cavity, but will not allow air out. Increasing air accumulation causes a rapid rise in intrathoracic pressure, which inhibits venous return and optimal function of the heart and lungs. This is a life-threatening disorder.

Iatrogenic Pneumothorax

Iatrogenic pneumothorax is a complication of medical or surgical procedures. It most commonly results from transthoracic needle aspiration, but can be caused by therapeutic thoracentesis, pleural biopsy, central venous catheter insertion, transbronchial biopsy, positive pressure mechanical ventilation, and inadvertent intubation of the right mainstem bronchus. Therapeutic thoracentesis is complicated by pneumothorax 30% of the time when performed by inexperienced clinicians, in contrast to only 4% of the time when performed by experienced clinicians.

Clinical Presentation

The clinical signs and symptoms of a pneumothorax include chest pain, dyspnea, and increased respiratory rate. On inspection, there may be an obvious asymmetry of the chest, as well as intercostal muscle retractions. Percussion may reveal chest hyperresonance, whereas auscultation may reveal a lack of breath sounds on the affected side.

Diagnosis

Chest x-ray or CT scan confirms the diagnosis of pneumothorax. On chest x-ray, a linear shadow of visceral pleura with lack of lung markings peripheral to the shadow may be observed, indicating a collapsed lung (see Fig. 21-8). A mediastinal shift toward the contralateral, undamaged lung may be apparent. Pulse oximetry and ABG analysis demonstrate hypoxemia; ABG analysis can also show varying degrees of acidosis, and hypercapnia, the occurrence of which depends on the extent of cardiopulmonary compromise at the time of collection.

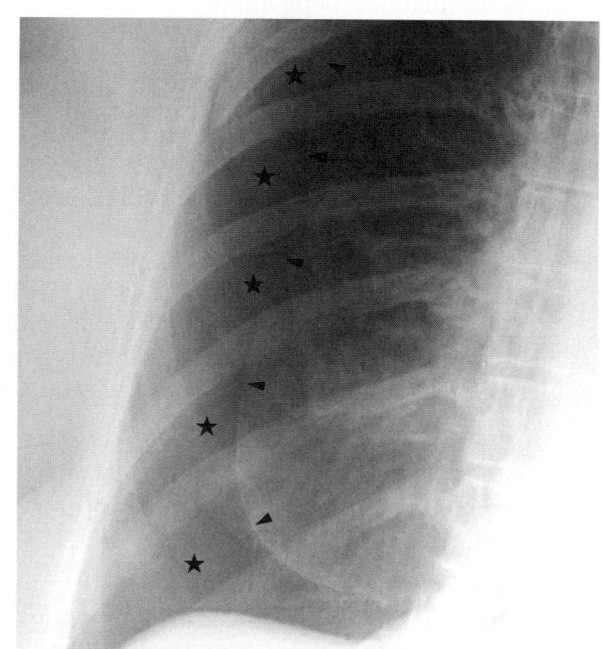

FIGURE 21-8. Chest x-ray showing pneumothorax. (From Weber, E. C. (2013). *Practical radiology*. Philadelphia, PA: F.A. Davis Company, with permission.)

Treatment

Treatment of an open traumatic pneumothorax requires a chest tube with suction on the affected side. The chest tube apparatus pulls the air out of the pleural cavity and allows the collapsed lung to reexpand. A tension pneumothorax is an emergency situation that requires a large bore needle inserted into the affected side to pull the air out of the chest to relieve the accumulated pressure on the mediastinal structures. Oxygen administration is also necessary for patients with a pneumothorax.

In some cases of spontaneous pneumothorax, a procedure called pleurodesis is performed to prevent reoccurrence. Pleurodesis intentionally causes chemical or surgical irritation of the layers of the pleural membrane. The irritation causes the visceral and parietal pleural membrane layers to adhere to each other and close off the pleural space. Those who are susceptible to a spontaneous pneumothorax should be cautioned to avoid cigarette smoking, high altitudes, unpressurized aircraft, and scuba diving.

Pleural Effusion

A **pleural effusion** is an abnormal collection of fluid within the pleural cavity that compresses lung tissue and inhibits lung inflation (see Fig. 21-9). It is commonly edematous fluid that accumulates within the pleural space because of heart failure, severe pulmonary

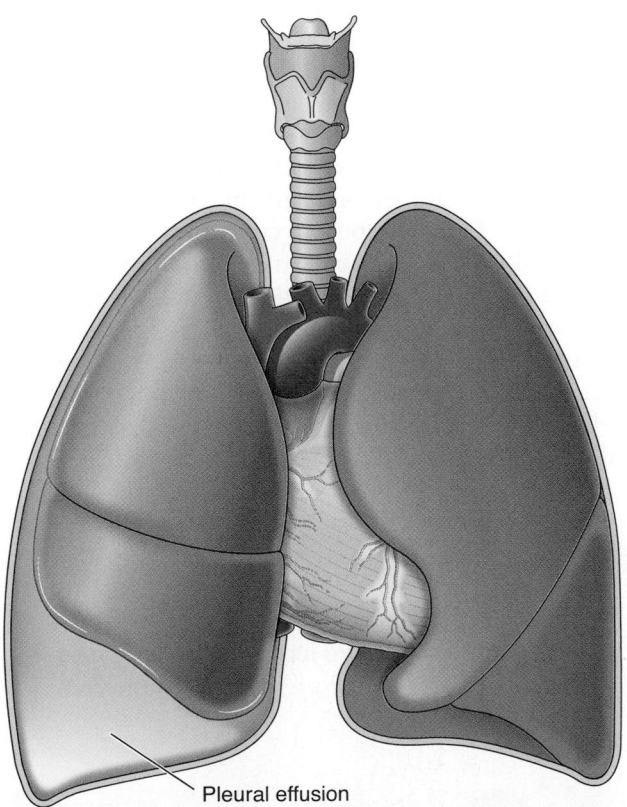

Pleural effusion

FIGURE 21-9. Pleural effusion. When fluid accumulates within the pleural space, it is called a pleural effusion. A pleural effusion presses against the lung tissue, inhibiting the lung's full expansion. The midline of the chest cavity deviates to the opposite side of the pleural effusion.

infection, or neoplasm. The fluid may be an exudate or transudate, purulent, lymph, or sanguinous (bloody). **Pleuritis** (also called **pleurisy**) is inflammation of the pleural membrane. This condition is common in infections that extend to the pleura.

Epidemiology

The estimated incidence of pleural effusion is 1.5 million cases per year, with most effusions caused by heart failure, malignancy, infections, and pulmonary emboli.

Etiology

Transudates are filtrates of the blood that accumulate within the pleural space because of an imbalance in the capillary forces: hydrostatic and oncotic pressure. Elevated hydrostatic pressure causes fluid to leak out of capillaries into the pleural space. Major etiologies of transudates are listed in Box 21-3.

In contrast, exudates are mainly caused by pleural or lung inflammation or infection. Less commonly, exudates come from impaired lymphatic drainage of the pleural space or from extension of inflammatory fluid from the peritoneal space. Common causes of exudates are listed in Box 21-4.

Pathophysiology

Normally, the pleural space contains approximately 1 mL of fluid used to lubricate the visceral and parietal pleural membranes. The pleural cavity should be free of any additional fluid or air. Pleural effusions result from disruption of the balance between hydrostatic and oncotic forces in the lung tissue. When hydrostatic pressure in the lung tissue greatly exceeds oncotic pressure, fluid leaks out of the pulmonary capillaries and cells into the pleural space, causing a pleural effusion.

Clinical Presentation

The most common signs of a pleural effusion are dyspnea, tachypnea, sharp pleuritic chest pain, dullness to

---

BOX 21-3. Transudative Pleural Effusion Etiologies

A transudate is a filtrate of the bloodstream that is non-infectious, clear, and low in protein content. Transudates develop because of high hydrostatic pressure within the capillaries and consequent fluid accumulation in the involved tissues.

- Atelectasis
- Cirrhosis
- Congestive heart failure
- Constrictive pericarditis
- Hypoalbuminemia
- Myxedema
- Nephrotic syndrome
- Peritoneal dialysis

BOX 21-4. Exudative Pleural Effusion Etiologies

An exudate is a cloudy, edematous fluid with high protein content. It is most commonly caused by an infectious, immunological, or inflammatory process.

- Asbestos exposure
- Chylothorax
- Collagen-vascular conditions
- Drug use
- Esophageal perforation
- Malignancy
- Meigs syndrome
- Pancreatitis
- Parapneumonic causes
- Postcardiac injury syndrome
- Radiation pleuritis
- Sarcoidosis
- Trauma
- Tuberculosis

percussion, and diminished breath sounds on the affected side. There is lack of breath sounds over the area of a pleural effusion. Percussion over the area demonstrates a flat, dull sound that indicates fluid blocking the normally resonant lung tissue. Tactile fremitus is decreased over a pleural effusion.

Diagnosis

Chest x-ray, CT scan, and ultrasound can all detect the presence of a pleural effusion. With large pleural effusions, mediastinal structures are pushed away from the side of pleural effusion on chest x-ray. Alternatively, on chest x-ray, if mediastinal structures are pushed toward the side of the effusion, this is usually because of an obstruction within the bronchus caused by malignancy or, less commonly, a foreign body.

Thoracentesis should be performed on pleural effusions to relieve pressure on the lungs and provide fluid for analysis. Laboratory testing helps distinguish pleural fluid transudates from exudates. The fluid is analyzed for blood, glucose, infectious material, WBCs, tumor markers, and other constituents that assist in the diagnosis.

CT angiography should be ordered if pulmonary embolism (PE) is suspected. If TB or a malignancy is suspected, biopsy of the lesion is necessary. Bronchoscopy is necessary if a lesion is suspected within a bronchiole. Thoracoscopy and thoracotomy are other diagnostic procedures that can allow biopsy of the pleural membrane.

Treatment

Treatment is aimed at the cause for the pleural effusion. Suction and drainage of a pleural effusion is usually necessary. Surgical intervention is most often required for effusions that cannot be drained adequately by needle or small-bore catheters.

Environmental Lung Disorders

Environmental lung diseases, known as pneumoconioses, result from occupational exposure to specific airborne agents or particulate air pollution. The most dangerous particles are those that reach the terminal small airways. Normally, inhaled particulate matter is phagocytosed by pulmonary macrophages. However, in pneumoconioses, macrophages are overwhelmed by a large quantity of dust or particles deposited because of environmental exposures. Also, large particles may resist dissolution by macrophages and persist within the lung tissue. Some of the most common environmental exposures are coal worker's pneumoconiosis, asbestosis, and silicosis.

Coal Worker's Pneumoconiosis

In coal worker's pneumoconiosis, also called anthracosis, the findings in the lung depend on the amount of exposure to coal dust. The disorder ranges from asymptomatic with little pulmonary dysfunction to complicated pneumoconiosis with progressive massive pulmonary fibrosis.

Coal worker's pneumoconiosis is characterized by coal particles of 1 to 2 mm in diameter and larger coal nodules in the lungs. These lesions are scattered throughout the lung fields and develop over the course of many years. On autopsy, intensely blackened lung tissue consisting of coal dust and collagen with necrotic centers are found. Coal dust that enters the lungs can neither be destroyed nor removed by the body. The particles are engulfed by alveolar macrophages and remain in the lungs, residing in the connective tissue or pulmonary lymph nodes. Macrophages release various products, including enzymes, cytokines, free radicals, and fibroblast growth factors, that cause inflammation and fibrosis.

The patient exhibits cough with gray sputum, wheezes, and dyspnea on exertion. Diagnosis involves chest x-ray, CT scan, sputum culture, and PFTs. Chest x-ray and CT scan demonstrate round dark opacities throughout the lungs. PFTs demonstrate hypoxemia, decreased FEV, and decreased total lung capacity as in obstructive disease. Treatment involves an occupational change that limits contact with coal dust, if possible, as well as oxygen, bronchodilators, and pneumococcal and influenza vaccine. Smoking cessation is critical.

 CLINICAL CONCEPT

Coal worker's pneumoconiosis can be considered both a fibrotic and obstructive lung disorder because it is associated with chronic bronchitis and emphysema.

 CLINICAL CONCEPT

Coal worker's pneumoconiosis is not limited to coal workers, as it is also present in the lungs of urban dwellers because of air pollution.

Asbestosis

Asbestos is a mineral crystal used by many manufacturers and industries. Workers exposed to asbestos include those in the mining, welding, shipyard, milling, painting, and construction fields. Asbestos causes pulmonary fibrosis that is related to the intensity and duration of exposure. This restrictive disease causes a decrease in all lung volumes. Asbestos exposure also increases susceptibility to lung cancer, particularly in smokers, with squamous cell carcinoma and adenocarcinoma being the most frequent types of cancer associated with asbestos. Mesothelioma, a type of tumor specifically associated with asbestos, is often present within the pleural membrane, but can also metastasize.

 CLINICAL CONCEPT

Cancers related to asbestos can develop decades after exposure.

Silicosis

Silica is a quartz crystal that, if inhaled, can cause pulmonary fibrosis. The major occupational exposures occur in mining, stonecutting, and industries using abrasives such as stone, clay, glass and cement, packing of silica flour, and quarrying, particularly of granite. The disease can occur after as little as 2 years of exposure to silica. Silicosis increases susceptibility to tuberculosis, and all patients exposed to silica should receive a Mantoux test. Talc dust, a type of silica, can also cause pulmonary fibrosis. Pleural and lung cancer have also been associated with exposure to talc dust.

Thoracic Cage Deformity

Thoracic cage deformity is a deviation in the vertebral column related to either structural changes or postural defects. The term *kyphoscoliosis* is used to describe the combination of a curve of the cervical spine (kyphosis) and twisting of the thoracic vertebral column (scoliosis).

A thoracic cage deformity such as kyphoscoliosis causes restrictive lung disease. The deformity causes rigidity of the chest wall and limited chest expansion that results in breathing difficulty, breathlessness on exertion, and hypoventilation. The ventilation of the lungs is diminished because of the distorted thoracic cage.

Clinical manifestations of kyphoscoliosis include a noticeable deformity with one shoulder or hip higher than the other and hunched posture. Diagnosis is made by a physical examination and confirmed by x-rays, CT scan, or MRI. With advancing age, the chest wall stiffens and degenerative changes in ligaments and joints aggravate the spinal deformity. Decreased ventilation leads to carbon dioxide retention and hypoxemia. Chronic hypoxia leads to pulmonary hypertension and right ventricular failure. Treatment of a thoracic cage deformity requires an orthopedic brace or surgical intervention. Early correction of spinal deformity can reverse the decreased lung capacity.

Idiopathic Pulmonary Fibrosis

IPF is a restrictive lung disease caused by repeated injury of lung tissue by an unidentified agent. The alveoli undergo repeated episodes of inflammation, also called alveolitis, that eventually involves fibroblastic proliferation and fibrotic changes. In IPF, an exaggerated fibrotic response occurs with consequent stiffening of lung tissue.

Patients with IPF present with dyspnea, tachypnea, crackles, and eventual cyanosis. The chest x-ray reveals a pattern of diffuse markings called a "ground glass" appearance in the lower lung fields. Later in the disease, nodules and a honeycomb lung pattern can be observed. Erythrocyte sedimentation rate is usually elevated, indicating inflammation. PFTs demonstrate restrictive lung disease changes, including reduced vital capacity, residual volume, increased FEV1, and decreased compliance. Evidence of airway obstruction is minimal. Hypoxemia is present, but PCO_2 is usually normal. Bronchoscopy is performed to obtain lung tissue biopsies and confirm the diagnosis. Collagen vascular disease, such as sarcoidosis, and pneumoconioses must be ruled out because these diseases often have a similar presentation.

Treatment for IPF aims to reduce inflammatory and fibrotic changes in the lungs. Treatment measures for right ventricular failure and pulmonary hypertension are usually necessary. Lung transplantation is commonly indicated.

Hypersensitivity Pneumonitis

Hypersensitivity pneumonitis is an immunologically mediated lung disorder caused by prolonged, intense exposure to inhaled organic dusts that act as antigens. Commonly, the organic dusts are made of bacterial spores, fungi, or animal proteins. Affected persons have an abnormally heightened sensitivity to the antigen that causes alveolar inflammation.

Signs and symptoms include acute attacks of dyspnea, cough, fever, and an elevated WBC count. Symptoms appear 4 to 6 hours after exposure, and prolonged exposure can lead to pulmonary fibrosis. PFTs demonstrate restrictive disease, and chest x-rays show nodular infiltrates. Farmer's lung, pigeon-breeder's lung, and air conditioner lung are specific forms of hypersensitivity pneumonitis. Corticosteroids are standard treatment for severely ill patients with all varieties of hypersensitivity pneumonitis.

Pathophysiology of Selected Pulmonary Vascular Disorders

Pulmonary edema, pulmonary embolism (PE), and pulmonary hypertension are disorders caused by a vascular problem in the lungs. Pulmonary edema is the manifestation of heart failure. PE is most commonly caused by venous thrombosis of the lower extremities. Chronic hypoxia stimulates pulmonary hypertension.

Pulmonary Edema

Pulmonary edema is the accumulation of fluid around the alveoli that inhibits oxygen transfer at the alveolar-capillary interface. It occurs when there is an increase in hydrostatic pressure in the capillary bed of the lungs. The most common cause of pulmonary edema is left ventricular heart failure (LVF). In LVF, the weakened left ventricle cannot eject all the blood within the chamber, causing blood to accumulate in the left ventricle. As a result, hydrostatic pressure builds backward into the left atrium, pulmonary veins, and, eventually, into the pulmonary capillaries. The high hydrostatic pressure within the pulmonary capillaries causes fluid from the blood to diffuse into the interstitial tissues.

The main symptom of pulmonary edema is severe respiratory distress. The patient exhibits extreme shortness of breath, which may be accompanied by pink frothy sputum. As pulmonary edema worsens, the lack of oxygen to the brain causes confusion and stupor. Coarse, loud crackles are heard on auscultation. Diagnosis is made by clinical presentation and a chest x-ray demonstrates congested pulmonary vasculature and infiltrates.

Treatment is aimed at decreasing hydrostatic pressure in the pulmonary capillaries, reducing the fluid in the pulmonary interstitium, and increasing oxygen content in the blood. Diuretic medications, oxygen administration, digitalis, and ACE inhibitors accomplish these goals. Diuretics enhance water loss from the bloodstream and thereby lessen edema in the lungs. Digitalis is used to enhance left ventricular function. ACE inhibitors can reduce the constant cycling of the RAAS that occurs in left ventricular failure.

Pulmonary Embolism

A PE is a clot that has traveled to the pulmonary arterial circulation and caused obstruction of arterial blood flow through the lungs. Usually the embolism has originated in the venous circulation as a deep vein thrombus in the leg or in the right side of the heart as an atrial thrombus. Thrombi also often form around central venous catheters and travel to the right side of the heart into the pulmonary artery.

PE is a leading cause of death because the clinical presentation is often vague and occurs without warning. Most cases are diagnosed at autopsy because the patient did not demonstrate symptoms.

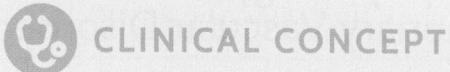 CLINICAL CONCEPT

At autopsy, 60% of hospitalized patients demonstrate existence of a PE, with 70% of these cases undiagnosed.

Pulmonary Hypertension

Pulmonary hypertension is abnormally high pressure within the pulmonary arteries. A normal pulmonary artery pressure is approximately 25 mm Hg. When pulmonary arterial pressure is greater than 25 mm Hg at rest or 30 mm Hg with exercise, pulmonary hypertension is present.

Etiology

There are two types of pulmonary hypertension. Primary pulmonary hypertension is a genetic disorder caused by abnormal structure of the pulmonary blood vessels. Secondary pulmonary hypertension is an increase in pulmonary artery pressure as a result of elevated pulmonary venous pressure, increased pulmonary blood flow, pulmonary vascular obstruction, or hypoxemia. Chronic obstructive pulmonary disease, collagen vascular disease, and recurrent pulmonary thromboemboli may be causes of secondary pulmonary hypertension.

Chronic hypoxia is a common cause of pulmonary hypertension because the lung response to decreased ventilation or hypoxia is pulmonary arterial vasoconstriction. Pulmonary arterial vasoconstriction causes increased pulmonary vascular resistance and increased workload of the right ventricle. Prolonged pulmonary hypertension causes the right ventricle to hypertrophy and fail. Failure of the right side of the heart caused by a pulmonary disorder is known as cor pulmonale.

As pulmonary hypertension progresses, right ventricular failure causes diminished cardiac output. The decreased cardiac output is particularly apparent during exercise. Symptoms include syncope, dyspnea on exertion, and fatigue.

Diagnosis

Pulmonary hypertension is diagnosed through x-rays, echocardiography, and Doppler ultrasonography. A right heart cardiac catheterization is done to obtain pulmonary arterial pressure. Transthoracic echocardiogram is the preferred test for screening for pulmonary hypertension. Complete PFTs should be obtained for any person with pulmonary hypertension. A CT scan of the lungs is also performed on those with abnormal PFTs. Individuals with a history of excessive daytime somnolence or witnessed apneas should be tested with overnight oximetry or polysomnogram to rule out pulmonary hypertension related to sleep-disordered breathing.

Treatment

Treatment for pulmonary hypertension focuses on vasodilation of the pulmonary arterial vessels, improving function of the right ventricle, and enhancing oxygenation. Supplemental oxygen and calcium channel blockers may be effective in the early stages of the disease. As pulmonary hypertension worsens, Epoprostenol, a pulmonary vasodilator, and Bosentan, a vasoconstriction antagonist, are frequently used. Sildenafil, a vasodilator, is also used to decrease pulmonary artery pressure in patients with right-sided heart failure and pulmonary hypertension.

Adult Respiratory Distress Syndrome

Adult respiratory distress syndrome (ARDS) is pulmonary dysfunction characterized by diffuse alveolar injury, pulmonary capillary damage, bilateral pulmonary infiltrates, and severe hypoxemia. It occurs in critically ill patients and is commonly a sequela to trauma, sepsis, drug overdose, massive transfusion, acute pancreatitis, or aspiration. Patients developing ARDS are critically ill, often with multisystem organ failure, and they may not be capable of providing historical information. Typically, the illness develops within 12 to 48 hours after an inciting event, although, in rare instances, it may take up to a few days

 CLINICAL CONCEPT

The most common risk factor for ARDS is sepsis, but multiple other risk factors exist, including direct lung injury, most commonly aspiration of gastric contents; systemic illnesses; and injuries.

One of the characteristics of ARDS is sudden progressive pulmonary edema. An inflammatory trigger initiates the release of cellular and chemical mediators.

The mediators damage the alveolar-capillary membrane and fluid leaks into the alveolar interstitial spaces. Alveoli collapse, small airways are narrowed, and lung compliance decreases. The lungs lose the ability to ventilate, and perfusion is diminished at the alveolar-capillary level, resulting in severe hypoxemia and hypercapnia. As hypoxemia progresses, there is a decreased level of consciousness, compensatory tachycardia, diminished peripheral circulation, diaphoresis, restlessness, and anxiety. As hypoxemia continues, the alveoli become fibrotic and lungs become stiff with dead air space. Crackles are a sign of fluid leaking into the pulmonary interstitium.

Diagnosis is based on clinical presentation and diagnostic studies. A defining feature of ARDS is arterial hypoxemia that does not improve with administration of oxygen. ABG levels demonstrating a PO_2 of 50 mm Hg or less and PCO_2 of 50 mm Hg or above are diagnostic; these values are also consistent with respiratory failure. Chest x-rays demonstrate pulmonary edema. Treatment includes mechanical ventilation to facilitate oxygenation of tissues and bronchodilators to open constricted airways.

 CLINICAL CONCEPT

Treatment of ARDS is often ineffective, making this disorder a major cause of death.

Chapter Summary

- Pulmonary disorders can be categorized according to the results of a PFT as obstructive or restrictive disease.
- A pneumothorax, also called a collapsed lung, occurs when air enters the pleural space and presses on lung tissue so that it cannot expand. A chest tube inserted to suction is the treatment of pneumothorax.
- A pleural effusion occurs when fluid enters the pleural space and hinders lung tissue from fully expanding. An effusion can be a transudate or an exudate. Thoracotomy is the treatment for pleural effusion.
- Major obstructive diseases include asthma and COPD, which are two of the most common diseases worldwide.
- Asthma is a chronic inflammatory disease with acute episodes of bronchospasm.
- Asthma medication consists of inhalers that contain beta-2 adrenergic agonists, which cause bronchodilation, and corticosteroids, which decrease inflammation.
- Each acute attack of asthma remodels the bronchioles to make them more susceptible to acute bronchospasm and inflammation.

- Status asthmaticus occurs when an asthma attack resists treatment and is potentially fatal.
- COPD is a combination of emphysema, chronic bronchitis, and asthma. Individuals can have COPD that has more features of emphysema or chronic bronchitis.
- Long-term cigarette smoking and exposure to second-hand smoke are primary causes of COPD.
- In emphysema, the alveoli are injured, cannot recoil, and become enlarged because they accumulate excessive carbon dioxide.
- In chronic bronchitis, the bronchioles are edematous and full of mucus, which obstructs oxygen from gaining entry into alveoli.
- Individuals with emphysema classically have a barrel chest, pursed lip breathing, and chronic hypercapnia.
- Individuals with chronic bronchitis classically have cyanosis, chronic hypoxia, and susceptibility to right ventricular failure.
- Chronic hypoxia causes pulmonary hypertension, which leads to right ventricular failure, also known as cor pulmonale.

- COPD is characterized by a decreased FEV during the first second of exhalation (FEV1). COPD prolongs the patient's exhalation phase.
- In patients with long-term COPD, the respiratory center becomes insensitive to carbon dioxide. The patient's drive to breathe is stimulated by hypoxia.
- High oxygen concentration can shut down the hypoxic drive to breathe for a patient with severe COPD. Sedatives, narcotics, and any drugs that suppress respiratory rate should be used with caution in patients with long-term COPD.
- OSA is the episodic cessation of breathing during sleep. OSA is associated with obesity and excess pharyngeal tissue mass that inhibits airflow.
- Most disorders caused by environmental exposures such as asbestosis, silicosis, and hypersensitivity pneumonitis cause restrictive lung disease.

- Coal worker's pneumoconiosis can be considered both a fibrotic and obstructive lung disorder because it is associated with chronic bronchitis and emphysema.
- Asbestosis increases susceptibility to lung cancer decades after initial exposure.
- Restrictive lung disease causes increased FEV1 because of the compressive forces of the stiffened lung tissue, whereas obstructive lung disease causes decreased FEV1.
- Collagen vascular diseases such as sarcoidosis cause fibrotic changes in the lungs.
- Deep venous thrombosis can cause a PE that obstructs perfusion of the lungs.
- Pulmonary edema is a consequence of left-sided heart failure.
- Sepsis is a risk factor for ARDS.

 ## Making the Connections

Pathophysiology	Signs and Symptoms	Assessment Findings	Diagnosis	Treatment
Asthma | Chronic inflammatory disorder that causes reversible bronchospasm because of bronchial hyperreactivity.				
	Wheezes, cough, dyspnea, chest tightness.	Wheezes, prolonged exhalations, rhonchi, retractions, and use of accessory muscles during breathing.	During an acute asthma attack, PFTs reveal slow, prolonged FEV1, decreased FEV1/FVC ratio, and decreased PEF on peak flow meter caused by bronchoconstriction, which decreases ability to inhale and exhale. Most apparent by measuring expiratory volume.	Adrenergic agonist bronchodilators and corticosteroid inhalers to counteract inflammation; if severe bronchospasm, add epinephrine and oral corticosteroid. Other types of medication include leukotriene antagonists, theophylline, and cromolyn sodium.
Chronic Obstructive Pulmonary Disease | A combination of emphysema, chronic bronchitis, and asthma. Bronchospasm, excessive mucus, edema, and fibrosis in the bronchioles. Also loss of lung elastic recoil, alveolar membrane injury, and smooth muscle hypertrophy.				
	Dyspnea, cough, and wheezes.	Wheezes, prolonged exhalations, rhonchi, barrel-shaped chest, and cyanosis. Right ventricular failure findings such as jugular venous distension, ascites, ankle edema, hepatosplenomegaly possible.	PFTs reveal slow, prolonged FEV1, FEV1/FVC ratio lower than 70%. Chest x-ray reveals hyperinflation of lungs and flattened diaphragm. Hyperinflation of lungs is caused by alveolar accumulation of carbon dioxide (CO_2).	Adrenergic agonist bronchodilators and corticosteroids via inhaler or anticholinergic-type bronchodilator and corticosteroids via inhaler, careful administration of oxygen, pulmonary rehab. Mechanical ventilation, if needed. Lung reduction surgery, if needed.

Continued

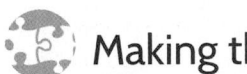 # Making the Connections–cont'd

Pathophysiology	Signs and Symptoms	Assessment Findings	Diagnosis	Treatment
Bronchiectasis | Abnormal and permanent dilatation of bronchi, fibrotic changes of bronchioles, and static, thick purulent secretions.				
	Dyspnea, cough, wheezes, sputum production, and hemoptysis.	Dyspnea, cough, and wheezes throughout lung fields.	CT scan; bronchography shows dilated, fibrotic airways. Difficulty with inhalation and exhalation of air shown by decreased. FEV1 /FEV. Sputum culture may show infectious agent.	Mucolytic agents; bronchodilators; oxygen, if needed; antibiotics, if needed; surgical excision of dilated airways may give relief; lung transplantation may be necessary.
Obstructive Sleep Apnea | Intermittent cessation of airflow from the nose and mouth during sleep. It is characterized by recurrent episodes of sleep apnea of 2 to 3 minutes in duration. The upper airway closes repeatedly during sleep.				
	Daytime sleepiness, snoring.	Snoring or apneic episodes during sleep. Obesity is common.	Polysomnography shows recurrent episodes of sleep apnea of 2 to 3 minutes in duration.	CPAP keeps airway open during sleep. Surgery may be needed to reduce pharyngeal tissues.
Pneumothorax | Presence of air in the pleural cavity that presses against an area of lung tissue and causes collapse of a large section or whole lobe of lung tissue.				
	Dyspnea, chest pain, increased respiratory rate.	Lack of breath sounds over area of pneumothorax, asymmetric chest expansion with inhalation, percussion of hyperresonance over area of pneumothorax.	Chest x-ray shows collapsed lung and air in the pleural space.	Chest tube attached to suction to pull air from pleural space and allow reexpansion of lung.
Pleural Effusion | Abnormal collection of fluid within the pleural cavity that can be either transudate or exudate. Fluid that accumulates within the pleural space can be caused by heart failure, severe pulmonary infection, or neoplasm.				
	Dyspnea, increased rate of breathing, pleuritic chest pain.	Lack of breath sounds over area of effusion, asymmetric chest expansion with inhalation, percussion of dullness over area of effusion.	Chest x-ray, ultrasound, or CT scan shows fluid in the pleural space that compresses lung tissue. Thoracocentesis allows fluid extraction for analysis.	Thoracotomy and chest tube attached to suction.
Coal Miner's Pneumoconiosis | Coal dust stimulates an inflammatory reaction in the lungs. The particles are engulfed by alveolar macrophages and remain in the lungs. Chronic bronchitis develops. The lungs eventually become fibrotic because of chronic inflammation.				
	Cough, dyspnea on exertion, wheezes.	Cough, dyspnea, and wheezes heard throughout lung fields. Sputum is gray.	Chest x-ray or CT scan reveals dark opacities caused by coal dust and macrophages within the lungs. PFTs reveal decreased FEV and total lung	Oxygen and bronchodilators to enhance ventilation. Smoking cessation. Pneumococcal and influenza vaccine to prevent lung infections.

Continued

Making the Connections—cont'd

Pathophysiology	Signs and Symptoms	Assessment Findings	Diagnosis	Treatment
			capacity. ABGs show hypoxemia. Patient can develop right ventricular failure caused by pulmonary hypertension that develops because of chronic hypoxia.	

Asbestosis | Inhalation of fine asbestos crystals from different types of manufacturing and inhaled in different occupations. Crystals stimulate a chronic inflammatory reaction with eventual fibrotic changes in the lungs.

Pathophysiology	Signs and Symptoms	Assessment Findings	Diagnosis	Treatment
	Dyspnea, cough. Symptoms occur decades after exposure.	Dyspnea, cough, crackles, wheezes across lung fields Patient may have signs of right ventricular failure such as jugular vein distension and hepatosplenomegaly. Finger clubbing.	Chest x-ray may show abnormalities such as areas of plaques of foreign matter. CT scanning is better to visualize areas of plaque. PFTs reveal a restrictive lung disease pattern. Susceptibility to malignancy is increased; may show on chest x-ray or CT scan.	Cease exposure. Treatment of symptoms. Oxygen. Surgery, if malignancy present. Smoking cessation.

Silicosis | Inhalation of fine quartz crystals from different types of manufacturing and inhaled in different occupations. Crystals stimulate a chronic inflammatory reaction with eventual fibrotic changes in the lungs.

Pathophysiology	Signs and Symptoms	Assessment Findings	Diagnosis	Treatment
	Dyspnea, cough. Symptoms occur decades after exposure.	Dyspnea, cough, crackles, wheezes across lung fields. Patient may have signs of right ventricular failure such as jugular vein distension and hepatosplenomegaly. Finger clubbing.	Chest x-ray may show abnormalities such as areas of plaques or foreign matter. CT scanning is better to visualize areas of plaque. PFTs reveal a restrictive lung disease pattern. Susceptibility to TB and malignancy is increased; may show on chest x-ray or CT scan. Mantoux test used for TB.	Cease exposure. Treatment of symptoms. Oxygen. Surgery, if malignancy present. Smoking cessation. Antitubercular drugs, if TB present.

Thoracic Cage Deformity | Severe deviation in the vertebral column related to either structural changes or defects.

Pathophysiology	Signs and Symptoms	Assessment Findings	Diagnosis	Treatment
	Postural abnormality.	Kyphoscoliosis or scoliosis. One hip higher than other or one shoulder higher than other. Decreased thoracic expansion.	Chest, neck, and thoracic x-ray. PFTs show restrictive lung disease. ABGs show hypoxemia and hypercapnia caused by poor gas exchange in restricted lungs.	Orthopedic bracing or surgery.

Continued

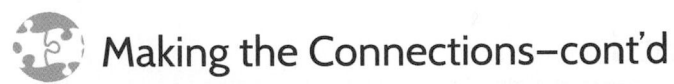

Making the Connections—cont'd

Pathophysiology	Signs and Symptoms	Assessment Findings	Diagnosis	Treatment

Idiopathic Pulmonary Fibrosis | A restrictive lung disease caused by repeated injury of lung tissue by some unidentified agent. The alveoli undergo repeated episodes of inflammation that eventually involves fibroblastic proliferation and fibrotic changes in lungs.

Pathophysiology	Signs and Symptoms	Assessment Findings	Diagnosis	Treatment
	Dyspnea, tachypnea, cough, and cyanosis.	Dyspnea, cough, tachypnea, crackles, and cyanosis.	Elevated ESR Serology tests are negative for immunological collagen vascular diseases. Hypoxemia on ABG Chest x-ray shows "ground glass" appearance of lungs. PFTs demonstrate restrictive disease.	Oxygen, Bronchodilators, Corticosteroids. Pulmonary vasodilators such as Epoprostenol, Bosentan, and Sildenafil. Treatment of right ventricular failure with diuretics may be necessary. Many treatments tend to fail and lung transplantation may be necessary.

Hypersensitivity Pneumonitis | An immunologically mediated lung disorder caused by prolonged, intense exposure to inhaled organic dusts that act as antigens. There is widespread alveolar inflammation.

Pathophysiology	Signs and Symptoms	Assessment Findings	Diagnosis	Treatment
	Acute attacks of cough, dyspnea, and fever.	Dyspnea, cough, fever, and an elevated WBC count.	PFTs demonstrate restrictive disease. Chest x-rays show nodular infiltrates.	Corticosteroid treatment.

Pulmonary Edema | Accumulation of fluid around the alveoli that inhibits oxygen transfer at the alveolar-capillary interface. An increase in hydrostatic pressure in the capillary bed of the lungs is caused by backward effects of LVF.

Pathophysiology	Signs and Symptoms	Assessment Findings	Diagnosis	Treatment
	Cough, dyspnea, or stridor may occur.	Cough, dyspnea, stridor, pink frothy sputum Coarse, loud crackles in both lung fields.	Chest x-ray. Cardiac catheter can show poor. LV ejection fraction lower than 40%. High pulmonary capillary wedge pressure is caused by backward pressure from left ventricle.	Oxygen. Diuretics to decrease fluid in lungs. Digitalis to enhance cardiac contractility ACE inhibitors to decrease RAAS effects in heart failure.

Pulmonary Embolus | A clot that has traveled to the pulmonary arterial circulation and caused obstruction of arterial blood flow through the lungs.

Pathophysiology	Signs and Symptoms	Assessment Findings	Diagnosis	Treatment
	Dyspnea, chest pain, increased respiratory rate.	Sudden respiratory distress, tachycardia.	V-Q scan shows decreased perfusion in area of embolism blocking circulation.	Anticoagulants, thrombolytic agents, pain medication; inferior vena cava filter can inhibit clot travel into the right heart and pulmonary artery.

Pulmonary Hypertension | Abnormally high pressure within the pulmonary arteries.

Pathophysiology	Signs and Symptoms	Assessment Findings	Diagnosis	Treatment
	Syncope, dyspnea on exertion, and fatigue.	Dyspnea on exertion; dizziness on exertion.	Transthoracic echocardiogram, CT scan, Doppler ultrasound, or cardiac catheterization can show evidence of	Vasodilators, calcium channel blockers, oxygen. Epoprostenol, a pulmonary vasodilator, and Bosentan, a

Continued

Making the Connections—cont'd

Pathophysiology	Signs and Symptoms	Assessment Findings	Diagnosis	Treatment
			high pulmonary artery pressure, right ventricular hypertrophy, or right ventricular failure.	vasoconstriction antagonist, are frequently used. Sildenafil, a vasodilator, is also used to decrease pulmonary artery pressure.

Adult Respiratory Distress Syndrome | Pulmonary dysfunction characterized by diffuse alveolar injury, pulmonary capillary damage, bilateral pulmonary infiltrates in critically ill patients. Commonly a sequela to trauma, sepsis, drug overdose, massive transfusion, acute pancreatitis, or aspiration.

Pathophysiology	Signs and Symptoms	Assessment Findings	Diagnosis	Treatment
Critically ill patient commonly in intensive care for another diagnosis.	Severe respiratory distress, coarse loud crackles across lungs. Tachycardia, elevated blood pressure.	ABGs show hypoxemia and hypercapnia. Chest x-ray shows pulmonary edema.		Treatment should focus on major etiologic disorders. Oxygen. Intubation and mechanical ventilation may be necessary.

Bibliography

Agnelli, G., & Becattini, C. (2010). Acute pulmonary embolism. *N Engl J Med, 363*(3), 266–274.

Anonymous. (2011). How to treat an asthma attack. *Am Fam Phys,* 84(1), 49–50.

Archer, S. L., & Michelakis, E. D. (2009). Phosphodiesterase type 5 inhibitors for pulmonary arterial hypertension. *N Engl J Med,* 361(19), 1864–1871.

Armstrong, C. (2012). ACP updates guideline on diagnosis and management of stable COPD. *Am Fam Phys,* 85(2), 204–205.

Barrett, K. E., Barman, S. M., Boitano, S., & Brooks, H. L. (2010). *Ganong's review of medical physiology.* 24th ed. New York: McGraw-Hill/ Lange Medical Series.

Beasley, R., Patel, M., Perrin, K., & O'Driscoll, B. R. (2011). High-concentration oxygen therapy in COPD. *Lancet,* 378(9795), 969–970.

Bel, E. H. (2013). Clinical practice. Mild asthma. *N Engl J Med,* 369(6), 549–557. doi: 10.1056/NEJMcp1214826. Erratum in: *N Engl J Med.* 2013 Nov 14;369(20):1970.

Ben-Chetrit, E., & Merin, O. (2010). Images in clinical medicine. Spontaneous tension pneumothorax. *N Engl J Med,* 2010, 362(12), e43.

Benich, J. J., 3rd, & Carek, P. J. (2011). Evaluation of the patient with chronic cough. *Am Fam Phys,* 84(8), 887–892.

Busse, W. W., Morgan, W. J., Gergen, P. J., et al. (2011). Randomized trial of omalizumab (anti-IgE) for asthma in inner-city children. *N Engl J Med,* 364(11), 1005–1015. doi: 10.1056/NEJMoa1009705.

Calhoun, W. J., Boushey, H. A., Ameredes, B. T., & Asthma Clinical Research Network BASALT Trial Investigators. (2013). Strategies for tailoring asthma treatment in adults—reply. *JAMA,* 309(2), 136–137.

Cayley, W. E., Jr. (2009). Should salmeterol be used for long-term asthma control? *Am Fam Phys.* 79(11), 957–958.

Chowdhury, B. A., & Dal Pan, G. (2010). The FDA and safe use of long-acting beta-agonists in the treatment of asthma. *N Engl J Med,* 362(13), 1169–1171. doi: 10.1056/NEJMp1002074. Epub 2010 Feb 24.

Crandall, M. A., & Mulvagh, S. L. (2010). 68-year-old woman with chronic cough and recurrent pleural effusions. *Mayo Clin Proceed,* 85(5), 479–482.

Dahlén, S. E., Dahlén, B., & Drazen, J. M. (2011). Asthma treatment guidelines meet the real world. *N Engl J Med,* 364(18), 1769–1770. doi: 10.1056/NEJMe1100937.

Decramer, M., Janssens, W., & Miravitlles, M. (2012). Chronic obstructive pulmonary disease. *Lancet,* 379(9823), 1341–1351.

Drazen, J. M. (2011). A step toward personalized asthma treatment. *N Engl J Med,* 365(13), 1245–1246. doi: 10.1056/NEJMe1102469. Epub 2011 Sep 26.

Evensen, A. E. (2010). Management of COPD exacerbations. *Am Fam Phys,* 81(5), 607–613.

Gershon, A. S., Warner, L., Cascagnette, P., Victor, J. C., & To, T. (2011). Lifetime risk of developing chronic obstructive pulmonary disease: a longitudinal population study. *Lancet,* 378(9795), 991–996.

Ghuman, M., Ludwig, M. J., & Anna, L. S. (2011). FPIN's clinical inquiries. Clinical indicators of obstructive sleep apnea. *Am Fam Phys,* 83(9), 3–4.

Gibson, P. G., McDonald, V. M., & Marks, G. B. (2010). Asthma in older adults. *Lancet,* 76(9743), 803–813.

Goldhaber, S. Z., & Piazza, G. (2011). Optimal duration of anticoagulation after venous thromboembolism. *Circulation.* 23(6), 664–667.

Gøtzsche, P. C., & Johansen, H. K. (2009). Alpha1-antitrypsin deficiency. *N Engl J Med,* 361(21), 2101–2102.

Grainge, C. L., Lau, L. C., Ward, J. A., et al. (2011). Effect of bronchoconstriction on airway remodeling in asthma. *N Engl J Med,* 364(21), 2006–2015. doi: 10.1056/NEJMoa1014350.

Gupta, A., Patel, B., Almoosa, K., & McKelvy, B. J. (2010). Recurrent spontaneous pneumothorax. *Cleveland Clin J Med,* 77(6), 345–347.

Hall, J. B., & Kress, J. P. (2011). *The burden of functional recovery from ARDS. N Engl J Med,* 364(14), 1358–1359.

Hancock, D. B., London, S. J., & CHARGE Pulmonary Function Working Group. (2011). Determinants of lung function, COPD, and asthma. *N Engl J Med*, 364(1), 86–87.

Hansel, T. T., Johnston, S. L., & Openshaw, P. J. (2013). Microbes and mucosal immune responses in asthma. *Lancet*, 381(9869), 861–873.

Hensley, M., & Ray, C. (2010). Sleep apnea. *Am Fam Phys*, 81(2), 195.

Herridge, M. S., Tansey, C. M., Matté, A., et al. (2011). Functional disability 5 years after acute respiratory distress syndrome. *N Engl J Med*, 364(14), 1293–1304.

Hokusai-VTE Investigators, Büller, H. R., Décousus, H., Grosso, M. A., et al. (2013). Edoxaban versus warfarin for the treatment of symptomatic venous thromboembolism. *N Engl J Med*, 369(15), 1406–1415. doi: 10.1056/NEJMoa1306638. Epub 2013 Aug 31. Erratum in: *N Engl J Med*. 2014 Jan 23;370(4):390.

Hopkins, T. G., Maher, E. R., Reid, E., & Marciniak, S. J. (2011). Recurrent pneumothorax. *Lancet*, 377(9777), 1624. doi: 10.1016/S0140-6736(11)60072-X.

Hurst, J. R., Vestbo, J., Anzueto, A., et al. (2010). Susceptibility to exacerbation in chronic obstructive pulmonary disease. *N Engl J Med*, 363(12), 1128–1138.

Jackson, D. J., Hartert, T. V., Martinez, F. D., Weiss, S. T., & Fahy, J. V. (2014). Asthma: NHLBI Workshop on the Primary Prevention of Chronic Lung Diseases. *Ann Am Thorac Soc*, 11 Suppl 3, S139–S145. doi: 10.1513/AnnalsATS.201312-448LD.

Johnson, J. D., & Theurer, W. M. (2014). A stepwise approach to the interpretation of pulmonary function tests. *Am Fam Phys*, 89(5), 359–366.

Kerstjens, H. A., Engel, M., Dahl, R., et al. (2012). Tiotropium in asthma poorly controlled with standard combination therapy. *N Engl J Med*, 367(13), 1198–1207. Epub 2012 Sep 2.

King, T. E., Jr. (2011). Smoking and subclinical interstitial lung disease. (2011). *N Engl J Med*, 364(10), 968–970.

King, T. E., Jr., Pardo, A., & Selman, M. (2011). Idiopathic pulmonary fibrosis. *Lancet*, 378(9807), 1949–1961.

Krafczyk, M. A., & Asplund, C. A. (2011). Exercise-induced bronchoconstriction: diagnosis and management. *Am Fam Phys*, 84(4), 427–434.

Lamela, J., & Vega, F. (2009). Immunologic aspects of chronic obstructive pulmonary disease. *N Engl J Med*, 361(10), 1024.

Laumbach, R. J. (2010). Outdoor air pollutants and patient health. *Am Fam Phys*, 81(2), 175–180.

Lazarus, S. C. (2010). Clinical practice. Emergency treatment of asthma. *N Engl J Med*, 363(8), 755–764. doi: 10.1056/NEJMcp1003469.

Lee, H., Kim, J., & Tagmazyan, K. (2013). Treatment of stable chronic obstructive pulmonary disease: the GOLD guidelines. *Am Fam Phys*, 88(10), 655–663.

Leung, C. C., Yu, I. T., & Chen, W. (2012). Silicosis. *Lancet*, 379(9830), 2008–2018.

Leuppi, J. D., Schuetz, P., Bingisser, R., et al. (2013). Short-term vs conventional glucocorticoid therapy in acute exacerbations of chronic obstructive pulmonary disease: the REDUCE randomized clinical trial. *JAMA*, 309(21), 2223–2231.

Li, J. T. (2009). Toward the optimal control of asthma. *Mayo Clin Proceed*, 84(8), 673–674.

Longo, D., Fauci, A., Kasper, D., et al. (2011). *Harrison's principles of internal medicine: volumes 1 and 2*. 18th ed. New York: McGraw-Hill.

Mador, M. J., & Sethi, S. (2013). Systemic inflammation in predicting COPD exacerbations. *JAMA*, 309(22), 2390–2391.

Marin, J. M., Agusti, A., Villar, I., et al. (2012). Association between treated and untreated obstructive sleep apnea and risk of hypertension. *JAMA*, 307(20), 2169–2176.

McGoon, M. D., & Kane, G. C. (2009). Pulmonary hypertension: diagnosis and management. *Mayo Clin Proceed*, 84(2), 191–207.

McPhee, S. J., & Hammer, J. (2009). *Pathophysiology of disease*. 6th ed. New York: Lange Medical Books/ McGraw-Hill Medical Publishing Division.

Meyer, G., Vicaut, E., Danays, T., et al. (2014). Fibrinolysis for patients with intermediate-risk pulmonary embolism. *N Engl J Med*, 370(15), 402–411. doi: 10.1056/NEJMoa1302097.

Moffatt, M. F., Gut, I. G., Demenais, F., et al. (2010). A large-scale, consortium-based genomewide association study of asthma. *N Engl J Med*, 363(13), 1211–1221. doi: 10.1056/NEJMoa0906312.

Murphy, D. M., & O'Byrne, P. M. (2010). Recent advances in the pathophysiology of asthma. *Chest*, 137(6), 1417–1426.

Nazir, T., & Punekar, S. (2010). Images in clinical medicine. Pneumothorax—an uncommon complication of a common procedure. *N Engl J Med*, 363(5), 462.

Nici, L., Lareau, S., & ZuWallack, R. (2010). Pulmonary rehabilitation in the treatment of chronic obstructive pulmonary disease. *Am Fam Phys*, 82(6), 655–660.

Niewoehner, D. E. (2010). Clinical practice. Outpatient management of severe COPD. *N Engl J Med*, 362(15), 1407–1416.

Pachman, D. R., Morrison, T. B., & Szostek, J. H. (2011). 84-year-old man with respiratory distress and abdominal distention. *Mayo Clin Proceed*, 6(2), e10–e13.

Peters, S. P., Kunselman, S. J., Icitovic, N., et al. (2010). Tiotropium bromide step-up therapy for adults with uncontrolled asthma. *N Engl J Med*, 363(18), 1715–1726.

Piazza, G., & Goldhaber, S. Z. (2010). Management of submassive pulmonary embolism. *Circ*. 122(11), 1124–1129.

Piazza, G., & Goldhaber, S. Z. (2011). Chronic thromboembolic pulmonary hypertension. *N Engl J Med*, 364(4), 351–360.

Pollart, S. M., Compton, R. M., & Elward, K. S. (2011). Management of acute asthma exacerbations. *Am Fam Phys*, 84(1), 40–47.

Pollart, S. M., & Elward, K. S. (2009). Overview of changes to asthma guidelines: diagnosis and screening. *Am Fam Phys*, 79(9), 761–767.

Price, D., Musgrave, S. D., Shepstone, L., et al. (2011). Leukotriene antagonists as first-line or add-on asthma-controller therapy. *N Engl J Med*, 364(18), 1695–1707. doi: 10.1056/NEJMoa1010846.

Price, D. B., Yawn, B. P., & Jones, R. C. (2010). Improving the differential diagnosis of chronic obstructive pulmonary disease in primary care. *Mayo Clin Proceed*, 85(12), 1122–1129.

Qaseem, A., Wilt, T. J., Weinberger, S. E., et al. (2011). Diagnosis and management of stable chronic obstructive pulmonary disease: a clinical practice guideline update from the American College of Physicians, American College of Chest Physicians, American Thoracic Society, and European Respiratory Society. *Annals of Intern Med*, 155(3), 179–191. doi: 10.7326/0003-4819-155-3-201108020-00008.

Raghu, G. (2012). Idiopathic pulmonary fibrosis: new evidence and an improved standard of care in 2012. *Lancet*, 380(9842), 699–701.

Ray, S. M., & Barger Stevens, A. R. (2013). Choosing the right inhaled medication device for COPD. *Am Fam Phys*, 88(10), 650, 652.

Risser, A., Donovan, D., Heintzman, J., & Page, T. (2009). NSAID prescribing precautions. *American Family Physician*, 80(12) 1371–1378.

Salvi, S. S., & Barnes, P. J. (2009). Chronic obstructive pulmonary disease in non-smokers. *Lancet*. 374(9691), 733–743.

Serisier, D. J., Martin, M. L., McGuckin, M. A., et al. (2013). Effect of long-term, low-dose erythromycin on pulmonary exacerbations among patients with non-cystic fibrosis bronchiectasis: the BLESS randomized controlled trial. *JAMA*, 309(12), 1260–1267.

Sethi, S., Mahler, D. A., Marcus, P., et al. (2012). Inflammation in COPD: implications for management. *Am J Med*, 125(12), 1162–1170.

Silverman, E. K., & Sandhaus, R. A. (2009). Clinical practice. Alpha1-antitrypsin deficiency. *N Engl J Med*, 360(26), 2749–2757.

Sin, D. D., & Park, H. Y. (2013). Steroids for treatment of COPD exacerbations: less is clearly more. *JAMA*, 309(21), 2272–2273.

Smith, L. J. (2010). Anticholinergics for patients with asthma? *N Engl J Med*, 363(18), 1764–1765. doi: 10.1056/NEJMe1009429. Epub 2010 Sep 19.

Soriano, J. B., Zielinski, J., & Price, D. (2009). Screening for and early detection of chronic obstructive pulmonary disease. *Lancet*, 374(9691), 721–732.

Stein, P. D., Dalen, J. E., & Matta, F. (2014). Underuse of vena cava filters in unstable patients with acute pulmonary embolism. *Am J Med*, 127(1), 6. doi: 10.1016/j.amjmed.2013.07.040. Epub 2013 Nov 14.

Sterk, P. J., & Sont, J. K. (2013). Strategies for tailoring asthma treatment in adults. *JAMA*, 309(2), 135–136.

Stupka, E., & deShazo, R. (2009). Asthma in seniors: Part 1. Evidence for underdiagnosis, undertreatment, and increasing morbidity and mortality. *Am J Med*, 122(1), 6–11.

Sveum, R., Bergstrom, J., Brottman, G., et al. (2012). Diagnosis and management of asthma. Retrieved from https://www.icsi.org/_asset/rsjvnd/Asthma.pdf

Tan, H., Sarawate, C., Singer, J., et al. (2013). Inflammatory biomarkers and exacerbations in chronic obstructive pulmonary disease. *JAMA*, 309(22), 2353–2361.

Tantisira, K. G., Lasky-Su, J., Harada, M., et al. (2011). Genomewide association between GLCCI1 and response to glucocorticoid therapy in asthma. *N Engl J Med*, 365(13), 1173–1183. doi: 10.1056/NEJMoa0911353. Epub 2011 Sep 26.

Tarlo, S. M., & Lemiere, C. (2014). Occupational asthma. *N Engl J Med*, 370(7), 640–649. doi: 10.1056/NEJMra1301758.

Torpy, J. M., Burke, A. E., & Glass, R. M. (2010). *JAMA* patient page. Chronic obstructive pulmonary disease. *JAMA*, 303(23), 2430.

Tschumperlin, D. J. (2011). Physical forces and airway remodeling in asthma. *N Engl J Med*, 364(21), 2058–2059. doi: 10.1056/NEJMe1103121.

van Dijk, W. D., & Käyser, S. C. (2014). Bronchodilator safety in chronic obstructive pulmonary disease: time to focus? *JAMA Intern Med*, 174(4), 647. doi: 10.1001/jamainternmed.2013.12708.

Verdoorn, B. P., & McDonald, F. S. (2011). 62-year-old woman with fever, dyspnea, pleuritic chest pain, and weight loss. *Mayo Clin Proceed*, 86(2), 152–155.

Vogelmeier, C., Hederer, B., Glaab, T., et al. (2011). Tiotropium versus salmeterol for the prevention of exacerbations of COPD. *N Engl J Med*, 364(12), 1093–1103.

von Mutius, E., & Drazen, J. M. (2010). Choosing asthma step-up care. *N Engl J Med*, 362(11), 1042–1043. doi: 10.1056/NEJMe1002058. Epub 2010 Mar 2.

Wahls, S. A. (2012). Causes and evaluation of chronic dyspnea. *Am Fam Phys*, 86(2), 173–182.

Washko, G. R., Hunninghake, G. M., Fernandez, I. E., et al. (2011). Lung volumes and emphysema in smokers with interstitial lung abnormalities. *N Engl J Med*, 364(10), 897–906.

Wechsler, M. E. (2009). Managing asthma in primary care: putting new guideline recommendations into context. *Mayo Clin Proceed*, 84(8), 707–717.

Wedzicha, J. A. (2011). Choice of bronchodilator therapy for patients with COPD. *N Engl J Med*, 364(12), 1167–1168.

Yancey, J. R., & Chaffee, D. (2014). The role of breathing exercises in the treatment of COPD. *Am Fam Phys*, 89(1), 15–16.

Yawn, B. (2009). The new asthma guidelines. *Am Fam Phys*, 79(9), 727–731.

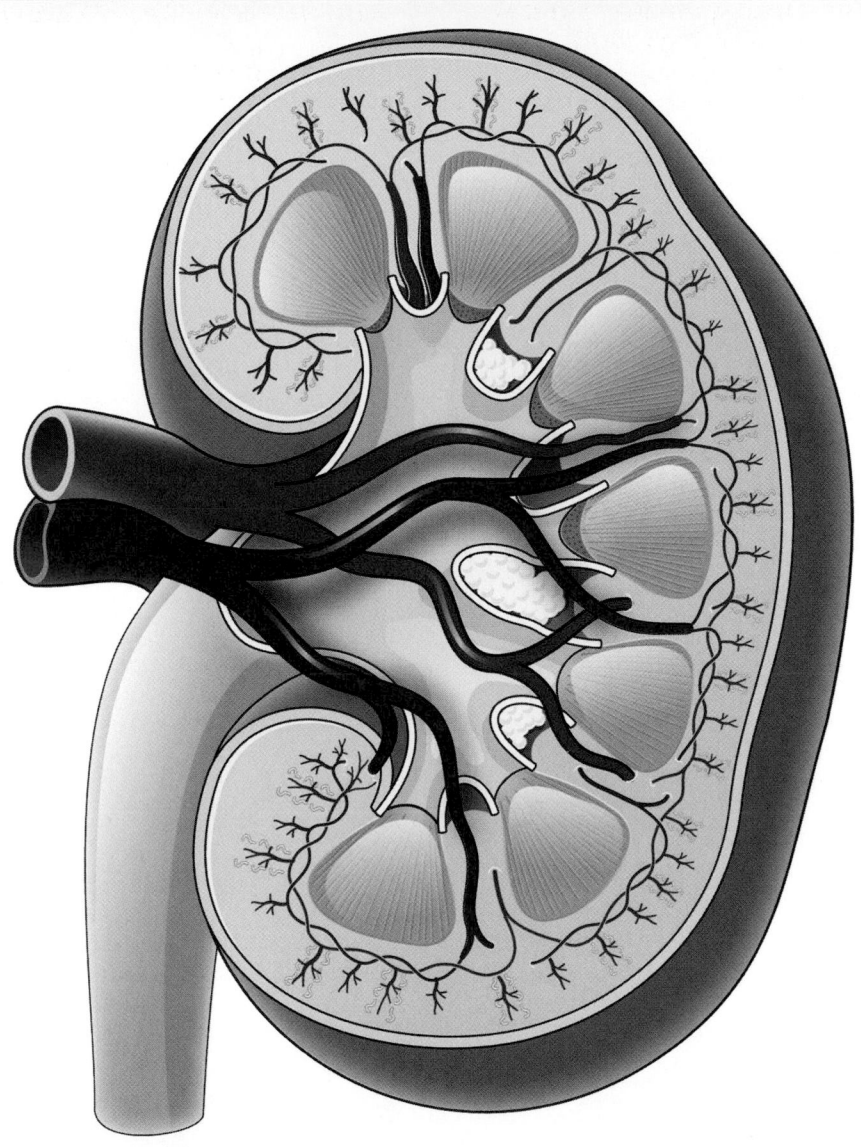

Chapters

Renal Disorders

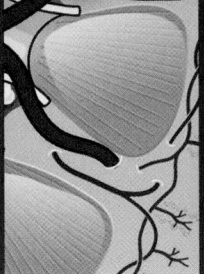

Key Terms

Acute kidney injury (AKI)

Acute tubular necrosis (ATN)

Albuminuria

Azotemia

Continuous renal replacement therapy (CRRT)

Costovertebral angle (CVA) tenderness

End-stage renal disease (ESRD)

Glomerular filtration rate (GFR)

Hematuria

Hemodialysis

Hydronephrosis

Intrarenal dysfunction

Nephrolithiasis

Nephrotic syndrome

Obstructive uropathy

Oliguria

Peritoneal dialysis (PD)

Postrenal dysfunction

Prerenal dysfunction

Proteinuria

Renal osteodystrophy

Urea

Uropathy

The kidneys are commonly recognized as the organs of excretion, because they filter the bloodstream of waste products and excrete urine. They also, however, perform many other functions that are essential for life. The kidneys play a major role in controlling blood pressure, regulating red blood cell (RBC) production, breaking down drugs, metabolizing hormones, synthesizing vitamin D, managing electrolytes, and balancing pH of the bloodstream. The kidney influences every system of the body, from brain to bone, and it is only in their failure that we can appreciate the kidney's multiple actions and far reaching effects on the body.

Epidemiology

The incidence of kidney disease continues to grow in the United States. According to a study by the National Institutes of Health (NIH), the number of individuals with **end-stage renal disease (ESRD)** increased from approximately 86,000 in the 1980s to 548,000 in 2008. The reason for this drastic increase is unclear; however, with the aging of the population, the incidence of ESRD is expected to grow more over the next 10 years. Although kidney dysfunction is seen in all ethnic groups, African Americans have the greatest incidence of kidney disease. Individuals with ESRD require hemodialysis or transplant, either of which consumes a large proportion of the health-care budget in the United States.

Basic Concepts of Renal Function

Renal function begins with blood flow to the renal vasculature. The kidneys receive 20% to 25% of the body's cardiac output. The glomerulus filters approximately 90 to 120 mL/min of blood, which is pushed through Bowman's capsule because of high hydrostatic pressure. The renal blood filtered per unit of time, known as the **glomerular filtration rate (GFR),** is directly related to renal perfusion. Disease processes that decrease blood pressure and renal perfusion result in a decreased GFR. As an individual ages, the normal GFR rate diminishes. Peak function of the kidneys occurs at age 30 years; for each year after, GFR decreases by 1 mL/minute until, by age 70 years, GFR is 70 mL/min. This reduction in GFR in the elderly adult can cause accumulation of toxins in the blood, particularly drug metabolites.

Excretory Functions

The basic unit of the kidney is the nephron, a sequence of tubes that filters the blood of waste and conserves the fluid and electrolytes that the body needs. Each nephron is surrounded by blood vessels where exchange of water and electrolytes occur between the blood and the tubule fluid. At the glomerular capillaries, the major mechanisms of the nephron—waste removal and water recycling—begin. The different sections of the nephron perform various functions in order to form the final product, which is a concentrated urine. Urine must contain all the waste products, electrolytes, metabolites, and nitrogenous compounds for excretion. At the same time, urine needs to be sparing of water; the kidney needs to conserve the water the body needs.

The Nephron

Renal blood flow through the glomerulus requires high hydrostatic pressure to push blood through the filtration process. There is an autoregulation of renal blood flow by the kidneys that maintains sufficient pressure to push blood through the glomeruli, whether blood volume is high or low.

As blood flows through the glomerulus and a membranous cap called Bowman's capsule, water and electrolytes leave the blood and pass into the proximal tubule. At this point, the glomerular filtrate is very dilute and contains a high amount of electrolytes, glucose, and metabolic waste products.

At the proximal tubule, approximately 60% of water is reabsorbed back into the bloodstream. As the tubule fluid travels through the various parts of the nephron, water and electrolytes such as sodium and potassium move to and from tubule fluid and blood. Within the next section of the nephron, called the loop of Henle, urea is secreted into the tubule fluid. **Urea** is a composite of nitrogenous waste that needs to be excreted. At this juncture within the nephron, the tubule fluid, which contains urea, starts to resemble the finished product: urine. Overall, the loop of Henle reabsorbs about 25% of filtered electrolytes, such as sodium, chlorine, potassium, calcium, and bicarbonate, and 15% of the filtered water. At the distal tubule, aldosterone acts to reabsorb more sodium and water into the bloodstream and secrete potassium into the tubule fluid. Here again, tubule fluid is further concentrated and the body saves water. Finally, at the collecting duct under the influence of antidiuretic hormone, the last amount of water needed by the body is reabsorbed from the tubule fluid back into the bloodstream. At this last stage, the highly concentrated tubule fluid is urine (see Fig. 22-1).

Acid-Base Balance

Normal body function is dependent upon acid-base balance, and the kidneys play a major role through regulation of bicarbonate and hydrogen reabsorption or secretion. Acids are produced during normal metabolic processes, requiring the physiologic response of buffering to maintain the physiologic pH of 7.35 to 7.45. The kidneys' role in maintaining acid-base balance involves excretion of excess hydrogen ions [$H+$] and formation of bicarbonate ions [HCO_3-].

Waste Elimination

During the cell's metabolic activity, waste products are accumulated. These waste products include such substances as urea, uric acid, creatinine, and drug metabolites. If not excreted in the urine, waste products become toxic to body tissues, particularly breakdown products of drugs. A reduction in renal function can prolong the effect of some medications, which can lead to adverse effects or toxicity.

Secretory Functions

The kidney has several unique secretory functions that are triggered by certain conditions in the body. Hypoxia and low blood volume are two such conditions.

Control of Blood Pressure

The major mechanism whereby the kidneys influence systemic blood pressure and blood volume is the renin-angiotensin-aldosterone system (RAAS).

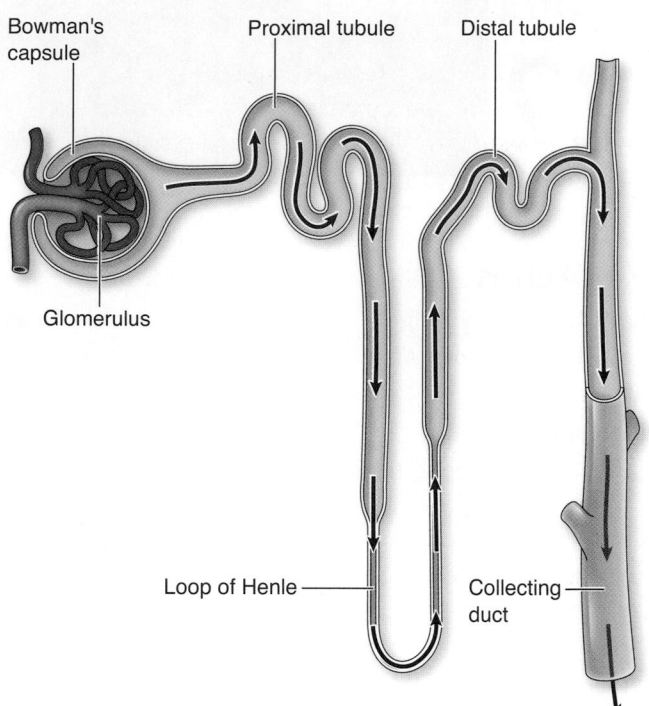

FIGURE 22-1. Basic functions of the nephron. The nephron's basic goal is to yield a concentrated urine that contains waste products. The blood and tubule fluid undergo a great deal of exchange before the tubule fluid becomes urine. The glomerulus is a tuft of capillaries from which blood is filtered at Bowman's capsule. The glomerulus allows substances out of the blood such as water, sodium, bicarbonate, acids, and urea. However, the glomerulus does not allow large proteins such as albumin out of the blood. At the proximal tubule, a large amount of water, sodium, and potassium are reabsorbed into the bloodstream. At the descending loop of Henle, a high amount of sodium is reabsorbed and urea is secreted from the blood into the tubule. Aldosterone, a hormone secreted by the adrenal gland, increases sodium and water reabsorption. In the distal tubule, sodium and water are reabsorbed from the tubule fluid into the bloodstream and urine is formed. If the body needs more water, antidiuretic hormone from the posterior pituitary works at the collecting duct to increase water reabsorption into the bloodstream for a more concentrated urine.

The RAAS contributes to sodium and water reabsorption into the bloodstream at the renal tubules and potassium excretion. A specialized region of the nephron called the juxtaglomerular apparatus is sensitive to sodium. These cells sense low sodium and, in response, secrete renin. Other triggers for renin secretion include decreased renal perfusion and increased sympathetic nervous system activity. The net effects of the RAAS activity are sodium and water reabsorption, potassium excretion, and arterial vasoconstriction.

Red Blood Cell Production

The kidney secretes erythropoietin, which stimulates synthesis of RBCs in the bone marrow. Erythropoietin is released in response to low oxygen levels in arterial blood. The kidney also secretes erythropoietin in response to anemia and reduced renal blood flow.

Vitamin D Synthesis and Calcium Balance

The kidneys synthesize components that comprise vitamin D. Without kidney function, vitamin D is inactive, which affects calcium absorption. In the gastrointestinal tract, calcium is absorbed with the facilitation of vitamin D. Without vitamin D, calcium absorption is diminished, which disrupts calcium balance in the bloodstream.

Glucose Homeostasis

The renal tubules reabsorb glucose from the glomerular filtrate up to the renal threshold of a blood glucose level of 180 mg/dL. If the blood glucose level is greater than the renal threshold, the excess glucose is excreted in the urine. Additionally, in states of prolonged fasting or starvation, the kidneys can create glucose from amino acids in the process known as gluconeogenesis. The kidneys are also responsible for the degradation of insulin. Patients with renal failure have decreased insulin clearance.

Basic Pathophysiologic Concepts of Renal Disorders

The kidneys are at risk for injury because they require a large blood flow in order to function and they process potentially toxic waste products. For the nephrons to work, the blood entering at the glomerulus needs to have high hydrostatic pressure. The kidneys are susceptible to ischemic injury if not provided with high blood flow. All tubule fluid from the nephrons must travel toward the renal pelvis and out the ureter. The nephrons need high pressure pushing tubule fluid out of the kidney without any stasis or backflow. The tubule fluid contains waste products that can be toxic to the fragile nephron cells. Many drug metabolites are particularly nephrotoxic. The nephron cells are at risk if urine outflow is not maintained. Any obstruction to urine outflow, also called obstructive **uropathy,** can cause urine to back up from the ureter into the renal pelvis and cause cellular injury.

The causes of kidney dysfunction are divided into three categories based upon the mechanism of injury:

1. **prerenal dysfunction:** caused by decreased blood flow and perfusion to the kidney.

2. **intrarenal dysfunction:** develops secondary to actual injuries to the kidney itself.
3. **postrenal dysfunction:** related to obstruction of urine outflow from the kidneys.

Prerenal Dysfunction

Prerenal dysfunction of the kidney describes pathophysiologic processes that affect GFR and are directly related to blood flow and renal perfusion (see Fig. 22-2). Any condition that directly or indirectly decreases renal perfusion may lead to prerenal dysfunction. Prerenal dysfunction occurs because of reduced cardiac output or severe hypovolemia (low blood volume). In any type of shock, the patient is vulnerable to prerenal dysfunction. Maintenance of a sufficiently high blood pressure is necessary for kidney function because glomerular filtration requires high hydrostatic pressure. Large blood loss from the body, as in hemorrhage, is a common cause of prerenal kidney injury caused by ischemia.

Intrarenal Dysfunction

Direct damage to renal tissue, as in trauma or toxic injury, causes nephron damage within the kidney itself, known as intrarenal dysfunction. This is most commonly caused by nephrotoxic medications, renal infections, or systemic illnesses that affect the kidney. Common

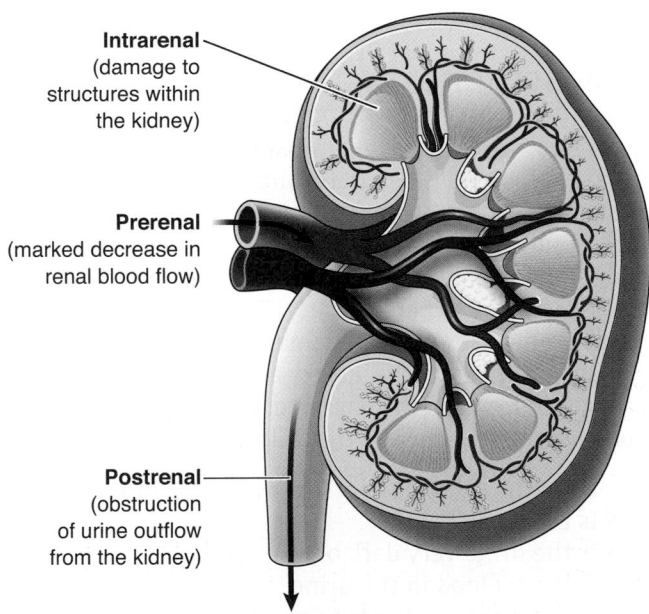

Intrarenal
(damage to structures within the kidney)

Prerenal
(marked decrease in renal blood flow)

Postrenal
(obstruction of urine outflow from the kidney)

FIGURE 22-2. There are three basic categories of renal dysfunction: prerenal, intrarenal, and postrenal. These are sometimes referred to as prerenal, intrarenal, or postrenal azotemia. Prerenal azotemia occurs in severe dehydration or hemorrhage; there is inadequate blood flow to optimally perfuse the kidney. The kidney is not the cause of prenatal azotemia; rather, a circumstance that decreases perfusion of the kidney is the source of the problem. In intrarenal azotemia, there is a problem intrinsically with the kidney, such as trauma to the kidney, infection, or nephrotoxic drugs. Postrenal azotemia occurs when urine outflow is obstructed. Urine needs to flow freely out of the kidney; if backed up, it is toxic to the nephrons. Prostate enlargement, kidney stones, kinked ureter, or tumors can cause postrenal azotemia.

examples include nephrotoxicity caused by nonsteroidal anti-inflammatory drugs (NSAIDs) and poststreptococcal glomerulonephritis. Both of these conditions cause direct injury to the kidney.

Postrenal Dysfunction

Postrenal dysfunction is caused by obstructive uropathy, a problem that prevents urine outflow from the kidney. A few conditions can cause this obstruction, including kidney stone or prostate gland hyperplasia. In postrenal kidney dysfunction, urine backs up within the ureter and into the kidney, which can lead to **hydronephrosis,** a fluid-filled swollen kidney. Urine is toxic to the nephron cells and urine stagnation increases risk of infection.

Acute Tubular Necrosis

Ischemia and hypoxia can damage the renal tubules and result in **acute tubular necrosis (ATN),** the most common cause of **acute kidney injury (AKI)**. With ischemia, there is sloughing of the cells of nephron tubules into the tubular lumen. The lumen becomes blocked, preventing fluid from flowing through them, thereby reducing urine formation. The blocked lumen further contributes to ischemic injury to cells lining the tubules, causing additional intrarenal injury. Unless this process is reversed, renal failure with permanent injury to the kidney will occur.

Assessment

The history and physical assessment for patients with renal disease includes determining exposure to any medications or substances that would be nephrotoxic. Additionally, any systemic illnesses or infections associated with renal damage need to be identified. Illnesses such as hypertension (HTN) and diabetes are important causes of renal damage.

Patients need to be asked about their pattern of urine excretion and the character of their urine. Typical questions would include the following:

- Does the urine have an unusual odor or color?
- Is the urine foamy?
- Is the urine very dark or tea-colored?
- Is there blood in the urine?
- Is there pain or burning on urination? Is there abdominal or flank pain on urination?
- Have you noticed any change in the amount of urine or the frequency of urination?

Risk Factors

Exposure to nephrotoxic agents is one of the greatest risks for the development of renal disorders. A list of current medications is needed. Specific questions concerning HTN and diabetes mellitus (DM) are important. The patient needs to describe the duration of the

ALERT! Long-term DM and HTN often lead to renal failure.

disorder, medications involved, and management of the disorders.

The patient should be asked about a recent streptococcal infection because poststreptococcal glomerulonephritis can occur. Patients who have had major surgery are at risk for altered renal function. Major surgery can reduce renal blood flow and lead to kidney injury. A reduction in renal blood flow is also a concern for patients who have had an acute myocardial infarction or heart failure. Renal ischemia commonly is a complication of severe heart failure.

Signs and Symptoms

The patient with renal failure generally has a variety of multisystemic symptoms, which are the result of reduced secretory and excretory functions of the kidney. The symptoms can include fatigue, weakness, nausea, constipation, abdominal pain, and confusion. Patients with renal calculi may have abdominal or flank pain in addition to hematuria. **Costovertebral angle (CVA) tenderness** is a classic sign of a kidney disorder, particularly infection (see Fig. 22-3).

The presence of blood (**hematuria**) or protein (**proteinuria**) in urine is often readily apparent to the patient. Urine looks pink or red when blood is present and foamy when it contains high levels of protein. Tea-colored urine often indicates bilirubin is in the urine,

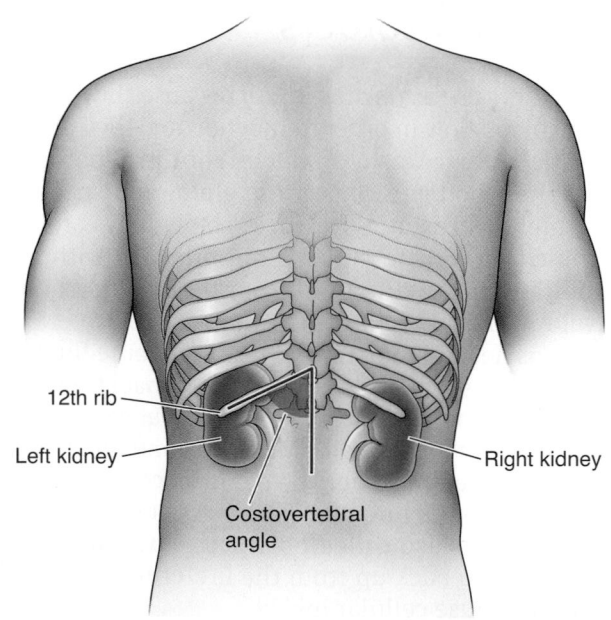

12th rib

Left kidney

Right kidney

Costovertebral angle

FIGURE 22-3. The kidney is located in the costovertebral angle (CVA) region. In physical examination, the examiner should firmly tap the CVA to assess its pain of kidney disorder. The pain of nephrolithiasis and pyelonephritis is commonly in the CVA region.

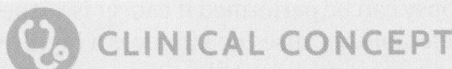

CLINICAL CONCEPT

Hematuria is most often a sign of renal calculi or an infection.

as occurs in jaundice. All these signs are an indication for further study.

Proteinuria, also called microalbuminuria, indicates that the urine contains proteins. Normal total protein excretion does not usually exceed more than 150 mg/day. Excess protein in the urine is abnormal and is usually an indication of glomerular injury. The glomerular capillaries should not filter out blood proteins; however, when injured they demonstrate extra permeability. Glomerular injury can occur in such disorders as glomerulonephritis, diabetes, and HTN.

Diagnosis

Renal function can be evaluated through examination of the urine and blood. Imaging studies can be performed to evaluate the anatomy of the kidneys and renal blood flow and visualize renal calculi, tumors, or cysts.

Urinalysis

Urinalysis is a basic examination of urine that includes a description of the character of the urine as well as biochemical and microscopic analysis. Normally, urine is odorless and clear or slightly hazy with a color ranging from yellow to amber. The color varies according to the concentration of solutes and water content of the urine. For example, a dehydrated person has an amber-colored urine, whereas a well-hydrated person has a light yellow urine, though urine color can vary with some medications or certain disorders. For example, hepatitis will cause a dark brown, tea-colored urine, caused by bile pigments.

Reagent strips, also called dipsticks, are used for analysis of the urine. Urinary pH should be close to a neutral pH of 7, but it does vary from acidic to basic. The specific gravity should be between 1.001 when dilute and 1.030 when highly concentrated. All of the biochemical tests that are measured by reagent strips should be negative in healthy individuals. If any of these tests are positive, they are suggestive of a variety of illness states (see Table 22-1).

The presence of glucose and ketones is indicative of diabetic ketoacidosis. A positive leukocyte esterase measures the amount of enzyme secreted by WBCs; a high amount is indicative of either a bladder or kidney infection. Crystals are often seen in the urine of patients with renal calculi. Casts are substances that are secreted into the nephron tubules and retain the shape of the tubules. They are made of protein or fats and can be benign or signify kidney disease.

Blood Urea Nitrogen

Azotemia is the increase of blood urea nitrogen (BUN) within the bloodstream. The normal level for BUN is 5 to 20 mg/dL. An elevated BUN can occur when there is a decrease in the GFR, which leads to accumulation of nitrogenous waste products in the blood. However, a high BUN level is not always an indicator of kidney dysfunction; it can result from dehydration, which highly concentrates the urea in the urine. A high BUN level can also occur in any condition that elevates the amount of nitrogen waste in the bloodstream. In extremely muscular individuals, there is high nitrogen in the bloodstream because of high muscle breakdown. The muscle cell proteins break down into amino acids, which are nitrogen compounds. Another cause of high BUN occurs in persons on high protein diets, as the large load of protein breakdown into amino acids raises nitrogen in the bloodstream. Because of the possible elevation

TABLE 22-1. Urine Analysis Using Reagent Strips		
Test	**Normal value**	**Common Etiology**
GLUCOSE	negative	If positive: hyperglycemia, diabetes
KETONES	negative	If positive: starvation or diabetic ketoacidosis
PROTEIN	negative or trace	Minimal: exercise or infection
		Moderate: polycystic kidney disease (PKD), infection, heart failure, diabetic kidney disease
		Marked: PKD, glomerulonephritis, diabetic kidney disease, nephrosis, lupus nephritis
BLOOD	negative	If positive: infection or kidney stone
BILIRUBIN	negative	If positive: hemolysis or liver disease
UROBILINOGEN	minimal	If high: liver disease
NITRITE	negative	If positive: urinary tract infection
LEUKOCYTE ESTERASE	negative	If positive: urinary tract infection

of BUN with nonrenal conditions such as dehydration, the clinician should not rely on BUN alone as an indicator of renal dysfunction.

Serum Creatinine

Creatinine is a muscle breakdown product that is practically completely filtered at the glomerulus. The normal range of serum creatinine is approximately 0.5 to 1.5 mg/dL. After it is filtered out of the bloodstream, it is not reabsorbed by the nephron tubules.

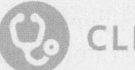

CLINICAL CONCEPT

Serum creatinine is a reliable indicator of kidney function.

Accumulation of serum creatinine indicates decreased filtering of creatinine at the glomerulus. There are exceptions to this rule in extremely muscular individuals and very frail individuals. Because serum creatinine is based on muscle tissue breakdown, serum creatinine can vary depending on the patient's muscle mass. A person who has an increased amount of muscle breakdown daily may have an abnormally high serum creatinine, whereas a frail individual will have a low amount of serum creatinine daily.

ALERT! Nephrotoxic antibiotics include the aminoglycosides. Whenever these are administered, serum levels of the medication and serum creatinine levels must be monitored.

Creatinine Clearance

Creatinine clearance is sometimes used to assess the GFR. The test requires measurement of both blood and urine creatinine and 24-hour urine volume. The amount of creatinine filtered at the glomerulus is the total amount of creatinine that appears in the urine. A decreased creatinine clearance indicates decreased GFR and impaired renal function. This can be caused by conditions such as renal disease or can result from lack of circulation to the kidney, which occurs in hypotension, heart failure, and shock. Increased creatinine clearance indicates there is more creatinine in the urine than normal. This can be seen in pregnant women, patients with diabetes mellitus, or those with large dietary protein intake.

Imaging Studies

Visualization of the kidneys through various imaging studies can provide valuable information about renal size and function. Renal ultrasound is used to determine the size of both kidneys. It can also be used in the diagnosis of hydronephrosis, renal cysts, tumors, and calculi. Intravenous pyelography is often used to diagnose renal stones. Abdominal x-rays can visualize radiopaque stones or nephrocalcinosis. Computed tomography (CT) scans can usually visualize stones if used with contrast media. Magnetic resonance imaging (MRI) is useful in those who cannot tolerate radiopaque contrast media.

Renal biopsy can be performed if cancer is suspected but is not preferable because the kidney is a highly vascular organ and a great amount of bleeding can occur.

ALERT! IV contrast-enhanced imaging studies should be avoided in patients with renal impairment because radiopaque dye can cause renal failure. Dehydration markedly increases this risk.

Treatment

In treating renal disease, regardless of the etiology, all of the functions regulated by the kidney need to be maintained. It is important to maintain fluid, electrolyte, and acid-base levels; control blood glucose; control blood pressure; and monitor RBC production. To accomplish this, patients usually need multiple medications to maintain physiologic homeostasis; sodium bicarbonate can help control metabolic acidosis, whereas beta blocker medications can control blood pressure. Epogen is a synthetic form of erythropoietin that can be used to stimulate RBC production. Diuretics can be used to stimulate water loss from the body. However, when these medications cannot reverse the imbalances of renal failure, dialysis is necessary. Indications for dialysis include persistent hyperkalemia, uncompensated metabolic acidosis, and fluid volume excess that is unresponsive to diuresis.

There are two types of dialysis: hemodialysis and peritoneal dialysis. When both kidneys are no longer functioning and the patient is in relatively good health, renal transplant may be considered.

Peritoneal Dialysis

In **peritoneal dialysis (PD),** the patient's peritoneum is filled with a dialysis solution that pulls wastes and extra fluid from the blood into the abdominal cavity. The dialysis solution, called the dialysate, contains certain electrolytes that cause diffusion of solutes and ultrafiltration of fluid from the blood to cross the peritoneal membrane. The process works based on the principle that diffusion of substances in water tends to move from an area of high concentration to an area of low concentration. After the fluid is instilled, it sits in the peritoneal cavity for a period, called a dwell time, of approximately 4 hours. After the dwell time, the solution is drained from the peritoneal cavity and discarded. PD is uncommon, but at times it is used as an alternative to hemodialysis. The process of draining and filling takes about 30 to 40 minutes. A typical schedule of PD requires approximately four exchanges a day, each with a dwell time of 4 to 6 hours.

Hemodialysis

Hemodialysis is a treatment during which the patient's blood is drawn out of the body at a rate of

200 to 400 mL/minute and passed through a device called a dialyzer. Commonly, a patient has an arterial-venous fistula created in the arm that can facilitate this process. For example, a tubular connection between the brachiocephalic artery and cephalic vein is often surgically implanted. Blood is drained from the brachiocephalic artery and pumped into a dialyzer, which removes excess solutes and fluid from the blood. The blood is then returned to the body via the cephalic vein. The dialysis solution is a sterile solution of electrolytes. Urea and other waste products, such as potassium and phosphate, diffuse into the dialysis solution. During the treatment, the patient's entire blood volume (about 5,000 mL) circulates through the machine every 15 minutes. Electrolytes, serum albumin, BUN, and serum creatinine are normalized during the dialysis procedure. The procedure is usually required at least three times a week for 4 to 6 hours each session.

Continuous Renal Replacement Therapy

Continuous renal replacement therapy (CRRT) is similar to hemodialysis; however, it is a slower process used for patients who are hemodynamically unstable and fluid overloaded. This continuous process takes smaller volumes of blood from the patient and filters it through a dialyzer over 24 hours.

Pathophysiology of Selected Disorders

Major pathophysiolgic conditions of the kidney include acute glomerulonephritis, nephrotic syndrome, nephrolithiasis, and pyelonephritis.

Acute Glomerulonephritis

Acute glomerulonephritis (AGN) is a renal disorder in which an immunological mechanism triggers inflammation that damages the membranes of the glomerulus. It can lead to significant illness because the glomerulus is the critical, initial region of every nephron unit that filters the blood. Damage to the glomerular capillaries causes a loss of vital substances, such as albumin, from the blood.

Epidemiology

AGN is the cause of 25% to 30% of all cases of ESRD. In cases that progress to ESRD, the disease course is fairly rapid. End-stage renal failure may occur within weeks or months of the onset of AGN. Most cases of AGN occur in patients aged 5 to 15 years; only 10% occur in patients older than 40 years. It predominantly affects males with a 2:1 male-to-female ratio.

Etiology

Poststreptococcal infection is the most common cause of AGN. Acute infection with group A beta-hemolytic streptococcus (GABHS) usually begins as pharyngitis

and then causes a secondary immunological reaction at the glomeruli. AGN can also occur after a skin infection with GABHS, known as impetigo. Although AGN most commonly develops because of streptococcal infection, it can also arise because of other types of bacterial, viral, fungal, or parasitic infections. AGN can follow infections such as rubella, mumps, Epstein-Barr virus, or cytomegalovirus. Autoimmune and immunological diseases also frequently cause AGN, such as systemic lupus erythematosus. Acute disease may progress to chronic disease, particularly in patients with other risk factors. The course of chronic glomerulonephritis is often gradual and silent. By the time of diagnosis, the patient is commonly already in the early stages of ESRD.

Pathophysiology

AGN begins with an antigen-antibody reaction. An antigen, such as streptococcus, enters the body and stimulates antibody synthesis. There are two theoretical explanations for the mechanism of disease. One theory claims that the antibodies attack the antigen, but also form antigen-antibody complexes that float freely in the bloodstream until they deposit within glomerular membranes. The other theory asserts that molecular mimicry occurs where the antibodies that are stimulated attack the antigen and mistakenly attack the glomerular membranes as well (see Fig. 22-4).

Regardless of mechanism, the antigen-antibody complexes damage the structure of the glomeruli and cause nephron dysfunction throughout the kidneys. Glomerular injury causes hyperpermeability of the

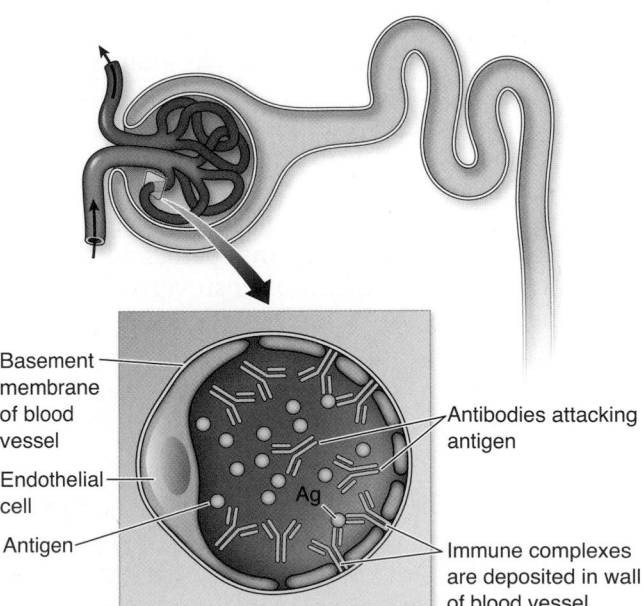

FIGURE 22-4. Glomerular damage in glomerulonephritis. The damage to glomerular membranes in glomerulonephritis is caused by antibodies. These antibodies are commonly activated by streptococcus bacteria. The antibodies combine with antigen and deposit as immune complexes within the kidney that are normally eliminated in the circulation. However, in glomerulonephritis, the immune complexes accumulate and cause inflammation and membrane damage.

capillaries, which allows loss of albumin and RBCs in the urine. The large loss of albumin from the bloodstream causes proteinuria, also called microalbuminuria. Because albumin content of the bloodstream decreases, diminished colloid oncotic pressure (COP) occurs throughout the body. According to Starling's Law of Capillary Forces, the decrease of COP causes an imbalance in hydrostatic and oncotic pressure. The low COP is overcome by hydrostatic pressure, which causes edema.

Also, because there is diminished glomerular filtration of the blood, there is diminished urine production. **Oliguria,** which is lack of sufficient urine production, develops as GFR decreases. The patient becomes hypervolemic and edematous, and blood pressure rises.

CLINICAL CONCEPT

A certain amount of urine production is necessary to excrete waste products. An inadequate amount of urine is termed oliguria. Oliguria is less than 400 mL of urine output per day or fewer than 20 mL of urine per hour.

Clinical Presentation

Acute glomerulonephritis has a classic presentation of sudden edema, hematuria, proteinuria, and HTN. The onset of clinical manifestations occurs approximately 7 to 21 days following a streptococcal infection. This is consistent with the time frame needed for antibody formation. As glomerular function decreases, urinary output decreases. As glomerular injury increases, hematuria and proteinuria increase. The patient develops puffiness of the eyelids and facial edema. The urine is dark because it contains RBCs; it has been described as cola-colored. Blood pressure may be elevated. Nonspecific symptoms include weakness, fever, abdominal pain, and malaise. The patient may complain of costovertebral angle tenderness.

CLINICAL CONCEPT

Edema in kidney disease is most prevalent in the periorbital region.

CLINICAL CONCEPT

Costovertebral angle tenderness is a classic symptom of kidney infection.

Diagnosis

Serum creatinine and BUN will be elevated because of kidney dysfunction and should be monitored during the course of treatment. Routine urinalyses will show low specific gravity of dilute urine caused by the inability of the kidneys to concentrate urine. In addition, urinalysis will show a large amount of protein and blood in the urine. Urine creatinine clearance will be low because dysfunctional kidneys do not excrete nitrogenous wastes. Creatinine accumulates in the blood. Additionally, serum studies that are diagnostically definitive include an elevated antistreptolysin O titer; a drop in C3 complement (an immune mediator); and cryoglobulins, which are large immune complexes. Serum albumin will be low because glomeruli are filtering albumin out of the blood into the tubules, then into the urine.

Treatment

The management of AGN is largely based upon clinical presentation and symptoms. Antibiotics, antipyretics, and analgesics are needed. With systematic manifestations, such as edema and elevated blood pressure, diuretics and antihypertensive agents may be indicated. Dietary restrictions of sodium and protein are also advised. Plasmapheresis may be used to rid the blood of antiglomerular antibodies. Immunosuppressants are also used in the treatment of AGN.

Nephrotic Syndrome

Nephrotic syndrome is a combination of clinical findings that occur when the glomerulus is damaged. When glomeruli are injured, they become hyperpermeable to proteins and other substances in the bloodstream. The blood becomes depleted of albumin and other large molecules as they enter into the nephron tubules and become excreted with the urine. Common causes of nephrotic syndrome include glomerulonephritis, DM, and autoimmune disease.

Epidemiology

Diabetic nephropathy is the most common type of nephrotic syndrome, with an incidence of 50 to 100 cases per million population per year. Native Americans, Latino Americans, and African Americans have a higher incidence than do Caucasians. There is a male predominance in the occurrence of nephrotic syndrome, as there is for chronic kidney disease in general. However, nephrotic syndrome secondary to systemic lupus erythematosus is more common in women.

Etiology

Three systemic diseases—DM, amyloidosis, and systemic lupus erythematosus (SLE)—are implicated in more than 90% of all cases of nephrotic syndrome. Other causes include immune-complex deposition disease, vasculitis, allergies, pre-eclampsia, morbid obesity, malignant HTN, and infections such as bacterial endocarditis and tuberculosis.

Pathophysiology

Glomerular damage occurs as a primary insult or secondary to one of the causes described. Structural changes that occur in the glomerulus include injury to the endothelial cells, derangement of the basement membrane, and damage to the epithelium. Massive **albuminuria** is a consequence of the glomerular damage. As albumin is lost in the vascular space, edema forms because of decreased colloidal osmotic pressure.

Clinical Presentation

Patients have albuminuria with consequent edema. Edema of the face is common, especially in the periorbital region. With severe albumin loss, edema of the lower extremities, pleural effusion, and ascites can develop. Patients also often present with hematuria and HTN.

Diagnosis

The workup for nephrotic syndrome includes urinalysis and blood tests for albumin, BUN, and serum creatinine. Urinalysis usually shows proteinuria and hematuria. Elevations in BUN and serum creatinine occur and are followed to assess renal function. The serum albumin level is classically low in nephrotic syndrome, below its normal range of 3.5 to 4.5 g/dL. Tests for hepatitis B and C, human immunodeficiency virus (HIV), and lupus, including antinuclear antibody (ANA), antidouble-stranded deoxyribonucleic acid (anti-dsDNA) antibodies, and complement, are commonly done when etiology of nephrotic syndrome is unclear. In immunological etiologies of nephrotic syndrome, complement is decreased in the bloodstream.

A 24-hour urine sample is collected for analysis. The urine can contain up to 3 grams of protein over 24 hours (normal is fewer than 150 mg/day). The urine also contains fatty casts caused by loss of lipoproteins at the glomerulus, which take on the shape of the tubules before excretion into urine. Renal ultrasonography and renal biopsy may be done when etiology is unclear.

Treatment

The patient with nephrotic syndrome needs to be vigilant of nutritional needs. The diet should provide adequate energy (caloric) intake and adequate protein (1 to 2 g/kg/d). However, supplemental dietary protein is of no proven value because it will be excreted. A low-sodium diet (fewer than 1,500 g/day) will help to limit fluid overload. Adequate fluid intake is essential but overhydration should be avoided.

Because albumin levels are low, it is important to recognize that there are less-binding sites for drugs. This will increase the amount of free active drug in the bloodstream. Also in nephrotic syndrome, immunoglobulins are lost to the urine as well. This increases susceptibility to infection. Medication regimens commonly include diuretics, anti-inflammatory agents, and, in certain cases, immunosuppressants. Angiotensin-converting enzyme (ACE) inhibitors are often used to control blood pressure.

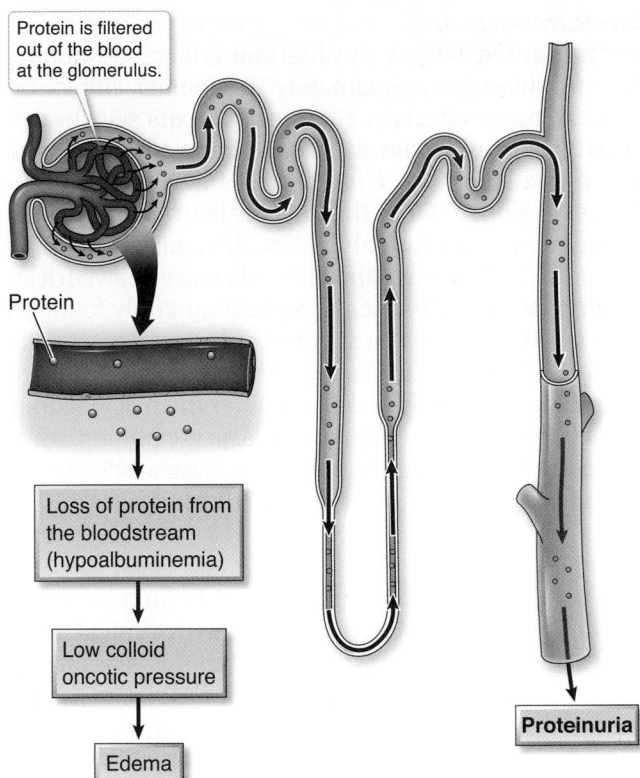

FIGURE 22-5. Nephrotic syndrome. In nephrotic syndrome, the glomerulus is damaged and allows proteins to be filtered out of the bloodstream. The major protein from the bloodstream that is lost is albumin; thus, hypoalbuminemia results. The loss of protein (albumin) in the bloodstream causes decreased colloid oncotic pressure, which leads to edema. Therefore, the signs of nephrotic syndrome are hypoalbuminemia, proteinuria, and edema.

Complications

As nephrotic syndrome progresses, hyperlipidemia may develop secondary to increased lipoprotein synthesis in the liver. As the liver increases synthesis of albumin to replenish the lost albumin in the urine, it also hypersynthesizes lipids. There is commonly an elevation in low-density lipoprotein (LDL) and triglycerides. Hyperlipidemia requires drugs that decrease liver synthesis of lipids such as statin drugs. With increased loss of protein in the urine, there is loss of antithrombin III and plasminogen, the body's natural thrombolytic substances. This increases the risk of thromboembolism and patients may require anticoagulants (see Fig. 22-5).

Nephrolithiasis

Nephrolithiasis is the formation of stones, also called calculi, in the kidney. Although stones can develop in other areas of the urological system, such as the ureter or bladder, kidney stones are most common. Although pain is a presenting sign with all types of renal calculi, characteristics vary based upon the stone's location.

Epidemiology

In the United States, the lifetime risk of developing nephrolithiasis is approximately 12% for men and 7% for women. Approximately 2 million patients seek health care for kidney stones each year. People living in the south and southwest United States have higher incidences of kidney stones than people living in other parts of the country because of the hot, dry climate.

Caucasians have nephrolithiasis more than African Americans, and the disease is predominately found in males. Kidney stones most commonly develop in adults aged 20 to 49 years, with a peak incidence at age 35 to 45 years old. A family history doubles the risk of kidney stones. Recurrence of nephrolithiasis is common. After suffering a kidney stone, individuals have a 52% chance of suffering another stone within 10 years.

Etiology

The exact cause of nephrolithiasis is unknown, but about 90% of patients who present with clinical manifestations have at least one metabolic risk factor: hypercalcemia, hyperoxaluria, hyperuricemia, hyperparathyroidism, or gout. In addition, low fluid intake is a significant risk factor because dehydration enhances kidney stone formation. There is a genetic predisposition with more than 30 genetic variations associated with renal calculi development. Differences in intestinal calcium absorption, renal calcium transport, and renal phosphate transport have all been attributed to genetic variation. In patients without specific metabolic or genetic risk factors, nephrolithiasis is attributed to dietary habits such as excessive calcium supplements and low fluid intake. Hypercalciuria and low fluid content of the urine are the most common predisposing factors that lead to nephrolithiasis (see Box 22-1).

Excessive bone resorption caused by immobility, bone disease, hyperparathyroidism, and renal tubular acidosis are all predisposing risk factors to calcium stone formation. Indinavir is a drug used for HIV infection that predisposes to calcium stones. Urinary tract infection and alkaline urine can predispose individuals to struvite stones, which are usually large.

 CLINICAL CONCEPT

Struvite stones commonly cause staghorn calculi, which can fill the entire renal pelvis (see Fig. 22-6).

Pathophysiology

The formation of renal calculi involves many different factors that include dietary and intestinal absorption factors, endocrine abnormalities, crystalline components in the blood, constituents of urine, pH of urine, urinary tract structures, and heredity.

BOX 22-1. Predisposing Factors of Nephrolithiasis

There are a wide number of predisposing factors for nephrolithiasis. Nephrolithiasis is usually caused by a number of different conditions that act together to cause precipitation of calculi in the kidney.

- Age greater than 40 years
- Male gender
- Certain medications (e.g., Sulfonamides, Indinavir, Acetazolamides)
- Dietary factors (e.g., purines, calcium, oxalate)
- Gastric bypass surgery
- Geographic location (hot, arid climates)
- Hypercalciuria
- Hyperparathyroidism
- Hyperuricemia
- High sodium diet
- Inflammatory bowel disease
- Inherited conditions (e.g., polycystic kidney disease, renal tubular acidosis)
- Low hydration/low urine volume
- Obesity
- Proteus urinary tract infection

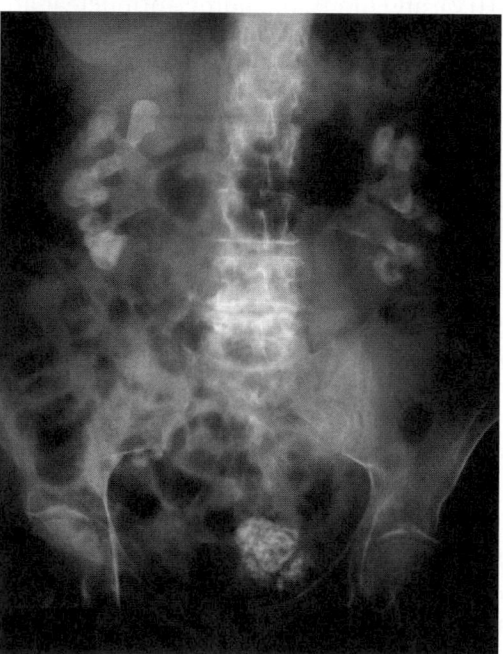

FIGURE 22-6. X-ray showing staghorn calculus. A staghorn calculus is a large calcification that occupies the renal pelvis. (*From Scott Camazine/Science Source.*)

The most common renal calculi are:

- calcium stones
- struvite (magnesium ammonium phosphate) stones
- uric acid stones
- cystine stones.

Seventy-five percent of renal calculi consist of calcium; most are composed of calcium oxalate. The cause for these stones is attributed to hyperabsorption of calcium and oxalate from the gastrointestinal tract.

Struvite stones account for 15% and are associated with chronic urinary tract infection and specific urine pH. Usual organisms include *Proteus, Pseudomonas,* and *Klebsiella* species; urine pH is typically alkaline, greater than 7. The bacteria possess the enzyme urease, which can react with urea in the urine to form ammonia and carbon dioxide. Ammonia makes the urine alkaline.

Uric acid stones account for 6% of renal calculi and are associated with high purine intake, malignancy, and gout. Purines are derived from the DNA of animal cells or cancer cells. High purine levels in the bloodstream occur with high ingestion of meats or whenever there is high cellular breakdown, as in treatment of malignancy. Approximately 25% of patients with uric acid stones have gout, which is caused by hyperuricemia.

Cystine stones account for 2% of renal calculi and arise because of failure of renal tubular reabsorption of cystine, an amino acid, into the blood. Urine becomes supersaturated with cystine, with resultant crystal deposition.

There are three main theories regarding the formation of renal calculi. The first theory proposes that there is supersaturation of the urine by stone-forming crystalline constituents. Crystals can act as a nucleus, upon which more crystalline constituents settle and build into a calculus. Depending on where it is formed, in the renal pelvis or ureter, the calculus becomes impacted in a site in the ureter as it passes along with urine toward the urinary bladder.

The second theory proposes that there is a deposition of calcium phosphate, a normal compound from breakdown of bone, onto an area of tubule cell membranes in the renal papilla, an area of kidney that empties into the minor calyx. The calcium phosphate compound collects layers of collagenous material and cellular debris, at which point it is called a Randall plaque, within the subepithelial membrane. The plaque collects layers of crystalline elements, becomes a calculus, and eventually erodes through the urothelium of the renal pelvis to enter the ureter.

The third theory suggests that persons with nephrolithiasis have a deficiency of one or all proteins that inhibit stone formation. The kidney is supposed to secrete three types of stone-inhibitors: nephrocalcin, Tamm-Horsfall mucoprotein, and uropontin.

Regardless of etiology or composition, a renal calculus flows into the ureter, becomes impacted, and causes an obstruction. As the stone travels down the ureter, it scrapes against the ureter's membrane, causing minor bleeding into the urine and intense pain. The ureter spasms around the stone, causing a colicky type of pain. Obstruction of urine can lead to increased pressure within the kidney. Based upon the degree of obstruction, the stone can cause backpressure into the renal pelvis, a condition called hydronephrosis.

Hydronephrosis occurs when edema and distention of the renal pelvis interferes with renal blood flow and function (see Fig. 22-7). Prolonged hydronephrosis causes compression of the kidney tissue, ischemia, and irreversible kidney damage.

Clinical Presentation

Pain is the major symptom of nephrolithiasis. The pain is described as renal or ureteral colic because it occurs in waves. It is also described as acute, excruciating pain in the flank and upper outer quadrant of the abdomen on the affected side, and it is often accompanied by radiating pain into the lower abdomen and groin (see Fig. 22-8). The patient is commonly bent over and cannot find a comfortable position. Pain related to

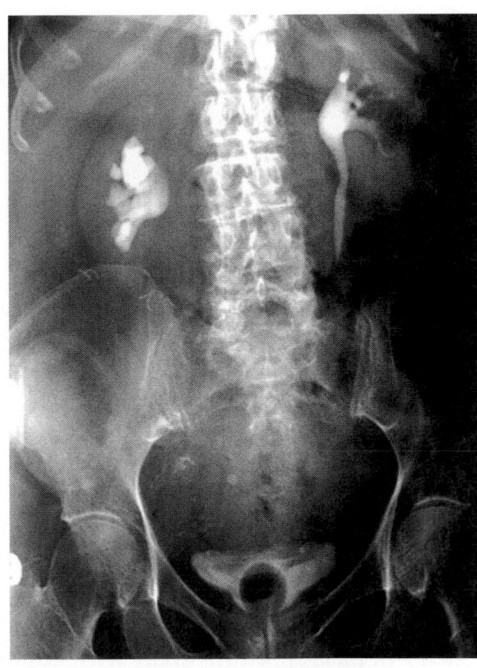

FIGURE 22-7. X-ray showing swelling of the renal pelvis termed hydronephrosis. It can develop in cases of severe obstruction of urine outflow. *(From Living Art Enterprises, LLC/Science Source.)*

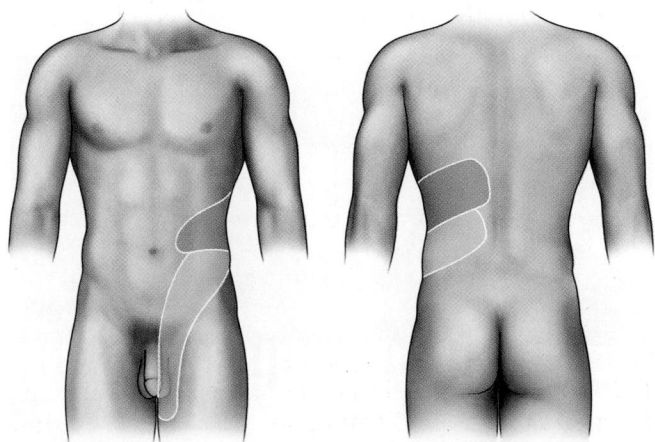

FIGURE 22-8. Pain of nephrolithiasis usually begins in the costovertebral angle region of the back and radiates around into the abdomen and down into the groin.

distention of the renal pelvis and calyx causes a dull, deep ache in the flank or back that may vary in intensity. This type of pain is often associated with increased intake of fluids that distends the calyx. Because of the intensity of the pain, the patient often presents with cool, clammy skin; nausea; and vomiting. Hematuria is often noted because of damage caused by obstruction or movement of the stone.

 CLINICAL CONCEPT

Flank pain with radiation into the groin, hematuria, and crystalluria are classic signs of nephrolithiasis.

Diagnosis

The clinical presentation may be similar with varying types of stones; therefore, a definitive diagnosis requires stone analysis. Kidney stones can vary from the size of the head of a pin to the size of a piece of gravel or larger (see Fig. 22-9). Routine urine analyses are conducted, along with analysis of any stone fragments. Urinalysis provides data related to hematuria, infection, urine pH, and presence of crystals. Additional diagnostic studies that may be indicated include x-rays, intravenous pyelography, abdominal ultrasonography, retrograde urography, and CT scanning.

Treatment

The approach to definitive treatment is based upon symptom management, as well as the type and composition of the renal calculi. Pain relief is a priority because of the excruciating nature of the pain that interferes with activities of daily living. Antibiotics may be necessary if urinary tract infection is present. Most renal stones will pass spontaneously with administration of large amounts of fluid to increase urine volume. Patients are instructed to drink at least 3 liters of fluid a day and strain all urine. If the patient cannot pass the stone, lithotripsy is often used. In lithotripsy, sound waves break up the stone into smaller particles

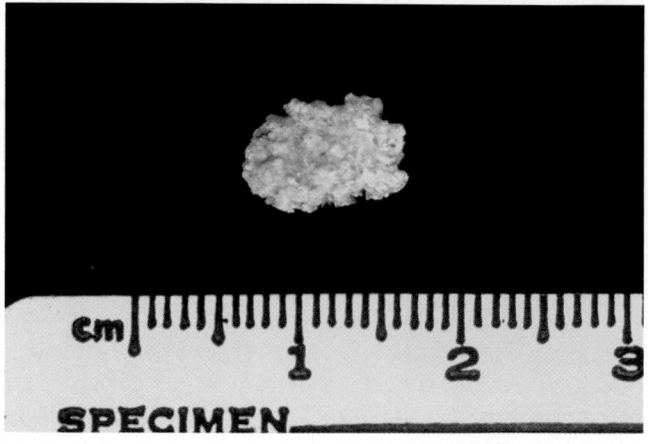

FIGURE 22-9. Kidney stone. *(From Southern Illinois University/Science Source.)*

to facilitate passage. If lithotripsy is unsuccessful, cystoscopic surgery may be necessary.

A major treatment goal in the patient with nephrolithiasis is to prevent recurrence, and this is largely dependent upon determining the stone composition. Dietary changes may be necessary. Alteration of the pH of urine with medications, such as thiazide diuretics or specific types of antibiotics, may be necessary to reduce the risk of stone formation. Calcium phosphate, calcium carbonate, and magnesium phosphate stones develop in alkaline urine; when this occurs, the urine is kept acidic. Uric acid, cystine, and calcium oxalate stones precipitate in acidic urine; in this situation, the urine should be kept alkaline or less acidic than normal. Meat and cranberry juice can keep the pH of urine acidic. A diet rich in citrus fruits, legumes, and vegetables raises the pH and produces urine that is more alkaline.

Complications

Infection is one complication that may develop related to damage to renal tissue and urinary stasis. With a urinary tract infection, there is a risk for pyelonephritis or urosepsis. Although uncommon, with bilateral stones, renal damage caused by scarring from stone formation may lead to acute or chronic renal failure (CRF). Hydronephrosis is a serious complication that occurs because of complete obstruction of urine outflow that causes urine to back up into the renal pelvis and destroy kidney tissue.

Pyelonephritis

Pyelonephritis is an infection of the renal pelvis and interstitium. It can be either acute or chronic, and is most often secondary to bacteria, fungus, or virus.

Epidemiology

Pyelonephritis is a very common infection occurring in more than 250,000 individuals per year in the United States. Approximately 200,000 persons are hospitalized annually for this infection. The incidence is higher in young women, commonly related to lower urinary tract infection. The rate increases in the older male and is attributed to increased incidence of prostatitis. Approximately 20% to 30% of pregnant women develop pyelonephritis.

Etiology

There are numerous causes of pyelonephritis, and many of them are related to an obstruction somewhere in the renal system, also referred to as an obstructive uropathy. Any kind of obstructive uropathy predisposes individuals to urinary tract infection. Whenever there is obstructed outflow of urine, the stagnant urine acts as a medium for bacterial growth, which can ascend into the kidney to cause pyelonephritis.

An anatomic abnormality called vesicoureteral reflux is a common predisposing factor for pyelonephritis.

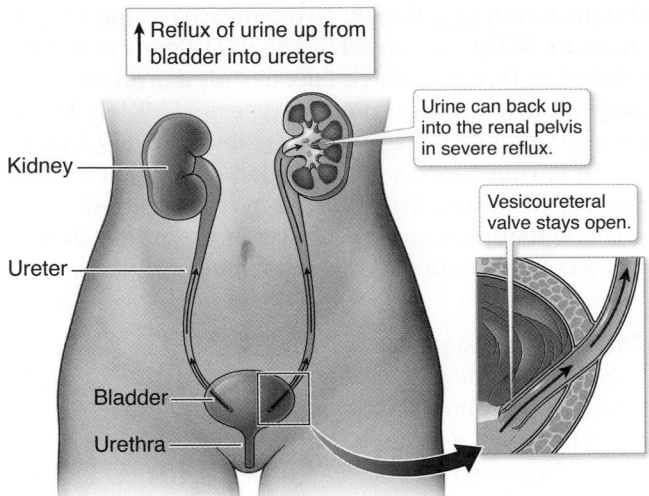

Reflux of urine up from bladder into ureters

Urine can back up into the renal pelvis in severe reflux.

Kidney

Ureter

Vesicoureteral valve stays open.

Bladder

Urethra

FIGURE 22-10. Vesicoureteral reflux (VUR). Urine should flow in one direction—down from the kidneys, through the ureters, to the bladder. VUR is the abnormal flow of urine from the bladder back up into the ureters.

Reflux of urine occurs from the bladder into the ureter. The refluxed urine acts as a medium for bacterial growth, which leads to ascending bacterial infection (see Fig. 22-10). Neurogenic bladder is another condition that predisposes individuals to ascending bacterial infection and pyelonephritis. Neurogenic bladder occurs in patients with conditions such as multiple sclerosis, spinal cord injury, or transection of pelvic parasympathetic nerves. Because of the lack of neurological control of the bladder, there is an inability to completely empty the bladder and urine retention is common. The retained urine acts as a medium for bacterial growth and ascending infection leads to pyelonephritis.

Another risk factor for pyelonephritis is urological instrumentation with catheters or cystoscopes. Instruments can introduce pathogens into the bladder during these procedures. Lastly, pregnancy increases the risk of pyelonephritis, partly because of obstruction by the enlarged uterus and partly because of ureteral relaxation secondary to elevated progesterone levels.

Pathophysiology

The pathophysiology of pyelonephritis varies based upon whether the condition is acute or chronic. With acute pyelonephritis, an inflammatory process develops, usually secondary to infection. Most often the infection ascends from the lower urinary tract and is associated with gram-negative bacteria. Less frequently, the infection is from the bloodstream, and is most often secondary to a staphylococcus aureus infection.

Chronic pyelonephritis occurs because of repeated kidney infection. Because of recurrent infections and inflammatory processes, permanent changes develop in the renal tissue that increase susceptibility to infection. Any deformity, scar, or fibrotic tissue can cause reflux of urine or stagnant urine that leads to growth of microorganisms and an infectious process.

Clinical Presentation

The clinical presentation of acute pyelonephritis includes fever, chills, flank or groin pain, costovertebral angle tenderness, urinary frequency, and dysuria. Flank or costovertebral angle pain can be mild or severe, but the patient usually feels a general malaise. Nausea and vomiting commonly accompany this disorder. Hematuria is present in 30% to 40% of patients. The patient may or may not present with signs of lower urinary tract infection such as dysuria, urgency, and frequency. Symptoms can develop gradually and can be present for weeks before the patient seeks health care. In patients with chronic pyelonephritis, the clinical manifestations may be more subtle; patients present with urinary frequency, dysuria, and flank pain, with HTN possibly accompanying these symptoms. Chronic pyelonephritis may present more insidiously, particularly with unilateral involvement. As renal function declines because of this disorder, polyuria, nocturia, and proteinuria are common.

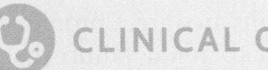

CLINICAL CONCEPT

Costovertebral tenderness, fever, and pyuria are classic signs of pyelonephritis.

Diagnosis

In both acute and chronic processes, urine cultures are important in the diagnosis of pyelonephritis. The most common bacteria that cause acute pyelonephritis is uropathogenic *Escherichia coli*. Others include *Staphylococcus saprophyticus*, *Proteus mirabilis*, and *Klebsiella pneumoniae*. On dipstick urinalysis, almost all patients with acute pyelonephritis have significant pyuria, which is defined as greater than 20 WBCs per high power field [hpf].

A positive leukocyte esterase test is found with presence of WBCs in the urine. The nitrite test can be used for bacteriuria and is usually positive, though it may be falsely negative in the presence of diuretic use, low dietary nitrate, or organisms that do not produce nitrate reductase, such as *Enterococcus, Pseudomonas,* or *Staphylococcus.* Gross hematuria usually does not occur in pyelonephritis and is more common with cystitis, calculi, cancer, glomerulonephritis, tuberculosis, trauma, and vasculitis. Microscopic hematuria may be present in patients with uncomplicated acute pyelonephritis, but other causes also should be considered, particularly calculi. Proteinuria is expected (up to 2 g/day). When it exceeds 3 g/day, glomerulonephritis should be considered.

Imaging studies such as intravenous pyelogram (IVP) are preferably ordered after acute pyelonephritis has resolved. An IVP can be used to identify urinary tract abnormalities that can predispose the patient to infection. CT scan and ultrasound imaging studies may or may not demonstrate findings. CT urography is becoming a useful test that outlines the detailed structure of urological organs. Urological procedures such as cystoscopy can demonstrate bladder and urethral disorders.

In females, pelvic exam should be done to rule out gynecological problems.

Treatment

Acute pyelonephritis is usually treated with 2 weeks of antibiotic therapy based upon identification of the specific microorganism by urine culture. If symptoms recur, repeat urine cultures are recommended at 1 and 4 weeks after completion of the antibiotic regimen. During exacerbations of chronic pyelonephritis, antibiotics are administered. If some type of obstruction is found to be the underlying cause of the recurrent infections, the obstruction must be relieved for cure. Treatment of chronic pyelonephritis includes management of an infectious process and prevention of further renal function deterioration.

Complications

With appropriate treatment of acute pyelonephritis, long-term complications are rare. Chronic renal insufficiency deteriorating to renal failure may develop in the patient with chronic pyelonephritis. It is estimated that 10% to 20% of ESRD is secondary to chronic pyelonephritis.

Polycystic Kidney Disease

Polycystic kidney disease is a genetic disorder that affects the kidneys and other organs. Because of the development of cysts in the renal tissue, renal function is impaired. Cysts also develop in other organs of the body, such as the liver.

Epidemiology

Polycystic kidney disease (PKD) affects approximately 250,000 to 500,000 people in the United States. The most common type is autosomal dominant polycystic kidney disease (ADPKD), one of the most common inherited disorders. It is the most common hereditary cause of renal disease in adults and accounts for 6% to 8% of patients on dialysis in the United States. Almost all people who inherit the ADPKD gene will develop renal cysts by the age of 30 years.

The disease can also be inherited because of a recessive gene; this form is referred to as autosomal recessive polycystic kidney disease (ARPKD). This is a much less common form because both parents must carry the gene in order for an individual to develop the disorder. There is a 5% to 10% incidence of ARPKD with no family history, and this is attributed to a sporadic type of gene mutation. The disease caused by ARPKD is less severe than ADPKD, and the mean age of renal failure in affected patients is 74 years.

Etiology

Autosomal dominant polycystic kidney disease is categorized as either ADPKD 1 or ADPKD 2, depending on the mutation of either of two genes. The majority of cases are ADPKD 1 caused by the PKD 1 gene mutation located at 16p13.3, which encodes for a protein called polycystin 1. The less common type is ADPKD 2, which involves a mutation at 4q21-22 called the PKD 2 gene, which encodes for a protein called polycystin 2. Both polycystin 1 and 2 are involved in renal epithelial cell cycle regulation and intracellular transport of calcium. ADPKD 1 is a more severe disease than ADPKD 2.

Pathophysiology

Polycystic kidney disease leads to formation of fluid-filled cysts in both kidneys. The renal epithelial cell cycle becomes dysfunctional, leading to hyperplasia of renal epithelial cells. The hyperplastic cells cause an outpocketing of the nephron tubule walls, with the formation of cysts that fill with fluid derived from glomerular filtrate. The cystic structures have continual hyperplastic growth and proliferate within the kidney. Glomerular filtrate accumulates in the cysts, and the surrounding normal renal tissue is compressed and damaged. As cysts increase in number and size, the kidneys enlarge. Fibrotic changes occur in the kidneys with time. The cystic structures also develop blood vessels. The blood vessels are extremely fragile and susceptible to rupture, which causes leakage of blood into the cysts. With the entry of blood, the cystic walls stretch, causing excruciating pain. Cysts often rupture into the renal calyces, causing gross hematuria.

Aside from cystic kidneys, patients with PKD are also susceptible to disorders of other organs. Cysts can form in the liver, pancreas, and spleen. Diverticula, which are saccular structures that form in the intestinal wall, often occur in the colon. Heart valve problems such as mitral valve prolapse commonly develop, causing heart murmur. The patient with PKD also has a susceptibility to cerebral aneurysms, which are weak pouches that form in the walls of the cerebral arteries. The cerebral aneurysms often rupture, causing hemorrhagic stroke, which is often fatal. Polycystic kidney disease also increases susceptibility to renal carcinoma.

Clinical Presentation

Patients with PKD usually present with pain caused by the pressure associated with fluid accumulation in the cysts. Because of stagnation of fluid within the cysts, uric acid and calcium crystals can precipitate and renal calculi can develop, which cause obstruction. The patient presents with the pain of renal colic and hematuria in these cases. Stagnation of fluid also increases susceptibility to infection. Costovertebral angle tenderness, fever, and pyuria occur if pyelonephritis develops. In addition, cysts place pressure on kidney blood vessels, which activates the RAAS. In this situation, the patient will present with hypervolemia and HTN. If cerebral aneurysm is present, HTN can trigger a hemorrhagic stroke. The patient with PKD can demonstrate various symptoms, depending on the involvement of other organs, such as the colon, liver, spleen, and pancreas. Thoracic aortic aneurysm is also a common problem in patients with PKD.

Diagnosis

Ultrasonography and abdominal CT scans are used to diagnose PKD. In 80% to 90% of people with PKD, cysts are detectable via CT scanning by the age of 20 years. Magnetic resonance imaging (MRI) is the best diagnostic study that can visualize cysts in the kidneys and extrarenal organs. MRI can also rule out renal carcinoma. Genetic testing can be used to determine the type of disease. Serum chemistry profiles should include calcium and uric acid levels. Urinalysis shows microalbuminuria. Magnetic resonance angiography should be used to investigate the possibility of cerebral aneurysms.

Treatment

Because there is no definitive treatment for management of PKD, treatment is primarily supportive, with the goal to delay disease progression. Control of associated urinary tract infections and HTN are integrated into the treatment plan. Angiotensin-converting enzyme (ACE) inhibitors or angiotensin receptor blockers are commonly used to control blood pressure. Reversing metabolic imbalances associated with ESRD is necessary. Such conditions as hyperkalemia, hypocalcemia, and metabolic acidosis require treatment. Urinary tract infections are common in PKD and antibiotic treatment is needed. Large cysts of the kidney can be surgically decompressed if the patient endures severe pain. Hemodialysis is necessary because of ESRD. Patients are usually eligible for kidney transplant. Development of cysts in the liver, hepatomegaly, and liver failure can occur in PKD. Patients may require liver transplant.

Goodpasture's Syndrome

Goodpasture's syndrome is an immunological disease of the kidney. Some experts refer to the disorder as antiglomerular basement membrane (anti-GBM) disease. The disorder is an acute, rapidly progressive type of glomerulonephritis caused by circulating antibodies. These antibodies are directed against an antigen intrinsic to the glomerular basement membrane.

Epidemiology

Goodpasture's syndrome is an uncommon disorder that affects 1% to 2% of the U.S. population annually. This autoimmune disease affects the kidney and, sometimes, the lungs. It is more common in Caucasians than African Americans. Most commonly, young adults from age 20 to 30 years, as well as older adults aged 60 to 70 years, develop the disease. Among young adults, men are more likely to develop the disease. Among older adults, women are predominantly affected compared with men. From 60% to 80% of patients have clinically apparent manifestations of pulmonary and renal disease, 20% to 40% have renal disease alone, and fewer than 10% have disease that is limited to the lungs.

Etiology

Goodpasture's syndrome is an autoimmune disease of unknown etiology. Autoantibodies are developed against the collagen in glomerular membranes and alveolar membranes. There is a strong genetic predisposition in Goodpasture's syndrome, and persons with the specific tissue type HLA-DR15 are more susceptible than others. Pulmonary involvement is influenced by factors that increase the permeability of the alveolar-capillary membrane. These factors include:

- increased capillary hydrostatic pressure
- high concentrations of inspired oxygen
- bacteremia
- endotoxemia
- exposure to volatile hydrocarbons
- upper respiratory infections
- tobacco smoking
- cocaine inhalation
- exposure to heavy metal dusts.

Pathophysiology

In Goodpasture's syndrome, autoantibodies develop against a specific type of collagen within the glomerular and alveolar membranes and initiate an inflammatory process. Direct immunofluorescence techniques demonstrate linear deposition of immunoglobulins in the glomerular and alveolar membranes. Persons with tissue type HLA-DR2, HLA-DR, and HLA-B7 are at high risk for the disorder in the kidney and lungs. T cells play a key role in the initiation of the disorder. T cells assist B cells to secrete immunoglobulins that attack kidney and lung membranes. Glomerular inflammation causes decreased nephron function. The ability of the kidneys to filter blood and excrete urine is impaired. Autoantibody attacks on alveolar membranes cause diminished gas exchange and inflammatory changes in the lungs.

Clinical Presentation

The patient with Goodpasture's syndrome presents with nonspecific symptoms of malaise, chills, and fever. Along with pulmonary involvement, dyspnea, pleuritic chest pain, cough, and hemoptysis are common initial signs. Massive pulmonary hemorrhage is possible, which is a medical emergency. Renal manifestations include hematuria, edema, high blood pressure, and eventually renal failure. On physical examination, there is tachypnea, tachycardia, cyanosis, pulmonary crackles, and HTN.

Diagnosis

Blood tests are available to determine the presence of antiglomerular basement membrane (anti-GBM) antibodies. Radioimmunoassays or enzyme-linked immunosorbent assays for anti-GBM antibodies should be performed. Positive results should be confirmed by a Western blot test. The titer of anti-GBM antibodies can be used to monitor the severity of disease and efficacy of treatment. Antineutrophilic cytoplasmic antibodies can also develop, and a titer for this antibody is commonly done. Urinalysis demonstrates proteinuria, hematuria, and RBC casts. On the complete blood count, anemia may be observed secondary to pulmonary bleeding. There is leukocytosis, elevated BUN, and serum creatinine. Kidney biopsy may be necessary, but is preferably avoided because the kidney is a highly vascular organ and severe bleeding is common. Chest x-ray shows bilateral hilar lymphadenopathy and consolidations throughout both lung fields. Pulmonary function testing will reveal a restrictive disease pattern.

Treatment

Plasmapheresis is a process of filtering the blood that can remove anti-GBM and other antibodies. Immunosuppressants can be used to stop further production of antibodies. Various pulmonary treatments may be needed, depending on the disorder. Dialysis or kidney transplantation may be indicated if disease deteriorates to ESRD. Anti-GBM disease can occur in the newly transplanted kidney as well.

Acute Kidney Injury

AKI, previously called acute renal failure, is related to an abrupt insult to the kidney that causes a rapid decrease in renal filtration function. Because of this decline in function, there is an accumulation of nitrogenous waste products in the body. With appropriate interventions, normal renal function can return, usually within 2 weeks to 3 months of the initial precipitating event.

Epidemiology

AKI occurs in 5% to 7% of hospitalized patients yearly in the United States. In critical care units, up to 67% of patients have AKI. AKI also develops postoperatively in approximately 1% of general surgery cases.

Etiology

There are various causes of AKI, but the major reason it occurs is because of reduced renal blood flow that, in turn, reduces GFR. As renal function decreases, there is an accumulation of nitrogenous wastes and impairment of fluid and electrolyte balance. AKI is frequently superimposed on other conditions affecting the patient. There are three classifications of AKI:

1. prerenal
2. intrinsic
3. postrenal.

Approximately 60% of patients suffer AKI because of prerenal disorders. Decreased blood flow is the major cause of prerenal AKI and is usually reversible with timely treatment. This type of AKI can occur anytime there is an extreme drop in blood volume. Various shock states, including hypovolemic, cardiogenic, and septic shock, which result in decreased renal perfusion, lead to prerenal AKI. Prolonged renal hypoperfusion will cause damage of the nephron tubule epithelial cells, a condition known as acute tubular necrosis (ATN).

Intrinsic causes of are associated with actual damage to kidney tissue, often associated with nephrotoxic agents, infectious processes, trauma, or obstruction of nephron tubules. A common cause of AKI is ATN caused by nephrotoxic agents. Common nephrotoxic agents include NSAIDs, aminoglycoside antibiotics, and radiopaque dye used in imaging studies. Infectious processes such as glomerulonephritis or pyelonephritis can cause intrinsic AKI. Obstruction of nephron tubules can occur in disorders that cause excretion of a large amount of breakdown products from hemoglobin, myoglobin, or purines. These breakdown products in need of excretion can overwhelm the nephron tubules. For example, hemoglobinuria is seen in transfusion reactions and other hemolytic disorders. Myoglobinuria can occur in severe muscle trauma or extreme exertion. Excessive purines within the bloodstream occur when there is massive tumor or cellular destruction. For example, in chemotherapy, large amounts of cellular deterioration occurs; tumor cell breakdown releases purines, which are DNA breakdown products. These can overwhelm the nephron tubules.

Postrenal AKI develops secondary to obstruction of urine outflow. Obstruction can occur in nephrolithiasis, ureteral stricture, prostatic hyperplasia, or bladder disorders. Approximately 5% of AKI cases are caused by postrenal etiologies.

Pathophysiology

Decreased glomerular filtration of the blood in AKI leads to azotemia, high serum creatinine, and fluid retention. AKI can be divided into four phases:

1. initial
2. oliguria
3. diuresis
4. recovery.

The initial phase usually last hours or days and is determined as the time from the precipitating insult until the time of initial manifestations of AKI. The oliguric phase is associated with a significant decrease in GFR, as well as retention of urea, potassium, sulfate, and creatinine. Urine formation is usually decreased during this time and is accompanied by signs of fluid overload. The nephrons are filled with WBCs and inflammation occurs. In the diuretic phase, the kidneys are beginning to recover from the initial insult. Healing occurs and fibrotic tissue may begin to form in regions of damaged nephrons. The urine output is high; however, it may not be sufficiently concentrated or diluted. Urine may be isosthenuric, which means it has the same osmolarity as the bloodstream. This indicates that the kidney is not excreting urine containing all waste products from the bloodstream. The recovery phase is the time needed for final repair of renal damage, and usually starts with the onset of increased urine output. During this phase, nephrons that are healthy compensate for those nephrons that are damaged. The undamaged nephrons demonstrate hyperfiltration and hypertrophic changes and can perform normal clearance of solutes from the bloodstream. During the recovery phase, urine is appropriately concentrated, inflammation is diminished, and renal function returns to normal. This stage can last months and scar tissue is apparent in regions of kidney damage.

Clinical Presentation

The patient's clinical presentation is influenced by the cause of AKI. For example, AKI caused by autoimmune disease will present with different symptoms than AKI because of renal trauma. However, regardless of etiology, AKI causes oliguria and fluid overload. Nitrogenous waste builds up in the blood and signs and symptoms of uremia occur, such as encephalopathy, anemia, hyperkalemia, metabolic acidosis, thrombocytopenia, and neuromuscular irritability. As urine output decreases, signs of fluid overload occur such as edema of the face and extremities. Pulmonary edema can develop, causing respiratory distress. As renal function returns, the patient demonstrates a diuresis phase, with urine output increasing to 1 to 2 liters per day and resolution of hypervolemia.

Diagnosis

Urinalysis, serum electrolytes, serum creatinine, BUN, arterial blood gases, and complete blood count are used in the diagnosis of AKI. Radiographic imaging may be used to assess for any type of obstructive process or changes in the kidneys' size and structure. A renal biopsy may be used to evaluate for intrarenal etiology of AKI.

Treatment

Treatment of the underlying cause of AKI directs the management plan. With prerenal AKI, fluid administration is indicated. Once the patient develops oliguria, diuretics such as furosemide (Lasix) may be used cautiously. Electrolytes are monitored; with hyperkalemia, cardiac monitoring is necessary. In patients who do not have rapid resolution of the AKI, continuous renal replacement treatment (CRRT) or hemodialysis may be indicated. CRRT is a blood purification process that occurs over 24 hours within a critical care setting, whereas hemodialysis is an intermittent process occurring a few times a week.

Chronic Renal Failure

CRF is an irreversible, progressive disease process. Gradual in onset, the disease may develop over months to years, with 90% to 95% of the nephrons affected. CRF usually progresses to ESRD; as CRF progresses, kidney function deteriorates to the point that the kidney is unable to excrete waste products or control volume status, making dialysis or a kidney transplant the only options to support life.

Epidemiology

Incidence of CRF continues to increase in the United States. This increase is partially explained by the increase in the prevalence of DM and HTN, the two most common causes of chronic kidney disease. It is estimated that almost 8% of adults 20 years old and older have some evidence of CRF based upon a severely reduced GFR. The highest incidence rate of ESRD occurs in older adults. A recent study demonstrated that the prevalence of CRF is 37% among patients older than 70 years. The incidence of CRF is significantly greater in the African American population, which may be attributed to increased HTN in this population. A wide number of genetic mutations have been discovered that correlate with increased predisposition to CRF. Genetic predisposition, secondary illness, lifestyle, and environmental factors all contribute to the development of CRF. Mortality rate for patients with CRF is high; patients with late stage CRF have more than a 75% mortality rate. According to the 2011 U.S. Renal Data System, the life expectancy for healthy 60-year-old individuals is approximately 20 years, whereas the life expectancy of a 60-year-old on hemodialysis is approximately 4 years. Mortality rates for patients over age 65 with ESRD are 6 times greater than the general population.

Etiology

There are numerous causes of CRF, with DM, HTN, glomerulonephritis, and polycystic kidney disease as leading etiologies (see Box 22-2).

BOX 22-2. Causes of Chronic Renal Failure

There are many different etiologies and risk factors for CRF. Many different conditions can lead to CRF. The two most common are DM and HTN.

- Family history of kidney disease
- Age greater than 60 years
- Atherosclerosis
- Bladder obstruction
- Chronic glomerulonephritis
- Congenital kidney disease
- Diabetes
- HTN
- Systemic lupus erythematosus
- Overexposure to some toxins
- Sickle cell disease
- Nephrotoxic medications

Pathophysiology

CRF can have an insidious onset based upon etiology. The rate of nephron deterioration differs according to etiology, and can range from several months to many years. According to the National Kidney Foundation, the progression of CRF usually occurs in five stages:

- Stage 1: kidney damage with normal or increased GFR (greater than 90 mL/min)
- Stage 2: mild reduction in GFR (60 to 89 mL/min)
- Stage 3: moderate reduction in GFR (30 to 59 mL/min)
- Stage 4: severe reduction in GFR (15 to 29 mL/min)
- Stage 5: kidney failure (GFR lower than 15 mL/min).

Glomerular filtration of the bloodstream is accomplished by approximately 1 million nephrons in each kidney. The body has more than double the number of nephrons necessary for maintenance of normal GFR (90 to 120 mL/min); therefore, normal filtration of the blood is possible with only one kidney. The kidney is a resilient organ because of its huge number of nephrons. With mild kidney damage, which occurs in stages 1 and 2, no filtration problems usually occur. The patient is usually asymptomatic and blood and urine tests may appear normal. This occurs because the functioning nephrons compensate for the damaged nephrons. Hyperfiltration and hypertrophy of the functioning nephrons maintain normal kidney function.

In stage 3, there is diminished renal function, and symptoms start to become apparent because fewer than 50% of nephrons are functioning. In this stage, there is moderate reduction in GFR, serum creatinine and BUN begin to rise, and creatinine clearance starts to decrease. The functioning nephrons start to become unable to compensate for the lost nephrons. The damaged nephrons start to undergo fibrosis and glomerulosclerosis is apparent on renal biopsy. In stage 4, a state of renal insufficiency becomes apparent. Nephrons start to become overwhelmed and GFR is lower than 20% of normal. The kidney's health is precarious in this stage. The patient must restrict dietary protein because remaining healthy nephrons have difficulty removing nitrogenous wastes from the bloodstream. Finally, in stage 5, renal failure develops and GFR falls to lower than 5% of normal. At this stage, nephrons cannot accomplish complete filtration of the bloodstream. The kidney's varied function, such as erythropoietin synthesis, blood pressure maintenance, and acid-base balance, are lost. As a consequence, fluid, electrolyte, and acid-base imbalances occur and effects on other organ systems become apparent. ESRD occurs with widespread effects of uremia. The term "uremia" actually means urine in the bloodstream. The kidneys deteriorate in function and begin to atrophy. Dialysis and renal transplant are the only options for survival.

Clinical Presentation

In CRF, accumulation of nitrogenous wastes causes systemwide symptoms. The brain cannot function in a high nitrogenous environment and encephalopathy occurs—confusion, disorientation, or stupor and coma. Platelets and RBCs lyse because of the blood's high nitrogen content, resulting in thrombocytopenia and anemia. Thrombocytopenia causes bruising and spontaneous bleeding, whereas anemia causes severe fatigue, weakness, and dyspnea. Metabolic acidosis and electrolyte imbalances have varying effects. Hyperkalemia can cause life-threatening cardiac dysrhythmias and extreme muscle weakness. Because the kidneys cannot activate vitamin D, calcium absorption from the gastrointestinal tract decreases, causing hypocalcemia, which in turn can cause neuromuscular irritability, tetany, and seizures. Hypocalcemia also stimulates the parathyroid glands to release parathyroid hormone (PTH), which causes bone breakdown. This bone demineralization process is referred to as **renal osteodystrophy.** Bone mineral density is diminished and fracture susceptibility increases.

Diagnosis

A CBC with differential, serum electrolytes, serum creatinine, total albumin, BUN, and urinalysis will demonstrate abnormalities of renal failure. Normochromic normocytic anemia is seen in chronic kidney disease caused by lack of erythropoietin. Sodium, potassium, bicarbonate, and other electrolytes will be elevated in the bloodstream. Hyperkalemia may cause cardiac dysrhythmias, requiring ECG monitoring. BUN and creatinine levels will be elevated because all nitrogenous wastes are accumulating in the bloodstream. When 50% of nephrons are dysfunctional, serum creatinine rises to approximately double the normal blood level. Patients will have hypoalbuminemia caused by glomerular damage, which causes loss of protein. Proteinuria is a classic sign of renal dysfunction. Serum calcium, vitamin D, and PTH levels will be abnormal. Hyperphosphatemia occurs because of hypocalcemia. Renal ultrasound and other imaging studies may be indicated. Other more disease-specific blood tests may be done according to etiology of renal failure.

Urinalysis will likely show protein, RBCs, and WBCs, as these will all be lost in the urine. A 24-hour urine collection for protein and creatinine clearance will show excessive loss of protein. However, a single urine specimen can be used to calculate the protein-to-creatinine ratio, which allows reliable approximation of total 24-hour urinary protein excretion. The calculation usually shows protein loss greater than 2 grams in the urine.

Noninvasive renal imaging studies such as x-ray, ultrasound, CT, and MRI can show any intrarenal masses, cysts, or calcium stones. Intravenous contrast-enhanced studies should be avoided in renal failure.

Treatment

Fluid and electrolyte management are critical to the management of patients with CRF. Blood pressure management and erythropoietin-stimulating medications are usually administered. Hyperphosphatemia can be treated with dietary phosphate binders and dietary phosphate restriction. Hypocalcemia can be treated with calcium supplements that contain vitamin D. Hypervolemia can be reduced using diuretics. Metabolic acidosis can be reversed with bicarbonate administration. Once the GFR is lower than 10 to 20 mL/min (normal 90 to 120 mL/min), dialysis is initiated, and the patient will be evaluated for a kidney transplant.

Complications

In ESRD, there are bodywide adverse effects (see Fig. 22-11). As the disease progresses and other systems are involved, the patient may develop respiratory compromise related to fluid overload, HTN, and uremic coma. Without definitive treatment, usually dialysis or transplantation, death will occur.

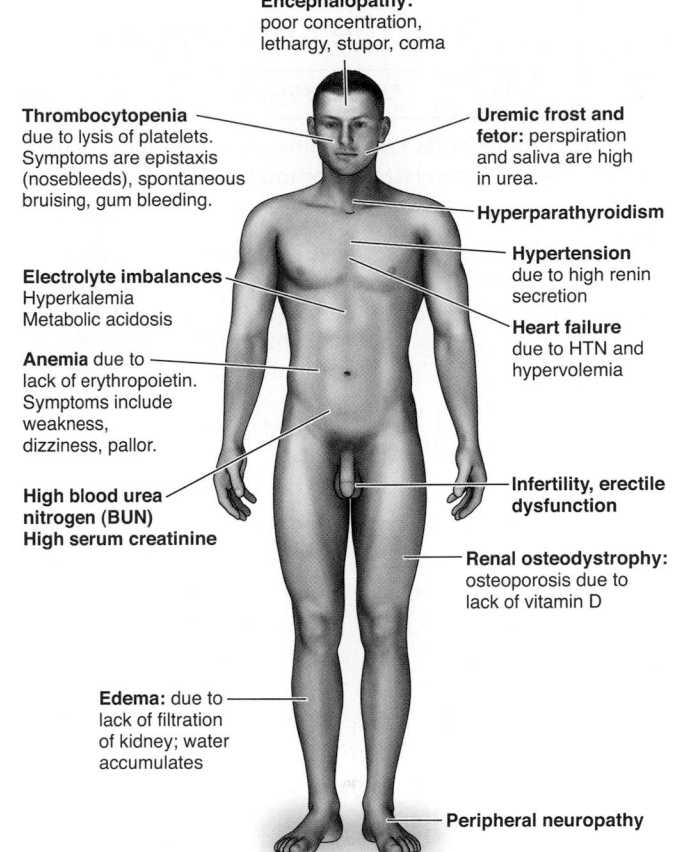

Encephalopathy: poor concentration, lethargy, stupor, coma

Thrombocytopenia due to lysis of platelets. Symptoms are epistaxis (nosebleeds), spontaneous bruising, gum bleeding.

Uremic frost and fetor: perspiration and saliva are high in urea.

Hyperparathyroidism

Hypertension due to high renin secretion

Electrolyte imbalances Hyperkalemia Metabolic acidosis

Heart failure due to HTN and hypervolemia

Anemia due to lack of erythropoietin. Symptoms include weakness, dizziness, pallor.

High blood urea nitrogen (BUN) High serum creatinine

Infertility, erectile dysfunction

Renal osteodystrophy: osteoporosis due to lack of vitamin D

Edema: due to lack of filtration of kidney; water accumulates

Peripheral neuropathy

FIGURE 22-11. Widespread complications of ESRD.

Chapter Summary

- Between 1980 and 2009, the prevalence rate of ESRD has increased 600%. The majority of these persons are over age 60—and with the aging of the population, the incidence of renal disorders is expected to increase.

- African Americans have the greatest incidence of kidney disease.

- The renal blood filtered per unit of time is known as the GFR.

- With age, GFR decreases; this raises the risk of medication toxicity.

- Kidney dysfunction is divided into three categories based upon the mechanism of injury: prerenal dysfunction, intrinsic renal dysfunction, and postrenal dysfunction.

- Postrenal dysfunction can lead to hydronephrosis; swelling of the renal pelvis, and compression of nephrons.

- ATN occurs when there is ischemia of the kidney. It is the most common cause of AKI.

- Azotemia is the increased amount of urea in the blood.

- Serum creatinine is used to indicate kidney function.

- Oliguria is fewer than 400 mL of urine output per day.

- In acute glomerulonephritis, an immunological reaction triggers inflammation that damages the membranes of the glomerulus.

- Nephrotic syndrome is caused by glomerular injury and causes hypoalbuminemia, edema, and proteinuria.

- Pyelonephritis is an infection of the kidney that causes fever, chills, and costovertebral angle tenderness.

- Nephrolithiasis causes colicky pain in the back, which radiates to the groin, hematuria, and crystalluria.

- The most common type of kidney stone is made of calcium oxalate.

- Hydronephrosis is the swelling of the renal pelvis that can occur with obstructive uropathy.

- AKI is most often caused by ischemia of the kidney, which is reversible.

- CRF causes widespread systemic symptoms such as anemia, HTN, metabolic acidosis, hyperkalemia, azotemia, hypocalcemia, and hyperphosphatemia.

- ESRD occurs when there is 5% to 10% nephron function.

Making the Connections

Pathophysiology	Signs and Symptoms	Assessment Findings	Diagnostic Tests	Treatment

Glomerulonephritis | Most commonly caused by group A beta-hemolytic streptococcal (GABHS) antibodies that develop against the antigen (strep); for unknown reasons, antibodies attack glomerular membranes (molecular mimicry theory). Other theory asserts that antigen-antibody complexes develop and deposit in glomerular membranes, causing inflammation.

	Back pain (costovertebral angle tenderness). Edema (commonly periorbital). Fever. Cola-colored urine. Malaise.	HTN. Proteinuria. Hematuria. Edema (periorbital region common).	Elevated serum creatinine and elevated BUN is caused by kidney dysfunction. Urinalysis shows a large amount of protein and blood. Urine is dilute because the kidney is not concentrating urine. Urine 24-hour creatinine clearance is low because creatinine is not being filtered by dysfunctional kidneys. Streptolysin antibody titer demonstrates antibodies are present against GABHS. Cryoglobulin titer indicates antigen-antibody complexes are present. Complement in the blood is low and is depleted because immune reaction uses up complement.	Antibiotics, antipyretics, and analgesics are needed. With systematic manifestations such as edema and elevated blood pressure, diuretics and antihypertensive agents may be indicated. Dietary restrictions of sodium and protein are also advised. Plasmapheresis may be used to rid the blood of antiglomerular antibodies. Immunosuppressants are also used in the treatment.

Nephrotic Syndrome | Any disorder that causes glomerular injury. When glomeruli are injured, they become extrapermeable and allow proteins to filter out of blood. Albumin leaves the blood and is excreted in the urine called proteinuria or albuminuria. Hypoalbuminemia causes edema. Glomerulonephritis caused by infection or immunological inflammatory disease are causes of nephrotic syndrome.

	Edema, especially of periorbital region and face.	Edema of the face is common, especially in the periorbital region. HTN. With severe albumin loss, edema of lower extremities, pleural effusion, and ascites can develop.	Albuminuria. Hypoalbuminemia. Hematuria. Hyperlipidemia. Hypertriglyceridemia. Elevated serum creatinine and BUN. 24-hour urine collection shows greater than 3 grams of protein /dL. Antinuclear antibodies may be positive if etiology is an autoimmune disease.	Diet low in sodium. Adequate protein and fluid. Diuretics, anti-inflammatory agents, and immunosuppressants may be necessary.

Continued

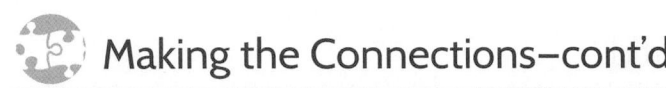 Making the Connections–cont'd

Pathophysiology	Signs and Symptoms	Assessment Findings	Diagnostic Tests	Treatment
Nephrolithiasis | The formation of calculi in the kidney, which can cause obstructive uropathy. Calculi are commonly composed of calcium.				
	Severe back pain with radiation into the groin. Severe abdominal pain. Chills.	Costovertebral angle tenderness. Hematuria. Crystalluria.	Blood may show high calcium, uric acid, or purines, depending on the etiology of nephrolithiasis. Elevated blood pressure and tachycardia are caused by pain. Urinalysis shows RBCs and crystals. Intravenous pyelogram, retrograde urography, abdominal x-ray, CT, or ultrasound can show calculi.	Intravenous fluid. Analgesics. Strain urine. Increase oral fluid intake greater than 3 liters/day. Lithotripsy. Cystoscopic surgery.
Pyelonephritis | Infection of the upper urinary tract, commonly caused by an ascending lower urinary tract infection.				
	Back pain. Fever. Malaise. Chills. Dysuria. Frequency.	Costovertebral angle tenderness. Fever.	Elevated WBC count. Microscopic hematuria. Pyuria. Bacteruria. Proteinuria.	Antibiotics.
Polycystic Renal Disease | Disease causing multiple cysts in the kidneys and dysfunction caused by genetic mutation at 16p13 and 4q21-22.				
	Back pain. Fever (if infection).	Costovertebral angle tenderness, if infection. Hematuria.	Hematuria. Crystalluria. Bacteruria. Ultrasound or CT scan can show cysts within kidneys.	Supportive treatment of symptoms. Hemodialysis. Renal transplant.
Goodpasture's Syndrome | An autoimmune disease where the kidney nephrons and pulmonary alveolar membranes are attacked as an antigen.				
	Malaise, chills, fever, dyspnea, pleuritic chest pain, cough, and hemoptysis. Massive pulmonary hemorrhage possible.	Renal manifestations include hematuria, edema, and high blood pressure. Pulmonary symptoms include tachypnea, cyanosis, and pulmonary crackles.	Elevated serum creatinine, BUN, WBC count. Antiglomerular basement membrane antibody titer (immunoassay and Western blot). Antineutrophilic cytoplasmic antibody titer. Chest x-ray shows bilateral hilar lymphadenopathy and diffuse consolidations. Urinalysis shows hematuria, proteinuria, and RBC casts.	Immunosupressants. Plasmapheresis. Dialysis. Renal transplant.

Continued

Making the Connections—cont'd

Pathophysiology	Signs and Symptoms	Assessment Findings	Diagnostic Tests	Treatment
			Pulmonary function test reveals restrictive disease.	

Acute Kidney Injury (AKI) | Reversible failure of the kidneys caused by prerenal, intrarenal, or postrenal disorders. Prerenal AKI is most commonly renal ischemia caused by decreased blood volume. Intrarenal AKI is most commonly caused by nephrotoxic drugs, immune disorder, or infection. Postrenal AKI is most commonly caused by obstructive uropathy as with nephrolithiasis or prostate hyperplasia.

Pathophysiology	Signs and Symptoms	Assessment Findings	Diagnostic Tests	Treatment
	Edema of the face and extremities. Lack of urine output initially. Dyspnea if pulmonary edema present. Confusion, sleepiness, stupor, or coma if nitrogenous wastes are high. Easy bruising if thrombocytopenia develops. Fatigue, weakness, palpitations if anemia present. Muscle spasms possible if hypocalcemia present.	Oliguria. Fluid overload. Edema in the face and extremities. Pulmonary edema can develop, causing respiratory distress. Hypervolemia leads to HTN. Signs of uremia can develop such as encephalopathy, hyperkalemia, metabolic acidosis, thrombocytopenia, and neuromuscular irritability. As renal function returns, the patient demonstrates a diuresis phase, with urine output increasing to 1 to 2 liters per day and resolution of hypervolemia.	Urinalysis, serum electrolytes, serum creatinine, BUN, arterial blood gases, and CBC. Radiographic imaging may be used to assess for any type of obstructive process or changes in size and structure of the kidneys. Renal biopsy may be used to evaluate for intrarenal etiology.	Diuretics. Cardiac monitor. Hemodialysis or CRRT in unstable patients.

Chronic Renal Failure | Deterioration of 90% to 95% of nephrons. ESRD. Kidneys cannot filter nitrogenous wastes nor excrete fluid.

Pathophysiology	Signs and Symptoms	Assessment Findings	Diagnostic Tests	Treatment
	Confusion, stupor, or coma caused by high nitrogenous wastes affecting brain. Bruising caused by thrombocytopenia. Fatigue and dyspnea on exertion caused by anemia. Edema caused by fluid overload. Lack of urine output. Muscle spasms or seizures caused by hypocalcemia. Amenorrhea, male and female infertility caused by lack of excretion of sex hormones. Sex hormones negatively feed back to organs.	High blood pressure. Oliguria. Edema. Pallor. Dyspnea. Muscle spasms or seizure.	Hyperkalemia. Hypoalbuminemia. Hyperphosphatemia. Hypocalcemia. Urinalysis shows proteinuria, RBCs, and WBCs. Elevated serum creatinine and BUN. Arterial blood gases show metabolic acidosis. Complete blood count shows anemia. Ultrasound, x-ray, CT, magnetic resonance imaging can show kidney size, masses, stones, or cysts. A renal biopsy may be used to evaluate for intrarenal etiology.	Hemodialysis. Renal transplant.

Bibliography

Abbasi, M., Chertow, G., & Hall, Y. (2010). End-stage renal disease. *Am Fam Phys*, 82(12), 1512–1515.

Barrett, K. E., Barman, S. M., Boitano, S., & Brooks, H. L. (2010). *Ganong's review of medical physiology*. 23rd ed. New York: McGraw-Hill/ Lange Medical Series.

Baumgarten, M., & Gehr, T. (2011). Chronic kidney disease: detection and evaluation. *Am Fam Phys*, 84(10), 1138–1148.

Bellomo, R., Kellum, J. A., & Ronco, C. (2012). Acute kidney injury. *Lancet*, 380(9843), 756–766.

Chandrashekar, K. B., Fulop, T., & Juncos, L. A. (2012). Medical management and prevention of nephrolithiasis. *Am J Med*, 125(4), 344–347.

Choudhury, D. (2010). Acute kidney injury: current perspectives. *Postgrad Med*, 122(6), 29–40.

Colgan, R., Williams, M., & Johnson, J. R. (2011). Diagnosis and treatment of acute pyelonephritis in women. *Am Fam Phys*, 84(5), 519–526.

Coritsidis, G. N., Linden, E., & Stern, A. S. (2011). The role of the primary care physician in managing early stages of chronic kidney disease. *Postgrad Med*, 123(5), 177–185.

Coyne, D. W. (2014). Anemia in chronic kidney disease: treating the numbers, not the patients. *JAMA Intern Med*, Mar 3. doi: 10.1001/jamainternmed.2013.13305.

de Boer, I. H. (2012). Chronic kidney disease—a challenge for all ages. *JAMA*, 308(22), 2401–2402.

FHN Trial Group, Chertow, G. M., Levin, N. W., Beck, G. J., et al. (2010). In-center hemodialysis six times per week versus three times per week. *N Engl J Med*, 363(24), 2287–2300.

Frassetto, L., & Kohlstadt, I. (2011). Treatment and prevention of kidney stones: an update. *Am Fam Phys*, 84(11), 1234–1242.

Hall, P. M. (2009). Nephrolithiasis: treatment, causes, and prevention. *Cleveland Clin J Med*, 76(10), 583–591.

Hallan, S. I., Matsushita, K., Sang, Y., et al. (2012). Age and association of kidney measures with mortality and end-stage renal disease. *JAMA*, 308(22), 2349–2360.

Himmelfarb, J., & Ikizler, T. A. (2010). Hemodialysis. *N Engl J Med*, 363(19), 1833–1845.

Hsu, T. W., Liu, J. S., Hung, S. C., et al. (2014). Renoprotective effect of renin-angiotensin-aldosterone system blockade in patients with predialysis advanced chronic kidney disease, hypertension, and anemia. *JAMA Intern Med*, 174(3), 347–354.

Kellum, J. A., Bellomo, R., & Ronco, C. (2012). Kidney attack. *JAMA*, 307(21), 2265–2266. doi: 10.1001/jama.2012.4315.

Kodner, C. (2009). Nephrotic syndrome in adults: diagnosis and management. *Am Fam Phys*, 80(10), 1129–1134.

Kucirka, L. M., Grams, M. E., Lessler, J., et al. (2011). Association of race and age with survival among patients undergoing dialysis. *JAMA*, 306(6), 620–626. doi: 10.1001/jama.2011.1127.

Kurella Tamura, M., & Winkelmayer, W. C. (2012). Treated and untreated kidney failure in older adults: what's the right balance? *JAMA*, 307(23), 2545–2548.

Lameire, N. H., Bagga, A., Cruz, D., et al. (2013). Acute kidney injury: an increasing global concern. *Lancet*, 382(9887), 170–179.

Longo, D. L., Fauci, A. S., Kasper, D. L., et al. (Eds.). (2011). *Harrison's principles of internal medicine*. 18th ed. New York: McGraw-Hill.

Mitka, M. (2013). Nephrologists question ACP's kidney disease guidelines. *JAMA*, 310(22), 2387–2388. doi: 10.1001/jama.2013.282671.

Nicolle, L. E. (2012). Minimum antimicrobial treatment for acute pyelonephritis. *Lancet*, Jun 20. Epub ahead of print.

O'Connor, N. R., & Corcoran, A. M. (2012). End-stage renal disease: symptom management and advance care planning. *Am Fam Phys*, 85(7), 705–710.

Park, M., & Hsu, C. Y. (2014). An ACE in the hole for patients with advanced chronic kidney disease? *JAMA Intern Med*, 174(3), 355–356. doi: 10.1001/jamainternmed.2013.12176.

Parker, B. D., & Ix, J. H. (2009). Renal disease. In S. J. McPhee & J. Hammer, *Pathophysiology of disease* (6th ed.). New York: Lange Medical Books/ McGraw-Hill Medical Publishing Division.

Pearle, M. S. (2012). Shock-wave lithotripsy for renal calculi. *N Engl J Med*, 367(1), 50–57. doi: 10.1056/NEJMct1103074.

Rahman, M., Shad, F., & Smith, M. C. (2012). Acute kidney injury: a guide to diagnosis and management. *Am Fam Phys*, 86(7), 631–639.

Rajaian, S., & Kekre, N. S. (2009). Images in clinical medicine. Staghorn calculus. *N Engl J Med*, 361(15), 1486. doi: 10.1056/NEJMicm0805190.

Rivera, J. A., O'Hare, A. M., & Harper, G. M. (2012). Update on the management of chronic kidney disease. *Am Fam Phys*, 86(8), 749–754.

Roumelioti, M. E., & Unruh, M. (2014). Update in nephrology: evidence published in 2013. *Ann Intern Med*, Apr 10. doi: 10.7326/M14-0263. Epub ahead of print.

Salant, D. J. (2010). Goodpasture's disease—new secrets revealed. *N Engl J Med*, 363(4), 388–391.

Sethi, S., & Fervenza, F. C. (2012). Membranoproliferative glomerulonephritis—a new look at an old entity. *N Engl J Med*, 366(12), 1119–1131.

Sharp, V. J., Barnes, K. T., & Erickson, B. A. (2013). Assessment of asymptomatic microscopic hematuria in adults. *Am Fam Phys*, 88(11), 747–754.

Tanner, G. A. (2009). Kidney function. In R. A. Rhoades & D. R. Bell, *Medical physiology: principles for clinical medicine*. Philadelphia, PA: Walters Kluwer/Lippincott Williams & Wilkins.

Thomas, L. D., Elinder, C. G., Tiselius, H. G., Wolk, A., & Akesson, A. (2013). Ascorbic acid supplements and kidney stone incidence among men: a prospective study. *JAMA Intern Med*, 173(5), 386–338. doi: 10.1001/jamainternmed.2013.2296.

Thorsteinsdottir, B., Swetz, K. M., Feely, M. A., Mueller, P. S., & Williams, A. W. (2012). Are there alternatives to hemodialysis for the elderly patient with end-stage renal failure? *Mayo Clin Proceed*, 87(6), 514–516.

United States Renal Data System. (2012). 2011 Annual data report. Retrieved from http://www.usrds.org/adr.aspx

Watnick, S., & Morrison, G. (2010). Kidney disease. In S. J. McPhee & M. A. Papadakis, *2010 Current medical diagnosis & treatment*. New York: Lange Medical Books/ McGraw-Hill Medical Publishing Division.

Worcester, E. M., & Coe, F. L. (2010). Clinical practice. Calcium kidney stones. *N Engl J Med*, 363(10), 954–963. doi: 10.1056/NEJMcp1001011.

bibliography

Urological Disorders

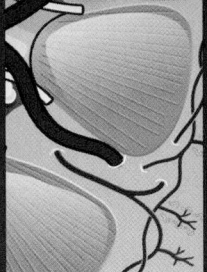

Key Terms

Hydronephrosis

Hydroureter

Interstitial cystitis (IC)

Micturition reflex

Obstructive uropathy

Oliguria

Proteinuria

Pyelonephritis

Urinary casts

Urolithiasis

Urosepsis

Urological disorders are those pathophysiologic conditions that affect the lower urinary tract, specifically the ureters, bladder, and urethra. In males, the prostate is also considered part of the urological system. Normal urological function is integral to healthy renal function. Healthy kidneys require the free, unencumbered flow of urine out of the body—**obstructive uropathy** refers to any condition that blocks such free flow of urine from the body. A severe obstructive uropathy can cause backflow of urine into the kidney, which leads to hydronephrosis, a condition that potentially causes kidney failure. Early recognition and treatment of urological disorders are keys to preventing renal dysfunction.

Epidemiology

Lower urinary tract infection (UTI) is the most common urological disorder. Approximately 6 million visits to primary care clinicians each year is for UTI. Lower UTI, also referred to as cystitis, is a very common condition in women. Up to 40% of women in the United States aged 20 to 40 years have endured a lower UTI. Young adult women, particularly those in the childbearing years, are 30 times more likely to suffer a lower UTI compared with young adult men. Although lower UTI is a frequent condition among women, it is rare in males. The incidence of UTI in males is approximately 5 to 8 per 10,000 population in the United States. A lower UTI in a young adult male should prompt the clinician to investigate the urological system further.

Another common urological problem is urinary obstruction. The most common causes of urinary obstruction are **urolithiasis** and benign prostatic hyperplasia (BPH). Both of these conditions are more common in males. The lifetime prevalence of urolithiasis is approximately 12% for men and 7% for women in the United States. BPH occurs in up to 14 million men per year; the majority are older than age 50.

Basic Concepts of Urological Function

The nephron, the basic unit of the kidney, acts to filter the blood at the glomerulus, reabsorb water at the tubules, secrete urea into the tubule fluid, reabsorb water at the collecting duct, and form a concentrated urine that passes out into the renal pelvis and ureter. Normal urine production in an adult depends on hydration. Adequate hydration is essential for optimal kidney function. The kidney needs to excrete at least 400 mL of urine per day to rid the body of wastes; any amount less than 400 mL per day is termed **oliguria.**

Adequate urine volume and unimpeded urine outflow from the body are essential for kidney health. Urine outflow depends on adequate pressure from the glomerulus into the nephron tubules, peristalsis of the ureters, and the effects of gravity. Adequate hydration enhances the volume of the blood filtered at the glomerular capillaries; this, in turn, increases flow of tubule fluid through the nephrons. Ureteral peristalsis moves urine from the renal pelvis down into the urinary bladder, where it is collected before urination (also called micturition). Passing urine, emptying the bladder, and urination involve involuntary and voluntary neuromuscular control of the structures in the lower urinary tract (see Fig. 23-1).

Neuromuscular Control of the Bladder

The detrusor muscle is the major muscle of the bladder; its fibers are arranged in spiral, longitudinal, and circular layers. This arrangement of muscle fibers allows the bladder to expand as it fills and to expel urine when it contracts. The sympathetic (adrenergic) and parasympathetic (cholinergic) autonomic nerves innervate the detrusor muscle. Sympathetic nerves, specifically alpha-adrenergic fibers, relax the detrusor muscle while they tighten the internal sphincter of the bladder neck; these actions allow filling of the bladder. The

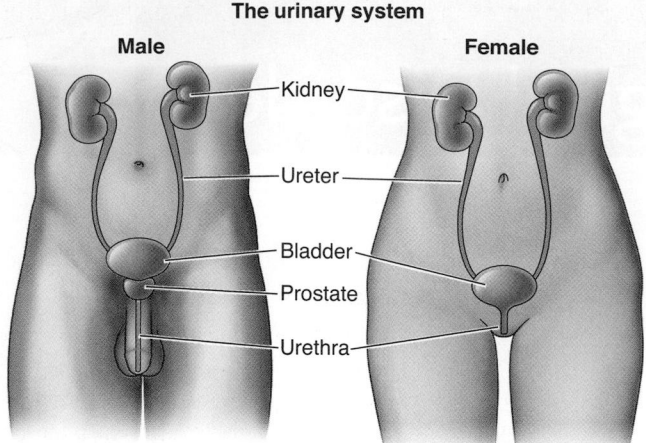

The urinary system

Male   Female

- Kidney
- Ureter
- Bladder
- Prostate
- Urethra

FIGURE 23-1. The anatomy of the urological system.

stretching of the bladder signals the parasympathetic nervous system to contract the detrusor muscle and relax the internal sphincter, actions that enable the bladder to expel urine through the urethra. The urethral sphincter, a voluntarily controlled muscle, has to be relaxed for urine to exit the bladder. Urination is both autonomically and voluntarily controlled.

The urinary bladder usually holds 300 to 400 mL of urine. As urine accumulates, the wall of the bladder thins as it stretches, allowing the bladder to contain increasing amounts of urine without a significant rise in interior pressure. The urge to urinate usually starts when the stretched bladder reaches approximately 25% of its volume. When the amount of urine reaches 100% of the urinary bladder's capacity, the voluntary external urethral sphincter cannot remain closed and urine is expelled.

The Micturition Reflex

Micturition is a term that is synonymous with urination. The **micturition reflex,** which is a reflex involving the spinal cord and cortex of the brain, controls voiding. It involves nerve impulses traveling from the urinary bladder to the spinal cord and impulses passing from the spinal cord to the bladder. Neurons in the spinal cord coordinate this reflex, but the cerebral cortex can override it, thereby enabling conscious control of micturition. When the bladder wall stretches to accommodate the increasing volume of urine, the parasympathetic nerves in the reflex arc respond by stimulating the detrusor muscle in the bladder wall to contract. At the same time, the spinal cord sends nerve impulses up to the cerebral cortex, thereby allowing a conscious decision about whether it is appropriate to void. If voiding is not appropriate, the cerebral cortex initiates impulses that travel back down the spinal cord to inhibit the reflex arc, thereby preventing micturition. These impulses play a significant role in inhibiting micturition by keeping the external urinary sphincter contracted. When micturition is appropriate, impulses from the cerebral cortex stimulate the micturition reflex. The spinal cord nerves allow the external urinary sphincter to relax, thereby allowing urine to be expelled through the urethra.

Basic Pathophysiologic Concepts of Urological Function

In order to understand the pathophysiology of urological disorders, certain terminology and urinary functions need to be described.

Obstructive Uropathy

Obstruction is one of the most common pathophysiologic problems that occur in the urinary tract. Renal calculi, also known as kidney stones, are the most common cause of urinary obstruction in young and middle-aged men. After age 60 years, urinary obstruction is most common in men secondary to benign prostatic hyperplasia (BPH). In young and middle-aged women, kidney stones, gynecological surgery, pregnancy, and cancers of pelvic organs are important etiologies of obstruction.

Obstruction of the urinary tract at any level eventually results in elevation of intraluminal ureteral pressure. With prolonged obstruction, ureteral peristalsis is overcome and increased hydrostatic pressures are transmitted directly to the nephron tubules. As pressures in the proximal tubule and Bowman space increase, glomerular filtration rate (GFR) decreases. After 12 to 24 hours, if complete obstruction is not relieved, a depressed GFR is maintained and there is a decrease in renal blood flow. With continued obstruction, renal blood flow progressively falls, resulting in ischemia and incremental nephron loss. Obstructive uropathy can lead to obstruction of urine at the kidney, backup of urine into the kidney, and kidney failure. Recovery of GFR depends on the duration and level of obstruction, preobstruction blood flow, and coexisting medical illness or infection.

Hydronephrosis and Hydroureter

Hydronephrosis is the distention of the renal calyces and pelvis as a result of obstruction of the outflow of urine distal to the renal pelvis, whereas **hydroureter** is the dilation of the ureter caused by obstruction. Hydronephrosis can cause kidney tissue damage; microscopic changes consist of dilation of the nephron tubules and flattening of the tubular epithelium. The renal calyces become enlarged and edematous. In children, the major causes of obstructed urine flow are anatomic abnormalities such as vesicoureteral reflux, urethral stricture, or stenosis. In comparison, calculi are the most common cause of obstruction in young adults, whereas BPH or pelvic neoplasms are primary causes in older patients.

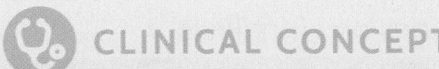

CLINICAL CONCEPT

Acute hydronephrosis is a short-term condition and, when corrected, allows full recovery of renal function. Chronic hydronephrosis, however, is a situation in which the loss of function is irreversible even with correction of the obstruction.

Assessment

A complete history regarding the patient's present illness, past illnesses and surgeries, current medications, allergies, environmental exposures, and family history is necessary. The patient's daily diet, exercise routine, and occupation should also be noted. If a urological problem is suspected, the clinician should focus on symptoms concerning the patient's urinary frequency; pain quality, location, and duration; urine control; nocturia; and the color and amount of urine per day.

Signs and Symptoms

Disorders of urological function present with similar signs and symptoms, including dysuria, frequency, urgency, and hesitancy. Table 23-1 provides a description and common causes of these signs and symptoms.

Diagnosis

The diagnostic studies used to investigate urological conditions include macroscopic or dipstick urinalysis, microscopic urinalysis, urine culture and sensitivity, serum electrolytes, and complete blood count (CBC) with differential. Specific procedures such as cystoscopy, intravenous pyelography (IVP), and urodynamic testing are used when diseases such as bladder cancer, urolithiasis, or **interstitial cystitis (IC)** are suspected.

Urinalysis
In addition to history and physical examination, a urinalysis is needed if a urological disorder is suspected. Proper collection of the urine is necessary to decrease the possible contaminants that could alter the results. A clean-catch midstream urine specimen is used for macroscopic and microscopic urinalysis. A macroscopic

observation of the urine refers to that which is visible with the naked eye.

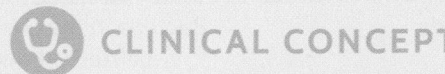

CLINICAL CONCEPT

A clean-catch midstream urine specimen limits the number of contaminants; it is not a sterile specimen.

The physical appearance of the urine is inspected, and a dipstick test is performed on the specimen. The examiner notes the amount, color, clarity, and cloudiness of the urine, as well as any other visible characteristics, such as the presence of blood or sediments. Abnormalities in color, clarity, and cloudiness may suggest conditions such as dehydration, infection, liver disease, protein loss, or muscle breakdown (rhabdomyolysis). Medications can change the color of urine. A quick analysis can be accomplished using a chemical-coated dipstick on the urine sample. The dipstick can grossly detect glucose, ketones, blood, bilirubin, protein, leukocyte esterase, and nitrites. A microscopic laboratory analysis of urine is more accurate than the dipstick method. Table 23-2 lists the constituents of a laboratory urinalysis.

Urine Culture and Sensitivity
A urine culture reveals whether or not bacteria is growing in the urine. For clean-catch samples that have been properly collected, cultures with greater than 100,000 colony-forming units (CFU)/mL of one type of bacteria usually indicate infection. For samples collected using a technique that minimizes contamination, such as a sample collected with a urinary catheter, results as low as 1,000 microorganism CFU/ml may be considered significant. In such cases, the laboratory will often perform additional tests to identify the specific strain of bacteria, as well as susceptibility testing to determine the most appropriate antibiotic treatment. A culture that is reported as "no growth in 24 or 48 hours" usually indicates that there is no infection.

Serum Electrolytes
Serum levels of sodium, potassium, chloride, bicarbonate ion, calcium, and phosphate need to be reviewed when urological problems are present. A urological problem can cause abnormalities in nephron function, and this can alter electrolyte excretion and reabsorption.

TABLE 23-1. Common Signs and Symptoms of Urological Dysfunction

Sign or Symptom	Description	Common Cause
Dysuria	Pain and burning on urination	UTI
Frequency	An abnormally high amount of times that the patient needs to urinate	UTI, BPH, urological obstruction, IC
Hesitancy	Interrupted flow of a urinary stream	BPH
Urgency	A feeling that urination will occur imminently	UTI, BPH, IC

TABLE 23-2. Abnormal Laboratory Findings on Urinalysis

Urinalysis Finding	Description	Common Cause
Bacteriuria	Bacteria in the urine that can be visualized on microscopy	UTI or asymptomatic bacteriuria (ASB)
Bilirubinuria	Bilirubin in the urine	Liver disorders Excessive hemolysis
Crystalluria	Crystals or pieces of a kidney stone in the urine; commonly calcium or uric acid	Nephrolithiasis or urolithiasis
Glucosuria	Glucose in the urine	Uncontrolled diabetes mellitus (DM)
Hematuria	Blood in the urine	UTI Nephrolithasis or urolithiasis Urological malignancy
Ketonuria	Ketones in the urine	Fasting Starvation Uncontrolled DM
Leukocyte esterase	WBCs in the urine	UTI or ASB
Nitrites	Bacteria in the urine	UTI or ASB
Proteinuria (microalbuminuria)	A condition in which urine contains an abnormal amount of protein. Normally urine should contain no more than 200 mg of protein per liter.	Glomerular injury Kidney dysfunction caused by diabetes Kidney dysfunction caused by high blood pressure Inflammation of the kidneys
Pyuria	WBCs (neutrophils) in the urine	UTI or ASB
Urinary casts	Cylindrical mucoprotein structures produced by the nephron tubules that appear in the urine. Various casts found in urine sediment include hyaline, waxy, granular, fatty, crystal, RBC, WBC, bacterial, and epithelial.	Nephrotic syndrome Dehydration Vigorous exercise Diuretics Tubular necrosis Autoimmune disorders Pyelonephritis Other kidney diseases

CBC With Differential

To diagnose infection, a white blood cell (WBC) count is necessary. An elevated WBC count is present with upper UTI or **pyelonephritis.** A lower UTI is a confined, localized infection and should not raise WBC count.

Imaging Studies

Imaging studies can include an x-ray of the abdomen to exclude masses in the pelvis or abdomen. An intravenous pyelogram (IVP) can be used to study the function of the urological system and highlight areas of the kidney and ureter. An IVP is often used to investigate the presence of renal or urological stones.

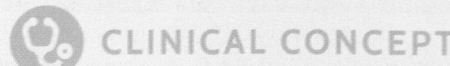 CLINICAL CONCEPT

It is important to ask the patient about allergies before an IVP, because some patients can be allergic to the dye that is used for this procedure.

Ultrasound studies can be used to examine the kidneys and bladder. For example, small, portable ultrasound devices can help determine the extent of bladder over-filling or distention. Cytoscopy, an invasive study that uses a scope inserted into the urethra and bladder, can provide direct visualization of the bladder. During this procedure, dye can be injected into the bladder and ureters to highlight the anatomy. Cystoscopy can also be used to biopsy bladder tumors, and cystoscopic surgical procedures can also be performed.

Urodynamic studies help to evaluate the bladder's neuromuscular status. Studies are done during both bladder filling and emptying. This testing can determine if the bladder can fully expand and the actual process of voiding to determine if the bladder can contract properly.

Treatment

Treatment of urological disorders depends upon the etiology of the particular disorder. For example, antibiotics will be used for an infection. For renal calculi, treatment involves pain medication, increased fluid intake (more than 3 liters/day of water), and straining of the urine. Lithotripsy may be necessary. Cystoscopic surgery may be required for urolithiasis or tumors of the bladder. Surgical procedures are commonly used for BPH and bladder cancer. Medication, surgery, and Kegel exercises are most commonly used to treat urinary incontinence.

Pathophysiology of Selected Urological Disorders

The major urological disorders include lower UTI; asymptomatic bacteriuria (ASB); interstitial cystitis (IC); urolithiasis, also commonly called nephrolithiasis; bladder cancer; and urinary incontinence.

Lower Urinary Tract Infections

Lower UTIs account for 1% to 3% of all visits to family clinicians. The patient commonly presents with pain and burning on urination, as well as urinary frequency and urgency. If the infection persists, the symptoms can progress to cloudy, strong-smelling urine and hematuria. An untreated lower UTI can put the patient at risk for an ascending UTI that can result in pyelonephritis, which is kidney infection.

Epidemiology
Lower UTI is the reason for 6 to 7 million primary care visits per year. Lower UTIs are more prevalent in women than men. In women, a lower UTI is commonly referred to as cystitis. The majority of women with lower UTI are young adults aged 20 to 40 years old. It is estimated that approximately 50% of all women will have a UTI at some point in their lifetime. Conversely, men have a much lower prevalence of UTI. A lower UTI is rare in a young adult male and requires further investigation of the urological system. However, after age 60, BPH is a common cause of UTI in men.

 CLINICAL CONCEPT

Women are at higher risk for lower UTI than men because of the anatomical proximity of the rectum to the female urethra.

Risk Factors
Factors that increase susceptibility to UTI in women include improper perineal hygiene; tight, restrictive clothing; and use of irritating bath products. Sexual intercourse increases a woman's risk of UTI, and use of contraceptive diaphragms and spermicides are also known to increase susceptibility. Pregnancy commonly causes ASB, which is defined as bacteria in the urine with no symptoms. Pregnancy and ASB increase a woman's risk for pyelonephritis, especially at the end of the second trimester and the beginning of the third trimester.

UTIs in older males are generally associated with urinary tract obstruction caused by enlargement of the prostate gland. Lower UTI in men before the age of 50 years is uncommon.

In both males and females, other risk factors for UTI include dehydration, urinary catheterization, diabetes, bladder cancer and cancer in tissues adjacent to the bladder, and cancer treatments.

Etiology
The etiologic organism that most commonly causes lower UTI is *Escherichia coli* (*E. coli*), which originates from the bowel. This organism causes approximately 75% to 90% of all urinary infections. *Proteus, Pseudomonas, Streptococci, Enterococci, Staphylococcus epidermidis, Staphylococcus saprophyticus*, and *Klebsiella* are other organisms of etiologic significance. In nosocomial infections, multidrug-resistant bacterial organisms often cause UTI.

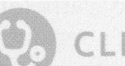 **CLINICAL CONCEPT**

E. coli is commonly transmitted from the rectum to the urethra in women.

Pathophysiology
A healthy urinary tract is sterile and bacterial flora are normally confined to the urethral opening. In women, the anatomic proximity of the rectum and urinary tract enable bacteria to colonize the urethra easily. However, urine contains high osmolarity, urea, and organic acids that diminish bacterial viability in the bladder. Any obstruction of urinary outflow decreases the bladder's resistance to bacterial infection. Stagnant urine is a good medium for bacterial growth. Continual free outflow of urine clears bacteria from the body. Immunoglobulin A (IgA), secreted by WBCs in the urinary tract, also prevents adherence of bacteria to the bladder wall. However, many women are nonsecretors of IgA, which decreases their ability to combat bacterial invasion of the bladder.

When host defenses are overcome, urine can act as a medium for bacterial growth. *E. coli*, a bacteria found in the bowel, causes 70% to 95% of upper and lower UTIs. *Staphylococcus saprophyticus, Klebsiella, Proteus, Pseudomonas,* and *Enterococcus faecalis* are also uropathogenic bacteria. Uropathogenic bacteria can adhere, proliferate, and resist host defenses when in the bladder. The bacteria frequently have resistant outer capsules that can resist the acid in the urine. The bacteria can also secrete hemolysins and cytotoxic necrotizing factor (CNF), which can enhance their migration up to the bladder.

Proteus mirabilis, another bacterium from the bowel, secretes urease, which decreases the acidity of urine and enhances its ability to invade the bladder. The bacteria are flagellated and swarm in large groups when migrating up to the bladder. The bacteria also change the pH of the urine, which enhances formation of struvite staghorn calculi in the kidney. *Proteus* UTI is most commonly associated with urinary instrumentation or catheterization.

Interference with urinary outflow occurs in such conditions as chronic voluntary suppression of urination, sexual intercourse, urinary tract obstruction, instrumentation of the urinary tract, use of catheters not drained to gravity, and vesicoureteral reflux. Frequent emptying of the bladder is necessary for health of the urinary tract. Instrumentation of the urinary tract with a cystoscope or catheter increases risk of bacterial introduction into the bladder. Sexual intercourse and use of the diaphragm contraceptive increase the urethra's exposure to bacteria. Vesicoureteral reflux commonly occurs in young female children. The condition is caused by an anatomical abnormality at the junction where the ureter enters the bladder. This anatomical anomaly allows urine to reflux up toward the kidney, which increases risk of UTI. *Candida albicans*, a fungal pathogen that colonizes the vaginal area, can also cause UTI. Risk factors for *Candida* UTI are diabetes mellitus, antibiotic use, and urinary catheters.

Although common, UTIs are not a serious disease in women unless they are associated with urinary obstruction or pregnancy. In males, UTIs are very uncommon and the cause should be thoroughly investigated. Prostatitis and epididymitis are associated with lower UTI in young adult males. In young men, risk factors for lower UTI include anal intercourse, intercourse with an infected female, lack of circumcision, and human immunodeficiency virus (HIV) infection. The most common reason for infection in older males is stasis of urine caused by obstruction of the urethra because of BPH.

Nosocomial (hospital-acquired) UTI is often associated with urinary catheterization and multidrug-resistant pathogens. Polymicrobial infections that are resistant to antibiotics are common nosocomial UTIs. Urosepsis, bacterial invasion of the bloodstream, can be a complication of UTI in older adults, particularly those with long-term indwelling urinary catheterization.

Clinical Presentation

Most of the time, the history reveals the classic UTI symptoms of frequency, pain or burning on urination (dysuria), urgency, and occasionally hematuria. UTI symptoms are caused by the inflammation and edema of the urethra and bladder. Frequency is the need to urinate many times a day. Commonly in UTI, the bladder does not completely empty and urinary retention causes frequent small amounts of urine flow. Urgency is the sensation that urination is imminent and can cause frequent trips to the bathroom only to yield small amounts of urine. Rarely, there might be suprapubic tenderness. Severe infections can cause bladder spasms; in men, these spasms can produce severe referred pain in the glans penis. Usually there are no changes noted in the physical examination.

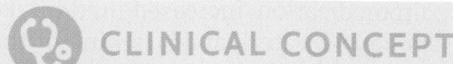

CLINICAL CONCEPT

Lower UTI does not cause fever. Fever should prompt the clinician to suspect pyelonephritis.

Diagnosis

Urinalysis and urine culture are used to diagnose lower UTI. A urinalysis using a dipstick usually shows some red blood cells (RBCs); positive leukocyte esterase, which indicates WBCs; and nitrates, which indicate bacteria. On microscopic urinalysis, neutrophils, RBCs, and bacteria are present in a clean-catch midstream specimen of urine. On a urine culture, infection is indicated by a colony count of bacteria greater than 10^5/mL. However, colony count of bacteria as low as 1,000/ml may be cause of significant infection.

Treatment

The usual treatment for lower UTI is an antibiotic. The specific antibiotic can be determined by culture and sensitivity testing. Nitrofurantoin and/or trimethoprim-sulfamethoxazole are commonly prescribed. Fluoroquinolones may also be used. Phenazopyridine (Pyridium) may be prescribed for urinary tract pain relief. Hydration to accentuate unidirectional clearance of bacteriuria is also part of recommended treatment. Some studies have shown that cranberry juice can decrease the risk of UTI because it lessens the adherence of bacteria to the bladder wall.

ALERT! If a patient is ordered phenazopyridine, let the patient know that one of the side effects of the medication is that it can turn urine red.

Complications

Urosepsis, a condition caused by bacteremia, is a serious complication of UTI. Patients with urosepsis are acutely and severely ill with symptoms of fever, chills, confusion, disorientation, and hypotension. Bacterial endotoxins are responsible for the clinically observable effects of the bacteremia in the host. Elderly individuals, catheterized patients, and those who are immunocompromised are particularly susceptible to urosepsis. Obstruction within the urinary tract increases an individual's susceptibility. Elderly males with BPH are at increased risk.

Asymptomatic Bacteriuria

ASB refers to two consecutive urine cultures growing more than a colony count of 100,000 bacteria in a patient lacking symptoms of a UTI. It is a common disorder, with varying prevalence by age, sex, sexual activity, and the presence of genitourinary abnormalities. It is more common in women than men. In healthy women,

CHAPTER 23 Urological Disorders 517

the prevalence of bacteriuria increases with age, from about 1% in females 5 to 14 years of age to more than 20% in women at least 80 years of age.

E. coli is the most common organism isolated from patients with ASB. Other infecting organisms include *Enterobacteriaceae, Pseudomonas aeruginosa, Enterococcus* species, and group B streptococcus. Organisms isolated in patients with ASB are influenced by patient variables: healthy persons commonly have *E. coli,* whereas nursing home residents with a urinary catheter are more likely to have multidrug-resistant bacteria. Enterococcus species and gram-negative bacilli are common in men.

Among patients with ASB, treatment with antibiotics has not been found to improve patient outcomes. For this reason as well as increased antimicrobial resistance, it is important to refrain from treating patients with ASB unless there is evidence of potential benefit. Women who are pregnant should be screened for ASB in the first trimester and, if positive, treated.

Interstitial Cystitis

IC is a syndrome characterized by urgency and frequency of urination, feeling of bladder fullness, and pain. Painful bladder syndrome (PBS) is a term often used synonymously with IC. This syndrome is diagnosed primarily on the basis of symptoms, as there is no known etiology and pathophysiology is unclear.

Epidemiology
Ninety percent of those affected with IC are women, and the average age of onset is 40 years; most are Caucasian. Prevalence rates vary among different countries. In the United States, IC has a prevalence of 6 to 7 cases per 10,000 women, whereas reports from Europe indicate a prevalence of 1.8 cases per 10,000 women, and only 0.3 to 0.4 cases per 10,000 women in Japan.

Etiology/Risk Factors
The etiology of IC is unknown, but proposed causes include infection with an undetermined pathogen, autoimmunity, toxicity caused by an environmental substance, or neurogenic hypersensitivity at the spinal cord segment that innervates the bladder.

Patients with IC frequently report prior gynecological surgery, history of UTIs, and/or childhood bladder problems. IC is often associated with inflammatory bowel disease, systemic lupus erythematous, irritable bowel syndrome, fibromyalgia, and atopic allergy.

Pathophysiology
The pathophysiology of IC is unclear. There are two different types of IC based on histological findings; nonulcerative and ulcerative. In nonulcerative IC, the bladder wall shows small tears and hemorrhages when the bladder is distended. There is a thinning of bladder mucosa, and fibrosis is found in the deeper layers of the bladder wall. In ulcerative IC, a lesion called a Hunner ulcer is present on histological examination of the bladder wall. The inner bladder surface is erythematous and may contain one or more ulcerations surrounded by inflammation. These ulcers become apparent only after overdistention of the bladder on urodynamic testing.

Clinical Presentation
Patients with IC report chronic pelvic pain, perineal pain, dysuria, a sense of fullness of the bladder, urinary urgency, and frequency. In severe IC, a patient may feel the need to urinate more than 50 times a day and endure many episodes of nocturia. The bladder usually has normal size and capacity. The pain begins during bladder filling and is relieved by emptying the bladder. Symptoms may occur daily or weekly or may be constant and unrelenting for months or years and then resolve spontaneously with or without therapy. The disorder commonly occurs in a pattern of remissions and exacerbations.

Diagnosis
To diagnose IC, an infectious cause of symptoms needs to be excluded with urinalysis and urine culture. In women, endometriosis needs to be ruled out, which requires hysteroscopy and laparoscopy. In men, prostate disease should be ruled out. Patients require cystoscopy, urine cytology, and biopsy of suspicious bladder lesions to rule out bladder cancer. Cystoscopy can confirm the erythema, tears, and ulcerations of the bladder walls. A cystoscopy examination with bladder distention under anesthesia, with or without bladder biopsy, is a diagnostic procedure. Urodynamic studies can evaluate bladder sensation and neuromuscular function.

Treatment
In IC, there is no one treatment that is used for all situations. Pelvic floor rehabilitation and bladder training programs are usually attempted first. Kegel exercises are recommended, and the patient is advised to gradually increase voiding intervals over a course of weeks. Certain foods have been known to aggravate symptoms of IC. The patient is advised to avoid tomatoes, chocolate, spicy foods, alcohol, coffee, and vinegar.

If dietary and behavioral therapies are ineffective, the clinician usually attempts drug therapy. Anticholinergic agents such as oxybutynin and tolterodine can be used to treat the urinary frequency component of the condition, but these agents can cause urinary retention, impair bladder emptying, and may exacerbate pelvic pain.

Various pharmacological agents may be used to alleviate symptoms, such as antihistamines, tricyclic antidepressants, analgesics, and anti-inflammatory agents. Also, a medication called pentosan polysulfate sodium has been shown to be effective in some persons with IC. This medication may not show its effects until 6 months of treatment.

At times, patients report relief of IC after hydrodistention of the bladder, which is done during diagnostic evaluation. Intravesical instillation therapy with dimethyl sulfoxide (DMSO) has also been effective. In intravesical therapy, the clinician instills medication directly into the bladder using a catheter. This therapy may require several episodes of instillation before it is effective. Transurethral intradetrusor muscle injection of botulinum toxin in conjunction with hydrodistention of the bladder have proven effective in some cases. Transcutaneous electrical nervous stimulation (TENS) has also shown some success. Electrodes can be placed over the sacral nerve region or suprapubic area. If all treatments fail to provide relief, surgical techniques may be attempted. Surgical fulguration, laser treatment and resection of ulcerations in the bladder, can be attempted. In the most severe cases of unrelieved pain, cystectomy can be done.

Urolithiasis

Urolithiasis is the condition of calculi that are formed or located anywhere in the urinary system. The term *nephrolithiasis* (renal calculus) refers to stones that are in the kidney, whereas *ureterolithiasis* refers to stones that are in the ureter. Cystolithiasis (vesical calculi) refers to stones that form or have passed into the bladder.

Epidemiology

Urolithiasis affects an estimated 240,000 to 720,000 people in the United States annually. This estimate consists of persons who have suffered more than one incident of stone in the urinary system. A history of stone disease is more common in Caucasians compared with African Americans, and more common in males compared with females. Population estimates of the incidence of urolithiasis range from 1 to 3 per 1,000 in men to 0.6 to 1.0 per 1,000 in women. Incidence increases among men in their 20s and peaks in the late 50s. In women, the incidence rate is approximately equal across all age groups. Reoccurrence of the formation of calculi is common, with 35% at 5 years and 52% at 10 years after the initial incident.

Etiology/Risk Factors

Genetics, diet, metabolic abnormalities, and structural abnormalities in the urinary tract can lead to urolithiasis (see Box 23-1). Having a family member with kidney stones is a strong risk factor. Lack of adequate hydration also contributes to stone formation. A low fluid intake, with a subsequent low volume of urine production, produces high concentrations of stone-forming solutes in the urine.

Another contributing factor to the formation of stones is diet. Diets that are high in animal protein, sodium, and calcium can lead to urolithiasis. Stones can be a result of excessive consumption of certain minerals or faulty metabolism of minerals. The following are the four main types of renal calculi:

1. calcium stones
2. struvite (magnesium ammonium phosphate) stones
3. uric acid stones
4. cystine stones.

BOX 23-1. Conditions Leading to Urolithiasis

There are various conditions that increase susceptibility to kidney stone formation. A condition involving kidney stones is referred to as urolithiasis when a stone is impacted within the ureter or bladder.

Biliary cirrhosis
Chronic dehydration
Cystinuria
Distal renal tubular acidosis
Ehlers-Danlos syndrome
Hypercalciuria
Hyperoxaluria
Hyperparathyroidism (hypercalcemia)
Lesch-Nyhan syndrome
Marfan syndrome
Multiendocrine neoplasm
Polycystic kidney disease
Sjögren's syndrome

Calcium Stones. Calcium is the most common component of urological stones, and hypercalciuria is the most common metabolic abnormality found in urolithiasis. Some cases of hypercalciuria are related to increased intestinal absorption of calcium, which is associated with excess dietary calcium and overactive calcium absorption mechanisms; some are related to excess resorption of calcium from bone, such as in hyperparathyroidism; and some are related to an inability of the renal tubules to properly reabsorb calcium in the glomerular filtrate, such as in renal-leak hypercalciuria.

Struvite Stones. Struvite stones are composed of a combination of magnesium, ammonium phosphate, and carbonate apatite and can grow to occupy the entire pelvis of the kidney, called a staghorn calculus. Struvite stones occur when urea is split into ammonia, bicarbonate, and carbonate ions by urease-producing organisms, especially *Proteus mirabilis*. Other organisms that cause struvite stones include *Haemophilus influenzae*, *Staphylococcus aureus*, and *Yersinia enterocolitica*. Factors that predispose individuals to struvite stone formation include anatomical abnormalities in the urinary tract, neurological disorders of the bladder, and indwelling catheters.

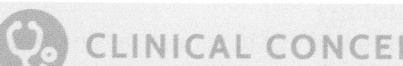 CLINICAL CONCEPT

Patients with spinal cord injuries are particularly vulnerable to the formation of struvite stones; 8% of these patients form stones, 98% of which are struvite stones.

Uric Acid Stones. Foods high in animal proteins contain a high amount of purines, which break down into uric acid. Meats increase the amount of uric acid in the bloodstream, which can then precipitate out of solution at the kidney and form uric acid stones.

Cystine Stones. Cystine stones are uncommon. They are associated with a genetic disorder associated with the faulty metabolism of the amino acid, cystine.

Pathophysiology

Urolithiasis occurs because of supersaturation of the urine with stone-forming salts as a result of chemical, metabolic, or genetic causes. Stones in the bladder can also occur as a result of stasis of urine, repeated UTIs, urinary obstruction, or neurogenic bladder. Intraureteral stones cause pressure proximal to the stone in the ureter, which causes spasm. Spasms of the ureter occur because of obstruction at one of four sites:

1. ureteropelvic junction, where the ureter attaches to the kidney.
2. midureter at the level of the iliac vessels.
3. posterior aspect of the pelvis in women, at the point the ureter crosses the broad ligament.
4. ureterovesical jct, which is where the ureters connect with the bladder.

An IVP reveals the stone location, outline of the kidney, and ureteral flow of urine. A stone slowly travels down the ureter, pushed by urine flow. It shears off some of the ureteral mucosa, which causes superficial bleeding of the membrane. The stone causes a buildup of pressure and spasms proximally within the ureter that causes intense pain. Low urine flow slows the passage of the stone, which is why increased hydration is recommended to increase urine volume. Lack of urine passage can cause backward accumulation of pressure into the renal pelvis, causing hydronephrosis, which is swelling of the renal pelvis. Backward accumulation of urine is toxic to nephrons and can result in kidney failure.

 CLINICAL CONCEPT

Dehydration is a significant contributor to urolithiasis and incidence of the disorder is greater in regions with hot climates.

Clinical Presentation

Diagnosis of urolithiasis is most often based on the patient's history because there are distinct symptoms. The physical examination frequently does not reveal significant findings.

History. The patient suspected of urolithiasis should fully describe his or her pain. The characteristics of the pain in urolithiasis are distinctive and often the basis of diagnosis. Pain should be completely assessed, including location, onset, duration, characteristics, radiation, and aggravating factors, including any treatment that relieves the pain. Current medications, including over-the-counter medications and herbal supplements, should be assessed because some drugs can predispose individuals to stone formation. Past medical history and family history of kidney stones are key because there is a strong genetic predisposition and repeat episodes of kidney stones are common. Any disorders that increase susceptibility to hypercalcemia or hyperuricemia are important, as calcium and uric acid are common components of stones. Patients with hyperparathyroidism or malignancy often have hypercalcemia and hypercalciuria, whereas patients with gout have hyperuricemia. Frequent UTIs or any possible cause of urinary stasis should be investigated because these are risk factors.

Signs and Symptoms. Patients typically present with costovertebral angle pain, also called flank pain, or abdominal pain when the kidney stone is high in the urinary tract in the ureter. The pain of urolithiasis is regarded as severe and intermittent. Rather than lying still, patients usually constantly move in an effort to control the pain. The distinctive pain, referred to as renal colic, can be associated with nausea, vomiting, fever, hematuria, pyuria, crystalluria, and painful urination. Renal colic typically comes in waves lasting 20 to 60 minutes, beginning in the flank or lower back and often radiating to the groin or genitals. The patient usually describes the pain as severe. The patient may be able to painfully pass a kidney stone or stone particles with high urine flow. The stone should be analyzed for composition.

Diagnosis

The diagnosis of urolithiasis is made on the basis of information obtained from the history and physical examination, as well as urinalysis and imaging studies. The patient's description of the pain is key in the diagnosis because renal colic is distinctive. Urinalysis will be positive for blood, and will often show crystals. Serum analysis for electrolytes, calcium, and uric acid is important. IVP is more sensitive in detecting urolithiasis than abdominal x-rays of the kidneys, ureters, and bladder, which miss stones that are not opaque to x-ray. Computed tomography (CT) scans visualize stones. A confirmation of urolithiasis is made on passing of the stone, surgical recovery of the stone, or by radiological imaging. Stone analysis, together with serum and 24-hour urine metabolic evaluation, can identify the cause of the stone in more than 95% of patients.

Treatment

Patients are advised to increase hydration (more than 3 liters of water/day) in order to attempt to pass the stone in the urine. Patients should also strain urine to catch the stone for analysis. Pain medications such as opioids are usually necessary. Pharmacological intervention is specific to the type of stone. Diuretics such as hydrochlorothiazide can limit calcium excretion into urine. The patient may require extracorporeal shock wave lithotripsy to enable passing of the stone. Lithotripsy uses sound waves to break up a stone into smaller pieces so they may be passed more easily. Cystoscopic surgery may be needed if the stone does not pass.

Bladder Cancer

Although not a common disorder, cancer of the bladder is the most common type of urological cancer. Specifically, transitional cell carcinoma (TCC) is the most common form of bladder cancer, accounting for 90% of cases. Other less common types of bladder cancer include squamous cell carcinoma and adenocarcinoma.

Epidemiology

In the United States, approximately 72,000 persons suffered bladder cancer in 2013 and more than 15,000 died from the disorder. Bladder cancer is 3 times more common in males than females. There is a greater prevalence of bladder cancer in Caucasians compared with African Americans. The highest incidence of bladder cancer is in men aged 60 years and older. Among women, incidence is highest after age 70 years.

Etiology

Up to 80% of bladder cancers are related to environmental exposure, with cigarette smoking the major risk factor. The degree of risk is directly proportional to the number of pack-years of the patient. A smoker has up to 6 times the risk of bladder cancer compared with nonsmokers. Occupational exposure is another major risk factor for bladder cancer. Use of various organic chemicals, such as naphthalene, benzidine, and aniline, are associated with bladder cancer. Chronic exposure to diesel exhaust, rubber, and petroleum products have also been associated with bladder cancer. Analgesics containing phenacetin and sustained low doses of the chemotherapeutic agent cyclophosphamide are also risk factors, as is radiotherapy to the pelvis.

In developing countries, particularly the Middle East, bladder cancer is commonly caused by a parasitic infection caused by *Schistosoma haematobium*. The eggs of the parasite are found within the bladder wall.

Patients with spinal cord injuries who require a long-term indwelling urinary catheter have 16 to 20 times greater risk of developing bladder cancer than the general population.

Genetic mutations can also cause bladder cancer. Mutations of the tumor suppressor gene *p53*, found on chromosome 17, are associated with high-grade bladder cancer, whereas mutations of the tumor suppressor genes *p15* and *p16*, found on chromosome 9, are associated with low-grade and superficial tumors. The retinoblastoma (*Rb*) oncogene is also associated with bladder cancer.

Pathophysiology

The most common type of bladder cancer, TCC, arises from the bladder's interior surface. Growth of this form of cancer often involves the development of a tumor that protrudes into the bladder lumen and, if untreated, eventually penetrates the basement membrane and then continues into the bladder muscle, where it can metastasize. Nearly 90% of transitional cell bladder tumors exhibit this type of disease process. The remaining 10% of TCCs are less invasive and referred to as carcinoma in situ or nonmuscle invasive bladder cancer. This is a flat, superficial tumor that spreads along the bladder's surface. Bladder tumors are categorized according to their invasiveness. Low grade tumors are commonly polyplike tumors that grow from the superficial layers of the bladder, whereas the most severe types of tumors invade the muscle wall. Commonly, bladder tumors consist mainly of TCC with small areas of squamous cell and adenocarcinoma.

Clinical Presentation

The cardinal feature of bladder cancer is painless, intermittent, gross hematuria. Other symptoms include frequency, pain, and burning on urination, as well as the sensation of incomplete bladder emptying. Some types of bladder cancer present similarly to a UTI with urgency, frequency, and dysuria. Usually located deep within the bladder, bladder cancer rarely presents as a palpable mass.

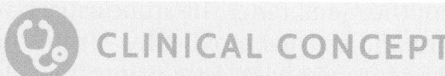

CLINICAL CONCEPT

Assumption of a UTI, especially in women, is a common cause of a delayed diagnosis of bladder cancer.

Diagnosis

Often the first suspicion of bladder cancer occurs because a urinalysis using a standard dipstick or microscopic evaluation shows RBCs in the urine. A microscopic urinalysis should be repeated to confirm the presence of RBCs and exclude other causes of hematuria. There are some bladder tumor antigen tests; however, these have high false positive and false negative results.

Cystoscopy is the gold standard for evaluating unexplained hematuria. It is the best diagnostic procedure for detecting bladder lesions and is definitive when combined with transurethral biopsy. Abdominal CT scan with contrast is the preferred imaging investigation when evaluating high risk patients with gross painless hematuria and patients suspected of having invasive tumors. Abdominal and pelvic ultrasound combined with cystoscopy may be used in lower risk patients such as young women with unexplained hematuria.

ALERT! Painless hematuria is usually the only sign of bladder cancer. Because of this, no amount of hematuria is too small to require further investigation.

Treatment

Surgical treatment involves a transurethral resection of the tumor. Chemotherapy and radiation therapy are also used to eradicate the tumor or reduce tumor size. Radical cystectomy with urinary diversion may be necessary for very large invasive tumors.

Urinary Incontinence

Many persons endure urinary incontinence silently and do not seek medical attention. The majority are women. Many are reticent to admit to the disorder because of embarrassment. Therefore, prevalence is difficult to determine.

Epidemiology

In the United States, 10 million persons endure urinary incontinence. The majority of this population are women. Female incontinence in the United States increases with age from 20% to 30% during young adulthood to almost 50% in elderly women. The prevalence of daily incontinence in older men is 2% to 11%. Urinary incontinence occurs in 30% of men who have had surgery for prostate disease. Urinary incontinence affects 50% to 84% of elderly persons in long-term care facilities.

Etiology/Risk Factors

There are different etiologies of incontinence (see Table 23-3). Increasing age, pregnancy, childbirth, obesity, diabetes, stroke, and neurological impairment have been identified as risk factors. Prostate disease and its treatments are significant risk factors in men.

Pathophysiology

The most common type of urinary incontinence is stress incontinence in women. This occurs because of loss of muscle support in the pelvic floor. Menopause, multiple episodes of childbirth, aging of the musculature, immobility, and surgery such as hysterectomy can cause weakness of the pelvic muscles. Low estrogen levels of menopause contributes to the pelvic muscle weakness.

Overactive bladder (OAB) (also called urge incontinence) is another type of urinary incontinence that is mainly caused by detrusor muscle overactivity. The exact mechanism for OAB is unclear. Proposed etiologies include neurological impairment, urothelium and suburothelium dysfunction, as well as IC. Obesity and COPD can also contribute to OAB. In men, the most common cause of OAB is prostate surgery. Bladder sphincter dysfunction occurs after nerves are disrupted in surgery.

Overflow incontinence results from chronic overdistention and urinary retention in the bladder. The detrusor muscle of the bladder wall loses strength and elasticity. BPH is the most frequent cause in men. Failure of the detrusor muscle caused by damage of the pelvic spinal nerves can also cause this type of incontinence. Pelvic surgery, trauma, compression of spinal nerves, tumor, or infection can be the cause.

Another type of incontinence referred to as neurogenic bladder is associated with spinal cord disorders that cause peripheral nerve weakness, as well as sympathetic and parasympathetic nerve dysfunction. The spinal cord nerves are insensitive to bladder filling and muscles cannot contract to release the urine.

TABLE 23-3. Types of Incontinence

Type of Incontinence	Description
Stress incontinence	Involuntary leakage of urine as abdominal pressure rises, which typically occurs during coughing and sneezing. The leakage occurs because of either poor pelvic support or to weakness in the urethral sphincter.
Urge incontinence also called Overactive bladder (OAB)	Detrusor muscle overactivity is the cause of the urine leakage. The cause is unclear but IC is thought to be the etiology in some patients. The patient complains of feelings of urgency and frequency of urination many times a day.
Overflow incontinence	Chronic overdistention and urinary retention in the bladder results in overflow incontinence. BPH, which obstructs urine outflow, is the most frequent cause in men. Failure of the detrusor muscle caused by damage of the pelvic spinal nerves can also cause this type of incontinence.
Neurogenic bladder	This disorder is the result of an interruption of the sensory nerve fibers between the bladder and the spinal cord or the afferent nerve tracts to the brain. Chronic overdistention of the bladder occurs.
Functional incontinence	Inability to hold urine caused by CNS problems such as stroke, psychiatric disorders, prolonged immobility, dementia, or delirium.
Mixed incontinence	Combination of stress incontinence and OAB.

Functional incontinence is the inability to hold urine because of prolonged immobility, CNS lesions such as stroke, delirium, or psychiatric disorders such as dementia.

A type of incontinence categorized as mixed incontinence is a combination of stress incontinence and OAB.

Clinical Presentation

Patients with incontinence should be assessed with a thorough history, physical examination, and urinalysis. A gynecological exam should be performed on women.

History. A thorough health history is necessary regarding any systemic illnesses, past surgeries, UTIs, or other urinary problems. The patient will report loss of urine with straining or coughing. Alternatively, the patient can report an inability to hold urine and/or repetitive feelings of urinary urgency throughout the day. It is important to ask about use of absorbent pads or sanitary napkins because these are useful to quantify urine loss.

Signs and Symptoms. The patient's report of urinary loss should prompt further investigation. Physical examination may or may not reveal signs of a disorder that is causative of urinary incontinence. A complete neurological examination is particularly important. All possible causes and contributing factors need to be ruled out such as central nervous system problems, diabetes, spinal cord compression, urinary tract anomalies, UTI, cystocele, and nephrolithiasis. The patient may be asked to keep a voiding diary or complete a specific questionnaire regarding urinary symptoms.

Diagnosis

A simple urinary cough test may be diagnostic. Asking the patient to forcefully cough with a full bladder in the standing position can demonstrate urinary incontinence. Mobility and strength of the bladder sphincter can be assessed with a cotton swab test in which a sterile cotton swab lubricated with lidocaine is inserted transurethrally into the bladder. The patient is asked to cough, and the angle of the cotton swab can indicate if stress incontinence is present.

X-ray of the kidney, ureter, and bladder is essential. Ultrasound, CT scan, and IVP can rule out kidney stones or urological anomalies. However, urodynamic testing and cystoscopy may be necessary. Measurement of postvoid residual volume in the bladder is needed.

Treatment

Nonsurgical treatments for incontinence in women include electrostimulation, medical devices, and local estrogen therapy, though the effectiveness of these treatments is inconclusive. Kegel exercises can improve pelvic muscle strength, and bladder training can reduce urge incontinence and stress incontinence.

Urethral occlusive devices are available that can be inserted into the urethral meatus and prevent incontinence for several hours. Incontinence pessary devices that are inserted into the vaginal canal to support the pelvic floor are also available. If long-term catheterization is necessary, a suprapubic catheter may be preferable to a transurethral catheter. Procedures called transvaginal tape and transobturator vaginal tape are minimally invasive surgeries that have shown some success for stress incontinence. Anticholinergic drugs such as oxybutynin can be used to treat OAB syndrome. These drugs diminish bladder activity and allow retention of urine. Antidepressants, alpha-adrenergic blockers, and antispasmodic medications have shown some success. Intradetrusor muscle injection of botulinum toxin is being used when all pharmacological agents fail.

Chapter Summary

- Lower UTI is one of the most common problems presented to primary care clinicians.

- The classic symptoms of a lower UTI include dysuria, frequency, and urgency.

- Lower UTI is common in young adult women, but rare in young adult men.

- In males over age 60, BPH frequently causes lower UTI.

- In elderly persons, particularly those in long-term care facilities, lower UTI can lead to urosepsis.

- *E. coli* is the most common pathogen that causes lower UTI.

- Urinalysis is the diagnostic test used most often to determine the presence of infection, blood, or crystals in the urine.

- An abdominal x-ray of the area encompassing the kidneys, ureter, and bladder (KUB) can be used to diagnose many conditions.

- Classic signs and symptoms of nephrolithiasis and urolithiasis include flank pain that radiates into the groin, hematuria, and crystalluria.

- The most common type of calculi in urolithiasis is calcium oxalate. Other types of calculi are uric acid, struvite, and cystine.

- An IVP can show structure and function of the urinary tract. It can outline the presence of calculi in the urological system.

- IC (also called PBS) is a urological disorder with an unknown etiology that causes chronic pelvic pain, perineal pain, dysuria, a sense of fullness of the bladder, urgency, and urinary frequency.

- Cystoscopic investigation is often the most definitive diagnostic procedure for urological disorders.
- Urodynamic studies obtain information about the bladder as it fills and empties.
- Painless, gross hematuria is frequently the only sign of bladder cancer.

- TCC is the most common type of bladder cancer.
- There are different types of urinary incontinence: stress, overflow, urge (OAB), neurogenic, functional, and mixed incontinence.

 ## Making the Connections

Pathophysiology	Signs and Symptoms	Assessment Findings	Diagnostic Testing	Treatment
Lower UTI | Invasion of the bladder mucosa by bacteria, typically *E. coli,* which usually inhabits bowel.				
	Dysuria, frequency, urgency, general fatigue, and malaise. Urine often has a cloudy appearance and can have foul odor.	No physical examination findings.	Urinalysis and culture and sensitivity tests will reveal the bacterial etiology and appropriate antibiotic.	Antibiotics used to eradicate the organism. Increase fluids to enhance flushing out infectious material from the bladder. Phenazopyridine (Pyridium) may be used for urinary tract pain.
Asymptomatic Bacteriuria | A chronic condition of 100,000 bacterial count in the urine without patient symptoms.				
	No symptoms.	No physical findings.	Urinalysis and culture and sensitivity tests will reveal the bacterial etiology.	No antibiotics recommended if no symptoms are present.
Interstitial Cystitis | The pathology of IC is not well understood. Two different types of IC—nonulcerative and ulcerative. In nonulcerative IC, the bladder wall shows thinning, small tears, and hemorrhages. In ulcerative IC, a Hunner ulcer, erythema, and inflammation is found on the inner bladder wall.				
	Urgency, frequency, and discomfort. Pelvic pain.	No physical findings.	Filling cystometry used to assess detrusor muscle function when bladder is full.	Dietary changes and Kegel exercises. Bladder training Amitriptyline, analgesic, anti-inflammatory, anticholinergic agents, pentosan polysulfate sodium, DMSO intravesical therapy, or surgery may be required.

Continued

Making the Connections–cont'd

Pathophysiology	Signs and Symptoms	Assessment Findings	Diagnostic Testing	Treatment
Urolithiasis | Kidney stone formation in the urinary tract. Stones occur because of supersaturation of the urine with stone-forming salts. Anatomical abnormalities in the urinary tract predispose to stone formation. Urease-producing bacteria can increase susceptibility to formation of struvite stones.				
	Severe back and flank pain radiating into the groin. Severe abdominal pain occurs if stone is high in ureter. Frequency, urgency, and dysuria may or may not be present.	Low grade fever may be present, as well as costovertebral angle tenderness, hematuria, crystalluria.	Microscopic hematuria and crystalluria. IVP and CT scan useful to visualize stones.	Conservative management includes analgesics, high fluid intake, low animal protein diet, and low sodium intake. Extracorporeal shock wave lithotripsy or surgery may be necessary. Straining of urine necessary.
Bladder Cancer | TCC of superficial wall of inner bladder is most common type of cancer. Less commonly, squamous cell or adenocarcinoma of the bladder.				
	Microscopic to frank hematuria.	No physical assessment findings. Blood may be apparent in the urine.	Urinalysis and urine cytology may show cancer cells; cystoscopy shows bladder tumor.	Laser ablation of tumor, intravesical chemotherapy, or radical surgery is required for advanced tumors.
Urinary Incontinence | Several different types. (1) Stress incontinence caused by pelvic muscle weakening. (2) Urge incontinence (OAB) caused by spasms of detrusor muscle. (3) Overflow incontinence caused by obstructive uropathy. (4) Neurogenic incontinence caused by loss of spinal nerve function. (5) Functional incontinence caused by dementia, delirium, immobility, stroke, or psychiatric problems. (6) Mixed urinary incontinence has features of stress incontinence and OAB.				
	Leakage of urine or complete inability to hold urine.	Inability to suppress urination with leakage of urine.	Full serum metabolic panel; CBC, electrolytes, BUN, creatinine. Urinalysis, urine culture. Urinary cough test. Cotton swab test. Urodynamic evaluation of bladder filling or voiding phase. Some patients may require cystoscopy.	Pelvic floor exercises (Kegel exercises), bladder training, estrogen treatment are used for stress incontinence. Vaginal ring pessaries for pelvic organ prolapse may be tried for stress incontinence. A surgical procedure referred to as transvaginal or transobturator vaginal tape (TVT surgery) is used for stress incontinence. Anticholinergic, antidepressant, and antispasmodic drugs are used for OAB. Patients with neurogenic bladder often require long-term urinary catheterization; suprapubic catheters may be preferable.

Bibliography

Barry, M. J., Meleth, S., Lee, J. Y., et al. (2011). Effect of increasing doses of saw palmetto extract on lower urinary tract symptoms: a randomized trial. *JAMA, 306*(12), 1344–1351. doi: 10.1001/jama.2011.1364.

Cayley, W. E., Jr. (2013). Are cranberry products effective for the prevention of urinary tract infections? *Am Fam Phys, 88*(11), 745–746.

Colgan, R., & Williams, M. (2011). Diagnosis and treatment of acute uncomplicated cystitis. *Am Fam Phys, 84*(7), 771–775.

Drekonja, D. M., Rector, T. S., Cutting, A., & Johnson, J. R. (2013). Urinary tract infection in male veterans: treatment patterns and outcomes. *JAMA Int Med, 173*(1), 62–68.

Drugs for urinary tract infections. (2014, February 26). *JAMA, 311*(8), 855–856. doi: 10.1001/jama.2014.972.

French, L. M., & Bhambore, N. (2011). Interstitial cystitis/painful bladder syndrome. *Am Fam Phys, 83*(10), 1175–1181.

Hooton, T. M. (2012). Clinical practice. Uncomplicated urinary tract infection. *N Engl J Med, 366*(11), 1028–1037.

Jepson, R., Craig, J., & Williams, G. (2013). Cranberry products and prevention of urinary tract infections. *JAMA, 310*(13), 1395–1396. doi: 10.1001/jama.2013.277509.

Keller, D. L. (2011). Ultrasensitive culture in urinary tract infection diagnosis. *Am Fam Phys. 84*(3), 250.

Khandelwal, C., & Kistler, C. (2013). Diagnosis of urinary incontinence. *Am Fam Phys, 87*(8), 543–550.

Kodner, C. M., & Thomas Gupton, E. K. (2010). Recurrent urinary tract infections in women: diagnosis and management. *Am Fam Phys, 82*(6), 638–643.

Lee, J. H., Gomez, S., & Jankowski, T. A. (2011). FPIN's clinical inquiries: hormone therapy for postmenopausal women with urinary incontinence. *Am Fam Phys, 84*(1), 1–2.

McNicholas, T., & Kirby, R. (2012). Benign prostatic hyperplasia and male lower urinary tract symptoms. *Am Fam Phys, 86*(4), 359–360.

Meng, M. V., Stoller, M. I., & Walsh, T. (2010). Urologic disorders. In S. J. McPhee & M. A. Papadakis, *Current medical diagnosis & treatment 2010.* New York: McGraw-Hill/Lange Medical Series.

Mody, L., & Juthani-Mehta, M. (2014). Urinary tract infections in older women: a clinical review. *JAMA, 311*(8), 844–854. doi: 10.1001/jama.2014.303.

Peleg, A. Y., & Hooper, D. C. (2010). Hospital-acquired infections due to gram-negative bacteria. *N Engl J Med, 362*(19), 1804–1813.

Saint, S., Greene, M. T., Kowalski, C. P., et al. (2013). Preventing catheter associated urinary tract infection in the United States: a national comparative study. *JAMA Int Med, 173*(10), 874–879. doi: 10.1001/jamainternmed.2013.101.

Sarma, A. V., & Wei, J. T. (2012). Clinical practice. Benign prostatic hyperplasia and lower urinary tract symptoms. *N Engl J Med, 367*(3), 248–257.

Schultz, H. J., & Edson, R. S. (2011). Cystitis treatment in women, circa 2011: new role for an old drug. *Mayo Clin Proceed, 86*(6), 477–479.

Seminerio, J. L., Aggarwal, G., & Sweetser, S. (2011). 26-year-old man with recurrent urinary tract infections. *Mayo Clin Proceed, 86*(6), 557–560.

Sharp, V. J., Barnes, K. T., & Erickson, B. A. (2013). Assessment of asymptomatic microscopic hematuria in adults. *Am Fam Phys, 88*(11), 747–754.

Sharp, V. J., Takacs, E. B., & Powell, C. R. (2010). Prostatitis: diagnosis and treatment. *Am Fam Phys, 82*(4), 397–406.

Simati, B., Kriegsman, B., & Safranek, S. (2013, May 15). FPIN's clinical inquiries. Dipstick urinalysis for the diagnosis of acute UTI. *Am Fam Phys, 87*(10), Online.

Stapleton, A. E., Dziura, J., Hooton, T. M., et al. (2012). Recurrent urinary tract infection and urinary *Escherichia coli* in women ingesting cranberry juice daily: a randomized controlled trial. *Mayo Clin Proceed, 87*(2), 143–150.

Trautner, B. W. (2013). New perspectives on urinary tract infection in men. *JAMA Int Med, 173*(1), 68–70.

U.S. Preventive Services Task Force. (2010). Screening for asymptomatic bacteriuria in adults: reaffirmation recommendation statement. *Am Fam Phys, 81*(4), 505.

Wang, B. S. (2013). Assessing catheter-associated urinary tract infection. *Lancet, 381*(9877), 1535–1536.

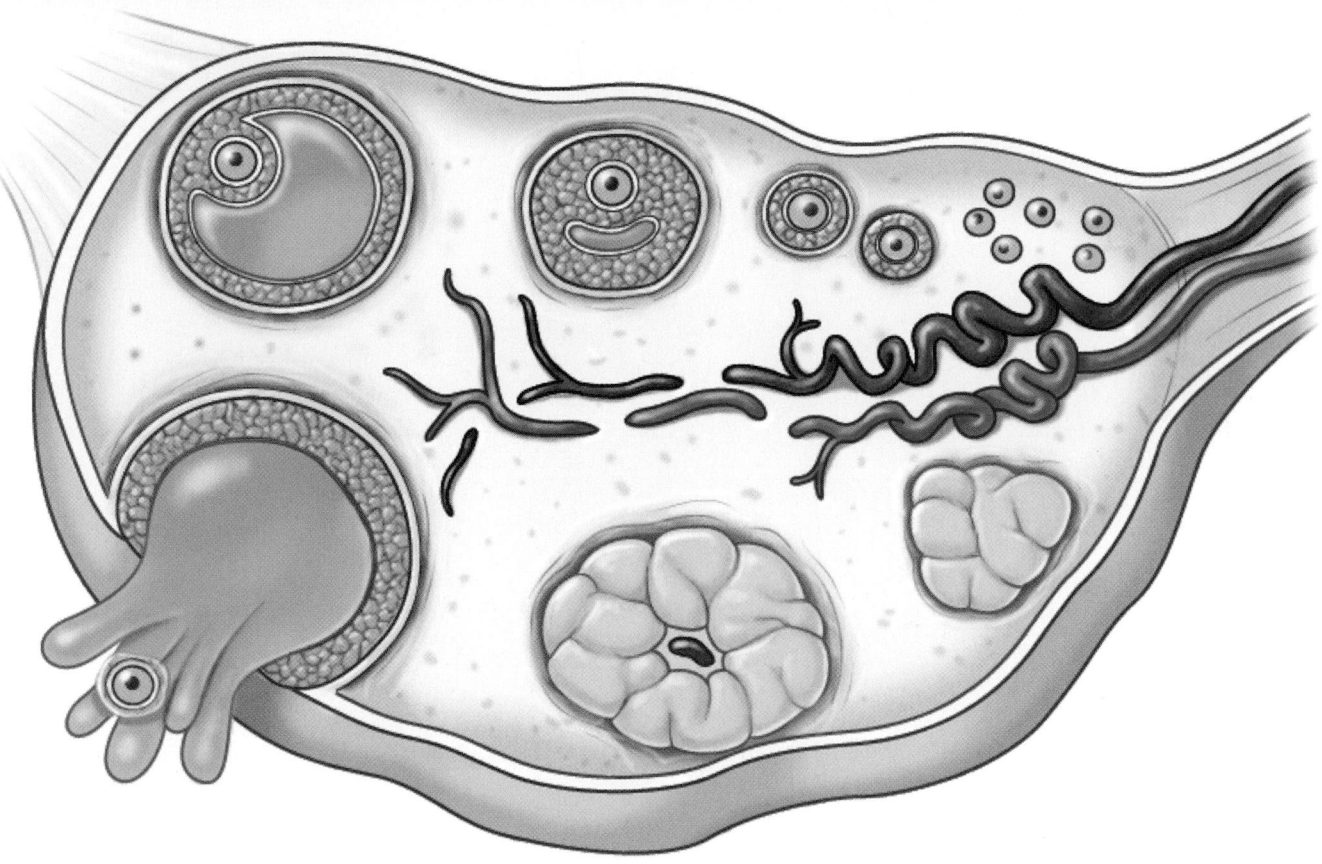

Chapters

Endocrine Disorders

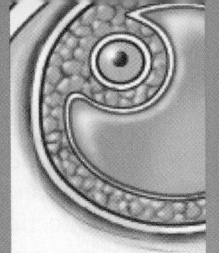

Key Terms

Acromegaly
Adenohypophysis
Addison's disease
Adrenal insufficiency
Adrenocorticotropic hormone (ACTH)
Cortisol
Cushing's disease
Cushing's syndrome
Diabetes insipidus

Exophthalmos
Goiter
Goitrogen
Graves' disease
Growth hormone (GH)
Hypophysis
Hypothalamic-pituitary-hormone axis
Mineralocorticoid
Myxedema

Neurohypophysis
Pheochromocytoma
Prolactin (PRL)
Syndrome of inappropriate antidiuretic hormone (SIADH)
Thyroid-stimulating hormone (TSH)
Thyroxine
Tropic hormone

The endocrine glands are a unique group of organs that secrete chemical messengers known as hormones. In the endocrine system, there is a set sequence of hormone secretion from organ to organ. In most sequences, the hypothalamic portion of the brain secretes a releasing factor that stimulates the pituitary gland. The pituitary, also called the master gland, has widespread effects on the body. With effects on growth, reproduction, fluid balance, and metabolism, the pituitary is involved in all endocrine organ sequences. After the pituitary is stimulated, it releases a substance referred to as a **tropic hormone** that targets an endocrine organ. The target endocrine organ then secretes a hormone that acts on the body and causes a physiologic effect. The sequence of endocrine organ function is termed the hypothalamic-pituitary-hormonal axis.

Endocrine gland hormones include thyroxine, **cortisol,** epinephrine, growth hormone (GH), parathyroid hormone (PTH), and antidiuretic hormone (ADH). These well-known hormones keep the body in homeostatic balance and are kept in check by a unique endocrine feedback system. After the appropriate physiologic action by the target organ is achieved, the endocrine system can shut off the effect. Conversely, the endocrine system keeps the sequence cycling if the target organ action is not achieved.

When the endocrine system dysfunctions, there is an imbalance of hormones that can cause hyperfunction or hypofunction of the target organs. Dysfunction can occur at the hypothalamus, pituitary, or endocrine gland itself. In this chapter, dysfunction of the pituitary, thyroid, adrenal, and parathyroid glands will be discussed. For dysfunction of the pancreas, testes, and ovaries, see the chapters on diabetes, female reproductive systems, and male reproductive systems, respectively.

Epidemiology

Some endocrine diseases are common, such as diabetes mellitus (DM), whereas others, such as pheochromocytoma, are rare (see Chapter 25: Diabetes Mellitus and the Metabolic Syndrome, for more details on DM). Thyroid disease is another prevalent endocrine disorder, particularly among middle-aged women. The thyroid is in control of the body's metabolism and has widespread effects on multiple body systems. Hypothyroidism occurs in 4.6% of the population in the United States. Iodine is an integral constituent of thyroid hormone. In areas of the world where iodine deficiency is prevalent, the number of individuals with thyroid disease is much higher. Worldwide, approximately 1 billion people are at risk for hypothyroidism because of iodine deficiency.

Like the thyroid, the adrenal gland, which secretes cortisol, has widespread effects on the body. Cushing's syndrome, a disorder caused by an excess of cortisol, has been estimated at 13 cases per 1 million individuals per year in the United States. Of these cases, approximately 70% are caused by a pituitary **adrenocorticotropic hormone (ACTH)**-secreting tumor, 15% to an adrenal gland tumor, and another 15% caused by administered corticosteroids or a cancerous lesion that secretes ACTH. Females are affected more often than males, with an incidence of 5 to 1. The average age of those affected is between 25 and 40 years old.

In contrast, Addison's disease, a hypofunction of the adrenal gland, is rare. The reported incidence of Addison's disease is 5 or 6 cases per million per year in the

United States. More females are affected with Addison's disease, with a female to male ratio of 3 to 1. There are numerous causes of hypoadrenalism, including malignancy and infectious disease. It can occur in persons of any age, but it is most common in people aged 30 to 50 years old.

Pituitary dysfunction is uncommon, and symptoms can be gradual and subtle. Because the pituitary is the master gland that controls all other endocrine functions, when it becomes dysfunctional it sets off multiple endocrine abnormalities. The annual incidence of pituitary neoplasms varies from 1 to 7 cases per 100,000 population worldwide. A pituitary neoplasm is the most common type of intracranial tumor.

Basic Concepts of Endocrine Function

There is a unique relationship between the hypothalamus, pituitary, and endocrine glands. The hypothalamus, the coordinating center of the endocrine system, consolidates signals derived from thoughts, feelings, autonomic function, environmental cues, and peripheral endocrine feedback. The hypothalamus secretes a releasing factor that delivers precise signals to the pituitary gland. In turn, the pituitary gland releases a specific tropic hormone that stimulates a specific endocrine target organ. The regulatory link between the hypothalamus, pituitary gland, and endocrine target organ is the **hypothalamic-pituitary-hormone axis;** this fundamental control system exists with all endocrine organs. The pituitary, also called the **hypophysis,** has two distinct sections: The anterior pituitary is called the **adenohypophysis** and the posterior pituitary is referred to as the **neurohypophysis.** The hypothalamus and pituitary gland are in communication with each other via specialized neurovascular tissue called the hypothalamus-hypophyseal portal system.

The Pituitary as Master Gland

The pituitary, a pea-sized organ located in the center of the brain, is called the master gland because it regulates all the body's endocrine glands. It can be compared with a dispatcher because, in response to a signal from the hypothalamus, it releases one of its many tropic hormones. The anterior pituitary secretes **growth hormone (GH), prolactin (PRL),** adrenocorticotropic hormone (ACTH), **thyroid-stimulating hormone (TSH),** follicle-stimulating hormone (FSH), and luteinizing hormone (LH). The hypothalamus synthesizes ADH and oxytocin (OXT), which are stored and released by the posterior pituitary. ADH is also called arginine vasopressin (AVP), and GH is also called somatotropin.

The Feedback System

As a result of pituitary stimulus, an endocrine gland secretes a specific hormone. After the hormone is secreted,

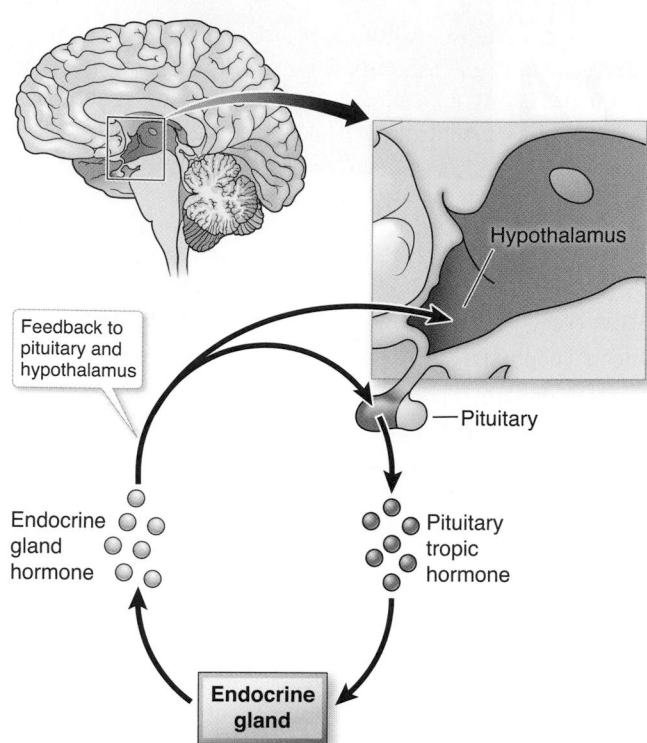

FIGURE 24-1. The hypothalamic-pituitary-endocrine gland axis feedback mechanism.

the pituitary senses the level in the bloodstream. This unique feature of the endocrine gland is called a feedback system (see Fig. 24-1). The pituitary interprets the level of hormone as normal, high, or low and then responds by either rereleasing the tropic hormone or ceasing tropic hormone release, thereby maintaining a normal hormone level. Feedback control, both negative and positive, is a fundamental feature of the endocrine system. Negative feedback regulates each of the hypothalamic-pituitary-hormone axes, a process that maintains hormone levels within a narrow range.

For example, when an individual is running in a marathon, the hypothalamus receives signals from the body that the muscles and organs have extra metabolic needs. The hypothalamus secretes corticotropin-releasing factor (CRF), which stimulates the pituitary gland. The pituitary gland secretes ACTH which, in turn, stimulates the adrenal gland to secrete the hormone cortisol. As cortisol levels in the bloodstream rise, the pituitary senses the increased level and shuts off the stimulus to the adrenal gland; this is an example of the endocrine negative feedback system.

The Regulation of Endocrine Gland Receptors

Pituitary hormones act on receptors located on endocrine glands to secrete hormones. The reactions of the receptors on endocrine glands vary depending on the amount of stimulation by these pituitary hormones. For instance, prolonged, excessive stimulation of an endocrine gland often results in receptor insensitivity and may decrease its number of receptors in a process known as a downregulation of receptors. Conversely, upregulation of receptors is an increase in the number of receptors and their sensitivity. The most common reason for upregulation is a reduction in the receptor stimulation by hormones. An example of downregulation occurs when an individual takes an excessive, prolonged dose of glucocorticoid drugs. The pituitary senses the high blood level of glucocorticoids and, as a result, it does not need to secrete ACTH. There is no need to stimulate the adrenal gland because natural glucocorticoids are unnecessary; the body is receiving more than enough exogenous glucocorticoids. As a result, the adrenal gland downregulates its receptors and becomes less sensitive to ACTH stimulation.

Basic Pathophysiologic Concepts of Endocrine Dysfunction

Endocrine dysfunction occurs when the hypothalamus-pituitary-hormone axis is disrupted. Endocrine disease can be divided into three major types of conditions:

1. hormone deficiency
2. hormone excess
3. hormone resistance.

Most examples of hormone deficiency occur because of glandular destruction caused by autoimmunity, infection, inflammation, infarction, or tumor infiltration. The endocrine cells are damaged and cannot synthesize any hormone. An example is autoimmune destruction of the pancreatic islet cells in type 1 DM. Damaging autoantibodies render pancreatic cells nonfunctional, which results in complete insulin deficiency.

Syndromes of hormone excess are mainly caused by tumor growth, autoimmune disorders, or genetic mutations that cause excessive function of endocrine cells. For example, Graves' disease is an autoimmune disease that causes overproduction of thyroid hormone. In this disease, autoantibodies form that mimic TSH. These autoantibodies excessively stimulate the thyroid gland to release elevated levels of thyroxine. Elevated thyroxine causes multiple systemic effects, such as atrial fibrillation, tremulousness, hot flashes, and muscle weakness.

Hormone resistance syndromes are mainly caused by genetically inherited defects that produce dysfunctional membrane receptors. These disorders are characterized by defective hormone action at the receptor despite the presence of elevated hormone levels. A common example of resistance to a hormone is type 2 DM. Despite the pancreatic secretion of high levels of insulin, cells throughout the body are insensitive to insulin in this type of diabetes.

Types of Endocrine Dysfunction

Endocrine gland dysfunction can be divided into two categories: hypofunction and hyperfunction. Hypofunction of an endocrine gland occurs when there is an inadequate amount of hormone secreted by the gland. Hyperfunction of an endocrine gland occurs when there is an excessive amount of hormone secreted by the gland.

Dysfunction of an endocrine gland can be caused by any of the organs in the hypothalamus-pituitary-hormone axis. Endocrine gland hypofunction or hyperfunction can be caused by the hypothalamus, pituitary, or the endocrine gland itself. Hypothalamic or pituitary origin of endocrine dysfunction is uncommon. When the endocrine dysfunction is caused by the pituitary, it means that the pituitary is either excessively secreting its tropic hormone or releasing insufficient tropic hormone. If the etiology of the disorder lies with the endocrine gland itself, then the gland is secreting either excessive or insufficient amounts of hormone. Endocrine gland disorders are commonly caused by an autoimmune, inflammatory, neoplastic, or vascular disease of the gland.

Endocrine dysfunction can also be referred to as a primary, secondary, or tertiary disorder:

- Primary disorder: dysfunction caused by the endocrine gland itself.
- Secondary disorder: dysfunction caused by abnormal pituitary activity.
- Tertiary disorder: dysfunction caused by a hypothalamic origin.

For example, if an individual has hypothyroidism because of autoimmune destruction of the thyroid gland itself, this would be a case of primary hypothyroidism. If hypothyroidism occurs because of lack of secretion of TSH by the pituitary gland, this would be a case of secondary hypothyroidism. If hypothyroidism occurs because of lack of secretion of releasing factor by the hypothalamus, this would be a case of tertiary hypothyroidism.

Role of Autoimmunity in Endocrine Dysfunction

Many endocrine disorders occur because of autoimmunity, which itself occurs when the body manufactures antibodies against its own tissues. The cause for these autoantibodies is unknown, but they trigger inflammation in organs they target. In the endocrine system, autoimmunity can cause either hypofunction or hyperfunction of the gland.

Role of Neoplasia in Endocrine Dysfunction

Another common cause of endocrine dysfunction is neoplasia, or tumor formation. Tumors can be a source of excess hormones and cause hyperfunction of the gland. They can also interfere with hormone production and cause hypofunction. A pituitary tumor can cause dysfunction in multiple organs because of the wide array of endocrine glands under its control.

 CLINICAL CONCEPT

Pituitary tumors can cause such problems as growth disturbances, electrolyte imbalances, and infertility. They classically cause visual disturbances because of their proximity to the optic chiasm in the brain.

Some cancers cause development of paraneoplastic disorders. These are disorders where, for an unknown reason, the cancer cells have the ability to secrete an endocrine hormone; for example, specific types of lung cancer often secrete ACTH.

Assessment

To evaluate a patient for an endocrine disorder, the clinician needs to perform a complete history and physical examination, as well as specific types of diagnostic studies. The patient's risk factors, present symptomatology, and physical signs of disease are key parts of the complete assessment. Symptoms commonly involve multiple body systems, and a high index of suspicion is needed.

The patient's complaints regarding the present illness are most important in the history, as endocrine disorders often cause a change in metabolic function that may present in subtle ways. Also, endocrine symptoms overlap with signs of other diseases that can confound the clinical picture. For example, in hyperthyroidism, the patient's chief complaint may be heart palpitations, which can lead to multiple cardiovascular diagnostic procedures versus thyroid investigation.

When symptoms are multisystemic, the clinician should look at the whole patient picture and recognize that an endocrine disorder may cause a syndrome, a constellation of symptoms from different systems. Symptoms reported by the patient from different body systems are often part of one endocrine gland dysfunction syndrome. Thyroid diseases, for example, are exhibited by abnormalities of the cardiovascular, musculoskeletal, and reproductive systems. Atrial fibrillation, nervousness, hot flashes, muscle weakness, and menstrual irregularities constitute some of the changes that occur in hyperthyroidism. These symptoms arise from dysfunction of different body systems and may be mistakenly treated separately instead of as one syndrome.

Endocrine dysfunction commonly has an effect on mood and behavior as well. Often the presenting symptoms are misinterpreted as emotional or psychological distress. In hypothyroidism, for example, the patient may describe lack of energy and excessive sleepiness, which is often misinterpreted as depression.

Family history is also very important because many endocrine disorders are genetic in origin. Thyroid disease, for example, is often seen among members of the same family. Diabetes is also familial.

Occupational and environmental exposures are also key pieces of information. Many chemical compounds are endocrine disruptors that interfere with pathways within the endocrine system. Over-the-counter and prescription medications, as well as possible toxic exposures, should be reviewed.

Risk Factors

Each endocrine gland has different risk factors for dysfunction, but major risk factors for endocrine disease include genetic predisposition, radiation exposure, medications, and pollutants.

Genetic predisposition is a known risk factor for many endocrine disorders, particularly thyroid disorders. For example, Graves' disease, hyperfunction of the thyroid, is more common in individuals with *6p* and *20q* mutations.

Radiation exposure has been strongly linked to endocrine disorders. Radiation can trigger cancerous transformation of cells in the body; for example, irradiation of the head and neck, particularly in childhood, increases the susceptibility to thyroid cancer later in life.

Many medications can increase an individual's susceptibility to endocrine dysfunction. Lithium, phenothiazines, and glucocorticoids are some examples that affect the pituitary and adrenal glands.

Pollutants in the environment that cause endocrine gland dysfunction are being increasingly recognized. These substances, called endocrine disruptors, include environmental contaminants such as heavy metals, drug metabolites, and organic hydrocarbon compounds (see Box 24-1).

BOX 24-1. Endocrine Gland Disruptors

Endocrine disruptors, also referred to as hormonally active agents, are manmade substances in the environment that interfere with the natural hormones in the body. These agents are widely dispersed in the environment and are shown to accumulate in the body. One endocrine disruptor under intense investigation is bisphenol A (BPA), which is commonly found in plastic bottles such as water bottles and baby bottles; dental materials; and the linings of metal food cans. Studies have found that BPA can exert estrogenlike effects on males and females. Laboratory animals exposed to low levels of BPA have elevated rates of diabetes, mammary and prostate cancers, decreased sperm count, reproductive problems, early puberty, obesity, and neurological problems.

Signs and Symptoms

To diagnose an endocrine disorder, the clinician needs to be vigilant of physical manifestations of hormone deficiency or excess. Most endocrine organs are not easily accessible on physical examination. The most accessible endocrine gland is the thyroid, and commonly a small lesion is nonpalpable. Astute clinical skills and knowledge of the patient's baseline level of health are important because endocrine abnormalities can be difficult to distinguish from nonspecific physical findings; for example, a patient with the hyperadrenalism of Cushing's disease may present with excessive body fat, striae, hypertension, and muscle weakness. These findings on physical examination may not be distinguished as signs of a single endocrine disorder.

Diagnosis

Immunoassays or blood levels of hormones are the most important diagnostic tool in endocrine disorders. Most hormone measurements are based on samples of blood plasma.

Urinary hormone levels are useful for some conditions. Urinary collection over 24 hours often can provide useful information in the analysis of metabolic function. With any urinary collection, a measurement of urine creatinine is needed to provide information about the patient's renal function. A 24-hour urine cortisol level is an example of a test that provides a measurement of biologically active hormones.

The normal ranges of hormones are commonly affected by gender, age, or circadian rhythm. Cortisol values increase 5-fold between midnight and dawn, female reproductive hormones vary with the menstrual cycle, and estrogen and testosterone levels vary according to age.

Suppression tests are used when endocrine hyperfunction is suspected. An example is the dexamethasone suppression test, which is used to diagnose Cushing's syndrome. Dexamethasone, a potent corticosteroid, is administered and should decrease the adrenal gland's activity. If the dexamethasone does not suppress adrenal secretion of cortisol, the adrenal gland is hyperactive.

Stimulation tests such as the ACTH stimulation test are commonly used to assess endocrine hypofunction. The ACTH stimulation test assesses the adrenal gland response in patients suspected of adrenal insufficiency.

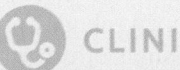 CLINICAL CONCEPT

Normally, the adrenal gland should be stimulated by ACTH, but a hypofunctioning adrenal gland will not be stimulated by administration of ACTH.

Ultrasound is commonly used to investigate thyroid masses. The thyroid specifically binds to iodine for synthesis of thyroxine, and radioactive iodine uptake is used for thyroid imaging. Fine needle aspiration biopsy is commonly used when investigating thyroid nodules. Computed tomography (CT) and magnetic resonance imaging (MRI) are used to investigate tumors or masses in all endocrine organs.

Treatment

Hormone replacement therapy is used with hormone deficiency. Most common replacement treatments include glucocorticoids, thyroid hormone, sex steroids, GH, and vasopressin (also called ADH). Dosage schedules attempt to mimic physiologic hormone production.

Suppression of hormone overproduction is accomplished medically or surgically. An example of medical suppression involves the use of bromocriptine, a dopamine agonist, in pituitary prolactinomas. Surgical procedures are used to excise growths or tumors of endocrine organs. Transsphenoidal surgery, a procedure that uses the sphenoid sinus to gain access to the pituitary gland, is used in removal of pituitary tumors. Radiation is used either as a primary therapy or as an adjunct treatment in endocrine tumors. Radioactive iodine ablation therapy is commonly used in hyperfunctioning thyroid disease. For specific information on diagnostic studies and treatment, see the sections on specific disorders as they are covered in this chapter.

Pathophysiology of Selected Endocrine Disorders

Each endocrine gland disorder can be categorized according to its hypoactivity or hyperactivity. Epidemiology, etiology, pathophysiology, clinical presentation, and treatment all differ according to which gland is dysfunctioning and whether the gland is secreting either a low amount of hormone or excessive amount of hormone.

Pituitary Gland Disorders

The pituitary gland, as the master gland, affects many different organ systems when it is dysfunctional. The side effects of the gland's dysfunction vary according to the individual's age. Growth defects are the major problem in children, whereas in adults there are a wide number of organ disorders.

Hypopituitarism

Hypopituitarism, also known as pituitary insufficiency, is the hyposecretion of one or more of the pituitary hormones. In the United States, approximately 2 to 8 in 100,000 adults per year present with symptoms attributed to pituitary tumors. Congenital hypopituitarism occurs very rarely, affecting approximately 1 in 3,500 infants per year.

Etiology. There are many possible etiologies for hypopituitarism, including pituitary tumor, complications following brain surgery, or radiation of a brain tumor. Complete and sudden loss of pituitary function is most often caused by trauma, ischemia, infarction, or hemorrhage. Sheehan's syndrome is pituitary ischemia and infarction that develops after childbirth because of severe hemorrhage. Empty sella syndrome, a condition caused by compression of the pituitary gland by brain tissue herniation, is also a cause of hypopituitarism. Panhypopituitarism, a rare disorder, is the complete loss of all the pituitary hormones.

Pathophysiology. There are many different tropic hormones secreted by the pituitary gland; therefore, dysfunction of the gland can cause multisystemic problems. Hormones secreted by the anterior pituitary include the following:

- Thyrotropin, or TSH
- Gonadotropins, or FSH and LH
- Somatotropin, or GH
- Corticotropin, or ACTH
- Prolactin or PRL.

The posterior pituitary does not produce its own hormones; it stores hormones. The hypothalamus produces anti-diuretic hormone (ADH) (also referred to as AVP) and oxytocin (OXT). These two hormones are released into the hypothalamic-hypophyseal tract to the posterior pituitary, where they are stored. From the posterior pituitary they are released into the circulation when needed.

In hypopituitarism, tropic hormone production is reduced and, in turn, target gland hormone production is decreased. Normally, low levels of target gland hormone feedback to the pituitary gland increases tropic hormone production. However, in hypopituitarism, the pituitary gland is dysfunctional and the response is absent or inadequate. This results in secondary failure of the target endocrine glands.

Some cases of congenital hypopituitarism are associated with mutations in the *PIT1, LHX3,* and *LHX4* genes. Mutations in these genes cause multiple pituitary hormone deficiencies, leading to lack of GH, PRL, and TSH. The lack of these hormones causes bodywide effects, such as growth failure, weakness, diminished muscle mass, poor bone density, poor memory, and depression. In women, amenorrhea, infertility and deficient lactation also occur.

In adults, a pituitary adenoma is the most common cause of hypopituitarism. A pituitary adenoma is a benign, epithelial neoplasm that can compress pituitary tissue or interfere with the delivery of hypothalamic hormones to the pituitary gland. The etiology of the adenoma is unknown.

Another intracranial tumor associated with hypopituitarism is a craniopharyngioma. This is a benign neoplasm that can develop close to the pituitary gland or in the pituitary stalk. It causes pressure on the pituitary gland, which renders the gland nonfunctional.

Sheehan's syndrome, which can occur after childbirth, is another cause of hypopituitarism. During pregnancy, the pituitary gland enlarges because of hyperplasia and hypertrophy of the cells that produce prolactin (PRL). PRL is the hormone that stimulates lactation in the postpartum period. When there is a large loss of blood during childbirth or afterward in the postpartum period, the pituitary can become ischemic. The hemorrhage severely reduces blood supply to the pituitary, causing ischemia, infarction, and necrosis of the gland. The degree of necrosis correlates with the severity of the hemorrhage. Women who suffer Sheehan's syndrome develop widespread endocrine gland failure because of the many tropic hormones that originate in the pituitary. Because ACTH, TSH, FSH, LH, ADH, and PRL are diminished; the effects of Sheehan's syndrome include adrenal insufficiency, hypothyroidism, amenorrhea, diabetes insipidus (DI), and inadequate lactation.

Pituitary apoplexy is the sudden destruction of the pituitary tissue caused by infarction or hemorrhage into the gland. Traumatic brain injury is the most common cause, but it can occur in patients with DM, pregnancy, sickle cell anemia, anticoagulation, or increased intracranial pressure.

Empty sella syndrome, another cause of hypopituitarism, occurs when the meningeal membrane that surrounds the brain herniates into the sella turcica, a bony area where the pituitary gland sits in the brain. The herniation of this membrane flattens the pituitary against bone and pituitary insufficiency results. Empty sella syndrome can be caused by increased intracranial pressure, radiation, or trauma.

In some physiologic or psychological conditions, hypothalamic function can be impaired, thereby decreasing stimulation of the pituitary. Poor nutrition can reduce the hypothalamic secretion of gonadotropin-releasing hormone (GnRH) which, in turn, decreases stimulation of pituitary secretion of follicle-stimulating hormone (FSH) and lutenizing hormone (LH). Other causes of hypothalamic dysfunction include excessive stress, emotional disorders, changes in body weight, habitual exercise, anorexia, bulimia, heart failure, renal failure, and certain medications.

Clinical Presentation. The signs and symptoms of pituitary insufficiency are dependent upon which tropic hormones are not secreted. The symptoms are secondary endocrine gland deficiencies. For example, if a pituitary adenoma interferes with ACTH secretion, secondary adrenal insufficiency symptoms develop. These symptoms include severe hypotension, weakness, and weight loss. The onset of hypopituitarism is often gradual over a period of years, but rapid onset can occur. The most serious concerns are adrenal insufficiency, hypothyroidism, and **diabetes insipidus (DI),** the last of which occurs because of lack of posterior pituitary secretion of ADH.

The problems that arise because of hypopituitarism depend upon the age of onset. The infant mainly exhibits growth failure. Clinical presentation in the neonate and infant include dwarfism, developmental delay, various visual and neurological symptoms, seizure disorder, and a number of congenital malformations.

Adults with hypopituitarism have different clinical manifestations according to the specific hormones that are deficient. Adults often exhibit gradual symptoms of hypothyroidism, adrenal insufficiency, and ADH deficiency. The clinical presentation may be weakness, weight loss, and hypotension caused by adrenal insufficiency; or weight gain, sluggishness, and depression caused by hypothyroidism. Lack of ADH causes excessive urination and dehydration, a syndrome known as DI.

When hypopituitarism is acute, the patient presents in a rapidly deteriorating state of hypotension, severe dehydration, neurological deficits, and abnormalities in electrolyte levels, glucose levels, body temperature, and heart rate.

Diagnosis. Hypopituitarism causes low tropic hormone levels and, as a result, low corresponding endocrine organ hormone levels in the bloodstream. Hypothalamic releasing factors normally stimulate the pituitary to secrete tropic hormones; however, in hypopituitarism, there is no response from the pituitary. The diagnosis is made by finding low serum levels of pituitary tropic hormones, such as TSH, ACTH, FSH, LH, GH, PRL, and ADH, and low corresponding endocrine organ hormones, such as thyroxine (T4), cortisol, and estrogen.

The corticotropin stimulation test, which evaluates the hypothalamic-pituitary-adrenal axis, can distinguish hypopituitarism from primary adrenal insufficiency. This test measures serum cortisol levels before and after administration of ACTH. Normally, the cortisol level should rise 30 to 60 minutes after ACTH administration in those with normal adrenal function. A low cortisol level that fails to rise after ACTH administration is seen in primary adrenal insufficiency.

CT and MRI scan are also used, particularly when pituitary tumor or empty sella syndrome is suspected. Imaging studies are interpreted in combination with serum levels of tropic hormones.

Treatment. Treatment for hypopituitarism varies depending on which tropic hormones are lacking. Hormone replacement and surgical excision of tumor, if present, are the treatment measures.

Diabetes Insipidus

DI is a disorder of hypopituitarism that originates in the posterior pituitary, also called the neurohypophysis. The disorder involves ADH, and there are two categories of disease: central DI, which occurs because of a lack of secretion of ADH from the posterior pituitary, and nephrogenic DI, which occurs when the kidney fails to respond to ADH.

Central DI is uncommon in the United States, with a prevalence of 4 cases per 100,000 population. Nephrogenic DI is less common, with a prevalence of 0.4 per 100,000 persons, and can be inherited as an X-linked

disorder; it can also be acquired because of medications or renal disease.

Etiology. The etiology of central DI includes tumors such as craniopharyngiomas or head trauma that causes injury of the posterior pituitary or the hypothalamichypophyseal tract. Other causes include pituitary surgery, inflammatory disorders, infection, or exposure to chemical toxins. Nephrogenic DI is often caused by nephrotoxic drugs such as lithium, obstructive uropathy, ischemia of the kidney, hypokalemia, or hypocalcemia.

Pathophysiology. Whether there is decreased ADH secretion from the posterior pituitary gland or an insensitive ADH receptor in the kidney, the same pathophysiologic process occurs. The nephron does not perform antidiuresis, meaning that the nephron does not reabsorb water from the tubule fluid. As a consequence, the body loses high amounts of water in the urine, causing polyuria and highly dilute urine. The bloodstream loses water, which concentrates its sodium content, causing hypernatremia, polyuria, dilute urine, and dehydration.

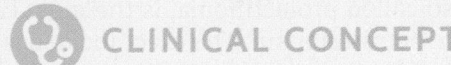

CLINICAL CONCEPT

A syndrome known as psychogenic polydipsia can present similarly to DI. In psychogenic polydipsia, the patient drinks excessive amounts of water and therefore has excessive, very dilute urine.

Clinical Presentation. The symptoms associated with DI, regardless of etiology, are those of dehydration and hypernatremia. The patient will report frequent urination and thirst. In addition, because of dehydration, neurological problems can occur, including confusion, disorientation, myoclonus, seizures, and, in severe cases, coma. These neurological changes are potentially reversible with adequate hydration and hormone replacement.

Diagnosis. Differentiating DI from other causes of polyuria requires blood glucose testing, as well as analyzing urine for glucose, specific gravity, osmolality, and sodium. It is necessary to obtain serum osmolality and sodium levels at the same time urinary testing is performed. Central DI can be distinguished from nephrogenic DI by the administration of ADH. If the kidney responds to ADH, then the problem is lack of secretion of ADH by the posterior pituitary, and the diagnosis is central DI. If administration of ADH does not concentrate the urine, then the kidney is resistant to ADH, and the diagnosis is nephrogenic DI.

To distinguish psychogenic polydipsia from DI, patients must be put on fluid restriction. If after fluid restriction urine osmolality is increased, the disorder is psychogenic polydipsia; however, following fluid restriction, if polyuria and a dilute urine still occur, the diagnosis is DI, either central or nephrogenic.

> **ALERT!** Because polyuria and dehydration occur in both DM and DI, it is important to measure serum glucose to differentiate DM from DI. Serum glucose is elevated in DM, but not in DI.

Treatment. The treatment for central DI is administration of ADH. Surgical treatment of some pituitary causes of DI may be required. Supportive treatment measures and the use of nonsteroidal anti-inflammatory agents (NSAIDs) are used for the patient with nephrogenic DI. Indomethacin, an NSAID, has been successful in nephrogenic DI, though the mechanism is unclear.

Hyperpituitarism

Hyperpituitarism, or primary hypersecretion of pituitary hormones, is rare in children and adults. Pituitary adenoma is the most common cause of hyperpituitarism. The adenoma is often a tumor producing either PRL, ACTH, TSH, or GH, though a PRL-producing adenoma, also called prolactinoma, is the most common cause of hyperpituitarism. The exact incidence of prolactinomas in the general population is not clearly established. In some research studies, the tumor accounts for approximately 25% to 30% of all pituitary adenomas, with the highest incidence in females younger than 20 years old.

A GH-secreting pituitary adenoma is rare. Incidence is estimated to be 3 to 4 cases per million population per year in the United States. In children, a GH-secreting tumor causes gigantism, whereas in adults, it causes acromegaly.

Pathophysiology. A pituitary adenoma is caused by a genetic mutation on chromosome 11q13 in 15% to 40% of cases. Most pituitary adenomas secrete a specific hormone that produces a characteristic clinical presentation. Overall, prolactinomas are the most common pituitary adenoma encountered in childhood; they cause symptoms secondary to excess PRL, which causes antiestrogenic and antiandrogenic effects. In the female, menstrual abnormalities, amenorrhea, galactorrhea, vaginal dryness, and osteopenia occur. In males, hypogonadism, decreased libido, erectile dysfunction, and infertility occur. The prolactinoma can also cause symptoms secondary to the space-occupying effects of the tumor itself. Large tumors can cause headache, dizziness, and visual disturbances because of proximity to the optic nerve chiasm. The tumor can also compress pituitary tissue, reducing the gland's ability to secrete other hormones.

In children, ACTH-producing adenomas, also called corticotropinomas, are commonly observed before puberty, although they occur in people of all ages. They are more prevalent in females. The tumor secretes

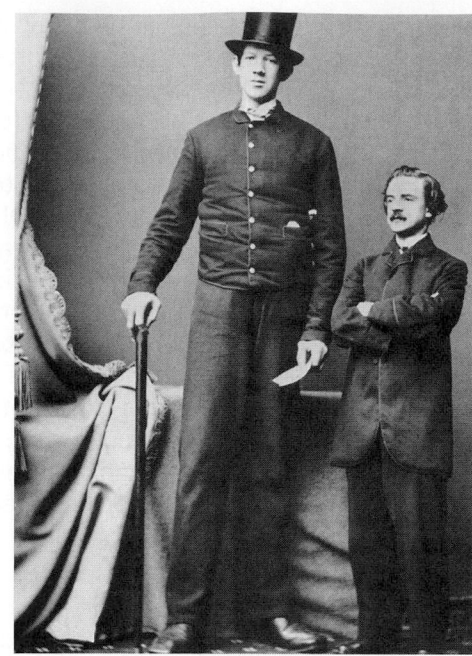

FIGURE 24-2. Gigantism of hyperpituitary function. *(From Science Source.)*

excessive ACTH that stimulates excess cortisol secretion from the adrenal gland. The affected individual has all the features of Cushing's syndrome, which is covered later in this chapter.

GH-secreting adenomas, also called somatotropinomas, are uncommon but can cause gigantism in children (see Fig. 24-2). In children, GH stimulates the growth plates of long bones, which results in excessive longitudinal growth. The affected individual grows to heights of 7 feet or more. The individual often suffers from other endocrine or genetic conditions that negatively impact overall health. Gigantism can occur as an isolated disorder or it can be a feature of other conditions such as multiple endocrine neoplasia (MEN) type 1, McCune-Albright syndrome, neurofibromatosis, or tuberous sclerosis.

In adults, excessive GH stimulates a gradual growth of certain bones such as the jaw, hands, and feet called **acromegaly.**

Clinical Presentation. Prolactinoma is the most common type of pituitary adenoma. Most pediatric cases occur in adolescence, predominately in females. Females with these tumors present with amenorrhea and galactorrhea, whereas males present with gynecomastia and hypogonadism. Somatotropinomas are rare but cause gigantism in children. Individuals exhibit tall stature, moderate obesity, large hands and feet, coarse facial features, cardiac hypertrophy, and endocrine disorders such as hypogonadism, diabetes, and hyperprolactinemia.

In adults, excess GH results in acromegaly. Symptoms of acromegaly develop slowly and gradually, taking years to decades to become apparent (see Fig. 24-3). Signs include overgrowth of the jaw and facial bones;

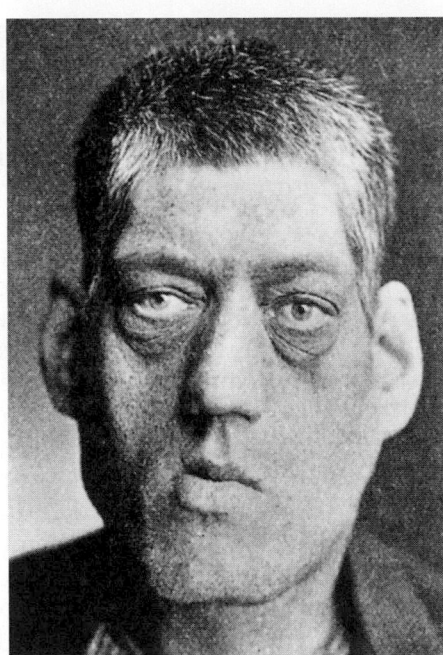

FIGURE 24-3. Acromegaly from hyperpituitary function. *(From SPL/Science Source.)*

enlarged hands and feet; organ overgrowth, including tongue enlargement (macroglossia) and hypertrophy of the heart, thyroid, liver, and kidneys; insulin resistance; and increased risk of colon polyps. The patient may also suffer the effects of the pressure of the pituitary tumor against brain tissue, which can result in headaches and visual impairment.

ACTH-secreting adenomas often present in pre-pubescent children. ACTH stimulates the adrenal gland to produce excess cortisol, and the presentation is called Cushingoid appearance. The signs include obesity; stunted growth; swollen face, called moon facies; acne; ruddy complexion; hirsutism; fat in the posterior neck area, called buffalo hump; and striae, also known as stretch marks. TSH-secreting adenomas are rare but can present with signs and symptoms of hyperthyroidism, including nervousness, tremulousness, palpitations, weight loss, visual disturbances, headaches, and hyper-sensitivity to heat.

Diagnosis. Hyperpituitarism causes high tropic hor-mone levels and, as a result, high corresponding en-docrine organ hormone levels in the bloodstream. The diagnosis is made by finding high serum levels of pituitary tropic hormones, particularly GH and PRL. Other tropic hormones, such as ACTH and TSH, and corresponding endocrine organ hormone levels can also be high. CT and MRI scans are used when pituitary tumor is suspected. Imaging studies are interpreted in combination with serum levels of tropic hormones.

Treatment. Treatment requires medications that block GH and surgical excision of any pituitary tumor. In pro-lactinoma, bromocriptine is a medication that blocks secretion of PRL and can shrink tumors. For treatment

of corticotropin-secreting pituitary tumors, transsphe-noidal surgery is usually required with medication. Adrenal enzyme inhibitors, such as ketoconazole, are prescribed to block formation of adrenal hormones. In somatotropin-secreting tumors, a medication called oc-treotide is used to suppress excessive growth-hormone secretion. A dopamine agonist, such as bromocriptine, is used in addition to octreotide to shrink tumors. Alternatively, a GH receptor antagonist, Pegvisomant, has shown some success when used for 3 months.

Syndrome of Inappropriate Antidiuretic Hormone

Syndrome of inappropriate antidiuretic hormone (SIADH) secretion is a common condition in patients who sustain brain injury or those who undergo neu-rosurgery for brain disorders. The syndrome is char-acterized by hyponatremia and hypo-osmolality of the blood that result from excessive secretion or action of ADH.

Epidemiology. Acute brain injury is one of the most common triggers of SIADH, though few studies have demonstrated the exact incidence or prevalence of the disorder. However, in one investigation of patients with traumatic brain injury and subarachnoid hemorrhage, 5% of patients demonstrated SIADH after surgery.

Etiology. There are numerous causes of SIADH, includ-ing nervous system disorders such as stroke and meningitis, neoplastic causes such as lung and colon cancer, and pulmonary diseases such as emphysema and pneumonia. SIADH can also be drug-induced or a side effect of brain surgery or brain injury.

Pathophysiology. ADH is synthesized by the hypo-thalamus and transmitted via nerve tracts to the posterior pituitary, where it is stored and secreted. Essential for fluid balance in the body, ADH stimulates reabsorption of water at the collecting duct of the nephron. SIADH causes excess water reabsorption into the bloodstream. This excess water creates hyper-volemia, dilutional hyponatremia and highly concen-trated urine.

Clinical Presentation. Patients with SIADH may com-plain of symptoms related to fluid volume overload and hyponatremia, including fatigue, weakness, confusion, and headache. The physical examination of the hypona-tremic patient may be normal, but if hyponatremia is severe or rapid in onset, findings include myoclonus, slowed reflexes, seizures, problems with gait and bal-ance, nystagmus, dysarthria, dysphagia, and coma.

Diagnosis. To diagnose SIADH, measurements of sodium, electrolytes, and water of the blood and urine are most important. Diagnostic tests include urine-specific gravity, urine osmolality, hematocrit, and plasma osmolality. In SIADH, hyponatremia, elevated urine osmolality, excessive urine sodium, and decreased serum osmolality are found.

Treatment. Treatment of SIADH requires slow replacement of sodium and excretion of water. Furosemide, which increases excretion of free water, has been used along with hypertonic saline in severe cases. Older tetracycline antibiotics have a unique nephrogenic DI effect and can be used to counteract SIADH. ADH receptor antagonists, such as conivaptan or tolvaptan, can also be used.

Thyroid Disorders

The thyroid gland is a 2-inch, butterfly-shaped gland located in the neck. The hormones of the thyroid gland, triiodothyronine (T3) and **thyroxine** (T4), have a wide range of physiologic effects. Thyroxine is the regulator of body metabolism, which influences almost every body system. Thyroid dysfunction presents as either hypothyroidism or hyperthyroidism, both of which are more likely in women than men. The thyroid is easily examined, but normally should not be palpable in the neck. An enlarged thyroid can occur in hypofunction or hyperfunction. Primary thyroid disorders, where the thyroid gland itself is dysfunctional, are the most common type of disease.

Goiter

A **goiter** is an enlargement of the thyroid gland with or without symptoms of thyroid dysfunction. When there are no symptoms of thyroid disease, the enlargement is referred to as a nontoxic goiter. Excess pituitary TSH can stimulate enlargement of the thyroid gland and cause goiter formation. Alternatively, if iodine levels are decreased in the body, thyroid hormone synthesis is diminished. Iodine is a necessary component in the synthesis of thyroid hormone. Low iodine levels cause low thyroid hormone manufacture, which the pituitary senses and then attempts to compensate for by increasing TSH, which incites goiter formation.

 CLINICAL CONCEPT

Iodine deficiency is a problem for many persons in developing countries. It is estimated that across the world 1 billion persons are at risk for iodine deficiency.

Enlargement of the thyroid gland can also occur from **goitrogens,** which are foods or other substances that promote thyroid gland enlargement. Goitrogens are in medications such as lithium, phenytoin, and rifampin. When individuals take these medications, thyroid hormone levels need to be monitored.

Hypothyroidism

Hypothyroidism occurs when there are insufficient levels of the thyroid hormones T3 and T4. Primary hypothyroidism, where the thyroid gland itself is not secreting T3 and T4, is the predominant type of hypothyroidism, affecting approximately 95% of patients. In a minority of individuals, secondary hypothyroidism is the cause, where the pituitary is not secreting sufficient TSH; this, in turn, causes low T3 or T4 synthesis.

Epidemiology. Hypothyroidism occurs in approximately 4% of the population per year in the United States. The frequency of hypothyroidism, goiters, and thyroid nodules increases with age. Approximately 6% of women and 2.4% of males older than age 60 have hypothyroidism; in addition, as many as 20% of adults over age 80 have some form of hypothyroidism. Generally, thyroid disease is much more common in females than males, with prevalence reports of 2 to 10 times higher in females. Caucasians have a higher incidence of hypothyroidism than African Americans. Lymphocytic thyroiditis (also called Hashimoto's thyroiditis) is the most common cause of hypothyroidism. The postpartum period is particularly a time of high incidence of thyroiditis, with 10% of women suffering the disorder in the 2 to 12 months after pregnancy.

Etiology. Hypothyroidism is a common endocrine disorder resulting from deficiency of thyroid hormone. It usually is a primary process in which the thyroid gland produces insufficient amounts of thyroid hormone. Hashimoto's thyroiditis, an autoimmune disorder, is the most common cause of hypothyroidism. Risk factors include age older than 50 years, female gender, pregnancy, autoimmune disease, radiation to the neck, family history, and certain drugs, including radioactive iodine, amiodarone, interferon alpha, interleukin, and lithium.

Pathophysiology. Hashimoto's thyroiditis occurs from autoimmune destruction of the thyroid gland. Biopsy of thyroid tissue reveals a high number of lymphocytes in the thyroid gland. There are TSH receptor antibodies present as well. When these antibodies bind to the TSH receptor, there is an absence of the normal response of T3 and T4 synthesis and secretion. Other antibodies associated with this condition include antithyroglobulin antibody and antithyroperoxidase antibody. Antithyroperoxidase (anti-TPO) antibodies are the hallmark of the disorder.

Hypothyroidism may also occur as a congenital condition. Cretinism is the result of thyroid hormone deficiency during embryonic development and early neonatal life. The child exhibits short stature, intellectual disability, and other metabolic disorders. The incidence of this is 1 in 5,000 in the Caucasian population and 1 in 32,000 in the African American population.

Clinical Presentation. Adult patients with hypothyroidism take on an altered appearance because of a combination of factors. Reduction in the conversion of carotene to vitamin A causes hypercarotenemia, which gives skin a yellow-orange tint. A puffy face occurs because of accumulation of sodium and water from protein/polysaccharide complex deposits. A characteristic hoarse voice also develops.

Lack of thyroid hormone causes a decrease in the body's various metabolic activities. Reduced levels of low-density lipoprotein (LDL) receptors in the liver lead to elevations in cholesterol and triglycerides. Anemia occurs from decreased hematopoiesis. Reduced kidney function causes decreased clearance of medications and increased susceptibility to drug toxicity. Alterations in pulmonary function leads to hypercapnia and hypoxia. Over time, an increased risk of cardiomegaly develops. The longer the hypothyroid condition lasts, the more profound the effects.

The effects of the reduced levels of T3 and T4 are seen in all body systems. Constitutional symptoms include cold intolerance, weight gain, lethargy, and fatigue. Other symptoms include memory deficits, poor attention span, muscle cramps, constipation, decreased fertility, puffy face, hair loss, and brittle nails (see Fig. 24-4). In the adult, severe hypothyroidism is called **myxedema.**

Subclinical hypothyroidism, which is common in elderly individuals, can cause subtle neuropsychiatric problems such as disorientation, depression, and pseudodementia (see Box 24-2 for more details).

Diagnosis. Diagnosis of hypothyroidism requires a TSH blood level. Also, free T3 and T4 levels are necessary. A high TSH level with low T3 and T4 is diagnostic of primary hypothyroidism. There is low hormone secretion by the thyroid gland that constantly signals the pituitary to secrete TSH. Early in hypothyroidism, T3 may be normal; however, free T4 level is low. Blood is also tested for the presence of thyroid autoantibodies referred to as antithyroglobulin (anti-Tg) and antithyroperoxidase (anti-TPO) antibodies. These antibodies indicate autoimmune destruction of the thyroid gland. A high TSH level with normal T3 and T4 levels indicate mild or subclinical hypothyroidism. In secondary

> ### BOX 24-2. Subclinical Hypothyroidism
>
> Subclinical hypothyroidism is a disorder in which thyroid function is only mildly low, so that the blood level of thyroxine (T4) remains within the normal range, but the blood level of TSH is elevated, indicating mild thyroid failure. Individuals can suffer mild symptoms of hypothyroidism such as fatigue, difficulty losing weight, and depression. Subclinical hypothyroidism can be treated with a single daily dose of thyroxine. This treatment requires monitoring of the thyroid hormone levels in the blood over several months. Recent studies suggest that treatment is warranted, especially if the blood TSH level is above 10 mU/L.

hypothyroidism, TSH and T4 will be low because the pituitary gland is the cause of inadequate thyroid function. Most likely, if the pituitary is not secreting TSH, other tropic hormones will also be deficient. A complete blood count, serum metabolic profile, serum creatinine and liver enzymes are needed. Anemia, hyponatremia, and hyperlipidemia are commonly found in hypothyroidism. A PRL level is sometimes elevated in the setting of increased TRH and TSH.

Ultrasound is used to visualize any nodules in the thyroid along with a fine needle biopsy to take tissue samples. However, in hypothyroidism, thyroiditis is usually the etiology without presence of nodules. The use of color Doppler flow ultrasound will demonstrate decreased vascular flow in hypothyroidism.

The American Thyroid Association recommends thyroid screening tests in women at age 35 and every 5 years thereafter; however, other organizations differ in their recommendations. The American College of Physicians recommends screening women aged 50 and older who have one or more clinical features of the disorder.

Treatment. Treatment for primary hypothyroidism includes replacement hormone therapy with levothyroxine and surgical intervention, if necessary.

> **ALERT!** When hypothyroidism is untreated it can progress to myxedema coma, which is a serious illness with a high mortality rate. There are severe hypothyroid symptoms as well as susceptibility to SIADH, hypoglycemia, and hyponatremia. If left untreated, the symptoms will progress to confusion and coma.

Hyperthyroidism

Hyperthyroidism, sometimes referred to as thyrotoxicosis, is an excessive secretion of the thyroid hormones T3 and T4. The most common etiology is **Graves' disease,** an autoimmune stimulation of the thyroid gland.

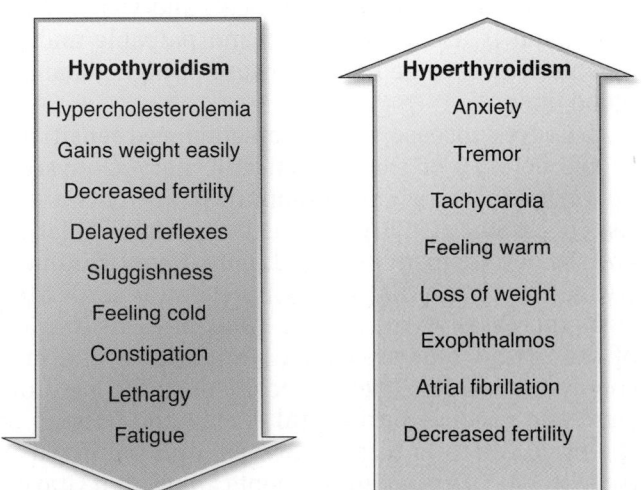

Hypothyroidism	Hyperthyroidism
Hypercholesterolemia	Anxiety
Gains weight easily	Tremor
Decreased fertility	Tachycardia
Delayed reflexes	Feeling warm
Sluggishness	Loss of weight
Feeling cold	Exophthalmos
Constipation	Atrial fibrillation
Lethargy	Decreased fertility
Fatigue	

FIGURE 24-4. Signs and symptoms of thyroid disorder.

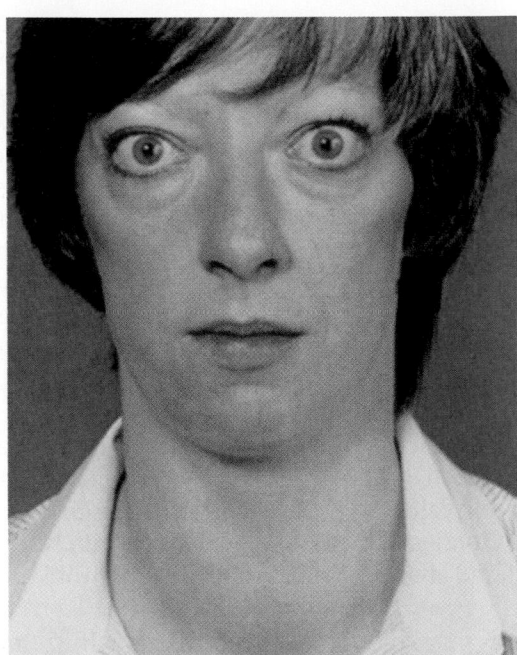

FIGURE 24-5. Graves' ophthalmopathy, also called exophthalmus. Graves' disease is an autoimmune disorder causing hyperthyroidism. The eyes develop an inflammatory disorder that affects the orbit around the eye, characterized by upper eyelid retraction, edema, conjunctivitis, and bulging eyes. *(From Biophoto Associates/Science Source.)*

time. Women are more often affected with Graves' ophthalmopathy than men.

Thyroid dermopathy, also called pretibial myxedema, refers to skin changes in the lower legs. Because of accumulation of glycosaminoglycans, the skin becomes thickened and develops a nonpitting edema. Myxedema can be seen in hypothyroidism or hyperthyroidism.

Diagnosis. To diagnose hyperthyroidism or Graves' disease, blood tests that include TSH, T3, T4, antithyroglobulin, and antithyrotropin receptor antibody are necessary. Ultrasound with color-Doppler evaluation should be performed as a first step in all patients who are hyperthyroid. Radioactive iodine scanning and measurements of iodine uptake are useful in differentiating the causes of hyperthyroidism. In Graves' disease, the radioactive iodine uptake is increased and the uptake is diffusely distributed over the entire gland.

Treatment. Treatment involves ablation of the hyperactive thyroid through the use of antithyroid hormone medication such as propylthiouracil (PTU), radioactive iodine treatment, or surgery. Radioactive iodine is taken up by the gland and suppresses its activity. Alternatively, PTU can suppress the thyroid function or the gland is surgically removed. After the gland is rendered inactive, replacement thyroid hormone (levothyroxine) is needed for life.

Thyrotoxic Crisis

Thyrotoxic crisis, also call thyroid storm, is an intense, overwhelming release of thyroid hormones that exerts an intense stimulus on the metabolism. This is a life-threatening condition most commonly precipitated by surgery, trauma, or infection. Thyrotoxic crisis is a rare disorder. Approximately 1% to 2% of patients with hyperthyroidism progress to thyrotoxic crisis. Patients typically have high fever, tachycardia, nausea and vomiting, tremulousness, agitation, and psychosis. Late in the progression of disease, patients may become stuporous or comatose with hypotension. Diagnostic and treatment procedures are similar to those for hyperthyroidism.

> **ALERT!** Thyrotoxic crisis is a medical emergency. Heart failure and pulmonary edema can develop rapidly and cause death.

Thyroid Nodules

Most thyroid nodules are asymptomatic, but they can cause hypothyroidism or hyperthyroidism. Individuals with thyroid nodules will occasionally report complaints of dysphagia, dysphonia, and pain caused by the structural pressure created by the nodule.

A single thyroid nodule is associated with an increased risk of malignancy, whereas multiple nodules are often benign, though the presence of any nodule must be carefully evaluated to rule out neoplastic disease (see Box 24-3). A TSH assay, T3, and T4 levels are needed. Antithyroperoxidase antibody and antithyroglobulin antibody tests are needed.

Ultrasound-guided fine needle aspiration biopsy is the most useful diagnostic test to rule out a malignant thyroid nodule. A technetium scan, using a radioactive isotope, is also used to differentiate malignant from benign nodules. The technetium scan identifies nodules as hot, warm, or cold according to their uptake of radioactive isotope. A hot nodule is a hyperfunctioning tumor, a warm nodule indicates normal tissue, and a cold nodule is hypofunctional tissue that is sometimes malignant. Surgical intervention is the treatment for a thyroid nodule that is malignant or obstructive.

> ### BOX 24-3. Characteristics Associated With Malignant Thyroid Nodule
>
> Factors suggesting a malignant thyroid nodule include the following:
>
> - Age younger than 20 years or older than 70 years
> - Male sex
> - Associated symptoms of dysphagia or dysphonia
> - History of neck irradiation
> - Firm, hard, or immobile nodule
> - Presence of cervical lymphadenopathy.

Parathyroid Gland Disorders

The parathyroid glands are four pea-sized glands nestled within the thyroid tissue of the neck. The glands produce and secrete PTH in response to a low serum calcium level. PTH promotes calcium reabsorption in the renal tubules and the release of calcium from bone. It also promotes vitamin D production by the kidney, which helps to maintain normal calcium levels within the body. Many of the effects seen in parathyroid disorders are related to alterations in calcium levels.

Hypoparathyroidism

Hypoparathyroidism is a very rare disorder. The etiology of primary hypoparathyroidism most often is trauma or inadvertent damage or removal of the parathyroid glands during thyroid surgery. However, neck irradiation, autoimmune disease, many different genetic disorders, and metal toxicity can cause primary parathyroid gland insufficiency. Fetal alcohol syndrome and many other congenital disorders can also cause diminished parathyroid gland function. Secondary hypoparathyroidism, which is the lack of pituitary parathyroid-stimulating hormone, can occur because of any primary disease that causes hypercalcemia. The high calcium levels send feedback to the pituitary gland to diminish parathyroid-stimulating hormone.

The symptoms associated with hypoparathyroidism are the result of insufficient PTH secretion and the resultant decrease in serum calcium levels. There is often a concomitant increase in phosphate levels, because low PTH lessens phosphate excretion by the kidney.

The most serious symptoms of primary hypoparathyroidism are the result of low levels of calcium. The patient can present with muscle cramps, irritability, tetany, and convulsions. Hypocalcemia also causes a carpal spasm known as Trousseau's sign and facial muscle twitch called Chvostek's sign. Diagnostic tests include serum PTH, calcium, phosphate, and vitamin D levels. Treatment includes replacement of PTH and normalizing serum calcium and vitamin D levels.

Hyperparathyroidism

Hyperparathyroidism is excessive secretion of PTH that affects calcium homeostasis in the body. The prevalence has been reported to be approximately 21 cases per 100,000 persons annually. The average age of those affected is between 52 and 56 years, and women are affected more often than men.

Pathophysiology. In approximately 85% of cases, primary hyperparathyroidism is caused by an adenoma. The growth in the parathyroid gland causes excessive secretion of PTH with resulting high levels of calcium in the blood. Any disorder that causes hypocalcemia can cause stimulation of the parathyroid gland and resultant hyperparathyroidism.

Clinical Presentation. The systemic effects of hyperparathyroidism are related to excessive levels of calcium.

The most common effects of hypercalcemia include muscle weakness, poor concentration, neuropathies, hypertension, kidney stones, metabolic acidosis, osteopenia, pathological fractures, and constipation. Neuropsychiatric manifestations are also common and may include depression, confusion, or subtle cognitive deficits. Increased calcium can increase gastric acid secretion, and persons with hyperparathyroidism may have a higher prevalence of peptic ulcer disease. Physical examination findings are usually insignificant. Examination may reveal muscle weakness and depression. A palpable neck mass is not commonly found.

Diagnosis. Blood testing for PTH levels is required for diagnosis. An elevated PTH level with an elevated ionized serum calcium level is diagnostic of primary hyperparathyroidism. A radiolabeled sestamibi scan and ultrasound are also used to detect parathyroid tumors.

Treatment. Treatment involves reducing elevated serum calcium levels through the use of diuretics, calcitonin, and bisphosphonates. Vitamin D should also be administered. Surgical intervention is also frequently needed.

Adrenal Gland Disorders

The adrenal gland consists of two parts: the cortex and medulla. The cortex secretes corticosteroids, also called glucocorticoids; androgens; and mineralocorticoids, mainly aldosterone. The medulla secretes epinephrine and norepinephrine. Corticosteroids, mainly cortisol, assist the body in dealing with stress; they stimulate gluconeogenesis to increase blood sugar, mobilize fat stores, and break down proteins. However, long-term secretion of corticosteroids has negative effects on the body, such as suppression of the immune system and breakdown of bone. **Mineralocorticoids** from the adrenal gland, mainly aldosterone, assist in fluid and electrolyte balance. As in other endocrine feedback systems, a pituitary hormone stimulates the adrenal gland; in turn, the hypothalamus stimulates the pituitary. Hypothalamic CRF provokes pituitary ACTH, which in turn stimulates the adrenal gland. Disorders of the adrenal gland mainly consist of adrenal overactivity or adrenal insufficiency. The major disorder of adrenal overactivity is Cushing's syndrome, whereas the most common disorder of adrenal insufficiency is Addison's disease.

Adrenal Insufficiency

Adrenal insufficiency can occur because of decreased ACTH from the pituitary gland or dysfunction of the adrenal gland, causing decreased cortisol secretion. Primary adrenal insufficiency, which is failure of the adrenal glands, is also called **Addison's disease.** This rare disorder, with a prevalence of 39 to 60 cases per million people, most often occurs because of autoimmune destruction of the adrenal glands, which accounts for 80% of cases.

Etiology. Adrenal insufficiency is most commonly caused by autoimmune destruction of the adrenal gland caused by two types of antibodies: adrenal cortex antibodies and antibodies to the steroid enzymes. These antienzyme antibodies prevent the conversion of precursor hormones to the adrenal hormones, potentially leading to adrenocortical failure. Patients with autoimmune adrenal insufficiency may also have autoantibodies to other organs, such as the thyroid gland and gastric parietal cells. This is referred to as autoimmune polyglandular syndrome. Autoimmune adrenal insufficiency may also be associated with pernicious anemia, vitiligo, atrophic gastritis, and alopecia.

Other causes of adrenal insufficiency include tuberculosis of the adrenal gland, adrenal hemorrhage and infarction, human immunodeficiency virus infection, radiation therapy, and surgery. Secondary adrenal insufficiency is often the result of tumors of the pituitary gland or because of prolonged administration of corticosteroid drugs.

Pathophysiology. Gradual autoimmune destruction of the adrenal gland leads to a decreased cortisol response to stress and reduced cortisol reserve. As the glandular destruction increases, there is less cortisol available, and this can lead to adrenal crisis (see Box 24-4).

When patients are administered prolonged corticosteroid treatment beyond 4 to 5 weeks, there is negative feedback suppression of CRH and ACTH. As a result, the adrenal gland can down-regulate its receptors and undergo glandular atrophy. With atrophy, there is a decreased ability to secrete natural cortisol. When corticosteroid therapy is abruptly stopped or there is an episode of severe trauma or stress, the hypothalamic-pituitary-adrenal axis is not able to respond appropriately. The patient will then develop symptoms of adrenal insufficiency; in the case of high stress, surgery, or infection, the patient may develop adrenal crisis (see Fig. 24-6).

ALERT! When administering corticosteroids to patients, the smallest dose should be used for a short period of time. Long-term corticosteroid administration can cause decreased secretion of natural cortisol and atrophy of the adrenal gland.

Clinical Presentation. In primary adrenal insufficiency, both parts of the adrenal gland, the cortex and medulla, secrete deficient amounts of hormones. The adrenal cortex secretes diminished glucocorticoids; mainly cortisol. The adrenal cortex secretes diminished mineralocorticoids, mainly aldosterone. As in other endocrine feedback mechanisms, the pituitary gland senses the low hormone level. The pituitary, in response, secretes ACTH. Uniquely, when ACTH is excessively secreted, melanocyte-stimulating hormone (MSH)

BOX 24-4. Adrenal Crisis

Lack of sufficient levels of corticosteroids in conjunction with increased need because of stress, trauma, infection, or surgery increases the risk of developing an adrenal crisis. Patients will present with severe abdominal pain, high fever, weakness, confusion, nausea, and vomiting. Diagnostic studies will show hyponatremia, hyperkalemia, leukocytosis, and hypoglycemia. This is a life-threatening condition. If not treated appropriately, profound hypotension, organ failure, and coma can occur.

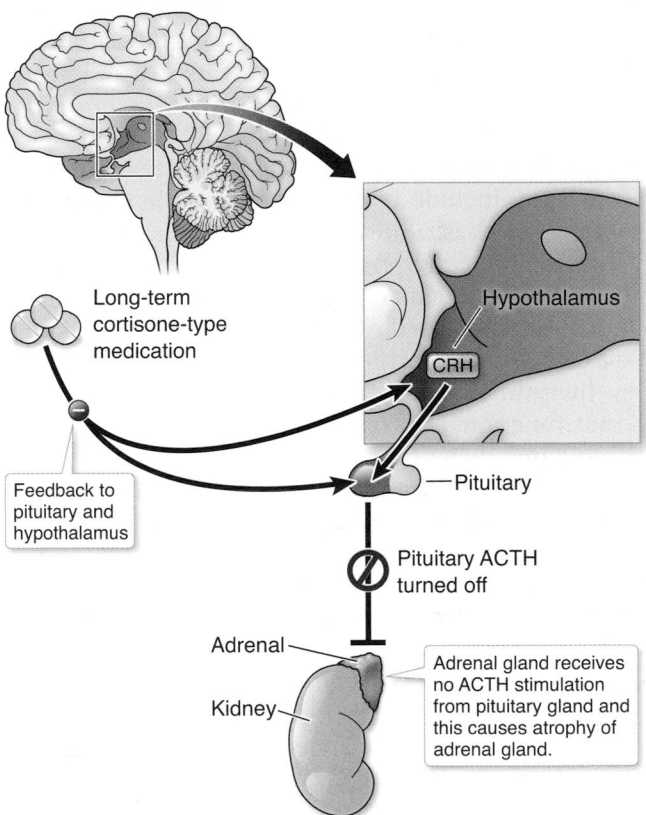

FIGURE 24-6. Effects of excess corticosteroid medications on the adrenal gland. Long-term use of corticosteroids can cause adrenal gland atrophy. (1) Excess corticosteroid medications in the bloodstream will be sensed by the hypothalamus and pituitary gland. (2) The hypothalamus will cease release of corticotropin-releasing hormone (CRH). (3) The pituitary will then not be stimulated by CRH and cease secreting ACTH. (4) The adrenal gland will not receive sufficient stimulation from the pituitary and eventually cells will atrophy.

is triggered as well because both ACTH and MSH have the same precursor. The adrenal gland is provoked, and MSH stimulates melanocytes. The stimulated melanocytes give patients a tanned appearance. However, the stimulated adrenal gland cannot yield sufficient amounts of corticosteroids or mineralocorticoids.

The development of adrenal insufficiency is often gradual. The initial symptoms are nonspecific symptoms of weakness, hypotension, lethargy, easy fatigue, anorexia, nausea, and vomiting. Some patients have episodes of hypoglycemia.

Electrolyte imbalances occur from mineralocorticoid (aldosterone) deficiency. Aldosterone normally functions to stimulate the nephron to reabsorb sodium and water into the bloodstream and excrete potassium. In the absence of aldosterone, these functions do not occur. There is loss of sodium and water with retention of potassium. Patients experience hyponatremia, hyperkalemia, and dehydration. The physiologic response to this electrolyte imbalance is an increase in secretion of ADH by the posterior pituitary. ADH stimulates water reabsorption at the nephron; consequently, this water volume increase predisposes the patient to fluid volume overload.

Other symptoms of adrenal insufficiency include personality changes, inability to concentrate, and emotional lability. In women, there is loss of pubic and axillary hair and amenorrhea.

Diagnosis. Laboratory tests that indicate adrenal insufficiency include hyponatremia and hyperkalemia caused by lack of aldosterone. The rapid ACTH test is used to diagnose adrenal insufficiency by assessing the adrenal cortex's capacity to produce cortisol. The patient is administered ACTH, after which there should be a rise in blood cortisol level to 2 to 5 times its basal level within 15 to 30 minutes. If this occurs, adrenal cortex function is normal; if there is no rise in cortisol, adrenal insufficiency is diagnosed.

Abdominal CT scan may be normal or may show bilateral enlargement of the adrenal glands in patients with Addison's disease because of tuberculosis, fungal infections, adrenal hemorrhage, or infiltrating diseases involving the adrenal glands. Alternatively, adrenal atrophy may be the cause of adrenal insufficiency; this will be apparent on CT scan.

Treatment. The patient needs replacement doses of glucocorticoid and mineralocorticoid daily. This is commonly achieved with 100 mg or more of hydrocortisone per day and 9-alpha-fludrocortisone in doses of 0.05 to 0.10 mg per day or every other day. Patients may need to be advised to increase salt intake in hot weather. Surgery may be necessary if there is an adrenal tumor or mass.

Parenteral steroid coverage should be used in times of major stress, trauma, or surgery and during any major procedure. In stress situations, the normal adrenal gland output of cortisol is approximately 250 to 300 mg in 24 hours. This amount of hydrocortisone should be given, preferably by continuous infusion.

Cushing's Syndrome

Cushing's syndrome, also called hyperadrenalism or hypercortisolism, is an endocrine disorder caused by high levels of cortisol in the blood. There are two terms that connote different sources of hyperadrenalism: Cushing's syndrome and Cushing's disease.

Cushing's disease refers to a tumor of the pituitary gland that produces large amounts of ACTH that results in excessive cortisol production. **Cushing's syndrome** is hyperadrenalism that is caused by a hyperactive adrenal gland that secretes excessive cortisol. Alternatively, excessive cortisol can occur because of certain cancers that secrete inappropriate ACTH or prolonged use of corticosteroid drugs such as prednisone or dexamethasone. Cushing's syndrome is more common than Cushing's disease; the most common source of the syndrome is excessive use of corticosteroid drugs.

Epidemiology. Cushing's syndrome is diagnosed in an estimated 10 to 15 persons per million each year. It is more common in women than in men, with a female-to-male ratio of 8:1. Although it can occur at any age, it is most often seen in people between the ages of 20 and 50 years. It is characterized by excessive levels of glucocorticoids and their physiologic effects.

Etiology. Pituitary adenomas are the most common cause of Cushing's disease. Pituitary adenomas cause excessive secretion of ACTH from the anterior pituitary gland. ACTH then stimulates the adrenal cortex to produce excessive adrenal corticosteroids. If large, the adenoma can put pressure on the pituitary and cause decreased production of other anterior pituitary hormones (TSH, FSH, LH, GH, and PRL) and the posterior pituitary hormone ADH. Nelson syndrome is a disorder caused by a large ACTH-secreting pituitary tumor. It usually occurs in patients who undergo removal of the adrenal glands without pituitary irradiation; the pituitary secretes excessive ACTH in an attempt to raise corticosteroids, but there is no adrenal gland. There is no feedback to the pituitary from the adrenal gland to shut off the ACTH secretion. Cushing's syndrome can occur because of a few different etiologies. The syndrome can be caused by adrenal neoplasms, which include adrenal adenoma, adrenal carcinoma, and adrenal hyperplasia. The Carney complex is a genetic disorder that includes hyperplasia of the adrenal gland, which causes Cushing's syndrome. McCune-Albright syndrome is a rare cause of hyperfunction of the adrenal glands that leads to Cushing's syndrome and precocious puberty. Cushing's syndrome can also be caused by secretion of ACTH from tumors of the lung or other cancers. Ectopic ACTH is commonly secreted by oat cell or small-cell carcinoma of the lung or by carcinoid tumors.

Administration of exogenous steroids can lead to the development of Cushing's syndrome. Cushing's syndrome symptoms can occur with the administration of oral, injected, or inhaled steroids. This is likely the most common cause of Cushing's syndrome; however, many cases are not reported and prevalence is unknown.

Pathophysiology. Patients with Cushing's disease have diffuse hyperplasia of the cells of the anterior pituitary, which is responsible for the production and secretion of ACTH. The hyperplasia may be caused by excess secretion of CRH by the hypothalamus or because of an adenoma of the pituitary. The constant secretion of ACTH stimulates hyperplasia of the adrenal glands. Interestingly, the precursor of ACTH is also the precursor of MSH, which causes melanin pigmentation of the skin.

Under normal conditions, there is a circadian rhythm of ACTH secretion; throughout the day, ACTH and cortisol rise and fall in a predictable pattern. However, this pattern is absent in Cushing's disease. Instead, ACTH secretion is excessively released in a random pattern. Also, the negative feedback signal to the pituitary is blunted with persistently high ACTH levels.

In times of stress, ACTH is released; this stimulates adrenal secretion of cortisol. In response to stress, there should be a spike in the level of ACTH. However, in Cushing's disease, ACTH is excessive, yet there is no rise in ACTH level in response to stress. Therefore, patients with Cushing's disease need to be carefully monitored for complications associated with lack of appropriate ACTH secretion in response to stressors such as trauma, surgery, or infection. For example, the patient with Cushing's disease undergoing surgery may need to have ACTH or cortisol administered preoperatively.

In Cushing's syndrome caused by an adrenal tumor, cortisol secretion is also random and episodic. However, there is an intact negative feedback response by the pituitary. The pituitary gland senses excessive levels of cortisol, leading to reduced ACTH production. The reduced ACTH stimulus of the adrenal gland often causes atrophy of the adrenal gland.

Clinical Presentation.

The clinical features of cortisol excess are initially subtle, but easily recognizable when the patient's pictures from several years ago are compared with the patient at present. Weight gain is evident, with a redistribution of body fat to the face, trunk, and abdomen. Patients develop a characteristic rose-colored, puffy face called "moon facies," as well as extra subcutaneous fat in the cervicothoracic area called "buffalo hump." There is an increase in the waist-to-hip circumference ratio, with apple-shaped fat distribution. Over time, the patient develops *Acanthosis nigricans*, or a darkening of the skin at friction sites such as under the breasts, the belt line, and the neck. Increased subcutaneous fat deposits, particularly in the abdomen, lead to the development of purple stretch marks called striae. There is easy bruising and poor wound healing. Women will also demonstrate hirsutism, which is male pattern hair growth.

Elevated cortisol levels are associated with enhanced gluconeogenesis, which is glucose production by the liver. Cortisol also blocks the action of insulin, decreasing the body's utilization of glucose, which means that the patient will have hyperglycemia.

Additionally, excess cortisol inhibits bone formation and accelerates bone reabsorption, which leads to the development of osteopenia, osteoporosis, and an increased risk of bone fracture.

Cortisol's anti-inflammatory effects suppress the normal response to infection and injury. This occurs from reduced formation of inflammatory mediators such as thromboxanes, prostaglandins, and prostacyclins. Cortisol also suppresses the formation of antibodies and inhibits the migration of white blood cells (WBCs) to sites of inflammation. These effects immunosuppress the patient with Cushing's syndrome.

Patients with elevated cortisol levels often have elevated blood pressure, though the mechanism is unclear. It may be caused by excess sodium and water retention or increased vascular responsiveness to catecholamines (see Fig. 24-7).

Diagnosis.

The laboratory abnormalities associated with Cushing's syndrome include elevated WBC count greater than 11,000/mm^3, hyperglycemia, and hypokalemia. High cortisol levels cause elevated WBCs, glucose release from the liver, and a mineralocorticoid effect at the kidney causing potassium excretion. The diagnosis of Cushing's syndrome caused by overproduction of cortisol requires the demonstration of inappropriately high blood or urine cortisol levels. Diagnostic

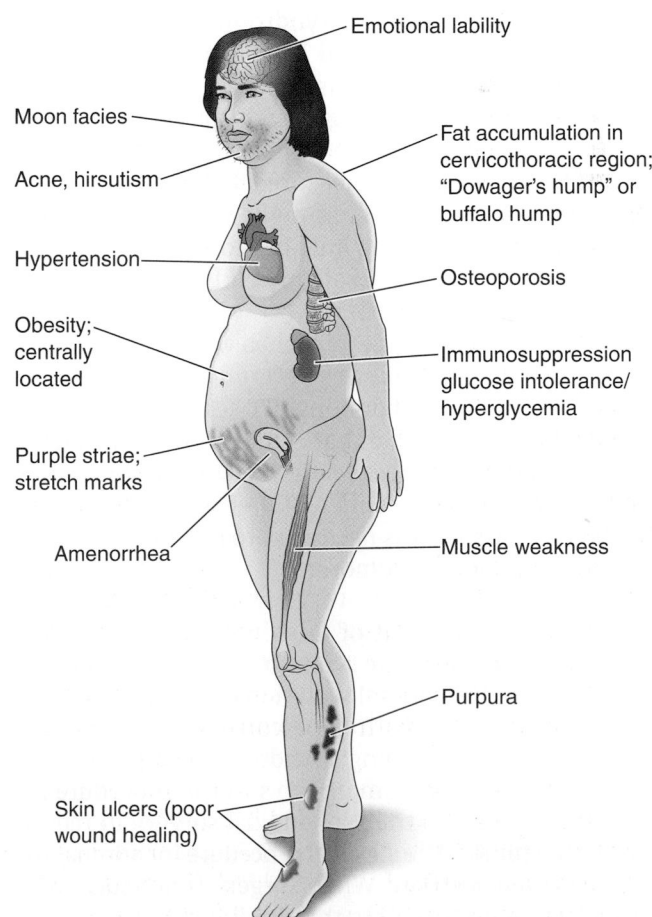

FIGURE 24-7. The widespread effects of Cushing's syndrome.

tests include 24-hour urinary, blood, and salivary cortisol levels, which should all show an excess level of cortisol in Cushing's syndrome.

The dexamethasone suppression test is administered to test the interactions of the hypothalamic-pituitary-adrenal axis. The test requires administration of 1 mg of dexamethasone at 11 p.m. with subsequent measurement of cortisol level at 8 a.m. In healthy individuals, the serum cortisol level should be suppressed at a level lower than 1.8 mcg/dL. However, in Cushing's syndrome, there is no suppression of cortisol and a high level, greater than 3 mcg/dL, is present.

When results from the dexamethasone suppression test cannot confirm diagnosis of Cushing's syndrome with certainty, the dexamethasone-CRH test is administered. It combines a 48-hour dexamethasone suppression test with CRH stimulation. Dexamethasone is given 8 times starting at 8 a.m. throughout 2 days. Then, CRH is administered intravenously 6 hours after the last dose of dexamethasone. Plasma cortisol and ACTH levels are obtained at 15-minute intervals for 1 hour. In healthy individuals, there should be no cortisol in the blood at first, but then an increase in cortisol parallel to ACTH level should occur. However, an elevated cortisol value unrelated to ACTH and greater than 1.4 mcg/dL identifies Cushing's syndrome. The problem is caused by an adrenal source of excessive cortisol.

Salivary cortisol level measurement is another laboratory test for Cushing's syndrome. It is a practical test that can be completed by the patient at home, whereas other laboratory tests require hospitalization. The saliva is collected at night by the patient over a few nights as designated by the clinician. The cortisol content of the saliva is then measured. In healthy patients, the salivary cortisol level at night should be at a low level of fewer than 1.3 ng /mL. In those with Cushing's syndrome, a high level of salivary cortisol, greater than 1.3 ng/mL, will be present.

Once the diagnosis is established with the laboratory tests, the next step requires determining the etiology by imaging studies. Abdominal CT scan of the adrenal glands and a contrast-enhanced MRI of the pituitary may reveal the presence of a tumor. Octreotide scintigraphy can rule out ectopic ACTH-secreting tumors in the body. Chest x-ray is necessary to rule out an ACTH-secreting pulmonary tumor.

Treatment. Treatment of Cushing's syndrome is directed by the cause of the syndrome. In general, therapy should reduce the cortisol secretion to normal to reduce the risks associated with hypercortisolism. The treatment of choice for Cushing's syndrome is surgical resection of the causative tumor. The surgical procedure for Cushing's disease is transsphenoidal surgery to reduce a pituitary tumor. The surgical procedure for adrenal tumors is adrenalectomy. When surgery is not successful or cannot be used, agents that inhibit steroidogenesis such as ketoconazole have been used.

Pheochromocytoma

Pheochromocytoma is an extremely rare tumor of the adrenal medulla that secretes norepinephrine and epinephrine, also referred to as catecholamines. The etiology of pheochromocytoma tumors is unknown; however, they cause excessive stimulation of alpha-adrenergic and beta-adrenergic receptors in the body. The symptoms caused by overstimulation of adrenergic receptors include severe hypertension, tremors, increased cardiac contractility, cardiac arrhythmias, and elevated heart rate. A pheochromocytoma is associated with a hypertensive crisis that is characterized by severely elevated blood pressure, altered mental status, focal neurological signs and symptoms, and seizures. Possible neurological complications include stroke caused by cerebral infarction or intracerebral hemorrhage. Collection of a 24-hour urine that is analyzed for an excessive amount of catecholamine metabolites is the most useful diagnostic test. An MRI of the abdomen to visualize the adrenal gland is also necessary. Surgical removal of the tumor and adrenergic blocker medications are treatment measures.

Multiple Endocrine Neoplasia

There are several syndromes of MEN, but the most common is called MEN 1. MEN 1 is caused by a defective tumor suppressor gene at *11q13* that allows tumor growth in several different endocrine glands. The endocrine glands most frequently involved are the parathyroid gland, pituitary gland, and pancreas. Parathyroid tumors cause excessive bone breakdown with resulting hypercalcemia and osteopenia. Pancreatic islet cell tumors called insulinomas and gastrinomas occur in 75% of the patients. These tumors lead to disturbed glucose metabolism, gastric hyperacidity (Zollinger-Ellison syndrome), peptic ulcer disease, and diarrhea. The effects seen from pituitary adenomas are related to excessive secretion of GH, PRL, and ACTH. The clinical presentation of MEN depends on the specific hormone that is secreted excessively. Although the symptoms do not often appear until the patient is about 40 years of age, abnormal hormone levels may be seen as early as age 14 years. Surgical removal of tumors, medical antagonists of the excess hormones, and supportive therapies are treatment measures.

Pineal Gland Dysfunction

The pineal gland is a neuroendocrine gland located in the brain near the hypothalamus. This gland contains sympathetic neurons that travel to the retina. Upon stimulation, the pineal gland converts sympathetic input into hormonal output by producing melatonin with the phases of the light-dark cycle. The gland releases melatonin with darkness, which facilitates sleep. Pineal tumors represent about 1% of all brain tumors in adults. A pineal tumor is mainly problematic because of the pressure it places on adjacent brain tissue. They often compress parts of the brain that drain cerebrospinal fluid (CSF), causing a buildup of pressure called hydrocephalus. Symptoms include headache, nausea and vomiting, seizures, memory disturbances, and visual changes. Hydrocephalus can be treated by placement of a ventriculo-peritoneal shunt, which is a long tube placed within one of the CSF-containing spaces of the brain; it is then passed under the skin to the abdominal cavity to provide a pathway for CSF drainage and absorption in the abdomen.

Chapter Summary

- The endocrine system is made up of glands that produce and secrete hormones.
- The endocrine feedback mechanism is the most important and unique property of the system.
- Hormones are regulated by the pituitary gland and hypothalamus. The hypothalamus secretes releasing factors that stimulate the pituitary. The pituitary secretes tropic hormones that stimulate a target endocrine gland to secrete its hormone. As the level of this hormone rises in the circulation, the hypothalamus and the pituitary gland shut down secretion of their hormones, which in turn slows the secretion by the target gland. This mechanism is disrupted in endocrine disorders and results in either hyperfunction or hypofunction of the gland.
- The pituitary gland is called the master gland because it controls all the endocrine glands.
- The pituitary gland secretes GH, TSH, ACTH, PRL, FSH, and LH.
- When an endocrine gland dysfunctions, the condition is a primary disease. For example, a tumor of the thyroid gland that secretes excessive hormone is a primary disorder of the thyroid gland.
- When the pituitary gland dysfunctions, the problem is a secondary disease. For example, ACTH deficiency causes adrenal insufficiency secondary to pituitary dysfunction, or termed secondary adrenal insufficiency.
- Hyperpituitarism of the child will cause gigantism, excessive growth of the long bones and organs, whereas hyperpituitarism of the adult causes acromegaly, which results in coarsening of facial features; enlarged jaw, hands, and feet; and organ dysfunction.
- A pituitary adenoma that secretes PRL is the most common type of pituitary tumor.
- Hypopituitarism of the posterior pituitary causes DI, which is a lack of ADH that causes polyuria, dehydration, and thirst. ADH is also referred to as AVP.

- Excessive secretion of ADH by the posterior pituitary causes syndrome of inappropriate ADH (SIADH), which causes hypervolemia, dilutional hyponatremia, and edema.
- Hypothyroidism, commonly caused by Hashimoto's thyroiditis, causes classic signs of cold sensitivity, sluggishness, excessive fatigue, weakness, weight gain, constipation, slowed mentation, and depression.
- Myxedema coma occurs because of long-standing, untreated hypothyroidism and has an associated mortality rate of 30% to 40%.
- Hyperthyroidism, commonly caused by Graves' disease, causes classic signs of heat sensitivity, weight loss, tremulousness, palpitations, insomnia, and ophthalmoplegia.
- Thyroid storm, also called thyrotoxic crisis, is a severe discharge of thyroid hormone triggered by infection or stress, which can cause hypertension, heart failure, and pulmonary edema.
- Adrenal gland hyperactivity causes high cortisol levels, which presents as Cushing's syndrome—a classic presentation of moon facies, buffalo hump, obesity, hirsutism, and striae.
- Adrenal insufficiency causes Addison's disease, which classically presents with loss of weight, weakness, and severe hypotension.
- Adrenal crisis is a life-threatening condition that causes profound weakness, severe abdominal pain, fever, and shock.
- Pheochromocytoma is a rare tumor of the adrenal medulla that secretes epinephrine and causes hypertensive crisis and cardiac arrhythmias.
- MEN 1 is a disorder caused by tumor growth in the parathyroid, pancreas, and pituitary glands.
- Pineal gland tumors compress adjacent brain tissue, causing buildup of CSF, visual disturbances, seizures, and headache.

Making the Connections

Disorder and Pathophysiology	Signs and Symptoms	Physical Assessment Findings	Diagnostic Testing	Treatment
Hypopituitarism | Low pituitary hormones such as low ACTH, GH, TSH, FSH, or LH, commonly caused by a pituitary adenoma.				
	In child: dwarfism and small stature. In adult: deficiency of many tropic hormones causes a wide variety of endocrine gland deficiency symptoms.	In child: short stature or mental retardation. In adult: a variety of findings, depending on tropic hormone deficit.	The corticotropin stimulation test evaluates the hypothalamic-pituitary axis. ACTH is administered to assess its effect on the adrenal gland. A normal result causes elevated cortisol and decreases ACTH. If ACTH is high, there is a disorder of hyperpituitarism. CT and MRI may show mass or pituitary enlargement.	GH replacement and other tropic hormones are used, if deficient. Replacement needed for life.
Diabetes Insipidus | Lack of ADH from the posterior pituitary, which causes lack of water reabsorption at the nephron and consequent water loss.				
	Polydipsia (thirst). Polyuria.	Signs of dehydration: poor skin turgor, low BP, concentrated urine, and dry mucous membranes.	Low ADH level. CT/MRI scan of head looks for pituitary tumor.	Replacement hormone treatment is given with AVP.
Hyperpituitarism | High pituitary hormones, often caused by tumor, commonly prolactinoma, which secretes excess PRL; this hormone stimulates lactation.				
	In child: gigantism and organomegaly. In adult: acromegaly, which has subtle symptoms of coarsening of facial features; if prolactinoma is present, symptoms include gynecomastia, galactorrhea, amenorrhea, headache, or visual disturbances caused by tumor near the optic chiasm.	If tumor is prolactinoma: galactorrhea, amenorrhea, visual impairment, may have high blood pressure, arrhythmias, and thyroid or adrenal enlargement, depending on the hormone excess.	Measurements of tropic hormones such as ACTH, PRL, FSH, LH, or TSH to look for elevations of levels of any pituitary hormones. CT and MRI scans of head are provided to look for pituitary tumor.	Bromocriptine inhibits PRL if prolactinoma is present. Surgery is used for pituitary tumor.

Continued

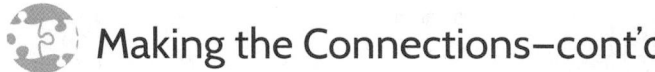

Making the Connections–cont'd

Disorder and Pathophysiology	Signs and Symptoms	Physical Assessment Findings	Diagnostic Testing	Treatment
Syndrome of Inappropriate Antidiuretic Hormone (SIADH) | Excess ADH is caused by brain trauma or a variety of other etiologies. It causes excess water reabsorption at the nephron and consequent dilution of electrolytes such as dilutional hyponatremia.				
	Confusion, seizures, nausea, vomiting.	Patient may have no significant physical findings.	Dilutional hyponatremia is caused by excess water in the bloodstream. Highly concentrated urine is caused by excess reabsorption of water from the nephrons. High ADH level is present. Low serum osmolarity (dilute blood) is present. High urine osmolality (concentrated urine) is present. CT/MRI may show pituitary mass.	ADH antagonists; conivaptan or tolvaptan are used. Furosemide is used to diminish the water content of blood. Tetracyclines can decrease the ADH effect on the kidney. Surgery performed, if warranted.
Hypothyroidism | There is a lack of sufficient thyroid hormone released by the thyroid gland.				
	In child: cretinism. In adult: sluggishness, weight gain, sensitivity to cold, constipation, depression.	Enlarged thyroid or nodule. If myxedema present: puffy face, periorbital edema, interstitial tibial edema.	In primary hypothyroidism, TSH level is high. T3 and T4 are low. There may be thyroid antibodies causing autoimmune disease (called Hashimoto's thyroiditis). Antithyroid peroxidase antibodies are present. Antithyroglobulin antibodies are present. Ultrasound may show mass or cyst. Radioactive iodine scan shows slow function of gland.	Levothyroxine (replacement thyroid hormone). Surgery to remove thyroid if nodule present.
Hyperthyroidism | Excess secretion of thyroid hormone by thyroid gland occurs.				
	Weight loss, sensitivity to heat, palpitations, tremor, nervousness, restlessness, diaphoresis.	Enlarged thyroid or nodule, exophthalmos, tremor, lower limb weakness, atrial fibrillation, audible bruit over thyroid gland caused by high blood flow over gland.	In primary hyperthyroidism, TSH level is low. T3, T4 will be elevated because of hyperactive gland. Thyroid antibodies often cause hyperthyroidism (called	Surgery is used to remove thyroid or radioactive iodine medication is used to ablate the gland. PTU can suppress gland activity.

Continued

Making the Connections—cont'd

Disorder and Pathophysiology	Signs and Symptoms	Physical Assessment Findings	Diagnostic Testing	Treatment
			Graves' disease). Antithyroid peroxidase antibodies are present. Antithyroglobulin antibodies are present. Ultrasound may show mass or cyst. Radioactive iodine scan shows hyperactive gland.	

Adrenal Insufficiency | This condition causes lack of cortisol, which is often caused by autoimmune destruction of the adrenal gland, called Addison's disease.

Disorder and Pathophysiology	Signs and Symptoms	Physical Assessment Findings	Diagnostic Testing	Treatment
	Feeling faint when standing from seated position; weight loss, weakness.	Orthostatic hypotension, tanned appearance.	Elevated ACTH and decreased cortisol, androgen, and aldosterone levels in primary adrenal insufficiency (caused by adrenal gland itself). Hyponatremia and hyperkalemia is caused by low aldosterone. An abdominal CT scan may show mass or atrophy of adrenal gland.	Replacement of ACTH or cortisol depending on cause of hypoadrenal function.

Cushing's Syndrome | Excess cortisol causes characteristic bodily changes.

Disorder and Pathophysiology	Signs and Symptoms	Physical Assessment Findings	Diagnostic Testing	Treatment
	Weight gain in central region of body, puffy face called "moon facies," easy bruising, striae, hirsutism, fat in cervico-thoracic region called "buffalo hump."	Moon facies, buffalo hump, hirsutism, striae, central obesity, high blood pressure, low bone density.	Low ACTH and high cortisol, androgen, and aldosterone levels occur in primary hyperadrenalism. Dexamethasone suppression test shows high natural cortisol levels are nonsuppressible. Dexamethasone–corticotropin-releasing hormone test shows high cortisol despite efforts to suppress it. Elevated 24-hour urine cortisol and catecholamines are present. Abdominal CT scan may show tumor or enlarged adrenal gland.	Surgery performed if adrenal tumor is present. Administration of Ketoconazole suppresses cortisol (mechanism unclear).

Continued

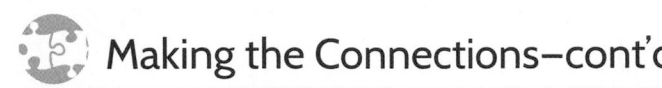

Making the Connections—cont'd

Disorder and Pathophysiology	Signs and Symptoms	Physical Assessment Findings	Diagnostic Testing	Treatment
Hyperparathyroidism | Excess PTH is secreted by the parathyroid, often caused by adenoma.				
	Bone demineralization causing pain, increased fracture risk. Muscle weakness. Hypercalcemia causes constipation.	May not show any physical findings.	High PTH level, hypercalcemia, low bone density, sestamibi scan of parathyroid glands to rule out adenoma. Ultrasound of parathyroid glands to check for cysts, masses, gland enlargement.	Calcium and vitamin D for bone building. Bisphosphonates, which inhibit osteoclast activity. Calcitonin, which inhibits bone breakdown. Increased water intake to prevent kidney stones.
Hypoparathyroidism | There is a lack of PTH secreted by parathyroid glands.				
	Muscle spasms, tetany, seizures.	Chvostek's and Trousseau's sign, which are present in hypocalcemia.	Hypocalcemia caused by lack of PTH. Sestamibi scan and ultrasound to look for masses or cysts of parathyroid glands.	Replacement of PTH.
Pheochromocytoma | Tumor of the adrenal medulla that secretes excess catecholamines: norepinephrine and epinephrine.				
	Palpitations, tremor, altered mental status, seizure, and possible focal neurological signs of stroke such as slurred speech or weakness.	Severe hypertension, tachycardia, cardiac arrhythmias. May have signs of stroke: weakness of an extremity, facial droop, slurred speech.	24-hour urine for catecholamines. CT or MRI scan of abdomen to look for adrenal tumor.	Adrenergic blockers. Surgery to remove tumor.
Multiple Endocrine Neoplasia (MEN) 1 | Tumors are found within endocrine glands; particularly pancreas, parathyroid, and pituitary. Pancreatic insulinoma and gastrinoma are common.				
	Symptoms depend on the endocrine gland affected. Parathyroid tumor causes osteopenia, bone pain, or susceptibility to fractures. Pancreatic tumors can cause excessive gastric acid production, causing ulcer pain or diarrhea. Pituitary tumors cause visual disturbances resulting from pressure on the optic chiasm and may oversecrete PRL, causing galactorrhea or gynecomastia in the male.	Physical findings depend on the endocrine gland affected. Parathyroid tumor causes bone pain and a susceptibility to fractures. Pituitary tumors can cause visual disturbances and may oversecrete PRL, causing galactorrhea or gynecomastia in the male.	Blood levels of hormones commonly involved: PTH, PRL, GH, ACTH. Blood level of gastrin and insulin.	Hormone antagonists, depending on which hormone is oversecreted. Surgery to remove tumors.

Continued

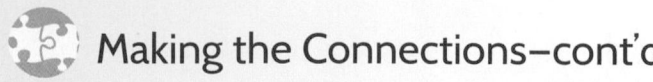 Making the Connections–cont'd

Disorder and Pathophysiology	Signs and Symptoms	Physical Assessment Findings	Diagnostic Testing	Treatment
Pineal Tumor | A neuroendocrine gland that secretes melatonin located near hypothalamus. Enlargement of the gland or tumor places pressure on adjacent brain tissue.				
	Headache, nausea and vomiting, seizures, memory disturbances, and visual changes.	Often there are no physical findings. Disturbed vision may be present.	CT/MRI of head is used to look for tumor.	Surgical removal of tumor. Ventriculo-peritoneal shunt to decrease blockage of CSF.

Bibliography

Barrett, K. E., Boitano, S., Barman, S. M., & Brooks, H. L. (2012). *Ganong's review of medical physiology.* 24th ed. New York: Lange/McGraw-Hill.

Colucci, R., Jimenez, R. E., Farrar, W., et al. (2012). Coexistence of Cushing syndrome from functional adrenal adenoma and Addison disease from immune-mediated adrenalitis. *J Am Ost Assoc,* 112(6), 374–379.

Cooper, D. S., & Biondi, B. (2012). Subclinical thyroid disease. *Lancet,* 379(9821), 1142–1154.

DeHerder, W. W. (2012). Familial gigantism. *Clinics (Sao Paulo),* 67(S1), 29–32. Retrieved from http://www.ncbi.nlm.nih.gov/pmc/articles/PMC3328828/. doi: 10.6061/clinics/2012 (Sup01)06.

Donangelo, I., & Braunstein, G. D. (2011). Update on subclinical hyperthyroidism. *Am Fam Phys,* 83(8), 933–938.

Endocrine-disrupting chemicals: how much of a health threat? (2013, March 2). *Lancet,* 381(9868), 700. doi: 10.1016/S0140-6736(13)60564-4.

Fleseriu, M., & Petersenn, S. (2012). Medical management of Cushing's disease: what is the future? *Pituitary,* Jun 7. Epub ahead of print, vol 15 issue 3 pages 330–341.

Franklyn, J. A., & Boelaert, K. (2012). Thyrotoxicosis. *Lancet,* 379(9821), 1155–1166.

Iglesias, P., & Díez, J. J. (2011). Chronic anemia as first clinical manifestation of a prolactin-secreting pituitary macroadenoma in a male patient. *Am J Med,* 124(6), e3-4.

Klibanski, A. (2010). Clinical practice. Prolactinomas. *N Engl J Med,* 362(13), 1219–1226.

Lake, M. G., Krook, L. S., & Cruz, S. V. (2013). Pituitary adenomas: an overview. *Am Fam Phys,* 88(5), 319–327.

Longo, D. L., Kasper, D. L., Jameson, J. L., et al. (2011). *Harrison's principles of internal medicine.* 18th ed. New York: McGraw-Hill.

Marcocci, C., & Cetani, F. (2011). Clinical practice. Primary hyperparathyroidism. *N Engl J Med,* 365(25), 2389–2397.

McDermott, M. T. (2012). Hyperthyroidism. *Ann Int Med,* 157(1), ITC1–1.

McPhee, S., Papdakis, M., & Rabow, M. W. (2012). *Current medical diagnosis and treatment.* 51st ed. (Lange's Current Series). New York: McGraw-Hill.

Mitka, M. (2012). Endocrine Society seeks better testing to determine endocrine disruptor health risks. *JAMA,* 308(6), 556–557. doi: 10.1001/jama.2012.8816.

Pantalone, K. M., & Nasr, C. (2010). Approach to a low TSH level: patience is a virtue. *Cleveland Clin J Med,* 77(11), 803–811.

Pluta, R. M., Burke, A. E., & Golub, R. M. (2011). *JAMA* patient page. Cushing syndrome and Cushing disease. *JAMA,* 306(24), 2742.

Ponto, K. A., & Kahaly, G. J. (2012). Autoimmune thyrotoxicosis: diagnostic challenges. *Am J Med,* 125(9), S1. doi: 10.1016/j.amjmed.2012.05.011.

Redberg, R. F. (2013). My thyroid story. *JAMA Int Med,* 173(19), 1769. doi: 10.1001/jamainternmed.2013.9279.

Van Durme, C. M., Kisters, J. M., van Paassen, P., van Etten, R. W., & Tervaert, J. W. (2011). Multiple endocrine abnormalities. *Lancet,* 378(9790), 540.

Willard, D. L., Leung, A. M., & Pearce, E. N. (2014). Thyroid function testing in patients with newly diagnosed hyperlipidemia. *JAMA Int Med,* 174(2), 287–289. doi: 10.1001/jamainternmed.2013.12188.

Diabetes Mellitus and the Metabolic Syndrome

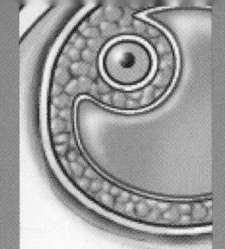

Key Terms

Alpha-glucosidase inhibitors
Amylin
Biguanides
Diabetic ketoacidosis (DKA)
eAG
Gestational diabetes mellitus (GDM)
Glycogenesis
Gluconeogenesis
Glucosuria
Glycated hemoglobin (A1c)
Glycemic index

Glycogenolysis
Hyperglycemia
Hyperinsulinism
Hyperosmolar hyperglycemic syndrome (HHS)
Hypoglycemia
Impaired glucose tolerance (IGT)
Incretin
Insulin
Islets of Langerhans

Ketonemia
Ketonuria
Metabolic syndrome
Oral glucose tolerance test (OGTT)
Postprandial
Prediabetes
Preprandial blood glucose
Postprandial glucose
Sulfonylureas
Thiazolidinediones

Diabetes mellitus (DM), a disorder of carbohydrate metabolism, is characterized by high levels of blood glucose resulting from the body's inability to produce or utilize insulin. The chronic high levels of blood glucose that occur in diabetes predispose the affected individual to cardiovascular disease, renal damage, peripheral vascular disease, and disorders of the eyes and nervous system. Diabetes is a leading cause of blindness, renal failure, and lower extremity amputation.

Because of an increased susceptibility to these long-term complications, there is increased morbidity and mortality among diabetic individuals. The risk of death in persons with diabetes is approximately twice as high as that in individuals who do not have diabetes.

According to the American Diabetes Association (ADA), there are four major categories of DM:

1. type 1
2. type 2
3. gestational diabetes
4. other specific types of diabetes.

The classification of diabetes has changed many times over the years as research has revealed more about the underlying pathological processes involved in this disorder. Each type of diabetes is caused by a different pathophysiologic mechanism and every individual who is diabetic requires an individualized treatment regimen.

Incidence of diabetes has reached epidemic proportions in the United States and is continuing to increase within the population. It is essential that clinicians across all health-care settings understand the pathophysiology of diabetes because they will undoubtedly encounter patients with this disorder.

Epidemiology

In the United States, diabetes affects an estimated 25.8 million people, or approximately 8% of the population. Prevalence increases with age; 26.9% of persons 65 years or older have diabetes compared with 13.7% of those 40 to 59 years old. The incidence of diabetes is increasing worldwide, a trend that has been parallel with a rise in obesity within the population (Fig. 25-1). Obesity and sedentary behavior, which have steadily increased in incidence in the last decade, are major risk factors for diabetes.

Among ethnic groups, Hispanics and African Americans are almost twice as likely to develop diabetes as non-Hispanic Caucasians. Native Americans are 2.2 times as likely to have diabetes as non-Hispanic Caucasians of similar age.

The Centers for Disease Control and Prevention (CDC) estimates that diabetes affects more than 1 in 4 people older than age 65 years in the United States; at current rates of diagnosis, prevalence will increase 165% by the year 2050.

 CLINICAL CONCEPT

Risk of death in persons with diabetes is approximately twice as high as that in individuals who do not have diabetes.

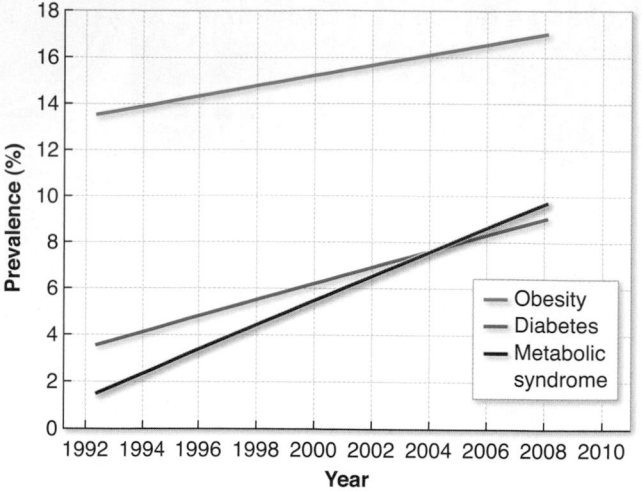

FIGURE 25-1. The prevalence of obesity has paralleled the rise in diagnosis of diabetes and metabolic syndrome

Basic Concepts of Carbohydrate Metabolism

Dysfunctional carbohydrate metabolism is the major pathophysiologic process and cause of complications in diabetes. To understand how diabetes affects carbohydrate metabolism, it is necessary to have basic knowledge of normal and impaired glucose regulation as well as action of insulin and other glucose-regulating hormones.

Normal Blood Glucose Regulation

Ingested carbohydrates, which are broken down into monosaccharides in the intestine, are the major source of glucose in the bloodstream. Glucose is a major energy source for cell function. Before glucose can be utilized for energy, it must be transported through the plasma membrane into the cytoplasm of the cells. However, glucose is a large molecule that cannot diffuse freely across the plasma membrane; it requires a process termed facilitated diffusion, which is an insulin-supported process that occurs at the cell's plasma membrane.

Insulin is a hormone produced by the beta cells of the **islets of Langerhans;** specialized tissue within the pancreas. After eating, glucose is absorbed into the bloodstream at the intestine. The rise in blood glucose stimulates the pancreas to release insulin; this, in turn, causes rapid uptake, storage, and use of glucose by almost all cells of the body (Fig. 25-2).

After eating, there is a synchronous physiologic rise and fall of insulin and glucose in the bloodstream. The rate of cellular uptake of glucose is controlled by the rate of insulin secretion by the pancreas (Fig. 25-3).

After absorption into cells, glucose can either be used for energy production, be stored in the form of glycogen, or be converted into fat. All cells can store some glucose in the form of glycogen, but the liver and muscle cells can store the largest amounts.

Glycogenesis is the process of glycogen formation. In cells, glucose is stored as glycogen to a saturation

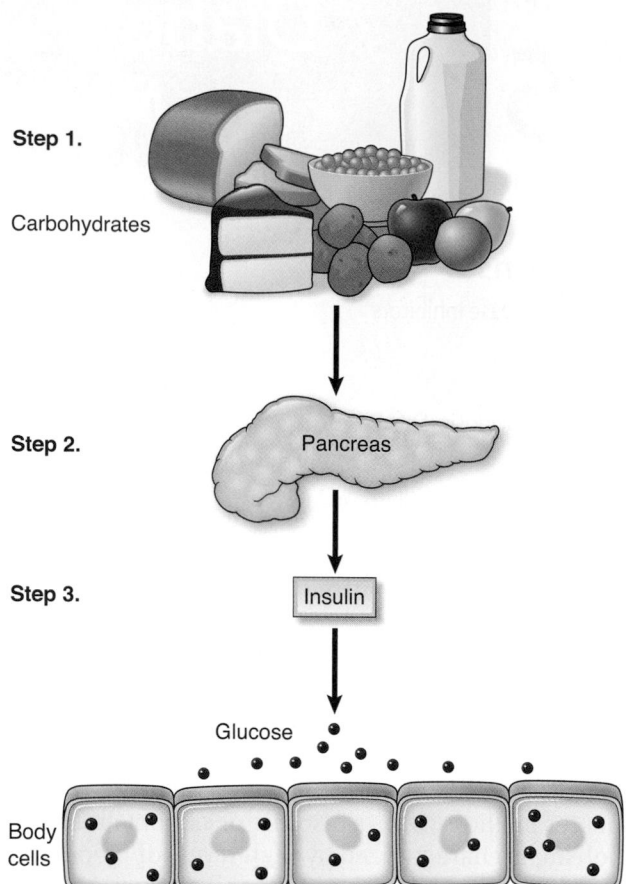

FIGURE 25-2. Glucose stimulation of normal pancreatic insulin secretion. (1) Carbohydrate ingestion leads to glucose absorption from the gastrointestinal system. (2) Glucose in the bloodstream stimulates the pancreatic islet beta cells to secrete insulin. (3) Insulin facilitates cellular uptake of glucose.

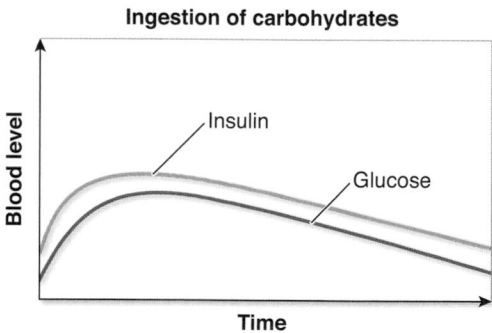

FIGURE 25-3. Synchronous physiologic rise and fall of insulin and glucose in the bloodstream after carbohydrate ingestion.

point—an amount sufficient to supply cells with energy for 12 to 24 hours. Cells require glucose for energy; during periods of starvation, the body is capable of producing glucose through the processes termed *glycogenolysis* and *gluconeogenesis*.

Glycogenolysis is the breakdown of the body's stored glycogen to yield glucose (Fig. 25-4). This process occurs when the body does not have sufficient circulating blood glucose from carbohydrate ingestion. The hormones epinephrine, released from the adrenal gland, and glucagon, released from the pancreas, can activate the enzymatic breakdown of glycogen. A well-nourished person who is

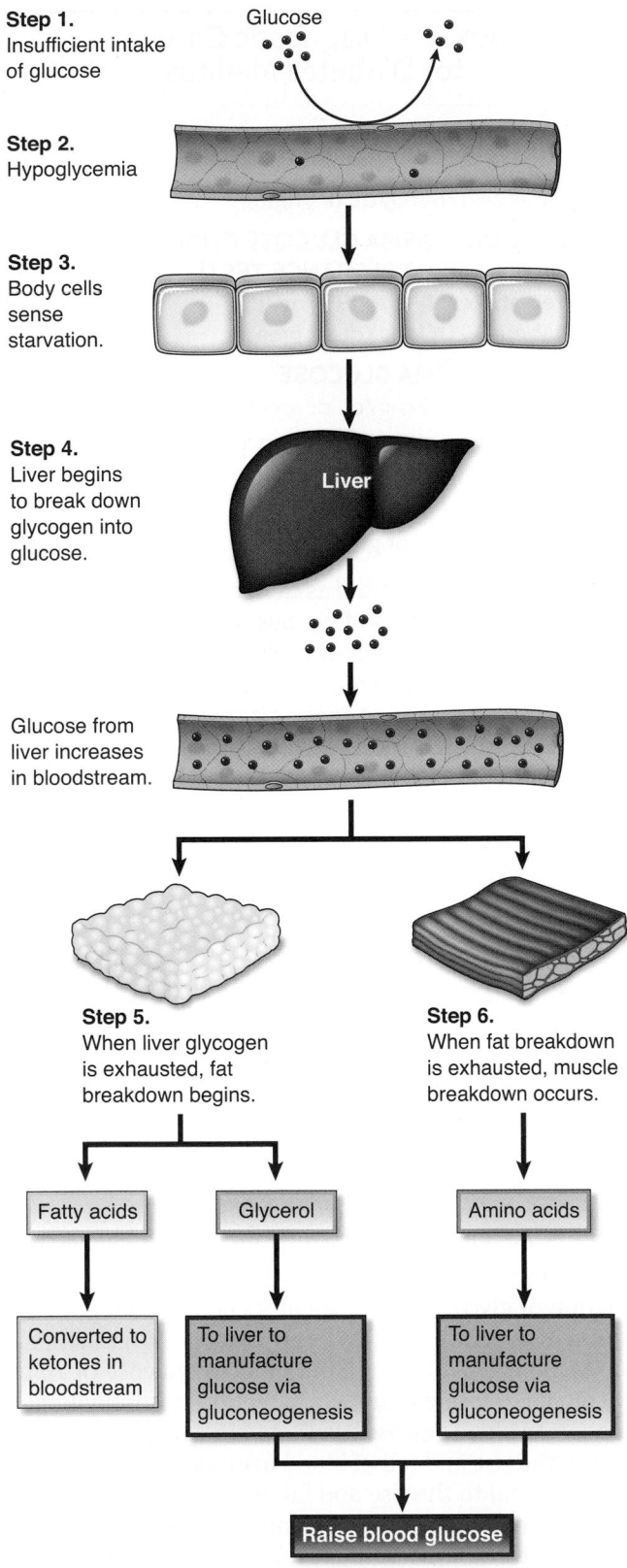

Step 1.
Insufficient intake
of glucose

Glucose

Step 2.
Hypoglycemia

Step 3.
Body cells
sense
starvation.

Step 4.
Liver begins
to break down
glycogen into
glucose.

Liver

Glucose from
liver increases
in bloodstream.

Step 5.
When liver glycogen
is exhausted, fat
breakdown begins.

Step 6.
When fat breakdown
is exhausted, muscle
breakdown occurs.

Fatty acids   Glycerol   Amino acids

Converted to
ketones in
bloodstream

To liver to
manufacture
glucose via
gluconeogenesis

To liver to
manufacture
glucose via
gluconeogenesis

Raise blood glucose

FIGURE 25-4. Glucose regulation during prolonged fasting or starvation. (1) Insufficient intake of glucose. (2) Hypoglycemia develops in the bloodstream. (3) Body cells sense starvation. (4) Liver is activated to break down its storage form of glucose called glycogen. (5) When glycogen is exhausted, fat breakdown occurs. Fat breaks down into fatty acids and glycerol. Fatty acids are converted to ketones, whereas glycerol goes to the liver for manufacture of glucose via hepatic gluconeogenesis. (6) When fat sources are depleted, muscle breakdown begins. Muscle proteins break down into amino acids, which go to the liver and manufacture glucose via gluconeogenesis. The process of hepatic gluconeogenesis raises blood glucose.

fasting can rely on the breakdown of glycogen stores for 12 to 24 hours.

Blood Glucose Maintenance in Starvation

During times when fasting is prolonged or starvation occurs, glycogen stores in the liver will be depleted. The liver then can synthesize glucose by another process: **gluconeogenesis** (Fig. 25-4). In gluconeogenesis, amino acids and fats are converted into glucose. Fats are mobilized from stored adipose tissue and broken down into two components: fatty acids and glycerol. The glycerol is used in gluconeogenesis, but fatty acids are not; instead, the fatty acids accumulate in the bloodstream.

As fatty acids accumulate, they are converted into acetoacetic acid, beta-hydroxybutyric acid, and acetone, three substances referred to as ketoacids or ketones (Fig. 25-4). Ketone accumulation in the bloodstream is known as ketosis or ketoacidosis. Ketones in the bloodstream cause the breath, saliva, and sweat to take on a fruity odor. High levels of ketones affect the brain, causing poor concentration and, at times, confusion and disorientation. **Diabetic ketoacidosis (DKA)** is a condition that develops in those with no insulin reserves, such as those with uncontrolled type 1 diabetes. Individuals with type 1 diabetes often present with DKA when first diagnosed; DKA is a critical condition requiring immediate treatment.

Along with fats, proteins are used to manufacture glucose in gluconeogenesis. Proteins are mobilized mainly from muscle tissue by cortisol, a hormone produced by the adrenal gland. Proteins are broken down into amino acids, which become depleted of nitrogen by the liver. Therefore, during periods of starvation, adipose tissue and muscle tissue are utilized to manufacture glucose (Fig. 25-4). Consequently, prolonged starvation causes depletion of fat stores and muscle mass.

Impaired Blood Glucose Maintenance

In a healthy person, blood glucose concentration is narrowly controlled and must be maintained at sufficiently high levels for cellular nutrition. Brain function is reliant solely on glucose; therefore, blood glucose levels must not decline to very low levels. Most cells can utilize proteins or fats for energy if carbohydrates are unavailable, but glucose is the only nutrient utilized by the brain. Very low levels of blood glucose cause a condition termed **hypoglycemia.**

Although it is vital that blood glucose levels are sufficiently high for cellular nutrition, it is also important that blood glucose levels do not rise to extremely high levels. An abnormally high blood glucose level is referred to as **hyperglycemia.** Blood glucose values corresponding to hyperglycemia are diagnostic of DM.

Normal blood glucose concentration in a fasting person is approximately 70 mg/dL with an upper limit of 100 mg/dL. Hypoglycemia occurs when blood glucose levels fall to lower than 70 mg/dL. After a meal containing carbohydrates, blood glucose normally rises to a maximum level of approximately 200 mg/dL. A fasting

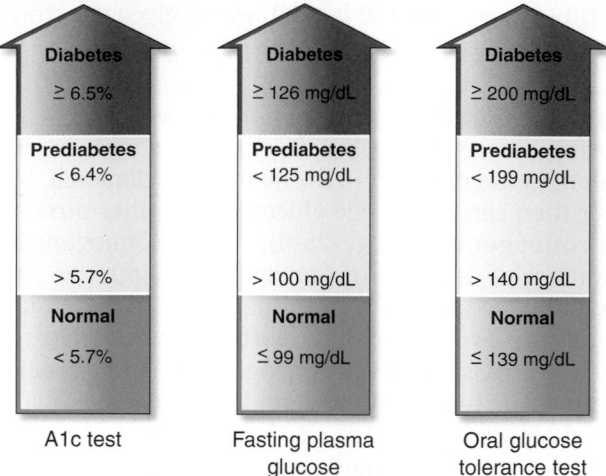

FIGURE 25-5. The ADA suggests the following values in the diagnosis and management of diabetes. *(Source: www.diabetes.org/diabetes-basics/diagnosis. Last accessed July 8, 2015.)*

BOX 25-1. Diagnostic Criteria for Diabetes Mellitus

FASTING BLOOD GLUCOSE
- **Prediabetes:** 100 to 125 mg/dL
- **Diabetes:** 126 mg/dL or greater

TWO-HOUR PLASMA GLUCOSE DURING OGTT* (ORAL GLUCOSE TOLERANCE TEST)
- **Prediabetes:** 140 to 199 mg/dL
- **Diabetes:** 200 mg/dL or greater

RANDOM PLASMA GLUCOSE
- **Diabetes:** 200 mg/dL or greater

A1c (USED FOR DIAGNOSIS OR TRACKING GLUCOSE CONTROL)
- **Prediabetes:** 5.7% to 6.4%
- **Diabetes:** 6.5% or greater

Values above can be used as categories when repeated on two different days of venous blood drawn (except for random sample of plasma glucose). Fasting glucose and A1c test can be paired on the same day; if both are in the diabetes range, diagnosis is confirmed.

*OGTT based on loading dose of 75 G. To convert values to millimoles, multiply by 0.05551. Values in the categories are slightly different in the World Health Organization classification.
(Source: American Diabetes Association. (2012). Standards of medical care in diabetes–2012. *Diabetes Care*, 35 (Suppl 1), S11–S63; Inzucchi, S. E. (2012). Diagnosis of diabetes. *N Engl J Med*, 367(6), 542–550.)

---

blood glucose level of 100 mg/dL to 125 mg/dL is referred to as **impaired glucose tolerance (IGT)** or a condition called **prediabetes** (Fig. 25-5). Persons with prediabetes have blood glucose levels higher than normal but not high enough to be classified as diabetes. A fasting blood glucose level greater than or equal to 126 mg/dL is considered diabetes. Fasting is defined as an 8-hour lapse of eating or drinking.

A blood glucose level measured after eating is termed a **postprandial** glucose level. A postprandial blood glucose level greater than 140 mg/dL and lower than 200 mg/dL is also considered IGT or prediabetes. Postprandial blood glucose levels greater than or equal to 200 mg/dL are consistent with diabetes (Box 25-1).

Role of Insulin in Regulation of Blood Glucose

Immediately after ingestion of a carbohydrate meal, the glucose that is absorbed into the blood stimulates the pancreas to release insulin. Within seconds, circulating insulin binds to cell surface membrane receptors, making cells permeable to glucose. Insulin causes rapid uptake, storage, and use of glucose by almost all tissues of the body, particularly muscle, adipose tissue, and liver cells. In nonexercising muscle, the glucose that enters is stored as glycogen. Exercising muscle, however, does not require much insulin, because the contractile tissue is highly permeable to glucose. Brain cells, highly reliant on glucose for function, also do not require insulin for glucose entry.

Insulin has several effects on the liver. One of insulin's most important effects is to facilitate glucose storage in the liver in the form of glycogen. Insulin promotes glycogen formation and inactivates the enzymes that break down glycogen. When the quantity of glucose entering the liver cells is more than can be stored as glycogen, insulin promotes the conversion of excess glucose into fatty acids, which in turn become stored as adipose tissue.

In many ways, insulin decreases the utilization of fat stores by the body and is considered a "fat sparer." First, by enhancing the body's use of glucose, insulin inhibits the body's use of fats for energy. Second, insulin inhibits the action of lipase, the enzyme that causes hydrolysis of fat. Insulin also inhibits liver enzymes that activate gluconeogenesis and inhibits the breakdown of body proteins. In addition to increasing cellular permeability to glucose, insulin enhances cellular permeability to amino acids. It inhibits muscle tissue from breaking down and promotes the building of muscle, storage of fat, and formation of glycogen. Because of its body-building functions, insulin is referred to as an anabolic hormone.

At the normal fasting level of blood glucose of 70 to 90 mg/dL, the rate of insulin secretion is minimal. Ideally, when blood glucose levels remain within the normal range, the rise and fall of blood insulin concentration is proportional to the rise and fall in blood glucose. However, if blood glucose concentration suddenly increases by 2 to 3 times the normal level and is kept at this level for a prolonged time, insulin secretion increases dramatically. Insulin concentration increases almost 10-fold within 3 to 5 minutes after sudden elevation of blood glucose. However, this initial high rate of secretion is not maintained and, in 5 to 10 minutes, insulin concentration drops. After 15 minutes of a high blood glucose level, insulin secretion rises a second time and reaches a new plateau in 2 to 3 hours, at a rate of secretion greater than the initial phase (Fig. 25-6).

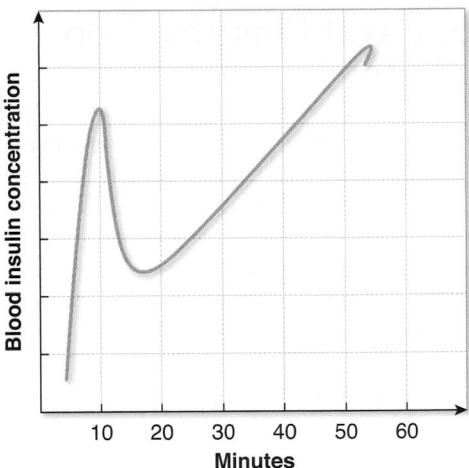

FIGURE 25-6. After a sudden increase in blood glucose to 2 to 3 times normal, plasma insulin concentration increases. There is an initial rapid surge in insulin concentration and then a delayed but higher and continuing increase in concentration beginning 15 to 20 minutes later. (Adapted from Guyton, A. C., & Hall, J. E. (2011). *Textbook of medical physiology.* Philadelphia, PA: W.B. Saunders Co.)

A condition termed **hyperinsulinism** can occur when body cells are resistant to insulin. In this disorder, the pancreas attempts to compensate for the body's cellular resistance to insulin by overworking and increasing secretion, which increases the level of insulin in the blood to high levels. This increased secretion of insulin can compensate for cellular resistance for many years, with maintenance of normal glucose levels. However, with time, cellular insulin resistance usually worsens or pancreatic secretion ability declines; blood glucose levels then begin to rise.

Alternatively, excessive pancreatic secretion of insulin without any body cell insulin resistance can cause hyperinsulinism. The excessive insulin causes severely low blood glucose levels, a condition referred to as hyperinsulinemic hypoglycemia. Congenital hyperinsulinism can occur in infants and young children. In adults, severe hyperinsulinemic hypoglycemia is often caused by an insulinoma, an insulin-secreting tumor of the pancreas.

Other Major Glucose-Regulating Hormones

The pancreas and other organs moderate blood glucose levels by responding to states of hyperglycemia or hypoglycemia. The pancreas does not only respond to high blood glucose levels; it is also stimulated by hypoglycemia. Glucagon and somatostatin are other hormones secreted by the pancreas that regulate blood glucose levels. Endocrine glands such as the adrenal gland can also secrete glucose-regulating hormones. Cortisol and epinephrine can stimulate pancreatic secretion of insulin or provoke the breakdown glycogen in the liver, thereby lowering or raising blood glucose levels. The gastrointestinal tract secretes hormones called incretins, which slow the gastrointestinal absorption of carbohydrates. In response to a meal, incretins slow the rise of blood glucose.

Glucagon. Glucagon, a hormone secreted by the alpha cells of the pancreatic islets of Langerhans, has several functions that counteract insulin action. It can be referred to as a hyperglycemic hormone because it works to increase the concentration of glucose in the bloodstream. The major effects of glucagon include breakdown of glycogen stores in the liver (glycogenolysis) and activation of gluconeogenesis in the liver. In gluconeogenesis, glucagon enhances the rate of amino acid uptake by the liver and their conversion to glucose. Both of these processes increase blood glucose concentration and make more glucose available to the body cells. Glucagon also activates lipase, the enzyme that breaks down adipose tissue into fatty acids and inhibits storage of fat in the liver.

Glucagon secretion is regulated by blood glucose concentration. A rise in blood glucose concentration inhibits glucagon secretion and a fall in blood glucose stimulates its secretion (Fig. 25-7). Severely low levels of blood glucose, as in hypoglycemia, increase glucagon secretion several-fold. This high amount of glucagon then greatly increases the output of glucose from the liver through glycogenolysis and gluconeogenesis, making more glucose available to body tissues (Fig. 25-8).

> ### 🩺 CLINICAL CONCEPT
>
> In severe hypoglycemia, glucagon can be administered as an injectable medication to raise blood glucose levels.

Somatostatin. The delta cells of the islets of Langerhans within the pancreas secrete the hormone somatostatin. After ingestion of food, the secretion of somatostatin is stimulated by the increase in glucose, amino acids, and fatty acids within the bloodstream. Somatostatin diminishes the secretion of insulin and glucagon and

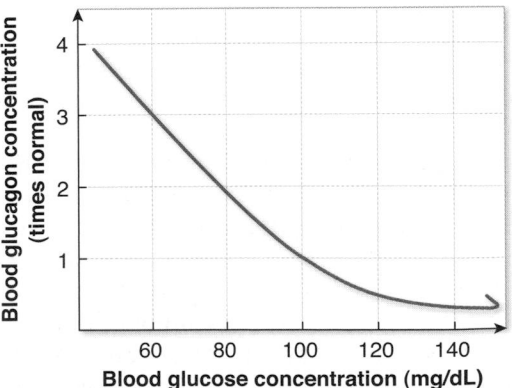

FIGURE 25-7. Approximate blood glucagon concentration at different blood glucose levels. When blood glucose levels are severely low, glucagon levels are high. When blood glucose levels are normal or high, glucagon levels are low. (Adapted from Guyton, A. C., & Hall, J. E. (2011). *Textbook of medical physiology.* Philadelphia, PA: W.B. Saunders Co.)

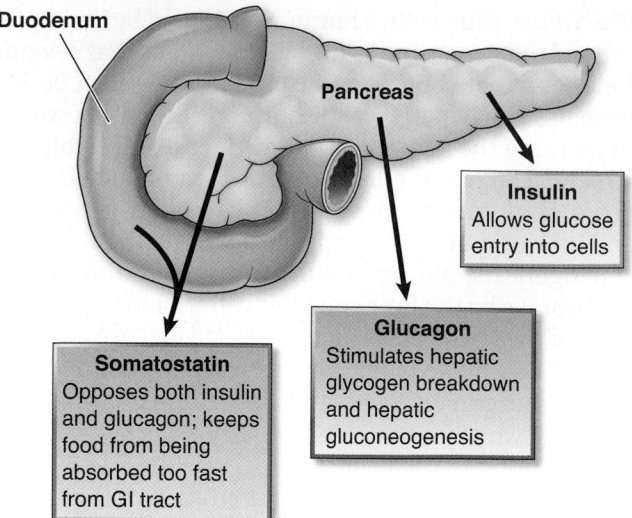

FIGURE 25-8. Major hormones involved in regulation of blood glucose concentrations.

decreases the activity of the gastrointestinal tract (Fig. 25-8). Diminished insulin and glucagon decreases cellular uptake of glucose, amino acids, and fatty acids. Slowing the activity of the gastrointestinal tract prolongs the period of time over which food nutrients are absorbed into the blood. Through these activities, somatostatin prevents rapid exhaustion of nutrients and extends the period of time that ingested nutrients are available.

Gastrointestinal Glucose-Regulating Hormones. Several gastrointestinal hormones stimulate insulin secretion, including gastrin, secretin, cholecystokinin, gastric inhibitory peptide (GIP), and glucagonlike peptide-1 (GLP-1). GIP and GLP-1 are also called **incretins.** All of these hormones are released in the gastrointestinal tract after ingestion of a meal. They cause an anticipatory increase in the blood insulin in preparation for the glucose, amino acids, and fatty acids to be absorbed from the meal. In addition to stimulating insulin, GLP-1 suppresses glucagon secretion during hyperglycemia, delays gastric emptying, slows gut motility, and enhances satiety. All these activities of GLP-1 attempt to bring high levels of glucose down to normal.

Endocrine Glucose-Regulating Hormones. The other hormones that either directly increase insulin secretion or enhance the glucose stimulus for insulin secretion include growth hormone, cortisol, epinephrine, progesterone, and estrogen. Prolonged secretion of any one of these hormones can lead to prolonged stimulation of insulin-secreting pancreatic beta cells and eventual exhaustion. Diabetes often occurs as a secondary condition in endocrine disorders that cause hypersecretion of hormones. For example, diabetes occurs in individuals affected by Cushing's disease, which is a condition caused by a hyperfunctioning adrenal gland that secretes extremely high levels of cortisol.

Etiology and Classification of Diabetes

DM is classified according to the etiologic process that causes the disorder. Assigning a type of diabetes to an individual often depends on the clinical signs and symptoms at diagnosis. Many diabetic individuals do not fit easily into a single category.

The classification of diabetes has changed numerous times over the years. Many classifications used in the past are now obsolete, including juvenile-onset DM, insulin-dependent DM, noninsulin dependent DM, adult-onset DM, and maturity-onset DM. As our knowledge base has broadened regarding the pathology of diabetes, the classification of diabetes has changed.

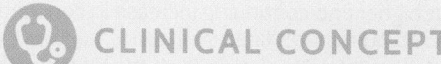

CLINICAL CONCEPT

For the clinician, it is more important to understand the pathogenesis of the disease process rather than categorize the patient.

According to the American Diabetes Association (ADA), the majority of cases of DM fall into type 1, type 2, other specific types, and gestational diabetes (Table 25-1). In addition, some experts describe an intermediate form of diabetes termed latent autoimmune diabetes of adults (LADA) or type 1.5 diabetes. LADA is a slowly, progressive form of diabetes with features of both type 1 and type 2 diabetes.

TABLE 25-1. Classifying Diabetes Mellitus

Category/ Subcategory of	Etiology
Type 1 diabetes Type 1 Immune-mediated	Autoantibody destruction of insulin-secreting beta cells within islets of Langerhans of the pancreas
Type 1 Idiopathic	Unknown etiology
Type 2 diabetes	Cellular resistance to insulin with or without pancreatic beta cell exhaustion
GDM (gestational diabetes mellitus)	Any degree of glucose intolerance during pregnancy
Other specific types of DM	Various disorders: genetic defects, maturity onset diabetes of the young, pancreatic disease, endocrine disorders, drug-induced diabetes, infections

(Adapted from the American Diabetes Association. (2011). Diagnosis and classification of diabetes mellitus. Retrieved from http://care.diabetesjournals.org/content/27/suppl_1/s5.full on July 8, 2015.)

It is also important for the clinician to be familiar with the classification termed prediabetes, which describes impaired glucose tolerance (IGT) that develops before diabetes. Despite the many different classifications, most experts focus on the two major classifications: type 1 DM and type 2 DM.

Type 1 diabetes accounts for only 5% to 10% of all cases of diabetes and has two subcategories: immune-mediated type 1 diabetes and idiopathic type 1 diabetes. Both kinds of type 1 diabetes are caused by a deficiency of insulin caused by complete or partial pancreatic beta cell failure. Immune-mediated type 1 diabetes is caused by immunological destruction of the insulin-secreting beta cells within the islets of Langerhans of the pancreas. Those with idiopathic type 1 diabetes have no evidence of autoimmune pancreatic damage and the cause of this form of diabetes is unknown. Approximately 90% of individuals with type 1 diabetes have the immune-mediated form.

Type 2 diabetes is mainly characterized by cellular resistance to insulin, which can eventually cause pancreatic beta cell exhaustion. For unknown reasons, in this form of diabetes body cells are insensitive to the effects of insulin and, therefore, do not allow entry of glucose. Type 2 diabetes accounts for 90% to 95% of all cases of diabetes. This form of diabetes often goes undiagnosed for many years because hyperglycemia develops slowly and individuals do not exhibit the classic symptoms in the early stages. Formerly thought to be an adult disease, type 2 diabetes is now increasingly diagnosed in children and adolescents.

Gestational diabetes mellitus (GDM) is defined as any degree of glucose intolerance that occurs during pregnancy. It complicates approximately 4% of all pregnancies in the United States and can cause maternal and fetal complications.

There are other causes of DM, such as diseases of the pancreas, endocrine disorders, specific genetic defects, infections, and drug-induced diabetes. These are categorized as "other specific types of diabetes." Such types of diabetes account for 1% to 5% of all diagnosed cases.

Pathological Mechanism of Type 1 Diabetes Mellitus

Type 1 diabetes is classified as either an immune-mediated disease or an idiopathic disorder, which has no known cause. Immune-mediated type 1 diabetes, the most common form, is caused by deficient insulin resulting from T cell-mediated autoimmune destruction of the insulin-secreting beta cells of the pancreas. The individual has circulating autoantibodies to islet cells, insulin, and enzymes involved in insulin production. This form of the disease also has a strong genetic influence. Among affected individuals, the rate of beta cell damage is variable, being rapid in mainly infants and children and slow mainly in adults. The presenting sign of this type of diabetes is often ketoacidosis, particularly in children. Many affected adults retain some beta cell function to prevent ketoacidosis for many years, but eventually become dependent on exogenous insulin for survival. Often, individuals with immune-mediated type 1 diabetes are susceptible to other autoimmune disorders.

Idiopathic Type 1 Diabetes

Idiopathic type 1 diabetes has no known etiology. Affected individuals are deficient in insulin but have no evidence of pancreatic cell autoimmune damage. This form of diabetes is inherited and occurs mostly in those of African and Asian ethnicity. Because of insulin deficiency, individuals with this form of diabetes can develop ketoacidosis.

Clinical Manifestations of Type 1 Diabetes

Initial symptoms of type 1 diabetes include the classic triad of polydipsia (constant thirst), polyuria (excessive urination), and polyphagia (increased appetite). The individual may also complain of visual disturbances. Inability to concentrate, fatigue, weakness, and a general feeling of malaise may be experienced before the initial diagnosis. A history of chronic *Candida* infection of the genital tract may also be the male or female patient's initial complaint. Physical examination in the patient with new onset type 1 diabetes may be unremarkable unless there is an infection present. Often, DKA is the presenting sign of those with type 1 diabetes.

Pathological Mechanism of Type 2 Diabetes

Insulin resistance is the major pathophysiologic process that causes type 2 diabetes. Pancreatic insulin deficiency, to a lesser degree, is also involved in its pathogenesis. The insensitivity of body cells to insulin causes the pancreas to attempt to compensate by secreting increasing amounts of insulin. Greater-than-normal amounts of pancreatic insulin are required to produce a normal biological response, causing the pancreas to overwork. Eventually, the pancreas becomes exhausted and cannot continue to secrete insulin in amounts commensurate with glycemic levels. Blood glucose levels climb as the pancreas dysfunctions and cells continually resist insulin. There is no immunological damage of the pancreas and the exact cause for insulin resistance is unknown.

Obesity is a major contributing factor to the development of type 2 diabetes. Fat cells are particularly resistant to insulin; the greater the adiposity of an individual, the greater the insulin resistance.

Risk of developing this form of diabetes increases with age, obesity, and lack of physical activity. It also occurs frequently in women who endured gestational diabetes when pregnant and in individuals affected by hypertension and dyslipidemia.

BOX 25-2. What Is Metabolic Syndrome?

The American Heart Association (AHA) and the National Heart, Lung, and Blood Institute (NHLBI) recommend that the metabolic syndrome be identified as the presence of three or more of these components:

- **Elevated waist circumference:**
  - Men: equal to or greater than 40 in. (102 cm)
  - Women: equal to or greater than 35 in. (88 cm)
- **Elevated triglycerides:** equal to or greater than 150 mg/dL
- **Reduced HDL cholesterol:**
  - Men: lower than 40 mg/dL
  - Women: lower than 50 mg/dL
- **Elevated blood pressure:** equal to or greater than 130/85 mm Hg
- **Elevated fasting glucose (IGT):** equal to or greater than 100 mg/dL.

(Adapted from What Is Metabolic Syndrome? Retrieved from http://www.heart.org/HEARTORG/Conditions/More/MetabolicSyndrome/Metabolic-Syndrome_UCM_002080_SubHomePage.jsp on July 8, 2015.)

Glucose intolerance or type 2 diabetes is also part of a constellation of disorders termed **metabolic syndrome.** Persons with metabolic syndrome have hypertension, dyslipidemia, hyperinsulinism, centralized or "apple-shaped" obesity, glucose intolerance, and a predisposition to type 2 diabetes. Metabolic syndrome increases the risk of coronary artery disease and other diseases related to arteriosclerosis, such as stroke and peripheral vascular disease. The syndrome has become increasingly common in the United States, with 50 million Americans affected by the disorder (see Box 25-2).

In type 2 diabetes, insulin resistance frequently improves with weight reduction, increased physical activity, and pharmacological treatment of hyperglycemia. Many individuals affected by type 2 diabetes do not require exogenous insulin and are adequately treated with oral antidiabetic medications.

There is a strong genetic predisposition associated with type 2 diabetes, more so than with type 1 diabetes. Ketoacidosis seldom occurs in this form of diabetes, but a similar disorder termed **hyperosmolar hyperglycemic syndrome (HHS)** can develop.

Clinical Manifestations of Type 2 Diabetes

The clinical manifestations of type 2 diabetes are similar to those of type 1 diabetes: polyuria, polydipsia, and polyphagia. These three classic symptoms occur because of the same pathological process as in type 1 diabetes—the development of hyperglycemia caused by deficient insulin action. Hyperglycemia causes intracellular fluid shifts, resulting in polydipsia and excessive diuresis at the kidney that causes polyuria. With lack of glucose entry, cells sense starvation, resulting in polyphagia.

DKA is not typically a feature of type 2 diabetes because of the presence of some insulin. However, it can occur in type 2 diabetes as pancreatic insulin secretion capacity dwindles. The pancreas is able to secrete insulin, albeit erratically, in most individuals with type 2 diabetes. The presence of insulin allows for some glucose uptake by the cells and inhibits breakdown of fat, thereby preventing the development of ketoacids. Insulin protects the individual from developing overt DKA; however, the acute complication of HHS can develop if blood glucose climbs to high levels.

Other Types of Diabetes

Some forms of diabetes do not fit into the classification of type 1 or type 2. These forms of diabetes are caused by a primary injury, illness, or defect; glucose intolerance is a secondary effect. Genetic defects of the pancreatic beta cell have been identified that cause hyperglycemia before age 25 years. These disorders are referred to as maturity-onset diabetes of the young and are characterized by deficient insulin secretion with minimal or no deficiency in insulin action. The most common form is associated with gene mutations on chromosome 12 and chromosome 7.

ALERT! HHS causes severe dehydration, confusion, stupor, and possibly coma.

Gestational Diabetes Mellitus

Diabetes or any degree of glucose intolerance that develops during pregnancy is referred to as gestational diabetes mellitus (GDM), which is diagnosed regardless of whether the patient requires insulin or only diet modification. It affects approximately 4% of all pregnant women in the United States and occurs more frequently in African Americans, Hispanics, and Native Americans. GDM requires treatment to normalize maternal blood glucose levels in order to avoid complications in the infant. In the absence of treatment, GDM can cause fetal defects, premature delivery, and hypoglycemia in the newborn, and large-for-gestational-age infants.

The etiology of GDM is unclear, but the high hormone levels secreted during pregnancy create cellular insulin resistance. Women are at high risk for GDM if they are obese, hypertensive, had GDM in a previous pregnancy, gave birth to a large infant (heavier than 9 lbs.) or an infant with a birth defect, or had a stillbirth in the past. Also, pregnant women with glucose in the urine during their prenatal checkup require screening for GDM (see Box 25-3). Commonly, pregnant women are screened for GDM with an oral glucose tolerance test (OGTT) during the second trimester, and ultrasounds are performed more frequently to assess the size of the fetus in GDM.

High levels of estrogen, the major hormone that sustains pregnancy, can cause cellular insensitivity to insulin and consequent hyperglycemia. Hyperglycemia and insulin resistance make the maternal pancreas overwork to secrete more insulin in order to compensate. A pregnant woman with GDM may need three times the normal amount of insulin secretion from her pancreas. Insulin is a large molecule and does not cross the placenta; however, glucose does cross the placenta. Because the mother has hyperglycemia, the fetus develops high blood glucose levels. This glucose stimulates the fetus' pancreas to synthesize extra insulin in order to bring down blood glucose levels.

Without treatment, in uncontrolled GDM, the constant high maternal blood glucose levels cause high fetal blood glucose levels. Because these high glucose levels are excessive and more than the fetus needs for normal growth, extra glucose is stored as fat in the fetus. The extra fat synthesized in the fetus often leads to large-for-gestational-age newborns, known as macrosomia. Macrosomia increases the risk for the maternal complication of cephalopelvic disproportion, where the neonate is too large to naturally pass through the birth canal. The infant can also suffer shoulder dystocia at delivery, where the infant's shoulders are too large to pass through the birth canal. Nerve damage or fracture can occur in these cases, but most deliveries are accomplished by caesarian section. Also, because of the extra insulin made by the fetus' pancreas, newborns may develop very low blood glucose levels. Neonatal hypoglycemia often occurs shortly after birth in GDM. Lastly, studies show newborns who are born with excess insulin are at risk for obesity and type 2 diabetes as they become older.

Gestational diabetes is usually transient and resolves after pregnancy. However, about two-thirds of women with GDM are at high risk for GDM in future pregnancies. In some women, the stress of pregnancy provokes the development of a permanent condition of diabetes. Studies show that about 50% of women who endure gestational diabetes will develop type 2 diabetes within the first 5 years after delivery.

Diagnosis of Diabetes Mellitus

Blood Glucose Levels in Diabetes

Diagnosis of all types of diabetes is based on the same venous blood glucose parameters. The gold standard laboratory test used to diagnose diabetes is a fasting plasma glucose level. A fasting plasma glucose level greater than 126 mg/dL on 2 separate days confirms the diagnosis. A random plasma glucose greater than 200 mg /dL that is repeated on more than one occasion is also diagnostic of the disorder.

The **oral glucose tolerance test (OGTT)** is also a procedure used to diagnose diabetes. During an OGTT, an individual ingests a specific amount of carbohydrate-rich soda (75 gram glucose load) and then has blood glucose measured 2 hours later. After 2 hours, if the patient registers a postprandial blood glucose level of 140 to 199 mg/dL, prediabetes is diagnosed. If the measurement is greater than or equal to 200 mg/dL, diabetes is diagnosed.

The **glycated hemoglobin (**termed **A1c)** test can be used to diagnose diabetes and assess blood glucose control over the preceding 3 months. A A1c value of greater than 6.5% is diagnostic of diabetes, and a value between 5.7% and 6.4% is considered prediabetes. The ADA allows for A1c testing paired with fasting plasma glucose on the same day. If values of both are in the diabetic range, the diagnosis is confirmed. Another test, called the **eAG,** is the average glucose over the last few months measured in mg/dL. The ADA recommends an eAG of lower than 154 mg/dL.

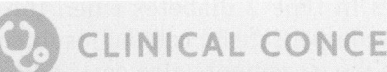
CLINICAL CONCEPT

In the general population, screening for diabetes is recommended every 3 years beginning at age 45. However, it is important for clinicians to recognize that type 2 diabetes is increasingly diagnosed in young adults, children, and adolescents.

Urine Testing in Diabetes

During hyperglycemia of uncontrolled diabetes, blood filtered by the kidney contains a high level of blood glucose. At the nephrons of the kidney, glucose is reabsorbed back into the bloodstream to a certain threshold and the remaining unreabsorbed glucose remains within the tubule fluid. The tubule fluid continues further onward within the nephron to become urine containing residual glucose. Glucose in the urine is termed **glucosuria.**

A urine dipstick test or urinalysis will reveal glucosuria, which is indicative of uncontrolled diabetes. Also, ketones in the blood, which are filtered at the kidney, can appear in the urine. Urine that contains ketones is termed **ketonuria.** If ketonuria exists, a urine dipstick or urinalysis will reveal positive ketones, which can be indicative of prolonged fasting or uncontrolled diabetes. Urine testing can also be used to monitor treatment effectiveness, but should not be relied upon for diagnostic purposes.

Islet Cell Autoantibodies

Several types of autoantibodies can be detected at the onset of immune-mediated type 1 diabetes. Islet cell, insulin, and insulin receptor autoantibodies are immunological markers that can be used for diagnostic purposes. The most commonly measured autoantibody level is that of islet cell autoantibodies (ICAs). The presence of this autoantibody can assist in the diagnosis of type 1 diabetes and differentiate type 1 from type 2 diabetes. In nondiabetics, the presence of ICAs indicates increased risk for subsequent development of type 1 diabetes.

C-Peptide Test

The C-peptide test is used to detect if there is natural insulin secretion from the pancreas. When the pancreas secretes insulin, it also releases C-peptide. A C-peptide test can differentiate between type 1 and type 2 diabetes.

In type 1 diabetes, C-peptide levels can evaluate if an individual has residual pancreatic beta cell function. Low or absent C-peptide levels are consistent with type 1 diabetes. With type 2 diabetes, the test may be ordered to monitor the status of the pancreatic beta cells and insulin production over time. A high C-peptide level indicates high insulin production by the pancreas, which occurs in type 2 diabetes when the pancreas overworks to compensate for cellular insulin resistance.

C-peptide measurements also can be used in conjunction with blood insulin and glucose levels to help diagnose the cause of hypoglycemia and monitor its treatment. It can distinguish between excessive natural insulin production and excessive exogenous insulin administration as the cause for hypoglycemia. Administration of excessive exogenous insulin suppresses natural insulin released from the pancreas. If excessive exogenous insulin is administered, the blood will contain a high insulin level and low or absent C-peptide level.

In cases of pancreatectomy (removal of part of the pancreas) or pancreatic islet cell transplants, C-peptide levels may be monitored to verify natural insulin production and function of the pancreas.

Complications of Diabetes Mellitus

In all types of diabetes, acute and long-term complications are possible. Acute complications occur early in the course of the disease and are often the first sign of the disorder. Long-term complications occur mainly because of chronic episodes of hyperglycemia, which can occur in poorly controlled diabetes.

Acute complications result from either extreme hyperglycemia or severe hypoglycemia. In any type of diabetes, lack of insulin hinders cellular uptake of glucose and can result in severe hyperglycemia, or accumulation of excessively high levels of glucose in the bloodstream. Individuals with severe hyperglycemia develop a constellation of symptoms and require emergency treatment and hospitalization.

One of the most serious acute complications caused by severe hyperglycemia is diabetic ketoacidosis (DKA), which occurs mainly in type 1 diabetes and is not a common occurrence in type 2 diabetes. In type 2 diabetes, severe hyperglycemia usually causes hyperosmolar hyperglycemic syndrome (HHS). Both DKA and HHS. can be life-threatening disorders and are often the first sign of diabetes for many individuals.

The other serious acute complication of all types of diabetes is hypoglycemia, a severely low blood glucose level. Hypoglycemia causes a constellation of symptoms, can be life-threatening, and requires emergency treatment. Both acute hyperglycemia and hypoglycemia-provoked complications of diabetes are short-term systemic effects that are reversible with treatment.

There are also long-term systemic complications from prolonged uncontrolled diabetes. Most of these complications are caused by chronic hyperglycemia and the damaging effect that glucose has on the arteries and arterioles. The retina, kidney, cardiovascular, peripheral vascular, and nervous systems are affected. These complications are usually irreversible and are the cause for much of the increased morbidity and mortality that accompanies diabetes.

Hypoglycemia

Hypoglycemia can occur because of excessive exogenous insulin, inadequate food intake, stress, excessive physical activity, infection, illness, alcohol abuse, drug interactions, surgery, and excess insulin or oral antidiabetic medication.

A fall in blood glucose triggers a cascade of compensatory mechanisms that attempt to return the body to a state of normoglycemia, which is normal glucose level in the bloodstream. When blood glucose levels fall to hypoglycemic levels (lower than 70 mg/dL), the hypothalamic region of the brain and portal vein of the liver sense the drop in glucose. These glycemic sensors initiate a compensatory response mainly involving the adrenal gland, pancreas, and liver. Epinephrine and glucagon are

<table>
<tr><td>

BOX 25-4. Signs and Symptoms of Hypoglycemia

- sweating
- hunger
- dizziness
- nervousness
- tremulousness
- irritability
- headache
- heart palpitations
- confusion
- disorientation
- inability to concentrate
- seizures
- stupor or loss of consciousness

</td><td>

BOX 25-5. "Quick Fix" Snacks for Counteracting Hypoglycemia

- 2 or 3 glucose tablets
- $\frac{1}{2}$ cup (4 ounces) of any fruit juice
- $\frac{1}{2}$ cup (4 ounces) of a regular (not diet) soft drink
- 1 cup (8 ounces) of milk
- 5 or 6 pieces of hard candy
- 1 or 2 teaspoons of sugar or honey

PATIENT ADVICE
After ingesting one of the above snacks, wait 15 minutes and check the blood glucose level again to make sure that it is no longer too low. If it is still too low, repeat these steps until blood glucose is at least 70 mg/dL. Then, if it will be an hour or more before your next meal, have a snack.

</td></tr>
</table>

(Source: Hypoglycemia remedy recommended by the NIH National Institute of Diabetes.)

released, causing activation of the sympathetic nervous system and rise in blood glucose. Activation of the sympathetic nervous system is responsible for most of the initial signs and symptoms of hypoglycemia, which include sweating, hunger, dizziness, nervousness, tremulousness, irritability, headache, and heart palpitations. In addition, confusion, disorientation, inability to concentrate, seizures, and loss of consciousness can occur (see Box 25-4).

As hypoglycemia continues, epinephrine and glucagon promote glycogenolysis and gluconeogenesis in the liver. Usually, the liver can sustain blood glucose levels for 12 hours or more, unless glucose demand is increased by strenuous exercise, illness, or starvation. In times of extreme need, the kidney can also act as a source of glucose through gluconeogenesis. Muscle protein, triglycerides, and fat tissue are broken down to supply the liver and kidney with amino acids and glycerol as sources for gluconeogenesis. As hypoglycemia progresses, cortisol and growth hormone are released to further stimulate the liver and sustain glucose output.

Hypoglycemia can also present as unexplained night sweats or a clouded mental state upon arising in the morning. Nocturnal hypoglycemia can present as sleep disturbances, vivid nightmares, morning headache, chronic fatigue, or depression.

Those with long-term diabetes need to understand that they may be affected by autonomic dysfunction that causes hypoglycemia unawareness. Autonomic neuropathy, a possible side effect of diabetes, can cause dysfunction of the compensatory sympathetic response to low blood glucose. The patient fails to experience the warning signs of hypoglycemia, such as tachycardia and nervousness, and can endure the condition, unknowingly, until suffering loss of consciousness.

Managing Hypoglycemia
Individuals with diabetes need to be educated about the possible signs and symptoms of hypoglycemia and develop an action plan. Ingestion of fast-acting carbohydrates

such as commercially available glucose tablets or gels, juices, soft drinks, or candy will remedy an acute episode of hypoglycemia. The suggested amount of carbohydrate consumption in hypoglycemia is 15 grams. Five grams of carbohydrate will increase blood glucose by approximately 15 mg/dL. Foods rich in fat will delay carbohydrate absorption and should be avoided. If after 15 minutes, blood glucose is still less than 70 mg/dL and symptoms have not diminished, an additional dose of 15 grams is recommended. The glycemic response to hypoglycemia is transient; therefore, a snack or meal is advised after correction of hypoglycemia (see Box 25-5).

Intravenous glucose (25 grams) may be necessary if hypoglycemia is severe or if the individual is unable to take oral carbohydrates. A 1 mg dose of glucagon by subcutaneous injection is an alternative; however, intravenous injection of 50 mL of 50% dextrose is a more rapid—and preferred—remedy.

Frequent episodes of hypoglycemia can eventually blunt the compensatory responses and hormone counterregulation of low blood glucose levels. If an individual endures repetitive episodes of hypoglycemia, the clinician should reassess the patient's dietary intake, dosage, and timing of insulin or antidiabetic medication administration, as well as the blood glucose testing procedure. The bedtime glucose level is usually predictive of subsequent hypoglycemia developing during sleep.

ALERT! Hypoglycemia is a life-threatening medical emergency that requires urgent treatment.

Somogyi Effect and Dawn Phenomenon
Individuals on insulin therapy can experience nocturnal hypoglycemia, which is usually a consequence of excessive insulin dosage or peaking of insulin action during sleep. During the night, while the patient is asleep,

hypoglycemia stimulates hepatic breakdown of glycogen and gluconeogenesis, which raise blood glucose. Epinephrine, growth hormone, cortisol, and glucagon are all released in response to hypoglycemia, which raise blood glucose further. This results in a raised blood glucose level, allowing for the development of hyperglycemia by early morning.

Upon arising, the patient's fasting blood glucose measurement is within the hyperglycemic range. A hyperglycemic fasting morning glucose measurement may be confusing to the patient and clinician. Therefore, morning hyperglycemia should raise suspicion of nighttime hypoglycemia. This syndrome of nocturnal hypoglycemia with rebound morning fasting hyperglycemia is known as the Somogyi effect, named after the physician who investigated the phenomenon.

A bedtime glucose measurement is usually predictive of the possibility of subsequent hypoglycemia developing during sleep. Reduction of insulin dosage, rescheduling of insulin administration, or changing the type of insulin should rectify the nocturnal hypoglycemia and resultant fasting morning hyperglycemia.

Morning fasting hyperglycemia can also be related to nocturnal elevations of growth hormone, which raises blood glucose. This syndrome occurs without nocturnal hypoglycemia and is known as the dawn phenomenon. Diabetics who have little endogenous insulin and, therefore, little capacity to bring glucose into the cells are mainly affected by this phenomenon. During the night, peaks of growth hormone slow the cellular utilization of glucose, allowing the glucose level to rise in the bloodstream. These effects result in a morning fasting hyperglycemic blood glucose measurement.

Individuals with serious fluctuations in blood glucose should be advised to test bedtime and early morning hour blood glucose to detect either the dawn phenomenon or the Somogyi effect. If the blood glucose level is low between 2 a.m. and 4 a.m., nocturnal hypoglycemia is present and the Somogyi effect should be suspected. If the blood glucose level is normal or high between 2 a.m. and 4 a.m., it is likely the dawn phenomenon.

To remedy the Somogyi effect or dawn phenomenon, the clinician needs to reevaluate the patient's insulin or antidiabetic medication regimen, meal times, and exercise patterns.

Short-Term Acute Complications of Type 1 Diabetes

The classic signs of type 1 diabetes are excessive thirst (polydipsia), frequent urination (polyuria), and increased appetite (polyphagia).

Polydipsia and Polyuria

Hyperglycemia in all types of diabetes causes multiple adverse short-term (adjective) systemic effects. High numbers of glucose molecules are solutes that raise the osmolarity of the bloodstream. The bloodstream is the extracellular fluid compartment that requires specific osmolarity to limit fluid from shifting out of the compartment. Hyperglycemia raises osmotic pressure within the extracellular compartment and alters fluid balance at the capillary-cell interfaces throughout the body. As osmotic pressure rises within the extracellular compartment, a gradient develops that moves intracellular fluid into the bloodstream. High osmolarity in the bloodstream causes a shift of water out of the cells and interstitial compartments into the extracellular fluid compartment (see Fig. 25-9). The result is cellular dehydration, which causes the individual to perceive thirst. This constant fluid shift from cells into the bloodstream creates polydipsia and polyuria (Fig. 25-10).

Polyuria also occurs because of the effect of hyperglycemia at the kidney nephrons. When the kidney filters hyperglycemic blood, high glucose levels develop within the fluid of nephron tubules. At the nephron, fluid within the tubules is reabsorbed in order to concentrate the urine. However, nephron tubules have a threshold for the amount of glucose they can reabsorb back into the bloodstream. Reabsorption of glucose occurs to a maximum level and then excess glucose remains within the tubule fluid. When blood glucose

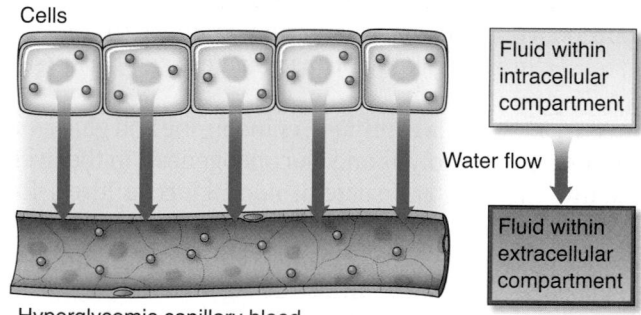

FIGURE 25-9. Osmotic gradient that causes fluid shifts in hyperglycemia from intracellular to extracellular compartment.

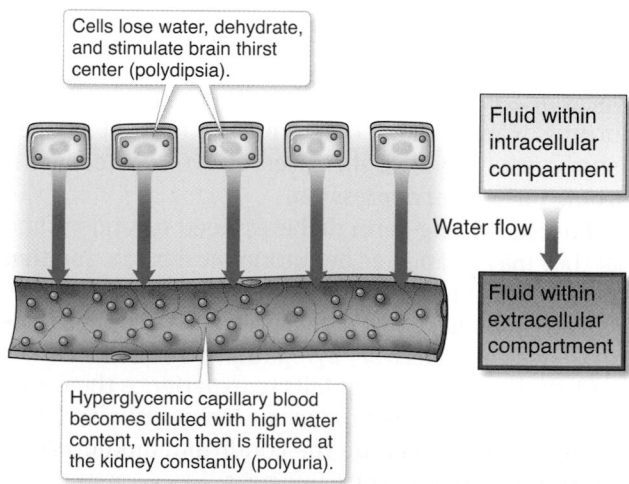

FIGURE 25-10. Cellular dehydration from hyperglycemia. In hyperglycemia, fluid from the body cells move into the capillaries. The cellular dehydration causes thirst, called polydipsia. The water that moves into the bloodstream causes high water content that has to be eliminated; this causes excessive urination, called polyuria.

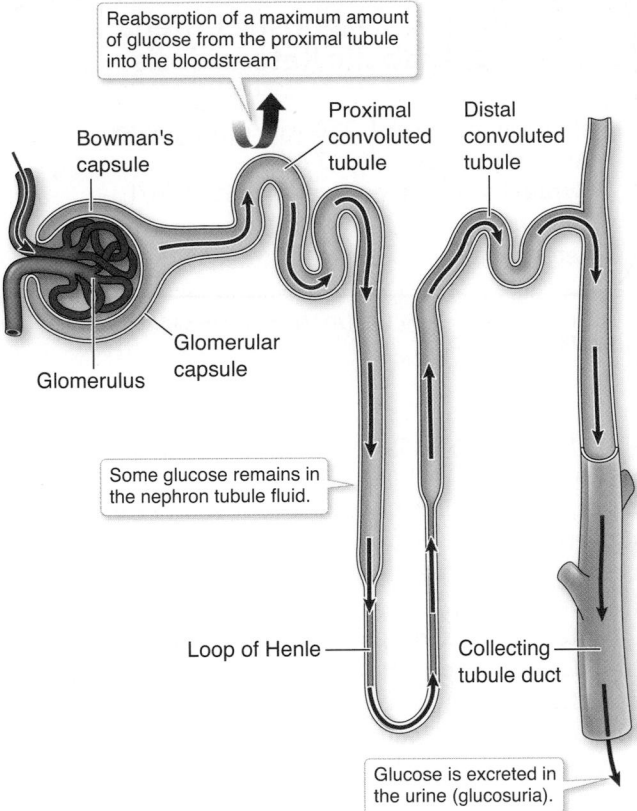

Reabsorption of a maximum amount of glucose from the proximal tubule into the bloodstream

Bowman's capsule

Proximal convoluted tubule

Distal convoluted tubule

Glomerulus

Glomerular capsule

Some glucose remains in the nephron tubule fluid.

Loop of Henle

Collecting tubule duct

Glucose is excreted in the urine (glucosuria).

FIGURE 25-11. Acute effects of hyperglycemia at the nephron. Glucose is filtered out of the blood at the glomerulus. Glucose is then reabsorbed back into the bloodstream at the proximal tubule to a maximum threshold. Some glucose is left in the nephron tubule because the blood cannot reabsorb all of it. Glucose remains in the tubule fluid and is then eliminated in the urine, called glucosuria.

reaches between 300 and 500 mg/dL, glucosuria often develops. High glucose in the tubule fluid sets up an osmotic gradient that pulls water from the cells lining the tubules into the urine. The nephron tubule cells lose water to the tubule fluid, which becomes urine. The osmotic gradient creates excess water in the urine, increasing the amounts and frequency of urination as well as glucosuria (see Fig. 25-11).

Blurred Vision. Blurring of vision can occur because of the accumulation of glucose in the aqueous fluid of the eye. Aqueous fluid is a filtrate of blood; in uncontrolled diabetes, blood is hyperglycemic. The high glucose changes the osmolarity of the aqueous fluid, which bathes the cornea and changes the refraction of light coming into the eye.

Electrolyte Imbalances. Electrolyte imbalances can occur with fluid shifts in uncontrolled diabetes. Water shifting from the intracellular fluid compartment into the bloodstream can dilute the blood, causing dilutional hyponatremia. Potassium within the cells also moves out with the fluid into the bloodstream, creating an intracellular depletion of potassium and a *false* level of either normokalemia or hyperkalemia in the blood. With

insulin treatment, this false level of normokalemia or hyperkalemia in the blood may become true hypokalemia after potassium ions move back into the cells.

Polyphagia. A third classic symptom of type 1 and type 2 diabetes is polyphagia. In uncontrolled type 1 diabetes, the individual typically has increased appetite with an incongruous loss of weight. Because insulin is deficient, the body's cells are not receiving glucose. As a response, the body cells perceive that starvation is occurring, which has several physiologic consequences.

When the body senses starvation, compensatory processes are activated to increase blood glucose levels (Fig. 25-12). Glycogen stores within the organs, mainly the liver, are broken down to release glucose into the bloodstream. However, this "assistive" glucose release by the liver is detrimental because the blood is already high in glucose related to the lack of insulin. The liver will also attempt to compensate for the cellular starvation by synthesizing glucose from noncarbohydrate sources. Hepatic glucose is manufactured through the process of gluconeogenesis. In gluconeogenesis, the liver can synthesize glucose from proteins and fats. Breakdown of muscle, fat, and triglycerides supply the liver with amino acids and fatty acids for gluconeogenesis.

As a consequence of hepatic glycogenolysis and gluconeogenesis, blood glucose levels rise higher. Therefore, in diabetes, the liver attempts to assist the body to deal with the cellular lack of glucose; however, its actions add to the existing problem of hyperglycemia.

As the body continues to sense starvation, adipose tissue is broken down and the individual experiences weight loss. In the absence of insulin, as in type 1 diabetes, the breakdown of fat known as lipolysis develops because of activation of the enzyme lipase. Stored triglycerides are broken down into fatty acids that circulate in the bloodstream. Excess fatty acids in the bloodstream are taken up by the liver to promote cholesterol synthesis, glucose production, and the formation of ketones. The promotion of cholesterol synthesis contributes to the enhanced development of atherosclerosis in diabetes. Hepatic glucose production further increases hyperglycemia, and the formation of ketones begins when fatty acids are taken up by liver cell mitochondria. Mitochondria oxidize the fatty acids to yield large amounts of acetoacetic acid, some of which is used by body cells, with the excess converted into beta-hydroxybutyric acid and acetone which are ketones.

Ketones accumulate in the bloodstream as well as other body fluids, such as the urine, saliva, and sweat. The individual with uncontrolled diabetes can develop **ketonemia,** ketonuria, ketone breath, and ketone body odor, which can be identified as a fruity odor. If ketones accumulate to high levels, DKA can occur.

Diabetic Ketoacidosis. It is important to note that ketone formation is a consequence of lipolysis, which occurs in the absence of endogenous insulin; therefore,

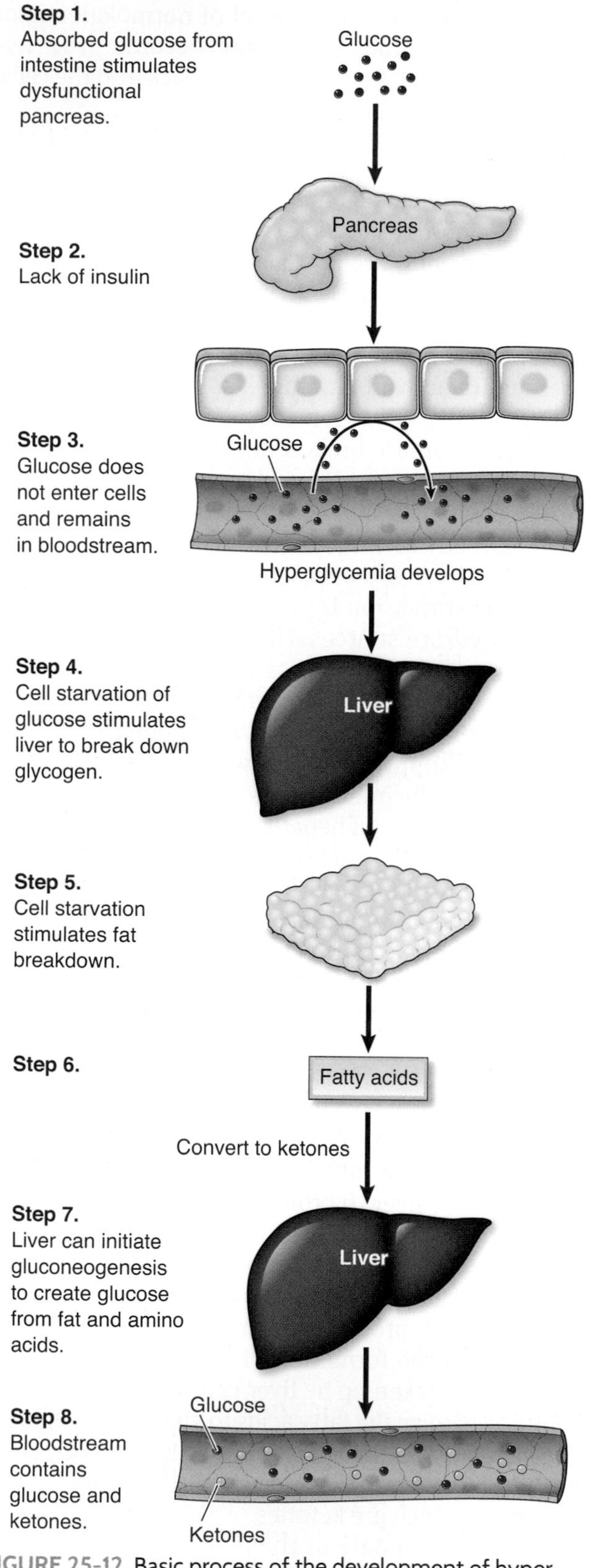

Step 1.
Absorbed glucose from intestine stimulates dysfunctional pancreas.

Glucose

Step 2.
Lack of insulin

Pancreas

Step 3.
Glucose does not enter cells and remains in bloodstream.

Glucose

Hyperglycemia develops

Step 4.
Cell starvation of glucose stimulates liver to break down glycogen.

Liver

Step 5.
Cell starvation stimulates fat breakdown.

Step 6.

Fatty acids

Convert to ketones

Step 7.
Liver can initiate gluconeogenesis to create glucose from fat and amino acids.

Liver

Step 8.
Bloodstream contains glucose and ketones.

Glucose

Ketones

FIGURE 25-12. Basic process of the development of hyperglycemia and ketones in DM. (1) Ingestion of glucose causes a rise in blood glucose, which stimulates the dysfunctional pancreas. (2) The pancreas does not secrete insulin. (3) Glucose cannot enter body cells, hyperglycemia develops, and cells stimulate the body to go into starvation mode. (4) The liver starts to break down its storage of glycogen. (5) Fat starts to break down after glycogen storage is exhausted. (6). Fats break down into fatty acids, which are converted into ketones. (7) Liver initiates gluconeogenesis, making glucose from amino acids and fats, which raises blood glucose. (8) Finally, blood contains high glucose and ketones.

BOX 25-6. Diagnostic Criteria for Diabetic Ketoacidosis

- **Blood glucose level:** 250 mg/dL or greater
- **Arterial pH:** lower than 7.3
- **Serum bicarbonate:** lower than 15 mEq/L
- ketonuria
- ketonemia

(Adapted from Trachtenberg, D. E. (2005). Diabetic ketoacidosis. *Am Fam Phys*, 71(9), 1705–1730.)

it mainly occurs in type 1 diabetes. Ketone formation seldom occurs in type 2 diabetes because, in most cases, there is some endogenous insulin available that prevents lipolysis. However, if pancreatic beta cell failure occurs in type 2 diabetes, ketone formation and DKA can occur.

Ketones are strong acids that accumulate in the blood, alter blood pH, and cause metabolic acidosis, specifically DKA. Severe nausea, vomiting, and profound dehydration can occur in DKA. The severe hyperosmolarity of the blood and the consequent loss of intracellular fluid in the brain can cause coma. Diagnostic criteria for DKA includes a blood glucose level greater than or equal to 250 mg/dL, arterial pH lower than 7.3, serum bicarbonate (HCO3−) lower than 15 mEq/L, and ketonuria and ketonemia (see Box 25-6). Often, individuals with type 1 diabetes do not recognize their symptoms until they experience DKA and seek health care in this emergency state.

In DKA, the lungs attempt to rid the body of acid by hyperventilating to release carbon dioxide (CO_2). Hyperventilation decreases the CO_2 content of blood, which in turn lessens the hydrogen (H+) concentration of the bloodstream (see Fig. 25-13).

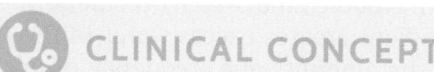 **CLINICAL CONCEPT**

The characteristic rapid, deep respirations exhibited by the patient in DKA are called Kussmaul's breathing.

Managing DKA. Many patients with diabetes die of DKA each year. Most patients with DKA present with polyuria, polydipsia, polyphagia, weakness, abdominal pain, Kussmaul's respirations, nausea, and vomiting. The patient may be lethargic, stuporous, or comatose. Signs of dehydration such as dry mucous membranes, tachycardia, and hypotension are found. Often the patient has ketone breath, ketonuria, and ketone body odor. Common causative factors of DKA include new onset of diabetes, noncompliance with insulin treatment, the stress of infection, myocardial infarction, or alcohol abuse.

Selected patients with mild DKA who are alert and able to take oral fluids may be treated in the emergency department and discharged after stabilization. Patients

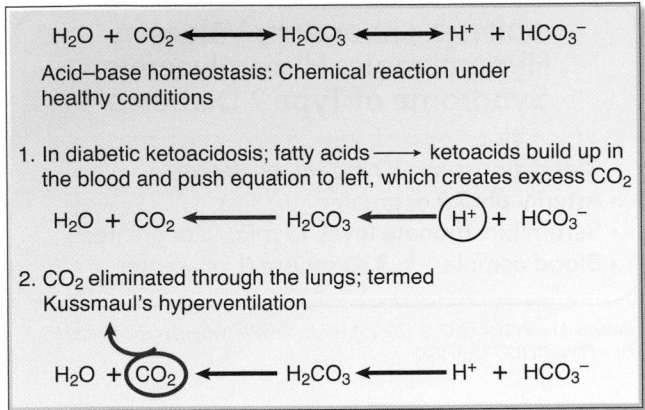

FIGURE 25-13. The chemistry of hyperventilation in DKA. DKA causes acid (H+) to build up in the blood. The excess H+ causes production of excess carbon dioxide (CO_2). The CO_2 is eliminated via the lungs in Kussmaul's hyperventilation.

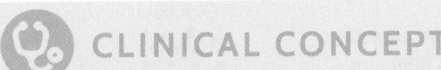

CLINICAL CONCEPT

During treatment for DKA, intravenous insulin is administered until the blood glucose diminishes to lower than 250 mg/dL.

in DKA should have blood glucose evaluated every 1 to 2 hours until stabilized. Blood urea nitrogen (BUN), serum creatinine, serum sodium, potassium, and bicarbonate levels also should be monitored frequently. Urine should be checked for ketones and glucose periodically. Cardiac monitoring is necessary with significant electrolyte imbalances. Patients with severe DKA should be admitted to an intensive care clinical setting.

Fluid replacement is essential to counteract the dehydration and hyperosmolarity caused by hyperglycemia. Intravenous insulin is administered until the blood glucose diminishes to lower than 250 mg/dL. The patient can be switched to subcutaneous insulin to maintain blood glucose in the range of 150 to 200 mg/dL.

Before treatment, serum potassium levels may appear normal or elevated. This is usually a falsely high potassium level, because intracellular potassium moves into the extracellular compartment in acidosis. H+ ions replace the intracellular potassium (K+), which displaces K+ into the bloodstream. As insulin is administered and acidosis is diminished, K+ moves back into the cellular compartment, which then reveals the true blood levels of potassium as hypokalemia, which is why potassium supplementation is necessary in DKA.

Serum sodium levels may appear falsely low because of dilution of excess fluid in the bloodstream, a condition known as dilutional hyponatremia. Sodium levels usually normalize with correction of blood glucose levels.

Cerebral edema is a severe complication that can develop in DKA. The patient may present to the emergency department in this severe state or may develop this during treatment of DKA. Early signs are headache, confusion, and lethargy. Papilledema, which is swelling of the optic disc; hypertension; and hyperpyrexia may also occur. In more severe cases, seizures, pupillary changes, and respiratory arrest from brainstem pressure may occur. There is a 70% mortality rate once severe symptoms of cerebral edema develop. To prevent this potentially fatal event, the clinician needs to be careful to not overhydrate the patient and the blood glucose level should be decreased slowly during treatment.

Short-Term Acute Complications of Type 2 Diabetes

Patients with type 2 diabetes usually do not exhibit DKA; however, a disorder called hyperosmolar hyperglycemic syndrome (HHS) can occur. Cells resist insulin, causing critically high plasma glucose levels.

Hyperosmolar Hyperglycemia Syndrome

The major short-term complication of type 2 diabetes is HHS, characterized by severe hyperglycemia, hyperosmolarity, and dehydration. In some cases, mild ketonemia and ketonuria can be present.

In type 2 diabetes, because of cellular insulin resistance, glucose is not absorbed into the cells. Hyperglycemia develops as a result and sets up an osmotic gradient as it does in type 1 diabetes. The hyperosmolarity of the blood causes intracellular fluid to move into the extracellular compartment. Extracellular fluid volume increases and cellular dehydration occurs.

Simultaneously, the cells are not absorbing glucose and begin to sense starvation. As in type 1 diabetes, the body enters starvation mode with hepatic glycogen breakdown and activation of gluconeogenesis. These mechanisms attempt to compensate for cellular starvation. As a result, with cells continually resisting the glucose, blood glucose levels rise higher (Fig. 25-14).

Because insulin is present in type 2 diabetes, ketones are not commonly formed. Ketone formation is a result of fat breakdown and insulin counteracts lipolysis. Therefore, the presence of insulin in type 2 diabetes blocks fat breakdown and the consequent formation of ketones (Fig. 25-14).

Concurrently, an early event in HHS is glucosuric diuresis. At the nephron, the glucose–rich blood is filtered and the glucose reabsorption threshold is exceeded, causing high levels of glucose to remain in the tubule fluid. The high osmolarity created by the glucose in the tubule fluid pulls water into the tubule. This is an osmotic diuresis resulting in extra water excreted in the urine. As in type 1 diabetes, glucosuria and dehydration occur.

Thirst and polyuria are the initial complaints caused by these pathological processes. If water intake is insufficient to counteract the water loss, hypovolemia, dehydration, and hyperosmolarity of the bloodstream develop. A mild metabolic acidosis can be present in some individuals with nonketotic HHS. The laboratory parameters include blood glucose greater than or equal to 600 mg/dL, arterial pH less than or equal to 7.3, serum bicarbonate level less than or equal to

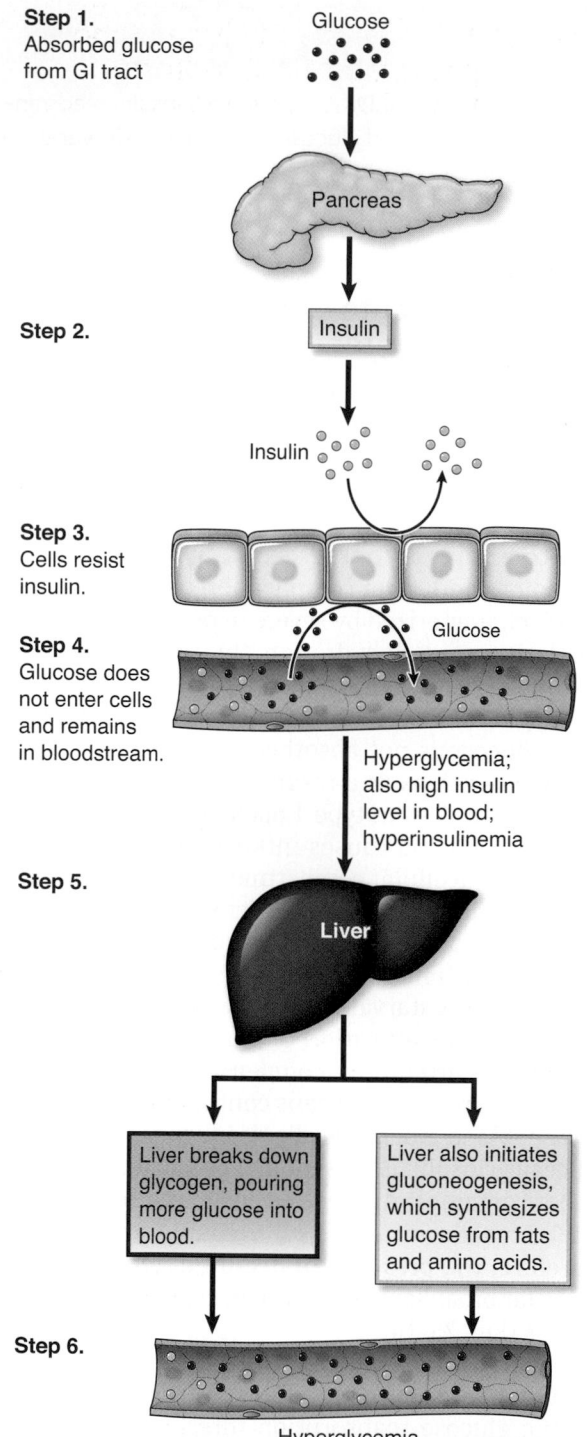

Step 1.
Absorbed glucose from GI tract

Glucose

Pancreas

Step 2.

Insulin

Insulin

Step 3.
Cells resist insulin.

Step 4.
Glucose does not enter cells and remains in bloodstream.

Glucose

Hyperglycemia; also high insulin level in blood; hyperinsulinemia

Step 5.

Liver

Liver breaks down glycogen, pouring more glucose into blood.

Liver also initiates gluconeogenesis, which synthesizes glucose from fats and amino acids.

Step 6.

Hyperglycemia

FIGURE 25-14. Development of hyperglycemia and hyperosmolarity in type 2 diabetes. (1) Glucose is absorbed from the gastrointestinal tract. (2) The pancreas is stimulated to secrete insulin. (3) Body cells resist insulin and glucose cannot enter cells. (4) Glucose accumulates in the blood (hyperglycemia) and insulin builds up in the blood, called hyperinsulinemia. (5) Cell starvation stimulates the liver to break down glycogen storage and initiate gluconeogenesis. (6) The blood develops hyperglycemia and hyperosmolarity. Fat is not broken down in the presence of insulin; therefore, ketone formation is minimal.

15 mEq/L, and blood osmolarity greater than or equal to 320 mOsm/L (see Box 25-7).

This syndrome can develop insidiously over days to weeks. Anorexia, weight loss, weakness, visual

---

> **BOX 25-7. Laboratory Values in Hyperosmolar Hyperglycemic Syndrome of Type 2 Diabetes**
>
> - **Blood glucose:** 600 mg/dL or greater
> - **Arterial ph:** 7.3 or greater
> - **Serum bicarbonate level:** 15 mEq/L or greater
> - **Blood osmolarity:** 320 mOsm/L or greater

(Adapted from Stoner, G. D. (2005). Hyperosmolar hyperglycemic state. *Am Fam Phys*, 71(9), 1723–1730.)

disturbances, poor tissue turgor, tachycardia, and confusion are common complaints. Seizure and neurological disturbances can occur. Approximately 25% of patients present in coma because of the effect of blood hyperosmolarity on the brain.

Clinical Manifestations of HHS. HHS is manifested by blood glucose levels greater than 600 mg/dL and extremely high blood osmolarity levels in patients with type 2 diabetes. Common precipitating factors include infection, noncompliance with diet or medication, new onset type 2 diabetes, substance abuse involving alcohol or cocaine, or coexisting diseases. In type 2 diabetes, the most common cause of hyperosmolar hyperglycemia is infection; pneumonia, urinary tract infection, or sepsis. Severe stresses such as myocardial infarction, stroke, or pulmonary embolus can also precipitate uncontrolled glycemic control. Although some insulin is present in type 2 diabetes, it is not sufficient to control extremely high levels of blood glucose.

Dehydration is the major pathophysiologic mechanism that causes complications in HHS. When blood glucose rises to a high level, blood osmolarity rises. Osmotic diuresis causes constant loss of water in the urine, which concentrates the electrolytes in the bloodstream, resulting in increased serum osmolarity that can be calculated using the following equation:

$$2 \times Na+ \ (mEq/L) + \frac{plasma \ glucose \ (mg/dL)}{18}$$
$$= serum \ osmolarity$$

Serum osmolarity levels greater than 320 mOsm/kg are associated with HHS.

As in DKA, serum potassium levels may appear normal or falsely high because of the shift of K+ from the intracellular compartment into the extracellular compartment. As rehydration and insulin treatment ensues, potassium returns to the intracellular compartment. Serum potassium levels then decrease as the K+ ions move back into the cells. Therefore, hypokalemia results from HHS, and K+ replacement is usually necessary in the treatment plan.

HHS presents with signs of profound dehydration; hypotension; rapid, thready pulse; and changes in mental status from lethargy to coma. Abdominal distension can occur because of gastroparesis, which resolves with rehydration. Seizures are possible if blood osmolarity reaches severely high levels (see Box 25-8).

Management of HHS. Treatment of HHS includes IV rehydration, electrolyte replacement, and IV insulin. Adequate fluids should be administered first. If insulin is administered before fluids, extracellular water will move intracellularly, worsening hypotension and possible hypovolemic shock. IV insulin should be given after rehydration stabilizes the patient's osmolarity; it can be administered until blood glucose reaches 300 mg/dL, at which time subcutaneous insulin can be initiated. The precipitating cause of HHS should be corrected and patients should be cared for in an intensive care setting.

Long-Term Complications of DM

Long-term DM of any type can lead to multiple serious complications (see Table 25-2 and Fig. 25-15). Chronic

> ### BOX 25-8. Symptoms of Hyperosmolar Hyperglycemic Syndrome in Type 2 Diabetes
>
> - extreme hyperglycemia
> - rapid, thready pulse
> - hypotension
> - profound dehydration
> - polydipsia
> - polyuria
> - confusion, disorientation, stupor, possible seizures or coma

hyperglycemia is the major pathophysiologic mechanism that causes most of the complications. In treating diabetes, it is difficult to mimic the physiologic control of blood glucose achieved by endogenous,

TABLE 25-2. Systemic Long-Term Complications of Diabetes

Body System	Complication	Pathological Process	Signs and Symptoms
Arterial	Accelerated atherosclerosis	Arterial plaque buildup, narrowing of arteries, with possible plaque disruption and thrombotic or embolic obstruction of arterial blood flow	Pain caused by ischemia of any organ system that results from blockage of arterial circulation Hypertension
Cardiac	Coronary artery disease	Coronary artery plaque buildup, narrowing of arteries, with plaque disruption and emboli, resulting in angina pectoris or myocardial infarction	Chest pain due to ischemia (angina) Dyspnea Myocardial infarction (often silent; without classic signs and symptoms) Sudden death possible because of cardiac arrest
Cerebrovascular	Stroke Transient ischemic attack	Arteriosclerosis of cerebral arteries or carotid arteries causing emboli or thrombi to block circulation to brain	Dizziness, disorientation, hemiparesis or hemiparalysis, cranial nerve dysfunction, possible aphasia
Peripheral vascular	Peripheral arterial disease of lower extremities	Arterial plaque buildup, narrowing of arteries, and obstruction of arterial blood flow in lower extremities	Pain of lower extremity due to ischemia (intermittent claudication) Weak or absent pulses Paresthesias in feet Pallor of lower extremity Coolness to palpation of lower extremity Poor wound healing which may lead to amputation
Retina	Retinopathy	Narrowing of retinal arteries, hemorrhages, exudates	Vision impairment with possible blindness
Kidneys	Nephropathy	Damage to glomeruli and renal arterial circulation	Microalbuminuria Renal insufficiency Possible renal failure

Continued

TABLE 25-2. Systemic Long-Term Complications of Diabetes—cont'd

Body System	Complication	Pathological Process	Signs and Symptoms
Peripheral nervous system	Peripheral neuropathy; mainly sensory/motor to less extent	Damage to endoneurial arterial circulation that decreases blood flow to nerves, particularly sensory nerves of lower extremity	Loss of sensation in feet, paresthesias of feet, foot deformities (Charcot joint), gait disturbance
Autonomic nervous system	Autonomic neuropathy	Damage to endoneurial arterial circulation, which decreases blood flow to autonomic nerves; dysfunction of sympathetic and parasympathetic nervous systems	Postural hypotension Gastroparesis Bladder and bowel dysfunction Anhidrosis (sweat gland dysfunction) Lack of sympathetic nervous symptoms in hypoglycemia ("hypoglycemia unawareness")
Immune system	Immunosuppression	WBCs dysfunction in high glucose environment	Susceptibility to infections, gangrene Poor wound healing (particularly lower extremities)
Reproductive system	*Candida vaginitis* *Candida balanitis*	Glycogen accumulation within vaginal cells Susceptibility to infection	*Candida vulvovaginitis*; pruritus, vaginal discharge *Candida balanitis*; pruritic rash in uncircumsized males
	Gestational diabetes	IGT in pregnancy	Fetal defects, premature delivery, large for gestational age newborn
Dermatological system	Skin ulceration, susceptibility to *Staphylococcal* infection, and poor wound healing *Necrobiosis lipoidica diabeticorum* *Acanthosis nigricans* Lipoatrophy and lipohypertrophy Intertriginous *Candida* infection	Skin ulceration: anhidrosis, dry skin, prolonged wound healing caused by immunosuppression *Necrobiosis lipoidica diabeticorum*: unknown etiology *Acanthosis nigricans*: unknown etiology Lipoatrophy and lipohypertrophy can occur at sites of repeated insulin injection	Skin breakdown with susceptibility to infection caused by staphylococcal colonization of skin, immunosuppression, and poor wound healing *Necrobiosis lipoidica diabeticorum*: ulcerated lesions commonly on legs *Acanthosis nigricans*: hyperpigmented, velvety macular lesions usually located on the neck, axilla, or extensor surfaces of arms Lipoatrophy and lipohypertrophy: soft-tissue damage at injection sites Intertriginous *Candida* infection: papular; pruritic papular, or macular rash between folds of skin
Psychological/emotional effects	Anxiety Depression Eating disorders "Insulin purging" Denial of the disorder termed "psychological insulin resistance"	Stress, misinterpretation of the disease process, and lack of appropriate coping skills	Excessive worrying Feelings of sadness Feelings of loss Anhedonia Withdrawal "Insulin purging" (underdosing or omitting doses of insulin) Weight loss and excessive concern about weight gain Frequent episodes of poor glycemic control Excessive exercising Noncompliance with recommended insulin injection administration

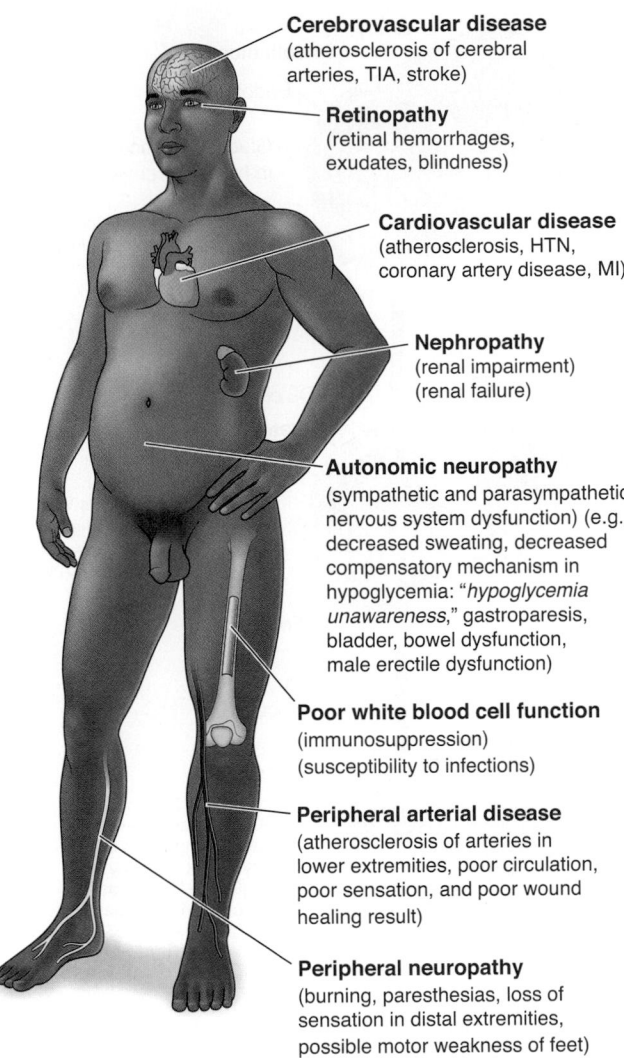

Cerebrovascular disease
(atherosclerosis of cerebral
arteries, TIA, stroke)

Retinopathy
(retinal hemorrhages,
exudates, blindness)

Cardiovascular disease
(atherosclerosis, HTN,
coronary artery disease, MI)

Nephropathy
(renal impairment)
(renal failure)

Autonomic neuropathy
(sympathetic and parasympathetic
nervous system dysfunction) (e.g.,
decreased sweating, decreased
compensatory mechanism in
hypoglycemia: "*hypoglycemia
unawareness*," gastroparesis,
bladder, bowel dysfunction,
male erectile dysfunction)

Poor white blood cell function
(immunosuppression)
(susceptibility to infections)

Peripheral arterial disease
(atherosclerosis of arteries in
lower extremities, poor circulation,
poor sensation, and poor wound
healing result)

Peripheral neuropathy
(burning, paresthesias, loss of
sensation in distal extremities,
possible motor weakness of feet)

FIGURE 25-15. Systemic long-term complications of diabetes.

natural insulin. Episodic elevation of blood glucose commonly occurs despite the most stringent treatment regimens.

Postprandial hyperglycemia has been found to be the most damaging of all blood glucose fluctuations. The risk of complications increases in relation to duration of chronic hyperglycemia, usually becoming apparent after years of this disorder. There is also a probable genetic susceptibility for the development of certain complications because there is variability in individual development of complications despite comparable levels of glycemic control.

Chronic hyperglycemia is the major cause of damage to the small and large arterial vessels. Vascular damage, termed angiopathy, is a major cause of the long-term complications in diabetes. The exact pathological mechanism responsible for this damage is not yet fully elucidated.

Regardless of theory, the pathological mechanism of hyperglycemia involves damage of the endothelial cells, as well as the lining of the arterioles and arteries. Hyperglycemic damage to the smallest arterial blood vessels occurs initially, with arterial vessels of the retina, nutrient arterial vessels of the neurons, and arterial vessels

surrounding the nephrons primarily demonstrating this endothelial damage. Eventually, diabetic retinopathy, diabetic neuropathy, and diabetic nephropathy develop. Injury of retinal arteries can be seen on dilated fundoscopic examination. Neuron damage causes sensory and motor peripheral nerve dysfunction. Injured autonomic nerves, also called autonomic neuropathy, causes dysfunction of the parasympathetic and sympathetic nervous system. Impaired arterial vessels of the nephron cause renal insufficiency and failure. Injury to larger diameter arterial vessels, termed macrovascular angiopathy, may be demonstrated by coronary artery disease, cerebrovascular disease, and peripheral vascular disease. In addition to arterial vessel damage, hyperglycemia causes white blood cells (WBCs) to function less efficiently. This negative effect on WBCs causes immunosuppression, poor wound healing, and increased susceptibility to infection.

Diabetes as an Atherosclerosis Accelerator. Cardiovascular disease is the number-one cause of mortality, and acute cardiac events occur 2 to 4 times more often in diabetic individuals than in the general population. One of the major reasons for this high mortality rate in individuals with diabetes is that chronic hyperglycemia causes damage to the endothelial lining of artery walls. Endothelial injury is the initiating event of arteriosclerosis. Macrovascular and microvascular angiopathy are terms used for the injury to large arterial vessels and small arterial vessels, respectively.

The exact pathological mechanism of vascular injury in diabetes is yet to be explained, but several theories exist. Each theory describes how a specific biochemical change caused by hyperglycemia affects the endothelium.

There are four major biochemical abnormalities that result in vascular damage:

- activation of the polyol pathway
- increased formation of advanced glycation end-products (AGEs)
- activation of protein kinase C (PKC)
- activation of reactive oxygen species (ROS).

Although each plays a role in the vascular injury of diabetes in a distinctive manner, these pathways have an underlying commonality. All the biochemical abnormalities caused by hyperglycemia of diabetes result in oxidative stress caused by overproduction of mitochondrial ROS, also called free radicals.

Polyol Pathway Theory. The polyol pathway theory asserts that in cells that do not require insulin for entry of glucose, such as brain and exercising muscle cells, intracellular hyperglycemia activates an enzyme termed aldose reductase. An enzymatic reaction ensues, which transforms glucose into polyol sorbitol. Intracellular sorbitol causes osmotic cellular damage of endothelial cells and consequent vascular dysfunction. Also, constant activation of the enzymatic reaction of aldose reductase to form sorbitol causes oxidative stress and the overproduction of damaging ROS.

Glycation Theory. The pathogenesis of vascular injury also involves the advanced glycation end-product (AGE) theory. During episodes of hyperglycemia, glucose damages the endothelial cell membranes through the process of glycation. In glycation, glucose chemically attaches to the amino acids of the proteins that make up the endothelial membranes. The degree of glycation is directly related to the level of blood glucose. There are a variety of harmful extracellular and intracellular products of glycation that have been termed AGE products. Extracellular AGE products alter endothelial cell protein function, whereas intracellular AGE products alter endothelial cell gene expression. As a result of damage, endothelial permeability increases, coagulation activity is enhanced, cytokines and growth factors are released, and fibroblast and smooth muscle cells proliferate within the walls of arteries. The net result of these AGE-induced changes is oxidative stress and abnormal vascular function of the endothelium.

Protein Kinase C Theory. The protein kinase C (PKC) theory describes PKC as an important intracellular signaling molecule that regulates many vascular functions, including endothelial permeability, endothelial activation, and growth factor signaling. In the PKC theory, pathological activation of PKC occurs in diabetes, specifically in blood vessels from the retina, kidney, and nerves. The activation of PKC has several effects, including production of vascular endothelial growth factor (VEGF), which is implicated in diabetic retinopathy. PKC also stimulates endothelin, a potent vasoconstrictor, and inhibits nitric oxide, a potent vasodilator. PKC enhances production of coagulant molecules and proinflammatory cytokines. Oxidative stress, coagulation of blood, vascular damage, and disordered vascular proliferation are the end results of PKC activation.

Reactive Oxidation Theory. All the pathways involved in the pathogenesis of vascular injury have a common denominator: the activation of reactive oxygen species (ROS), which are also known as free radicals. The ROS theory asserts that regardless of the biochemical pathways involved, hyperglycemia of diabetes causes oxidative stress on the endothelium. The oxidation of glucose releases free radicals that damage the endothelial cell membranes; this causes extensive vascular injury and blood vessel dysfunction.

Resultant Endothelial Injury. Regardless of the etiologic mechanism, chronic hyperglycemia in diabetes is known to cause endothelial injury; this, in turn, activates inflammation. Inflammation brings WBCs, inflammatory mediators, and platelets to the site of endothelial injury. Lipid and macrophage deposition within the injured area causes the eventual formation of foam cells, precursors to atherosclerotic plaque. Simultaneously, in response to injury, endothelial membranes secrete endothelin. Endothelin inhibits arterial vasodilation and promotes vascular smooth muscle proliferation. This narrows the diameters of arterial vessels, increasing the risk of hypertension in individuals with

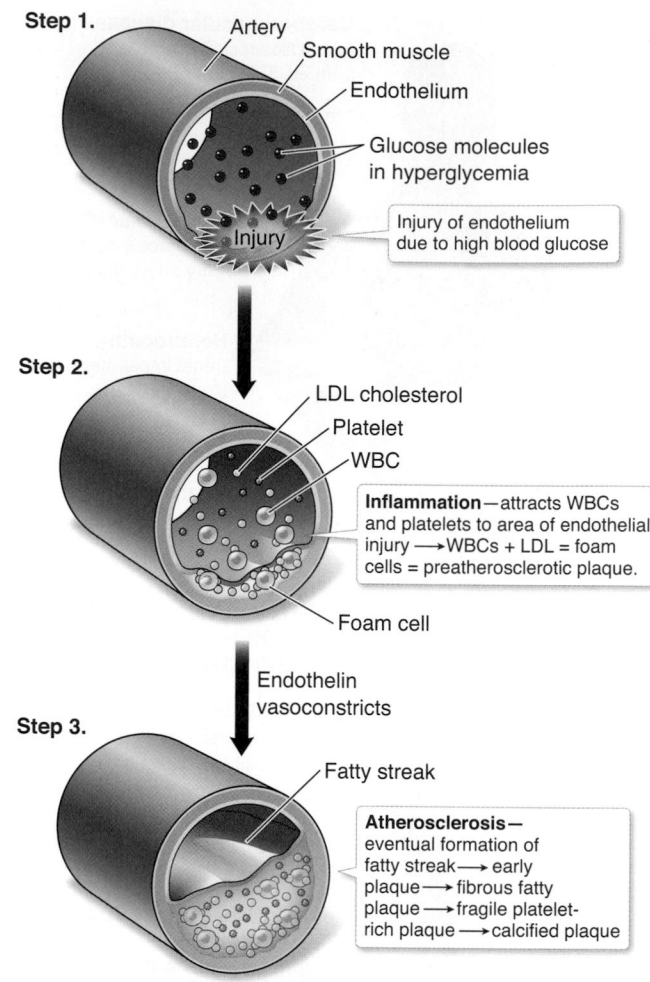

Step 1.
Artery
Smooth muscle
Endothelium
Glucose molecules in hyperglycemia
Injury of endothelium due to high blood glucose
Injury

Step 2.
LDL cholesterol
Platelet
WBC
Inflammation—attracts WBCs and platelets to area of endothelial injury ⟶WBCs + LDL = foam cells = preatherosclerotic plaque.
Foam cell

Endothelin vasoconstricts

Step 3.
Fatty streak
Atherosclerosis— eventual formation of fatty streak⟶ early plaque ⟶fibrous fatty plaque ⟶fragile platelet-rich plaque ⟶calcified plaque

Narrowed vasoconstricted artery with atherosclerosis= Result

FIGURE 25-16. Diabetes as an atherosclerosis accelerator. (1) High glucose in the bloodstream damages the endothelial lining of the artery. (2) Inflammation of the artery lining attracts WBCs, platelets, and inflammatory mediators to the site. WBCs take in LDLs, which are in the bloodstream and form foam cells. Endothelial cells secrete endothelin, which is a potent vasoconstrictor. (3) Foam cells eventually form a fatty streak, which is early atherosclerotic plaque. Atherosclerotic plaque eventually matures into calcified plaque. The results of high glucose in the bloodstream are atherosclerotic plaque formation and vasoconstriction.

diabetes (Fig. 25-16). Every arterial blood vessel is susceptible to injury, and the sequela are most evident in coronary, cerebral, and retinal arteries; glomerular capillaries; and arteries of the lower extremity. Compared with nondiabetic individuals, persons with diabetes have a greater susceptibility to myocardial ischemia (MI), myocardial infarction, stroke, visual impairment, renal impairment, and peripheral vascular disease caused by the endothelial injury of hyperglycemia.

Peripheral Neuropathy of Diabetes. Distal symmetric polyneuropathy, a neural dysfunction of the sensorimotor nerves in the lower extremities, is one of the most common complications of diabetes. It is theorized that hyperglycemia damages the endoneurial arterioles, the small nutrient arterioles that supply the nerves with blood. As a result of the lack of blood flow, the nerves undergo demyelination and axonal degeneration. The fragile small caliber sensory nerve fibers of the lower extremities usually demonstrate this damage first. Peripheral neuropathy of diabetes most commonly presents as sensory loss in the feet and progresses proximally up the lower extremity. Symptoms of burning, pain, and paresthesias of the feet may be reported by individuals. A motor neuropathy can also present as pain accompanied by motor weakness. Individuals may develop a gait disturbance from the lack of sensorimotor capacity in the feet.

The sensory and motor neuronal disruption can also lead to abnormal muscle mechanics and structural changes in the foot, including hammer toe, claw toe deformity, prominent metatarsal heads, and neuropathic joint disease or Charcot joint. Charcot joint is demonstrated by instability of joints and deformity, commonly occurring in metatarsal and tarsal joints of the feet. This complication usually occurs in older adults with many years of long-standing diabetes.

Peripheral neuropathy also blunts pain sensation for the individual with diabetes. The pain associated with serious inflammatory conditions and MI or infarction may not be perceived. Silent MI is particularly common in those with diabetes and concomitant coronary artery disease. Because pain may not be a chief complaint, individuals with diabetes have atypical presentations of disease processes.

Individuals with long-standing diabetes can develop autonomic neuropathy. This involves dysfunction of the sympathetic and cholinergic nervous systems. The mechanism of injury likely involves the endoneurial arterioles, which supply the nerves, similar to peripheral neuropathy. The dysfunction of these two major involuntary nervous systems have systemwide effects. Autonomic neuropathy affecting the cardiovascular system may cause resting tachycardia and postural hypotension. The gastrointestinal system demonstrates parasympathetic dysfunction by gastroparesis, a gastric emptying abnormality. The individual with gastroparesis suffers anorexia, nausea, vomiting, early satiety, and abdominal bloating. Bowel dysfunction can occur, presenting as alternating bouts of diarrhea and constipation.

Bladder problems can develop as a result of parasympathetic dysfunction, including autonomic bladder complications such as the inability to sense a full bladder and diminishing bladder contractility. As bladder contractility decreases, urine retention occurs, which increases the risk of urinary tract infection. Bladder and bowel incontinence can also result from sympathetic neuropathy. Erectile dysfunction and female sexual dysfunction are also side effects of autonomic neuropathy.

In addition, autonomic neuropathy can mask the signals of hypoglycemia in the patient who is diabetic. In hypoglycemia, a nondiabetic individual receives symptoms signaling blood sugar is dangerously low, including sweating, tachycardia, headache, lack of concentration ability, irritability, pallor, and tremors. These symptoms occur because of the sympathetic stress response and the brain cell's lack of glucose. However, these warning signals of hypoglycemia may not occur in person with diabetes because of autonomic dysfunction. Autonomic neuropathy blunts the individual's ability to perspire, which is a necessary mechanism of heat regulation. Tachycardia and tremors may not occur because of the lack of sympathetic neuron discharge. The diabetic patient may suffer from episodes of hypoglycemia unawareness to the point of loss of consciousness.

In addition, lack of sweating can cause:

- heat intolerance in warm weather
- problems during exercise, as heat release from the body is blocked
- anhidrosis leading to dry skin, which increases the risk of skin breakdown in the feet.

ALERT! Anhidrosis, decreased blood flow, and lack of sensation in the feet together dramatically increase the susceptibility to foot ulcers.

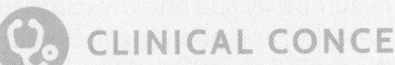

CLINICAL CONCEPT

Elderly individuals are particularly susceptible to hyperthermia and heat stroke because of autonomic neuropathy.

Lack of appropriate sympathetic and parasympathetic nervous system responses also contributes to atypical clinical presentation of disease processes. The individual with diabetes who is experiencing a concomitant condition such as acute abdomen, myocardial infarction, inflammatory disease, or infection may not present with expected symptoms. Autonomic neuropathy alters cardiovascular, bronchial, gastrointestinal, and genitourinary responses to illness.

Susceptibility to Infection. Individuals with diabetes have a greater susceptibility to infection than the general population. T cells and WBC phagocytic function are detrimentally affected by the hyperglycemic environment of the bloodstream. WBCs become less able to fight infection, resulting in a level of immunosuppression.

Hyperglycemia caused by poor glycemic control is a factor for the colonization of certain microorganisms. Individuals with poor glycemic control have an increased colonization of staphylococcus aureus on the skin, which increases susceptibility to wound infection. Pneumonia, urinary tract infection, and skin and soft-tissue infections are more common in the diabetic population, as are tuberculosis and fungal infections.

Candida (yeast) is a frequent cause of infection of the genital tract and also commonly develops within intertriginous skinfolds. Chronic *Candida vaginitis* may be a presenting feature of diabetes before other signs. *Candida* infection is common in diabetes because with hyperglycemia, the vaginal cells become glycogen rich. High glucose changes the pH of the vaginal canal, making it more conducive to proliferation of *Candida* organisms.

> ### 🩺 CLINICAL CONCEPT
>
> Both males and females can have *Candida* infection of the genital tract caused by diabetes.

Diabetes as a Cause of Lower Extremity Amputation.

Diabetic foot complications are the most common cause of nontraumatic lower extremity amputation in the United States and worldwide. Foot complications are also the most frequent cause of hospitalization in patients with diabetes. With long-term exposure to hyperglycemia, the nerves and arterial vessels of the lower extremity are damaged, with the most distal nerves and arterial vessels affected initially.

Peripheral neuropathy and microvascular injury lead to a loss of sensation and poor circulation in the feet. In addition, the inhibitory effects of hyperglycemia on WBCs cause increased risk of infection in the lower extremities. All of these factors contribute to the risk of nonhealing wounds and infections in the lower extremities of patients with diabetes.

It is important to understand that individuals with diabetes can sustain a minor foot injury without sensory perception of the wound. However, minor skin injury can rapidly develop into an infected foot ulcer caused by peripheral neuropathy, poor circulation, and WBC dysfunction, which decreases the efficiency of wound healing (Fig. 25-17). Poorly healing wounds can lead to deeper tissue infection and the complication of gangrene, a bacterial infection that can develop in wounds with poor circulation. In gangrene, Clostridium, a gas-producing bacterium, invades the ischemic tissue of the foot and causes tissue necrosis. The infection can spread upward into the more proximal regions of the lower extremity.

Osteomyelitis, infection of the bone, can develop if an infection such as *Staphylococcus aureus*, a common bacterial inhabitant of the skin, extends deep into lower level tissue. Osteomyelitis and gangrene are often the complications that necessitate amputation in the individual with diabetes (see Fig. 25-18).

Careful examination of the diabetic foot is the most effective measure to prevent lower extremity amputation. Meticulous neurological and vascular assessment of the feet are needed on a regular basis. Examination of foot sensation using light touch over noncallused areas is recommended (see Fig. 25-19). During the examination, it is important to have the patient close his or her eyes so as not to visually detect the regions the examiner is testing. The neurological exam of the lower extremities should include testing the Achilles tendon reflex, light sensation, sense of toe position, and vibration sense. Regular podiatric care is also recommended,

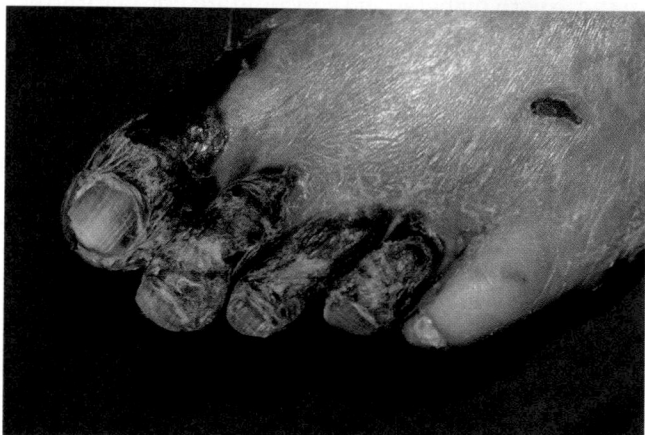

FIGURE 25-18. Osteomyelitis and gangrene of the diabetic foot. *(From Scott Camazine/Science Source.)*

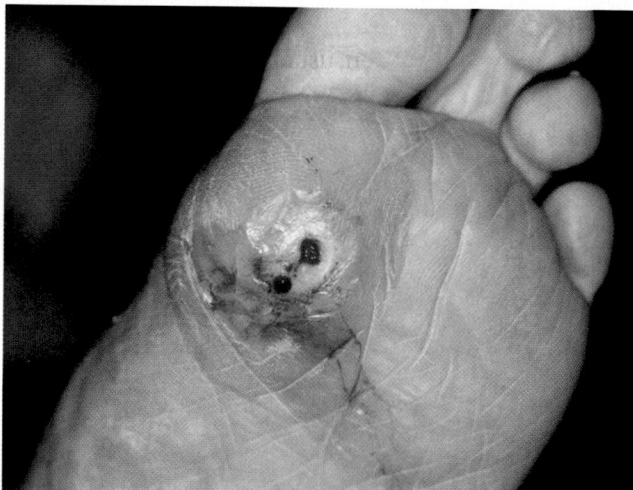

FIGURE 25-17. Diabetic foot ulcer. *(From Roberto A. Penne-Casanova / Science Source.)*

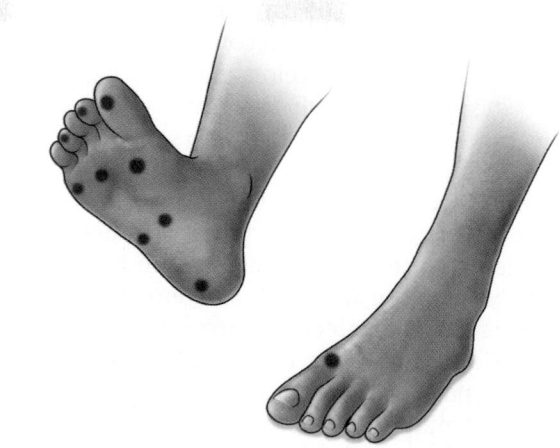

FIGURE 25-19. Sensory testing of the feet in diabetes. *(Adapted from U.S. Department of Health & Human Services (DHHS).)*

because sensory loss may prevent the individual with diabetes from performing safe care.

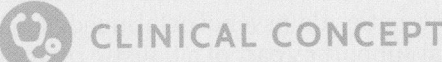

CLINICAL CONCEPT

Because of sensory loss in the feet, individuals with diabetes need specialized foot care by a podiatrist.

Diabetic Retinopathy as a Cause of Blindness. Diabetes is one of the leading causes of blindness in adults. The hyperglycemia of poorly controlled diabetes damages the fragile retinal artery endothelium. Endothelial injury incites inflammation, which attracts WBCs and platelets to the sites. Products of inflammation eventually occlude the small caliber retinal arterioles and capillaries, causing retinal ischemia. Injured endothelium becomes extrapermeable, allowing fluid to leak into the tissue, resulting in edema. Blindness is the end result of years of retinal circulatory damage caused by exposure to high blood glucose. Concomitant hypertension accelerates damage to the retina. Clinical signs of retinopathy are microaneurysms, hemorrhages, macular edema, exudates, and "cotton wool spots" (infarcted regions of the retina from prolonged ischemia) evident on fundoscopic examination. Later in the course of disease, during the stage called proliferative retinopathy, proliferation of new retinal artery branches emerge from the optic disc region (see Fig. 25-20). It is theorized that hypoxia of the retinal tissue stimulates endothelial secretion of VEGF, which causes the proliferation of new blood vessels in a process called neovascularization. These new fragile arterial branches grow in between the internal surface of the retina and vitreous gel. Rupture of these vessels pulls the retinal layer away from the aqueous gel, which causes the patient to see floaters and flashes of light, as well as experience visual disturbances. Proliferative retinopathy increases the risk of retinal detachment.

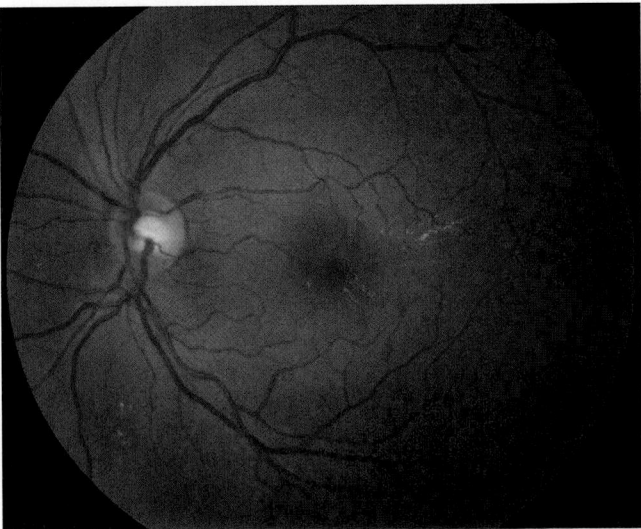

FIGURE 25-20. Changes of the retina in diabetic retinopathy. *(From Paul Whitten /Science Source.)*

The development of retinopathy depends on the duration of diabetes and degree of glycemic control. There is a probable genetic susceptibility as well. After initial signs and symptoms of retinopathy are detected, progression to a more advanced form of the disease occurs within 5 years if untreated. Routine nondilated eye examinations are inadequate to detect diabetic retinopathy. Periodic, regular fundoscopic and complete ophthalmological examinations are advised. Laser photocoagulation therapy, used to treat retinopathy, has decreased the development of blindness among individuals with diabetes.

Diabetic Nephropathy as a Cause of Renal Failure. Diabetes is the leading cause of end-stage renal disease in adults. Microscopic glomerular injury is the initial mechanism that causes kidney dysfunction in diabetes. Hyperglycemia of poorly controlled diabetes damages the glomerular capillaries, causing them to become hyperpermeable, allowing albumin to be filtered out of the blood. Under healthy conditions, the glomerulus should not filter any significant amount of protein out of the blood. Glomerular injury becomes apparent when small amounts of albumin from the bloodstream leak into the urine in microalbuminuria. Standard urinalysis dipstick tests cannot detect this minute amount of albumin in the urine, and frank proteinuria develops after years of glomerular damage is sustained. Proteinuria typically increases as renal function decreases.

In diabetic nephropathy, the glomerular basement membrane (GBM) thickens and the renal vasculature demonstrates atherosclerotic changes. Factors that trigger thickening of the GBM include glycosylation endproducts, angiotensin II, growth hormone, and insulinlike growth factor. The thickened glomerular walls eventually cause glomerular hypertension and obliteration of the glomerular capillary lumens. If enough glomeruli are affected, glomerulosclerosis, a cause of renal dysfunction, results. Renal dysfunction leads to constant renin secretion, which increases blood pressure. The renal impairment is a source of hypertension, which further damages glomeruli and worsens renal function; the damage then continues in a cyclical manner. Diabetic retinopathy, also worsened by hypertension, usually precedes the complication of nephropathy.

Dermatological Complications of Diabetes. The most significant skin manifestations of diabetes are prolonged wound healing and skin ulceration, but less serious skin lesions are also common in diabetes. Pigmented pretibial papules known as diabetic skin spots are hyperpigmented areas on the legs that develop because of minor trauma in the tibial region. *Necrobiosis lipoidica diabeticorum* is a rare disorder that develops in a similar manner; however, atrophy and ulceration also occur within the lesions. *Acanthosis nigricans* are a conglomeration of tiny, hyperpigmented, velvety macular lesions usually located on the neck, axilla, or extensor surfaces in individuals with insulin resistance and diabetes. Lipoatrophy and lipohypertrophy can occur at sites of insulin injection but are not common with the use of human insulin. Dry skin and pruritus are common complaints of individuals with diabetes because of the anhidrosis of autonomic neuropathy.

 CLINICAL CONCEPT

To prevent lipoatrophy and lipohypertrophy, rotation of insulin injection sites between the abdomen, deltoid, and thigh is recommended.

Psychological and Emotional Aspects of Diabetes. Depression is two times more common in persons with diabetes than in the general population. Guilt and discouragement are emotions frequently expressed by individuals with diabetes, despite their best efforts to manage the condition. Many patients tend to view their blood glucose measurements, weight, and A1c values as a report card of their ability to control the disease. Individuals with poor glycemic control often blame themselves and feel powerless and angry about their inability to manage the disease process.

Anxiety is also a common emotional response of patients affected by diabetes. Many patients find it stressful to manage a chronic disease because it requires preplanning of diet and exercise, precautions with traveling, and self-administration of scheduled medication. Unlike other diseases, the responsibility for management of diabetes lies with the patient. Patients are often worried about their ability to maintain adequate glycemic control and fear long-term complications. Some patients cite specific concerns, such as fear of hypoglycemia, needles, problems with pregnancy, complications, or weight gain. Anxiety particularly affects those suffering infection and poor circulation of the lower extremity. Inadequate wound healing increases the diabetic individual's risk of gangrene and amputation. Many patients in this situation worry about the prospect of amputation.

Denial is common among many individuals with diabetes. Many affected individuals refuse to comply with insulin administration. Clinicians refer to this as psychological insulin resistance. This is particularly common in persons with type 2 diabetes who initially obtain good glycemic control with oral medications and later in the course of the disease require insulin. Many patients in this situation view taking insulin as a loss of control and refuse to comply with medical advice. Some patients worry that taking insulin will rob their lives of spontaneity, make travel and dining out difficult, and place restrictions on their lifestyle. Others refuse to take insulin because they worry about the threat of hypoglycemia and weight gain. The clinician should not imply that the addition of insulin is because of the patient's inability to control glucose or failure of oral medication. Insulin treatment should not be depicted in negative terms or as punishment for poor glycemic

control. At the time of diagnosis, the clinician should discuss the likelihood that insulin will be needed for optimal control of blood glucose as the disease progresses. In addition, clinicians should periodically assess the patient's psychosocial needs and provide emotional support as part of a holistic treatment plan.

Eating Disorders and Diabetes. Eating disorders are pervasive among adolescents, particularly females. Studies have shown that many young women with type 1 diabetes have a heightened risk for food bingeing and bulimia (vomiting or using laxatives to avoid weight gain).

Often, upon initial diagnosis of type 1 diabetes, an individual presents with symptoms that include weight loss; this occurs because of the deficiency of insulin, lack of cellular glucose uptake, and consequent breakdown of fats. Among some individuals, this weight loss may be perceived as a desirable effect of diabetes.

After diagnosis, to obtain optimal glycemic control, the individual with type 1 diabetes must adhere to strict dietary, exercise, and insulin regimens. After optimal glycemic control is established, weight gain often occurs because of the anabolic effects of insulin. Insulin inhibits fat breakdown, enhances cellular uptake of glucose, and blocks hepatic glucose production.

Individuals with diabetes often find this weight gain undesirable and associate it with insulin administration. To initiate weight loss, the diabetic individual with an eating disorder administers less insulin despite glycemic needs. Studies show that one-third to one-half of young women with type 1 diabetes may engage in this practice, known as *insulin purging.* These individuals often completely omit dosages of insulin, endure frequent episodes of hyperglycemia, and allow the body to enter starvation mode to enhance fat breakdown.

ALERT! Eating disorders should be suspected in patients with recurrent DKA or chronically poor glycemic control.

These individuals are at increased risk for DKA or HHS. Ultimately, the prolonged exposure to hyperglycemia damages organs and increases risk of long-term complications in these patients.

Treatment of Diabetes

Managing diabetes requires an understanding of the extremes of poor glycemic control— hypoglycemia versus hyperglycemia (see Fig. 25-21). In both types of diabetes, individuals on insulin are susceptible to hypoglycemic episodes; blood glucose should be maintained within a narrow range of 70 to 140 mg/dL regardless of food intake or physical activity. In mild hypoglycemia with a blood glucose level lower than 60 mg/dL, the individual experiences hunger, irritability, palpitations, pallor, nervousness, headache, and an inability to concentrate. As hypoglycemia worsens, tachycardia, hypertension or

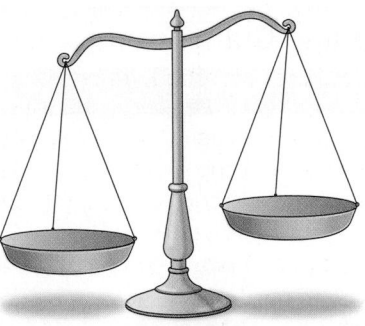

Diabetes

Hypoglycemia	Hyperglycemia
Blood glucose too low; symptoms: nervousness or tremors, diaphoresis, pallor, weakness, inability to concentrate, irritability, headache, tachycardia, syncope, coma	Blood glucose too high; symptoms: blurry vision, polyuria, polydipsia, polyphagia, weight loss, confusion, weakness, nausea, vomiting, ketone breath, coma, *DKA or hyperosmolar hyperglycemic syndrome*
Possible etiologies: too much insulin or antidiabetic medication excessive exercise lack of eating drug interactions alcohol use extreme stress illness infection	**Possible etiologies:** inadequate insulin (endogenous or exogenous) insulin resistance infection ingestion of excess carbohydrates low physical activity drug interactions "Somogyi effect"

FIGURE 25-21. The extremes of poor glycemic control in diabetes.

hypotension, diaphoresis, slurred speech, blurred vision, and syncope can occur. If blood glucose falls to extremely low levels, such as 30 mg/dL or lower, seizure and coma are possible.

Insulin excess is the most common cause of hypoglycemia; however, other causative factors are alcohol use, drug interactions, strenuous physical activity, inadequate dietary intake, or carbohydrate malabsorption. Beta-adrenergic blockers and sulfonylureas are drugs that increase the risk of hypoglycemia.

ALERT! Beta-adrenergic blockers will mask the symptoms of hypoglycemia in patients with diabetes.

Beta-adrenergic blockers blunt the process of hepatic glycogenolysis and mask the symptoms of hypoglycemia. Beta-adrenergic blockers counteract the hypoglycemia warning signs of tremor, tachycardia, and other symptoms of sympathetic nervous system activation. Critical illnesses such as liver, renal, or heart failure; serious infection; and sepsis also increase the risk of hypoglycemia or hyperglycemia. In diabetes, any major stress, including emotional strain, can cause erratic variations in blood glucose and necessitate altered glycemic control measures.

Individuals with type 1 or type 2 diabetes can delay or prevent complications by maintaining near-normal blood glucose levels. Strict glycemic control is the goal of all forms of treatment. Aggressive control of lipids and blood pressure also assist to counteract the development of complications. The individual with diabetes should try to avoid large fluctuations in blood glucose levels. The clinician uses three major indices to guide and evaluate treatment efficacy:

- A1c level
- fasting blood glucose level
- postprandial blood glucose level.

Diabetes involves a delicate balancing act in blood glucose control: prevention of hypoglycemia versus hyperglycemia.

Lifestyle Modifications

A diagnosis of diabetes often provokes a patient to review his or her lifestyle. Diet, exercise, and habits such as use of alcohol or smoking need to be assessed to find areas where the patient needs modification. Often diet and exercise alone can control diabetes.

Diet

Maintaining ideal body weight is an important factor in diabetes because obesity causes insulin resistance. Patients with newly diagnosed diabetes should consult with a nutritionist or diabetes educator to identify individualized daily calorie recommendations, preferred food choices, daily menus, cooking recommendations, and exercise regimens. A diet low in sugar and carbohydrates is advised, with carbohydrates comprising about 50% of daily caloric intake. Each gram of carbohydrate contains 4 calories.

To achieve optimal glycemic control, carbohydrate counting is one method that is advised. For example, an individual who is diabetic is on a 1,600-calorie diet and aims to consume 50% of total calories from carbohydrates. This would be a total of 800 calories of carbohydrate. To calculate how many grams of carbohydrate this is equal to, take 800 calories divided by 4 calories/gram. This is equal to 200 grams of carbohydrate spread out over the day. For examples of how many grams of carbohydrates are in some common foods, see Table 25-3.

The individual's recommended total daily calorie intake is determined based on the patient's gender, body mass index (BMI), goal weight, physical activity level, and body-build. A schedule for meals and snacks can be determined based on the patient's medication regimen and daily routine. A nutritionist or diabetes educator can advise which foods and how many servings per day are recommended.

Because the patient who is diabetic is at increased risk of cardiovascular disease, a low-fat, low-sodium diet is also recommended. It should consist of:

- Total fats: 25% to 30% of total calories
  - Saturated fats: less than i 7% of total calories

TABLE 25-3. Different Carbohydrate Sources and Gram Count

Food	Amount	Carb Grams	Food	Amount	Carb Grams
1% Fat milk	1 cup	12	Yogurt fruited	1 cup	40
Bran Chex	2/3 cup	23	Yogurt fruit	1 cup	19
Frosted Flakes	3/4 cup	26	Raisin Bran	3/4 cup	28
Fruit juice	1/2 cup	15	Bread/toast	1 slice	15
Banana	1/2	15	Sugar	1 tsp.	4
Pancake syrup	2 Tbsp.	30	Pancakes-4	2	15
Low-fat granola	1/2 cup	30	Sugar-free syrup	2 Tbsp.	4

(Source: Treatment of Diabetes. Retrieved at http://www.endocrineweb.com/diabetes/treatment.html on July 8, 2015.)

- ○ Monounsaturated fats: less than i 10% of total calories
- ○ Polyunsaturated fats: less than i 10% of total calories
- Cholesterol: less than 200 mg daily
- Sodium to: less than 2300 mg per day (1500 mg if hypertension present).

Overall, the diabetic diet should consist of approximately 50% carbohydrates, 30% fats (as previously categorized), and 20% protein. The total calorie count is calculated according to how much weight loss is desired or if weight maintenance is the goal. To maintain weight, patients with diabetes should have a diet that has approximately 35 calories per kg of body weight per day (or approximately 16 calories per pound of body weight per day). To lose weight, the nutritionist would recommend a lower total daily calorie count depending on the individual patient's goal.

Glycemic Index

A diet can also be devised that takes glycemic index into consideration. The **glycemic index** measures how a carbohydrate-containing food raises blood glucose. Carbohydrate-containing foods with a low glycemic index include dried beans and legumes, most vegetables, most fruit, and whole grain breads and cereals. As a general rule, the more processed a food, the higher the glycemic index. A low glycemic index diet combines low glycemic index foods with high glycemic index foods. Some nutritionists can be consulted about this strategy. Portion sizes are still relevant for managing blood glucose, as well as for losing or maintaining weight. Research shows that both the amount and the type of carbohydrate in food affect blood glucose levels. Studies also show that the total amount of carbohydrate in food, in general, is a stronger predictor of blood glucose response than the glycemic index.

Exercise

Exercise is beneficial for individuals with diabetes because contractile muscle activity enhances cellular uptake of glucose, and contracting muscle cells do not require insulin for glucose entry, which is why individuals with diabetes can lower their blood glucose levels with vigorous physical activity. In addition, exercise builds collateral blood vessels in the heart and large muscle groups, raises high-density lipoprotein (HDL) cholesterol, reduces obesity, and lowers blood pressure. Collateral blood vessel growth, elevated HDL cholesterol levels, and reduced blood pressure are advantageous cardiovascular effects that counteract coronary artery and peripheral vascular disease, which are major complications of diabetes. Exercise also counteracts obesity, which is a major cause of insulin resistance.

ALERT! Strenuous muscle activity lowers blood glucose which can lead to hypoglycemia.

However, individuals with diabetes must remember that strenuous muscle activity will reduce blood glucose levels, which can lead to hypoglycemia. To reduce risk for hypoglycemia, insulin doses should be reduced before vigorous physical activity. Exercise should be scheduled 1 to 2 hours after a meal or when insulin is not at peak levels. The individual should ingest carbohydrate snacks during sustained exercise and vigilantly monitor blood glucose. Delayed hypoglycemia can occur for 6 to 15 hours, or as long as 24 hours, after strenuous exercise. Postexercise delayed hypoglycemia is a result of increased glucose uptake of skeletal muscle, heightened insulin sensitivity of skeletal muscle, and depletion of hepatic glycogen stores. The replenishment of hepatic glycogen stores may require higher carbohydrate intake in the ensuing hours after exercise.

The individual who performs vigorous exercise should carry glucose tablets or gel and a diabetic identification bracelet or card. He or she should also exercise with a partner who is aware of the possibility of hypoglycemia. A glucagon kit may be necessary to keep as a precaution for episodes of hypoglycemia.

Proper foot care is essential for athletic individuals with diabetes. Vigilant inspection of foot surfaces is important after exercise because peripheral neuropathy can hinder the sensation of lesions. Autonomic neuropathy can cause heat intolerance, lack of perspiration, dependent edema, orthostatic hypotension, and hypoglycemic unawareness with exercise. Because individuals with diabetes are at increased risk for coronary artery and peripheral vascular disease, a periodic cardiology consultation is advisable before beginning a regular vigorous exercise routine.

Aerobic exercise activities benefit individuals with diabetes. Strength training with light weights and high repetitions is recommended for young persons, but not for older patients or those with long-standing diabetes. Both clinicians and patients need to be aware of the risks of strenuous exercise. Meticulous attention to blood glucose monitoring, diet, insulin, and medication are particularly important for athletic individuals with diabetes.

Health Maintenance

Diabetes increases the risk of cardiovascular disease, so periodic measurement of serum lipids and blood pressure are advised. Ideal goals to prevent cardiovascular disease in diabetes include maintaining the following levels:

- Blood pressure: lower than or equal to 120/80 mm Hg
- Low-density lipoprotein (LDL) cholesterol: lower than or equal to 100 mg/dL
- HDL cholesterol: greater than or equal to 60 mg/dL
- Triglycerides: lower than or equal to 150 mg/dL.

Periodic cardiac assessment should include exercise testing and identification of risk for autonomic neuropathy. Exercise tolerance testing, also known as stress testing, is key because silent MI and infarction can occur in diabetes. Smoking increases susceptibility to cardiac and peripheral vascular disease and cessation methods should be advised. Diabetic individuals should aim for an ideal body weight and learn how to maintain it.

Because an increased risk of infection is present with diabetes, individuals should receive flu vaccine annually and, depending on age, pneumococcal vaccine every 5 years. Patients need to understand that infection can cause changes in glycemic levels. The possibility of blood glucose fluctuations requires more frequent blood glucose monitoring during illness.

ALERT! Infection can cause significant fluctuations in blood glucose. Frequent blood glucose monitoring is important during illness.

Foot care is a key element in the prevention of complications. Individuals need to understand the possible loss of sensation and their vulnerability to foot ulcers. Well-fitting shoes, dry socks, and daily foot inspection are essential. Those with long-term diabetes should have regular podiatric care.

Older patients with diabetes and those with long-term disease need to be aware of the possibility of visual problems and complications of the eye. Annual ophthalmological examination, including a dilated fundoscopic examination, is recommended.

Urine glucose and ketones should be checked during periodic physical examinations. Clinicians also need to check for microalbuminuria, which may be an early warning sign of nephropathy.

BOX 25-9. Recommended Blood Glucose Values in Diabetes

- **Preprandial:** 90 to 130 mg/dL
- **Postprandial:** lower than 180 mg/dL
- **Bedtime:** 100 to 140 mg/dL

Patient Self-Monitoring of Blood Glucose

All individuals with diabetes need to have a blood glucose measuring device known as a glucometer. Use of a glucometer requires thorough patient education so that lifetime blood glucose testing becomes part of the patient's daily routine. Clinicians should demonstrate use of the device and have the patient give a return demonstration to ensure understanding. These devices require a drop of blood obtained by a lancet. The sample of blood obtained from a finger or forearm is placed on a clinical testing strip and inserted into the glucometer. The device then evaluates the glucose level within the blood droplet. Blood glucose levels should be evaluated twice to several times per day, depending on the clinician's recommendation. Commonly, clinicians recommend measurement of blood glucose before eating, known as **preprandial blood glucose;** 2 hours after eating, known as **postprandial glucose;** and at bedtime. The individual needs to be aware of the parameters indicating adequate control of blood glucose (see Box 25-9).

Many types of glucometers have memory of daily glucose values and the patient can have the clinician review the glucometer readings for periodic assessment of glucose control.

Basics of Insulin Therapy

The goal of insulin therapy is to mimic physiologic control of blood glucose levels through basal and postprandial levels of insulin. Basal insulin levels occur during fasting, whereas postprandial insulin levels occur after eating a meal. To mimic physiologic control of glucose, insulin regimens must closely mimic pancreatic secretory patterns without causing hypoglycemia. Conventional insulins and insulin analogues are the two types of insulin available. There are short-, intermediate-, and long-acting forms of both types of insulin. Often, the combined use of these types of insulin can be used to simulate fasting and postprandial pancreatic insulin.

Conventional Insulins. Used for many years, conventional insulins are synthetic human insulins. These include:

- **Regular:** rapid-acting, short duration
- **NPH:** intermediate-acting, longer duration
- **Lente:** intermediate-acting, longer duration
- **Ultralente:** long-acting, long duration.

For an in-depth comparison of the different insulins, see Table 25-4.

Regular and NPH human insulin are the most commonly used preparations.

TABLE 25-4. Pharmacokinetics of Conventional Insulins and Insulin Analogues

Insulin	Classification	Onset of Action (hr)	Peak of Activity (hr)	Duration (hr)
Regular insulin (Novolin R) (Humulin R)	Rapid-acting conventional insulin	$\frac{1}{2}$ to 1 hour	2 to 6 hours	3 to 8 hours
Aspart insulin (Novolog) Lispro insulin (Humalog)	Rapid-acting analogue insulin	Less than $\frac{1}{2}$ hour	1 hour	3 to 4 hours
NPH (Novolin N) (Humulin N)	Intermediate-acting conventional insulin	2 to 4 hours	4 to 10 hours	10 to 20 hours
Lente (Novolin L) (Humulin L)	Intermediate-acting conventional insulin	3 to 4 hours	4 to 12 hours	10 to 20 hours
Ultralente (Humulin U)	Long-acting conventional insulin	6 to 10 hours	Dose dependent	16 to 20 hours
Glargine insulin (Lantus) Detemir insulin (Levemir)	Long-acting analogue insulin	2 to 3 hours 6 to 8 hours	None (steady level)	24 hours 6 to 24 hours depending on dosage

A mixture of 70% NPH human insulin and 30% regular human insulin (Novolin 70/30, Humulin 70/30) is available in vials, cartridges, and prefilled syringes.

(Adapted from White, J. R., Campbell, R. K., & Hirsch, I. B. (2003). Novel insulins and strict glycemic control. *Postgrad Med*, 113(6), 30–36.)

Insulin Analogues. Although fairly effective in reducing blood glucose levels, conventional insulins cannot mimic normal physiologic insulin secretion. Insulin analogues, synthetic preparations with a slightly different structure than human insulin, have pharmacokinetic profiles that closely approximate physiologic endogenous insulin secretion. The analogues include:

- **Lispro (Humalog):** rapid-acting
- **Aspart (NovoLog):** rapid-acting
- **Glargine (Lantus):** long-acting
- **Detemir (Levemir):** long-acting.

As compared with regular insulin, insulin lispro has a more rapid onset of action, an earlier peak effect, and a shorter duration of action. It reaches peak activity 0.5 to 2.5 hours after injection. Therefore, insulin lispro should be injected 15 minutes before a meal as compared with regular insulin, which is injected 30 to 60 minutes before a meal.

Insulin aspart has a rapid onset of action (20 minutes) and a shorter duration of action (3 to 5 hours) than regular human insulin. It reaches peak activity 1 to 3 hours after injection. Insulin glargine has a slower onset of action (70 minutes) and a longer duration of action (24 hours) than regular human insulin. Its activity does not peak. Detemir insulin also has a duration of action of 24 hours and slow onset of action.

The Right Insulin for the Right Patient. An individualized insulin regimen is devised according to the patients' specific needs for glucose control. The basal-prandial insulin regimen, also called basal-bolus, is a common type of treatment for optimal glycemic control. This regimen uses a once-daily injection of a long-acting insulin to control the fasting plasma glucose level (basal insulin) and boluses of a rapid-acting insulin for postmeal glucose elevations (prandial insulin). A once-daily injection of

NPH can be used as a basal level of insulin supplemented by regular insulin bolus injections after meals. The clinician prescribes the dosages and approximate times when the patient should administer these insulins. There is also a premixed combination of 70% NPH human insulin and 30% regular human insulin (Novolin 70/30, Humulin 70/30) available for this type of regimen.

The basal-prandial analogue insulin regimen has been found to closely approximate normal physiologic insulin patterns and is becoming the preferred treatment. It combines a rapid acting insulin, such as lispro, with a longer-acting insulin analogue, such as glargine (see Fig. 25-22).

Clinicians individualize insulin treatment regimens based on the patient's age, lifestyle, self-reported

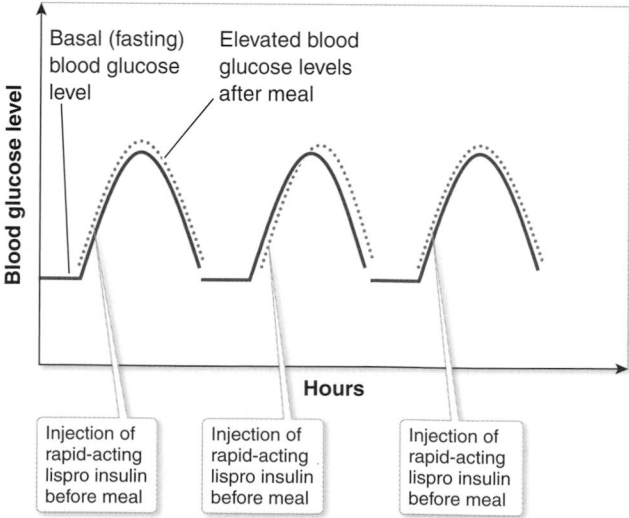

FIGURE 25-22. Example of a basal-prandial insulin analogue injection regimen for strict glycemic control. The patient is administered rapid-acting insulin (lispro) before each meal for postprandial control of blood glucose elevations and once a day is administered a long-acting insulin (glargine) for basal control of blood glucose.

symptoms, existence of concomitant conditions, and history of glycemic control. Insulin dosage, route of administration, and times for administration need to be tailored to patient needs. Insulin can be injected subcutaneously via a syringe or a penlike device or administered at a steady rate via a programmable pump (see Box 25-10). The subcutaneous tissue of the abdomen, upper arm, or thigh are recommended injection sites and should be rotated. Some insulin suspensions require refrigeration. Alternative forms of insulin such as inhalers, sublingual tablets, and transdermal insulin patches are in development.

Patient education regarding proper insulin injection is required. Family members or significant others should ideally be taught the technique as well. Early in insulin treatment, the clinician and patient must closely monitor daily preprandial, postprandial, bedtime, and possibly early morning blood glucose levels. The clinician reviews the various blood glucose values, evaluates the patient's condition, and may revise insulin dosage until appropriate glycemic control is reached.

Oral Antidiabetic Agents in Management of Type 2 Diabetes

Treatment of type 2 diabetes is a stepwise approach that begins with lifestyle modification. Oral antidiabetic agents are initiated when lifestyle modifications prove insufficient to maintain glycemic control. If monotherapy with an oral antidiabetic agent cannot control blood glucose levels, combinations of oral medications are often effective. If oral medications alone do not control blood glucose, insulin is often added to the oral medication regimen.

A wide array of different types of oral antidiabetic agents are available. Different categories of drugs have different mechanisms of action and pharmacokinetics. Although monotherapy can be effective in some individuals, combination therapy is more often indicated. Because of this, there are many available medications that are presynthesized combinations of different classes of drugs. The following are the categories of available oral antidiabetic agents:

- Insulinotropic agents, also called insulin secretagogues
  ○ Subcategories: sulfonylureas, meglitinides
- Biguanides
- Thiazolidinediones
- Alpha-glucosidase inhibitors
- Incretin mimetics
- Amylin mimetics
- DPP-4 inhibitors
- SGLT2 inhibitors.

See Table 25-5 for a detailed breakdown of the different categories of oral antidiabetic agents.

BOX 25-10. How Does an Insulin Pump Work?

An insulin pump is an external device that continuously delivers rapid-acting insulin to the body through a small cannula placed under the skin. About the size of a cell phone, it can be hidden under clothing or worn on the waistband.

Before a patient can use an insulin pump, the clinician must assess the patient and determine appropriate insulin dosages. The patient must have an adequate understanding of the disease process and learn how to program the pump. Patient education with a diabetes educator or the clinician are necessary before patient use.

Insulin pumps are programmed by the user to continuously deliver small doses of rapid-acting insulin between meals or overnight during fasting. This dose is called a basal insulin level. At meals, the user programs an extra dose of insulin, called a bolus, to cover the increase in blood glucose. This insulin regimen most closely mimics how a healthy pancreas functions in a person without diabetes.

ADVANTAGES OF USING AN INSULIN PUMP
Some advantages of using an insulin pump instead of insulin injections are:

- Using an insulin pump allows elimination of individual insulin injections.
- Insulin pumps deliver insulin more accurately than injections.

- Insulin pumps often improve A1c levels.
- Using an insulin pump usually results in fewer fluctuations in blood glucose levels.
- Using an insulin pump makes diabetes management easier—if blood glucose level is high, extra insulin can be delivered by pushing a button on the pump.
- Insulin pumps allow individuals to be more flexible about when and what they eat.
- Using an insulin pump eliminates unpredictable effects of intermediate- or long-acting insulin.
- Insulin pumps allow the individual to exercise without having to eat large amounts of carbohydrates.

DISADVANTAGES OF USING AN INSULIN PUMP
The disadvantages of using a pump are that it can:

- cause weight gain
- cause DKA if the cannula is dislodged and doesn't deliver insulin for hours
- be expensive
- be bothersome because the individual is attached to the pump most of the time
- require a hospital stay or maybe a full day in the outpatient center to be trained.

(Source: American Diabetes Association. Insulin pumps. Retrieved from http://www.diabetes.org/living-with-diabetes/treatment-and-care/medication/insulin/how-do-insulin-pumps-work.html on July 8, 2015.)

TABLE 25-5. Oral Antidiabetic Agents

Oral Antidiabetic Agent Generic and (Brand) Name	Classifications	Action	Indications/Usage
Glimepiride (Amaryl) Glipizide (Glucotrol) Glyburide (DiaBeta) Chlorpropamide (Diabinese)	Sulfonylureas (insulinotropic)	Stimulates pancreas to secrete insulin	Type 2 diabetes; patient must have the ability to secrete natural endogenous insulin
Metformin (Glucophage or Fortamet)	Biguanide	Sensitizes cells to insulin; inhibits hepatic glucose production; lowers cholesterol, triglycerides, and LDLs; raises HDLs	Type 2 diabetes; patient with mainly insulin resistance; hyperinsulinism; patients with metabolic syndrome
Acarbose (Precose or Miglitol)	Alpha-glucosidase inhibitor	Blocks enzyme that assists in intestinal absorption of carbohydrates	Type 2 diabetes; patient with insulin resistance, metabolic syndrome, or pancreatic beta cell dysfunction
Pioglitazone (Actos) Rosiglitazone (Avandia)	Thiazolinedione (also called glitazones)	Counteracts insulin resistance by sensitizing cells to insulin, reduces glucose production by liver	Type 2 diabetes; patient with mainly insulin resistance; hyperinsulinism; patients with metabolic syndrome
Repaglinide (Prandin) Nateglinide (Starlix)	Meglitinides (insulinotropic)	Stimulates pancreas to secrete insulin	Type 2 diabetes; patient must have the ability to secrete natural endogenous insulin
Sitagliptin (Januvia)	DPP-4 inhibitor	Inhibits the enzyme dipeptidyl peptidase-4 that destroys GLP-1 and GIP and thereby increases the levels and activity of both hormones. As a result, blood glucose levels fall.	Type 2 diabetes
SGLT2 inhibitor: canagliflozin (Invokana) dapagliflozin (Farxiga)	SGLT2 inhibitor	SGLT2 inhibitors: inhibit reabsorption of glucose at the kidney	Type 2 diabetes

Insulinotropic Agents

Insulinotropic agents stimulate pancreatic beta cells to secrete insulin and are used in type 2 diabetes. These agents require that individuals have some endogenous pancreatic insulin reserve. Sulfonylureas and meglitinides are the two types of medications under this category.

Sulfonylureas. **Sulfonylureas** are the oldest oral antidiabetic medications and have long been the cornerstone of type 2 diabetes treatment. Chlorpropamide (Diabinese) is the only first generation drug still used. There are three second generation drugs:

- Glipizide (Glucotrol)
- Glyburide (Micronase, Glynase, DiaBeta)
- Glimepiride (Amaryl).

Sulfonyureas are generally taken once or twice daily before meals. They have similar effects in reducing blood glucose but differ in side effects, duration of action, and interactions with other drugs. Hypoglycemia and weight gain are two common side effects. Allergy to sulfa is a contraindication to use of these drugs. Alcohol use is also contraindicated with some sulfonylureas. Sulfonylureas have no effect on triglycerides or cholesterol.

The majority of sulfonylureas undergo renal elimination. For example, chlorpropamide should not be used in patients with renal dysfunction (20% is excreted unchanged in the urine), and the active metabolites of glyburide can accumulate in patients with a creatinine clearance lower than 30 mL/min. Glipizide is preferred in patients with moderate to severe renal dysfunction. Compared with other oral antidiabetic medications, the sulfonylureas are the least expensive.

Meglitinides. Meglitinides, like sulfonylureas, stimulate the pancreatic beta cells to secrete insulin. Repaglinide (Prandin) and nateglinide (Starlix) are rapid-acting drugs with short duration of action that are taken before each meal. Meglitinides lower postprandial hyperglycemia. A possible side effect is hypoglycemia.

Biguanides

Biguanides are insulin sensitizers that make body tissues less resistant to endogenous insulin. Metformin (Glucophage) is the only biguanide approved for use in the United States by the U.S. Food and Drug Administration (FDA). It lowers blood glucose by making body cells more sensitive to insulin and decreases the amount of glucose produced by the liver. Metformin also decreases triglyceride concentrations, LDL cholesterol, total cholesterol, and body weight; it also increases HDL cholesterol. It can be taken once or twice a day.

When used as monotherapy, metformin has not been associated with hypoglycemia. However, gastrointestinal disturbances such as nausea, abdominal pain, bloating, anorexia, metallic taste, and diarrhea are common side effects. Additionally, asymptomatic subnormal B_{12} levels may occur. A rare condition termed lactic acidosis can occur with the use of metformin; therefore, patients presenting with vague, flu-like illness should be assessed for presence of lactic acidosis. Metformin is contraindicated in patients with renal or hepatic dysfunction, congestive heart failure, or history of alcohol abuse. Additionally, patients undergoing procedures requiring radiographic contrast media should have metformin discontinued before the procedure, withheld 48 hours postprocedure, and should not be restarted until the patient's renal function has been evaluated as normal.

Thiazolidinediones

Rosiglitazone (Avandia) and pioglitazone (Actos) are the two FDA-approved thiazolidinediones for use in the United States. **Thiazolidinediones** act by sensitizing skeletal muscle and adipose tissue to insulin and blocking hepatic gluconeogenesis. When used as monotherapy, both rosiglitazone and pioglitazone have not been associated with hypoglycemia but can cause weight gain and raise blood lipid levels. Rosiglitazone raises HDL, but it may also slightly raise LDL cholesterol with minimal effect on triglyceride concentrations. In comparison, pioglitazone raises HDLs, has minimal effect on LDLs, and decreases triglyceride concentrations.

Rosiglitazone and pioglitazone should be used with caution in patients with advanced congestive heart failure. It is also important to note that pioglitazone may decrease the concentration of oral contraceptives, so patients taking pioglitazone and oral contraceptives should be informed of this potential interaction. Additionally, thiazolidinediones may cause resumption of ovulation in premenopausal anovulatory women.

The clearance of rosiglitazone and pioglitazone is decreased in patients with moderate to severe liver disease. Thus, liver function should be monitored every 2 months for 1 year, then periodically thereafter.

Alpha-Glucosidase Inhibitors

There are two alpha-glucosidase inhibitors: acarbose (Precose) and miglitol (Glyset). **Alpha-glucosidase inhibitors** block the action of alpha-glucosidase enzymes at the brush border of the intestine. The inhibition slows the breakdown of dietary carbohydrates, which decreases postprandial glucose concentrations.

Acarbose and miglitol have minimal effect on cholesterol and body weight. Gastrointestinal adverse events are common, including abdominal pain, diarrhea, and flatulence. Acarbose, eliminated by the liver, may cause elevations in liver function tests; it is recommended to monitor hepatic enzymes every 3 months for 1 year, then periodically thereafter. In contrast, miglitol is excreted primarily by the kidneys, and should be used with caution in moderate to severe renal failure.

It is important to note that pancreatic enzyme tablets will reduce effectiveness of acarbose and miglitol. Also, patients taking alpha-glucosidase inhibitors should not use table sugar or soft drinks (sucrose) to raise blood glucose during hypoglycemic events because these will be ineffective. Milk, apple juice, orange juice, or glucose tablets should be used to reverse hypoglycemia instead because the absorption rates of sucrose and other complex carbohydrates are drastically reduced with the administration of alpha-glucosidase inhibitors.

Incretin Mimetics (GLP Agonist, GIP Agonist)

The term *incretin* refers to an insulin-stimulating factor found in the gastrointestinal tract. In response to food, incretin factors are produced by the gastrointestinal tract and stimulate pancreatic insulin secretion. Incretins include glucagon-like peptide (GLP-1) and GIP (gastric inhibitory polypeptide). Incretins also preserve pancreatic cell mass and enhance the proliferation of pancreatic cells.

Incretin dysfunction results in significant postprandial hyperglycemia as manifested in IGT and type 2 DM. Studies show that GLP-1 is reduced in patients who are obese with insulin-resistant type 2 DM. Standard meal tests in patients with type 2 diabetes have decreased GLP-1 responses and decreased insulin secretion as compared with patients without diabetes. These lower GLP-1 levels are thought to be caused by impaired secretion and decreased response of the incretin.

Exenatide. Exenatide (Byetta) is an incretin mimetic agent that has multiple mechanisms of action resulting in better glycemic control in diabetics. There are advantageous immediate and delayed effects of this drug. The immediate effects include glucose-dependent insulin secretion, suppression of postprandial high glucagon levels, and delayed gastric emptying. The delayed effects include weight loss and improved beta cell mass and function.

The most striking feature of this drug is glucose-dependent insulin secretion, meaning that it stimulates insulin secretion mainly in the postprandial period. Because its insulin-stimulating action is glucose-dependent, insulin secretion rises and falls in synchrony with blood glucose. This is similar to the physiologic rise and fall of insulin in response to glucose.

In addition, exenatide decreases postprandial glucagon secretion, which further augments its antidiabetic effect. Blocking postprandial glucagon decreases hepatic glucose production, which reduces the patient's insulin requirements. It does not impair normal glucagon response to hypoglycemia. Additionally, exenatide slows gastric emptying, thereby delaying absorption of carbohydrates into the bloodstream. This leads to a feeling of satiety and fullness, resulting in decreased appetite, which may manifest as loss of weight. Exenatide also reduces postprandial triglyceride levels.

At the cellular level, exenatide promotes the growth and development of pancreatic beta cells and improves their life span and function. In addition, it promotes nerve growth factor and may rejuvenate degenerating neurons, which is valuable in diabetic neuropathy.

Adverse drug reactions are few and mild to moderate in severity. These include dizziness, jitteriness, headache, uneasiness, nausea, vomiting, diarrhea, dyspepsia, and a decrease in appetite. When combined with a sulfonylurea, hypoglycemia can occur. Because exenatide is available only as an injectable, allergic reactions at the injection site are possible.

Exenatide is recommended as an adjunct to metformin or sulfonylureas in the dose of 5 µg subcutaneously twice a day within 60 minutes of morning and evening meals. It is important to remember that it is not indicated in type 1 DM or DKA and that it is not an insulin substitute. It is not recommended for diabetics with end-stage renal disease (creatinine clearance lower than 30 mL/min) and severe gastrointestinal disease like gastroparesis. It is yet to be studied in pregnant or lactating mothers.

Amylin Mimetics

Pramlintide (Symlin) is an injectable antidiabetic medication indicated for patients with type 2 or type 1 diabetes using insulin who have not achieved desired glucose control. It is a synthetic form of human **amylin,** a naturally occurring pancreatic hormone that, with insulin, helps to control glucose during the postprandial period. Naturally occurring amylin slows gastric emptying and suppresses glucagon secretion, which diminishes hepatic glucose production and controls appetite. In patients with diabetes, amylin, much like insulin, is absent or deficient.

Pramlintide slows nutrient absorption in the GI tract, inhibits glucose synthesis by the liver, promotes a feeling of satiety and fullness, and suppresses appetite. It limits postprandial rise in blood glucose and can lead to weight loss. Most adverse events are gastrointestinal in nature, such as nausea and vomiting. The drug is administered by subcutaneous injection at mealtimes and eliminated by the kidney.

Pramlintide and insulin should be administered as separate injections and should never be mixed. Adverse events associated with pramlintide include an increased risk of insulin-induced severe hypoglycemia. Proper patient selection and an initial 50% reduction in mealtime insulin are critical to safe and effective use of Pramlintide.

DPP-4 Inhibitors

Sitagliptin (Januvia) and saxagliptin (Onglyza) are oral drugs that reduce blood glucose levels in patients with type 2 diabetes. These drugs inhibit the enzyme dipeptidyl peptidase-4 (DPP-4), which is an enzyme that destroys the gastrointestinal incretin hormones GLP-1 and GIP. In response to food, the incretin hormones GLP-1 and GIP are released from the intestine, and their levels increase in the blood. GLP-1 and GIP stimulate the pancreas to secrete insulin and block the release of glucagon. Drugs that inhibit DDP-4, in turn, block enzymatic breakdown of GLP-1 and GIP, allowing these hormones to remain in circulation for a longer amount of time.

The net effect of increased release of GLP-1 and GIP is to reduce blood glucose levels. Therefore, DDP-4 inhibitors, by increasing the amounts of GLP-1 and GIP, reduce blood glucose levels. Hypoglycemia and gastrointestinal disturbances are the possible adverse side effects.

SGLT2 inhibitors

Sodium glucose cotransporter 2 (SGLT2) inhibitors are another class of oral antidiabetic medications for type 2 diabetes. SGLT2 is a protein that enhances glucose reabsorption in the proximal tubule of the nephron. SGLT2 inhibitors block glucose reabsorption into the bloodstream at the kidney, enhance glucose excreted in the urine, and diminish levels of glucose in the bloodstream. Drugs in this class include canagliflozin (Invokana®) and dapagliflozin (Farxiga®). This class of drug is informally referred to as a "glucoretic" medication.

Chapter Summary

- DM is a complex metabolic disease that causes decreased glucose absorption into body cells.
- The disease has reached epidemic proportions in the United States. There are mainly two types of diabetes: type 1 DM and type 2 DM.

- In type 1 diabetes, there is a deficiency of insulin. In type 2 diabetes, body cells resist insulin. Both types result in glucose accumulation in the bloodstream.
- Metabolic syndrome is a constellation of disorders that increase the risk of cardiovascular disease and DM:

apple-shaped obesity, hypertension, insulin resistance (prediabetes), and hyperlipidemia.

- In uncontrolled DM, hyperglycemia has a wide range of acute and long-term effects on the body.

- The classic acute symptoms of DM are polydipsia, polyuria, and polyphagia.

- As glucose is prevented from entering body cells, hyperglycemia develops.

- A fasting plasma glucose of 126 mg/dL or greater is diagnostic of DM.

- An A1c of 6.5% or greater or a random glucose of 200 mg/dL or greater are also diagnostic of DM.

- In type 1 DM, cells "sense" starvation and the body goes into starvation mode, where the liver and fat tissue liberate glucose and fatty acids, respectively, causing development of DKA–a life-threatening complication that requires emergency treatment.

- With chronic hyperglycemia, the arteries throughout the body are damaged. Arterial injury incites a cascade of effects that lead to widespread arteriosclerosis. Coronary arteriosclerosis leads to early myocardial infarction. Retinal artery damage leads to blindness. Damage to the fragile glomerular capillaries causes kidney failure. Peripheral arteriosclerosis leads to ischemic stroke and ischemic necrosis of the lower extremities.

- The lower extremities suffer lack of circulation, decreased sensation, and increased susceptibility to infection, all of which increases the risk of gangrene and amputation.

- In the management of DM, the patient must carefully monitor blood glucose, diet, and exercise daily.

- There are various types of insulin and oral antidiabetic agents that can stave off the harmful effects of diabetes.

Making the Connections

Disorder and Pathophysiology	Signs and Symptoms	Physical Assessment Findings	Diagnostic Testing	Treatment
Type 1 Diabetes				
Immune-Mediated Type 1 Diabetes | Autoimmune destruction of insulin-secreting pancreatic islet beta cells occurs. Without insulin, glucose cannot enter cells. Cells "sense" starvation, and complications such as liver synthesis of glucose and fat breakdown into fatty acids are set in motion. Cellular dehydration occurs. Fatty acids become ketones and hyperglycemia worsens.				
Idiopathic Type 1 Diabetes | No autoimmune aspect is present; pancreatic beta cell dysfunction occurs for an unknown reason. Same pathophysiologic mechanism occurs as above.				
	Polydipsia. Polyuria. Polyphagia. Weight loss. Weakness. Fatigue. Vision disturbances. Infection possible.	No significant findings except in cases of infection or DKA. Possible visual impairment. If in DKA: fever, abdominal pain, nausea, vomiting, dehydration, possible decreased level of consciousness.	Fasting blood glucose: 126 mg/dL or greater. Random blood glucose: 200 mg/dL or greater. A1c: 6.5% or greater. Glucosuria: excess glucose cannot be reabsorbed by the kidney and it spills into urine. Ketonuria: ketones in urine are caused by a high amount of fatty acids (ketoacids) in the bloodstream.	Insulin replacement.

Continued

Making the Connections–cont'd

Disorder and Pathophysiology	Signs and Symptoms	Physical Assessment Findings	Diagnostic Testing	Treatment
Type 2 Diabetes | Insulin resistance of body cells and pancreatic dysfunction occurs.				
	Polydipsia. Polyuria. Polyphagia. Weight loss. Weakness. Fatigue. Vision disturbances. Infection possible.	Obesity and hypertension common findings.	Fasting blood glucose: 126 mg/dL or greater. Random blood glucose: 200 mg/dL or greater. A1c: 6.5% or greater. Glucosuria: excess glucose cannot be reabsorbed by the kidney and it spills into urine. Hyperlipidemia common. Metabolic syndrome common. Hyperinsulinemia.	Oral antidiabetic medications, injectable diabetic medications, or insulin.

Bibliography

American Diabetes Association. (2012). Diagnosis and classification of diabetes mellitus. *Diabetes Care,* 35(S1), S64–S71. Retrieved from http://care.diabetesjournals.org/content/35/Supplement_1/S64.extract. doi: 10.2337/dc12-s064.

American Diabetes Association. (2014). *Summary of revisions to the 2014 Clinical Practice Recommendations: revisions to the standards of medical care in diabetes–2014.* Retrieved from http://care.diabetesjournals.org/content/37/Supplement_1/S14.full.pdf+html

Antonetti, D. A., Klein, R., & Gardner, T. W. (2012). Diabetic retinopathy. *N Engl J Med,* 366(13), 1227–1239.

Brodovicz, K. G., Engel, S. S., & Thornberry, N. A. (2013). Glucagon-like peptide 1-based drugs and pancreatic safety. *JAMA Int Med,* 173(19), 1842–1843. doi: 10.1001/jamainternmed.2013.8138.

Campbell, R. K., Cobble, M. E., Reid, T. S., & Shomali, M. E. (2010). Distinguishing among incretin-based therapies. Pathophysiology of type 2 diabetes mellitus: potential role of incretin-based therapies. *J Fam Pract,* 59(9 Suppl 1), S5–S9.

Canadian Diabetes Association Clinical Practice Guidelines Expert Committee, Bowering, K., & Embil, J. M. (2013, April). Foot care. *Can J Diabetes,* 37(Suppl 1), S145–S149. doi: 10.1016/j.jcjd.2013.01.040. Epub 2013 Mar 26.

Cheng, J., Zhang, W., Zhang, X., et al. (2014). Effect of angiotensin-converting enzyme inhibitors and angiotensin II receptor blockers on all-cause mortality, cardiovascular deaths, and cardiovascular events in patients with diabetes mellitus: a meta-analysis. *JAMA Int Med,* 174(5), 773–785. doi: 10.1001/jamainternmed.2014.348.

Cordts, S. (2012). Self-monitoring of blood glucose in patients with type 2 diabetics not using insulin. *Am Fam Phys,* 85(9), 866–867.

Dunkler, D., Dehghan, M., Teo, K. K., et al. (2013). Diet and kidney disease in high-risk individuals with type 2 diabetes mellitus. *JAMA Int Med,* 173(18), 1682–1692.

Eckel, R. H., Alberti, K. G., Grundy, S. M., & Zimmet, P. Z. (2010). The metabolic syndrome. *Lancet,* 375(9710), 181–183.

Edwards, J. L., & Kirt, B. L. (2011). Case report: patient with ketoacidosis and impaired insulin secretion. *Am Fam Phys,* 83(3), 232.

Emerging Risk Factors Collaboration, Di Angelantonio, E., Gao, P., Khan, H., et al. (2014). Glycated hemoglobin measurement and prediction of cardiovascular disease. *JAMA,* 311(12), 1225–1233. doi: 10.1001/jama.2014.1873.

Erlich, D. R., Slawson, D. C., & Shaughnessy, A. F. (2014). "Lending a hand" to patients with type 2 diabetes: a simple way to communicate treatment goals. *Am Fam Phys,* 89(4), 256, 258.

Everett, C. M., Thorpe, C. T., Palta, M., et al. (2014). The roles of primary care PAs and NPs caring for older adults with diabetes. *JAAPA,* 27(4), 45–49. doi: 10.1097/01.JAA.0000444736.16669.76.

Florez, J. C. (2014). Insights from monogenic diabetes and glycemic treatment goals for common types of diabetes. *JAMA,* 311(3), 249–251. doi: 10.1001/jama.2013.283981.

Freeman, J. S. (2010a). A physiologic and pharmacological basis for implementation of incretin hormones in the treatment of type 2 diabetes mellitus. *Mayo Clin Proceed,* 85 (12 Suppl), S5–S24.

Freeman, J. S. (2010b). Managing hyperglycemia in patients with type 2 diabetes mellitus: rationale for the use of dipeptidyl peptidase-4 inhibitors in combination with other oral antidiabetic drugs. *J Am Osteo Assoc,* 110(9), 528–537.

Garber, A. J. (2012). Hypoglycaemia: a therapeutic concern in type 2 diabetes. *Lancet,* 379(9833), 2215–2216.

Geller, A. I., Shehab, N., Lovegrove, M. C., et al. (2014). National estimates of insulin-related hypoglycemia and errors leading to emergency department visits and hospitalizations. *JAMA Int Med*, 174(5), 678–686. doi: 10.1001/jamainternmed.2014.136.

Gemechu, F. W., Seemant, F., & Curley, C. A. (2013). Diabetic foot infections. *Am Fam Phys,* 88(3), 177–184.

Gionfriddo, M. R., McCoy, R. G., & Lipska, K. J. (2014). The 2013 American Association of Clinical Endocrinologists' diabetes mellitus management recommendations: improvements needed. *JAMA Int Med*, 174(2), 179–180. doi: 10.1001/jamainternmed.2013.12971.

Gonzalez, J. S., Fisher, L., & Polonsky, W. H. (2011). Depression in diabetes: have we been missing something important? *Diabetes Care*, 34(1), 236–239.

Hamaty, M. (2011). Insulin treatment for type 2 diabetes: when to start, which to use. *Cleveland Clin J Med,* 78(5), 332–342.

Hanson, M. (2014). Understanding the origins of diabetes. *JAMA*, 311(6), 575–576. doi: 10.1001/jama.2014.2.

Himpens, J. (2014). Bariatric surgery for diabetes control in overweight people. *Lancet Diabetes Endocrinol.* 2014 Apr 7. pii: S2213-8587(14)70019-1. doi: 10.1016/S2213-8587(14)70019-1. Epub ahead of print.

Huang, E. S., Laiteerapong, N., Liu, J. Y., et al. (2014). Rates of complications and mortality in older patients with diabetes mellitus: the diabetes and aging study. *JAMA Int Med*, 174(2), 251–258. doi: 10.1001/jamainternmed.2013.12956.

Hunt, D. (2009). Diabetes: foot ulcers and amputations. *Am Fam Phys*, 80(8), 789.

Inzucchi, S. E. (2012). Diagnosis of diabetes. *N Engl J Med*, 367(6), 542–550.

Ismail-Beigi, F. (2012). Clinical practice. Glycemic management of type 2 diabetes mellitus. *N Engl J Med,* 366(14), 1319–1327.

Kim, C. (2010). Gestational diabetes: risks, management, and treatment options. *Int J Womens Health*, 7(2), 339–351.

Kripke, C. (2009). Dipeptidyl-peptidase-4 inhibitors for treatment of type 2 diabetes. *Am Fam Phys*, 79(5), 372.

Lambert, M. (2012). ADA releases revisions to recommendations for standards of medical care in diabetes. *Am Fam Phys*, 85(5), 514–515.

Lavery, L. A., Hunt, N. A., Lafontaine, J., et al. (2010). Diabetic foot prevention: a neglected opportunity in high-risk patients. *Diabetes Care*, 33(7), 1460–1462. 61.160.

Lipska, K. J., & Krumholz, H. M. (2014). Comparing diabetes medications: where do we set the bar? *JAMA Int Med*, 174(3), 317–318. doi: 10.1001/jamainternmed.2013.13433.

Lipska, K. J., & Montori, V. M. (2013). Glucose control in older adults with diabetes mellitus—more harm than good? *JAMA Int Med*, 173(14), 1306–1307. doi: 10.1001/jamainternmed.2013.6189.

Maclennan, P. A., McGwin, G., Jr., Heckemeyer, C., et al. (2014). Eye care use among a high-risk diabetic population seen in a public hospital's clinics. *JAMA Ophthalmol,* 132(2), 162–167. doi: 10.1001/jamaophthalmol.2013.6046.

Mitka, M. (2013a). New drugs improve glycemic control in type 2 diabetes, but improving heart health remains elusive. *JAMA*, 310(14), 1435–1436. doi: 10.1001/jama.2013.279038.

Mitka, M. (2013b). Study: exercise may match medication in reducing mortality associated with cardiovascular disease, diabetes. *JAMA*, 310(19), 2026–2027. doi: 10.1001/jama.2013.281450.

Palalau, A. I., Tahrani, A. A., Piya, M. K., & Barnett, A. H. (2009). DPP-4 inhibitors in clinical practice. *Postgraduate Med*, 121(6), 70–100.

Pan, A., Lucas, M., Sun, Q., et al. (2010). Bidirectional association between depression and type 2 diabetes mellitus in women. *Arch Int Med*, 170(21), 1884–1891.

Pan, A., Lucas, M., Sun, Q., et al. (2011). Increased mortality risk in women with depression and diabetes mellitus. *Arch Gen Psych*, 68(1), 42–50.

Patel, P., & Macerollo, A. (2010). Diabetes mellitus: diagnosis and screening. *Am Fam Phys,* 81(7), 863–870.

Perreault, L., Pan, Q., Mather, K. J., et al. (2012). Effect of regression from prediabetes to normal glucose regulation on long-term reduction in diabetes risk: results from the Diabetes Prevention Program Outcomes Study. *Lancet*, 379(9833), 2243–2251.

Pickup, J. C. (2012). Insulin-pump therapy for type 1 diabetes mellitus. *N Engl J Med,* 366(17), 1616–1624.

Prasad, H., Ryan, D. A., Celzo, M. F., & Stapleton, D. (2012). Metabolic syndrome: definition and therapeutic implications. *Postgrad Med*, 124(1), 21–30.

Ricci, C., Gaeta, M., Rausa, E., Macchitella, Y., & Bonavina, L. (2014). Early impact of bariatric surgery on type II diabetes, hypertension, and hyperlipidemia: a systematic review, meta-analysis and meta-regression on 6,587 patients. *Obes Surg*, 24(4), 522–528. doi: 10.1007/s11695-013-1121-x.

Ritsinger, V., Malmberg, K., Mårtensson, A., et al. (2014). Intensified insulin-based glycaemic control after myocardial infarction: mortality during 20 year follow-up of the randomised Diabetes Mellitus Insulin Glucose Infusion in Acute Myocardial Infarction (DIGAMI 1) trial. *Lancet Diabetes Endocrinol.* 2014 May 12. pii: S2213-8587(14)70088-9. doi: 10.1016/S2213-8587(14)70088-9. Epub ahead of print.

Roett, M. A., Liegl, S., & Jabbarpour, Y. (2012). Diabetic nephropathy—the family physician's role. *Am Fam Phys*, 85(9), 883–889.

Scheen, A. J. (2014). Personalising metformin therapy: a clinician's perspective. *Lancet Diabetes Endocrinol.* 2014 Mar 19. pii: S2213-8587(14)70064-6. doi: 10.1016/S2213-8587(14)70064-6. Epub ahead of print.

Scheen, A. J., & Paquot, N. (2012). Gliptin versus a sulphonylurea as add-on to metformin. *Lancet,* 380(9840), 450–452.

Skyler, J. S., & Sosenko, J. M. (2013). The evolution of type 1 diabetes. *JAMA,* 309(23), 2491–2492. doi: 10.1001/jama.2013.6286.

Tabák, A. G., Herder, C., Rathmann, W., Brunner, E. J., & Kivimäki, M. (2012). Prediabetes: a high-risk state for diabetes development. *Lancet*, 379(9833), 2279–2290.

The Diabetes Control and Complications Trial Research Group. (1993). The effect of intensive treatment of diabetes on the development and progression of long term complications in insulin-dependent diabetes mellitus. *N Engl J Med,* 329(14), 977–986.

Torpy, J. M., & Golub, R. M. (2011). *JAMA* patient page. Diabetes. *JAMA,* 305(24), 2592.

United Kingdom Prospective Diabetes Study Group (UKPDS). (1998). Intensive blood glucose control with sulphonylureas or insulin compared with conventional treatment and risk of complications in patients with type 2 diabetes (UKPDS 33). *Lancet,* 352, 837–853.

United States Department of Health & Human Services (DHHS). (2000). *Health Resources and Services Administration. Lower Extremity Amputation Prevention Program (LEAP Program). Diabetic Foot Screening Test publications.* Washington, DC: USDHHS.

Vijan, S. (2013). Diabetes: treating hypertension. *Am Fam Phys*, 87(8), 574–575.

Wareham, N. J. (2014). The long-term benefits of lifestyle interventions for prevention of diabetes. *Lancet Diabetes Endocrinol,* Apr 3. pii: S2213-8587(14)70074-9. doi: 10.1016/S2213-8587(14)70074-9. Epub ahead of print.

Westerberg, D. P. (2013). Diabetic ketoacidosis: evaluation and treatment. *Am Fam Phys,* 87(5), 337–346.

Williams, S. L., Haskard-Zolnierek, K. B., Banta, J. E., et al. (2010). Serious psychological distress and diabetes care among California adults. *Int J Psych Med,* 40(3), 233–245.

Wolpert, H. A. (2010). Continuous glucose monitoring—coming of age. *N Engl J Med,* 363(4), 383–384.

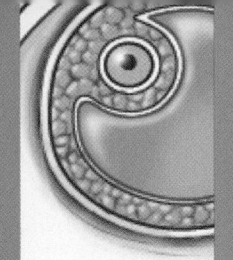

Disorders of the Female Reproductive System

Key Terms

Amenorrhea

Beta-human chorionic gonadotropin (b-HCG)

Carcinoembryonic antigen 125 (CA-125)

Colposcopy

Corpus luteum

Culdoscopy

Dysfunctional uterine bleeding (DUB)

Dysmenorrhea

Endometrium

Follicle-stimulating hormone (FSH)

Gonadatropic hormone

Gravidity

Hysteroscopy

In vitro fertilization (IVF)

Laparoscopy

Liquid-based cytology (LBC)

Lutenizing hormone (LH)

Menarche

Menopause

Menorrhagia

Menstrual cycle

Myometrium

Papanicolaou smear

Parity

Premenstrual syndrome (PMS)

Thelarche

Vulvovaginitis

Disorders of the female reproductive system can have broad effects on a woman's overall health. Hormonal fluctuations influence the way women demonstrate disease, and distinct changes occur in a woman's body at puberty, childbearing, and menopause. These changes endow women with the potential for different types of disorders than men. Menstrual disorders are the most common reason women seek the attention of a healthcare provider, whereas childbirth is the most common reason women seek emergency medical treatment.

Epidemiology

During the reproductive years of a woman's life there are many reasons to seek the attention of a health-care provider. Common disorders include painful menstrual periods, termed dysmenorrhea, and **dysfunctional uterine bleeding (DUB).** Dysmenorrhea affects 25% of women and up to 90% of adolescents. DUB, which causes excessive uterine blood loss called **menorrhagia,** occurs in approximately 5% of women aged 30 to 49 years annually. **Premenstrual syndrome (PMS),** which causes headache, mood swings, insomnia, and other symptoms, occurs in 90% of all women at some time during their reproductive years. A disorder of the menstrual cycle affects nearly 100% of all women at some point during their lifetime.

Basic Concepts of Female Reproduction

The female reproductive organs consist of the ovaries, uterus, fallopian tubes, vagina, and breasts (see Fig. 26-1).

The ovaries produce estrogen and progesterone; at puberty, the female begins to secrete these hormones in cyclical phases that trigger ovulation and confer fertility. Estrogen and progesterone make the uterus suitable for the growth of a fertilized egg in pregnancy. Each month the female reproductive system undergoes a series of changes called the **menstrual cycle.** The cycle consists of distinct hormonal, ovarian, and uterine changes. Each month, the female body readies the uterus for pregnancy by proliferation of the endometrial layer. When pregnancy does not occur, the uterus sheds the endometrial tissue and yields blood during menstruation. A woman's menstrual cycle usually occurs monthly from approximately age 13 years to age 55 years. At menopause, the ovary degenerates, no longer undergoes ovulation, and fertility wanes.

The female breast is also somewhat affected by monthly hormonal changes. However, it is during pregnancy that the breast undergoes transformation. Because the pituitary releases prolactin (PRL), the breast glands become active and lactation occurs.

The Menstrual Cycle

Female reproductive potential comes to fruition at puberty, with the activation of the hypothalamic-pituitary-ovarian axis. The hypothalamus secretes gonadotropic-releasing hormone (GnRH) that, in turn, stimulates the pituitary to release two gonadotropic hormones: **follicle-stimulating hormone (FSH)** and **luteinizing hormone (LH)**. These **gonadotropic hormones** activate ovarian secretion of estrogen and progesterone, which leads to maturation of the reproductive organs.

Female reproductive function begins at **menarche,** the first episode of menstrual bleeding. This bleeding,

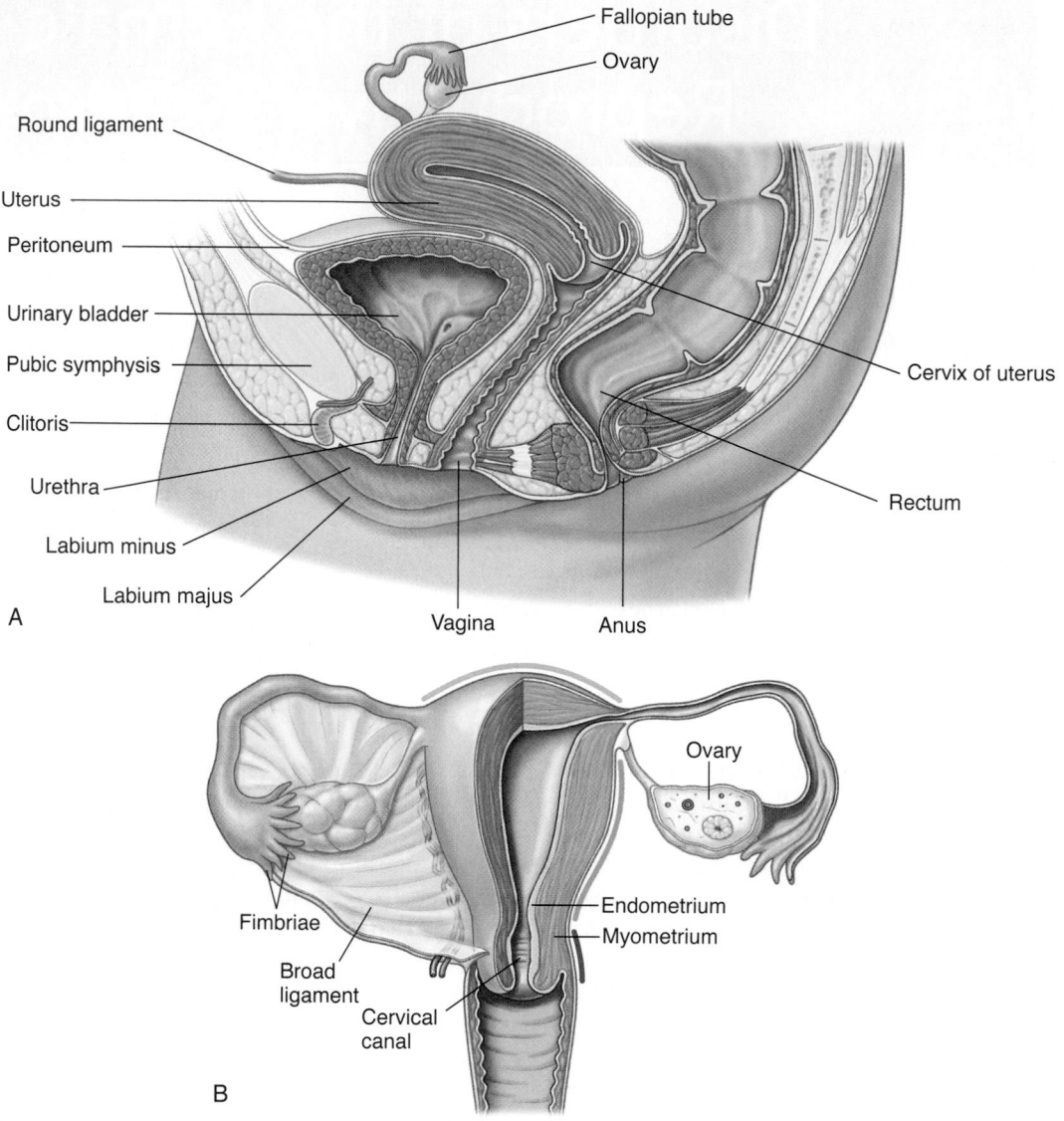

FIGURES 26-1a and 26-1b. The female reproductive system. (From Thompson, G. S. (2013). *Understanding anatomy and physiology.* Philadelphia, PA: F.A. Davis Company, with permission.)

which occurs on a monthly basis, can last anywhere between 2 and 7 days. At menarche, the ovary starts to release an ovum and the menstrual cycle is initiated. At about the same time, the female also experiences the development of breast buds, called **thelarche.** The female adolescent experiences puberty at this time with accelerated skeletal growth and pubic and axillary hair development.

The menstrual cycle consists of a natural rise and fall of estrogen and progesterone with corresponding changes in the ovary and uterus. During the cycle, an ovum is released from the ovary and the uterine lining proliferates to prepare for implantation of a fertilized egg. If fertilization does not occur, the uterine lining is shed, causing menses.

The menstrual cycle lasts approximately 28 days, beginning with the first day of menstrual bleeding and ending just before the next menstrual period. The first part of the cycle is termed the follicular phase and is characterized by increased pituitary

gland production of FSH. FSH stimulates estrogen secretion by the ovary and initiates development of an ovum that rises to the surface at a region called the Graafian follicle (mature follicle). At a peak level of FSH, the pituitary releases LH, resulting in ovulation, which is defined as the release of an ovum from the ovary. The ovum travels from the ovary to the uterus via the fallopian tube (see Fig. 26-2).

After ovulation, remnants of the Graafian follicle on the ovary surface form a region referred to as the **corpus luteum,** which produces progesterone (see Fig. 26-3). This hormone supports the ovum's implantation in the uterine wall and inhibits FSH and LH production. After 14 days, the corpus luteum degenerates if fertilization does not occur and progesterone levels decline. Following progesterone decline, FSH and LH levels begin to rise before the onset of the next menstrual period. If the ovum is fertilized, the corpus luteum continues to secrete progesterone for 5 to 9 weeks to support the pregnancy.

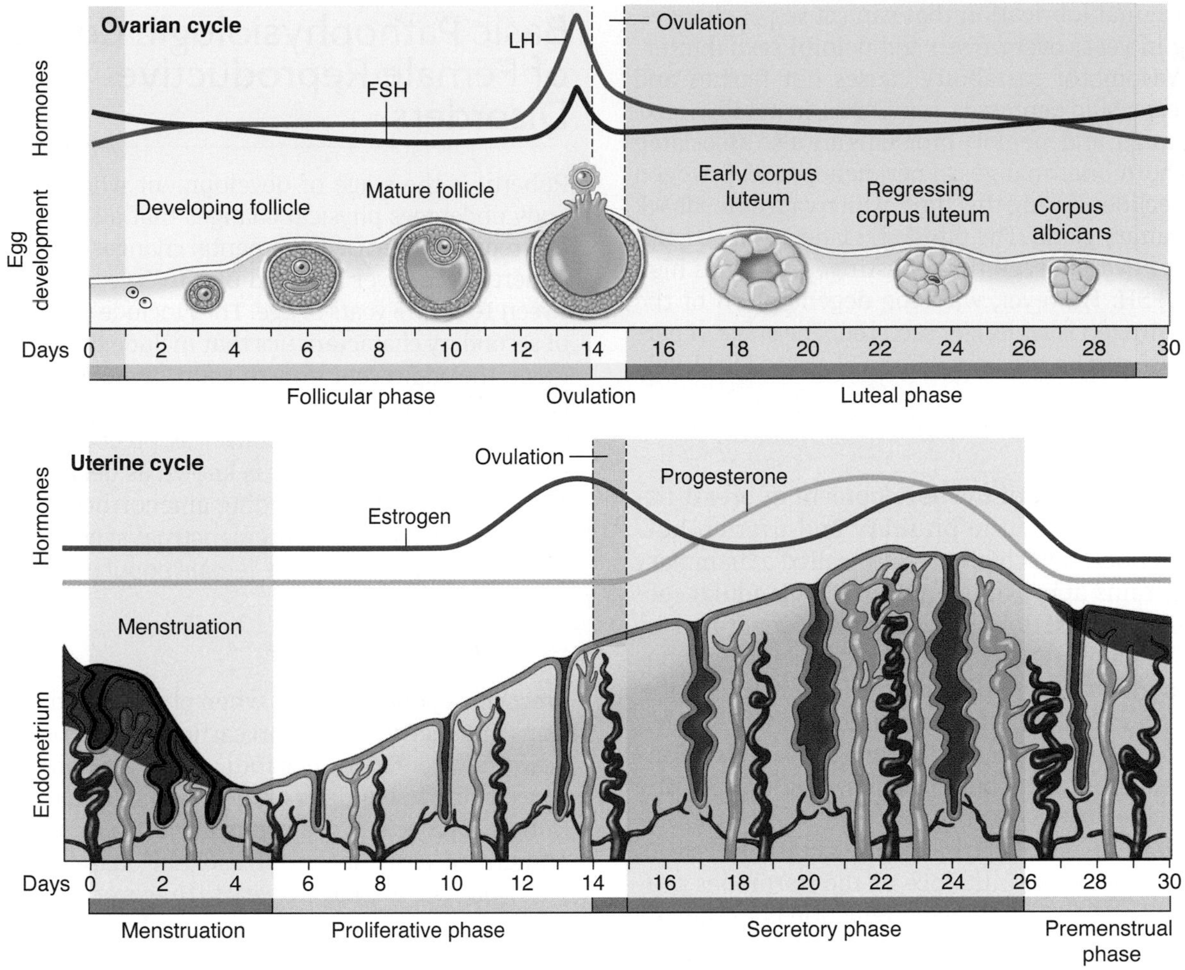

Ovarian cycle

Hormones

LH   Ovulation

FSH

Egg development

Developing follicle   Mature follicle   Early corpus luteum   Regressing corpus luteum   Corpus albicans

Days 0 2 4 6 8 10 12 14 16 18 20 22 24 26 28 30

Follicular phase   Ovulation   Luteal phase

Uterine cycle

Hormones

Ovulation

Progesterone

Estrogen

Menstruation

Endometrium

Days 0 2 4 6 8 10 12 14 16 18 20 22 24 26 28 30

Menstruation   Proliferative phase   Secretory phase   Premenstrual phase

FIGURE 26-2. Hormonal, ovarian, and uterine changes of the menstrual cycle. (From Thompson, G. S. (2013). *Understanding anatomy and physiology*. Philadelphia, PA: F.A. Davis Company, with permission.)

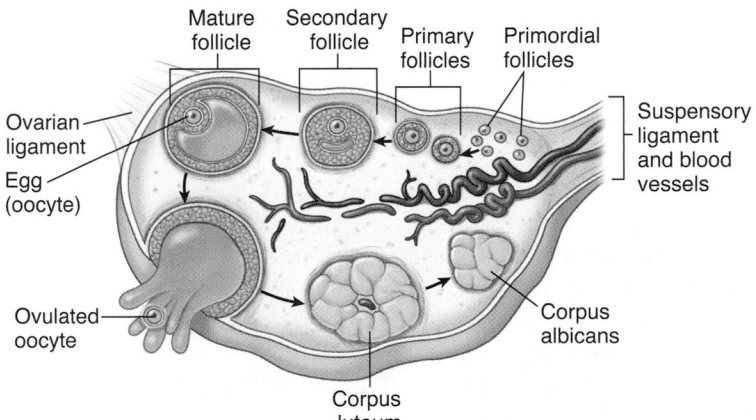

Mature follicle   Secondary follicle   Primary follicles   Primordial follicles

Ovarian ligament

Egg (oocyte)

Suspensory ligament and blood vessels

Ovulated oocyte

Corpus luteum

Corpus albicans

FIGURE 26-3. The corpus luteum. (From Thompson, G. S. (2013). *Understanding anatomy and physiology*. Philadelphia, PA: F.A. Davis Company, with permission.)

Female fertility requires health of the ovaries, fallopian tubes, uterus, vagina, and external genitalia. In addition, the endocrine hormones, particularly estrogen and progesterone, need to be secreted and released at appropriate times during the menstrual cycle. Stress, infection, lesions of the reproductive organs, endocrine hormone disruption, and cardiopulmonary and renal disorders can lead to reproductive organ dysfunction. Ectopic pregnancy and sexually transmitted diseases can also cause dysfunction of reproductive organs.

Menopause

Menopause is the permanent cessation of menstrual cycles caused by normal, physiologic degeneration of the ovaries and the decline of estrogen levels. In the time frame before menopause, called perimenopause, there is a gradual decline in hormone production; this decline can last several years and cause physiologic changes that include erratic menses, atrophic vaginitis, and vasomotor instability. Atrophic vaginitis is a marked decrease in natural vaginal lubrication that can cause pH changes, resulting in yeast overgrowth and painful sexual intercourse. Vasomotor instability causes hot flashes and night sweats. Mild depressive symptoms, irritability, anxiety, insomnia, and memory problems are also associated with the hormonal changes of perimenopause. Estrogen sharply declines during this time, which causes feedback to the pituitary gland. The pituitary gland, in an attempt to increase ovarian secretion of estrogen, secretes high levels of FSH. However, with the degeneration of the ovaries, estrogen is no longer secreted. The stage of perimenopause can be confirmed by an elevated FSH level.

The Breast

Thelarche, the onset of the development of breast tissue, is stimulated by the pituitary and ovarian hormones at puberty. Each breast, also called a mammary gland, contains approximately 15 to 25 glandular sections called breast lobules, which are separated by Cooper ligaments. Each lobule is composed of a tubuloalveolar gland and adipose tissue. Each lobule drains into a lactiferous duct, which empties onto the nipple's surface. Lactiferous ducts form large dilated regions called the lactiferous sinuses, which store milk during lactation (see Fig. 26-4).

Proliferation of breast tissue and lactation occur in pregnancy under the influence of the hormones prolactin (PRL) and oxytocin. Milk production is stimulated by PRL, whereas milk release is stimulated by oxytocin.

The breast can develop masses, cysts, or infection. Many women have fibrocystic breasts, which contain benign movable, tender, compressible masses that change in size with the menstrual cycle. Fibrocystic breast changes do not increase the susceptibility to breast cancer.

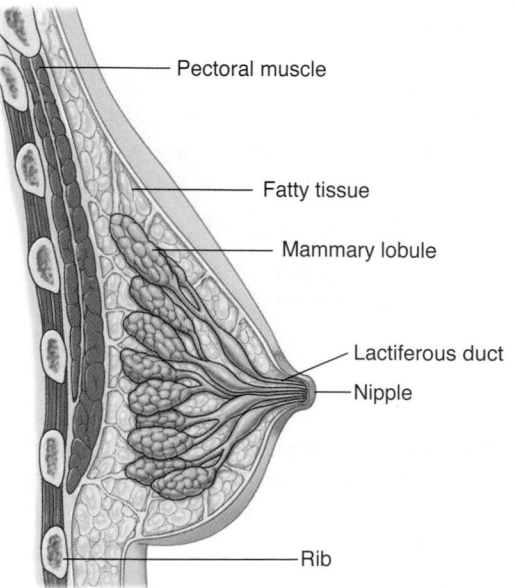

FIGURE 26-4. Anatomy of the breast. (From Thompson, G. S. (2013). *Understanding anatomy and physiology.* Philadelphia, PA: F.A. Davis Company, with permission.)

Basic Pathophysiologic Concepts of Female Reproductive Disorders

Puberty is the stage of development when the female body undergoes physical changes that allow for fertility and reproduction. Developmental changes in girls during puberty occur over a period of 3 to 5 years, usually between 10 and 15 years of age. They include the occurrence of secondary characteristics that include breast development, the adolescent growth spurt, the onset of menarche, and beginning of fertility. Early development of these reproductive changes is known as precocious puberty, whereas late development is known as delayed puberty. Menstrual disorders, including amenorrhea, dysmenorrhea, menorrhagia, and premenstrual syndrome (PMS), affect a large percent of the female population.

Precocious Puberty

Precocious puberty occurs when physical and hormonal signs of puberty occur at an earlier age than considered normal. Recently studies indicate that normal puberty is occurring in children earlier than in the past. Traditionally precocious puberty was defined as the development of early secondary sexual characteristics in girls younger than age 8 years. However, studies from 1977 to 2010 show that there has been a steady decrease in the age of puberty in girls, particularly in African American girls, with some reaching puberty as early as age 6 years. Many experts assert that precocious puberty should be redefined as the appearance of any sign of secondary sexual maturation in Caucasian girls younger than 7 years, and in African American girls younger than 6 years. The incidence of precocious puberty is estimated to be 1 per 5,000 to 10,000 children in the United States per year.

There are two types of precocious puberty: central precocious puberty and peripheral precocious puberty. Central precocious puberty is the early maturation of the hypothalamic-pituitary-ovarian axis; children with the disorder demonstrate the full range of physical and hormonal changes of puberty that are gonadotropin-dependent. Peripheral precocious puberty, less common than central precocious puberty, is gonadotropin-independent. The cause is the release of estrogen because of problems with the ovaries, adrenal glands, or pituitary gland.

When evaluating children with premature development of secondary sexual characteristics, precocious pseudopuberty should be excluded. Precocious pseudopuberty is a gonadotropin-independent disorder in which there is an increased production of sex hormones independent of the pituitary secretion of gonadotropin. Excess circulating estrogen from the adrenal gland or ingested sources of estrogen cause the secondary sexual development in precocious pseudopuberty.

Delayed Puberty

In females, delayed puberty is diagnosed when secondary sex characteristics have not appeared by age 13 years. Short stature commonly accompanies delayed puberty. In 95% of cases, delayed puberty is inherited; in these cases, delayed puberty is called constitutional growth delay (CGD). In CGD, the onset of puberty occurs later than average, but the individual reaches normal stature and sexual maturity by adulthood. Other common causes of delayed puberty include chronic illness, eating disorders, strenuous exercise, and drug or alcohol abuse.

Infertility

Female infertility, male infertility, or a combination of the two affects millions of couples in the United States, with an estimated 10% to 15% of couples classified as infertile. To be classified as infertile, a couple must have been trying to conceive with frequent, unprotected intercourse for at least a year with no success. In 40% to 50% of infertility cases, female infertility is the cause. In women, factors that can disrupt fertility include hormonal disorders, polycystic ovarian syndrome, primary ovarian failure, fallopian tube disorders, endometriosis, cervical disorders, and uterine tumors or adhesions. Box 26-1 covers other risk factors for female infertility.

Ovulation disorders account for infertility in 25% of infertile couples. These can be caused by disruptions in the regulation of reproductive hormones by the hypothalamus or the pituitary gland, or by problems in the ovary itself. The pituitary gland produces the two hormones responsible for stimulating ovulation each month, FSH and LH, in a specific pattern during the menstrual cycle. Excess physical or emotional stress or a very high or very low body weight can disrupt this pattern and affect ovulation. The main sign of this problem is irregular or absent periods.

Specific diseases of the pituitary may be the cause of infertility, although these are less common. In polycystic ovary syndrome (PCOS), complex changes occur in the hypothalamus, pituitary, and ovary, resulting in overproduction of androgens and causing the ovary to not release ova or produce insufficient progesterone, both of which are needed for pregnancy.

Premature ovarian failure (POF) is a disorder usually caused by an autoimmune response, where the body develops antibodies against ovarian tissue. It results in the loss of ova and decreased estrogen production.

Fallopian tube damage can also prevent pregnancy. When fallopian tubes become damaged or blocked, they keep sperm from getting to the egg or close off the passage of the fertilized egg into the uterus. Causes of fallopian tube damage or blockage can include inflammation of the fallopian tubes (salpingitis); previous ectopic pregnancy, in which a fertilized egg becomes implanted and starts to develop in a fallopian tube instead of in the uterus; or previous abdominal or pelvic surgery.

Endometriosis and its treatment can put a woman at risk for infertility because the extra tissue growth—and subsequent surgical removal of it—can cause scarring, which impairs fertility.

Cervical obstruction, also called cervical stenosis, can be caused by an inherited malformation or damage to the cervix. In cervical obstruction, the malformed or damaged cervix cannot produce adequate mucus for sperm mobility and fertilization. In addition, the cervical opening may be closed, preventing any sperm from reaching the egg.

Benign polyps or tumors (fibroids or leiomyomas) in the uterus, common in women aged 30 to 45 years, can impair fertility by blocking the fallopian tubes or by disrupting implantation.

Scarring or adhesions within the uterus also can disrupt implantation, and some women born with uterine abnormalities, such as an abnormally shaped uterus, can have problems becoming or remaining pregnant.

BOX 26-1. Risk Factors for Female Infertility

- **Older age:** After age 32 years, the quantity and quality of a woman's eggs begin to decline.
- **Smoking:** Tobacco smoking ages ovaries prematurely and increases risk of miscarriage and ectopic pregnancy.
- **Excessive use of caffeine:** Excessive use is considered consumption of more than 900 mg/day (greater than 6 cups coffee/day).
- **Excessive use of alcohol:** Excessive use increases risk of ovulation disorders and endometriosis.
- **Sexually transmitted disease:** STDs can cause fallopian tube damage.
- **Obesity:** Obesity can cause disruption of the hypothalamic-pituitary-ovarian axis.
- **Underweight:** Being underweight can cause disruption of the hypothalamic-pituitary-ovarian axis.

Menstrual Disorders

Common menstrual disorders include amenorrhea, dysmenorrhea, and PMS. The etiology of amenorrhea is considered pregnancy until proven otherwise. Dysmenorrhea and PMS are two of the most common reasons that women seek gynecological care.

Amenorrhea

Amenorrhea is the absence of menstrual periods. Primary amenorrhea is diagnosed if the onset of menses does not occur by age 15. Secondary amenorrhea is diagnosed, if after menses has occurred, there is an absence of menses for more than 3 months. Pregnancy is the most common cause of amenorrhea; therefore, the patient should be tested for pregnancy whenever there is a missed menstrual period. Anovulation and irregular menstrual periods are common for up to 2 years after menarche and for 1 to 2 years before menopause. There are many types of menstrual disorders (see Table 26-1).

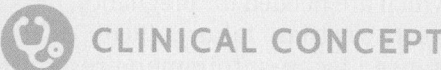

CLINICAL CONCEPT

The **beta-human chorionic gonadotropin (b-HCG)** blood test confirms pregnancy. It should be done on any woman who has missed a menstrual period.

Amenorrhea can be caused by disorders of the uterus or vagina, or the ovary's lack of ovulation. Many causes of primary amenorrhea are congenital and go unrecognized until puberty. An imperforated hymen, which is an obstructive membrane that exists within the vagina, can also be a cause of amenorrhea. Often, genital tract anomalies or the absence of reproductive organs become apparent at puberty.

Mayer-Rokitansky-Kuster -Hauser syndrome (MRKH) is an anomaly of the genital tract where the uterus is absent and the vagina is foreshortened. Because the ovaries function normally and produce estrogen, breasts are normal in shape and contour. MKRH syndrome accounts for 15% of primary amenorrhea cases and is second to Turner syndrome as the most common cause of primary amenorrhea.

TABLE 26-1. Possible Causes of Menstrual Disorders

Menstrual disorders vary according to the age at menarche, regularity of menstrual cycles, duration and volume of bleeding, and presence of pain.

Menstrual Disorder	Possible Causes
PRIMARY AMENORRHEA Lack of development of menses by age 15	• Delay that may be normal if puberty characteristics, such as breast development, are present by age 13 years • Birth defects of the female reproductive system • Genetic disorder • Lack of an opening in the membrane at the entrance of the vagina (imperforate hymen) • Problem with the hypothalamus or pituitary gland • Ovarian failure
SECONDARY AMENORRHEA Lack of menses for more than 3 months	• Drastic weight loss • Eating disorders • Pregnancy • Stress and anxiety • Significant weight gain or obesity • Hormonal imbalance, such as with polycystic ovarian syndrome • Endocrine disorders such as thyroid disease or pituitary disease/tumor • IUD • Excessive exercise • primary ovarian failure (POF) • Menopause, which is normal for women older than age 45 years • Use of birth control pills and other contraceptives • Uterine scarring, usually from procedures such as D&C
MENORRHAGIA Excessive menstrual bleeding; total loss of greater than 80 mL of blood; menses that last greater than 7 days	• Hormonal imbalance • Leiomyoma of uterus • Adenomyosis of uterus • Uterine polyp • Endometriosis • Ovarian disorder • IUD • Pregnancy (miscarriage) • Cancer • Inherited bleeding disorder • Medications (such as anticoagulant)

TABLE 26-1. Possible Causes of Menstrual Disorders–cont'd

Menstrual Disorder	Possible Causes
METRORRHAGIA Excessive uterine bleeding, both at the usual time of menstrual periods and at more frequent intervals	• Hormonal imbalance • Leiomyoma of uterus • Adenomyosis of uterus • Uterine polyp • Endometriosis • Ovarian disorder • IUD • Pregnancy (miscarriage) • Cancer • Inherited bleeding disorder • Medications (such as anticoagulant)
OLIGOMENORRHEA Irregular periods with long spans of time between periods	• Hormonal imbalance • Leiomyoma of uterus • Adenomyosis of uterus • Uterine polyp • Endometriosis • Ovarian disorder • Pregnancy (miscarriage) • Cancer
DYSMENORRHEA Painful menstrual periods	• Hormonal imbalance • IUD • Leiomyoma of uterus • Adenomyosis of uterus • Ovarian cyst • Pelvic inflammatory disease or infection • Cancer • Endometriosis

Asherman's syndrome, which is a lack of the uterine endometrial lining, can be a cause of secondary amenorrhea. This syndrome can occur after a surgical procedure called a dilation and curettage (D&C), which is performed after a miscarriage, delivery, or medical abortion. The endometrium can become scarred with adhesion formations within the uterine cavity. In the extreme, the whole uterine cavity can become occluded by scar tissue. Scarred endometrium fails to respond to estrogen, does not regenerate monthly, and cannot support a pregnancy.

Alternatively, disorders of ovulation can be the cause of amenorrhea. Hypothalamic or pituitary dysfunction can prevent the ovary from releasing an egg. Stress can commonly cause disturbance of the hypothalamic-pituitary-ovarian axis.

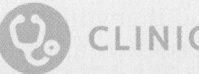 CLINICAL CONCEPT

A woman can miss several menstrual periods because of stress. Menstrual periods can also be lost for several months following dysfunction of the hypothalamic-pituitary-ovarian axis, which can occur after discontinuation of hormonal contraceptives.

Primary Ovarian Failure (POF) can be idiopathic, secondary to chemotherapy or radiation therapy, or autoimmune in origin. Hypergonadotropic hypogonadism is another ovarian disorder that causes amenorrhea. Elevated levels of FSH and LH characterize this syndrome with low estrogen production. The most common example of hypergonadotropic hypogonadism is found in Turner syndrome, which is caused by a 45X karyotype. Clinical manifestations of Turner syndrome include a webbed neck, short stature, broad shieldlike chest, anomalous auricles, and hypoestrogenemia, resulting in sexual immaturity. Gonadal dysgenesis, the lack of development of the ovaries, also causes high FSH and LH and low estrogen levels; it is caused by a mosaic karyotype with an abnormal X chromosome, with loss of part of an X chromosome or translocation, or with a normal karyotype (46,XX) and undeveloped, streak ovaries.

In the postpartum period, hemorrhage can cause pituitary necrosis, also known as Sheehan's syndrome. This syndrome causes lack of pituitary function, which can cause amenorrhea and decreased lactation.

PCOS is a common condition that can cause amenorrhea. In this disease, the ovary cannot release an egg each month. The follicles develop to the point of releasing an egg, but the egg remains under the ovary's surface. This causes the formation of multiple regions of unreleased egg on the ovarian surface, which appear as multiple fluid-filled cysts. In PCOS, the patient is commonly obese with high androgen levels and abnormalities of insulin level.

Functional hypothalamic amenorrhea is caused by excessive exercise, eating disorders, and chronic disease. The hypothalamus does not liberate gonadotropic-releasing factor, and in turn the pituitary does not release FSH or LH. As a result, there is failure of the ovaries to produce estrogen or release ova.

Hyperprolactinemia is a pituitary cause of amenorrhea in the presence of normal puberty. Often caused by a prolactin-secreting pituitary adenoma (prolactinoma), it raises PRL levels in the bloodstream and inhibits estrogen release by the ovaries. Aside from prolactinoma, high PRL can occur as a consequence of breastfeeding; psychoactive medications, such as haloperidol, phenothiazines, amitriptyline, benzodiazepines, cocaine, and marijuana.

Dysmenorrhea

Dysmenorrhea is painful menstruation associated with release of prostaglandins in ovulatory cycles. The severity of pain is related to the duration and amount of menstrual flow. Up to 75% of 15- to 25-year-old women experience dysmenorrhea. The chief symptom is cramping pelvic pain with radiation into the groin, back, and legs. Anorexia, nausea, diarrhea, headache, and syncope may accompany painful menstruation. The pain usually begins when prostaglandins are released, usually within the first 48 hours of menstruation; the pain rarely persists more than 2 days.

Women with dysmenorrhea produce a greater amount of prostaglandin F, which is a uterine muscle stimulant and vasoconstrictor. To diagnose dysmenorrhea, all possible pelvic pathological conditions must be excluded. Primary dysmenorrhea is the diagnosis if there is no associated pathology in the reproductive tract. Secondary dysmenorrhea is diagnosed if there is a pathological cause for painful menstruation, such as fibroid tumor. A thorough medical history and pelvic examination are required. Oral contraceptives, which stop ovulation and decrease prostaglandin synthesis and myometrial contractility, can relieve dysmenorrhea. Nonsteroidal anti-inflammatory drugs (NSAIDs), such as ibuprofen, are particularly effective in dysmenorrhea. Low-fat diets, regular exercise, local application of heat, massage, and relaxation techniques are other recommended measures.

Premenstrual Syndrome and Premenstrual Dysphoric Disorder

PMS is the occurrence of distressing physical, emotional, and behavioral changes that interfere with activities of daily living during the luteal phase of the menstrual cycle. It is estimated that 50% or more of women experience mild to moderate PMS, with 5% to 10% experiencing severe to disabling symptoms.

PMS is thought to result from an abnormal tissue response to levels of neurotransmitters that exist during the time before the menses. Because treatment with selective serotonin receptor inhibitors (SSRIs) has been successful, it is thought that PMS is a disorder of decreased synaptic serotonin levels. Fluctuating levels of endorphins, estrogen, and progesterone have been implicated as triggers as well. Alternatively, nutritional deficiency of magnesium or calcium may be causative of PMS.

Emotional symptoms such as depression, anger, irritability, and fatigue have been reported as the most prominent signs, with physical symptoms such as bloating, water retention, and headache.

 CLINICAL CONCEPT

A more severe form of PMS is premenstrual dysphoric disorder (PMDD). The symptoms of PMDD include markedly depressed mood, marked anxiety, tension, marked affective lability, persistent irritability or anger, difficulty concentrating, easy fatigability, food cravings, hypersomnia or insomnia, and a subjective sense of being overwhelmed. PMDD interferes with work or school, social activities, and relationships.

Diagnosis of PMS is based on health history. Treatment focuses on education and self-help techniques. Dietary changes such as increased intake of complex carbohydrates, fiber, and water, as well as decreased intake of caffeine, alcohol, sugar, and animal fat, are suggested. Medications such as SSRIs are frequently prescribed.

Assessment

The assessment of women for reproductive disorders requires a thorough history and physical examination. The patient should be asked about any history of disease, such as diabetes and endocrine, hematologic, cardiovascular, pulmonary, or renal disorders. Systemic disorders can have an effect on the female's reproductive organs. For example, diabetes increases susceptibility to vaginal candida infection, von Willebrand disease increases menstrual blood loss, and thyroid problems can cause amenorrhea or excessive menstrual blood loss. Questions regarding abdominal and pelvic pain are essential. Ask the patient to identify the site of pain and its quality. Is it sharp, dull, or cramping? Continuous or intermittent? Ask when the pain occurs and if anything relieves or worsens it. Ask about breast masses, pain, tenderness, or galactorrhea (milk discharge).

Ask the patient about her last menstrual period (LMP), duration of each menstrual period, and how often periods occur. Other questions include:

- Is there pain with menstruation?
- How much blood loss occurs with each period?

CLINICAL CONCEPT

The volume of blood loss is a difficult estimation, but you can ask the patient to identify the number of tampons or pads used per day in order to roughly gauge blood loss. Saturation of a tampon or pad per hour is excessive menstrual blood loss.

Pregnancies are dated in weeks, starting from the first day of a woman's LMP. If menstrual periods are regular and ovulation occurs on day 14 of the menstrual cycle, conception takes place about 2 weeks after the LMP. A woman is therefore considered to be 6 weeks pregnant 2 weeks after the first missed period. The estimated date of childbirth can be calculated using Naegele's rule: adding 1 year to the LMP, subtracting 3 months, and adding 7 days. Childbirth occurs approximately 40 weeks after the LMP.

The history of pregnancy and childbirth is integral to the assessment of reproductive organs. Has the patient been pregnant before and, if so, what kind of delivery occurred: vaginal or caesarian section? Identifying the patient's gravidity and parity are important to note. **Gravidity** is the number of times a woman has been pregnant. **Parity** is the number of times a woman has given birth to a fetus past 24 weeks in gestation.

CLINICAL CONCEPT

The adult female patient who has not had a pregnancy is referred to as nulliparous, whereas the adult female who has had multiple pregnancies is referred to as multiparous. A woman carrying her first pregnancy is called a primigravida, and after delivery she would be called a primiparous woman.

CLINICAL CONCEPT

In a patient history, a woman may be described in terms of gravidity and parity. For example, a woman described as "gravida 2, para 2" (sometimes abbreviated to G2 P2) has had two pregnancies and two deliveries after 24 weeks, and a woman who is described as "gravida 2, para 0" (G2 P0) has had two pregnancies, neither of which survived to a gestational age of 24 weeks.

Sexual history is also an important part of a woman's health assessment. Depending on the patient's age, the age of menarche or menopause is important. Also, it is critical to ask if safe sex is practiced and if birth control is used. If so, what type of birth control is used? The patient should be asked about homosexuality versus

heterosexuality and number of sexual partners. The number of sexual partners is significant, as multiple partners increases susceptibility of sexually transmitted disease. The patient should be asked if there is pain with intercourse, also called dyspareunia. Also, is there bleeding after intercourse? If the patient is perimenopausal, questions about hot flashes, night sweats, and vaginal dryness are indicated.

Family history is significant, as some reproductive disorders are genetic. A history of breast cancer in a first-degree relative is particularly important. The BRCA gene is an inherited genetic mutation that increases the risk of breast, ovarian, and other cancers. Many women are being increasingly tested for the mutation. Social habits such as smoking and the use of alcohol, drug, and caffeine are important to document. Behaviors such as exercise regimen and diet should also be assessed. Women who exercise excessively, underweight athletes, and those with eating disorders frequently endure amenorrhea. In addition, current medications, particularly hormonal drugs and oral contraceptives, are important to note in the history. Ask about over-the-counter medications as well as vitamins and herbal supplements.

A thorough physical examination of women older than age 18 years, or sexually active girls, includes a pelvic and breast examination, Pap smear, and digital rectal exam. The adolescent should be assessed for childhood growth and development, including height, weight, and age at thelarche and menarche. Assessment of the patient's Tanner stage by inspection of the breast tissue and pubic hair is indicated (see Fig. 26-5). In adolescents, ascertaining the age of the patient's mother and sisters at menarche is recommended because the age at menarche in family members can occur within a year of the age in others.

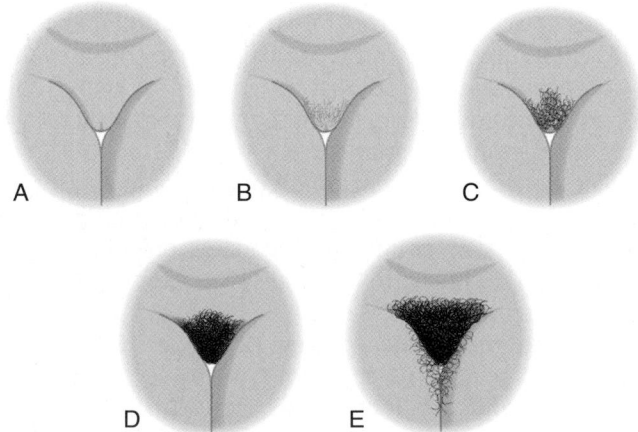

FIGURE 26-5. Tanner stages of female development. A, Preadolescent. No pubic hair, just fine body hair similar to hair on abdomen. B, Sparse growth of long, downy hair; straight or slightly curled mainly along labia. C, Darker, coarser, curlier hair that spreads over pubic symphysis. D, Hair is coarse, curly, and covers more area. E, Adult. Hair may spread over medial surfaces of thighs, but not over abdomen. (From Ward, S., & Hisley, S. (2009). *Maternal-child nursing care, enhanced revised reprint.* Philadelphia, PA: F.A. Davis Company, with permission.)

Diagnosis

The diagnostic studies performed for assessment of female reproductive disorders depend on the patient's symptoms and suspected condition. Some common diagnostic studies include bone age, bone density, thyroid function, PRL levels, adrenal function, and sex hormones, as well as estrogen and progesterone levels. Serum levels of FSH, LH, estradiol, testosterone, thyroid-stimulating hormone, thyroxine, and HCG are also commonly measured. At times, a karyotype needs to be performed, as well as magnetic resonance imaging (MRI) of the pituitary gland.

The **Papanicolaou smear,** also called Pap smear, Pap test, or cervical smear, is a common screening test used in gynecology to detect cellular changes associated with cervical cancer. An anal Pap smear is an adaptation of the procedure to screen and detect anal cancers. In performing a Pap smear, a pelvic examination using a speculum is required. Cells from the outer opening of the cervix (exocervix) and the inner surface of the cervix (endocervix) are sampled. The cells are then microscopically examined to look for abnormalities. Another method that can be used in place of a Pap smear, called **liquid-based cytology (LBC),** can detect cervical cell changes, cervical cancer, and the presence of human papilloma virus (HPV).

A clinician performing a **colposcopy** examines the cervix using a colposcope, which provides an illuminated, magnified view of the cervix and the tissues of the vagina and vulva. The main goal of colposcopy is to detect early signs of cervical cancer and allow for a biopsy of the tissue.

Culdoscopy visualizes the fallopian tubes and ovaries using a type of endoscope with a light that can be inserted into the vaginal canal. In an ectopic pregnancy, bleeding commonly occurs into the cul-de-sac, which is a region of the peritoneal cavity behind the uterus. The culdoscope can be inserted into the vagina and then into the region posterior to the cervix to reach this area. In a culdocentesis, the culdoscope is used to search for blood in the cul-de sac. Blood found in this region can diagnose ectopic pregnancy.

The beta-human chorionic gonadotropin (b-HCG); is a hormone produced during pregnancy that is made by the developing embryo after conception and later by the placenta. This is the most accurate test used to diagnose pregnancy.

Carcinoembryonic antigen 125 (CA-125) is a biomarker associated with various disorders, including uterine fibroids, endometriosis, pelvic inflammatory disease, and cirrhosis, as well as pregnancy and normal menstruation. Certain cancers, including ovarian, endometrial, peritoneal, and fallopian tube, also can cause CA-125 to be released into the bloodstream. A CA-125 blood level is often used to rule out ovarian cancer.

Common pelvic diagnostic procedures include a transabdominal or transvaginal ultrasound, hysterosalpingography, hysteroscopy, and laparoscopy. Transvaginal ultrasound visualizes the ovaries, fallopian tubes, and uterus using sound waves. This test is commonly used to evaluate the ovaries for masses or cysts. Hysterosalpingography is an image study that uses radiopaque dye to outline the uterine cavity and fallopian tubes. **Hysteroscopy** visualizes the interior of the uterus using a specialized thin telescopic type device. The scope is inserted into the uterus via the vagina. A **laparoscopy** requires a small surgical incision in the abdominal surface for insertion of a specialized scope that allows internal visualization of the reproductive organs. A surgeon can visualize endometriosis, scarring, masses, cysts, or anatomic abnormalities of the organs.

Proctoscopy is a procedure in which an instrument called a proctoscope is used to examine the anal cavity, rectum, or sigmoid colon. These areas of the body may contain metastatic lesions from the female genital tract. The proctoscope has a hollow barrel through which another instrument may be inserted to take a biopsy of a small amount of tissue. Air may be injected through the proctoscope to help make viewing easier. Similar instruments—the sigmoidoscope and colonoscope—may be used to visualize more proximal parts of the bowel.

Mammography is a specialized x-ray that visualizes breast tissue and is used as a screening tool. The goal of mammography is the early detection of breast cancer, typically through detection of characteristic masses or microcalcifications. Digital mammography and ultrasound-guided fine needle biopsy of breast masses are procedures used when breast cancer is suspected.

Treatment

The treatment for reproductive disorders depends on the cause of the condition. For the adolescent with constitutional delay and anovulation, the goal is stimulation of ovulatory cycles. Estrogen-progestin therapy, which is commonly available in oral contraceptives, can stimulate ovulation. Commonly, oral contraceptives are prescribed to induce ovulation and regulate menstruation in any age female with oligomenorrhea.

Hormone replacement therapy (HRT) or estrogen therapy alone is also used to alleviate severe menopausal symptoms such as hot flashes, night sweats, and vaginal dryness. HRT is reserved for those who have severe symptoms or those with hysterectomy-induced menopause. Health-care providers have to weigh the risk and benefits of HRT, as risks include cardiac disease, stroke, venous thrombus, and breast, ovarian, and uterine cancer.

Hypothalamic amenorrhea is most common in patients who exercise to excess or have eating disorders, caloric restriction, and psychogenic stress. Hypothalamic amenorrhea is best treated using behavioral modification and a multidisciplinary team approach, depending on the root cause.

Symptomatic hyperprolactinemia from a pituitary disorder should first be treated by dopamine agonists such as bromocriptine (Parlodel) and cabergoline

(Dostinex). Surgery or radiation of the pituitary may be indicated.

Patients with hyperprolactinemia associated with medications such as antipsychotics and metoclopramide should consider discontinuation or switching of the causative medication.

Premature ovarian failure (POF) after puberty occurs in 1% of adult women. Treatment should be decided on an individual basis. Some patients may require estrogen replacement therapy (ERT) for hot flashes and other symptomatic menopausal issues. No medications or therapies have been found to induce normal cycling; its occurrence is sporadic, spontaneous, and not inducible.

Fertility drugs, which regulate or induce ovulation, are the main treatment for women who are infertile because of ovulation disorders. In general, they work like the natural hormones FSH and LH to trigger ovulation. Using fertility drugs increases chances of multiple pregnancies. There are several fertility drugs for abnormal LH and FSH production. These drugs include clomiphene citrate, gonadotropins, human menopausal gonadotropin, FSH, HCG, metformin, and aromatase inhibitors.

Reproductive assistance or **in vitro fertilization (IVF)** is a highly effective technique that involves retrieving mature eggs from the female, fertilizing them with sperm in a petri dish in a laboratory, and implanting the embryos in the uterus 3 to 5 days after fertilization. IVF is recommended for a number of disorders that cause infertility, including bilateral salpingitis, endometriosis, unexplained infertility, cervical factor infertility, and ovulation disorders. IVF increases the chances of multiple births because multiple fertilized eggs are implanted into the uterus to increase the chances that at least one will develop into an embryo.

Dilatation and Curretage (D&C) is a common surgical procedure that refers to the dilation of the cervix and surgical removal of the lining of the uterus or contents of the uterus by scraping (curettage). A D&C can be used for diagnostic purposes as well as treatment.

A hysterectomy is the surgical excision of a woman's uterus. This procedure can be done via an abdominal incision or via the vaginal canal. A total hysterectomy is the removal of the ovaries, fallopian tubes, and uterus. A partial hysterectomy usually leaves the ovaries in place.

Endometrial ablation is a procedure that uses a hysteroscope and curettage device to remove the uterine endometrial lining. It eliminates hyperplastic layers of endometrium and menstrual bleeding. This procedure is often used for women instead of a hysterectomy.

Several surgical procedures use a laparotomy approach, which is a small abdominal or pelvic incision and insertion of a scope to visualize and operate on the reproductive organs. Many reproductive disorders involve use of the laparotomy, such as tissue removal of endometriosis or pelvic adhesions with laser or ablation procedures, tubal ligation, tubal reversal surgery (microscopic) to reconnect fallopian tube integrity, dilation of a fallopian tube, or creation of a new tubal opening.

Cryosurgery (cryotherapy) is the application of extreme cold to destroy abnormal or diseased tissue. Cryosurgery is done after a colposcopy confirms the presence of abnormal cervical cells. It is most commonly used for treatment of cervical lesions such as precancerous cells or cervicitis.

Conization of the cervix is the excision of a cone-shaped or cylindrical wedge from the cervix that includes all or a portion of the endocervical canal. It is used for the definitive diagnosis of squamous or glandular intraepithelial lesions, for excluding microinvasive carcinomas, and for conservative treatment of cervical intraepithelial neoplasia (CIN).

Uterine artery embolization is a procedure mainly used to suppress growth of uterine fibroid tumors. It involves use of a specialized x-ray called a fluoroscope to guide the delivery of small particles into the uterine artery via a catheter. The procedure cuts off blood flow to areas of the uterus where there are fibroid tumors; it is effective in 90% of patients.

Pathophysiology of Selected Female Reproductive Disorders

The common female reproductive disorders encountered in the clinical setting will be discussed in the next sections. For uterine, cervical, ovarian, and breast cancer, see Chapter 40: Cancer.

Disorders of the Uterus

Endometritis

The **endometrium** of the uterus is the inner lining that varies in thickness throughout the menstrual cycle. The uterus is a sterile environment with the cervix acting as a barrier to ascending infection. Infection of the endometrium, called endometritis, can occur in association with instrumentation of the uterus, abortion, childbirth, pelvic inflammatory disease, or an implanted intrauterine device (IUD). Endometritis often occurs in conjunction with inflammation of the fallopian tubes (salpingitis), ovaries (oophoritis), and pelvic peritoneum (pelvic peritonitis).

Endometritis is usually caused by more than one microorganism; it is most commonly caused by an ascending infection from the vagina. It also occurs in 70% to 90% of cases of salpingitis. Endometritis is an uncommon occurrence after vaginal childbirth, at a rate of 1% to 3%, but more common with caesarian section, depending on the circumstances necessitating surgery. Microorganisms such as *Gonococcus, Chlamydia trachomatis, Enterococcus,* and several strains of anaerobic bacteria are the most common causes of endometritis. The endometrium can be acutely or chronically affected by infection. In acute infection, white blood cells and bacterial organisms invade the endometrial layer. In chronic infection, plasma cells and T lymphocytes are found in the endometrial layer and deeper. Symptoms usually include abnormal vaginal bleeding, uterine tenderness, fever, and malodorous discharge. Endocervical cultures should be obtained for gonorrhea and chlamydia when appropriate. Blood cultures and urinalysis are necessary to rule out extension of the infection into the blood or urinary tract. Ultrasound and computed tomography (CT) scans may be needed if retained tissue of pregnancy is the cause of the infection. Antibiotic therapy is indicated and usually can thoroughly eradicate the condition.

Endometriosis and Adenomyosis

Endometriosis is the growth of endometrial tissue outside the uterus (see Fig. 26-6). The most common sites are the ovaries, uterine ligaments, rectovaginal septum, pelvic peritoneum, umbilicus, vagina, vulva, and appendix. Endometrial tissue in these sites responds to hormone fluctuations in the same way as uterine endometrium. Bleeding can occur at these sites monthly. Endometriosis commonly causes infertility, dysmenorrhea, and pelvic pain.

A related disorder, adenomyosis, occurs when the endometrial tissue grows inside the muscular layer of the uterus. In adenomyosis, the endometrium, in response to hormone fluctuations, bleeds within the muscle wall of the uterus, causing menorrhagia, dysmenorrhea, dyspareunia (pain with sexual intercourse), and pelvic pain.

Approximately 10% to 15% of women have endometriosis; in addition, 80% of women with pelvic pain have endometriosis. There may be a genetic cause of endometriosis because first-degree relatives frequently have the disease. The cause of endometriosis is unclear, but there are several theories:

- **Regurgitation/implantation theory:** This suggests that menstrual blood containing fragments of endometrium are forced up through the fallopian tubes and into the peritoneal cavity.
- **Metaplastic theory:** This suggests that during embryonic development, immature endometrial tissue spreads over a wider area than normal; during adulthood, it matures and functions like misplaced endometrium.

- **Vascular or lymphatic theory:** This suggests that some endometrial tissue breaks away and metastasizes to other locations in the pelvis.
- **Immunological dysfunction:** This suggests displaced endometrial tissue may trigger an autoimmune reaction. Immunoglobulins attack the endometrial tissue and cause inflammation.
- **Environmental toxicity:** Some studies have shown an association between dioxin (an herbicide) exposure and endometriosis.

Pelvic pain in the reproductive years is a common presentation of endometriosis. There are usually no physical examination findings. Definitive diagnosis of endometriosis can only be accomplished through laparoscopy. Other helpful tools are ultrasonography, MRI, and serum CA-125. Treatment involves pain relief, endometrial tissue suppression, and surgery. NSAIDs are often prescribed for pain relief, as well as oral contraceptives, continuous progestogen, danazol (androgen), or long-acting GnRH to inhibit pituitary gonadotropin and suppress ovulation. Surgery involving cautery, laser ablation, and excision techniques via laparoscopy are used to treat endometriosis.

Endometrial Polyps

An endometrial polyp is a mass that protrudes into the endometrial cavity. These polyps can be of varying size, from as small as a pencil eraser to as large as a golf ball. They are neoplastic growths of the endometrium of unknown etiology. They are usually benign, but coexistence of atypical endometrial hyperplasia or adenocarcinoma is common. Growth of endometrial polyps has been associated with tamoxifen, which is used to prevent breast cancer in some women. Polyps may be asymptomatic or cause abnormal bleeding if they ulcerate or undergo necrosis. They most often develop in women between the ages of 40 and 60 years and are a frequent cause of intermenstrual or excessive menstrual bleeding. Diagnosis is made by hysteroscopy or curettage and biopsy. Surgical excision is the treatment.

Leiomyomas

Uterine leiomyomas are commonly referred to as fibroid tumors and are the most common benign tumors in humans. As many as 3 out of 4 women have uterine fibroid tumors sometime during their lives; however, the majority are asymptomatic and undiagnosed. The etiology of fibroid tumors is unknown, but they tend to be familial, and those who take oral contraceptives have a lesser rate of fibroid tumor than those who do not take them. Fibroid tumors can be small or large enough to distort the shape of the uterus. The tumors are sharply circumscribed, firm growths that are most commonly found in the **myometrium** (see Fig. 26-7). They are composed of smooth muscle and connective tissue in a distinctive swirled pattern when seen on biopsy.

Leiomyomas can be asymptomatic or cause abnormal vaginal bleeding, bladder compression, dysmenorrhea, back pain, or infertility. Excessive menstrual

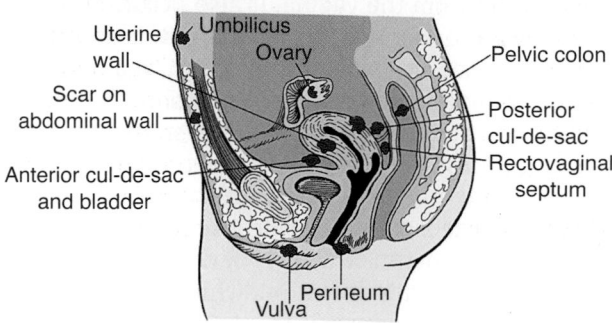

FIGURE 26-6. Sites of endometriosis. (From Williams, L., & Hopper, P. (2011). *Understanding medical-surgical nursing. 4th ed.* Philadelphia, PA: F.A. Davis Company, with permission.)

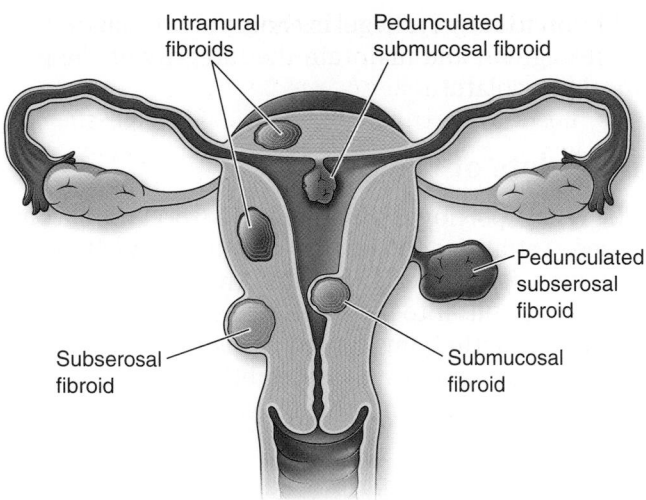

Intramural fibroids

Pedunculated submucosal fibroid

Pedunculated subserosal fibroid

Subserosal fibroid

Submucosal fibroid

Fibroid uterus

FIGURE 26-7. Sites of leiomyomas of the uterus.

bleeding can occur that causes anemia. Malignant transformation of leiomyoma to leiomyosarcoma is rare, with a rate of fewer than 1%. There is usually more than one fibroid tumor and they can increase in size because of estrogen stimulation and with pregnancy. Transabdominal and transvaginal ultrasound are the diagnostic procedures most commonly used to diagnose uterine fibroids. MRI can be used to visualize the tumors. CT scan can also be used, but cannot sharply visualize these tumors unless they are calcified.

Most leiomyomas regress with menopause, but if the tumor causes intolerable pain or bladder compression, surgical excision of the tumor, also called myomectomy, can be performed. Hypothalamic GnRH can be given to suppress growth of fibroid tumor. Alternatively, a procedure called uterine artery embolization can obstruct blood supply to a fibroid tumor and diminish its growth.

Dysfunctional Uterine Bleeding

Dysfunctional uterine bleeding (DUB) is abnormal uterine bleeding caused by a disturbance of the menstrual cycle. The diagnosis of DUB can indicate an excessive loss of blood from the uterus or it can indicate lack of normal menstruation at cyclical periods. It is estimated that 5% of women aged 30 to 49 years seek medical care for DUB each year. Although DUB may occur at any time during the reproductive years, it is most common in adolescents at the beginning of their menses and in women approaching menopause.

Anovulatory cycles (failure to ovulate) are the most common cause of DUB. Anovulation may be a sign of physiologic menopause, progesterone deficiency, polycystic ovarian syndrome (PCOS), immaturity of the hypothalamic-pituitary axis, or primary ovarian failure (POF). Other conditions associated with lack of ovulation include hyper- or hypothyroidism, obesity, pregnancy, or estrogen-secreting ovarian tumors. Stress can also cause disruption of the hypothalamic-pituitary axis, leading to DUB.

Anovulatory DUB can be demonstrated as a condition of missed periods, prolonged intervals between menses, more frequent periods than normal, or excessive menstrual blood loss. It is commonly caused by progesterone deficiency or estrogen excess. In the absence of progesterone, unopposed estrogen causes the uterine endometrial layer to proliferate with increased vascularity and glandular development. A lack of ovulation and absence of progesterone allows for excessive uterine endometrial accumulation without menstrual shedding of the tissue. A thick layer of endometrium accumulates with no stimulus for menstruation; consequently, amenorrhea occurs. Eventually, the excessive endometrial layer does break down and the woman experiences an irregular menstrual cycle and flow irregularities, such as menorrhagia, metrorrhagia, menometrorrhagia, intermenstrual spotting, and oligomenorrhea.

In ovulatory DUB, excessive bleeding occurs cyclically and is thought to originate from defects in the control mechanisms of menstruation. In women with ovulatory DUB, there is an increased rate of blood loss resulting from endometrial vascular vasodilatation, decreased vascular tone, and excessive prostaglandins. Women suffer heavy menstrual blood loss, up to three times normal. Large menstrual blood loss often causes anemia and interferes with daily activity.

DUB is made by history and clinical examination. In DUB, pregnancy must first be ruled out by serum beta-HCG. A complete blood count is necessary to rule out anemia caused by gynecological blood loss. Because bleeding can always be caused by coagulation disorders, blood samples for platelet and coagulation factors are drawn. If any endocrine disorders are suspected, these blood tests are also drawn. Transabdominal and transvaginal ultrasound can rule out uterine masses or lesions. Hysteroscopy can be used if uterine lesions are suspected. Endometrial biopsy, CT, or MRI scans are sometimes needed.

Treatment goals involve control of bleeding and hormonal regulation with either progestin-estrogen therapy or progesterone-only treatment. If the patient has not had a menstrual period for 3 or more months, most clinicians will administer progesterone. This will stimulate endometrial breakdown and menses will occur. Conversely, if there is excessive uterine bleeding causing DUB, danazol is used. This medication decreases estrogen and increases androgens, which causes endometrial atrophy and reduced menstrual loss of blood. Alternatively, GnRH stimulants may be used to inhibit menses and allow for rebuilding of red blood cell mass. Another medication, tranexamic acid, is an antifibrinolytic drug that inhibits plasminogen. It diminishes fibrinolytic activity within endometrial vessels to prevent excessive bleeding. Total or partial ablation of the endometrium or hysterectomy are surgical procedures sometimes used for DUB in women who are older than reproductive age.

Uterine Prolapse

Uterine prolapse is the protrusion of the uterus into the vaginal canal that occurs when supportive ligaments of the pelvic floor are stretched (see Fig. 26-8).

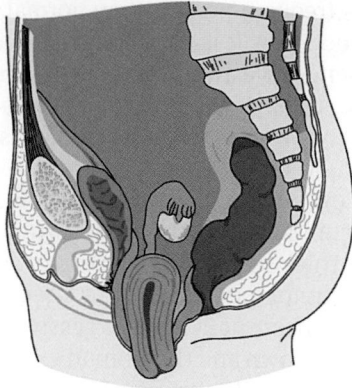

FIGURE 26-8. Uterine prolapse. (From Williams, L., & Hopper, P. (2011). *Understanding medical-surgical nursing. 4th ed.* Philadelphia, PA: F.A. Davis Company, with permission.)

It commonly occurs in multiparous women because childbirth is accompanied by pelvic wall distention and ligament relaxation. It may also occur with pelvic masses or neurological conditions. Prolapse can be categorized as first, second, or third degree, depending on how far into the vaginal canal the uterus protrudes. In first-degree prolapse, the cervix protrudes into the vaginal canal slightly, whereas in third-degree prolapse the prolapsed cervix can be seen protruding through the exterior of the vaginal opening. Perineal irritation and discomfort are the symptoms of uterine prolapse. A pessary is a supportive device that can be inserted to readjust the uterus's position. Alternatively, surgical intervention can repair the ligaments and readjust the uterus's position.

Cystocele, Rectocele, and Enterocele

A cystocele is the herniation of the urinary bladder into the vaginal canal. It occurs when the muscle support for the bladder is weakened and the bladder sinks below the uterus. It appears as a bulge through the vaginal canal, commonly leading to symptoms of frequency, urgency, and perineal pressure. Stress incontinence can occur at times of lifting, coughing, straining, sneezing, and laughing.

A rectocele is the herniation of the rectum into the vaginal canal. This also occurs because of perineal muscle weakening and appears as a bulge in the vaginal canal.

An enterocele is a herniation of intestine within the area between the uterosacral ligaments posterior to the cervix; these can weaken and form a hernia sac in which the small bowel protrudes. It can cause a feeling of pressure in the perineum, a dull aching sensation, and low backache.

For each of these herniations, surgical intervention is necessary. A surgical intervention using a transvaginal mesh material to repair pelvic organ prolapse has been used. Some women have experienced adverse side effects, such as pelvic pain and inflammation, from this procedure. It is currently being evaluated by the FDA; however, alternate surgical procedures that do not use synthetic mesh are recommended. In addition to surgery, Kegel exercises are recommended to strengthen and maintain the integrity of the perineal musculature.

Disorders of the Cervix

The visible portion of the cervix, or exocervix, is composed of stratified squamous epithelium, which is continuous with the vaginal wall. The endocervix, the canal that leads into the uterine cavity, is composed of columnar epithelium that contains mucus-secreting glands. Blockage of a mucus-secreting gland in the endocervix can cause a nabothian cyst, a common benign cyst requiring no treatment (see Fig. 26-9).

The junction of the exocervix squamous epithelium and mucus-secreting glandular endocervix cells is called the transformation zone. This zone is the area that is sampled during a Papanicolaou smear and examined during colposcopy to rule out cervical cancer. The Papanicolaou smear, also called Pap smear and Pap test, is a screening test used to detect potentially precancerous and cancerous processes of the cervix (see Box 26-2).

Normal cervix   Nabothian cysts on the cervix

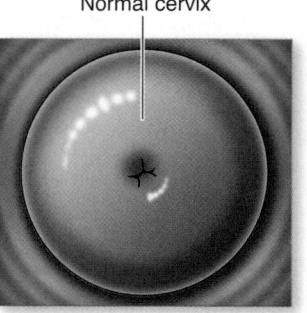 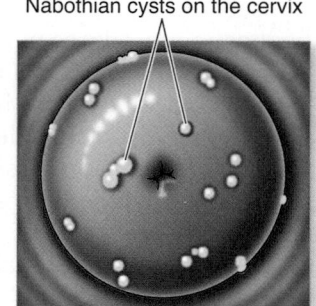

FIGURE 26-9. Nabothian cyst.

BOX 26-2. Pap Smear Guidelines

According to the National Cancer Institute in 2012:

- Cervical cancer screening, which includes the Pap test and human papillomavirus (HPV) testing, is an essential part of a woman's routine health care because it can detect cancer or abnormalities that may lead to cancer of the cervix.
- Current guidelines recommend that women should have a Pap test every 3 years beginning at age 21 years. These guidelines further recommend that women ages 30 to 65 years should have HPV and Pap cotesting every 5 years or a Pap test alone every 3 years.
- Women with certain risk factors may need to have more frequent screening or to continue screening beyond age 65 years. Women who have received the HPV vaccine still need regular cervical screening.

(Adapted from National Cancer Institute. (2014). *Pap and HPV testing.* Retrieved from http://www.cancer.gov/cancertopics/factsheet/detection/Pap-HPV-testing.)

In taking a Pap smear, a speculum is used to open the vaginal canal and allow the collection of cells from the outer region of the cervix and the endocervix. The cells are examined under a microscope to look for cervical intraepithelial neoplasia (CIN) (also called cervical dysplasia). The test is used for early detection of precancerous changes and cervical cancer. The test may also detect infections and abnormalities in the endocervix and endometrium. In women who are 30 years and older, a HPV test should be combined with the Pap smear. Both cervical cancer and HPV can be detected by a procedure called liquid-based cytology (LBC) (ThinPrep®).

To report Pap smear results, most laboratories in the United States use a set of categories called the Bethesda system. HPV results are reported as simply positive or negative. The Bethesda system categories range from benign inflammatory changes to malignant cancer (see Table 26-2) (For further detail on cervical cancer, see Chapter 40: Cancer).

Cervicitis

Some degree of inflammation of the cervix is found in most women and is of little clinical significance. The cervix is exposed to endogenous vaginal aerobic and anaerobic organisms, such as *Streptococci*, *Enterococci*, *E. coli*, and *Staphylococci*. However, clinically important organisms include human immunodeficiency virus (HIV), gonococci, *Trichomonas vaginalis*, *Chlamydiae*, HPV, and herpes simplex virus. These organisms are dangerous because of the potential of ascending endometrial infection, systemic infection, pregnancy-related complications, cancer predisposition, or sexual transmission. Chlamydia trachomatis is the organism most commonly associated with cervicitis.

Cervicitis is characterized by inflammatory cells, erosion, and epithelial changes, and may be culture positive or culture negative for a specific microorganism. Some inflammatory changes can resemble precancerous lesions, which is why a Pap smear is important. Signs of cervicitis include an erythematous, edematous cervix

with a large amount of purulent discharge. Diagnosis is based on clinical pelvic examination, colposcopy, Pap smear, and, if necessary, biopsy. Colposcopically guided laser treatment of abnormal epithelium is treatment.

Cervical Polyps

Polyps are erythematous lesions that protrude through the cervical os. They are usually a result of benign, inflammatory changes of the endocervix. They are usually asymptomatic but may cause postcoital bleeding. Most are benign, but they should nevertheless be removed and biopsied.

Disorders of the Vagina and External Genitalia

One of the most common disorders of the female reproductive tract is vulvovaginitis. *Candida albicans* is a common cause of inflammation of the vulva and vaginal tract. Inflammation is common, whereas cancer of the vulva is a very rare condition.

Vulvodynia

Vulvodynia is pain of the vulva characterized as burning, irritation, or stinging. Causes of vulvodynia include chronic yeast infection, chemical irritation, or drug effects (particularly prolonged use of topical steroids), irritation from elevated levels of urine calcium oxalate, immunoglobulin A deficiency, genital herpes, and dermatoses such as lichen planus. Diagnosis is made by history and physical examination. Treatment is aimed at symptom relief and elimination of the suspected cause.

Vulvar Cancer

Vulvar cancer is a rare disease in which malignant cancer cells form in the tissues of the vulva over a period of many years. A precancerous condition called vulvar intraepithelial neoplasia can progress to vulvar cancer. Risk factors include human papillomavirus infection and older age. Possible signs of vulvar cancer include

TABLE 26-2. Classification System for Papanicolaou Smears

Different systems in which Pap smears can be described and classified. The columns describe the cellular change, CIN system category, and Bethesda system category.

Dysplasia/Neoplasia	CIN	Bethesda System
Benign	Benign	Negative for intraepithelial lesion or malignancy
Benign with inflammation	Benign with inflammation	Negative for intraepithelial lesion of malignancy, ASC-US
Mild dysplasia	CIN 1	Low grade SIL, ASC-H
Moderate dysplasia	CIN 2	High grade SIL
Severe dysplasia and carcinoma in situ (CIS)	CIN 3	High grade SIL
Invasive cancer	Invasive cancer	Invasive cancer

ASC-US: atypical squamous cells of undetermined significance
SIL: squamous intraepithelial lesion
ASC-H: cannot rule out high grade SIL
(Adapted from National Cancer Institute/National Health Institutes. (2014). Cervical Cancer Screening. Retrieved from http://www.cancer.gov/cancertopics/pdq/screening/cervical/HealthProfessional/page2.)

bleeding, itching, palpable mass, and tenderness in the vulvar area. Diagnostic tests and procedures include pelvic exam, biopsy, cystoscopy, proctoscopy (visualization of the anus and rectum), intravenous pyelogram, CT scan, and MRI. The four types of treatment are laser therapy, surgery, radiation, and chemotherapy.

Vaginitis

Vaginitis, also called **vulvovaginitis,** is inflammation of the vagina characterized by discharge, burning, itching, redness, and edema of vaginal tissue. Pain often occurs with urination or sexual intercourse. The disorder can be caused by many different agents, depending on the patient's age. Before menarche, vaginitis is most often caused by poor hygiene, intestinal parasites, or presence of foreign bodies. The most common causes of vaginitis in women of childbearing age are bacterial vaginosis (40% to 45%), vaginal candidiasis (20% to 25%), and trichomoniasis (15% to 20%). Vaginitis in postmenopausal women occurs because of vaginal atrophy resulting from diminishing estrogen levels.

Bacterial vaginosis is the most common cause of vaginitis, accounting for 50% of cases. It is caused by an overgrowth of organisms such as *Enterococcus, Gardnerella vaginalis, Mobiluncus* species, *Mycoplasma hominis,* and *Peptostreptococcus* species. Most organisms are anaerobic bacteria that inhabit the bowel as normal flora. The organisms spread from the rectum into the vaginal canal.

Candida, also referred to as yeast, is natural flora within the vagina in as many as 50% of women. However, in vaginal candidiasis there is an overgrowth of the organism caused by a disruption in the vaginal pH, glycogen content of vaginal cells, or other vaginal environmental change. Factors that can disrupt vaginal conditions include oral contraceptive use, IUD use, young age at first intercourse, increased frequency of intercourse, receptive cunnilingus, diabetes, HIV or other immunocompromised states, long-term antibiotic use, and pregnancy.

Trichomonas vaginalis is an oval-shaped flagellated protozoan called a trichomonad that is 15 mm long, the size of a leukocyte. These organisms primarily infect vaginal epithelium; less commonly, they infect the endocervix, urethra, and Bartholin glands. Trichomonads are transmitted sexually and can be identified in as many as 80% of male partners of infected women.

Because symptoms of burning, discharge, and itching are common for many different kinds of vaginal infections, precise identification of the pathogen is essential for treatment. Specific culture and sensitivity testing is required. Studies that may be performed in cases of suspected vaginitis include saline wet mount (also called whiff test), pH testing, culture, nucleic acid amplification testing, and a number of other second-line tests.

Candida albicans, a most common cause of vaginitis, requires a specific diagnostic procedure called a potassium hydroxide (KOH) saline-wet mount smear. A small amount of vaginal mucus is placed on a slide with two drops of saline and a small amount of KOH. KOH destroys the vaginal epithelial cells, allowing for visualization of the buds and hyphae that are characteristic of *Candida*.

Trichomonas infection and bacterial vaginosis can be diagnosed using the whiff test. Vaginal discharge is placed on a slide with 10% KOH solution. A positive test result is the release of an amine (fishy) odor after the addition of KOH to the discharge.

The pH of vaginal secretions can also be tested using litmus paper. In bacterial vaginosis the vaginal pH is 5.0 to 6.0; in vaginal candidiasis, pH is lower than 4.5; and in *T. vaginalis* infection, pH is 5.0 to 7.0. Other tests using the polymerase chain reaction to identify the specific organism are performed by using swabs of the cervix or vagina or by collecting a urine sample.

Candida infections are commonly treated with fluconazole vaginal applicator cream or a similar antifungal preparation. Trichomonas is treated with oral metronidazole, and sex partners of the infected woman should be treated as well. Bacterial vaginosis is treated with the oral or applicator gel form of metronidazole.

Measures to prevent future vaginal infections include proper perineal hygiene, avoidance of feminine deodorants and douches, and avoidance of tight undergarments.

Atrophic Vaginitis. Atrophic vaginitis is inflammation of the vagina that occurs after menopause or after removal of the ovaries. Estrogen deficiency causes diminished growth of vaginal epithelium, making the tissue susceptible to irritation. Itching, burning, and dyspareunia are symptoms. Local estrogen application can be used as treatment.

Bartholin Cyst and Abscess

The Bartholin glands—small, spherical structures at the entry to the vagina—release secretions that enhance lubrication and mobility of sperm. When the ducts of these glands become obstructed, the glandular fluid accumulates and becomes infected. Abscesses can form and cause extremely tender cysts. Treatment includes antibiotics, local application of moist heat, and surgical incision and drainage. Asymptomatic cysts require no treatment.

Disorders of the Ovary

The most common disorder of the ovary is a follicular cyst. Each month, women are at risk for a follicular cyst when an ovum comes to the surface of the ovary but is not ejected. In polycystic ovarian syndrome, many cysts form on the ovary's surface, but anovulation occurs each month. Cancer must be ruled out when any type of ovarian mass is present, cystic or solid.

Premature Ovarian Failure

POF is the cessation of ovarian function in a woman younger than age 40 years. The condition, also known as primary ovarian insufficiency and hypergonadotropic hypogonadism, results from underfunctioning ovaries or a deficiency in the number of follicles in the ovaries. POF occurs in approximately 1% of the female population. Approximately 10% to 28% of women with primary amenorrhea, and 4% to 18% of those with secondary amenorrhea, have POF. At puberty, there are 300,000 to 400,000 follicles within the ovary available for ovulation. During the monthly menstrual cycle, several ova come to the ovary's surface for ovulation; however, only one is released. The degeneration of those that did not release an egg play an important role in the hypothalamic-pituitary-ovarian axis by secreting regulatory hormones such as estradiol. In POF there is a reduced follicle number that leads to disruption of the process of follicular growth and ovulation. Many genetic mutations cause diminished follicle number. Autoimmunity and enzyme deficiencies also cause POF. The most common symptoms of POF include infertility, irregular menstrual cycles, hot flashes, night sweats, irritability, poor concentration, decreased libido, dyspareunia, and vaginal dryness.

Women with POF usually do not have physical signs unless POF is part of another endocrine or congenital disorder such as Turner syndrome, hypothyroidism, or Addison's disease. Physical examination may demonstrate atrophic vaginitis resulting from an estrogen deficiency. A pelvic examination may be normal; however, some may have ovarian enlargement. Patients with Turner syndrome have characteristic physical signs such as short stature, webbed neck, and shieldlike chest. Patients with Addison's disease may have premature gray hair, vitiligo, or increased pigmentation of the gums or the skinfolds. They might also have loss of axillary and pubic hair because of reduced ovarian and adrenal androgen production. Thyroid enlargement may be present resulting from Hashimoto thyroiditis. To diagnose POF, an FSH level is most important, as this will be elevated. LH, estradiol, and serum levels of endocrine hormones; cortisol; thyroid hormone; and PRL levels may be abnormal. A karyotype and ovarian ultrasound are needed. CT scan and an MRI of the brain are also necessary to rule out pituitary tumor. All women with POF should receive cyclical hormone therapy with estrogens and progestins to relieve the symptoms of estrogen deficiency and maintain bone density.

Benign Ovarian Cysts

Benign ovarian cysts are commonly functional cysts (see Fig. 26-10). In ovulating women, these cysts are commonly follicular or corpus luteum cysts, which are caused by normal physiologic events. For ovulation to occur, the ovary normally develops a follicle that matures and contains an ovum. The mature follicle, called a Graafian follicle, is located on the ovary's surface and resembles a small cyst. The Graafian follicle containing the ovum normally ruptures and ejects the ovum in a process known as ovulation. When the follicle does not eject the ovum, the result is a follicular cyst; these cysts are usually asymptomatic and require no treatment, because they regress or rupture spontaneously within a few months. However, at times a follicular cyst, although benign, can become large and cause back pain, painful intercourse, chronic abdominal pain, and menstrual irregularities.

A corpus luteum cyst is another type of functional cyst that can occur after ovulation. The corpus luteum is the structure formed by the empty Graafian follicle after ovulation. Under normal conditions, the corpus luteum degenerates. However, a corpus luteum cyst can form because of bleeding inside the corpus luteum 2 to 4 days postovulation. These cysts typically cause symptoms, particularly if they rupture. Symptoms include dull pelvic pain and amenorrhea, followed by irregular or heavy bleeding. Rupture of the cyst occurs during days 20 to 26 of the menstrual cycle. A negative b-HCG test is needed to exclude the possibility of pregnancy, and ultrasound confirms the diagnosis. Laparotomy may be necessary to remove the cyst.

Ovarian Torsion

In ovarian torsion, also known as adnexal torsion, the ovary is twisted and blood flow is obstructed. An enlarged ovary caused by a mass or cyst is most susceptible to torsion. Ovarian torsion is usually unilateral, most likely on the right side. The enlarged ovary will weigh more than normal and dangle lower from the fallopian tube. The ovary can then twist and pinch off arterial and venous vessels. With obstructed blood flow, the ovary can undergo ischemia and infarction.

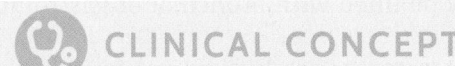

CLINICAL CONCEPT

Approximately 50% to 60% of cases of torsion of the ovary are associated with an ovarian mass.

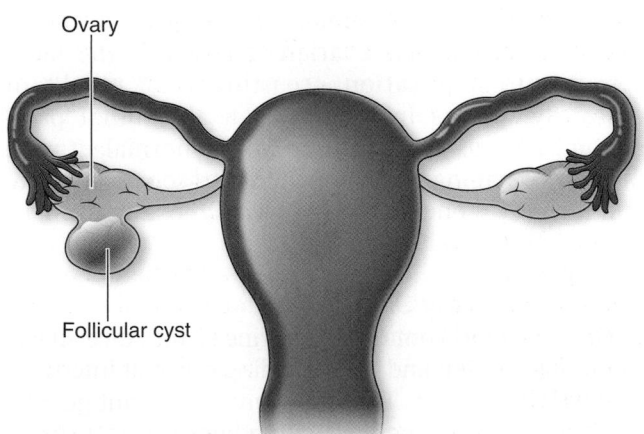

FIGURE 26-10. Ovarian cyst. A follicular cyst can form from an unreleased ovum from the ovarian surface.

The patient with ovarian torsion has unilateral, sudden severe abdominal pain radiating to the pelvis, groin, and thigh. It is most commonly described as sharp and occurs when the patient is active. Nausea and vomiting occur in the majority of patients, which often confounds the clinical picture and leads to a search for a gastrointestinal problem. Abdominal tenderness may or may not be present. In addition, an ovarian mass may or may not be palpable. Clinical examination must exclude possible diagnoses of appendicitis, gastroenteritis, ectopic pregnancy, pelvic inflammatory disease, and ruptured corpus luteum. A pregnancy test is necessary to rule out ectopic pregnancy. Ultrasound with color Doppler analysis is the best diagnostic procedure because it can show structural and vascular changes of the ovary. Laparotomy and surgical removal of the involved ovary is the most common treatment.

ALERT! Ovarian torsion is a gynecological emergency that can present similarly to appendicitis. A pregnancy test is necessary to rule out ectopic pregnancy.

Teratoma of the Ovary

Teratoma of the ovary (also called dermoid cyst) is a cystic mass that has a characteristic composition. Teratomas are made up of various types of embryonic tissue, including epidermal, dermal, bone, and glandular tissue. The interior of the cystic mass is often lined with squamous epithelium and usually contains many sebaceous and sweat glands. Hair and teeth are commonly present within the cyst. Occasionally, the cyst wall may be lined with bronchial or gastrointestinal cells.

Most teratomas are benign and form in the peritoneum or ovaries. They account for 10% to 20% of all ovarian tumors and are bilateral in 8% to 14% of cases.

Teratomas become symptomatic when a complication is present; otherwise, they can be silent. Complications include ovarian torsion, ovarian rupture, infection, hemolytic anemia, and malignant degeneration. Torsion of the ovarian teratoma is the most significant complication, occurring in 3% to 11% of cases. Symptoms include sudden abdominal pain, abdominal mass or swelling, and abnormal uterine bleeding. Imaging studies such as ultrasound, CT scan, and MRI are frequently used to diagnose teratomas. Surgical excision is required.

Polycystic Ovary Syndrome

PCOS is the most common endocrine disturbance affecting young women and is the leading cause of infertility in the United States. This autosomal dominant genetic disorder is often associated with other endocrine disorders. PCOS most commonly affects females between puberty and 30 years of age.

The etiology of PCOS involves a dysfunctional hypothalamic-pituitary-ovary axis. High serum concentrations of androgenic hormones, such as testosterone, androstenedione, and dehydroepiandrosterone sulfate, are found in these patients. In PCOS, multiple cysts develop on the ovary because of multiple areas of follicular cyst formation. Ova develop within the ovary, come to the ovary's surface, and form a follicular cyst; however, they are not released from the ovarian surface. There is no ovulation, and thus no release of eggs from the surface. The ovarian surface develops multiple areas of unreleased ova that resemble multiple cysts.

Clinical manifestations include amenorrhea or dysfunctional uterine bleeding, hirsutism, and infertility. Approximately 38% of women with PCOS are obese. Women with PCOS often have androgen excess, anovulation, and hyperinsulinemia, which is caused by cellular resistance to insulin. Possible late sequela of the disorder include dyslipidemia, diabetes, hypertension, and endometrial carcinoma.

PCOS can be part of metabolic syndrome. Diagnosis of PCOS is based on evidence of androgen excess, chronic anovulation, and inappropriate gonadotropin secretion. Tests for impaired glucose tolerance are recommended. Treatment involves reversal of androgen excess, stimulating cyclic menstruation, restoring fertility, and ameliorating endocrine disturbances. Insulin sensitizers are recommended to decrease the insulin resistance and prevent diabetes and heart disease. Progesterone therapy is recommended to oppose estrogen's effects on the endometrium and initiate monthly menstrual bleeding. For infertility, clomiphene, which stimulates egg production, is used to facilitate ovulation. For those who desire contraception, low-dose oral contraceptives are suggested.

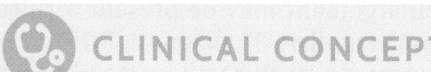 **CLINICAL CONCEPT**

Because PCOS may be associated with metabolic syndrome, patients with the disorder should be checked for hypertension, hyperlipidemia, hyperinsulinemia, and glucose intolerance.

Ectopic Pregnancy

Ectopic pregnancy occurs when a fertilized ovum implants outside the uterus. Although 98% of ectopic pregnancies occur within the fallopian tube, implantation can occur in the cervix, ovary, upper uterus, or peritoneum (see Fig. 26-11). The prevalence is estimated at 25 cases per 1,000 pregnancies. The cause of ectopic pregnancy is slow ovum transport, which may result from decreased fallopian tube motility or distorted tubal structure. Past infection and scarring of the fallopian tube are the most common causes of ectopic pregnancy. Risk factors for ectopic pregnancy include pelvic inflammatory disease, therapeutic abortion, tubal ligation, previous ectopic pregnancy, intrauterine exposure

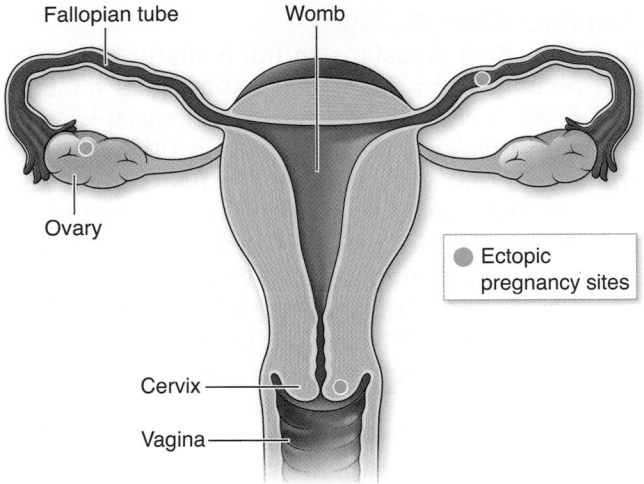

FIGURE 26-11. Possible sites of ectopic pregnancy.

to diethystilbesterol (DES), infertility, and use of fertility drugs, progestin-only oral contraceptives, or levonorgestrel (also called the morning-after pill).

In a tubal pregnancy, the embryo implants in the wrong place, eventually grows to a size that cannot be accommodated by the region, and then ruptures the tissue surrounding it. Most commonly the embryo implants in a fallopian tube, develops to a certain size that cannot be accommodated by the tubule diameter, stretches the tubal walls, and ruptures the fallopian tube.

The classic signs of ectopic pregnancy are pain, vaginal bleeding, and amenorrhea. Rupture of the fallopian tube causes intense lower abdominal pain, bleeding into the abdomen, and referred shoulder pain from bleeding into the abdominal cavity. It is frequently misdiagnosed as an acute abdominal disorder such as appendicitis. Physical examination may reveal adnexal tenderness or adnexal mass. Culdocentesis, extraction of fluid in the area called the cul-de-sac behind the vaginal canal, reveals blood if rupture has occurred. Low levels of HCG are found. Pelvic ultrasound demonstrates an empty uterine cavity and gestational sac outside the uterus. Treatment requires a laparoscopic salpingostomy to remove the ectopic pregnancy if rupture has not occurred and a salpingectomy if rupture has occurred. This is followed by a course of Methotrexate, a chemotherapeutic agent, to eliminate residual pregnancy tissue. Close monitoring of HCG levels is necessary until pregnancy is completely resolved.

ALERT! A diagnosis of ectopic pregnancy should be considered whenever a woman of reproductive age complains of abdominal or pelvic pain. It is a gynecological emergency and the leading cause of maternal mortality in the first trimester.

Disorders of the Breast

The majority of breast masses are benign; fibrocystic breast disease is the most common condition of the breasts. Frequently, a singular breast cyst, called a fibroadenoma, develops that has to be differentiated from cancer.

Fibrocystic Breast Disease

Fibrocystic breast disease, the most common disorder of the breast, is present in 1 in 3 women between 35 and 50 years old in the United States. It presents as benign nodular, granular breast masses that are most prominent during the progesterone-dominant phase of the menstrual cycle. During this phase, tenderness, vascular engorgement, and cystic distension are the symptoms.

Fibrocystic breast disease is largely benign, but certain variants of the disease—including proliferative, epithelial cysts with atypical cells—can increase the risk of breast cancer. Diagnostic studies include ultrasound, mammogram, and needle aspiration of a cyst for histological examination. Danazol, a weak androgen, has been effective in some cases. Use of a supportive bra and avoidance of foods with methylxanthines such as coffee, cola, tea, and chocolate is recommended.

Fibroadenoma

Fibroadenoma, a benign breast mass, is commonly found in premenopausal women, 25 to 45 years old (see Fig. 26-12). Fibroadenomas are benign tumors composed of fibrotic tissue and epithelial cells. Multiple or complex fibroadenomas may indicate a slightly increased risk for breast cancer. The relative risk of patients with fibroadenomas is approximately twice that of patients of similar age without fibroadenomas.

A fibroadenoma is a singular, rubbery, round, movable mass. A small percentage of women have multiple

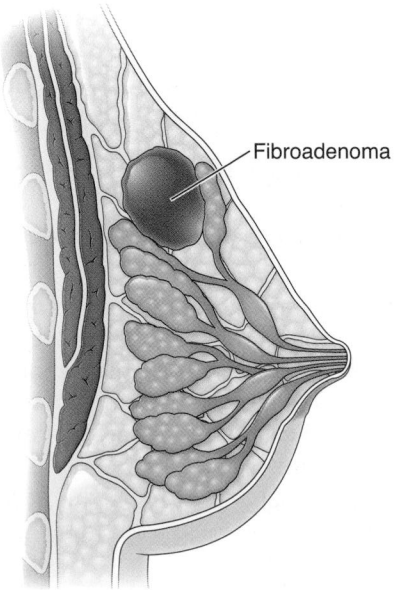

FIGURE 26-12. A fibroadenoma is a benign mass of the breast.

fibroadenomas. There are usually no symptoms; however, biopsy or excision is needed to exclude the possibility of cancer.

Mastitis

Mastitis, inflammation of the breast, most frequently occurs during the postpartum period with lactation. It is most often caused by an ascending infection from the nipple to interior ductal structures. The most common pathogens are *Staphylococcus* and *Streptococcus*. Mastitis infection usually occurs during the early weeks of breastfeeding and is indicated by the breast becoming hard, inflamed, and tender. Without treatment, a breast abscess can form, which requires incision and drainage. Treatment of mastitis includes application of heat or cold compresses, analgesics, antibiotics, and a supportive bra.

Galactorrhea

Galactorrhea is the secretion of breast milk in a non-lactating breast, which can result from vigorous nipple stimulation, exogenous hormones, internal hormone imbalance, local chest infection, or trauma. A pituitary tumor that produces large amounts of PRL will cause galactorrhea (see Chapter 24: Endocrine Disorders). Diagnosis includes investigating hormone levels and performing a CT scan or MRI of the head.

Mammary Duct Ectasia

Mammary duct ectasia is an inflammatory disorder that occurs within the terminal subareolar ducts of the breast. It is common in postmenopausal women. For unclear reasons, the ducts become filled with cellular debris that irritate the duct walls. A small, calcified, palpable mass forms in the central area of the nipple. Fibrous thickening of the surrounding breast tissue can cause dimpling of the breast with nipple inversion. Nipple discharge may be present. A biopsy is usually performed to rule out malignancy. Surgical excision of the affected, dilated subareolar ducts is indicated.

Reactions to Breast Augmentation

Surgical augmentation of the breast has been one of the most common cosmetic surgical procedures in the past 25 years. Silicone gel encased in polyurethane were popularly used implants in the past. However, some studies found that silicone implants may be associated with adverse immunological side effects. Also, trauma to silicone implants caused rupture with leakage of silicone gel into surrounding tissue. Currently, implants filled with saline solution are used alternatively. Treatment for the side effects of the leaked silicone involves surgical removal of the breast implants.

Chapter Summary

- The female reproductive system includes the uterus, cervix, ovaries, fallopian tubes, and breasts. Estrogen and progesterone cause monthly menstrual cyclical changes in these tissues. Estrogen increases cellular growth of the endometrium, whereas progesterone enhances the shedding of endometrium, called menstruation.

- Menarche is the time of the first menstrual period. Thelarche is the time of the development of breast tissue. Menopause is the end of menstrual cycles.

- Amenorrhea, regardless of the cause, requires a b-HCG pregnancy test.

- Tanner stages depict the phases of development in puberty.

- There are several different kinds of menstrual dysfunction: Amenorrhea is the absence of menstruation, dysmenorrhea is painful menstruation, menorrhagia is the loss of excess blood during menstruation, oligomenorrhea indicates there is a lengthy amount of time between periods.

- An ovum is developed and brought to the ovary's surface within a follicle. When the ovum is not released, a benign, follicular ovarian cyst can develop. It usually resolves on its own.

- The corpus luteum, which is the empty follicle on the ovary's surface after the egg is released, can develop a cyst that causes abdominal pain. It usually resolves on its own.

- An ovarian cyst can cause torsion of the ovary, which causes acute abdominal pain and requires surgery.

- Polycystic ovarian syndrome is largely a hormonal disorder that causes amenorrhea and infertility. Patients often suffer from metabolic syndrome as well.

- A teratoma is a tumor of the ovary that contains distinctive tissue: teeth, hair, skin, and different glandular tissue.

- Leiomyomas, also known as fibroid tumors, are common benign growths within the uterus.

- Endometritis can occur from an ascending sexually transmitted disease.

- Endometriosis is a common disorder where endometrial tissue grows in regions outside the uterus.

- DUB is abnormal uterine bleeding caused by a disturbance of the menstrual cycle. Anovulatory cycles are the most common cause.

- Uterine prolapse, cystocele, rectocele, and enterocele can occur with weakening of the pelvic muscles.

- Cervicitis is found in most women because of ascending vaginal aerobic and anaerobic bacteria is benign.
- Cervical cancer is squamous cell carcinoma.
- HPV is known to be a cause of cervical cancer.
- A Pap smear, which includes HPV testing, is the screening test recommended for sexually active women. A standard set of terms, called the Bethesda system, is used to report Pap test results.
- Vaginitis is most commonly caused by *Candida albicans*, trichomonas, or bacterial vaginosis. Each requires different types of medication.

- Vaginal atrophy after menopause can cause vaginitis.
- Ectopic pregnancy most commonly occurs in the fallopian tube, causes acute abdominal pain, and requires immediate surgical treatment.
- Fibrocystic breasts are common, change in size with a woman's menstrual cycle, and are not a precursor to cancer.
- Fibroadenoma is a singular, benign, movable, discrete breast mass.
- Mastitis is infection of the breast, which is common in the postpartum period.

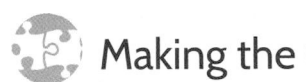 Making the Connections

Disorder and Pathophysiology	Signs and Symptoms	Physical Assessment Findings	Diagnosis	Treatment
Endometritis | An infection of the endometrial layer of the uterus caused by an ascending infection from the vagina.				
	Fever, malaise, pelvic pain, and malodorous vaginal discharge.	Fever. Abdominal and pelvic tenderness. Abnormal vaginal discharge.	Culture of the discharge will determine microorganism. Blood cultures will show if infection has entered the bloodstream. Urinalysis is used to look for infection.	Antibiotic treatment.
Endometriosis | A growth of endometrial tissue outside the uterus.				
	Painful menstruation.	No physical assessment findings.	Laparoscopy is the standard procedure used for visualizing the endometrial tissue in inappropriate locations.	Surgical excision of endometrial tissue.
Leiomyoma of Uterus | A benign smooth muscle tumor growth within the uterine muscle wall.				
	Painful menstruation.	May be able to palpate mass on pelvic exam.	Laparoscopy and hysteroscopy are the standard procedures used that can visualize leiomyomas.	Surgical excision of tumor. Uterine artery embolization to diminish circulation to the tumor.
DUB | A lack of menstrual bleeding that is most often caused by anovulatory cycles. DUB can cause excessive bleeding at irregular intervals.				
	Missed periods or prolonged intervals between menses.	No physical assessment abnormalities.	Hysteroscopy can visualize if there are any lesions inside the uterus that could cause irregular menses. FSH, LH, estrogen, and progesterone levels are sometimes drawn to assess the hormonal cycle.	Progesterone or HRT is the most common treatment that resets the regularity of the menstrual cycle.

Continued

Making the Connections—cont'd

Disorder and Pathophysiology	Signs and Symptoms	Physical Assessment Findings	Diagnosis	Treatment
Uterine Prolapse | Protrusion of the uterus into the vaginal canal that occurs when supportive ligaments of the perineum are stretched and there is loss of pelvic muscle strength. Cystocele: Protrusion of the bladder into the vaginal canal. Rectocele: Protrusion of the rectum into the vaginal canal.				
	May feel back pain or pressure in vaginal canal or on bladder or toward rectum.	On pelvic exam, visualization of a protrusion of the uterus into the vaginal canal.	Laparoscopy can visualize uterus, bladder, or rectum displacement.	Surgical reinforcement of the ligaments and pelvic muscles.
Cervicitis | A disorder that is commonly caused by infection or inflammation of the cervix.				
	Patient may have no symptoms.	Abnormal cervical discharge.	Culture of cervical discharge is taken. Pap smear and HPV testing occurs. Colposcopy directly inspects the cervical surface.	Kegel exercises advised. Antibiotics or periodic observation is used to check for dysplastic development. If squamous cell carcinoma is present, cancer treatments are instituted.
Vaginitis | An infection of the vaginal canal with *Candida*, trichomonas, or bacterial vaginosis.				
	Itching and vaginal discharge Can be a white thick discharge or fishy odor of discharge.	Vaginal erythema and discharge.	Potassium hydroxide wet mount, whiff test, vaginal pH.	Antibiotic, metronidizole for trichomonas or antifungal agent for *Candida* treatment.
POF | Dysfunction of the hypothalamic-pituitary-ovarian axis. Lack of development of follicles for ovulation.				
	Amenorrhea. Infertility. May have other endocrine or congenital disorder such as Turner syndrome (45XO), hypothyroidism, or Addison's disease. Turner syndrome symptoms are webbed neck, short stature, and shield-like chest.	May or may not have physical examination findings. Depends on etiology of disorder.	FSH will be elevated because of a lack of ovarian production of estrogen, which feeds back to pituitary-stimulating FSH. Other hormones may be abnormal, depending on the etiology of POF. Thyroid, cortisol, and PRL hormones may be abnormal. CT and MRI of the brain are used to look for a pituitary tumor. Karyotype is used to check for Turner syndrome (45 XO) or other genetic disorder.	Hormone treatment to stimulate ovulation.

Continued

Making the Connections–cont'd

Disorder and Pathophysiology	Signs and Symptoms	Physical Assessment Findings	Diagnosis	Treatment
Ectopic Pregnancy | This is growth of an embryo outside the uterus, most commonly in the fallopian tube.				
	Acute abdominal pain, nausea, vomiting.	Abdominal tenderness, abdominal rigidity, abdominal mass palpation possible.	Transvaginal or pelvic ultrasound is the best test to visualize an ectopic pregnancy. Laparoscopy may be necessary if ultrasound does not show the ectopic pregnancy.	Surgical excision Removal of the fallopian tube common.
Functional Ovarian Cyst | Growth composed of the remains of a Graafian follicle that has not ejected the ovum, or remains of the corpus luteum that did not degenerate.				
	Abdominal pain.	Abdominal or pelvic mass palpable.	Transvaginal or pelvic ultrasound is the best test to visualize an ovarian cyst. Laparoscopy may be necessary.	Surgical excision.
Torsion of the Ovary | A twisting of the ovary that obstructs arterial flow. Usually occurs only if the ovary is enlarged or if a large cyst is present.				
	Intense abdominal pain, nausea, vomiting.	Abdominal or pelvic mass palpable.	Transvaginal or pelvic ultrasound is the best test to visualize an ovarian cyst. Laparoscopy may be necessary.	Surgical excision.
Polycystic Ovarian Syndrome | A hormonal imbalance of androgen and estrogen that causes amenorrhea and infertility. Ova can develop and come to the ovary's surface but are not released. Multiple ova under the surface resemble multiple cysts.				
	Amenorrhea. Infertility. Hirsutism. Obesity.	Patient commonly has metabolic syndrome; hypertension, glucose intolerance, hyperlipidemia, and central obesity.	Laparoscopy to visualize ovaries and hormone levels; androgens, FSH, LH, estrogen, and progesterone are performed. Patient has high androgens and an imbalance of other hormones.	Insulin sensitizers are recommended to decrease the insulin resistance and prevent diabetes and heart disease. Progesterone therapy is recommended to oppose estrogen's effects on the endometrium. Clomiphene is administered when pregnancy is desired.

Continued

Making the Connections–cont'd

Disorder and Pathophysiology	Signs and Symptoms	Physical Assessment Findings	Diagnosis	Treatment
Teratoma of the Ovary | Ovary develops large cystic growth containing embryonic tissue that forms hair, teeth, and other kinds of tissue.				
	Abdominal and pelvic pain. Back pain.	Abdominal or pelvic mass may be palpable.	Transvaginal or pelvic ultrasound can visualize the growth. Laparoscopy also can visualize growth.	Surgical excision.
Fibrocystic Breasts | This is not a pathological condition; breasts have multiple, mobile, tender cysts that change in size with menstrual cycle.				
	Patient has breast tenderness during menstruation.	Clinical breast exam reveals multiple, movable, compressible cysts throughout breast tissue bilaterally.	Mammogram to rule out any cancerous growths.	No treatment. Advise decreased coffee, tea, chocolate, or cola. Supportive bra.
Fibroadenoma of Breast | A singular mass that develops within the breast tissue, which is usually benign.				
	Discrete, movable, rubbery mass.	Discrete, movable, rubbery mass on clinical breast exam.	Biopsy can demonstrate the lesion as benign or malignant.	Surgical excision.
Mastitis | Infection of the breast caused by staphylococcus or streptococcus ascending from the skin to the duct and glands.				
	Tender, erythematous nipple area, usually during breastfeeding.	Tender, erythematous nipple area in a breastfeeding mother.	Mammogram can visualize malignancy. Clinical examination is usually sufficient.	Antibiotic.

Bibliography

Barnhart, K. T. (2009). Clinical practice. Ectopic pregnancy. *N Engl J Med*, 361(4), 379–387.

Berkowitz, Z., Saraiya, M., & Sawaya, G. F. (2013). Cervical cancer screening intervals, 2006 to 2009: moving beyond annual testing. *JAMA Intern Med*, 173(10), 922–924. doi: 10.1001/jamainternmed.2013.368.

Biggs, W. S., & Demuth, R. H. (2011). Premenstrual syndrome and premenstrual dysphoric disorder. *Am Fam Phys*, 84(8), 918–924.

Bleyer, A., & Welch, H. G. (2012). Effect of three decades of screening mammography on breast-cancer incidence. *N Engl J Med*, 367(21), 1998–2005. doi: 10.1056/NEJMoa1206809.

Bulun, S. E. (2009). Endometriosis. *N Engl J Med*, 360(3), 268–279.

Bulun, S. E. (2013). Uterine fibroids. *N Engl J Med*, 369(14), 1344–1355.

Cardoso, I. C., & Araujo, M. M. (2011). Precocious puberty in an eight-year-old girl. *Am Fam Phys*, 83(4), 455–456.

Caronia, L. M., Martin, C., Welt, C. K., et al. (2011). A genetic basis for functional hypothalamic amenorrhea. *N Engl J Med*, 364(3), 215–225.

Centers for Disease Control and Prevention. (2014). Human papilloma virus: making sense of your PAP and HPV tests.

Retrieved from http://www.cdc.gov/sTd/hpv/pap/default.htm#table2

Crochet, J. R., Bastian, L. A, & Chireau, M. V. (2013). Does this woman have an ectopic pregnancy?: the rational clinical examination systematic review. *JAMA*, 309(16), 1722–1729. doi: 10.1001/jama.2013.3914.

Cuzick, J., Sestak, I., Bonanni, B., et al. (2013). Selective oestrogen receptor modulators in prevention of breast cancer: an updated meta-analysis of individual participant data. *Lancet*, 381(9880), 1827–1834. doi: 10.1016/S0140-6736(13)60140-3. Epub 2013 Apr 30.

Davis, J. D., & Harper, A. L. (2011). FPIN's clinical inquiries: treatment of recurrent vulvovaginal candidiasis. *Am Fam Phys*, 83(12), 1482–1484.

Dawson, S. J., Tsui, D. W., Murtaza, M., et al. (2013). Analysis of circulating tumor DNA to monitor metastatic breast cancer. *N Engl J Med*, 368(13), 1199–1209.

De Vos, M., Devroey, P., & Fauser, B. C. (2010). Primary ovarian insufficiency. *Lancet*, 376(9744), 911–921.

de Ziegler, D., Borghese, B., & Chapron, C. (2010). Endometriosis and infertility: pathophysiology and management. *Lancet*, 376(9742), 730–738.

D'Hooghe, T., & Tomassetti, C. (2014). Surgery for ectopic pregnancy: making the right choice. *Lancet*, 383(9927),

1444–1445. doi: 10.1016/S0140-6736(14)60129-X. Epub 2014 Feb 3.

Endres, J., Graber, M. A., & Dachs, R. (2013). Does screening mammography lead to overdiagnosis of invasive breast cancer? *Am Fam Phys*, 87(6), 408–409.

Feldman, S. (2011). Making sense of the new cervical-cancer screening guidelines. *N Engl J Med*, 365(23), 2145–2147.

Fontaine, P. L., Saslow, D., & King, V. J. (2012). ACS/ASCCP/ASCP guidelines for the early detection of cervical cancer. *Am Fam Phys*, 86(6), 501, 506–507.

Gillison, M. L., Broutian, T., Pickard, R. K., et al. (2012). Prevalence of oral HPV infection in the United States, 2009–2010. *JAMA*, 307(7), 693–703. doi: 10.1001/jama.2012.101. Epub 2012 Jan 26.

Giudice, L. C. (2010). Clinical practice. Endometriosis. *N Engl J Med*, 362(25), 2389–2398.

Goodwin, S. C., & Spies, J. B. (2009). Uterine fibroid embolization. *N Engl J Med*, 361(7), 690–697.

Gordon, C. M. (2010). Clinical practice. Functional hypothalamic amenorrhea. *N Engl J Med*, 363(4), 365–371.

Gradison, M. (2012). Pelvic inflammatory disease. *Am Fam Phys*, 85(8), 791–796.

Hainer, B. L., & Gibson, M. V. (2011). Vaginitis. *Am Fam Phys*, 83(7), 807–815.

Hampton, T. (2013, March 6). NIH panel: name change, new priorities advised for polycystic ovary syndrome. *JAMA*, 309(9), 863. doi: 10.1001/jama.2013.1236.

Harris, R., & Kinsinger, L. (2013). Screening mammography: the goal is changing. *Am Fam Phys*, 87(4), 246–247.

Hauk, L. (2012). American College of Obstetricians and Gynecologists updates breast cancer screening guidelines. *Am Fam Phys*, 85(6), 654–659.

Hicks, C. W., & Rome, E. S. (2010). Menstrual manipulation: options for suppressing the cycle. *Cleveland Clin J Med*, 77(7), 445–453.

Hill, D. A. (2009). New guidelines: fewer Pap tests for women older than 30 years and less aggressive treatment for adolescents. *Am Fam Phys*, 80(2), 131.

Hughes, I. A. (2013). Releasing the brake on puberty. *N Engl J Med*, 368(26), 2513–2515. doi: 10.1056/NEJMe1306743.

Jensen, J. R., Morbeck, D. E., & Coddington, C. C. (2011). Fertility preservation. *Mayo Clin Proceed*, 86(1), 45–49.

Juckett, G., & Hartman-Adams, H. (2010). Human papillomavirus: clinical manifestations and prevention. *Am Fam Phys*, 82(10), 1209–1213.

Kahn, J. A. (2009). HPV vaccination for the prevention of cervical intraepithelial neoplasia. *N Engl J Med*, 361(3), 271–278.

Kim, J. J., Sharma, M., & Ortendahl, J. (2013). Optimal interval for routine cytologic screening in the United States. *JAMA Intern Med*, 173(3), 241–242.

Klein, D. A., & Poth, M. A. (2013). Amenorrhea: an approach to diagnosis and management. *Am Fam Phys*, 87(11), 781–788.

Krishnaiah, P. B., Nunes, N. L., & Safranek, S. (2012). FPIN's clinical inquiries. Screening mammography for reducing breast cancer mortality. *Am Fam Phys*, 85(2), 176–183.

Kruszka, P. S., & Kruszka, S. J. (2010). Evaluation of acute pelvic pain in women. *Am Fam Phys*, 82(2), 141–147.

Kuehn, B. M. (2011). Group advises clinicians to routinely screen women for sexual assault history. *JAMA*, 306(10), 1072. doi: 10.1001/jama.2011.1240.

Kuehn, B. M. (2012). USPSTF: taking vitamin D and calcium doesn't prevent fractures in older women. *JAMA*, 308(3), 225–226. doi: 10.1001/jama.2012.7955.

Kuncharapu, I., Majeroni, B. A., & Johnson, D. W. (2010). Pelvic organ prolapse. *Am Fam Phys*, 81(9), 1111–1117.

Lambert, M. (2012). ACS releases updated guidelines on cancer screening. *Am Fam Phys*, 86(6), 571, 576–577.

Longo, D., Fauci, A., Kasper, D., et al. (2011). *Harrison's principles of internal medicine.* 18th ed. New York: McGraw-Hill.

Mac Bride, M. B., Rhodes, D. J., & Shuster, L. T. (2010). Vulvovaginal atrophy. *Mayo Clin Proceed*, 85(1), 87–94.

Manson, J. E., Chlebowski, R. T., Stefanick, M. L., et al. (2013). Menopausal hormone therapy and health outcomes during the intervention and extended poststopping phases of the Women's Health Initiative randomized trials. *JAMA*, 310(13), 1353–1368. doi: 10.1001/jama.2013.278040.

Nabel, E. G. (2013). The Women's Health Initiative—a victory for women and their health. *JAMA*, 310(13), 1349–1350. doi: 10.1001/jama.2013.278042.

National Cancer Institute (NCI) of National Institutes of Health (NIH). Pap and HPV testing. Retrieved from http://www.cancer.gov/cancertopics/factsheet/detection/Pap-HPV-testing 2015 July 8.

National Cancer Institute (NCI) of National Institutes of Health (NIH). Cervical cancer screening. Description of the evidence. Retrieved from http://www.cancer.gov/cancertopics/pdq/screening/cervical/HealthProfessional/page2 2015 July 8.

Palefsky, J. M., Giuliano, A. R., Goldstone, S., et al. (2011). HPV vaccine against anal HPV infection and anal intraepithelial neoplasia. *N Engl J Med*, 365(17), 1576–1585. doi: 10.1056/NEJMoa1010971.

Palmert, M. R., & Dunkel, L. (2012). Clinical practice. Delayed puberty. *N Engl J Med*, 366(5), 443–453.

Radosh, L. (2009). Drug treatments for polycystic ovary syndrome. *Am Fam Phys*, 79(8), 671–676.

Rao, S. S., Singh, M., Parkar, M., & Sugumaran, R. (2008a). Health maintenance for postmenopausal women. *Am Fam Phys*, 78(5), 583–591.

Rao, S. S., Singh, M., Parkar, M., & Sugumaran, R. (2008). Information from your family doctor. Menopause: what you should know. *Am Fam Phys*, 78(5), 593–594.

Riley, M., Dobson, M., Jones, E., & Kirst, N. (2013). Health maintenance in women. *Am Fam Phys*, 87(1), 30–37.

Roehm, E. (2014). Hormone therapy use and outcomes in the Women's Health Initiative trials. *JAMA*, 311(4), 417. doi: 10.1001/jama.2013.285154.

Salzman, B., Fleegle, S., & Tully, A. S. (2012). Common breast problems. *Am Fam Phys*, 86(4), 343–349.

Schrager, S., Falleroni, J., & Edgoose, J. (2013). Evaluation and treatment of endometriosis. *Am Fam Phys*, 87(2), 107–113.

Shuster, L. T., Bundrick, J. B., & Litin, S. C. (2012). Clinical pearls in women's health. *Mayo Clin Proceed*, 87(1), 89–93.

Smith, N. L., Blondon, M., Wiggins, K. L., et al. (2014). Lower risk of cardiovascular events in postmenopausal women taking oral estradiol compared with oral conjugated equine estrogens. *JAMA Intern Med*, 174(1), 25–31. doi: 10.1001/jamainternmed.2013.11074.

Stewart, E. A. (2012). Uterine fibroids and evidence-based medicine—not an oxymoron. *N Engl J Med*, 366(5), 471–473.

Sweet, M. G., Schmidt-Dalton, T. A., Weiss, P. M., & Madsen, K. P. (2012). Evaluation and management of abnormal uterine bleeding in premenopausal women. *Am Fam Phys*, 85(1), 35–43.

Tria Tirona, M. (2013). Breast cancer screening update. *Am Fam Phys*, 87(4), 274–278.

Utz, A. L., Schaefer, P. W., & Snuderl, M. (2010). Case records of the Massachusetts General Hospital. Case 20-2010. A 32-year-old woman with oligomenorrhea and infertility. *N Engl J Med*, 363(2), 178–186.

Vadaparampil, S. T., Malo, T. L., Kahn, J. A., et al. (2014). Physicians' human papillomavirus vaccine recommendations, 2009 and 2011. *Am J Prev Med,* 46(1), 80–84. doi: 10.1016/j.amepre.2013.07.009.

Van Horn, L., & Manson, J. E. (2008). The Women's Health Initiative: implications for clinicians. *Cleveland Clin J Med,* 75(5), 385–390.

Van Voorhis, B. (2009). A 41-year-old woman with menorrhagia, anemia, and fibroids: review of treatment of uterine fibroids. *JAMA,* 301(1), 82–93.

Vinay Kumar, V., Abbas, A., Fausto, N., & Aster, J, (2010). *Robbins & Cotran pathologic basis of disease.* 8th ed. Philadelphia, PA: Elsevier.

Wesolowski, R., & Budd, G. T. (2010). A young woman with a breast mass: What every internist should know. *Cleveland Clin J Med,* 77(8), 537–546.

Wilkinson, J. E. (2011). Effect of mammography on breast cancer mortality. *Am Fam Phys,* 84(11), 1225–1227.

Wilson, R. D., Langlois, S., American Congress of Obstetricians and Gynecologists, The Society of Obstetricians and Gynecologists of Canada, and The Society of Gynecologic Oncologists of Canada. (2012). Genetic considerations for a woman's annual gynaecological examination. *J Ob Gyn Canada,* 34(3), 276–284.

Yaqub, F. (2013, August). MKRN3 and central precocious puberty. *Lancet Diabetes Endocrinol,* 1 (Suppl 1), s15. doi: 10.1016/S2213-8587(13)70041-X. Epub 2013 Jun 13.

Yonkers, K. A., O'Brien, P. M., & Eriksson, E. (2008). Premenstrual syndrome. *Lancet,* 371(9619), 1200–1210.

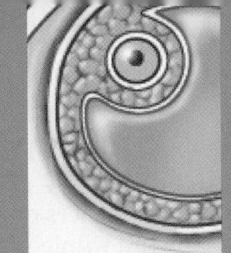

Disorders of the Male Reproductive System

Key Terms

Benign prostatic hyperplasia (BPH)
Cryptorchidism
Digital rectal examination (DRE)
Erectile dysfunction (ED)
Hematocele
Hydrocele
Hypospadias

Orchiectomy
Orchitis
Paraphimosis
Peyronie's disease
Phimosis
Priapism
Prostate surface antigen (PSA)

Spermatic cord
Teratogens
Testicular dysgenesis syndrome (TDS)
Varicocele
Vas deferens
Vasectomy

The male reproductive system can be divided into its external organs and internal organs. External organs include the penis, scrotum, and urethra, whereas internal organs include the testis, epididymis, vas deferens, seminal vesicles, ejaculatory ducts, prostate, and bulbourethral glands (see Fig. 27-1).

The testes are the male's sex-determining organs because of their essential functions. Each testicle contained within the scrotum produces testosterone, the hormone that endows humans with male characteristics and allows synthesis of spermatozoa. The duct system of the male reproductive system, which includes the ejaculatory ducts, epididymis, vas deferens, and penis, work together to mobilize and eject sperm. The glands, which include the seminal vesicles, prostate, and bulbourethral glands, add fluid to the sperm, which is necessary to transport them in the fertilization process. In order to deliver sperm for fertilization, the penis has the ability to modify its structure to become erect. This is accomplished through vascular dilation and engorgement of erectile tissue, which includes the corpus cavernosum and corpus spongiosum. Dysfunction of any of the hormonal, glandular, ductile organs or erectile tissue of the male reproductive system can cause problems for sexuality and fertility.

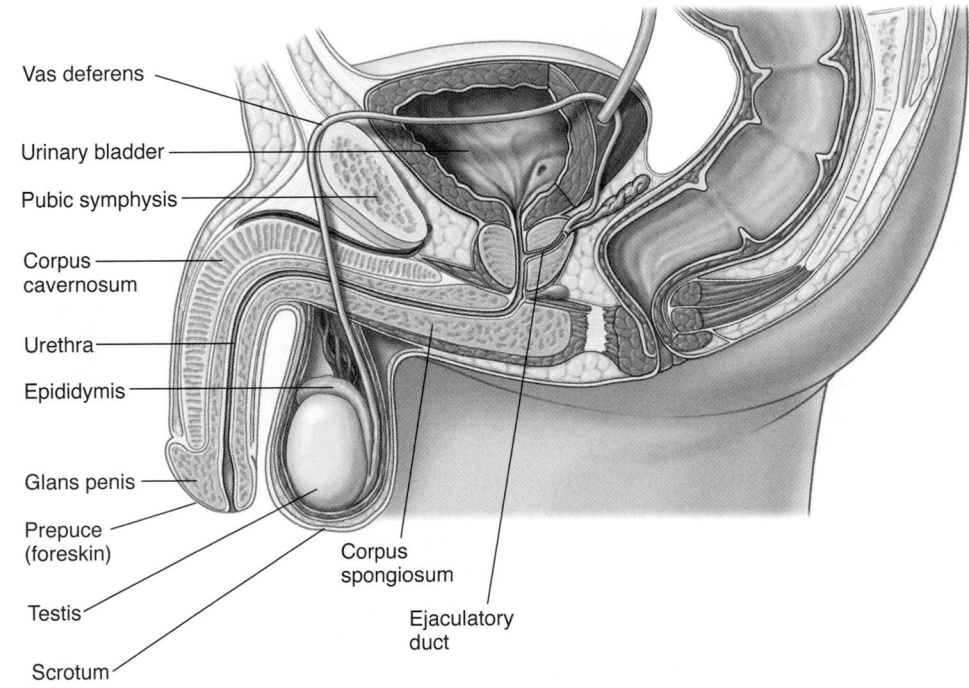

FIGURE 27-1. The male reproductive system. (From Thompson, G. S. (2013). *Understanding anatomy and physiology.* Philadelphia, PA: F.A. Davis Company, with permission.)

Vas deferens
Urinary bladder
Pubic symphysis
Corpus cavernosum
Urethra
Epididymis
Glans penis
Prepuce (foreskin)
Testis
Scrotum
Corpus spongiosum
Ejaculatory duct

Epidemiology

Disorders of reproductive organs can occur throughout the whole life span of a male. At birth, cryptorchidism and hypospadias are two of the most common congenital abnormalities of the male newborn. **Cryptorchidism** is caused by undescended testes, where the testicle remains within the abdomen or inguinal canal. **Hypospadias** is a disorder caused by an abnormally positioned urethral orifice of the penis. Cryptorchidism affects 2% to 9% of all newborn boys and 1% to 3% of boys at 3 months of age. Prematurely born males have a higher prevalence of cryptorchidism. For unknown reasons, there has been an increase in the frequency of hypospadias by 100% to 200% over the last 20 years. In young adult males, testicular cell tumors are the most common neoplasm, whereas prostate cancer is the overall leading cancer in older males. Among Caucasians, there has been a significant increase in the incidence of testicular cancer, with present figures being 2 to 3 times higher than 30 to 40 years ago. The American Cancer Society estimates that about 8,400 new cases of testicular cancer are diagnosed annually in the United States. The lifetime chance of developing testicular cancer is about 1 in 300 and the risk of dying is very low—about 1 in 5,000.

An estimated 1 in 6 Caucasians and 1 in 5 African Americans will develop prostate cancer in their lifetime, with the likelihood increasing with age. The American Cancer Society estimates that 217,730 new cases of prostate cancer are diagnosed annually.

In Western societies, as many as 15% of all couples experience infertility problems, with rough estimates indicating that male reproductive dysfunction is responsible in at least 50% of these cases. Failure of the reproductive system affects a significant proportion of males and is of concern, not only on an individual basis, but also for society, where the financial burden of medical management is substantial.

Basic Concepts of Male Reproductive Function

Male sexuality, spermatogenesis, fertilization ability, and hormonal regulation are the major functions of the male reproductive organs. The most important organs that determine male sexuality are the testes, which synthesize testosterone and generate spermatozoa. Genes on the Y chromosome enable male gonads to become testes. Therefore, the father determines the gender of the fetus. The development of testes occurs during the first trimester of gestation of the male fetus. The testes develop within the abdomen and descend into the inguinal canal by the time of birth. The descent of the testes into the scrotum occurs within the first few months of the newborn's life. The testes should completely descend into the scrotal sac by the end of the first year.

During childhood testosterone levels remain steady until puberty, when a surge in testosterone level occurs, between ages 10 and 13. When a male reaches puberty, the hypothalamus begins secretion of gonadotropin-releasing hormone (GnRH), which affects the pituitary gland. The anterior pituitary is stimulated to secrete luteinizing hormone (LH) and follicle-stimulating hormone (FSH); these hormones are part of a hypothalamic-pituitary-endocrine gland feedback system (see Fig. 27-2). LH stimulates the Leydig cells of the testes to secrete testosterone, enabling the development of male secondary sexual characteristics

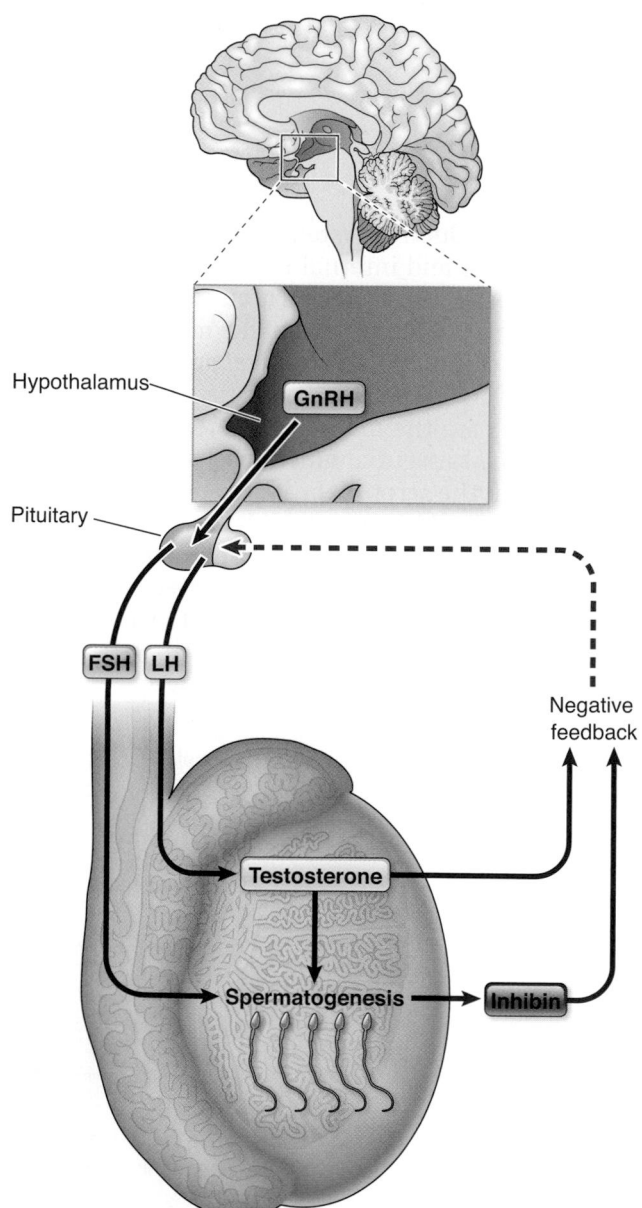

FIGURE 27-2. Endocrine control of testicular function. The hypothalamus secretes GnRH, which stimulates the pituitary to secrete LH and FSH. LH promotes testosterone secretion by the Leydig cells of the testes. Testosterone (T) is used in the synthesis of sperm. FSH promotes spermatogenesis by the Sertoli cells. Inhibin is a hormone that sends feedback to the pituitary to turn off spermatogenesis. Testosterone sends feedback to the pituitary and hypothalamus to turn off LH and GnRH. In the epididymis, spermatids mature into sperm cells.

and spermatogenesis. In this negative feedback system, high levels of testosterone inhibit LH secretion and low levels of testosterone stimulate LH. The FSH secreted by the pituitary stimulates the Sertoli cells of the seminiferous tubules to synthesize spermatozoa. The Sertoli cells also secrete a hormone called inhibin. High inhibin levels send feedback to the pituitary to decrease FSH levels. In contrast, low inhibin levels send feedback to the pituitary to increase FSH secretion by the pituitary.

During spermatogenesis, the process of meiosis causes each sperm cell to contain 23 chromosomes. Each spermatozoa is a gamete with half the number of human chromosomes. When the sperm fertilizes the female's ovum, a full set of chromosomes is attained in the fertilized egg.

Millions of sperm travel daily from the seminiferous tubules to the epididymis, an organ that sits atop each testis (see Fig. 27-3). The seminiferous tubules also produce the seminal fluid used for sperm motility. Within the epididymis, sperm undergo maturation and are stored for weeks.

The **vas deferens** are tubules that ascend from the epididymis on top of each testicle and pass into the urinary bladder. The vas deferens is part of the **spermatic cord** that suspends the testicle from the abdomen into the inguinal region. The vas deferens and seminal vesicle combine to form the ejaculatory duct, which passes into the penis. The structure and function of these tubules need to be normal for male fertility. A **vasectomy** is a procedure in which the vas deferens tubule is cut and consequently blocks sperm delivery to the penis for fertilization. Vasectomy is the most popular form of surgical birth control in the United States, with a rate of 10 per 1,000 men undergoing the procedure.

The prostate is a gland that sits below the urinary bladder and encircles the urethra. The prostate secretes an alkaline fluid that combines with seminal fluid to form the semen that promotes sperm motility. In addition, the prostate secretes **prostate surface antigen (PSA),** which can be used in the assessment of prostatic structure and function. The prostate gland naturally enlarges with age.

The bulbourethral glands, also called Cowper's glands, are two pea-sized glands located below the prostate that secrete a lubricating fluid that coats the urethra during sexual arousal. Semen, needed for sperm motility, is a combination of fluids secreted by the seminal vesicle, prostate, and bulbourethral glands.

Erectile function of the penis requires adequate circulation and autonomic neurological control. The penis consists of spongy tissue called the corpus spongiosum and corpus cavernosum. Vasodilation of the pudendal branches of the hypogastric artery allows for penile erection and ejaculation. The penile artery is a branch of the pudendal artery that vasodilates with sexual stimulation. The dorsal artery, a branch off the penile artery, provides for engorgement of the glans during erection, whereas the bulbourethral artery supplies the bulb and corpus spongiosum. The cavernous artery causes swelling of the corpus cavernosum and is principally responsible for erection. Neural control is provided by both the sympathetic and parasympathetic nervous systems. Parasympathetic nerves transmitted via the sacral spinal cord allow for penile erection. Sympathetic innervation, which arrives via the lumbar spinal cord to the penis, allows for ejaculation.

Male fertility depends on the quantity of semen, sperm count, morphology of sperm, motility of sperm, adequate circulation, intact hormonal regulation, neurological control, and normal anatomical structure of the male sex organs. Inadequacy of any of these qualities or functions can cause male reproductive system disorders.

Basic Concepts of Male Reproductive Dysfunction

Anatomical anomalies, urinary tract problems, sexually transmitted infections (STIs), trauma, injury, and infertility are the major causes for males to seek health care involving the reproductive system.

Infertility

Fertility problems often provide the impetus for investigation into male reproductive disorders (see Box 27-1). Low sperm count is commonly found as a cause of

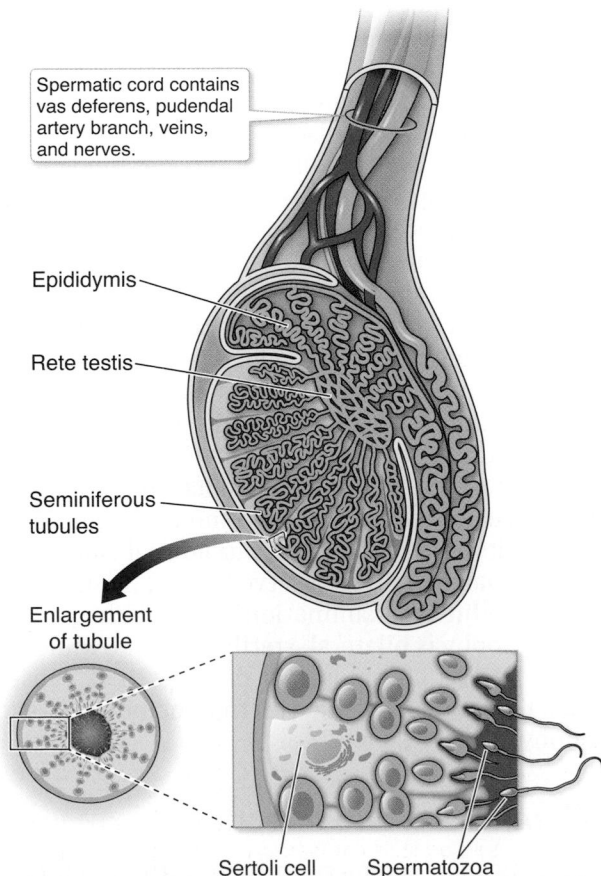

Spermatic cord contains vas deferens, pudendal artery branch, veins, and nerves.

Epididymis

Rete testis

Seminiferous tubules

Enlargement of tubule

Sertoli cell   Spermatozoa

FIGURE 27-3. The testicular sac.

infertility. It is believed that in many males a genetic cause is responsible for poor spermatogenesis. Microdeletions of the Y chromosome are genetic mutations that are associated with a significant proportion of male infertility cases. Androgens, mainly testosterone, dihydrotestosterone, and a functional androgen receptor (AR), are crucial for male sexual differentiation, secondary sex characteristics at puberty, and sperm maturation. The gene for the AR is on the X chromosome at Xq11-12. An absent or dysfunctional AR gene in otherwise healthy 46XY individuals causes androgen insensitivity syndrome, undermasculinization, and decreased spermatogenesis. Presently, over 300 different AR gene mutations have been discovered.

Erectile dysfunction (ED), also called impotence, is another cause of male infertility. There are many underlying physical and psychological causes of ED. Physiologic conditions that reduce blood flow to the penis or those that cause nerve damage are etiologic factors of ED.

Anatomical Abnormalities

Cryptorchidism is a condition of undescended testicles, where the testes remain high in the inguinal canal or abdominal cavity. Full descent of the testes into the scrotal sac should occur by age 1. The testes need to be in the scrotal sac, which is anatomically located external to the body's core. The distance from the body facilitates lower-than-normal body temperature, which is necessary for healthy sperm production.

Another common anatomical abnormality that can cause infertility is hypospadias. In hypospadias, the urethral orifice is located on the ventral or underside of the penis instead of the glans. When the urethral orifice is on the dorsal or anterior side of the penis, this is called epispadias.

Other anatomical disorders involve the foreskin of the penis. **Phimosis** occurs when the foreskin is too constricted and cannot easily retract from the penis. **Paraphimosis** occurs when the foreskin is in a permanently retracted position behind the tip of the penis.

Peyronie's disease is an inflammatory vasculitis of unknown etiology where the penis takes on a curvature, primarily in middle-aged and elderly men. Men with severe Peyronie's disease may develop scar tissue in the corpora cavernosum that impedes blood flow.

Traumatic injury of the testicles can cause disorders known as varicocele, hematocele, or hydrocele. These conditions can cause swelling of the scrotum, overheating of the testes, lack of blood flow, and interruption of sperm production. If untreated, these disorders can cause permanent male reproductive dysfunction.

Torsion of the testes can occur as a consequence of trauma to the groin; it can also arise without history of injury. In this disorder, the spermatic cord, which suspends the testes, twists and disrupts circulation to the testicle. Torsion of the testes is common in children and adolescents and is considered a urological emergency.

Testicular atrophy is observed as small, intrascrotal testes on clinical examination of the male genitalia. When atrophy is bilateral, sterility results. Klinefelter syndrome is a chromosomal disorder that causes a constellation of abnormalities that includes testicular atrophy.

Inflammation and Infection

STIs of the male commonly present with lesions on the penis as well as discharge. Frequently urination is painful and there are signs of disease on the genitalia. The chancre of syphilis is an inflammatory ulcerlike lesion on the male genitalia. Condyloma are wartlike lesions that can be signs of syphilis or human papilloma virus (HPV). Herpes genitalis presents as small, tender vesicular lesions. STIs often ascend into organs above the testes and cause prostatitis and epididymitis (see Chapter 28: Sexually Transmitted Diseases). **Orchitis,** or inflammation of the testes, may be bilateral or unilateral. It is most commonly caused by a bacterial infection or mumps virus.

Precocious Puberty

During childhood a male can exhibit precocious puberty. A boy is considered to have precocious puberty if secondary male sexual characteristics are evident before the age of 9 years. In the healthy boy, growth during puberty accounts for about 15% to 20% of his adult height. This growth occurs before the fusion of the bone growth plates. In precocious puberty, bone growth plate fusion occurs early and results in a reduced adult height. In addition, there is apparent adult development of the male genitalia and presence of axillary and pubic hair. Evaluation of puberty development occurs through use of Tanner staging (see Fig. 27-4).

Delayed Puberty

When a teenage boy lacks testicular enlargement and has little or no pubic hair at age 14 years, he is considered to have delayed puberty. One of the most common causes of delayed puberty is lack of hormonal secretion by the anterior pituitary. However, systemic illnesses such as inflammatory bowel disease and chronic renal failure can also contribute to delayed puberty.

Clinical presentation in delayed puberty includes a small penis and testes, scant pubic and axillary hair, persistent high-pitched voice, gynecomastia, and long arms and legs caused by delayed bone growth plate closure.

Other Common Causes of Male Reproductive Dysfunction

Prostate gland dysfunction can cause male reproductive and urological problems. The prostate gland can be palpated through the rectal wall in the male. Prostatitis is often caused by an STI, and prostatic hyperplasia is a normal consequence of aging. Prostate cancer, the second-most common type of cancer in men, can be lethal if not discovered early in the course of the disease.

Priapism is an abnormally prolonged erection of the penis in the absence of stimulation. It can be extremely painful and may last several hours. Among the known causes of priapism is the drug sildenafil and the vasoocclusive crisis of sickle cell anemia.

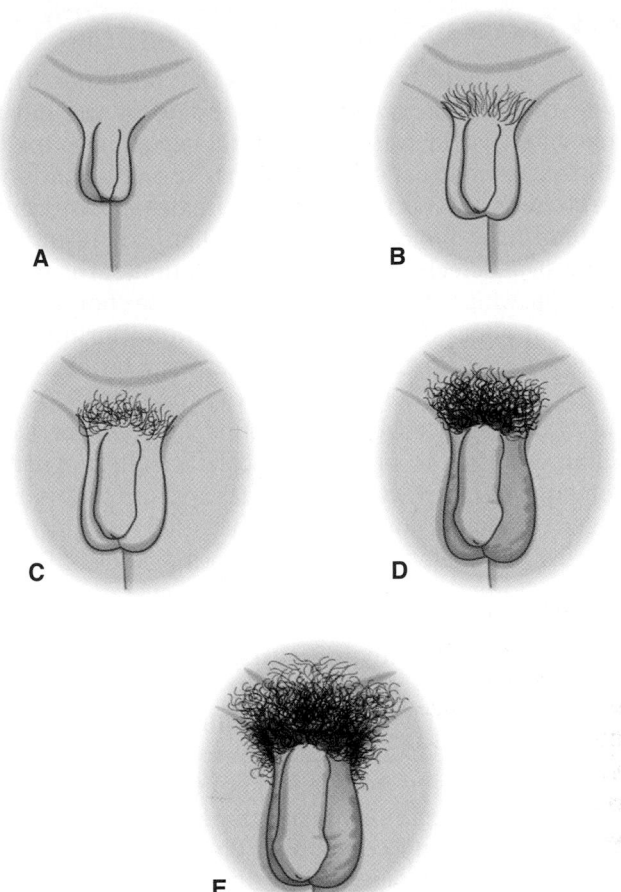

FIGURES 27-4a through 27-4e. Male Tanner stages. (A) No pubic hair except for fine body hair similar to that on abdomen. Penis, testes, and scrotum are same size and proportions as in childhood. (B) Sparse growth of long, slightly pigmented, downy hair, straight or only slightly curled, chiefly at the base of the penis. Slight or no enlargement of the penis. Testes larger, scrotum larger, somewhat reddened and altered in texture. (C) Darker, coarser, curlier hair spreading sparsely over the pubic symphysis. Larger penis, especially in length. Testes and scrotum further enlarged. (D) Coarse and curly hair, as in adult; area covered greater than in stage 3, but not as great as in adult. Penis further enlarged in length and breadth, with development of glans. Testes and scrotum further enlarged; scrotal skin darkened. (E) Hair same as adult in quantity and quality, spreading to medial surfaces of thighs but not up over abdomen. Penis now adult in size and shape. Testes and scrotum now adult in size and color. (From Dillon, P. (2007). *Nursing health assessment.* 2nd ed. Philadelphia, PA: F.A. Davis Company, with permission.)

Assessment of Male Reproductive Disorders

To diagnose reproductive disorders in a male patient, the clinician needs to inquire about risk factors, present symptoms, lifestyle, and past health history. Inquiry regarding the practice of safe sex is significant. Present and past health history are also important because systemic diseases often affect male reproductive function. A complete physical assessment, which includes prostate, testicular, and rectal examination, as well as tests to rule out hernia, is necessary.

Risk Factors

There are a number of risk factors that predispose the male to reproductive disorders. Some of the most important risk factors involve fetal exposure to toxic substances, also called teratogens, during gestation. **Teratogens** are substances that cause the development of abnormal cell masses during fetal growth, resulting in physical defects in the fetus. Formation of the male genitalia, which is dependent upon male sex hormones, occurs at about 8 to 12 weeks gestation. During this early time of pregnancy, a woman can be exposed to any number of teratogens. From the late 1940s to early 1970s, an estrogenic compound, diethylstilbestrol (DES), was used to prevent miscarriages in pregnant women. Later on it was found that exposure to this estrogen compound during gestation caused reproductive disorders for male and female offspring. Sons of DES-treated mothers had increased risk of several male reproductive disorders, such as cryptorchidism, urethral abnormalities, epididymal cysts, and testicular hypoplasia. Potential adverse effects of estrogenic compounds on male reproductive function have been reinforced by the fact that several compounds used in industry, agriculture, or in the home act as estrogen-like compounds and cause male hormone disruption. Polychlorinated biphenyl compounds are examples of these estrogen-like compounds found in plastics. Growing evidence indicates an increase in the incidence of male reproductive problems, such as genital abnormalities, testicular cancer, reduced semen quality, and infertility. Together, these male reproductive problems may reflect the existence of one common entity, a **testicular dysgenesis syndrome (TDS).** Studies suggest that TDS is a result of disruption of embryonal programming and gonadal development during fetal life and may be causally linked to endocrine disruptors.

Other than endocrine disruptors, radiation is known to cause abnormal male sexual development and lack of spermatogenesis. For this reason, the testes should be covered with a lead apron during x-ray procedures. Recent data also show that cigarette smoking has a negative impact on sperm count as well as seminal fluid volume. Studies show that decreased sperm counts are found among sons of mothers who smoked more than 10 cigarettes per day during pregnancy. Spermatogenesis can also be negatively affected by overheating of the testes. Tight undergarments or hot baths can diminish sperm production.

Many studies focus on erectile dysfunction (ED) as a predominant male reproductive health disorder. Evidence suggests that lifestyle risk factors for ED are similar to those for cardiovascular disease and diabetes. These conditions include atherosclerosis, hypertension, obesity, metabolic syndrome, and smoking. Other risk factors for ED include low testosterone levels, Peyronie's disease, enlarged prostate, certain medications, alcoholism and other substance abuse, and neurological disorders. The brain also plays a key role in triggering the series of physical events that cause an erection, starting with feelings of sexual excitement. A number of psychological disorders can interfere with sexual feelings and cause ED. These include depression, anxiety, high stress, fatigue, or relationship problems.

Age is consistently associated with increased risk of male reproductive health problems, including ED and prostatic hyperplasia. Although some older men may consider poorer reproductive health a consequence of the aging process, changes caused by age are treatable.

Risk of male reproduction problems occurs with malformations of the male genitalia. The most common malformation, cryptorchidism, can predispose men to testicular cancer. The exact cause of testicular cancer is unknown. Factors that increase a man's risk for testicular cancer include genetic predisposition, abnormal testicle development, and Klinefelter syndrome. Other possible causes of male reproductive system cancers include exposure to certain chemicals, radiation, human immunodeficiency virus (HIV), and HPV.

Trauma can also predispose individuals to reproductive disorders such as hydrocele, hematocele, varicocele, and torsion of the testes. For this reason, males who participate in competitive sports are encouraged to wear protective gear. Unprotected sexual activity can also increase the risk of infection, which leads to male reproductive dysfunction. Urethritis, prostatitis, and epididymitis can be caused by sexually transmitted infections (STIs) such as syphilis, gonorrhea, and herpes genitalis. Mumps virus predisposes the male to orchitis, which can lead to infertility.

Signs and Symptoms

The male patient with suspected reproductive disorders should have a complete physical examination with focus on the lower pelvis, inguinal, and scrotal region. When examining the male infant, the clinician should inspect and palpate the scrotal sac. The scrotum should contain palpable testes by the end of the first year of life.

In childhood, torsion of the testes is a common disorder. Testicular torsion is seen most frequently in the 12- to 18-year-old age group, but it can occur at any age, including in newborns.

During adolescence, males usually go through puberty from approximately age 11 years through 15 years. Patients age 9 years or younger may exhibit signs of precocious puberty, whereas patients aged 14 years or older may demonstrate delayed puberty. To assess the patient for stage of puberty, the patient's pelvic and inguinal region should be compared with the Tanner stages.

In males with Klinefelter syndrome, a genetic disorder, signs include small penis; small testicles; diminished pubic, axillary, and facial hair; sexual dysfunction; enlarged breast tissue; tall stature; abnormal body proportions (long legs, short trunk); learning disabilities; and a single crease in the palm. These patients have a karyotype that demonstrates an extra X chromosome as XXY.

In older males, swelling of the scrotum often indicates hydrocele, hematocele, or varicocele. The patient may complain of heaviness in the scrotal area.

Painless enlargement of a testicle is diagnostic of testicular cancer. Swollen inguinal lymph nodes, a palpable lump, and a scrotal sac that does not transilluminate are signs of cancer.

To assess the prostate gland, a **digital rectal examination (DRE)** is necessary. In prostatitis, the gland feels boggy and is tender. In **benign prostatic hyperplasia (BPH),** the enlargement is firm, painless, and generalized. Lesions of prostate cancer are hard, painless, and unmovable. The patient with an enlarged prostate will commonly complain of urinary symptoms such as frequency, hesitancy, and diminished urine stream. Urethritis, prostatitis, and epididymitis can occur in an STI. The patient may demonstrate swollen inguinal lymph nodes and a lesion on the external genitalia or penile discharge.

Diagnosis

Because the testes are endocrine glands, diagnostic testing often involves a hormonal analysis for FSH, LH, and testosterone levels. Provocative testing of the hypothalamic-pituitary-gonadal axis can be done with a GnRH stimulation test. A normal response to this test would be elevated levels of FSH and LH. A lack of response to GnRH stimulation is indicative of pituitary failure; in contrast, a marked elevation in FSH and LH is suggestive of lack of responsiveness of the testes to produce testosterone.

When a hereditary disorder is suspected, gene testing can be done. A karyotype can confirm disorders such as Klinefelter syndrome, which is caused by an extra X chromosome. If cancer is suspected, the biomarkers alpha-fetoprotein and beta-human chorionic gonadotropin (b-HCG) are frequently elevated in testicular cancer. A DRE and the PSA blood test are used when prostate cancer is suspected. However, the PSA has to be carefully evaluated in conjunction with other diagnostic tests because its elevation does not always indicate cancer. Computed tomography (CT) scan and biopsy are necessary to confirm the diagnosis of cancer. The clinician also performs a DRE with suspected prostate enlargement. Urine flow studies, ultrasound, or cystoscopy may be needed to differentiate prostate cancer from BPH. Squamous cell carcinoma of the penis, associated with HPV, is a rare cancer found mainly in uncircumcised males.

Males with STIs will often present with inflammatory, vesicular, or wartlike lesions of the genitalia and penile discharge. Swollen inguinal lymph nodes often can be palpated. Culture of the lesions and discharge can reveal such pathogens as gonorrhea, syphilis, herpes genitalis, HPV, or Chlamydia. Urinalysis and urine culture may also reveal the infecting microorganism. Because STIs increase one's susceptibility to HIV infection, HIV testing should be done.

There are certain laboratory tests necessary to diagnose infertility. Semen must be analyzed for sperm number, morphology, and motility. The normal quantity of semen is 1.5 to 5 mL; optimally, it should contain 50 to 250 million sperm per mL.

Common Treatments for Male Reproductive Disorders

Anatomical anomalies such as cryptorchidism, phimosis, hypospadias, and epispadias require surgical treatment. Hydrocele, varicocele, and torsion of the testes also require surgical intervention.

Treatment of STI depends on the microorganism involved. Some STIs are asymptomatic in males but cause symptoms in the female. Antibiotic medication and patient education regarding safe sex are the interventions for the STIs causing urethritis, prostatitis, and epididymitis. Importantly, the patient should be advised to inform sexual partners of the need for treatment as well.

Surgical intervention is often needed for prostate disorders. BPH often causes hyperplastic cell growth around the urethra, which interferes with urination. The hyperplastic tissue of BPH often requires transurethral surgical resection. However, medications can also be used to relieve the pressure of the prostate on the urethra.

Surgical excision of the prostate may be required if cancer is present. When radical prostatectomy is done, pelvic lymph nodes are removed and examined. Radiation in the form of an implant or external beam delivery is commonly necessary. Antiandrogenic hormone chemotherapy may also be required.

When testicular cancer is diagnosed, **orchiectomy,** which is removal of the testicle, and radiation are the common treatment procedures. Chemotherapy or bone marrow transplant may be required. Because treatment causes sterility, freezing of sperm before treatment is commonly done for future procreation.

Disorders of the Male Reproductive System

The common disorders of the male reproductive system include BPH, ED, and prostate cancer. These problems mainly occur in older age males. Testicular cancer is a disorder of young adult males as is testicular torsion, varicocele, hydrocele, and hematocele.

Benign Prostatic Hyperplasia

BPH is characterized by excessive cell growth of the prostate gland, a physiologic change of aging. Approximately 14 million men have symptoms associated with BPH annually. The prevalence of BPH in Caucasian and African American men is similar, though the disorder tends to be more severe and progressive in

African American men. Men older than age 50 years have roughly a 50% chance of developing BPH; by age 80 years, about 80% to 90% of men are diagnosed with BPH. The etiology of BPH is testosterone-sensitive cellular proliferation and lack of cellular apoptosis in the prostate gland.

The prostate is a walnut-sized gland that is located anterior to the rectum and below the urinary bladder. The urethra runs through its middle and connects with the penile urethra. The gland is composed of different kinds of cellular sections called the peripheral, central, anterior, and transition zones. BPH originates in the transition zone, which surrounds the urethra. Cellular proliferation encroaches on the urethra and causes obstruction of urine flow from the bladder (see Fig. 27-5).

The main function of the prostate gland is secretion of an alkaline fluid that comprises approximately 70% of the seminal volume. The secretions produce lubrication and nutrition for the sperm, and the alkaline fluid in the ejaculate helps to neutralize the acidic vaginal environment. The prostatic urethra is a conduit for semen and closes off the bladder neck during sexual climax in order to prevent retrograde ejaculation (ejaculation resulting in semen being forced backwards into the bladder).

The diagnosis of BPH is often based on the patient signs and symptoms (see Box 27-2). The patient needs to urinate frequently during the day or night but voids only small amounts of urine with each episode. Also, the patient reports the sudden urges to urinate, incomplete emptying of the bladder, interruptions in the flow of urine, and the loss of small amounts of urine. The patient is susceptible to lower urinary tract infection because of retained urine in the bladder, which provides a medium for bacterial growth.

To physically assess the patient for BPH, the clinician performs a DRE. The posterior wall of the prostate

---

BOX 27-2. Signs and Symptoms of Benign Prostatic Hyperplasia

There are several symptoms that are characteristic of BPH. Usually these occur in males over age 50 years old.

- Dribbling of urine
- Frequency
- Hesitancy
- Retention of urine in bladder
- Straining to urinate
- Weak urinary stream
- Urgency

---

can be palpated through the anterior wall of the rectal vault (see Fig. 27-6). On physical examination, the hyperplastic prostate is enlarged, smooth, firm, and nontender. A PSA blood test should be done to rule out prostate cancer. However, a diagnosis of prostate cancer cannot be based solely on PSA testing because the test has a high false positive rate. Urine flow studies, ultrasound, and cystoscopy are other diagnostic tests that may be needed.

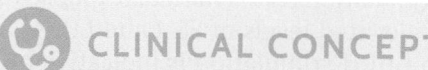

CLINICAL CONCEPT

At age 50, men should begin having yearly exams for BPH and prostate cancer, which include DRE and PSA testing.

There are medical and surgical treatments for BPH. The two primary drug classes used for BPH are alpha-blockers and 5-alpha-reductase inhibitors. Alpha-blocker drugs

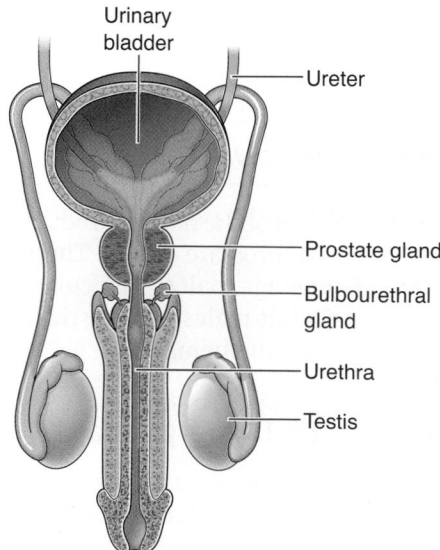

FIGURE 27-5. Cross section of the prostate gland, urinary bladder, and urethra in BPH. The prostate gland surrounds the male urethra; with hyperplasia, the prostate can encroach on the urethra, causing obstruction to urinary flow.

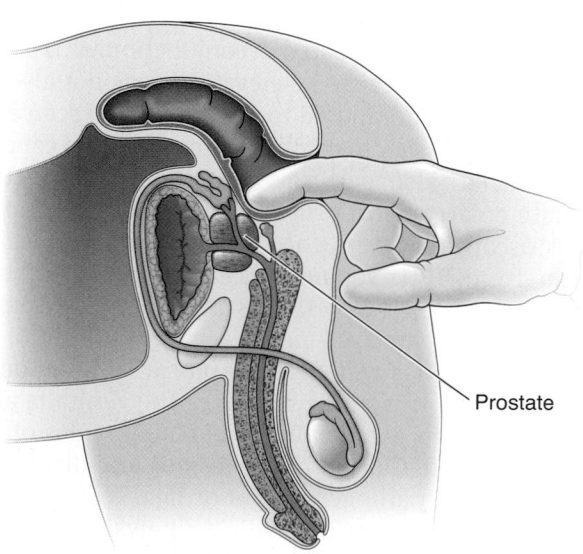

FIGURE 27-6. DRE. The clinician can use DRE to assess the prostate gland, which can be palpated through the rectal wall.

relax smooth muscles, especially in the bladder neck and prostate. Alpha-blockers help relieve BPH symptoms, but they do not reduce the size of the prostate. However, they can help improve urine flow and reduce risk of bladder obstruction. They are often the first choice, especially for men with smaller prostates. A typical alpha-blocker is tamsulosin (Flomax®).

The 5-alpha-reductase inhibitors are drugs that block the conversion of testosterone to dihydrotestosterone, the male hormone that stimulates the prostate. These drugs are for men with significantly enlarged prostates. In addition to relieving symptoms, they increase urinary flow and may even help shrink the prostate. However, patients may have to take these drugs for up to 6 to 12 months to achieve full benefits. Finasteride (Proscar®) is an example of a 5-alpha-reductase inhibitor.

Because alpha-blockers and 5-alpha-reductase inhibitors work in different ways, combinations of the two types of drugs may control symptoms in select patients more effectively than either drug alone. Women should not handle crushed or broken finasteride tablets when they are or may potentially be pregnant. Because of the ability of type II 5-alpha-reductase inhibitors such as finasteride to inhibit conversion of testosterone to dihydrotestosterone, finasteride may cause abnormalities of the external genitalia of a male fetus when administered to a pregnant woman.

CLINICAL CONCEPT

5-alpha-reductase inhibitor drugs decrease PSA levels, which may mask the presence of prostate cancer.

ALERT! Women should not handle finasteride tablets when they are or may potentially be pregnant.

Surgical treatment of BPH involves transurethral needle ablation (TUNA) or transurethral resection of the prostate (TURP). In both of these procedures, the obstructive prostatic tissue is excised so that the urethra can allow free flow of urine.

Erectile Dysfunction

Disorders such as ED and female sexual dysfunction are becoming increasingly more important as a result of the aging of the population, direct-to-consumer mass marketing of pharmaceuticals, and new therapies. Sexual dysfunction is highly prevalent in men and women. Complete ED is defined as (1) the total inability to obtain or maintain an erection during sexual stimulation and (2) the absence of nocturnal erections. In the landmark Massachusetts Male Aging Study (MMAS) of 1987–2004, a community-based survey of men aged 40 to 70 years,

52% of the respondents reported some degree of erectile difficulty. However, complete ED was only reported by 10% of the respondents. Extrapolating the MMAS data to the American population, an estimated 18 to 30 million men are affected by ED annually.

ED is essentially a vascular disease. It is often associated with other vascular diseases and conditions such as diabetes, hypertension, and coronary artery disease. Diabetes is a well-recognized cause of ED, with approximately 50% of diabetic men experiencing the condition. Diabetes causes endothelial damage and neurological impairment, which leads to circulatory and structural changes in penile tissues. For erection to occur, dilation and engorgement of the penis is required. Arterial insufficiency, defective smooth muscle relaxation, inadequate pudendal neurological control, and lack of engorgement of the corpora cavernosum and spongiosum tissues are the effects of diabetes, and these conditions together cause dysfunction of the penis. Additionally, ED is often an adverse effect of many commonly prescribed medications. Some drugs such as antidepressants and antihypertensive agents can cause ED. Men with sleep disorders commonly experience ED. Another important consideration is the patient's hormonal status. Hypogonadism that results in low testosterone levels adversely affects libido and erectile function. There are a wide array of possible causes of ED (see Box 27-3).

Most patients with ED have multiple etiologic factors, so assessing how much each is contributing to the

BOX 27-3. Causes of Erectile Dysfunction

The following are common causes of ED, which most commonly occurs in middle-aged and elderly males.

- Alcoholism and other forms of substance abuse
- Atherosclerosis
- Certain prescription medications
- Diabetes
- Fatigue
- Heart disease
- High blood pressure
- Low testosterone
- Mental health conditions such as depression and anxiety
- Metabolic syndrome
- Multiple sclerosis
- Obesity
- Parkinson's disease
- Peyronie's disease; development of scar tissue inside the penis
- Stress
- Surgeries or injuries that affect the pelvic area or spinal cord
- Tobacco use
- Treatments for prostate cancer or enlarged prostate

problem is difficult. Because of the various possible causes of ED, a thorough general health and sexual history is necessary to correctly identify the specific etiology in an individual. It is difficult to assess the prevalence of ED. Often, clinicians do not complete a sexual history; therefore, it is believed that ED is underdiagnosed. Conversely, it is believed that ED is overdiagnosed as a result of intense mass-media marketing efforts directed toward men and women regarding sexual expectations. To diagnose ED, patients may be submitted to laboratory studies; however, in many cases, treatment is based on the patient's subjective symptoms.

Laboratory diagnostic tests include an evaluation of the patient's hormone status, particularly if the symptom is diminished or absent libido. Patients who demonstrate any signs of diminished secondary sexual characteristics should have an endocrine evaluation that consists of measuring morning serum testosterone levels. A measurement of LH and, in some instances, prolactin is obtained if the patient has evidence of pituitary dysfunction or cases of low serum testosterone levels. Hemoglobin A1c, serum chemistry studies, lipid profiles, thyroid hormones, and prostate-specific antigen levels should be obtained to assess general health. A urinalysis looking for red blood cells, white blood cells, protein, and glucose is also important. Following completion of this phase, the clinician should be able to determine the patient's medical status, to identify and characterize the type of dysfunction, and to determine the need for additional testing such as penile or pelvic blood flow studies, nocturnal penile tumescence testing, or other blood tests. There are many imaging studies that can be used to diagnose ED, but these are rarely performed.

Mechanical devices, implants, and injectable medications are available for ED; however, oral phosphodiesterase (PDE) inhibitor medication is the most commonly prescribed treatment. Sildenafil (Viagra), tadalafil (Cialis), and vardenafil (Levitra) are PDE inhibitors. These drugs block the release of PDE in the corpus cavernosum of the penis. Blocking the enzyme PDE enhances the effects of nitric oxide, the natural chemical that produces vasodilation and relaxation of smooth muscles in the penis.

ALERT! PDE inhibitors, such as sildenafil, are absolutely contraindicated in patients taking nitrates. PDE inhibitors potentiate the vasodilatory effects of the nitrate-based medication, resulting in a severe drop in BP.

Testicular Torsion

Testicular torsion most commonly occurs in adolescents, although it can occur at any age, even prenatally, in the male. Anatomically, the testicle is covered by a fibrous tissue called the tunica vaginalis, which is

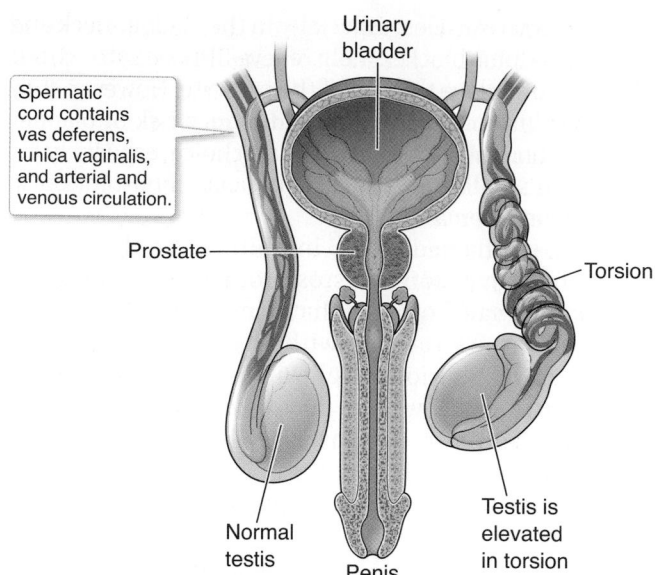

FIGURE 27-7. Testicular torsion is an acute, painful disorder where the spermatic cord twists and cuts off circulation to the testicle. Upon examination, the affected testicle will be elevated up toward the abdomen because of shortening of the spermatic cord.

contained—along with the vas deferens—in a spermatic cord that attaches to the anterior two-thirds of the testicle (see Fig. 27-7). In some patients, there is a congenital anatomic anomaly of high attachment of the tunica vaginalis that allows the testicle to rotate freely. This congenital abnormality is present in approximately 12% of males. Testicular torsion can obstruct blood flow to the testicle, which can lead to ischemia and infarction of the testicle; this is why testicular torsion is a urological emergency: delay in diagnosis and treatment can lead to loss of the testicle.

Symptoms include sudden onset of severe unilateral scrotal pain. Torsion can occur during activity or rest; it is related to trauma in 4% to 8% of cases. Scrotal swelling, erythema, abdominal pain, nausea, and vomiting are other symptoms. The diagnosis of testicular torsion is based on symptoms and clinical presentation. Laboratory tests and imaging studies usually are not necessary. The patient should go directly to surgery without any delay to perform diagnostic studies. If there is uncertainty regarding the diagnosis, radionuclide scan of the testicles or ultrasonography can be helpful to assess blood flow and to differentiate torsion from other conditions. Emergency detorsion surgery is the treatment. There are few complications if detorsion surgery is implemented within 6 hours of pain; however, loss of the testicle can occur if surgery is delayed for 12 to 24 hours.

Testicular Cancer

Testicular tumors are the most common cancer in males between the ages of 15 and 35 years in the United States. Approximately 9,000 new cases are diagnosed annually.

The lifetime chance of developing testicular cancer is about 1 in 300, and the risk of dying is very low—about 1 in 5,000. The incidence of testicular cancer is 5-fold higher in Caucasians than in African Americans; however, African Americans tend to present with more severe disease and have a much worse prognosis. The risk for the disease is higher in first-degree relatives of cancer patients than in the general population.

The most common type of testicular cancer is a germ cell tumor, which is a cellular neoplasm inside the testes. Germ cell tumors are classified as either a seminoma or nonseminoma, based on cellular derivation. Seminomas originate in the germinal epithelium of the seminiferous tubules. About half of germ cell tumors of the testis are seminomas.

In patients with cryptorchidism, the risk of developing a testicular germ cell tumor is increased 4-fold to 8-fold. Other risk factors include family history, infertility, prior testicular cancer, HIV infection, and environmental exposures. Exposure to DES in utero, Agent Orange, and numerous industrial chemicals increase cancer risk. Also, studies have shown a genetic risk of testicular cancer; 80% of testicular tumors have one or more copies of the short arm of chromosome 12.

A painless swelling, nodule, or mass lesion of one testicle is the most common presenting symptom. On the physical exam, the mass cannot be separated from the testis. Dull ache or heavy sensation in the lower abdomen also could be presenting symptoms. Patients who experience a hematoma with trauma should undergo evaluation to rule out testicular cancer.

A complete history and physical examination is needed for diagnosis. On physical exam, a cancer is palpable as a solid, immobile, nontender mass in the scrotum. Diagnostic tests include a chemistry profile, complete blood count, and the serum tumor markers alpha-fetoprotein (AFP) and b-HCG. Ultrasound, CT scan, and lymph node examination are usually done, and biopsy of the testicular mass is necessary. Staging of testicular cancer follows the tumor, node, metastasis system (see Chapter 40: Cancer). Treatment involves orchiectomy; radiation and chemotherapy also may be necessary. Because 45% to 55% of testicular cancer patients are infertile after therapy, those patients who wish to preserve fertility are offered semen cryopreservation before treatment.

Testicular cancer has one of the highest cure rates of all cancers: greater than 90%; that rate increases to essentially 100% if it has not metastasized. Even for the relatively few cases in which malignant cancer has spread widely, chemotherapy offers a cure rate of at least 85%.

Varicocele, Hematocele, and Hydrocele

A **varicocele** is a dilatation of the veins within the scrotum. Approximately 15% to 20% of the healthy fertile male population is estimated to have asymptomatic varicoceles. However, varicoceles are often the cause of infertility and are discovered when the male patient is trying to conceive with lack of success. Alternatively, the patient may report scrotal pain or heaviness. Careful physical examination remains the primary method of varicocele detection. An obvious varicocele is often demonstrated by a swollen scrotum and palpated by the examiner as a "bag of worms." If physical examination findings are uncertain, high-resolution color-flow Doppler ultrasonography is the diagnostic method of choice. Acute problems such as torsion of the testes or hernia need to be ruled out because they also cause a swollen scrotum. Also, abdominal or pelvic mass lesions should be ruled out because they can obstruct testicular blood flow and present as a varicocele. Microsurgical repair is the treatment.

Hydrocele is a collection of serous fluid in the scrotum that causes swelling and a feeling of heaviness. **Hematocele** is a collection of blood in the scrotum that causes the same symptoms. Hydrocele and hematocele are often caused by trauma or infection of the testes. Edema fluid or ruptured blood vessels cause each, respectively. The scrotum can be transilluminated with a penlight to aid in diagnosis. Ultrasound of the scrotum is also used. Allowing the body to reabsorb the fluid or blood requires watchful waiting as treatment. If absorption does not occur, surgical evacuation of fluid may be necessary.

Chapter Summary

- The male reproductive system is an endocrine feedback system of the hypothalamus that produces GnRH, which stimulates the anterior pituitary to secrete FSH and LH. FSH stimulates spermatozoa production by the testes. LH stimulates testosterone secretion by the testes.

- The most important organs that determine male sexuality are the testes, which synthesize testosterone and generate spermatozoa. The testes need to lie away from the body because optimal spermatogenesis requires temperatures cooler than the core body temperature.

- Puberty can be assessed using criteria set forth by the Tanner stages. Precocious puberty in males occurs when secondary sexual characteristics develop before age 9 years. Delayed puberty in males occurs when sexual development is not occurring by age 14 years.

- Cryptorchidism is the disorder where the testes remain in the abdomen or high in the inguinal canal and do not descend into the scrotum. The testes should lie within the scrotum by the end of the first year in the infant. Untreated cryptorchidism is a risk factor for testicular cancer.

- Hypospadias and epispadias are anatomical anomalies of the penis. The urethral opening is on the posterior side of the penis in hypospadias and the urethral opening is on the anterior side of the penis in epispadias.
- Hydrocele, varicocele, and hematocele are disorders of the scrotum that can occur with trauma.
- Torsion of the testes is an acute condition caused by twisting of the testicle on the spermatic cord. It is extremely painful and a medical emergency.
- BPH is a condition that commonly occurs in men older than 50 years. Physiologically, the prostate enlarges with age. BPH can obstruct the urethra and cause urinary symptoms that include urgency, frequency, hesitancy, weak urinary stream, and urinary tract infection.
- BPH can be treated with medication or transurethral surgery.
- Testicular cancer, although rare, is the most common cancer in males between ages 15 and 35 years. It is highly treatable.

- Prostate cancer is the most common cancer in men older than age 50. DRE and PSA testing are two screening procedures that can be used to prevent this cancer. Men older than age 50 years should have a prostate exam yearly.
- The PSA test has a high rate of false positive results for prostate cancer. Diagnosis of prostate cancer cannot be based solely on PSA test results.
- From adolescence to middle age, STIs cause significant acute and chronic pain, infertility, and contagious disease. Many STIs are silent in the male but symptomatic in the female.
- ED, once a taboo subject, is now freely discussed in the media and there is raised awareness among male patients regarding available treatment. Men with atherosclerosis and diabetes commonly have ED. Nitrates are contraindicated with use of medications for ED.

 ## Making the Connections

Disorder and Pathophysiology	Signs and Symptoms	Physical Assessment Findings	Diagnostic Testing	Treatment
Cryptorchidism | Undescended testes that remain in the abdomen or within the inguinal canal.				
	Infertility.	Lack of palpable testes in the scrotum.	CT scan of pelvis and abdomen.	Surgery to bring testes down into scrotum.
Hypospadias/Epispadias | Penile orifice misplaced either above or below the glans penis.				
	Difficult urination.	Penile orifice apparently misplaced.	Clinical examination.	Surgery to place urethral opening in the tip of the penis.
Testicular Torsion | Testicular tunica vaginalis twisted and obstructing blood flow to testes.				
	Acute pain in the scrotum.	Erythema, swelling, and tenderness of scrotum.	Clinical exam.	Surgery; testicular removal may be necessary.
ED | Inability of the penis to achieve erection.				
	Infertility.	None.	Patient history.	PDE inhibitor medications such as sildenafil cause vascular vasodilation in the penis.
BPH | Increased cellular growth and size of prostate gland with urethral obstruction; this is a normal physiologic change of aging.				
	Urinary frequency, urgency, hesitancy, straining to urinate, weak stream, nocturia, susceptibility to urinary tract infection.	Enlarged prostate palpable on DRE.	DRE; clinician palpates enlarged prostate. PSA blood test shows elevated PSA level. CT scan shows enlarged prostate.	Alpha-blocker medications, 5-alpha-reductase inhibitors, TURP, TUNA, or radical resection of prostate.

Continued

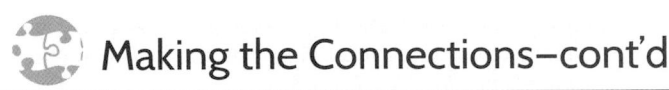

Making the Connections—cont'd

Disorder and Pathophysiology	Signs and Symptoms	Physical Assessment Findings	Diagnostic Testing	Treatment
Testicular Cancer | Most common cancer type is germ cell seminoma; neoplastic growth of the seminiferous tubule cells.				
	Swelling or mass in testes within scrotum.	Swelling or mass in testes within scrotum.	Elevated AFP, and beta-hCG. Biopsy.	Surgery. Radiation. Chemotherapy.
Hydrocele, Hematocele, Varicocele | Varicocele is a condition of distended veins and lack of blood drainage of the testes. Hydrocele is fluid in the scrotal sac, causing swelling of the scrotum. Hematocele is a collection of blood in the scrotal sac.				
	Heaviness and swelling in scrotum.	Swelling in scrotum.	Ultrasound shows fluid or enlarged vessels in the scrotum.	Surgery to drain fluid from scrotum.

Bibliography

Abreu, A. P., Dauber, A., Macedo, D. B., et al. (2013, June 27). Central precocious puberty caused by mutations in the imprinted gene MKRN3. *N Engl J Med,* 368(26), 2467–2475. doi: 10.1056/NEJMoa1302160. Epub 2013 Jun 5.

Anic, G. M., & Giuliano, A. R. (2011). Genital HPV infection and related lesions in men. *Prev Med,* 53(Suppl 1), S36–S41.

Andriole, G. L., Bostwick, D. G., Brawley, O. W., et al. (2010). Effect of dutasteride on the risk of prostate cancer. *N Engl J Med,* 362(13), 1192–1202.

Anothaisintawee, T., Attia, J., Nickel, J. C., et al. (2011). Management of chronic prostatitis/chronic pelvic pain syndrome: a systematic review and network meta-analysis. *JAMA,* 305(1), 78–86. doi: 10.1001/jama.2010.1913.

Barkin, J. (2011). PSA and the family physician. *Canadian J Urol,* 18(Suppl), 20–23.

Beckman, T. J., & Litin, S. C. (2010). Clinical pearls in men's health. *Mayo Clin Proceed,* 85(7), 668–673. doi: 10.4065/mcp.2010.0164.

Bill-Axelson, A., Holmberg, L., Garmo, H., et al. (2014). Radical prostatectomy or watchful waiting in early prostate cancer. *N Engl J Med,* 370(10), 932–942. doi: 10.1056/NEJMoa1311593.

Brosman, S. (2010). Erectile dysfunction. Retrieved from http://emedicine.medscape.com

Carel, J. C., & Léger, J. (2008). Clinical practice. Precocious puberty. *N Engl J Med,* 358(22), 2366–2377.

Chang, H. J. (2011). Lower abdominal swelling and scrotal enlargement. *JAMA,* 306(15), 1709–1710.

Croswell, J., & Sikorski, C. (2011). Screening for testicular cancer. *Am Fam Phys,* 84(4), 451–452.

DiIorio, C., Steenland, K., Goodman, M., et al. (2011). Differences in treatment-based beliefs and coping between African American and white men with prostate cancer. *J Comm Health,* 36(4), 505–512.

Edwards, J. L. (2008). Diagnosis and management of benign prostatic hyperplasia. *Am Fam Phys,* 77(10), 1403–1410.

Goodman, A., Schorge, J., & Greene, M. F. (2011). The long-term effects of in utero exposures—the DES story. *N Engl J Med,* 364(22), 2083–2084. Epub 2011 Apr 20.

Heidelbaugh, J. J. (2010). Management of erectile dysfunction. *Am Fam Phys,* 81(3), 305–312.

Hitzeman, N., & Molina, M. (2011). Screening for prostate cancer: prostate-specific antigen testing is not effective. *Am Fam Phys,* 83(7), 802–804.

Information From Your Family Doctor. (2010). Erectile dysfunction. *Am Fam Phys,* 81(3), 313.

Inman, B. A., Sauver, J. L., Jacobson, D. J., et al. (2009). A population-based, longitudinal study of erectile dysfunction and future coronary artery disease. *Mayo Clin Proceed,* 84(2), 108–113.

Jacobsen, S. J., Jacobson, D. J., McGree, M. E., et al. (2012). Sixteen-year longitudinal changes in serum prostate-specific antigen levels: the Olmsted county study. *Mayo Clin Proceed,* 87(1), 34–40.

Jones, C. U., Hunt, D., McGowan, D. G., et al. (2011). Radiotherapy and short-term androgen deprivation for localized prostate cancer. *N Engl J Med,* 365(2), 107–118.

Kumar, V., Abbas, A. K., Fausto, N., & Aster, J. (2010). *Robbins and Cotran pathologic basis of disease.* 8th ed. Philadelphia, PA: Elsevier.

Longo, D. L., Kasper, D. L., Jameson, J. L., et al. (2011). *Harrison's principles of internal medicine.* 18th ed. New York: McGraw-Hill.

McNicholas, T., & Kirby, R. (2012). Benign prostatic hyperplasia and male lower urinary tract symptoms. *Am Fam Phys,* 86(4), 359–360.

Miner, M., Nehra, A., Jackson, G., et al. (2014). All men with vasculogenic erectile dysfunction require a cardiovascular workup. *Am J Med,* 127(3), 174–182. doi: 10.1016/j.amjmed.2013.10.013. Epub 2013 Nov 1.

Mitka, M. (2012). Endocrine Society seeks better testing to determine endocrine disruptor health risks. *JAMA,* 308(6), 556–557.

Mohan, R., & Schellhammer, P. F. (2011). Treatment options for localized prostate cancer. *Am Fam Phys,* 84(4), 413–420.

Prostate cancer: who should be treated? (2011). *Am Fam Phys,* 84(4), 424.

Resnick, M. J., Koyama, T., Fan, K. H., et al. (2013). Long-term functional outcomes after treatment for localized prostate cancer. *N Engl J Med, 368*(5), 436–445. doi: 10.1056/NEJMoa1209978.

Rim, S. H., Hall, I. J., Fairweather, M. E., et al. (2011). Considering racial and ethnic preferences in communication and interactions among the patient, family member, and physician following diagnosis of localized prostate cancer: study of a US population. *Int J Gen Med, 4,* 481–486. Epub 2011 Jun 17.

Rudkin, S., & Kazzi, A. (2010). Hydrocele: treatment & medication. Retrieved from http://emedicine.medscape.com

Rupp, T., & Zwanger, M. (2010). Testicular torsion. Retrieved from http://emedicine.medscape.com.

Sachdeva, K., Javeed, M., Makhoul, I., Jana, B, & Curti, B. (2010). Testicular cancer. Retrieved from http://emedicine.medscape.com

Sarma, A. V., & Wei, J. T. (2012). Clinical practice. Benign prostatic hyperplasia and lower urinary tract symptoms. *N Engl J Med, 367*(3), 248–257. doi: 10.1056/NEJMcp1106637. Review. No abstract available. Erratum in: *N Engl J Med.* 2012 Aug 16;367(7):681.

Screening for testicular cancer: reaffirmation recommendation statement. (2011). *Am Fam Phys, 84*(4), 444–445.

Sharp, V. J., Takacs, E. B., & Powell, C. R. (2010). Prostatitis: diagnosis and treatment. *Am Fam Phys, 82*(4), 397–406.

Shaw, J. (2008). Diagnosis and treatment of testicular cancer. *Am Fam Phys, 77*(4), 469–474.

Simmons, M. N., Berglund, R. K., & Jones, J. S. (2011). A practical guide to prostate cancer diagnosis and management. *Cleveland Clin J Med, 78*(5), 321–331.

Sina, A., & Alizadeh, F. (2011). Concealed male epispadias: a rare form of penile epispadias presenting as phimosis. *Urol Jrnl, 8*(4), 328–329.

Tangen, C. M., Goodman, P. J., & Thompson, I. M., Jr. (2013). Survival in the prostate cancer prevention trial. *N Engl J Med, 369*(20), 1968. doi: 10.1056/NEJMc1311498.

Terris, M., & Rhee, A. (2010). Prostate cancer—metastatic and advanced disease. Retrieved from http://emedicine.medscape.com

Tiemstra, J. D., & Kapoor, S. (2008). Evaluation of scrotal masses. *Am Fam Phys, 78*(10), 1165–1170.

Traish, A. M., Miner, M. M., Morgentaler, A., & Zitzmann, M. (2011). Testosterone deficiency. *Am J Med, 124*(7), 578–587. doi: 10.1016/j.amjmed.2010.12.027.

Trojian, T. H., Lishnak, T. S., & Heiman, D. (2009). Epididymitis and orchitis: an overview. *Am Fam Phys, 79*(7), 583–587.

Walsh, P. C. (2010). Chemoprevention of prostate cancer. *N Engl J Med, 362*(13), 1237–1238.

Xu, J., Dailey, R. K., Eggly, S., Neale, A. V., & Schwartz, K. L. (2011). Men's perspectives on selecting their prostate cancer treatment. *J Natl Med Assoc, 103*(6), 468–478.

Sexually Transmitted Diseases

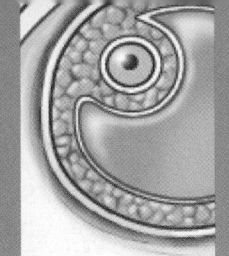

Key Terms

Buboe

Chancre

Chlamydia trachomatis

Condyloma acuminata

Condyloma lata

Gummas

Herpes simplex virus (HSV)

Human papilloma virus (HPV)

Hutchison teeth

Jarisch-Herxheimer reaction

MSM

Neisseria gonorrhoeae

Pelvic inflammatory disease (PID)

Polymerase chain reaction (PCR)

Sexually transmitted disease (STD)

Syphilis

Tabes dorsalis

Treponema pallidum

Urethritis

A **sexually transmitted disease (STD),** also termed sexually transmitted infection or venereal disease, is an infection that is transmitted between humans by means of sexual behavior, including vaginal intercourse, oral sex, and anal sex. A person with an STD is infected and may potentially infect others, with or without showing signs of disease. Some STDs can also be transmitted via blood, reuse of intravenous drug needles, childbirth, and breastfeeding.

STDs affect both men and women. In pregnant women, STDs can have adverse effects on the fetus. In terms of transmission, STDs are highly contagious, so prevention and screening are important interventions, particularly in the teen and young adult populations.

Most STDs are treated with antibiotics and behavior modification. However, some STDs, such as human immunodeficiency virus (HIV) infection, can cause significant morbidity and mortality.

Epidemiology

STDs are a major public health challenge in the United States. According to the Centers for Disease Control and Prevention (CDC), as of 2013 there are eight common STDs. Human papilloma virus (HPV) is the most common STD; other prevalent STDs are trichomoniasis, Chlamydia, gonorrhea, herpes simplex virus 2 (HSV2), hepatitis B (HBV), HIV, and syphilis. In total, the CDC estimates that there are approximately 20 million new cases of STDs each year, which cost the U.S. health-care system $16.4 billion annually. There are approximately 110 million persons with STDs in the United States.

Yet, there are large disparities in the incidence of STDs by race and age. CDC surveillance data from 2010 show much higher rates of reported STDs among some racial or ethnic minority groups than among Caucasians. This is consistent with other data sources showing marked STD disparities in some minority populations. A range of factors contributes to these disparities, including poverty, lack of access to health care, and an already high prevalence of STDs in communities, all of which can increase a person's risk of infection with each sexual encounter.

In the United States, 67% of gonorrhea cases occur in African Americans, even though they represent only 14% of the U.S. population. The gonorrhea rate among Hispanics is twice that of Caucasians. American Indians /Alaska natives have STD rates 4 times that of Caucasians.

Regardless of race, 50% of STDs occur in the 15- to 24-year-old age group. In this age group, the incidence of STDs among males and females is similar. The CDC estimates that HPV accounts for the majority of newly contracted STDs. Primary care clinicians are urged to screen young adults for STDs when possible. Undetected and untreated STDs increase a person's risk for HIV infection, which can be present with no symptoms for a lengthy period of time.

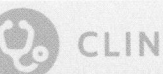 **CLINICAL CONCEPT**

Untreated gonorrhea and Chlamydia often cause **pelvic inflammatory disease (PID)** in women, a condition that can cause infertility. Each year, STDs cause at least 24,000 women in the United States to become infertile.

Untreated syphilis can lead to serious long-term complications, including brain, cardiovascular, and organ damage. Syphilis in pregnant women can also result in congenital syphilis (syphilis among infants), which can cause stillbirth, death soon after birth, and, in children who survive, physical deformity and neurological complications. Untreated syphilis in pregnant women results in infant death in up to 40% of cases. Studies suggest that individuals with gonorrhea, Chlamydia, or syphilis are at increased risk for HIV. Frequently, individuals are infected with more than one STD at the same time.

Basic Concepts of Sexual Disease and Dysfunction

Common STDs include Chlamydia and gonorrhea, which are easily treatable. Early diagnosis and treatment are important to prevent complications. For example, gonorrhea can cause PID, which can lead to infertility. Chlamydia can cause conjunctivitis in the newborn that is delivered vaginally. It is also important to recognize that an individual with an STD should be tested for other STDs. For example, syphilis is often found with HIV infection and gonorrhea is often found with Chlamydia infection. Some STDs are completely curable and leave no complications. However, STDs such as HIV, syphilis, and HBV are associated with widespread systemic complications that include cardiac and neurological problems, immunosuppression, and liver failure.

Etiology

STDs can be caused by bacteria, viruses, fungi or parasites. There are more than 20 types of STDs, including:

- Chlamydia
- gonorrhea
- herpes simplex virus (HSV)
- HIV/acquired immune deficiency syndrome (AIDS)
- human papilloma virus (HPV)
- HBV
- syphilis.

Each organism causes different signs and symptoms, and each type of infection requires specific diagnostic and treatment interventions.

Risk Factors

Sexual activity is the risk factor for STDs, as STDs can be transmitted during any type of sexual exposure, including vaginal, anal, and oral sexual practices. Adolescents and young adults are at highest risk for contraction of STDs. In addition, persons with multiple sex partners and men who have sex with men **(MSM)** are at high risk for STDs. MSM who also take part in illicit drug use (particularly methamphetamine use) are at increased risk for STDs. Some STDs can be prevented with the use of a condom during sexual activity, although others, such as HSV2, merely require close skin-to-skin contact for transmission. Blood-to-blood transmission is also a risk factor; STDs can be transmitted from person to person during sharing of unsterile needles used for intravenous drug use. Some practices, such as tattooing and piercing,

can transmit HIV or HBV if needles are unsterile. STDs are commonly transplacentally transmitted from mother to child during gestation or passed to the newborn during childbirth or breastfeeding.

Pathophysiology

There are different pathological mechanisms for each type of STD. Organisms that cause STDs may have localized effects, systemic effects, or both. An organism such as herpes simplex may exert an effect mainly on the reproductive tract or, as in the case of syphilis, an organism may cause multiple organ pathology. It is important to note that the presence of an STD increases an individual's susceptibility to HIV. Organisms that cause genital tract ulcers, such as HSV or syphilis, are highly associated with the transmission of HIV. HIV causes a decreased immune response, which in turn allows the STD to flourish. STDs that cause a vaginal or urethral discharge, such as Chlamydia or gonorrhea, are also associated with higher transmission rates of HIV. There is a synergistic effect noted in the combined exposure to certain STDs along with exposure to HIV.

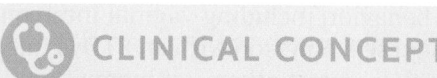

CLINICAL CONCEPT

The presence of an STD should alert the clinician to test for HIV. HIV increases susceptibility to other STDs.

Clinical Presentation

In women, STDs can be classified as either lower tract infections—those that affect the vulva, vagina, and cervix—or upper tract infections—those that affect the uterus, fallopian tubes, and the ovaries. Purulent vaginal discharge or bleeding and pelvic or abdominal pain and tenderness are commonly signs of an STD in women. Some STDs can cause external lesions that are apparent during pelvic examination, whereas others can remain dormant and unobservable. STDs can lead to occlusion of the fallopian tubes, which can cause ectopic pregnancy or infertility. Some STDs can be transmitted to the fetus during pregnancy or intrapartum period, causing perinatal loss, neonatal infection, low birth weight of the newborn, or preterm labor.

In men, STDs commonly cause inflammation of the urethra termed **urethritis,** which consists of burning upon urination and a thick or watery discharge leaking from the opening in the penis. The infectious process can ascend to the testicles (orchitis), prostate (prostatitis), or epididymis (epididymitis), causing tenderness and pain.

Diagnosis

The diagnosis of an STD requires a laboratory procedure that can demonstrate growth of the suspected etiologic organism. These laboratory procedures vary according to the suspected organism. For example, HIV infection requires antibody testing or viral ribonucleic acid (RNA) levels, which require a blood sample and specific immunoassay procedures. The diagnosis of gonorrhea, however, requires a specific type of agar that can grow cultures of the bacteria.

In lieu of cultures, the diagnostic test called **polymerase chain reaction (PCR)** is increasingly being used. In the diagnosis of STDs, PCR is used to detect the deoxyribonucleic acid (DNA) or RNA of a microorganism in a cell sample. PCR is highly sensitive and can detect minute quantities of microorganism DNA or RNA. PCR can also reveal the number of microorganisms in a cell sample. For example, the number of HIV viral particles can be quantified by PCR early after contraction of the virus. PCR can reveal the presence of viral RNA before antibody appears in the blood. Other diagnostic techniques will be discussed in subsequent sections of this chapter.

Treatment

Treatments for different STDs vary; however, most require an antimicrobial drug. In addition, education regarding contagion, transmission, and prevention of the infection is necessary. Different therapies will be discussed in subsequent sections of this chapter.

Pathophysiology of Sexually Transmitted Diseases

STDs can be caused by a number of different bacteria, viruses, and parasites. Each type of infection presents differently and causes distinct symptoms.

Bacterial Infections

The most common bacterial microorganisms that cause STDs include Chlamydia, gonococcus, and syphilis. Chlamydia is often a silent infection, whereas gonorrhea and syphilis have evident symptoms.

Chlamydia

Chlamydia trachomatis infection is a widespread disease that does not cause many signs or symptoms. Often this infection is present along with other STDs, particularly gonorrhea. *C. trachomatis* infection can affect the cervix, urethra, fallopian tubes, uterus, rectum, nasopharynx, and epididymis; it is the most commonly reported bacterial STD in the United States and a leading cause of infertility in women. *C. trachomatis* also causes conjunctivitis or pneumonia in neonates born vaginally to infected mothers.

Epidemiology. Chlamydia is one of the most common STDs in the United States. Females have higher rates of infection than males. It is estimated that 3 million individuals within the sexually active population have been infected at some point in their lives. Approximately 4 million cases of Chlamydial infection are reported per year in the United States, with an overall prevalence of 5% in the population. Sexually active adolescent girls have a higher prevalence rate of 10%. African American females, aged 18 to 26 years, have a prevalence rate of Chlamydia infection as high as 14%. In females with gonorrhea, prevalence of Chlamydia infection is 17%. Approximately 100,000 neonates are exposed to Chlamydia at childbirth each year.

Risk Factors. Unprotected sexual activity is the major risk factor for Chlamydial infection. Vaginal, anal, or oral sexual practices can transmit this bacterial infection. In addition, contraction of neonatal infection can occur as an infant is delivered vaginally from an infected mother. Two-thirds of infants born to mothers with Chlamydia develop conjunctivitis or pneumonia. Specific risk factors for Chlamydial infection include multiple sexual partners, a new sexual partner, lack of barrier contraceptive, and coinfection with another STD.

Etiology. C. trachomatis is a gram-negative, obligate intracellular bacteria that can only live inside a host's cells. Obligate intracellular bacteria cannot reproduce outside their host cell, meaning that the organism's life cycle is entirely dependent on host cell resources.

Pathophysiology. C. trachomatis causes cervicitis, urethritis, PID, and a type of conjunctivitis known as inclusion conjunctivitis. The bacteria invades mucosal epithelium and its incubation period is 1 to 3 weeks. The most common initial infection affects the columnar epithelial cells present on the cervix. Upon infection, the initial inflammation reaction attracts neutrophils, followed by lymphocytes, macrophages, plasma cells, and eosinophils. The release of cytokines and interferon by white blood cells maintain the inflammation reaction. Infection stimulates both antibody-mediated and cellular immune responses demonstrated by the presence of secretory immunoglobulin A (IgA), circulatory immunoglobulin M (IgM), immunoglobulin G (IgG) antibodies, and T cells.

Chlamydia bacteria can have two types of presentation depending on its environment. In the extracellular environment, Chlamydia inclusion bodies (also called elementary bodies) are found. Inclusion bodies are inactive Chlamydia infectious particles, similar to spores. When Chlamydia gains entry into a host cell, the inclusion body protects the bacteria from phagocytosis by white blood cells. The Chlamydia bacterium then uses host cell energy to reproduce. After a sufficient amount of Chlamydia have formed, some transform back into inclusion bodies, exit the cell, and infect others.

Clinical Presentation Chlamydia is a silent infection without symptoms in approximately 50% of infected males and 80% of infected females. In women, it can present as inflammation of the cervix on pelvic examination. The infection sometimes causes a mucopurulent cervicitis in females and urethritis in males, which alerts the patient of the need for treatment. From the cervix the bacteria can easily ascend upward into the uterus and infect the fallopian tubes, termed salpingitis; this infection can cause obstruction and scarring of the fallopian tubes and lead to infertility.

In males, up to 50% of nongonococcal urethritis can be attributed to Chlamydia. Aside from infecting the cervix in the female and urethra in the male, Chlamydia can infect the rectum or the pharynx, depending on sexual practices. Without early diagnosis, ascending infection can result in PID in women and is the most common cause of epididymitis in men younger than 35 years. Of women with PID, 5% to 10% develop peritonitis and perihepatitis, also called Fitz-Hugh-Curtis syndrome. Fibrotic adhesions develop around the liver and cause right upper quadrant tenderness of the abdomen.

Chlamydial infection develops in 60% of newborns who are delivered vaginally to infected mothers. Newborns can develop inclusion conjunctivitis, which presents as mucopurulent discharge of the eyes. The inflammation of the conjunctiva begins between 7 and 12 days after birth. *C. trachomatis* is one of the most common causes of pneumonia in the newborn and can cause blindness.

Diagnosis. The lack of reported symptoms caused by silent infection makes clinical assessment difficult. It also contributes to the delay in treatment. Because the disease is prevalent among adolescents and young adults, raising awareness and screening in this population is important.

Chlamydial infection causes inflammation of the cervix with fragile epithelial lesions that bleed easily. Frequently, a mucopurulent discharge can be visualized at the cervical opening (cervical os) on pelvic examination. External signs are usually not visible to the infected woman; however, many times, slight vaginal bleeding after intercourse can be indicative of the infection.

There are several methods for laboratory analysis and diagnosis of Chlamydia. Endocervical, rectal, urethral, and oropharyngeal secretions can be cultured. It is important to be sure to sample cells from the endocervix in women and 1 to 2 cm deep into the urethra in men. A urine sample can also reveal the microorganism. An HIV test should be performed, and in women a Pap smear should be done. Women should also be given a pregnancy test because certain treatments for Chlamydia are contraindicated in pregnancy. Tissue culture, PCR, direct fluorescent antibody (DFA), and enzyme-linked immunosorbent assay (ELISA) are the laboratory tests used to identify Chlamydia. A direct DNA probe test on urine can also be used. In addition, an RNA test can be used on liquid cytology Pap smear samples.

In the newborn with *C. trachomatis* conjunctivitis, discharge from the eye can be sampled and cultured. Chlamydial inclusion bodies found in the cells of the sample are diagnostic.

Treatment. The CDC recommendations for treatment of Chlamydia STD include antibiotics and patient education. Tetracycline, Amoxicillin, or Erythromycin are commonly used for Chlamydia infection. For assurance of cure, a repeat diagnostic test should be done 3 weeks after initial treatment. A positive test is usually not a failure of treatment, but a sign of noncompliance or reinfection. Reinfection often occurs if the sexual partner is not treated. It is important the infected person make sexual partners aware of the diagnosis and need for treatment. Newborns are treated with erythromycin ophthalmic ointment at birth to prevent Chlamydia conjunctivitis.

Gonorrhea

Neisseria gonorrhoeae is a bacterial organism that infects mucous membranes by sexual transmission. Infections can cause cervicitis, proctitis, urethritis, PID, conjunctivitis, and pharyngitis. Complications include ectopic pregnancy, infertility, and increased susceptibility to HIV. During vaginal delivery, newborns can contract gonorrhea and develop conjunctivitis, which may lead to blindness.

Epidemiology. *N. gonorrhoeae* infection is a prevalent STD, with an estimated 200 million new cases annually worldwide. It is a reportable disease in the United States, with approximately 700,000 cases annually. Because it is an underdiagnosed disease, prevalence may be as much as 50% higher than reported. The rate of gonorrhea is higher in African Americans compared with Caucasians. There is a high prevalence of infection in the rural, southeastern United States, as well as in urban areas.

Incidence of gonorrhea in men is similar to that of women, at 128 per 100,000. The major age group affected consists of individuals who are 19- to 24-year-olds. It is transmitted through sexual contact; however, infected untreated mothers can also transmit the disease to their newborns. Incidence of gonorrhea in children usually indicates sexual abuse and should be reported.

Risk Factors. The major risk factor associated with gonorrheal infection is sexual contact. Multiple sex partners, male homosexuality, and lack of condom protection are also risk factors. Perinatal transmission to the newborn during vaginal childbirth can cause an eye infection. Gonorrhea commonly causes neonatal conjunctivitis, a mucopurulent eye infection called ophthalmia neonatorum, which is treatable with antibiotics. Sepsis is also possible in the infected newborn. MSM have the highest rate of carrier status and frequently contract antibiotic-resistant strains of gonococcus. Untreated gonorrhea can result in epididymitis in men and PID in women. *N. gonorrhoeae* and *C. trachomatis* account for most cases of epididymitis in men younger than 35 years. In women, infection can be followed by salpingitis, resulting in scarring of the fallopian tubes, infertility, or ectopic pregnancy.

Pathophysiology. *N. gonorrhoeae* is a gram-negative, diplococcal bacterium. It is spread by sexual contact, including vaginal, anal, and oral sex, or through vertical transmission during childbirth. It mainly affects human columnar epithelium, making any mucous membrane susceptible to infection. It is commonly transmitted to individuals in combination with HIV and Chlamydia.

The gonococcal organism has unique characteristics that enhance its virulence. The gonococcal surface has pili, which are hairlike appendages that allow the bacteria's attachment to mucosal surfaces. They are adherent to mucosal membranes, particularly the cervix, urethra, and conjunctiva of the eye.

The gonococcal organisms are resistant to many of the body's defense mechanisms because of their genetic mutation ability. Gonococcal organisms carry antibiotic-resistance genes, most notably penicillinase-coding genes. Therefore, most gonococcal organisms can resist penicillin, and many strains are becoming resistant to quinolones. The gonococcal organism also has frequent mutation of surface protein-coding genes that allows transformation in its appearance to the immune system. The surface antigens change, elude host immune processes, and easily result in reinfection of the host.

Retrograde spread of gonorrhea from the cervix into the uterus, fallopian tubes, and abdomen can lead to PID, gonococcal peritonitis, and perihepatitis known as Fitz-Hugh-Curtis syndrome.

Gonococcal conjunctivitis can occur in adults, as well as children, following direct transfer of organisms by hand-eye contact. Gonococcal conjunctivitis can lead to blindness. Neonatal gonococcal disease of the eyes, called ophthalmia neonatorum, can occur at childbirth.

Uniquely, changes in the vaginal pH that occur during menses, pregnancy, and the postpartum period make the vaginal environment more suitable for the growth of gonococcus and provide increased access to the bloodstream. This allows disseminated gonococcal infection that can affect the skin, joints, heart, and meninges.

Clinical Presentation. Ninety percent of infected men and 50% of infected women complain of symptoms with gonococcal infection. Men develop dysuria 2 to 5 days after exposure, often followed by copious purulent discharge. Women will often be asymptomatic or report a purulent vaginal discharge, dysuria, genital pruritus, and occasional vaginal spotting. Abdominal pain usually indicates PID. Asymptomatic urethral and cervical infections are present in 10% to 50% of cases. Gonococcal infection of the conjunctiva can result in blindness. Also, gonococcal infection of the bloodstream can lead to arthritis, meningitis, or myocarditis. Reiter's syndrome is an autoimmune disorder commonly triggered by a gonococcal infection. In this disorder, arthritis, conjunctivitis, uveitis, cervicitis, penile balanitis, and urethritis occurs. The knee and sacroiliac joints are often involved.

Diagnosis. Purulent exudate can be sampled and cultured for identification of the microorganism and antibiotic sensitivity. In the female, it is very important to collect the specimen from the endocervix with a large swab. In the male, the swab should be inserted 1 to 2 cm into the urethra. Urine culture can demonstrate urethral gonococcus in men. With cervical or urethral infection, anal culture should also be sampled. If pharyngeal gonococcus infection is suspected, a throat culture is also necessary. Gram stain and culture are commonly used, but molecular testing that includes DNA probe and PCR methods are simpler screening methods. One swab can test for more than one STD. Patients suspected of having gonorrhea should also be checked for HIV, Chlamydia, HBV, herpes simplex, and syphilis; in addition, women should receive a pregnancy test.

Treatment. Treatment should be based on analysis of the microorganism's specific antibiotic sensitivity. If the patient has not been tested for Chlamydia, the CDC recommends treating for Chlamydia at the same time as gonorrhea. There is a strain of quinolone-resistant gonococcal bacteria in the high risk population. For this reason, the CDC recommends not to use quinolone, but instead a different antibiotic, in the MSM population or those individuals who have HIV. Persons infected with gonorrhea are advised to notify sexual partners of the need for treatment.

Infants can become infected from cervical or vaginal exudates during delivery. The infection manifests itself after 2 to 5 days as sepsis or ophthalmia neonatorum. Sepsis can include meningitis and rhinitis. Symptoms improve with prompt antibiotic treatment.

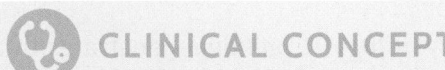

CLINICAL CONCEPT

In order to prevent gonorrheal ophthalmia neonatorum, most states mandate use of erythromycin or tetracycline ointment in the eye of the newborn at birth as prophylaxis. The antibiotics also prevent chlamydia eye infection.

Syphilis

Syphilis is an infectious disease caused by the bacterial organism ***Treponema pallidum,*** a spirochete. Syphilis is transmissible by sexual contact, transplacentally from mother to fetus in utero, via blood product transfusion, and occasionally through breaks in the skin that come into contact with infectious lesions. Syphilis has many different presentations; in advanced stages, it affects almost every body system, making it known as "the great impostor."

Epidemiology. Syphilis was a common infection before the invention of penicillin in the 1940s. Following the introduction of penicillin, syphilis incidence greatly declined, reaching its lowest point in the year 2000 with

2.1 cases per 100,000. Since then, rates have been increasing, primarily because of an increased incidence among MSM. Men are affected more frequently than women, with a male-to-female incidence ratio of approximately 6 to 1. The incidence rate of syphilis is highest in people aged 25 to 29 years (8.9 per 100,000). African Americans are affected more frequently than Caucasians, with an incidence 5.6 times higher than the incidence in Caucasians.

Etiology. Syphilis is caused by *T. pallidum*, which is a long, spiral-shaped bacterium called a spirochete. The bacterium enters the body via mucous membranes, transplacentally to a fetus, or through blood-to-blood transfer. The organism can survive only briefly outside of the body; transmission almost always requires direct contact with the infectious lesion.

Risk Factors. People considered at high risk for syphilis include persons who engage in high-risk sexual behavior, persons diagnosed with other STDs, those who exchange sex for drugs, intravenous drug abusers, and incarcerated adults. In addition, the fetus can be infected transplacentally in pregnant women.

> ### CLINICAL CONCEPT
>
> Patients who have syphilis should be tested for HIV, hepatitis B, gonorrhea, HPV, herpes simplex, chlamydia, h.ducreyi and hepatitis C. There is an estimated 2- to 5-fold increased risk of acquiring HIV when syphilis is present.

Pathophysiology *T. pallidum* penetrates intact mucous membranes and, within a few hours, enters the lymphatics and bloodstream. The incubation period from time of exposure to development of a primary lesion can range from 10 to 90 days.

There are four specific phases of syphilis infection: primary, secondary, latent, and tertiary. In the primary phase, syphilis bacteria enter the host through mucous membranes or a break in the skin. At the point of contact, treponema organisms multiply. Two to ten weeks after contact, the primary manifestation becomes apparent: a sore known as a **chancre** (see Fig. 28-1). The chancre is usually on the external genitalia, and it heals within about a week. As it heals, *T. pallidum* organisms enter the bloodstream.

After 2 to 10 weeks, the secondary stage develops, in which a rash develops all over the body. Bacteria disseminate throughout the lymphatics and bloodstream and tissue injury occurs. Invasion of the tissues occurs with cellular changes that include endothelial injury, called endarteritis, and infiltrates that contain numerous plasma cells, macrophages, and T cells.

Both primary and secondary syphilis are highly infectious states, during which spirochetes can be recovered

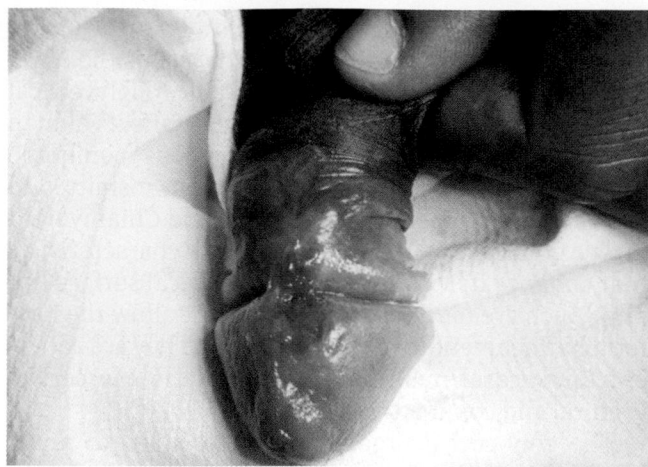

FIGURE 28-1. Chancre lesion of primary syphilis. *(Courtesy of CDC.)*

from lesions and the bloodstream. After the lesions of secondary syphilis heal, there is a latent period, during which time one-third of infected persons heal spontaneously, another third remain asymptomatic, and another third progress to tertiary syphilis. During latent disease, granulomas called **gummas,** which consist of macrophages, plasma cells, and T cells, form in many different organs. The granulomatous lesions interfere with organ function and can be found in the skin, bones, liver, heart, and brain. Aortic valve deformity and aortic aneurysm are common forms of cardiovascular syphilis. Some of the granulomatous lesions cause ulceration and necrosis of tissue.

Tertiary syphilis is the stage of degenerative changes in various organs of the body. Lesions in the neurological system commonly cause mental status changes, as well as vision and hearing disorders. Neurosyphilis can cause meningitis, stroke, paresis, and dementia. Aortic arteritis and neurological degeneration are disorders characteristic of tertiary syphilis.

> ### CLINICAL CONCEPT
>
> The treponema microorganism is evident in the bloodstream throughout the infection, which can span decades. A low level of antibodies stay in the blood for months to years after the disease has been treated.

Clinical Presentation. The primary stage of syphilis, demonstrated by a skin lesion called a chancre, is the most clinically observable sign of the infection. The chancre, usually located in the genital area weeks after sexual contact, starts as a papule and becomes an ulcerlike lesion. This lesion often goes unnoticed by the infected person because it is painless. The primary lesion usually is associated with regional lymphadenopathy that may be unilateral or bilateral. Inguinal lymph nodes are enlarged, firm, mobile, and painless, without overlying skin changes.

After this chancre heals, a rash, appearing as erythematous maculopapular lesions over all areas of the body, becomes observable in some individuals. Uniquely, the rash can appear on the palms of the hands and soles of the feet. This nonpruritic rash is often the first visible sign of illness to the patient. The rash can also present as pustular or mixed lesions. Patchy areas of alopecia may occur. Systemic symptoms of secondary syphilis include malaise, sore throat, headache, fever, anorexia, and, rarely, the stiff neck of meningitis. Gastrointestinal dysfunction, arteritis, hepatitis, proctitis, arthritis, and optic neuritis can also occur. Commonly, **condyloma lata,** wartlike lesions, can be found in the genital region.

After the body rash fades, there is a latent asymptomatic period that can last for years. Gradual damage to organs with formation of granulomas (gummas) develops during latent syphilis. Tertiary syphilis occurs when there are granulomatous lesions in the neurological system. These lesions commonly cause mental status changes, as well as vision and hearing disorders. Neurosyphilis can cause meningitis, stroke, paresis, and dementia. The patient can be referred to as suffering from syphilitic insanity. **Tabes dorsalis** is the term used for syphilitic involvement of the posterior columns of the spinal cord that causes ataxia and sensory changes in the limbs. The Argyll Robertson pupil is a neurological phenomenon in syphilis that causes a nonreactive pupil.

Syphilis can also be transmitted by the mother to her fetus. This transmission occurs when the placenta is beginning to function, at 10 to 15 weeks gestation. *T. pallidum* crosses the placenta, where it can cause miscarriage or stillbirth. Even if the fetus is born alive, there are often signs of congenital syphilis, such as **Hutchison teeth,** saddle nose, and various neurological manifestations. There is a 100% chance of transmission if the mother has early syphilis, because it is at that time that the spirochetes can pass through the placenta. If the mother has been infected for a long time, transmission is less likely.

Diagnosis. Various tests are available for the diagnosis of syphilis. Serological tests are most commonly used and search for treponemal antigen or antibodies in the blood. The serological tests used are called the venereal disease research laboratory (VDRL), rapid plasma reagin (RPR), ICE syphilis recombinant antigen test, and fluorescent treponemal antibody (FTA-ABS) test. The results are expressed in terms of antibody levels, or titers. It is recommended that all pregnant women be tested for syphilis at the first prenatal visit.

Unlike other infections, which show a decline in titers or become nonreactive with effective treatment, syphilis antibody-specific tests usually remain reactive for life. Therefore, treponemal-specific test titers are not useful for assessing treatment efficacy.

The enzyme immunoassay (EIA) test is used to screen large numbers of individuals and can be used at any stage during syphilis.

PCR testing for syphilis can be used for diagnosis during the primary syphilis stage, but it displays only moderate sensitivity in blood from secondary syphilis.

Lumbar puncture for analysis of CSF should be done in patients suspected of suffering from neurosyphilis. All patients tested for syphilis should also be tested for HIV infection.

CT scanning and magnetic resonance imaging (MRI) of the head and body may be used to document the complications of tertiary syphilis.

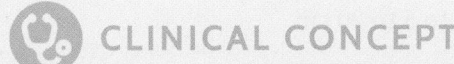

CLINICAL CONCEPT

An antibody titer against syphilis remains reactive for life.

Treatment. The treatment of syphilis depends on whether the infection is in the primary, secondary, latent, or tertiary stage. Often, a patient is being treated because of a positive screening test and has no history of an infection and no signs and symptoms of syphilis. Usually, the clinician chooses to err on the side of caution by treating for a higher level of involvement. Benzathine penicillin, administered intramuscularly, is the single drug of choice in the treatment of syphilis. A phenomenon called the **Jarisch-Herxheimer reaction** can occur during treatment. This occurs when large numbers of bacteria are killed by antibiotic all at once, causing a large release of bacterial endotoxins. Fever, chills, myalgias, and exacerbation of skin lesions occur.

Lymphogranuloma Venereum, Chancroid, and Granuloma Inguinale

Lymphogranuloma venereum (LGV), chancroid, and granuloma inguinale, once uncommon in the United States, are increasingly diagnosed in HIV-infected individuals. Chancroid is thought to be transmitted through casual sexual contact, mostly from prostitutes. For this reason, one infected woman can infect several men. Uncircumcised men are most vulnerable. LGV and granuloma inguinale are both more prevalent in tropical climates. Recently, the incidence of LGV has been increasing among MSM.

Pathophysiology. Chancroid is caused by a short, compact, gram-negative streptobacillary rod, *Haemophilus ducreyi*. LGV is caused by *C. trachomatis*, and granuloma inguinale by Klebsiella granulomatis (previously called *Calymmatobacterium granulomatis*). *C. trachomatis* is an obligate intracellular bacterial organism that can only live and reproduce within the cells of the host. *K. granulomatis* is a gram-negative bacterium that contains cytoplasmic granules called Donovan bodies. Granuloma inguinale is also called Donovanosis.

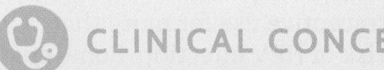

CLINICAL CONCEPT

The FTA-ABS is a first test that becomes positive in early syphilis. When this test is positive in the newborn, it provides good evidence of congenital syphilis.

Clinical Presentation. The chancrelike lesion of chancroid is soft in contrast to the more solid chancre of syphilis. *H. ducreyi* enters through a break in the skin in the genital area. Incubation of 3 to 10 days produces a papule that soon ulcerates. The ulcer of chancroid is painful, as opposed to the chancre of syphilis. Lymphadenopathy of the inguinal lymph nodes is common. These enlarged lymph nodes are called **buboes.**

LGV presents in three stages, similar to syphilis. The first stage is a painless induration at the point of entry. After this resolves, the second stage of inguinal lymphadenopathy occurs. The enlarged lymph nodes called buboes develop sinuses that yield drainage of purulent discharge. The third stage consists of anogenitorectal syndrome where proctocolitis, perirectal abscesses, and fistulas develop. Granuloma inguinale also presents as a painless indurated papule. Over months or years, it enlarges to 5 to 20 cm.

Diagnosis. All patients who have genital ulcers should be evaluated with a serological test for syphilis and a diagnostic evaluation for genital herpes. In settings where chancroid is prevalent, a test for *H. ducreyi* should also be performed. In addition, there are high rates of HIV infection among patients who have chancroid in the United States and other countries. Other laboratory tests that should be done include VDRL test or RPR, PCR assays for *H. ducreyi* and HSV2, and HIV antibodies because patients with LGV may also have contracted other STDs.

Specific tests for evaluation of genital ulcers include syphilis serology and either a dark-field examination or direct immunofluorescence test for *T. pallidum*; culture or antigen test for HSV; and culture for *H. ducreyi*. Diagnosis for LGV is made with identification of *C. trachomatis*. Laboratory diagnosis for granuloma inguinale is made by scraping the lesion and examining scraped cells under a microscope; stained K. granulomatis are observed and identified.

Nucleic acid amplification and PCR testing can be used to confirm diagnosis more accurately and more rapidly than other laboratory tests.

Treatment. Antibiotic treatment is used for all three of these infections. Ulcerated lesions usually improve symptomatically within 3 days. If no clinical improvement is evident, the clinician must consider whether the diagnosis is correct, the patient is coinfected with another STD, the patient is infected with HIV, the patient was noncompliant with treatment, or the *H. ducreyi* strain is resistant to the antibiotic. The time required for complete healing depends on the size of the ulcer; large ulcers might require more than 2 weeks. Clinical resolution of the fluctuant lymphadenopathy lesions or buboes is slower than resolution for ulcers and might require needle aspiration or incision and drainage.

Viral Infections

Human Papilloma Virus

Human papilloma virus (HPV) is a DNA virus in which approximately 70 distinct genetic types have been

---

> ## BOX 28-1. **Cancers Caused by Human Papilloma Virus**
>
> The percentages of cancers caused by oncogenic HPV are as follows:
>
> - cervical cancer: 100%
> - anal cancer: 90%
> - vulvar cancer: 40%
> - vaginal cancer: 40%
> - oropharyngeal cancer: 12%
> - oral cancer: 3%.

---

identified. Several types of these are considered to be cancer-causing (oncogenic) viruses (see Box 28-1).

Epidemiology. HPV infection is the most common sexually transmitted infection in the world. The incidence of HPV infection has dramatically increased during the past 20 years. There are 6 million new cases of HPV infection per year in the United States with a prevalence of 20 million cases annually. Approximately half of HPV cases occur in females aged 15 to 24 with the highest incidence in the 20- to 24-year-old age group. Anogenital warts, also called condylomata acuminata, are the characteristic manifestations of HPV infection. The annual incidence of anogenital warts is estimated between 500,000 and 1 million cases, with similar rates in males and females. Approximately two-thirds of individuals who have sexual contact with an infected partner develop genital warts.

HPV is detected in more than 95% of cases of cervical cancer. In the United States, 2.5 million women are estimated to have a cytological diagnosis of low-grade cervical cancer precursor annually. HPV has also been implicated in anal, vulvar, vaginal, rectal, oropharyngeal, and laryngeal cancers.

Etiology/Risk Factors. There are several types of HPV that affect humans. HPV types 6 and 11 account for the genital wart infection, condyloma acuminata. Types 16, 18, 31, 33, and 51 are more commonly found in cervical cancer. According to some sources, when the most sensitive detecting tests are used, it shows that 80% of young women are infected with HPV. Some infections can be transient and cleared by the host's immune responses. Infection rate correlates with multiple partners, early onset of sexual activity, and high frequency of different sexual partners. Patients who are immunosuppressed and those with HIV infection are at higher risk for HPV infection. Smoking and oral contraceptive use for more than 5 years also increase the risk of HPV infection. Some studies show that there is an increased prevalence of anogenital warts during pregnancy. Anal cancer caused by HPV is most common in MSM. Anal cancer caused by HPV is most common in MSM. MSM should have yearly HPV pap smears.

Pathophysiology HPVs integrate their DNA into the genetic material of the host cell. Humans are the only carriers of HPV, and the virus can live outside the body for many months. HPV reproduction occurs in keratinocytes found at the skin surface and mucous membranes. Cells containing the virus are ultimately shed into the environment. Infection occurs when mucosal epithelial cells in the host are exposed to HPV through a break in the epithelial barrier, as would occur during sexual intercourse or after minor skin abrasions. Viral genes transform the mucosal cells into benign genital warts or preneoplastic types of warts. HPV proteins inactivate the host's tumor suppressor proteins, thereby resulting in unregulated host cell proliferation and malignant transformation. HPV particles are released as a result of degeneration of desquamating cells. Although HPV is highly contagious and can lead to cancer, the immune system is capable of clearing the virus. Therefore, not all cases of HPV lead to cancer.

Clinical Presentation. **Condyloma acuminata** are fleshy growths, either single or in multiple clusters, around the vagina or anus or on the penis (see Fig. 28-2). They are easily visible with the naked eye. They seem to enlarge during pregnancy under the influence of hormones.

Diagnosis. Condyloma acuminata diagnosis is made by clinical observation. Biopsy of the lesions and DNA identification techniques can be used to detect the viral genome. It is important to sample cervical, anal, vulvar, or vaginal lesions. ELISA for IgG associated with HPV can also be done. Because HPV infection is often associated with other STDs, other diagnostic tests for HIV, HBV, hepatitis C, herpes virus simplex, Chlamydia, syphilis, and gonococcus should be done. Pap smear is important to screen women for cervical cancer. Pap smear can catch early dysplasia or more serious changes in the cells of the cervix. Colposcopy allows a closer look at cells that are suspicious of cancer. Cone biopsy can sample cells for histological evaluation. Anal Pap smear should be done annually on MSM.

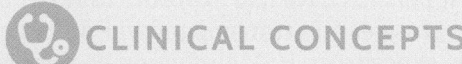

CLINICAL CONCEPTS

Women diagnosed with HPV are strongly advised to have a Pap smear every year, and to have any suspicious lesions removed.

Treatment. There is no cure for HPV, because it is a viral infection. Condyloma acuminata can be treated with application of topical podophyllin, trichloroacetic acid, or laser surgery. Although these treatments can reduce the appearance of the warts, the virus remains in the person's body. Most persons need multiple treatments.

Treatment of cervical dysplasia and cancer is treated according to the level of invasion. Cryosurgery of the cervix and total hysterectomy are common treatments. Treated women require a follow-up Pap smear every 3 years. There is no reported risk to fertility from HPV. There is a possibility of papilloma infection in the pharynx of children born of mothers with extensive genital warts.

CLINICAL CONCEPT

A vaccine called Gardasil® is available that offers protection against HPV. The vaccine has demonstrated nearly 100% efficacy in preventing precancerous lesions of the cervix and vagina. Vaccination of school-aged girls and boys is recommended.

Herpes Simplex Virus

Herpes simplex virus (HSV) causes genital herpes. These viruses are capable of causing both acute and latent viral infections. During the acute phase, the virus is highly proliferative and symptomatic, causing vesicular lesions on the skin. However, during the latent phase of the infection, the viral DNA remains in the neuron's nucleus in a dormant state, when no viral proteins are produced. During this dormant state, the immune system does not detect the virus; however, the virus can reactivate at a later time, causing symptoms. At times of immunosuppression, the virus commonly reactivates.

There are two herpes viruses: herpes simplex type 1 (HSV1) and herpes simplex type 2 (HSV2). HSV1 most commonly causes oral "cold sores" and HSV2 most

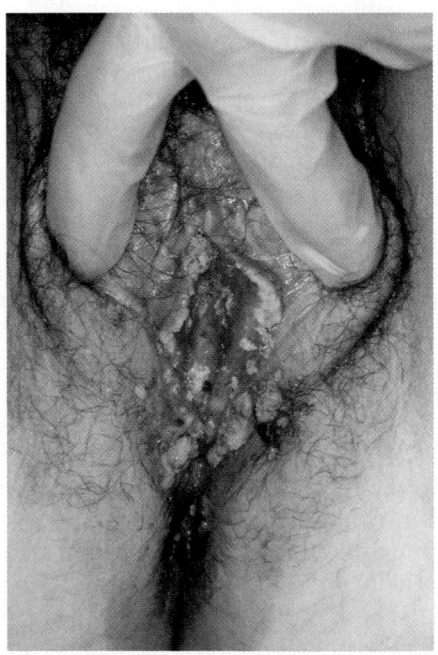

FIGURE 28-2. Genital warts caused by HPV. *(Courtesy of CDC/ Joe Millar.)*

commonly causes genital infection transmitted through sexual activity. However, either virus can cause infection in either region. In the literature, when the term genital herpes is used, this indicates an HSV2 infection.

Epidemiology. The prevalence of genital HSV infection worldwide has increased over the last several decades, making it a major public health concern. It is estimated that 50 million persons are infected annually. Most persons have had exposure to HSV1 by adulthood, as it is readily transmitted via oral secretions. However, exposure to HSV2 infection begins at puberty and is correlated with level of sexual activity. HSV2 infection is more common in women than men. Also, HSV2 can be transmitted to the neonate at childbirth because of contact with maternal genital lesions. It is important to recognize that the presence of HSV2 infection in children can be a sign of sexual abuse. Most persons who have HSV2 infection are not aware that they are infected, so they can transmit the virus during sexual contact. Genital herpes is a lifelong viral illness, with exacerbations when symptoms are present and remissions when symptoms are absent.

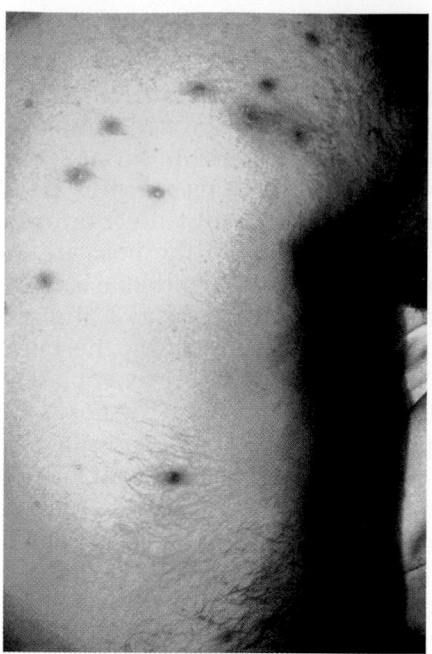

FIGURE 28-3. Genital herpes. *(Courtesy of CDC.)*

 CLINICAL CONCEPT

HSV2 can be transmitted during symptomatic and asymptomatic periods.

Pathophysiology. Humans are the only carriers of HSV, which is a DNA virus. The features of HSV infection are skin invasion, neurological involvement, dormancy, and reactivation. HSV1 or HSV2 virus enters the mucosa or injured epithelium at the site of contact. Close skin contact, mucosa secretions, or saliva can transmit HSV. The virus reproduces within the skin, causing blisters and ulceration, but travels rapidly to the dorsal ganglion of sensory nerves. In the neurons, the virus either (1) replicates and travels back to the skin, where it produces blisters, or (2) becomes dormant until later reactivation. The time from initial contraction to infection is 6 to 7 days. The virus usually remains dormant within the trigeminal or sacral spinal nerves. During times of low immunity or stress, reactivation often occurs.

Clinical Presentation. Classic manifestations of HSV infection include local tenderness, burning, and erythema, followed by eruption of vesicles that rupture into painful ulcers covered with yellow exudates (see Fig. 28-3). The patient may have fever and lymphadenopathy in the region of lesions. Crusting of ulcerative lesions occurs after several days. New lesions appear through the first week, peaking between 8 to 10 days. Dysuria, urethritis, meningitis, and pharyngitis can be the symptoms, depending on the site of infection. Lesions are commonly observable on the external genitalia and perineal area of both males and females. However, lesions can also appear within the vaginal canal and cervix. Recurrences of herpes infection are usually similar in symptomatology, but have a much shorter duration.

Diagnosis. To diagnose HPV infection, a swab samples the lesion exudate, which is then cultured on specialized media called a Tzanck smear. Serological testing, which demonstrates HSV antibody levels in the blood, can also be used. However, a rise in antibody titer does not occur during recurrences of HSV infection. Therefore, the test is generally not useful for the diagnosis of HSV relapse. Detection of HSV DNA in clinical specimens is possible with PCR techniques. PCR can detect viral shedding during symptomatic or asymptomatic phases. Currently there is no recommendation for universal screening of the population for HSV infection.

Treatment. There is no cure for HSV. The antiviral medication, acyclovir, is used to treat the infection. Treatment is aimed at reducing symptoms and the extent of outbreak. Importantly, treatment can prevent infection from mother to fetus. The CDC recommends treatment with antiviral medication 3 times a day for 7 to 10 days.

Herpes infection is usually self-limited, except when pregnancy occurs and a fetus is involved. In women, during a herpetic attack, the cervix is almost always involved. Neonatal HSV infection can occur transplacentally to the fetus. More often, however, the mother transmits the infection during delivery as the neonate passes through the birth canal. Maternal transmission of HSV to the neonate can occur whether the mother is symptomatic or asymptomatic at the time of birth. Herpes encephalitis or meningitis is the feared complication in the newborn.

Pelvic Inflammatory Disease

Pelvic inflammatory disease (PID) is the most serious STD in women; 85% of the cases occur in women of childbearing age. Any infection ascending from the vagina and cervix to the internal upper reproductive organs, including the uterus, fallopian tubes, or ovaries, is considered PID. Women who are most at risk include those who have a history of multiple sex partners, past STDs, intrauterine device use, or failure to use contraceptive methods. Women who have had a dilatation and curettage (D&C), abortion by vacuum curettage, or hysterosalpingogram are at increased risk.

Pathophysiology. The majority of cases of PID are caused by *N. Gonorrhoeae* or *C. trachomatis*. Less commonly, PID is caused by aerobic and anaerobic organisms, such as *G. vaginalis*, *Prevotella* sp., *H. influenzae*, *E. coli*, *S. agalactiae*, *S. pyogenes*, *S. pneumoniae*, Cytomegalovirus, *M. hominis*, and *U. urealyticum*.

The two phases involved in PID are (1) infection of vagina or cervix and (2) upward ascent of the infection into the uterus, fallopian tubes, and ovary. Inflammation of the vaginal canal, sexual activity, and disruption of the balance of flora in the vagina allow the microorganisms to reach the internal organs. Inflammation resulting from *N. gonorrhoeae* and *C. trachomatis* infections makes the fallopian tubes susceptible to invasion by anaerobic organisms. When the causative organism is *N. gonorrhoeae*, exudates from the fallopian tubes may enter the peritoneum, causing pelvic peritonitis. The uterus, fallopian tubes, and ovaries can become fixed by pelvic inflammatory adhesions. Fallopian tubes and ovaries often adhere to the posterior uterus or are prolapsed in the cul-de-sac; this disrupts the position of the uterus, causing dyspareunia, chronic pelvic pain, and infertility. Peritoneal involvement may result in perihepatitis or Fitz-Hugh-Curtis syndrome, a disorder that causes adhesions of the outer liver.

C. trachomatis salpingitis is usually asymptomatic, which is why universal screening has been recommended for women younger than age 25 years. The organism can attach to sperm, which ascend to the fallopian tube and cause cell injury and scarring of the tube by destroying the cilia. The ciliated cells of the fallopian tubes are very important in moving an ova into the uterus; interference with their function can lead to infertility.

Clinical Presentation. When a woman of childbearing age presents with such symptoms as lower abdominal pain, pelvic tenderness, or possible genital tract infection or inflammation, further investigation is necessary (see Box 28-2). If uterine and adnexal tenderness are present and if pain with cervical motion exists, the diagnosis of PID should be considered.

PID presents as an acute, chronic, or silent infection. The acute presentation, which is characterized by the classic pelvic pain and possibly fever or chills, is the more common presentation and is more apt to be treated. The causative organism in the acute type of PID is most often

---

BOX 28-2. Diagnoses to Exclude When PID Is Suspected

When pelvic or abdominal pain is part of the clinical presentation, PID and the following conditions must be ruled out:

- ectopic pregnancy
- acute appendicitis
- ruptured ovarian cyst
- endometritis
- endometriosis
- septic abortion
- tubo-ovarian abscess.

N. gonorrhoeae. The silent type, which is usually caused by Chlamydia, has a more insidious presentation and is often misdiagnosed as a mild salpingitis; thus, it is not treated as aggressively. Because of its unrecognized, silent presentation, it may account for up to 40% of infertility cases involving tubal dysfunction. In chronic PID, inflammation of the walls of the fallopian tubes leaves scars, which then create problems for egg transport.

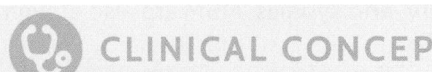
CLINICAL CONCEPT

If there is exquisite tenderness of the cervix on a pelvic examination, this is often called a Chandelier sign, which is pathognomonic for PID.

Diagnosis. PID can be difficult to diagnose. A general health and sexual history is essential, as are a physical examination and pelvic examination. A pregnancy test is also required because ectopic pregnancy is possible. Specific symptoms and laboratory test findings are usually the sources used to diagnose PID (see Box 28-3). Imaging studies usually do not contribute much to the diagnosis. MRI may visualize thickened, inflamed fallopian tubes, uterus, and ovaries. Transvaginal ultrasound might visualize some inflammation of the ovaries, uterus, and fallopian tubes. Laparoscopic examination of the abdomen and pelvic region may be necessary.

ALERT! Any woman presenting with abdominal or pelvic pain should have a pregnancy test to rule out ectopic pregnancy.

Treatment. According to CDC guidelines, clinicians may treat a patient with PID as an outpatient or an inpatient. The decision to hospitalize the patient depends on certain criteria (see Box 28-4). Regardless of place of treatment, the patient with PID is treated with high dose antibiotics.

BOX 28-3. Diagnosing Pelvic Inflammatory Disease

Pelvic or lower abdominal pain, in combination with the following signs and symptoms, strengthen the diagnosis of PID:

- oral temperature of 101°F
- abnormal vaginal or cervical mucopurulent discharge
- presence of white blood cells (on microscopic survey of vaginal secretions)
- elevated erythrocyte sedimentation rate
- elevated C-reactive protein
- laboratory documentation of gonococcus or Chlamydia.

BOX 28-4. Criteria for Hospitalization in PID

The following criteria can be used when deciding whether or not to hospitalize a patient with suspected PID:

- when diagnosis is uncertain
- if surgical emergencies cannot be excluded
- if a pelvic abscess is suspected
- if the woman is pregnant
- if the patient is a minor
- if the patient's condition is severe, such as high fever, nausea, or vomiting
- if the patient is unable to follow or tolerate an outpatient regimen, or if clinical follow-up is not possible within 72 hours of starting treatment.

Chapter Summary

- Female adolescents and young adult women are at increased risk of infection with HPV, Chlamydia, gonorrhea, HIV, and syphilis. MSM are also at high risk for these STDs.

- *Chlamydia trachomatis* is the most common cause of an STD. It causes cervicitis, urethritis, PID, and a type of conjunctivitis known as inclusion conjunctivitis. It is usually a silent, asymptomatic disease.

- Gonorrheal infections can cause cervicitis, proctitis, urethritis, PID, conjunctivitis, and pharyngitis. Complications include ectopic pregnancy, infertility, and increased susceptibility to HIV. Strains are becoming increasingly resistant to antibiotics.

- Syphilis infection occurs in four stages: primary, secondary, latent, and tertiary. Syphilis has many different presentations and in advanced stages it can appear as many other diseases, making it known as "the great impostor." The classic lesion of syphilis is the painless chancre. Granulomas, called gummas, develop in different organs. Syphilis infection can span several decades. Syphilis increases susceptibility to HIV infection.

- Lymphogranuloma venereum (LGV) and granuloma inguinale are both more prevalent in tropical climates. MSM are at increased risk for LGV. Classic signs of disease are buboes, which are enlarged inguinal lymph nodes.

- HPV infection is a precursor to cervical, anal, rectal, oropharyngeal, and laryngeal cancer. Condyloma acuminata are the genital warts that occur in HPV infection. There is no cure, but there is a vaccine available.

- Genital herpes, commonly referred to as HSV2, is a lifelong viral illness, with periods of exacerbations when symptoms are present and remissions when symptoms are absent. It is important to understand that HSV2 can be transmitted during symptomatic and asymptomatic periods.

- The majority of cases of PID are caused by *N. gonorrhoeae* or *C. trachomatis*. Women with abdominal or pelvic pain should have a pregnancy test to rule out ectopic pregnancy. Complications associated with PID are ectopic pregnancy and infertility.

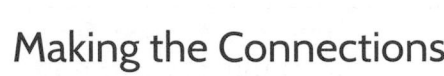

Making the Connections

Disorder and Pathophysiology	Signs and Symptoms	Physical Assessment Findings	Diagnostic Testing	Treatment

Bacterial Infections

Chlamydia | An obligate intracellular microorganism that reproduces in the cells of the host. Chlamydia can protect itself from the host's immune system by converting into a sporelike inclusion body.

	Signs and Symptoms	Physical Assessment Findings	Diagnostic Testing	Treatment
	Often asymptomatic in both males and females. Female: possible vaginal bleeding/discharge. Male: possible urethritis.	Female: pelvic exam shows friable cervix and discharge. Male: painful urination and discharge from meatus.	Culture in special medium. Characteristic inclusion body found in cervical cells.	Antibiotics.

Gonorrhea | Gonococcus is a gram-negative diplococcal microorganism that invades mucosal epithelium. It is highly virulent because of pili that attach to mucosa. Organism has a high mutation ability.

	Signs and Symptoms	Physical Assessment Findings	Diagnostic Testing	Treatment
	Often asymptomatic in both males and females. Females: purulent vaginal discharge can occur. Males: urethritis can occur.	If symptomatic, purulent discharge. Female: inflamed cervix. Male: painful urination, discharge from penile meatus.	Culture on special medium. Gram stain slide on microscope. PCR testing can identify organism DNA.	Antibiotics are curative.

Syphilis | A bacterial spirochete, *T. pallidum*, that can infect the body and remain dormant for decades. It invades mucous membranes or can be transferred to the fetus through placenta. It forms granulomas called "gummas" that disrupt body organs.

	Signs and Symptoms	Physical Assessment Findings	Diagnostic Testing	Treatment
	Primary stage: painless chancre on the external genitalia Often not readily apparent. Secondary stage: rash appears on body, palms, and soles of feet. Tertiary stage: neurological and cardiovascular complications become apparent.	Painless ulcerated lesion at site of inoculation. Maculopapular rash all over body, including palm of hands and soles of feet. Late stages cause neurological problems such as ataxia, stroke, and dementia.	Dark-field microscope (observe spirochetes). VDRL: positive. RPR: positive. Fluorescent treponemal antibodies: absorbed. PCR testing can detect organism DNA.	Benzathine penicillin intramuscular injection.

LGV, Chancroid, Granuloma Inguinale | LGV is caused by *C. trachomatis*; chancroid is caused by *H. ducreyi*; and granuloma inguinale by *K. granulomatis*.

	Signs and Symptoms	Physical Assessment Findings	Diagnostic Testing	Treatment
	Soft chancre; enlarged inguinal nodes called buboes.	Ulcer at site of inoculation. Enlarged inguinal lymph nodes called buboes.	Microorganisms are found via culture. Scraping the lesion and examining scraped cells under microscope; stained bacteria are observed and identified. Nucleic acid amplification and PCR testing used.	Antibiotics are curative.

Continued

Making the Connections–cont'd

Disorder and Pathophysiology	Signs and Symptoms	Physical Assessment Findings	Diagnostic Testing	Treatment
Viral Infections				
Herpes Simplex Virus | Genital herpes can be caused by HSV1 or HSV2. Viruses invade skin and remain dormant in neurological tissue. Remissions and exacerbations of lesions can occur.				
	May be asymptomatic or painful recurrent blisters.	Blisters in pelvic area.	Viral culture of scrapings of blisters.	Antivirals such as acyclovir can only diminish symptoms; they are not curative. They can also be taken as prophylactic treatment.
HPV | These genital warts can increase the risk of cervical cancer. HPV infection can occur in other areas predisposing to cancer: anal, rectal, oropharyngeal, or laryngeal cancer.				
	Fleshy wart growths, usually in pelvic area.	Painless fleshy papules in and around genitalia or anal region.	Clinical evaluation. HPV: Pap smears to identify types.	Podophyllin, laser ablation. Trichloroacetic acid application. Not curative but can decrease appearance of warts. Frequent Pap test is needed to prevent cervical cancer.
PID | Most common causes are *N. gonorrhea* and *C. trachomatis*. The microorganisms ascend from the vagina into the uterus, fallopian tubes, and ovaries.				
	Lower abdominal pain, fever, chills, myalgias.	Cervical motion tenderness Abdominal or pelvic tenderness on palpation.	Pelvic exam shows tenderness of cervix. Specific criteria for PID.	Oral or IV antibiotics.

Bibliography

Bolan, G. A., Sparling, P. F., & Wasserheit, J. N. (2012). The emerging threat of untreatable gonococcal infection. *N Engl J Med,* 366(6), 485–487.

Brill, J. R. (2010). Diagnosis and treatment of urethritis in men. *Am Fam Phys,* 81(7), 873–878.

Coutinho, B., Baranowski, U., & Miller, E. (2008). Male patient with a genital ulceration. Primary syphilis. *Am Fam Phys,* 77(2), 215–216.

de Vries, H. J. (2014). Sexually transmitted infections in men who have sex with men. *Clinical Dermatol,* 32(2), 181–188. doi: 10.1016/j.clindermatol.2013.08.001.

Dietrich, A., Gauglitz, G. G., Pfluger, T. T., Herzinger, T., & Braun-Falco, M. (2014). Syphilitic aortitis in secondary syphilis. *JAMA Dermatol,* Mar 5. doi: 10.1001/jamadermatol.2013.9537. Epub ahead of print.

Douglas, J. M. (2009). Penicillin treatment of syphilis: clearing away the shadow on the land. *JAMA,* 301(7), 769–771.

Duncan, S., & Duncan, C. J. (2012). The emerging threat of untreatable gonococcal infection. *N Engl J Med,* 366(22), 2136.

Fantasia, H. C. (2013). Updated treatment guidelines for gonorrhea infections. *Nurs Womens Health,* 17(3), 231–235. doi: 10.1111/1751-486X.12037.

Golden, M. R., & Wasserheit, J. N. (2009). Prevention of viral sexually transmitted infections—foreskin at the forefront. *N Engl J Med,* 360(13), 1349–1351.

Gradison, M. (2012). Pelvic inflammatory disease. *Am Fam Phys,* 85(8), 791–796.

Hampton, T. (2008). Researchers seek ways to stem STDs: "alarming" STD rates found in teenaged girls. *JAMA,* 299(16), 1888–1889.

Johnson, B. K. (2013). Sexually transmitted infections and older adults. *J Gerontol Nurs,* 39(11), 53–60.

Juckett, G., & Hartman-Adams, H. (2010). Human papillomavirus: clinical manifestations and prevention. *Am Fam Phys,* 82(10), 1209–1213.

Kirkcaldy, R. D., Bolan, G. A., & Wasserheit, J. N. (2013). Cephalosporin-resistant gonorrhea in North America. *JAMA,* 309(2), 185–187. doi: 10.1001/jama.2012.205107.

Kumar, V., Abbas, A. K., & Fausto, N. (2011). *Robbins and Cotran pathologic basis of disease.* 8th ed. Philadelphia, PA: Elsevier/Saunders.

Lin, K. W., & Ramsey, L. (2008). Screening for chlamydial infection. *Am Fam Phys,* 78(12), 1349–1350.

Longo, D., Fauci, A., Braunwald, E., et al. (Eds.). (2011). *Harrison's principles of internal medicine.* 18th ed. New York: McGraw-Hill.

Lopaschuk, C. C. (2013). New approach to managing genital warts. *Can Fam Phys,* 59(7), 731–736.

Martin, R. D., & Spics, L. A. (2011). Recognizing syphilis in an HIV-infected patient. *Nurse Pract,* 36(12), 7–11. doi: 10.1097/01.NPR.0000407608.77194.2f.

Mayor, M. T., Roett, M. A., & Uduhiri, K. A. (2012). Diagnosis and management of gonococcal infections. *Am Fam Phys,* 86(10), 931–938.

Meyers, D., Mattei, P. L., Beachkofsky, T. M., Gilson, R. T., & Wisco, O. J. (2012). Syphilis: a reemerging infection. *Am Fam Phys,* 86(5), 433–440.

Meyers, D., Wolff, T., Gregory, K., et al. (2008). USPSTF recommendations for STI screening. *Am Fam Phys,* 77(6), 819–824.

Millett, G. A., Peterson, J. L., Flores, S. A., et al. (2012). Comparisons of disparities and risks of HIV infection in black and other men who have sex with men in Canada, UK, and USA: a meta-analysis. *Lancet,* 380(9839), 341–348. Epub 2012 Jul 20.

Mishori, R., McClaskey, E. L., & WinklerPrins, V. J. (2012). *Chlamydia trachomatis* infections: screening, diagnosis, and management. *Am Fam Phys,* 86(12), 1127–1132.

Paavonen, J. (2012). Chlamydia trachomatis infections of the female genital tract: state of the art. *Ann Med,* 44(1), 18–28. doi: 10.3109/07853890.2010.546365. Epub 2011 Feb 1.

Plavchan, J. (2013). Testing options for the detection of gonorrhea and Chlamydia. *Am Fam Phys,* 88(5), 290–291.

Roett, M. A., Mayor, M. T., & Uduhiri, K. A. (2012). Diagnosis and management of genital ulcers. *Am Fam Phys,* 85(3), 254–262.

Ruhl, C. (2013). Update on Chlamydia and gonorrhea screening during pregnancy. *Nurs Womens Health,* 17(2), 143–146. doi: 10.1111/1751-486X.12023.

Schlecht, H. P. (2012). Oral human papillomavirus infection: hazard of intimacy. *JAMA,* 307(7), 724–725. doi: 10.1001/jama.2012.117. Epub 2012 Jan 26.

Senior, K. (2012). Chlamydia: a much underestimated STI. *Lancet Infect Disease,* 12(7), 517–518.

Smith-McCune, K. (2014). Choosing a screening method for cervical cancer: Papanicolaou testing alone or with human papillomavirus testing. *JAMA Intern Med,* May 5. doi: 10.1001/jamainternmed.2014.1368. Epub ahead of print.

Soper, D. E. (2010). Pelvic inflammatory disease. *Obstet Gyn,* 116(2 Pt 1), 419–428.

Trojian, T. H., Lishnak, T. S., & Heiman, D. (2009). Epididymitis and orchitis: an overview. *Am Fam Phys,* 79(7), 583–587.

Tronstein, E., Johnston, C., Huang, M. L., et al. (2011). Genital shedding of herpes simplex virus among symptomatic and asymptomatic persons with HSV-2 infection. *JAMA,* 305(14), 1441–1449. doi: 10.1001/jama.2011.420.

Turner, R. (2012). Strategies to prevent gonorrhoea reinfection in men. *Nurs Stand,* 26(30), 35–39.

Turner, R., Brown, L., Davidson, C., & Roberts, C. (2014). Diagnosis, treatment and prevention of gonorrhoea. *Nurs Stand,* 28(27), 37–41. doi: 10.7748/ns2014.03.28.27.37.e8336.

Vall-Mayans, M., Caballero, E., & Sanz, B. (2009). The emergence of lymphogranuloma venereum in Europe. *Lancet,* 374(9686), 356.

Van de Perre, P., & Nagot, N. (2012). Herpes simplex virus: a new era? *Lancet,* 379(9816), 598–599.

Wasserman, S., Vallie, Y., & Bryer, A. (2011). The great pretender. *Lancet,* 377(9781), 1976.

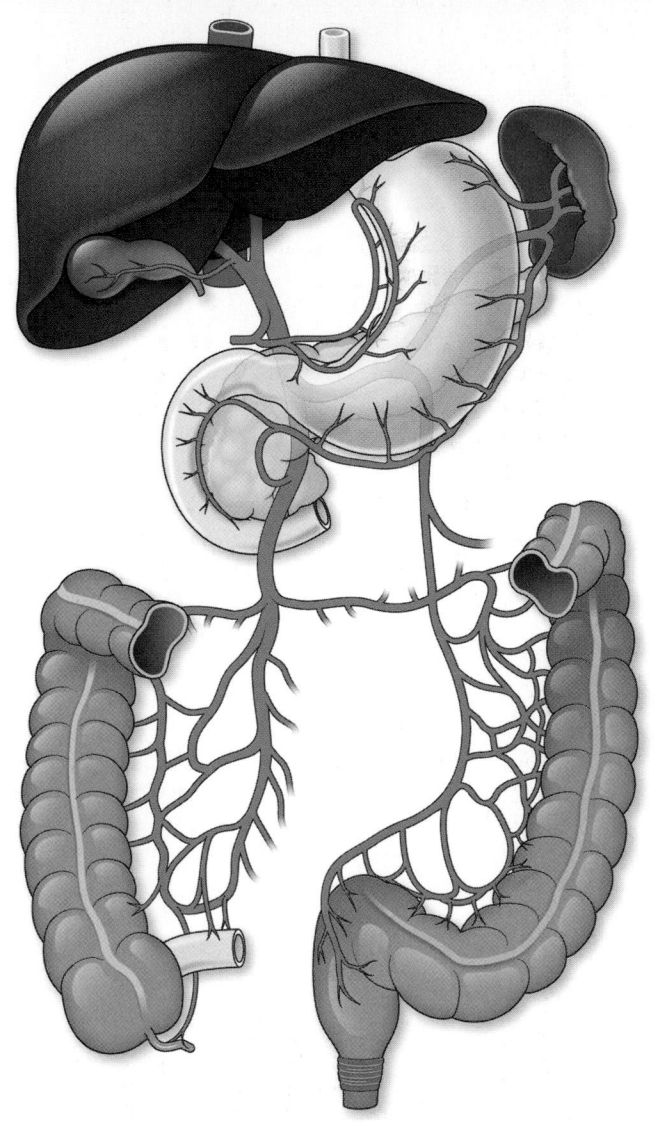

Chapters

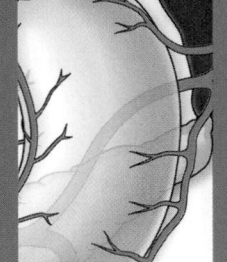

Key Terms

Achalasia
Barrett's esophagus
Borborygmi
Celiac disease
Dyspepsia
Dysphagia
Enterohepatic circulation
Gastroesophageal reflux disease (GERD)

Gastroparesis
Hematemesis
Hiatal hernia
Laparotomy
Melena
Odynophagia
Paralytic ileus

Peptic ulcer disease (PUD)
Peritoneal lavage
Peritonitis
Steatorrhea
Thrush
Upper gastrointestinal bleed (UGIB)
Villi

Gastrointestinal (GI) disease can take many forms and affects people across the world in both industrialized and undeveloped countries. GI disorders are among the most common disorders encountered within the U.S. population; however, because many individuals self-medicate using over-the-counter medications, many disorders go unreported and undiagnosed.

The GI tract can be divided into upper and lower segments. The esophagus, stomach, and small intestine comprise the upper GI tract (see Fig. 29-1). These organs have the primary role of food and fluid digestion and absorption of essential nutrients, vitamins, and minerals. Any alteration in upper GI organ function can cause indigestion, malabsorption, malnutrition, or dehydration, all of which have profound effects on the whole body.

Epidemiology

One of the major disorders of the upper GI tract is **gastroesophageal reflux disease (GERD).** This disorder is diagnosed if a person has esophagitis more than a few times a week. GERD occurs in all ages, most commonly in infants and in persons older than age 40 years. Approximately 25% to 40% of Americans experience GERD at some point in their lives.

A disorder that can be associated with esophagitis and GERD is **peptic ulcer disease (PUD).** In the United States, PUD affects approximately 4.5 million people annually. Approximately 10% of the U.S. population has evidence of a duodenal ulcer. If PUD goes untreated, there is the possibility that acute GI bleeding can occur. This potentially life-threatening abdominal emergency is a common cause of hospitalization, affecting 100,000 individuals annually in the United States.

The GI disorder that affects the most people across the world is gastroenteritis, although most cases are undiagnosed, unreported, and treated by affected individuals themselves. Most cases are caused by a virus that lasts 1 to 2 days. However, in many parts of the world, gastroenteritis is a potentially lethal condition.

Basic Concepts of Esophageal, Stomach, and Small Intestine Function

Disorders of the upper GI tract involve the esophagus, stomach, and small intestine. These organs are responsible for the major digestion and absorption of vital nutrients. Dysfunction of any of the upper GI organs can lead to malnutrition and dehydration.

Esophagus

The esophagus is a tubelike structure extending from the pharynx to the stomach that lies behind the trachea in the thorax. Two sphincters are located at each end of the esophagus: the upper esophageal sphincter (UES) and the lower esophageal sphincter (LES), also known as the cardiac sphincter. Both are contracted in their resting state and open in response to nerve stimulation.

The UES directs food and liquids into the esophagus and prevents their aspiration into the airway. The epiglottis is a membrane that closes over the trachea during eating to prevent food from entering the respiratory system. In the esophagus, ingested food moves down by peristalsis. Peristalsis occurs by the contraction and relaxation of the muscle of the esophagus, innervations by the sensory neurons, and moisture from the mucosal membranes. The peristaltic waves continue to the LES, where the vagus nerve stimulates the opening of the sphincter and the bolus is pushed into the stomach cavity.

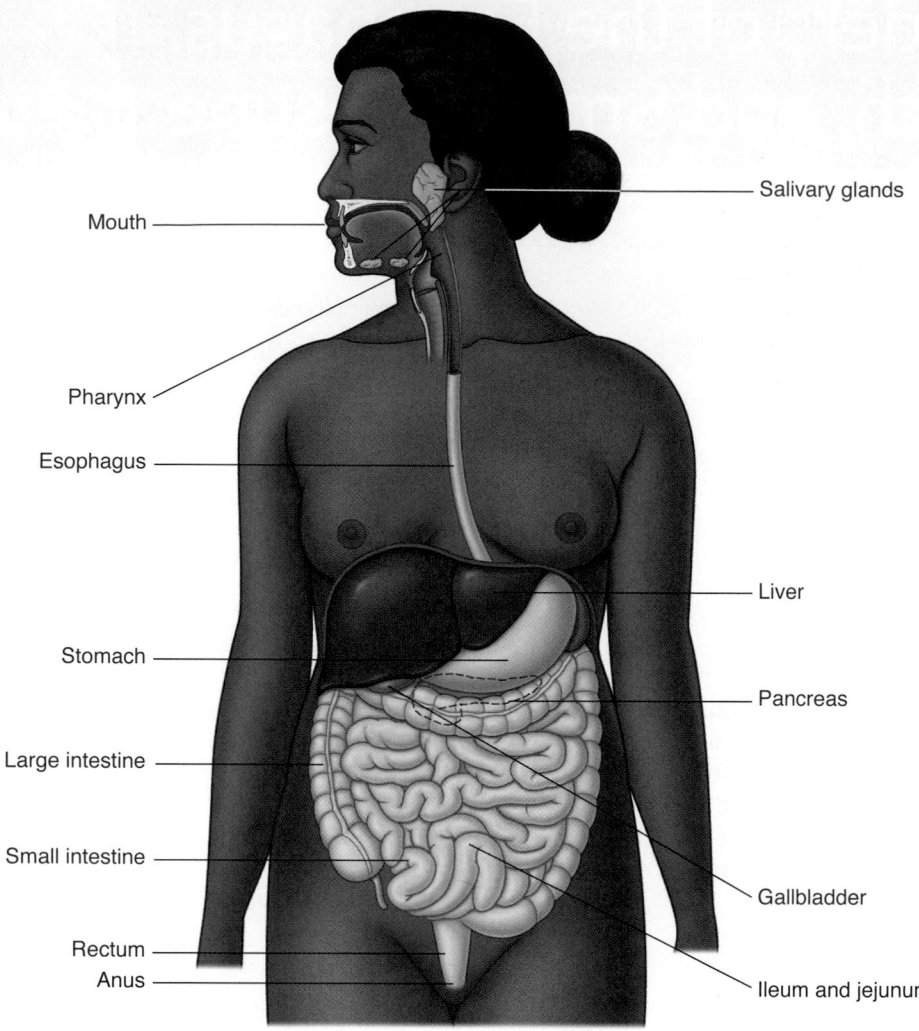

Mouth

Pharynx

Esophagus

Stomach

Large intestine

Small intestine

Rectum

Anus

Salivary glands

Liver

Pancreas

Gallbladder

Ileum and jejunum

FIGURE 29-1. The upper GI system.
(From Thompson, G. S. (2013). *Understanding anatomy and physiology.* Philadelphia, PA: F.A. Davis Company, with permission.)

Stomach

The stomach is located in the upper part of the abdomen and consists of three portions: the fundus, the uppermost portion of the stomach; the body, the center and largest part of the stomach; and the pylorus, the lower portion of the stomach. There are two sphincters that help regulate the inflow and outflow of stomach contents—the LES, located between the lower esophagus and the stomach, and the pyloric sphincter, which separates the stomach from the duodenum.

The digestive process in the stomach consists of three phases:

1. cephalic phase
2. gastric phase
3. intestinal phase.

The cephalic phase occurs in response to a sensory stimulus, such as the sight, smell, or taste of food. In this phase, there is activation of the vagal nerve, secretion of acetylcholine, and parasympathetic motor response. To follow this, cells prepare for the second phase of digestion, the gastric phase. As part of this preparation, histamine and gastrin are released from stomach cells. The gastric phase starts as food or fluids enter the stomach, stimulating the activity of mucous and gastric acid from stomach secretory cells. Gastric goblet cells secrete mucus and parietal cells secrete hydrochloric acid (HCL) and intrinsic factor. Intrinsic factor is necessary for the absorption of vitamin B_{12} in the small intestine. HCL sterilizes and breaks down food, mainly proteins and carbohydrates.

Within the parietal cells the proton pump regulates synthesis of acid. Acid is stimulated by acetylcholine, histamine, or gastrin. Acetylcholine, histamine, and gastrin bind to receptors on the parietal cells; this triggers the action of the proton pump, which elevates the stomach's hydrogen (H^+) ion concentration.

Chief cells secrete pepsinogen, which in the acidic environment converts to pepsin, an enzyme utilized for protein digestion. The stomach's cells are capable of secreting 1,500 mL of gastric secretions a day while maintaining an acidic pH of 1.5 to 2.0 because of HCL. To counteract the acid in the stomach, gastric mucosal cells secrete prostaglandin E2 (PGE2), a lipid-rich molecule, which exerts a strong protective effect. PGE2 stimulates gastric mucus production and pancreatic bicarbonate secretion, which reduce the effects of HCL.

To digest proteins, G cells, located in the pylorus, secrete gastrin. G cells are endocrine-like cells that increase gastric motility, stimulate secretions from parietal and chief cells, and trigger the release of bile from the gallbladder and enzymes from the pancreas. The bile and pancreatic enzymes enter the digestive system via the common bile duct into the duodenum.

The stomach's peristaltic function enables the mixing of food and digestive enzymes. Food is broken down into small particles and enzymatically liquefied to form chyme. Chyme is then propelled toward the pyloric sphincter and into the duodenum for the final stages of digestion. This is the beginning of the third stage of digestion, the intestinal phase.

Small Intestine

The small intestine is the largest GI organ, measuring approximately 20 feet long, and its primary function is absorption and digestion. The duodenum marks the beginning of the small intestine, followed by the jejunum, ileum, and ileocecal valve.

The mucosal lining of the small intestine is covered with thousands of tiny fingerlike projections known as **villi;** each villus contains goblet cells, whose functions are to release digestive enzymes, secrete mucus, and absorb nutrients. A unique characteristic of the small intestine is the presence of microvilli, located on the villi's epithelial cells. This double set of villi is known as the brush border. The combination of the villi and microvilli double the surface area, significantly increasing the small intestine's absorptive capacity (see Fig. 29-2).

The final phase of the digestive process, the intestinal phase, includes neural and hormonal responses. The neural response, the enterogastric reflex, is responsible

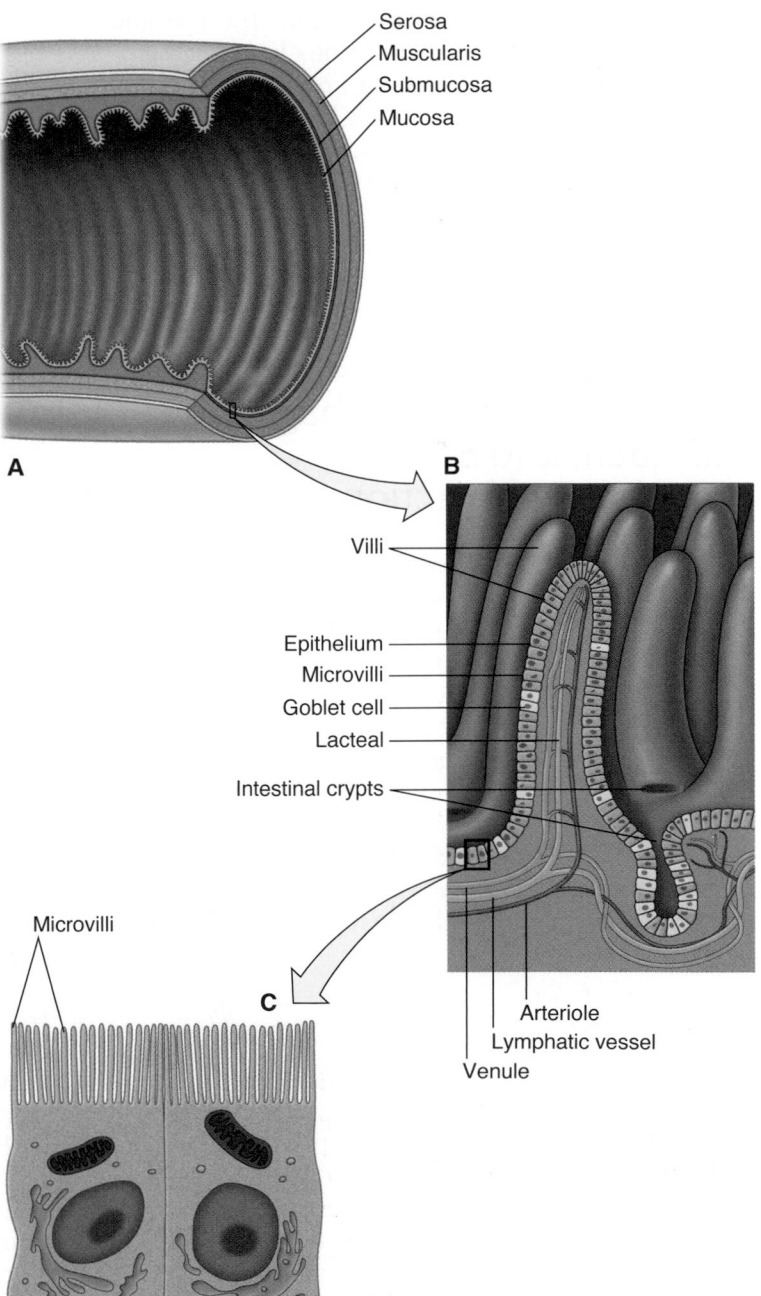

FIGURE 29-2. (A) The intestinal lining contains circular folds that slow the progress of chyme and its contact with the mucosa. On top of the circular folds are projections called villi. (B) The villi are covered by absorptive epithelial cells as well as mucus-secreting goblet cells. An arteriole, a venule, and a lymph vessel called a lacteal fill the core of each villus. Pores at the base of the villi, called intestinal crypts, contain goblet cells that secrete mucus that helps the passage of food. They also serve as sites for rapid cellular growth, producing new cells to replace those shed from the cell. (C) Epithelial cells covering the villi have a brush border of ultrafine microvilli. Besides further increasing the absorptive area, the microvilli produce digestive enzymes. (From Thompson, G. S. (2013). *Understanding anatomy and physiology.* Philadelphia, PA: F.A. Davis Company, with permission.)

for the opening of the pyloric sphincter. This reflex is stimulated by intestinal distention and decreases gastric motility and acid production.

In the duodenum, bile from the liver, enzymes from the pancreas, and chyme from the stomach come together to complete the digestive process. Both the duodenum and jejunum contain receptors that sense acidity, osmotic pressure, and such products of digestion as fats and peptides. Secretin, a hormone secreted by the intestine, inhibits gastric secretion. Gastric emptying into the duodenum is decreased if the duodenal pH is lower than 3.5. Acidic stomach contents enter the duodenum gradually at a rate that allows for neutralization by pancreatic bicarbonate.

The primary function of the middle section of the intestine, the jejunum, is absorption. Nutrients such as amino acids, glucose, iron, calcium, and the fat-soluble vitamins A, D, E, and K are absorbed in the jejunum.

The primary function of the ileum—the last and longest segment of the small intestine—is the reabsorption of vitamin B_{12} and the return of bile acids to the liver. The return of bile acids to the liver from the ileum is termed the **enterohepatic circulation** process. Bile acids are recycled by this process. The gastroileal reflex stimulates the opening of the ileocecal valve, which controls the release of digestive contents into the large intestine.

Basic Pathophysiologic Concepts of the Esophagus, Stomach, and Small Intestine Dysfunction

The functions of the GI tract are to ingest, digest, absorb, and eliminate. An alteration in the ingestion process where contents cannot progress from one area of the GI tract to subsequent areas creates motility dysfunction. Normal movement of gastric contents through the digestive tract is necessary for digestion and absorption of nutrients. Contents that progress too quickly fail to be adequately broken down, which results in malabsorption; in contrast, contents that move too slowly often cause nausea and vomiting. Inflammation, as well as structural and cellular abnormalities, in any of the GI structures will also have a direct effect on motility and absorption.

Assessment

The history and physical examination of the patient provide information for initial evaluation of an upper GI disorder. In general, with regard to the GI tract, the patient should be questioned about swallowing, indigestion, eructation (belching), and abdominal pain. Has there been any weight loss or anorexia? If pain is present it needs to be fully explored regarding onset, location, and duration. Is the pain a burning, gnawing feeling, as occurs in esophagitis? Does the pain occur with or between meals? Is the pain relieved by food, as in peptic ulcer? Are there nocturnal symptoms, as in GERD?

If nausea or vomiting is a problem, the clinician should review the onset of nausea, triggering factors, the time frame in regard to eating, and if vomiting occurs. Does the emesis contain blood, mucus, or bile? Does it have a coffee-ground appearance, as occurs in upper GI bleeding? Does the patient take NSAIDs or aspirin? How much coffee does the patient drink? What other medications are taken? Does the patient take antacids, proton pump inhibitors (PPIs) such as lansoprazole (Prevacid), or histamine-2 receptor blockers such as ranitidine (Zantac), and how often? The patient's medication list can often be responsible for GI symptoms or reveal information about symptoms. Questioning the patient about alcohol use and smoking is also important, as these are often causative of GI irritation. The clinician needs to ask about bowel movements. Has there been any diarrhea, as in malabsorptive diseases? Is there any bleeding or dark stools, as in GI bleeding?

One of the major risk factors for upper GI problems is the use of nonsteroidal anti-inflammatory drugs (NSAIDs), including aspirin. These medications are often associated with gastric irritation and erosion and can be the cause of peptic ulcer disease (PUD). Alcohol use and smoking are associated with esophagitis, peptic ulcer, and esophageal cancer. Alcohol abuse, the etiology of cirrhosis of the liver, can also cause problems for the upper digestive tract. Upper GI bleeding is often caused by esophageal varices, which occur in cirrhosis. Frequent heartburn can cause GERD, which is a precursor of Barrett's esophagus, a precancerous change of the esophagus. Patients who are bulimic have frequent vomiting episodes that can cause esophageal tears, called Mallory-Weiss syndrome or Boerhaave syndrome. Immunosuppressed individuals are susceptible to esophagitis caused by *Candida* infection.

Diagnosis

Often esophageal or upper GI pain cannot be immediately distinguished from cardiac chest pain, so an acute coronary event needs to be ruled out before exploration of a GI disorder. If the patient has upper GI bleeding, hemodynamic stabilization of the patient is necessary; a nasogastric aspirate can be used to investigate the source of bleeding. If the stomach contains bile but no blood, upper GI bleeding is less likely. If the aspirate reveals clear gastric fluid, a duodenal site of bleeding may be possible.

The most accurate method of diagnosing upper GI tract disorders is upper endoscopy. The endoscope can be used to diagnose, take a biopsy of tissue, and treat upper GI problems. Videocapsule endoscopy is an alternative if conventional endoscopy cannot be used. This vitamin-sized capsule contains a camera; when swallowed, it travels through the digestive tract, taking pictures of the internal GI tract.

Upper GI barium x-rays, also called an upper GI series, are often done to highlight the anatomy of the upper GI tract. The patient is instructed to swallow barium, a radiopaque substance; barium allows visualization of the esophagus, stomach, and duodenum. Clinicians can also visualize the patient's ability to swallow by using fluoroscopic x-ray procedures. Esophageal manometry studies are often performed to measure the strength of the esophageal sphincter muscles. Manometry is performed using a special nasogastric tube that is passed from the nostril to the stomach.

Helicobacter pylori studies are done when peptic ulcer is suspected. Antibodies to *H. pylori* can be measured in the blood. Using an endoscope, a gastric mucosal biopsy can be sampled and tested for *H. pylori.* Fecal antigen testing identifies active *H. pylori* infection in the stool. Urea breath tests detect active *H. pylori* infection by analyzing the breath.

If there is bleeding, type and crossmatch of the patient's blood is necessary. Other laboratory tests that are commonly performed include complete blood count (CBC), electrolytes, blood urea nitrogen (BUN), serum creatinine, liver function tests, prothrombin time/ partial thromboplastin time, and international normalized ratio (INR). A gastrin level is done to rule out Zollinger-Ellison syndrome (ZES), which causes peptic ulcers. Amylase and lipase levels are also checked to exclude a pancreatic disorder or perforation of an organ.

Treatment

Any disorder that includes bleeding, such as esophageal varices and perforated ulcer, requires primary hemodynamic stabilization. Patients with occasional indigestion should take antacids and make lifestyle modifications such as weight loss if obese, decreased alcohol and coffee intake, and smoking cessation, if appropriate. Esophagitis that occurs more often can be treated with PPIs such as lansoprazole (Prilosec) for 4 to 8 weeks. Some clinicians suggest PPIs or histamine-2 receptor antagonists such as cimetidine (Tagamet) for patients with ulcerlike symptoms. These agents decrease gastric acid production by inhibiting the proton pump mechanism and blocking histamine-2 receptors in gastric parietal cells. Some clinicians use gastroprokinetic agents such as cisapride (Propulsid) for patients with dysmotility type symptoms such as nausea and bloating.

Patients with upper GI bleeding caused by esophageal varices often require balloon tamponade, which is the insertion of a catheter with an inflatable balloon on the tip. A special catheter called a Sengstaken-Blakemore tube is inserted into the esophagus to exert pressure on the esophageal veins. Pressure from the balloon on the vessels can alleviate the bleeding. Surgery is needed in patients with a perforated viscus, such as in perforated duodenal ulcer, perforated gastric ulcer, and Boerhaave syndrome (esophageal rupture). Surgery may involve a laparoscopic procedure to suture bleeding vessels in the esophagus, stomach, or duodenum; it might also involve cutting the vagus nerve to the stomach to cease acid stimulation. Endoscopic surgery is another type of treatment that can be used in upper GI bleeding to ligate bleeding vessels or inject sclerosing agents.

Disorders of the Esophagus, Stomach, and Small Intestine

Disorders of each organ within the upper GI tract are different because of their distinct composition and function. The esophagus mainly undergoes inflammation. Although tumor growth is uncommon, stricture, spasm, or diverticula can occur. The stomach commonly undergoes inflammation or ulceration. Tumor growth is rare in the stomach. The small intestine disorders are mainly those of inflammation or obstruction, which can cause severe malabsorption, dehydration, and malnutrition.

Disorders of the Esophagus

The initial section of the GI tract, the esophagus, can undergo specific types of defects and alterations. The mechanism of the esophagus is to propel food and fluid from the mouth to the stomach. A series of contractions and relaxations within the esophageal tract create peristalsis, which facilitates the movement of food to the stomach. Alterations of esophageal motility, inflammation, or obstruction within the esophagus will result in the person's inability to effectively swallow.

Dysphagia

Dysphagia, also known as difficulty swallowing, is a term that is widely used with disorders of the esophagus. A wide range of causes result in dysphagia, making incidence difficult to report. Dysphagia is associated with the lack of a gag reflex, as occurs in degenerative neurological diseases and stroke. In stroke, 50% to 70% of individuals are affected by decreased gag reflex and dysphagia. In diseases such as myasthenia gravis or amyotrophic lateral sclerosis, dysphagia and loss of gag reflex are late signs that can cause death.

Etiology. Dysphagia most often occurs because of neuromuscular dysfunction; however, structural abnormalities of the esophagus are causes as well. Zenker's diverticulum is a weakening in the wall of the esophagus that causes an outpouching or sac where food can accumulate. Food accumulates within the sac and fills to create an obstructive mass in the esophagus that interferes with swallowing. Esophageal strictures, rings, or tumors can also cause dysphagia. A Schatzki ring is a constrictive muscular band of esophageal tissue. This congenital abnormality is often found in the distal esophagus. Thin membranous webs of tissue can also form in the esophagus and cause dysphagia. In Plummer-Vinson syndrome, patients have trouble swallowing because of congenital or acquired webs of tissue in the upper esophagus. Another cause of dysphagia is an esophageal stricture, which is an abnormal thinning or narrowing of the esophagus. Strictures can occur as a result of chronic esophagitis, GERD, tumors, Barrett's esophagus, inflammatory disorders such as scleroderma, or congenital abnormality. **Achalasia** is an esophageal motility problem that involves the smooth muscle of the esophagus. There is incomplete relaxation of the LES, as well as increased muscular tone. It is characterized by lack of peristalsis of the esophagus.

Pathophysiology. Dysphagia frequently begins with difficulty swallowing solid foods and progresses to the inability to swallow liquids. An individual may complain of feeling as though the food gets stuck, and frequent attempts to swallow are necessary for movement of food. Structural abnormalities of the esophagus such as diverticula, stricture, webs, and rings cause mechanical problems of swallowing. Food becomes obstructed because of the anatomic abnormality. Damage or dysfunction of cranial nerves IX, X, or XII can also cause inability to swallow solids or liquids. These nerves can become dysfunctional in stroke, spinal cord injury, degenerative neurological diseases, and trauma.

The esophagus lies posterior to the trachea, creating a high risk for aspiration. Any time there is altered motility of the esophagus, there is an increased risk of food or fluids entering the trachea rather than the esophagus, known as aspiration. The inhaled contents will follow the path of the trachea and eventually lodge within the sterile environment of the respiratory system, leading to an infection called aspiration pneumonia. Individuals with the greatest risk for aspiration pneumonia are those with a history of a stroke, trauma to the upper spinal cord, brain injury, or someone who is receiving enteral feedings.

> ### CLINICAL CONCEPT
>
> Aspiration pneumonia is demonstrated by the presence of pulmonary crackles, an elevated white blood cell (WBC) count, and fever. It most commonly occurs in the right lung.

Clinical Presentation. In dysphagia, the patient may exhibit evidence of cranial nerve dysfunction. If there is a unilateral facial droop, cranial nerve VII is dysfunctional. In a patient with an absent gag reflex, the tongue and uvula may be deviated to one side, which indicates dysfunction of cranial nerves IX, X, and XII. Regurgitation of food or fluids is associated with esophageal impairment; patients will have pooling of food or liquid in the back of the throat, and individuals may have drooling of food from one side of the mouth. Frequent coughing while eating is indicative

of dysphagia and places the person at a high risk for aspiration. Painful swallowing, or **odynophagia,** may occur as efforts to swallow are ineffective and necessitate repeated attempts to swallow.

> ### 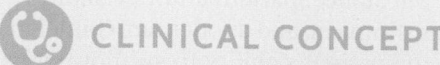 CLINICAL CONCEPT
>
> To assess the gag reflex, ask the patient to open the mouth and say "ah." The uvula and soft palate should rise as the patient vocalizes. In addition, the uvula should be in the midline position.

Diagnosis and Treatment. An upper GI series, also called a barium swallow test, is a specialized x-ray used to diagnose dysphagia. This fluoroscopic procedure demonstrates the patient's ability to swallow. The presence of aspiration pneumonia can be confirmed with a conventional chest x-ray. An individual with dysphagia can be trained to swallow during rehabilitation. Often the patient requires pureed foods and thickened fluids. Individuals with a neurological impairment of the esophagus will require enteral nutrition, which is composed entirely of liquid and has a high caloric content. This form of nutrition is given through a tube that transports the food into the stomach or intestine (see Fig. 29-3).

Esophagitis

Esophagitis is an acute or chronic inflammation of the esophagus. This condition most commonly arises

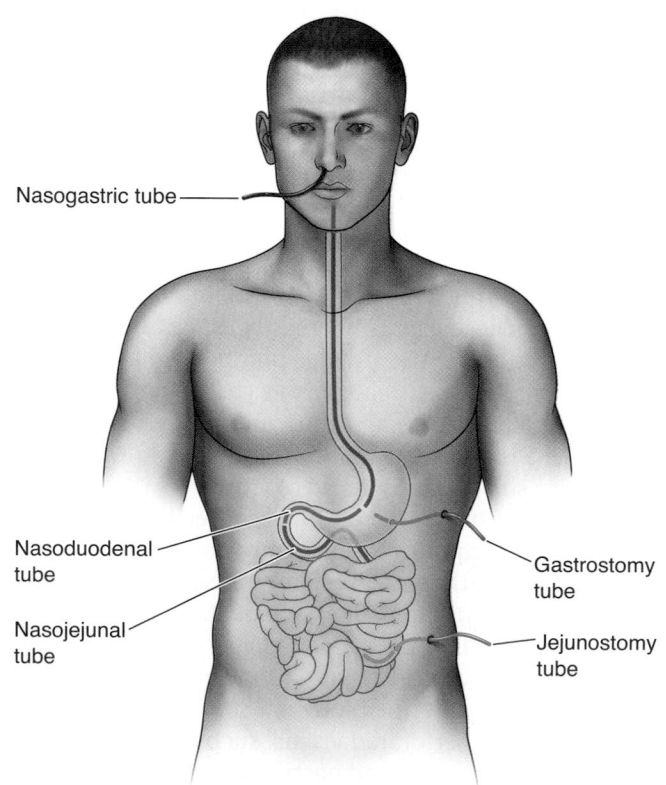

FIGURE 29-3. Individual receiving an enteral feeding.

from an irritation to the mucosa of the esophageal lining by refluxed acid. It can also be caused by the fungal organism, *Candida albicans*, in immunosuppressed individuals.

Esophagitis is a disorder that can occur occasionally, or it can be a more serious condition that occurs frequently and is diagnosed as GERD. Generally, 33% to 44% of the population endure esophageal reflux symptoms at some time during a month. However, up to 10% of people have daily symptoms, which indicates a diagnosis of GERD. *Candida* esophagitis, also called **thrush,** is the most common type of infectious esophagitis.

Etiology. Acute esophagitis occurs from an infection, chemical ingestion, medications, excessive vomiting, or occasional episodes of acid reflux. Obesity, pregnancy, smoking, alcohol, fatty foods, and coffee increase susceptibility to esophagitis. Some medications, such as calcium antagonists, anticholinergics, NSAIDs, and bisphosphonates, increase susceptibility to esophagitis. Chronic esophagitis is most often associated with the presence of poorly controlled GERD. Major predisposing factors for *Candida* esophagitis include antibiotic use, radiation therapy or chemotherapy, hematologic malignancies, and acquired immune deficiency syndrome (AIDS). Other conditions associated with an increased incidence of *Candida* esophagitis include esophageal stasis, alcoholism, malnutrition, and advanced age.

Pathophysiology. Esophagitis occurs as a result of an irritation to the squamous epithelium, the protective lining of the esophagus. The body responds to the injury by initiating the inflammatory process. Edema will occur as a result of vasodilation. Pain is associated with the erosion, or destruction, of the epithelium. The area of injury is repeatedly irritated as the contractions of peristalsis and the progression of food or fluids move through the esophagus. A risk for esophageal obstruction exists with severe esophageal inflammation because the edema and inflammation can block foods from being swallowed. In addition, chronic irritation to the esophagus can lead to ulcerations, scarring, or strictures.

Thrush often begins as an infection in the mouth. *Candida* is yeast that is considered as part of the normal flora of the oral cavity. When a person is immunosuppressed, overgrowth of *Candida* in the mouth is common. This condition is commonly found in neonates, individuals with AIDS, and those receiving chemotherapy, immunomodulators, or long-term antibiotic therapy. If thrush is not quickly identified or properly treated, the infection can progress into the esophagus, causing *Candida* esophagitis.

H. pylori are aggressive bacteria that invade the lining of the stomach, leading to PUD. *H. pylori* resists acid and burrows under the stomach mucosa. In GERD, acid and *H. pylori* constantly reflux upward into the esophagus. The esophageal epithelial mucosa becomes severely irritated by acid, and *H. pylori* can cause ulceration in the lower esophageal cells. Other organisms that can cause esophagitis include herpes simplex, varicella zoster, cytomegalovirus, and human immunodeficiency virus. A growing body of evidence is showing that HPV can also infect the esophagus.

Chemical or corrosive esophagitis can occur with ingestion of household chemicals. Many chemicals consist of strong alkali or acid components that are corrosive to the esophagus's lining. The caustic action of the ingested chemicals often leads to perforation and bleeding of the esophageal lumen. Vomiting should not be induced because of the risk for additional injury to the esophagus as the corrosive agents are expelled.

Chronic use of NSAIDs or aspirin can cause drug-induced ulcerations of the esophagus. Additional medications that may be irritating to the esophageal lining include antibiotics, chemotherapy, bisphosphonates, and potassium. Individuals should be encouraged to drink adequate amounts of water with these medications to ensure that the pills have not lodged against the wall of the esophagus. As these medications dissolve, they may become corrosive to the esophageal lining.

The process of vomiting causes irritation to the epithelium of the esophagus as acidic gastric contents are forcefully expelled. The combination of the pressure of the expulsion and the acidity of gastric contents can lead to erosion of the esophagus and deterioration of the LES. Recurrent vomiting, as seen with eating disorders or pregnancy, can lead to esophagitis.

Mallory-Weiss syndrome, which is a vertical tear in the lower esophagus, can occur with forceful, frequent bouts of vomiting. This may lead to esophageal bleeding and hematemesis. Boerhaave syndrome, a transmural rupture of the esophagus, can occur because of excessive, forceful vomiting or because of instrumentation of the esophagus. Severe hematemesis occurs with loss of an extensive amount of blood.

Clinical Presentation. In esophagitis, the most common complaint is a burning sensation in the throat or midsternal chest. Dysphagia, odynophagia, and heartburn are other symptoms associated with esophagitis. A complaint of a sore throat or tongue and white patches on the tongue, palate, or buccal mucosa are hallmark signs of thrush. Hematemesis, nausea, and vomiting can also occur.

Diagnosis and Treatment. The diagnosis and severity of esophagitis can be ascertained with endoscopy, which allows for visualization of ulcerations or perforations and provides the option to obtain a biopsy of the affected area. Barium studies can also be used in the diagnosis. Treatment of esophagitis is primarily focused on treating the inflammation and relieving symptoms. The clinician should advise lifestyle changes such as smoking cessation, alcohol limitation, reduced caffeine intake, and avoidance of NSAIDs and aspirin. Pharmacological treatment includes histamine-2 receptor blockers such as ranitidine or PPIs such as omeprazole for 4 to 8 weeks. Sucralfate is a viscous adhesive substance that can augment the stomach's protective lining. In *Candida* infection, antifungal agents such as fluconazole can be used. Surgery can be done when lifestyle and pharmacological management has been ineffective.

Gastroesophageal Reflux Disease

GERD is the most common and most costly GI disorder in the United States. Over 700,000 persons are hospitalized with GERD per year. However, many persons with GERD self-medicate with over-the-counter drugs, so there are many unreported cases. Approximately 20% of the U.S. population experiences GERD at least once per week. GERD is most common in infants and those older than age 40 years.

Etiology. A functional or mechanical problem that decreases muscular tone of the LES is the most common cause of GERD. Relaxation of the LES allows for regurgitation of stomach contents into the esophagus. Different conditions, foods, and medications can cause decreased strength of the LES (see Box 29-1).

Pathophysiology. In GERD, the LES is weak and allows the contents of the stomach to reflux up into the esophagus. The stomach contents are acidic; when refluxed upward, they irritate the esophageal squamous epithelium. Although the LES is dysfunctional in GERD, **gastroparesis,** which is the delayed emptying of gastric contents into the duodenum, is also a problem. Gastroparesis causes increased gastric distention that leads to increased pressure within the stomach against the LES. Any cause of increased gastric or intra-abdominal pressure can place tension on the LES. Obesity and pregnancy, for example, commonly cause GERD. A hiatal hernia also interferes with the closure of the LES, resulting in a reflux of gastric secretions into the esophagus.

In GERD, the esophageal epithelial cells are not able to withstand the acidity of the refluxed stomach

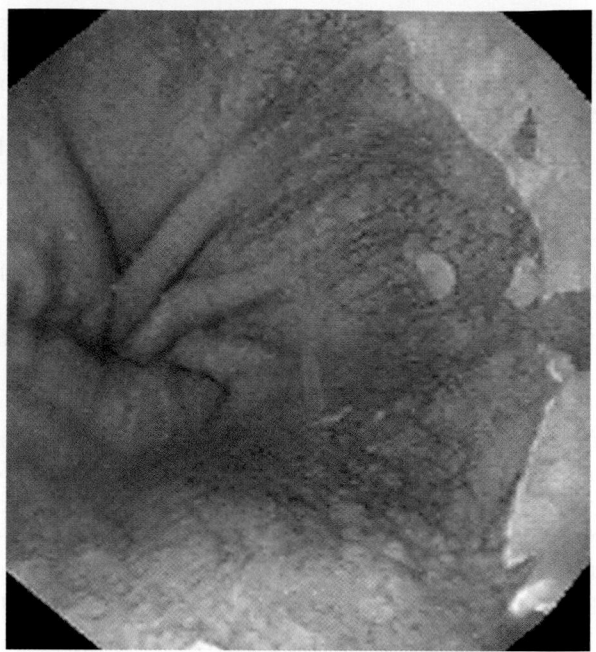

FIGURE 29-4. Endoscopic view of Barrett's esophagus. *(Courtesy of H. Worth Boyce, MD.)*

contents. The gastric acid can quickly erode the protective mucosal epithelial layer and lead to ulceration of the esophagus. Repeated injury to the epithelial layer commonly causes metaplasia, the change of esophageal epithelial cells into stomachlike columnar epithelium. The metaplastic cellular change at the gastroesophageal junction, called **Barrett's esophagus,** is a precancerous change of cells (see Fig. 29-4).

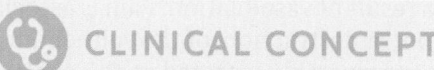
CLINICAL CONCEPT

Barrett's esophagus requires periodic endoscopic examination to check for dysplastic cell changes.

Clinical Presentation. The most frequent symptoms associated with GERD are dysphagia, heartburn, epigastric pain, and regurgitation. Frequent heartburn may also be described as acid indigestion or **dyspepsia.** Individuals often describe regurgitation as a bitter taste in their mouth. Respiratory complaints, such as chronic dry cough, asthma, and aspiration pneumonia, are also associated with the presence of GERD. Individuals frequently complain of increased pain following the ingestion of certain foods, such as those that have a high fat content and take longer to digest, thereby causing delayed gastric emptying and increased gastric distention. Postural positioning, such as lying flat or bending over, will also aggravate GERD. These positions will cause increased pressure from the stomach to the LES, forcing the LES to weaken, resulting in reflux of gastric content.

In severe cases of GERD, an individual may present with complaints of weight loss, frequent cough,

---

BOX 29-1. Causes of LES Dysfunction

Certain conditions, substances, foods, or medications can weaken or hinder closure of the LES:

- alcohol
- chocolate
- coffee
- fatty meals
- medications, including anticholinergics, beta-agonists, calcium channel blockers, nitrates, and hormones such as progesterone
- nicotine
- obesity
- pregnancy.

aspiration pneumonia, GI bleeding, or anemia. Any of these symptoms carry an increased cause for concern because they represent a progression of the disease. The GI bleeding is related to chronic irritation of the mucosal tract and erosion into the cellular layer. Anemia may be related to blood loss or nutritional deficits. A frequent cough and repeated episodes of aspiration pneumonia are indicative of the progression of GERD further up the esophageal tract. GERD with aspiration can occur while the patient is asleep; the regurgitation of acidic contents into the lungs can often stimulate nocturnal asthma attacks.

Diagnosis and Treatment. The most effective diagnostic tools for GERD are endoscopy and manometry. Through an endoscope, the clinician can visualize the esophageal mucosa. Manometry can determine the pressure at the LES. Ambulatory 24-hour pH testing can be done to confirm acid reflux in patients with atypical presentations or when endoscopy fails to reveal reflux. Barium studies (also called upper GI series) can outline the esophageal tract and highlight any erosions or ulcers. If GERD has been present for 5 years or more, a biopsy should be done to screen for the presence of Barrett's esophagus.

Treatment for GERD is focused on lifestyle changes. These include eating small, frequent meals to prevent abdominal distention; not lying down for 2 to 3 hours following a meal; losing weight in those who are obese; and smoking cessation. The clinician should also review the patient's medications because the side effects of some can cause LES dysfunction.

Pharmacological treatments of GERD focus on decreasing the acidity levels of gastric secretions and improving the function of the LES. PPIs, histamine-2 receptor antagonists, and antacids are commonly prescribed.

Fundoplication is the surgical procedure used when other treatments have failed. During fundoplication surgery, the fundus, which is the upper curve of the stomach, is wrapped around the esophagus and sutured into place. This surgery strengthens the LES to block acids from refluxing up into the esophagus. Recently, an esophageal sphincter device composed of magnets, called the LINX® Reflux Management System, has shown to be successful in alleviating reflux in many patients. However, follow-up studies are needed to determine its long-term safety.

Upper Gastrointestinal Bleed

The presence of bleeding in the esophagus, stomach, or duodenum is classified as an **upper gastrointestinal bleed (UGIB).** The bleeding can occur from a lesion, erosion, ulceration, varicosed vein, or tear to the GI lining. The incidence of UGIB is approximately 100 cases per 100,000 population per year. Bleeding from the upper GI tract is 4 times more common than bleeding from the lower GI tract, and mortality rates from UGIB are 6% to 10% overall.

Etiology. Several disorders, such as PUD, esophageal varices, Mallory-Weiss syndrome, Boerhaave syndrome, esophageal cancer, and hemorrhagic gastritis, can cause UGIB. The morbidity of GI bleeding is directly associated with the amount of blood loss.

Pathophysiology. UGIB can be classified as chronic or acute. An acute bleed is associated with a rupture, tear, or perforation in the esophageal or gastric lining, resulting in blood loss. The severity of clinical symptoms is associated with the amount of blood lost; for example, a large blood loss causes sudden hypotension and hypovolemia. An acute UGIB can quickly develop into hypovolemic shock. A chronic bleed is the result of a small tear or opening in the GI tract that causes a gradual, small amount of blood loss. A chronic bleed causes complaints of fatigue, low hemoglobin, and low iron levels. Slow UGIB often leads to iron deficiency anemia. The stool contains blood in chronic blood loss, a condition referred to as **melena.**

Clinical Presentation. Classic symptoms of UGIB include hematemesis, melena, and occult blood. **Hematemesis** is vomitus with bright red bloody streaks or a dark coffee ground appearance. The presence of bright red blood indicates a current bleed. Melena is bloody stool with a characteristic black tarry appearance. Occult blood is the presence of blood in the stool that is not visible. Individuals experiencing a slow, chronic GI bleed may have vague symptoms of fatigue and lethargy. Pain may or may not be present.

A sudden or massive UGIB may present with rapid onset of anxiety, dizziness, weakness, shortness of breath, or change in mental status. Tachycardia and tachypnea will occur because of decreased cardiac output. The skin will be pale and clammy as a result of the body's effort to shut down peripheral blood flow.

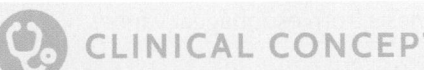
CLINICAL CONCEPT

In hematemesis, blood that has a coffee ground appearance indicates the blood has mixed with the stomach's acid. If bright, red blood is apparent, there is current bleeding occurring from a blood vessel.

Diagnosis and Treatment. A slow GI bleed may reveal low hemoglobin and low iron levels, which confirm the presence of anemia. A stool guaiac test, also known as a fecal occult blood test (FOBT), can determine the presence of blood in a stool sample. BUN levels will be elevated secondary to decreased fluid volume and the absorption of blood proteins into the small intestine. Diagnostic tests include endoscopy, CBC, and stool samples for occult blood. A videocapsule endoscopy can visualize the entire GI tract, including the walls of the small intestine. However, it does not offer the option to obtain biopsy or perform any surgical repair, as compared with traditional endoscopic procedures.

Treatment for an acute GI bleed includes rapid fluid replacement, insertion of a nasogastric tube to prevent abdominal distention from accumulation of blood, and administration of blood transfusions. Laparoscopy and surgical repair at the site of the bleeding is often done for acute episodes with large amounts of blood loss. A chronic UGIB is primarily treated with PPIs such as omeprazole for 4 to 8 weeks. Sucralfate is a viscous adhesive medication that can be used to augment the gastric lining if ulceration is present.

Esophageal Varices

Esophageal varices are engorged varicose veins that develop in the lower third of the esophagus because of portal vein hypertension in the liver. Cirrhosis of the liver is the major cause of esophageal varices.

Etiology. Portal vein hypertension, which occurs in liver disease, is the cause for the development of esophageal varices. Alcoholic and viral cirrhosis of the liver are the major diseases associated with esophageal varices.

CLINICAL CONCEPT

In long-term alcohol abuse, individuals often suffer hematemesis from esophageal varices.

Pathophysiology. The portal vein of the liver drains all the venous blood from the GI system before the blood enters the inferior vena cava. Liver disease, most often cirrhosis, causes congestion and high pressure within the portal vein. The pressurized portal vein develops backup pressure into the veins of the GI system. Collateral veins develop in an attempt to decrease pressure within the portal vein. Collaterals develop, particularly around the lower esophagus. The esophageal veins, in turn, take on the pressure of the portal vein and gradually take on more pressure as conditions in the liver worsen. The pressurized, engorged esophageal veins eventually become enlarged and protrude into the esophageal lumen. The venous pressure weakens the esophageal venous walls, creating the risk for rupture. When rupture occurs, bleeding into the esophagus, hematemesis, and hemorrhage occurs (see Fig. 29-5).

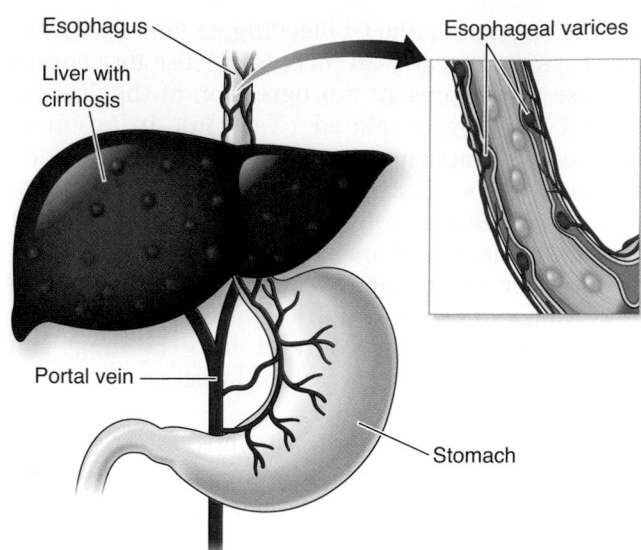

FIGURE 29-5. Esophageal varices. In portal hypertension, which is high pressure within the portal vein, backup or venous pressure occurs, causing the veins at the base of the esophagus to become dilated and fragile. The veins are termed esophageal varices and they are susceptible to rupture and bleeding.

Clinical Presentation. The patient with esophageal varices usually presents with symptoms of cirrhosis of the liver. The patient will have jaundice, nausea, vomiting, weight loss, dark urine, and abdominal distention because of liver dysfunction. The primary clinical symptoms of esophageal varices include hematemesis and melena if there is a slow leak of blood from the veins. However, the esophageal veins often rupture and cause major hemorrhage. In the event of hemorrhage, the patient will present with bright red blood in the vomitus, hypotension, tachycardia, abdominal pain, and confusion. The clinical presentation is an acute UGIB with massive blood loss.

CLINICAL CONCEPT

Ten percent of episodes of UGIB are caused by bleeding from esophageal varices. Esophageal varices have fragile membranes, so rupture with hemorrhage is common. In patients with long-term cirrhosis, there is a 60% to 70% chance of esophageal variceal bleeding.

Diagnosis and Treatment. Ultrasound can be used to diagnose portal hypertension in cases of esophageal varices. In addition, CT and MRI can be used if ultrasound findings are inconclusive. Diagnosis of esophageal varices is confirmed with endoscopy. Treatment is focused on the prevention of a rupture. Beta-adrenergic blockers and isosorbide mononitrate will help decrease blood pressure, thereby decreasing portal hypertension. Ruptured esophageal veins require immediate surgical treatment and often carry a poor prognosis.

An esophageal tamponade is the insertion of a specialized nasogastric tube, known as the Sengstaken-Blakemore tube, which is inflated in the esophagus to cause direct pressure on the area of an acute bleed. Vasopressin, somatostatin, and octreotide are strong vasoconstrictors that can be administered intravenously to control the bleeding. Surgical repair, such as sclerotherapy, vein ligation, or banding of the vein, are common treatments.

> **ALERT!** UGIB caused by esophageal varices requires emergency medical treatment.

Esophageal Cancer

Esophageal cancer is a disease that has changed over the last few decades. Previously an incurable squamous cell carcinoma with a protracted painful course, it is now more commonly an adenocarcinoma with curable treatment. The incidence of esophageal carcinoma is approximately 3 to 6 cases per 100,000 persons. In the United States in 2013, the American Cancer Society estimates approximately 18,000 new cases of esophageal cancer with approximately 15,000 fatalities. Males are affected more than females and persons over age 65 have the highest risk. Higher numbers of African American males are affected by squamous cell carcinoma than Caucasian males. However, Caucasian males have a higher rate of adenocarcinoma compared with African American males.

Etiology. There are two types of cancer of the esophagus: squamous cell carcinoma and adenocarcinoma. In the past, 90% to 95% of esophageal cancer in the United States was caused by squamous cell carcinoma located in the middle esophagus. However, the incidence of adenocarcinoma of the distal esophagus and gastroesophageal junction has progressively increased in the United States. Currently, adenocarcinoma accounts for more than 70% of all new cases of esophageal cancer. GERD is the primary risk factor for adenocarcinoma of the esophagus.

In squamous cell carcinoma, cancer cells invade the lining of the esophagus. Chronic alcohol consumption and tobacco use are risk factors for squamous cell carcinoma. Drinking whiskey is associated with a higher incidence of cancer than other alcoholic beverages.

The presence of adenocarcinoma, the most common form of esophageal cancer, occurs in the glandular tissues in the distal esophagus near the junction of the esophagus and the stomach. Primary risk factors associated with adenocarcinoma include Barrett's esophagus, chronic GERD, and tobacco use.

A genome study has identified susceptible gene loci on chromosomes 5q11, 6p21, 10q23, 12q24, and 21q22. Persons with mutations of the tumor suppressor gene *TP 53* and Barrett's esophagus develop adenocarcinoma. The findings suggest that there is involvement of both genes and environment in the development of esophageal cancer.

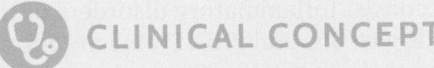

> **CLINICAL CONCEPT**
>
> The risk of esophageal adenocarcinoma among patients with Barrett's esophagus has been estimated to be 30 to 60 times that of the general population.

Pathophysiology. Chronic irritation of the epithelial cells that line the esophagus causes chronic cellular injury. Commonly, the irritation is caused by acid from GERD. In GERD, a metaplastic change often occurs at the lower esophagus, called Barrett's esophagus. From metaplasia, over time, the cells become dysplastic and gradually turn into adenocarcinoma. The proliferation of cancerous cells is apparent with alterations in the size, shape, function, and density of cells. The reproduction of multiple abnormal cells leads to the development of tumor growth and the potential for metastasis of cancerous cells to other parts of the body.

Clinical Presentation. The clinical symptoms of esophageal cancer are similar to other disorders of the esophagus. Dysphagia is the most common complaint, but it is usually not present until the disease is in the advanced stages. The inability to swallow is initially noted with solids, and eventually progresses to liquids and saliva. Weight loss and change of eating patterns frequently occurs in response to dysphagia. The inability to effectively swallow increases the risk of aspiration pneumonia. Additional complaints include chest pain or a burning sensation behind the sternum. The area and size of the cancer can cause pressure on nerves, leading to such symptoms as hiccups, hoarse voice, pain at the back of the throat, chronic cough, and odynophagia (painful swallowing). Difficulty breathing can arise if the pressure on nerves limits the rise and fall of the diaphragm.

Diagnosis and Treatment. Diagnosis is confirmed with endoscopy, barium study, and tissue biopsy. An endoscopic ultrasound is commonly done to visualize the depth of the tumor. A computed tomography (CT) scan or bronchoscopy may be performed to identify areas of metastasis. Treatment involves surgical resection, laser therapy, photodynamic treatment, chemotherapy, and radiation. An esophagectomy can be done via endoscope or open abdominal surgery. The use of chemotherapy before and after surgical treatment for individuals with adenocarcinoma has shown an increase in survival rates. Enteral feeding is frequently needed to meet nutritional needs. The overall 5-year survival rate for esophageal cancer is approximately 20% to 25%.

Disorders of the Stomach

Gastric dysfunction can be caused by structural problems, inflammatory disorders, and neoplasms of the stomach. Structural problems include hiatal hernia and pyloric stenosis. Inflammatory disorders of the stomach include gastritis and PUD. Stomach cancer is a rare type of cancer in the United States, but its incidence is rising for unclear reasons.

Hiatal Hernia

A hernia is a protrusion of an organ into surrounding tissue as the result of an anatomical defect in the barrier that normally contains it. A **hiatal hernia** occurs as a result of part of the stomach pushing up through the opening in the diaphragm and protruding into the thoracic cavity (see Fig. 29-6). Hiatal hernia is a very common disorder; however, many are undiagnosed, asymptomatic, and discovered incidentally. They become more common with advanced age, and incidence significantly increases after age 60 years. Seventy percent of cases occur in persons over age 70.

Etiology. There are two types of hiatal hernias: a sliding hiatal hernia, also referred to as a direct hernia, and a paraesophageal hernia, or rolling hiatal hernia. The sliding type of hernia is the most common, accounting for 90% to 95% of cases. Any cause of increased intra-abdominal pressure can cause hiatal hernia; for example, obesity and pregnancy are major risk factors for hiatal hernia.

Pathophysiology. The esophageal hiatus is the opening in the diaphragm that allows the esophagus and vagus nerve to connect with the stomach. With age, the opening within the diaphragm weakens and widens, and the stomach is able to protrude upward through the aperture into the thorax. The fundus of the stomach pushes upward into the thoracic cavity, which prevents the LES from properly closing, thereby allowing reflux of gastric contents into the esophagus; this creates esophagitis or GERD.

A sliding hiatal hernia can easily protrude above the diaphragm when the person is lying supine. When the person stands, the hernia slides back into the abdominal cavity. A paraesophageal hernia is the protrusion of only the fundus part of the stomach into the thorax while the gastroesophageal junction stays below the diaphragm. This type of hernia is less common and has a higher risk for complications because the fundus of the stomach pushes into the thorax cavity and remains above the diaphragm. This leads to the potential for gastritis, ulcer formation, or strangulation of the herniated portion of the stomach.

Clinical Presentation. Clinical symptoms of sliding hiatal hernia usually occur as a result of esophagitis or GERD, which include dysphagia, substernal burning, belching, and epigastric discomfort. A paraesophageal hernia rarely has symptoms associated with reflux because

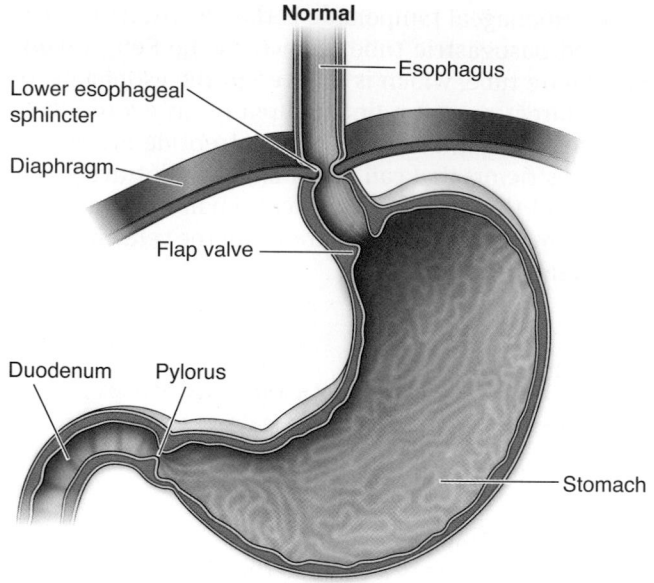

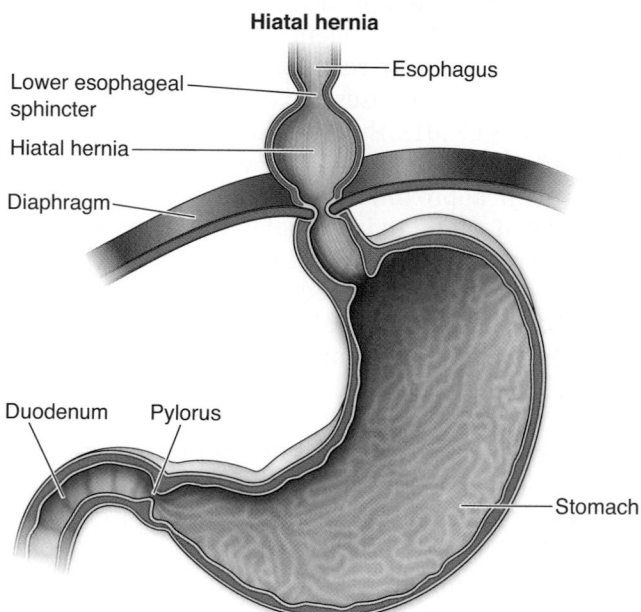

FIGURE 29-6. Hiatal hernia. A hiatal hernia occurs when part of the stomach protrudes up through the diaphragmatic opening in the chest. This allows acid from the stomach to reflux back up into the esophagus.

the gastroesophageal junction remains below the diaphragm. The pain is associated with strangulation of the hernia and presents as acute chest pain or dysphagia.

Diagnosis and Treatment. The diagnosis of a hiatal hernia is easily confirmed with endoscopy or an upper GI barium x-ray. Treatment aims to prevent reflux and accumulation of acid contents in the esophagus. Lifestyle changes that assist in treatment include weight loss, small meals, coffee limitation, and smoking cessation. Individuals should also refrain from lying down after eating. Sleeping with the head of the bed elevated or the use of two pillows will help to decrease gastric reflux. Pharmacological agents such as histamine-2 blockers (e.g., ranitidine) or PPIs (e.g., omeprazole) relieve symptoms of hiatal hernia associated with GERD. Surgical repair called laparoscopic fundoplication can decrease episodes of reflux and may be needed if symptoms do not respond to other treatments.

Pyloric Stenosis

Pyloric stenosis is a constriction of the pyloric sphincter, the muscular valve that connects the stomach to the duodenum. The narrowing of this region impairs the movement of gastric contents into the small intestine. In infants, this is a congenital abnormality. Adults develop pyloric stenosis secondary to an ulceration or fibrosis of tissue surrounding the pyloric sphincter. The incidence of infantile pyloric stenosis is 2 to 4 per 1,000 live births. It occurs most commonly in Caucasian newborns and has a 4 to 1 incidence in males compared with females. This is an uncommon condition in the adult.

The role of the pyloric sphincter is to control the release of gastric contents from the stomach into the duodenum. The stenosis, or inadequate opening, of the pyloric sphincter delays the emptying of the gastric contents, causing gastroparesis (distended stomach). Pyloric stenosis can develop into pyloric obstruction, which occurs when the stenosis becomes severe and the passage through the sphincter is blocked. The accumulation of food and fluids in the stomach leads to abdominal pain and distention. Nausea and vomiting are common symptoms. Weight loss, dehydration, and electrolyte imbalances also can occur. The abdomen will be firm upon palpation, particularly over the pylorus, and visible peristalsis may be noted. Projectile vomiting of undigested food eaten a few hours earlier is associated with a pyloric obstruction. Diagnosis is confirmed with x-ray, upper GI series, and ultrasound. Surgical repair is necessary, with a resulting good prognosis.

Acute Gastritis

Acute gastritis, also known as erosive gastritis, is an inflammation in the lining of the stomach. It can be caused by a number of medications and factors such as infection, allergy, acute stress, bile reflux, alcohol abuse, radiation, and direct trauma. Chronic use of aspirin, NSAIDs, or corticosteroids commonly cause gastritis. These medications suppress the inflammatory response and irritate the stomach lining by blocking gastric mucus production. They are known to frequently cause GI bleeding or PUD.

The wall of the stomach consists of layers: an inner mucosal lining, a middle muscle layer, and an outer serous coat. Inflammation associated with acute gastritis is limited to the mucosa layer. An irritant to the mucosa, such as an NSAID, triggers an inflammatory response. With inflammation, WBCs rush to the area and increase the blood supply, causing edema. The swelling creates increased pressure within the tissue layers, causing pain. NSAIDs are prostaglandin inhibitors; prostaglandins cause the pain in inflammation, but also stimulate the production of gastric mucus. Although NSAIDs relieve the inflammation, they deplete the gastric mucus. By eradicating prostaglandins, NSAIDs impair the stomach's protective mechanism. Without mucus, the gastric lining is exposed to acidic contents that increases the pain.

Clinical symptoms include complaints of heartburn, nausea, and epigastric pain. Diagnosis is based on history, physical examination, and endoscopy; treatment is focused on the cause of injury. Acute gastritis will typically heal within a few days when causative agents are removed. Antacids, histamine-2 receptor antagonists, or PPIs are prescribed for gastritis.

CLINICAL CONCEPT

Chronic use of NSAIDs will diminish the formation of gastric mucus which can lead to gastritis and peptic ulcer disease.

Chronic Gastritis

Chronic gastritis, also known as nonerosive gastritis, is associated with an underlying disease or severe infection. The presence of the *H. pylori* bacterium is the most common cause of chronic gastritis, which usually affects the fundus of the stomach. It is different than acute gastritis because it causes atrophy of the glandular stomach lining, a condition called atrophic gastritis.

H. pylori bacterium attacks the mucosal layer of the stomach wall. If the mucosal wall is eroded it is unable to repair or regenerate cells. The death of chief cells and parietal cells diminishes the production of pepsin, HCL, and intrinsic factor. With low HCl levels, gastrin is repeatedly secreted in efforts to increase acid production. HCl is constantly stimulated and destroys mucosal cells. Erosion of the mucosa occurs, which enhances the environment for replication of *H. pylori*. A vicious cycle of bacterial replication and cellular tissue death occurs. The total destruction of parietal cells eventually leads to achlorhydria, which is a marked reduction in acid secretion. Atrophy of the gastric wall and loss of HCl results. Additionally, there is an insufficient level of intrinsic factor, which decreases the body's ability to absorb vitamin B_{12}, causing pernicious anemia.

CLINICAL CONCEPT

Chronic gastritis is a precursor for the development of stomach cancer.

Symptoms associated with chronic gastritis include burning or gnawing epigastric pain, nausea, weight loss, anorexia, and hematemesis. Diagnosis is confirmed with endoscopy and a biopsy of the affected tissue. Antibiotics will be prescribed to eradicate the *H. pylori*. Antacids, PPIs, or histamine-2 blockers may be indicated to decrease the acid level in the stomach. Replacement of vitamin B_{12} will be required.

Peptic Ulcer Disease

Peptic ulcer disease (PUD) is an inflammatory erosion in the stomach or duodenal lining. Ulceration occurs 4 times more often in the duodenum than in the stomach. Approximately 4.5 million persons are affected annually in the United States, and approximately 10% of the U.S. population has evidence of a duodenal ulcer at some time in their lives. The hospitalization rate for PUD is approximately 30 patients per 100,000 cases. The incidence of PUD is equal in males and females.

Etiology. The most frequent causes of PUD are the bacteria *H. pylori* and the use of NSAIDs. Stress, alcohol abuse, excessive caffeine, and smoking are additional risk factors. Though most adults are colonized with the *H. pylori* bacteria, it is unclear exactly how the bacterium is contracted or transmitted. However, not all persons colonized by *H. pylori* develop ulcer disease. Genetic susceptibility is believed to play a role in PUD development. NSAIDs cause PUD because they counteract prostaglandin E secretion, the major stimulant of gastric mucus production, and diminish the stomach's protective layer. Persons have a high risk of ulcer when NSAIDs are used and *H. pylori* is present.

Duodenal ulcers commonly occur in the region termed the duodenal bulb, the upper portion of the duodenum near the pyloric sphincter, because of its proximity to the highly acidic gastric contents of the stomach. Individuals with a first-degree relative diagnosed with a duodenal ulcer are three times more likely to develop one, indicating a genetic predisposition. However, the most significant risk factor is the presence of *H. pylori*. Additional risk factors include alcoholic cirrhosis, pancreatitis, hyperthyroidism, and chronic obstructive pulmonary disease. Stressful conditions such as severe burns, sepsis, CNS trauma, and severe hypotension can also cause peptic ulcer.

Pathophysiology. The underlying pathophysiology of PUD is hypersecretion of HCL, ineffective GI mucus production, and poor cellular repair. These abnormalities lead to the erosion of the mucous membrane in the stomach or duodenum. In PUD, the protective mechanisms of the intestinal mucosal barrier are damaged by *H. pylori*, which are helically shaped, gram-negative bacteria that secrete the enzyme urease. Urease breaks down urea, which is a normal component of stomach mucus, into carbon dioxide and ammonia (NH_3). The ammonia is converted to ammonium (NH_4) by accepting a proton (H^+) from HCL; the acid is then neutralized. This neutralization of acid protects the integrity of the *H. pylori* colony. The ammonia produced is toxic to the epithelial cells of the stomach and duodenum. Intestinal cell damage also occurs because of other products of *H. pylori*, such as proteases, cytotoxins, and phospholipases.

The erosion in the mucosal lining of the stomach or duodenum permits the diffusion of HCL into the stomach wall and blood vessels. This stimulates an inflammatory response with the release of prostaglandins and histamine. Prostaglandins trigger the stomach cells to release additional mucus and bicarbonate in an attempt to neutralize the acid.

However, the parietal cells keep releasing histamine and HCL, substances that are required for normal digestion. The HCL irritates and destroys the stomach lining as it continues to trigger inflammation. Histamine causes vasodilation and stimulates the release of pepsin, a proteolytic enzyme, and gastrin, a hormone that stimulates acid, which together damage the unprotected stomach lining. Cellular repair can occur, but repeated episodes of elevated gastric acidity will cause scarring and fibrosis of the GI lining. Fibrosis prevents the reproduction of healthy cells, thereby decreasing the mucus and bicarbonate production to protect the gastric lining.

Ulcers can vary in size from millimeters to centimeters; depending on the depth of penetration into the cellular layer, the worn area may be classified as an erosion or as an ulcer (see Fig. 29-7). If the superficial layer of the gastric mucosa is affected and does not extend into the muscularis layer, it is considered to be an erosion. An ulcer extends beyond the mucosa and into the muscularis layer.

Clinical Presentation. The main symptom of gastric and duodenal ulcers is epigastric, abdominal pain. Episodes of pain occur between meals, about 2 to 3 hours after eating. The pain is described as an intense, burning, and gnawing sensation that can be slightly relieved by food and can be strong enough to awaken a person from sleep.

If ulceration progresses to perforation of the stomach or intestinal wall, symptoms include sudden, excruciating abdominal pain, abdominal rigidity, pale skin, hematemesis, and cold sweat.

Diagnosis. Identifying the characteristics, region, and timing of the abdominal pain are important in determining the diagnosis. The pain of PUD is distinct because it occurs when the stomach is empty. An upper GI series can be used to visualize an ulcer. All suspected

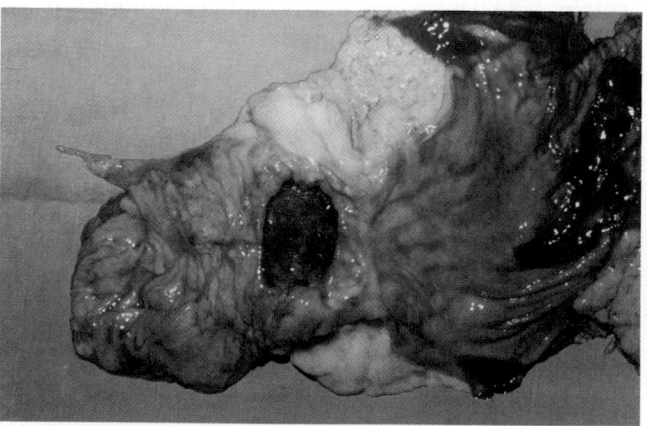

FIGURE 29-7. A peptic ulcer is an area of severe irritation, inflammation, and erosion in the duodenum. A gastric ulcer is a similar lesion in the stomach. *(From Biophoto Associates/Science Source.)*

cases of PUD need to be screened for the presence of *H. pylori*; a blood sample tested for the presence of antibodies to *H. pylori* is the most common method of diagnosis. An endoscopy should be done to determine the location and severity of the ulceration, in addition to obtaining a tissue biopsy to rule out cancer.

A urea breath test is also highly accurate in detecting *H. pylori*. Patients swallow urea with radiolabeled carbon 14. After 10 to 30 minutes, the detection of radioactive carbon dioxide in the patient's exhaled breath indicates that the urea was split, indicating the presence of *H. pylori* bacteria. A stool antigen test can also detect the presence of *H. pylori*.

Treatment. The focus of treatment is to identify the underlying cause and reduce acid levels in the GI tract. This requires interrupting the stimulation of histamine, gastrin, and pepsin. Antibiotics are frequently prescribed to eradicate the *H. pylori* bacteria. Antacids will lower the gastric acid level and decrease the production of pepsin. Histamine-2 antagonists will inhibit the release of histamine and decrease the production of acid. PPIs and anticholinergic medications can also hinder the acid secretion by parietal cells.

Lifestyle changes are necessary to decrease the risk of relapse during the healing process. The goal is to neutralize the acid level and promote healing of the gastric mucosa. Individuals should make an effort to avoid caffeine, alcohol, and tobacco because they stimulate acid production. Foods that are spicy, high in fat, or are acidic in nature should also be avoided.

In severe cases, surgical removal of the affected area may be necessary. A gastroduodenostomy, also known as Billroth I, is the removal of the distal portion of the stomach; the remainder of the stomach is then directly connected to the duodenum. The benefit of surgery is the removal of the parietal cells, which are responsible for release of HCL.

A gastrojejunostomy, also known as Billroth II, is the removal of the lower stomach, with the remaining portion of the stomach connected to the jejunum. This surgery eliminates the gastrin-producing properties of the lower stomach and the duodenum.

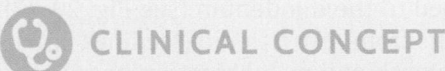

CLINICAL CONCEPT

There is a 90% chance that an ulcer with *H. pylori* can be cured if patients take the full dose of recommended antibiotics. However, patients need to continue taking the medication even when symptoms may have subsided.

Zollinger-Ellison Syndrome

ZES is a rare disorder that occurs in fewer than 1% of patients with duodenal or gastric ulcers. It is most commonly caused by a gastrin-secreting tumor (gastrinoma) of the pancreas. The tumor may alternatively be located in the duodenum, lymph nodes, or other site.

In ZES, there is constant secretion of gastrin from a tumor. Gastrin stimulates the proliferation of parietal cells, which yield excessive HCL. The high level of HCL eventually leads to ulceration of the GI mucosa. ZES may occur sporadically or as part of an autosomal-dominant familial syndrome called multiple endocrine neoplasia type 1 (MEN type 1). The pathophysiology of cellular destruction is similar to that of PUD with erosion of the mucosa and constant HCl secretion.

Clinical symptoms are similar to those of a peptic ulcer, although more severe. Common complaints include abdominal pain, diarrhea, nausea, vomiting, weight loss, fatigue, and GI bleeding. Complications include hemorrhage secondary to ulcer perforation and obstruction related to inflammation.

Hypergastrinemia can be detected in serum blood tests and through a fasting serum gastrin level. CT scan or magnetic resonance imaging (MRI) scan can visualize the tumor. PPIs also can be used because these medications inhibit the activity of the parietal cells and decrease their ability to manufacture acid. Surgical removal of the pancreatic tumor or a gastrectomy, which is the removal of all or a portion of the stomach, is frequently required.

Bariatric Surgery

Obesity is a public health problem that has reached epidemic proportions in the United States. Up to two-thirds of the U.S. population is overweight, and half of the people in this group can be classified as obese. Obesity is defined as a body mass index (BMI) greater than 30 (for more information about obesity see Chapter 5). Obesity is associated with increased risk of many disorders, including cardiovascular disease, diabetes, cancer, sleep apnea, and arthritis. For those who are morbidly obese, with a BMI of greater than 40, diet and exercise are recommended as primary treatment. However, when conservative treatment has proven unsuccessful, bariatric surgery can significantly reduce morbidity and mortality associated with obesity. Long-term studies show that patients who undergo bariatric surgery have successful weight loss, less cardiovascular events, improved glucose control, and, in some cases, amelioration of diabetes. The most common types of bariatric surgery include the following:

- gastric bypass (also called Roux-en-Y gastric bypass)
- gastric banding
- sleeve gastrectomy
- biliopancreatic diversion with duodenal switch.

Gastric Bypass. In gastric bypass, the stomach is stapled so that it becomes a smaller sac. Then part of the jejunum is brought up to connect with this area of stomach, bypassing the whole duodenum and part of the jejunum. The duodenum and jejunum are left as blind tracts. A gastric bypass creates a stomach of approximately 20 mL in volume, which gives the patient a feeling of fullness after eating a small meal. The bypass also creates some intentional malabsorption because it detours

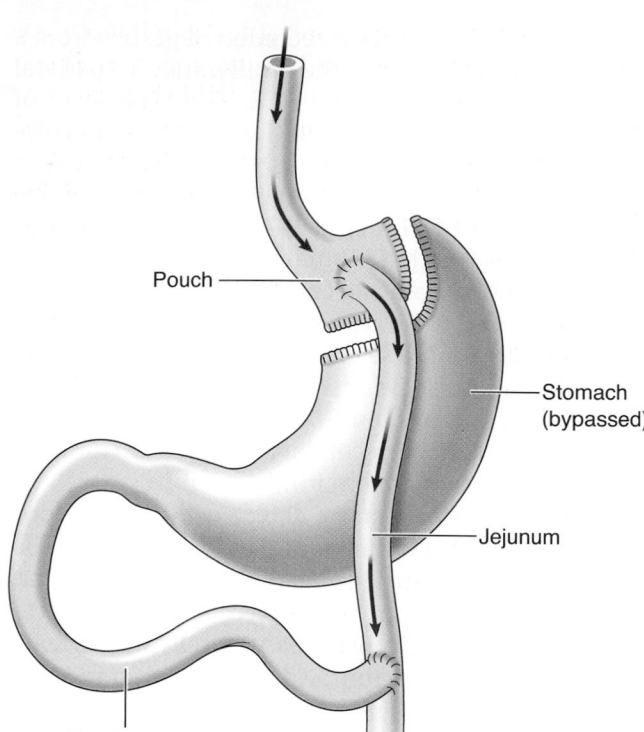

FIGURE 29-8. Gastric bypass surgery, also called roux-en-Y bypass, is a procedure that decreases the size of the stomach and attaches a small portion of small intestine directly to the stomach. The major portion of the stomach is bypassed and some small intestinal length is unused.

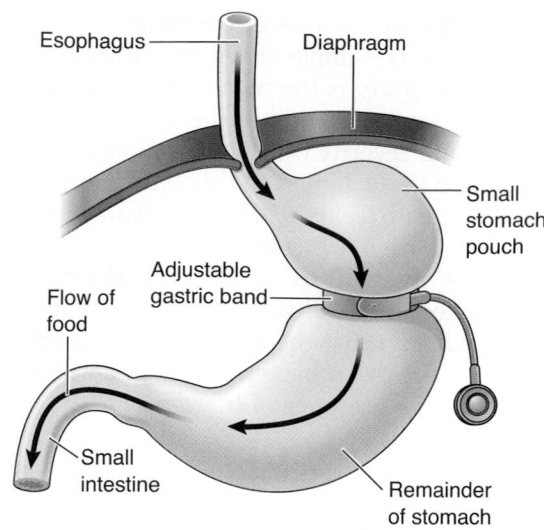

FIGURE 29-9. In gastric band surgery, a band is placed around the upper stomach to decrease its size and capacity. The volume of food allowed in the small stomach is restricted. The band can be adjusted according to the patient's needs.

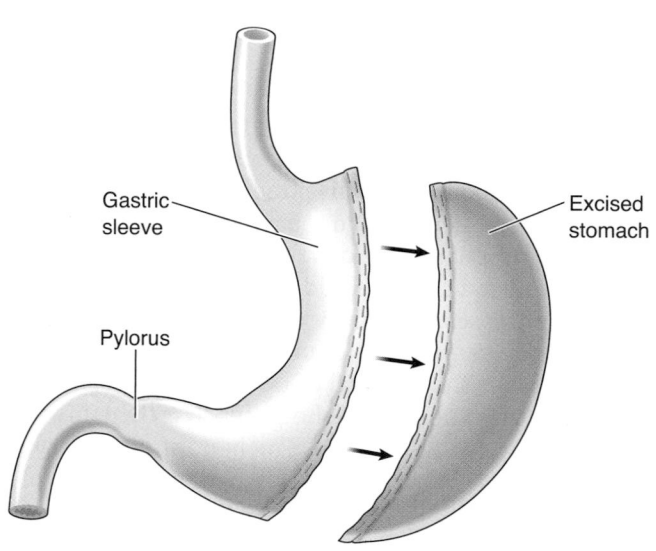

FIGURE 29-10. A vertical sleeve gastrectomy requires vertical stapling of the stomach and reduces its size to 15% of normal size. The remaining 85% is removed from the abdomen at the time of surgery.

around the distal stomach and the entire duodenum; it also varies the length of the jejunum. Patients are prescribed vitamins and minerals and are advised about dietary changes to avoid malnutrition (see Fig. 29-8).

Gastric Banding. Gastric banding involves placing an inflatable band around the upper portion of the stomach to restrict the amount of food the individual can consume (see Fig. 29-9). The inflatable gastric band is connected to a tube that is brought out through the skin to a port. Using the port, the band can be gradually tightened during a slow period of treatment, which is about 1 to 2 years for weight loss. Patients are advised about dietary changes to accommodate the smaller stomach.

Sleeve Gastrectomy. Sleeve gastrectomy involves subtotal gastrectomy, where the stomach is reduced to about 15% to 20% of its original size (see Fig. 29-10). Compared with other bariatric procedures, sleeve gastrectomy is the more physiologic treatment, because it does not involve malabsorption, abnormal tracts, blind tracts, or the placement of a foreign body.

Biliopancreatic Diversion. Biliopancreatic diversion with duodenal switch involves a 75% gastrectomy, resulting in a tubular stomach. The distal end of the ileum

is attached to the duodenum (see Fig. 29-11). Weight loss occurs from restriction of feedings because of the small stomach and malabsorption because the procedure detours around the jejunum. There is an optional appendectomy and cholecystectomy. Compared with other bariatric surgery, in this procedure there is less malabsorption of fats and proteins.

Results of Bariatric Surgery. Results of studies of gastric bypass procedures demonstrate that patients lose an average of 69% of their excess weight by 12 months and 83% at 24 months postsurgery. Studies show weight loss after gastric banding has been 50% to 60% of excess body weight over approximately 2 years. Patients followed after sleeve gastrectomy have been found to lose

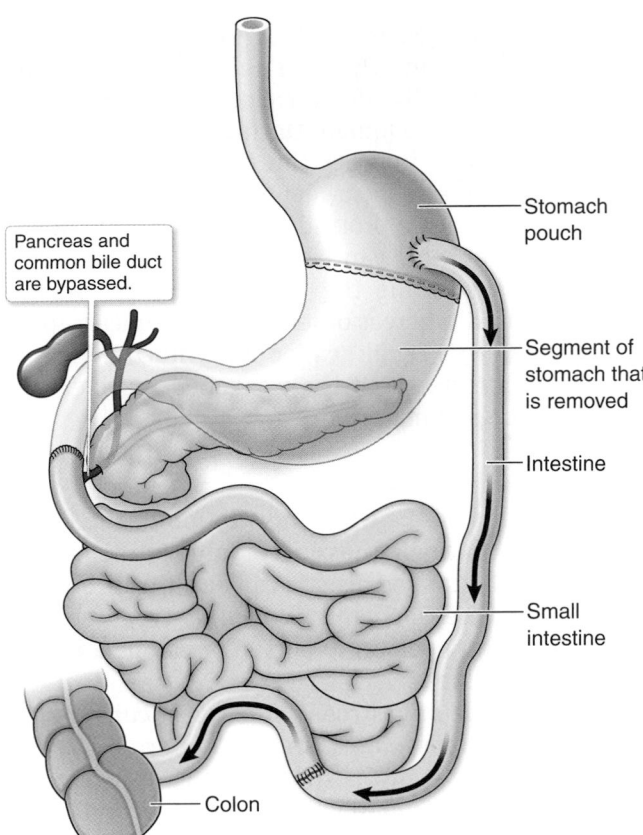

Pancreas and common bile duct are bypassed.

Stomach pouch

Segment of stomach that is removed

Intestine

Small intestine

Colon

FIGURE 29-11. In biliopancreatic diversion, the stomach size is decreased and the intestine is attached to the segment of stomach. The procedure bypasses the pancreas and common bile duct.

33% to 83% of their excess weight after a period of 6 months to 3 years. In contrast, biliopancreatic diversion has resulted in 75% to 85% of excess body weight loss by 18 months.

Dumping Syndrome

Dumping syndrome is caused by rapid gastric emptying. This is a common complication following any surgical procedure that removes part or all of the stomach, such as bariatric surgery. Poorly digested material enters the intestine before its breakdown in the stomach. The material tends to be hypertonic, causing a shift of fluid out of the intestinal cells into the intestinal lumen. The fluid shift reduces blood volume, creates hypotension, and stimulates the sympathetic nervous system to increase heart rate. The abdomen becomes distended because of the ingested contents and the fluid shift into the jejunum. Peristalsis and intestinal motility increase in response to the abdominal distention. The pancreas releases excess insulin in response to gastric fullness and increased peristalsis, creating a risk for hypoglycemia.

Clinical Presentation. The clinical presentation of dumping syndrome has two phases, early and late. The early phase occurs within 30 minutes of eating. Abdominal cramping, nausea, hyperactive bowel sounds,

diarrhea, tachycardia, diaphoresis, and palpitations are common symptoms during the early phase. These symptoms are associated with the fluid shift that occurs from the bloodstream into the small intestine and the decrease in blood volume. The late phase occurs 2 to 3 hours after eating, and clinical presentation includes epigastric fullness, syncope, palpitations, and symptoms associated with hypoglycemia.

The epigastric discomfort of dumping syndrome is the result of excess fluid volume in the stomach pushing upward upon the diaphragm. The risk for hypoglycemia is related to the pancreatic release of excessive amounts of insulin stimulated by gastric fullness.

Diagnosis and Treatment. Endoscopy and upper GI series will show a partial stomach. Dietary management is the focus of treatment. Frequent, small feedings are recommended to decrease the volume ingested at one time. The patient should be prescribed a low-carbohydrate, high-protein, high-fat diet. Simple carbohydrates should be eliminated as they increase intestinal osmolarity. Drinking fluids in between mealtime rather than with food consumption is an alternative to reduce rapid filling of the intestine. Medications that delay gastric emptying may be prescribed.

Disorders of the Small Intestine

The small intestine is the main part of the intestinal tract that absorbs nutrients. A long length and distinctive villous mucosal epithelium allow it to have a great amount of surface area. Different kinds of disorders affect the small intestine. A loop of intestine can herniate through a weak muscle in the abdominal wall. Inflammation of the intestine can occur because of ingestion of pathogens. Autoimmune and allergic reactions can cause inflammation of the mucosal lining of the small intestine, leading to malabsorption.

Hernia

A hernia is a protrusion of a section of the small intestine through a weakened abdominal wall muscle. As much as 10% of the population develops some type of hernia during their lifetime. More than a half million hernia operations are performed in the United States each year. Males have a higher rate of hernia than females.

Etiology. There are several different types of hernia: umbilical, inguinal, obturator, femoral, or incisional (see Figure 29-12). The most common is an inguinal hernia, which occurs when a loop of the small intestine protrudes down into the inguinal canal in the groin. Its occurrence is significantly higher in males because of the anatomical location of the scrotal sac. Between the scrotum and abdominal cavity there is a gap in the membranes that allow displacement of the intestines. It is most likely to occur before the first year of life or in the later stages of puberty. Inguinal hernias can also develop with advanced age as abdominal muscles

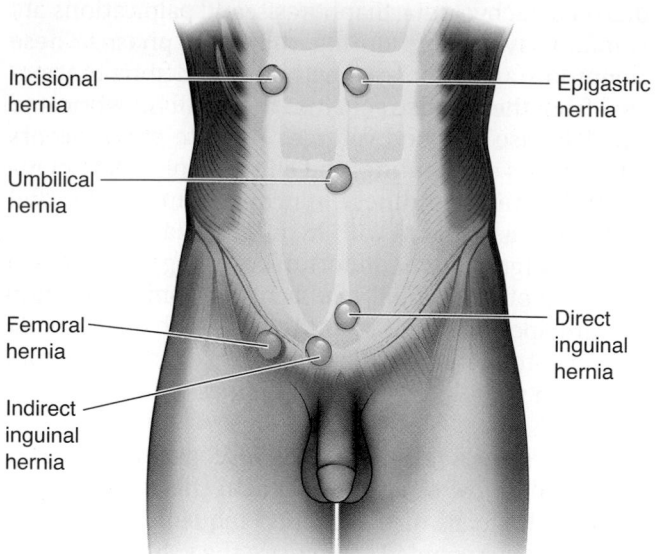

FIGURE 29-12. There are several types of hernias. These weakened areas in the abdominal muscle wall allow protrusion of intestine just under the skin. On physical examination, there is a bulge in the abdominal or inguinal region. A hernia can become incarcerated when a section of intestine is strangled or squeezed by the abdominal muscle wall. Intestinal contents cannot move forward in an incarcerated hernia, which this requires immediate treatment.

weaken. Risk factors include positive family history for inguinal hernia, obesity, ascites, pregnancy, heavy lifting, chronic cough, or chronic constipation.

Pathophysiology. The pathophysiologic processes of all types of hernias are similar. They differ based on the location of the protrusion of the loop of bowel. An inguinal hernia is directly related to the anatomical location of the scrotum and weak abdominal muscle wall. The pressure within the intestines pushes against the lower abdominal wall, eventually forcing the weakened area to separate, permitting protrusion of the intestine into the inguinal canal. It is possible that a severe herniation could extend into the entire scrotal sac. Hernias can be reducible, incarcerated, or strangulated. In a reducible hernia, the loop of bowel can be pushed back into normal position with manual pressure. Incarceration occurs when the loop of intestine becomes trapped in between muscle fibers. Strangulation of a hernia occurs when blood supply to the incarcerated loop of intestine is obstructed and at risk for ischemia.

Clinical Presentation. Clinical symptoms and severity will be dependent upon the location and degree of the protrusion of intestine. The patient may be asymptomatic or have pain near the hernia site. Coughing or straining can cause the herniation to protrude and induce pain. If the hernia is pressing toward the bladder, urinary frequency or incomplete emptying of the bladder can occur. Pain occurs if strangulation of the hernia occurs with intestinal ischemia.

Diagnosis and Treatment. Diagnosis is based on the patient's history and the physical examination. The patient can usually demonstrate the bulging of the hernia in the abdomen. During the examination, the clinician will instruct the patient to cough or strain; this will raise intra-abdominal pressure, which will make the hernia protrude, thus confirming diagnosis. Some hernias can be manually reduced with gentle pressure while the patient is placed in the supine position, whereas others require surgical repair. A surgical hernia repair, called a herniorrhaphy, involves reinforcement of the weakened muscle with synthetic surgical material.

Gastroenteritis

Gastroenteritis occurs from an irritation to the lining of the stomach, small intestine, or large intestine by a pathogen or toxin. The disease can occur from a virus, bacteria, parasite, or chemical toxin. Gastroenteritis is transmitted from person to person or can be a water- or foodborne illness.

The incidence of gastroenteritis is difficult to estimate because most cases are not reported. In the United States, as many as 100 million cases occur per year, with several million health-care visits and thousands of hospitalizations. Children account for more than 1.5 million outpatient visits. According to the Centers for Disease Control and Prevention, probably more than 21 million cases a year and nearly 50% of foodborne outbreaks in adults are caused by norovirus, the most common etiologic agent of gastroenteritis.

Etiology. Norovirus is highly contagious and transmitted through the fecal-oral route or through close contact. In children, rotavirus is a common etiologic agent that is also transmitted via the fecal-oral route. Some bacterial organisms, such as *Enterotoxigenic Escherichia coli*, *Salmonella*, *Shigella*, and *Clostridium difficile,* can cause severe illness with bloody diarrhea. Parasites such as Ameba and Giardia can cause dysentery, which is a severe diarrheal condition with dehydration. Box 29-2 details organisms that cause gastroenteritis. Individuals that have close contact, such as those in nursing homes, day-care centers, cruise ships, and dormitories, are at increased risk for viral or bacterial gastroenteritis.

Pathophysiology. Infectious microorganisms are usually responsible for acute gastroenteritis and are often contracted via the oral route. These microorganisms cause diarrhea by adherence to the mucosa, invasion into the mucosal layer, or toxin production. The end result of most microbial infections is increased fluid to shift into the lumen of the intestine, to a point where the excessive amount of fluid cannot be adequately reabsorbed. This fluid shift results in watery, small intestinal contents that pass into the large intestine and are then excreted as diarrhea. The fluid shift also can cause dehydration and loss of

BOX 29-2. Common Organisms That Cause Gastroenteritis

Viral, bacterial, and parasitic microorganisms most commonly cause gastroenteritis.

VIRAL (APPROXIMATELY 70% OF CASES OF GASTROENTERITIS)
- adenovirus
- coronavirus
- norovirus
- parvovirus
- rotavirus.

BACTERIAL (15% TO 20% OF CASES OF GASTROENTERITIS)
- *Bacillus cereus*
- *Campylobacter jejuni*
- *Clostridium difficile*
- *Clostridium perfringens*
- *E. coli*–Enterohemorrhagic O157:H7, enterotoxigenic, enteroadherent, enteroinvasive
- *Listeria*
- *M. avium-intracellulare,* immunocompromised
- *Providencia*
- *Salmonella*
- *Shigella*
- *Vibrio cholera*
- *Vibrio parahaemolyticus*
- *Vibrio vulnificus*
- *Yersinia enterocolitica.*

PARASITIC (10% TO 15%)
- *Amebiasis*
- *Cryptosporidium*
- *Cyclospora*
- *Giardia lamblia.*

FOOD-BORNE TOXIGENIC DIARRHEA
- preformed toxin: *Staphylococcus aureus, Bacillus cereus*
- postcolonization: *Vibrio cholera, Clostridium perfringens, enterotoxigenic E. coli, Aeromonas.*

electrolytes and nutrients. Gastroenteritis diarrheal illness can occur by different mechanisms:

- Osmotic diarrhea occurs because of an increase in the osmotic load presented to the intestinal lumen because of diminished absorption.
- Inflammatory diarrhea occurs when the mucosal lining of the intestine is inflamed, edematous, and unable to reabsorb fluid or nutrients.
- Secretory diarrhea occurs when an organism stimulates the intestine to secrete fluid and mucus.
- Motility diarrhea is caused by intestinal neuromuscular disorders.

Pathogens or toxins either act directly on the intestinal epithelium, causing inflammation and malabsorption, or

stimulate secretory mechanisms that produce watery diarrhea. The epithelium of the microvilli, which provides the surface area of the small intestine, is often the target of the infectious agent. The virus or bacteria attaches to the epithelium and impairs the small intestine's ability to absorb carbohydrates, fats, fluids, or electrolytes. Sometimes the infectious agent secretes a toxin that irritates the intestinal membrane. The infectious agent or its toxin stimulates inflammation of the GI tract and destruction of the epithelial lining. The villi are often damaged, which decreases the absorptive ability of the intestinal brush border. With lack of absorption, intestinal contents become hypertonic compared with the surrounding intestinal cells. An osmotic exchange of fluids and salts occurs at the intestine, resulting in water entry into the intestine. An osmotic diarrhea occurs, producing watery stool and loss of electrolytes. A secretory diarrhea can also result if microorganisms stimulate the intestine to produce mucus and fluids. In any of the mechanisms, excess water and essential electrolytes are lost from the GI tract. Dehydration and electrolyte imbalance are the result of any type of gastroenteritis.

Clinical Presentation. The primary clinical presentation is nausea, vomiting, abdominal cramping, and diarrhea. If the gastroenteritis is associated with a virus, symptoms can usually persist between 12 and 72 hours. A bacterial form of gastroenteritis will produce symptoms until the causative agent is eradicated. Hyperactivity of the intestine produces intestinal cramping as well as high-pitched bowel sounds, known as **borborygmi.** Hyponatremia and hypokalemia can occur as a result of fluid loss, as well as acid-base imbalances of metabolic acidosis or alkalosis. Individuals must be closely monitored for dehydration.

Diagnosis and Treatment. Diagnosis is aimed at identifying the causative factor. Stool cultures can be tested for WBCs, parasites, ova, or bacteria. Treatment is aimed at relieving symptoms and preventing transmission. Medical management is focused on resting the bowel and providing fluid replacement. Medications to suppress the vomiting and the diarrhea may be indicated. Antibiotics are routinely ordered if gastroenteritis is identified as bacterial.

ALERT! Children and elderly individuals are at high risk of dehydration in gastroenteritis. Often hospitalization is needed to administer intravenous fluids to replace losses.

Celiac Disease

Celiac disease, also known as sprue and gluten-sensitive enteropathy, is a condition that occurs from a hypersensitivity reaction to gluten, a by-product of wheat, barley, and rye. The cause is unknown but it is considered an autoimmune disease. It occurs in 1% of the American population; however, many individuals with the disorder go undiagnosed, as another 3 million people in the United States are estimated to be affected. Onset of celiac disease can appear in young children as foods are being introduced into the diet. In adults, celiac disease can occur between age 20 and 50 years.

Etiology. In celiac disease, a gluten-derived peptide called gliadin damages the intestinal mucosa in persons with genetic predisposition to this disease. The exact etiology is unknown, but T cells predominate in an autoimmune inflammatory reaction against intestinal villi. There is a higher prevalence in those with a first-degree relative, such as a parent or sibling, with celiac disease, type 1 diabetes, or Down syndrome. More than 90% of affected persons have the cell surface marker HLA-DQ2.5.

Pathophysiology. The pathophysiology of celiac disease is related to an autoimmune, inflammatory process that destroys the intestinal villi. This destruction leads to a decreased surface area, causing atrophy of the intestinal wall. The atrophy creates a flattened appearance of the intestinal villi, greatly reducing the absorptive and transport properties of the small intestine. The decreased surface area impairs the absorption of all nutrients, vitamins, minerals, electrolytes, and bile salts.

The inability to digest carbohydrates leads to a buildup of gases within the intestinal system, causing abdominal bloating and diarrhea. The inability to absorb proteins impairs the body's ability to build and maintain muscle tone, causing muscle wasting. When fats are not absorbed, vitamins A, D, E, and K are not absorbed, causing fat to be excreted in the stool. **Steatorrhea** is the loss of fat in the stool; with steatorrhea, stool is light colored and soft. Deficiency of vitamin A will cause visual disturbances, particularly difficulty with vision in diminished light, a condition called night blindness. Vitamin D is necessary for the absorption of calcium. With vitamin D deficiency, calcium absorption is diminished and hypocalcemia occurs. Hypocalcemia causes symptoms such as muscle spasms and tetany; it also stimulates parathyroid hormone (PTH). PTH causes breakdown of bone with resulting osteomalacia and susceptibility to fractures. Vitamin E, which protects cellular membranes, is also not absorbed. Red blood cells and platelet membranes become excessively fragile, leading to hemolysis, anemia, and thrombocytopenia. Deficiency of vitamin K causes defective clotting mechanisms, leading to spontaneous bleeding and bruising. In addition, iron is not absorbed, causing iron deficiency anemia.

Clinical Presentation. There are numerous clinical symptoms associated with celiac disease, mainly caused by malabsorption of essential nutrients, vitamins, and minerals. Weight loss occurs early in the disease and, if diarrheal illness occurs, dehydration is also common. Initial symptoms are fatigue, abdominal pain, bloating,

or steatorrhea. As the disease progresses, symptoms associated with vitamin deficiencies will present, including anemia, high incident of fractures or bone pain, abnormal growth, bruising, poor skin turgor, and dehydration.

Diagnosis and Treatment. A serology celiac panel can determine if an immune reaction to gluten is present. Affected individuals show a positive antibody titer of IgA antitissue transglutaminase (IgA TTG). If the results of this test are positive, a biopsy of the duodenum or jejunum is necessary. Treatment of celiac disease is aimed at making dietary changes. A consultation with a nutritionist to identify and eliminate gluten products in the diet is recommended. The patient frequently needs vitamin replacement. If the immune response is extreme, corticosteroids may be prescribed.

Short-Bowel Syndrome

The average length of the small intestine is 600 cm. Short-bowel syndrome is a result of any disease, traumatic injury, vascular accident, or other pathology that leaves fewer than 200 cm of small intestine, which is approximately one-third of the size of the normal small intestine. Studies show that, in the United States, approximately 10,000 to 20,000 patients receive total parenteral nutrition for short-bowel syndrome per year.

Etiology. Intestinal abnormalities that may require a partial removal of the small intestine include Crohn's disease, trauma to the bowel, strictures, tumors, radiation enteritis, mesenteric ischemia, strangulated hernia, and volvulus. Short-bowel syndrome can also occur because of congenital defects.

Pathophysiology. Short-bowel syndrome is directly associated with the amount of bowel that is remaining, the segment of the intestine that was removed, the health of the remaining intestine, and the functioning ability of the ileocecal valve. The ileum is the largest segment of the small intestine; it is responsible for absorption of fluids, electrolytes, fats, carbohydrates, proteins, vitamin B_{12}, and the return of bile to the liver. Removing any part of the ileum reduces the GI absorptive surface and can lead to nutritional deficiencies.

In short-bowel syndrome, the remaining intestine gradually adapts to the changes. The remaining intestinal villi increase in number and enlarge to accommodate the need for increased absorption. It is necessary for individuals with small-bowel syndrome to receive enteral nutrition during the postoperative period until the intestine adapts sufficiently to adjust to oral feedings.

Clinical Presentation. Short-bowel syndrome is divided into three phases:

1. acute phase
2. adaptation phase
3. maintenance phase.

The acute phase presents with symptoms of dehydration, electrolyte imbalance, weight loss, loss of folic acid, fat-soluble vitamins A, D, E, and K, and vitamin B_{12}. These signs and symptoms are related to the small intestine's inability to absorb nutrients because of lost surface area and length. Fluid loss can be 6 to 8 liters per day. Malnutrition can rapidly develop, leading to muscle wasting, fatigue, skin irritation, and anemia. The acute phase lasts up to 3 months, followed by the adaptation phase, which may last 12 to 18 months. During this phase, the body begins to adjust by lengthening the microvilli, which creates an increased surface area for reabsorption. During the maintenance phase, the patient accommodates diet to the changed intestine, focusing on what amount of oral intake can be consumed without causing nausea, vomiting, or diarrhea.

Diagnosis and Treatment. The most definitive diagnostic test for short-bowel syndrome is a barium contrast x-ray series. This allows for visualization and measurement of the small intestine. Abdominal CT scan with contrast and ultrasound may also be done. If the length of the bowel is fewer than 200 cm, short-bowel syndrome is confirmed. Treatment goals are to slowly increase fluid and nutrient intake. The need for enteral or total parenteral nutritional replacement to meet caloric and nutritional demands may be required. Oral intake should be encouraged with a trial-and-error approach of slowly adding new food into the diet. Medications such as somatropin, which is a synthetic form of growth hormone, can stimulate intestinal cell proliferation. Teduglutide, an analog of glucagon-like peptide, can be used to enhance the absorptive ability of the remaining intestinal mucosa. PPIs and histamine-2 blockers can reduce the effect of acid on the intestine. Lomotil, codeine, and Imodium are used to reduce diarrhea. Octreotide, a somatostatin analog, is used in cases of severe diarrhea.

Small Bowel Obstruction

A small bowel obstruction (SBO) can be acute or chronic and partial or complete. An acute obstruction has a sudden onset that can occur with adhesions or a herniation of the bowel, whereas a chronic obstruction is often seen with inflammatory disease or tumors. A partial obstruction decreases the flow of intestinal content through the bowel, whereas a complete obstruction prevents passage of all contents and fluid through the bowel and is considered a surgical emergency.

Etiology. The major cause of SBO is postsurgical adhesions (60%), followed by malignancy, Crohn's disease, and hernias. Postoperatively, surgeries that most often cause adhesions are appendectomy, colorectal surgery, and gynecological and upper GI procedures.

Pathophysiology. Adhesions are bands of connective tissue that form between tissues and organs, often as a result of injury during surgery. In the abdomen, adhesions commonly bond sections of intestine together. The adhesions cause obstruction and interfere with the intestine's normal function. Intestinal contents cannot move forward through the bowel. At the point of obstruction, there is increased peristalsis and mucus accumulation that worsen the blockage.

Clinical Presentation. The presentation of intestinal symptoms is directly related to the severity of the obstruction. The larger the obstruction, the more dramatic the symptoms. Abdominal distention, pain, nausea, vomiting, and hyperactive bowel sounds occur. Abdominal distention occurs proximal to the site of obstruction from the accumulation of chyme and intestinal gases. Pain is sharp, cramping, and intermittent, occurring with the contractions of hyperactive peristalsis. Pain that is continuous and steadily increases in severity is associated with a strangulation of the intestine. This indicates ischemia or necrosis of the intestinal lumen and requires emergency surgery. Nausea and vomiting can cause fluid and electrolyte depletion, which could potentially lead to dehydration, hypotension, or hypovolemic shock. Diarrhea is present with a partial obstruction because liquid intestinal contents can leak around an obstruction in the lumen.

Diagnosis and Treatment. Abdominal x-ray provides visualization of the area of obstruction and severity of the blockage (see Fig. 29-13). X-ray will show excessive gas in the area of intestine proximal to the obstruction. CT and ultrasound can also be used to identify the obstruction. A nasogastric tube is inserted to decompress

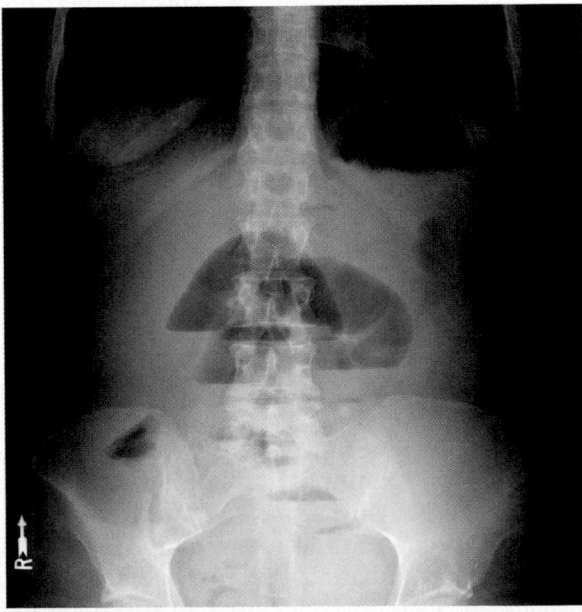

FIGURE 29-13. In SBO, there are specific findings on an abdominal x-ray. Areas that are filled with air or gas will appear black and fluid lines will be gray in color. Areas the x-ray cannot penetrate, such as an obstruction, will appear white. (From Weber, E.C. (2013). *Practical radiology.* Philadelphia, PA: F.A. Davis Company, with permission.)

the bowel and remove the accumulation of fluid within the bowel. Intravenous fluids are given to assure adequate fluid and electrolyte balance. The majority of partial SBOs can resolve with medical treatment. Pain management, antiemetic medications, and antibiotics are frequently necessary. Complete obstructions usually require surgical intervention.

Peritonitis

The peritoneal membrane is the serous membrane that surrounds the abdominal cavity and covers the organs. **Peritonitis** is the inflammation of the peritoneal membrane caused by bacterial infection or leakage of intestinal contents into the peritoneal cavity. The peritoneal cavity is a sterile environment and can become contaminated with intestinal or organ rupture. The overall incidence of peritonitis is unclear because it can be caused by a wide number of conditions.

Etiology. Peritonitis is widespread irritation of the peritoneal membrane. The condition most often occurs when organ rupture introduces bacteria, bile, acids, or enzymes into the sterile peritoneal environment. Less often, peritonitis is caused by hematogenous spread of infection from bacteremia. Most often, intestinal perforation allows *E. coli*, anaerobic bacteria, and other microorganisms to spill into the peritoneal cavity and cause abdominal sepsis. A perforated gallbladder or a lacerated liver can cause bile to enter the peritoneal cavity; gastric acid from a perforated ulcer can also leak into the peritoneal cavity. Peritonitis can also result from traumatic injury. Women can endure peritonitis from an infected fallopian tube or a ruptured ovarian cyst.

Pathophysiology. Peritonitis is classified according to whether or not perforation of an organ has occurred. Primary peritonitis is limited to the inflammation of the peritoneum; there is no perforation of any organ. Secondary peritonitis is associated with trauma or is secondary to an infection from surrounding organs, such as appendicitis, pancreatitis, bowel obstruction, ischemic bowel disease, or the perforation of a peptic ulcer. A rupture from these areas will release bacteria into the peritoneal cavity. The contamination of the bacteria into the peritoneum causes a movement of fluid from intravascular spaces into the peritoneal cavity, called a peritoneal fluid shift. The excess fluid creates peritoneal edema but decreases blood volume and increases the risk of hypovolemic shock. In addition, these fluid shifts can lead to electrolyte imbalances.

Secondary complications of peritonitis include paralytic ileus, abdominal abscess, cardiac arrhythmias, and shock. An abdominal abscess is an area of purulent exudate that accumulates in a small cavity surrounded by inflammation. A **paralytic ileus** is the decrease or absence of intestinal motility that occurs during peritonitis. The body responds to peritonitis by decreasing peristalsis and shifting blood flow to the area of injury. Blood is shifted to the bowel or abdomen, causing a decrease in circulating blood volume, resulting in hypotension. Cardiac arrhythmias can occur because of electrolyte imbalances, which result from the fluid shift or from the loss of absorption because of reduced GI motility. The decrease or absence of peristalsis stops the movement of undigested material through the intestinal tract. As this content lies in the intestine, it continues to ferment, producing gas and swelling within the intestine. There is a high risk for intestinal perforation, septicemia (bloodstream infection), and shock if emergency treatment is not provided.

Clinical Presentation. In peritonitis, there is a classic triad of symptoms: abdominal pain, abdominal rigidity, and rebound tenderness. Abdominal pain occurs with any movement of inflamed tissues. The patient wants to remain still with peritoneal inflammation so as not to disturb any peritoneal contents, because even a cough will usually cause abdominal pain in the patient with peritonitis. The patient's abdominal musculature is contracted in peritonitis; when palpated, the abdomen is rigid, a sign called involuntary guarding. Rebound tenderness occurs as the clinician palpates the abdomen.

Fluid shifts occur in peritonitis with fluid moving into the peritoneum from the bloodstream. As the infection and fluid shifts progress, the patient will present with symptoms associated with severe hypotension or shock—tachycardia, tachypnea, clammy skin, decreased or absent bowel sounds, and oliguria. Electrolyte imbalances will occur because of the shift of intravascular fluid into the peritoneum. Fever occurs if the peritonitis is related to an infection.

CLINICAL CONCEPT

Assess for rebound tenderness by having the patient lie supine with knees slightly flexed. Place one hand with fingers pointing down into the right lower quadrant of the abdomen. Apply a gradual and deep pressure, followed by a quick release of the hand. If the patient experiences pain upon the release of the pressure, it indicates rebound tenderness.

Diagnosis and Treatment. Diagnosis is initially based upon physical examination, laboratory findings, and an x-ray. A WBC count will be markedly elevated (greater than 11,000 cells/uL) with a high neutrophil count, whereas an x-ray will show air or fluid in the abdominal cavity. A paracentesis is a procedure where a sample of peritoneal fluid is withdrawn and analyzed; ultrasound can be used to guide the paracentesis. Peritoneal fluid with neutrophil count greater than 500 cells/uL is an indicator of peritonitis. The diagnosis can be confirmed with CT scan or emergency surgical **laparotomy,** which is a surgical incision through the abdomen into the peritoneal cavity. On abdominal x-ray, free air under the diaphragm may be present if there is perforation of the intestine or organ. Treatment consists of **peritoneal lavage,** which is a sterile cleansing of the peritoneum.

Intravenous fluids are necessary to replace fluids and electrolytes, as well as prevent cardiac arrhythmias and dehydration. Large doses of intravenous antibiotics should be administered to limit the spread of infection. Decompression of the GI tract occurs with the insertion of a nasogastric tube. Intestinal abscesses can be drained percutaneously or surgically removed.

Chapter Summary

- Disorders such as achalasia, Zenker's diverticulum, esophageal stricture, stroke, and neuromuscular disease can cause dysphagia, which is a risk factor for aspiration pneumonia.
- Check the patient's gag reflex, tongue, and uvula position to assess for dysphagia.
- Hiatal hernia is a common disorder that increases susceptibility to acid reflux and esophagitis.
- GERD is a common disorder that can lead to metaplasia of the lower esophageal epithelium and Barrett's esophagus.
- PUD is most commonly caused by *H. pylori* and NSAIDs.
- PPIs are drugs used to treat GERD and PUD.
- Chronic gastritis causes achlorhydria and is a risk factor for stomach cancer.
- There are four major types of bariatric surgery that have been successful in treating morbid obesity.
- Bariatric surgery can effectively decrease susceptibility to hypertension, diabetes, coronary artery disease, sleep apnea, and arthritis.
- Dumping syndrome is caused by rapid gastric emptying. This is a common complication following any

surgical procedure that removes part or all of the stomach.
- Short-bowel syndrome, which causes malabsorption, can occur after any surgical procedure that removes a large segment of the intestine.
- Gastroenteritis is commonly caused by pathogens contracted via the oral route, or through water- or foodborne illness. This diarrheal illness can cause dehydration. Norovirus is the most common cause of gastroenteritis.
- Celiac disease is a condition that occurs from a hypersensitivity reaction to gluten, a by-product of wheat, barley, and rye. Although the cause is unknown, it is considered an autoimmune disease.
- Abdominal hernia is the protrusion of a loop of intestine through the abdominal muscle wall. It can become strangulated, which causes ischemia of the intestine.
- Adhesions are the most common cause of SBO. There are characteristic patterns on the abdominal x-ray that indicate bowel obstruction.
- Peritonitis causes extreme abdominal pain, guarding, and rebound tenderness. It can cause a paralytic ileus, which is a lack of peristaltic activity in the intestine.

 ## Making the Connections

Disorder and Pathophysiology	Signs and Symptoms	Physical Assessment Findings	Diagnostic Testing	Treatment
Dysphagia | Difficulty swallowing related to structural or neurological impairment.				
	Pooling of liquids in the back of the throat. Frequent coughing while eating. Repeated attempts to swallow.	Assess gag reflex, tongue, and uvula to check for dysphagia. Poor gag and deviated tongue and uvula indicate dysphagia. Drooling of food or liquids may be a sign of dysphagia.	Elevated WBC count is present with aspiration pneumonia. Swallow test, barium swallow, and esophagography shows the patient's swallowing ability.	Keep head elevated greater than 60° while eating. Provide small, frequent meals. Pureed and thick liquids are necessary because these are easiest to swallow.

Continued

Making the Connections–cont'd

Disorder and Pathophysiology	Signs and Symptoms	Physical Assessment Findings	Diagnostic Testing	Treatment
		Abnormal lung sounds such as crackles are indicative of aspiration pneumonia. Elevated temperature indicates aspiration pneumonia.		A powder called "thick it" should be added to fluids.
Esophagitis | Inflammation of the esophagus caused by reflux of gastric acid that injures the esophageal squamous epithelium.				
	Patient complains of burning sensation in the throat, painful swallowing, or substernal or epigastric pain.	No significant physical assessment signs.	If chronic esophagitis, endoscopy is used to determine the cause.	Instruct the patient to avoid eating or drinking items that have an extreme temperature or spiciness. Decrease inflammation and relieve symptoms through antacids such as PPIs.
GERD | Inability of the LES to completely close; the opening permits the reflux (backflow) of acid contents from the stomach up into the esophagus. The epithelium of the esophagus can become metaplastic; this condition is called Barrett's esophagus.				
	Patient complains of burning sensation in the throat, painful swallowing, or substernal or epigastric pain. Increased pain is present after eating acidic or spicy foods. Dry cough is present. Nocturnal asthma can be caused by GERD.	No particular physical assessment findings.	Endoscopy. Barium swallow (upper GI series). Esophageal manometry will show pressure within the LES. Ambulatory 24-hour pH testing. Biopsy of lower esophageal cells to look for metaplastic changes if suspect Barrett's esophagus or check for dysplasia.	Keep head elevated greater than 60° while eating. Provide small, frequent meals. Encourage weight loss. Encourage smoking cessation. Administer PPIs to decrease stomach acid and give esophagus time to heal. Periodic endoscopic examination is necessary to check for development of Barrett's esophagus.
UGIB | An area in the esophagus, stomach, or duodenum that is bleeding small, moderate, or large amounts. Most common causes of UGIB are esophageal varices and PUD.				
	Fatigue. Anemia. Abdominal pain. Rapid pulse. Syncope. Shortness of breath. Decreased urine output.	Hematemesis; blood in vomitus. sometimes referred to as "coffee ground" emesis. Melena; tarry, dark stool caused by blood in stool. Hypotension.	Decreased hemoglobin and hematocrit caused by bleeding. Decreased plasma volume because of fluid loss with bleeding. Increased BUN caused by dehydration. Positive FOBT.	Treatment is specific to the cause of bleeding. Surgical repair is performed of esophageal varices or perforated ulcer in the stomach or duodenum. Blood transfusions. Rapid intravenous fluid infusion.

Continued

Bibliography

Altahawi, F., Alraiyes, A. H., & Alraies, M. C. (2011). Unmasking gastric cancer. *Cleveland Clin J Med*, 78(9), 606–608. doi: 10.3949/ccjm.78a.10129.

Anderson, W. D., & Strayer, S. M. (2013). Evaluation of nausea and vomiting: a case-based approach. *Am Fam Phys*, 88(6), 371–379.

Anvari, M. (2008). Endoscopic treatments for gastro-oesophageal reflux disease. *Lancet*, 371(9617), 965–966.

Barrett, K. E., Barman, S. M., Boitano, S., & Brooks, H. L. (2012). *Ganong's review of medical physiology*. 24th ed. New York: Lange/McGraw-Hill.

Biere, S. S., van Berge Henegouwen, M. I., et al. (2012). Minimally invasive versus open oesophagectomy for patients with oesophageal cancer: a multicentre, open-label, randomised controlled trial. *Lancet*, 379(9829), 1887–1892.

Boeckxstaens, G. E., Zaninotto, G., & Richter, J. E. (2013). Achalasia. *Lancet*, Jul 16. doi:pii: S0140-6736(13)60651-0. 10.1016/S0140-6736(13)60651-0. Epub ahead of print.

Bok, K., & Green, K. Y. (2012). Norovirus gastroenteritis in immunocompromised patients. *N Engl J Med*, 367(22), 2126–2132.

Bull-Henry, K., & Al-Kawas, F. H. (2013). Evaluation of occult gastrointestinal bleeding. *Am Fam Phys*, 87(6), 430–436.

Cardwell, C. R., Abnet, C. C., Cantwell, M. M., & Murray, L. J. (2010). Exposure to oral bisphosphonates and risk of esophageal cancer. *JAMA*, 304(6), 657–663.

Carlsson, L. M., Peltonen, M., Ahlin, S., et al. (2012). Bariatric surgery and prevention of type 2 diabetes in Swedish obese subjects. *N Engl J Med*, 367(8), 695–704.

Cartwright, S. L., & Knudson, M. P. (2008). Evaluation of acute abdominal pain in adults. *Am Fam Phys*, 77(7), 971–978.

Case, D. J., & Baron, T. H. (2010). Flexible endoscopic management of Zenker diverticulum: the Mayo Clinic experience. *Mayo Clin Proceed*, 85(8), 719–722.

Chang, J. Y., Talley, N. J., Locke, G. R., 3rd, et al. (2011). Population screening for Barrett esophagus: a prospective randomized pilot study. *Mayo Clin Proceed*, 86(12), 1174–1180.

Chason, R. D., Reisch, J. S., & Rockey, D. C. (2013). More favorable outcomes with peptic ulcer bleeding due to *Helicobacter pylori*. *Am J Med*, 126(9), 811–818.e1. doi: 10.1016/j.amjmed.2013.02.025. Epub 2013 Jul 3.

Di Sabatino, A., & Corazza, G. R. (2009). Coeliac disease. *Lancet*, 373(9673), 1480–1493.

Dixon, J. B., le Roux, C. W., Rubino, F., & Zimmet, P. (2012). Bariatric surgery for type 2 diabetes. *Lancet*, 379(9833), 2300–2311.

Ebell, M. H. (2010). Diagnosis of gastroesophageal reflux disease. *Am Fam Phys*, 81(10), 1278.

Fasano, A., & Catassi, C. (2012). Clinical practice. Celiac disease. *N Engl J Med*, 367(25), 2419–2426. doi: 10.1056/NEJMcp1113994.

Forman, D., & Pisani, P. (2008). Gastric cancer in Japan—honing treatment, seeking causes. *N Engl J Med*, 359(5), 448–451.

Ganz, R. A., Peters, J. H., Horgan, S., et al. (2013). Esophageal sphincter device for gastroesophageal reflux disease. *N Engl J Med*, 368(8), 719–727. doi: 10.1056/NEJMoa1205544.

Gralnek, I. M., Barkun, A. N., & Bardou, M. (2008). Management of acute bleeding from a peptic ulcer. *N Engl J Med*, 359(9), 928–937.

Green, P. H. (2009). Mortality in celiac disease, intestinal inflammation, and gluten sensitivity. *JAMA*, 302(11), 1225–1226.

Guirguis-Blake, J. (2008). Medical treatments in the short-term management of reflux esophagitis. *Am Fam Phys*, 77(5), 620.

Hartgrink, H. H., Jansen, E. P., van Grieken, N. C., & van de Velde, C. J. (2009). Gastric cancer. *Lancet*, 374(9688), 477–490.

Hvid-Jensen, F., Pedersen, L., Drewes, A. M., Sørensen, H. T., & Funch-Jensen, P. (2011). Incidence of adenocarcinoma among patients with Barrett's esophagus. *N Engl J Med*, 365(15), 1375–1383.

Jacobs, D. O. (2012). Bariatric surgery—from treatment of disease to prevention? *N Engl J Med*, 367(8), 764–765.

Kahrilas, P. J. (2008). Clinical practice. Gastroesophageal reflux disease. *N Engl J Med*, 359(16), 1700–1707.

Khan, M. A., John, B. K., Lashner, B. A., & Kirby, D. F. (2010). Difficulty swallowing solid foods; food 'getting stuck in the chest'. *Cleveland Clin J Med*, 77(6), 354–363.

Khushalani, N. (2008). Cancer of the esophagus and stomach. *Mayo Clin Proceed*, 83(6), 712–722.

Knox, M. A. (2011). Should we screen patients for Barrett's esophagus? No: the case against screening. *Am Fam Phys*, 83(10), 1148, 1150.

Kripke, C. (2012). Medical management vs. surgery for gastroesophageal reflux disease. *Am Fam Phys*, 82(3), 244.

Lacy, B. E., Weiser, K., Chertoff, J., et al. (2010). The diagnosis of gastroesophageal reflux disease. *Am J Med*, 123(7), 583–592. doi: 10.1016/j.amjmed.2010.01.007. Epub 2010 May 20.

Lau, J. Y., Barkun, A., Fan, D. M., et al. (2013). Challenges in the management of acute peptic ulcer bleeding. *Lancet*, 381(9882), 2033–2043. doi: 10.1016/S0140-6736(13)60596-6.

Leffler, D. (2011). Celiac disease diagnosis and management: a 46-year-old woman with anemia. *JAMA*, 306(14), 1582–1592.

Longo, D., Kasper, D., Fauci, A., Hauser, S., & Jameson, J. L. (2011). *Harrison's principles of internal medicine*. 18th ed. New York: McGraw-Hill.

Loyd, R. A., & McClellan, D. A. (2011). Update on the evaluation and management of functional dyspepsia. *Am Fam Phys*, 83(5), 547–552.

Ludvigsson, J. F., Montgomery, S. M., Ekbom, A., Brandt, L., & Granath, F. (2009). Small-intestinal histopathology and mortality risk in celiac disease. *JAMA*, 302(11), 1171–1178.

Mazzoleni, L. E., Francesconi, C. F., & Sander, G. B. (2011). Mass eradication of *Helicobacter pylori*: feasible and advisable? *Lancet*, 378(9790), 462–464.

Mingrone, G., Panunzi, S., De Gaetano, A., et al. (2012). Bariatric surgery versus conventional medical therapy for type 2 diabetes. *N Engl J Med*, 366(17), 1577–1585.

Mitka, M. (2012). Bariatric surgery continues to show benefits for patients with diabetes. *JAMA*, 307(18), 1901–1902.

[No authors listed]. (2010). Summaries for patients. Benefits and risks of continuing aspirin in patients with peptic ulcer bleeding. *Ann Int Med*, 152(1), I–20.

Orloff, M., Peterson, C., He, X., et al. (2011). Germline mutations in MSR1, ASCC1, and CTHRC1 in patients with Barrett esophagus and esophageal adenocarcinoma. *JAMA*, 306(4), 410–419.

Oxentenko, A. S., Bundrick, J. B., & Litin, S. C. (2011). Clinical pearls in gastroenterology 2011. *Mayo Clin Proceed*, 86(11), 1104–1108.

Padwal, R., Klarenbach, S., Wiebe, N., et al. (2011). Bariatric surgery; a systematic review of clinical and economic evidence. *J Gen Int Med*, 26(10), 1183–1194.

Schauer, P. R., Kashyap, S. R., Wolski, K., et al. (2012). Bariatric surgery versus intensive medical therapy in obese patients with diabetes. *N Engl J Med*, 366(17), 1567–1576.

Schroeder, R., Garrison, J. M., Jr., & Johnson, M. S. (2011). Treatment of adult obesity with bariatric surgery. *Am Fam Phys*, 84(7), 805–814.

Shah, M. A., & Ajani, J. A. (2010). Gastric cancer—an enigmatic and heterogeneous disease. *JAMA*, 303(17), 1753–1754.

Shaheen, N. J., Sharma, P., Overholt, B. F., et al. (2009). Radiofrequency ablation in Barrett's esophagus with dysplasia. *N Engl J Med*, 360(22), 2277–2288.

Sharma, P. (2009). Clinical practice. Barrett's esophagus. *N Engl J Med*, 361(26), 2548–2556.

Spechler, S. J. (2011). Pneumatic dilation and laparoscopic Heller's myotomy equally effective for achalasia. *N Engl J Med*, 364(19), 1868–1870.

Spechler, S. J. (2013). Barrett esophagus and risk of esophageal cancer: a clinical review. *JAMA*, 310(6), 627–636. doi: 10.1001/jama.2013.226450.

Srygley, F. D., Gerardo, C. J., Tran, T., & Fisher, D. A. (2012). Does this patient have a severe upper gastrointestinal bleed? *JAMA*, 307(10), 1072–1079.

Strayer, S. M. (2011). Should we screen patients for Barrett's esophagus? Yes: men with long-standing reflux symptoms should be screened with endoscopy. *Am Fam Phys*, 83(10), 140, 1142, 1147.

Temmerman, J. C. (2012). Effects of bariatric surgeries on obesity and comorbidities. *Am Fam Phys*, 86(3), 218, 222.

Torpy, J. M., Lynm, C., & Glass, R. M. (2010). *JAMA* patient page. Stomach cancer. *JAMA*, 303(17), 1771.

van der Windt, D. A., Jellema, P., Mulder, C. J., Kneepkens, C. M., & van der Horst, H. E. (2010). Diagnostic testing for celiac disease among patients with abdominal symptoms: a systematic review. *JAMA*, 303(17), 1738–1746.

van Zanten, S. V. (2009). Dyspepsia and reflux in primary care: rough DIAMOND of a trial. *Lancet*, 373(9659), 187–188.

Wee, E. W. (2013). Evidence-based approach to dyspepsia: from *Helicobacter pylori* to functional disease. *Postgrad Med*, 125(4), 169–180.

Wilkins, T., Khan, N., Nabh, A., & Schade, R. R. (2012). Diagnosis and management of upper gastrointestinal bleeding. *Am Fam Phys*, 85(5), 469–476.

Wong, T., Tian, J., & Nagar, A. B. (2010). Barrett's surveillance identifies patients with early esophageal adenocarcinoma. *Am J Med*, 123(5), 462–467. doi: 10.1016/j.amjmed.2009.10.013.

Common Disorders of the Large Intestine

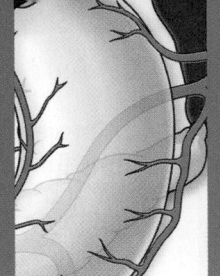

Key Terms

Acute abdomen
Acute colonic pseudo-obstruction
Anastomosis
Appendicitis
Borborygmi
Cathartic colon
Colectomy
Colostomy
Diverticula

Diverticulitis
Diverticulosis
Fecal impaction
Hematochezia
Hemorrhoids
Ileostomy
Inflammatory bowel disease (IBD)
Irritable bowel syndrome (IBS)
McBurney's point

Melena
Murphy's sign
Obstipation
Peritonitis
Pseudopolyp
Skip lesions
Stoma
Toxic megacolon
Volvulus

The normal function of the intestinal tract is to propel digested food forward, absorb nutrients and water, and finally excrete waste and indigestible contents. Inflammation, irritation, infection, obstruction, and certain medications can all interfere with the normal function of the large intestine. Inflammatory bowel disease (IBD) hinders adequate absorption of nutrients and causes pain in the affected individual throughout life. IBD produces extremely painful intestinal lesions visible on colonoscopy; in contrast, irritable bowel syndrome (IBS) causes similar abdominal pain but has no clear etiology or apparent pathology.

Obstruction of the large bowel can occur abruptly and cause sudden, severe abdominal pain; this condition requires prompt intervention. Inflammation of the intestine commonly causes a tender abdomen, intense pain, and fever for the patient, a syndrome known as acute abdomen, which is a surgical emergency. Obstructive neoplasms, diverticulitis, and twisting of the intestine can lead to a serious, potentially lethal complication known as peritonitis. Appendicitis—inflammation of a vestigial part of the intestine—can lead to perforation if not diagnosed promptly. Perforation of the bowel and peritonitis are the major concerns of clinicians treating disorders of the large intestine.

Epidemiology

Disorders of the large intestine can be classified as either alterations in the integrity of the gastrointestinal (GI) wall or alterations in motility. Alterations in the integrity of the GI wall can occur anywhere along the large bowel; they can be caused by IBD, such as Crohn's disease and ulcerative colitis (UC), and inflammatory conditions, such as appendicitis and diverticulitis. IBD affects an

estimated 1 to 2 million people in the United States, with an incidence of 70 to 150 cases per 100,000 individuals.

Common disorders that cause alterations in motility include IBS, bowel obstruction, and intestinal herniation. Between 30% and 45% of all GI conditions are caused by intestinal motility disorders, with up to 30 million Americans affected per year. Colonic motility dysfunction caused by malignancy occurs most commonly in the elderly population. Approximately 60% of large bowel obstructions (LBOs) are caused by malignancies, 20% are caused by diverticular disease, and 5% are the result of colonic volvulus. There is no clear pathological cause of IBS, but it is prevalent in people aged 20 to 40 years, affecting women 3 times more often than men. Dysfunctional colonic motility may be caused by diet or an autonomic imbalance called acute colonic pseudo-obstruction.

Basic Concepts Regarding Function of the Large Intestine

There are a number of different kinds of large intestine disorders. To understand the pathophysiology of intestinal dysfunction, knowledge of the normal functions of the intestine is required.

Structure of the Large Intestine

The large intestine is a hollow tube approximately 1.5 m in length and 6 to 7 cm in diameter. It works to absorb water and salt and to store feces until defecation. The large intestine is made up of the cecum; ascending, transverse, descending, and sigmoid colon; rectum; and anal canal.

The cecum is a blind pouch that projects downward at the junction of the ileum portion of the small intestine and the colon. The appendix, which is approximately 2.5 cm in length, arises from the cecum and has no apparent function. The illeocecal and rectosigmoid (O'Beirne) sphincters control the flow of contents through the large intestine. The ileocecal sphincter, also called the iliocecal valve, located at the junction of the ileum and the cecum allows approximately 500 to 700 mL of fluid waste to flow through it every day. The ascending colon arises from the cecum on the right side of the abdomen and curves to the left just under the liver, where it becomes the transverse colon. The transverse colon, the largest portion of the bowel, lies beneath the stomach and spleen. The portion under the liver is called the hepatic flexure, whereas the portion beneath the spleen is called the splenic flexure. Throughout the ascending and transverse colon, a large amount of water and electrolytes is absorbed from the intestinal contents. The descending colon passes down through the upper back portion of the abdomen and along the side of the left kidney. Within the descending colon, there is also a large amount of water reabsorption. It continues into the S-shaped sigmoid colon that sits in the pelvis. At the sigmoid, intestinal contents are solid and are slowed up in their forward progress by the rectosigmoid sphincter, which controls the movement of wastes from the sigmoid colon into the rectum. The rectum is a 6- to 8-inch length of bowel that functions as a holding site for feces until excretion through the anal canal (see Fig. 30-1).

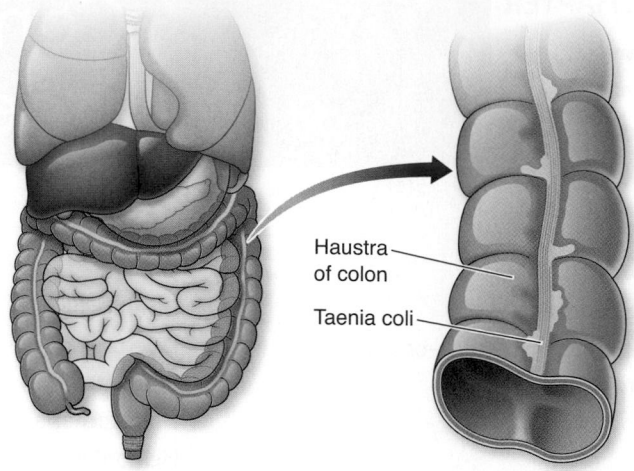

FIGURE 30-2. Haustra and taenia coli of the large intestine. Haustra, pouchlike formations of the wall of the large intestine, are formed by circular muscle fibers called taenia coli that are 1 to 2 cm apart.

The large intestine is composed of longitudinal and circular muscle layers. The longitudinal layer is made up of three long muscle bands called taenia coli. These muscle bands are shorter than the colon, producing a gathered appearance, much like the way a skirt is gathered at the waist. The circular muscle layer separates the colon into segments termed haustra, which gives the large intestine its characteristic appearance (see Fig. 30-2).

Structure of the GI Wall

The GI wall begins below the upper one-third of the esophagus and has five layers:

1. inner
2. middle
3. circular
4. longitudinal
5. outer.

The inner layer, also known as the mucosa, is composed mainly of goblet cells and columnar epithelial cells. Goblet cells produce mucus to lubricate the intestine and protect it from injury. Columnar epithelial cells absorb fluid and electrolytes. The mucosal layer constantly replicates, and approximately 250 grams of mucosal epithelial cells are shed every day in the stool.

The middle layer, also known as the submucosal layer, contains connective tissue, blood vessels, nerves, and cellular structures responsible for secreting digestive enzymes. Below the submucosa are muscle layers. The circular and longitudinal muscle layers facilitate the forward peristaltic movement of intestinal contents along the colon. Finally, the outer layer, also known as the peritoneum, is loosely attached to the entire outer wall of the intestine; it is the largest serous membrane in the body (see Fig. 30-3).

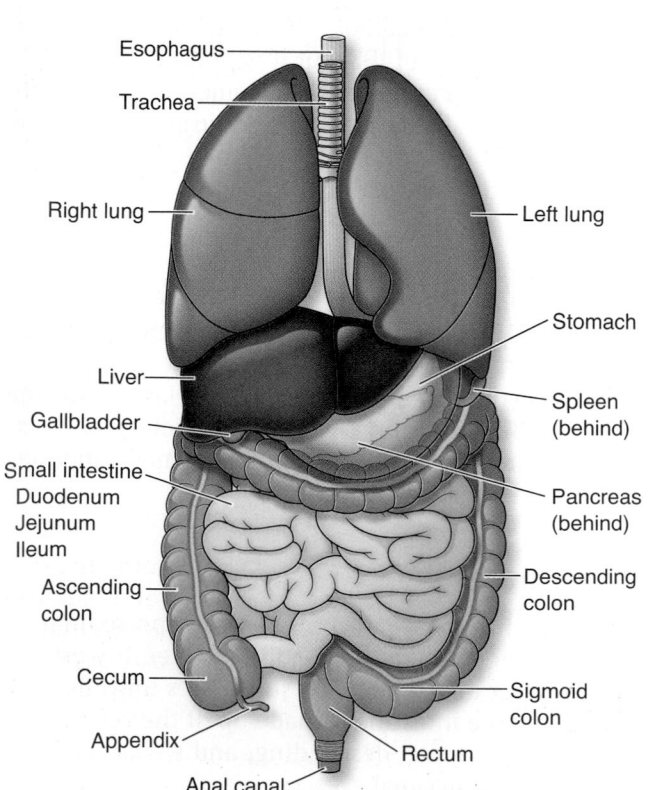

FIGURE 30-1. Anatomy of the GI system.

and the rectum, which stimulates defecation. The hormones gastrin and cholecystokinin participate in the stimulation of this reflex. Epinephrine is an inhibitor of this reflex, as can be seen in the fact that during the fight-or-flight response, when levels of epinephrine are high, the urge to defecate is suppressed.

Neural Control of GI Tract

Neural control of the large intestine is generally directed by the autonomic nervous system as well as the nerves that compose the enteric nervous system, which lies entirely in the wall of the GI tract. Neurons in the wall of the GI tract consist of two networks: the myenteric and the submucosal plexuses. Both are aggregates of ganglionic cells that extend along the length of the GI wall.

The myenteric plexus controls the motility of the entire gut, as it extends all the way down the intestinal wall. The submucosal plexus innervates each segment of the GI tract separately and controls local motility and secretory functions as well as absorption. The myenteric plexus regulates both motor and secretory activity.

Extrinsic parasympathetic innervation occurs through the vagus nerve, passing through the pelvic nerves and extending from the cecum to the first part of the transverse colon. This innervation is responsible for the rhythmic contraction of the colon. The internal anal sphincter is usually maintained in a state of contraction; however, when the rectum is distended, the reflex is stimulated to relax. The intrinsic nerve plexuses provide the major innervation to the internal anal sphincter, which also receives sympathetic stimulation to maintain contraction and then parasympathetic stimulation, which stimulates relaxation when the rectum is full and stretched.

The external anal sphincter is innervated by branches of nerves from the sacral division of the spinal cord. This is sympathetic stimulation from the celiac and the superior mesenteric ganglia. The sympathetic stimulation of the large intestine is responsible for modulating reflexes, conveying somatic sensations of fullness and pain, participating in the defecation reflex, and constricting blood vessels. The blood supply to the large intestine is provided through branches of the superior and inferior mesenteric arteries.

Absorption Within the Large Intestine

The surface of the large intestine is smooth, and one of its main functions is the absorption of water and electrolytes—mainly sodium and chloride. Sodium is actively absorbed, whereas chloride follows passively down an electrochemical gradient. Water follows osmotically.

Most of the digestion and absorption of food and nutrients takes place in the small intestine. As such, the large intestine does not secrete any digestive enzymes.

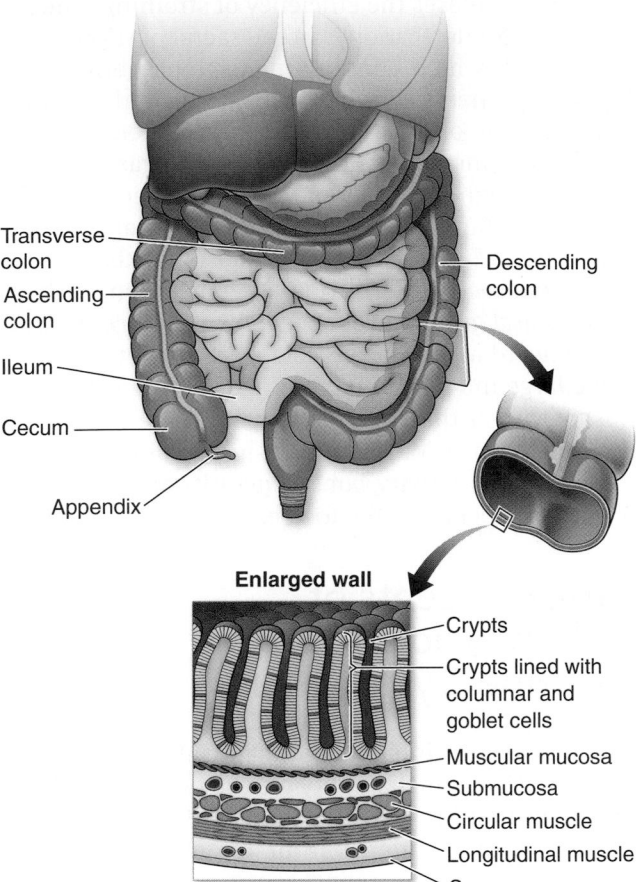

FIGURE 30-3. The mucosal lining of the large intestine is a large surface area that can absorb water and nutrients. There is a large presence of goblet cells that secrete mucus. Smooth muscles within the wall perform peristalsis to keep intestinal contents moving forward.

Labels: Transverse colon, Ascending colon, Ileum, Cecum, Appendix, Descending colon

Enlarged wall labels: Crypts, Crypts lined with columnar and goblet cells, Muscular mucosa, Submucosa, Circular muscle, Longitudinal muscle, Serosa

Colonic Motility

The movements in the large intestine can be classified as two types: haustrations and propulsions. Haustrations are segmental mixing or kneading movements that shuffle the contents back and forth among the haustra. This increases the contact time with the mucosa to facilitate the absorption of water and electrolytes and allow time for bacteria to accumulate. The circular muscles contract and relax at different sites, creating a shuffling effect. This is the primary type of movement in the colon, which is initiated by the autonomic nerves within the smooth muscle cells.

Propulsions, or propulsive mass movement, generally occur after meals. A large segment of the colon (greater than 20 cm) contracts as one unit, moving fecal contents forward. A series of these movements lasts approximately 10 to 30 minutes and occurs several times per day. After contents arrive at the rectum, defecation is initiated by one of these movements. Within the anal canal, there are voluntary muscles that allow self-control of defecation.

The gastrocolic reflex initiates propulsion of the entire colon, usually during or after eating. This causes the fecal mass to pass rapidly into the sigmoid colon

It secretes alkaline mucus, which coats and protects the mucosa from chemical and mechanical injury. This alkalinity neutralizes acids produced by local bacteria fermentation. There is less absorption in the large intestine than the small intestine, because of the smaller amount of surface area in the large intestine.

The electrochemical gradient established by sodium movement enhances the diffusion of serum potassium from the capillaries in the lumen. As more sodium is absorbed, more potassium is lost.

Aldosterone responds when sodium is low or potassium is high. Aldosterone increases the membrane permeability to sodium, and it increases both the diffusion of sodium into cells and its active transport into interstitial fluid. By the time that the mass gets to the sigmoid colon, it consists entirely of wastes and is now called feces. Feces is made up of water, food residue, unabsorbed GI secretions, shed epithelial cells, bile pigments, and bacteria.

Microorganisms in the colon are responsible for the breakdown of proteins that were not digested or absorbed in the small intestine. These resulting amino acids are broken down by bacteria, which leaves ammonia. This ammonia is carried to the liver and is converted to urea. The majority (95%) of the bacteria in the large intestine are anaerobes. Bacteria contribute to one-third of the bulk of solid feces. The most common organisms are bacteroides, *Clostridia, Anaerobic lactobacilli*, and *E. coli.*

At birth, the large intestine is sterile. By 3 to 4 weeks after birth, normal flora is established. The microorganisms of the colon do not have any digestive or absorptive function. However, they do play a part in the metabolism of bile salts by helping to absorb bile and remove toxic metabolites. Microorganisms also function in the metabolism of estrogens, androgens, and lipids. They convert unabsorbed carbohydrates into absorbable organic acids. Finally, microorganisms in the large intestine aid in the metabolism of various nitrogenous substances and drugs and also protect against infection.

Defecation

Defecation is controlled by the internal and external anal sphincters. The urge to defecate occurs with the movement of feces into the sigmoid colon and the rectum. When food enters the stomach, mass movements occur in the colon by means of the gastrocolic reflex. This is most evident after the first meal of the day. Nerve endings in the rectum become stretched, sending a signal to the sacral cord, which then reflexively sends them back to the descending and sigmoid colon, rectum, and anus. The internal anal sphincter is innervated to relax, which creates the urge to defecate.

This reflex can be overridden by voluntary contraction of the external anal sphincter, which then reduces the urge to defecate. Stress or pain can inhibit defecations and, possibly, lead to constipation. Defecation is facilitated by squatting or sitting, because this straightens out the angle between the rectum and the anal canal and increases the efficiency of straining. The reflex center for defecation is in the sacral portion of the spinal cord, which contains parasympathetic nerve fibers. These nerves produce contraction of the rectum and relaxation of the internal anal sphincter.

At times, instead of feces, intestinal gas or flatus passes through the intestine. The gas that is passed originates from either of two sources: swallowed air (can be up to 500 mL per meal) and the gas that is produced from bacterial fermentation in the colon. Rushing of fluids and gurgling sounds, known as **borborygmi,** can be heard as the gas percolates through the lumen of the large intestine. Eructation, or burping, removes most of the gas that is swallowed, but some of it passes into the intestine. Most of the gas in the colon is a result of the bacterial activity, but the quantity and the nature of the gas depends on the food eaten.

Basic Concepts of Pathophysiology of Large Intestine Dysfunction

Alterations in the integrity of the intestinal wall or disruptions of intestinal motility are the pathophysiologic conditions that can affect the large intestine. Intestinal motility disorders range from frequent spasmodic, repetitive abnormal intestinal contractions to loss of intestinal motility called paralytic ileus. Inflammatory conditions include appendicitis, diverticulitis, and IBD.

Intestinal Motility Dysfunction

Any alteration in the transit of foods and secretions in the digestive tube may be considered an intestinal motility disorder. This would include an obstructive lesion, intestinal pseudo-obstruction (Ogilvie syndrome), IBS, fecal incontinence, and constipation.

An obstructive lesion in the large intestine causes ineffective intestinal propulsion and characteristic signs of dilated tubular loops of intestine related to the obstruction on image studies, such as abdominal x-ray. Common causes of obstruction include a cancerous mass, benign polyps, diverticular disease, adhesions, volvulus, incarcerated hernia, or intussusception.

In a condition referred to as **acute colonic pseudo-obstruction,** the patient undergoes the same symptoms of intestinal nonpropulsion—abdominal distention and cramping caused by gas collection in the bowel. However, there is no obstructive lesion. The etiology of pseudo-obstruction is thought to involve dysfunctional changes in the neuromuscular system of the intestine.

Commonly used drugs such as tricyclic antidepressants can interfere with intestinal motility. Drugs that have anticholinergic effects cause constipation (see Box 30-1). Narcotic bowel syndrome, which causes decreased intestinal motility, is commonly observed in patients who abuse opiates for chronic pain. Endocrine disorders such as myxedema can also cause slowed colonic motility or pseudo-obstruction. Laxatives, including purgatives and cathartic agents, are agents taken to induce bowel movements or to loosen the stool, which are most often taken to treat constipation. Laxatives work to increase the movement of fecal matter along the colon. Certain stimulant, lubricant, and saline laxatives are used to evacuate the colon for rectal or bowel examinations and may be supplemented by enemas under certain circumstances.

Sufficiently high doses of laxatives cause diarrhea. Some laxatives combine more than one active ingredient to produce a combination of the effects. Laxatives may be oral or in suppository form. Chronic use of laxatives is not recommended because it can lead to lack of natural colonic motility. **Cathartic colon** is the anatomical and physiologic change in the colon that occurs with chronic use of stimulant laxatives. Excessive laxative use is defined as more than 3 times per week for at least 1 year. Signs and symptoms of cathartic colon include bloating, a feeling of fullness, abdominal pain, and incomplete fecal evacuation. Radiological studies show an atonic and redundant colon. Chronic use of stimulant laxatives can lead to serious medical consequences, such as fluid and electrolyte imbalance, steatorrhea, protein-losing gastroenteropathy, osteomalacia, and vitamin and mineral deficiencies. When the drug is discontinued, radiographic and functional changes in the colon may only partially return to normal because of drug-induced neuromuscular damage to the colon.

Constipation is a common problem, especially in the elderly. Problems occur when severe constipation causes fecal impaction and obstipation. **Fecal impaction** occurs when hard stool that cannot be passed is lodged in the sigmoid colon and rectum. Commonly, a patient can develop liquid stools that pass around a fecal impaction. In **obstipation,** there is the sensation to defecate but no passage of stool, liquid, or gas from the colon.

Inflammation of the Bowel

Aside from motility disorders, inflammation of the colon's interior can occur. Appendicitis is one of the most common inflammatory conditions of the GI tract.

The appendix, a small tubular appendage off the cecum that has no function, can become filled with indigestible contents and become inflamed. Appendicitis causes intense abdominal pain and requires surgery.

Abdominal pain also occurs in **irritable bowel syndrome (IBS)**. Patients experience frequent episodes of abdominal pain, bloating, and abdominal distention. There are also bouts of constipation and diarrhea; however, there is no pathological change within the interior of the bowel and etiology is unclear.

Inflammatory Bowel Disease (IBD), in contrast, is caused by pathological changes in the wall of the colon. UC and Crohn's disease, both types of IBD, cause severe abdominal pain, diarrhea, bloody stools, and weight loss. The bowel mucosa is friable, edematous, ulcerated, scarred, and bleeding. There are some extraintestinal symptoms such as fever, dermatological lesions, weight loss, and arthralgias.

Diverticulitis is another inflammatory disorder of the colon. Diverticuli are weak areas that form pouches off the wall of the large intestine. Commonly, these pouches become filled with stagnant intestinal contents, leading to obstruction and inflammation of the bowel wall.

Assessment

The clinician should obtain a complete patient history, recording information about the following:

- abdominal pain, cramping, nausea or vomiting, excessive gas, and rectal fullness
- frequency, amount, and timing of normal defecation and any recent change
- amount, consistency, and color of stool
- type of diet, use of laxatives or enemas, and drug use.

When interviewing the patient, it is important to distinguish complete bowel obstruction from partial obstruction, which is associated with passage of some gas or stools. Partial obstruction is a less urgent condition than complete obstruction. It is important that the clinician ask about the patient's current and past medical history, including current medications. With a large bowel obstruction (LBO), the patient may complain of abdominal distention, nausea, vomiting, cramping, and colicky abdominal pains. An abrupt onset of symptoms makes an acute obstructive event, such as volvulus, a likely diagnosis. Obstruction that dilates the colon causes vague, abdominal cramps; anorexia; and, late in the disorder, vomiting. LBO may be accompanied by fever or leukocytosis. A history of chronic constipation, long-term laxative use, and straining at stools implies diverticulitis or malignancy. Changes in the patient's caliber of stool and dark color can suggest malignancy as well. Dark stools may contain blood, which is a condition called **melena.** When weight loss accompanies changes in stool, the likelihood of malignancy increases. A history of recurrent left lower quadrant (LLQ) abdominal pain over several years is consistent with diverticulitis, diverticular stricture, or similar disorder. Intense abdominal pain may indicate peritonitis. In **peritonitis,** the inflamed peritoneum is highly sensitive and any movement of the abdominal contents causes pain.

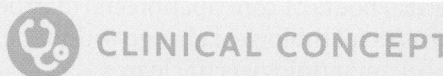 **CLINICAL CONCEPT**

Colicky pain, intense abdominal pain that occurs in waves, is often a characteristic of large bowel disorders.

Physical Examination

The physical examination of the abdomen should be done in the order of inspection, auscultation, percussion, and palpation. The abdomen may appear distended if filled with gas because of obstruction. When auscultating the abdomen, bowel sounds may be normal early in the course of the disorder, but may become quiet or rushing as time passes. Percussion of the abdomen may reveal tympany, a high-pitched sound, if there is a gas-filled bowel. Palpation of the abdomen may reveal tenderness, rigidity, and involuntary guarding, which are signs of inflammation of the peritoneal membrane. An abdomen that is tender and showing signs of inflammation of the peritoneal membrane is referred to as an **acute abdomen.** Signs of acute abdomen include involuntary guarding and rebound tenderness (see Table 30-1).

During the physical exam, it is important that the clinician palpate the tender area of the abdomen last. Any disruption of abdominal contents will cause pain in peritonitis. Patients want to lie as still as possible when being examined because movement causes pain. Right lower quadrant (RLQ) tenderness is commonly caused by appendicitis, whereas LLQ tenderness is commonly associated with diverticulitis. Upper right quadrant (URQ) tenderness elicited by palpation is called **Murphy's sign,** which is commonly caused by cholecystitis, an inflammation of the gallbladder. A rectal examination may elicit pain in disorders such as appendicitis. A digital exam may also demonstrate hard stool in the rectum with fecal impaction. A stool sample should be obtained for fecal occult blood testing (FOBT). In female patients, a pelvic examination is needed to rule out a gynecological source of pain; for example, ectopic pregnancy or ovarian cysts can cause abdominal pain that appears similar to GI pain.

Evaluation of the inguinal and femoral regions should be an integral part of the examination in a patient with suspected LBO. Incarcerated hernias represent a frequently missed cause of bowel obstruction. In particular, colonic obstruction is often caused by a left-sided inguinal hernia with the sigmoid colon incarcerated in the hernia (see Fig. 30-4).

TABLE 30-1. Signs of Acute Abdomen on Physical Examination	
ABDOMINAL PAIN	Waves of sharp constricting pain that take the breath away. Pain is worsened by movement.
INVOLUNTARY GUARDING	The patient's abdominal muscles contract with palpation.
ABDOMINAL RIGIDITY	The abdomen is stiff to the touch.
REBOUND TENDERNESS	When the examiner deeply palpates the abdomen, pain is felt by the patient as the examiner lifts his or her hand.

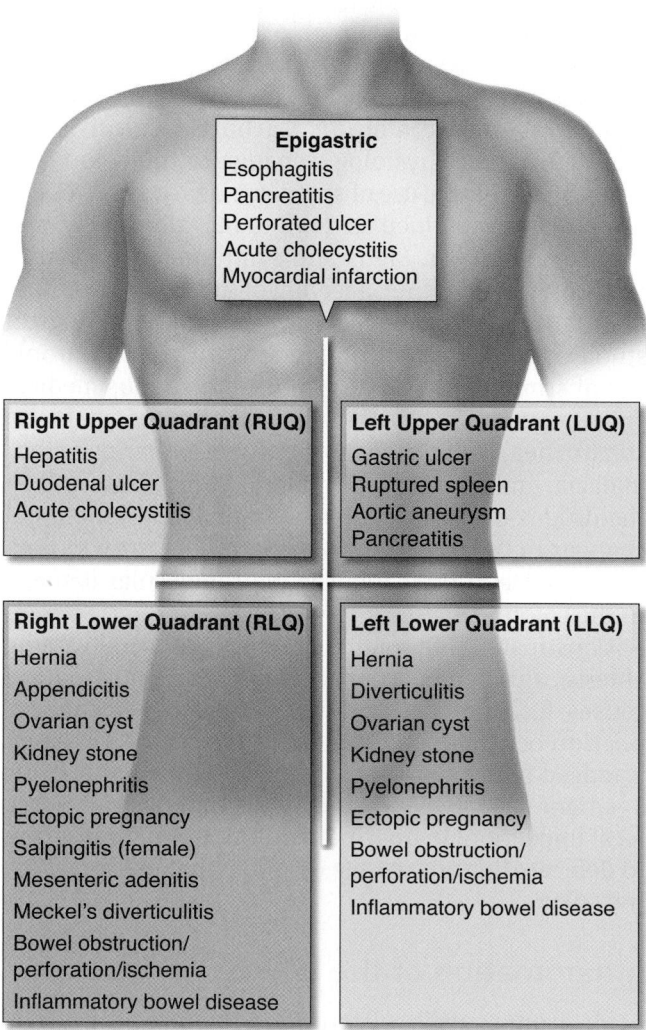

Epigastric
Esophagitis
Pancreatitis
Perforated ulcer
Acute cholecystitis
Myocardial infarction

Right Upper Quadrant (RUQ)
Hepatitis
Duodenal ulcer
Acute cholecystitis

Left Upper Quadrant (LUQ)
Gastric ulcer
Ruptured spleen
Aortic aneurysm
Pancreatitis

Right Lower Quadrant (RLQ)
Hernia
Appendicitis
Ovarian cyst
Kidney stone
Pyelonephritis
Ectopic pregnancy
Salpingitis (female)
Mesenteric adenitis
Meckel's diverticulitis
Bowel obstruction/perforation/ischemia
Inflammatory bowel disease

Left Lower Quadrant (LLQ)
Hernia
Diverticulitis
Ovarian cyst
Kidney stone
Pyelonephritis
Ectopic pregnancy
Bowel obstruction/perforation/ischemia
Inflammatory bowel disease

FIGURE 30-4. Causes of acute abdomen by abdominal quadrant in which pain is felt.

ALERT! Women with acute abdomen require a pelvic exam and pregnancy test to rule out ectopic pregnancy.

Diagnosis

One of the simplest diagnostic studies that can be performed is a FOBT. Blood in the stool, termed melena, can be detected in such disorders as bleeding peptic ulcer or bowel malignancy. Laboratory studies can demonstrate dehydration and electrolyte imbalance. A complete blood count, serum chemistry, and urinalysis should also be conducted. A decreased hemoglobin (Hgb) and hematocrit (Hct) can indicate iron deficiency anemia, which often develops in chronic GI bleeding. An elevated serum amylase can indicate a perforated organ or pancreatitis. A chest x-ray can demonstrate free air under the diaphragm, which indicates perforation of the intestine or a hollow organ. Abdominal x-rays can clearly show shadows of the dilated, obstructed bowel. Contrast studies using barium or gastrografin can highlight the bowel anatomy. Radiological signs of bowel obstruction include bowel distention and the presence of multiple gas-fluid levels on supine and erect abdominal x-rays. Contrast barium enema, GI series, or computed tomography (CT) scan can be used to define the level of obstruction, determine whether the obstruction is partial or complete, and help define the cause of the obstruction. Flexible colonoscopy can visualize the large bowel up to the cecum.

CLINICAL CONCEPT

- FOBT or stool guaiac tests can detect blood in the stool. Accuracy is highest after completion of three tests at three different times.
- A chest x-ray can show free air under the diaphragm when there is perforation of the bowel or abdominal organ. Air under the diaphragm from perforation of the bowel commonly causes shoulder pain.

Treatment of Large Intestine Disorders

In general, a diet high in fiber is recommended for bowel health. However, when there is an obstructive lesion or acute inflammation, resting the bowel is necessary. Intravenous fluid, nothing-by-mouth (NPO) orders, analgesics, and antipyretics are used in appendicitis, diverticulitis, and IBD. Antibiotics, corticosteroids, and immunosuppressants are used in IBD. Surgical intervention is commonly used to relieve a bowel obstruction. In most patients, the obstructing lesion is surgically excised; if necessary, a colostomy

or ileostomy is then performed. An **ileostomy** or **colostomy** is a reversible or irreversible surgical procedure where the healthy end of the intestine is brought out of the abdomen through an incision in the anterior abdominal wall. In ileostomy, the ileum of the small intestine is surgically brought out to the exterior abdominal wall. In colostomy, the colon is similarly brought out to the anterior abdomen. The opening, called a **stoma,** allows for excretion of intestinal contents into an attached collection appliance. Alternatively, endoscopically placed expandable stents can be used to relieve LBO.

CLINICAL CONCEPT

Pain is a valuable diagnostic clue in cases of acute abdomen. The location of pain can assist in diagnosis. Opiates are often withheld until a diagnosis is made.

Pathophysiology of Specific Disorders of the Large Intestine

The large intestine can undergo many different kinds of pathophysiologic conditions. Inflammation, perforation, structural problems, and acute abdominal processes all present in different ways and require various kinds of medical or surgical treatment.

Inflammatory Bowel Disease

IBD includes Crohn's disease, also called regional enteritis, and ulcerative colitis (UC). Both Crohn's disease and UC are chronic, incurable diseases that can occur at any age, but they are more prevalent in the young adult.

Crohn's Disease

Crohn's disease is a chronic, transmural inflammatory process of the bowel that often leads to fibrosis and obstructive symptoms; it can affect any part of the GI tract from the mouth to the anus. The most common location is the terminal ileum and ascending right colon.

Prevalence is approximately 7 cases per 100,000 population in the United States. Urban areas have a higher prevalence of IBD than rural areas, and individuals of upper socioeconomic classes have a higher prevalence than persons of lower socioeconomic classes. The rate of Crohn's disease in women is 1.1 to 1.8 times higher than that in men. The peak of onset occurs between age 15 and 30 years, and a second peak occurs between age 60 and 80 years. However, most cases begin before age 30 years, and approximately 20% to 30% of all patients with Crohn's disease are diagnosed before age 20 years.

Etiology. There is no known cause of Crohn's disease. Etiologic theories involve genetic, immunological, infectious, and environmental influences that contribute to an overactive inflammatory response to unknown triggers. When both parents have Crohn's, there is a 50% chance that their children will have the disease. Although an association has been established between Crohn's disease and high consumption of refined sugars and saturated fats, no conclusive dietary etiology has been identified. Also, smoking has been strongly linked to the development of the disorder. Psychological and psychosocial stress factors can precipitate exacerbations. It has also been proposed that infection with *Mycobacterium paratuberculosis*, *Pseudomonas*, or *Listeria* may be causative of Crohn's disease. A diet high in fatty foods has also been implicated as an etiologic agent.

Risk factors include genetic predisposition, ethnicity, and cigarette smoking. An individual has a high risk of Crohn's disease if a family member has the disease. Caucasians are affected more often than African Americans. Those of Ashkenazi Jewish ethnic background are particularly at high risk. Urban living has also been associated with Crohn's disease. There is an increasing amount of information about Crohn's disease and mutated genes on several different chromosomes. Mutations within the *NOD2* gene, also known as the *IBD1* gene or *CARD-15* gene, have been shown to confer susceptibility to Crohn's disease. The *NOD2* gene, which is found on chromosome 16, regulates intracellular immune responses to bacterial products. Approximately 25% of Caucasian children have the *NOD2* gene, compared with only 2% of African American and Hispanic children. Other regions linked to IBD are the *IBD3* gene on chromosome 6 and *IBD5* gene on chromosome 5. A protective gene, termed the *IL23R* gene, has recently been discovered. Individuals with a mutated *IL23R* gene have a susceptibility to Crohn's disease. Another recent discovery is a single nucleotide polymorphism in the *ATG16L1* gene, which predisposes individuals to Crohn's disease. Research regarding genetic mutations and susceptibility to IBD continues to evolve. It is most likely a disorder caused by a combination of genetic and immunological factors.

Pathophysiology. Crohn's disease characteristically affects the entire thickness of the bowel wall and all layers of the submucosa. The mucosa is chronically inflamed and contains a high number of immunoglobulins, T cells, and macrophages. T cells attract nonspecific inflammatory cells, especially neutrophils, which play a major role in tissue damage. This response produces cytokines, growth factors, antibodies, and proteases, which all contribute to continual tissue destruction. The lesions are visible as edematous, reddish-purple areas in a segmental pattern. There are areas of disease separated by healthy areas, referred to as **skip lesions.**

Lymph nodes in the submucosa are enlarged. Small superficial ulcerations with deep fissures penetrate the bowel and lead to fistulas and abscesses. Anal fissures are common; ulceration of the perianal area can result from chronic diarrhea. Characteristic lesions, known as crypt abscesses, are composed of polymorphonuclear

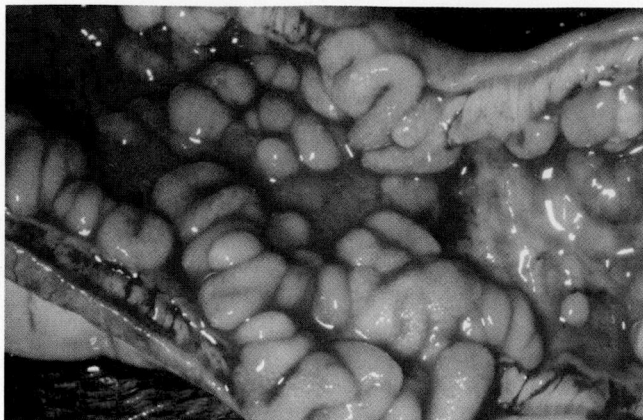

FIGURE 30-5. Inflammatory cobblestoning found in Crohn's disease. *(From Biophoto Associates/Science Source.)*

leukocytes, lymphocytes, red blood cells, and cellular debris. The bowel mucosa develops granulomas; this is exhibited as an effect called cobblestoning. Secondary infections occur, leaving scarred and fibrotic tissue, narrowing of the lumen, thickening of the bowel wall, and shortening of the colon (see Fig. 30-5).

Occasionally toxic megacolon occurs in Crohn's disease. **Toxic megacolon** is the extreme dilation of a segment of the diseased colon, commonly the transverse colon. It causes complete obstruction and impaired absorption of fluids and electrolytes. In toxic megacolon, life-threatening perforation and peritonitis can result.

Clinical Presentation. The patient usually complains of episodes of diarrhea and abdominal pain. The typical presentation of Crohn's disease occurs in remissions and exacerbations. The clinician should focus on associated GI symptoms, such as appearance of stool, blood in the stool, number of stools per day, and aggravating or alleviating factors.

Malabsorption and nutritional deficiencies are a prominent sign of Crohn's disease with resultant anemia and fatigue. There is impaired absorption of fats, folic acid, iron, calcium, and vitamins A, B_{12}, C, D, E and K. Electrolytes, trace elements, and minerals are lost through diarrhea, including sodium, potassium, magnesium, zinc, and copper. The patient can become anemic from loss of blood in the stool, as well as dehydrated from loss of fluid in the stool. The patient's weight is important as many affected by Crohn's disease suffer malabsorption. Laxative or antibiotic use, dietary intake of certain foods, and emotional stress can stimulate an exacerbation.

Signs and Symptoms. The signs and symptoms of Crohn's disease include abdominal tenderness, increased bowel sounds, steady progressive weight loss, anorexia, nausea, vomiting and diarrhea, pallor, and, in acute exacerbations, fever. Severe bouts can cause intestinal obstruction with accompanying signs of borborygmi, abdominal distention, and tympany on percussion.

Aside from intestinal symptoms, Crohn's disease can cause arthritis, uveitis, cheilitis, and dermatological problems. Hepatic or bile duct inflammation can also occur. Cheilitis is an inflammatory lesion of the lips, commonly in the corners of the mouth. Canker sores, also called aphthous ulcers, may develop as well. Uveitis is the inflammation of the middle layer of the eye where circulation is provided to the retina. Retinal detachment can result from uveitis. Dermatological lesions, referred to as erythema nodosum, can develop; they are tender, red nodules commonly occurring on the shins.

Diagnosis. A diagnosis of IBD is based on clinical signs and symptoms and endoscopic, radiological, and histological criteria. Distinguishing between Crohn's disease and UC can be a challenge because of their similar presenting symptoms; however, a colonoscopy can differentiate the disorders (see Table 30-2).

Colonoscopy with terminal ileoscopy and biopsy is central to the diagnosis of Crohn's disease. Biopsies should be taken of both the inflamed and normal tissues for pathological analysis. Capsule endoscopy can be used to study the whole length of the GI tract. Otherwise, upper GI and lower GI studies need to be performed as well as upper endoscopy and colonoscopy. Upper and lower GI contrast studies with gastrografin are used in diagnosis. Barium has been replaced by gastrografin as a contrast media because it is nontoxic if the intestine is perforated. CT scans and magnetic resonance imaging (MRI) scans are also used in diagnosis.

Treatment. Management of Crohn's disease includes consuming adequate fluids and a balanced diet, along with a multivitamin supplement. Chronic diarrhea in Crohn's disease responds well to antidiarrheals, such as loperamide, diphenoxylate with atropine, and tincture of opium. Patients with terminal ileal disease may not absorb bile acids normally, which can lead to secretory diarrhea in the colon. These patients may benefit from bile acid sequestrants, such as cholestyramine. Abdominal cramps may be reduced with propantheline dicyclomine or hyoscyamine. 5-aminosalicylic acid derivative medications, such as sulfasalazine, are used to reduce the inflammation brought on by the immune reaction. Immunosuppressives and antibiotics are also used to diminish the inflammation. Corticosteroids are used to treat flare-ups of moderate-to-severe disease, but are not indicated for maintenance therapy.

Although most patients with Crohn's disease require surgical intervention during their lifetime, surgery does not cure the disorder. Between 75% and 80% of persons with Crohn's disease require surgery within 20 years of the onset of symptoms. Many require multiple procedures. Within 1 year after surgery, 20% to 30% of patients experience a recurrence of disease. Every attempt at conserving the bowel is made in the surgical approach to Crohn's disease. However, repeated intestinal resection is common and its complication, short-bowel syndrome, can occur.

Ulcerative Colitis

Like Crohn's disease, UC is an IBD, and they each present with similar symptoms and pathophysiologic changes of the intestine. However, UC solely involves the large intestine, whereas Crohn's disease can affect any area of the GI tract. UC can also lead to cancer.

Incidence of UC is 10 to 12 cases per 100,000 people in the United States per year. It is 3 times more common than Crohn's disease and it is more frequent in Caucasians than in African Americans or Hispanics. Incidence is reported to be 2 to 4 times higher in Ashkenazi Jews and slightly more common in women than in men. There is a peak age of onset at age 15 to 25 years and another peak at age 55 to 65 years, although the disease can occur in people of any age. Approximately 20% to 25% of all cases of UC occur in people aged 20 years or younger.

Etiology. There is no known cause of UC; however, like Crohn's disease, etiologic theories involve genetic, immunological, and environmental influences that contribute to an overactive inflammatory response to unknown triggers. It is thought that genetically susceptible individuals produce an immune reaction against intestinal bacteria that predisposes them to colonic inflammation. Serum and mucosal autoantibodies against intestinal epithelial cells are found in UC. Sulfate-reducing bacteria, which produce sulfides, are found in large numbers in patients with UC. There is also a decreased amount of *Klebsiella* bacteria in the ileum of patients with UC compared with normal. Nonsteroidal anti-inflammatory drug (NSAID) use is

TABLE 30-2. Differences Between Ulcerative Colitis and Crohn's Disease

Ulcerative Colitis	Crohn's Disease
Only affects the large intestine	Affects anywhere in the GI tract; mouth to anus
Affects from rectum continually upward into colon	Affects GI tract with skip lesions; healthy tissue interrupted by areas of diseased tissue
Only affects upper layers of instestinal wall (mucosa and submucosa)	Affects the whole thickness of the intestinal wall (transmural)
Pseudopolyps seen on examination of the colon	Cobblestoning seen on examination of the colon
No fistula or anal fissure formation	Anal fistula and anal fissure formation
Predipoases to colon cancer	Does not characteristically predispose to cancer

higher in patients with UC compared with normal, and one-third of patients with an exacerbation of UC report recent NSAID use. Milk consumption has also been found to exacerbate the disorder. Psychological and psychosocial stress factors also precipitate exacerbations.

Risk factors include genetic predisposition, family history, ethnic background, and use of the drug isotretinoin. An individual has a high risk of developing ulcerative colitits if a family member has suffered the disease. Those of Ashkenazi Jewish ethnic background have a particularly high risk. There is conflicting information as to whether use of the acne medication isotretinoin (Accutane®) can increase the risk of IBD. Some research has suggested a link, whereas other studies have found no such evidence. Studies are complicated by the fact that individuals treated with acne are also treated with tetracycline class antibiotics. There is controversy as to whether tetracyclines also play a part in the development of UC.

IBD is a multifactorial disease that involves a combination of different gene mutations. Some of the same genes that are involved with UC are also associated with Crohn's disease.

Pathophysiology. A variety of immunological changes have been documented in UC. Cytotoxic T cells accumulate in the wall of the diseased colonic segment. Also, there are an increased number of B cells and plasma cells, with increased production of immunoglobulin G and immunoglobulin E. Microscopically, there is an acute and chronic inflammatory infiltrate of the intestinal wall with formation of crypt abscesses. These findings are accompanied by a discharge of mucus from the goblet cells, the number of which is reduced as the disease progresses. The ulcerated areas become covered by granulation tissue, which leads to the formation of inflammatory areas of protruding growths termed **pseudopolyps.** Pseudopolyps and continuous areas of inflammation in the large intestine are characteristic of UC (see Fig. 30-6).

In severe cases of UC, there can be damage to the nerves in the intestinal wall, resulting in colonic dysmotility, dilation, and eventual infarction and gangrene. This condition causes toxic megacolon, which predisposes the area to perforation. Chronic and severe cases of UC can be associated with areas of precancerous changes. Colon cancer develops in 3% to 5% of patients with the disorder, and the risk increases as the duration of disease increases. The risk of colonic malignancy is higher in cases in which onset of the disease occurs before the age of 15 years.

Clinical Presentation. As in Crohn's disease, the patient suffering from UC usually describes episodes of diarrhea and abdominal pain in the history. The disease has a pattern of remissions and exacerbations, with approximately 15% of patients requiring hospitalization.

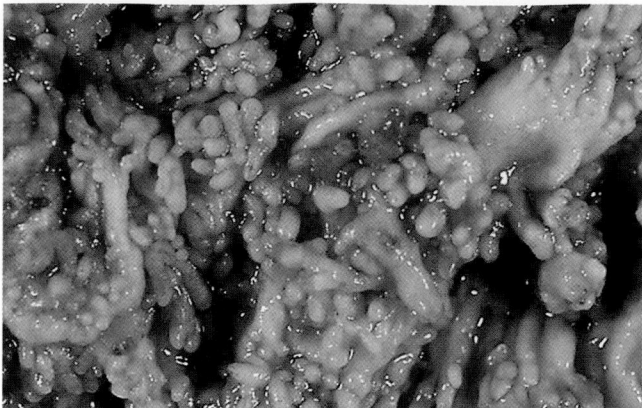

FIGURE 30-6. Pseudopolyps in UC. *(Photograph by Ed Uthman, MD: http://web2.airmail.net/uthman/index.html.)*

The clinician should focus on associated GI symptoms, such as the characteristics of pain, appearance of stool, blood in the stool, number of stools per day, and aggravating or alleviating factors. Colicky, abdominal pain is usually described. The patient with UC can have more than 20 stools per day and a fluid loss of 500 to 2,000 mL over 24 hours. The patient's weight is important, as many affected by UC suffer malabsorption. Severe dehydration and anemia can occur, especially in the elderly population. Emotional stress, laxative or antibiotic use, or dietary intake of certain foods can incite an exacerbation.

Physical Examination. An exacerbation of UC is marked by severe abdominal pain and tenderness, abdominal guarding, fever, leukocytosis, and abdominal distention. Aside from intestinal symptoms, UC is associated with various other manifestations. These include ocular problems, such as uveitis, as well as the dermatological disorders pyoderma gangrenosum and erythema nodosum. Arthritis and pleuritis are common. Inflammatiom of the liver and bile ducts can also occur.

Diagnosis. It is important to distinguish UC from Crohn's disease. Although both have the same symptomatology, there are some specific characteristic features of each (see table 30-2). For example, pseudopolyps are involved in UC, but not Crohn's disease. Crohn's disease impacts the whole thickness of the intestinal wall, whereas UC only invades the mucosal surface. Colonoscopy and biopsy are the most significant diagnostic studies.

Treatment. UC has similar treatment to Crohn's disease. It involves corticosteroids and anti-inflammatory agents, such as sulfasalazine, in conjunction with antidiarrheal agents and rehydration. Immunosuppressive agents and antibiotics are used to combat inflammation. When medical treatment is ineffective alone, surgery is performed. Surgical options include colostomy and ileostomy.

> **ALERT!** Severe UC or Crohn's disease can cause toxic megacolon, which is a medical emergency.

Large Bowel Obstruction

The inability of intestinal contents to move through the large intestine is referred to as an intestinal obstruction or large bowel obstruction (LBO). Obstructions may be partial or complete, acute or chronic, and reversible or irreversible. Approximately 10% to 15% of bowel obstructions occur in the large intestine, whereas the majority of LBOs occur in the sigmoid section of the bowel. LBO has a high mortality rate if diagnosis and treatment are not commenced within the first 24 hours.

Epidemiology

Approximately 20% of patients who present to the hospital with abdominal pain are suffering from bowel obstruction. The epidemiology of LBO depends on the cause of the disorder. Approximately 50% to 60% of all cases of LBO in the United States are caused by cancer of the colon or rectum, 20% are caused by diverticular disease, and up to 5% result from a volvulus. The prevalence of LBO increases with age. Sigmoid and cecal volvulus most commonly occur in individuals aged 60 years and older. Individuals older than age 60 are also at increased risk for acute colonic pseudo-obstruction of the large intestine, especially following surgery or severe medical illness.

Etiology

The etiology of an LBO can be classified as mechanical or nonmechanical. A mechanical obstruction physically blocks the movement of material through the intestines. Mechanical blockage may be caused by scar tissue from prior surgery (adhesions), benign or malignant tumors, abdominal hernia, a swallowed foreign body, a gallstone that migrated into the intestine, bolus of undigested food, intussusception, volvulus, stricture, or diverticula.

Nonmechanical causes stem from certain intestinal conditions, such as a disruption of the peristalsis caused by weakness of muscles of the intestinal wall (dysmotility syndrome or pseudo-obstruction) or paralysis of the bowel wall (paralytic ileus). In older individuals or in the bedridden, feces can become hardened into a solid mass and obstruct the bowel (fecal impaction). Also in the elderly population, peristaltic contractions can cease causing air and secretions to collect in the bowel. The bowel appears to be obstructed but is actually dilated. The condition is called acute colonic pseudo-obstruction or Ogilvie syndrome.

Abdominal surgery, appendectomy, gynecological surgery, hernia, bowel tumors, diverticular disease, and digestive disturbances put individuals at higher risk for intestinal obstruction. Adhesions that form after these surgeries account for a high number of LBOs. A mass lesion in the bowel and diverticular disease obstruct the intestine more than any other disorder. Diverticula, which are pouches formed in a weak bowel wall, can fill with intestinal contents and become a mass obstruction.

Pathophysiology

Mechanical LBO refers to an obstruction that causes the bowel to become dilated proximal to the obstruction. The main result of an obstruction is abdominal distention, intestinal mucosa inflammation, and the loss of fluids and electrolytes.

Distention is aggravated by the swallowing of gases such as air. This distention of the bowel results in an increase in peristalsis in an effort to excrete intestinal contents through the obstruction. As the distention progresses and pressure rises within the bowel, the bowel's ability to absorb fluids is impaired, and there is decreased blood flow to the bowel, causing ischemia. If the obstruction is not resolved, perforation of the bowel wall may occur. Perforation of the bowel leads to the spilling of fecal material into the peritoneal cavity, causing peritonitis. Bowel inflammation and ischemia can result in increased permeability of the bowel's mucosa that facilitates bacterial invasion, infection, and fluid and electrolyte imbalances. Endotoxins released by invading bacteria can cause circulatory shock that may result in death.

With nonmechanical obstruction, motility through the intestine is impaired. This can be caused by weakness of intestinal peristalsis, also known as paralytic ileus. Ileus can result from neurological disease, acute colonic pseudo-obstruction, metabolic disturbances, ischemia of the bowel, or infection of an abdominal organ.

Clinical Presentation

The history of the patient depends on whether a complete or a partial bowel obstruction has occurred. With a complete intestinal obstruction, the individual will report an inability to produce a bowel movement or pass gas. Abdominal pain is the major complaint. Nausea and vomiting usually accompany small intestinal obstruction but are not usually present in LBO. For those with a partial obstruction, gas or bowel movements are possible, but abdominal pain and distention are consistently present. The clinician should focus on questions regarding the characteristic of stool; the quality of pain, which may be colicky and cramping; and the ability to pass gas. In a complete obstruction, a rectal exam will reveal no feces in the rectum, unless obstruction is caused by fecal impaction. In fecal impaction, diarrhea may occur if the intestinal contents pass around the obstruction. If the obstruction enlarges, the abdominal pain can become more continuous. Sweating, anxiety, and restlessness also occur.

Signs and Symptoms. Clinical manifestations of LBO depend on the position and amount of bowel involved in the obstruction, as well as the interference with the blood supply. Cardinal manifestations of an LBO are abdominal pain, abdominal distention, tenderness, and rigidity upon examination.

In a partial obstruction, bowel sounds are high pitched or tympanic; patients may continue to have flatus or diarrhea. In a complete obstruction, bowels sounds are absent. In the presence of bowel perforation, signs of infection and shock become evident as the bowel contents contaminate the peritoneal cavity.

 CLINICAL CONCEPT

In a partial obstruction, auscultation of the abdomen reveals high-pitched bowel sounds. In a complete obstruction or paralytic ileus, bowels sounds are absent.

Diagnosis. Such radiological studies as abdominal x-ray and CT or MRI scan are most commonly used to diagnose LBO. The abdominal x-ray can reveal a distended colon with loops of dilated bowel readily apparent. If a perforation has occurred, there is commonly free air visualized under the diaphragm. The CT scan with contrast dye is useful to confirm a mechanical obstruction and its extent. A colonoscopy may be needed if other tests are ineffective. Diagnostic laboratory results include elevated white blood cell (WBC) count and electrolyte imbalance.

 CLINICAL CONCEPT

Serum amylase levels are elevated with perforation of the bowel or organ.

Treatment

The treatment of the LBO depends on the cause and type of obstruction, as well as whether it is acute or chronic. The overall management of the LBO includes fluid replacement, prophylactic antibiotic therapy, intestinal decompression, and surgical consultation. For intestinal decompression, a nasogastric tube is inserted into the stomach or a colorectal tube through the rectum to relieve pressure from the obstruction.

With acute obstruction, medical management is focused on maintaining fluid and electrolyte balance and preventing shock. Resting the bowel and using pharmacological agents, such as high doses of dexamethasone, are methods to treat inflammation, nausea, and pain.

A complete obstruction usually requires surgical intervention to remove the diseased or nonfunctioning segment of intestine. Some surgical procedures remove the dysfunctional area of large intestine and then reattach the healthy ends together. The connection between the two ends is called an **anastomosis.** Alternatively, an endoscopic stent may be inserted to expand a blocked area of bowel. In some cases, surgical resection of the bowel, known as a **colectomy,** and a colostomy are necessary. If obstruction is the result of adhesions, laparoscopic surgery can be performed.

 CLINICAL CONCEPT

A colostomy is a surgical procedure that brings one end of the large intestine out through the abdominal wall where a stoma is created.

ALERT! Laxative or motility agents are contraindicated in complete bowel obstruction. These agents can worsen symptoms as they stimulate the bowel to propel contents forward against an obstruction in the bowel.

Appendicitis

Appendicitis is an inflammation of the vermiform appendix, which is a blind-ended, pouchlike area that protrudes from the cecum where the small intestine meets the large intestine. In humans, the appendix is a vestigial organ—a structure that has lost all of its original function through the process of evolution. It is believed that it once contained important bacterial flora that helped digest cellulose. Appendicitis is one of the most common causes of acute abdomen. If left untreated, the appendix can rupture, causing peritonitis.

Appendicitis usually develops between childhood and young adulthood, but it can occur at any age. In the United States, the incidence is 10 cases per 100,000 population per year. The median age of appendectomy is 22 years. Perforation of the appendix happens most often in children and the elderly. There is a low mortality rate of 0.2% to 0.8%, which is caused by the complications of the disease rather than the surgery. The mortality rate in children ranges from 0.1% to 1%; in patients older than age 70 years, the rate rises above 20%, primarily because of a delay in diagnosis.

Etiology

It is hypothesized that appendicitis results from a nearby blockage, commonly caused by stool or fecalith (calcified feces). Blockage of the appendix often occurs when neighboring mesenteric lymph nodes become inflamed in response to a viral or bacterial infection and compress the appendix. Abdominal trauma can initiate an inflammatory response that results in inflammation of the appendix. Alternatively, appendicitis can occur if the appendix becomes twisted or occluded by bowel adhesions.

The incidence of appendicitis is lower in cultures who consume a diet high in dietary fiber. Dietary fiber is thought to decrease the viscosity of feces, decrease bowel transit time, and discourage formation of fecaliths, which predispose individuals to obstructions of the appendiceal lumen. Having a family history of appendicitis increases risk for the disorder, especially in males, and having cystic fibrosis also seems to put a child at higher risk.

Pathophysiology

There are two major initiating events for appendicitis:

1. Narrowing of the appendix lumen because of an obstruction that results in ischemia and a compromised blood supply to the region.
2. Development of a medium for bacterial growth as normal mucous secretions remain trapped behind the lumen because of narrowing. These trapped secretions add to the increasing intraluminal pressure and distention.

As a result of these two events, the protective mucosa layer of the appendix becomes compromised as luminal bacteria multiply and attack the wall of the appendix, causing inflammation. This inflammation, in combination with tissue ischemia, leads to necrosis and perforation of the appendix. With perforation, the contents of the appendix, which include bacteria, WBCs, and mucus, spill into the peritoneal cavity, leading to peritonitis.

Clinical Presentation

The individual with appendicitis complains of vague pain in the abdomen, which usually starts in the umbilical or epigastric region. The pain usually increases in severity over time and localizes to the RLQ. The pain increases with any jarring movements, coughing, or taking deep breaths. Nausea, vomiting, anorexia, fever, and chills are reported. Constipation or diarrhea and abdominal bloating are usually present.

 CLINICAL CONCEPT

On average, the time period from onset of vague umbilical pain to the localized RLQ pain of acute appendicitis takes 1 to 3 days.

Signs and Symptoms

Typical manifestations of appendicitis include abdominal pain that originates in the umbilical region radiating to the RLQ, also known as **McBurney's point.** The pain becomes more severe and localized as the appendix becomes more inflamed. Rebound tenderness in the RLQ is apparent on physical examination (see Table 30-3). Positive psoas sign, Rovsing's sign, and obturator sign are indicative of appendicitis, which can be elicited on physical examination (see Fig. 30-7). As the pain increases, the affected individual often guards the RLQ by being immobile and drawing the legs up in the fetal position to relieve tension on the abdominal muscles. Abdominal distention and low-grade fever are usually present.

TABLE 30-3. Signs of Appendicitis on Physical Examination

Rebound tenderness	The examiner deeply palpates the abdomen; upon release of the hand, the patient feels intense pain.
Psoas sign	Elicited by asking the supine patient to actively flex the right thigh at the hip. If abdominal pain results, this is positive for psoas sign.
Rovsing's sign	Can be elicited when the examiner palpates the LLQ of the abdomen. If pain in the patient's RLQ develops, this is positive for Rovsing's sign.
Obturator sign	Can be elicited when internal and external rotation of the patient's flexed right hip causes pain in the RLQ.

ALERT! It is important for females with abdominal pain to have a pregnancy test and pelvic exam to rule out ectopic pregnancy.

Diagnosis

A clinical diagnosis of appendicitis is based on a combination of physical examination findings, abdominal x-ray, CT scan, abdominal ultrasound, elevated C-reactive protein, and elevated WBC count. An ultrasound will not visualize a normal appendix, only one that is inflamed and edematous. An abdominal x-ray is usually not informative unless there is a calcium stone present within the appendix. Urinalysis is necessary to rule out a kidney stone or pyelonephritis, which can present similarly to appendicitis. High 5-HIAA, a breakdown product of serotonin, may be evident in the urine in appendicitis. The appendix contains many serotonin-producing cells. A pelvic exam and beta-HCG blood test should be done on all females of childbearing age to rule out ectopic pregnancy or other gynecological disorder.

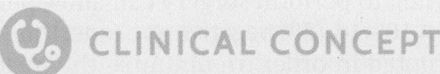 **CLINICAL CONCEPT**

The CT scan yields the most accurate information in the diagnosis of appendicitis.

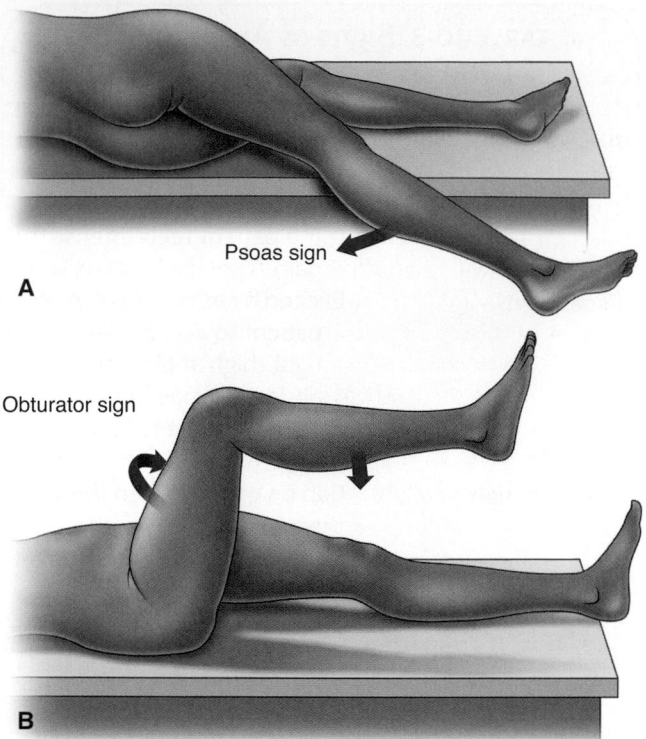

A Psoas sign

Obturator sign

B

FIGURE 30-7. Signs indicative of appendicitis. (A) Psoas sign indicates irritation to the iliopsoas group of hip muscles and indicates an inflamed appendix, which lies within the region. It is elicited by passively extending the thigh of a patient lying on his side with knees extended. If abdominal pain results, it is a positive psoas sign. (B) To elicit an obturator sign, the patient lies on his or her back with the hip and knee both flexed at 90°. The clinician holds the patient's ankle with one hand and knee with the other hand. The clinician rotates the hip by moving the patient's ankle away from the patient's body while allowing the knee to move only inward. This is flexion and internal rotation of the hip. Pain in the RLQ that radiates into the groin occurs if appendicitis is present.

Treatment

Early treatment with antibiotics that are effective against gram-negative bacteria should be initiated preoperatively and administered up to at least 48 hours postoperatively. Laxatives should be avoided; in addition, pain medications should be avoided before diagnosis of appendicitis as these can mask diagnostic signs. Continuous monitoring for peritonitis and IV therapy to restore or maintain fluid and electrolyte balance is essential. In acute appendicitis, effective pain management in conjunction with surgical removal of the appendix through laparoscopic surgery is the primary treatment. The surgeon's goal is to selectively operate on patients with true appendicitis and to minimize the negative appendectomy rate. The surgeon wants to avoid performing unnecessary surgery; however, waiting to perform surgery can allow perforation to occur. A 10% to 15% negative appendectomy rate has been accepted in order to minimize the incidence of perforated appendicitis with its increased morbidity. Often patients who have mesenteric adenitis, defined as swollen mesenteric lymph nodes, present with signs

and symptoms exactly like appendicitis; these patients undergo negative appendectomies.

Irritable Bowel Syndrome

IBS is a GI disorder characterized by abdominal pain and altered bowel activity in the absence of specific pathology. No specific motility or structural disorders of the intestine or bowel have been shown. The layman's terms for IBS are colitis, irritable colon, or spastic colon. This chronic and relapsing motility disorder affects the intestinal tract. Common findings related to IBS include abdominal discomfort and alterations in elimination, such as diarrhea and constipation, or a combination of the two. IBS is not linked to long-term mortality, but it negatively affects one's quality of life. IBS should not be confused with inflammatory bowel disease (IBD).

As much as 20% of the adult population, or one in five Americans, has symptoms of IBS, making it one of the most common disorders seen in primary care. It occurs more often in women than in men, and it usually begins before the age of 35 years. In the United States, there is a lower prevalence of IBS in Hispanics and Asians. The role of different cultural influences is unclear.

Etiology

The cause of IBS is unknown, but many theories exist regarding the diarrhea and constipation associated with the disease (see Box 30-2).

Risk factors for IBS include female gender, age under 40 years, family history, stress, and, possibly, history of traveler's diarrhea. IBS may also be related to consumption of dairy, wheat, fructose, or sorbitol. Although there is no definitive proof that any of these dietary items cause IBS, they may trigger symptoms.

Pathophysiology

In IBS, despite unclear etiology, there is an alteration in GI motility linked to central nervous system-directed motor functions of the bowel. Peristaltic waves are either slowed or increased in intensity as they push food through the intestine. Patients also have greater visceral pain sensitivity. There is no evidence of inflammation or pathological changes in the intestinal mucosa. The intestine appears normal in all diagnostic studies.

Clinical Presentation

The main manifestations of IBS are chronic abdominal pain lasting for at least 6 months and a change in normal bowel patterns to constipation, diarrhea, or both. The abdominal pain is often caused by eating and relieved by bowel movement. Other associated manifestations may include anxiety, flatulence, mucus in stools, nausea and vomiting, and abdominal distention. The patient commonly reports a stressor in his or her life. The physical examination is normal in IBS.

Certain signs of IBS are referred to as "alarm" symptoms; these require specific diagnostic testing such as colonoscopy. These alarm symptoms include weight

BOX 30-2. IBS: Many Theories of Etiology

There is no clearly understood etiology of IBS; many different theories exist.

1. Up to one-third of patients with IBS may have altered colonic transit. In those with constipation, delayed colonic motility may be the etiology, whereas those with diarrhea may suffer from accelerated colonic transit.
2. Infectious gastroenteritis can cause IBS. Infection with *Giardia lamblia* has been shown to lead to an increased prevalence of IBS. In a historic cohort study of patients with *G. lamblia* infection as detected by stool cysts, the prevalence of IBS was 46.1% as long as 3 years after exposure, compared with 14% in controls.
3. The brain's limbic system, which mediates emotion and autonomic response, enhances bowel motility and reduces gastric motility to a greater degree in patients who are affected with IBS compared with normal. Limbic system abnormalities, as demonstrated by positron emission tomography, have been described in patients with IBS and in those with major depression.
4. The hypothalamic-pituitary axis may be involved in the origin of IBS. Motility disturbances correspond to an increase in hypothalamic corticotropin-releasing factor production in response to stress.
5. Small-bowel bacterial overgrowth provokes the symptoms of bloating and gaseous distention in patients with IBS.
6. Bloating and distention may also occur from intolerance to dietary constituents. Reflex-mediated small-bowel gas clearance is more impaired by ingestion of lipids in patients with IBS than in patients without the disorder. Other studies have suggested that poorly absorbed short-chain carbohydrates, in the form of fructose and fructans, may create symptoms among patients with IBS.

loss, iron deficiency anemia, and family history of GI illness such as colon cancer or celiac sprue. Other symptoms that should prompt clinicians to order diagnostic studies are rectal bleeding, nocturnal symptoms, and age over 50 years.

Diagnosis

The diagnosis of IBS is commonly made by the patient's description of signs and symptoms. In some patients, such as those with rectal bleeding, more in-depth diagnostic studies are completed. The diagnostic tests that are commonly performed to rule out other underlying disease processes or structural abnormalities include stool samples for ova and parasites, occult blood, and culture and sensitivity to assess for inflammation or infection. A complete blood count with differential and erythrocyte sedimentation rate are performed routinely to rule out anemia, infection, or inflammation. Transglutaminase antibody testing should be completed to rule out celiac sprue. Thyroid hormone testing is needed to rule out hypo- or hyperthyroidism. Hydrogen breath testing can exclude the possibility of lactose or fructose intolerance. An upper endoscopy and colonoscopy can identify any structural or functional abnormalities, although none are usually present. Abdominal CT scan can exclude the possibility of tumor, obstruction, or pancreatic disease. Finally, GI motility is evaluated through either an upper GI series or a barium enema. Rarely, manometry or an electromyogram may be used to measure pressure changes in the intestinal lumen caused by spasms. All diagnostic studies are usually negative.

Treatment

The primary goals of management are to regulate bowel movements, relieve abdominal pain, and decrease stress. These goals are achieved through pharmacological interventions, dietary alterations, and lifestyle changes to manage the symptoms.

Bulk-forming laxatives are often prescribed to decrease the number of bowel movements and increase consistency. Antidiarrheals, such as loperamide (Imodium) and lomotil, are frequently prescribed. Anticholinergic and antispasmodic medications help decrease intestinal motility and abdominal pain. Antidepressants have been prescribed to reduce the anxiety linked with IBS.

Patients can keep a food diary to keep track of symptoms in relation to foods. Dietary management for IBS includes modification of dietary intake to reduce the incidence of diarrhea and constipation, identification of food intolerances, and the exclusion of wheat bran, lactose, fructose, and sorbitol. The avoidance of gas-producing foods and beverages that contain caffeine is also recommended. Although IBS is not regarded as a gluten enteropathy, a gluten-free diet does reduce symptoms in many patients with IBS. Stress reduction is key to successful management of IBS. Lifestyle changes, such as regular exercise, behavioral management, and relaxation techniques, can decrease stress and facilitate coping with IBS.

Diverticular Disease

The two disorders associated with diverticular disease are diverticulosis and diverticulitis. In **diverticulosis,** the bowel wall has multiple weakened areas that form small outpouchings called diverticula. In diverticulitis, there is inflammation of these weakenings in the wall. **Diverticula** can collect intestinal contents and form a colonic obstruction. Most diverticula are found in the sigmoid and descending colon. Diverticula often become inflamed, at which point the condition becomes **diverticulitis.**

Epidemiology

Asymptomatic diverticulosis is a common condition that increases with age. Of patients with diverticulosis, 80% to 85% remain asymptomatic. The risk of developing diverticulosis before age 40 years is lower than 5%; however, this percentage rises to greater than 65% by age 85 years. Approximately 15% to 20% of those with diverticulosis develop diverticulitis, and 15% to 25% of those with diverticulitis develop complications leading to surgery, including abscess formation, intestinal rupture, peritonitis, and fistula formation. Patients with diverticulitis who do not undergo surgery have a recurrence rate of 20% to 35%. The disease occurs equally in males and females. The mean age at presentation with diverticulitis appears to be about age 60 years.

Etiology

The etiology of diverticular disease is associated with two main factors: weakness of the bowel wall and increased intraluminal pressure. Diverticulitis occurs when intestinal contents block the diverticulum, thus cutting off the blood supply and providing an environment conducive to the formation of infection.

The most significant risk factor for diverticular formation is a diet low in fiber. Diverticulosis is very common in Western countries and is thought to be associated with lack of dietary fiber and obesity. There are also genetic factors, as those with a family history tend to have an increased risk of disease.

Pathophysiology

Weakness in the bowel musculature can occur where branches of the blood vessels enter the colonic wall, thus creating areas for bowel protrusion during periods of increased intra-abdominal pressure. These entry points for blood vessels are the areas where diverticula develop (see Fig. 30-8). When the bowel does not drain

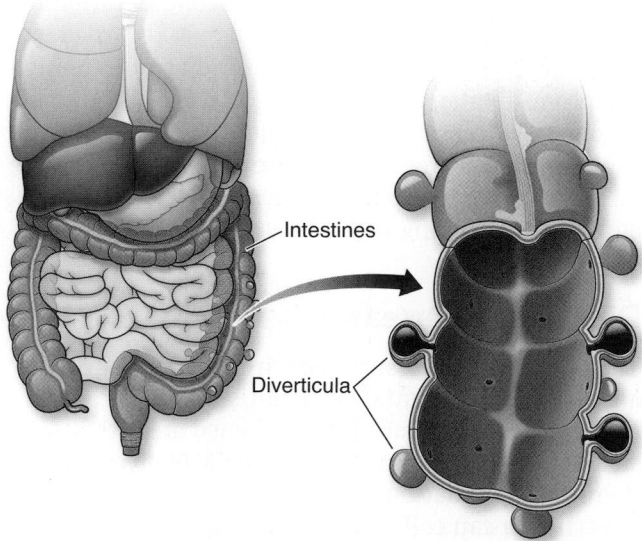

FIGURE 30-8. In diverticulosis, there are small, weakened areas in the wall of the colon. The weak areas bulge and create pouches that can become impacted and inflamed. Once inflamed, the condition is called diverticulitis.

effectively, intestinal contents can become trapped, collect and form a mass, and cause obstruction and irritation, thereby leading to diverticulitis. Chronic diverticulitis can cause scarring and narrowing of the bowel lumen.

Clinical Presentation

The signs and symptoms of diverticular disease are dependent on the severity of the inflammation and where it occurs in the bowel. There may be dull, episodic, or steady left quadrant or midabdominal pain. Acute lower abdominal pain, fever, and tachycardia may also be present. There are usually alterations in bowel habits, including constipation, diarrhea, increased flatulence, anorexia, and low-grade fever.

The patient with diverticulosis may have no signs of the disorder on physical examination. If diverticulitis exists, the patient classically has LLQ abdominal tenderness, fever, and nausea. Traces of occult blood may be found in the stool. Patients with right-sided diverticular disease can have RLQ tenderness of the abdomen similar to appendicitis. Pain of diverticular disease of the transverse colon can simulate pain of peptic ulcer or pancreatitis.

Diagnosis

Diagnostic studies include abdominal x-ray, lower GI series, CT scan, and MRI. Colonoscopy can also visualize the location of diverticula within the colon. CT scan is the recommended diagnostic procedure for diverticulitis.

Treatment

Dietary modification may help with strategies to prevent constipation, including adequate fluid and fiber intake. Diverticulitis may require resting the colon by NPO, insertion of an NG tube, and total parenteral nutrition (TPN). Opioids may be required for pain, but morphine should be avoided because it can cause colon spasm.

During acute episodes of diverticulitis, broad-spectrum antibiotics and intravenous therapy may be needed. Surgery may be required when complications include hemorrhage, obstruction, abscesses, or perforation. A temporary colostomy may be used to help with healing and allow the bowel to rest.

Volvulus

A **volvulus** is a twisting of the large intestine around a point of attachment in the abdomen. Neonates are most often affected by a volvulus caused by congenital abnormality; however, more than 40% of cases occur at older ages. Sigmoid volvulus, the most common type found in adults, is responsible for 10% to 15% of LBO cases and is mainly a disease of elderly men.

The sigmoid colon is weighed down because of chronic constipation and a high fiber diet; this makes it most susceptible to volvulus. The weight of the sigmoid colon increases its susceptibility to twisting on the mesentery. Volvulus of the intestine results in bowel obstruction and ischemia of the bowel. Venous and lymphatic vessel obstructions usually occur, causing bowel edema and possible GI bleeding. Lymphatic congestion causes the formation of enlarged mesenteric lymph nodes or ascites caused by accumulation of lymphatic fluid. The intestinal lumen accumulates gas and fluid up to the point of obstruction. The large volume of gas and fluid can place pressure on the intestinal wall, cutting off circulation. This can lead to ischemia and infarction of the intestinal wall. Perforation and necrosis of the affected intestinal wall can occur.

The symptoms of volvulus include bilious vomiting, abdominal pain (colicky at first, then steady), anorexia, blood and mucus in the stool, abdominal tenderness, and, eventually, shock. The most definitive tests are upper and lower barium GI contrast studies. Surgical correction is the treatment, often by laparoscopy. It is most important to recognize the diagnosis early before infarcted bowel occurs.

Hemorrhoids

Hemorrhoids are dilated, swollen venous blood vessels in the lower rectum. They are among the most common causes of lower intestine pathology. The prevalence of symptomatic hemorrhoids is estimated at 4.4% in the general population of the United States. This is a low estimate because only one-third of individuals affected with hemorrhoids seek medical attention. Many affected persons self-medicate with over-the-counter preparations. The prevalence of hemorrhoids increases with age, with a peak in persons aged 45 to 65 years.

Hemorrhoids are mainly caused by decreased venous return and venous pooling in the blood vessels of the rectum. Hemorrhoids can be likened to varicose veins in the perianal region. High venous pressure in the rectal region is commonly caused by constipation and straining during defecation, high pressure within the portal vein of the liver, anal intercourse, pregnancy, prolonged sitting, and aging of support structures in the recto-anal region. In addition, lack of fiber in the diet causes chronic constipation, which leads to hemorrhoids. In pregnancy, the gravid uterus places high pressure on the inferior vena cava, leading to hemorrhoids.

Hemorrhoids generally cause symptoms when they become inflamed, thrombosed, or prolapsed. Hemorrhoid symptoms usually depend on the location, whether they are internal or external blood vessels. Internal hemorrhoids lie inside the rectum. Straining or irritation when passing stool can damage the hemorrhoid's fragile surface and cause it to bleed. Bleeding from hemorrhoids, exhibited as small amounts of bright red blood from the rectum, is called **hematochezia.** Commonly, straining at defecation pushes an internal hemorrhoid through the anal meatus; this is known as a prolapsed hemorrhoid. External hemorrhoids are more superficial, just under the skin around the anus. When irritated, external hemorrhoids can itch or bleed. Sometimes blood may pool in an external hemorrhoid and form a thrombosed hemorrhoid, resulting in severe pain, swelling, and inflammation.

Diagnosis requires digital rectal exam, anoscopy, flexible sigmoidoscopy, or colonoscopy. Conservative treatments involve use of over-the-counter hemorrhoid cream or suppository containing hydrocortisone, or use of pads containing witch hazel or a numbing agent. Minimal invasive procedures are commonly performed to treat hemorrhoids; these include rubber band ligation, sclerotherapy, or coagulation techniques that use laser or infrared light. Stapled hemorrhoidectomy is needed in some cases.

Chapter Summary

- The order of physical examination techniques used in abdominal assessment should be inspection, auscultation, percussion, and palpation.
- Any disorder that causes sudden, severe acute abdominal pain and tenderness is referred to as an acute abdomen.
- IBD includes Crohn's disease and UC.
- Crohn's disease can occur anywhere throughout the whole GI tract.
- Crohn's disease causes malabsorption, dehydration, arthritis, uveitis, cheilitis, and dermatological problems. Hepatic and bile duct inflammation can also occur. It is characterized by transmural inflammation with skipped areas of the intestine.

- UC is an inflammatory disease limited to the surface of the large intestine. Pseudopolyps and continuous areas of inflammation in the large intestine are characteristic.
- UC predisposes individuals to colon cancer.
- Severe Crohn's disease or UC can cause toxic megacolon, which is a medical emergency.
- IBS is a condition of abnormal bowel activity with no organic pathology and unknown etiology.
- LBO is most commonly caused by cancer or tumor of the colon.
- A colostomy is a surgical procedure that brings one end of the large intestine out through the abdominal wall where a stoma is created.

- Appendicitis begins with vague pain in the umbilical region, which increases in severity over time and localizes to the RLQ.
- Appendicitis causes peritoneal inflammation, demonstrated by rebound tenderness at McBurney's point in the RLQ.
- In diverticulosis, the bowel wall has multiple weakened areas that form small outpouchings called diverticula. In diverticulitis, there is inflammation of these weakenings in the wall, which most commonly cause LLQ tenderness.
- A volvulus is a twisting of large intestine that can cause ischemia and infarction of the intestinal wall.
- Hemorrhoids are swollen blood vessels in the lower rectum that can bleed, become thrombosed, or become prolapsed. Treatment involves either conservative topical treatment or minimally invasive surgical procedures.

 ## Making the Connections

Disorder and Pathophysiology	Signs and Symptoms	Physical Assessment Findings	Diagnostic Testing	Treatment
Crohn's Disease | Inflammation of any part of the GI tract from mouth to anus; involves the whole thickness of the intestine's wall, characteristic skip lesions, cobblestone mucosa, and anal fistulas. This may be an autoimmune disorder.				
	Abdominal pain. Chronic diarrhea with bleeding or mucus. Malabsorption causes weight loss. Symptoms come in remissions and exacerbations.	Abdominal tenderness, fever, anal fistulas possible. Weight loss.	Colonoscopy can visualize the inflamed areas of the intestine. Biopsy will show the inflammation of the whole wall of the intestine.	Aminosalicylates decrease the inflammation and enhance remission. Corticosteroids decrease the inflammation. Immunosuppressives are used to diminish an autoimmune process.
UC | Inflammation of the large bowel; involves the mucosal layer of intestine and characteristic pseudopolyps, which are areas of intense inflammation. This may be an autoimmune disorder. It predisposes individuals to colon cancer.				
	Abdominal pain. Chronic diarrhea with bleeding or mucus. Malabsorption causes weight loss. Remissions and exacerbations.	Abdominal tenderness, fever; stool may contain blood, pus, and mucus; weight loss.	Colonoscopy can visualize the inflamed areas of the intestine. Biopsy will show the inflammation of the mucosa of the intestine.	Aminosalicylates decrease the inflammation and enhance remission. Corticosteroids decrease the inflammation. Immunosuppressives are used to diminish an autoimmune process.
LBO | These obstructions can be caused by mechanical, vascular, or neurogenic disorders and can be complete or partial. The bowel dilates proximal to the obstruction. Causes include diverticular disease, volvulus, hernia, and neoplasm.				
	Acute or chronic colicky lower abdominal pain, distention, tenderness, and rigidity caused by buildup of pressure and gas proximal to obstruction.	Abdominal tenderness, distention. High-pitched bowel sounds auscultated if a partial obstruction. Lack of bowel sounds if a complete obstruction.	Abdominal. X-ray shows a classic pattern of gas and bowel distention. X-ray may show free air under the diaphragm if perforation occurs. Elevated WBC count and serum amylase levels occur with inflammation and perforation.	Volume replacement of the bloodstream caused by loss of large amount of water in fluid shifts intraintestinally. Prophylactic antibiotic therapy is used to prevent bacteremia if perforation allows spill of bacteria into the peritoneum.

Continued

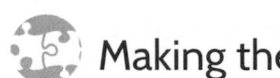

Making the Connections–cont'd

Disorder and Pathophysiology	Signs and Symptoms	Physical Assessment Findings	Diagnostic Testing	Treatment
				Gastric decompression allows gas out from the intestine. Insertion of a stent or colectomy may be necessary. Dexamethasone is used to diminish inflammation. Motility agents can only be used if the patient has a partial obstruction evidenced by passage of gas.

Appendicitis | Condition caused by narrowing of the appendix lumen from obstruction. Inflammation of the wall of the appendix develops. Inside the appendix, there is development of a medium for bacterial growth.

Disorder and Pathophysiology	Signs and Symptoms	Physical Assessment Findings	Diagnostic Testing	Treatment
	Acute abdominal pain, fever, constipation, abdominal pain originating in the umbilicus and radiating to the RLQ.	Abdominal tenderness at McBurney's point. Rebound tenderness caused by peritoneal inflammation. Abdominal rigidity, also called involuntary guarding.	CT scan is the best image study to visualize an inflamed appendix. Abdominal ultrasound can demonstrate an inflamed appendix. Elevated WBC count is caused by inflammation.	Antibiotics to prevent bacteremia. IV therapy for fluid replacement. Surgery to remove appendix.

IBS | Modification in GI motility that is linked to alteration in central nervous system-directed motor function of the bowel. Enhanced visceral sensitivity exists, as well as no inflammation.

Disorder and Pathophysiology	Signs and Symptoms	Physical Assessment Findings	Diagnostic Testing	Treatment
	Acute or chronic colicky abdominal pain lasting 6 months or more.	Complaints of abdominal cramping and pain. Constipation or diarrhea.	Stool samples to rule out other causes of pathology. Sigmoidoscopy to visualize large bowel up to sigmoid. Complete blood count shows no WBC elevation. Upper GI series shows no abnormality. Lower GI series shows no abnormality.	Anticholinergic and antispasmodic medications to decrease the irritability of the colon.

Diverticular Disease | Weakness in bowel wall musculature, which allows protrusion of small outpouchings or sacs called diverticula. Diverticula can become infected (called diverticulitis) or inflamed or can fill with intestinal contents and cause an obstructive mass.

Disorder and Pathophysiology	Signs and Symptoms	Physical Assessment Findings	Diagnostic Testing	Treatment
	Chronic dull LLQ episodic or steady pain OR acute pain,	Pain and tenderness in LLQ, abdomen, fever.	Elevated WBC count caused by inflammation.	Colon needs rest. NPO status allows colon to rest.

Continued

Making the Connections–cont'd

Disorder and Pathophysiology	Signs and Symptoms	Physical Assessment Findings	Diagnostic Testing	Treatment
fever, constipation, or diarrhea.			Sigmoidoscopy to visualize the lower bowel.	Nasogastric tube relieves gas accumulation. Pain relievers are used. Surgery after acute episode passes, and encourage increased fiber in diet.
Volvulus | A twisting of the intestine that cuts off the circulation to the intestinal wall.				
	Abdominal pain. Vomiting, abdominal distention.	Abdominal tenderness. Vomiting. Abdominal distention.	Lower GI series can visualize the twisted segment of bowel.	Laparoscopic surgery to unwind the intestine or perform colectomy.
Hemorrhoids | Enlarged, inflamed blood vessels at the rectal-anal region.				
	Rectal pain, loss of small amount of bright red blood per rectum (hematochezia).	Hematochezia. Thrombosis within a prolapsed vein at the anal meatus.	Digital rectal exam. Sigmoidoscopy, or colonoscopy if other pathology suspected.	Topical corticosteroid cream to decrease the inflammation. Minimally invasive procedures that decrease circulation to the veins causing the hemorrhoid.

Bibliography

Abraham, C., & Cho, J. H. (2009). Inflammatory bowel disease. *N Engl J Med,* 361(21), 2066–2078.

Adams, S. M., & Bornemann, P. H. (2013). Ulcerative colitis. *Am Fam Phys,* 87(10), 699–705.

Anderson, W. D., & Strayer, S. M. (2013). Evaluation of nausea and vomiting: a case-based approach. *Am Fam Phys,* 88(6), 371–379.

Atnip, S., & Schaffer, J. I. (2011). A unique approach to severe constipation. *Urologic Nurs,* Nov-Dec, 31(6), 348–350.

Bao, J., Lopez, J. A., & Huerta, S. (2013). Acute abdominal pain and abnormal CT findings. *JAMA,* 310(8), 848–849. doi: 10.1001/jama.2013.276158.

Camilleri, M. (2012). Peripheral mechanisms in irritable bowel syndrome. *N Engl J Med,* 367(17), 1626–1635.

Danese, S., & Fiocchi, C. (2011). Ulcerative colitis. *N Engl J Med,* 365(18), 1713–1725.

Ebell, M. H. (2008a). Diagnosis of appendicitis: part 1. History and physical examination. *Am Fam Phys,* 77(6), 828–830.

Ebell, M. H. (2008b). Diagnosis of appendicitis: part 2. History and physical examination. *Am Fam Phys,* 77(8), 1153–1155.

Halpert, A. D. (2010). Importance of early diagnosis in patients with irritable bowel syndrome. *Postgrad Med,* 122(2), 102–111. doi: 10.3810/pgm.2010.03.2127.

Hammond, N. A., Nikolaidis, P., & Miller, F. H. (2010). Left lower-quadrant pain: guidelines from the American College of Radiology appropriateness criteria. *Am Fam Phys,* 82(7), 766–770.

Jackson, P. G., & Raiji, M. T. (2011). Evaluation and management of intestinal obstruction. *Am Fam Phys,* 83(2), 159–165.

Johansen, M. (2013). Absence of abdominal pain does not rule out diagnosis of IBS. *Am Fam Phys,* 87(5), 307–310.

Katz, S. (2013). My treatment approach to the management of ulcerative colitis. *Mayo Clin Proceed,* 88(8), 841–853. doi: 10.1016/j.mayocp.2013.05.001.

Khalili, H., Ananthakrishnan, A. N., Konijeti, G. G., et al. (2013). Physical activity and risk of inflammatory bowel disease: prospective study from the Nurses' Health Study cohorts. *BMJ,* 347, f6633. doi: 10.1136/bmj.f6633.

Kim, Y. G., & Jang, B. I. (2013). The role of colonoscopy in inflammatory bowel disease. *Clin Endo,* 46(4). 317–320. doi: 10.5946/ce.2013.46.4.317. Epub 2013 Jul 31.

Kumar, A., Auron, M., Aneja, A., et al. (2011). Inflammatory bowel disease: perioperative pharmacological considerations. *Mayo Clin Proceed,* 86(8), 748–757. doi: 10.4065/mcp.2011.0074.

Li, C. H., Chen, C. H., & Chou, J. W. (2011). Intestinal obstruction caused by small bowel volvulus. *Am J Med,* 124(11), e3–4.

Lichtenstein, G. R., Hanauer, S. B., Sandborn, W. J., & Practice Parameters Committee of American College of Gastroenterology. (2009). Management of Crohn's disease in adults. *Am J Gastro,* 104(2), 465–483.

Longo, D. L., Kasper, D. L., Jameson, J. L., et al. (2011). *Harrison's principles of internal medicine.* 18th ed. New York: McGraw-Hill.

Mason, R. J. (2011). Appendicitis: is surgery the best option? *Lancet,* 377(9777), 1545–1546. doi: 10.1016/S0140-6736(11)60623-5.

McCutcheon, T. (2013). The ileus and oddities after colorectal surgery. *Gastro Nurs,* 36(5), 368–375; quiz 376–377. doi: 10.1097/SGA.0b013e3182a71fdf.

Mills, S., von Roon, A. C., Tekkis, P. P., & Orchard, T. R. (2011). Crohn disease. *Am Fam Phys,* 83(12), 1479–1481.

O'Connor, E. S., Leverson, G., Kennedy, G., & Heise, C. P. (2010). The diagnosis of diverticulitis in outpatients: on what evidence? *J Gastro Surg,* 14(2), 303–308.

Oxentenko, A. S., Bundrick, J. B., & Litin, S. C. (2011). Clinical pearls in gastroenterology 2011. *Mayo Clin Proceed,* 86(11), 1104–1108.

Pimentel, M., Lembo, A., Chey, W. D., et al. (2011). Rifaximin therapy for patients with irritable bowel syndrome without constipation. *N Engl J Med,* 364(1), 22–32.

Shah, S. S., Gaffney, R. R., Dykes, T. M., & Goldstein, J. P. (2013). Chronic appendicitis: an often forgotten cause of recurrent abdominal pain. *Am J Med,* 126(1), e7–8. doi: 10.1016/j.amjmed.2012.05.032. Epub 2012 Nov 20.

Shim, K. N., Moon, J. S., Chang, D. K., et al. (2013). Guideline for capsule endoscopy: obscure gastrointestinal bleeding.

Clin Endo, 46(1), 45–53. doi: 10.5946/ce.2013.46.1.45. Epub 2013 Jan 31.

Soriano, A., & Davis, M. P. (2011). Malignant bowel obstruction: individualized treatment near the end of life. *Cleveland Clin J Med,* 78(3), 197–206. doi: 10.3949/ccjm.78a.10052.

Spiegel, B. M., Farid, M., Esrailian, E., Talley, J., & Chang, L. (2010). Is irritable bowel syndrome a diagnosis of exclusion?: a survey of primary care providers, gastroenterologists, and IBS experts. *Am J Gastro,* 105(4), 848–858.

Tack, J. (2011). Antibiotic therapy for the irritable bowel syndrome. *N Engl J Med,* 364(1), 81–82.

Tyson, R. L. (2010). Diagnosis and treatment of abdominal angina. *Nurse Pract,* 35(11), 16–22; quiz 22-3. doi: 10.1097/01.NPR.0000388938.08875.99.

Vons, C., Barry, C., Maitre, S., et al. (2011). Amoxicillin plus clavulanic acid versus appendectomy for treatment of acute uncomplicated appendicitis: an open-label, non-inferiority, randomised controlled trial. *Lancet,* 377(9777), 1573–1579. doi: 10.1016/S0140-6736(11)60410-8.

Wilkins, T., Embry, K., & George, R. (2013). Diagnosis and management of acute diverticulitis. *Am Fam Phys,* 87(9), 612–620.

Wilkins, T., Jarvis, K., & Patel, J. (2011). Diagnosis and management of Crohn's disease. *Am Fam Phys,* 84(12), 1365–1375.

Wilkins, T., Pepitone, C., Alex, B., & Schade, R. R. (2012). Diagnosis and management of IBS in adults. *Am Fam Phys,* 86(5), 419–426.

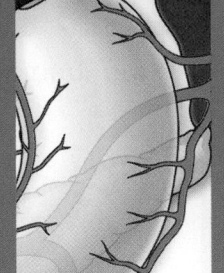

Key Terms

Asterixis	Enterohepatic recycling	Jaundice
Bilirubin	Gluconeogenesis	Nonalcoholic fatty liver disease (NALFD)
Caput medusa	Glycogenesis	Nonalcoholic steatohepatitis (NASH)
Cholestasis	Glycogenolysis	Portal hypertension
Cirrhosis	Hepatitis	Spider angioma
Conjugated bilirubin	Hepatocytes	Steatorrhea
Conjugation	Hyperbilirubinemia	Steatosis
Deamination	Icterus	Unconjugated bilirubin

The liver is the largest internal organ in the body, weighing 1,500 grams in the average adult. Metabolically complex, it functions simultaneously as an accessory organ of digestion, an endocrine organ, a hematologic organ, and an excretory organ. Its cells have a distinctive regenerative capacity that enables it to function until approximately 80% of its cells are destroyed.

Liver disease can be caused by hepatocellular injury, obstructive injury, or both cellular and obstructive injury. Because of the liver's abundant blood reserve and regenerative capability, symptoms of liver dysfunction may not become evident until the hepatocytes are severely damaged or bile outflow is significantly obstructed.

Because of the liver's complex metabolic functions, liver disease often results in systemic, life-threatening complications, regardless of whether the disease is primary or secondary or is manifested by acute or chronic symptoms.

Epidemiology

Worldwide, hepatitis is one of the most common pathological conditions of the liver. Acute hepatitis is commonly the result of infection with one of several types of viral agents, but the clinical presentations of the various types of the illness are very similar. In 5% of hepatitis B (HBV) cases and 85% of hepatitis C (HCV) cases, the patient is unable to produce an immune response to clear the liver of the virus, leading to a chronic infectious condition that may predispose the patient to hepatocellular cancer. In most of the world, HBV and HCV are the common causes of **cirrhosis,** whereas in the United States, alcoholism is the predominant cause. Chronic liver disease and cirrhosis result in about 35,000 deaths each year in the United States. Cirrhosis

is the ninth leading cause of death in the United States and is responsible for 1.2% of all deaths in the United States, with many patients dying from the disease in their fifth or sixth decade of life.

Each year, 2,000 additional deaths are attributed to liver failure, which may be caused by viral hepatitis, drugs such as acetaminophen, toxins, autoimmune hepatitis, Wilson disease, or a variety of less common etiologies. Patients with liver failure have a 50% to 80% mortality rate unless they have liver transplantation.

Basic Concepts of Liver Function

The liver is located in the right upper quadrant (RUQ) of the abdomen, immediately beneath the diaphragm. A thick connective tissue called Glisson's capsule, which contains nerves, lymph, and blood vessels, covers the liver. When the capsule is stretched, the distention gives rise to the RUQ pain associated with liver disease and allows lymphatics to leak fluid into the peritoneal space; this produces ascites, also known as peritoneal edema.

The liver is a vascular organ and has a dual blood supply from the hepatic artery, which is a branch of the aorta, and the portal vein, which drains the veins of the gastrointestinal tract. These vessels supply the liver with approximately 1,500 mL of blood per minute. The hepatic artery delivers 25% of the blood, whereas the portal vein supplies 75% of the blood. The liver synthesizes and secretes bile for fat digestion into the hepatic duct. Along with the pancreatic duct, the hepatic duct empties into the common bile duct, which carries bile into the intestine (see Fig. 31-1).

Hepatocytes, the functional cells of the liver that are capable of regeneration, excrete metabolic substances into small channels called canaliculi. These

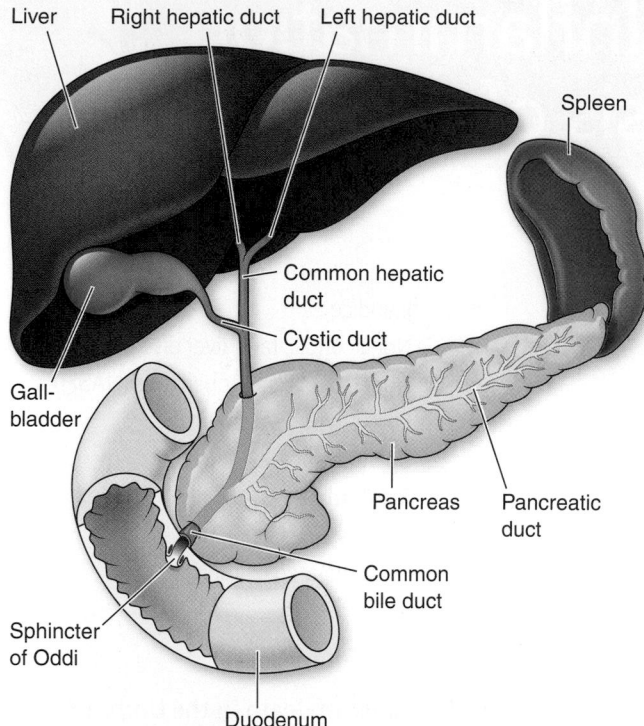

FIGURE 31-1. Gross anatomy of the liver and common bile duct. Note how the hepatic duct, cystic duct, and pancreatic duct come together to form the common bile duct. The common bile duct empties into the small intestine.

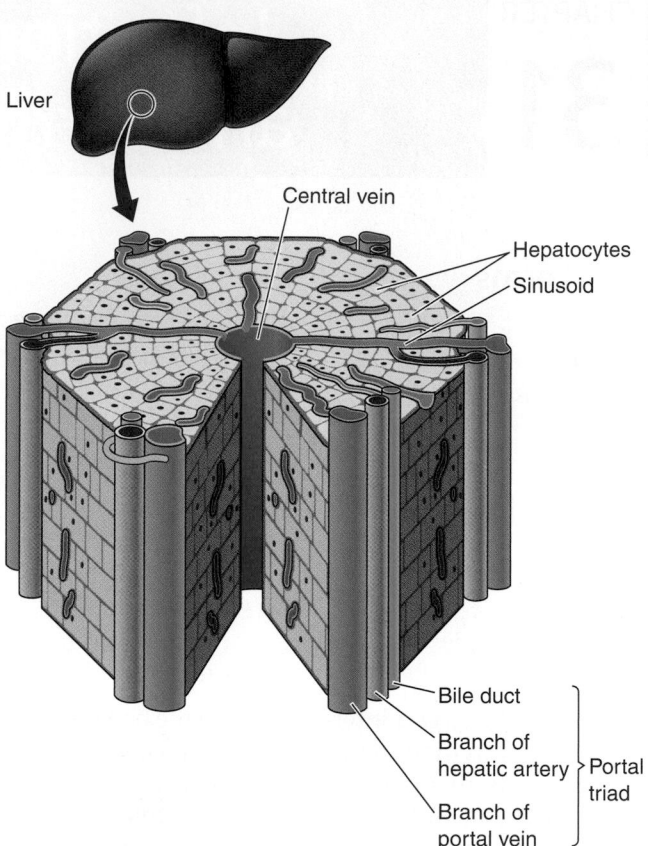

FIGURE 31-2. Cellular anatomy of a liver lobule.

canaliculi are responsible for conduction of bile to the hepatic duct. Sinusoids are vascular spaces located between the hepatocytes that contain a mixture of venous and arterial blood from the hepatic artery and portal vein. Kupffer cells, specific macrophages of the liver, line the sinusoids and protect the body by detoxifying the bloodstream. The liver is histologically divided into lobules; each lobule contains a branch of arterial and venous blood vessel and a portion of bile duct—known as a portal triad (see Fig. 31-2).

Normal Hepatic Physiology

The liver serves as a digestive organ, an organ of metabolism, and a hematologic, endocrine, and excretory organ. It also plays an important role in filtration and detoxification of the bloodstream. Any damage to the liver cells will result in hindrance of these important functions.

Digestion

As an accessory organ of digestion, the liver is responsible for bile salt secretion to aid in fat digestion in the small intestine. Bile, a yellow-green alkaline fluid, is formed in the hepatocytes; some is stored in the gallbladder for later use, whereas other bile salts continue to the ileum and colon for excretion. Some bile salts are reabsorbed from the ileum into the portal vein, return to the liver, and become secreted again in a process called **enterohepatic recycling** (see Fig. 31-3).

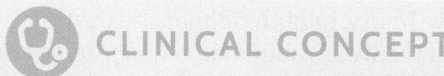

CLINICAL CONCEPT

High amounts of bile salts in the bloodstream can cause pruritus.

Bilirubin Metabolism

One of the liver's most important functions is the conversion of bilirubin into bile. **Bilirubin,** a yellow-colored compound, is derived from the breakdown of aged red blood cells (RBCs). Hemoglobin in the RBCs breaks down into heme and globin; heme is then further broken down into iron and porphyrin. The porphyrin fraction is converted into biliverdin, which rapidly changes into free or **unconjugated bilirubin.** Unconjugated bilirubin travels to the liver. For the body to excrete bilirubin in the bile, it has to be water-soluble. Through the process of **conjugation** in the liver, bilirubin is transformed into a water-soluble form. **Conjugated bilirubin** goes on to be excreted in the bile. Some conjugated bilirubin in the distal ileum and colon is converted to urobilinogen by bacteria. Most urobilinogen is reabsorbed from the GI tract into the bloodstream and then excreted in urine. Urobilinogen gives urine its yellow color. Some urobilinogen continues on in the GI tract where bacteria convert it to stercobilinogen, which is then excreted in the feces (see Fig. 31-4).

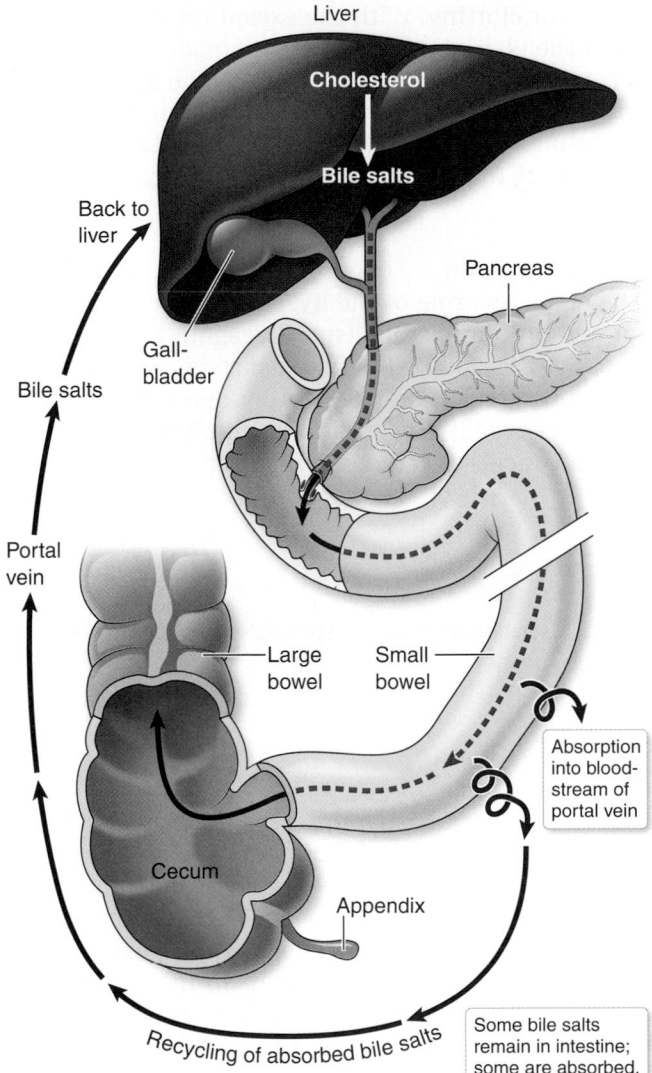

FIGURE 31-3. Bile secretion and enterohepatic recycling of bile salts. Bile salts are formed from cholesterol and secreted into the small intestine to aid fat digestion. Ninety percent of bile salts are reabsorbed into the blood and recycled via enterohepatic circulation.

🩺 CLINICAL CONCEPT

Unconjugated bilirubin is also referred to as indirect bilirubin in diagnostic studies, whereas conjugated bilirubin is also referred to as direct bilirubin.

Fat and Protein Metabolism

The liver secretes bile into the intestine, which breaks down fats efficiently and rapidly. After bile acts on fats in the intestine, they are broken down into triglycerides. These are absorbed into the portal vein and enter the liver, where they are further broken down into fatty acids, cholesterol, and glycerol. The liver is a major producer of cholesterol.

The liver is capable of both synthesizing and breaking down protein. In its role as a manufacturer of protein, the liver produces most of the body's albumin,

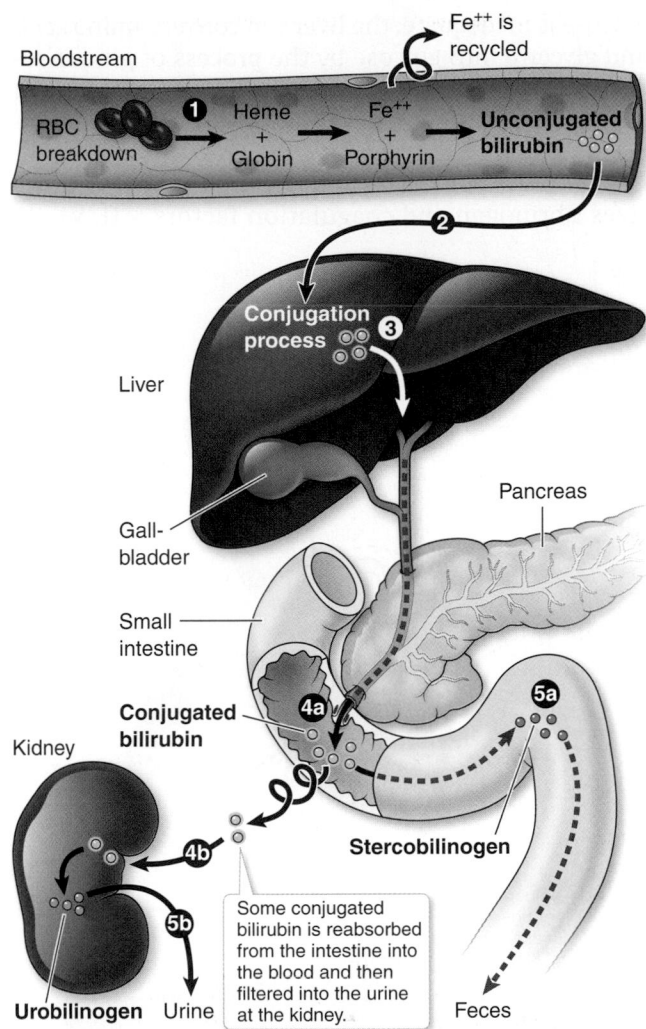

FIGURE 31-4. Conjugation of bilirubin and excretion. (1) RBCs are broken down into iron (Fe++) and protein called porphyrin. Porphyrin is converted to biliverdin, which is further transformed into bilirubin. Iron becomes recycled. Bilirubin needs to be excreted. (2) Bilirubin in the blood enters the liver. (3) The liver conjugates the bilirubin. (4a) Some conjugated bilirubin enters the intestine, (4b) whereas some continues on in the bloodstream. (5a) Some conjugated bilirubin remains in the intestine and is converted into stercobilinogen, which is then excreted in the feces, (5b) whereas other conjugated bilirubin is absorbed by the kidney and is converted into urobilinogen, which gives urine its yellow color.

which exerts colloid oncotic pressure within the bloodstream. In breaking down protein, the liver performs **deamination**—a process that removes nitrogen from proteins and converts it to ammonia (NH_3). Ammonia is absorbed into the bloodstream, becomes integrated into urea, and is then excreted by the kidneys in urine.

Carbohydrate Metabolism

The liver stores glucose as glycogen through the function termed **glycogenesis.** Because of glycogenesis, the liver can store large amounts of glucose that can be used when the body needs energy. When the body is enduring starvation or undergoing high stress, catecholamines stimulate the breakdown of glycogen in a process called **glycogenolysis.** If the body's store of glucose is inadequate, the liver can convert amino acids and glycerol into glucose by the process of **gluconeogenesis** (see Fig. 31-5).

Hematologic Role

As part of its hematologic function, the liver synthesizes fibrinogen and coagulation factors I, II, VI, IX, and X for clotting. With the exception of factor VIII, all of the elements of clotting are made by the hepatocytes. Prothrombin is produced by the liver with the assistance of vitamin K and bile. Vitamin K, which is essential for clotting, is a fat-soluble vitamin. Without any of these components, there is great risk of bleeding.

Endocrine Role

The endocrine role of the liver involves regulation of fat and protein metabolism. Glucagon, which is produced by the alpha cells of the pancreas, acts mainly in the liver and stimulates hepatic glycogenolysis and gluconeogenesis; it also stimulates lipolysis, converting free fatty acids to ketones in the liver.

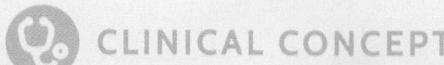

CLINICAL CONCEPT

Administration of glucagon stimulates the liver to secrete glucose from its glycogen stores.

Detoxification

The liver plays an active role in the detoxification of ingested substances and drugs. After a substance is ingested, it is absorbed by the GI system and then passes into the portal vein. The portal vein brings all absorbed substances through the liver, where the detoxification processes called biotransformation and the first pass effect occur. Through these processes, substances are broken down by the liver into detoxified metabolites before reaching the systemic circulation (see Fig. 31-6). In the metabolism of drugs, the liver enzymatically processes the compounds by the cytochrome P450 system, which is a diverse group of enzymes that catalyze the oxidation of many different organic substances, metabolites, hormones, and toxic chemicals.

Biotransformation and the first pass through the liver greatly reduce the bioavailability or concentration of available drug in the bloodstream. The liver transforms drugs into inert compounds that are excreted into the bile and eliminated via the GI tract.

CLINICAL CONCEPT

Hepatocyte injury disrupts the liver's detoxification activity, which results in excess accumulation of drugs, hormones, or metabolites in the blood, tissues, or organs.

Other Functions

The liver stores vitamins A, D, and B_{12}; iron-rich ferritin; and copper, all of which are necessary for

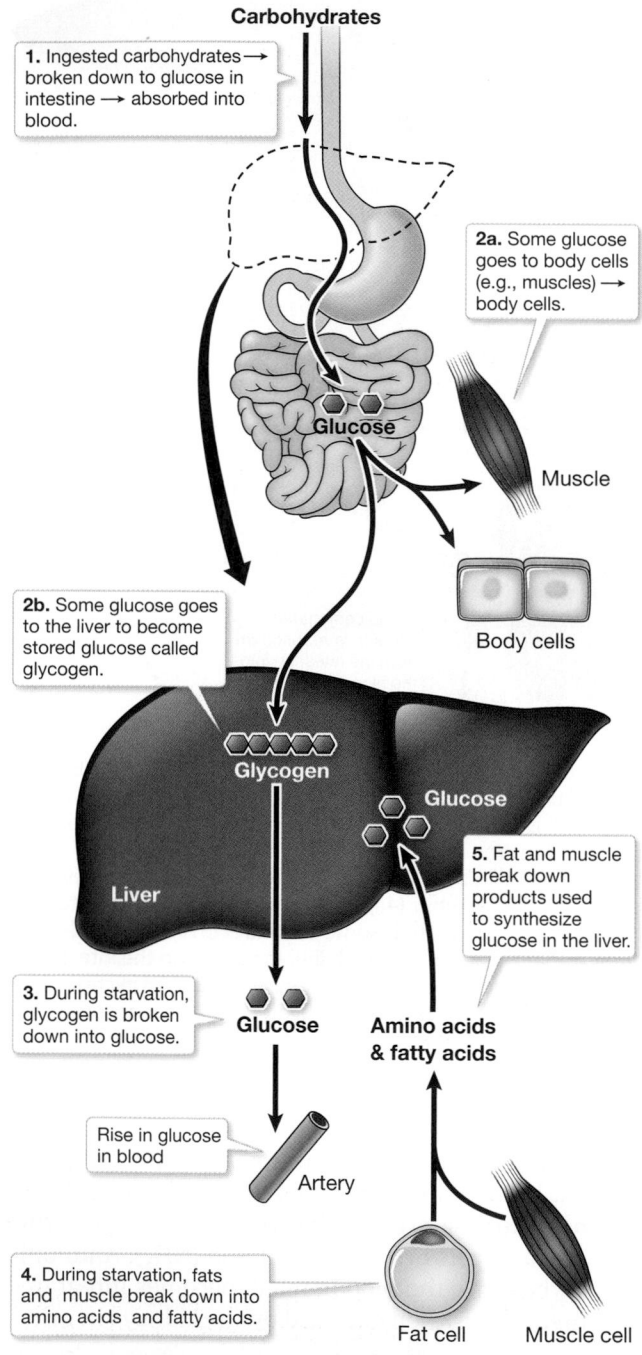

Carbohydrates

1. Ingested carbohydrates → broken down to glucose in intestine → absorbed into blood.

2a. Some glucose goes to body cells (e.g., muscles) → body cells.

Glucose

Muscle

2b. Some glucose goes to the liver to become stored glucose called glycogen.

Body cells

Glycogen

Glucose

Liver

5. Fat and muscle break down products used to synthesize glucose in the liver.

3. During starvation, glycogen is broken down into glucose.

Glucose   **Amino acids & fatty acids**

Rise in glucose in blood

Artery

4. During starvation, fats and muscle break down into amino acids and fatty acids.

Fat cell   Muscle cell

FIGURE 31-5. Role of the liver in carbohydrate metabolism. (1) Ingested carbohydrates are broken down into glucose in the intestine; glucose is then absorbed into blood. (2a) Some glucose goes to body cells such as muscles, (2b) whereas other glucose goes to the liver to synthesize glycogen, called glycogenesis. (3) During starvation or fasting, glycogen in the liver is broken down in a process called glycogenolysis. (4) When glycogen stores are exhausted, muscle and fat break down to form amino acids and fatty acids. (5) Amino acids and fatty acids are then used by the liver to make glucose in a process called gluconeogenesis.

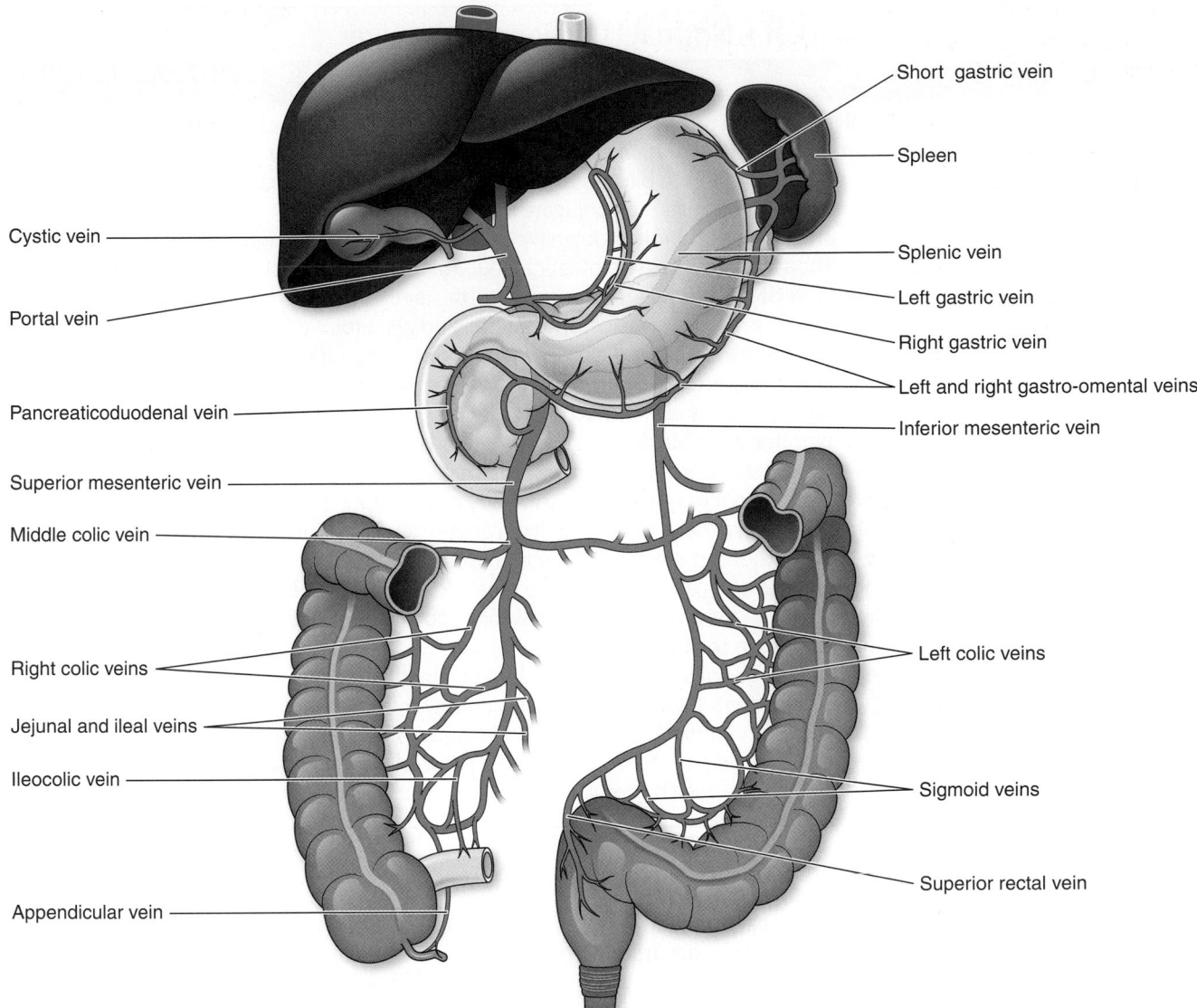

FIGURE 31-6. Detoxification of blood via the portal vein. Drainage of the veins of the gastrointestinal organs enter the portal vein, which carries blood to the liver. The hepatic portal vein is a blood vessel that drains blood from the gastrointestinal tract and spleen and brings it into the liver. This blood is rich in nutrients that were extracted from food, which the liver processes; it also filters toxins that may have been ingested with the food. The liver receives about 75% of its blood through the hepatic portal vein, with the remainder coming from the hepatic artery. The blood leaves the liver and travels to the heart via the hepatic veins and the inferior vena cava.

efficient cellular functions. The liver also produces insulin-like growth factor 1, a polypeptide protein hormone that plays an important role in childhood growth and has anabolic effects in adults. The liver synthesizes thrombopoietin, the hormone that regulates the production of platelets by the bone marrow. The liver also synthesizes angiotensinogen, a hormone that takes part in the renin-angiotensin-aldosterone system, which maintains blood pressure. The liver is responsible for immunological protection; the reticuloendothelial system of the liver contains B lymphocytes and immunoglobulins and also acts as a filter for antigens carried to it via the portal system (see Table 31-1).

Basic Pathophysiologic Concepts of Liver Dysfunction

Liver dysfunction occurs by either cholestasis, which is caused by bile flow obstruction; hepatocellular injury, which is a result of inflammation; or a mixture of both. The consequences of liver disease are related to failure of the liver's main functions: synthesis, metabolism, detoxification, storage, or clearance.

Hyperbilirubinemia and Jaundice

Jaundice, yellowing of the skin and sclera, is the key symptom of liver disease. **Hyperbilirubinemia,** a high

TABLE 31-1. Normal Functions of the Liver

Function	Description
Digestion	The liver manufactures bile and secretes it into the hepatic duct, which enters the common bile duct and, in turn, empties into the intestine for digestion of fats.
Bilirubin conjugation	To convert bilirubin into bile, it has to be made water-soluble (conjugation). In the liver, glucuronic acid is used to conjugate bilirubin.
Fat metabolism	In the intestine, fat is broken down by bile into triglycerides. Triglycerides are then absorbed across the gastrointestinal mucosa into the bloodstream. All venous blood from the GI tract flows into the liver's portal vein. In the liver, triglycerides are further broken down into fatty acids, cholesterol, and glycerol.
Protein metabolism	The liver synthesizes and breaks down protein and manufactures albumin. Proteins are broken down (referred to as deamination) into ammonia, which is then absorbed into the bloodstream and excreted in urine.
Carbohydrate metabolism	In the liver there is a buildup of glucose, which is stored in the form of glycogen (glycogenesis). There is also breakdown of glycogen by the liver when the body needs it (glycogenolysis). When the body needs more glucose, gluconeogenesis, which is the synthesis of glucose from amino acids and fats, occurs in the liver,
Hematologic role	The liver synthesizes coagulation factors using vitamin K.
Endocrine role	Pancreatic glucagon acts at the liver to break down glycogen. Glucagon also stimulates lipolysis. With fat breakdown, there is formation of fatty acids. Fatty acids are converted into ketones in the liver.
Detoxification	The portal vein brings all substances absorbed by the gastrointestinal system into the liver, which then detoxifies substances through biotransformation and first pass effects.
Other functions	The liver stores vitamin A, D, B_{12}, iron, and copper. The liver produces B lymphocytes. The liver synthesizes angiotensinogen, which has a role in the RAAS. The liver synthesizes thrombopoietin, which stimulates platelet production in bone marrow.

amount of bilirubin in the bloodstream, causes jaundice, also called **icterus**. Hyperbilirubinemia occurs because of one of three specific etiologies:

- excessive RBC hemolysis
- hepatocellular injury
- bile duct obstruction.

These causes are referred to as prehepatic, intrahepatic, and posthepatic jaundice, respectively (see Fig. 31-7).

Increased hemolysis of RBCs causes breakdown of hemoglobin into heme and globin. Heme breaks down

further into iron and a protein called porphyrin. Porphyrin breaks down into biliverdin, which is then converted to bilirubin in the bloodstream. Therefore, a high amount of RBC breakdown leads to hyperbilirubinemia. The liver processes bilirubin to make it water-soluble during conjugation. If there is a large amount of hemolysis, bilirubin levels can overwhelm the liver, and some bilirubin can go without being conjugated, which is why prolonged hemolysis increases both conjugated and unconjugated bilirubin concentrations. This type of jaundice is referred to as prehepatic jaundice.

In hepatocellular injury, the liver cannot conjugate bilirubin at all, and there is an accumulation of unconjugated bilirubin in the bloodstream. This type of jaundice, referred to as intrahepatic jaundice, is commonly the result of inflammation of the liver.

In bile duct obstruction, the liver can conjugate the bilirubin but the bile duct does not allow its excretion, resulting in increased levels of conjugated bilirubin circulating in the bloodstream. This is referred to as posthepatic jaundice, and it commonly occurs because of gallstones or tumors that obstruct the common bile duct.

Hepatocyte Inflammation and Infection
Inflammation of the liver is most often caused by a virus, drugs or toxic substances, or excessive alcohol use. The most common viruses that infect the liver are hepatitis virus A, B, C, D, and E. Other viruses include

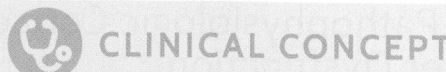

CLINICAL CONCEPT

An example of prehepatic jaundice is exhibited in physiologic jaundice of the newborn. In this disorder, the breakdown of RBCs causes accumulation of bilirubin in the bloodstream. The newborn develops jaundice because its immature liver cannot effectively conjugate the bilirubin. Conjugated and unconjugated bilirubin are both found in the newborn's bloodstream. The infant becomes temporarily jaundiced until RBCs are processed by the immature liver, which takes a few days.

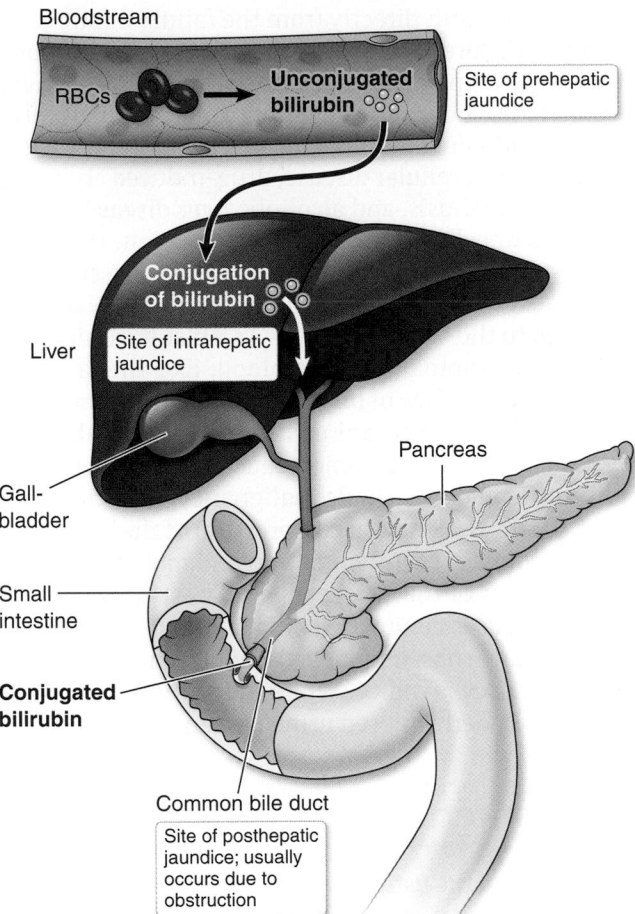

Bloodstream

RBCs

Unconjugated bilirubin

Site of prehepatic jaundice

Conjugation of bilirubin

Liver

Site of intrahepatic jaundice

Gall-bladder

Pancreas

Small intestine

Conjugated bilirubin

Common bile duct

Site of posthepatic jaundice; usually occurs due to obstruction

FIGURE 31-7. Sites of jaundice. (1) Prehepatic jaundice occurs when there is an overwhelming amount of hemolysis occurring in the body. With overwhelming hemolysis, there is an abundance of bilirubin, and all bilirubin cannot be processed by the liver. Because the bilirubin is backing up into the bloodstream and has not entered the liver, it is called prehepatic jaundice. (2) Intrahepatic jaundice occurs when the liver is having problems conjugating the bilirubin, resulting in only a portion becoming conjugated. This is referred to as an intrahepatic problem, so it is called intrahepatic jaundice. (3) Posthepatic jaundice occurs when the bilirubin has been conjugated and fully processed by the liver. The bilirubin, however, is not backing up because there is an obstruction in the bile duct—either in the hepatic duct or common bile duct. Bilirubin that has already left the liver cannot get to the bile duct for secretion, so this is called posthepatic jaundice.

cytomegalovirus and Epstein-Barr virus. Viral hepatitis usually begins as an acute syndrome that involves liver enzyme elevation and hyperbilirubinemia. Acute infection with a hepatitis virus may result in conditions ranging from subclinical disease to self-limited symptomatic disease to fulminant hepatic failure. Common changes in the liver with hepatitis include infiltration of white blood cells (WBCs) and increased permeability of hepatocyte cell membranes. When viral hepatitis lasts longer than 6 months, it can become a chronic, long-term inflammatory condition. Chronic hepatic inflammation increases the risk of hepatocellular cancer.

In toxic hepatitis, the liver is affected by drugs or toxic substances (see Box 31-1). Acetaminophen is one

---

BOX 31-1. Common Causes of Hepatic Inflammation

The following agents can directly injure hepatocytes:

DRUGS
- acetaminophen
- acetylsalicylic acid (aspirin)
- allopurinol
- captopril
- carbamazepine
- diazepam
- erythromycin
- estrogen
- halothane
- methotrexate
- methyldopa
- oral contraceptives
- phenobarbital
- phenytoin
- sulfonamides
- tetracycline.

TOXINS
- carbon tetrachloride
- ethyl alcohol
- kava (herb)
- trichloroethylene
- toluene
- wild mushrooms (some).

VIRUSES
- coxsackie virus
- cytomegalovirus
- Epstein-Barr virus
- hepatitis viruses A, B, C, D, E.

of the most common causes of toxic hepatitis. There are specific enzymes in the liver that detoxify substances in the blood, called the cytochrome P450 system. Activation of some enzymes in the cytochrome P450 system can lead to oxidative stress; this injures hepatocytes and bile duct cells, which leads to accumulation of bile acid inside the liver. This accumulation causes liver damage, which involves dysfunction of liver macrophages (also called Kupffer cells) and activation of stellate cells. Activation of stellate cells leads to fat and collagenous tissue accumulation. Alternatively, many chemicals can damage cellular mitochondria. Dysfunctional mitochondria diminish energy production within the liver, thereby slowing the many metabolic functions of the liver. Mitochondrial dysfunction also causes release of oxidizing free radicals, further injuring hepatic cells.

Alcohol is a common cause of long-term, chronic liver disease. With chronic inflammation, stellate cells within the liver are stimulated to synthesize collagen and fibrotic tissue. Other classical histological features of the disease include bile duct damage, lymphoid follicles or aggregates, and macrovesicular steatosis. Steatosis is the infiltration of fat in the liver. Fatty liver is a characteristic change in alcohol abuse.

Nonalcoholic fatty liver disease (NAFLD) and **nonalcoholic steatosis (NASH)** are also common pathophysiologic conditions of the liver. Although the etiology is unclear, the patient usually has comorbidities of obesity, hypertriglyceridemia, or diabetes. The liver becomes infiltrated with fat and fibrotic tissue. NAFLD is a major cause of cirrhosis.

Severe cases of hepatocellular injury may progress to fulminant hepatic failure, which is acute liver failure complicated by hepatic encephalopathy—involvement of the brain. Hepatic encephalopathy is exhibited by lethargy, confusion, and, in extreme cases, stupor and coma. The encephalopathy of fulminant hepatic failure is attributed to increased permeability of the blood-brain barrier and brain swelling. Cerebral edema is a potentially fatal complication of fulminant hepatic failure.

Bile Duct Obstruction

Biliary obstruction refers to the blockage of any duct that carries bile from the liver to the small intestine (see Fig. 31-8). The major signs and symptoms of biliary

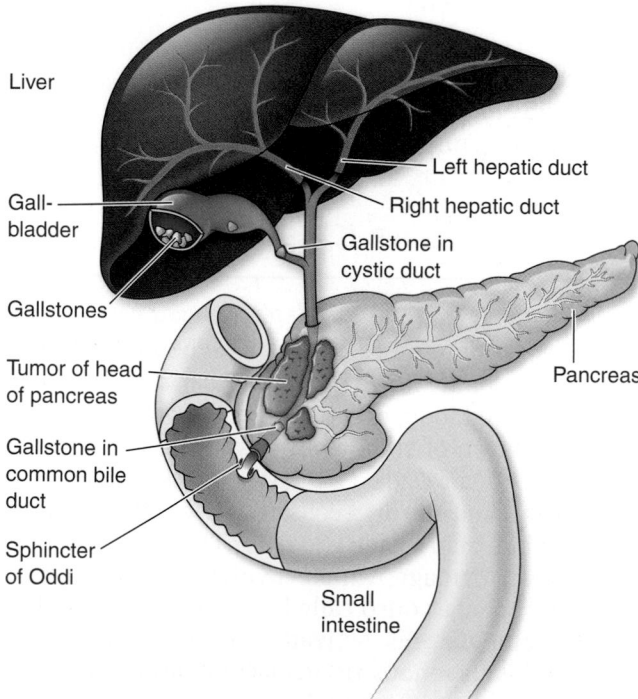

Liver

Gall-
bladder

Gallstones

Tumor of head
of pancreas

Gallstone in
common bile
duct

Sphincter
of Oddi

Left hepatic duct

Right hepatic duct

Gallstone in
cystic duct

Pancreas

Small
intestine

FIGURE 31-8. Common causes of bile obstruction. The most common causes of bile duct obstruction are gallstones and tumor of the head of the pancreas. In cholelithiasis, a gallstone commonly lodges in the cystic duct, which causes backup of pressure and bile in the gallbladder, resulting in cholecystitis. A gallstone can also travel out of the cystic duct and lodge in the common bile duct, which causes backup of bile into the liver and then into the bloodstream, causing jaundice. A tumor of the head of the pancreas also commonly leads to obstruction of the common bile duct. This causes bile to backup into the liver and blood, leading to jaundice.

obstruction result directly from the failure of bile to be excreted. Failure of bile to reach the ducts for excretion causes a backup of bile, also referred to as **cholestasis**. Intrahepatic cholestasis generally occurs at the level of the hepatocyte or biliary canalicular membrane. Causes include hepatocellular disease, drug-induced cholestasis, biliary cirrhosis, and alcoholic liver disease.

In hepatocellular disease, interference in the three major steps of bilirubin metabolism—uptake, conjugation, or excretion—usually occurs. Excretion is usually impaired to the greatest extent. As a result, conjugated bilirubin accumulates in the blood. Extrahepatic obstruction to the flow of bile may occur within the ducts or secondary to external compression. Overall, gallstones are the most common cause of biliary obstruction. Other causes include malignancy, infection, and biliary cirrhosis. External compression of the ducts may occur secondary to inflammation and malignancy.

Regardless of the cause, physical obstruction of the bile duct causes conjugated bilirubin to accumulate in the blood and subsequent deposition in the skin which, in turn, causes jaundice. When bilirubin is filtered by the kidneys, dark-colored urine is seen.

Assessment

Assessment of the patient with liver dysfunction requires a thorough history, complete physical examination, and use of laboratory tests and diagnostic procedures. Risk factors for liver disease should also be investigated (see Box 31-2).

History

In the history, the clinician should focus on the etiology of disease, the patient's appetite, digestion, exercise tolerance, and bowel changes. The patient with liver

---

BOX 31-2. Risk Factors for Liver Disease

The following conditions increase susceptibility to liver disease:

- alcohol abuse, excessive
- certain medications
- gastric bypass surgery
- HBV or HCV, chronic
- high cholesterol
- high triglycerides
- iron overload
- malnutrition
- metabolic syndrome
- obesity
- toxins, chemicals
- weight loss, rapid
- Wilson disease.

dysfunction often reports extreme fatigue, abdominal pain, weakness, anorexia, nausea, vomiting, abdominal bloating, changes in bowel habits, and weight loss. Interestingly, smokers often lose their taste for tobacco. Because the liver may not be secreting bile for fat digestion, the patient may complain of **steatorrhea,** which are defined as light-colored, soft stools. Jaundice and dark urine are signs of bilirubin accumulation in the bloodstream. Accumulation of bile salts in the bloodstream often causes pruritus, or itching of the skin.

Signs and Symptoms

In the physical examination, RUQ tenderness may be present. Hepatomegaly may be palpated on abdominal examination. Hyperbilirubinemia occurs and, because of bilirubin's affinity for elastin fibers, the skin and sclera become yellow. The presence of jaundice in the sclera indicates a minimum level of 3.0 mg/dL of serum bilirubin. Other sites to examine for jaundice are under the tongue and, in persons of color, the mucous membranes of the mouth. Examination of the skin may show spider angioma, caput medusa over the abdomen, and palmar erythema. **Spider angioma** are fine capillaries that fan out from a central point on the skin's surface (see Fig. 31-9). Caput medusa are obvious dilated veins over the umbilical area of the abdomen. Ascites is common in liver disease and can be confirmed by eliciting "shifting dullness" in the abdomen. Steatorrhea can occur when bilirubin is not excreted into the intestine. Dark urine can occur in liver disease because of the backup of bilirubin into the bloodstream that is filtered at the kidney. Box 31-3 details classic signs of liver disease.

Diagnostic Tests

The initial battery of tests for liver function include liver enzymes, serum alanine transaminase (ALT), serum aspartate transaminase (AST), alkaline phosphatase, direct and indirect bilirubin, albumin, and prothrombin levels (see Table 31-2). The pattern of abnormalities enables the differentiation between hepatocellular

> ### BOX 31-3. Classic Signs of Liver Disease
>
> The following signs and symptoms occur anytime there is hepatocyte injury or obstruction of bile excretion:
>
> - anorexia
> - ascites
> - dark urine
> - hepatomegaly
> - hyperbilirubinemia
> - jaundice
> - RUQ tenderness
> - splenomegaly
> - steatorrhea.

and cholestatic disease and determination of acute or chronic stages. A hepatitis serology panel is done that includes specific laboratory data regarding hepatitis A, B, C, D, or E (see Table 31-3). Autoimmune markers help in determining biliary cirrhosis. Diagnostic imaging uses ultrasound tomography, computed tomography (CT) scans, and magnetic resonance imaging (MRI). Liver biopsy is the gold standard test for diagnosing the stages and severity of liver disease, predicting prognosis, and monitoring therapy.

Treatment

Treatment for liver disorders includes control of symptoms and supportive care with rest and small, high-calorie, high-protein meals. The patient should avoid alcohol or any drugs, unless prescribed. Hepatitis has some treatment regimens that include interferon, nucleoside analogues, protease inhibitors, and other antiviral agents. Patients with encephalopathy should be monitored in an intensive care setting. As encephalopathy progresses, maintenance of the airway and circulation requires frequent assessment. Careful attention should be paid to fluid management and hemodynamics. Monitoring of metabolic parameters, surveillance for infection, maintenance of nutrition, and prompt recognition of gastrointestinal bleeding are crucial. Coagulation parameters, complete blood cell count (CBC), and metabolic panel should be checked frequently. Serum aminotransferases and bilirubin are generally measured daily to follow the course of infection. Liver transplantation, in selected cases, is an option if the patient has fulminant hepatic failure.

Select Pathophysiologic Disorders of the Liver

The dysfunction of the liver is caused by either damage to hepatocytes or blockage of bile flow. Interference with bile outflow causes backup of bilirubin into the bloodstream, which is manifested as jaundice. Commonly

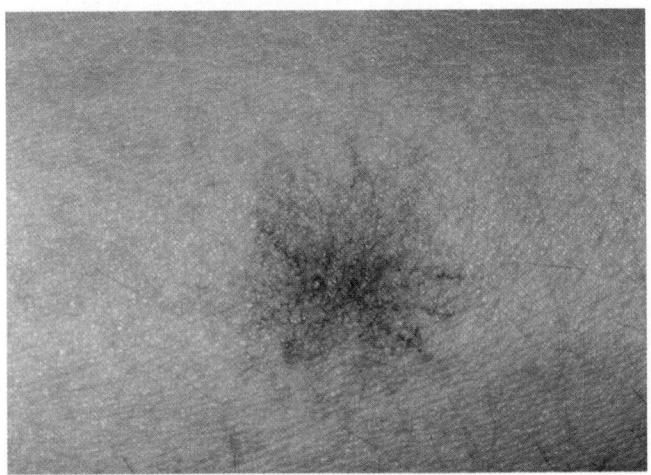

FIGURE 31-9. Spider angioma. *(From SPL/Science Source.)*

TABLE 31-2. Diagnostic Test Results in Different Types of Liver Disease

Test	Normal Levels	Abnormality
AST	5 to 40 U/mL	Elevated in alcoholic liver disease
ALT	5 to 35 U/mL	Elevated in liver disease
Alkaline phosphatase	35 to 150 U/mL	Elevated in hepatitis and liver disease
Bilirubin, indirect	Less than 0.8 mg/dL	Elevated unconjugated bilirubin occurs in Gilbert's disease
Bilirubin, total	Less than 1.0 mg/dL	Elevated bilirubin causes jaundice in hepatitis
PT	11.5 to 14 sec	Prolonged suggests hepatic dysfunction
Serum albumin	3.5 to 5.5 g/dL	Decreased indicates hepatic dysfunction
Serum globulin	2.5 to 3.5 g/dL	Elevated in autoimmune hepatitis
γ-Glutamyl transpeptidase	10 to 48 U/mL	Large elevation in alcoholic liver disease

TABLE 31-3. Viral Hepatitis Diagnostic Tests

After a patient is diagnosed with viral hepatitis, it is important to clarify which kind of hepatitis virus is causing the infection. The laboratory tests used to diagnose the different types of hepatitis virus infections are shown in this table.

Test	HAV	HBV	HCV
Alkaline phosphatase	Elevated	Elevated	Elevated
Aminotransferase	Elevated	Elevated	Elevated
Anti-HCV antibodies			Diagnostic of HCV infection
Bilirubin	Elevated	Elevated	Elevated
HBsAg		Diagnostic of HBV infection	
Immunoglobulin M anti-HAV virus antibody	Diagnostic of acute HAV infection		
Immunoglobulin M anti-HBcAg antibodies		Diagnostic of acute HBV infection	
Prothrombin		Prolonged	Prolonged
Viral assay	HAV RNA viral assay	HBV DNA viral assay	HCV RNA viral assay

hepatocyte damage leads to fatty degeneration of the liver, which terminates in a fibrotic change of the liver known as cirrhosis.

Acute Hepatitis

Hepatitis is a systemic infection affecting the liver, usually caused by one of five viral agents:

1. hepatitis A (HAV)
2. hepatitis B (HBV)
3. hepatitis C (HCV)
4. hepatitis D (HDV)
5. hepatitis E (HEV).

With the exception of HBV, which is caused by a deoxyribonucleic acid (DNA) virus, all the others are ribonucleic (RNA) viruses. Nonviral hepatitis results from exposure to toxic chemicals or certain drugs. Other viruses that can cause inflammation of the liver are cytomegalovirus and EBV. Generally, all types of hepatitis produce similar clinical manifestations, ranging from mild symptoms to fulminant infections or chronic progressive liver disease.

Hepatitis A Virus

HAV is usually caused by ingestion of contaminated food or water or contracted from person to person by unsanitary conditions. The virus is able to live on surfaces at room temperature, but is killed by cooking food thoroughly. HAV is absorbed by the intestine and travels to the liver, where it damages the hepatocytes. It mainly causes a mild disease with no complications.

There is a low incidence of HAV infection in the United States because there are high standards of sanitation and hygiene. Between 1995 and 2006, reported HAV incidence declined by 90% to the lowest rate ever recorded—1.2 cases per 100,000 population. The greatest decline in incidence in the United States was seen after

1999 because some states required routine vaccination of children with HAV immunization. In accordance with these findings, in 2006, the Centers for Disease Control and Prevention (CDC) recommended an expansion of routine HAV vaccination to include all children in the United States aged 12 to 23 months. HAV vaccination has made HAV infection uncommon. HAV infection is endemic in Asia, Africa, Mexico, and South America.

Etiology. HAV is an RNA virus that uses its own RNA polymerase to achieve replication of its viral parts in the hepatocyte. HAV is contracted through the fecal-oral route, although isolated cases of parenteral transmission have been reported. HAV is resilient and can remain viable for many years. Boiling water is an effective means of destroying it; chlorine and iodine are similarly effective.

Risk factors that increase susceptibility to HAV infection are a weak immune system, living in unsanitary conditions, institutionalization, foreign travel to a country where HAV is endemic, male homosexuality, and illicit parenteral drug use. Eating food that has been in contaminated water, such as seafood, fruits, and vegetables, is a major risk factor.

Pathophysiology. Uptake of HAV and viral replication occurs within hepatocytes. After entry into the cell, viral RNA is converted into DNA by polymerase enzymes. Viral proteins are synthesized, and assembled virus particles are shed into the biliary tree and excreted in the feces. HAV can be found in bile, stool, and blood. Person-to-person contact is the most common means of transmission and is generally limited to close contacts. The period of greatest contagion of HAV is during the first 14 to 21 days after infection, when jaundice has not yet occurred. After exposure to the virus, antibodies to HAV of the immunoglobulin (Ig) M class can be detected in blood. The antibody response persists for several months. After acute illness, anti-HAV antibodies of the IgG class remain detectable. IgG antibodies endow immunity to prevent repeat infection.

Clinical Presentation. Patients with HAV infection report fever, abdominal pain, mild flulike symptoms of nausea and vomiting, fatigue, malaise, myalgias, arthralgias, and mild headache. Anorexia and loss of taste for food may also be reported. Smokers often lose their taste for tobacco. The clinician should ask questions regarding the patient's possible exposure to HAV and also inquire about his or her occupation, living conditions, diet, and recent travel or exposure to others who travel. The patient may have contracted HAV through food eaten weeks in the past; however, a dietary history is difficult to track.

Signs and Symptoms Flulike symptoms are commonly present, and the physical examination may demonstrate hepatomegaly and jaundice. Jaundice occurs in most (70% to 85%) adults. Stool may have a pale appearance, and dark urine and pruritus may accompany jaundice. Children who acquire HAV usually do not develop jaundice and are mildly symptomatic.

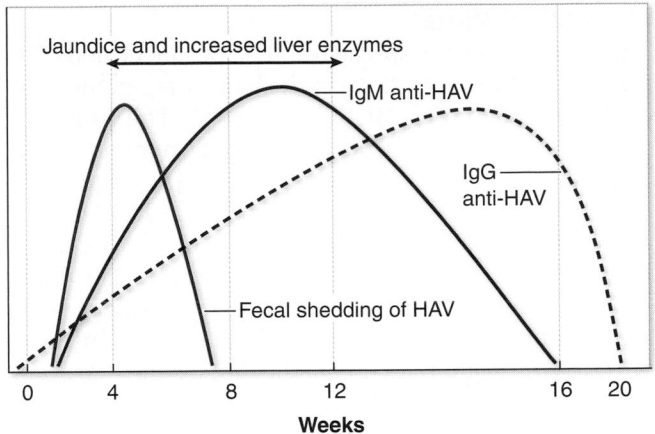

FIGURE 31-10. HAV infection. HAV is an infection spread by the fecal-oral route. After contraction of HAV, the virus is shed in the feces. Jaundice and increased liver enzymes become apparent after approximately 2 weeks. The first antibodies to develop against HAV are immunoglobulin (Ig) G antibodies. IgG antibodies against HAV are formed in large amounts later and remain elevated for more than 20 weeks.

Diagnosis. HAV has an incubation period of 2 to 4 weeks, and liver enzymes will rise after the first 4 weeks. HAV is apparent in the stool early, within the first 2 to 4 weeks. HAV RNA appears in the blood up to 2 weeks before clinical illness develops. IgM antibodies against HAV appear after the first 4 weeks, and IgG antibodies rise after 8 to 12 weeks. Diagnosis is usually based on antibodies, specifically the anti-HAV of IgM class. IgG anti-HAV antibodies remain elevated and provide long-term immune protection (see Fig. 31-10).

Treatment. Treatment is supportive and does not change the course of the disease. Rest and good nutrition are important, along with avoidance of alcohol and acetaminophen. Good hygiene is also necessary. HAV vaccine endows immunity with one dose. Passive immunization with HAV Ig is also available for contacts of patients with HAV infection. This immunization is a short-term, rapid dose of protective antibodies given to family members and close contacts before exposure or during the early incubation period. For postexposure prophylaxis, HAV Ig can be administered as late as 2 weeks after contact. HAV vaccine is available for all who want or need prevention before exposure.

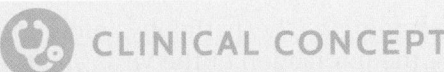

CLINICAL CONCEPT

A very small proportion of patients develop a relapse of HAV weeks to months after acute infection. Rarely, cholestatic hepatitis characterized by jaundice, pruritus, and liver test abnormalities can persist for up to a year postinfection. However, even when these complications occur, HAV infection is self-limited and does not progress to chronic liver disease.

Hepatitis B Virus

HBV is a stable virus spread by blood products, body fluids, or sexual contact. Once in the bloodstream, the virus produces viral proteins in the hepatocyte. The virus does not directly kill the cell, but the host's own immune system attacks hepatocytes when the viral antigens are encountered on the surface. Individuals carry HBV for life, and hepatocellular carcinoma (HCC) can occur because of the chronic inflammation caused by the virus.

HBV infection is a global problem, with an estimated one-third of the world's population infected with it. An estimated 200,000 new cases of HBV occur annually in the United States, and 1 to 1.25 million people are carriers. HBV disease accounts for 5% to 10% of cases of chronic, end-stage liver disease and 10% to 15% of cases of HCC. The prevalence is low in persons younger than 12 years, but increases in those older than 12 years; this statistic is associated with the initiation of sexual contact, which is the major mode of transmission. In the United States, an estimated 5,000 persons die per year from chronic HBV.

Etiology. HBV is an extremely resilient virus capable of withstanding extreme conditions. It can survive when stored for years at temperatures below zero and for weeks at temperatures over 110°F. Certain hepatitis viral antigens are significant when following the progress of the viral infection. Hepatitis surface antigen (HBsAg) is a protein found on its outer surface that can be used to measure the number of viral particles. The antibody to this protein is anti-HBsAg. The protein expressed by the viral DNA is called HBV core antigen (HBcAg) and its corresponding antibody is anti-HBcAg. The e antigen, HBeAg, comes from the core and is a marker of active viral replication. The best indication of active viral replication is the presence of HBV DNA in the serum.

Risk factors include non-Hispanic black ethnicity, cocaine use, high number of sexual partners and unprotected sexual activity, sexually transmitted infection, human immunodeficiency virus positive status, handling of blood products, intravenous drug use and use of unsterile needles, men who have sex with men, household contact with someone with HBV, and hemodialysis. Also, travel to regions with high rates of HBV, such as Africa, Central and Southeast Asia, and Eastern Europe, places a person at risk (see Box 31-4). Perinatal transmission is possible; in addition, oral passage of the virus is uncommon, but possible.

Pathophysiology. The pathophysiology of HBV is caused by the interaction of the virus and the human immune system. The immune system attacks HBV and causes liver injury. Activated CD4+ and CD8+ cells react against HBV proteins located on the surface of infected hepatocytes, and an immunological reaction occurs. Four different stages have been identified in the viral life cycle of HBV.

- **Stage 1:** In the first stage, the incubation period, there are no signs or symptoms; however, the

---

BOX 31-4. High-Risk Populations for HBV Infection

The following persons are at high risk for development of HBV infection:

- foreign travelers to countries with endemic hepatitis
- health-care providers
- household contacts of persons with HBV
- men who have sex with men
- patients on hemodialysis
- persons who use intravenous drugs or illicit drugs
- persons with HCV
- persons with a history of sexually transmitted infections
- persons with multiple sex partners
- persons with human immunodeficiency virus
- prison inmates.

---

patient can pass the virus to others. The duration of this stage is approximately 2 to 4 weeks. For newborns, the virus can incubate for years. Active viral replication is occurring during this stage without elevation in the liver enzyme (aminotransferase levels).
- **Stage 2:** In the second stage, an inflammatory reaction of the hepatocytes occurs. The patient may experience flulike symptoms and jaundice begins to develop. HBeAg, HbsAg, and HBV DNA can be detected in the bloodstream. Liver enzymes begin to increase. The duration of this symptomatic stage is approximately 3 to 4 weeks.
- **Stage 3:** In the third stage, the immune system reacts against the infected hepatocytes and HBV. Viral replication slows. The HBV DNA levels are lower or undetectable, and liver enzyme levels decrease to normal.
- **Stage 4:** In the fourth stage, the virus cannot be detected and antibodies to HBsAg, HBcAg, and HBeAg have been produced.

The production of antibodies against HBsAg confers long-term protective immunity and can be detected in patients who have recovered from HBV or in those who have been vaccinated. Antibody to HBcAg is only detected in those with actual previous infection with HBV. Those with vaccination do not obtain the HBcAg in the vaccine. The HBcAg blood test can be used to differentiate persons who have contracted the disease from those who have undergone vaccination. Only those who have endured the disease have circulating HBcAg in the bloodstream.

In the patient's lifetime, HBV antigens and HBV DNA can persist and recur in extrahepatic sites, such as the lymph nodes, bone marrow, spleen, and pancreas. However, the virus does not appear to harm tissue in these organs.

The final stage of HBV disease is cirrhosis. Patients with cirrhosis and HBV are likely to develop HCC. This stage may occur after many years of chronic disease.

Clinical Presentation. The patient with HBV presents to the clinician after a prolonged incubation period of 2 to 6 months, during which the patient is asymptomatic. When symptomatic, the patient presents with a flulike syndrome, anorexia, RUQ or epigastric pain, jaundice, pruritus, dark urine, and light-colored stools. The clinician should encourage the patient to disclose his or her HBV status to contacts because of contagion. Contacts can obtain hepatitis B immunoglobulin (HBIg), which can provide rapid passive immunity against HBV.

During the patient's recovery, symptoms gradually subside. The course is variable and may run from a moderate illness to fulminant hepatitis. Patients with chronic HBV can be healthy carriers without any evidence of active disease.

Signs and Symptoms. The patient presents with fever, flulike symptoms, jaundice, and hepatomegaly. Splenomegaly, lymphadenopathy, spider angioma, and palmar erythema may be evident. Jaundice can last for months. Patients with severe cases of infection may present with signs of hepatic encephalopathy—somnolence, confusion, stupor, or coma.

Diagnosis. Diagnosis of HBV is usually made by the presence of HBsAg in the bloodstream. However, the level of HBsAg in the bloodstream is not correlated with the severity of disease. Indeed, some with low titers have severe disease, whereas high titers can be present with mild disease. HBeAg blood levels are present during the time of active replication of the virus. HBeAg is most closely monitored during the convalescent phase. Tests for detection of HBV DNA in the liver and bloodstream are also available. To distinguish between acute and chronic infection, IgM- versus IgG-type antibodies are assessed. Anti-HBc antibodies are IgM-type antibodies that are present in acute infection, whereas IgG-type anti-HBc antibodies are present in chronic infection. Liver enzymes and bilirubin levels are elevated in active disease. Serum albumin, prothrombin time (PT), and coagulation factors also should be monitored over the course of the disease (see Fig. 31-11).

Treatment. Treatment is symptomatic and is usually supportive with rest. The patient should be encouraged to eat small, high-calorie, high-protein meals. Currently, interferon alfa and drugs that inhibit viral polymerase, such as lamivudine, telbivudine, adefovir, entecavir, and tenofovir, are used to treat HBV. Prevention is the key to disease control. HBV vaccine is recommended for all people. During the course of the disease, close contacts of the patient can receive HBIg for short-acting immediate immunity. For unvaccinated individuals who are exposed to HBV, postexposure prophylaxis with a combination of HBIg and HBV vaccine is recommended.

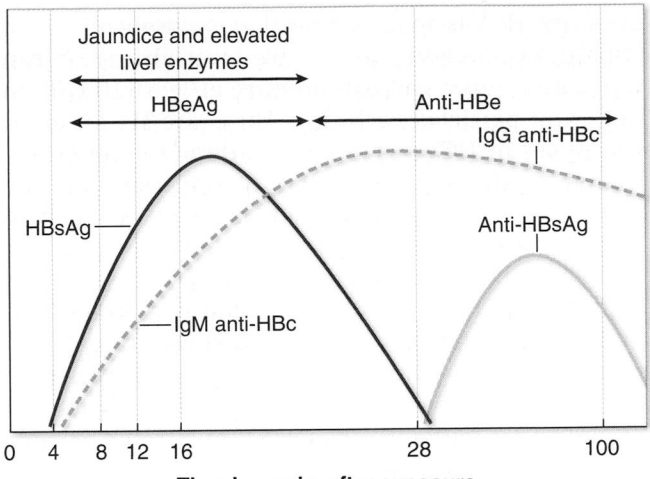

FIGURE 31-11. HBV infection. HBV is an infection spread by blood or body fluids. After contraction of HBV, jaundice and increased liver enzymes become apparent after approximately 4 weeks. Hepatitis B surface antigen (HBsAg) and hepatitis B antigen (HBeAg) rise in the blood after approximately 4 weeks. The first antibodies to develop against HBV are immunoglobulin (Ig) M type antibodies against HBcAg. Later in the course of disease, IgG antibodies against HBcAg are formed. Antibodies against HBV antigen and HBV surface antigen develop much later in the course of disease.

CLINICAL CONCEPT

Most individuals with HBV do not recover completely. Patients who are of advanced age and have serious underlying medical conditions may have a prolonged course and suffer severe disease. Some patients with acute HBV go on to endure chronic HBV. This is common in infants, those affected by Down syndrome, patients on long-term hemodialysis, and those who are immunosuppressed and HIV-positive. Persons who have suffered HBV become carriers of inactive HBV.

Hepatitis C

HCV is a virus that targets hepatocytes and B lymphocytes. Acute HCV infection is usually mild and chronic hepatitis occurs in at least 75% of patients. The mode of transmission is via blood as in intravenous drug use; sexual transmission is not as likely. HCV can live dormant in the patient for years before symptoms develop.

HCV is a global public health problem and a major cause of both acute and chronic viral hepatitis. The World Health Organization estimates that 170 million individuals worldwide are infected with HCV. According to the CDC, an estimated 1.8% of the U.S. population is positive for HCV antibodies. This corresponds to an estimated 2.7 million people with active HCV infection nationwide. Infection caused by HCV accounts for 20% of all cases of acute hepatitis, an estimated 30,000 new acute infections, and 8,000 to 10,000 deaths each year in the United States.

Etiology. HCV is an RNA virus that is closely related to hepatitis G, dengue, and yellow fever viruses. It can replicate rapidly and can produce at least 10 trillion new viral particles each day. There are six different genotypes of HCV; each has a different severity, response to therapy, and mode of transmission. The major HCV genotype worldwide is genotype 1, which accounts for 40% to 80% of all isolates. Genotype 1 is thought to be associated with severe liver disease and a high risk of HCC. Genotypes 1a and 1b are prevalent in the United States, whereas in other countries, genotype 1a is less frequent. HCV genotype 1 does not respond to therapy as well as other genotypes. Genotypes 2a and 2b are found in 10% to 15% of affected persons in the United States and have good response to therapy. Other genotypes are more common in affected persons of other countries.

CLINICAL CONCEPT

There are many different genotypes of HCV caused by the virus' great potential to mutate.

Transmission of HCV occurs mainly via blood. People who inject illegal drugs with nonsterile needles or who use cocaine with shared straws are at highest risk for HCV. The screening of donated blood for HCV antibody has decreased the risk of transfusion-associated HCV to fewer than 1 case in 230,000 donations. Health-care providers can contract HCV via needlestick injuries or other occupational exposures. Needlestick injuries in the health-care setting result in a 3% risk of HCV transmission. Nosocomial patient-to-patient transmission may occur by means of contaminated instruments, such as a colonoscope, dialysis equipment, or surgical tools. HCV may also be transmitted via tattooing, sharing razors, and acupuncture. The use of disposable needles for acupuncture, which is standard practice, has eliminated this transmission route. Uncommon routes of transmission of HCV, which affect fewer than 5% of the individuals at risk, include high-risk sexual activity and maternal-fetal transmission. Co-infection with HIV type 1 appears to increase the risk of both sexual and maternal-fetal transmission of HCV. Casual household contact and contact with the saliva of those infected are uncommon modes of transmission.

Pathophysiology. After contraction of HCV, the incubation period can vary from 2 weeks to 8 months. During this time, the patient is asymptomatic and can spread the virus. Although replication of HCV is rapid, it is imperfect. RNA polymerase, an enzyme critical in HCV replication, allows for inaccurate copying of the virus, generating a large number of mutant viruses known as HCV quasispecies; these pose a major challenge to vaccine development. HCV RNA

BOX 31-5. Signs and Symptoms of Viral Hepatitis

The following are classic signs and symptoms that occur in viral hepatitis infections:

- anorexia
- arthralgias
- fatigue
- fever
- myalgias
- nausea and vomiting
} Flulike illness
- dark urine
- hepatomegaly
- jaundice
- RUQ tenderness
- splenomegaly
- steatorrhea
- weight loss.

---

can be detected weeks to months before antibody development and remains detectable indefinitely. After contraction of the virus there is a strong response by cytotoxic T lymphocytes and helper T cells. In most infected people, viremia is accompanied by hepatic inflammation and fibrosis. Acute HCV becomes chronic in 70% of patients.

Clinical Presentation. The patient history may include apparent risk factors for HCV, such as intravenous drug use. Patients usually present with low-grade fever, nausea, vomiting, fatigue, malaise, jaundice, anorexia, and weight loss. Physical examination signs are similar to other types of viral hepatitis (see Box 31-5). Some people may be asymptomatic, but most patients progress to a chronic illness or a carrier state. The course of disease is widely erratic, with wide fluctuations in liver enzymes. HCV remains one of the causes of end-stage liver disease.

Diagnosis. Diagnostic testing for HCV involves the recombinant immunoblot assay. A positive immunoblot assay result is defined as the detection of antibodies against two or more antigens. HCV RNA assay and HCV genotyping should be performed as well. Genotyping can predict the likelihood of response and duration of treatment. Patients with genotypes 1 and 4 are generally treated for 12 months, whereas 6 months of treatment is sufficient for other genotypes. Liver biopsy is done when diagnosis is uncertain. In addition, CBC with differential, bilirubin level, liver function tests, thyroid function studies, screening tests for co-infection with HIV or HBV, and screening for alcohol abuse and drug abuse should be performed. The CBC demonstrates thrombocytopenia in approximately 10% of patients. Low thyroxine levels are found in approximately 10% of patients as well (see Fig. 31-12).

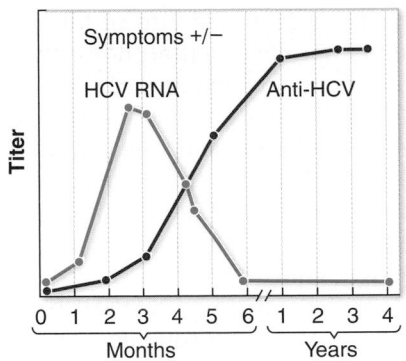

FIGURE 31-12. HCV infection. Most patients with chronic HCV infection are asymptomatic or may have nonspecific symptoms for months. The HCV ribonucleic acid (RNA) assay indicates virus particles in the bloodstream. HCV RNA develops within the bloodstream approximately 1 to 2 months after contraction of the virus. Antibodies against HCV develop late in the course of infection, months to years later.

Treatment. Treatment is supportive, and most cases resolve without sequela. Patients with acute HCV appear to have an excellent chance of responding to 6 months of standard therapy with interferon. Pegylated interferon-A by intramuscular injection once weekly accompanied by administration of riboflavin orally twice daily is used, but there are serious side effects and the therapy is expensive. Interferon in combination with protease inhibitors such as tenofovir has proven to be effective treatment for HCV. A prototype vaccine has not been developed because of rapid HCV viral mutations. Immunoglobulin is ineffective in preventing HCV and is not recommended for postexposure prophylaxis. Health-care personnel who sustain a needlestick injury involving an HCV-infected patient should undergo HCV RNA assay immediately and then every 2 months for 6 months. If positive, treatment should be commenced.

 CLINICAL CONCEPT

Chronic hepatitis with HCV is common. After acute infection, the persistence of HCV-RNA levels demonstrates chronic infection. Biopsy samples of the liver reveal chronic liver inflammation, and cirrhosis develops in 20% to 50% of patients. Liver failure and HCC can eventually result. HCC occurs in 11% to 19% of patients.

Hepatitis D and Hepatitis E
HDV is a defective RNA virus that requires the helper function of HBV for its replication, expression, and duration. It accelerates the progress of liver disease in those with HBV. HDV can either infect a person simultaneously with HBV or superinfect a person who is already infected with HBV. Similar to HBV, its mode of transmission is parenteral drug use or sexual contact.

HEV is clinically similar to HAV, which is spread by the oral-fecal route. It is the most common cause of hepatitis in India, Asia, Africa, and Central America, and its actions are similar to those of HAV. Serological testing for HEV infection is not routinely available.

Chronic Hepatitis
Chronic hepatitis occurs as a result of the progression of acute hepatitis. Hepatitis is considered chronic when inflammation and necrosis of hepatic tissue continues for 6 months or longer. Most cases of chronic hepatitis are from autoimmune diseases, drug toxicity, or progression of HBV or HCV. After acute HCV, 85% to 90% of affected individuals suffer chronic infection. Chronic HCV accounts for over 40% of cases of chronic liver disease and patients undergoing liver transplantation. Clinical and laboratory features that suggest progression of acute hepatitis to chronic hepatitis include continual weight loss, anorexia, fatigue, and persistent hepatomegaly. Liver function tests and bilirubin remain elevated for over 6 months.

Chronic hepatitis predisposes a patient to cirrhosis or carcinoma of the liver. Patients with chronic active hepatitis caused by HBV or HCV are considered carriers and may transmit the disease. Treatment for chronic hepatitis is mainly supportive. Patients with end-stage disease may require a liver transplant.

Autoimmune Hepatitis
Autoimmune hepatitis, also called idiopathic hepatitis, is a chronic disorder characterized by inflammation, fibrosis, and necrosis of the liver. In this form of hepatitis, there is no preceding virus or exposure to toxic agents. The hepatic tissue shows evidence of cell-mediated immunological attack with lesions composed of cytotoxic T cells, antinuclear antibodies, and rheumatoid factor. Lymphocytes of patients with this disorder are sensitized to hepatic cell membrane proteins, react against liver cells, and cause hepatocyte destruction. Patients often respond favorably to anti-inflammatory and immunosuppressive agents.

Toxic Hepatitis
Liver injury can follow the inhalation, ingestion, or parenteral administration of some pharmacological and chemical agents. Exposure to certain drugs, such as isoniazid and acetaminophen, or chemicals, such as carbon tetrachloride or vinyl chloride, cause toxic hepatitis. Liver damage may be rapid after contact, depending on the amount of exposure or drug dosage. Most individuals with nonviral hepatitis recover, but some may develop chronic liver damage.

Nonalcoholic Fatty Liver Disease
NAFLD affects 20% to 30% of the U.S. population and is one of the most common causes of chronic liver disease in the United States. The etiology is unclear; however, hepatocytes exhibit an accumulation of triglycerides. In some patients, fatty liver is accompanied by hepatic

inflammation and scarring of the liver, the condition called non-alcoholic steatohepatitis (NASH). NASH is the most extreme form of NAFLD, and is regarded as a major cause of cirrhosis of the liver.

Among different ethnic groups, African Americans have the lowest rate of NAFLD. The incidence of NASH occurs in 2% to 3% of the general population. Up to 20% of patients with NASH progress to cirrhosis and its complications.

Etiology. The condition most commonly associated with NAFLD is metabolic syndrome, a combination of hyperlipidemia, insulin resistance, and obesity. Other risk factors include diabetes mellitus, protein malnutrition, hypertension, and sleep apnea. Obesity is the most apparent risk factor, with NAFLD risk increasing as individuals' weight increases in the population.

Various drugs, such as amiodarone, tamoxifen, and methotrexate, can cause NAFLD (see Box 31-6). Metabolic abnormalities—such as galactosemia, glycogen storage diseases, homocystinuria, celiac disease, Wilson disease, and tyrosinemia—are also associated with the disorder.

Pathophysiology. NAFLD is linked to metabolic syndrome: insulin resistance, obesity, and hyperlipidemia. Insulin resistance and obesity play important roles in establishing the disease. Under normal conditions, insulin enhances free fatty acid storage in adipose tissue. However, when insulin resistance occurs, storage of fat is shifted to nonadipose tissues, such as the liver. Insulin resistance and obesity also result in decreased levels of adiponectin, which inhibits liver gluconeogenesis and suppresses lipogenesis. Therefore, decreased levels of adiponectin increases gluconeogenesis and enhances lipogenesis in the liver. These processes lead to an accumulation of glucose and fat in the liver.

A small amount of fat accumulation within the liver is of no consequence. However, when 5% to 10% of the liver contains fat, this is **steatosis,** also called fatty degeneration. Steatosis is the abnormal accumulation of lipids within a cell. In hepatic steatosis, excess lipid accumulates in vesicles that displace the cytoplasm of the hepatocyte. A small amount of fat accumulation within a cell is not detrimental; however, large accumulations can disrupt cellular organelles, and in severe cases the cell can rupture. When the vesicles are large enough to distort the nucleus, the condition is known as macrovesicular steatosis; otherwise, the condition is known as microvesicular steatosis. Most patients with NAFLD have microvesicular steatosis and are reported to have a benign clinical course.

A serious complication of NAFLD is nonalcoholic steatohepatitis (NASH). This complication theorizes that the development of NASH is the result of two types of liver injury, referred to as a two-hit process. With the initial hit, macrovesicular steatosis occurs; this alters the metabolic pathways of uptake, synthesis, degradation, and secretion of free fatty acids within the liver cell. Ultimately, the alteration leads to accumulation of a large amount of lipids in the hepatocytes. Mitochondrial dysfunction occurs because of the large accumulation of fat inside the cell. With mitochondrial dysfunction comes the release of free radicals. These free radicals make the liver susceptible to a second hit, which results in inflammation and progression of liver damage. Proinflammatory cytokines, such as tumor necrosis factor, are believed to play an important role in the progression of liver damage to cirrhosis. NASH cirrhosis is a risk factor for development of hepatocellular carcinoma (HCC).

Clinical Presentation. Individuals with a mild case of NAFLD commonly have no noticeable symptoms, though there has been a correlation with morbid obesity. Most often individuals come to the attention of the clinician because of abnormal liver enzymes on a routine physical exam.

Individuals with NASH usually have obvious liver impairment. Symptoms include fatigue, weakness, loss of appetite, nausea, RUQ abdominal pain, spiderlike blood vessels, yellowing of the skin and eyes (jaundice), ascites, ankle edema, and mental confusion.

Diagnosis. When making the diagnosis of NAFLD, the clinician must rule out all other possible causes of liver disease, such as alcoholism or primary diseases that cause secondary NAFLD. All potentially reversible and treatable causes of fatty liver must be excluded. Serological tests must rule out the possibility of HAV, HBV, or HCV.

There are no biomarkers or blood tests yet developed that can diagnose NAFLD with absolute accuracy. Fatty liver can be detected using noninvasive testing such as ultrasound, CT scan, or MRI. However, these tests are most accurate when more than 33% of the liver consists of fat. Liver biopsy is a key test in the diagnosis of NASH, but false negative results are possible if the sample is not obtained from a representative area of the liver with high fat content. Clinicians should assume that the patient with elevated liver enzymes, metabolic syndrome, or type 2 diabetes also has probable NAFLD.

BOX 31-6. Drugs Associated With NAFLD

The following drugs can potentially damage hepatocytes and initiate the development of NAFLD:

- amiodarone
- antiviral drugs (nucleoside analogues)
- aspirin, (as part of Reye's syndrome in children)
- corticosteroids
- methotrexate
- tamoxifen
- tetracycline.

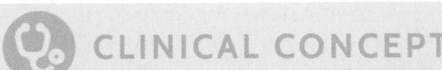

CLINICAL CONCEPT

There is an NAFLD fibrosis score consisting of age, hyperglycemia, body mass index (BMI), platelet count, albumin level, and ratio of AST to ALT. This assessment tool is available for NAFLD diagnosis and helps to avoid liver biopsies.

Treatment. Treatment is aimed at each component of metabolic syndrome. The patient should be advised about a diet and exercise plan with a goal of ideal BMI for the individual. Weight loss of 1 to 2 pounds per week is advisable. In more than 80% of cases, improvements in NASH have been shown with weight loss. Liver enzymes can decrease to normal levels with loss of as little as 4% to 5% of body weight. If a traditional low-calorie diet is unsuccessful, bariatric surgery is recommended for patients with morbid obesity.

Because insulin resistance is a common feature of NAFLD, insulin sensitizers are recommended. Biguanides such as metformin and glitazones such as pioglitazone have been found to lower liver enzymes, enhance cellular insulin sensitivity, and improve histological findings in NAFLD.

Lipid-lowering agents are recommended; however, close monitoring for liver toxicity is essential.

Alcoholic Liver Disease

Chronic and excessive ingestion of alcohol is a major cause of liver disease. Alcohol is the most commonly used drug in the United States, and 14 million adults meet the diagnostic criteria for alcohol abuse. Alcoholic hepatitis is an acute disorder that causes a distinct syndrome of reversible and transient symptoms; it can resolve if ingestion of alcohol ceases, but long-term effects often remain. Alcoholic liver disease, also known as alcoholic cirrhosis, is a pathological condition that develops over a long period of time and is permanent. It can be diagnosed by the presence of histopathological changes in the liver.

In the United States, alcoholic liver disease affects more than 2 million people, or approximately 1% of the population. This, however, is believed to be a low estimate because individuals commonly will not admit to heavy alcohol use. Alcohol is directly hepatotoxic; between 10% and 20% of alcohol abusers develop alcoholic hepatitis. There is no known genetic predisposition, but alcohol abuse tends to run in families. Alcoholism and alcoholic liver disease are more common in minority groups, particularly among Native Americans, than other nationalities. In alcoholic cirrhosis of the liver, there is severe functional impairment and the prognosis is poor, with a mortality rate of nearly 60% at 4 years after diagnosis.

Etiology. The time it takes to develop alcoholic liver disease is dependent on the amount of alcohol consumed.

Alcohol contained in one beer or 4 ounces of wine contains approximately 12 grams of alcohol. Alcoholic liver disease usually develops in men who ingest greater than 60 to 80 grams of alcohol per day for 10 years, whereas for women this amount is 20 to 40 grams per day for 10 years. Ingestion of 160 grams per day is associated with a 25-fold increased risk of developing alcoholic liver disease.

Pathophysiology. Alcohol is a potent toxin to hepatocytes. Hepatocytes can sustain injury and regenerate but have a low tolerance for repeated damage. Repeated bouts of alcoholic hepatitis will lead to alcoholic liver disease. Steatosis is the initial cellular change that takes place with excessive, chronic alcohol abuse. Fatty liver develops in every individual who consumes more than 60 g/day of alcohol. Chronic ingestion of ethanol inhibits the oxidation of fatty acids in the liver. Fat accumulates in and around hepatocytes as constant alcohol use occurs, and this fat accumulation within the hepatocyte disrupts the integrity of the organelles. Nuclear disruption causes death of the hepatocytes. Disrupting the mitochondria leads to free radical release and inflammation.

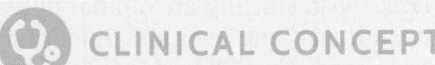

CLINICAL CONCEPT

A distinctive histological sign of alcoholic hepatitis found on biopsy is the Mallory body—a filamentous structure composed of keratin within a swollen hepatocyte. After fatty liver develops, large areas of hepatocyte injury, necrosis, inflammation, and fibrosis occur. When the liver demonstrates fibrosis and scar tissue, the disorder is referred to as cirrhosis.

About 50% of alcoholic hepatitis patients will progress to alcoholic liver disease and cirrhosis with poor prognosis for recovery. If alcohol use ceases, alcoholic hepatitis can resolve slowly over weeks to months, sometimes without permanent sequelae but often with residual cirrhosis.

Clinical Presentation. The diagnosis of alcoholic liver disease requires an accurate history of alcohol amount and duration. The condition is frequently discovered by a primary care provider in a routine examination of a patient for an unrelated matter. It is common for the patient not to admit to an excessive amount of alcohol use. Sensitive inquiry is required by the provider. Alcohol use assessment tools exist that ask standard, validated questions of the patient. Both the health-care provider and patient can review these questions together to assess alcohol use. Clues to the presence of alcoholism include a history of multiple motor vehicle accidents, convictions for driving while intoxicated, and poor interpersonal relationships. Alcoholism exhibits a genetic predisposition, and a history of alcoholism in a close relative may also indicate that a patient is at risk.

Signs and Symptoms. Patients with acute alcoholic hepatitis typically present with mild, nonspecific symptoms of RUQ pain, nausea, malaise, and low-grade fever. Jaundice and darkened urine may be present because of liver dysfunction and bilirubin accumulation in the bloodstream. The liver is usually enlarged, often with mild hepatic tenderness. The short-term prognosis is good, and no specific treatment is required.

In contrast, individuals with severe alcoholic hepatitis are at high risk of death. The patient may present with signs of severe liver dysfunction, such as hepatic encephalopathy—confusion, disorientation, or stupor. There may be coagulation dysfunction, which causes spontaneous bruising and bleeding. Hyperbilirubinemia may be present and cause jaundice. The patient may exhibit gastrointestinal bleeding via hematemesis.

Liver disease caused by chronic alcohol abuse is more common than acute alcoholic hepatitis. Patients exhibit signs of liver impairment, such as hepatomegaly and splenomegaly, and signs of portal hypertension, such as esophageal varices and ascites. Esophageal varices are apparent on endoscopy. Ascites is demonstrated by bulging flanks with shifting abdominal dullness with the patient in the supine position. Spider angiomata, proximal muscle wasting, altered hair distribution, and gynecomastia may also be observed.

A person who uses alcohol heavily may come to medical attention because of another medical illness that requires abstention of alcohol as part of recovery. The patient may not admit to alcohol abuse or recognize the abuse. Frequently during this time, alcohol abusers develop withdrawal symptoms of restlessness, mood disturbance, tremors called delirium tremens, and, possibly, seizures.

Diagnosis. Patients with alcoholic liver disease are often identified through abnormal diagnostic study results. Modest elevation of liver enzymes accompanied by hypertriglyceridemia, hypercholesterolemia, and, at times, hyperbilirubinemia are present. In alcoholic cirrhosis specifically, AST and ALT liver enzymes are elevated from 2- to 7-fold. Hypoalbuminemia and coagulation disturbances indicate severe liver dysfunction. Ultrasound of the liver is useful to detect fatty infiltration of the liver. Liver biopsy can confirm alcoholic liver disease.

Treatment. Cessation of alcohol use and proper nutrition constitute the treatment for alcoholic hepatitis. Patients should be on a high-protein, low-fat, low-sodium diet. However, if hepatic encephalopathy is present, the diet should not be high in protein. Supplemental vitamins and minerals, including folate and thiamine, are recommended. Patients with coagulation dysfunction should receive vitamin K parenterally. Short-term use of glucocorticoids may be part of treatment.

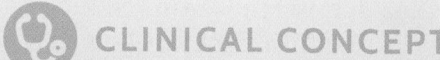

CLINICAL CONCEPT

Cirrhosis of the liver and liver failure may be the outcome of alcoholic liver disease. Patients with alcoholic hepatitis may have improvement of liver function if there is 6 months of abstinence from alcohol. If cirrhosis develops, they can be considered for liver transplantation if they remain committed to sustained abstinence.

Cirrhosis and Liver Failure

Cirrhosis and chronic liver failure are leading causes of morbidity and mortality in the United States, with the majority of cases attributed to excessive alcohol consumption and viral hepatitis. Cirrhosis often is a silent and gradual disease; most patients remain asymptomatic until a late stage of liver impairment marked by ascites, spontaneous bacterial peritonitis, hepatic encephalopathy, or variceal bleeding from portal hypertension. The liver becomes irreversibly damaged with collagen and connective tissue infiltration. Cirrhosis, the final stage of liver injury, can be caused by many different etiologies (see Box 31-7).

Cirrhosis of the liver is the third most common cause of death in people ages 45 to 65 years, after heart disease and cancer. Established cirrhosis has a 10-year mortality of 34% to 66%, largely dependent on the cause of the cirrhosis; alcoholic cirrhosis has a worse prognosis. There is a higher incidence of cirrhosis in men than in women.

Etiology. The most common causes of cirrhosis of the liver are HCV, alcoholic liver disease, and NAFLD. HCV often causes chronic inflammation, which leads to cirrhosis or liver cancer.

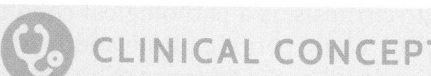

CLINICAL CONCEPT

HCV is the major cause of cirrhosis of the liver in the United States. Alcohol abuse, the major cause of cirrhosis in years past, is second to HCV.

BOX 31-7. Most Common Causes of Cirrhosis in the United States

- alcoholic liver disease
- chronic HBV
- chronic HCV
- NALFD
- NASH.

Source: National Institutes of Health. National Institute of Diabetes and Digestive and Kidney Diseases (NIDDK), Retrieved from http://digestive.niddk.nih.gov/ddiseases/pubs/cirrhosis/ on July 8, 2015.)

Alcohol is a direct hepatotoxin and its effect on the liver is dose dependent. NAFLD is a disease with unclear etiology that involves excessive fat accumulation in the liver. Persons with NAFLD have one or more of the following risk factors: obesity, diabetes, or hypertriglyceridemia. The incidence of NAFLD is increasing, with up to one-third of Americans affected. About 2% to 3% of Americans have NASH, and it is estimated that 10% of patients with NASH will ultimately develop cirrhosis. NAFLD and NASH are anticipated to have a major impact on the U.S. public health over the next decade.

Pathophysiology. In cirrhosis, the liver undergoes structural changes and fails to function. Stellate cells, which usually produce the extracellular matrix of the liver, become activated by cell injury. The cells produce an abundant amount of collagenous fibrous tissue, which interferes with hepatocyte function. Stellate cells also exert a constrictive effect on the liver's portal venous system. Collagen infiltration increases liver density and changes the liver's structural architecture. On autopsy, the liver is severely scarred and distorted in shape (see Fig. 31-13). The progression of liver injury to cirrhosis usually occurs over years. Portal hypertension, an elevated pressure within the portal vein, is a key pathophysiologic change associated with cirrhosis.

Portal Hypertension. A significant pathophysiologic occurrence in cirrhosis is the increased resistance within the portal vein termed **portal hypertension.** The portal vein drains the venous circulation of the GI system. The intestine, spleen, pancreas, stomach, and esophagus have venous networks that drain into the portal vein, which empties into the inferior vena cava. As cirrhosis develops, large veins develop collateral branches that initially decrease pressure within the portal vein. However, as cirrhosis worsens, pressure within the portal vein increases, causing backup of pressure to the GI veins and collaterals. Dilated, superficial veins become visible around the umbilicus, a sign referred to as **caput medusa.** Increased venous pressure builds

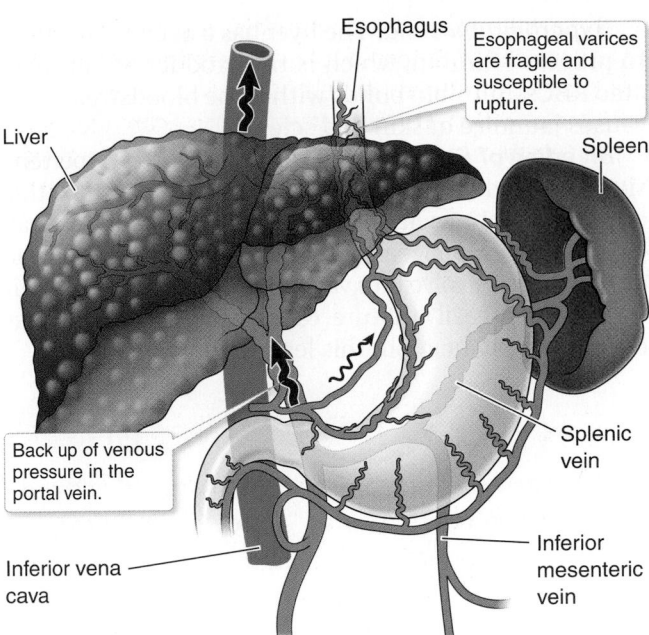

FIGURE 31-14. Portal hypertension. High blood pressure within the portal vein is referred to as portal hypertension. This heightened venous pressure causes backup of pressure within all the veins of the gastrointestinal system. The veins at the lower end of the esophagus become distended and are referred to as esophageal varices. The vein walls become fragile and tend to rupture, causing bleeding in the form of hematemesis.

within the vascular beds of the GI system, producing splenomegaly, esophageal varices, rectal varices, and eventually ascites. The esophageal veins and rectal veins are fragile submucosal veins that are prone to rupture; ruptured esophageal veins can cause vomiting of blood (hematemesis), whereas ruptured rectal veins can cause rectal bleeding (see Fig. 31-14).

Decreased Detoxification Capability. Patients on medications may experience the toxic effects of drugs caused by lack of liver metabolism in cirrhosis. Nitrogenous wastes accumulate in the blood, causing high NH_3 levels; this increases susceptibility to encephalopathy. Lethargy, confusion, and inability to concentrate are initial signs of encephalopathy. Stupor and coma are late signs.

Decreased Bile Synthesis. Diminished synthesis of bile by the cirrhotic liver will cause problems with fat digestion. Undigested fat in the digestive system leads to steatorrhea. Excretion of undigested fat eventually causes decreased fat-soluble vitamins A, D, E, and K.

Decreased Albumin Synthesis. Decreased synthesis of albumin by the liver causes nutritional deficiency and decreased colloid oncotic pressure. According to Starling's Law of Capillary Forces, decreased colloid oncotic pressure will allow hydrostatic pressure to go unbalanced. Hydrostatic pressure causes edema, which is most apparent in the peritoneal cavity as ascites. Edema can occur in the pulmonary system, causing impaired pulmonary function. Pleural effusions and the diaphragmatic elevation caused by massive ascites may alter the ventilation-perfusion ratio.

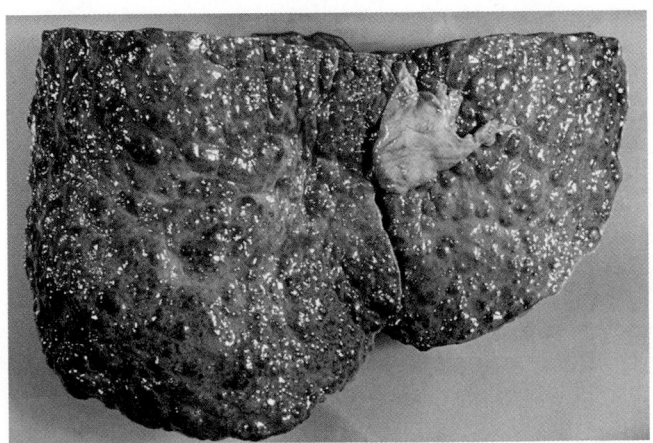

FIGURE 31-13. Cirrhosis of the liver. *(From Biophoto Associates/Science Source.)*

Hyperbilirubinemia. The liver has a decreased ability to process bilirubin, which is the product of degenerated RBCs. Bilirubin builds within the bloodstream and causes jaundice of skin and sclera.

Bleeding of Esophageal Varices. In portal hypertension, venous drainage backs up within the GI system; this causes congestion within the spleen, as well as intestinal, gastric, and esophageal veins. Esophageal veins become distended and evolve into varicose veins. Because of their fragility, they easily rupture, causing bleeding at the gastroesophageal junction; this leads to hematemesis.

 CLINICAL CONCEPT

In hematemesis, blood mixed with gastric fluids and acid is often referred to as "coffee ground emesis" because of its appearance.

Coagulopathy. Lack of synthesis of coagulation factors occurs as cirrhosis develops. In addition, patients may have thrombocytopenia from hypersplenism caused by portal hypertension. A prolonged PT is a lab test that indicates clotting deficiency. The patient can exhibit spontaneous bruising, nosebleeds, and hematemesis. Bleeding of the dilated varices in the esophagus and rectum often occurs.

 CLINICAL CONCEPT

Patients with cirrhosis may have spontaneous bleeding or bruising caused by low coagulation factors.

Osteoporosis. Osteoporosis is common in patients with liver disease caused by malabsorption of vitamin D and decreased calcium ingestion. The rate of bone resorption exceeds bone formation in cirrhosis.

 CLINICAL CONCEPT

Low vitamin D causes lack of calcium absorption from the GI tract, leading to bone demineralization.

Hepatic Encephalopathy. The development of encephalopathy in patients with cirrhosis is associated with a grave prognosis. Encephalopathy is an alteration of mental status and cognitive function in the presence of liver failure. Patients can exhibit confusion, personality change, or stupor. Gastrointestinal toxins and nitrogenous wastes, such as NH_3 that are not removed by the liver, affect the brain. Patients exhibit symptoms from confusion and disorientation to stupor and coma. **Asterixis,** which is a flapping tremor of the hands, may be present with hepatic encephalopathy. Cerebral edema can occur in severe encephalopathy; in addition, brain herniation is a serious complication.

 CLINICAL CONCEPT

Asterixis is elicited by having the patients extend their arms and bend the wrists backward. In this maneuver, patients with hepatic encephalopathy have a sudden forward movement of the wrist, known as a "liver flap."

Spontaneous Bacterial Peritonitis. Spontaneous bacterial peritonitis may develop in patients with alcoholic hepatitis and ascites, especially in those with concomitant gastrointestinal bleeding. Bacterial translocation is the presumed mechanism with GI bacterial flora traversing from the intestine into the mesenteric lymph nodes, ascitic fluid, and bloodstream. The most common organisms are *E. coli*, *Streptococcus viridans*, *Staphylococcus aureus*, and *Enterococcus*.

Iron Overload. As many as 50% of patients with alcoholic liver disease have increased hepatic iron content. This excess deposition of iron may play a significant role in the progression of alcoholic liver damage. Occasionally, this excessive iron deposition leads to hemochromatosis.

Anemia and Thrombocytopenia. Anemia may result from folate deficiency, hemolysis, or hypersplenism. Thrombocytopenia usually is secondary to hypersplenism and decreased levels of thrombopoietin.

 CLINICAL CONCEPT

Thiamine and folic acid deficiency are common in alcoholic cirrhosis of the liver.

Hepatorenal Syndrome. Hepatorenal syndrome (HRS) is a type of renal failure that occurs in approximately 10% of patients with cirrhosis. For unclear reasons, the kidney vessels undergo vasoconstriction; progressive impaired renal function then occurs. HRS is often seen in patients with a large amount of ascites.

Clinical Presentation. Some patients with cirrhosis are completely asymptomatic and have a normal life expectancy. Other individuals have a multitude of the most severe symptoms of end-stage liver disease and have a poor prognosis (see Fig. 31-15). Common signs and symptoms of cirrhosis are caused by decreased hepatic synthetic function, decreased detoxification capabilities of the liver, or portal hypertension.

In the history, the patient should be asked about risk factors for HBV and HCV, as these infections can lead to chronic hepatitis and cirrhosis. The patient should also be asked about possible exposures to hepatotoxic substances or chronic use of alcohol. Obesity, diabetes, and hypertriglyceridemia are often present in those with NAFLD. The patient may present with symptoms

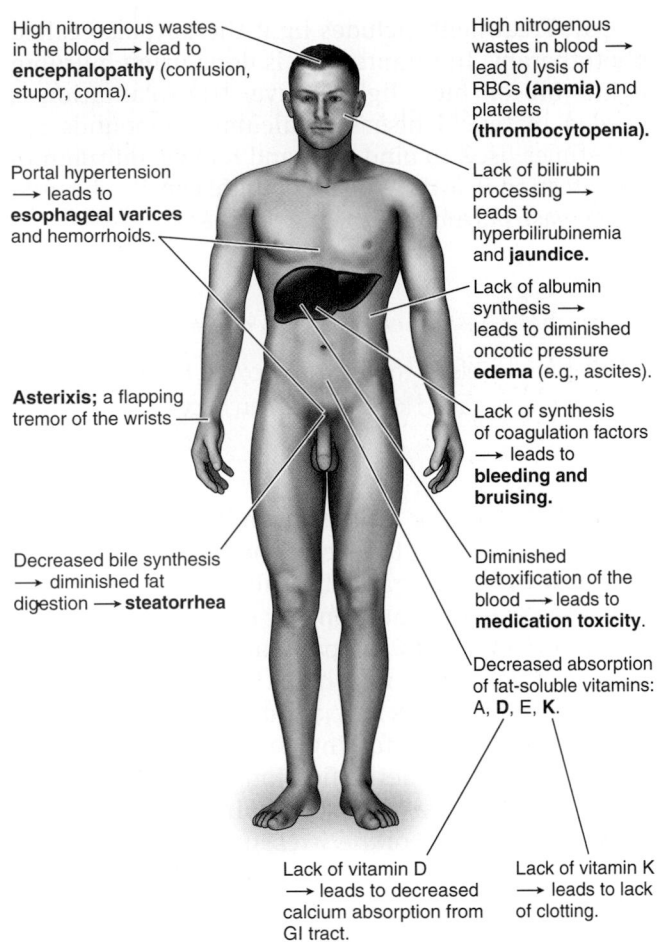

High nitrogenous wastes in the blood → lead to **encephalopathy** (confusion, stupor, coma).

High nitrogenous wastes in blood → lead to lysis of RBCs **(anemia)** and platelets **(thrombocytopenia).**

Portal hypertension → leads to **esophageal varices** and hemorrhoids.

Lack of bilirubin processing → leads to hyperbilirubinemia and **jaundice.**

Lack of albumin synthesis → leads to diminished oncotic pressure **edema** (e.g., ascites).

Asterixis; a flapping tremor of the wrists

Lack of synthesis of coagulation factors → leads to **bleeding and bruising.**

Decreased bile synthesis → diminished fat digestion → **steatorrhea**

Diminished detoxification of the blood → leads to **medication toxicity**.

Decreased absorption of fat-soluble vitamins: A, **D**, E, **K**.

Lack of vitamin D → leads to decreased calcium absorption from GI tract.

Lack of vitamin K → leads to lack of clotting.

FIGURE 31-15. The widespread effects of liver failure.

of severe liver dysfunction such as jaundice, steatorrhea, and darkened urine. Some patients may present with symptoms of portal hypertension, such as ascites and hematemesis caused by esophageal varices.

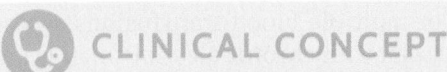

CLINICAL CONCEPT

Signs of portal vein hypertension include ascites, splenomegaly, esophageal varies, caput medusa and hemorrhoids.

Signs and Symptoms. Patients with cirrhosis usually complain of fatigue, anorexia, and weight loss. Dermatological manifestations of cirrhosis include jaundice, spider angiomata, skin telangiectasias, palmar erythema, and finger clubbing. Pruritus often develops because of accumulation of bile salts in the bloodstream, and muscle wasting and ascites are common because of protein loss. Males may develop gynecomastia and impotence. Loss of axillary and pubic hair is noted in both men and women. Signs of portal hypertension, such as ascites and caput medusa, are often present.

Diagnosis. Early in cirrhosis, laboratory tests can be normal. With progression, however, many different abnormalities become apparent. Platelet count is often reduced early in disease, which is caused by hyper-

splenism of portal hypertension. Serum bilirubin can be elevated with jaundice exhibited by the patient. PT is often prolonged, and liver enzymes are elevated. Patients may be anemic if there is gastrointestinal blood loss from esophageal varices or bone marrow suppression of RBC synthesis by alcohol. Liver biopsy shows the characteristic histopathological changes of cirrhosis.

Treatment. Abstinence of alcohol is the cornerstone of therapy in patients who have cirrhosis caused by excessive alcohol ingestion. Good nutrition and management of complications of cirrhosis is necessary. Glucocorticoids or other anti-inflammatory drugs, such as anti-tumor necrosis factor agents, are used. Liver transplantation is offered to those patients who have abstained from alcohol for 6 months or more and show evidence of commitment to an alcohol-free lifestyle.

Biliary Cirrhosis

Biliary cirrhosis is a cholestatic disease where bile production is dysfunctional. It occurs more often in women than men, mainly in the fifth or sixth decade of life. It can be a primary disorder with unknown etiology or it can be secondary to another disorder. Prolonged obstruction of the intrahepatic or extrahepatic biliary system causes biliary cirrhosis.

Pathophysiology. Inflammation and fibrous destruction of the intrahepatic bile ductules are the tissue evidence of primary biliary cirrhosis (PBC). The exact etiology is unknown; however, an autoimmune mechanism is theorized because the condition is often associated with other autoimmune disorders. There are four developmental stages for PBC:

- **Stage I:** inflammation of the portal triads and destruction of small and medium bile ducts
- **Stage II:** inflammation progresses with a decrease in bile ducts
- **Stage III:** destruction of liver cells, fibrotic tissue taking over hepatic cells, and loss of intralobular bile ducts
- **Stage IV:** development of micronodular or macronodular cirrhosis.

In secondary biliary cirrhosis, there is chronic destruction of larger hepatic ducts from prolonged obstruction by postoperative adhesions or gallstones. Unrelieved blockage of the extrahepatic bile ducts will cause bile stasis with areas of necrosis. The portal bile ducts enlarge with infiltration of the surrounding tissue with WBCs. The fibrotic ducts then expand and rupture with bile exuding into the necrotic tissue, forming "lakes of bile." The liver tissue regenerates into a nodular cirrhosis with loss of metabolic and chemical function.

Clinical Presentation. In the early stages, most patients are asymptomatic; if biliary cirrhosis is found at this stage, it is usually during a routine screening, when the patient's alkaline phosphatase level returns elevated.

Patients commonly exhibit jaundice; steatorrhea; pruritus, especially of the palms; and elevated lipid levels that lead to xanthelasmas, which are cholesterol deposits around the eyes. Signs and symptoms of portal hypertension and ascites develop as the disease advances. Osteomalacia, with accelerated osteoporosis, occurs as the disease progresses because of decreased vitamin D absorption. Raynaud's phenomenon and esophageal motility disorder are common.

Diagnosis. An elevation of liver enzymes is identified in most patients with PBC, but significant elevations of immunoglobulin levels (mainly IgM) are usually the most prominent findings. Lipid levels and cholesterol levels may be increased, with an increased high-density lipoprotein fraction. An increased erythrocyte sedimentation rate is another finding. As the disease progresses to cirrhosis, an elevated bilirubin level, a prolonged PT, and a decreased albumin level can be found. The increased bilirubin level is an ominous sign of disease progression, and liver transplantation must be considered. The hallmark of this disease is the presence of anti-mitochondrial antibodies (AMAs) in the blood. AMAs can be found in 90% to 95% of patients with PBC.

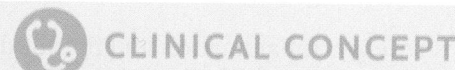

CLINICAL CONCEPT

AMAs are key findings in the diagnosis of PBC.

Treatment. Administration of the drug ursodiol, in doses of 13 to 15 mg/kg per day, reduces serum alkaline phosphatase and aminotransferase levels in PBC. The drug does not cure or prevent progression of advanced disease, but improves symptoms and histological features; this allows the patient to survive longer. Otherwise, the only cure is a liver transplant.

Crigler-Najjar Syndrome
Crigler-Najjar syndrome is a disease caused by deficiency of the enzyme glucuronyl transferase, which is used to conjugate bilirubin in the liver. Type I Crigler-Najjar syndrome is very rare; it is found in neonates who have a complete absence of the enzyme because of inherited gene mutations from both parents. Infants born with the syndrome rarely live beyond childhood, and the only treatment is a liver transplant. Type II Crigler-Najjar syndrome is more common; it is caused by a gene mutation inherited from a parent carrier. The patient has a reduced amount of glucuronyl transferase enzyme. Patients live into adulthood with elevated serum bilirubin levels. Kernicterus encephalopathy caused by excessive bilirubin in the blood can occur when the patient is under stress.

Diagnostic tests used to evaluate liver function include liver enzymes, conjugated bilirubin, total bilirubin, and unconjugated bilirubin in blood and liver

biopsy. Treatment includes light therapy, also called phototherapy. In infants, this is done using bilirubin lights (bili or 'blue' lights). Liver transplantation is needed in type I disease. Calcium compounds are sometimes used to bind with and remove bilirubin in the intestine. The drug phenobarbital can also be used to decrease bilirubin in the bloodstream.

CLINICAL CONCEPT

If bilirubin levels in the blood become too high, brain damage, also called kernicterus, can occur.

Gilbert's Syndrome. Gilbert's syndrome is caused by decreased activity of the enzyme glucuronyl transferase, which conjugates bilirubin in the liver. Because of a genetic mutation, the disease is present in approximately 5% of the population. This is a mild, chronic disorder in which patients have elevated serum bilirubin levels and jaundice during periods of stress, infection, or fasting. Individuals may have problems with liver detoxification of certain drugs. In Gilbert's syndrome, hyperbilirubinemia usually resolves with removal of the stressful event. Treatment is unnecessary.

Hemochromatosis. Hemochromatosis is a genetic disorder that is caused by an accumulation of iron in the liver from excessive absorption of iron from the intestine. Primary hemochromatosis is the most common genetic disorder in the United States, affecting an estimated 1 of every 200 to 300 Americans. Secondary hemochromatosis is a side effect of excessive RBC breakdown associated with thalassemia, sideroblastic anemia, or multiple blood transfusions. Occasionally, it may be seen with chronic alcoholism. It is more common in Caucasians than African Americans and affects more men than women. Symptoms are often seen in men between the ages of 30 and 50 years and in women older than age 50 years. The liver is the primary site of iron storage; with accumulation of iron, the organ enlarges. Diagnosis includes high serum ferritin, serum transferrin, and free iron levels. Patients often demonstrate fatigue, hepatomegaly, skin hyperpigmentation, arthritis, and erectile dysfunction. Treatment involves chelation with deferoxamine. If left untreated, cirrhosis can develop.

Wilson Disease. Wilson disease is a rare, inherited metabolic disorder characterized by excessive copper deposits in the liver, brain, and eye. Excessive copper in the liver leads to fibrosis and destruction of the hepatocytes. The patient may develop hepatitis, fatty deposits in the liver, and encephalopathy. The patient demonstrates symptoms of hepatic dysfunction: jaundice, ascites, and prominent abdominal veins, spider nevi, palmar erythema, and hematemesis.

Commonly, there is difficulty speaking, tremor, arthritis, excessive salivation, clubbing, ataxia, mask-like facies, clumsiness, and personality changes. Diagnosis is made by identification of copper rings in the cornea called Kayser-Fleischer rings, low levels of a serum copper transport protein (ceruloplasmin), and increased levels of hepatic and urinary copper. Treatment involves chelation with penicillamine. If left untreated, Wilson disease leads to cirrhosis and liver failure.

Chapter Summary

- The liver is a multifunctional organ that synthesizes albumin and coagulation factors, detoxifies the blood, and enables fat digestion. It also stores glucose, vitamins, and minerals.

- The liver conjugates bilirubin to make it water-soluble. Conjugated bilirubin is also called direct bilirubin. Unconjugated bilirubin is also called indirect bilirubin.

- The breakdown of RBCs, hepatocellular dysfunction, and obstructed bile release can lead to bilirubin in the bloodstream. These conditions are referred to as prehepatic, intrahepatic, and posthepatic jaundice.

- Hyperbilirubinemia leads to jaundice, a yellowing of skin and sclera.

- The most common causes of liver dysfunction are HCV virus, alcohol abuse, and NAFLD.

- The hepatitis viruses include hepatitis A, B, C, D, and E.

- HAV causes the mildest disease, is spread solely by the fecal-oral route, is self-limiting, and leads to no complications.

- There are vaccines available to prevent HAV and HBV. Presently there is treatment for HCV but no vaccine.

- HBV and HCV cause hepatocellular dysfunction, lead to chronic infection, and are spread by blood and body fluids.

- HBV and HCV are often present with human immunodeficiency virus and both can lead to HCC.

- HDV is spread mainly by blood containing HBV, and HEV–similar to HAV–is spread by the fecal-oral route.

- To diagnose hepatitis, a hepatitis laboratory test can reveal hepatitis viral antigen and antibody levels.

- Alcohol abuse is second to HCV as the main cause of cirrhosis of the liver.

- Before cirrhosis, the liver undergoes the process of steatosis, the accumulation of fat.

- The changes of cirrhosis of the liver include hepatocyte necrosis, connective tissue infiltration, fibrosis, and buildup of scar tissue throughout a shrunken liver.

- NAFLD is associated with metabolic syndrome, hyperlipidemia, obesity, and insulin resistance.

- NAFLD, the most common form of liver disease in the United States, can lead to a more severe form of the disease called NASH; this, in turn, can cause cirrhosis and hepatocarcinoma.

- In cirrhosis, the patient exhibits characteristic signs and symptoms, such as jaundice, poor fat digestion, diminished coagulation factor synthesis, and inefficient detoxification of the blood.

- Portal hypertension is a complication of cirrhosis that can lead to life-threatening side effects.

- Esophageal varices caused by portal hypertension result in hematemesis.

- There are very few treatments for liver disease, and liver transplantation is often the only alternative.

Making the Connections

Disorder and Pathophysiology	Signs and Symptoms	Physical Assessment Findings	Diagnostic Testing	Treatment
HAV | HAV is usually caused by ingestion of contaminated food or water or contracted from person to person by unsanitary conditions. HAV is absorbed by the intestine and travels to the liver, where it damages the hepatocytes.				
	Fatigue, nausea, vomiting, anorexia, malaise, abdominal pain, fever, myalgias, headache, jaundice, dark urine, light-colored stools.	RUQ tenderness, hepatomegaly, jaundice.	Fecal HAV is demonstrated in the first 4 weeks. Blood shows IgM anti-HAV antibodies during the first 4 weeks, IgG anti-HAV antibodies at 8 to 12 weeks, elevated liver enzymes in first 4 weeks, and elevated serum bilirubin, WBC, and prolonged PT for 4 weeks. No chronic disease is present.	Supportive, including rest. Nutrition includes small high-caloric meals, no alcohol. Patient should have no acetaminophen. Patient should be on enteric precautions. HAV Ig can be administered to contacts for temporary immunity. For long-term immunity, administration of HAV vaccine is necessary.
HBV | HBV is a stable virus spread by blood products, body fluids, or sexual contact. Once in the bloodstream, the virus produces viral proteins in the hepatocyte. The virus does not directly kill the cell, but the host's own immune system attacks hepatocytes when the viral antigens are encountered on the surface.				
	Fatigue, vomiting, anorexia, malaise, abdominal pain, fever, myalgias, headache, jaundice, dark urine, light-colored stools.	RUQ tenderness, hepatomegaly, jaundice. More severe signs include splenomegaly, lymphadenopathy, spider angioma, palmar erythema, and encephalopathy.	Blood shows positive HBsAg, HB DNA, HBeAg, HBcAg, and anti-HBc IgM antibodies. Blood shows anti-HBc IgG antibodies in chronic infection. Elevated liver enzymes, serum bilirubin, WBC, and prolonged PT are present. A HBV carrier state is possible and chronic long-term disease can lead to HCC.	Supportive, including rest. Nutrition includes small high-caloric meals, with no alcohol or acetaminophen. Patient needs to be on blood and body fluid precautions. For temporary immunity for contacts, HBIg can be administered. For long-term immunity, HBV vaccine should be administered.
HCV | HCV is an RNA virus that can replicate rapidly and can produce at least 10 trillion new viral particles each day. There are six different genotypes of HCV caused by mutation capability, and each has different severity and response to therapy. Symptoms can take 2 weeks to 8 months to appear and can lead to chronic infection and hepatocellular cancer.				
	Fatigue, vomiting, anorexia, malaise, abdominal pain, fever, myalgias, headache, jaundice, dark urine, light-colored stools.	RUQ tenderness, hepatomegaly, jaundice. More severe signs include splenomegaly, lymphadenopathy, spider angioma, palmar erythema, and encephalopathy.	HCV can live dormant in the body for lengthy time frames before signs and symptoms develop. Blood shows positive HCV RNA assay, anti-HCV antibodies, elevated liver enzymes, high serum bilirubin, high WBC, and prolonged PT. Low thyroxine is present.	Supportive, including rest. Nutrition includes small high-caloric meals. No alcohol, no acetaminophen. Patient must be on strict blood and body fluid precautions. No vaccine is available.

Continued

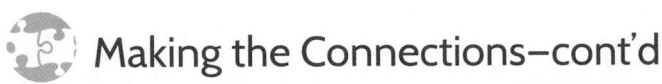

Making the Connections—cont'd

Disorder and Pathophysiology	Signs and Symptoms	Physical Assessment Findings	Diagnostic Testing	Treatment
Alcoholic Liver Disease | Alcohol is a potent toxin to hepatocytes. Repeated alcohol abuse leads to steatosis, which is the replacement of hepatocytes with fat. Chronic ingestion of ethanol inhibits the oxidation of fatty acids in the liver. Fat accumulates in and around hepatocytes and disrupts the integrity of the organelles. Nuclear disruption causes death of the hepatocytes. With time, large areas of hepatocyte injury, necrosis, inflammation, and fibrosis develop. When the liver demonstrates fibrosis and scar tissue, the disorder is referred to as cirrhosis.	Fatigue, vomiting, anorexia, malaise, abdominal pain, fever, myalgias, headache, jaundice, dark urine, light-colored stools. Hematemesis possible because of esophageal varices. Hepatic encephalopathy: confusion, lethargy, stupor.	RUQ tenderness, hepatomegaly, and jaundice. Signs of portal hypertension, which include ascites, caput medusa, esophageal varices, and rectal hemorrhoids. Proximal muscle wasting, altered hair distribution, asterixis, and gynecomastia. Hepatic encephalopathy signs. Delirium tremens. Seizure possible.	Blood shows elevated liver enzymes, high serum bilirubin, high WBC, prolonged PT, hypertriglyceridemia, hypercholesterolemia, and hypoalbuminemia. Ultrasound of liver. Liver biopsy.	Supportive, including rest. Nutrition includes small high-caloric meals with low protein. No alcohol, no acetaminophen. Folate, thiamine, vitamin K. If cessation of alcohol, consideration for liver transplant.
Cirrhosis and Liver Failure | Cirrhosis is the term for fibrotic changes of the liver. Hepatocytes are severely injured, dysfunctional, and are replaced by fibrotic tissue. Liver is scarred and shrunken.	Anorexia, nausea, weight loss, steatorrhea, dull abdominal pain, jaundice, dark urine. Signs of hepatic encephalopathy. Bleeding tendencies, pruritus, osteoporosis, musty odor to breath, ascites, signs of portal hypertension. HRS possible.	Enlarged, firm nodular liver on palpation. Jaundice, palmar erythema, spider angiomas, skin telangiectasia, clubbing of fingers, caput medusa, splenomegaly, testicular atrophy, gynecomastia in males, ascites. Hematemesis possible because of portal hypertension.	Elevated liver enzymes, high serum bilirubin, high WBC, prolonged PT, hypertriglyceridemia, hypercholesterolemia, hypoalbuminemia. Ultrasound of liver. Liver biopsy.	Remove underlying cause of cirrhosis or fibrosis. Good nutrition with vitamins. Rest, and avoidance of exposure to toxins/chemicals or infections. No alcohol or sedatives. Low protein diet for encephalopathy. Diuretics for edema. Paracentesis for ascites. Ligation of bleeding varices.
Biliary Cirrhosis | Inflammation of the liver with cholestasis. Bile secretion is disrupted and hepatocytes become necrotic. Etiology is autoimmune disease. Eventually fibrotic changes develop in the liver; cirrhosis is the end result.	Asymptomatic early in disease. Later signs include fatigue, anorexia, weight loss, pruritus, xanthelasma, steatorrhea, muscle wasting, ascites, spider angioma, and loss of axillary and pubic hair.	No signs early jaundice, ascites, osteoporosis. Xanthelasma, muscle wasting, ascites, spider angioma, loss of axillary and pubic hair. Advanced disease shows signs of	Elevated liver enzymes, elevated alkaline phosphatase, elevated lipids, high serum bilirubin, high immunoglobulins, high erythrocyte sedimentation rate, prolonged PT, decreased albumin. AMAs are present.	Ursodiol. Liver transplant.

Making the Connections–cont'd

Disorder and Pathophysiology	Signs and Symptoms	Physical Assessment Findings	Diagnostic Testing	Treatment
	Advanced disease shows signs of portal hypertension, jaundice, or ascites.	portal hypertension and jaundice.		

Crigler-Najjar Syndrome Type I and II | Genetic syndrome of a deficiency of the enzyme glucuronyl transferase, which is used to conjugate bilirubin in the liver. Bilirubin accumulates in the blood. Kernicterus (brain damage) caused by excessive bilirubin in the blood can occur when the patient is under stress.

Disorder and Pathophysiology	Signs and Symptoms	Physical Assessment Findings	Diagnostic Testing	Treatment
	Type I: severe hyperbilirubinemia and brain damage and death. Type II: no symptoms usually. Jaundice can occur when body is under stress.	Type I: usually fatal. Type II: jaundice.	Blood shows elevated liver enzymes, high unconjugated bilirubin, and high total bilirubin.	Calcium compounds can bind bilirubin and aid in excretion. Phototherapy aids in the breakdown and excretion of bilirubin. Phenobarbital can lower bilirubin levels. Liver transplant performed in severe disease.

Gilbert's Disease | Decreased amount of glucuronyl transferase is made by the liver.

Disorder and Pathophysiology	Signs and Symptoms	Physical Assessment Findings	Diagnostic Testing	Treatment
	Often asymptomatic. Abdominal cramps, anorexia, fatigue, and jaundice with severe stress on body.	Jaundice with severe stress on body.	High unconjugated bilirubin levels when body is under stress.	No treatment needed.

Hemochromatosis | Primary hemochromatosis is a genetic disorder that is caused by an accumulation of iron in the liver from excessive absorption of iron from the intestine. Secondary hemochromatosis is caused by excessive RBC breakdown in hemolytic anemias and thalassemia.

Disorder and Pathophysiology	Signs and Symptoms	Physical Assessment Findings	Diagnostic Testing	Treatment
	May be asymptomatic or may exhibit fatigue, arthralgias, skin hyperpigmentation, or erectile dysfunction.	Hepatomegaly. Hyperpigmentation of skin (bronze). Arthritis.	High iron levels in body. High serum ferritin and transferrin. Genetic testing.	Periodic phlebotomy. Chelation with deferoxamine.

Wilson Disease | Autosomal recessive genetic disorder of copper metabolism that causes excessive deposition of copper in the liver, brain, and other tissues.

Disorder and Pathophysiology	Signs and Symptoms	Physical Assessment Findings	Diagnostic Testing	Treatment
	Signs of hepatic dysfunction: jaundice, ascites and prominent abdominal veins, spider nevi, palmar erythema, digital clubbing, hematemesis. Difficulty speaking, tremor, arthritis, excessive salivation, ataxia, masklike facies, clumsiness, personality changes.	Jaundice, ascites, prominent abdominal veins, clubbing, erythema of palms, Kayser-Fleischer rings of the cornea; green-gold in color. Difficulty speaking, tremor, arthritis, excessive salivation, ataxia, masklike facies, clumsiness, personality changes.	Low ceruloplasmin levels, high levels of urinary copper, liver biopsy shows high copper. CT and MRI of the brain.	Lifelong use of chelation agents such as penicillamine. Liver transplant.

Bibliography

Afdhal, N. H. (2012). Management of nonalcoholic fatty liver disease: a 60-year-old man with probable nonalcoholic fatty liver disease: weight reduction, liver biopsy, or both? *JAMA, 308*(6), 608–616.

Arora, S., Thornton, K., Murata, G., et al. (2011). Outcomes of treatment for hepatitis C virus infection by primary care providers. *N Engl J Med, 364*(23), 2199–2207.

Bernal, W., Auzinger, G., Dhawan, A., & Wendon, J. (2010). Acute liver failure. *Lancet, 376*(9736), 190–201.

Bossenbroek Fedoriw, K., & Rickett, K. (2013). FPIN's clinical inquiries. Screening for hepatocellular carcinoma in patients with hepatitis C virus infection. *Am Fam Phys,* 87(6), Online.

Carey, W. D. (2009). The prevalence and natural history of hepatitis B in the 21st century. *Cleveland Clin J Med,* 76 Suppl 3, S2–5.

Chung, R. T., & Baumert, T. F. (2014). Curing chronic hepatitis C—the arc of a medical triumph. *N Engl J Med, 370*(17), 1576–1578. doi: 10.1056/NEJMp1400986. Epub 2014 Apr 10.

Elgouhari, H. M., Abu-Rajab Tamimi, T. I., & Carey, W. (2009). Hepatitis B: a strategy for evaluation and management. *Cleveland Clin J Med,* 76(1), 19–35.

El-Serag, H. B. (2011). Hepatocellular carcinoma. *N Engl J Med,* 365(12), 1118–1127.

Forner, A., Llovet, J. M., & Bruix, J. (2012). Hepatocellular carcinoma. *Lancet,* 379(9822), 1245–1255.

Fowler, C. (2013). Management of patients with complications of cirrhosis. *Nurse Pract,* 38(4), 14–21; quiz 22–23. doi: 10.1097/01.NPR.0000427610.76270.45.

García-Pagán, J. C., Caca, K., Bureau, C., et al. (2010). Early use of TIPS in patients with cirrhosis and variceal bleeding. *N Engl J Med,* 362(25), 2370–2379.

Garcia-Tsao, G., & Bosch, J. (2010). Management of varices and variceal hemorrhage in cirrhosis. *N Engl J Med,* 362(9), 823–832.

Ginès, P., & Schrier, R. W. (2009). Renal failure in cirrhosis. *N Engl J Med,* 361(13), 1279–1290.

Gish, R. G. (2009). Hepatitis B treatment: current best practices, avoiding resistance. *Cleveland Clin J Med,* 76 Suppl 3, 14–19.

Harnois, D. M. (2012). Hepatitis C virus infection and the rising incidence of hepatocellular carcinoma. *Mayo Clin Proceed,* 87(1), 7–8.

Hitzeman, N., & Shen, S. J. (2012). Weight loss for patients with nonalcoholic fatty liver disease. *Am Fam Phys,* 86(5), 415–416.

Holmberg, S. D., Spradling, P. R., Moorman, A. C., & Denniston, M. M. (2013). Hepatitis C in the United States. *N Engl J Med,* 368(20), 1859–1861. doi: 10.1056/NEJMp1302973.

Jensen, D. M. (2011). A new era of hepatitis C therapy begins. *N Engl J Med,* 364(13), 1272–1274.

Kelso, L. A. (2008). Cirrhosis: caring for patients with end-stage liver failure. *Nurse Pract,* 33(7), 24–30.

Kim, C. H., & Younossi, Z. M. (2008). Nonalcoholic fatty liver disease: a manifestation of the metabolic syndrome. *Cleveland Clin J Med,* 75(10), 721–728.

Kourtis, A. P., Bulterys, M., Hu, D. J., & Jamieson, D. J. (2012). HIV-HBV coinfection—a global challenge. *N Engl J Med,* 366(19), 1749–1752. doi: 10.1056/NEJMp1201796.

Lee, H., Park, W., Yang, J. H., & You, K. S. (2010). Management of hepatitis B virus infection. *Gastro Nurs,* 33(2), 120–126.

Leise, M. D., Poterucha, J. J., Kamath, P. S., & Kim, W. R. (2014). Management of hepatic encephalopathy in the hospital. *Mayo Clin Proceed,* 89(2), 241–253. doi: 10.1016/j.mayocp.2013.11.009. Epub 2014 Jan 8.

Liang, T. J., & Ghany, M. G. (2014, May 22). Therapy of hepatitis C—back to the future. *N Engl J Med,* 370(21), 2043–2047. doi: 10.1056/NEJMe1403619. Epub 2014 May 4.

Liaw, Y. F., & Chu, C. M. (2009). Hepatitis B virus infection. *Lancet,* 373(9663), 582–592.

Limketkai, B. N., Mehta, S. H., Sutcliffe, C. G., et al. (2012). Relationship of liver disease stage and antiviral therapy with liver-related events and death in adults coinfected with HIV/HCV. *JAMA,* 308(4), 370–378.

Linas, B. P., Hu, H., Barter, D. M., & Horberg, M. (2014). Hepatitis C screening trends in a large integrated health system. *Am J Med,* 127(5), 398–405. doi: 10.1016/j.amjmed.2014.01.012. Epub 2014 Jan 28.

Liu, S., Cipriano, L. E., Holodniy, M., Owens, D. K., & Goldhaber-Fiebert, J. D. (2012). New protease inhibitors for the treatment of chronic hepatitis C: a cost-effectiveness analysis. *Ann Int Med,* 156(4), 279–290.

Longo, D. L., Kasper, D. L., Jameson, J. L., et al. (2011). *Harrison's principles of internal medicine.* 18th ed. New York: McGraw-Hill.

Machado, M. V., & Diehl, A. M. (2014). Liver renewal: detecting misrepair and optimizing regeneration. *Mayo Clin Proceed,* 89(1), 120–130. doi: 10.1016/j.mayocp.2013.10.009.

Mascitelli, L., Goldstein, M. R., & Grant, W. B. (2012). Why vitamin D status should be checked in patients with nonalcoholic fatty liver disease. *Mayo Clin Proceed,* 87(8), 808.

Matheny, S. C., & Kingery, J. E. (2012). Hepatitis A. *Am Fam Phys,* 86(11), 1027–1034.

McMahon, B. J., Block, J., Haber, B., et al. (2012). Internist diagnosis and management of chronic hepatitis B virus infection. *Am J Med,* 125(11), 1063–1067. doi: 10.1016/j.amjmed.2012.03.010.

Mitka, M. (2014). USPSTF advises HBV screening for US groups at high risk of infection. *JAMA,* 311(10), 1004. doi: 10.1001/jama.2014.2121.

Morris, K. (2011). Tackling hepatitis C: a tale of two countries. *Lancet,* 377(9773), 1227–1228.

Ollendorf, D. A., Tice, J. A., & Pearson, S. D. (2014). The comparative clinical effectiveness and value of simeprevir and sofosbuvir for chronic hepatitis C virus infection. *JAMA Intern Med,* May 5. doi: 10.1001/jamainternmed.2014.2151. Epub ahead of print.

Page, J. (2012). Nonalcoholic fatty liver disease: the hepatic metabolic syndrome. *J Am Acad Nurse Pract,* 24(6), 45–51. doi: 10.1111/j.1745-7599.2012.00716.x. Epub 2012 Apr 20.

Poordad, F., Lawitz, E., Kowdley, K. V., et al. (2013). Exploratory study of oral combination antiviral therapy for hepatitis C. *N Engl J Med,* 368(1), 45–53. doi: 10.1056/NEJMoa1208809.

Pozza, R. (2008). Clinical management of HIV/hepatitis C virus coinfection. *J Am Acad Nurse Pract,* 20(10), 496–505.

Rhee, E. J., Lee, W. Y., Cho, Y. K., Kim, B. I., & Sung, K. C. (2011). Hyperinsulinemia and the development of nonalcoholic fatty liver disease in nondiabetic adults. *Am J Med,* 124(1), 69–76.

Rockey, D. (2011). Treatment of hepatitis C by primary care providers. *N Engl J Med,* 365(10), 959–960.

Rosen, H. R. (2011). Clinical practice. Chronic hepatitis C infection. *N Engl J Med,* 364(25), 2429–2438.

Schiff, E. R. (2011). Diagnosing and treating hepatitis C virus infection. *Am J Man Care*, 17 Suppl 4, S108–115.

Selmi, C., Bowlus, C. L., Gershwin, M. E., & Coppel, R. L. (2011). Primary biliary cirrhosis. *Lancet*, 377(9777), 1600–1609.

Smith, B. D., Morgan, R. L., Beckett, G. A., et al. (2012). Hepatitis C virus testing of persons born during 1945 to 1965: recommendations from the Centers for Disease Control and Prevention. *Ann Int Med*, doi: 10.7326/0003-4819-157-9-201211060-00529.

Starr, S. P., & Raines, D. (2011). Cirrhosis: diagnosis, management, and prevention. *Am Fam Phys*, 84(12), 1353–1359.

Torrazza-Perez, E., & Carreno, N. (2010). Images in clinical medicine. Bleeding esophageal varices. *N Engl J Med*, 362(5), e13.

Tripodi, A., & Mannucci, P. M. (2011). The coagulopathy of chronic liver disease. *N Engl J Med*, 365(2), 147–156.

Udell, J. A., Wang, C. S., Tinmouth, J., et al. (2012). Does this patient with liver disease have cirrhosis? *JAMA*, 307(8), 832–842.

Wakim-Fleming, J. (2011). Hepatic encephalopathy: suspect it early in patients with cirrhosis. *Cleveland Clin J Med*, 78(9), 597–605.

Wilkins, T., Malcolm, J. K., Raina, D., & Schade, R. R. (2010). Hepatitis C: diagnosis and treatment. *Am Fam Phys*, 81(11), 1351–1357.

Wilkins, T., Tadkod, A., Hepburn, I., & Schade, R. R. (2013). Non-alcoholic fatty liver disease: diagnosis and management. *Am Fam Phys*, 88(1), 35–42.

Wilkins, T., Zimmerman, D., & Schade, R. R. (2010). Hepatitis B: diagnosis and treatment. *Am Fam Phys*, 81(8), 965–972.

Yang, J. D., Kim, B., Sanderson, S. O., et al. (2012). Hepatocellular carcinoma in Olmsted County, Minnesota, 1976–2008. *Mayo Clin Proceed*, 87(1), 9–16.

Yki-Järvinen, H. (2014). Non-alcoholic fatty liver disease as a cause and a consequence of metabolic syndrome. *Lancet Diabetes Endocrinol*, Apr 7. pii: S2213-8587(14)70032-4. doi: 10.1016/S2213-8587(14)70032-4. Epub ahead of print.

Gallbladder, Pancreatic, and Bile Duct Dysfunction

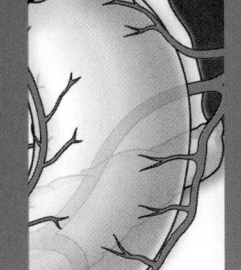

Key Terms

Acalculous cholecystitis
Ampulla of Vater
Biliary colic
Biliary sludge
Biliary stasis
Cholangitis

Cholecystectomy
Cholecystitis
Choledocholithiasis
Cholelithiasis
Cullen sign
Empyema

Grey Turner sign
Murphy's sign
Pancreatitis
Pseudocyst
Sphincter of Oddi

The gallbladder, pancreas, and biliary tract are key components of the gastrointestinal system. The liver manufactures bile, the major emulsifier of fats, and releases it into the hepatic duct, which leads to the common bile duct. The gallbladder stores bile until it is released into the cystic duct, which empties into the common bile duct. The pancreas has both endocrine and exocrine function. The endocrine portion of the pancreas produces insulin, glucagon, and somatostatin and releases them into the vascular system. The exocrine portion of the pancreas secretes the digestive enzymes lipase, amylase, trypsin, chymotrypsin, and bicarbonate and releases them into the pancreatic duct, eventually emptying into the common bile duct. The common bile duct is where the cystic, hepatic, and pancreatic ducts come together and is the major conduit that empties bile and digestive enzymes into the small intestine at the **ampulla of Vater.** The muscular valve at the ampulla of Vater is the **sphincter of Oddi** (Fig. 32-1).

Epidemiology

Gallbladder disease occurs frequently in the United States. **Cholelithiasis,** commonly known as gallstones, is the most frequent cause of gallbladder disease. **Cholecystitis,** which is inflammation of the gallbladder caused by cholelithiasis, is a very common cause of emergency medical care. The incidence of cholelithiasis is higher in women, at approximately 16%, than men, at approximately 8%. Mexican Americans have higher rates of gallstones than Caucasian Americans, but incidence is lower in African Americans.

Acute pancreatitis, chronic pancreatitis, and pancreatic cancer are the most common pancreatic disorders in the United States. Acute pancreatitis is a potentially lethal disease with an incidence of 4.5 to 79.8 per 100,000 persons/year worldwide. Approximately

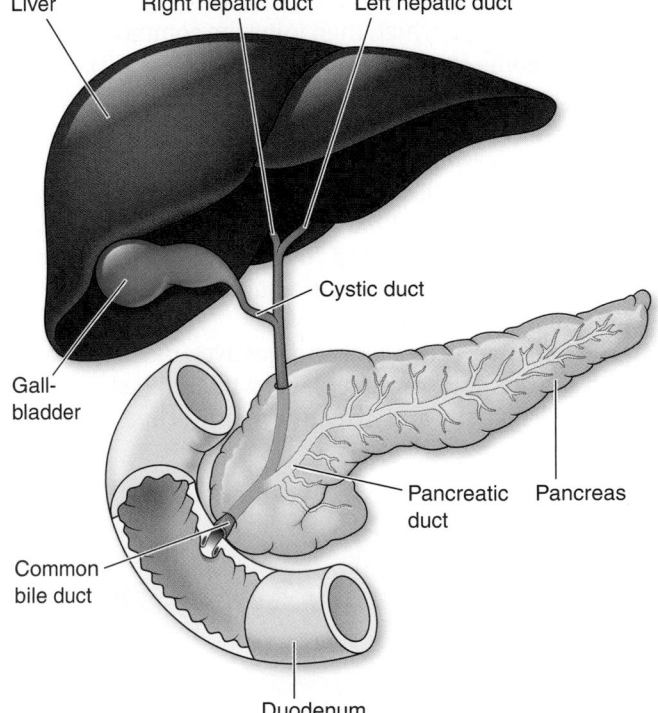

FIGURE 32-1. Anatomy of the gallbladder, pancreas, and biliary tract.

210,000 people are admitted to hospitals each year with acute pancreatitis in the United States. There is a 10% mortality rate associated with severe acute pancreatitis, with gallstones and alcohol abuse as the most common causes. Chronic pancreatitis occurs in 1.6 to 23 persons per 100,000/year worldwide, with alcoholism as the most common cause. Chronic pancreatitis in the United States results in more than 122,000 outpatient visits and more than 56,000 hospitalizations per year. Although the cause of pancreatic cancer is unclear, it is responsible for nearly 30,000 annual deaths and is the fourth most common cause of cancer death.

Basic Concepts of Gallbladder, Pancreas, and Biliary Function

Bile is manufactured by the liver and is composed of bile acids (80%), phospholipids (16%), and cholesterol (4%). It has two major functions: digestion and elimination. Bile emulsifies fats and facilitates absorption of fat-soluble vitamins, and it also carries waste products for elimination. One of the waste products contained in bile is bilirubin, which is processed by the liver and is a breakdown product of hemoglobin. Some bile is released into the hepatic duct, which travels into the common bile duct. Some bile is stored in the gallbladder.

The gallbladder is a hollow organ that sits just beneath the liver and is divided into three sections: fundus, body, and neck. The neck tapers and connects to the biliary tree via the cystic duct, which then joins the common hepatic duct to become the common bile duct (Fig. 32-2). When food containing fat enters the digestive tract, it stimulates the secretion of cholecystokinin (CCK) by the small intestine. In response to CCK, the gallbladder, which stores about 50 milliliters of bile, releases its contents into the duodenum. While in the gallbladder, bile can become highly concentrated, and cholesterol or bilirubin often precipitates out of solution and forms stones, also called calculi.

The pancreas produces the digestive enzymes lipase, which digests fats, and amylase, which digests carbohydrates. Trypsin and chymotrypsin, other enzymes

also manufactured by the pancreas, digest proteins. The pancreas also produces bicarbonate, which is a natural antacid. The pancreas is located behind the stomach and is surrounded by the duodenum, liver, and spleen. It is about 6 inches long and is shaped like a flat pear. The wide, medial portion, called the head of the pancreas, is located in the epigastric region behind the duodenum. The body and tail of the pancreas extends into the left hypogastric region. When food enters the stomach, pancreatic enzymes are triggered by the hormone secretin, which is produced by the intestine. The enzymes travel from the pancreatic duct into the common bile duct, which enters the small intestine at the ampulla of Vater. In the small intestine, pancreatic enzymes along with bile break down fats, proteins, and carbohydrates.

Basic Pathophysiologic Concepts of Gallbladder, Pancreas, and Biliary Dysfunction

Gallbladder, biliary tract, and pancreatic disorders may occur as primary or secondary disorders. Anatomical position and the function of both the gallbladder and pancreas create a situation where one organ's function influences another's function. Patients experiencing gallbladder or pancreatic dysfunction generally present with multiple metabolic disturbances. Nutritional disturbances and pain ranging from mild to severe are common. Disorders of the gallbladder, biliary tract, and pancreas have overlapping symptoms requiring careful assessment and management.

Gallbladder Dysfunction

Gallbladder motility disturbances and stasis of bile are the most common causes of obstruction, inflammation, and infection of the gallbladder. Motility disturbances causing stasis of bile generally precede gallstone formation. Three terms used in the discussion of gallbladder disease are cholelithiasis, cholecystitis, and **choledocholithiasis,** which is defined as stones in the common bile duct that can lead to backup of bile into the gallbladder and liver.

Figure 32-3 shows the differences between cholelithiasis, cholecystitis, and choledocholithiasis.

Biliary sludge is the precursor to gallstones. It is a combination of calcium bilirubinate, cholesterol crystals, and mucin. Motility disturbances contribute to the formation of biliary sludge. **Biliary stasis,** or delayed emptying of the gallbladder, leads to stone formation. Biliary sludge, biliary stasis, or gallstones can form if the gallbladder does not empty completely. When gallstones enter the cystic duct, **cholangitis,** which is obstruction and ductal inflammation, occurs. Gallstones can also enter and obstruct flow in the common bile duct or can move into the pancreas and cause pancreatitis, a potentially fatal inflammatory disorder.

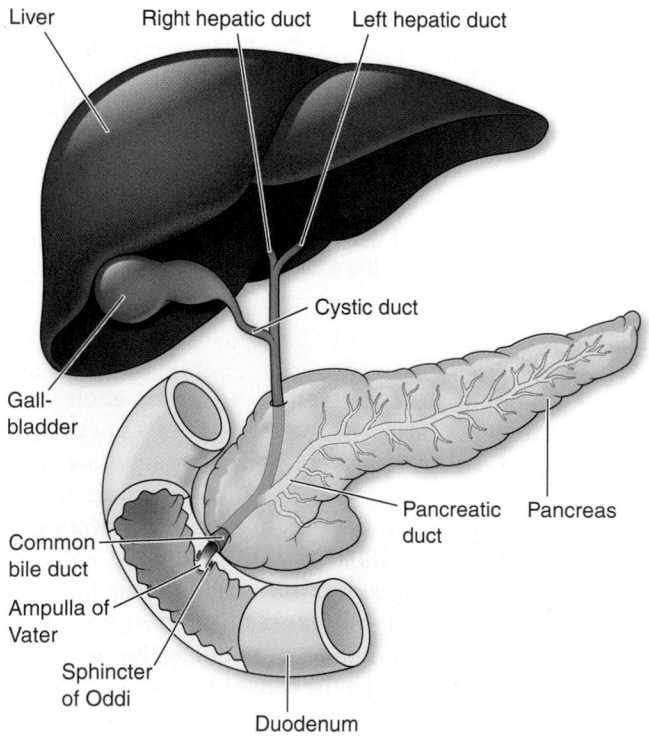

Liver   Right hepatic duct   Left hepatic duct

Cystic duct

Gall-
bladder

Common
bile duct

Ampulla of
Vater

Sphincter
of Oddi

Pancreatic
duct   Pancreas

Duodenum

FIGURE 32-2. The common bile duct, ampulla of Vater, and sphincter of Oddi.

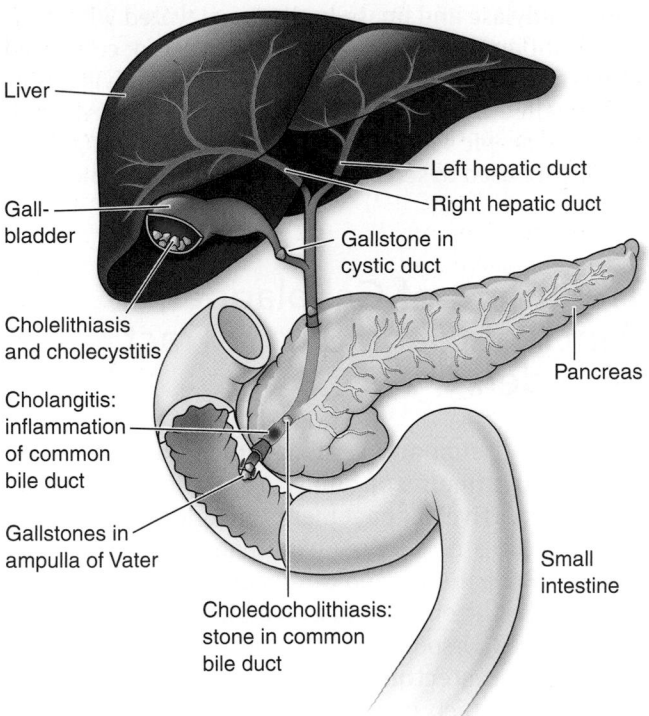

Liver

Gall-
bladder

Left hepatic duct

Right hepatic duct

Gallstone in
cystic duct

Cholelithiasis
and cholecystitis

Cholangitis:
inflammation
of common
bile duct

Pancreas

Gallstones in
ampulla of Vater

Small
intestine

Choledocholithiasis:
stone in common
bile duct

FIGURE 32-3. Location of common bile duct disorders.

Obstruction of the common bile duct hinders free flow of bile from the liver and can cause backup of bile constituents into the liver, leading to hepatic dysfunction. In common bile duct obstruction, hepatic conjugation of bilirubin is impeded, which in turn causes a backup of bilirubin and bile salts into the bloodstream. There are three types of gallstones:

1. **Cholesterol stones:** These are the most common stones formed in the gallbladder because of supersaturated cholesterol in bile. Eighty percent of all gallstones are made of cholesterol, whereas 20% are made of pigment stones.
2. **Black pigment stones:** These are small, hard gallstones composed of calcium bilirubinate and inorganic calcium salts. The formation of black pigment stones is related to alcoholic liver disease, chronic hemolysis, and aging.
3. **Brown pigment stones:** These are composed of calcium salts of unconjugated bilirubin, with small amounts of cholesterol and protein. They are often located in the bile ducts and cause obstruction and inflammation.

 CLINICAL CONCEPT

The most common causes of obstruction of the common bile duct are gallstones and tumor of the head of the pancreas. Obstruction of the common bile duct causes obstructive jaundice.

Biliary Colic

Biliary colic is a syndrome of pain associated with irritation of the gallbladder, commonly secondary to gallstones. The pain is steady, intense, and can last from 30 minutes to several hours. Nausea, vomiting, and right upper quadrant (RUQ) pain, right flank pain, or midchest pain can occur. The pain often radiates to the scapula and upper thoracic region. Additionally, although any type of food can precipitate the pain, fatty foods, in particular, incite pain.

Biliary colic is often associated with dilation of the biliary tract, elevation of plasma liver enzyme concentration, and elevation of serum bilirubin. Biliary colic is most frequently caused by obstruction of the common bile duct or the cystic duct by a gallstone. However, biliary colic can occur in the absence of gallstones or an identifiable cause. Acalculous biliary colic, which is pain without stones, can occur and be a consequence of dysfunction of the biliary tree and the sphincter of Oddi. Individuals can endure multiple bouts of biliary colic before severe pain and vomiting prompts them to seek health care.

Pancreatic Exocrine Dysfunction

The pancreas is both an endocrine and exocrine gland. As an endocrine gland, the pancreas secretes the hormones insulin, glucagon, and somatostatin. As an exocrine gland, the pancreas is a major gastrointestinal secretory organ that manufactures and releases key digestive enzymes that break down proteins, carbohydrates, and fats. Pancreatic exocrine dysfunction occurs when the pancreas does not secrete sufficient digestive enzymes. Without digestive enzymes, food is not broken down and malabsorption results. Malabsorption leads to deficiencies of essential nutrients and lack of fat absorption. Severe pancreatic insufficiency occurs in cystic fibrosis, chronic pancreatitis, and surgeries of the gastrointestinal system in which portions of the stomach or pancreas are removed. Certain gastrointestinal diseases, such as stomach ulcers, celiac disease, and Crohn's disease, as well as autoimmune disorders, such as systemic lupus erythematosus, may contribute to the development of pancreatic insufficiency.

Pancreatitis is inflammation of the pancreas that causes pancreatic insufficiency, malabsorption, and diabetes. Acute inflammation of the pancreas is usually a temporary condition and can be caused by gallstones, excessive alcohol consumption, high blood triglycerides, abdominal injury, and certain medications and toxins. The pancreas becomes vulnerable to its own digestive enzymes and undergoes autodigestion in inflammatory conditions. The pancreas can undergo chronic inflammation, a slow process that gradually destroys the gland and leaves it nonfunctional, fibrotic, and atrophied.

Assessment of Gallbladder, Pancreatic, and Biliary Tract Disorders

The clinical presentations of gallbladder, pancreatic, and biliary tract disorders are similar. Because of this, the patient's history is important, as it can assist the clinician in differentiating between them.

Risk Factors

Risk factors for gallbladder dysfunction are different than those for pancreatic and biliary tract disorders. Some of the major risk factors include age, female gender, estrogen level, low-calorie diets, fatty foods, and obesity. Pancreatic disorders affect men and women almost equally. Alcohol abuse and biliary tract disorders are the most common risk factors for pancreatic dysfunction.

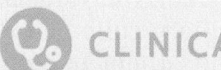 CLINICAL CONCEPT

Biliary tract disorders are most commonly caused by obstruction by a pancreatic tumor or gallstone.

Signs and Symptoms

Assessment of the patient for biliary disorders should include a complete history and physical examination. The clinician should focus on the location, timing, intensity, and quality of pain. Relieving and exacerbating factors should be noted. Nausea and vomiting often accompany biliary disorders. The patient may also report a feeling of fullness and abdominal distention may be present. The timing of nausea and vomiting in relation to the time of eating should be noted, as gallbladder disorders often present with pain after eating fatty foods. The clinician should also inspect the patient for jaundice of the skin and sclera and should monitor temperature and white blood cell (WBC) count as possible signs of infection. Abdominal assessment may reveal RUQ guarding and tenderness.

In pancreatic disorders, nausea, vomiting, and abdominal pain are common. Pain caused by pancreatic dysfunction often presents in the epigastric area, which may radiate to the back. Patients with biliary or pancreatic disorders may have changes in stool caused by fat malabsorption. Steatorrhea, or fat-containing stool, is soft and clay colored.

Diagnosis

There are specific laboratory tests and imaging studies designed to evaluate the gallbladder, pancreas, and biliary tract. Elevated WBC count, erythrocyte sedimentation rate (ESR), and C-reactive protein (CRP) are present in states of gallbladder or pancreatic inflammation. Liver function tests and bilirubin level may also be abnormal.

Serum amylase and lipase levels are elevated with pancreatic inflammation. Abdominal ultrasound; computed tomography (CT) scan; cholecystogram, which is sometimes called hydroxy iminodiacetic acid (HIDA) scan; and endoscopic retrograde cholangiopancreatography (ERCP) are used to screen for gallbladder and pancreatic disorders.

Treatment of Gallbladder, Pancreatic, and Biliary Tract Disorders

Surgery and supportive management are the most common treatments of biliary and gallbladder disorders. Supportive management includes intravenous fluids, nasogastric suction, pain management, and antibiotics. For patients who cannot endure surgery, medications that attempt to dissolve biliary stones can be administered. Ursodiol and chenodiol are such medications. **Cholecystectomy** is the surgical removal of the gallbladder, which is usually done via laparoscopy. In pancreatitis, the patient is usually placed on intravenous solution as well as on antibiotic and pain relievers. The goal is to rest the pancreas and gastrointestinal system. Nasogastric feedings or total parenteral nutrition may be needed if NPO status is prolonged. The patient's diet should be free of fat, caffeine, and alcohol. Pancreatic enzyme supplementation may be necessary with recovery. Pancreatic cancer commonly requires surgery called the Whipple procedure.

Disorders of the Gallbladder, Pancreas, and Biliary Tract

Biliary colic describes the typical pain experienced by individuals with gallbladder or pancreatic disease. Cholecystitis, which causes episodes of intense biliary colic, is one of the most common surgically treated disorders. Pancreatic disease is less common but can lead to serious complications.

Cholecystitis

Cholecystitis can occur as an acute or chronic disorder, with gallstones being the most common cause.

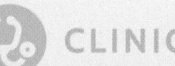 CLINICAL CONCEPT

Individuals can have gallstones for many years before they cause gallbladder inflammation.

An estimated 10% to 20% of Americans have gallstones, and as many as one-third of these individuals go on to develop acute cholecystitis. Cholecystectomy for either recurrent biliary colic or acute cholecystitis is the most common major surgical procedure performed by general surgeons, resulting in approximately 500,000 operations annually. Gallstones are 2 to 3 times more common in females than in males, resulting in a higher incidence of acute cholecystitis in females. **Acalculous cholecystitis** is inflammation of the gallbladder without stones; it is observed more often in elderly men.

> **ALERT!** Because epigastric pain with radiation to the shoulder is a common symptom, many patients can mistake an episode of acute cholecystitis for cardiac chest pain.

Etiology

Acute cholecystitis most often occurs because of biliary stasis and gallstones. Cholesterol calculi are the most common type of gallstones formed because of biliary stasis. Pigment stones that contain bilirubin can also develop in the gallbladder. Inflammation and spasms of the gallbladder can occur without the formation of stones. Highly concentrated bile without calculi can irritate the interior gallbladder mucosa and cause spasms of the gland. Acalculous cholecystitis can occur because of critical illness, major surgery, sickle cell disease, salmonella infections, acquired immune deficiency syndrome (AIDS), burns, sepsis, total parenteral nutrition, or prolonged fasting.

Individuals older than age 40 years, especially females with a family history of cholecystitis, are prone to the disorder. There are several classic risk factors that predispose individuals to cholecystitis (see Box 32-1).

Pathophysiology

Ninety percent of cases of cholecystitis are caused by gallstones that lodge in the cystic duct, called calculous cholecystitis; the other 10% of cases occur because of

---

BOX 32-1. Common Risk Factors of Cholecystitis

There are several risk factors that increase susceptibility to gallstone formation and cholecystitis, including:

- age greater than 40 years
- diet, if high-calorie, high-cholesterol
- estrogen
- female gender, particularly those who have had multiple pregnancies
- genetic predisposition
- obesity
- oral contraceptives
- rapid weight loss and yo-yo dieting.

---

acalculous cholecystitis. Obstruction of the cystic duct by gallstones causes distention of the gallbladder. As the gallbladder becomes distended, blood flow and lymphatic drainage are compromised, leading to mucosal ischemia and necrosis. The distention of the gallbladder irritates the nerves that innervate the wall, causing intense pain. As distention subsides, the pain wanes, leading to a pattern of spasmodic pain known as biliary colic.

The pathophysiology of acalculous cholecystitis is less clear. One theory suggests that this disorder begins with a noncontracting gallbladder, as bile can become highly concentrated and irritating in a gallbladder that does not contract. A gallbladder that remains noncontractile can be caused by either lack of organ response to CCK or prolonged fasting. Eating stimulates intestinal CCK; if an individual undergoes frequent fasting, the gallbladder lacks stimulus to contract and does not release bile.

The inflammatory process associated with acute cholecystitis can also occur because of bacterial infection that can progress to a purulent effusion of the gallbladder, called an **empyema.** *Escherichia coli*, *Streptococci*, and *Salmonella* are the most common bacteria involved.

Acalculous cholecystitis caused by infection is more serious than calculous cholecystitis because gangrene of the gallbladder wall, perforation, and empyema can all develop rapidly. In another condition called emphysematous cholecystitis, gas-forming bacterial organisms such as *Clostridia* can infect the gallbladder and cause gangrene and perforation of the gland.

Chronic cholecystitis can occur when the gallbladder becomes thickened, rigid, and fibrotic and functions poorly. This pathological change in the structure of the gallbladder results from repeated attacks of cholecystitis, calculi, or chronic episodes of irritation. Chronic cholecystitis commonly causes episodes of intense heartburn, eructations, flatulence, and indigestion. Repeated attacks of symptoms may occur and resemble acute cholecystitis.

Choledocholithiasis occurs when small gallstones pass from the gallbladder and cystic duct into the common bile duct. Stones remain in the common bile duct, causing obstruction, which causes backup of bile into the liver; this results in backup of bilirubin and bile salts in the bloodstream. Accumulation of bilirubin in the bloodstream results in jaundice, and backup of bile salts into the bloodstream causes pruritus (itching).

Clinical Presentation

The most common presenting symptom of acute cholecystitis is abdominal pain in the RUQ. The patient usually complains of anorexia, nausea, vomiting, eructations, heartburn, feeling full after eating, and, perhaps, fever. A key sign of cholecystitis with peritoneal inflammation is **Murphy's sign,** where the patient takes in a quick inspiration as the clinician palpates the RUQ. In some patients, the pain of cholecystitis radiates to the right shoulder or scapula. Although the pain may initially be described as spasmodic or colicky, it becomes constant in many cases.

Although patients with acalculous cholecystitis may present similarly, the condition commonly occurs in severely ill patients without a prior history of biliary colic. Patients with acalculous cholecystitis usually present with fever and sepsis, without history or physical examination findings consistent with acute cholecystitis.

Elderly patients, especially those with diabetes, may present with vague symptoms and without many classic findings. Pain and fever may be absent, and localized tenderness may be the only presenting sign. Elderly patients may also rapidly progress to complicated cholecystitis and rupture of the gland without warning.

Diagnosis

Laboratory tests used in cholecystitis include WBC count, ESR, CRP, liver enzymes, and bilirubin levels. Abdominal ultrasonography is the imaging study of choice for evaluating the gallbladder and biliary tree. Ultrasound can reveal the presence of stones, thickening of the gallbladder wall, and distention of the lumen. A cholecystogram can provide an assessment of gallbladder function. CT and ERCP are useful for gallbladder disorder when other studies are equivocal.

CLINICAL CONCEPT

ERCP can be used in both diagnosis and treatment; it may be used to perform ultrasonography, remove stones from the bile duct, or insert a bile duct stent.

Treatment

Laparoscopic cholecystectomy is the treatment of choice for symptomatic cholelithiasis and cholecystitis. This minimally invasive procedure has a low risk of complications and generally requires a hospital stay of fewer than 24 hours. The procedure is usually performed with four small incisions through which instruments are inserted. The gallbladder is freed either by electrosurgical or laser excision and is then withdrawn through one of the small incisions. Advantages of this technique include less postoperative pain than after laparotomy, which is open surgical investigation of the abdomen; small incisions; and more rapid return to daily activities. Incision length and the accompanying postoperative pain make open cholecystectomy more difficult for patients in terms of recovery.

CLINICAL CONCEPT

Not all patients are candidates for laparoscopic cholecystectomy, and there is always the risk that a laparoscopic cholecystectomy may be converted to a laparotomy or open cholecystectomy during the procedure.

When there is concern that stones may have moved into the common bile duct, intraoperative cholangiography and choledochoscopy may also be performed. This allows full exploration of the common bile duct. Occasionally, a transhepatic T tube may need to be placed in the common bile duct to decompress the biliary tree and decrease inflammation. The T tube is inserted to maintain patency of the duct and promote bile passage while the edema decreases. It can also be used in cases of biliary obstruction when obstructive jaundice is present. Excess bile is collected in a drainage bag secured below the surgical site.

After cholecystectomy, intracorporeal lithotripsy may be used to fragment retained stones in the common bile duct by pulsed laser or hydraulic lithotripsy applied through an endoscope directly to the stones. The stone fragments are removed by irrigation or aspiration. Retained stones may also be removed by basket retrieval through endoscopy or percutaneous transhepatic biliary approach.

Dietary Management. The dietary management of gallbladder disease involves avoiding food during an acute attack of cholecystitis. A nasogastric tube may be inserted to relieve nausea and vomiting. For patients who are able to eat, dietary fat intake may need to be limited, especially if the patient is obese. If bile flow is obstructed, fat-soluble vitamins, such as A, D, E, and K, and bile salts may need to be administered.

Medications. A narcotic analgesic may be required for pain relief during an acute attack of cholecystitis. Dilaudid is commonly administered in the emergency department as the patient is being evaluated for cholecystitis.

Oral medications to dissolve gallstones are indicated for patients who cannot tolerate surgery because of comorbid conditions. Ursodiol (Actigall) and chenodiol (Chenix) reduce the cholesterol content of gallstones, leading to their gradual dissolution. Patients with pruritus caused by accumulation of bile salts in the bloodstream may be given cholestyramine (Questran), which binds with bile salts to promote their excretion in the feces. The major adverse effects of medications used to treat biliary disease include diarrhea, abnormal liver function tests, and increased serum cholesterol.

Direct cholelitholysis therapy can also be used for treatment of gallstones. This approach involves the use of a cholesterol-dissolving agent directly infused into the gallbladder by a percutaneous transhepatic biliary catheter; it is indicated for symptomatic, high-risk patients whose gallbladder can be visualized by radiographic study.

ALERT! Rupture of an acutely inflamed gallbladder may result in acute pain that is transient and followed by relief of pain as contents are released from the distended, perforated gallbladder into the abdomen. It is critical to report this finding immediately to avoid sepsis.

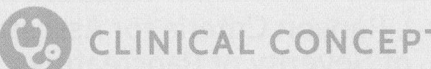 **CLINICAL CONCEPT**

If a narcotic analgesic is needed for pain management in biliary disorders, morphine and codeine are contraindicated because they can cause spasm of the biliary duct and sphincter of Oddi. Dilaudid is recommended in lieu of morphine or codeine.

Cancer of the Gallbladder

Gallbladder cancer is rare; however, when it does occur, it usually does so in individuals older than age 65 years. Manifestations of gallbladder cancer include intense pain and a palpable mass in the RUQ of the abdomen. Jaundice and weight loss are common. Gallbladder cancers spread by direct extension to the liver and metastasize via the blood and lymph system. The symptoms occur late in the disease process. Therefore, at the time of diagnosis, the cancer usually is generally too advanced to treat surgically. Ninety-five percent of patients with primary cancer of the gallbladder die within 1 year. Radical and extensive surgical interventions may be performed, but the prognosis is poor regardless of treatment.

Acute Pancreatitis

Acute pancreatitis is a serious disorder that is potentially lethal. Normally, the pancreas inhibits digestive enzymes from causing injury and destruction of the gland. However, the dysfunctional pancreas undergoes inflammation and cellular injury caused by the leakage of pancreatic digestive enzymes into the glandular parenchyma.

Worldwide, the incidence of acute pancreatitis ranges between 5 and 80 per 100,000 people, with the highest incidence recorded in the United States and Finland. The annual incidence of acute pancreatitis in Caucasians is 5.7 per 100,000 people, and in African Americans it is 20.7 per 100,000 people. The median age at onset depends on the etiology: The age of onset for alcohol-related pancreatitis is 39 years old and for biliary tract-related disease, 69 years old. Acute pancreatitis generally affects males more than females.

Etiology
The most common causes of pancreatitis are biliary tract disease and alcohol abuse. In biliary tract disease, the causative factor is obstruction of the pancreatic duct by a gallstone or other cause, with release of digestive enzymes within the gland parenchyma, followed by autodigestion. It has also been theorized that microlithiasis, defined as microscopic-size gallstones, can lodge at the ampulla of Vater, causing obstruction and backup pressure within the pancreas. In alcohol-related pancreatitis, ethanol causes intracellular accumulation of digestive enzymes and their premature activation and release.

Abdominal trauma causes clinical pancreatitis in 5% of cases. Pancreatic injury occurs more often in penetrating injuries, such as from knives and bullets, than in blunt abdominal trauma.

Several infectious diseases may cause pancreatitis, especially in children. Viral causes include mumps virus, coxsackievirus, cytomegalovirus, hepatitis virus, Epstein-Barr virus, echovirus, varicella-zoster virus, measles virus, and rubella virus. Bacterial causes include *Mycoplasma pneumoniae, Salmonella, Campylobacter,* and *Mycobacterium tuberculosis.* Pancreatitis has been associated with AIDS; however, this may be the result of opportunistic infections, neoplasms, lipodystrophy, or drug therapies.

Hypercalcemia from any cause can lead to acute pancreatitis. Such causes may include hyperparathyroidism, excessive doses of vitamin D, familial hypocalciuric hypercalcemia, and total parenteral nutrition. Hypertriglyceridemia can also cause pancreatitis. In surgical procedures that cause hypotension, acute pancreatitis can occur because of hypoperfusion and resulting ischemia. Also, following ERCP, hyperamylasemia and abdominal pain caused by pancreatitis is common.

Additional possible causes of pancreatitis include insecticides, methanol, organophosphates, and prescription drugs.

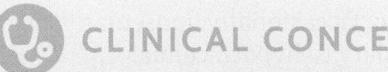 **CLINICAL CONCEPT**

Patients who engage in heavy drinking are commonly admitted with an acute exacerbation of chronic pancreatitis.

Pathophysiology
Acute pancreatitis is an inflammatory disease of the pancreas that can result from episodes of untreated cholecystitis caused by gallstones. A gallstone can lodge in the common bile duct and obstruct free flow of enzymes from the pancreas. The digestive enzymes then back up and perform autodigestion on the gland parenchyma and destroy the pancreatic cells. Autodigestion leads to severe damage to pancreatic cells, edema, vascular insufficiency, and ischemia of the gland.

Alcohol, drugs, and infectious agents can directly damage the cells of the pancreas. Alcohol and drug metabolites can reach the pancreas and cause premature activation of pancreatic enzymes. Ethanol or toxins can increase the permeability of ductules, allowing enzymes to reach the parenchyma and cause pancreatic damage. Ethanol also increases the protein content of pancreatic juice, decreases bicarbonate levels, and hinders trypsin inhibitor. Without trypsin inhibitor or bicarbonate, acids injure the gland and protein plugs block pancreatic outflow.

Acute pancreatitis is classified as either acute interstitial pancreatitis or acute hemorrhagic pancreatitis. Hemorrhagic pancreatitis can cause retroperitoneal blood accumulation. Chronic pancreatitis is characterized by permanent changes in pancreatic structure and persistent dysfunction even after the precipitating cause has been corrected. Necrotizing pancreatitis, which is the necrosis of cells, edema, and bleeding with loss of gland function, is the most severe condition and is associated with high morbidity and mortality.

After an episode of pancreatitis, both exocrine and endocrine functions of the pancreas can be impaired; with inflammation of the gland, the affected individual can become deficient in digestive enzymes and insulin.

Clinical Presentation

The classic symptom associated with acute pancreatitis is severe abdominal pain, which is characteristically dull, penetrating, and steady. Usually, the pain is sudden in onset and gradually intensifies in severity. Most often it is located in the epigastric region and radiates into the back. Nausea, vomiting, and diarrhea occur with accompanying anorexia. Fever, tachycardia, and hypotension commonly accompany the pain. Dyspnea and tachypnea may also occur because of irritation of the diaphragm.

On physical examination, abdominal tenderness, muscular guarding, and distention are observed in most patients; bowel sounds are often diminished or absent. Some patients exhibit jaundice. Patients with severe acute pancreatitis are often pale, diaphoretic, and lethargic. Occasionally, muscular spasms may be noted secondary to hypocalcemia.

Physical examination may also reveal Cullen sign and Grey Turner sign. The **Cullen sign** is a bluish discoloration around the umbilicus resulting from blood in the peritoneal cavity because of hemorrhagic pancreatitis. The **Grey Turner sign** is a reddish-brown discoloration along the flanks resulting from retroperitoneal blood dissecting along tissue planes. Erythematous skin nodules may result from subcutaneous fat necrosis; these are typically located on extensor skin surfaces. In addition, polyarthritis is occasionally seen.

Abnormalities on fundoscopic examination of the retina may be seen in severe pancreatitis. For example, Purtscher retinopathy is ischemic injury to the retina that is caused by blood clotting within the retinal vessels. It may cause temporary or permanent blindness.

Diagnosis

Establishing the severity of acute pancreatitis is critical to predict the patient's course and anticipate complications. Many scoring systems can predict morbidity and mortality. Ranson criteria include 11 characteristics (see Box 32-2). The five characteristics that are assessed at admission reflect the intensity of the inflammatory response, and the six characteristics evaluated during the initial 48 hours reflect the serious complications, including fluid shifts, cardiovascular instability, and end-organ failure. Patients with more than six positive criteria have an increased likelihood of pancreatic necrosis and infection and a high mortality rate.

BOX 32-2. Ranson Criteria for Assessment of Severity of Pancreatitis

It is difficult to assess the severity of acute and chronic pancreatitis. Several factors, referred to as the Ranson criteria, need to be considered to determine the need for hospitalization of the patient.

RANSON CRITERIA

On Admission
- age greater than 55 years
- WBC count greater than 16,000
- liver enzyme: lactic dehydrogenase greater than 600 U/L
- liver enzyme: aspartate aminotransferase greater than 120 U/L
- glucose greater than 10 mmol/L.

Within 48 Hours
- hematocrit fall greater than 10%
- blood urea nitrogen rise greater than 0.9 mmol/L
- calcium less than 2 mmol
- partial pressure of oxygen less than 60 mm Hg
- base deficit greater than 4
- fluid sequestration greater than 6 L.

Diagnostic testing involves blood work and noninvasive imaging. Blood work is used to categorize severity using the previously mentioned criteria and includes complete blood count, blood glucose level, blood urea nitrogen, serum calcium, lactic dehydrogenase, amylase, and lipase. The blood level of amylase is 10 to 20 times greater than normal in acute pancreatitis and is also an early response to injury. Serum lipase levels are usually elevated about 72 hours after the onset of symptoms. Noninvasive imaging studies include abdominal and endoscopic ultrasound, CT scan, and magnetic resonance cholangiopancreatography (MRCP).

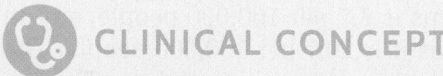

CLINICAL CONCEPT

Elevated serum lipase level is a key sign of acute pancreatitis.

Treatment

There is no proven therapy that directly ameliorates pancreatic inflammation. The main treatment goal for acute pancreatitis is to provide supportive care and minimize pancreatic stimulation. Treatment measures include fluid resuscitation, maintenance of optimal fluid balance, and close monitoring for signs of local systemic complications. Patients should not receive any oral fluids or food until abdominal pain and tenderness have subsided and bowel sounds have returned. Nasogastric suction is not necessary in mild pancreatitis, but it is recommended in the presence of vomiting and ileus. Therefore, careful monitoring is important to prevent associated fluid and electrolyte imbalances.

The patient should receive sufficient analgesic medication for pain control as abdominal pain may be intense. Dilaudid is commonly prescribed because it does not have gastrointestinal side effects. Neither total parenteral nutrition nor prophylactic antibiotic therapy is indicated in uncomplicated acute pancreatitis.

Hypovolemia can be caused by the exudation of fluid into the inflamed pancreatic retroperitoneal area and by the gastrointestinal fluid losses caused by vomiting and nasogastric suction. This fluid shift should be corrected promptly. Most patients with gallstone pancreatitis can undergo cholecystectomy. Patients with severe gallstone pancreatitis and evidence that gallstones are impacted at the ampulla of Vater often benefit from early ERCP, sphincterotomy, and stone extraction.

Patients who are still hypotensive after adequate volume replacement require placement of central catheters to allow more precise assessment and management of fluid and electrolyte requirements. The major indication for early surgical intervention is the presence of an acute abdomen. Intestinal perforation or necrosis, which sometimes mimics hemorrhagic acute pancreatitis, can be confirmed and corrected only when a laparotomy is performed.

Complications

Infected pancreatic necrosis should be suspected in patients who have moderate-to-severe acute pancreatitis; who have worsening symptoms after initial improvement; and who develop new fever, marked by leukocytosis, positive blood cultures, or other evidence of sepsis. If necrotic pancreatitis is suspected, an emergency abdominal CT scan with intravenous contrast enhancements should be performed.

Pancreatic pseudocysts occur in 10% to 20% of cases of acute pancreatitis. A **pseudocyst** is a circumscribed collection of fluid rich in pancreatic enzymes, blood, and necrotic tissue. Diagnosis is made most easily by abdominal ultrasound or CT scan. Small pseudocysts tend to resolve without treatment. Cysts that have been present for more than 6 weeks and are greater than 5 cm in diameter usually require treatment to prevent leakage and cellular injury.

Systemic Complications. The most important systemic complications of acute pancreatitis are cardiovascular, renal, and respiratory failure. Cardiovascular complications include profound hypotension.

Renal failure usually occurs as a result of hypovolemia and decreased renal perfusion. The prevention and treatment of pancreatitis-associated renal failure depends, to a large extent, on correcting fluid and electrolyte abnormalities. Mild and transient respiratory failure can occur as a result of splinting of respiration and atelectasis. In most cases, respiratory failure usually improves as the acute phase of pancreatitis ends. Some

patients progress to a more severe form of respiratory failure that resembles adult respiratory distress syndrome (ARDS). This poor prognostic sign is frequently associated with a complicated clinical course or death. Pancreatitis-associated ARDS results from injury to the alveolar membrane or degradation of surfactant by circulating enzymes, which may be released from the inflamed pancreas. Treatment is usually supportive because specific therapy for pancreatitis-associated ARDS has not been defined.

Chronic Pancreatitis

Chronic pancreatitis is defined as inflammation of the pancreas that does not heal and leads to permanent damage. Like acute pancreatitis, it occurs when digestive enzymes attack the pancreas and nearby tissues, causing episodes of pain.

Chronic pancreatitis often develops in people who are between the ages of 30 and 40 years. It is 3 times more common in African Americans compared with Caucasians. It has a bimodal incidence, with an early onset form at a median age of 19 years and a late onset form at 56 years. Alcohol-induced, chronic pancreatitis is more common in males, whereas hyperlipidemic-induced disease is more common in females. Hereditary pancreatitis can present in a person younger than age 30 years, but it might not be diagnosed for several years.

Etiology

The most common cause of chronic pancreatitis is long-term, heavy alcohol use and can be triggered by one acute attack that damages the pancreatic duct. Other causes of chronic pancreatitis include hereditary disorders, cystic fibrosis, hypercalcemia, hyperlipidemia, drugs, and autoimmune problems, such as Sjögren's syndrome. A diagnosis of hereditary pancreatitis is likely if the person has two or more family members with pancreatitis spanning more than one generation. Chronic pancreatitis has also been associated with primary biliary cirrhosis and renal tubular acidosis.

Pathophysiology

Chronic pancreatitis commonly results after several episodes of acute pancreatitis over the lifetime of the affected individual. Cellular injury is apparent with pancreatic fibrotic changes, which involve cellular release of growth factors, cytokines, and chemokines, leading to deposition of extracellular matrix and fibroblast proliferation. The pancreas ceases to function and develops scar tissue that requires patient supplementation of digestive enzymes and insulin.

Clinical Presentation

Most people with chronic pancreatitis experience upper abdominal pain, although some individuals have no pain at all. The pain may spread to the back, feel worse when eating or drinking, and become constant and disabling. In some cases, abdominal pain decreases as the condition worsens, most likely because the pancreas is no longer making digestive enzymes. Other symptoms include nausea, vomiting, weight loss, diarrhea, and steatorrhea. People with chronic pancreatitis often lose weight, even when their appetite and eating habits are normal. The weight loss occurs because the body does not secrete enough pancreatic enzymes to digest food and malabsorption of nutrients occurs.

Diagnosis

Serum amylase and lipase levels may be slightly elevated in chronic pancreatitis, but may be normal if pancreatic tissue is nonfunctional and fibrotic. Laboratory studies to identify causative factors of chronic pancreatitis include serum calcium and triglyceride levels. When common etiologies are not found, testing for genetic conditions such as cystic fibrosis should be done. Fecal studies can reveal steatorrhea, which is a manifestation of advanced chronic pancreatitis. Fecal chymotrypsin and human pancreatic elastase can be useful in confirming advanced chronic pancreatitis with exocrine insufficiency.

Abdominal x-ray may reveal pancreatic calcifications, considered pathognomonic of chronic pancreatitis, which are observed in approximately 30% of cases. CT scan often cannot decipher chronic pancreatitis. ERCP provides the most accurate visualization of the pancreatic ductal system and is regarded as the standard for diagnosing chronic pancreatitis. Magnetic resonance cholangiopancreatography (MRCP) provides information on the pancreatic parenchyma and adjacent abdominal viscera. Endoscopic ultrasonography can show characteristic calcifications in the pancreas with chronic inflammation. Biopsy of the pancreas shows fibrotic changes, protein plugs, and calcifications.

Treatment

Treatment for chronic pancreatitis commonly requires hospitalization for pain management, IV hydration, and nutritional support. Nasogastric feedings may be necessary for several weeks if the person continues to lose weight. When a normal diet is resumed, synthetic pancreatic enzymes may be prescribed if the pancreas does not secrete enough of its own. The enzymes should be taken with every meal to help the person digest food and regain some weight. The next step is to plan a diet that is low in fat and that includes small, frequent meals. Drinking plenty of fluids and limiting caffeinated beverages is also important. People with chronic pancreatitis are strongly advised not to smoke or consume alcoholic beverages, even if the pancreatitis is mild or in the early stages.

Complications

People with chronic pancreatitis who continue to consume large amounts of alcohol may develop sudden bouts of severe abdominal pain. As with acute pancreatitis, ERCP is used to identify and treat complications associated with chronic pancreatitis, such as gallstones, pseudocysts, and narrowing or obstruction of the ducts. Chronic pancreatitis also can lead to calcification of the pancreas, which means the pancreatic tissue hardens from deposits of insoluble calcium salts. Surgery may be necessary to remove part of the pancreas. In cases involving persistent pain, surgery or other procedures are sometimes recommended to block the nerves in the abdominal area that cause pain.

When pancreatic tissue is destroyed in chronic pancreatitis and the insulin-producing cells of the pancreas, called beta cells, have been damaged, diabetes may develop. Persons with a family history of diabetes are more likely to develop the disease. If diabetes occurs, insulin or oral antidiabetic medications are needed to keep blood glucose at normal levels. A health-care provider works with the patient to develop a regimen of medication, diet, and frequent blood glucose monitoring.

Cancer of the Pancreas

The incidence of pancreatic cancer rises steadily with age and mortality is nearly 100%. Pancreatic cancer occurs in 6% of the population and is the tenth most common site for cancer. It is the fourth leading cause of cancer death. At the time of diagnosis, 52% of all patients have metastatic disease and 26% have regional spread. The relative 1-year survival rate for pancreatic cancer is only 24%, and the overall 5-year survival is 5%.

Etiology

The cause of pancreatic cancer is unknown; however, there are risk factors associated with the disease, including cigarette smoking, obesity, diabetes mellitus, and chronic pancreatitis. Consumption of nitrites, preservatives found in such processed meats as bacon, has also been associated with a higher risk of pancreatic cancer.

Approximately 5% to 10% of patients with pancreatic carcinoma have some genetic predisposition to developing the disease. Inherited disorders that increase the risk of pancreatic cancer include hereditary pancreatitis, multiple endocrine neoplasia, hereditary nonpolyposis rectal cancer, familial adenomatous polyposis and Gardner syndrome, familial atypical multiple mole melanoma syndrome, von Hippel-Lindau syndrome, and mutations in the *BRCA1* and *BRCA2* genes.

Pathophysiology

Cancer of the pancreas can arise from exocrine or endocrine cells. Most pancreatic tumors arise from exocrine cells in the ducts; these are referred to as ductal adenocarcinomas. Tumors arising in small ducts invade nearby glandular tissue, penetrate the covering of the pancreas, and extend into surrounding tissues.

Ductal adenocarcinomas can occur in the head, body, or tail of the pancreas. Tumors of the head of the pancreas quickly spread to obstruct the common bile duct and portal vein. Obstruction of the common bile duct causes bile to back up into the liver. Bile backup leads to bilirubin backup and accumulation in the bloodstream, causing jaundice. Jaundice usually brings the patient to the attention of a health-care provider.

Ductal adenocarcinomas can infiltrate the superior mesenteric artery, the vena cava, and the aorta. Cancer cells that enter the blood vessels can form emboli. Tumors of the body and tail of the pancreas infiltrate the posterior abdominal walls. Lymphatic invasion occurs early and rapidly and involves local and regional lymph nodes. Venous infection causes metastases to the liver. Tumors that metastasize to the peritoneum can obstruct veins and promote development of ascites.

Clinical Presentation

Cancer that arises in the head of the pancreas leads to bile duct obstruction, which causes jaundice (see Fig. 32-4), an early warning sign of cancer of the pancreas. However, cancer of the body and tail of the pancreas is generally asymptomatic for a lengthy amount of time. Symptoms present late when there is intraductal destruction and tumor invasion of adjacent tissue.

Often, vague back pain is an initial symptom. As the disease worsens, there is constant epigastric pain with radiation to the back. Back pain worsens when the patient assumes the supine position; often this causes intense nighttime abdominal pain. Nausea, vomiting, and accompanying anorexia are common.

Jaundice eventually develops when the common bile duct is obstructed. Darkening of urine, stool changes, and pruritus are often noticed by patients before clinical jaundice occurs. Steatorrhea occurs because of malabsorption of fat, and pruritus occurs because of bile salts in the bloodstream. Weight loss occurs because of malabsorption of all nutrients when pancreatic enzymes are no longer produced. Depression is common in patients with pancreatic cancer and may be the most prominent presenting symptom for some individuals.

The onset of diabetes mellitus can be associated with pancreatic cancer. Cancer can invade the beta cells of the pancreas, which secrete insulin. Pancreatic cancer should be considered in a patient older than age 70 years with a new diagnosis of diabetes without any other diabetic risk factors.

Migratory thrombophlebitis and venous thrombosis also occur with higher frequency in patients with pancreatic cancer and may be the first presentation.

Distant metastases are found in the cervical and other lymph nodes, the lungs, and the brain. In late stages, the patient may present with signs of portal vein hypertension, which include ascites, hepatomegaly, and splenomegaly. Most individuals die of hepatic failure, malnutrition, or systemic disease.

ALERT! A left supraclavicular lymph node, also called Virchow's node, may be enlarged in pancreatic cancer, also a palpable, edematous gallbladder, also called Courvoisier sign, may be found in pancreatic cancer.

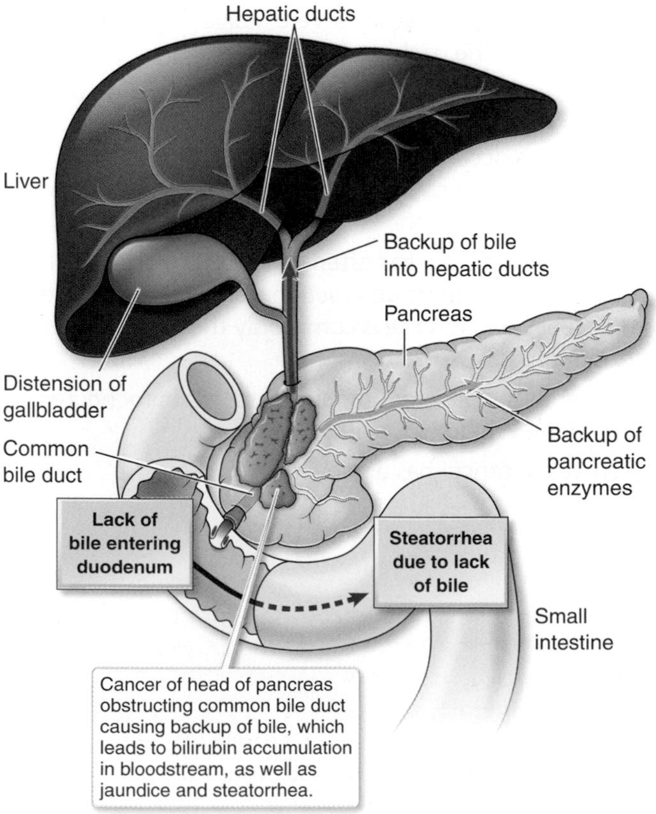

Diagnosis

Pancreatic cancer is often a silent disease until its late stages. Laboratory and imaging studies used to diagnose pancreatic cancer are the same as those used for acute and chronic pancreatitis. Jaundice does not become apparent until bilirubin backs up into the bloodstream because of an obstructed common bile duct. The most difficult clinical situation in which to diagnose pancreatic carcinoma is in the patient with underlying chronic pancreatitis. In such cases, imaging studies may show abnormalities that may not help to differentiate between pancreatic carcinoma and chronic pancreatitis. Abdominal CT scan is the standard imaging study used in pancreatic cancer and is often used to guide biopsy.

The carbohydrate antigen 19-9 (CA 19-9 antigen) is a tumor marker found in some cancer patients. It is also normally present within the cells of the biliary tract and can be elevated in acute or chronic biliary disease. However, about 5% to 10% of patients lack the enzyme necessary to produce CA 19-9; in such patients, monitoring the disease with this tumor marker is not possible. Carcinoembryonic antigen (CEA) is another tumor marker commonly found in gastrointestinal cancers; it is present in 40% to 45% of patients with pancreatic cancer.

Hepatic ducts

Liver

Backup of bile into hepatic ducts

Pancreas

Distension of gallbladder

Common bile duct

Lack of bile entering duodenum

Steatorrhea due to lack of bile

Backup of pancreatic enzymes

Small intestine

Cancer of head of pancreas obstructing common bile duct causing backup of bile, which leads to bilirubin accumulation in bloodstream, as well as jaundice and steatorrhea.

FIGURE 32-4. Cancer of the head of the pancreas.

Treatment

A laparotomy is performed, particularly if jaundice is present. Ultrasonography and CT scan may be needed to confirm the need for a laparotomy, especially in individuals without jaundice. Laparotomy is used to establish a definitive diagnosis, evaluate the extent of disease, and determine whether palliative bypass surgery is needed. Most individuals require palliative double bypass of the blocked bile ducts as well as gastrojejunostomy to prevent duodenal obstruction.

Candidates for surgery may undergo the Whipple procedure. This surgical intervention involves removal of the head of the pancreas as well as a portion of the bile duct, the gallbladder, and the duodenum. Occasionally, a portion of the stomach may also be removed. After removal of these structures, the remaining pancreas, bile duct, and duodenum are sutured back into the intestine.

Chapter Summary

- The liver produces and secretes bile for the digestion of fats; the gallbladder stores some of the bile. The liver releases bile into the hepatic duct, which continues on into the common bile duct.

- The gallbladder normally releases the bile into the cystic duct, which then continues into the common bile duct.

- Diminished gallbladder motility often causes bile stasis, which can develop into biliary sludge or cholesterol stones. The process of gallstone formation is called cholelithiasis.

- When cholesterol precipitates out of bile, it becomes a gallstone, also called a calculus.

- Bile stasis, biliary sludge, and gallstones often can irritate the gallbladder and cause cholecystitis.

- Women older than age 40 years are frequently affected by cholecystitis caused by cholelithiasis. Symptoms include RUQ abdominal pain, frequent indigestion, nausea, vomiting, eructations, and flatulence.

- Biliary colic is the term used to describe the type of pain that is caused by cholecystitis: a pain that increases to a peak, then wanes and decreases, giving temporary relief. This is referred to as colicky pain.

- The removal of the gallbladder, called laparoscopic cholecystectomy, is one of the most common surgical procedures performed.

- When a gallstone travels from the cystic duct into the common bile duct, it can cause common bile duct obstruction.

- Common bile duct obstruction causes backup of bile into the liver, which causes backup of bilirubin from the liver into the bloodstream. Hyperbilirubinemia causes jaundice, which is yellowing of the skin and sclera.

- When bile is blocked from getting into the intestine, fats are not digested, and steatorrhea (fat in stool) develops. Bile backs up into the liver, hyperbilirubinemia occurs, and bile salts accumulate in the bloodstream. Hyperbilirubinemia causes jaundice and high bile salts in the blood cause pruritus.

- The pancreas produces digestive enzymes and secretes them into the small intestine through the pancreatic duct for digestion of fats, proteins, and carbohydrates.

- Acute pancreatitis is a potentially lethal condition. The pancreatic enzymes back up into the gland and cause autodigestion.

- Alcohol abuse is the most common cause of pancreatitis. Gallstones or cystic fibrosis can also cause pancreatitis.

- Acute pancreatitis causes severe, epigastric pain that radiates into the back.

- Chronic pancreatitis causes gradual deterioration of the pancreas via autodigestion. Episodes of acute pain and symptoms occur. The patient suffers malabsorption from lack of digestive enzymes and eventual weight loss and malnutrition.

- Cancer of the pancreas often occurs in the head of the pancreas and causes obstruction of the common bile duct. Painless jaundice is commonly the first sign of this condition.

- Cancer of the pancreas requires a surgical procedure called the Whipple procedure.

- Pancreatic cancer has a poor survival rate.

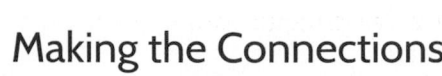 Making the Connections

Disorder and Pathophysiology	Signs and Symptoms	Physical Assessment Findings	Diagnostic Testing	Treatment
Cholelithiasis | The formation of gallstones, also called calculi, caused by precipitation of substances contained in bile, mainly cholesterol and bilirubin. Gallstones irritate the inner walls of the gallbladder, causing inflammation; this is referred to as cholecystitis.				
	The condition may be asymptomatic during the formation of the gallstones. Once formed, gallstones cause inflammation of the gallbladder, causing RUQ pain, indigestion, flatulence, eructations, nausea, and possibly vomiting. Pain builds up, then decreases, resulting in a biliary colic type of pain.	Murphy's sign: pain upon palpation of the RUQ of the abdomen.	Ultrasonography, CT scans, magnetic resonance imaging (MRI), and HIDA scans can show gallstones, inflamed gallbladder wall, bile stasis. or sludge. This can result in elevated WBC count, ESR, and CRP caused by inflammation. Total serum bilirubin and liver enzymes, aminotransferase, and alkaline phosphatase may be elevated if a gallstone causes obstruction of the common bile duct and backup of bile into the liver.	Laparoscopic surgical removal of gallbladder or open cholecystectomy. Narcotic for pain. If surgery is not an option, medications or lithotripsy can be used to dissolve the stones.
Cholecystitis | Inflammation of the gallbladder; it is generally associated with cholelithiasis, biliary sludge, or bile stasis.				
	The condition may be asymptomatic during the formation of the gallstones. Once formed, gallstones cause inflammation of the gallbladder, causing RUQ pain, indigestion, flatulence, eructations, nausea, and possibly vomiting. Pain builds up, then decreases, resulting in a biliary colic type of pain.	Murphy's sign.	Ultrasonography, CT scans, MRI, and HIDA scans can show gallstones, inflamed gallbladder wall, bile stasis, or sludge. This results in elevated WBC count, ESR, and CRP caused by inflammation. Total serum bilirubin and liver enzymes; aminotransferase, and alkaline phosphatase may be elevated if a gallstone causes obstruction of the common bile duct and backup of bile into the liver.	Laparoscopic surgical removal of gallbladder or open cholecystectomy. Narcotic for pain. If surgery is not an option, medications or lithotripsy can be used to dissolve the stones.

Continued

Making the Connections–cont'd

Disorder and Pathophysiology	Signs and Symptoms	Physical Assessment Findings	Diagnostic Testing	Treatment

Pancreatitis, Acute | A severe, life-threatening disorder associated with activated pancreatic enzymes secreted into the pancreatic tissue and surrounding tissue, causing inflammation and autodigestion.

| | Acute abdominal pain, nausea, vomiting. Abrupt onset; may follow a heavy meal or an alcoholic binge. Severe epigastric and abdominal pain that radiates to the back, which is aggravated when the person is lying supine and is relieved when the person is sitting and leaning forward. | Abdominal distention, hypoactive bowel sounds, tachycardia, hypotension. Cool, clammy skin and fever. Jaundice. | Elevated serum amylase and lipase occurs with pancreatic inflammation. Elevated blood glucose, urea nitrogen, calcium, and triglycerides. Elevated liver enzymes. Elevated bilirubin level. Urine amylase: elevated levels with pancreatic inflammation. Steatorrhea caused by lack of fat digestion because of decreased lipase in the intestine. ERCP, endoscopic ultrasound, MRCP. | Antibiotic prophylaxis, Dilaudid as pain reliever, and rest of the GI tract. Withholding of oral foods and fluid and institution of gastric suction to treat distention of the bowel and prevent further stimulation of the secretion of pancreatic enzymes. IV fluids and electrolytes to replace those lost from circulation and to combat hypotension and shock. |

Pancreatitis, Chronic | Characterized by progressive destruction of the pancreas by enzymes. Gradual autodigestion of the pancreas. Gradually fibrotic tissue replaces pancreatic tissue.

| | All symptoms associated with acute pancreatitis, although less severe. Episodic abdominal pain, nausea, and vomiting. Episodic epigastric and upper left quadrant pain, anorexia, nausea, vomiting, and flatulence. Steatorrhea; clay colored stool. | Episodes of abdominal tenderness, vomiting, abdominal distention, lack of bowel sounds, and jaundice. Steatorrhea; clay colored stool. | Elevated serum amylase and lipase occurs with pancreatic inflammation. Elevated blood glucose, urea nitrogen, triglycerides, and calcium. Elevated bilirubin level. Elevated liver enzymes. Urine amylase: elevated levels with pancreatic inflammation. Steatorrhea caused by lack of fat digestion because of decreased lipase in the intestine. ERCP, endoscopic ultrasound, MRCP, and CT scan. | Low-fat diet. Pancreatic enzymes may be needed. Insulin or antidiabetic medications are needed if the pancreas is not able to secrete insulin. |

Continued

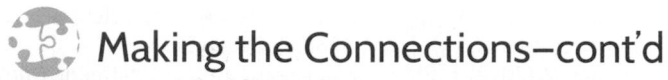 ## Making the Connections–cont'd

Disorder and Pathophysiology	Signs and Symptoms	Physical Assessment Findings	Diagnostic Testing	Treatment
Pancreatic Cancer | Neoplastic tumor that develops either in the head of the pancreas (most common) or the body or tail of the gland. Cancer of the head of the pancreas causes obstruction of the common bile duct, which causes backup of bile into the liver and backup of bilirubin into the bloodstream. This causes widespread destruction of the pancreas, with loss of pancreatic enzyme activity and metastasis to the liver.				
	When the tumor is in the head of the pancreas there are early symptoms, whereas if it is in the body or tail, cancer remains silent until there is severe organ involvement. Cancer of the pancreatic head causes obstructive jaundice, steatorrhea, nausea, vomiting, and backup of bile salts, which causes pruritus. Weight loss may be caused by lack of pancreatic enzymes and malabsorption of all nutrients.	Abdominal distention, hypoactive bowel sounds, and jaundice. Steatorrhea.	Elevated serum amylase and lipase occurs with pancreatic inflammation. Bilirubin and liver enzyme level. Urine amylase: elevated levels with pancreatic inflammation. Steatorrhea caused by lack of fat digestion because of decreased lipase in the intestine. Biomarkers: CEA and CA 19-9 (carbohydrate antigen). ERCP, MRCP. CT scan, and biopsy.	Whipple procedure: surgical excision of cancerous sections of the pancreas. Pain relief.

Bibliography

Albashir, S., & Stevens, T. (2012). Endoscopic ultrasonography to evaluate pancreatitis. *Cleveland Clin J Med, 79*(3), 202–206. doi: 10.3949/ccjm.79a.11092.

Baron, T. H. (2013). Managing severe acute pancreatitis. *Cleveland Clin J Med, 80*(6), 354–359. doi: 10.3949/ccjm.80gr.13001.

Bilimoria, K. Y., Chung, J., & Soper, N. J. (2013). Laparoscopic cholecystectomy, intraoperative cholangiograms, and common duct injuries. *JAMA, 310*(8), 801–802.

Bosmann, M., Schreiner, O., & Galle, P. R. (2009). Coexistence of Cullen's and Grey Turner's signs in acute pancreatitis. *Am J Med, 122*(4), 333–334.

Braganza, J. M., Lee, S. H., McCloy, R. F., & McMahon, M. J. (2011). Chronic pancreatitis. *Lancet, 377*(9772), 1184–1197.

Felicilda-Reynaldo, R. F. (2012). Oral gallstone dissolution therapies. *Medsurg Nurs, 21*(1), 41–43.

Frossard, J. L., Steer, M. L., & Pastor, C. M. (2008). Acute pancreatitis. *Lancet, 371*(9607), 143–152.

Hall, M. A. (2011, October). Chronic pancreatitis; an update for home care and hospice clinicians. *Home Healthcare Nurse, 29*(9), 562–570.

Hartwig, W., Werner, J., Jäger, D., Debus, J., & Büchler, M. W. (2013). Improvement of surgical results for pancreatic cancer. *Lancet Oncol, 14*(11), e476–485.

Hidalgo, M. (2010). Pancreatic cancer. *N Engl J Med, 362*(17), 1605–1617.

Jensen, R. T., & Delle Fave, G. (2011). Promising advances in the treatment of malignant pancreatic endocrine tumors. *N Engl J Med, 364*(6), 564–565.

Kessenich, C. R. (2011). Cholecystitis and HIDA scan. *Nurse Pract, 36*(9), 11–12. doi: 10.1097/01.NPR.0000403295.82092.20.

Lacovara, J. E. (2011). Whipple pancreatoduodenectomy surgery for the treatment of pancreatic cancer. *Medsurg Nursing, 20*(6), 337, 339.

Law, R., Bronner, M., Vogt, D., & Stevens, T. (2009). Autoimmune pancreatitis: a mimic of pancreatic cancer. *Cleveland Clin J Med, 76*(10), 607–615.

Li, D., Morris, J. S., Liu, J., et al. (2009). Body mass index and risk, age of onset, and survival in patients with pancreatic cancer. *JAMA, 301*(24), 2553–2562.

Longo, D. L., Kasper, D. L., Jameson, J. L., et al. (2011). *Harrison's principles of internal medicine.* 18th ed. New York: McGraw-Hill.

MacIntyre, J. (2011). Metastatic pancreatic cancer: what can nurses do? *Clin J Oncol Nurs, 15*(4), 424–428.

Mönkemüller, K., Vormbrock, K., & Kuhn, R. (2012). Case 32-2011: a man with recurrent pancreatitis. *N Engl J Med, 366*(7), 669–670.

Morse, B., Centeno, B., & Vignesh, S. (2014). Autoimmune pancreatitis: updated concepts of a challenging diagnosis.

Am J Med, May 14. pii: S0002-9343(14)00388-X. doi: 10.1016/j.amjmed.2014.04.033. Epub ahead of print.

Parsi, M. A., Stevens, T., Dumot, J. A., & Zuccaro, G., Jr. (2009). Endoscopic therapy of recurrent acute pancreatitis. *Cleveland Clin J Med*, 76(4), 225–233.

Patel, K., & Wong, T. (2013). ERCP: indications, complications and contraindications. *Gastrointestinal Nurs*, 11(2), 45–48.

Saccomano, S. J., & Ferrara, L. R. (2013). Evaluation of acute abdominal pain. *Nurse Pract*, 38(11), 46–53.

Selmi, C., Bowlus, C. L., Gershwin, M. E., & Coppel, R. L. (2011). Primary biliary cirrhosis. *Lancet*, 377(9777), 1600–1609. doi: 10.1016/S0140-6736(10)61965-4. Epub 2011 Apr 28.

Shah, U., & Shenoy-Bhangle, A. S. (2011). Case records of the Massachusetts General Hospital. Case 32-2011. A 19-year-old man with recurrent pancreatitis. *N Engl J Med*, 365(16), 1528–1536.

Stevens, T., Parsi, M. A., & Walsh, R. M. (2009). Acute pancreatitis: problems in adherence to guidelines. *Cleveland Clin J Med*, 76(12), 697–704.

Strasberg, S. M. (2008). Clinical practice. Acute calculous cholecystitis. *N Engl J Med*, 358(26), 2804–2811.

Sun, V. (2010). Update on pancreatic cancer treatment. *Nurse Pract*, 35(8), 16–22.

Thomas, S. (2013). Differentiating abdominal pain using Murphy's sign. *Pract Nurs*, 24(3), 141.

VanWoerkom, R., & Adler, D. (2009). Acute pancreatitis: review and clinical update. *Hosp Phys*, 45(1), 9.

Vincent, A., Herman, J., Schulick, R., Hruban, R. H., & Goggins, M. (2011). Pancreatic cancer. *Lancet*, 378(9791), 607–620. Epub 2011 May 26.

Wallace, M. (2009, February 2). Chronic pancreatitis. *Gastrointestinal Endoscopy*, 69(2), S117–120.

Warshaw, A. L. (2010). Improving the treatment of necrotizing pancreatitis—a step up. *N Engl J Med*, 362(16), 1535–1537.

Yegneswaran, B., & Pitchumoni, C. S. (2010). When should serum amylase and lipase levels be repeated in a patient with acute pancreatitis? *Cleveland Clin J Med*, 77(4), 230–231.

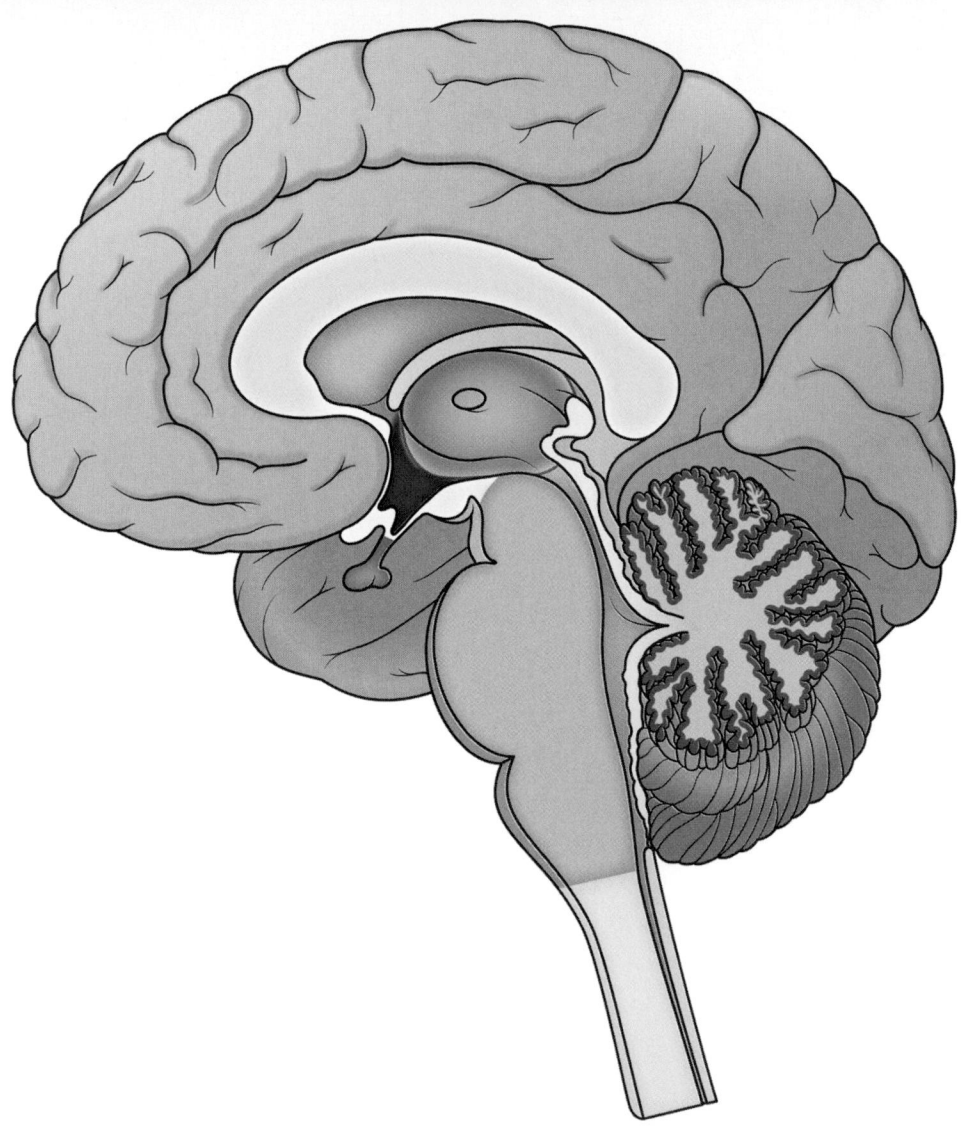

Chapters

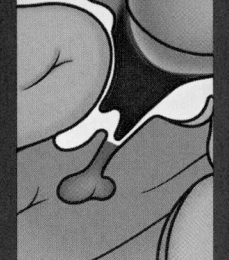

Key Terms

Anoxic encephalopathy

Aphasia

Cardioembolic event

Carotid stenosis

Cerebral infarction

Circle of Willis

Contralateral

Corticospinal tract

Cushing's Triad

Decussation

Expressive aphasia

Hemorrhagic stroke

Ipsilateral

Ischemic penumbra

Ischemic stroke

Lacunar infarct

Neurological deficit

Receptive aphasia

Spinothalamic tract

Subarachnoid hemorrhage

Transient ischemic attack (TIA)

Vertebral-basilar insufficiency (VBI)

The nervous system is an intricate web of fibers that enables the human body to interact with the environment. When these fibers are damaged, messages traveling to or from the brain or spinal cord may not reach their target destination. This can lead to numerous complications ranging from an inability to move to a constant struggle with intractable pain. There are various kinds of neurological disorders, and each disorder has an impact on a person's quality of life.

The most common cause of neurological disability is cerebrovascular disease; this involves disorders of the circulatory system of the brain, including cerebral ischemia and cerebral hemorrhage—the most common types of stroke. Both cause brain cell death and permanent neurological impairment.

Epidemiology

Stroke, also known as cerebrovascular accident (CVA), is the fifth leading cause of death in the United States and the leading cause of disability. Commonly, persons who sustain stroke are left with paralysis of one side of their body; in addition, 20% of individuals who suffer stroke die within 12 months. In the United States, someone has a stroke every 40 seconds, accounting for 780,000 incidents each year. The majority of persons who sustain stroke are age 65 years or older, and because of the rising number of elderly individuals in the population, the incidence of stroke is projected to be 1 million persons per year by the year 2050.

As with cardiovascular disease, men are at higher risk for cerebrovascular disease than women. Caucasian males have a stroke incidence of 62.8 per 100,000, with death being the final outcome in 26.3% of cases, whereas women have a stroke incidence of 59 per 100,000 and a death rate of 39.2%. The risk of

stroke for African Americans is about twice that of Caucasians.

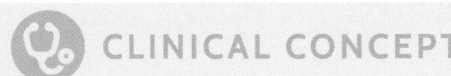

Although stroke often is considered a disease of elderly persons, 25% of strokes occur in persons younger than 65 years.

Basic Concepts of Cerebrovascular Structure and Function

The overall function of the nervous system is to detect, interpret, and respond to changes in the environment. It is important to review the basic concepts of cerebrovascular and neurological function before stroke can be understood.

Neuroanatomy and Neurophysiology

The nervous system is divided into two regions: the central nervous system (CNS), which consists of the brain and spinal cord, and the peripheral nervous system, which consists of cranial and spinal nerves. There is a section around the midline of the brain called the sensorimotor region; at this area, motor neurons descend down into the spinal cord and sensory neurons arrive up from the spinal cord.

Movement is dependent upon motor neurons that extend from the brain down into the spinal cord. Sensation such as pain, touch, and temperature enter the spinal cord from the periphery and ascend up into the brain. The motor and sensory neurons within the brain are called upper neurons and the neurons of the spinal cord are lower neurons. Sensory and motor neurons are located within the sensorimotor area of the brain adjacent to the central sulcus. The **corticospinal tract** is the major region of upper motor neurons that descend from the brain down into the spinal cord. The **spinothalamic tract** is the major region of sensory neurons that travel from the periphery up into the brain. The corticospinal nerves travel from the brain and cross over at the medulla before reaching the spinal cord. At the area referred to as the **decussation** in the medulla, upper motor neurons cross from one side of the brain to control the opposite side of the body (see Fig. 33-1). The spinothalamic tract originates in the spinal cord and crosses at some level within the spinal cord before arriving in the brain. This crossover of neurons causes any type of cerebral injury to manifest sensory and motor deficits on the contralateral side of the body.

CLINICAL CONCEPT

The majority of corticospinal and spinothalamic nerve fibers (80%) cross to the **contralateral** (opposite) side of the body and a small percentage of nerve fibers (20%) remain **ipsilateral** (same side).

The Central Nervous System

The brain can be separated into major regions: cerebrum, cerebellum, midbrain, pons, and medulla (see Fig. 33-2). The midbrain, pons, and medulla together form the brainstem. The cerebrum can be subdivided into lobes.

Cerebrum. The cerebrum makes up most of the brain tissue and is located in the uppermost region of the brain. It is divided into a right and left hemisphere, which are connected by the corpus callosum. The cerebrum is also divided into the frontal, parietal, temporal, and occipital lobes. Although each lobe has specific functions, there is some overlapping of responsibilities (see Box 33-1).

Hemispheric Specialization. The location of specific functions within the brain is described as complementary hemispheric specialization (see Fig. 33-3). The cerebral hemisphere associated with language comprehension skills and sequential-analytical processes is referred to as the categorical hemisphere; in most persons, this is the left hemisphere. The other, complementary hemisphere is referred to as the representational hemisphere; in most persons, this is the right hemisphere. It focuses more on recognition of faces, music, and visual spatial relationships than the other hemisphere.

Speech and Language Center. For most right-handed individuals, the left hemisphere is the categorical hemisphere. The left hemisphere contains

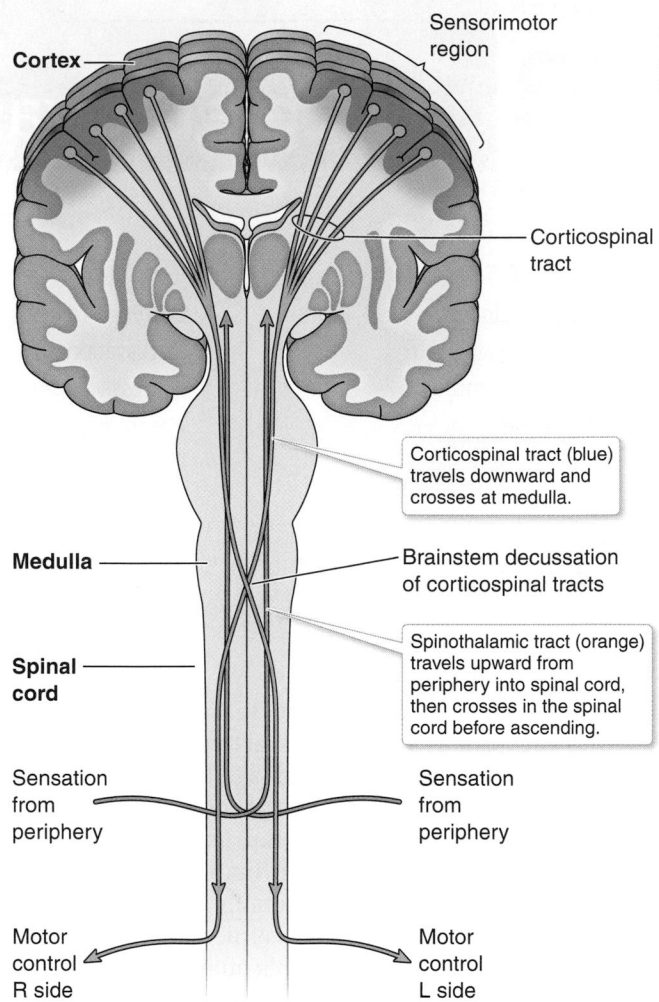

FIGURE 33-1. The sensorimotor region of the brain. Corticospinal tract neurons are motor neurons that travel from the brain into the spinal cord; they cross to the contralateral side of the medulla, an area called the decussation. Spinothalamic neurons are sensory neurons that arise from and travel up the spinal cord before crossing over to the contralateral side before reaching the brain.

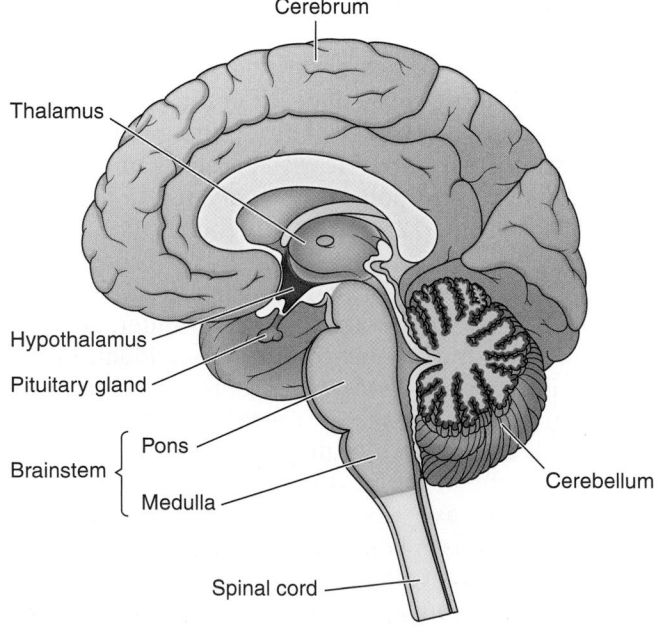

FIGURE 33-2. Major areas of the brain.

BOX 33-1. Brain Lobes and Responsibilities

The brain's four lobes each have their own unique responsibilities.

FRONTAL LOBE
- voluntary movements
- memory
- emotion
- social judgment
- decision making
- reasoning
- aggression

PARIETAL LOBE
- receiving and interpreting bodily sensations
- governing of proprioception, the awareness of one's body and body parts in space and in relation to each other

TEMPORAL LOBE
- hearing
- smelling
- learning
- memory
- emotional behavior
- visual recognition

OCCIPITAL LOBE
- analyzing and interpreting visual information

(Adapted from Thompson, G. S. (2013). *Understanding anatomy and physiology: a visual, auditory, interactive approach*. Philadelphia, PA: F.A. Davis.)

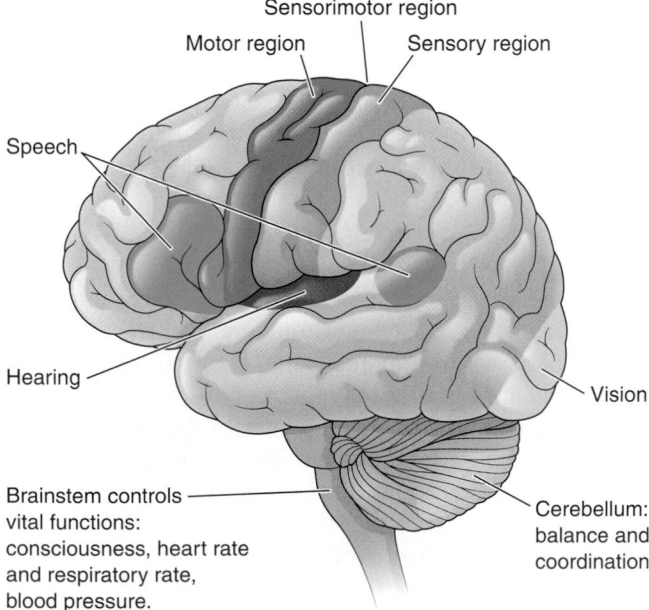

FIGURE 33-3. Functional areas of the brain.

areas for language comprehension, speech, and word formation. The ability to speak is controlled by a region called Broca's area; dysfunction of this area causes **expressive aphasia.** In expressive aphasia, the affected individual cannot make words, but he or she does understand what others are saying. Wernicke's area, which is connected to Broca's area, is critical for language comprehension; dysfunction of this area causes **receptive aphasia.** In receptive aphasia, the affected individual cannot understand words and can speak, but uses illogical language.

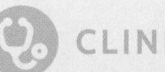
CLINICAL CONCEPT

Most individuals with damage to the left hemisphere develop **aphasia,** a disorder that makes it difficult to speak or understand language.

Brainstem. The brainstem is divided into three regions: the midbrain, pons, and medulla. These regions allow nerve fibers from the spinal cord to connect with the cerebrum. Damage to the brainstem can affect cranial nerve function, which includes changes in pupil size. The midbrain controls auditory and visual responses and modulates movement. The pons connects the cerebellum to the rest of the brain and controls arousal, sleep, and autonomic functions. The medulla oblongata, the "vital sign center," regulates vasomotor tone, cardiac, and respiratory functions.

ALERT! Damage to the brainstem can cause dysfunction of all vital signs and loss of consciousness.

Cerebellum. The cerebellum is located behind the pons and medulla and is responsible for smooth, coordinated movements. It also influences posture and equilibrium. Unlike the cerebrum, damage to one side of the cerebellum affects the ipsilateral (same) side of the body. Injury to the cerebellum leads to a variety of disorders depending on the affected region. Individuals may present with slurred speech and uncoordinated movements that are jerky and slow. Others may present with an ataxic gait (uncoordinated walking). The cerebellum also plays a role in motor learning. When a motor skill is learned, such as riding a bike, the cerebellum stores this information and later provides individuals with the ability to perform the skill without having to relearn it.

The cerebellum is perfused by the branches of the posterior cerebral artery, which derives blood flow from the basilar artery. The vertebral arteries bring blood up to the basilar artery. The vertebral arteries commonly succumb to arteriosclerosis with age. With arteriosclerosis, there is decreased perfusion of the basilar artery and posterior cerebral artery. Decreased blood flow within the posterior cerebral artery causes lack of blood supply to a lobe of cerebellum, thereby causing loss of coordination and ataxia. **Vertebral-basilar insufficiency (VBI)** is the syndrome that occurs when there

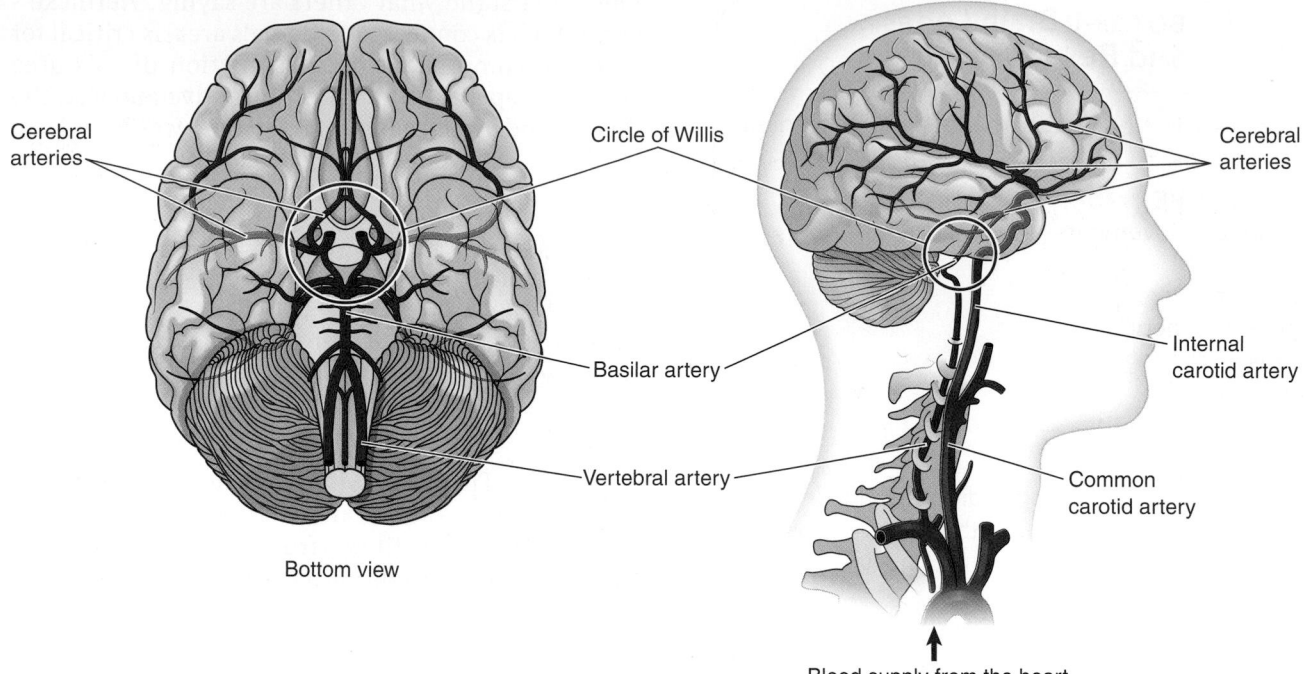

Cerebral arteries

Circle of Willis

Cerebral arteries

Basilar artery

Internal carotid artery

Vertebral artery

Common carotid artery

Bottom view

Blood supply from the heart

FIGURE 33-4. Vertebral-basilar circulation. The vertebral arteries travel up the neck, threaded through the vertical bones, and come together at the basilar artery, which flows into the circle of Willis.

is decreased vertebral and basilar artery blood flow and consequent decreased blood supply to the cerebellum (see Fig. 33-4).

Cerebrovascular Circulation

Brain cells have a high metabolic demand and require a constant supply of oxygen and nutrients. The cerebral blood supply arises from the vertebral and carotid arteries in the neck. The right and left vertebral arteries branch off the subclavian artery to supply the brain's posterior aspect. The left common carotid arises from the aortic arch; the right common carotid arises from the brachiocephalic artery. Both common carotids bifurcate to form the internal and external carotid arteries, and the right and left internal carotid arteries supply the brain's anterior and middle cerebral arteries. The anterior cerebral artery supplies the brain's frontal lobe. The middle cerebral artery supplies the lateral cortex, which is 80% of the brain's tissue. The route of the internal carotid artery into the middle cerebral artery is a common route of thrombi that reach the brain. Thrombi often arise from the aorta to the internal carotid artery, which flows into the middle cerebral artery.

The vertebral arteries are located on both posterior sides of the neck. The vertebral arteries unite to form the basilar artery, which bifurcates to form the posterior cerebral arteries. The anastomosis of the posterior cerebral arteries and the terminal branches of the internal carotids form the **circle of Willis.** Located at the base of the brain, the Circle of Willis provides collateral circulation in the event that one of the major cerebral vascular routes should occlude (see Fig. 33-5).

CLINICAL CONCEPT

The middle cerebral artery supplies a large area of brain tissue; when occluded, it causes deficit of a major region of the brain. Most strokes involve a branch of the middle cerebral artery.

ALERT! The circle of Willis is a frequent site of aneurysm formation. Aneurysms are susceptible to rupture, causing a hemorrhagic stroke.

Cranial Nerves

Cranial nerves arise from the brain and travel to places on the head, face, neck, and shoulders. There are 12 pairs of cranial nerves, numbered from I through XII, and they act as tiny antenna that sense changes in the brain. All of the cranial nerve tracts cross over to the opposite side of the body high in the brain before arising from the brainstem and connecting to their end organ. Cranial nerves that arise from the right side of the brain control the left side of the head, neck, and shoulders. Conversely, all cranial nerves that arise from the left side of the brain control the right side of the head, neck, and shoulders. The cranial nerves exit the brain tissue and come off the midbrain, pons, and medulla (see Fig. 33-6).

Cranial nerves have either motor or sensory functions; some have both. Cranial nerves are sensitive to changes in circulation of the brain and intracranial pressure. In conditions of stroke, tumor, or brain injury, the cranial nerves can become dysfunctional. When

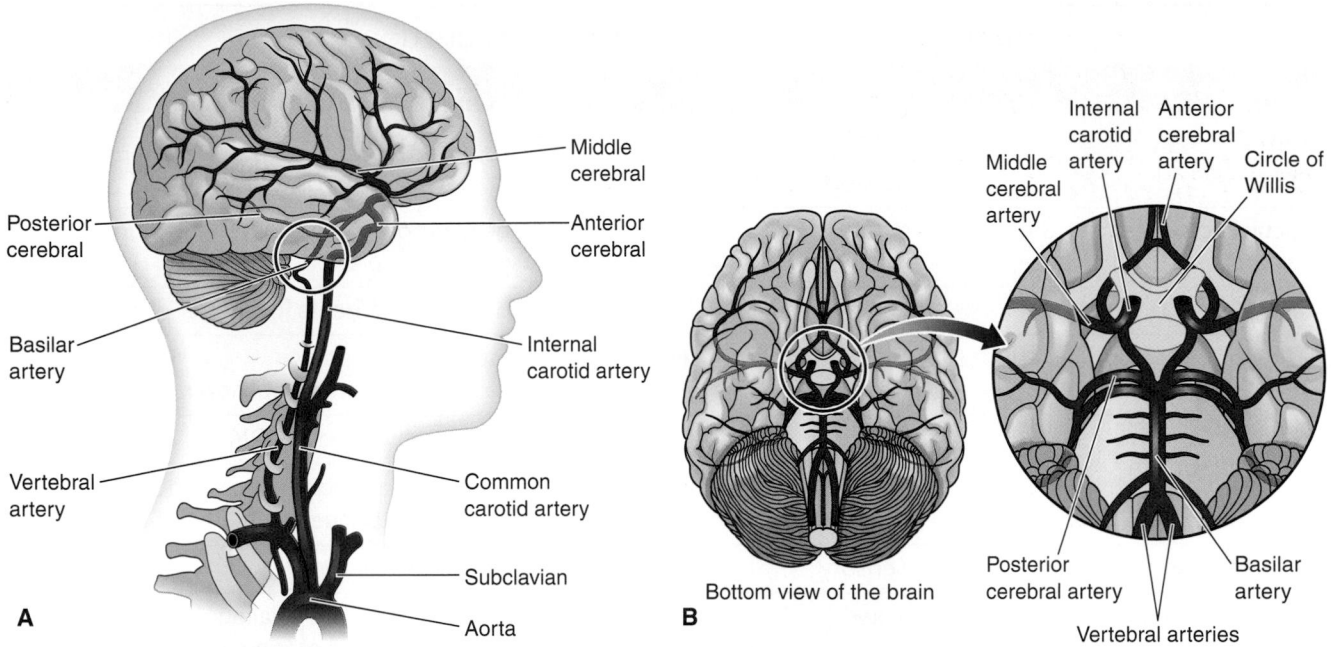

FIGURE 33-5. Circulatory routes from the neck to the brain include the internal carotid and vertebral arteries. (a) The common carotid artery divides into the internal carotid artery, which ascends into the circle of Willis. The vertebral arteries ascend up through the vertebrae and come together at the basilar artery, which flows into the circle of Willis. (b) The circle of Willis is a network of arteries at the underside of the brain. Major arteries that come off the circle of Willis include the middle cerebral artery, anterior cerebral artery, and posterior cerebral artery.

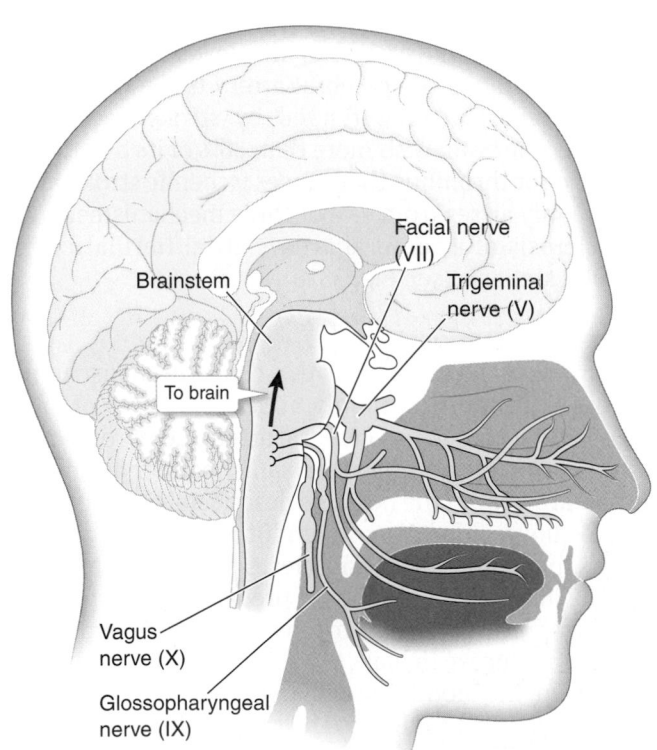

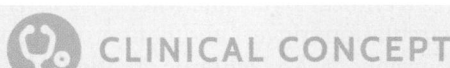

FIGURE 33-6. The cranial nerves have their origin deep in the brain. They cross over within the brain and arise off the midbrain, pons, and brainstem. They are imbedded in the brain and act as antenna that can sense changes in intracranial pressure. Symptoms of cranial nerve dysfunction can be assessed from examination of the eyes, face, mouth, throat, neck, and shoulders. Examples of the cranial nerves that come off the pons and brainstem include the trigeminal, facial, glossopharyngeal, and vagus nerves.

examining a patient, cranial nerve dysfunction commonly indicates that there is a disturbance within the opposite side of the brain. For example, when an individual suffers a stroke in the right cerebral hemisphere, there will be a left-sided facial droop caused by the dysfunction of cranial nerve VII, the facial nerve (see Table 33-1).

CLINICAL CONCEPT

Cranial nerve abnormalities are commonly a sign of increased intracranial pressure or dysfunction of a region of the brain.

Cerebral Metabolism

The brain is the most energy-consuming organ in the body, using 20% of the body's oxygen. Also, brain cells solely use glucose to function. Brain cell metabolism requires a continuous supply of oxygen and glucose. In hypoglycemic conditions, brain cells dysfunction, which can result in loss of consciousness. During times of starvation, the liver is capable of supplying the body with glucose through breakdown of glycogen and gluconeogenesis. Lack of cerebral blood flow causes cerebral hypoxia, which causes brain dysfunction. A lack of oxygen for as little as 10 seconds causes a loss of consciousness; a lack of oxygen for 5 minutes causes brain cells to die. Because brain cells are not capable of anaerobic metabolism, an alteration in oxygen supply can cause irreversible brain damage. Hypoxia or hypoglycemia can have a profound effect on the brain, often causing loss of consciousness and, in some cases, brain death.

TABLE 33-1. Cranial Nerves and Their Functions

Cranial Nerve	Type of Neuron	Basic Functions
I Olfactory	Sensory	Smell
II Optic	Sensory	Vision
III Oculomotor	Motor	Extraocular movements (EOMs) and pupil response
IV Trochlear	Motor	Extraocular movements (EOMs)
V Trigeminal	Mixed (motor and sensory)	Facial sensation Masseter muscle control of chewing
VI Abducens	Motor	Extraocular movements (EOMs)
VII Facial	Mixed (motor and sensory)	Facial expressions and taste over anterior two-thirds of tongue
VIII Auditory or Vestibulocochlear	Sensory	Hearing and equilibrium
IX Glossopharyngeal	Mixed (motor and sensory)	Elevation of pharynx in swallowing, taste over posterior one-third of tongue, and salivation
X Vagus	Mixed (motor and sensory)	Gag reflex and parasympathetic control of body
XI Accessory	Motor	Turn the head and shrug
XII Hypoglossal	Motor	Tongue movement

Basic Pathophysiologic Concepts of Cerebrovascular Disorders

A stroke is a specific type of brain injury caused by ischemia of brain tissue or hemorrhage of a cerebral blood vessel; it is a clinical syndrome whereby a disruption in cerebral circulation triggers abrupt neurological deficits that are permanent. An **ischemic stroke** is caused by a thrombus or embolus that lodges in a cerebral artery and blocks blood flow to the brain tissue. Ischemia of brain tissue leads to **cerebral infarction,** which is the death of brain cells. A **hemorrhagic stroke** is caused by rupture and hemorrhage of a cerebral artery, leading to compression of brain cells and loss of cerebral blood flow. Eighty-five percent of strokes are due to ischemia whereas 15% are hemorrhagic strokes (see Fig. 33-7).

Another kind of ischemic injury of the brain is called a **transient ischemic attack (TIA).** Many persons call this a "mini-stroke," which is an inaccurate label. A TIA is a disruption of cerebral circulation with neurological deficits that are reversible and last for fewer than 24 hours. In a TIA, the body naturally dissolves the clot that caused the ischemia, circulation returns, and there is no permanent neurological injury.

Ischemic Stroke

Ischemic strokes result from an obstruction in cerebral blood flow by a thrombus or embolus. The arterial vessels most commonly involved in ischemic stroke are the internal carotid and middle cerebral arteries. A clot commonly travels up the internal carotid artery into the middle cerebral artery and becomes lodged, causing ischemia of brain tissue. Ischemia leads to cerebral infarction. The middle cerebral artery is the most common cerebral artery affected by stroke because it supplies the brain with more than 80% of its blood flow.

A clot or thrombus that causes ischemic stroke most commonly arises from one of three mechanisms: arteriosclerosis of a cerebral artery, atrial fibrillation, or carotid stenosis (see Fig. 33-8).

Cerebral Arteriosclerosis

A thrombus is frequently the cause of an ischemic stroke. Thrombi commonly arise from areas of arteriosclerotic plaque in a cerebral artery. Cerebrovascular arteriosclerosis occurs in the same manner as any peripheral artery in the body. As described in the chapters on cardiovascular disease, endothelial injury usually starts the process of arteriosclerosis. Endothelial injury can be incited by a number of predisposing factors, including free radical injury, hypertension, hyperlipidemia, or glucose in diabetes. As arteriosclerotic plaque builds up, the blood vessel diameter decreases; this, in turn, lessens blood flow to the tissue. Alternatively, arteriosclerotic plaque often breaks and pieces of plaque become emboli. Either as a thrombus or embolus, a piece of plaque can lodge in an arteriole and obstruct blood flow. These mechanisms occur in cerebrovascular vessels, causing ischemia and infarction of brain tissue.

Atrial Fibrillation

Atrial fibrillation is another cause of ischemic stroke. In left-sided atrial fibrillation, the left atrium is quivering, not contracting sufficiently, and this leads to stasis of

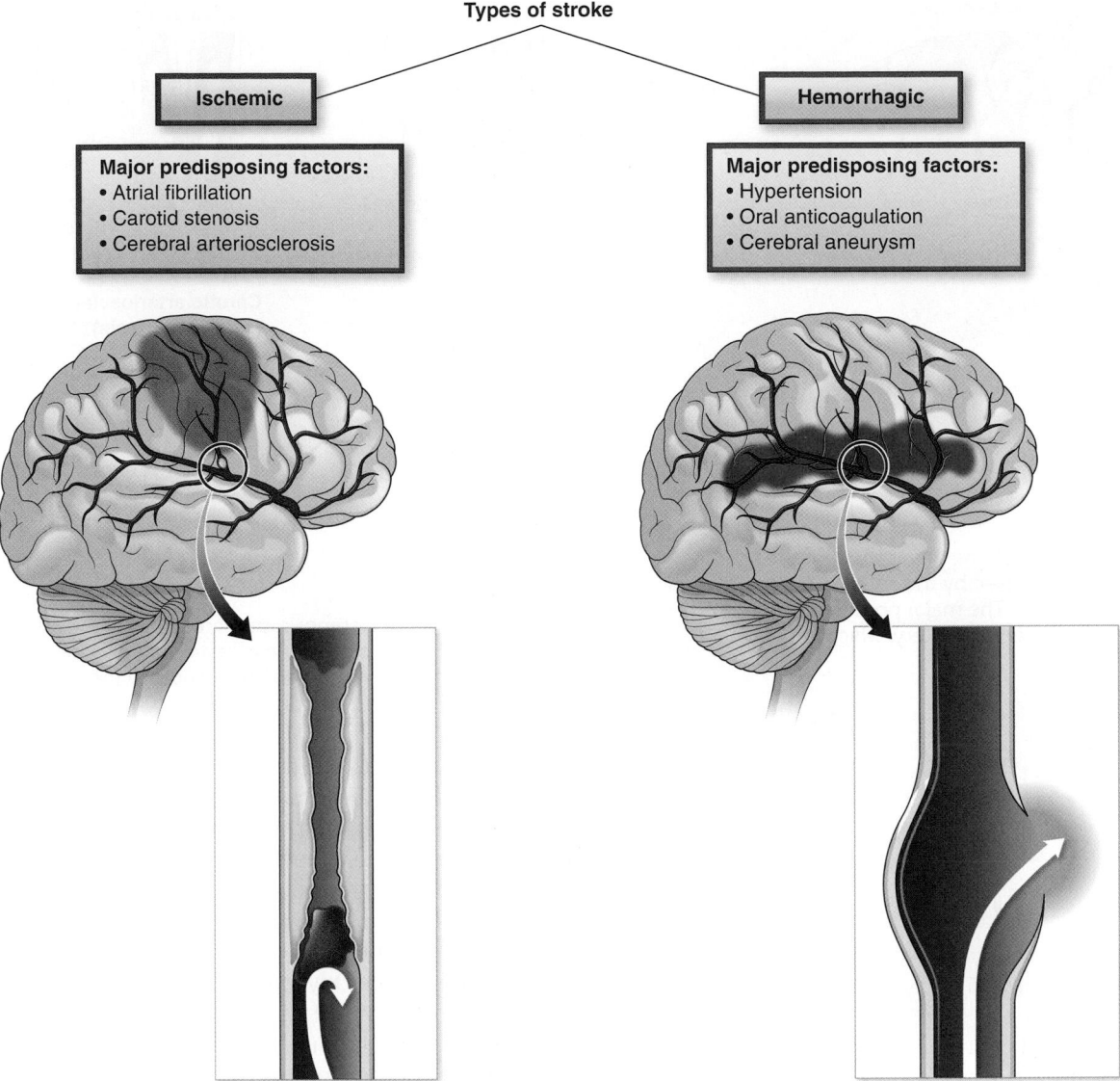

Types of stroke

Ischemic

Major predisposing factors:
• Atrial fibrillation
• Carotid stenosis
• Cerebral arteriosclerosis

Hemorrhagic

Major predisposing factors:
• Hypertension
• Oral anticoagulation
• Cerebral aneurysm

FIGURE 33-7. There are two types of stroke: ischemic and hemorrhagic. An ischemic stroke occurs when an obstruction blocks blood flow to the brain. A hemorrhagic stroke occurs when a vessel wall ruptures and bursts within the brain. Ischemic strokes are more common than hemorrhagic strokes.

blood in the chamber. Stasis of blood increases susceptibility of clot formation in the left atrium. Once formed, clots can travel from the left atrium to the left ventricle and into the aorta. From the aorta, the clot can ascend into the common carotid artery, to the internal carotid artery, and lodge in a cerebral vessel, most commonly the middle cerebral artery, which leads to brain tissue ischemia (see Fig. 33-9). If ischemia is prolonged, infarction of cerebral tissue and brain cell death occur. Brain cell death leads to loss of neurological functions; this is referred to as a **neurological deficit.** The travel of a clot from the left atrium to the brain is referred to as a **cardioembolic event.**

Carotid Stenosis
Arteriosclerosis of the carotid artery, called **carotid stenosis,** is also a common cause of ischemic stroke. In arteriosclerosis of the carotid artery, the lumen of the carotid artery narrows from plaque buildup. Normally, the endothelial lining of the carotid artery is smooth

and blood cells travel unencumbered. With carotid artery stenosis, the once smooth endothelial surface becomes irregular because of accumulated plaque. This rough surface promotes platelet adherence and aggregation, which leads to thrombus formation. Once formed, clots can stay in the narrowed carotid artery and cause obstruction of blood up to the brain. Alternatively, a clot can dislodge and travel up into a cerebral artery. Either scenario leads to obstructed blood flow to the brain and ischemic stroke (see Fig. 33-10).

ALERT! Left atrial fibrillation and carotid stenosis are the most common causes of ischemic stroke.

Ischemia and Ischemic Penumbra
Cerebral ischemia often occurs gradually and symptoms are progressive. The process of ischemia can appear over several hours and progress to maximal deficit

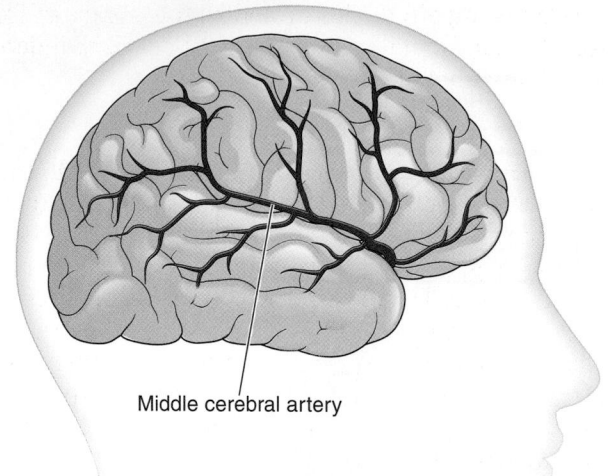

FIGURE 33-8. Parietal view of one hemisphere of the brain. Note the areas that are perfused by the anterior, posterior, and middle cerebral arteries. The major portion of the brain is perfused by the middle cerebral artery, which is involved in most strokes.

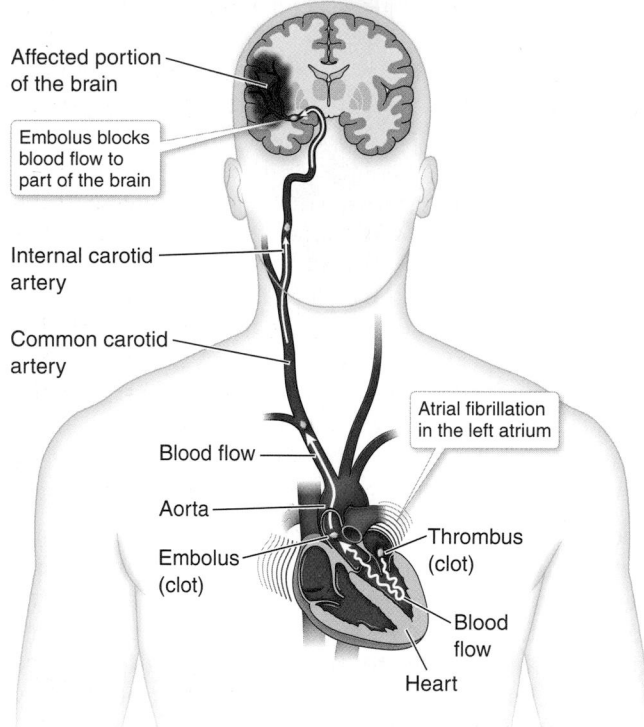

FIGURE 33-9. A thromboembolism can develop in the left atrium with atrial fibrillation. The clot travels from the left atrium to the left ventricle and up through the carotid artery to the middle cerebral artery. It then lodges in the middle cerebral artery and causes ischemia of the brain region.

over several days. The core area of tissue ischemia can increase over time. The survival of this area of ischemia is dependent upon collateral circulation and the length of time that the tissue is ischemic. Restoration of blood flow to the area is critical and can reverse some of the

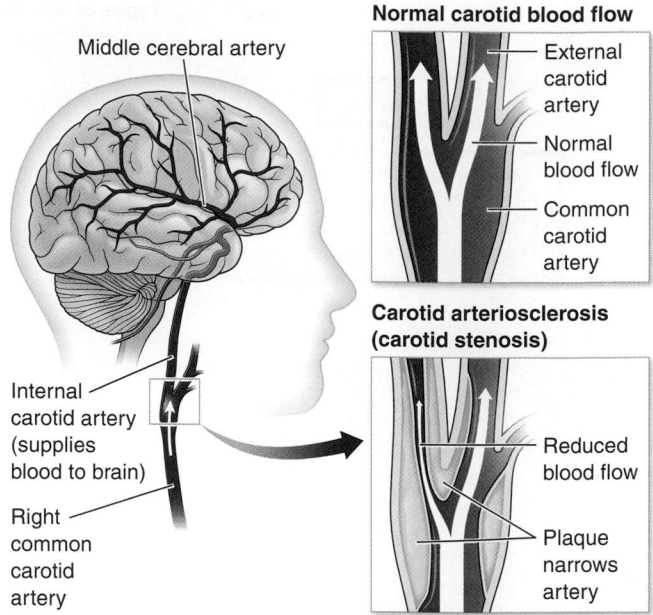

FIGURE 33-10. In carotid stenosis, the carotid artery is narrowed because of buildup of arteriosclerotic plaque. A piece of plaque or a clot can break off and travel up into the middle cerebral artery and cause ischemic stroke.

neurological dysfunction. Failure to restore blood flow results in the tissue becoming infarcted with consequent brain cell death. As the brain cells die, they are replaced by scar tissue called neuroglia (gliosis).

When a cerebral artery is occluded, cerebral perfusion pressure is diminished. Autoregulation of cerebral circulation is nonfunctional and is not able to restore blood flow to the area. Oxygen deprivation allows neurons in the core area of ischemia to progress to irreversible cerebral infarction in minutes. However, brain cells that lie at the perimeter of the stroke region are hypoperfused but are not irreversibly damaged. The perimeter around the core ischemic area is called the **ischemic penumbra.** The rapid reperfusion of this area is critical because, if left untreated, the penumbra will also succumb to ischemia and infarction.

Within the ischemic penumbra and surrounding brain tissue, cerebral edema occurs, which also contributes to hypoperfusion and further damage of brain cells. Lack of circulation causes lack of oxygen delivery to the brain tissue; this leads to a condition called **anoxic encephalopathy,** which causes decreased levels of consciousness. In cerebral edema, swelling brain cells are enclosed by the cranial bone with little room for expansion. Pressure that builds within the skull is directed downward toward the foramen magnum, the area where the spinal cord enters the brainstem. If cerebral edema causes pressure on the brainstem, the individual's level of consciousness and vital signs are affected, and there is potential for death (see Fig. 33-11). Pressure on the brainstem causes detrimental changes in respiratory rate, blood pressure, heart rate, and level of consciousness. The patient has a diminished level of consciousness with irregular respiratory rate, bradycardia, and hypertension. These changes in respiratory function,

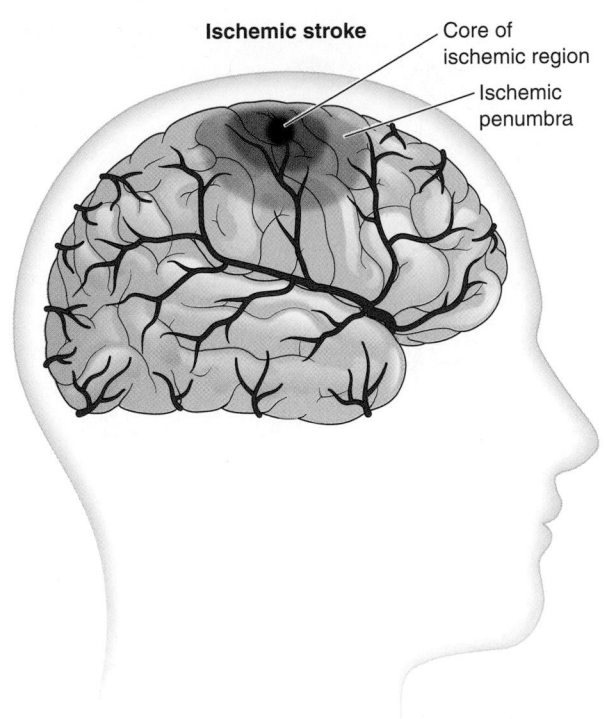

Ischemic stroke   Core of ischemic region

Ischemic penumbra

FIGURE 33-11. In ischemic stroke, there is a central core where the clot lodges and damages brain tissue. It is surrounded by the ischemic penumbra, which is brain tissue that is salvageable if reperfused.

heart rate, and blood pressure are known as **Cushing's triad**; when present, they are an ominous finding.

Glutamate

Neuronal injury has reversible and irreversible changes. Early changes involve the failure of cellular ion pumps. Movement of potassium across the cell membrane alters cell membrane action potentials. This causes depolarization of neuronal membranes and increased calcium ion influx. With this depolarization, there is increased release of neurotransmitters, such as glutamate, into the synaptic space.

Ischemia impairs cellular metabolism and leads to excessive glutamate receptor stimulation in the ischemic penumbra. Glutamate, an abundant excitatory neurotransmitter, opens cation channels and causes an influx of Na+ and Ca++, which is necessary for postsynaptic potentials to occur. Normally, the signaling for the uptake of Na+ and Ca++ is terminated by the synaptic reuptake of glutamate; increased intracellular levels of Na+ and Ca++ then return to normal. However, if the process is not reversed, persistent elevation of intracellular Ca++ activates degradative enzymes and results in cell death. During a stroke, ischemia impairs the normal mechanism for the removal of glutamate from the synapse. Sustained elevations of extracellular glutamate increase intracellular Ca++, lead to cellular death, and extend the stroke region (see Fig. 33-12). Progression to cellular death occurs through irreversible neuronal injury. As part of the process, mitochondrial

function is impaired. This promotes the release of free radicals that further alter cellular functions and damage cell membranes.

Transient Ischemic Attack

Approximately 50,000 Americans experience TIAs each year. TIAs were once considered benign events, but it is now understood that they are true medical emergencies that may signal impending stroke, with an estimated 20% to 25% of TIAs progressing to stroke. Therefore, rapid assessment and early intervention are imperative.

In TIAs, individuals present with temporary neurological symptoms that can last for several minutes to hours. In the past, TIAs lasting longer than 24 hours without interruption were termed reversible ischemic neurological deficits (RINDs). This term is no longer used. TIAs, as the name implies, are transient; neurological deficits commonly completely resolve within an hour. They are commonly caused by an embolus, which may arise from a clot that forms in an atherosclerotic lumen that suddenly dislodges, causing arterial occlusion. This leads to tissue anoxia and clinical presentation that is similar to stroke. However, in TIAs, the body's fibrinolytic system dissolves the occlusion and the focal deficits disappear in fewer than 24 hours.

A TIA may be most noticeable to bystanders, but not to the person enduring the transient neurological impairment. Confusion, disorientation, inability to communicate, and memory impairment affect the patient. Therefore, patients who report to the emergency room with signs of TIA are commonly brought in by another person. Often a TIA is resolved by the time the patient presents to the emergency department.

Small vessels in the brain can become occluded causing small areas of ischemic brain damage that often cause no major symptoms. Small areas in the brain that endure ischemia from occluded tiny blood vessels are called **lacunar infarcts**. These extremely small infarcts in the brain are often associated with hypertension, smoking, and diabetes.

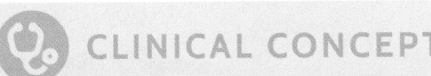

CLINICAL CONCEPT

To encourage individuals to seek immediate treatment, TIA is sometimes referred to as "brain attack." Lay persons also refer to them as mini-strokes.

Hemorrhagic Stroke. Hemorrhagic stroke occurs when a cerebral artery ruptures and can no longer bring blood to the brain tissue. The cerebral artery is commonly a branch of the middle cerebral artery deep within the brain tissue. A specific type of cerebral hemorrhage occurs when an arterial branch in the subarachnoid space ruptures; this event, called a **subarachnoid hemorrhage**, may be the result of head trauma or aneurysm rupture. The most common sites for cerebral aneurysm

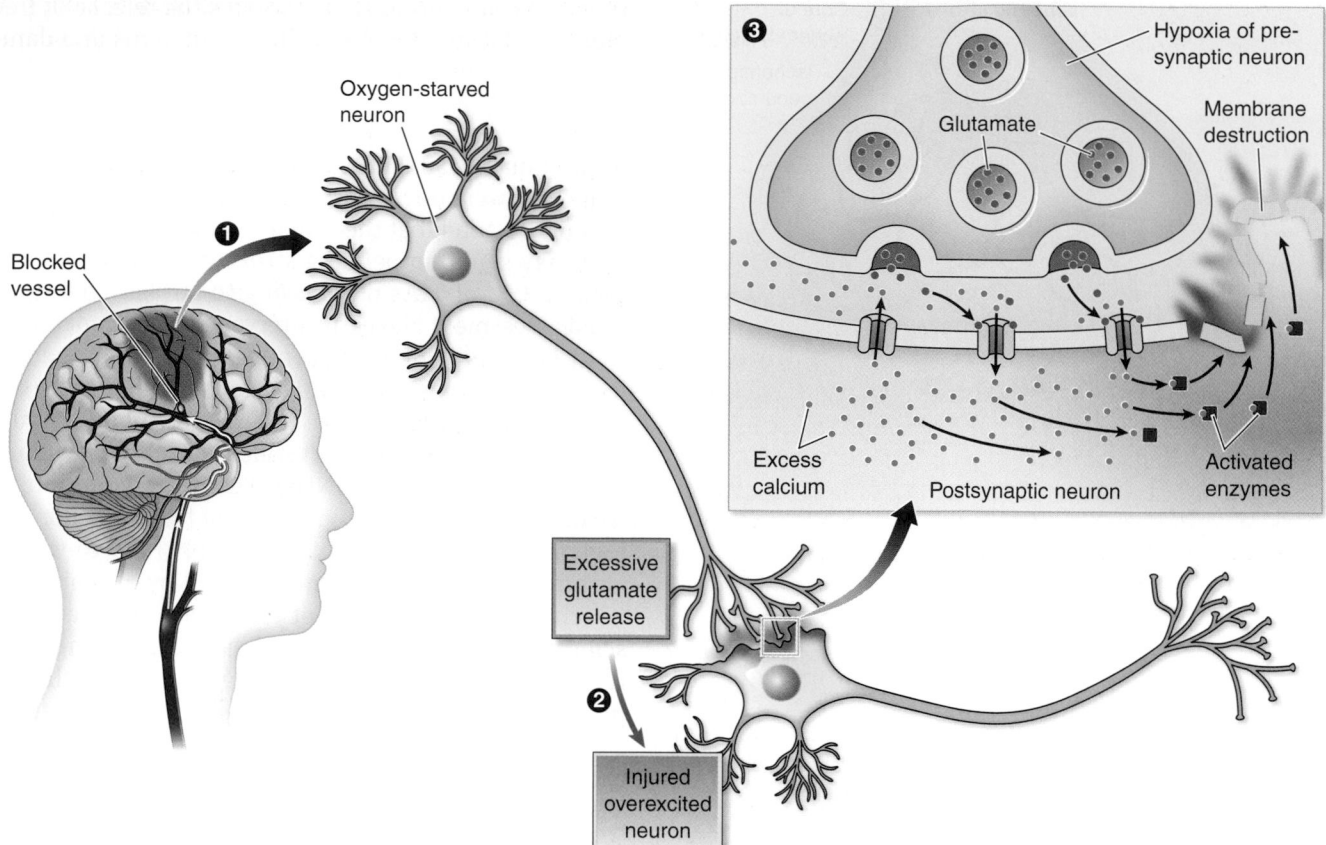

FIGURE 33-12. The effect of glutamate in ischemic stroke. (1) In ischemia, the hypoxic brain cells release excess glutamate. (2) The excess glutamate causes over-excitation of the postsynaptic neurons and triggers an influx of calcium. (3). This influx of calcium causes activation of enzymatic degeneration of brain cells.

are in those arteries that make up the circle of Willis within the subarachnoid space (see Fig. 33-13). An arteriovenous malformation (AVM) can also lead to the development of intracerebral bleeding. An AVM is a congenital abnormality that connects an artery with a vein within the brain tissue.

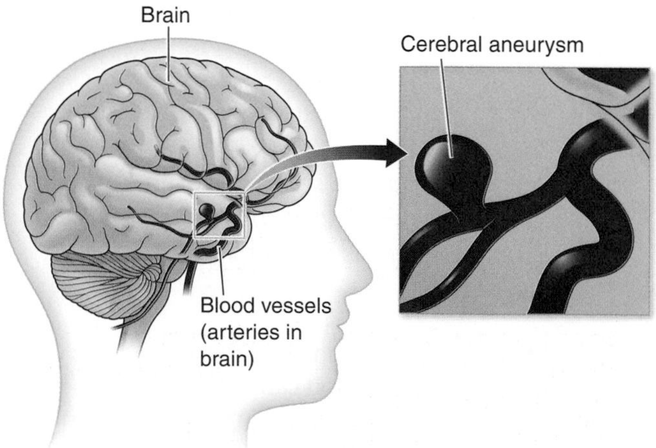

A hemorrhagic stroke is often caused by rupture of a large branch of the middle cerebral artery and creates severe brain damage. The major predisposing factor of hemorrhagic stroke is hypertension. A cerebral artery ruptures from excessive pressure and blood leaks into the brain, causing cerebral edema, increased intracranial pressure, and tissue destruction.

ALERT! A cerebral bleed can lead to brainstem herniation and death.

After rupture of a cerebral artery, blood flows into the brain tissue where it becomes compressed and often displaced. This compression leads to tissue ischemia and cerebral edema. Vasospasm of adjacent blood vessels occurs from exposure to blood, which subjects adjacent tissue to ischemia. In addition, the blood is chemically toxic to the brain cells. After a few days, the arterial bleeding ceases and a clot forms in the area of the bleed. As the clot resolves, the body reabsorbs the blood and it becomes smaller in size.

The recruitment of macrophages occurs as part of the physiologic and inflammatory response. The macrophages phagocytize both the hemorrhagic and

FIGURE 33-13. A cerebral aneurysm is a weakening in the wall of an artery that is susceptible to rupture. If the aneurysm ruptures it causes a cerebral hemorrhage. Cerebral aneurysms often develop on the circle of Willis in the brain. Because they resemble berries hanging off a tree, they are commonly called "berry aneurysms."

ischemic areas. The area is liquefied and a cavity is formed. Astrocytes form scar tissue that fills in the cavity.

Assessment of Cerebrovascular Disease

The risk factors for stroke are similar to those for cardiovascular disease. These include age greater than 65 years, male gender, arteriosclerosis, hyperlipidemia, diabetes mellitus, alcohol abuse, hypertension, smoking, obesity, and family history. African Americans, Hispanic Americans, and Native Americans have a higher rate of stroke than Caucasian Americans. The use of oral contraceptives is an additional risk factor, specifically for ischemic stroke, because oral contraceptives increase susceptibility to thrombus formation. Individuals with sickle cell disease are at increased risk for stroke because of possible vasoocclusive episodes in cerebral vessels (see Box 33-2).

Signs and Symptoms

Patients who suffer either ischemic or hemorrhagic stroke present with similar signs and symptoms. Because both types of stroke cause damage to the brain, neurological deficits are demonstrated. The area of the brain perfused by the middle cerebral artery is the most common region affected in either type of stroke.

In either kind of stroke, neurons within the left or right hemisphere become injured and die. Because of the anatomical crossover of nerve tracts at the medulla, patients present with neurological symptoms on the contralateral side of the cerebral hemisphere that is injured. Eighty percent of upper motor neurons cross over to the contralateral side of the body. However, 20% of the neurons remain on the ipsilateral side

---

BOX 33-2. Risk Factors for Stroke

The risk factors for stroke are similar to the risk factors for arteriosclerosis, coronary artery disease, and peripheral arterial disease.

- **High blood pressure:** High blood pressure, also called hypertension, can greatly increase the risk for stroke. Smoking cigarettes, eating a diet high in salt, and drinking too much alcohol can all raise blood pressure.
- **High blood cholesterol:** High blood cholesterol can build up fatty deposits (plaque) on blood vessel walls. These deposits can block blood flow to the brain, causing a stroke. Diet, exercise, and family history affect blood cholesterol levels.
- **Heart disease:** Common heart disorders can increase the risk for stroke. For example, coronary artery disease increases risk because plaque blocks the arteries that bring blood to the heart. Other heart conditions, such as heart valve defects; irregular heartbeat, including atrial fibrillation; and enlarged heart chambers, can cause blood clots that may break loose and cause a stroke.
- **Diabetes:** Having diabetes can increase risk of stroke and can make the outcome of strokes worse. The high blood glucose of uncontrolled diabetes causes endothelial injury and accelerates arteriosclerosis. Also high blood sugar tends to occur with high blood pressure and high cholesterol.
- **Overweight and obesity:** Being overweight or obese can raise total cholesterol levels, increase blood pressure, and promote the development of diabetes.
- **Previous stroke or transient ischemic attack (TIA):** If the patient has already had a stroke or a TIA, there is a greater chance that he or she could have a stroke in the future.
- **Sickle cell disease:** This is a blood disorder associated with ischemic stroke that mainly affects African American children. A stroke can happen if sickle cells get stuck in a blood vessel and clog blood flow to the brain. About 10% of children with sickle cell disease will have a stroke.
- **Tobacco use:** Smoking injures blood vessels and speeds up the hardening of the arteries. The carbon monoxide in cigarette smoke reduces the amount of oxygen blood can carry. Secondhand smoke can increase the risk of stroke for nonsmokers.
- **Alcohol use:** Drinking too much alcohol raises blood pressure, which increases the risk for stroke. It also increases levels of triglycerides, a form of cholesterol, which can harden arteries.
- **Physical inactivity:** Not getting enough exercise can lead to weight gain, which can lead to increased blood pressure and cholesterol levels. Inactivity also is a risk factor for diabetes.
- **Oral contraceptives:** Estrogenic component of oral contraceptives can increase susceptibility to clotting.
- **Family history:** Having a family history of stroke increases the chance of stroke.
- **Age and gender:** Stroke risk increases with age. For ages 65 years and older, men are at greater risk than women to have a stroke.
- **Race and ethnicity:** African Americans, Hispanic Americans, and American Indian/Alaska Natives have a greater chance of having a stroke than do non-Hispanic whites or Asian Americans.

(Adapted from Centers for Disease Control and Prevention. (2013). *Stroke: risk factors.* Retrieved from http://www.cdc.gov/stroke/risk_factors.htm.)

of the hemisphere. For example, patients who suffer ischemia in the left cerebral hemisphere will exhibit weakness or paralysis on the right side of the body. However, the patient has use of the 20% of ipsilateral neurons on the right side of the body that are retrained during the rehabilitation period (see Fig. 33-14).

Stroke manifestations occur as neurological deficits on one side of the body. Common symptoms of stroke include slurred speech, loss of gag reflex, facial droop, hemiparesis (weakness of extremities on one side of the body) or hemiplegia (paralysis; complete loss of function of extremities on one side of the body), vision loss in one or both eyes, and loss of sensation. Some patients have disorientation, confusion, and sleepiness, which can become stupor or coma.

Aphasia, a language disorder whereby individuals are unable to speak or understand the spoken word, is also a common presentation. In the majority of the population, language is a function of the left hemisphere. Two of the areas most critical for language that are usually found in the left hemisphere are Broca's area and Wernicke's area. Ischemic damage to the left hemisphere often results in aphasia. Damage to Broca's area usually causes expressive aphasia, whereas damage to Wernicke's area causes receptive aphasia. In expressive aphasia, individuals are unable to form words but can understand others. In receptive aphasia, however, individuals are unable to understand spoken words.

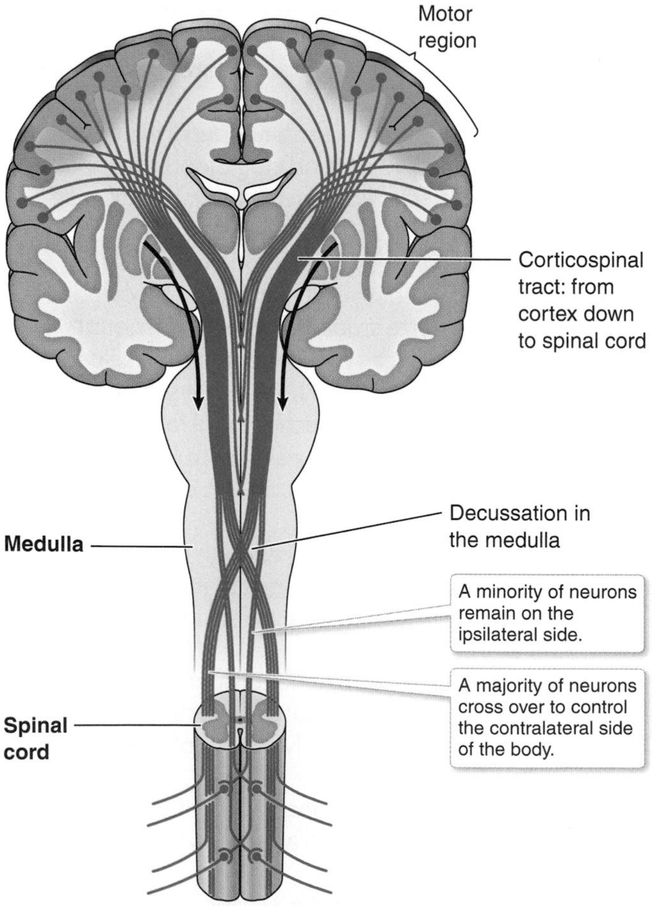

CLINICAL CONCEPT

The American Heart Association and American Stroke Association suggest using the acronym FAST to recognize signs of a stroke:

Facial droop
Arm weakness
Speech difficulty
Time to call 911.

Diagnosis

Any patient with a sudden change in neurological function should be assessed for a TIA or stroke. There is no reliable clinical presentation to distinguish between cerebral ischemia or hemorrhage. However, a slow progression of one-sided weakness or sensory loss and slurring of speech are more characteristic of ischemic stroke. Sudden headache, elevated blood pressure, and a depressed level of consciousness are more indicative of a hemorrhagic stroke.

Patient assessment needs to include neurological and cardiovascular examinations. This includes auscultation of carotid arteries for bruits, blood pressure in both arms, and ophthalmoscopic examination of the retina for changes associated with hypertension, such as arteriovenous nicking. Diagnostic testing needs to include electrocardiography, chest x-ray, blood work, and brain imaging studies. This testing should rule out other pathological processes with symptoms that could mimic stroke, such as hypoglycemia, hyperglycemia, vasculitis, migraine, seizure disorders, metabolic encephalopathy, recent head trauma, and tumors.

Computed Tomography

CT scans without contrast are often preferred during the acute phase of the stroke (see Fig. 33-15). The importance of CT scan is to identify or exclude hemorrhage as the etiology of the stroke. Once hemorrhage is eliminated, thrombolytic therapy can be given.

Cerebral ischemia may not be evident during the first 24 hours of the stroke. The use of contrast dye with CT scan can allow better visualization of ischemia. CT scans are also helpful in identifying the presence of abscesses, neoplasms, or other conditions that may mimic stroke symptoms.

Magnetic Resonance Angiography

Magnetic resonance angiography (MRA) can distinguish between cerebral hemorrhage and ischemia. The

FIGURE 33-14. The neurons of the corticospinal tract are motor neurons. The majority of corticospinal neurons cross at the medulla to the contralateral side of the spinal cord to control the opposite side of the body, but a minority of corticospinal neurons remain ipsilateral to control the same side of the body. The corticospinal tract is also called the pyramidal tract. The region of cross-over is called the decussation.

Motor region

Corticospinal tract: from cortex down to spinal cord

Medulla

Decussation in the medulla

A minority of neurons remain on the ipsilateral side.

A majority of neurons cross over to control the contralateral side of the body.

Spinal cord

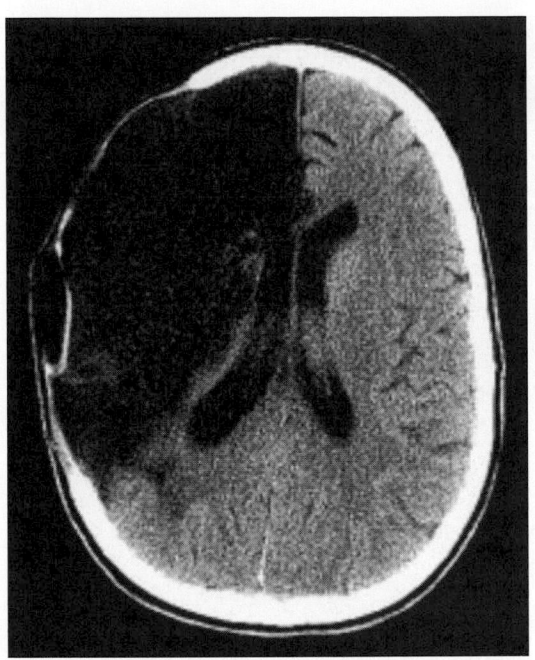

FIGURE 33-15. A CT scan showing stroke. *(From Science Source.)*

MRA can be used to determine the presence of a clot or aneurysm. Additional applications of MRA include diagnosing severe carotid artery occlusions.

National Institutes of Health Stroke Scale

The National Institutes of Health Stroke Scale (NIHSS) was developed as a way to quantify deficits attributed to a stroke and track the progress of treatment. The NIHSS is a graded neurological examination that evaluates visual fields, ataxia, speech, language, cognition, and motor and sensory function (see Table 33-2). Each section has a graded point scale based on level of function. The points are then added for a total score. Essentially, the higher the score, the greater the neurological deficit. A range of scores correlate with the patient's clinical presentation.

When the NIHSS score is used in combination with the size of the damaged area, as measured by the diffusion weighted imaging MRI (DWI-MRI), it is possible to assess the severity of stroke and identify the patients who have the greatest potential for recovery.

TABLE 33-2. National Institutes of Health Stroke Scale		
Category	**Scale**	**Score**
1A. LEVEL OF CONSCIOUSNESS (LOC) (alert, drowsy, etc.)	0 = alert 1 = drowsy 2 = not alert 3 = responds only with reflex motor or autonomic effects or totally unresponsive, flaccid, or areflexic	——
1B. LOC QUESTIONS (month, age)	0 = answers both correctly 1 = answers one correctly 2 = answers neither correctly	——
1C. LOC COMMANDS (open/close eyes; make fist/let go)	0 = performs both correctly 1 = performs one correctly 2 = performs neither correctly	——
2. BEST GAZE (eyes open, patient follows examiner's finger or face)	0 = normal 1 = partial gaze palsy 2 = forced deviation	——
3. VISUAL (introduce visual stimulus/threat to patient's visual field quadrants)	0 = no visual loss 1 = partial hemianopia 2 = complete hemianopia 3 = bilateral hemianopia	——
4. FACIAL PALSY (show teeth, raise eyebrows, squeeze eyes shut)	0 = normal 1 = minor paralysis 2 = partial paralysis 3 = complete paralysis	——
5A. MOTOR ARM, LEFT **5B. MOTOR ARM, RIGHT** (elevate arm to 90° if patient is sitting; 45° if patient is supine)	0 = no drift 1 = drift 2 = some effort against gravity 3 = no effort against gravity 4 = no movement	—— ——

Continued

TABLE 33-2. National Institutes of Health Stroke Scale–cont'd

Category	Scale	Score
6A. MOTOR LEG, LEFT 6B. MOTOR LEG, RIGHT (elevate leg 30° with patient supine)	0 = no drift 1 = drift 2 = some effort against gravity 3 = no effort against gravity 4 = no movement UN = amputation	_____ _____
7. LIMB ATAXIA (finger-nose; heel down shin)	0 = absent 1 = present in one limb 2 = present in two limbs UN = amputation	_____
8. SENSORY (pin prick to face, arm, trunk, and leg–compare side-to-side)	0 = normal 1 = mild-to-moderate sensory loss 2 = severe to total sensory loss	_____
9. BEST LANGUAGE (name item, describe a picture, read sentences)	0 = no aphasia 1 = mild-to-moderate aphasia 2 = severe aphasia 3 = mute, global aphasia	_____
10. DYSARTHRIA (evaluate speech clarity by patient repeating listed words)	0 = normal 1 = mild-to-moderate dysarthria 2 = severe dysarthria UN = physical barrier	_____
11. EXTINCTION AND INATTENTION (use information from prior testing to identify neglect or double simultaneous stimuli testing)	0 = no abnormality 1 = visual, tactile, auditory, spatial, or personal inattention 2 = profound hemi-inattention or extinction to more than one modality	_____

Score Range	Level of Neurological Impairment
Fewer than 5	Mild impairment
Between 5 and 15	Mild to moderate impairment
Between 15 and 25	Moderately severe impairment
Greater than 25	Very severe impairment

(Adapted from National Institutes of Health, NIH Stroke Scale. Retrieved from http://www.ninds.nih.gov/doctors/NIH_Stroke_Scale.pdf; Adams, H. P., Jr., Davis, P. H., Leira, E. C., et al. (1999). Baseline NIH Stroke Scale score strongly predicts outcome after stroke: A report of the Trial of Org 10172 in Acute Stroke Treatment (TOAST). *Neurology, 53*(1), 126–131.)

The DWI-MRI is an excellent tool that can detect small, evolving ischemic and infarcted areas. In addition to the NIHSS score and size of the ischemic or infarcted area, the time since the onset of symptoms is taken into account when assessing a patient. This information is combined into a 7-point scale. The best outcome is associated with scores of 5, 6, and 7, with 87% recovering. Scores of 3 and 4 have a 57% recovery rate. Only 7% of those with scores between 0 and 2 recover.

Treatment

Treatments differ for ischemic stroke and hemorrhagic stroke. Therefore, rapid diagnosis of the type of stroke that is occurring is extremely important for correct treatment initiation. A CT scan should be performed as soon as the patient enters the health-care facility. A DWI-MRI is a superior imaging device for identifying ischemic stroke; however, many medical settings do not have this technology. Once the CT scan or MRI determines whether there is an ischemic or hemorrhagic condition of the brain, rapid delivery of treatment can facilitate recovery.

Treatment begins with stabilization to prevent further brain injury. It is important to maintain a patent airway and to stabilize blood pressure and cardiac rhythm. Regulation of body temperature and blood glucose levels is also important. Blood glucose levels should be maintained below 200 mg/dL, whereas blood pressure should be maintained less than 130/80 mm Hg.

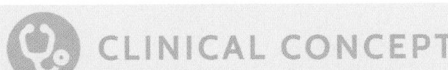 CLINICAL CONCEPT

After stroke, blood pressure should be slowly lowered if hypertension is present.

Treatment for Ischemic Stroke

Treatment for acute ischemic stroke utilizes intravenous thrombolysis, which dissolves the clot that is blocking arterial blood flow and allows for reperfusion to occur. It is important that this thrombolytic therapy be administered within 3-4.5 hours of symptom onset, because this provides the best chance for patient recovery and survival. Ideally, thrombolysis within 60 minutes shows best results. Studies show that for every 15-minute reduction of door-to-needle time, there is a 5% lower odds of in-hospital mortality.

Recombinant tissue-type plasminogen activator (rt-PA), often called a "clot-buster," is the thrombolytic agent most often used. Intravenous administration of rt-PA rapidly dissolves the clot that is causing the ischemia of brain tissue. However, not all ischemic stroke patients are candidates for rt-PA. There is a strict protocol that excludes patients who have a specific set of conditions, which includes susceptibility to bleeding. Despite following strict protocols, studies show 1 in 15 individuals develop hemorrhagic bleeds after thrombolytic treatment. It is important to identify the patients who will benefit the most from thrombolytic therapy. There are specific contraindications to thrombolytic therapy (see Box 33-3). If a patient receives rt-PA, there is a waiting period of 24 hours before long-term anticoagulant medication can be initiated.

Patients are usually treated with aspirin or another antiplatelet aggregation drug in the acute phase of ischemic stroke. Some patients are candidates for surgical thrombectomy, which is the mechanical removal of a clot from the occluded artery. A catheter called a stent-retriever can directly break up a clot and allow cerebral blood flow to resume. Thrombectomy is used on eligible patients who have persistent vessel occlusion despite treatment with IV rt-PA.

During the poststroke recovery, rehabilitation is initiated in an attempt to train neurons to develop new pathways for movement of extremities, maintain proper body alignment, and prevent muscle atrophy. Behavior modifications such as low cholesterol diet, smoking cessation, and weight loss are recommended. Antilipidemic medications such as statin drugs are usually prescribed to keep cholesterol levels low. Antiplatelet aggregators such as aspirin may be prescribed. Alternatively, anticoagulants such as warfarin (Coumadin) may be prescribed. Instead of warfarin, newer agents, such as Dabigatran (Pradaxa), Rivaroxaban (Xarelto), Apixaban (Eliquis), or Edoxaban (Savaysa) are easier to use for long term management of patients with ischemic stroke. These newer agents do not need monitoring and have more predictable therapeutic effects.

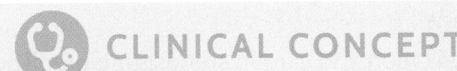 CLINICAL CONCEPT

Thrombolytic therapy has shown to be most effective if administered within 60 minutes of the onset of stroke symptoms.

Treatment for Cerebral Hemorrhage

Cerebral hemorrhage commonly occurs rapidly with associated loss of consciousness. Treatment involves first establishing hemodynamic stabilization. Intubation is commonly initiated with hyperventilation. Often intravenous mannitol or hypertonic saline is used to reduce cerebral edema. Reversal of any pre-existing anticoagulation is required. Blood pressure should be normalized and monitored. The patient's prognosis is dependent on the size of the hemorrhage.

Intracerebral hemorrhage can be surgically treated according to a strict protocol. There are various criteria used to establish that an intracerebral hemorrhage can be surgically treated. Patient age, comorbid conditions, size and location of the hemorrhage, and timing of the hemorrhage are involved in the decision to use surgery. Surgical procedures include craniotomy and hematoma evacuation under direct visual guidance. Also, endovascular therapy using coil embolization or microsurgical clipping of a cerebral aneurysm has shown to be effective. For surgical treatment, the cerebral vessel has to be in a location that is surgically accessible.

BOX 33-3. Thrombolytic Contraindications in Ischemic Stroke

Generally, thrombolytic drugs will not be given if the patient has:

- recent head injury
- bleeding problems
- bleeding ulcers
- pregnancy
- recent surgery
- taken blood-thinning medications such as Coumadin
- trauma
- uncontrolled high blood pressure.

Chapter Summary

- There are two major kinds of stroke: ischemic and hemorrhagic.
- Ischemic stroke is caused by a thrombus or embolus that lodges and obstructs cerebral blood flow.
- Hemorrhagic stroke is caused by rupture and bleeding of a cerebral artery within the brain.
- The most common cerebral artery affected by stroke is the middle cerebral artery.
- Ischemic stroke is often caused by an embolus that travels from the common carotid artery into the internal carotid artery to the middle cerebral artery.
- Ischemia of the cerebellum can be caused by vertebral-basilar arterial insufficiency.
- Hemorrhagic stroke is often caused by rupture of a cerebral aneurysm.
- Cerebral aneurysms are most commonly found on the circle of Willis within the subarachnoid space.
- A subarachnoid hemorrhage is a type of cerebral hemorrhage.
- African Americans, Hispanic Americans, and Native Americans have a higher risk of stroke than Caucasian Americans.
- Atrial fibrillation and carotid stenosis are predisposing factors for ischemic stroke.
- Hypertension is the major predisposing factor for hemorrhagic stroke.

- The motor neurons that originate in the brain and travel down into the spinal cord are within the corticospinal tract.
- The neurons of the corticospinal tract cross over at the decussation in the medulla.
- Ischemic or hemorrhagic injury of one side of the brain causes symptoms on the contralateral side of the body.
- One-sided weakness, loss of sensation of one extremity, facial droop, and slurring of speech are common signs of stroke.
- A transient ischemic attack (TIA) is a stroke-like syndrome that lasts minutes to hours and then resolves.
- A TIA is a major risk factor for stroke.
- A computed tomography scan is a diagnostic test that is required to differentiate an ischemic stroke from a hemorrhagic stroke.
- Early treatment can salvage the neurons within the ischemic penumbra in an ischemic stroke.
- Recombinant tissue plasminogen activator (rt-PA) is a thrombolytic agent that can be used to dissolve the thrombus in some patients with ischemic stroke.
- There are eligibility criteria and a 4 1/2 hour time frame in which rt-PA can be administered.
- Surgical thrombectomy is being increasingly used on eligible patients with ischemic stroke.

 ## Making the Connections

Disorder and Pathophysiology	Signs and Symptoms	Physical Assessment Findings	Diagnostic Testing	Treatment

Ischemic Stroke | An area of the brain undergoes ischemia and infarction.

Two main etiologies: (1) A thromboembolism commonly causes obstruction of a branch of a cerebral artery. Commonly, a piece of arteriosclerotic plaque breaks away from an area of carotid artery stenosis and travels up to a branch of the middle cerebral artery. (2) The left atrium undergoes atrial fibrillation with stasis of blood and clot formation. The clot travels from the left atrium into the left ventricle into the aorta and upward into the carotid artery into a cerebral artery.

| | Motor and sensory loss is evident on the opposite side of the body than the cerebral hemisphere undergoing the ischemia. Hemiparesis (weakness) or hemiplegia (paralysis) is observed. If the left hemisphere undergoes ischemia, most of those affected will suffer aphasia. | Hemiparesis or hemiplegia of limbs is observed on the opposite side of the cerebral hemisphere affected. Sensation is diminished on one side of body. Speech problems are evident if the cerebral ischemia is of the left hemisphere. | CT scan without contrast or MRI demonstrates area of injury. | Thrombolytic is administered if the ischemic stroke began fewer than 4.5 hours ago and the patient is eligible. Aspirin is given with anticoagulants to prevent further damage. Some patients are eligible for surgical thrombectomy. |

Continued

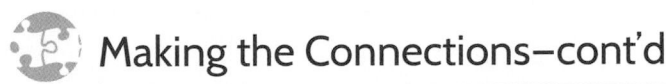

Making the Connections–cont'd

Disorder and Pathophysiology	Signs and Symptoms	Physical Assessment Findings	Diagnostic Testing	Treatment
Lacunar Infarct | Small blood vessel infarction associated with hypertension.				
	No symptoms or evidence of neurological changes are present.	No symptoms or evidence of neurological changes are evident.	CT scan or magnetic resonance imaging (MRI) demonstrates small area of infarction.	Aspirin or anticoagulant therapy is used to prevent further injury.
Transient Ischemic Attack | Ischemia of the brain that is caused by the same etiologies as ischemic stroke: thromboembolism from carotid stenosis or atrial fibrillation. Ischemia of the brain is caused by a thromboembolus that dissolves within 24 hours. The ischemia is reversible after the thrombus dissolves.				
	Motor and sensory loss is evident on the opposite side of the body than the cerebral hemisphere undergoing the ischemia. Hemiparesis (weakness) or hemiplegia (paralysis) is observed. If the left hemisphere undergoes ischemia, most of those affected will suffer aphasia.	Hemiparesis or hemiplegia of limbs is evident on the opposite side of the cerebral hemisphere affected. Loss of sensation on one side of body. Speech problems are evident if cerebral ischemia is of the left hemisphere. Gradually improving neurological examination Neuro exam is back to normal within 24 hours, with no remaining neurological deficits.	CT scan or MRI may not be helpful if ischemia area has resolved. Electrocardiogram. Carotid artery CT scan.	Aspirin or anticoagulant therapy is used to prevent reoccurrence. Carotid stenosis surgery called endarterectomy or treatment of atrial fibrillation may be done to prevent reoccurrence.
Hemorrhagic Stroke | Cerebral artery rupture occurs, which causes a large amount of blood to compress the brain tissue and cause brain death. Subarachnoid hemorrhage is one type of hemorrhagic stroke.				
	Motor and sensory loss is evident on the opposite side of the body than the cerebral hemisphere undergoing the hemorrhage. Hemiparesis (weakness) or hemiplegia (paralysis) is observed. If the left hemisphere undergoes hemorrhage, most of those affected will suffer aphasia. Subarachnoid hemorrhage causes severe headache with changing level of consciousness.	Sudden onset. Elevated blood pressure. Rapid deterioration of cognitive function. Motor and sensory loss on opposite side of the affected cerebral hemisphere. If the left hemisphere undergoes hemorrhage, most of those affected will suffer aphasia.	CT scan or MRI demonstrates specific area of bleeding in the brain. Over the following day, CT scans are done to evaluate bleeding into the brain.	Supportive care. Decrease cerebral edema with IV mannitol or hypertonic saline. Patient may need intubation and mechanical ventilation. Neurosurgery may be possible in some patients.

Bibliography

A Science Advisory From the American Heart Association/ American Stroke Association, del Zoppo, G. J., Saver, J. L., Jauch, E. C., & Adams, H. P., Jr., on behalf of the American Heart Association Stroke Council. (2009). Expansion of the time window for treatment of acute ischemic stroke with intravenous tissue plasminogen activator. *Stroke*, 40(8), 2945–2948. doi: 10.1161/STROKEAHA.109. 192535.

American Heart Association/American Stroke Association. (2015a). *Guidelines for the early management of adults with ischemic stroke. A guideline from the American Heart Association/American Stroke Association Stroke Council, Clinical Cardiology Council, Cardiovascular Radiology and Intervention Council, and the Atherosclerotic Peripheral Vascular Disease and Quality of Care Outcomes in Research Interdisciplinary Working Groups*. Retrieved from http://stroke .ahajournals.org/content/38/5/1655.full

American Heart Association/American Stroke Association. (2015b). *Guidelines for the management of aneurysmal subarachnoid hemorrhage. A guideline for healthcare professionals from the American Heart Association/American Stroke Association*. Retrieved from http://stroke.ahajournals.org/ content/43/6/1711

American Heart Association/American Stroke Association. (2015c). *Guidelines for the primary prevention of stroke. A guideline for healthcare professionals from the American Heart Association/American Stroke Association*. Retrieved from http://stroke.ahajournals.org/content/42/2/517 .full.pdf

American Heart Association/American Stroke Association. (2013). AHA/ASA publish advisory on oral antithrombotics for stroke prevention in nonvalvular atrial fibrillation. *Am Fam Phys*, 87(10), 732–733.

American Heart Association/American Stroke Association Stroke Council; Council on Cardiovascular Surgery and Anesthesia; Council on Cardiovascular Radiology and Intervention; Council on Cardiovascular Nursing; and the Interdisciplinary Council on Peripheral Vascular Disease. (2015). *Definition and evaluation of transient ischemic attack*. Retrieved from http://stroke.ahajournals.org/content/40/6/ 2276.full.pdf

Bangalore, S., Schwamm, L., Smith, E. E., et al. (2014). Secondary prevention after ischemic stroke or transient ischemic attack. *Am J Med*, Mar 26. pii: S0002-9343(14)00238-1. doi: 10.1016/j.amjmed.2014.03.011. Epub ahead of print.

Barrett, K. E., Barman, S. M., Boitano, S., & Brooks, H. L. (2010). *Ganong's review of medical physiology*. 24th ed. New York: McGraw-Hill/ Lange Medical Series.

Beck, R. A., & King, W. M., 4th. (2014). Apixaban (eliquis) for stroke prevention in atrial fibrillation. *Am Fam Phys*, 89(8), 672–675.

Bergman, D. (2011). Preventing recurrent cerebrovascular events in patients with stroke or transient ischemic attack: the current data. *J Am Acad Nurse Pract*, 23(12), 659–666. doi: 10.1111/j.1745-7599.2011.00650.x. Epub 2011 Jul 22.

Bos, D., Portegies, M. L., van der Lugt, A., et al. (2014). Intracranial carotid artery atherosclerosis and the risk of stroke in whites: the Rotterdam Study. *JAMA Neurol*, 71(4), 405–411. doi: 10.1001/jamaneurol.2013.6223.

Brouwers, H. B., Chang, Y., Falcone, G. J., et al. (2014). Predicting hematoma expansion after primary intracerebral hemorrhage. *JAMA Neurol*, 71(2), 158–164. doi: 10.1001/ jamaneurol.2013.5433.

Bruins Slot, K. M., & Berge, E. (2014). Factor Xa inhibitors vs warfarin for preventing stroke and thromboembolism in patients with atrial fibrillation. *JAMA*, 311(11), 1150–1151. doi: 10.1001/jama.2014.1403.

Carpenter, C. R., Keim, S. M., Milne, W. K., Meurer, W. J., Barsan, W. G.; Best Evidence in Emergency Medicine Investigator Group. (2010). Thrombolytic therapy for acute ischemic stroke beyond three hours. *J Emerg Med*, 40(1), 82–92. Epub 2010 Jun 25.

Coutts, S. B., Modi, J., Patel, S. K., et al. (2012). What causes disability after transient ischemic attack and minor stroke?: results from the CT and MRI in the triage of TIA and minor cerebrovascular events to identify high risk patients (CATCH) study. *Stroke*, 2012 Sep 13. Epub ahead of print.

Davis, L. L. (2013). Preventing stroke in patients with atrial fibrillation. *Nurse Pract*, 38(11), 24–31; quiz 31–32. doi: 10.1097/01.NPR.0000435781.73316.9c.

Ebinger, M., Winter, B., Wendt, M., et al. (2014). Effect of the use of ambulance-based thrombolysis on time to thrombolysis in acute ischemic stroke: a randomized clinical trial. *JAMA*, 311(16), 1622–1631. doi: 10.1001/ jama.2014.2850.

Fang, M. C., Perraillon, M. C., Ghosh, K., Cutler, D. M., & Rosen, A. B. (2014). Trends in stroke rates, risk, and outcomes in the United States, 1988–2008. *Am J Med*, Mar 25. pii: S0002-9343(14)00271-X. doi: 10.1016/j.amjmed .2014.03.017. Epub ahead of print.

Feigin, V. L., Forouzanfar, M. H., Krishnamurthi, R., et al. (2014). Global and regional burden of stroke during 1990–2010: findings from the Global Burden of Disease Study 2010. *Lancet*, 383(9913), 245–254. Review. Erratum in: *Lancet*. 2014 Jan 18;383(9913):218.

Fonarow, G. C., Smith, E. E., Saver, J. L., et al. (2011). Timeliness of tissue-type plasminogen activator therapy in acute ischemic stroke: patient characteristics, hospital factors, and outcomes associated with door-to-needle times within 60 minutes. *Circulation*, 123(7), 750–758. Epub 2011 Feb 10.

Fonarow, G. C., Zhao, X., Smith, E. E., et al. (2014). Door-to-needle times for tissue plasminogen activator administration and clinical outcomes in acute ischemic stroke before and after a quality improvement initiative. *JAMA*, 311(16), 1632–1640. doi: 10.1001/jama.2014.3203.

Giroud, M., Jacquin, A., & Béjot, Y. (2014). The worldwide landscape of stroke in the 21st century. *Lancet*, 383(9913), 195–197. No abstract available. Erratum in: *Lancet*. 2014 Feb 22;383(9918):696.

Grotta, J. C. (2014). tPA for stroke: important progress in achieving faster treatment. *JAMA*, 311(16), 1615–1617. doi: 10.1001/jama.2014.3322.

Longo, D., Fauci, A., Kasper, D., Hauser, S., & Jameson, J. (2011). *Harrison's principles of internal medicine*. 18th ed. New York: McGraw-Hill.

Mendelow, A. D., Gregson, B. A., Rowan, E. N., et al. (2013). Early surgery versus initial conservative treatment in patients with spontaneous supratentorial lobar intracerebral haematomas (STICH II): a randomised trial. *Lancet*, 382(9890), 397–408. doi: 10.1016/S0140-6736(13)60986-1. Epub 2013 May 29.

Mitka, M. (2014). New guidelines focus on preventing stroke in women. *JAMA*, 311(10), 1003–1004. doi: 10.1001/jama.2014.1775.

Morgenstern, L. B., Hemphill, J. C., Anderson, C., et al. (2010). Guidelines for the management of spontaneous intracerebral hemorrhage: a guideline for healthcare professionals from the American Heart Association/American Stroke Association. *Stroke*, 41 (2010), 2108–2129.

Perry, J. M., & McCabe, K. K. (2012). Recognition and initial management of acute ischemic stroke. *Emerg Med Clin N America*, 30(3), 637–657. doi: 10.1016/j.emc.2012.06.001.

Phillips, S., Stanley, L., Nicoletto, H., et al. (2012). Use of emergency department transcranial Doppler assessment of reperfusion after intravenous tPA for ischemic stroke. *J Emerg Med*, 42(1), 40–43.

Radecki, R. P. (2013). Acute ischemic stroke and timing of treatment. *JAMA*, 310(17), 1855–1856. doi: 10.1001/jama.2013.278893.

Reiffel, J. A. (2014). Atrial fibrillation and stroke: epidemiology. *Am J Med*, 127(4), e15–16. doi: 10.1016/j.amjmed.2013.06.002.

Sarraj, A., & Grotta, J. C. (2014). Stroke: new horizons in treatment. *Lancet Neurol*, 13(1), 2–3. doi: 10.1016/S1474-4422(13)70281-3.

Saver, J. L. (2014). Blood pressure management in early ischemic stroke. *JAMA*, 311(5), 469–470. doi: 10.1001/jama.2013.282544.

Vidale, S., Bellocchi, S., & Taborelli, A. (2013). Surgery for cerebral haemorrhage—STICH II trial. *Lancet*, 382(9902), 1401–1402. doi: 10.1016/S0140-6736(13)62211-4. Epub 2013 Oct 25.

Weant, K. A., & Baker, S. N. (2012). New windows, same old house: an update on acute stroke management. *Adv Emerg Nurs J*, 34(2), 112–121. doi: 10.1097/TME.0b013e3182542bce.

Chronic and Degenerative Neurological Disorders

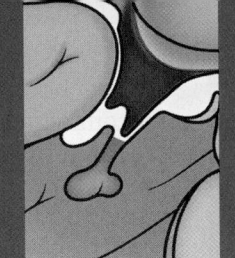

Key Terms

Acetylcholine

Ataxia

Athetosis

Aura

Basal ganglia

Chorea

Diencephalon

Dopamine

Gamma amino butyric acid (GABA)

Glutamate

Ictal period

Interictal period

Midbrain

Migraine

Myelin

Postictal period

Positron emission tomography (PET)

Seizure

Serotonin

Substantia nigra

Chronic and degenerative neurological disorders have a profound effect on patients and their caregivers. Some chronic neurological conditions, such as migraine headache and epilepsy, can be prevented and treated. In contrast, degenerative neurological disorders, such as Parkinson's disease and amyotrophic lateral sclerosis (ALS), are progressive in nature and slowly debilitating. With degenerative disorders, the patient has difficulty carrying out activities of daily living (ADLs), which impairs the patient's ability to function independently. Degenerative neurological disorders commonly require ongoing physical and occupational therapy to maximize function of the individual.

Epidemiology

Headaches, which are one of the most common disorders treated in the primary care and emergency clinical settings, account for 1% to 4% of all emergency department (ED) visits and are the ninth most common reason for a patient to consult a clinician. Clinicians classify 90% of headaches reported to them as muscle contraction or migraine headaches. Migraine headaches occur in more than 30 million people per year. Approximately 75% of all persons who experience migraines are women.

Seizure is a common, nonspecific manifestation of neurological injury and disease. It can appear as a temporary absence of attention, uncontrolled contractions of muscle groups, or whole body convulsion. Epilepsy is a disorder that causes chronic, unprovoked seizures that are often unpredictable. The lifetime likelihood of experiencing at least one epileptic seizure is about 9%, and the lifetime likelihood of receiving a diagnosis of epilepsy is almost 3%. However, the prevalence of active epilepsy is only about 0.8%.

Degenerative neurological diseases are those disorders that diminish neurological impulse transmission in

the body. The common result is lack of independent muscle contraction, postural imbalance, and loss of sensation and movement. Some degenerative disorders can also affect cognitive function. Parkinson's disease is one of the most common degenerative neurological disorders, affecting approximately 1% of individuals older than 60 years. The cause of Parkinson's disease is unknown, but the areas of the brain affected are clearly defined. Multiple sclerosis (MS) is an immune-mediated degenerative neurological disorder. Slowly, motor and sensory nerves are demyelinated, but remissions from the disease can occur. Prevalence estimates for MS in the United States vary from 58 to 95 per 100,000 population.

Basic Concepts of Neurological Function

The human nervous system is composed of the central nervous system (CNS) and peripheral nervous system (PNS). The CNS includes the brain and spinal cord, whereas the PNS includes the somatic nerves—motor and sensory types—and the autonomic nervous system (ANS). The CNS is composed of two types of neural cells: neurons and glial cells. Neurons transmit impulses, process information, and connect with other neurons. The nervous system can be likened to electrical circuits that control the body. Between the neurons are synapses—gaps between neurons through which information flows from one neuron to another. Glial cells provide structural support for the neurons and phagocytose foreign matter and cellular debris.

Neurons

There are three basic types of neurons: motor, sensory, and interneurons. The neuron has four major anatomical parts: dendrites, cell body, axon, and axon terminals.

Incoming signals from other neurons are received through its dendrites. The outgoing signal to other neurons flows along its axon. A neuron may have many thousands of dendrites, but it will have only one axon. The fourth distinct part of a neuron, the axon terminals, are located at the end of the axon. These are the structures that contain chemical substances called neurotransmitters.

Neurotransmitters

Some neuron-to-neuron connections are electrical synapses where an impulse travels to another neuron. However, at some neural synapses, axon terminals release chemical substances through which signals flow. Common neurotransmitters of the nervous system include acetylcholine, norepinephrine, serotonin, dopamine, gamma amino butyric acid (GABA), and glutamate.

Acetylcholine is found within the CNS, PNS, and ANS. It can act as either an excitatory or inhibitory neurotransmitter, depending on what neurons secrete it. For example, within the ANS, acetylcholine slows the heart rate, functioning as an inhibitory neurotransmitter. However, within the PNS, acetylcholine behaves as an excitatory neurotransmitter at neuromuscular junctions.

Serotonin, or 5-hydroxytryptamine, is a neurotransmitter chemically derived from tryptophan. It is primarily found in the gastrointestinal tract, platelets, and in the CNS. In the CNS, it is found primarily in the dorsal raphe region of the brainstem, and is thought to be a contributor to feelings of well-being.

Dopamine has many functions, including roles in:

- behavior and cognition
- voluntary movement
- motivation
- punishment and reward
- attention
- working memory
- learning.

Dopaminergic neurons are mainly located in the substantia nigra of the midbrain's basal ganglia region. Dysfunction of dopaminergic neurotransmission in the CNS has been implicated in a variety of neuropsychiatric disorders, including social phobia, Tourette's syndrome, Parkinson's disease, schizophrenia, neuroleptic malignant syndrome, attention deficit-hyperactivity disorder (ADHD), and drug and alcohol dependence.

Gamma amino butyric acid (GABA), the chief inhibitory neurotransmitter in the CNS, typically has a relaxing, antianxiety, and anticonvulsive effect on the brain. It also has an inhibitory effect on muscles, which decreases spasms and allows for muscle tone. Norepinephrine is an excitatory neurotransmitter in the brain and stress hormone within in the endocrine system. Stress activates a region of the brainstem called the locus coeruleus—the origin of most norepinephrine pathways in the brain. Neurons using norepinephrine project from the locus coeruleus to the cerebral cortex, limbic system, and the spinal cord.

Another neurotransmitter, **glutamate**, is considered to be a major mediator of excitatory signals in the CNS and is involved in cognition, memory, and learning. Glutamate is kept within the nerve terminal vesicles; after being released from the neuron, specific transporters must rapidly remove it from the extracellular space, as extracellular accumulation of glutamate causes brain cell injury and cell death (see Fig. 34-1).

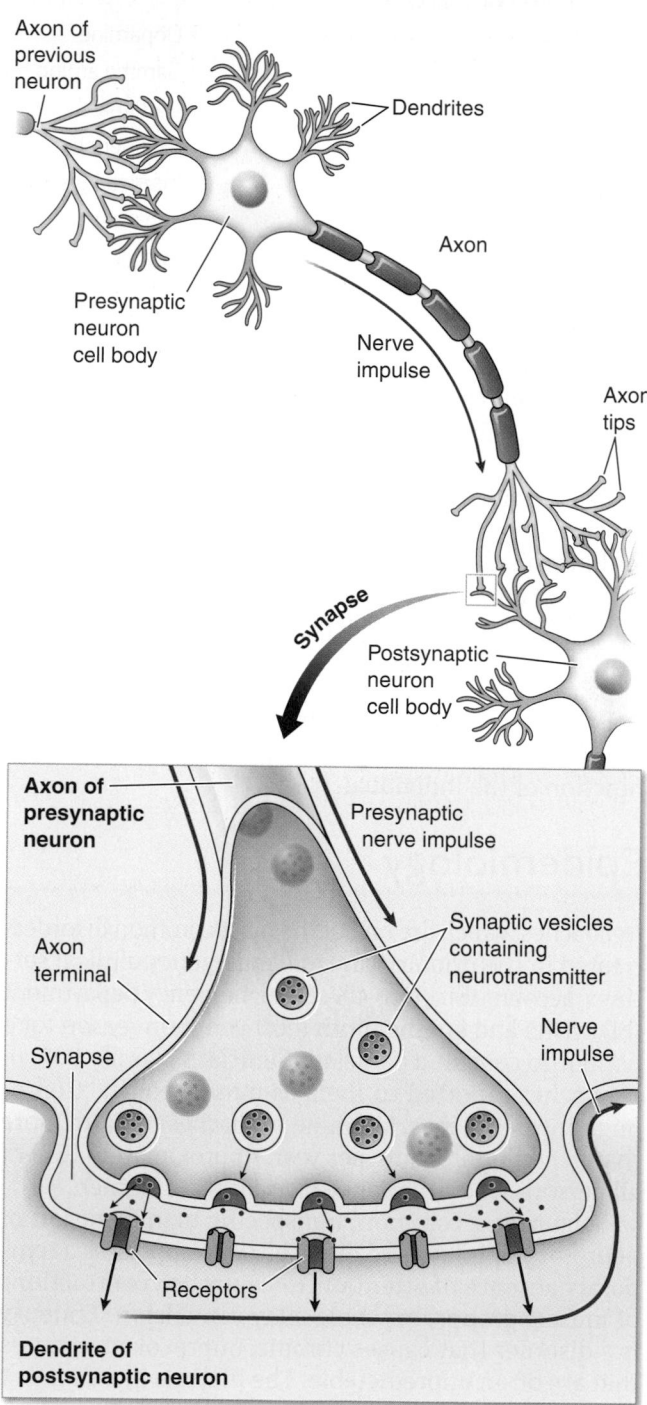

FIGURE 34-1. The neuron and transmission of impulses. (A) Neurons transmit impulses to each other in an orderly manner. Dendrites come off the cell body to pick up impulses and the impulse travels down the axon. (B) A synapse is a space between two neurons where neurotransmitters are secreted from a presynaptic neuron to a postsynaptic neuron. Neurotransmitters bind to receptors on the postsynaptic neuron, which stimulates an impulse.

Nerve Conduction

Neurons conduct impulses called action potentials that begin at the cell body and travel down the axon. This stimulates ions such as sodium (Na+), potassium (K+), and calcium (Ca++) to move across the membrane of the axon. Ions move back and forth across the axon membrane through ion channels that open and close (see Fig. 34-2). When ion channels open, charged particles such as Na+ flood across the membrane at a tremendous rate. When the concentration of ions on the inside of the neuron changes, the electrical property of the membrane changes. The influx of Na+ through ion channels during neurotransmission make the inside of the neuron more positive. This is called depolarization of the neuron. When this depolarization reaches a peak called a threshold, an action potential is generated. After depolarization, potassium channels of the neuronal membrane open, resulting in outward movement of potassium ions during a phase called repolarization. Repolarization refers to the return of the membrane potential to a negative value after the depolarization phase of an action potential.

Typically the repolarization phase of an action potential results in hyperpolarization, which is attainment of a membrane potential that is more negative than the resting potential (see Fig. 34-3). It is important that there is a refractory or resting period between impulses that provides time for the membrane to return to baseline levels. An excitatory phase (depolarization) and an inhibitory phase (repolarization) exists with each action potential—this keeps the impulse moving in a unidirectional manner. Impulses that do not maintain a systematic orderly, excitatory, inhibitory,

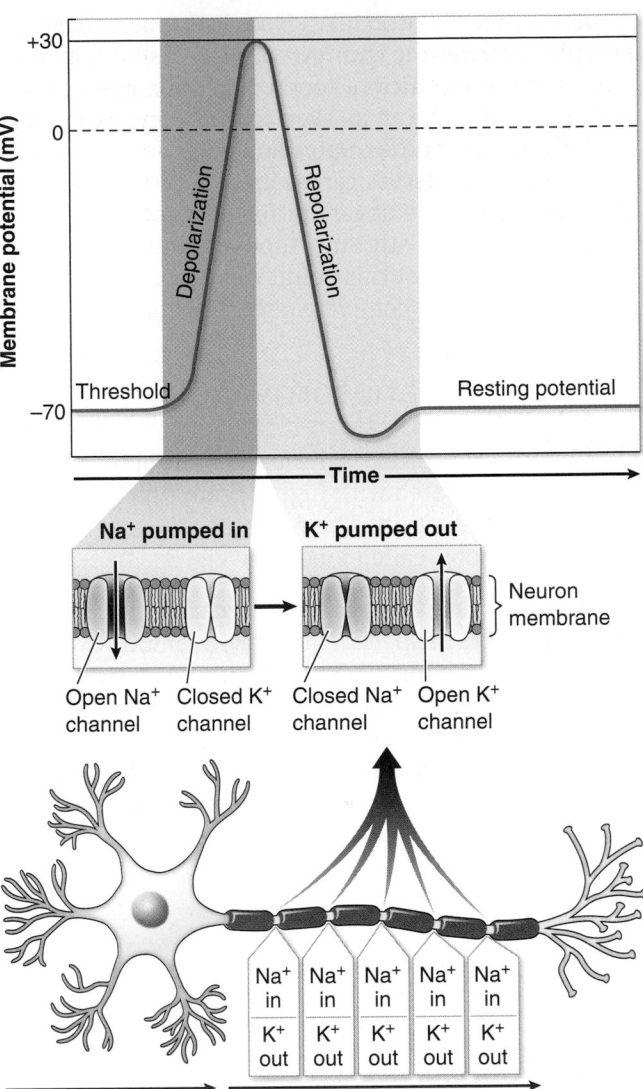

FIGURE 34-3. In neuron transmission, sodium (Na+) ion channels open and Na+ ions enter the cell membrane. The influx of Na+ through ion channels during neurotransmission makes the inside of the neuron more positive. This is called depolarization of the neuron. When this depolarization reaches a peak called a threshold, an action potential is generated. After depolarization, the neuronal membrane opens potassium channels, resulting in outward movement of potassium ions during a phase called repolarization.

and resting phase become irregular and chaotic, as occurs in seizure disorders.

Myelin

Myelin is a protective sheath that is formed around axons of some neurons in the nervous system. It acts as an insulator of the electrical signal that is conducted down the axon in neurotransmission, and is comparable with the insulation around an electrical wire. The myelin sheath contains a variety of fatty substances called lipids and is considered white matter. In the nervous system, neuron cell bodies are located within the gray matter, whereas axonal tracts and glial cells are within the white matter.

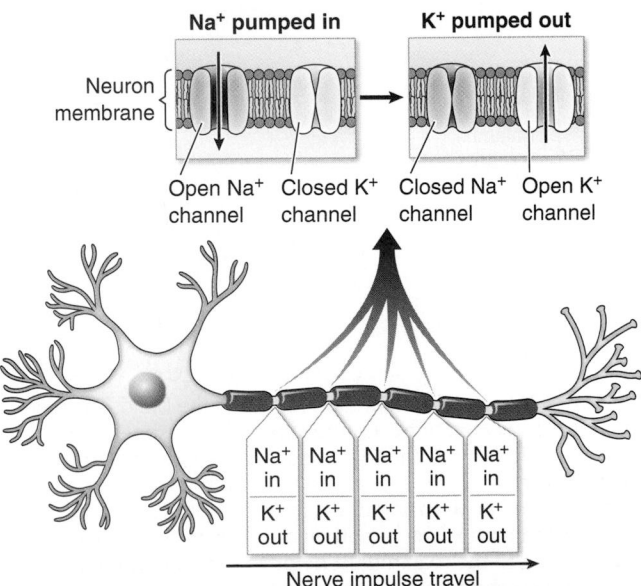

FIGURE 34-2. Ion channels across a neuron membrane. Neurons conduct impulses called action potentials that begin at the cell body and travel down the axon. This stimulates ions, such as sodium (Na+) and potassium (K+), to move across the axon's membrane. Ions move back and forth across the axon membrane through ion channels that open and close.

The way myelination takes place is through glial cells wrapping around the axons in a spiral fashion. Myelin allows for a rapid, efficient conduction of a nerve impulse down its axon. Without an even coating of myelin, nerve impulses can become disrupted and potential for conduction can be lost; nerves can eventually wither away. In disorders that cause degeneration of myelin, some regrowth is possible with time, though eventually myelin cannot regenerate; at this point, whole nerve degeneration occurs, causing complete nerve tract disruption.

Basic Neuroanatomy

The cerebrum, or cortex, is the largest part of the human brain; it is associated with higher brain functions such as thought and action. The cerebral cortex is divided into four sections, called lobes (see Fig. 34-4):

1. Frontal lobe: associated with reasoning, planning, parts of speech, movement, emotions, and problem solving
2. Parietal lobe: associated with movement, orientation, recognition, and perception of stimuli
3. Occipital lobe: associated with visual processing
4. Temporal lobe: associated with perception and recognition of auditory stimuli, memory, and speech.

Cerebellum

The cerebellum contributes to coordination, precision, and accuracy of movement. It receives input from sensory systems and from other parts of the brain and spinal cord, and integrates these inputs to fine-tune motor activity. Damage to the cerebellum causes lack of coordination, imbalance and a gait disturbance termed **ataxia**.

Diencephalon

The **diencephalon** is the posterior part of the forebrain that connects the midbrain with the cerebral hemispheres; it contains the thalamus and hypothalamus. The diencephalon relays sensory information between brain regions and controls many autonomic functions of the PNS. It also connects structures of the endocrine system with the nervous system and works in conjunction with limbic system structures to generate and manage emotions and memories (see Fig. 34-5).

Brainstem

The brainstem is responsible for basic vital life functions, such as breathing, heartbeat, and blood pressure. It is made up of the midbrain, pons, and medulla. The **midbrain** is involved in functions such as vision, hearing, eye movement, and body movement. The anterior part has the cerebral peduncle, which is a huge bundle of axons traveling from the cerebral cortex through the brainstem; these fibers, along with other structures, are important for voluntary motor function. The **basal ganglia** is a

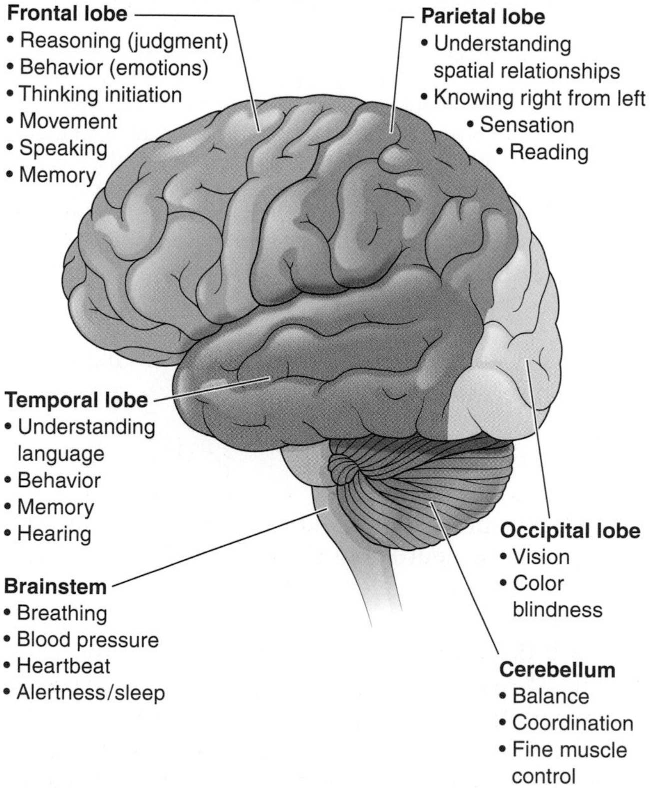

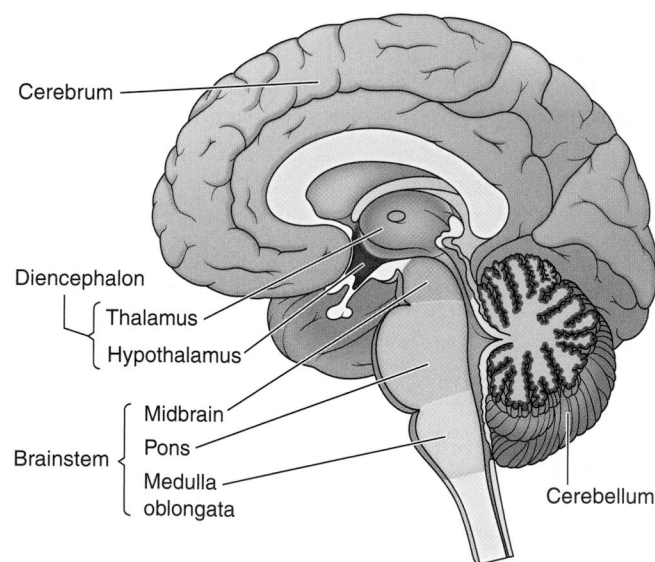

Frontal lobe
- Reasoning (judgment)
- Behavior (emotions)
- Thinking initiation
- Movement
- Speaking
- Memory

Parietal lobe
- Understanding spatial relationships
- Knowing right from left
- Sensation
- Reading

Temporal lobe
- Understanding language
- Behavior
- Memory
- Hearing

Brainstem
- Breathing
- Blood pressure
- Heartbeat
- Alertness/sleep

Occipital lobe
- Vision
- Color blindness

Cerebellum
- Balance
- Coordination
- Fine muscle control

FIGURE 34-4. Brain anatomy and functional areas.

FIGURE 34-5. The diencephalon region of the brain. The diencephalon is located between the cerebral hemispheres and the brainstem. It includes the thalamus and the hypothalamus. Nearly all sensory impulses travel through the thalamus, which sorts out the impulses and directs them to particular areas of the cerebral cortex. The hypothalamus is located in the midline area inferior to the thalamus. It helps to maintain homeostasis by controlling body temperature, water balance, sleep, appetite, and some emotions, such as fear and pleasure. Both the sympathetic and parasympathetic divisions of the ANS are under the control of the hypothalamus, as is the pituitary gland. The hypothalamus influences the heartbeat, the contraction and relaxation of blood vessels, hormone secretion, and other vital body functions.

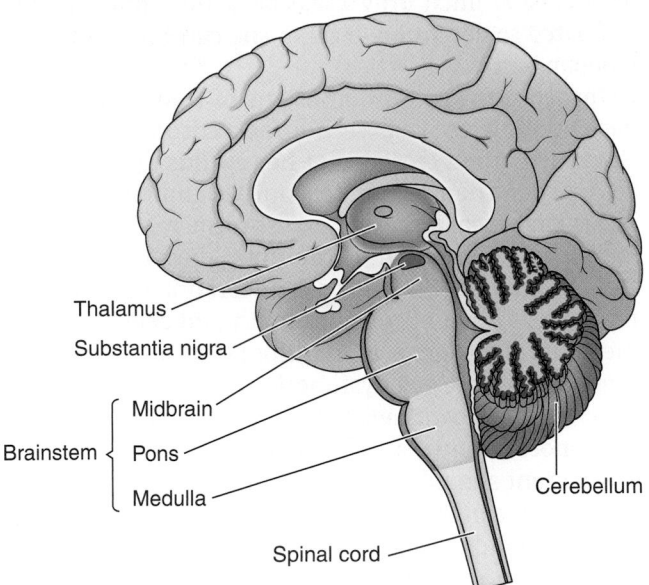

FIGURE 34-6. The components and functions of the brainstem. The brainstem is located in front of the cerebellum. It passes messages back and forth between the brain and other parts of the body. The cerebrum, cerebellum, and spinal cord are all connected to the brainstem, which has three main parts: the midbrain, pons, and medulla oblongata. The brainstem controls vital functions, including breathing, consciousness, cardiac function, involuntary muscle movements, and swallowing.

portion of the midbrain that modulates voluntary motor function and routine behaviors. The **substantia nigra** is a portion of the basal ganglia that synthesizes dopamine. The pons is involved in motor control and sensory analysis. For example, information from the ear first enters the brain in the pons. It has parts that are important for level of consciousness and sleep. Some structures within the pons are linked to the cerebellum and are involved in movement and posture. The medulla oblongata is part of the brainstem between the pons and spinal cord. It is responsible for maintaining vital body functions, such as breathing, sleep-wake cycles, blood pressure, and heart rate (see Fig. 34-6).

Basic Pathophysiologic Concepts of Neurological Dysfunction

The cellular causes of nervous system disorders commonly involve the sodium and potassium ion channels within the axonal tracts. The generation of an impulse is thwarted in ion channel disorders. In other disorders, the layers of myelin covering the axons are disrupted, which interferes with the smooth travel of impulses.

Ion Channel Disorders

Ion channel disorders, also called channelopathies, are responsible for a growing number of neurological diseases. Most are caused by mutations in ion channel genes or by auto-antibodies formed against ion channel

proteins. One example is epilepsy, a syndrome of repetitive synchronous firing of neuronal action potentials. Action potentials are normally generated by the opening of sodium channels and the inward movement of sodium ions down the intracellular concentration gradient. Depolarization of the neuronal membrane opens potassium channels, resulting in outward movement of potassium ions, repolarization, closure of the sodium channel, and hyperpolarization. Sodium or potassium channel subunit genes have long been considered candidate disease genes in inherited epilepsy; recently, such mutations have been identified. These mutations appear to alter the normal gating function of these channels, increasing the inherent excitability of neuron membranes in regions where the abnormal channels are expressed. Whereas the specific clinical manifestations of channelopathies are variable, one common feature is that manifestations tend to be intermittent or paroxysmal, as occurs in epilepsy, migraine headache, dysautonomia, and periodic paralysis.

Myelin and Myelin-Related Disorders

In demyelinating diseases, the myelin sheath around some axons is targeted. The most common demyelinating disease is Multiple Sclerosis (MS), which is suspected to be an autoimmune disease. After patches of myelin are taken off the axon, oligodendrocytes repair the damage, but also form scar tissue called gliotic plaques. These hard plaques then begin to interfere with the flow of electrical impulses that move through the axon. Some diseases such as Amyotrophic Lateral Sclerosis (ALS) have been found to cause demyelination of solely motor neurons, and others such as MS have demyelination of both sensory and motor neurons.

Assessment of the Neurological System

The clinician must carefully observe the patient during the history and physical when a neurological disorder is suspected, because neurological symptoms are often subtle.

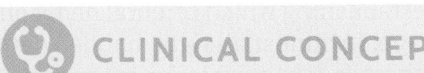

CLINICAL CONCEPT

Many neurological disorders are difficult to diagnose upon initial examination, because degenerative neurological diseases are progressive and the full picture of the disorder is not often apparent with early symptoms.

Assess vision, hearing, orientation, and cognitive ability first to assure that the patient can give an accurate history. If the patient is unconscious, the clinician should make an assessment based on the Glasgow Coma Scale, vital signs, and pupil response. The cause for the loss of consciousness must be sought, primarily through blood tests and imaging studies. (For more on the Glasgow Coma Scale, see Chapter 35: Brain and Spinal Cord Injury.)

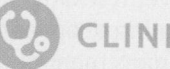 **CLINICAL CONCEPT**

If the patient is cognitively impaired, obtain the patient's history from the patient's parent, spouse, partner, or guardian, if able.

If the patient is conscious, note speech, demeanor, hygiene, and emotional state. Administration of the Mini-Mental Status Examination (MMSE) may be necessary if cognitive impairment is suspected. If this is not possible, mini-cognitive assessment through clock drawing can be used.

If there is any evidence of trauma, causation must be fully described. Have the patient describe pain, if present. When does the pain occur? Where is it located? Associated symptoms and aggravating and relieving factors should be assessed.

If the patient suffered a seizure, it needs to be fully characterized. Ask the patient about recent falls, dizziness, blackouts, and accidents. Although the patient often does not relate these events to a neurological disorder, they are significant signs. Also ask about loss of consciousness, sudden weakness in an extremity, or slurring of speech.

 CLINICAL CONCEPT

If the patient has been accompanied by someone who observed the incident, make sure to ask this person about loss of consciousness, extremity weakness, and slurring, as these symptoms are best described by a third party and not the patient.

Ask the patient about difficulty with range of motion, numbness, or sensation problems. Handedness is important in establishing which cerebral hemisphere controls language. In almost all right-handed persons, the left hemisphere is responsible for language. If the patient is taking any medication, it is necessary to evaluate any possible effects on the nervous system. Past medical and surgical history need to be assessed. For example, inquire about history of diabetes because it can lead to sensory or autonomic neuropathy. Past history of head trauma may be the cause of seizure disorder, and past history of transient ischemic attack (TIA) can be related to present stroke symptoms.

Family history should be assessed for any inheritable or contagious disease, and the patient should be asked about behavioral and social habits. Ask the patient about use of over-the-counter medication, alcohol, caffeine,

tobacco, and illicit drug use. The patient must also be evaluated to determine if he or she can carry out ADLs independently.

Inspect the head for any signs of trauma. Have the patient smile to observe if a facial droop is present. Have the patient close his or her eyelids tightly as you try to open them. A fundoscopic examination of the retina can reveal if there is excess intracranial pressure. Papilledema, swelling of the optic disc, can occur in stroke, tumor, or other causes of cerebral edema. Have the patient open his or her mouth and check to see if the uvula and tongue are midline; if they are deviated, there is probable gag dysfunction.

A full neurological examination, which includes sensory, motor, reflex, and balance functions, is needed. The patient should stretch out both arms where hands and fingers can be observed for tremor. Tremor, fasciculations, motor rigidity, or spasm should be noted. It is important to assess the patient's upper and lower motor strength. This can be quickly done by assessing the patient's bilateral grip strength and quadriceps strength against the clinician's resistance. With the patient's eyes closed, sensation to light touch with a cotton ball and pinpoint discrimination with a paper clip can be assessed. Sensation in the feet is most significant.

Examination of the patient's gait can reveal a lack of neurological integrity. The patient should be able to easily rise from a chair. Assess deep tendon reflexes of the upper and lower extremities, and evaluate the cranial nerves, which can reveal CNS problems. Assess the Babinski reflex, which is tested with stimulation of the sole of the foot. A negative Babinski reflex is normal in adults; the toes flex inward with stimulation of the sole of the foot. A positive Babinski reflex, where the patient has flaring of the toes in response to stimulation of the sole of the foot, indicates an upper motor neuron disorder.

 CLINICAL CONCEPT

An upper motor neuron disorder indicates that the source of the problem is in a neuron in the brain's area of motor control or along its path down into the spinal cord. A lower motor neuron disorder indicates the source of the problem is at the region where motor nerves exit the spinal cord (see Fig. 34-7).

Risk Factors

Risk factors vary across neurological disorders; some disorders have no known risk factors, whereas others have been linked with specific ones. For example, stroke is common in those with cardiovascular risk factors, including hypertension, hyperlipidemia, diabetes, tobacco use, and lack of exercise, but Myasthenia gravis (MG), ALS, and MS have no known risk factors. Head injury is a risk factor for intracranial bleeding, which

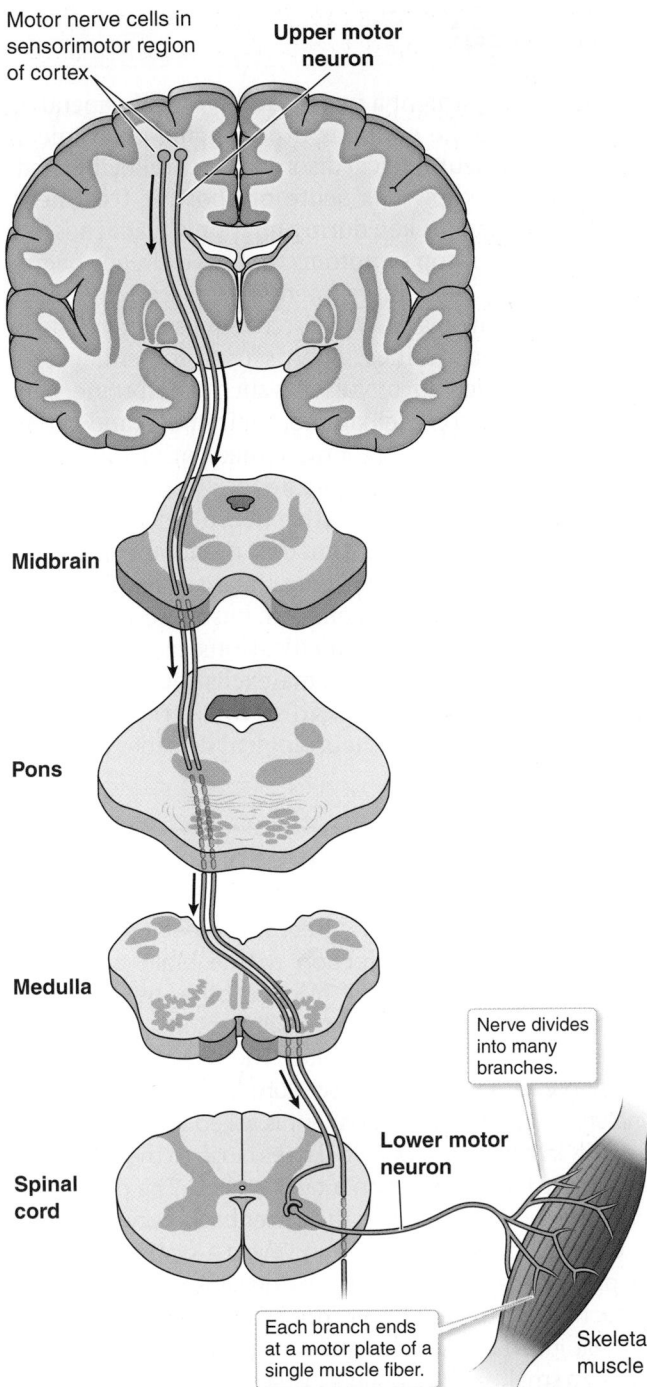

Motor nerve cells in sensorimotor region of cortex

Upper motor neuron

Midbrain

Pons

Medulla

Spinal cord

Nerve divides into many branches.

Lower motor neuron

Each branch ends at a motor plate of a single muscle fiber.

Skeletal muscle

FIGURE 34-7. Upper and lower motor neurons. The upper motor neuron cell bodies are located in the cortex in the brain's area of motor control. The lower motor neuron cell bodies are located in the spinal cord.

leads to neurological symptoms and places the patient at risk for seizures. Hormonal fluctuations increase susceptibility to migraine headaches. Severe upper respiratory infection can precede meningitis. Some medications can increase the risk of seizure, loss of consciousness, or confusion. Alcohol abuse and illicit drug use can also increase susceptibility to neurological symptoms such as seizure. Familial or genetic factors are sometimes the only conditions that predispose individuals to neurological disease. This is particularly true of Huntington's disease.

Signs and Symptoms

Signs and symptoms of degenerative neurological disease are often the only clues to diagnosis. Falls, accidents, and dizziness can be symptoms of neurological disease, which the patient may not think significant. Often a neurological disorder can present with mild and intermittent twitching, subtle weakness, or numbness in one extremity. Stroke often initially presents with numbness or weakness in one extremity, known as hemiparesis. MS can also present with sensory and motor symptoms similar to stroke. With disorders such as MS, the patient commonly presents to the clinician a number of times before the disorder can be diagnosed, as the symptoms are often subtle and confused with other diagnoses. Other neurological disorders may present with obvious gait disorder, rigid muscles, slowed motion, and loss of automatic movements, such as blinking and swinging the arms. Parkinson's disease commonly presents in this manner; in addition, patients commonly have a unique, characteristic resting tremor. The degenerative disorder of MG uniquely presents with ptosis of the eyelids.

Seizures, a symptom of epilepsy, can present in different ways depending on the type of epileptic disorder. A grand mal seizure presents with loss of consciousness and repetitive tonic and clonic muscle contractions; it is unmistakable as a seizure. However, an absence seizure is more difficult to diagnose because it simply presents as an episode of inattention.

Severe headache can also have different associated symptoms depending on the type of headache. For example, nausea and vomiting commonly accompany migraine headaches but not tension headaches.

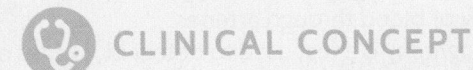

CLINICAL CONCEPT

Papilledema of the optic disc indicates elevated intracranial pressure.

Diagnosis

Researchers and clinicians use a variety of diagnostic imaging techniques and chemical and metabolic analyses to detect, manage, and treat neurological disease. Laboratory screening tests of blood, urine, or spinal fluid are used to help diagnose disease, better understand the disease process, and monitor levels of therapeutic drugs. Blood tests are also used to monitor levels of therapeutic drugs used to treat epilepsy and other neurological disorders.

Genetic testing of deoxyribonucleic acid (DNA) extracted from white cells in the blood can help diagnose Huntington's disease and other genetic diseases. Analysis of the cerebrospinal fluid that surrounds the brain and spinal cord can detect meningitis, acute and chronic inflammation, rare infections, and some cases of MS. Chemical and metabolic testing of the blood can indicate protein disorders, some forms of muscular dystrophy and other muscle disorders, and diabetes. Urinalysis can reveal abnormal substances in the urine or the presence or absence of certain proteins that cause diseases, including the mucopolysaccharidoses.

Genetic testing can help parents who have a family history of a neurological disease determine if they are carrying one of the known genes that cause the disorder or find out if their child is affected. Genetic testing can identify some neurological disorders in utero, such as spina bifida and Down syndrome. Amniocentesis, usually done between 14 and 16 weeks of pregnancy, tests a sample of the amniotic fluid in the womb for genetic defects. Chorionic villus sampling (CVS) is performed by removing and testing a very small sample of the placenta during early pregnancy. Uterine ultrasound is performed using a surface probe with gel. This noninvasive test can suggest the diagnosis of conditions such as chromosomal disorders. For other common diagnostic procedures used in neurological disorders, see Box 34-1.

Treatment

The type of treatment a patient receives will depend on whether or not he or she is experiencing a chronic or degenerative neurological disorder. Pain-relieving medications, also known as acute or abortive treatment, are types of drugs taken during migraine headaches and are designed to stop symptoms that have already begun. Alternatively, preventive medications can be taken regularly, often on a daily basis, to reduce the severity or frequency of migraines. Agents used for epilepsy or seizures include anticonvulsants such as valproate, lamotrigine, phenytoin, felbamate, topiramate, and carbamazepine. These are preventive medications meant to decrease susceptibility to seizure.

Treatments for degenerative neurological disorders such as MS and MG are aimed at modulating the autoimmune reaction underlying the disorder. For acute exacerbations, corticosteroids can hasten recovery from a given attack, but these medications cannot be used long term. In addition, plasma exchange can be used short term for severe attacks if steroids are contraindicated or ineffective. In neurological disorders such as

---

BOX 34-1. Diagnostic Procedures Used in Neurological Disorders

X-rays of the patient's chest and skull are often taken as part of a neurological work-up. *Fluoroscopy* is a type of x-ray that uses a continuous or pulsed beam of low-dose radiation to produce continuous images of a body part in motion. The fluoroscope (x-ray tube) is focused on the area of interest and pictures are either videotaped or sent to a monitor for viewing. A contrast medium may be used to highlight the images. Fluoroscopy can be used to evaluate the flow of blood through arteries.

Angiography is a test used to detect blockages of the arteries. A cerebral angiogram can detect the degree of narrowing or obstruction of an artery or blood vessel in the brain, head, or neck. It is used to diagnose stroke and to determine the location and size of a brain tumor, aneurysm, or vascular malformation.

Biopsy involves the removal and examination of a small piece of tissue from the body. Muscle or nerve biopsies are used to diagnose neuromuscular disorders and may also reveal if a person is a carrier of a defective gene that could be passed on to children. A small sample of muscle or nerve is removed under local anesthetic and studied under a microscope.

Brain scans are imaging techniques used to diagnose tumors, blood vessel malformations, or hemorrhage in the brain. These scans are used to study organ function, as well as injury or disease to tissue or muscle. Types of brain scans include CT, MRI, and positron emission tomography (PET).

Cerebrospinal fluid analysis involves the removal of a small amount of the fluid that protects the brain and spinal cord. The fluid is tested to detect any bleeding or brain hemorrhage, diagnose infection to the brain or spinal cord, identify some cases of MS and other neurological conditions, and measure intracranial pressure. The procedure is usually done in a hospital. The sample of fluid is commonly removed by a procedure known as a *lumbar puncture*, or spinal tap. The patient is asked to either lie on one side, in a ball position with knees close to the chest, or lean forward while sitting on a table or bed. The physician will locate a puncture site in the lower back, between two vertebrate, then clean the area and inject a local anesthetic. The patient may feel a slight stinging sensation from this injection. Once the anesthetic has taken effect, the physician will insert a special needle into the spinal sac and remove a small amount of fluid (usually about 3 teaspoons) for testing. Most patients will feel a sensation of pressure only as the needle is inserted.

A common after-effect of a lumbar puncture is headache, which can be lessened by having the patient lie flat. Risk of nerve root injury or infection from the puncture can occur but it is rare. The entire procedure takes about 45 minutes.

Computed tomography, also known as a CT scan, is a noninvasive, painless process used to produce rapid, clear two-dimensional images of organs, bones, and tissues. Neurological CT scans are used to view the brain and spine. They can detect bone and vascular irregularities, certain brain tumors and cysts, herniated discs, epilepsy, encephalitis, spinal stenosis (narrowing of the

BOX 34-1. Diagnostic Procedures Used in Neurological Disorders—cont'd

spinal canal), a blood clot or intracranial bleeding in patients with stroke, brain damage from head injury, and other disorders. Many neurological disorders share certain characteristics, and a CT scan can aid in proper diagnosis by differentiating the area of the brain affected by the disorder. An *intrathecal contrast-enhanced CT scan* is used to detect problems with the spine and spinal nerve roots.

Electroencephalography (EEG) monitors brain activity through the skull. EEG is used to help diagnose certain seizure disorders, brain tumors, brain damage from head injuries, inflammation of the brain and spinal cord, alcoholism, certain psychiatric disorders, and metabolic and degenerative disorders that affect the brain. EEGs are also used to evaluate sleep disorders, monitor brain activity when a patient has been fully anesthetized or loses consciousness, and confirm brain death.

Electromyography (EMG) is used to diagnose nerve and muscle dysfunction and spinal cord disease. It records the electrical activity from the brain and spinal cord to a peripheral nerve root (found in the arms and legs) that controls muscles during contraction and at rest. An EMG is usually done in conjunction with a *nerve conduction velocity* test, which measures electrical energy by assessing the nerve's ability to send a signal.

Electronystagmography describes a group of tests used to diagnose involuntary eye movement, dizziness, and balance disorders, as well as evaluate some brain functions. The test is performed at an imaging center. Small electrodes are taped around the eyes to record eye movements. If infrared photography is used in place of electrodes, the patient wears special goggles that help record the information. Both versions of the test are painless and risk-free.

Evoked potentials, also called evoked response, measure the electrical signals to the brain generated by hearing, touch, or sight. These tests are used to assess sensory nerve problems and confirm neurological conditions including MS, brain tumor, acoustic neuroma (small tumors of the inner ear), and spinal cord injury. Evoked potentials are also used to test sight and hearing (especially in infants and young children), monitor brain activity among coma patients, and confirm brain death.

Magnetic resonance imaging (MRI) uses computer-generated radio waves and a powerful magnetic field to produce detailed images of body structures including tissues, organs, bones, and nerves. Neurological uses include the diagnosis of brain and spinal cord tumors, eye disease, inflammation, infection, and vascular irregularities that may lead to stroke. MRI can also detect and monitor degenerative disorders such as MS and can document brain injury from trauma.

Functional MRI (fMRI) uses the blood's magnetic properties to produce real-time images of blood flow to particular areas of the brain. An fMRI can pinpoint areas of the brain that become active and note how long they stay active. It can also tell if brain activity within a region occurs simultaneously or sequentially. This imaging process is used to assess brain damage from head injury or degenerative disorders such as Alzheimer's disease and to identify and monitor other neurological disorders, including MS, stroke, and brain tumors.

Myelography involves the injection of a water- or oil-based contrast dye into the spinal canal to enhance x-ray imaging of the spine. Myelograms are used to diagnose spinal nerve injury, herniated discs, fractures, back or leg pain, and spinal tumors.

Positron Emission Tomography (PET) scans provide two- and three-dimensional pictures of brain activity by measuring radioactive isotopes that are injected into the bloodstream. PET scans of the brain are used to detect or highlight tumors and diseased tissue, measure cellular or tissue metabolism, show blood flow, evaluate patients who have seizure disorders that do not respond to medical therapy and patients with certain memory disorders, and determine brain changes following injury or drug abuse, among other uses.

A *polysomnogram* measures brain and body activity during sleep. It is performed over one or more nights at a sleep center.

Single photon emission computed tomography, a nuclear imaging test involving blood flow to tissue, is used to evaluate certain brain functions. The test may be ordered as a follow-up to an MRI to diagnose tumors, infections, degenerative spinal disease, and stress fractures.

Thermography uses infrared sensing devices to measure small temperature changes between the two sides of the body or within a specific organ. Also known as digital infrared thermal imaging, thermography may be used to detect vascular disease of the head and neck, soft tissue injury, various neuromusculoskeletal disorders, and the presence or absence of nerve root compression.

Ultrasound imaging, also called ultrasound scanning or sonography, uses high-frequency sound waves to obtain images inside the body. Neurosonography (ultrasound of the brain and spinal column) analyzes blood flow in the brain and can diagnose stroke, brain tumors, hydrocephalus (buildup of cerebrospinal fluid in the brain), and vascular problems. It can also identify or rule out inflammatory processes causing pain. It is more effective than an x-ray in displaying soft tissue masses and can show tears in ligaments, muscles, tendons, and other soft tissue masses in the back. Transcranial Doppler ultrasound is used to view arteries and blood vessels in the neck and determine blood flow and risk of stroke.

ALS, Guillain-Barré syndrome (GBS), and Huntington's disease, treatment is mainly supportive along with patient education.

Pathophysiology of Selected Chronic Neurological Disorders

Chronic neurological disorders vary in their severity. Migraine headache, a relatively benign form of neurological dysfunction, occurs episodically and leaves no residual neurological deficit. Epilepsy, in contrast, is a chronic neurological disorder that has major effects on the patient's life. Unpredictable, sudden episodes of seizure occur, usually with no lasting neurological deficit.

Epilepsy

Epilepsy is a chronic neurological disorder characterized by recurrent seizures. A **seizure** is a sudden, abnormal, disorderly discharge of neurons within the brain that is characterized by a sudden, transient alteration in brain function. A seizure may result in an altered level of consciousness as well as a number of motor, sensory, autonomic, and behavioral manifestations. Seizures have various clinical presentations depending on the specific part of the brain that is impacted by the abnormal impulse propagation. A seizure can present as a temporary disruption of the senses, a loss of consciousness, muscle spasms, or repetitive convulsions. Seizures can also occur as a symptom secondary to pathological conditions of the brain, such as tumor, CNS infection, stroke, head injury, metabolic imbalance, substance abuse, and acute alcohol withdrawal (see Box 34-2).

Epidemiology

Epilepsy, one of the most common chronic neurological conditions, affects more than 2.7 million people in the United States. The prevalence of epilepsy in the United States is 1% to 3%. It is most common in infants younger than 1 year of age and in adults older than 65 years. The occurrence of epilepsy during later childhood and early adulthood is less common. Epilepsy affects both genders and is seen in all racial and ethnic groups.

The annual incidence of seizures is approximately 100 per 100,000 individuals aged older than 60 years. Older adults have an increased risk of stroke and degenerative brain disorders such as Parkinson's disease; they are also more susceptible to metabolic disturbances and comorbid illnesses, which may explain why seizures are more commonly seen in this population.

Etiology

Epilepsy has no identifiable cause in about half of those who have the condition. In the other half, the condition may be traced to various factors (see Box 34-3). Head trauma is the most common cause in young adults, whereas stroke is the most common cause in the elderly.

Pathophysiology

Epilepsy is defined as a brain disorder characterized by a predisposition to seizures. Traditionally, the diagnosis

---

BOX 34-2. Common Etiologies of Seizure

Epilepsy
Brain neoplasms
Cerebrovascular disease
Congenital malformation
Degenerative brain disorders such as Alzheimer's disease
Environmental stimuli, such as blinking lights, loud noises, and certain music and odors
Genetic predisposition
Head trauma
Infections
Metabolic disturbances, such as hypoglycemia, hyponatremia, respiratory alkalosis
Perinatal injury (hypoxia)
Substance abuse
Withdrawal from alcohol or sedative-hypnotic drugs

BOX 34-3. Causes of Epilepsy

GENETIC INFLUENCE
Some types of epilepsy, which are categorized by your type of seizure, run in families, making it likely that there's a genetic influence. Researchers have linked some types of epilepsy to specific genes, though it's estimated that up to 500 genes could be tied to the condition. For most people, genes are only part of the cause, perhaps by making a person more susceptible to environmental conditions that trigger seizures. Some of the genes associated with epilepsy syndromes include 20q13.2, 19q12.1, 10q24, 6q24, Xq21–24.

HEAD TRAUMA
Severe, penetrating head trauma sustained during a car accident or other traumatic injury can cause epilepsy.

MEDICAL DISORDERS
Dementia is a leading cause of epilepsy among older adults, and disorders such as stroke and heart attack that result in damage to the brain can also cause epilepsy. Included in this are diseases that cause brain lesions, including meningitis, acquired immunodeficiency syndrome, and viral encephalitis.

PRENATAL INJURY
Before birth, babies are susceptible to brain damage caused by an infection in the mother, poor nutrition, or oxygen deficiencies. This can lead to cerebral palsy in the child. About 20% of seizures in children are associated with cerebral palsy or other neurological abnormalities.

DEVELOPMENTAL DISORDERS
Epilepsy can sometimes be associated with other developmental disorders such as autism and Down syndrome.

of epilepsy requires the occurrence of at least 2 unprovoked seizures 24 hours apart. Epileptic seizures commonly have no known etiology; however, in some cases, there is a causative agent (see Box 34-3). A seizure results when an abrupt imbalance occurs between the excitatory and inhibitory impulses within a region of cortical neurons in favor of a sudden-onset of hyperexcitability. Epileptogenesis refers to the transformation of a normal neuronal region into one that is chronically hyperexcitable. There is often a delay of months to years between an initial CNS injury, such as head trauma, stroke, or infection, and the first seizure. The injury appears to initiate a process that lowers the seizure threshold in the affected region; spontaneous seizure activity then becomes a chronic occurrence.

There are two major types of seizures: focal and generalized. Focal seizures arise from a neuronal area localized within one cerebral hemisphere. Generalized seizures arise within a hemisphere and rapidly involve neurons distributed across both cerebral hemispheres.

Pathological mechanisms that provoke focal seizures are better understood than mechanisms of generalized seizures. Focal seizure activity can begin in a distinct region of the cerebral cortex, known as a seizure initiation phase, and then spread to neighboring regions in a seizure propagation phase. The initiation phase is characterized by two concurrent events in a section of neurons: high frequency bursts of action potentials and hypersynchronization. The bursting activity is caused by a relatively long-lasting depolarization of the neuronal membrane that results from an influx of extracellular Ca^{++}, which leads to the opening of voltage-dependent Na^+ channels, influx of Na^+, and generation of repetitive action potentials. This is followed by a hyperpolarization mediated by GABA receptors or K^+ channels, depending on the cell type. The synchronized bursts from a sufficient number of neurons result in a spike discharge on an electroencephalography (EEG).

Focal seizures can cause motor, sensory, autonomic, or psychic symptoms without impairment of cognition. For example, a patient having a focal seizure arising from the right primary motor cortex in the area controlling hand movement will note the onset of involuntary movements of the contralateral, left hand. These movements are typically clonic, repetitive, flexion/extension movements. Because the cortical region controlling the hand is immediately adjacent to the region for facial expression, the seizure may also cause abnormal movements of the face synchronous with movements of the hand. The EEG will show abnormal spike discharges in a very limited region over the related area of cerebral cortex.

There are different types of seizures that are classified according to the symptoms and EEG results (see Box 34-4).

Clinical Presentation

Obtaining an accurate detailed history of the characteristics of a seizure is critical in establishing an accurate diagnosis. In addition, it is important to ask about the presence of systemic illnesses, history of malignancy,

---

BOX 34-4. Epileptic Seizure Classification

Seizures are classified according to the International Classification of Epileptic Seizures into three broad categories:

GENERALIZED SEIZURES

- **Absence seizure:** Also known as petit mal seizure, an absence seizure involves a brief, sudden lapse of consciousness for 5 to 30 seconds. Absence seizures are more common in children than adults. The individual looks as though he or she is staring into space for a few seconds. Absence seizures can be subcategorized as typical and atypical. In typical absence seizures, the patient briefly loses awareness of surroundings. In atypical absence seizures, the patient has muscle spasms with the loss of awareness.
- **Tonic-clonic seizure:** In a tonic-clonic seizure, also known as grand mal seizure, the patient commonly vocalizes loudly before the seizure and loses consciousness. The patient has rhythmic jerking movements and stiffening of muscles that can last up to 5 minutes. Medical assistance is necessary. A seizure that continues for up to 30 minutes or a series of three tonic-clonic seizures is a medical emergency called status epilepticus.
- **Clonic seizure:** Clonic seizures consist of rhythmic jerking movements of the arms and legs, sometimes on both sides of the body. The patient often falls but consciousness is usually preserved.
- **Tonic seizure:** In a tonic seizure, there is a 20- to 30-second time period when the patient has stiffening of muscles. The patient often falls but consciousness is usually preserved.
- **Atonic seizure:** In an atonic seizure, the patient loses muscle tone for up to 15 seconds. Consciousness is often preserved during the seizure. The patient usually falls to the ground.
- **Myoclonic:** In a myoclonic seizure, there are brief shocklike jerks of muscles—rapid alternating contraction and relaxation of muscles. They can be singular movements or multiple that last a few seconds.

FOCAL SEIZURES

- **Simple:** In a simple focal seizure, which usually only involves one hemisphere of the brain, the patient does not lose consciousness. Symptomology is related to the area of the brain affected.
- **Complex:** In a complex focal seizure, the patient may experience an altered level of consciousness or lose consciousness completely. These seizures can start within a localized area of the brain but progress to both hemispheres, leading to cognitive, affective, and psychomotor symptoms.

UNCLASSIFIED SEIZURES

Unclassified seizures are seizures that cannot be identified as either generalized or focal.

history of head trauma, family history of neurological disorders, and medication, drug, and alcohol use. Seizures need to be completely described. An individual who has observed the patient's seizures is usually the best person to provide an accurate history. Factors preceding the seizure should be described. Precipitating factors or relieving factors regarding the seizure also need to be detailed.

CLINICAL CONCEPT

When a patient first experiences a seizure, the etiologic origin is sought. When the patient experiences more than one episode of seizure, however, a diagnosis of epilepsy becomes clearer.

Before a seizure, an individual may have unique sensations referred to as an **aura.** An aura often manifests as the perception of a strange light, an unpleasant smell, or confusing thoughts or experiences. When occurring, auras allow epileptics time to prepare for a seizure, which can help prevent injury to themselves and others. The episode of the seizure is often referred to as the **ictal period,** and the phase after completion of the seizure is referred to as the **postictal period.**

The postictal state, the altered state of consciousness that a person enters after experiencing a seizure, usually lasts between 5 and 30 minutes; however, it can last longer in the case of larger or more severe seizures. The postictal state is characterized by drowsiness, confusion, nausea, hypertension, headache, and other disorienting symptoms. Additionally, emergence from this period is often accompanied by amnesia or other memory defects. During this period, the brain recovers from the trauma of the seizure.

CLINICAL CONCEPT

If multiple seizures occur in a short time frame, the **interictal period** is the time frame between seizures, when brain activity is more normal.

During the history, the patient should be asked to describe auras, loss of consciousness, and any details recalled about the ictal and postictal states. Did the patient note any warning before the seizure? If so, what kind? If an observer was present, ask what happened during the seizure. If the patient has recollection of the seizure, a full description is necessary. It is important to ask how the patient felt after the seizure. How long did it take for the patient to get back to normal? How long did the seizure last? How frequent did the seizures occur? Were there any precipitating factors? Relieving factors? Did the patient respond to therapy?

A complete physical examination should be performed, including a comprehensive neurological assessment and mental status exam. The cranial nerves should be completely tested to obtain clues about intracranial pressure. Physiologic illness, metabolic disturbance, head trauma, and substance abuse are often causes for a seizure.

Diagnostic clues about a physical cause of the seizure should be sought during the physical examination. Focal neurological deficits may be present. These are specific neurologic impairments due to nerve, spinal cord or brain dysfunction. One sided extremity weakness is a common example of a focal neurologic deficit. Neurological deficits may be caused by a variety of medical conditions, such as head trauma, tumors, and stroke; various diseases such as meningitis and encephalitis; or as a side effect of medications or abused substances.

CLINICAL CONCEPT

A quick neurological assessment requires evaluation of vital signs, level of consciousness, pupil reaction, upper and lower extremity strength, and verbal response to a question.

Diagnosis

Laboratory studies are necessary to rule out substance abuse or physiologic illness as the cause of a seizure. A complete blood count (CBC), serum chemistry, liver enzymes, and other blood tests pertaining to a suspected clinical illness are necessary. Brain imaging studies, such as magnetic resonance imaging (MRI) and computed tomography (CT), are helpful, especially if the individual has focal neurological deficits, altered mental status, recent history of head trauma, headache, anticoagulant use, or fever.

Individuals with suspected seizures should have an EEG as part of their diagnostic work-up. Analysis of interictal discharges on the EEG can help to support a diagnosis of epilepsy, help to classify the epilepsy syndrome, and determine the cerebral hemisphere that gives rise to the seizure. Taking an EEG on an individual who is sleep-deprived will increase the sensitivity of the EEG.

CLINICAL CONCEPT

The presence of a normal EEG does not rule out a seizure disorder. Approximately 50% of individuals with epilepsy will not show any abnormalities on a single EEG.

Treatment

For nonepileptic seizures, treatment for the underlying condition is necessary. Such conditions as head trauma, stroke, metabolic imbalances, and CNS infection require different treatment modalities and are often reversible.

When there is no identifiable, reversible cause for the seizure, treatment involves the use of antiepileptic drugs. Drug treatment is usually initiated when the individual is experiencing acute or chronic seizures or has clear structural predisposition to seizures. A wide variety of medications with different mechanisms of action have been successful in enabling many patients to have relatively normal lives with less frequent seizures. The actions of antiepileptic agents commonly modify the activity of ion channels or neurotransmitters in the brain. The medications include phenytoin, valproic acid, carbamazepine, topiramate, zonisamide, ethosuximide, lacosamide, gabapentin, lamotrigine, and benzodiazepines. The goal of epilepsy treatment is the prevention of further seizures without adverse medication side effects.

For individuals with recurrent seizures that are refractory to medication or for individuals with a localized epileptic focus of their seizures, surgical management may be utilized. Debulking a brain tumor, evacuating a subdural hematoma, performing a parietal or temporal lobectomy, or placing a vagal nerve stimulator are all interventions in which epilepsy can be surgically treated.

ALERT! During a seizure, the most important goal is to protect the patient from injury. Move objects that could cause injury out of the way. Do not physically restrain the patient and do not put anything in his or her mouth. Also, because of the risk of postseizure vomiting, after the seizure has ended, place the patient on his or her left side and turn the head so that any emesis or oral secretions will drain out of the mouth and not be inhaled.

Headache

Headaches can be categorized as either a primary or secondary disorder. Primary headaches arise independent of any other medical illness or traumatic cause. Secondary headaches are caused by another primary condition, such as head injury or concussion; vascular problems, such as aneurysms or arteriovenous malformations; medication side effects; sinus disease; and tumors.

Primary Headache
The most common types of primary headaches are tension-type headaches (TTH), migraine headaches, and cluster headaches.

Tension-Type Headache. TTH, the most common type of primary headache, occurs in as many as 78% of persons. There are three subtypes as described by the International Headache Society:

1. infrequent episodic TTH, with headache occurring fewer than 1 day per month

2. frequent episodic TTH, with at least 10 headache episodes per month for at least 3 months
3. chronic TTH, with headaches occurring 15 or more days per month for longer than 3 months.

A TTH can last minutes to days. The pain is often described as bilateral with mild to moderate pressure. It does not worsen with physical activity and there is no associated nausea or vomiting. Some patients may complain of either photophobia (light sensitivity) or phonophobia (sensitivity to sound), but these symptoms are more commonly associated with migraine type headaches.

Pathophysiology. TTH can be primarily a central neurological disturbance, similar to migraine, or can occur as the result of increased cervical and pericranial muscle activity, such as that caused by flexion-extension injury of the neck, poor posture, or anxiety with increased clenching or grinding of the teeth. Electromyographic (EMG) studies have shown muscle contraction in patients with TTH; however, it is unclear if muscle contraction is causative.

Clinical Presentation. The patient often complains of a bandlike pain or diffuse pain over the head. Tight cervical and shoulder muscles commonly accompany headache. Other features of TTH include:

- stable pattern of headaches over many months or years
- family history of similar headaches
- normal physical exam
- headaches that are consistently triggered by hormonal cycle, specific foods, specific sensory input of light, odors, or other typical triggers.

Diagnosis. The diagnosis of TTH is based on clinical findings. Usually a TTH does not require laboratory testing or imaging studies if the physical examination is normal.

Treatment. Episodic TTHs are generally treated with simple analgesics such as acetaminophen, aspirin, and other nonsteroidal anti-inflammatory drugs (NSAIDs). Medications containing ergotamine, caffeine, barbiturates and codeine should be avoided. For those individuals with chronic headaches, a prophylactic approach using tricyclic antidepressants and serotonin receptor inhibitors has been used effectively. In conjunction with pharmacological intervention, relaxation therapy, biofeedback, and stress management have been associated with reducing the frequency of headaches.

Migraine Headache. **Migraine** headaches are periodic, throbbing headaches that are characterized by altered perceptions, nausea, and severe pain. Photophobia and phonophobia often accompany a migraine headache. An aura may precede the headache.

Approximately 28 million people in the United States suffer from migraine headaches, with a 1 year prevalence of 18.2% among females and 6.5% among males. Among migraine sufferers, 75% are women. The peak prevalence of migraine is between the ages of 25 and

55 years. Individuals with migraine often report it as disabling, as they can have difficulty being productive at home, work, and school.

Pathophysiology. Knowledge regarding migraine pathophysiology is incomplete, although research into the pathogenesis of migraine headache is ongoing. The current theory proposes four stages of migraine:

1. **prodrome:** neural hyperexcitability in the brain
2. **aura:** cortical spreading depression (CSD) occurs
3. **pain:** trigeminovascular complex activation accounting for the pain
4. **postdrome:** sensitization of the trigeminovascular complex persists.

In the first stage, or prodrome to the migraine headache, there is a significant hyperexcitability of neurons in the cerebral cortex, most notably the occipital region. Once the nerve cells have reached the threshold of excitability, CSD is initiated. CSD describes a wave of neuronal depolarization that spreads across the cerebrum. This mechanism triggers the aura of migraine and activates trigeminal nerve impulses to the brain. The activation of the trigeminal nerve impulses to the brain by CSD is thought to cause an inflammatory change in the pain-sensitive meninges. Brainstem regions that modulate sensory input to the trigeminal nerves include the locus coeruleus and dorsal raphe nucleus.

In the next stage, a throbbing type pain begins. Both serotonin and calcitonin gene-related peptides (CGRP) are thought to play a role in the pain of migraine. There are decreased levels of serotonin as well as elevated levels of CGRP present in migraineurs during an attack. CGRP is a potent vasodilator of cerebral and dural vessels. The exact role of serotonin in migraine is unclear, though it is known that stimulation of the serotonin receptors can alleviate a migraine. Data also support a role of dopamine; most migraine symptoms can be induced by stimulation of dopamine receptors.

The final postdromal stage of migraine is evident in some patients who present with continued pain on the top of the head, upper trunk, or limb with movement after the headache subsides. These residual pains are believed to be a result of the sensitization of the trigeminal system.

Clinical Presentation. When a migraine headache is suspected, a complete history and physical examination are necessary to exclude other causes of headache. The patient should be asked about events and feelings before the headache. A full description of the headache is necessary to diagnose migraine. Most migraine headaches have a common pattern of presentation described by the sufferer.

The most common presentation of migraine headache is a severe throbbing, one-sided headache that is accompanied by nausea, vomiting, photophobia, and phonophobia. It usually worsens with movements such as climbing stairs, jumping, or leaning over. Migraine headache is usually disabling to the sufferer and the

---

> ### BOX 34-5. Migraine Triggers
>
> Migraine headaches may be precipitated by any of the following:
>
> - emotions such as worry or stress
> - intake of foods containing nitrites, glutamate, aspartate, and tyramine, among other chemicals
> - hormone shifts, as with oral contraceptives and menstruation
> - activities such as excessive exercise
> - lack of sleep or fatigue
> - hunger with an associated drop in blood sugar.
>
> Other triggers of migraine may include medications such as nitroglycerin, histamine, reserpine, withdrawal from corticosteroids, and hydralazine. Some individuals will find that odors such as perfumes, smoke, and other strong odors can trigger their migraine attacks.

patient usually needs to lie down. Some migraine headaches may have a preceding aura. The patient should be asked to describe the actions and feelings before a migraine headache to decipher if an aura occurs and assess triggers of the headache (see Box 34-5 and Box 34-6). It is helpful for individuals to keep a diary of their headaches. This diary should include a description of the symptoms, frequency of the headaches, and any information that could assist in identifying triggers of the migraines. The physical examination is usually normal yet the patient is incapable of performing duties or concentrating.

Diagnosis. The diagnosis of migraine headache is usually based on clinical signs and symptoms. Some clinicians use imaging studies such as CT or MRI to exclude any other cause of headache when diagnosis is questionable. There are diagnostic criteria for migraine, which include a normal physical examination and specific signs and symptoms (see Box 34-7).

Treatment. Most drugs that are effective in the treatment of migraine headaches are NSAIDs, serotonin receptor agonists, and dopamine receptor antagonists. In general, an adequate dose should ideally be administered as soon as possible after onset of the headache. However, migraine therapy is individualized, and there is no one standard approach for all patients (see Box 34-8).

Cluster Headache. Cluster headaches are typically characterized by repetitive headaches that occur for weeks to several months at a time, followed by remission. This uncommon type of headache affects fewer than 1% of the population. The majority of sufferers are male, and peak age of onset is between ages 25 and 50 years.

Pathophysiology. It is theorized that vasodilation is responsible for the pain and the autonomic features of cluster headaches. Similar to the migraine headache, the trigeminovascular system appears to be activated,

---

BOX 34-6. Types of Migraine

There are various types of migraine headaches–mainly migraine without aura and migraine with aura. During the history, the patient should be asked to describe the whole experience of the disorder, which includes setting, feelings, and actions before the migraine, as well as the type of pain and duration of migraine and associated symptoms.

MIGRAINE WITHOUT AURA

Migraine without aura is the most common type of migraine and is characterized by a headache that lasts from 4 to 72 hours if untreated. It is usually described as a pulsating or pounding pain on one side of the head, usually frontotemporal. The pain is of moderate or severe intensity and is aggravated by physical activity. During the headache, the individual can have nausea and vomiting. Migraines without aura that occur more than 15 times per month for 3 months or longer are classified as chronic migraines.

MIGRAINE WITH AURA

Migraine with aura is characterized by focal neurological symptoms that precede the headache. Aura of migraine can be described by patients as loss of vision or visualization of flickering lights, zig-zag lines, or spots. An aura can include strange tastes in the mouth and odors. Some patients may also have numbness and tingling in the extremities. Those with familial hemiplegic migraine experience severe weakness in one side of the body.

Aura associated with migraine often develops over a period of 5 to 20 minutes and can last up to 1 hour; all symptoms of aura are completely reversible. Headache can either start with aura or follow the aura and is clinically the same as migraine without aura as previously described.

Some patients with migraine may also experience premonitory symptoms hours to 2 days before a migraine attack. These symptoms include fatigue, loss of concentration, neck stiffness, photophobia and phonophobia, nausea, blurred vision, yawning, or pallor.

OTHER TYPES OF MIGRAINE HEADACHE

Many other types of migraine exist, and they are typically named according to their unique feature. Among them are:

- typical aura with nonmigraine headache
- typical aura without headache
- familial hemiplegic migraine
- sporadic hemiplegic migraine
- basilar-type migraine, which includes symptoms of dysarthria, vertigo, tinnitus, diplopia, visual symptoms, ataxia, decreased level of consciousness, and bilateral paresthesias
- cyclical vomiting migraine (children)
- abdominal migraine (children).

BOX 34-7. Diagnostic Criteria for Migraine

MIGRAINE WITHOUT AURA

Migraine without aura is diagnosed after repeated attacks of headache lasting 4 to 72 hours in patients with normal physical examination, no other reasonable cause for the headache, and at least two features from the primary list and at least one from the secondary list:

Primary List
- unilateral pain
- throbbing pain
- aggravation by movement
- moderate or severe intensity.

Secondary List
- nausea/vomiting
- photophobia and phonophobia.

MIGRAINE WITH AURA

Migraine with aura is a recurrent disorder manifesting in attacks of reversible focal neurological symptoms that:

- develop gradually over 5 to 20 minutes
- last for fewer than 60 minutes.

Headache with the features of migraine without aura usually follows the aura symptoms; less commonly, the headache lacks the migraine's features or is completely absent.

(Adapted from *The International Classification of Headache Disorders*. 2nd edition, Cephalalgia 2004, 24 (Suppl 1), 1–160.)

---

explaining the patterns of pain. The hypothalamus is postulated to play a prominent role because there are alterations in the circadian rhythms during the cluster period. It is also theorized that the clinical features of cluster headaches can be explained by a lesion involving the cavernous sinus portion of the internal carotid artery. At this site, both the nociceptive and autonomic fibers that innervate the eye are in close proximity of each other. There is also evidence of a genetic role in the etiology of cluster headaches. A high percentage of men (86%) and women (60%) who experience cluster headaches are smokers.

BOX 34-8. Treatment of Migraine Headaches

In the past, NSAIDs and opiate analgesics have been effectively used in the treatment of migraine. A combination of butalbital, caffeine, and aspirin known as Fiorinal has also been used to effectively treat migraine headache. However, stimulation of serotonin receptors through the use of selective serotonin receptor agonists known as triptans has become the preferred migraine treatment for many sufferers.

Triptans are available in oral, nasal spray, and subcutaneous preparations and as parenteral medication. A triptan transdermal patch has also proven to relieve pain and associated migraine symptoms. In some cases, coadministration of a long-acting NSAID can reduce rates of headache recurrence. Ergo alkaloids, such as ergotamine and dihydroergotamine, are nonselective serotonin receptor agonists that are also effective. Dopamine antagonists such as droperidol are sometimes used to stop migraine headache and accompanying nausea and vomiting.

Transcranial magnetic stimulation (TMS) has been effective for migraine headache in persons older than 18 years old. TMS is a handheld device that releases a pulse of magnetic energy to the occipital region of the head.

PREVENTION

To prevent migraines, patients should be advised to avoid triggers such as lack of sleep, fatigue, stress, vasodilators, oral contraceptives, and dietary components such as wine. Patients who have frequent migraine headaches, such as five or more attacks per month, are candidates for preventive therapy. Preventive drugs should be taken daily and there is usually a 2- to 12-week lag period before an effect is seen. Preventive drugs include beta blockers such as propranolol, tricyclic antidepressants such as amitriptyline, and anticonvulsants such as valproate. *Clostridium botulinum* (Botox) injections into the scalp and temple have also been approved for preventive migraine therapy.

Clinical Presentation. In the patient history, cluster headaches are often described as excruciating, with deep continuous, intense, and debilitating pain. Some patients will have pain described as an "ice pick" that is stabbing and sharp in quality. The pain is unilateral and most commonly starts around the eye or the temple. Less commonly, the pain will start in the face, neck, or ear. It is typical to see ipsilateral redness in the eye, stuffy nose or rhinorrhea, sweating, and pallor. Individuals with cluster headaches will often be restless and unable to sit quietly when experiencing a headache. This is in sharp contrast to the patient with a migraine headache, who will often withdraw to a dark quiet room. A typical cluster headache may last between 15 minutes to 3 hours, and in 80% of cases they occur between 9 p.m. and 9 a.m.

The frequency of attacks depends on the type of cluster headache. If the individual is experiencing episodic cluster headaches, which is most common, he or she is likely to experience one to three attacks of periorbital pain per day for up to 3 months. Remission periods usually last between 6 and 12 months. The individual who experiences no real sustained remission is considered to have chronic cluster headaches.

 CLINICAL CONCEPT

With cluster headache, the patient describes intense pain, usually around the temple region of the head. Conjunctivitis and rhinorrhea with diaphoresis may be present. Otherwise, the physical examination is normal.

Diagnosis. The diagnosis of cluster headache is usually based on clinical signs and symptoms. Some clinicians use imaging studies such as CT or MRI to exclude any other cause of headache when diagnosis is questionable.

Treatment. A number of medications as well as administration of oxygen have been shown to be effective in cluster headache. Medications used in the treatment of cluster headache include triptans, dihydroergotamine, and octreotide. Prednisone, lithium, cyproheptadine, methysergide, and indomethacin have also been effectively used. Surgery involving the resection of part of the trigeminal nerve and nerve block of the greater occipital nerve have also been effective in rare cases.

Secondary Headaches

With secondary headaches, it is important to discern whether or not the headache is related to another medical condition. Some secondary causes, such as sinusitis, are easily treatable. However, the most serious secondary cause of headache is brain tumor.

Sinus Headache. The International Headache Society describes the acute sinus headache as occurring in conjunction with acute sinusitis; fever and rhinorrhea may also be present. The pain is caused by sinus pressure and can worsen when the patient leans over. The facial areas over the frontal and maxillary sinuses may be tender to palpation. Transillumination of the sinuses may show nontransparency. Sinus x-rays may be needed to confirm diagnosis. The usual treatment of sinus headache includes the use of antibiotics and nasal decongestants.

Headache Caused by Brain Tumors. Approximately 50% of individuals with brain tumors will experience a headache. The headaches are usually dull and constant, and may or may not have a throbbing quality. The location of the headache is commonly bifrontal, with worse pain on the same side as the tumor. However, generalized head pain has also been reported, perhaps because of an increase in intracranial pressure. Increased intracranial pressure may lead to the classic triad of headache, nausea, and papilledema. Cranial nerve testing may reveal abnormalities.

> **ALERT!** Patients with the following symptoms need further evaluation to rule out the possibility of a brain tumor:
>
> - abnormal neurological examination
> - change in prior headache patterns
> - worsening of headache with a change in body position, such as bending over, or with coughing, sneezing, or any maneuver that raises intrathoracic pressure or intracranial pressure
> - worsening headaches at night that awaken the patient from sleep.

Pathophysiology of Selected Neurodegenerative Disorders

Common major neurodegenerative disorders include Parkinson's disease, Amyotrophic Lateral Sclerosis (ALS), and Multiple Sclerosis (MS). They are all slowly progressive diseases that affect motor or sensory nerves, or both.

Parkinson's Disease

Parkinson's disease is a common neurodegenerative disorder affecting approximately 1.5 million people in the United States. The National Parkinson Foundation estimates that 60,000 new cases are diagnosed each year. This slow and progressive disorder is typically diagnosed in the fifth or sixth decade of life. However, approximately 10% of those with Parkinson's disease are younger than 40 years of age; these individuals are classified as having young-onset Parkinson's disease. In rare instances, Parkinson-like symptoms can appear in children and teenagers in a disorder known as juvenile parkinsonism; this disorder has a different clinical course from typical Parkinson's disease and is usually attributed to hereditary causes.

Parkinson's disease affects both men and women equally, and there is no evidence that it is more prevalent in different ethnic groups or in any particular geographic regions. The clinical course of the disorder is highly variable for each individual.

Etiology

Most cases of Parkinson's disease (85% to 90%) have unknown etiology. Genetics plays a relevant role in the etiology of familial Parkinson's disease, which is responsible for 10% of cases. A mutated protein called leucine-rich repeat kinase 2 (LRRK2) is a common cause of familial Parkinson's disease. The LRRK2 gene mutation is located at 12p11–p13. Exactly how the protein affects synaptic function remains unclear. Mutations are also found in other genes, including the parkin gene at 6q25–27 and the alpha-synuclein gene at 4q21–23. The parkin gene causes mitochondrial dysfunction, and the alpha-synuclein gene causes an accumulation of an abnormal protein called alpha-synuclein.

In addition to genetics, important risk factors of Parkinson's disease include advancing age as well as certain viral infections and chemical exposures. Injection of a street drug containing a meperidine analog can produce parkinsonian symptoms. Repeated exposure to other chemicals such as pesticides and repeated head trauma may provide an increased risk as well.

Pathophysiology

Pathologically, Parkinson's disease is mainly associated with progressive loss of dopamine-producing cells in the substantia nigra, which is within the basal ganglia of the midbrain. The basal ganglia modulates movements, such as posture, standing, walking, or writing. In the basal ganglia, acetylcholine and dopamine are the neurotransmitters that modulate the body's movements. Acetylcholine stimulates muscle movement, whereas dopamine has an inhibitory effect on movement. In Parkinson's disease, the depletion of dopamine creates an imbalance of these two neurotransmitters. The effects of unopposed acetylcholine is apparent in the tremor and abnormal spasmodic, muscle movements of Parkinson's disease. Signs of the disease do not become apparent until 50% to 80% of the substantia nigra is degenerated.

In Parkinson's disease, there is also an accumulation of an abnormal protein called alpha-synuclein found in structures called Lewy bodies in the brainstem, spinal cord, and regions of the cortex. It is still unclear how alpha-synuclein causes the disorder, but the accumulation of this protein is associated with neurodegeneration and cell death.

Pathology can also involve the ANS, which causes nonmotor symptoms such as orthostatic hypotension, sleep disturbances, gastrointestinal disturbances, and impaired thermoregulation.

Clinical Presentation

The triad of bradykinesia, resting tremor, and muscle rigidity are the classic manifestations of Parkinson's disease. Bradykinesia, defined as slowed movements, and akinesia, which is the absence of movement, commonly occur in this disorder. Initial manifestations may be apparent on one side of the body, but eventually the symptoms involve bilateral, symmetrical areas of the body. The resting tremor is often the first symptom. As the disease progresses and with further deterioration of the substantia nigra, individuals have progressive difficulty with automatic movements. Daily tasks such as walking, dressing, writing, eating, and others become difficult. There is postural imbalance and, at times, difficulty with initiation of movement. The onset of Parkinson's disease is typically slow and insidious; as the disease progresses, the classic symptomatology appears.

Tremor. The classic tremor of Parkinson's disease is a resting, "pill rolling" tremor of the hand and finger; this is often the first motor symptom of the disease. The tremor usually presents unilaterally and then becomes bilateral, often spreading to the legs and sometimes the head, jaw, and face. Interestingly, a resting tremor ceases when purposeful movement of the limb occurs.

CLINICAL CONCEPT

With Parkinson's disease, a tremor can appear as though the person is rolling a pill in his or her hand, which is why the term "pill-rolling" is used to describe the tremor.

Rigidity. Rigidity is often felt by the patient as a tightness or stiffness in the arms, legs, neck, and trunk and presents initially on one side of the body with a gradual progression to both sides. On physical exam, the most notable finding will be the cogwheeling or ratchety movement felt by the examiner when passively moving the affected body part. This cogwheeling movement is caused by co-contraction of agonist and antagonist muscles. Rigidity of muscles is also manifested in facial muscles, causing a facial masking or emotionless stare that typifies the expression often seen in Parkinson's disease. Individuals may also experience decreased blink rates; soft, monotonous, low-volume speech; and difficulty swallowing.

Bradykinesia. Bradykinesia, which is a state of slowed movements, can inhibit independent functioning. Early Parkinson's disease patients may first see the effect in distal muscles of the arms and legs. Patients may have difficulty initiating gait or rising from a chair. Bradykinetic manifestations of the upper extremities include decreased arm swing, handwriting micrographia, and decreased fine motor function. Patients may also experience akinetic episodes, which they may describe as being "frozen" in place.

Postural Instability. Postural instability caused by the loss of postural reflexes usually manifests at later stages of disease progression. Patients may take very quick and short steps forward or they may step backward rapidly and uncontrollably. This, coupled with truncal rigidity and decreased ability to make corrective adjustments in balance, increases the risk for falling.

Nonmotor Symptoms. Nonmotor symptoms can be classified into three categories:

1. nonmotor symptoms with ANS involvement
2. nonmotor symptoms without ANS involvement
3. neuropsychiatric symptoms including cognitive changes.

These symptoms can be very disabling as they often affect socialization, motivation, and quality of life.

A large majority (90%) of individuals with Parkinson's disease experience symptoms attributed to the neurodegenerative effects of the disease on the ANS. These symptoms include constipation, dysphagia, orthostatic hypotension, drooling, sexual dysfunction, abnormal sweating, and thermoregulation, as well as urinary and bladder dysfunction. Nonmotor symptoms without ANS involvement include speech disturbances; seborrheic dermatitis; sleep disorders, including restless leg syndrome, daytime sleepiness, insomnia, fatigue; and olfactory and visual dysfunction.

Neuropsychiatric symptoms such as depression are commonly associated with Parkinson's disease, with a prevalence as high as 40%. Although depression is often referred to as a nonmotor symptom, the cause of depression may be either endogenous, as a result of the neurodegeneration process related to the disease, or exogenous, resulting from variables such as age of onset, disease severity, and disability.

Cognitive dysfunction in Parkinson's disease can affect as many as 80% of individuals and range from decreased executive functioning ability to severe symptoms of dementia. Other neuropsychiatric symptoms include anxiety and apathy. The neuropsychiatric manifestations of Parkinson's disease are associated with worsening disability, poor quality of life, poorer outcomes, and increased caregiver distress.

Diagnosis

The diagnosis of Parkinson's disease is usually made on the basis of clinical symptomatology. There are no laboratory tests that identify the disorder; however, recent studies are focusing on the protein alpha-synuclein. Several studies have found a decreased amount of alpha-synuclein in the cerebrospinal fluid of patients with Parkinson's disease. Genetic testing is not generally used routinely, but is used in research studies. Mutations of the LRRK2 gene are currently under investigation as a diagnostic test. CT scan and MRI reveal normal results, but imaging of the brain dopamine system with **positron emission tomography (PET)** or single photon emission CT show reduced uptake of dopaminergic markers. A substantial and sustained response to dopamine medications also helps confirm the diagnosis.

Treatment

Treatment goals in Parkinson's disease are aimed at relieving symptoms and maximizing independence and mobility while preserving the individual's quality of life.

The cornerstone of treatment is dopamine replacement therapy. Levodopa (L-dopa), the metabolic precursor of dopamine, in combination with carbidopa, a peripheral decarboxylase inhibitor, are used together. Carbidopa inhibits peripheral metabolism of levodopa and allows more of the levodopa to act at the brain. Commonly, after years of levodopa, a diminishing response occurs. Dopamine agonists such as pramipexole and ropinirole can be used as adjuncts to levodopa. Monoamine oxidase (MAO)-B inhibitors such as rasagiline and selegiline can provide symptomatic benefit as monotherapy in early disease and as adjuncts to levodopa. Catechol-O-methyl transferase (COMT) is the enzyme that shuts down dopamine in the synapse. COMT inhibitors such as entacapone and tolcapone, are used to prolong the effect of dopamine in the synapse.

Anticholinergic medications can be used for the treatment of resting tremor, but they are not particularly effective for bradykinesia, rigidity, gait disturbance, or other features of advanced Parkinson's disease. Surgical procedures such as deep brain stimulation of the subthalamic nuclei or globus pallidum[C4] are available for a select group of individuals with advanced disease. Exercise therapy is often recommended for individuals and should be used as an adjunct to pharmacological therapies, as it has significant positive effects on functional independence, motor function, ADLs, and quality of life.

ALERT! Anticholinergic medications have many undesirable side effects such as dry mouth, double vision, lack of perspiration and poor heat dissipation, confusion, and lack of concentration ability.

Amyotrophic Lateral Sclerosis

ALS, which is often referred to as Lou Gehrig's disease, is a progressive neurodegenerative disorder that is characterized by a loss of upper and lower motor neurons and eventually results in respiratory failure. Symptoms include painless muscle weakness and atrophy.

The worldwide incidence of ALS ranges from 0.4 to 2.6 per 100,000 population per year. The prevalence of ALS is 6 per 100,000 individuals. In the United States, it is estimated that 20,000 individuals have ALS, and 5,000 Americans are diagnosed with the disease on an annual basis. In the United States, ALS affects Caucasians more than other racial and ethnic groups. It is usually diagnosed between 40 and 60 years of age with more men affected than women.

Etiology
The etiology of ALS is unknown, but there are some proposed risk factors, including heavy metal toxic effects, environmental and occupational exposures, cigarette smoking, repeated physical trauma, and participation in heavy physical activity such as professional athletics.

BOX 34-9. The FUS Gene and ALS

Recently, there has been growing interest in the FUS gene (also called *FUS/TLS* for "fused in sarcoma–translated in sarcoma" gene) found on chromosome 16. This gene programs for FUS protein, which is normally found inside the motor neuron cell nucleus, where it serves its primary function as a ribonucleic acid binding protein. Researchers have found that mutated FUS genes direct the manufacture of mutant FUS protein that forms characteristic yarn-like cytoplasmic inclusions in spinal motor neurons in both familial and sporadic cases of ALS. Because this has been noted in both types of ALS, there is growing interest regarding the FUS gene.

Two classifications of ALS have been described: familial (inherited) ALS and sporadic ALS. Approximately 5% to 10% of all cases of ALS are thought to be familial, with mutations in the superoxide dismutase gene 1 accounting for approximately 20% of familial ALS cases. Mutations in the TAR DNA-binding protein gene 43 and FUS gene occur in about 4% to 5% of the familial ALS cases (see Box 34-9). Altogether, mutations in specific genes have been identified in about 30% of familial ALS cases.

Pathophysiology
ALS is a rapidly progressive, neurodegenerative disease that destroys the motor neurons that control voluntary muscles. Upper motor neurons, which are motor neurons located in the brain, send messages to lower motor neurons located in the spinal cord, and then to different voluntary muscle groups. In individuals affected by ALS, both the upper and lower motor neurons become sclerotic and die. They can no longer send messages to the muscles. The muscles that are no longer receiving messages from the upper and lower neurons weaken and atrophy. Specific gene mutations, particularly of the FUS gene, are under investigation as the instigators of motor neuron death.

Eventually, the damage to the motor neurons becomes so great that the brain is unable to start or adequately control voluntary muscle movement. The progressive atrophy and paralysis of the muscles that control the patient's speech, swallowing, and breathing slowly become impaired. The affected muscles become progressively weaker until they reach paralysis. Ultimately, the patient will require artificial ventilation for respiratory failure or may choose a palliative care approach. Because ALS only damages motor neurons, the sensory neurons remain intact—the abilities to see, detect sensation, hear, taste, and smell are not affected. Cognitive ability also remains intact.

Clinical Presentation
The initial symptoms of ALS can include weakness in the upper and lower extremities, head drop, speech

changes, and dysphagia. Symptoms of upper motor neuron involvement include muscle spasticity, hyper-reflexia, and a positive Babinski reflex. Symptoms of lower motor neuron damage include muscle weakness, atrophy, cramping, and fasciculations.

Diagnosis

The diagnosis of ALS is usually made on the basis of clinical symptomatology. There are no laboratory tests that identify the disorder, no biomarkers for the condition, and findings on MRI and CT scan are unremarkable. EMG studies may be helpful to rule out muscle or neurological conditions that may mimic ALS. The value of PET scanning, functional MRI, and magnetic resonance spectroscopy in ALS is being studied.

Treatment

There is no cure for ALS. However, the medication riluzole (Rilutek) is believed to reduce the damage to motor neurons by decreasing the release of the excitatory neurotransmitter glutamate. The exact mechanism is not entirely understood. Other treatments for ALS are designed to manage symptoms of the disease and improve the quality of life. Medications to reduce fatigue, relieve muscle cramps, control spasticity, and reduce excessive oral secretions can be beneficial to patients. Gentle, low-impact aerobic activity and range-of-motion and stretching exercises can help to prevent painful muscle spasticity and contractures. When respiratory muscles weaken, the use of intermittent positive pressure ventilation may be used to ease the work of breathing during sleep. Decisions regarding patient preference for life-sustaining treatment, such as mechanical ventilation, versus palliative care approaches should be discussed soon after the diagnosis of ALS, and should be revisited on several occasions before respiratory failure occurs.

ALERT! Dysphagia resulting from ALS increases the patient's risk for aspiration of food and oral secretions.

ALERT! Dysfunction of the diaphragm muscle causes respiratory failure in ALS.

Multiple Sclerosis

MS is a chronic neurological disorder that affects the brain and spinal cord. It is a demyelinating disorder that results in inflammation and damage to the myelin and other cells within the CNS. This progressive condition eventually results in CNS damage and neurological disability. The disease is characterized by remissions and exacerbations.

The prevalence of MS worldwide is approximately 2.5 million individuals, and 400,000 individuals living in the United States have the disorder. It is most commonly diagnosed among young adults between 18 to 48 years of age, and affects women more often than men (2:1). MS is more likely to occur among individuals of northern European heritage, although people from African, Asian, and Hispanic ancestry also can develop the disorder. Prevalence is higher at greater distances from the equator and in countries with cooler climates, which has been suggestive of some environmental influences in its pathogenesis.

Etiology

Although the etiology of MS remains unknown, the damage to the myelin of the CNS and peripheral nerves is caused by an autoimmune inflammatory disorder. Several risk factors including genetic predisposition, viral or other infective process, trauma, or exposure to heavy metals may trigger the autoimmune response in MS.

Pathophysiology

It is theorized that activated T cells that have been abnormally sensitized to attack myelin cause the damage of MS. T cells damage the CNS myelin; this acts as a stimulant for more T cells to be activated and damage more myelin. Ultimately, demyelination of multiple areas of the CNS results.

The white matter tracts of the CNS are most commonly affected by the demyelination process. However, gray matter tracts can also be involved. There is a predilection for the optic nerves. Both sensory and motor neurons are affected. At times, the inflammatory phase can resolve and areas of demyelination can heal, allowing the disease to go into remission. Alternatively, areas of demyelination can remain damaged and turn to irreversible fibrotic scar tissue. These fibrotic areas of the myelin disrupt the conduction of impulses traveling throughout the nervous system, and this causes the various sensory and motor symptoms of MS.

Progressive deterioration without remissions can occur as a form of the disease known as primary progressive multiple sclerosis (PPMS). PPMS affects about 10% to 15% of individuals with MS.

Clinical Presentation

The most common symptoms of MS are weakness, numbness, tingling sensations, balance problems, blurred vision, and fatigue. The patient suffers both sensory loss and motor impairment. MS follows several different courses that are associated with particular symptoms, patterns of disability, and recommended treatments. About 85% of patients have the most common form of MS, the relapsing-remitting form. This consists of brief episodes, lasting anywhere between several weeks to 3 months, of various symptoms, occurring approximately every 1 to 3 years; these are followed by a complete or almost complete return to normal function. For these patients, the most common and early symptoms involve the eyes. Because the optic nerves are heavily covered with myelin, when those nerves are attacked, patients may experience a temporary distortion or loss of vision in one eye, impairment in color perception, or pain with eye movement. Individuals commonly present with sensory symptoms, such as numbness or paresthesias. Sensory symptoms and debilitating fatigue are often seen at the time of diagnosis. In addition to symptoms related to optic nerve degeneration, signs caused by damage to cerebellar nerves commonly present initially. The cerebellar symptoms include ataxia, tremor, and dysarthria.

Severe motor nerve damage typically occurs late in the disease. Motor symptoms include hemiparesis, paraparesis, and quadriparesis. Individuals with MS may have difficulty walking or performing tasks that require coordination. Spinal cord involvement may also lead to urinary and fecal incontinence and sexual dysfunction because these spinal tracts are heavily covered with myelin.

Individuals with MS are more likely to experience affective and cognitive symptoms than the general population. It is theorized that the neurobiological risk factors associated with MS contribute to the increased risk of depressive disorders and cognitive impairment among these patients. The lifetime risk for major depression in individuals with MS may be as high as 50%. Recent data suggests that 45% to 65% of individuals with MS experience some cognitive impairment. Although MS affects a variety of cognitive domains, recent memory, abstract reasoning, attention, and visual-spatial perception are most often affected. Immediate recall, long-term memory, and language skills seem to be the least disrupted in MS.

Dehydration or malnutrition can result because of swallowing difficulties or an inability to care for oneself. Individuals with MS have dysphagia in later stages of the illness, increasing the risk of aspiration pneumonia. Urinary retention and urinary sphincter dysfunction are common symptoms, placing the individual at a higher risk for urinary tract and kidney infections.

After several decades, approximately 50% of individuals with relapsing-remitting MS go on to develop secondary progressive MS, in which they have continually progressive deterioration and consequent disability.

> **ALERT!** In degenerative neuromuscular disorders, dysphagia occurs because of weakened esophageal muscles, which is why the assessment of the gag reflex is necessary before feeding a patient.

Diagnosis

MS cannot be diagnosed after only a single symptomatic episode, because symptoms are only clues. Diagnosis requires the appearance of lesions of demyelination detected on imaging studies and patient report of specific neurological deficits. The McDonald criteria, which includes specific neurological examination findings; MRI evidence; and patient symptoms are used to diagnose MS. Blood studies are usually normal. The clinician should perform blood work to help exclude conditions such as other autoimmune disorders, infections such as Lyme disease, endocrine abnormalities such as thyroid disease, and vitamin B12 deficiency. Cerebrospinal fluid may be evaluated for oligoclonal bands (OCBs) and immunoglobulin G (IgG), as well as for signs of infection. OCBs are found in 90% to 95% of patients with MS, and IgG is found in 70% to 90% of MS patients. Evoked potentials, which are recordings of the timing of CNS responses to specific stimuli, can be useful neurophysiological studies for evaluation of MS.

Treatment

Because MS is suspected to be an autoimmune disease directed against the CNS, available treatments involve preventing inflammatory cells from traveling across the blood-brain barrier. Immunomodulating agents reduce clinical attacks of new MS lesions, and they may have an impact on disability progression. Agents currently approved for use include interferon beta, glatiramer acetate, natalizumab, and fingolimod. These medications work better when treatment is started early during the course of MS. Although none of the medications can cure the disorder, they may reduce the number of days that a person suffers symptoms. Most importantly, they appear to reduce the accumulation of lesions within the CNS as seen on MRI findings. Corticosteroids can be used to reduce acute inflammation and expedite recovery from acute exacerbations of MS. They may be used for rescue therapy as monthly boosters in patients who respond poorly to the immunomodulators. Immunosuppressive agents can be used for their ability to suppress T-cell immune reactions. Novantrone is indicated for reducing neurological disability and the frequency of clinical relapses in patients. Methotrexate, cyclophosphamide, and azathioprine are commonly used. Amantadine is also used as a first-line drug to relieve symptoms of fatigue. Pharmacological treatment of spasticity includes Baclofen as a first-line drug. Tizanidine is an alpha-2–adrenergic agonist that is also used to treat spasticity.

Huntington Disease

Huntington disease (HD) is an inherited, progressively degenerative neurological disorder that results in involuntary motor symptoms, cognitive decline, and emotional and behavioral symptoms. It is an autosomal, dominant CNS disorder caused by cellular deterioration in specific areas of the basal ganglia and cortex. Currently, there is no treatment to halt or slow the progression of HD.

Estimates of the international prevalence of HD range from 4 to 8 in every 100,000 individuals. In the

United States, it is estimated that 30,000 individuals have HD. Because it is an autosomal dominant disorder, each child of a parent with HD has a 50% chance of inheriting the gene that causes the illness. Typically, symptoms appear between 30 and 50 years of age and can progress over 10 to 30 years. Duration of illness varies, with a mean of approximately 19 years. Pneumonia and cardiovascular disease are the most common primary causes of death.

Pathophysiology

HD is a genetic disorder caused by a single mutated gene on chromosome 4 that produces an abnormal repetition of the DNA bases cytosine, adenine, and guanine, leading to synthesis of a mutated form of the protein called huntingtin. The mutated protein collects within the cytoplasm of brain cells, but exactly how it causes the disease is unknown. It is linked to neurodegeneration in certain parts of the brain. This degeneration is evident in portions of the basal ganglia, caudate nuclei, and the globus pallidus. These structures, which are found deep within the brain, regulate coordinated movement and emotional expression. HD also affects the cerebral cortex and causes problems with perception, memory, and thinking.

Clinical Presentation

The early symptoms of HD disease vary greatly from person to person, but there are three common clinical manifestations:

1. involuntary motor symptoms
2. emotional and behavioral symptoms
3. cognitive symptoms.

Involuntary Motor Symptoms. The involuntary motor symptoms of HD include two components: dyskinesia, or excess movement, and the loss of voluntary movement. Movements in HD are described as **chorea,** which are brief, irregular, dancelike movements, and **athetosis,** which refers to twisting and writhing movements. Walking may become difficult and include odd postures and leg movements. When chorea is severe, there are thrashing motions referred to as ballismus. As HD progresses, dystonic, rigid postures may develop and eventually worsen, speech becomes slurred, and verbal communication and swallowing become progressively more difficult. In late-stage HD, maintaining adequate caloric and fluid intake becomes challenging because of dysphagia and the high caloric demands caused by worsening chorea movements.

Emotional and Behavioral Symptoms. Approximately 30% of individuals with HD develop a major depressive episode. Additionally, 10% of patients with HD develop episodes of mania in which irritability and elation are prominent. Other common behavioral symptoms of HD include anger and agitation. Delusions and hallucinations are less common but can occur.

Cognitive Symptoms. The early cognitive changes of HD include apathy, impaired mental flexibility, and slowed thought processing. Recognition memory is relatively spared. As HD progresses, the individual might have difficulty with remembering new information and making sound decisions and judgments.

Diagnosis

The discovery of the HD gene, at locus 14p16.3, has resulted in the development of a test that is able to detect the majority of individuals who are at risk for developing HD. In order to perform the genetic test, a small sample of blood is tested for the presence or absence of the HD gene mutation. No research has been able to identify a biomarker that accurately predicts onset of HD or disease progression.

Treatment

Presently, there is no satisfactory treatment available to stop or reverse the course of HD. However, there are some approaches that may help with the symptomatic management of the illness. Treatment of chorea with antipsychotic medications such as haloperidol and olanzapine may be symptomatically beneficial. Antidepressant medications have been used for the mood and behavioral symptoms of HD.

Palliative care approaches that focus on symptom management for individuals with HD have received increasing attention in the past several years. Physical and occupational therapies and regular exercise may help the person with HD feel better physically and emotionally. Speech therapy, swallowing interventions, and interventions that promote adequate nutrition and hydration are commonly utilized in the later stages of HD.

Guillain-Barré Syndrome

Guillain-Barré syndrome (GBS) is an acute peripheral neuropathy that leads to progressive limb weakness over the course of several days up to 4 weeks. Incidence worldwide is 1.3 cases per 100,000, with men being more frequently affected than women. There is a slight peak of incidence in adolescence and young adulthood, which may be caused by cytomegalovirus (CMV) infections and *Campylobacter jejuni (C. jejuni)*. It also occurs more often in the elderly population and may be a result of decreased immune suppressor mechanisms.

GBS is a postinfectious disease, with most of the patients having an antecedent infection of either the upper respiratory tract or gastroenteritis. These infections have resolved by the time of onset of the neuropathy. In many cases, the pathogen responsible for the antecedent infection is unidentified. However, the most common pathogens that result in GBS are *C. jejuni*, CMV, Epstein-Barr virus, and *Mycoplasma pneumonia*. The syndrome has also occurred after immunization with various types of vaccines.

Pathophysiology

The proposed pathogenesis for GBS is one in which a previous infection evokes an autoimmune response in the peripheral nerves. Most patients report an infectious illness in the weeks before onset. Many of the identified infectious agents are thought to stimulate the production of antibodies that attack the infectious agent as well as the body's normal myelin sheaths covering nerve axons. The cause of this cross reaction is unknown. Pathological findings include the infiltration of lymphocytes around spinal nerves exiting the spinal cord, peripheral nerves, and cranial nerves, followed by macrophage attack of myelin. This reaction results in defects in the conduction of electrical nerve impulses, with eventual absence of conduction causing flaccid paralysis of muscles. Recovery can occur with remyelination. However, in some patients, severe inflammation is followed by complete axonal destruction. Acute inflammatory demyelinating polyradiculoneuropathy is the most widely recognized form of GBS in Western countries, but there are subtypes known as acute motor axonal neuropathy (AMAN) and acute motor-sensory axonal neuropathy (AMSAN).

Clinical Presentation

The cardinal clinical presentation of GBS is one of progressive, usually symmetric muscle weakness accompanied by absent or depressed deep tendon reflexes. Paresthesias and numbness are usually the first symptoms. Symptoms usually manifest quickly over a period of several days and plateau at about 4 weeks. The weakness can vary from mild weakness in the lower limbs, causing difficulty walking, to nearly complete paralysis of all extremities and respiratory muscles, requiring the support of artificial ventilation.

Acute inflammatory demyelinating polyneuropathy (AIDP) involves distal muscle weakness of the lower extremities followed by more proximal muscles, trunk, upper extremities, and cranial nerves. This is a unique clinical presentation that characterizes GBS, and it is often referred to as ascending paralysis. Patients have sensory and motor nerve involvement. Seventy percent of patients with AIDP often experience autonomic dysfunction, most commonly manifested as tachycardia fluctuating with bradycardia, hypertension fluctuating with hypotension, urinary retention, ileus, and loss of sweating. Recovery from AIDP is often steady and occurs within a few weeks or months; however, little improvement can be expected in disabilities that linger beyond 2 years.

AMAN is a motor form of neuropathy in which tendon reflexes are absent, though some patients are hyperreflexic during the early recovery phase. Autonomic dysfunction is rare in this subgroup. AMSAN is similar to AMAN, but very rare. It is associated with severe illness and slow recovery.

Treatment

There are two facets of treatment for GBS. The first is supportive, because GBS can have life-threatening sequelae. The second goal of treatment is to lessen the nerve damage.

Supportive care is of utmost importance in GBS, as 30% of patients develop neuromuscular respiratory failure requiring mechanical ventilation. Continuous hemodynamic monitoring is also required, especially in patients with autonomic involvement. Prophylaxis for deep vein thrombosis, physical and occupational therapy, and psychological support are also necessary when caring for these patients. Treatment with immunomodulating agents can lessen nerve damage. Intravenous immunoglobulin, corticosteroids, and plasmapheresis (plasma exchange) have been used with some success. Cerebrospinal fluid filtration is a newer treatment that has had similar results to plasmapheresis.

Myasthenia Gravis

MG is a relatively uncommon autoimmune neuromuscular disorder that can occur at any age. It has a prevalence of 100 to 200 per million worldwide, with 10 to 20 new cases per million each year. Prevalence has increased over the past 50 years, likely because of better recognition of the disease, aging of the population, and the longer life span of affected persons.

Pathophysiology

MG is an autoimmune disease caused by the loss of functioning acetylcholine (Ach) receptors in the neuromuscular junction. Most individuals with MG test positive for Ach receptor antibodies (see Fig. 34-8). Some individuals with the disorder have no detectable levels of antibodies against Ach receptors; this is known as seronegative MG. There is compelling evidence that there is also an antibody-mediated autoimmune component in this form of the disorder, but no tests have been able to detect antibodies in this form.

Normally, in a healthy individual, a nerve impulse releases Ach at the neuromuscular junction, where it travels across to reach Ach receptors that are concentrated in the folds of the muscle endplate. The muscle contracts when enough of the receptor sites have been activated by the Ach. In MG, there is as much as an 80% reduction in the number of Ach receptor sites because of the deterioration caused by Ach receptor antibodies. The end result of this process is inefficient neuromuscular transmission, which is manifested as muscle weakness and easy fatigability. Commonly, the extraocular muscles, such as those that control eyelids, are first affected in myasthenia and may be the predominant manifestation of the disorder. This is commonly manifested as ptosis of the eyelids. It is unknown why there is a predilection for ocular muscles.

Pathological Autoimmune Mechanism. The mechanism of the body's immunological attack on Ach receptors is not understood. MG can be considered a B cell- or T cell-mediated disease. It is known that the antibodies against Ach receptors are IgG immunoglobulins derived from

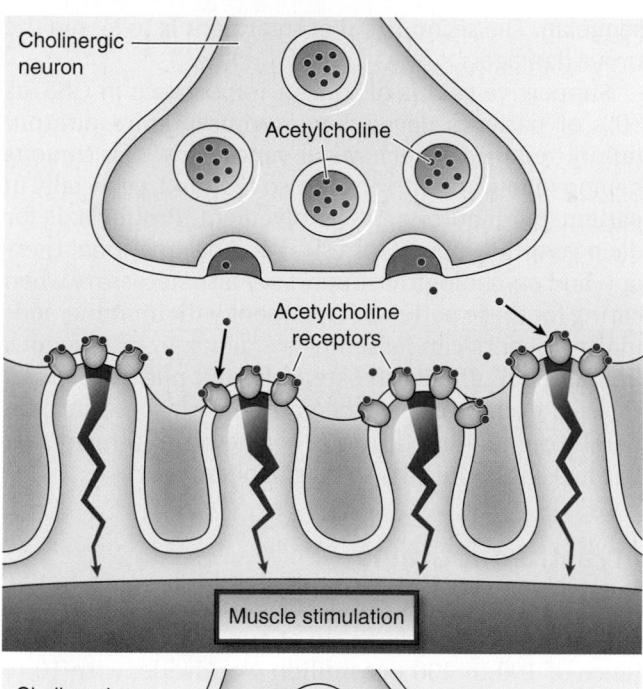

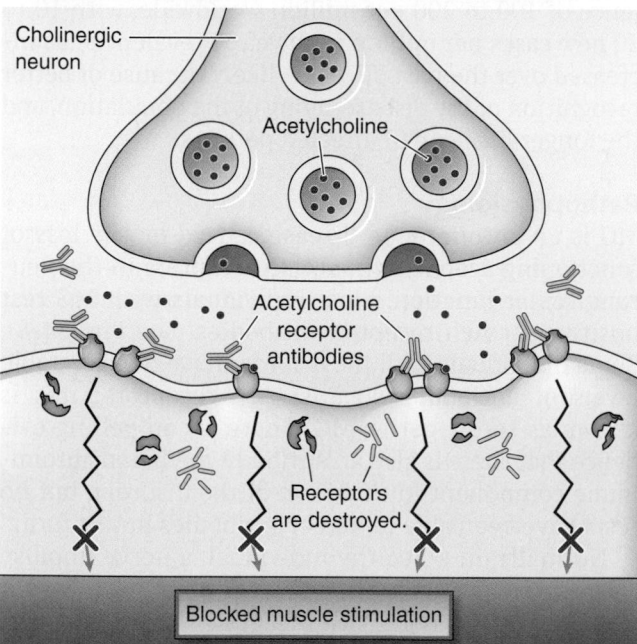

FIGURE 34-8. Myasthenia gravis. MG is a neuromuscular disorder caused by autoantibodies that destroy acetylcholine (Ach) receptors at neuromuscular junctions. As the disease progresses, increasing numbers of Ach receptors are destroyed, which decreases the ability of Ach to stimulate muscle. In MG, there is progressive weakness of the muscle. Fatal consequences can result when respiratory or swallowing muscles are weakened.

B cells. However, the importance of T cells in the pathogenesis of MG is becoming increasingly apparent. The thymus is the central organ in T cell-mediated immunity, and thymic abnormalities such as thymic hyperplasia or thymoma are well recognized in myasthenic patients. Approximately 70% of patients with MG have hyperplasia of the thymus gland. It is also likely that genetic factors contribute to the development of the disorder. Patients with MG frequently have other immune-mediated diseases such as rheumatoid arthritis, Graves' disease, and a family history of autoimmune disorders.

Clinical Presentation

MG can present in one of two ways: in an ocular form or a generalized form. In the ocular form of the disease, the muscle weakness occurs only in the eyelids and extraocular muscles. In the generalized form, the weakness involves a combination of limb, esophageal, and respiratory muscles, as well as involvement of their ocular muscles.

Ptosis and diplopia will be the presenting symptoms in as many as half of those diagnosed with MG. In addition, 50% of patients who present with ocular symptoms are likely to develop generalized disease within 2 years. Approximately 15% of patients will develop speech and esophageal symptoms, including dysarthria, dysphagia, and fatigable chewing. Very few patients will present with only limb weakness.

The cardinal feature of MG is a fluctuating skeletal muscle weakness, often with true muscle fatigue. The fatigue is seen as a worsening of muscle contractile force, not a sense of tiredness in the muscle. This is most notably seen with repetitive motion, such as blinking, walking, or even talking. For example, after only a few minutes of constant talking, the voice can become slurred with increased difficulty in forming words. After resting, the voice can return to normal. However, this cycle can be repeated if constant talking continues.

Early in the disease, the symptoms of weakness can fluctuate throughout the day. Muscle strength may be best in the morning hours and decrease throughout the day. As the disease progresses, the symptom-free periods shorten and symptoms become constant along a continuum of mild to severe. Factors that worsen myasthenic symptoms include emotional stress, concurrent illness, hypo- or hyperthyroidism, hormonal fluctuations, and increases in body temperature. MG can eventually lead to myasthenic crisis (see Box 34-10).

CLINICAL CONCEPT

It is important to assess respiratory function and gag reflex in patients affected with severe MG, because the diaphragm, intercostal muscles, and swallowing muscles can be affected.

ALERT! Aspiration and respiratory failure are major causes of death in severe MG and other neurodegenerative diseases.

Diagnosis

The diagnosis of MG can be established with clinical and serological testing. Edrophonium (Tensilon) testing is an option for those patients who present with ptosis or ocular symptomatology. Edrophonium is an acetylcholinesterase inhibitor; these medications

BOX 34-10. Myasthenic Crisis

Myasthenic crisis is weakness resulting from MG that is severe enough to cause respiratory failure necessitating ventilator support. Precipitating factors include infection, surgery, and tapering of immunosuppression, or it can be a spontaneous event. The patient in crisis experiences severe respiratory muscle weakness that increases risk for aspiration. The individual with an exacerbation of MG symptomatology must be closely monitored in an intensive care unit for respiratory failure. The patient's forced vital capacity and negative inspiratory force are monitored every 2 to 4 hours. Although arterial blood gases can be monitored, they are not a sensitive measure of respiratory muscle weakness.

diminish the enzyme that destroys Ach at neuromuscular junctions. Edrophonium allows more Ach to remain in the synapses for a longer period of time.

This enhanced Ach effect improves the neuromuscular weakness. Approximately 30 to 45 seconds after intravenous edrophonium is given, there is a noticeable improvement of strength in the muscle groups affected, with the effect lasting up to 10 minutes. Other useful diagnostic tests include serum Ach receptor antibodies and EMG.

Treatment

Pharmacological treatment of MG includes acetylcholinesterase inhibitors, corticosteroids, and immunosuppressive therapy. Physostigmine is a commonly used acetylcholinesterase inhibitor. If rapid treatment is warranted, therapeutic options include intravenous immune globulin, plasmapheresis, or plasma exchange, which removes Ach receptor antibodies from the circulation. Thymectomy is recommended for patients with a thymoma. The chance for remission of symptoms is 1.5 to 2 times higher for individuals who have the surgery compared with those who do not. Some medications, such as aminoglycoside antibiotics, can exacerbate symptoms of MG and should be avoided.

Chapter Summary

- The neuron has four major anatomical parts: dendrites, cell body, axon, and axon terminals.
- Incoming signals from other neurons are received through its dendrites. The outgoing signal to other neurons flows along its axon. Some axons are myelinated, covered with a lipid-rich substance that acts as insulation and keeps impulses travelling smoothly in one direction.
- An upper motor neuron disorder indicates that the source of the problem is in the brain's area of motor control: the sensory-motor cortex. A lower motor neuron disorder indicates that the source of the problem is at the region where motor nerves exit the spinal cord.
- A positive Babinski reflex in an adult indicates upper motor neuron dysfunction.
- Disorders of ion channels are responsible for a growing number of neurological diseases. Most are caused by mutations in ion channel genes or by autoantibodies formed against ion channel proteins.
- If a patient is unconscious, the clinician should make an assessment based on the Glasgow Coma Scale, vital signs, and pupil response.
- Epilepsy is a chronic neurological disorder characterized by recurrent seizures. A seizure is a sudden, abnormal, disorderly discharge of neurons within the brain that is characterized by a sudden, transient alteration in brain function. There are different types of seizures, including generalized, tonic-clonic, and absence seizures.
- Before a seizure, an individual may have unique sensations referred to as an aura.

- The most common types of primary headaches are tension-type headaches, migraine headaches, and cluster headaches.
- A TTH is the most common type of primary headache, occurring in as many as 78% of persons.
- Migraine headache is a severe, throbbing, one-sided headache that is accompanied by nausea, vomiting, photophobia, and phonophobia. Migraine headache is usually disabling to the sufferer. Some migraine headaches may have a preceding aura.
- Cluster headaches are repetitive headaches that occur for weeks to several months at a time, followed by remission. It is accompanied by rhinorrhea and conjunctivitis. Vasodilation is responsible for the pain and the autonomic features of cluster headaches.
- Parkinson's disease is mainly associated with progressive loss of dopamine-producing cells in the substantia nigra, which is within the basal ganglia of the midbrain. The basal ganglia modulates movements, such as posture, standing, walking, or writing.
- Resting tremor, bradykinesia, and muscle rigidity are the classic signs of Parkinson's disease.
- ALS is a progressive neurodegenerative disorder that is characterized by a loss of upper and lower motor neurons.
- HD is a neurodegenerative, genetic disorder caused by a single mutated gene on chromosome 4 that programs the manufacture of an abnormal protein called huntingtin that collects within brain neurons. Clinical manifestations include movement disturbances such as athetosis, chorea, and ballismus.

- In degenerative neuromuscular disorders, dysphagia occurs because of weakened esophageal muscles; because of this, assessment of the gag reflex is necessary before feeding a patient with a degenerative neuromuscular disorder.
- GBS is an acute peripheral neuropathy that leads to progressive limb weakness over the course of several days up to 4 weeks. This ascending paralysis often occurs after an infection or vaccine.
- MG is an autoimmune disease caused by autoantibodies that attack acetylcholine receptors in the neuromuscular junction. The first symptom of the disorder is often ptosis. As the day progresses, patient muscle weakness increases.

 Making the Connections

Disorder and Pathophysiology	Signs and Symptoms	Physical Assessment Findings	Diagnostic Testing	Treatment
Epilepsy | Abnormal electrical discharge of neurons in the brain, an imbalance of neurotransmitters, or both. Ion channel abnormalities causing hyperexcitability of regions of brain neurons.				
	Generalized seizure: loss of consciousness and tonic-clonic contractions of muscle. Postictal memory loss. Absence seizure: loss of attentiveness for period of time. Before a seizure, an individual may have unique sensations referred to as an aura.	Generalized: loss of consciousness, involuntary muscle contractions, autonomic symptoms, postictal vomiting common. Absence: loss of attentiveness.	Most patients have a normal EEG when not having a seizure. EEG is abnormal during seizure. Brain imaging may exhibit the cerebral hemisphere seizure origin. Metabolic panel is used to rule out electrolyte imbalances or toxicities.	Anticonvulsant medications to prevent seizures. Safety measures during seizure activity such as adjusting environment to prevent patient injury. After seizure, patient placed on side to prevent aspiration.
Tension Headache | Pericranial and cervical muscle tension.				
	Band of pain around head. Cervicothoracic muscle stiffness.	Normal physical exam.	Diagnosis mainly based on symptoms.	Tylenol, aspirin or NSAIDs).
Migraine Headache | Hyperexcitability of neurons; cortical spreading depression; trigeminal nerve complex activation, dural blood vessel sensitivity. Ion channel abnormalities may be associated.				
	Commonly lasts 4 to 72 hours. May or may not be accompanied by an aura. Nausea, vomiting, photophobia, and phonophobia are common.	Normal physical exam.	Normal lab tests and imaging studies. Specific criteria for diagnosis of a migraine headache.	NSAIDs to decrease inflammation. Triptans and ergot alkaloids, which are serotonin agonists. Avoidance of triggers.
Cluster Headache | Activation of the trigeminovascular system. The hypothalamus is postulated to play a prominent role because there are alterations in the circadian rhythms during the cluster period. It may be caused by a lesion involving the cavernous sinus portion of the internal carotid artery.				
	Stabbing, unilateral headache. Nasal discharge, tearing of the eye, pallor, and perspiration over one side of the face.	Rhinorrhea, tearing of the eye, sweating, and pallor over one side of the face.	Diagnosis mainly based on symptoms.	Different trials of medications, including triptans, dihydroergotamine, octreotide, prednisone, lithium, cyproheptadine, methysergide, and indomethacin.

Continued

Making the Connections–cont'd

Disorder and Pathophysiology	Signs and Symptoms	Physical Assessment Findings	Diagnostic Testing	Treatment
Parkinson's Disease | Progressive loss of dopamine-producing cells, especially in the substantia nigra of the basal ganglia that modulates movement and posture.				
	Bradykinesia, resting "pill rolling" tremor, and muscle "cogwheel" rigidity.	Stiff posture, muscle stiffness, blank expression, gait disturbances. "Freezing" episodes where individual cannot initiate movement, micrographia, slowed movements, depression, cognitive disturbance. Autonomic disturbances.	Diagnosis mainly based on symptoms. Normal lab tests and imaging studies. Genetic susceptibility and current research regarding accumulation of mutated protein in brain. Significant symptom improvement with trial of levodopa indicates Parkinson's disease.	Levodopa-carbidopa medications to replace dopamine in the brain and decrease peripheral effects of dopamine. Dopamine agonists. Catechol-O-methyl transferase inhibitors to decrease breakdown of dopamine. Anticholinergic drugs to balance acetylcholine effects.
ALS | Progressive neurodegenerative disorder characterized by a loss of upper and lower motor neurons.				
	Gradual loss of control of muscles.	Muscle weakness and atrophy, dysarthria dysphagia. Sensation intact.	Normal lab tests and imaging studies.	No cure. Riluzole (Rilutek). Supportive and palliative care.
MS | Autoimmune, demyelinating disorder that results in inflammation and damage to the myelin and other cells within the CNS, ANS, and peripheral nervous system.				
	Ocular and cerebellar symptoms often are initially present. Vision disturbances and gait and balance problems often are initial symptoms.	Motor and sensory weakness. Visual problems. Incoordination and gait disturbance (ataxia).	Condition cannot be diagnosed after only a single symptomatic episode. Symptoms are clues to diagnosis; however, diagnosis requires the appearance of demyelination lesions detected on imaging studies. McDonald criteria are used to diagnose. EMG and evoked potential tests are also used.	Immunomodulators and immunosuppressives to decrease autoantibody effects. Corticosteroids to decrease inflammation.
HD | Autosomal-dominant neurological disorder; genetic mutation on chromosome 4 that codes for huntingtin protein; causes progressive lack of muscle control.				
	Involuntary motor symptoms, cognitive decline, and emotional/behavioral symptoms.	Motor control deficits. Chorea, athetosis, ballismus, and cognitive impairment.	Presymptomatic blood test for the presence of the mutated HD gene.	Supportive treatment.
GBS | Postinfectious disease with resulting neuropathy; ascending paralysis, previous infection evokes an autoimmune response in the peripheral nerve, can occur postimmunization also.				
	Progressive, usually symmetric, ascending muscle weakness	Motor and sensory deficits, distal to proximal, starting	Clinical examination is only diagnostic modality.	May require temporary mechanical ventilation, intravenous

Continued

Making the Connections–cont'd

Disorder and Pathophysiology	Signs and Symptoms	Physical Assessment Findings	Diagnostic Testing	Treatment
accompanied by absent or depressed deep tendon reflexes, paresthesias, and numbness.		in lower limbs and moving upward.		immunoglobulin, corticosteroids, or plasmapheresis (plasma exchange).
MG | Autoimmune antibodies directed against muscle acetylcholine receptors.				
	Muscle weakness; often manifests as ptosis or easy fatigability.	Muscle weakness; ptosis of eyelids; worsens as day continues.	EMG. Edrophonium (Tensilon) testing.	Acetylcholinesterase inhibitors such as Physostigmine, to allow more acetylcholine to remain in the synapse. Corticosteroids and immunosuppressive therapy to decrease effects of autoantibodies.

Bibliography

Ahlskog, J. E. (2011). Cheaper, simpler, and better: tips for treating seniors with Parkinson disease. *Mayo Clin Proceed,* 86(12), 1211–1216.

Armstrong, C., American Academy of Neurology, & American Headache Society. (2013). AAN/AHS update recommendations for migraine prevention in adults. *Am Fam Phys,* 87(8), 584–585.

Aronin, N., & Moore, M. (2012). Hunting down huntingtin. *N Engl J Med,* 367(18), 1753–1754.

Barrett, K. E., Barman, S. M., Boitano, S., & Brooks, H. L. (2010). *Ganong's review of medical physiology.* 23rd ed. New York: McGraw-Hill/Lange Medical Series.

Berger, J. R. (2011). Functional improvement and symptom management in multiple sclerosis: clinical efficacy of current therapies. *Am J Man Care,* 17 (Suppl 5), S146–153.

Brück, W., Gold, R., Lund, B. T., et al. (2013). Therapeutic decisions in multiple sclerosis: moving beyond efficacy. *JAMA Neurol,* 70(10), 1315–1324.

Calabresi, P. A. (2011). Inflammation in multiple sclerosis—sorting out the gray matter. *N Engl J Med,* 365(23), 2231–2233.

Carroll, W. M. (2010). Oral therapy for multiple sclerosis—sea change or incremental step? *N Engl J Med,* 362(5), 456–458. Epub 2010 Jan 20.

Chang, H. J., & Zuccotti, G. (2011). Frontal headache. *JAMA,* 306(3), 317–318. doi: 10.1001/jama.2011.994.

Chataway, J., & Miller, D. H. (2011). Multiple sclerosis—quenching the flames of inflammation. *Lancet,* 378(9805), 1759–1760. Epub 2011 Oct 31.

Cohen, J. A., Barkhof, F., Comi, G., et al. (2010). Oral fingolimod or intramuscular interferon for relapsing multiple sclerosis. *N Engl J Med,* 362(5), 402–415. Epub 2010 Jan 20.

Compston, A., & Coles, A. (2008). Multiple sclerosis. *Lancet,* 372(9648), 1502–1517.

Deuschl, G., & Agid, Y. (2013). Subthalamic neurostimulation for Parkinson's disease with early fluctuations: balancing the risks and benefits. *Lancet Neurol,* 12(10), 1025–1034.

Deutch, A. Y. (2013). Parkinson's disease redefined. *Lancet Neurol,* 12(5), 422–423.

Devinsky, O. (2011). Sudden, unexpected death in epilepsy. *N Engl J Med,* 365(19), 1801–1811.

Dunckley, T., Huentelman, M. J., Craig, D. W., et al. (2007). Whole-genome analysis of sporadic amyotrophic lateral sclerosis. *N Engl J Med,* 357(8), 775–788.

Edvinsson, L., & Linde, M. (2010). New drugs in migraine treatment and prophylaxis: telcagepant and topiramate. *Lancet,* 376(9741), 645–655.

Fernandez, H. H. (2012a). Nonmotor complications of Parkinson disease. *Cleveland Clin J Med,* 79 (Suppl 2), S14–18.

Fernandez, H. H. (2012b). Updates in the medical management of Parkinson disease. *Cleveland Clin J Med,* 79(1), 28–35.

Fox, E. J. (2010). Emerging oral agents for multiple sclerosis. *Am J Man Care,* 16(8 Suppl), S219–226.

Gazewood, J. D., Richards, D. R., & Clebak, K. (2013). Parkinson disease: an update. *Am Fam Phys,* 87(4), 267–273.

Gilmore, B., & Michael, M. (2011). Treatment of acute migraine headache. *Am Fam Phys,* 83(3), 271–280.

Giovannoni, G., Comi, G., Cook, S., et al. (2010). A placebo-controlled trial of oral cladribine for relapsing multiple sclerosis. *N Engl J Med,* 362(5), 416–426. Epub 2010 Jan 20.

Guirguis-Blake, J. (2010). Effectiveness of acupuncture for migraine prophylaxis. *Am Fam Phys,* 81(1), 29.

Hainer, B. L., & Matheson, E. M. (2013). Approach to acute headache in adults. *Am Fam Phys,* 87(10), 682–687.

Hauser, S. L. (2008). Multiple lessons for multiple sclerosis. *N Engl J Med,* 359(17), 1838–1841.

Hoppitt, T., Calvert, M., Pall, H., Rickards, H., & Sackley, C. (2010). Huntington's disease. *Lancet*, 376(9751), 1463–1464.

Kiernan, M. C., Vucic, S., Cheah, B. C., et al. (2011). Amyotrophic lateral sclerosis. *Lancet*, 377(9769), 942–955. Epub 2011 Feb 4.

Kuehn, B. M. (2011a). Imaging helps to identify early changes associated with Huntington disease. *JAMA*, 305(2), 138.

Kuehn, B. M. (2011b). New model system offers clues to ALS. *JAMA*, 306(14), 1534.

Kuehn, B. M. (2011c). Scientists probe strategies to repair neuron damage in multiple sclerosis. *JAMA*, 305(9), 871–872, 874.

Kwan, P., Schachter, S. C., & Brodie, M. J. (2011). Drug-resistant epilepsy. *N Engl J Med*, 365(10), 919–926.

Loder, E. (2010). Triptan therapy in migraine. *N Engl J Med*, 363(1), 63–70.

Lomen-Hoerth, C., & Messing, R. O. (2010). Nervous system disorders. In S. J. McPhee & J. Hammer, *Pathophysiology of disease* (6th ed.). New York: Lange Medical Books/ McGraw-Hill Medical Publishing Division.

Longo, D. L., Kasper, D. L., Jameson, J. L., et al. (2011). *Harrison's principles of internal medicine*. 18th ed. New York: McGraw-Hill.

Loy, C. T., Lownie, A., & McCusker, E. (2010). Huntington's disease. *Lancet*, 376(9751), 1463.

Lucchinetti, C. F., Popescu, B. F., Bunyan, R. F., et al. (2011). Inflammatory cortical demyelination in early multiple sclerosis. *N Engl J Med*, 365(23), 2188–2197.

Mitka, M. (2009). New guidelines suggest ways to optimize treatment, care of patients with ALS. *JAMA*, 302(21), 2303–2304.

Nicholas, R., & Rashid, W. (2013). Multiple sclerosis. *Am Fam Phys*, 87(10), 712–714.

Palm-Meinders, I. H., Koppen, H., Terwindt, G. M., et al. (2012). Structural brain changes in migraine. *JAMA*, 308(18), 1889–1897. doi: 10.1001/jama.2012.14276.

Pelletier, D., & Hafler, D. A. (2012). Fingolimod for multiple sclerosis. *N Engl J Med*, 366(4), 339–347.

Pickett, H., & Blackwell, J. C. (2010). FPIN's clinical inquiries. Acupuncture for migraine headaches. *Am Fam Phys*, 81(8), 1036–1037.

Ramagopalan, S. V., & Ebers, G. C. (2008). Genes for multiple sclerosis. *Lancet*, 371(9609), 283–285.

Rawlins, M. (2010). Huntington's disease out of the closet? *Lancet*, 376(9750), 1372–1373.

Rudick, R. A. (2011). Multiple sclerosis, natalizumab, and PML: helping patients decide. *Cleveland Clin J Med*, 78 (Suppl 2), S18–23.

Rudick, R. A., & Trapp, B. D. (2009). Gray-matter injury in multiple sclerosis. *N Engl J Med*, 361(15), 1505–1506.

Scherder, E., & Statema, M. (2010). Huntington's disease. *Lancet*. 2010 Oct 30;376 (9751), 1464.

Silberstein, S. D. (2008). Recent developments in migraine. *Lancet*, 372(9647), 1369–1371.

Singer, C. (2012). Comprehensive treatment of Huntington disease and other choreic disorders. *Cleveland Clin J Med*, 79 (Suppl 2), S30–34.

Singer, C. (2012). Managing the patient with newly diagnosed Parkinson disease. *Cleveland Clin J Med*, 79 (Suppl 2), S3–7.

Tarsy, D. (2012). Treatment of Parkinson disease: a 64-year-old man with motor complications of advanced Parkinson disease. *JAMA*, 307(21), 2305–2314.

Thompson, A., & Polman, C. (2009). Improving function: a new treatment era for multiple sclerosis? *Lancet*, 373(9665), 697–698.

Venna, N., Gonzalez, R. G., & Zukerberg, L. R. (2011). Case records of the Massachusetts General Hospital. Case 39-2011. A woman in her 90s with unilateral ptosis. *N Engl J Med*, 365(25), 2413–2422.

Weaver-Agostoni, J. (2013). Cluster headache. *Am Fam Phys*, 88(2), 122–128.

Wexler, A. (2010). Stigma, history, and Huntington's disease. *Lancet*, 376(9734), 18–19.

Yancey, J. R., Sheridan, R., & Koren, K. G. (2014). Chronic daily headache: diagnosis and management. *Am Fam Phys*, 89(8), 642–648.

Zinman, L., & Cudkowicz, M. (2011). Emerging targets and treatments in amyotrophic lateral sclerosis. *Lancet Neurol*, 10(5), 481–490. doi: 10.1016/S1474-4422(11)70024-2.

Zwibel, H. L., & Smrtka, J. (2011). Improving quality of life in multiple sclerosis: an unmet need. *Am J Man Care*, 17 (Suppl 5), S139–145.

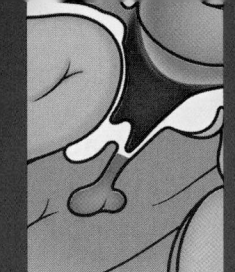

CHAPTER 35

Brain and Spinal Cord Injury

Key Terms

Acceleration-deceleration injury
Areflexia
Cauda equina
Concussion
Conus medullaris
Coup-contrecoup injury
Cushing's triad

Cytotoxic cerebral edema
Diffuse axonal injury (DAI)
Glasgow Coma Scale (GCS)
Intracranial pressure (ICP)
Monro-Kellie doctrine
Neurogenic shock
Postconcussion syndrome

Spinal shock
Transtentorial herniation
Traumatic brain injury (TBI)
Uncal herniation
Vasogenic cerebral edema

Traumatic brain injury (TBI) is sudden physical damage to the brain. The damage can result from a closed head injury, such as that caused by the head impacting an external unmovable object or surface, which can occur during falls and motor vehicle accidents. The damage can also result from a penetrating brain injury, such as that caused by a bullet or knife piercing the skull. Contact sports often cause TBI in the form of concussion. TBI can cause a diminished or altered state of consciousness that can result in alteration of cognitive abilities or physical functioning.

Traumatic spinal cord injury (SCI) is damage to the spinal cord that results in loss of mobility or sensation. In most cases, the spinal cord remains intact, but the damage causes loss of nerve function below the area of injury.

Epidemiology

Approximately 1.5 million patients are diagnosed with TBI in the United States annually. However, the actual incidence is higher because many persons who suffer TBI do not seek health care. Annually, approximately 50,000 deaths are attributed to TBI and another 235,000 people are hospitalized. Falls contribute to the greatest number of TBI-related injuries (28%), with motor vehicle collisions (20%) close behind. Other common causes include violence and sports injuries. Males are affected by TBI more than females, with a ratio of 3 to 1. Persons ages 15 through 24 are the most common victims of fatal TBI.

The cost of TBIs in the United States is estimated at $48.3 billion annually: $31.7 billion in hospitalization costs and another $16.6 billion in costs associated with fatalities. The Centers for Disease Control and Prevention (CDC) estimates the total cost of acute care and

rehabilitation for TBI victims in the United States is $9 to $10 billion per year—a number that does not include indirect costs to families and society.

Basic Concepts in Neurovascular Physiology

The brain sits inside of a rigid protective skull surrounded by meningeal membranes and cerebrospinal fluid (CSF). Broad anatomical regions of the brain have been mapped. However, functions of some regions of the brain still remain unknown.

Cerebral Anatomy and Physiology

The cerebrum of the brain consists of four lobes:

1. Frontal lobes: These are responsible for consciousness, judgment, and emotional responses. These processes comprise executive function, which controls how individuals react to the world.
2. Temporal lobes: These are responsible for hearing ability and memory acquisition. The center for speech is predominantly found in the left cerebral hemisphere.
3. Parietal lobes: These are responsible for sensory discrimination, such as touch perception and manipulation of objects.
4. Occipital lobes: These control vision.

The brainstem contains the vital sign center that controls respirations, heart rate, and blood pressure. It also contains the reticular activating system, which is responsible for the sleep-wake cycle and levels of alertness.

Intracranial Pressure

The bones of the skull form a rigid cranial compartment that contains brain tissue (80%), CSF (10%), and blood volume (10%). The pressure of these three elements must remain balanced to maintain normal **intracranial pressure (ICP).** ICP—the pressure inside the skull, brain tissue, and CSF—is normally 7 to 15 mm Hg in the resting, supine adult. Changes in ICP occur because of volume changes in either the brain tissue, cerebral blood flow, or CSF. To maintain normal ICP, any increase in the volume of any one of the components must be compensated by a decrease in the volume of another. For example, as a slow-growing brain tumor increases the volume of brain tissue, the CSF production is slowed to compensate and maintain normal ICP. Once the volume of the brain tumor exceeds the volume of the CSF reduction, ICP increases. This concept of maintaining normal pressure within the cranium is known as the **Monro-Kellie doctrine** (see Fig. 35-1).

When the compensating mechanisms are totally exhausted, ICP will increase as demonstrated by the volume-pressure curve in Figure 35-2. The ICP is maintained until a maximum point is reached. At this point, it takes only a small amount of volume increase to cause a large increase in ICP.

> **CLINICAL CONCEPT**
>
> Increased ICP is directly related to increased mortality in patients with TBI.

Normal state — ICP normal

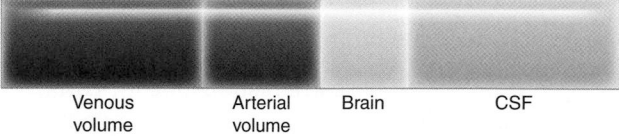

| Venous volume | Arterial volume | Brain | CSF |

Compensated state — ICP normal

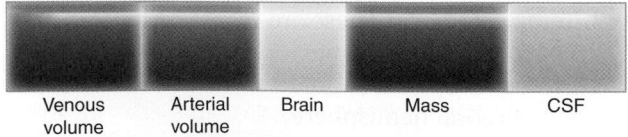

| Venous volume | Arterial volume | Brain | Mass | CSF |

Decompensated state — ICP elevated

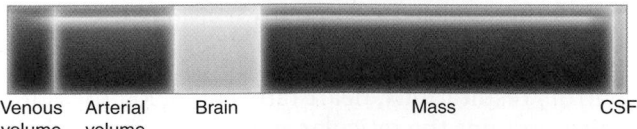

| Venous volume | Arterial volume | Brain | Mass | CSF |

FIGURE 35-1. The Monro-Kellie doctrine states that an increase in one compartment of the brain is compensated by a decrease in other compartments of the brain. An example of this is how the growth of a brain mass will cause compensatory decreases in cerebral spinal fluid and venous compartments.

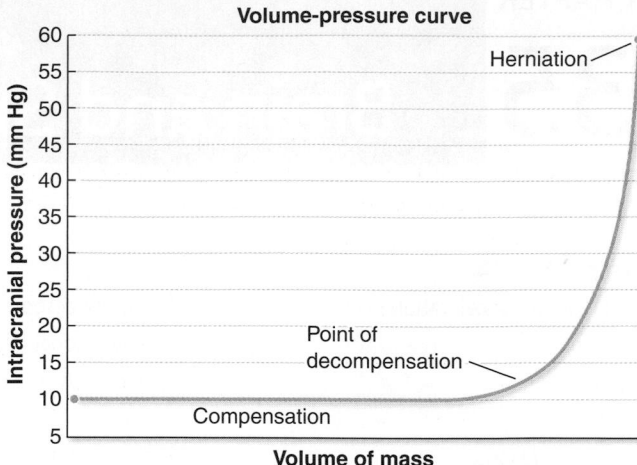

Volume-pressure curve

FIGURE 35-2. The volume-pressure curve in ICP. As the volume of an expanding mass in the brain increases, ICP rises until compensatory mechanisms are overcome. The point of decompensation is reached when further expansion of the brain mass causes a steep rise in ICP. The final result is herniation of the brain.

Level of Consciousness

Consciousness is associated with self-awareness and the ability to interact with the environment; this active process is the result of neuronal activity within the brain. Content of consciousness refers to the cognitive function and is mediated by the cerebral cortex. Consciousness itself, however, is not located within specific areas of the brain, and maintaining consciousness depends upon interconnected neural pathways within the brain. This includes the upper brainstem, the reticular activating system, and their interaction with the cerebral hemispheres. Whenever there is an alteration in the interconnected pathways, there can be a change in the level of consciousness (LOC). The change is measured by patient responses to stimulation or to the environment, and includes communication, emotional responses, and appropriate gestures.

An individual's LOC is a measure of his or her arousability and reaction to the environment. An individual's consciousness can be described on a continuum. Alertness is the highest LOC, where the individual is awake and fully interactive with the environment. Lethargy is a state in which the individual is sleepy but can be aroused easily. An obtunded person is more difficult to arouse. An obtunded or stuporous individual in a lower LOC is difficult to arouse and has little or no interaction with the environment. Coma, where the individual is in a sleeplike state and has no interaction with the environment, is the lowest LOC.

> **CLINICAL CONCEPT**
>
> Signs of increasing intracranial pressure include headache, vomiting, and decreasing level of consciousness.

Basic Pathophysiologic Concepts of Brain and Spinal Cord Injury

Although brain injury can occur because of different mechanisms, there are certain pathophysiologic alterations that result regardless of the etiology. These include changes in ICP and LOC.

Mechanisms That Increase ICP

Mechanisms that increase the volume of one or more of three compartments—circulation, brain tissue, and CSF—will increase ICP (see Fig. 35-1). Cerebral edema is a common cause of increased ICP. Major causes of cerebral edema include trauma, hemorrhage, tumor, inflammation, and ischemia. Trauma causes a shearing stress on the brain that leads to **vasogenic cerebral edema.** In this form of edema, the pores of the brain's capillaries open wide, allowing proteins and fluids to leak from the blood into the tissues.

Cerebral hemorrhage creates another form of cerebral edema. A ruptured cerebral vessel creates a pool of blood that forms a space-occupying lesion within the closed cranium. The collection of blood is toxic to brain cells and places pressure against brain tissue, which rapidly increases ICP. In the case of a brain tumor, the excess cancerous tissue changes the equilibrium of the ICP's components. When brain tissue increases, CSF and circulation decrease to maintain normal ICP. However, at some point, circulation and CSF cannot sufficiently diminish to counterbalance the brain tissue expansion. This is when ICP increases and symptoms become apparent. Brain tumor also compresses blood flow, which causes venous congestion and increased hydrostatic pressure, resulting in edema. Alternatively, when there is an inflammatory condition present in the brain, the permeability of capillary membranes increases and allows fluid to flow out into the tissue, creating edema.

Another kind of edema, **cytotoxic cerebral edema,** forms with cerebral ischemia or hypoxia which, if not reversed, results in brain cell death. Ischemia leads to anaerobic metabolism within brain cells and failure of ion pumps; this leads to cellular swelling. Cellular swelling increases the volume of brain tissue, which increases ICP. Also, when there are low oxygen levels or high carbon dioxide levels in the brain, a reflexive cerebral vasodilation is initiated. This increases the brain's blood volume, leading to increased ICP.

> **ALERT!** Compression of the jugular vein with tracheostomy ties or tight cervical collars reduces blood flow from the brain, resulting in increased venous blood volume within the brain. This can lead to increased ICP. Care must be taken to avoid this in patients with TBI.

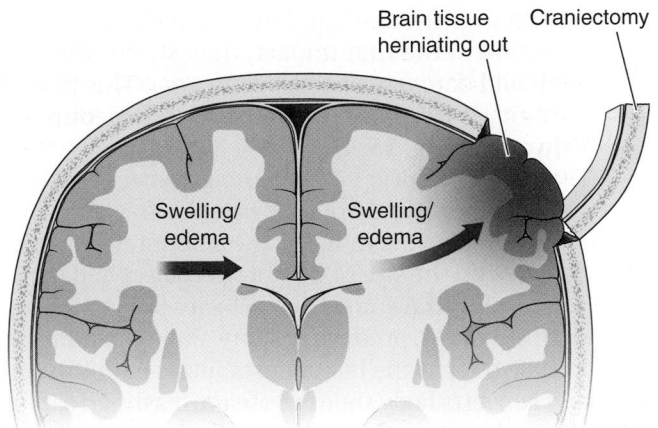

FIGURE 35-3. Open craniectomy allowing brain tissue decompression. Decompressive craniectomy is a neurological procedure in which part of the skull is removed to allow a swelling brain room to expand without being squeezed. It is performed on victims of TBI.

Mechanisms That Decrease ICP

Decreasing volume of any one of the three compartments—brain tissue, CSF, or circulation—will decrease the ICP (see Fig. 35-1). For example, externally draining CSF via a catheter placed in the ventricles will lower ICP. Blood volume can also be reduced by lowering blood pressure. A low carbon dioxide level will vasoconstrict cerebral arteries, reducing the volume of blood delivered to the brain. Removing brain tissue, such as occurs in a lobectomy, will likewise decrease volume and ICP.

Another method to decrease ICP is a decompressive craniectomy, in which a section of the skull is removed, creating an opening in the closed space of the skull and allowing expansion of the brain. This allows the ICP to increase without the danger of compressing brain tissue (see Fig. 35-3).

Mechanisms of Injury

TBI is the result of external forces that are transferred directly or indirectly to the brain. There are four mechanisms that can result in skull or brain injuries:

1. Blunt trauma: This occurs when an object hits the skull forcefully, causing fractures of the skull and damage to the underlying brain. Examples of blunt trauma include being struck in the head with a baseball or being a passenger in a motor vehicle accident whose head hits the dashboard.
2. Acceleration-deceleration: When the skull stops abruptly, as in a motor vehicle accident, the brain continues to move forward, rotating within the skull and causing shearing of brain tissue against the skull's rough interior edges. This movement is referred to as **acceleration-deceleration** and causes stretching and shearing of neural axons, resulting in diffuse axonal injuries. In acceleration-deceleration, the brain

bounces off the skull and moves in the opposite direction of the first impact, then strikes the skull and damages the opposite area. This type of injury is referred to as a **coup-contrecoup injury** (see Fig. 35-4).

3. Penetrating injury: When a foreign object penetrates the skull and brain, the skull is fractured and brain tissue is injured. The amount of damage depends on the size of the foreign object and the velocity it is traveling. High velocity projectiles, such as bullets, produce a cavity along the primary missile tract as the bullet destabilizes brain tissue and converts body fluids to steam, blasting apart a channel and creating extensive brain damage. Penetrating trauma causes an increase in infection as the foreign body disrupts the meningeal layers and carries external debris, such as gunpowder and pieces of skull and hair, into the brain. A penetrating injury usually causes a skull fracture which ruptures the middle meningeal artery and leads to an extensive arterial bleed in the epidural space.

4. Blast injury: The extent of injury caused by explosions depends on the type and amount of explosive material and the distance between the individual and the blast. One blast of an explosive can produce multiple effects on the body. A primary injury results from the detonation of explosives that produce a pressure wave that is particularly destructive to gas-filled structures of the body, such as the lungs and inner ears. This wave can produce an acceleration-deceleration injury within the skull. A secondary injury causes penetrating and blunt injuries from flying debris and bomb fragments. Tertiary injuries occur when individuals are thrown by the blast, resulting in blunt trauma. Quaternary injuries are related to burns, inhalation of gases, and angina that result from the experience.

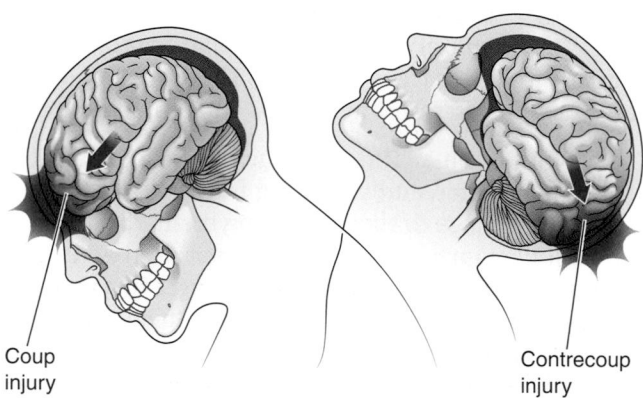

FIGURE 35-4. Acceleration-deceleration injury. This type of traumatic head injury, also called coup-contrecoup injury, occurs as a whiplash accident when the brain bounces back and forth inside the skull. The coup injury happens when the head stops abruptly because of an impact and the brain then crashes into the skull. The contrecoup injury occurs when the brain then bounces inside the skull and impacts the opposite side of the skull.

Coup injury

Contrecoup injury

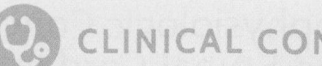 **CLINICAL CONCEPT**

Shaken baby syndrome is an example of a coup-contrecoup injury. "Coup" refers to the site of first impact, whereas "contrecoup" refers to the injury site opposite the impact area.

ALERT! All polytrauma patients should be treated as if there is a spinal cord injury until proved otherwise. Spinal immobilization is required in all trauma patients.

Brain Death

When ICP is not lowered, the brain tissue is compressed and forced downward in the skull to become herniated or displaced to another region of the brain. The most common type of herniation is a **transtentorial herniation,** also called **uncal herniation.** Part of the temporal lobe (the uncus) is forced through the tentorial notch—the opening in the sheet of tissue between the temporal lobe and cerebellum (see Fig. 35-5). This brain tissue compression results in death to brain tissue. If the herniation compresses vital centers of the brainstem, death ensues. Vital centers of the brainstem control heart rate, respiratory rate, blood pressure, and LOC, referred to as brainstem reflexes. Brain death is the irreversible end of all brain activity (see Box 35-1).

Neurological Assessment of TBI

Initial assessment of neurovascular injury involves determining the injury's cause and severity. This assessment provides information that determines the type of treatment.

Severity of Injury

Accurately assessing the severity of injury determines the individual's eventual physical, cognitive, psychosocial, and functional recovery. The **Glasgow Coma Scale (GCS),** which is used to assess the severity of brain injury (see Box 35-2), incorporates both LOC and orientation. It is determined by rating three areas: eye opening, verbal response, and motor response. The GCS was designed to be used as a noninvasive bedside tool capable of charting a patient's LOC over time, indicating improvement or decline in a patient's condition. The lowest GCS score is a 3, which indicates absence of all activity, and the highest score is 15, indicating a person opens eyes spontaneously, is oriented, and obeys commands.

Normal position
of brain tissue

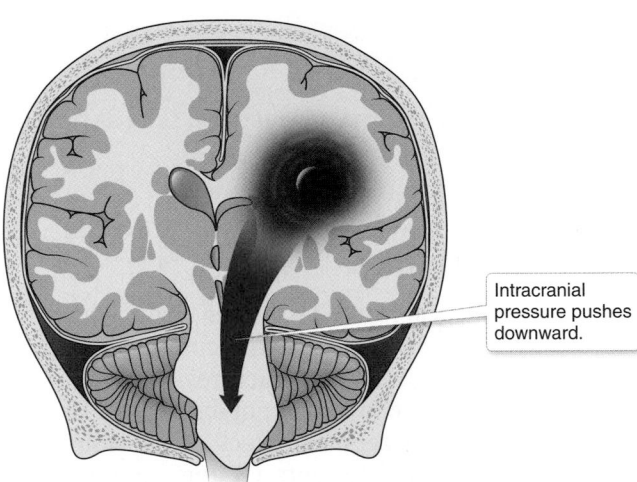

Brainstem: controls
vital functions
(consciousness,
heart rate, BP,
respiratory rate)

Foramen
magnum

Intracranial
pressure pushes
downward.

FIGURE 35-5. Uncal herniation. The skull is a rigid structure that houses the brain and related structures; it cannot accommodate expansion of the tissues and fluid within. Should there be swelling or bleeding within the brain tissue or cranial cavity, ICP pushes brain tissue downward. This is a critical condition because it places pressure on the brainstem, the center of all vital functions.

BOX 35-1. Brain Death

The cardinal findings of brain death are coma, absence of brainstem reflexes, and apnea. Before determination of brain death, patients must have normal temperatures and be free of drugs that depress brain activity, such as barbiturates and alcohol. Only a neurologist or neurosurgeon can determine a patient's brain death. Ancillary tests to confirm brain death include electroencephalogram, cerebral angiogram, and nuclear cerebral flow study. Repeated EEGs will reveal no brain activity for at least 30 minutes. A cerebral angiogram and nuclear cerebral blood flow study that show complete absence of intracranial blood flow can be used to confirm the diagnosis of brain death.

BOX 35-2. Glasgow Coma Scale

EYE OPENING RESPONSE
- spontaneous—open with blinking at baseline: **4 points**
- to verbal stimuli, command, speech: **3 points**
- to pain only (not applied to face): **2 points**
- no response: **1 point**

VERBAL RESPONSE
- oriented: **5 points**
- confused conversation, but able to answer questions: **4 points**
- inappropriate words: **3 points**
- incomprehensible speech: **2 points**
- no response: **1 point**

MOTOR RESPONSE
- obeys commands for movement: **6 points**
- purposeful movement to painful stimulus: **5 points**
- withdraws in response to pain: **4 points**
- flexion in response to pain (decorticate posturing): **3 points**
- extension response in response to pain (decerebrate posturing): **2 points**
- no response: **1 point**

CLASSIFICATION
- severe head injury: score of 8 or fewer
- moderate head injury: score of 9 to 12
- mild head injury: score of 13 to 15

(Center for Disease Control and Prevention. Retrieved from http://www.cdc.gov/masstrauma/resources/gcs.pdf. Last accessed July 8, 2015; Teasdale, G. & Jennet, B. (1974). Assessment of coma and impaired consciousness. *Lancet* 2(7872):81-4. Teasdale, G. & Jennet, B. (1976). Assessment and prognosis of coma after head injury. *Acta Neurochir,* 34(1-4):45-55.)

Severity of TBI is described by the GCS score in three categories:

- 3 to 8 points: severe injury
- 9 to 12 points: moderate injury
- 13 to 15 points: mild injury.

The severity of brain injury is determined after the patient has been fully resuscitated and any drugs or alcohol have cleared the patient's system, usually at 24 to 48 hours postinjury.

Other indices of severity of injury are duration of unconsciousness and post-traumatic amnesia (PTA). Both longer periods of unconsciousness and duration of PTA are associated with decreased functional recovery.

Patients with severe TBI are generally unconscious at least 24 hours and have PTA that lasts longer than

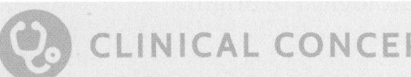

CLINICAL CONCEPT

PTA duration is a better predictor of cognitive function 2 years postinjury than length of coma.

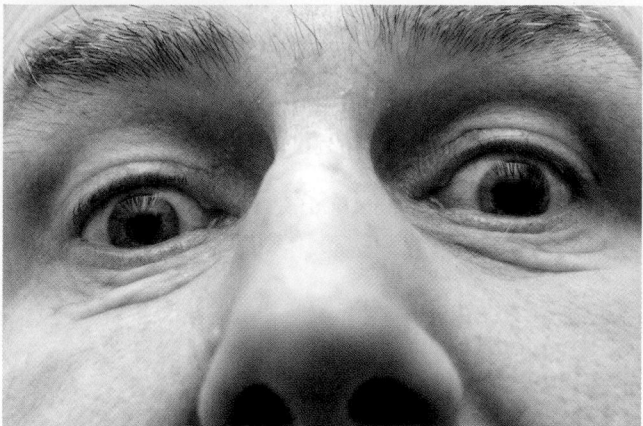

FIGURE 35-6. Pupil size alteration after head injury.
(From SPL/Science Source.)

7 days, usually 1 to 4 weeks. Patients with moderate TBI are unconscious between 1 and 24 hours and have PTA duration of 1 to 7 days. Patients with mild TBI may or may not experience unconsciousness; if they do, it will be for less than an hour. PTA duration for a mild TBI is fewer than 24 hours.

Clinical Manifestations of ICP

As ICP increases within the skull, cranial nerves and brain tissue are compressed. Early signs of increasing ICP include headache, caused by direct compression of brain tissue; vomiting, caused by compression of the vomiting center in the medulla; and decreasing LOC, caused by compression of the reticular activating system.

Pressure on the third cranial nerve (oculomotor) caused by an uncal herniation will produce an altered response of the pupil to light and alter the pupil's size (see Fig. 35-6). If the ICP continues to rise and causes significant pressure on the brainstem, a triad of symptoms called **Cushing's triad** occurs. These late signs consist of hypertension with a widened pulse pressure (difference between systolic and diastolic pressures), slowed heart rate, and abnormal respiratory patterns.

ALERT! Rising intracranial pressure can affect the brainstem causing symptoms known as CUSHING's TRIAD: Bradycardia, hypertension (with wide pulse pressure), and erratic respiratory rate.

Content of consciousness refers to the brain's cognitive function. A declining content of consciousness results in confusional states where a person is unable to maintain a coherent stream of thought or action. There are many causes of confusion, both neurological and nonneurological in origin.

Declining Levels of Consciousness

Declining LOC involves reduced responsiveness to stimuli, which exists on a continuum that ranges from drowsiness to stupor and finally coma. All levels except coma involve being able to arouse the person to respond; however, each level requires more effort and results in less response.

The difference between consciousness and unconsciousness can be determined by eye opening. People who are able to respond to stimulation by opening their eyes are not in a coma. Patients in a vegetative state can open their eyes and are not comatose, though they are not aware of their environment. Individuals who progress up to a minimally responsive state are slowly gaining awareness of their environment.

A return of the sleep-wake cycle is the first sign that a patient is slowly improving. Patients who have a GCS of 6 or lower are considered to be comatose. The longer the patient is not responsive to stimuli, the poorer the prognosis. After 30 days, patients who do not open their eyes in response to stimulation have a poor prognosis.

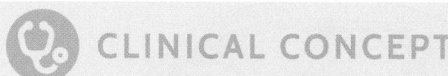

CLINICAL CONCEPT

Treat all patients in coma or vegetative state as if they are able to hear their surroundings.

Diagnostic Studies

Computed tomography (CT) scan, the test of choice for acute TBI, demonstrates areas of acute bleeding and pressure on the brain's vital structures.

Serial CT scans over a number of days can be used to follow hemorrhage size, mass effect, or CSF volume in more seriously injured patients. CT angiography (CTA) uses a dye to highlight the larger blood vessels of the brain or neck. These pictures are two dimensional, but advanced technology enables viewing as three-dimensional images so that traumatic aneurysms, vascular dissections, or occlusions can be seen. This is particularly necessary for skull fractures.

Magnetic resonance imaging (MRI) examines the brain's deeper structures. It may be used in mild TBI during the evaluation of persistent symptoms, showing subtle areas of edema or microhemorrhage. MRI is also indicated in patients with more severe TBI to gain a more detailed picture of the brain's deeper structures. The utility of MRI is limited because of its many contraindications, including retained metal fragments and internal pumps or pacemakers. Electroencephalogram (EEG) uses scalp electrodes to monitor the brain's electrical activity. In addition to evaluating seizures, EEG can be used therapeutically to determine the depth of drug-induced coma.

Treatment of TBI

Most patients with mild TBI will improve within 3 to 6 months without any interventions. Patients and families need education regarding expected symptoms and reasonable coping mechanisms. Promotion of adequate sleep can help minimize symptoms. Daily headaches benefit from prophylactic medications, including antidepressants, antiepileptics, and migraine-type medications. Patients should be counseled that overuse, defined as greater than 6 doses per week, of over-the-counter medications such as ibuprofen or naproxen sodium may exacerbate headache by leading to rebound headaches. For the same reason, narcotics should be avoided.

Cognitive therapy has not shown to improve outcomes in most cases of mild TBI. It is considered if neuropsychiatric testing demonstrates significant cognitive deficits. Games that test memory, hand-eye coordination, and concentration can be useful. Patients should also be encouraged to journal or keep detailed notes if memory is an issue.

Patients with moderate to severe TBI are admitted to an intensive care unit. Many require short-term mechanical ventilation. There is potential for this level of injury to worsen, resulting in increased ICP. Therefore, frequent neurological assessment of the patient's LOC with pupil size and reactivity is necessary.

Pathophysiology of Selected Types of TBI

There are different kinds of traumatic brain injuries. Head injury can affect either a particular structure within the brain or the entire brain. Symptoms depend upon the location as well as the extent of the injury. Treatment varies according to the extent of brain tissue damage.

Diffuse Axonal Injury

Diffuse axonal injury (DAI) is one of the most common types of TBI. The damage occurs over a widespread area of brain tissue, mainly white matter, where axons are located. It is the major cause of unconsciousness and persistent coma after head trauma.

Etiology
DAI occurs when the brain moves back and forth in the skull, hitting into the cranial bone, as a result of coup-contrecoup injury. Motor vehicle accidents, sports-related trauma, violence, falls, and child abuse, such as shaken baby syndrome, are common causes of DAI.

Pathophysiology
DAI is characterized by diffuse swelling of neuronal axons, hemorrhage or laceration of the corpus callosum, and hemorrhages in the brainstem. Rapid stretch of axons damages the axonal structure, resulting in a loss of elasticity and impairment of transport of impulses. Calcium entry into damaged axons initiates activation of proteases, which causes further brain cell damage. Swollen, stretched axons may become disconnected. A DAI can also cause swelling in the brain. Swelling causes increased pressure in the brain and can cause decreased blood flow to the brain, as well as additional injury.

Clinical Presentation
DAI causes immediate loss of consciousness, and most patients (greater than 90%) remain in a persistent coma. A person with a mild or moderate DAI who is conscious may show signs of neurological impairment, depending upon which area of the brain is affected.

Diagnosis
DAI is difficult to detect using imaging studies, though MRI is the preferred test for diagnosis. CT scan is less sensitive to DAI, with many patients exhibiting a normal CT scan upon presentation. The degree of microscopic injury is considered to be greater than that seen on diagnostic imaging. DAI is suggested in any patient who demonstrates clinical symptoms disproportionate to CT scan findings.

Treatment
Immediate treatment involves neurovascular stabilization. The patient should be treated as if there is a cervical injury until this is ruled out. Measures such as IV mannitol and steroids should be implemented to reduce swelling of the brain. Surgery is not an option for those who have sustained a DAI. If the patient has sustained a mild or moderate DAI, rehabilitation should begin after the patient is stabilized and awake. Rehabilitation includes physical therapy, occupational therapy, and speech therapy. About 90% of survivors with severe DAI remain unconscious. The 10% that regain consciousness are often severely impaired.

ALERT! All patients with head injury should be treated as if there is also cervical spine injury until proven otherwise.

Concussion

A **concussion,** also called mild TBI, is a physiologic disruption in brain function caused by traumatic forces that may or may not involve loss of consciousness. It is manifested by temporary memory loss and alteration of mental state. The trauma initiates a cascade of metabolic changes in the brain. Not well investigated in the past, concussion has recently become an area of intense research. Concussion in sports activities, in particular, is the subject of many current research studies.

Most information about concussion comes from studies of injured athletes. In studies of high school athletes, concussion accounts for 8% to 11% of all injuries in football. The incidence rate in ice hockey is estimated at 12% of total injuries. In a survey of competitive college athletes engaged in all sports at a university in Ohio, 32% reported concussive symptoms after a blow to the head. Many cases of concussion go unreported because athletes do not want to suffer ineligibility for sports-related activity. Other individuals do not seek medical care for mild head injury, because they perceive the injury as unimportant. For these reasons, the true incidence of concussion is underestimated. A 24-hour reprieve from sports activity is mandatory after a concussion.

Etiology

Concussions result from a blow to the head or severe shaking of the head and neck. Contact sports activities, motor vehicle accidents, and shaken baby syndrome are common causes of concussion.

Simple concussions progressively resolve without complications, a process that can take only a few hours or last up to 10 days. Complex concussions consist of persistent symptoms that recur with exertion and are associated with conditions such as seizure, prolonged loss of consciousness (greater than 1 min), or prolonged impairment of cognitive function.

A previous concussion is a significant risk factor for sustaining another concussion. Studies show that the risk of sustaining a concussion is 4 to 5 times higher in patients who had at least one concussion in the past.

Pathophysiology

There are several different theories that attempt to explain the pathophysiology of concussion. All theories contain the following basic concepts:

1. Concussion may be caused by a direct blow to the head, face, neck, or elsewhere on the body that involves a traumatic force transmitted to the head.
2. Concussion results in an acute, short-term neurological dysfunction that resolves spontaneously.
3. Concussion results in neuropathological functional changes in the brain but no structural brain injury.
4. Concussion results in symptoms that may or may not involve loss of consciousness.
5. Concussion is typically associated with grossly normal structural neuroimaging studies.

Concussion occurs when traumatic impact causes sudden strain on the brain tissue from rotational or acceleration-deceleration forces. On a cellular level, the strain on neurons in the brain causes metabolic dysfunction, resulting in diffusion of intracellular potassium ions into the extracellular space. This stimulates release of excitatory amino acids, particularly glutamate. Glutamate accumulation is toxic to neurons and causes a temporary disruption of neuronal cell membranes. Glutamate overstimulates the neurons and causes the neuronal membranes to open their pores. From the extracellular space, sodium flows into the neuron membrane pores, followed by water. This is followed by temporary neuronal cellular swelling. Cellular ions stabilize, swelling resolves over time, and cellular homeostasis is returned, with no remaining structural changes in the brain.

Clinical Presentation

Concussions are characterized by an alteration in consciousness, such as being dazed, confused, or "seeing stars," or, less commonly, a brief loss of consciousness. Headache, dizziness, and flat affect are common initially. Lack of coordination and imbalance are also present. Both pretraumatic (retrograde) amnesia and posttraumatic (antegrade) amnesia can occur. Usually, the duration of amnesia is brief, lasting seconds to minutes, depending upon the injury.

Vomiting may suggest a significant brain injury with associated elevated ICP. Other signs of increased ICP include worsening headache, increasing disorientation, and changing LOC. If these symptoms are present, the possible causes of increasing ICP include subdural hematomas, epidural hematomas (EDHs), or some other type of intracranial hemorrhage.

Postconcussion syndrome is the persistence of symptoms for more than 3 weeks after the initial injury. The symptoms associated with this include headache, dizziness, imbalance, fatigue, irritability, insomnia, and concentration or memory difficulties.

Diagnosis

The initial assessment of an acute concussion should begin with cardiac and pulmonary stabilization: checking the airway, breathing, and circulation (ABCs). Cervical spine injury should be considered and the unconscious individual should be treated as having a potential cervical spine injury. Those with prolonged loss of consciousness should be transported rapidly to an appropriate medical facility. For the conscious individual suspected of having sustained a concussion, a thorough neurological examination should be performed, including assessment of orientation to person, place, and time. This should be followed by questions to test recent memory, because these are the most sensitive in diagnosing concussion. The ability to perform simple tasks and postural stability should be assessed also.

According to the American Association of Neurology (AAN), concussions can be divided into Grade 1, 2, or 3. In Grade 1, there is no loss of consciousness and mental status changes resolve in fewer than 15 minutes. In Grade 2, there is no loss of consciousness and mental status changes resolve in greater than 15 minutes. In Grade 3, the patient has a loss of consciousness.

The Glascow Coma Scale (GCS) is not an adequately sensitive instrument for mild traumatic head injury. There are a few different concussion assessment checklists available for sports-related injuries. The CDC recommends a concussion assessment toolkit based on the AAN guidelines to aid in the evaluation of a concussion. The tool assesses multiple cognitive, physical, and emotional symptoms initially and at 15 minutes and 30 minutes postinjury. The AAN tool can be found at http://www.cdc.gov/headsup/index.html.

Patients with a concussion usually do not require imaging unless one or more of the following conditions are present:

- physical evidence of trauma above the clavicles
- anticoagulation or coagulopathy
- age older than 60 years
- alcohol or drug intoxication
- neurological deficit
- persistent vomiting
- seizure or short-term memory deficit.
- history of alcoholism

A CT scan is normal in more than 90% of concussion patients. However, if headache does not resolve or the patient becomes disoriented or begins to show decreased LOC, medical evaluation is necessary.

Treatment

Most people recover after a concussion, but how quickly they improve depends on many factors. These factors include severity of the concussion, age, state of health before the concussion, and care after the injury. Rest is the most important treatment measure. Patients with concussions are advised to rest for the first 24 to 48 hours, up to 7 days with gradual return to regular activities as appropriate. The clinician should assess the patient for neurological deficits, including inspection of pupils, and assessment of orientation to time, place and person. Counting backwards by sevens or reciting the months in reverse order are common tests of cognition. Clinicians assess grip strength, leg strength, ability to speak clearly, gait, and postural stability. The patient should avoid physically demanding activity and not return to work, school or sports activity without conferring with a physician. The patient can be given a mild pain reliever such as acetaminophen. The CDC has specific 5 step treatment guidelines, called the Head's Up Program, regarding recovery from concussion. These can be found on the CDC website: http://www.cdc.gov/headsup/basics/return_to_sports.html.

Cerebral Contusion

A cerebral contusion is considered a bruise of the brain tissue that occurs with head trauma. Often a contusion consists of scattered areas of bleeding on the brain's surface, most commonly along the undersurface and the frontal and temporal lobes. Cerebral contusions typically result from coup-contrecoup injury. They may also occur with penetrating TBI.

Etiology

The most common causes of contusion include blows to the head from motor vehicle accidents, gunshots, blunt trauma force, falls, and assault. People at high risk are those with mobility problems, those who are active in high-impact contact sports, and people who are taking anticoagulants.

Pathophysiology

A combination of vascular and tissue damage occur in cerebral contusion, which is a coup-contrecoup injury of the brain. Most of the force of impact from a small, hard object tends to remain at the injury site, leading to a coup contusion. In contrast, impact from a larger object causes less injury at the impact site, and energy is dissipated at the opposite side of the brain because of head motion, called a contrecoup contusion. Cerebral edema typically develops around cerebral contusions within 48 to 72 hours after injury; it is problematic because the brain is contained within the skull, which is a bony cranial vault that gives little room for cellular expansion. The swollen brain tissue may become compressed against the bone, which then leads to brain cell damage. Also, if cerebral edema is severe, downward pressure may be placed on the brainstem and herniation of brain tissue is possible, which leads to death. Pressure on the brainstem can compress the oculomotor nerve (CNIII), which may be exhibited as a dilated pupil. Pressure on the brainstem also affects vital centers and the reticular activating system, exhibited as changes in vital signs and decreased LOC.

Clinical Presentation

The signs and symptoms of a contusion include severe headache, dizziness, vomiting, increased size of one pupil, and sudden weakness in an arm or leg. The person may seem restless, agitated, or irritable. Often, the person has memory loss. These symptoms can last for several hours to several weeks, depending on the severity of the injury. As the brain tissue swells, the person may feel increasingly drowsy or confused. Vital signs may show decreased heart rate and decreased respirations and hypertension, which are signs of pressure on the brainstem. These changes in vital signs require immediate medical attention. If the person is difficult to awaken or loses consciousness, this is a medical emergency.

Diagnosis

Immediate CT scan is needed when cerebral contusion is suspected. However, the true amount of neuronal damage in the injured region can be underestimated.

 CLINICAL CONCEPT

Postconcussion syndrome is the persistence of symptoms for more than 3 weeks after the initial injury; symptoms include headache, dizziness, fatigue, irritability, insomnia, and concentration or memory difficulties.

MRI scans have greater sensitivity for cerebral edema. Skull x-ray is necessary to look for fracture. Skull fracture commonly causes rupture of the middle meningeal artery, which results in epidural hematoma (EDH). Daily CT scans may be needed in the days following cerebral contusion to assess progression or resolution. Cerebral angiography is often performed to visualize blood vessel damage and possible aneurysms.

Treatment

Cardiopulmonary life-saving measures are the priority with any head injury. The patient should be assessed for ABCs, as well as treated and stabilized as if he or she has a cervical spinal injury. In the emergency setting, IV Mannitol is frequently used to decrease cerebral edema. Craniectomy may be performed where a piece of skull is removed to relieve the pressure on the brain cells. If cerebral hematoma is present, evacuation of the blood is performed through a craniotomy.

ALERT! Delayed enlargement of brain contusion or hematoma is the most common cause of clinical deterioration and death. Periodic neurological assessment is essential after head injury.

Intracranial Bleeding

Head trauma can cause three types of intracranial bleeds: EDH, subdural hematoma, or subarachnoid hemorrhage (SAH). Each condition presents in a distinct manner and each is treated differently. To understand intracranial bleeding, an understanding of the meningeal layers that protect the brain is necessary (see Fig. 35-7).

Epidural Hematoma

An EDH is a bleed in the space below the skull bone and above the dura mater (see Fig. 35-8). EDH occurs in 1% to 2% of all head trauma cases and in about 10% of patients who present with traumatic coma. Patients younger than 5 years and older than 55 years have an increased mortality rate. Patients younger than 20 years account for 60% of EDHs. EDH is the most serious complication of head injury.

An EDH is commonly a bleed caused by a skull bone fracture that lacerates the middle meningeal artery. Normally, the middle meningeal artery runs along the skull bone, so close to the bone that it leaves its impression upon the skull. With skull fracture, rupture of the artery causes a high amount of pressure (sounds better) rapid and voluminous arterial bleeding, which places high pressure on the brain tissue. A midline shift in the brain on imaging studies can be visualized within an hour of the injury.

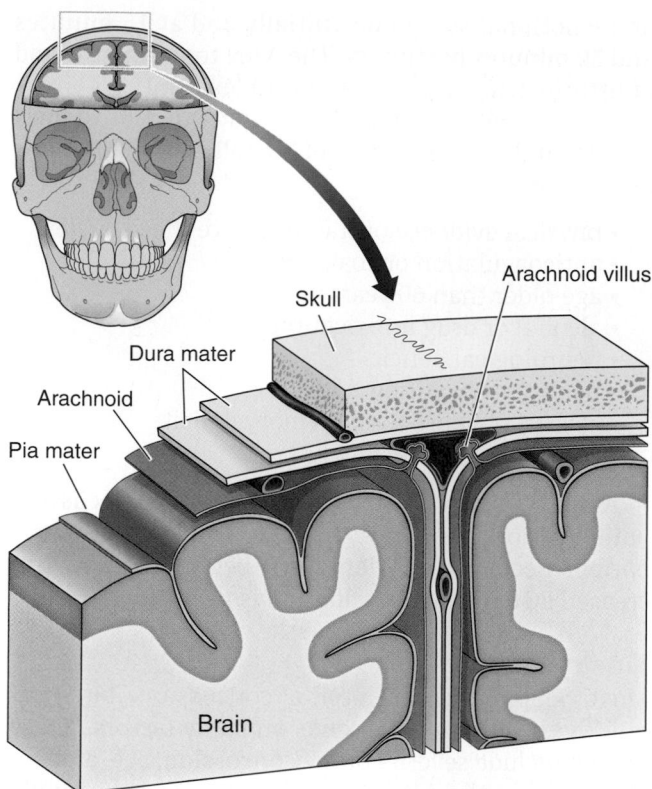

FIGURE 35-7. The meninges. The meninges are layers of membranes that envelop and protect the central nervous system. There are three meningeal membrane layers: the dura mater, arachnoid mater, and pia mater. Between each of the layers is a space. Between the skull bone and dura mater is the epidural space. Beneath the dura mater is the subdural space. Beneath the arachnoid membrane is the subarachnoid space. It is important to note that the middle meningeal artery runs very close to the skull bone above the dura mater. In skull fracture, the middle meningeal artery commonly ruptures and causes an EDH. There is a network of veins within the subdural space and head trauma often causes rupture of subdural veins, which causes a subdural hematoma. Also, note that the CSF is contained beneath the arachnoid membrane within the subarachnoid space.

Following injury, the patient may or may not lose consciousness. Other symptoms include severe headache, vomiting, and seizure. Patients may have a dramatically delayed deterioration. The patient can be conscious and talking, yet a minute later become apneic, comatose, and minutes from death. Cushing's triad of hypertension, bradycardia, and bradypnea are indicators of pressure on the brainstem. LOC may be decreased, with decreased or fluctuating GCS. Dilated, sluggish, or fixed

ALERT! A positive Babinski sign occurs when stimulation of the sole of the foot causes the toes to flare out. In the adult, the Babinski sign indicates upper neuron cortical dysfunction. The Babinski sign is normal in a newborn.

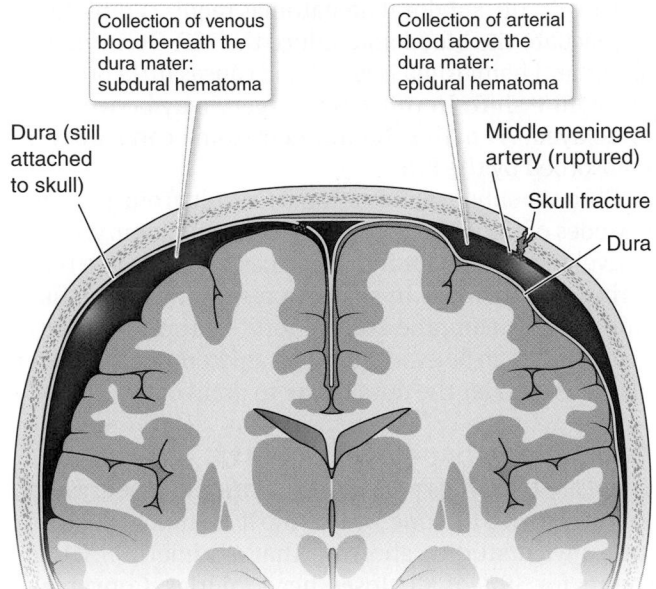

Collection of venous blood beneath the dura mater: subdural hematoma

Collection of arterial blood above the dura mater: epidural hematoma

Dura (still attached to skull)

Middle meningeal artery (ruptured)

Skull fracture

Dura

FIGURE 35-8. Epidural and subdural hematoma. An epidural or subdural hematoma can be caused by head trauma. An EDH is a collection of arterial blood above the dura mater that is caused by rupture of the middle meningeal artery. This is commonly associated with skull fracture. A subdural hematoma is a collection of venous blood that is beneath the dura mater. Both of these hematomas can place excessive pressure on the brain and cause neurological damage or death.

pupil(s), bilateral or ipsilateral to injury, suggest increased ICP or herniation. Signs of uncal herniation consist of coma, fixed and dilated pupils, and decerebrate posturing. Hemiplegia contralateral to the brain injury and a positive Babinski are present.

ALERT! Delayed recognition and diagnosis of epidural hematoma (EDH) is a major cause of death.

After severe head trauma, immediate CT scan and skull x-ray are necessary; skull x-ray commonly shows fractures, whereas CT scan will show evidence of bleeding into the epidural space. If bleeding has been prolonged, a midline shift in the brain tissue will be apparent (see Fig. 35-10).

This is a neurosurgical emergency requiring a craniotomy and surgical evacuation of the hematoma. The patient requires cardiopulmonary stabilization with airway and blood pressure control, as well as intubation for mechanical ventilation, IV access, oxygen, and cardiac monitoring. Hyperventilating the patient often can decrease ICP. Phenytoin provides prophylaxis against early posttraumatic seizure.

Subdural Hematoma

A subdural hematoma results from bleeding that accumulates in the space below the dura mater above the arachnoid membrane. The subdural hematoma occurs from tearing of bridging veins located in the subdural space. Acute subdural hematoma is the most common type of traumatic intracranial hematoma, occurring in 24% of patients who present in a coma. The bleeding from the subdural veins is slow but can accumulate with time to become substantial enough to place pressure on the brain tissue. An acute subdural hematoma occurs within 72 hours of head injury, whereas a subacute subdural hematoma can take several days to accumulate to levels that cause symptoms. Chronic subdural hematoma is one that has been present for up to 3 weeks.

Complete neurological examination is necessary. Neurological deficits are commonly not present until there is substantial bleeding into the subdural space. Repeat follow-up neurological examination is required in 2 to 5 days when subdural hematoma is suspected. Coagulation profiles are particularly important for patients taking anticoagulants as well as for alcoholics, who may

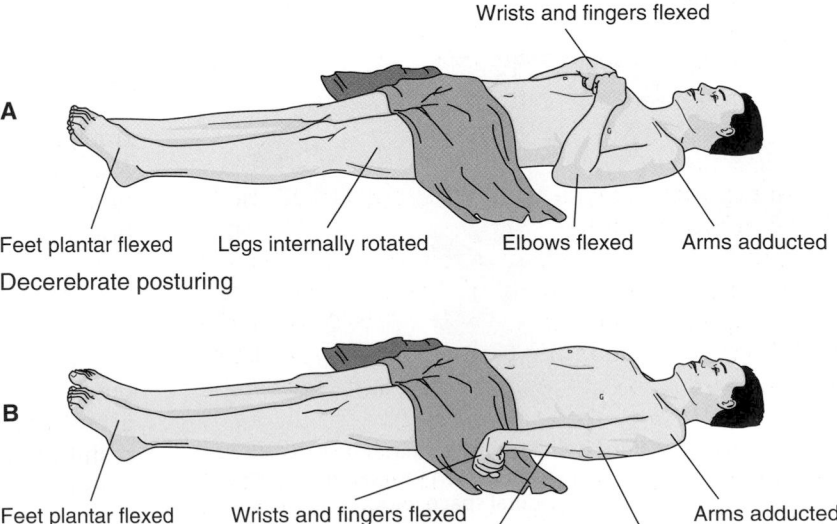

Decorticate posturing

Wrists and fingers flexed

A

Feet plantar flexed   Legs internally rotated   Elbows flexed   Arms adducted

Decerebrate posturing

B

Feet plantar flexed   Wrists and fingers flexed   Arms adducted

Forearms pronated   Elbows extended

FIGURE 35-9. Decorticate and decerebrate posturing in coma. Brain damage can result in coma. The patient can assume either decorticate (A) or decerebrate (B) postures depending on what part of the brain is damaged. Decorticate posture results from damage to the corticospinal tract, whereas decerebrate posture results from upper brainstem damage. In both postures, the patient exhibits extended, adducted legs with foot drop; a plantar flexion of the feet. In decorticate posture, the arms and wrists are flexed. In decerebrate posture, the arms are adducted and wrists are pronated.

Axial view
of brain

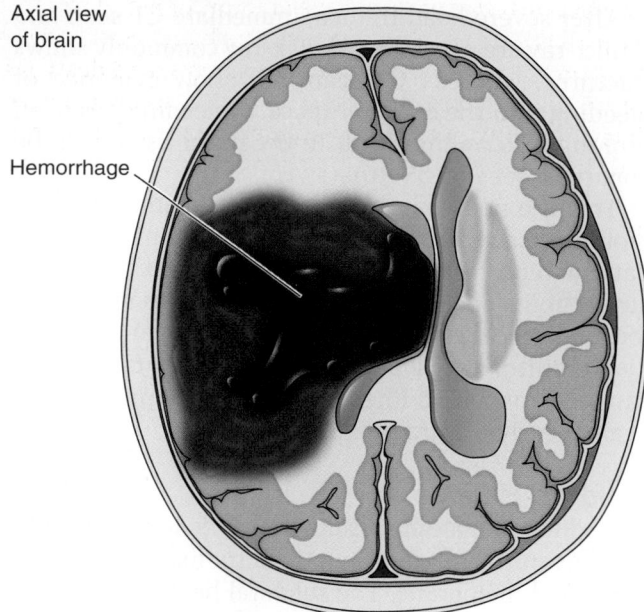

Hemorrhage

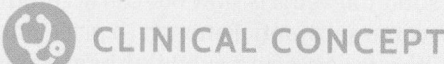

FIGURE 35-10. In space-occupying lesions, bleeding, and edema of the brain, a midline shift can occur. The pressure of the lesion pushes against the brain tissue.

> 🩺 **CLINICAL CONCEPT**
>
> Alcohol abuse increases the risk for development of subdural hematoma after head trauma.

have an associated coagulopathy placing them at high risk for subdural hematoma. CT scan and skull x-ray are therefore necessary. CT scan may or may not show apparent bleeding into the subdural space immediately after injury (see Fig. 35-11). Repeat CT scan is necessary in the next few days when subdural hematoma is suspected. If bleeding has been prolonged, a midline shift in the brain tissue will be apparent.

Dura **Subdural** Arachnoid
mater **hematoma** membrane

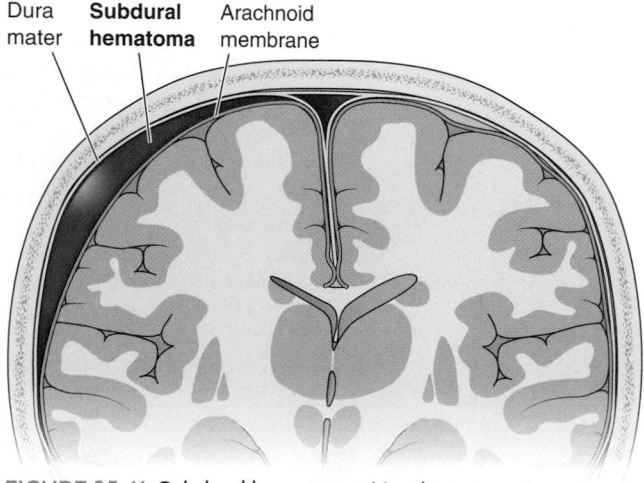

FIGURE 35-11. Subdural hematoma. Head trauma can cause a subdural hematoma, which occurs when veins rupture beneath the dura mater within the subdural space. Blood accumulates beneath the dura mater and above the arachnoid membrane. Accumulation of blood can place pressure on the brain, causing neurological damage

Large acute subdural hematomas require craniotomy to evacuate the blood and reduce the ICP. Occasionally, a subdural hematoma is small and causes little pressure or midline shift. In this case, surgery may be withheld or delayed. A small subdural hematoma can slowly be reabsorbed by the brain.

Chronic subdural hematomas result from multiple episodes of minor head trauma in close proximity. Alternatively, small subdural hematomas can fail to be reabsorbed and increase in size as a result of osmotic fluid shifts or membrane formation. Chronic subdural hematomas can be evacuated by craniotomy and catheter placement under the dura mater to drain out the blood.

Traumatic and Aneurysmal SAH

There are two types of SAH: traumatic and aneurysmal. Traumatic SAH is one of the most common head injuries, with studies showing that traumatic SAH accounts for 39% of all closed head injuries. Conversely, aneurysmal SAH is not a common disorder in the United States. The annual incidence is 6 to 16 cases per 100,000 population, with approximately 30,000 episodes occurring each year. Approximately 80% of cases of aneurysmal SAH occur in people aged 40 to 65 years, with 15% occurring in people aged 20 to 40 years.

> 🩺 **CLINICAL CONCEPT**
>
> Subdural hematoma can occur in the elderly after minor head trauma, particularly in those who are taking anticoagulants.

Etiology

Traumatic SAH results from tearing of the cerebral and meningeal vessels within the subarachnoid space of the brain. Causes include rotational-acceleration injury of the brain, stretching of the vertebral artery because of hyperextension of the neck, and sudden trauma to the carotid artery, which raises intra-arterial pressure in the brain. Skull fracture and cerebral contusion are commonly found with traumatic SAH. Posttraumatic cerebral vasospasm also occurs in traumatic SAH. Blood breakdown products within the subarachnoid space are believed to trigger vasospasm of cerebral arteries.

Cerebral aneurysms usually occur in the terminal portion of the internal carotid artery and the branching sites on the large cerebral arteries in the anterior portion of the circle of Willis. Aneurysms begin as small outpouchings through defects in the muscle layer of an artery wall. These defects are thought to expand as a result of pressure from pulsatile blood flow and blood turbulence, which is greatest at the arterial bifurcations. A mature aneurysm lacks the tunica media, which is replaced by connective tissue. The probability of rupture is related to the tension on the aneurysm wall. Cerebral aneurysms are often called saccular "berry aneurysms" because of the resemblance to a berry on a vine (see Fig. 35-12). There are certain conditions that increase one's risk for cerebral aneurysms (see Box 35-3).

Pathophysiology

Aneurysmal SAH and traumatic SAH have different etiologies, but the pathophysiologic mechanisms that cause brain damage are the same. The rupture of a

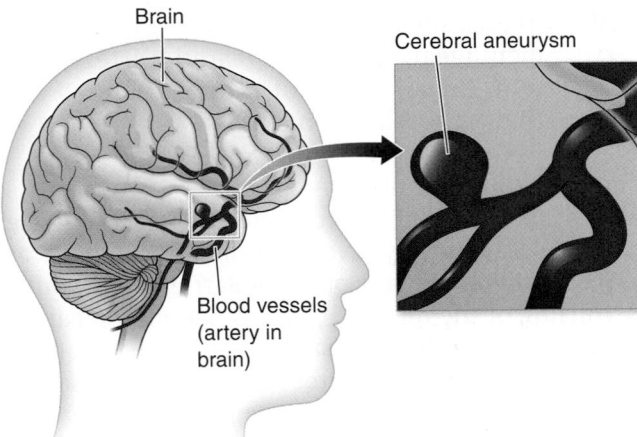

Brain

Cerebral aneurysm

Blood vessels (artery in brain)

FIGURE 35-12. A cerebral aneurysm is a weakening in a cerebral artery wall that bulges out and is susceptible to rupture.

BOX 35-3. Risk Factors for Cerebral Aneurysms

- aortic coarctation
- bacterial infections
- cerebral arteriovenous malformation
- cerebral atherosclerosis
- congenital conditions: persistent fetal circulation, hypoplastic/absent arterial circulation
- Ehlers-Danlos syndrome
- family history of stroke
- fibromuscular dysplasia
- fungal infections
- granulomatous angiitis
- hypertension
- Klippel-Trenaunay-Weber syndrome
- long-term analgesic use
- Marfan syndrome
- metastatic tumors to cerebral arteries: atrial myxoma, choriocarcinoma, undifferentiated carcinoma
- moyamoya disease
- Osler-Weber-Rendu syndrome
- persistent headache
- polycystic kidney disease
- pregnancy-induced hypertension
- pseudoxanthoma elasticum
- systemic lupus erythematosus
- vascular asymmetry in the circle of Willis

---

cerebral artery causes a large amount of blood to rapidly fill the subarachnoid space. The blood exerts pressure on the brain, irritates the meninges, and destroys brain cells in its path. SAH also causes an obstructive hydrocephalus, which is an accumulation of CSF within the brain. The buildup of blood and CSF creates a large amount of pressure that can lead to herniation of the brainstem and death.

Clinical Presentation

In up to 50% of aneurysmal SAH there are signs and symptoms that precede rupture of the cerebral aneurysm. Leakage of blood from a cerebral aneurysm can cause symptoms. Headache, dizziness, orbital pain, and diplopia can appear 10 to 20 days before rupture. Nuchal rigidity may be present. These symptoms may be ignored or thought to be related to a migraine syndrome. Cranial nerve dysfunction along with memory loss are present in 25% of patients.

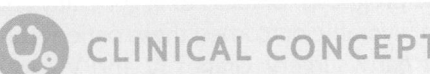

CLINICAL CONCEPT

The rupture of a subarachnoid cerebral aneurysm commonly causes a "thunderclap headache" and rapid decline of vital signs.

The circle of Willis is often the site of a cerebral aneurysm. The cranial nerves exit the brain adjacent to the circle of Willis, and a cerebral aneurysm or leakage of blood from a cerebral aneurysm can compress the cranial nerves. Oculomotor nerve dysfunction with pupil dilation can be exhibited, and vision loss can be caused by compression of the optic nerve. Hemiparesis can result from middle cerebral artery (MCA) aneurysm or ischemia. Patients may also have aphasia, hemineglect, or both.

In the assessment of SAH, clinicians commonly utilize a tool such as the Hunt and Hess grading system (see Box 35-4). Unfortunately in aneurysmal SAH often there are no outward signs of the impending rupture or hemorrhage, and death occurs within minutes of the event. Patients who suffer the sudden rupture of the aneurysm complain of "the worst headache of my life" just before unconsciousness. The patient is commonly found comatose and death quickly ensues.

Diagnosis

The diagnosis of SAH can be based on CT scan without contrast, cerebral angiogram, and lumbar puncture. CT scan is followed by lumbar puncture, which demonstrates blood in the CSF. A noncontrast CT followed by CT angiogram of the brain can rule out SAH with greater than 99% sensitivity.

Treatment

Current treatment recommendations involve management in an intensive care unit setting, because the

BOX 35-4. Hunt and Hess Grading Scale

The Hunt and Hess grading system grades SAHs as follows:

- grade 0: unruptured aneurysm
- grade I: asymptomatic or mild headache and slight nuchal rigidity
- grade Ia: fixed neurological deficit without acute meningeal/brain reaction
- grade II: cranial nerve palsy, moderate to severe headache, nuchal rigidity
- grade III: mild focal neurological deficit, lethargy, or confusion
- grade IV: stupor, moderate to severe hemiparesis, early decerebrate rigidity
- grade V: deep coma, decerebrate rigidity, moribund appearance.

In the Hunt and Hess system, the lower the grade, the better the prognosis. Grades I to III generally are associated with favorable outcomes; these patients are candidates for early surgery. Grades IV and V carry a poor prognosis. Survival correlates with the grade of SAH upon presentation. Reported figures include a 70% survival rate for Hunt and Hess grade I, 60% for grade II, 50% for grade III, 40% for grade IV, and 10% for grade V.

(Hunt, W. E., & Hess, R. M. (1968). Surgical risk as related to time of intervention in the repair of intracranial aneurysms. *J Neurosurgery, 28*(1), 14–20.)

patient requires hemodynamic stabilization. Breathing, blood pressure, and heart rate are maintained with consideration of the patient's neurological status. Additional medical management is directed toward the prevention and treatment of complications. Surgical treatment consists of clipping the berry aneurysm. Endovascular treatment is also often done. A catheter can insert thin wire coils into the aneurysm to block it off from blood flow.

Skull Fractures

The skull is prone to fracture in certain regions where the cranial bone has low density. Susceptible areas include the temporal bone, orbital fossa, base of the skull, and foramen magnum. Temporal bone fractures represent 15% to 48% of all skull fractures, whereas basilar skull fractures represent 19% to 21% of all skull fractures.

Etiology

Skull fracture occurs with a direct blow to the head or traumatic injury of the body, such as a fall, where the head hits an unmovable surface. Risk factors of skull fracture include motor vehicle accidents, contact sports activities, and falls.

Pathophysiology

Skull fractures are categorized as linear, depressed, or basilar, and may or may not involve injury to the brain tissue. Linear fracture, the most common type of fracture, does not affect brain tissue. Depressed fractures occur when an object fractures the skull with sufficient force to push bone fragments into the brain. Depressed fractures are commonly open fractures that involve underlying brain tissue. The temporal bone is the most commonly fractured bone of the skull. Basilar skull fractures, fractures at the base of the skull, occur in the temporal bone. Fractures that involve the temporal bone continue along the skull base with a pattern that follows the weakest points of the anatomy. The temporal bone encloses vital structures such as the inner ear organs, cranial nerves, meningeal membrane, carotid artery, and jugular vein. Injury to any of these structures can occur with temporal bone fracture.

Clinical Presentation

Basilar skull fractures occur most often along the middle fossa and may involve brain injury. Fractures in the middle fossa may produce Battle's sign, which is bruising of the mastoid process behind the ear on the affected side. There may also be a CSF leak from the ear or the nose. Fractures in the frontal fossa can result in periorbital ecchymosis referred to as raccoon eyes, edema, and CSF leak from the nose (see Fig. 35-13).

Diagnosis

To diagnose a skull fracture, an x-ray of the head is usually done, followed by a CT scan. MRI or magnetic resonance angiography (MRA) is of value for suspected vascular injury. Anyone with a head injury should have a complete neurological examination.

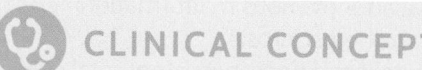

CLINICAL CONCEPT

After skull fracture, discharge from the nose or ear should be tested for beta-2-transferrin and glucose, which are diagnostic for CSF. Loss of CSF can cause headache, nausea, vomiting, and dizziness.

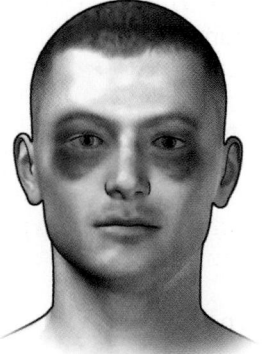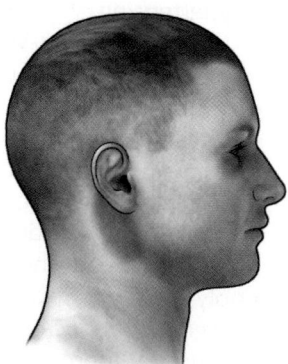

FIGURE 35-13. Signs of basilar skull fracture. Ecchymoses around both eyes ("raccoon eyes") and a bruise behind the ear ("Battle's sign") are key signs of basilar skull fracture.

Treatment

In skull fractures, treatment involves controlling pain, promoting healing, and preventing complications. The primary concern with skull fracture is potential TBI and epidural hematoma. Most linear skull fractures do not require specific treatment. If there are no complications of brain injury or epidural hematoma, the patient is treated for any external head wound and discharged with instructions to watch for late-developing signs of neurological deficit that may indicate a brain injury.

A linear skull fracture at the base of the skull can cause a tear in the meninges surrounding the brain. CSF, which is a clear or pink-tinged fluid, can leak from the nose (CSF rhinorrhea) or ear (CSF otorrhea). A concern is that the tear in the meninges may provide a path for infection; therefore, an antibiotic may be prescribed. A tear in the meninges can seal by itself in as little as 48 hours, but patients are nonetheless often admitted to the hospital for a brief period for observation.

In a depressed fracture, if bone fragments are dislodged, surgery may be required to align, elevate, or remove fragments. If the bone has not penetrated the meninges and there are no signs of brain injury, a full recovery can be expected. However, concussion symptoms may persist for months. Treatment is often determined by the depth of the depression, whether it is accompanied by an open wound, and the degree of accompanying brain trauma. Deep, open skull fracture is frequently accompanied by brain damage. Surgery to elevate the bone and remove any fragments is often required. Surgery may also be needed to treat bleeding inside the skull. In these cases, mild to severe impairment and disability caused by the brain injury can be expected. If cerebral bleeding or edema is present, the patient often requires a craniotomy or craniectomy, which removes a small section of skull bone to allow expansion of brain tissue.

Spinal Cord Injury

Spinal cord injury (SCI) results from compression, stretching, or laceration of the spinal cord following trauma. It can also occur from conditions that impair blood flow to the spinal cord. Injury to the spinal cord leads to temporary or permanent loss of normal sensory, motor, or autonomic function. These deficits are seen immediately following the injury. Further deterioration may occur as edema of the spinal cord develops.

Several factors affect morbidity and mortality following SCI: the patient's age at the time of injury, level of injury within the spinal cord, and the number of muscle groups affected. The degree of muscle weakness and sensory loss has the most impact on survival and early complication rates.

Epidemiology

According to the CDC, there are approximately 11,000 new spinal cord injuries diagnosed in the United States annually. The mean age at time of SCI is 26 years. Males are 4 times more likely than females to sustain an SCI.

Traumatic SCIs are preventable and numerous programs are aimed at reducing SCI incidence. The American Spinal Injury Association (ASIA) has collected in-depth information on a variety of prevention programs. The majority of these are based on the Think First program, whose mission is to prevent brain and spinal cord injuries through educating children, adults, and community leaders responsible for formulating public policy.

Basic Concepts in Spinal Cord Anatomy and Physiology

The spinal cord is an extension of the brain that travels through the base of the skull down through the vertebral bones of the back and terminates at the level of the first lumbar vertebrae. The end portion of the spinal cord is called the **conus medullaris.** The spinal nerves that continue down from it are referred to as the **cauda equina** (see Fig. 35-14). Vertebrae can be fractured by trauma, but unless the spinal cord within is injured, there will be no motor or sensory deficits. Like the brain, the spinal cord is surrounded by the meninges, which contain CSF.

In the spinal cord, the white matter surrounds the gray matter and contains ascending and descending neural tracts. The ascending tracts are sensory tracts that carry touch, pressure, vibration, position sense, pain, and temperature information to the brain. The tracts carrying pain and temperature cross over to the opposite side of the spinal cord, so that when the injury to the spinal cord is incomplete, damage to this tract causes loss of sensation on the opposite side of the body from the initial injury. The descending tracts are motor tracts that carry voluntary and involuntary motor commands down from the brain. Motor tracts from the brain also cross to the opposite side of the spinal cord (see Fig. 35-15).

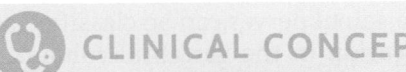
CLINICAL CONCEPT

The symptoms seen in SCI vary based on the neural tract that is injured. Injuries to the descending tracts result in motor deficits, whereas damage to the ascending tracts cause sensory deficits.

Within the gray matter are neuron cell bodies and their dendrites. These are located within three horns of the spinal cord (dorsal horn, ventral horn, and lateral horn) and are surrounded by white matter. The dorsal horn cells are sensory, the ventral horn cells are motor, and the lateral horn contains the cell bodies of the sympathetic and parasympathetic fibers.

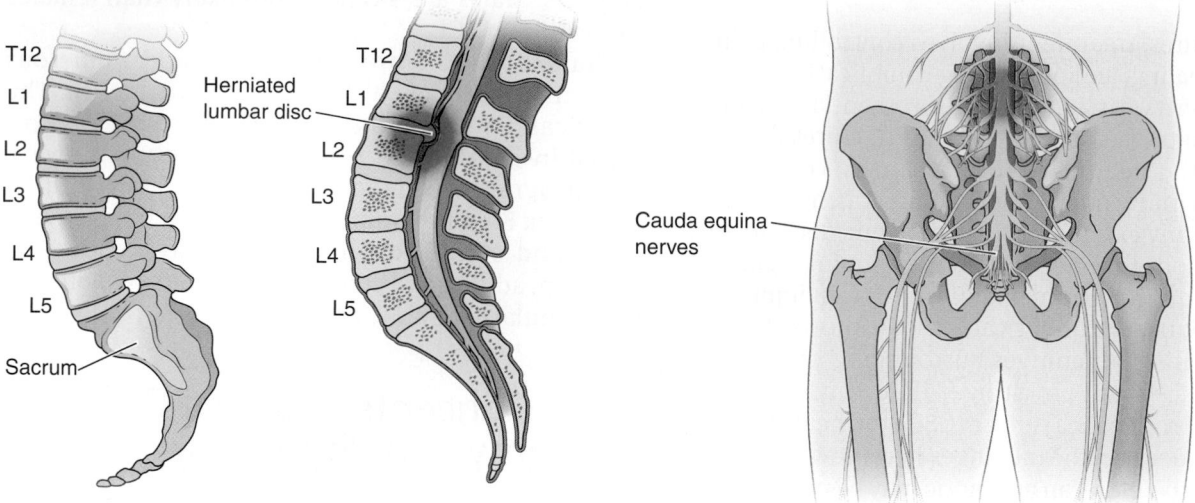

FIGURE 35-14. Cauda equina syndrome. In cauda equina syndrome, a herniated disc compresses the nerves that come off the bottom of the spinal cord, called cauda equina nerves. Symptoms include back pain radiating down the legs, weakness of legs, and bladder or bowel incontinence. This is a medical emergency.

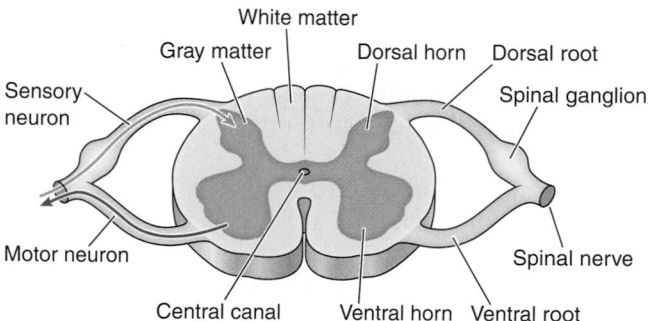

FIGURE 35-15. Cross section of the spinal cord. Spinal nerves contain sensory and motor components. In the spinal cord, the sensory nerves enter via the dorsal root and then synapse within the spinal cord. The motor nerves exit the spinal cord via the ventral root.

The spinal nerves that exit at each level of vertebrae control the sensation and motor response of specific areas of the body. The dermatome map (see Fig. 35-16) illustrates which vertebral level spinal nerve innervates which area of the body. The functions of the spinal nerves can be classified according to their location in the vertebral column. Cervical nerves in the neck provide movement and feeling in the neck, upper extremities, and upper trunk. The thoracic nerves supply the trunk and abdomen, whereas the lumbar nerves innervate the legs, bladder, and bowel; they are also responsible for sexual function.

Basic Pathophysiologic Concepts in SCI

Injury to the spinal cord can be primary or secondary and varies as to the mechanism of injury. A complete SCI indicates that there is no motor or sensory function below the site of injury. Preservation of some function occurs in an incomplete injury.

Primary Injury

Mechanical forces of trauma can immediately damage neurons and their supporting glial cells. Trauma can stretch or tear the spinal cord or cut off circulation, which interrupts the function of ascending and descending nerve tracts. The physical damage can result in immediate hemorrhage and neural cell death, which in turn creates an ischemic environment.

Secondary Injury

The ischemia caused by the primary injury initiates multiple secondary processes that worsen the damage over hours to weeks. The ischemia causes a cytotoxic edema similar to that found in TBI. An inflammatory reaction with endothelial injury is activated by the primary injury. Over time, these processes cause a cascade of tissue damage and scarring within the area of injured spinal cord, which inhibits regeneration of neurons.

Disruption of the neural tracts interrupts messages between the brain and the spinal cord below the level of injury. Unstimulated axons atrophy and a fluid-filled cyst forms within the spinal cord gray and white matter. This cyst occupies several segments above and below the primary injury site. Glial cells proliferate to form scar tissue.

Mechanisms of Injury

Hyperflexion injuries are often associated with sudden deceleration, such as that seen in high speed motor vehicle accidents and diving accidents. The extreme flexion disrupts the posterior longitudinal ligament, leading to vertebral body compressions. In milder cases, the spine is fairly stable and external orthosis (bracing) may be sufficient. However, in cases of severe flexion that affects both the anterior and posterior structures, surgery is necessary.

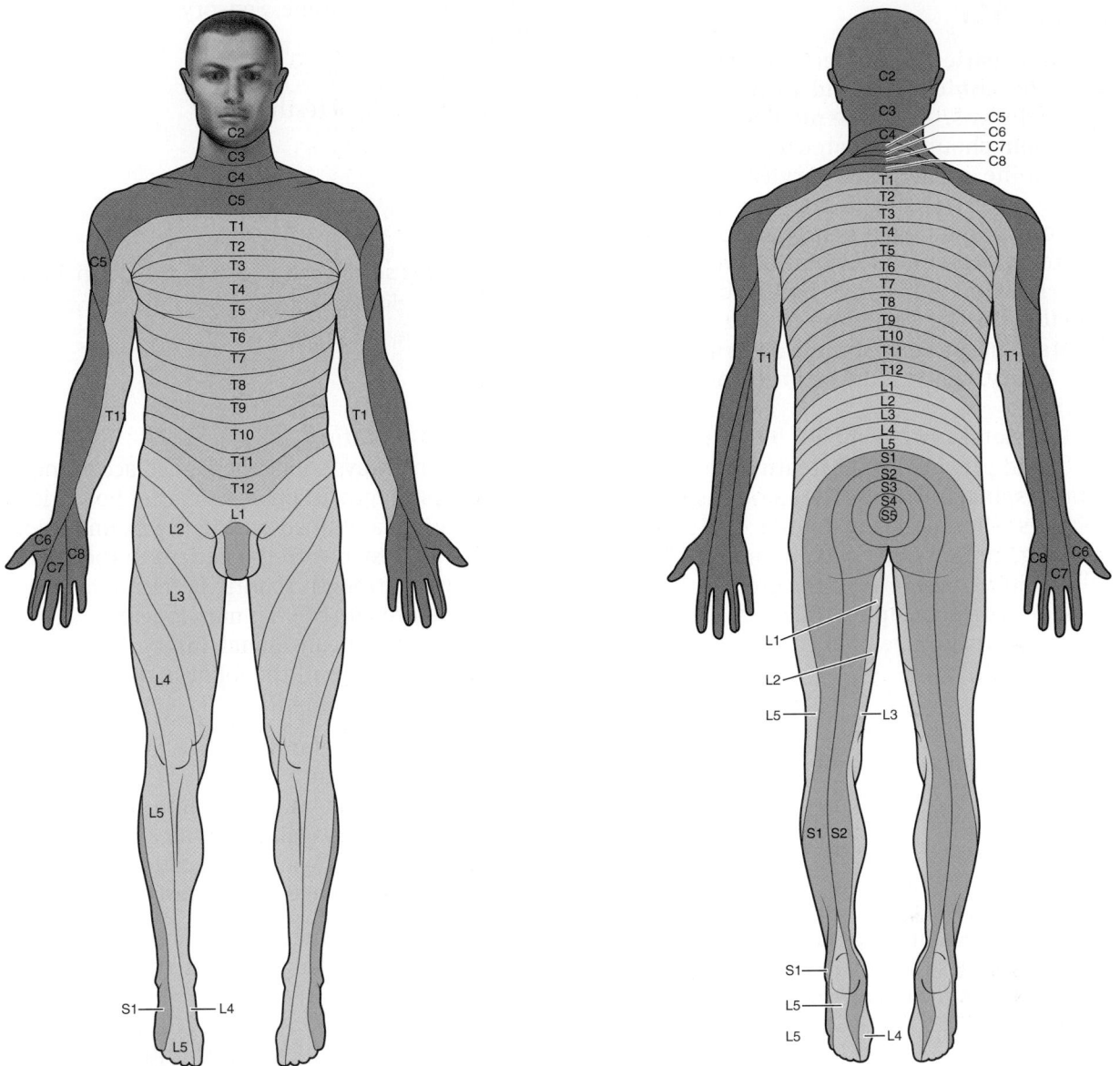

FIGURE 35-16. Dermatome map. A dermatome is an area of skin that is mainly supplied by a single spinal nerve. There are eight cervical nerves (C1 has no dermatome), 12 thoracic nerves, five lumbar nerves, and five sacral nerves. Each of these nerves carry sensory stimuli, including pain, from a particular region of skin to the spinal cord and up to the brain. Dermatomes can be used in physical examination of the patient to localize a region of neurological deficit.

Rotational injuries of the spinal column result from lateral flexion or extreme rotation of the spinal column. These injuries are typically unstable.

Hyperextension injuries typically result from falls or rear-end motor vehicle accidents and are most commonly seen in the lower cervical spine. If hyperextension is followed by forced flexion, often referred to as "whiplash," more severe injuries may result. Initial treatment may require a cervical collar and traction to realign the spine and reduce pressure on the spinal cord. Surgical decompression that relieves the stress on the spinal cord, as well as stabilization, is often required.

Axial loading or vertical compression occurs when overwhelming vertical force is applied to the vertebral body, causing burst fractures. Mechanically, fracture of the vertebral body and disruption of the posterior elements result from compressive forces. Treatment goals include realignment with traction, followed by bracing or surgical stabilization depending on the degree of instability.

Penetrating injury enters the spinal column and has direct spinal cord contact. Low velocity stab wounds cause actual spinal cord contact or vascular injury by the instrument or bony fragments, resulting in neurological deficit. Low-impact wounds are likely to cause incomplete injury and subsequently have a more favorable prognosis. In high velocity mechanisms, such as gunshots, damage is directly related to the amount of kinetic energy applied to the spinal cord as well as the extent of actual spinal cord trauma caused by the missile or bony compression. Missile injury is more likely to result in complete SCI.

Assessment in SCI

Initially, in trauma patients, a general survey is important. First, the clinician should focus on life-threatening conditions. Assessment of ABCs is a priority. The patient should be treated as if he or she has a cervical spine injury with cervical bracing while lying flat on a transfer board. The patient should be logrolled when each spinous process of the entire vertebral column is examined from the occiput to the sacrum. A history should focus on symptoms related to the vertebrae and motor or sensory deficits. The patient should describe the mechanism of injury, which indicates the potential for spinal injury.

The musculoskeletal system should be examined first to identify and provide initial treatment of potentially unstable spinal fractures. The spine and paravertebral tissues should be evaluated for pain, swelling, bruising, or possible malalignment. The skeletal level of injury is the level of the greatest vertebral damage on x-ray. Complete bilateral loss of sensation or motor function below a certain level indicates a complete SCI.

Pulmonary Evaluation

The clinician should evaluate respiratory rate, chest wall expansion, abdominal wall movement, cough, and chest wall and pulmonary injuries. Arterial blood gas (ABG) analysis and pulse oximetry are important. Injuries of C4 and above usually are associated with respiratory complications because C4 is the phrenic nerve that innervates the diaphragm. With high thoracic cord injuries, for example (injuries that occur from T2 through T4), vital capacity is 30% to 50% of normal, and cough is weak.

Hemorrhage, Hypotension, and Neurogenic Shock

In acute SCI, shock may be neurogenic, hemorrhagic, or both. **Neurogenic shock** occurs when SCI is above T6 because sympathetic nerves are affected. Sympathetic nervous system (SNS) dysfunction prevents the tachycardia and peripheral vasoconstriction that should normally counteract and characterize hemorrhagic shock. Therefore, it is important for the clinician to suspect hemorrhagic shock even when tachycardia is absent. Spinal cord injuries at C4 and above affect respiration ability. Injuries at T6 or above can cause sympathetic nervous system dysfunction causing hypotension and bradycardia.

Sensory Function Testing

In sensory function assessment, the clinician should test light touch, proprioception, vibration, and pain. The clinician can use a pinprick to evaluate pain sensation. The sensory dermatome map is used for this assessment. The patient's intact sensory level is determined by pinprick and light touch of the most caudal (lowest) dermatome. Sensory index scoring is as follows:

- 0: absent
- 1: impaired or hyperesthesia
- 2: intact.

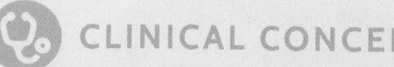 CLINICAL CONCEPT

In sensory index scoring, a score of zero is given if the patient cannot differentiate between the point of a sharp pin and the dull edge.

Motor Strength Testing

Muscle strength always should be graded according to the maximum strength attained, no matter how briefly that strength is maintained during the examination. The muscles are tested with the patient in the supine position. Muscle strength scoring is from 0/5 to 5/5. Normal muscle strength of 5/5 is muscle activity against resistance. The American Spinal Injury Association (ASIA) recommends use of the following scale for the assessment of motor strength in SCI:

- 0: no contraction or movement
- 1: minimal movement
- 2: active movement, but not against gravity
- 3: active movement against gravity
- 4: active movement against resistance
- 5: active movement against full resistance.

Motor level is determined by the most caudal muscles that have muscle strength of 3 or above while the segment above is normal (5/5).

Neurological Level and Extent of Injury

Neurological level of injury is the most caudal level at which motor and sensory levels are intact, with motor level assessed 0 to 5 and sensory level defined by a sensory score of 2. There are key muscles that should be tested on the ASIA assessment tool. A rectal examination is necessary to check motor function or sensation at the anal junction. The presence of either motor or sensory function is considered sacral-sparing. There are specific tests listed on the ASIA assessment tool that test the sacral nerve roots. The presence of sacral spinal nerve reflexes is a key factor because it is evidence of the integrity of spinal cord long tract fibers. Indication of the presence of sacral fibers is of significance in defining the completeness of the injury and the potential for some motor recovery.

The extent of injury is defined by the ASIA Impairment Scale using the following categories:

- A = Complete: No sensory or motor function is preserved in sacral segments S4–S5.
- B = Incomplete: Sensory, but not motor function is preserved below the neurological level and extends through sacral segments S4–S5.

- C = Incomplete: Motor function is preserved below the neurological level, and most key muscles below the neurological level have a muscle grade lower than 3.
- D = Incomplete: Motor function is preserved below the neurological level, and most key muscles below the neurological level have a muscle grade greater than or equal to 3.
- E = Normal: Sensory and motor functions are normal.

ASIA has established that the neurological level of injury is the most caudal level with normal sensory and motor function. For example, a patient with C5 injury has, by definition, abnormal motor and sensory function from C6 down. The ASIA method for classifying SCI is by identifying the intact neurological level. The ASIA classification uses the description of the neurological level of injury in defining the type of SCI, for example, "C8 ASIA A with zone of partial preservation of pinprick to T2" (see Table 35-1).

Diagnosis

When a SCI is suspected, x-rays are used to demonstrate alignment of the spinal column. In some cases, fractures can be seen. X-rays do not provide information regarding the spinal cord but do show injury or malalignment of the bones that may cause or aggravate injury to the spinal cord. Body size greatly impacts the quality of x-ray images. The cervical-thoracic junction is often not well-visualized in patients with short or muscular necks.

CT scans can evaluate the spinal anatomy in greater detail than traditional x-rays. Subtle fractures and soft tissue injury are more evident with this imaging technique. Technological advances in CT scanning can show the spinal column in three dimensions. CT scan can also provide information on the integrity of the vertebral and carotid arteries, which sometimes become occluded or dissected after cervical spine injury.

MRI can provide detailed pictures of the spinal cord, intervertebral discs, and CSF spaces. Trauma-related pathology seen on MRI includes herniated discs, spinal cord contusions, ligament integrity, and nerve root compression. Patients with cervical or high thoracic SCI should be carefully monitored for respiratory decompensation that may occur when they are placed in the supine position.

Myelography is an alternative for those with contraindications to MRI. It demonstrates obstructed CSF flow around the spinal cord or compression of the spinal cord, but is not able to demonstrate intrinsic spinal cord pathology. The test, which involves the injection of radiopaque dye into the CSF compartment, is performed through a lumbar puncture or a C1–2 puncture. X-rays or CT scans are then obtained of the spinal anatomy. Myelography involves some risk in the SCI patient that can exacerbate unstable injuries. Other potential complications of myelography include seizures, spinal cord puncture, and spinal headache.

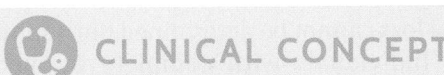

CLINICAL CONCEPT

According to ASIA, terms such as "paraplegia" and "quadriplegia" are considered obsolete.

Treatment

When treating a patient with SCI, attending to the ABCs of resuscitation takes precedence. The patient should be stabilized in the supine position with cervical bracing and spinal immobilization on a flat board, after which the patient should be transferred to a trauma care unit. After complete neurological examination, pain relievers and pneumatic compression stockings are needed to prevent thromboembolism. In addition, the patient needs wound care, warm intravenous fluid, oxygen, and urinary catheterization. Surgical decompression of the spinal cord is performed to preserve intact neurological function. Once the possibility of bleeding is excluded, low molecular weight heparin is administered. Treatment of neurogenic shock, which may include hypotension and bradycardia, is necessary.

TABLE 35-1. SCI and Loss of Function

Level of Injury	Loss of Function
Between C1 and C3	Unable to breathe without respirator Loss of bowel and bladder control Unable to move arms and legs
Between C4 and C7	Severe weakness in arms with no motor function or sensation in legs Loss of bowel and bladder control
Thoracic spine	Paralysis in legs but arms can still function Truncal instability Loss of bowel and bladder control
Lumbar sacral	Loss of bowel and bladder control Upper body strength and sensation normal Motor weakness or paralysis and sensory loss in hips and legs

(Adapted from: American Spinal Injury Association (ASIA). (2012). Assessment tool from the American Spinal Injury Association. Retrieved from http://www.asia-spinalinjury.org/.)

ALERT! The patient with SCI needs cervical bracing and should be logrolled when being examined or transferred for diagnostic tests.

Selected Pathophysiologic Disorders Related to SCI

Trauma to the spinal cord results in loss of function to the area distal to the trauma. However, an insult to one section of the cord leads to the development of **spinal shock,** which eventually resolves during the healing process.

Spinal Shock

Primary injury to the spinal cord results in a state of **areflexia,** which is demonstrated by flaccid muscles, paralysis, absence of sensation at and below the level of injury, and bowel and bladder dysfunction.

Loss of the anal reflex or bulbocavernosus reflex is the hallmark of spinal shock. Autonomic function (vasoconstriction and shivering) is also lost at the level of injury and below. The completeness of the SCI is indeterminable until spinal shock state abates. Return of the anal or bulbocavernosus reflex indicates the resolution of spinal shock, which usually occurs hours to weeks postinjury. The flaccidity of spinal shock is slowly replaced with spasticity and hyperreflexia in most patients.

The patient with spinal shock should first be hemodynamically stabilized with constant monitoring of blood pressure and electrocardiography. Systolic BP should be kept greater than 100 mm Hg and heart rate greater than 60 beats per minute. Motor assessment of the major muscle groups of upper and lower extremities should be tested periodically. It is important to note assymetrical movement of muscle groups or lack of motor ability. Differences in full strength, antigravity, and no movement should be noted. Periodic testing of the sensation of the extremities is also necessary. In patients with C4 injury or above, respiratory function and ABCs should be monitored. Mechanical ventilation is commonly needed. In patients with respiratory compromise, suctioning and respiratory physiotherapy are necessary. The patient in spinal shock is at high risk for deep venous thromboembolism; pneumatic compression devices can be used on the lower extremities. The patient should be kept in proper body alignment with splinting of extremities and have body position changed periodically, such as raising the head of the bed and going from bed to chair.

CLINICAL CONCEPT

The bulbocavernosus reflex is the contraction of the anal sphincter with squeezing of the glans penis or tugging on a Foley catheter. The presence of the reflex indicates intact S1, S2, and S3 nerves. In spinal shock there is loss of the reflex.

Neurogenic Shock

Although sometimes used interchangeably with spinal shock, neurogenic shock is a distinctly different condition that affects patients with SCI. It manifests in patients with injuries at the sixth thoracic vertebrae or above, resulting in the lack of normal sympathetic outflow from the T1–L2 region of the spinal cord. This means the SNS does not release norepinephrine, which results in a predominant parasympathetic effect, causing bradycardia. Without norepinephrine, blood vessels do not constrict, resulting in peripheral vasodilation. This allows blood to pool in the extremities, decreasing venous return to the heart and, eventually, reducing cardiac output and systemic blood pressure. The presence of bradycardia with hypotension differentiates neurogenic shock from hypovolemic shock. In hypovolemic shock, there is tachycardia in response to hypotension.

The patient with neurogenic shock should be hemodynamically stabilized with constant monitoring of blood pressure and electrocardiography. Measures used in the treatment of spinal shock are also necessary in neurogenic shock.

Complete and Incomplete SCI

SCI is classified by the degree of functional loss. Complete injuries result in the loss of all voluntary motor and sensory function below the level of injury. Accurate functional loss cannot be determined until spinal shock resolves. Individuals with complete or incomplete spinal injury are assessed and monitored, as described in spinal and neurogenic shock. With incomplete SCI, some motor or sensory function below the injury can remain intact. There are several types of syndromes associated with incomplete SCI.

Central Cord Syndrome

Central cord syndrome often occurs after hyperextension of the cervical spine that causes compression of the neurons within the center of the spinal cord. Because of the arrangement of the corticospinal nerve tracts within the spinal cord, there is greater motor dysfunction in the upper extremities than the lower extremities. Sensory and bladder function may or may not be intact. Partial to near-complete recovery can occur in younger, healthy patients. However, recovery is variable for those patients older than 50 years.

Anterior Spinal Artery Syndrome

This syndrome is associated with disruption of blood flow to the anterior two-thirds of the spinal cord, resulting in spinal cord ischemia and infarction. Injuries that cause anterior spinal artery syndrome include acute intervertebral disc herniation, bone fragments impinging on the anterior surface of the spinal cord, or disrupted aortic blood flow. The patient suffers paralysis, loss of sensation, and inability to discriminate pain and temperature. Because circulation remains intact in the dorsal columns of the spinal cord, proprioception, light touch, and vibration sense are undisrupted.

Brown-Séquard Syndrome

This type of incomplete SCI is commonly associated with penetrating injuries that lead to hemisection of the spinal cord, in which there is damage of ascending and descending neural tracts on one side of the spinal cord. The following symptoms can result from damage to the neuron tracts:

- Interruption of the lateral corticospinal tract causes ipsilateral (same side) paralysis and the presence of a Babinski sign on the side of the lesion.
- Interruption of dorsal spinal cord columns results in ipsilateral loss of tactile discrimination, vibratory sensation, and position sense (proprioception).
- Interruption of the lateral spinothalamic tract causes contralateral (opposite side) loss of pain and temperature sensation.

Horner's Syndrome

Horner's syndrome is associated with injuries at or above T1 that disrupt the cervical sympathetic tract of neurons. It is characterized by miosis (constricted pupil), anhidrosis (lack of sweat), and ptosis (drooping eyelid) on the affected side.

Conus Medullaris Syndrome

Conus medullaris syndrome occurs following injury to the lowest portion of the spinal cord (conus medullaris), particularly fractures of L1 and L2. The patient suffers urinary retention, erectile dysfunction, constipation, relaxed anal sphincter, sensory loss in inguinal area, loss of anal and bulbocavernosus reflexes, and motor weakness. Motor impairment varies but can include paralysis and muscle atrophy caused by spinal cord motor neuron involvement.

Cauda Equina Syndrome

Cauda equina syndrome results from compression of the bilateral nerve roots of the lumbosacral region. Motor and sensory losses are variable and depend on which nerve roots are affected. Incontinence is the major sign of this syndrome, which can follow fractures of the lower lumbar spine, sacrum, or acute herniated discs of the lower lumbar region.

Chapter Summary

- TBI is sudden physical damage to the brain that can result from a closed head injury, such as that caused by the head's impact with an external unmovable object or surface.
- Certain pathophysiologic alterations occur with brain injury, such as changes in ICP and LOC.
- There are three compartments to the brain: CSF, brain tissue, and blood. According to the Monro-Kellie doctrine, an increase in one compartment of the brain is compensated for by a decrease in other compartments.
- There are four mechanisms that can result in skull or brain injuries: blunt trauma, acceleration-deceleration (also called coup-contrecoup), penetrating trauma, and blast injury.
- When ICP increases, the brain tissue is compressed and forced downward in the skull to become herniated or displaced to another region of the brain. The most common type of herniation is a transtentorial (also called uncal) herniation.
- A decrease in the LOC is the earliest sign of neurological decline.
- Pressure on the brainstem will cause Cushing's triad: hypertension, bradycardia. and bradypnea.
- Pressure on the oculomotor nerve (CN III) causes pupils to become fixed and dilated.
- The GCS is used to assess brain injury severity. The GCS incorporates both LOC and orientation, and is determined by rating three areas: eye opening, verbal response, and motor response.
- DAI, often caused by the coup-contrecoup mechanism, is characterized by diffuse swelling of neuronal axons, hemorrhage or laceration of the corpus callosum, and hemorrhages in the brainstem. DAI commonly leads to coma.
- A concussion is a physiologic disruption in brain function that may or may not involve loss of consciousness. It is manifested by temporary memory loss and alteration of mental state. It leaves no permanent structural damage to the brain.
- A cerebral contusion is considered a bruise of the brain tissue that occurs with head trauma. Cerebral edema with increased ICP occurs, which causes loss of consciousness.
- An EDH is associated with skull fracture and rupture of the middle meningeal artery. Increased ICP can be caused by the bleeding.
- A subdural hematoma is caused by venous bleeding into the subdural space. This bleed can occur over a number of hours to days.
- A cerebral aneurysm is most commonly found on the circle of Willis.
- A SAH can be caused by trauma or rupture of a cerebral aneurysm.
- Leakage of a subarachnoid aneurysm can cause neurological deficits over a number of days. Alternatively, a SAH can be a sudden event that leads to bleeding into

the subarachnoid space, compression of brain tissue, and uncal herniation, which can cause death.

- Skull fractures are categorized as linear, depressed, or basilar and may or may not involve injury to the brain tissue. Periorbital ecchymosis, Battle's sign (bleeding in the mastoid region), CSF rhinorrhea, and otorrhea occur in basilar skull fracture.

- The symptoms seen in SCI vary based on the neural tract that is injured. Injuries to the descending tracts result in motor deficits, whereas damage to the ascending tracts cause sensory deficits.

- Primary injury to the spinal cord results in a concussive effect causing a state of areflexia, which is demonstrated by flaccid muscles, paralysis, absence of sensation at and below the level of injury, and bowel and bladder dysfunction.

- The ASIA assessment tool is used to evaluate SCI.

- With the ASIA classification system, the terms "paraparesis" and "quadriparesis" have become obsolete. Instead, the ASIA classification uses the description of the neurological level of injury in defining the type of SCI.

 ## Making the Connections

Disorder and Pathophysiology	Signs and Symptoms	Physical Assessment Findings	Diagnostic Testing	Treatment
BRAIN INJURY				
DAI	DAI is characterized by rapid stretch of axons that damages the axonal structure, resulting in a loss of elasticity and impairment of transport of impulses. Swollen, stretched axons may become disconnected. A DAI can also cause swelling in the brain. Swelling causes increased pressure in the brain and can cause decreased blood flow to the brain, as well as additional injury.			
	DAI results in immediate loss of consciousness, and most patients (greater than 90%) remain in a persistent comatose state. A person with a mild or moderate DAI who is conscious may show signs of neurological impairment, depending upon which area of the brain is most affected.	The patient may be comatose or exhibit specific neurological deficits that are related to the exact area of the brain injury. For example, those with injury in Broca's area of the brain will exhibit difficulty with speech. Others who suffer injury to the cerebral motor cortex will exhibit symptoms related to movement of extremities.	MRI is the preferred test for diagnosis. CT scan is less sensitive to DAI, with many patients exhibiting a normal CT scan upon presentation. The degree of microscopic injury usually is considered to be greater than that seen on diagnostic imaging.	Immediate treatment involves hemostabilization. The patient should be treated as if there is a cervical injury until this is ruled out. Measures should be implemented to reduce swelling of the brain, such as IV mannitol and steroids. Surgery is not an option for those who have sustained a DAI. If the patient has sustained a mild or moderate DAI, the rehabilitation phase will follow once the patient is stabilized and awake. About 90% of survivors with severe DAI are unconscious. The 10% that regain consciousness are often severely impaired.

Continued

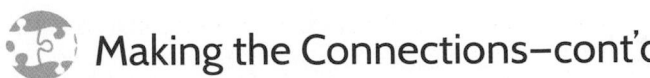
Making the Connections–cont'd

Disorder and Pathophysiology	Signs and Symptoms	Physical Assessment Findings	Diagnostic Testing	Treatment

Concussion | Concussion occurs when rotational or acceleration forces are applied to the brain, resulting in the shear strain of the tissue. On a cellular level, there is a disruption of neuronal membranes, resulting in an efflux of intracellular potassium ions into the extracellular space. This results in release of excitatory amino acids, particularly glutamate. Glutamate accumulation is toxic to neurons and temporarily causes a disturbance of surrounding neurons. Glutamate overstimulates the neurons and temporarily causes the neuronal membranes to open their pores. Sodium flows into the cell pores, followed by water, and temporary cellular swelling occurs. Depending on how much cellular swelling there is, resolution occurs over time with no remaining structural changes.

Alteration in consciousness, such as being dazed, confused, or "seeing stars"; or, less commonly, a brief loss of consciousness. Headache, dizziness and flat affect are common initially. Pretraumatic (retrograde) amnesia and posttraumatic (antegrade) amnesia can occur. Usually, the duration of amnesia is brief (seconds to minutes), depending upon the injury. Vomiting may suggest a significant brain injury with associated elevated ICP. Other signs of increased ICP include worsening headache, increasing disorientation, and changing LOC. Postconcussion syndrome is the persistence of symptoms for more than 3 weeks after the initial injury; symptoms include headache, dizziness, fatigue, irritability, insomnia, and concentration or memory difficulties.	Temporary disorientation. Amnesia for events before and just after the injury. Flat affect. Vomiting. Imbalance caused by dizziness.	Check ABCs. Cervical spine injury should be considered and the unconscious individual should be treated as having a potential cervical spine injury. Thorough neurological examination should be performed, including assessment of orientation to person, place, and time. The ability to perform simple tasks and postural stability should also be assessed. The CDC recommends a concussion assessment toolkit based on the American Academy of Neurology (AAN) guidelines to aid in the evaluation of a concussion. The tool assesses multiple cognitive, physical, and emotional symptoms initially and at 15 minutes and 30 minutes postinjury; it can be found at http://www.cdc.gov/headsup/index.html. Imaging is not normally required unless one or more of the following	Cognitive and physical rest are recommended. Bedrest, fluids, and a mild pain reliever such as acetaminophen may be prescribed. Ice may be applied to strains or superficial bruises to relieve pain and decrease swelling. No return to play or vigorous activity is recommended while signs or symptoms of a concussion are present. At least 24-hour reprieve. Experts recommend that those who suffer concussion should not return to playing sports on the same day as the injury. If the patient wants to sleep, wake the patient every quarter hour for the first 2 hours, then every half hour for the following 2 hours, then hourly for the following 12 hours. When awakened, ask the patient some simple questions to confirm orientation to time, place, and person.

Continued

Making the Connections–cont'd

Disorder and Pathophysiology	Signs and Symptoms	Physical Assessment Findings	Diagnostic Testing	Treatment
			conditions are present: • physical evidence of trauma above the clavicles • anticoagulation or coagulopathy • age older than 60 years • alcohol or drug intoxication • neurological deficit • persistent vomiting • seizure or short-term memory deficit. • history of alcoholism A CT scan is normal in more than 90% of concussion patients. However, if headache does not resolve or patient becomes disoriented or begins to show decreased LOC, hospitalization is necessary.	Assess grip strength, ability to speak clearly, gait, and postural stability. If any neurological deficit is noted, a medical evaluation should be immediately obtained.

Cerebral Contusion | A combination of vascular and tissue damage leads to cerebral contusion, similar to bruise of the brain. A contusion is often a coup-contrecoup type of injury. Cerebral edema typically develops around cerebral contusions within 48 to 72 hours after injury. Cerebral edema is problematic because the swollen brain tissue may become compressed against the bone, which then leads to brain damage. Also, if cerebral edema is severe, uncal herniation of brain tissue is possible, which can lead to death.

| | Severe headache, dizziness, vomiting, increased size of one pupil, or sudden weakness in an arm or leg may be present. Individual may seem restless, agitated, or irritable. Often, the person may have memory loss. These symptoms can last for several hours to several weeks, depending on the severity of the injury. As the brain tissue swells, the person may feel increasingly drowsy or confused. If the person is difficult to awaken or loses consciousness, immediate medical attention should be sought. | Neurological examination may show neurological deficits such as weakness in one extremity. Patient may seem irritable or restless. Memory loss is common. These symptoms can last for several hours to several weeks, depending on the severity of the injury. As the brain tissue swells, the person may feel increasingly drowsy or confused. | Immediate CT scan is needed, though the true volume of neuronal damage in the contused tissue can be underestimated. MRI scans have greater sensitivity for cerebral edema. Skull x-ray is necessary to look for skull fracture, which is commonly associated with EDH. Serial CT scans over the days following cerebral contusion are used to assess progression or resolution. Cerebral angiography is often performed to visualize blood vessel damage and possible aneurysms. | Life-saving measures are the priority with any head injury. The patient should be assessed for airway, breathing, and circulation. The patient needs to be treated and stabilized as if he or she has a cervical spinal injury. In the emergency setting, IV mannitol is frequently used to decrease cerebral edema. Surgical resection of the contused brain tissue is indicated when the patient has brain swelling that increases the ICP above an acceptable degree. Craniectomy may be performed where a piece of skull is |

Continued

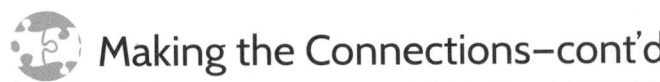

Making the Connections–cont'd

Disorder and Pathophysiology	Signs and Symptoms	Physical Assessment Findings	Diagnostic Testing	Treatment
				removed to relieve the pressure on the brain cells. If cerebral hematoma is present, evacuation is performed through a craniotomy.

EDH | Rupture of the middle meningeal artery into the epidural space; bleeding into the space between the cranial bone and dura mater (layer of meninges) can rapidly place pressure on the brain.

Disorder and Pathophysiology	Signs and Symptoms	Physical Assessment Findings	Diagnostic Testing	Treatment
	Patient may have no notable symptoms and deny need for medical attention. Possible loss of consciousness, severe headache, vomiting, and seizure may be present. Patients may have dramatically delayed deterioration. The patient can be conscious and talking, yet a minute later be apneic, comatose, and minutes from death.	Decreased LOC, with decreased or fluctuating GCS, may be present. Dilated, sluggish, or fixed pupil(s), bilateral or ipsilateral to injury, suggest increased ICP or herniation. If the ICP rises and causes significant pressure on the brainstem, Cushing's triad occurs: bradycardia, bradypnea, and hypertension. In coma, patients take on decerebrate or decorticate posturing. Positive Babinski sign is observed whenever the upper motor neurons are involved.	Complete neurological examination is performed, including GCS. Immediate CT scan and skull x-ray are necessary. Skull x-ray commonly shows fractures, whereas the CT scan will show evidence of bleeding into the epidural space. If bleeding has been prolonged, a midline shift in the brain tissue will be apparent. A decrease in LOC is the earliest sign of neurological decline.	This is a neurosurgical emergency requiring a craniotomy and surgical evacuation of the hematoma. The patient requires hemodynamic stabilization with airway and blood pressure control. The patient also needs intubation for mechanical ventilation, IV access, oxygen, and cardiac monitoring. Hyperventilating the patient often can decrease ICP. Phenytoin provides prophylaxis against early posttraumatic seizure.

Subdural Hematoma | A subdural hematoma results from bleeding that accumulates below the dura mater but above the arachnoid membrane. The subdural hematoma occurs from tearing of subdural bridging veins. Venous bleeding is slow but can accumulate with time to become substantial enough to place pressure on the brain tissue. An acute subdural hematoma occurs within 72 hours of head injury, whereas a subacute subdural hematoma can take several days to accumulate to levels that cause symptoms. Chronic subdural hematoma is one that has been present for up to 3 weeks.

Disorder and Pathophysiology	Signs and Symptoms	Physical Assessment Findings	Diagnostic Testing	Treatment
	Patients may have headache, nausea, vomiting, and exhibit neurological deficits such as: • confused or slurred speech • difficulty with balance or walking • lethargy or confusion • loss of consciousness • seizure • slurred speech	Patients may exhibit neurological deficits such as: • confused or slurred speech • difficulty with balance or walking • lethargy or confusion • loss of consciousness • seizure • slurred speech • visual disturbances • weakness of an extremity.	Complete neurological examination is performed, including GCS. Immediate CT scan and skull x-ray is performed. CT scan may or may not show evidence of bleeding into the subdural space. If bleeding has been prolonged, a midline shift in the brain tissue will be apparent.	Large acute subdural hematomas require craniotomy to evacuate the lesion and reduce the ICP. Occasionally, a subdural hematoma is small and causes little pressure or midline shift. In this case, surgery may be withheld or delayed. A small subdural hematoma can slowly

Continued

Making the Connections—cont'd

Disorder and Pathophysiology	Signs and Symptoms	Physical Assessment Findings	Diagnostic Testing	Treatment
	• visual disturbances • weakness of an extremity.	Cushing's triad indicates brainstem dysfunction; bradycardia, bradypnea, and hypertension. Positive Babinski sign is observed whenever upper motor neurons are involved.	Repeat neurological examination and CT scan in the following days are necessary if subdural hematoma is suspected.	be reabsorbed by the brain. Chronic subdural hematomas can be evacuated by craniotomy and catheter placement under the dura to drain out the blood.

SAH | Aneurysmal SAH and traumatic SAH have different etiologies; however, the pathophysiologic mechanisms that cause brain damage are the same: The rupture of a cerebral artery causes a large amount of blood to rapidly fill the subarachnoid space. The blood exerts pressure, irritates the meninges, and destroys brain cells in its path. SAH also causes an obstructive hydrocephalus, which is an accumulation of CSF within the brain. The buildup of blood and CSF place a large amount of pressure that can lead to herniation of the brainstem and death.

	Patients describe the worst headache they have ever experienced. Dizziness, orbital pain, diplopia, nuchal rigidity, memory loss, one-sided body weakness, or difficulty with speech may be observed. Often no outward signs of the impending hemorrhage are evident, and either coma or death occurs within minutes after an aneurysmal SAH.	Oculomotor nerve dysfunction with pupil dilation can be exhibited. The pupil, extraocular movements, or vision can be disturbed by compression of the oculomotor nerve. Vision loss can be caused by compression of the optic nerve. If the brainstem is injured, Cushing's triad—hypertension, bradycardia, and bradypnea—occur. Positive Babinski sign if upper motor neurons are involved.	Complete neurological examination, including GCS. Immediate CT scan. CTA. Lumbar puncture. Hunt and Hess Grading Scale (see Box 35-4).	The patient requires hemodynamic stabilization. Breathing, blood pressure, and heart rate are maintained with consideration of the patient's neurological status. Surgical treatment consists of clipping the ruptured berry aneurysm or catheter insertion of thin wire coils into the aneurysm to block it off from blood flow. In traumatic SAH, evacuation of blood and prophylactic antibiotics are necessary. Craniotomy or craniectomy may be needed if intracranial bleeding or swelling is a problem.

Skull Fracture | Skull fractures are categorized as linear, depressed, or basilar, and may or may not involve injury to the brain tissue. Linear fracture, the most common type of fracture, does not affect brain tissue. Depressed fractures occur when an object fractures the bone with sufficient force to push fragments into the brain; these are commonly open fractures that involve underlying brain tissue. The temporal bone is the most commonly fractured bone of the skull. Basilar fractures, fractures at the base of the skull, occur in the temporal bone.

	Bruising, headache, edema, rhinorrhea (nasal CSF discharge), or otorrhea (ear CSF discharge) may be present.	Basilar skull fractures may produce "Battle's sign," which is bruising of the mastoid process behind the ear on the affected side.	Complete neurological examination, including GCS. Skull x-ray. CT scan.	Linear fractures need little treatment except pain relief and instructions to check for any late-developing neurological deficits.

Continued

Making the Connections—cont'd

Disorder and Pathophysiology	Signs and Symptoms	Physical Assessment Findings	Diagnostic Testing	Treatment
	LOC is variable according to the area of injury.	There may also be a CSF leak from the ear. Fractures in the frontal fossa can result in periorbital ecchymosis, referred to as "raccoon eyes," edema, and CSF leak from the nose.	MRA if vascular injury is suspected.	Depressed fracture may require surgery and prophylactic antibiotics. Craniotomy or craniectomy may be needed if intracranial bleeding or swelling is a problem.

SCI

Spinal Shock | A traumatic, concussive effect on the spinal cord causing a state of areflexia. Mechanical forces of trauma can immediately destroy neurons and their supporting cells (glial cells), stretch or shear vasculature, and interrupt descending nerve tracts.

Disorder and Pathophysiology	Signs and Symptoms	Physical Assessment Findings	Diagnostic Testing	Treatment
	Flaccid muscles, paralysis, absence of sensation at and below the level of injury, plus bowel and bladder dysfunction. Late-developing muscle spasticity and hyperreflexia. In cervical injury, the inspiratory and expiratory muscles are weakened, impairing cough mechanisms. Thoracic injuries from T1 to T12 involve varying degrees of loss of abdominal and intercostal muscles.	Demonstrated by flaccid muscles, paralysis, absence of sensation at and below the level of injury, plus bowel and bladder dysfunction. Loss of the bulbocavernosus reflex is the hallmark of spinal shock. Loss of shivering and vasoconstriction at the level of injury also occurs. Flaccidity is slowly replaced with spasticity and hyperreflexia.	Blood pressure monitoring. Cardiac monitoring. CT scan. MRI. Deep tendon reflex tests. Bulbocavernosus reflex check. Motor assessment tests major muscle groups of the upper and lower extremities. Subtle differences can be difficult to determine. Differences in full strength, antigravity, and no movement should be visible. Noticing asymmetrical or absent limb movement is critical. Tests of proprioception, pain, and temperature for all extremities are recommended. If pulmonary function is affected, as in injuries to C4 and above, pulmonary function testing, ABGs, and oxygen saturation are tested.	Hemostabilization and spinal stabilization and immobilization. Oxygen. Maintain systolic blood pressure greater than 100 mm Hg with adequate fluid and vasopressor support. Maintain heart rate greater than 60 beats per minute with vasopressors and atropine as necessary. Veno-embolism prevention. Splinting of extremities to maintain normal alignment. Progressive mobilization: head of bed elevated, out of bed to chair. If pulmonary function involved—mechanical ventilation. Suctioning and chest physiotherapy can clear secretions, resolve atelectesis, and improve oxygenation.

Neurogenic Shock | Mechanical forces of trauma can immediately destroy neurons and their supporting cells, stretch or shear vasculature, and interrupt descending nerve tracts. Injuries at the sixth thoracic vertebrae or above cause lack of normal sympathetic outflow from the T1–L2 region of the spinal cord. Lack of norepinephrine from the SNS results in the parasympathetic

Continued

Making the Connections—cont'd

Disorder and Pathophysiology	Signs and Symptoms	Physical Assessment Findings	Diagnostic Testing	Treatment

system causing bradycardia. Also, blood vessels do not constrict, resulting in peripheral vasodilation. Blood pools in the extremities, decreasing venous return to the heart, which reduces cardiac output and systemic blood pressure.

Disorder and Pathophysiology	Signs and Symptoms	Physical Assessment Findings	Diagnostic Testing	Treatment
	Flaccid muscles, paralysis, absence of sensation at and below the level of injury, plus bowel and bladder dysfunction. Late-developing muscle spasticity and hyperreflexia. In cervical injury, the inspiratory and expiratory muscles are weakened, impairing breathing and cough mechanisms. Thoracic injuries from T1 to T12 involve varying degrees of loss of abdominal and intercostal muscles.	Bradycardia, hypotension. Flaccid muscles, paralysis, absence of sensation at and below the level of injury, plus bowel and bladder dysfunction. Flaccidity is slowly replaced with spasticity and hyperreflexia.	Blood pressure and cardiac monitoring, along with CT scan, MRI, and testing of deep tendon reflexes. Bulbocavernosus reflex check. Motor assessment tests major muscle groups of the upper and lower extremities. Subtle differences can be difficult to determine. Differences in full strength, antigravity, and no movement should be visible. Noticing asymmetrical or absent limb movement is critical. Tests of proprioception, pain, and temperature for all extremities are recommended. If pulmonary function is affected, as in injuries to C4 and above, pulmonary function testing, ABGs, and oxygen saturation are tested.	Hemostabilization and spinal stabilization and immobilization. Oxygen. Maintain systolic blood pressure greater than 100 mm Hg with adequate fluid and vasopressor support. Maintain heart rate greater than 60 beats per minute with vasopressors and atropine as necessary. Veno-embolism prevention. Splinting of extremities to maintain normal alignment. Progressive mobilization: head of bed elevated, out of bed to chair. If pulmonary function involved—mechanical ventilation. Suctioning and chest physiotherapy can clear secretions, resolve atelectesis, and improve oxygenation.

Complete or Incomplete SCI | Same as above; if there is cervical injury at or above C4, the diaphragm is paralyzed, impairing breathing and cough mechanisms. Thoracic injuries from T1 to T12 involve varying degrees of loss of abdominal and intercostal muscles. SCI at T6 or above causes sympathetic nervous system dysfunction.

Disorder and Pathophysiology	Signs and Symptoms	Physical Assessment Findings	Diagnostic Testing	Treatment
	Flaccid muscles, paralysis, absence of sensation at and below the level of injury, plus bowel and bladder dysfunction. Late-developing muscle spasticity and hyperreflexia. In cervical injury, the inspiratory and expiratory muscles are weakened, impairing breathing and cough mechanisms. Thoracic injuries from T1 to T12 involve varying degrees of	Bradycardia, hypotension. Flaccid muscles, paralysis, absence of sensation at and below the level of injury, plus bowel and bladder dysfunction. Flaccidity is slowly replaced with spasticity and hyperreflexia.	Blood pressure monitoring. Cardiac monitoring. CT scan. MRI. Deep tendon reflex tests. Bulbocavernosus reflex check. Motor assessment tests major muscle groups of the upper and lower extremities. Subtle differences can be difficult to determine. Differences in full strength, antigravity, and no	Hemostabilization and spinal stabilization and immobilization. Oxygen. Maintain systolic blood pressure greater than 100 mm Hg with adequate fluid and vasopressor support. Maintain heart rate greater than 60 beats per minute with vasopressors and atropine as necessary. Veno-embolism prevention. Splinting of extremities to

Continued

Making the Connections—cont'd

Disorder and Pathophysiology	Signs and Symptoms	Physical Assessment Findings	Diagnostic Testing	Treatment
	loss of abdominal and intercostal muscles.		movement should be visible. Noticing asymmetrical or absent limb movement is critical. Tests of proprioception, pain, and temperature for all extremities are recommended. If pulmonary function is affected, as in injuries to C4 and above, pulmonary function testing, ABGs, and oxygen saturation are tested.	maintain normal alignment. Progressive mobilization: head of bed elevated, out of bed to chair. If pulmonary function involved—mechanical ventilation. Suctioning and chest physiotherapy can clear secretions, resolve atelectasis, and improve oxygenation.

Bibliography

Albert, T., Beuret Blanquart, F., Le Chapelain, L., et al. (2012). Physical and rehabilitation medicine (PRM) care pathways: "Spinal cord injury." *Ann Phys Rehab Med*, 55(6), 440–450. doi: 10.1016/j.rehab.2012.04.004.

American Spinal Injury Association (ASIA). (2012). Assessment tool from the American Spinal Injury Association. Retrieved from http://www.asia-spinalinjury.org/

Armstrong, C. (2014). Evaluation and management of concussion in athletes: recommendations from the AAN. *Am Fam Phys*, 89(7), 585–587.

Bergman, K., & Bay, E. (2010). Mild traumatic brain injury/concussion: a review for ED nurses. *J Emerg Nurs*, 36(3), 221–230. doi: 10.1016/j.jen.2009.07.001.

Bergman, K., Given, B., Fabiano, R., et al. (2013). Symptoms associated with mild traumatic brain injury/concussion. *J Neurosci Nurs*, 45(3), 124–132. doi: 10.1097/JNN.0b013e31828a418b.

Boninger, M. L., Brienza, D., Charlifue, S., et al. (2012). State of the Science Conference in Spinal Cord Injury Rehabilitation 2011: introduction. *Spinal Cord*, 50(5), 342–343. doi: 10.1038/sc.2012.13.

Bulger, E. M., May, S., Brasel, K. J., et al. (2010). Out-of-hospital hypertonic resuscitation following severe traumatic brain injury: a randomized controlled trial. *JAMA*, 304(13), 1455–1464.

Chittiboina, P., Cuellar-Saenz, H., Notarianni, C., Cardenas, R., & Guthikonda, B. (2012). Head and spinal cord injury: diagnosis and management. *Neurologic Clin*, 30(1), 241–276.

Cooper, D. J., Rosenfeld, J. V., Murray, L., et al. (2011). Decompressive craniectomy in diffuse traumatic brain injury. *N Engl J Med*, 364(16), 1493–1502.

Courtine, G., van den Brand, R., & Musienko, P. (2011). Spinal cord injury: time to move. *Lancet*, 377(9781), 1896–1898.

Decuypere, M., & Klimo, P., Jr. (2012). Spectrum of traumatic brain injury from mild to severe. *Surg Clin N Amer*, 92(4), 939–957.

DeKosky, S. T., Ikonomovic, M. D., & Gandy, S. (2010). Traumatic brain injury—football, warfare, and long-term effects. *N Engl J Med*, 363(14), 1293–1296.

de Ribaupierre, S. (2011). Trauma and impaired consciousness. *Neurologic Clin*, 29(4), 883–902.

Diaz, A. L., & Wyckoff, L. J. (2013). NASN position statement: concussions—the role of the school nurse. *NASN Sch Nurse*, 28(2), 110–111.

El Masri, W. S., & Kumar, N. (2011). Traumatic spinal cord injuries. *Lancet*, 377(9770), 972–974.

Emery, C. A., Kang, J., Shrier, I., et al. (2010). Risk of injury associated with body checking among youth ice hockey players. *JAMA*, 303(22), 2265–2272.

Freund, P., Weiskopf, N., Ashburner, J., et al. (2013). MRI investigation of the sensorimotor cortex and the corticospinal tract after acute spinal cord injury: a prospective longitudinal study. *Lancet Neurology*, 12(9), 873–881. doi: 10.1016/S1474-4422(13)70146-7. Epub 2013 Jul 2.

Hampton, T. (2011). Traumatic brain injury a growing problem among troops serving in today's wars. *JAMA*, 306(5), 477–479.

Hunt, W. E., & Hess, R. M. (1968). Surgical risk as related to time of intervention in the repair of intracranial aneurysms. *J Neurosurg*, 28(1), 14–20.

Jamault, V., & Duff, E. (2013). Adolescent concussions: when to return to play. *Nurse Pract*, 38(2), 16–22; quiz 22–23. doi: 10.1097/01.NPR.0000425825.82811.

Mac Donald, C. L., Johnson, A. M., Cooper, D., et al. (2011). Detection of blast-related traumatic brain injury in U.S. military personnel. *N Engl J Med*, 364(22), 2091–2100.

Marco, S., & Pistoia, F. (2010). Defining consciousness: lessons from patients and modern techniques. *J Neurotrauma*, 27, 771–773.

McPhee, S. J., & Papadakis, M. A. (2011). *2011 Current medical diagnosis & treatment*. 50th ed. New York: McGraw-Hill/Lange Medical Series.

Mitka, M. (2010). Reports of concussions from youth sports rise along with awareness of the problem. *JAMA*, 304(16), 1775–1776.

Mott, T. F., McConnon, M. L., & Rieger, B. P. (2012). Subacute to chronic mild traumatic brain injury. *Am Fam Phys*, 86(11), 1045–1051.

National Guidelines Clearing House. (2009). Early acute management in adults with spinal cord injury: a clinical practice guideline for health-care professionals. Retrieved from http://www.guideline.gov/browse/by-topic.aspx

Ropper, A. (2011). Brain injuries from blasts. *N Engl J Med*, 364(22), 2156–2157.

Savica, R., Parisi, J. E., Wold, L. E., Josephs, K. A., & Ahlskog, J. E. (2012). High school football and risk of neurodegeneration: a community-based study. *Mayo Clin Proceed*, 87(4), 335–340.

Scorza, K. A., Raleigh, M. F., & O'Connor, F. G. (2012). Current concepts in concussion: evaluation and management. *Am Fam Phys*, 85(2), 123–132.

Servadei, F. (2011). Clinical value of decompressive craniectomy. *N Engl J Med*, 364(16), 1558–1559.

Snyder, E. Y., & Teng, Y. D. (2012). Stem cells and spinal cord repair. *N Engl J Med*, 366(20), 1940–1942.

Stuart, B., Mandleco, B., Wilshaw, R., Beckstrand, R. L., & Heaston, S. (2012). Mild traumatic brain injury: are ED providers identifying which patients are at risk? *J Emerg Nurs*, 38(5), 435–442. doi: 10.1016/j.jen.2011.04.006.

Valentine, V., & Logan, K. (2012). Cognitive rest in concussion management. *Am Fam Phys*, 85(2), 100–101.

van Middendorp, J. J., Hosman, A. J., Donders, A. R., et al. (2011). A clinical prediction rule for ambulation outcomes after traumatic spinal cord injury: a longitudinal cohort study. *Lancet*, 377(9770), 1004–1010.

Zafonte, R. (2011). Diagnosis and management of sports-related concussion: a 15-year-old athlete with a concussion. *JAMA*, 306(1), 79–86. Epub 2011 May 31.

Psychobiology of Behavioral Disorders

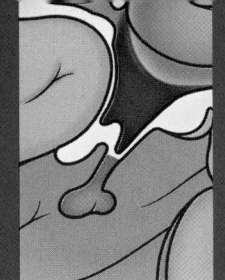

Key Terms

Agnosia

Amnesia

Amygdala

Anomia

Apathy

Apraxia

Attention deficit-hyperactivity
   disorder (ADHD)

Benzodiazepine (BNZ)

Bipolar disorder

Cognitive behavioral therapy (CBT)

Delirium

Dementia

Gamma amino butyric acid (GABA)

Generalized anxiety disorder (GAD)

Interpersonal psychotherapy

Kindling theory

Limbic system

Locus coeruleus

Major depressive disorder (MDD)

Mini-Mental Status Exam (MMSE)

Monoamine oxidase inhibitors (MAOIs)

Neocortex

Panic attack

Posttraumatic stress disorder (PTSD)

Psychosis

Selective serotonin reuptake inhibitors
   (SSRIs)

Serotonin

Serotonin-norepinephrine reuptake
   inhibitors (SNRIs)

Sundowning

Tricyclic antidepressant (TCAs)

Psychiatry, the study of the mind, attempts to explain human thoughts, emotions, and behaviors. As our base of scientific knowledge has expanded over the years, clinical psychiatry has undergone significant changes in theory, practice, and treatment. For example, psychiatric illnesses in the 17th and 18th century were explained in terms of evil spirits, in which persecution and isolation of the patient were customary treatment modalities. In the 19th century, Freud emphasized how the environment and past traumas influenced the individual's psyche. Although this was an advancement in the theory of mental illness, treatment modalities were lacking. Isolation and restraint were customary treatments, and the idea of chemical sedation was first introduced.

The late 20th century introduced psychobiology, a field of neuroscience that analyzes how biological processes influence mood, cognitive activity, and behavior. Emphasis turned toward neuroanatomy and neurobiology, and psychiatry began to focus on the function of the brain's naturally occurring chemical mediators—the psychoactive neurotransmitters. Since then, research has flourished regarding how specific neurotransmitters from certain areas of the brain influence mental processes such as cognition, mood, memory, perception, fear, addiction, pain, and anger.

In the latter part of the 20th century, psychiatry became increasingly focused on neurotransmitters, particularly how they could be biologically manipulated to treat disorders. Now, in the 21st century, psychiatry is emerging as psychobiology, a neuroscience where diagnosis and treatment of mental illness focuses on brain neurochemistry. Our knowledge base in psychobiology is growing because of increasing psychopharmacological investigation and advancements in neuroimaging technology. Twenty-first century clinical psychiatry is based on an expanding field of psychobiology, an area of study that encompasses neuroanatomy, neurophysiology, and new discoveries in genetics. The field of psychogenomics is creating a novel way of looking at susceptibility to mental illness and addiction. This field of genetic discoveries will likely characterize 21st century psychiatry.

Epidemiology

Research in psychiatric epidemiology shows that mental disorders are common throughout the United States, affecting tens of millions of people each year, and that only a fraction of those affected receive treatment. Women and men have the same likelihood of developing mental illness over the course of their lifetime, though women report symptoms and seek treatment more than men. The highest prevalence of mental disorders occur in those aged 30 to 44 years. Out of all of those affected by mental illness, only 36% receive treatment. Although mental disorders are widespread in the population, seriously debilitating mental illness is prevalent in about 6% of individuals.

Basic Concepts of Psychobiology

Major areas of the brain that are associated with behavior and emotional responses include the hypothalamus, neocortex, and limbic system. The autonomic nervous system (ANS) and endocrine organs also influence our thoughts, behaviors, reactions, and emotions. In turn, our thoughts, behavior, reactions, and emotions can influence the ANS via a mind-body connection. The study of psychobiology focuses on the unique connection between brain, body function, and behavior.

Neuroanatomy and Psychobiology

The current theory of psychobiology specifically concentrates on the interaction between the limbic system and the neocortex. The **limbic system** refers to a central rim of cortical tissue within the cerebral hemisphere (see Fig. 36-1). It includes specific structures, such as the amygdala and hippocampus, and is surrounded by the **neocortex,** a highly developed area of the cerebrum. The limbic system, in conjunction with the hypothalamus, regulates some autonomic responses, sexual behavior, rage, and fear. The **amygdala** is also responsible for memories that provoke fear and anger. The neocortex's role is to modify the limbic system responses, which tend to be impulsive and reactive. The neocortex's actions are described as executive decision making, judgment, and insight in response to stressors.

The cerebral cortex is involved in processing and integrating information received from other areas of the brain. In addition, motor and sensory function in certain areas of the cerebral cortex, referred to as the association cortex, is responsible for higher cognitive functioning. This area is concerned with language acquisition, abstract and symbolic thought, long-term memory, and other cognitive functions. The prefrontal lobes of the cerebral cortex are involved with personality, decision making, and insight.

Major Psychoactive Neurotransmitters

The major neurotransmitters that are released by the brain's neurons are serotonin (5-hydroxytriptamine), norepinephrine, and dopamine. **Serotonin** has several actions related to mood and behavior. Decreased serotoninergic activity is associated with depression and is seen in bipolar disorders. Serotonin is also involved in the inhibition of the transmission of painful stimuli. A reduction in catecholamines, particularly norepinephrine, is related to depression. The activity of norepinephrine is referred to as noradrenergic activity. Dopamine has been studied because of its role in movement disorders such as Parkinson's disease, but it also plays a major role in behavior and addiction. It is theorized that an excessive level of dopaminergic stimulation is related to the development of schizophrenia. Enhanced dopaminergic activity is also experienced as a positive reward response in a patient with an addiction.

Gamma amino butyric acid (GABA) is another psychoactive neurotransmitter. Neurons that produce GABA are called GABAergic neurons; these have chiefly inhibitory action at receptors.

Genetics and the Environment

Research studies have been conducted on monozygotic and dizygotic twins regarding mental illness, and researchers commonly conclude that the interaction of genetics and environment is responsible for mental illness. In some disorders, genetics plays a particularly significant role. For example, a patient with depression usually has someone in the family who suffers from depression. In **attention deficit-hyperactivity disorder (ADHD),** familial and twin studies have demonstrated a hereditary risk of 60% to 90%. Alternatively, studies show that exposure to environmental toxins such as nicotine in utero increases the risk of developing ADHD. Children whose mothers smoked during pregnancy are almost twice as likely to develop ADHD as those whose mothers were nonsmokers. It is theorized that early exposure to nicotine alters neuronal maturation and brain structure in the fetus.

Basic Pathophysiology Concepts of Behavioral Disorders

As brain anatomy and physiology have been studied in relation to behavioral disorders, specific alterations in psychobiology have been identified. Because of

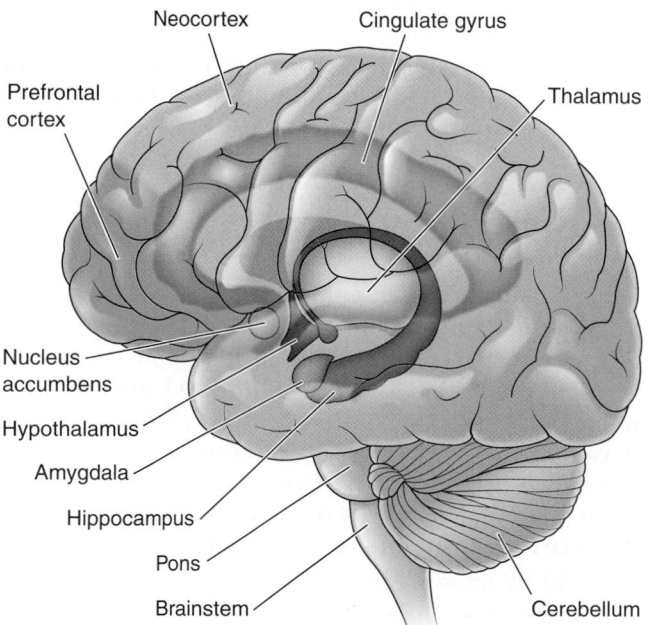

FIGURE 36-1. The limbic system. The limbic system is a complex set of structures that lies on both sides of the thalamus, just under the cerebrum. It includes the hypothalamus, hippocampus, amygdala, and several other nearby areas. It appears to be primarily responsible for our emotional life and the formation of memories.

breakthroughs in neuroscience and improvements in imaging technology, actual changes of brain structure and function can be visualized in some mental disorders. Imaging studies are used to assist in the diagnosis of patients with certain psychiatric disorders. Psychobiology is an emerging science, and the following theories and research findings are becoming the basis for treatments.

Kindling Theory and Bipolar Disorder

Neurons in the brain become active when stimulated, and the **kindling theory** asserts that if neurons are stimulated too frequently, they become overly sensitive to further stimulation. The theory was originally applied to epilepsy to explain that repeated seizures made the brain sensitive to lower levels of stimulation, and therefore to more seizures. Interestingly, the kindling theory has recently been applied to bipolar disorder. The rapid cycling between the manic and depressive stages that characterize bipolar disorder stimulates neurons, and the neurons become sensitized so that progressively less stimulation is needed to evoke a response from them. The more frequently the cycling occurs, the more sensitized or vulnerable the brain becomes for repeated episodes. This rapid cycling affects approximately 20% to 30% of patients who are diagnosed with bipolar disorder. Therefore, the kindling theory has been applied to both bipolar disorder and epilepsy. There is a similar hyperexcitability of neurons in both disorders. For this reason, antiepileptic drugs, which decrease neuron excitability, have a mood stabilizing effect on persons with bipolar disorder.

Alterations in the Prefrontal Cortex

Alterations in dopaminergic and noradrenergic activity in the prefrontal cortex have been linked to several behavioral disorders, including frontotemporal lobe dementia, Parkinson's dementia, and ADHD. Examination of single photon computed emission tomography (SPECT) has demonstrated decreased metabolic activity in the prefrontal area in patients with ADHD. The prefrontal cortex is the area that normally would exert control over the limbic system, and decreased activity in this area is consistent with the loss of executive function and poor impulse control seen in individuals with ADHD. It also provides a rationale for the use of medications that increase dopaminergic and noradrenergic activity in the prefrontal cortex in the treatment of ADHD.

Changes in the prefrontal cortex are also associated with bipolar disorder. Magnetic resonance imaging (MRI) and computed tomography (CT) scans have indicated that the prefrontal cortex is smaller in patients with bipolar disorder than in patients who do not have the condition.

Other Anatomical Alterations

Neuroimaging studies of the brain have demonstrated both cerebral atrophy and enlarged ventricles in patients who have schizophrenia. Additionally, changes have been identified in the white matter of the temporal and occipital lobes of patients with schizophrenia. White matter consists of myelinated neuronal tissue, so changes in white matter have the potential to alter neuronal function and neurotransmitter activity.

Alterations in Brain Physiology and Neurotransmitters

The integrated actions of the cortex and the hypothalamus are responsible for the physiologic responses to normal daily life. The ANS and hypothalamus work together to maintain homeostasis. However, in clinical depression or repeated episodes of severe persistent stress, this relationship can be altered.

When a patient experiences the physiologic stress response, there is enhanced activation of the hypothalamic-pituitary-adrenal (HPA) axis and the sympathetic nervous system (SNS). The result is that excessive amounts of both cortisol and catecholamines are produced. These increases have specific physiologic effects, such as increased heart rate, blood pressure (BP), and elevated blood glucose levels. Behavioral changes and changes in appetite accompany the high levels of cortisol and catecholamines. Over time, elevated cortisol levels can inhibit the serotonergic activity within the brain and lead to depressed mood.

Psychiatric Assessment

Psychiatric assessment involves obtaining information about psychological and physical symptoms as well as all current medications, supplements, and substance abuse. Because there are physical symptoms associated with behavioral disorders, patients need to be evaluated to rule out medical conditions that may also have similar symptomatology. For example, anxiety includes physiologic arousal of the SNS, resulting in restlessness, irritability, trembling, and increased heart rate. Similar symptoms are seen in hyperthyroidism, hypoglycemia, complex partial seizures, and caffeine intoxication. Therefore, medical conditions associated with the behavioral symptoms must be ruled out before diagnosis of mental illness is made.

Behavioral disorders are complex phenomena and diagnosis can be challenging. Specific criteria for diagnosing behavioral disorders are contained in the *Diagnostic and Statistical Manual of Mental Disorders,* which is published by the American Psychiatric Association and is currently in its fifth edition (*DSM-5*). Also, screening tools such as the Mini-Mental Status Exam (MMSE), Beck Depression Inventory, CAGE questionnaire, and Geriatric Depression Scale are commonly used to assess mental disorders.

Mini-Mental Status Exam

The **Mini-Mental Status Exam, (MMSE)** the most commonly used psychiatric test in clinical practice, is a brief questionnaire used to screen for cognitive impairment or dementia. It is also used to follow the course of cognitive changes in an individual over time, making it an effective way to document an individual's response to treatment. The MMSE includes simple questions and problems in a number of areas: orientation, short-term memory, basic arithmetic, language use, comprehension, and basic motor skills. The test can be administered in 10 minutes or fewer and numerical scores can be calculated to show whether the patient's cognition is normal or is slightly, moderately, or severely impaired. Although the MMSE has shown efficacy in the diagnosis of severe dementia in many individuals, the assessment tool has been criticized for its inaccuracy in individuals with less than high school education and low literacy. Studies have also shown that the MMSE has limited utility for diagnosing minimal cognitive impairment, which occurs in early stages of dementia. Because of the shortcomings of the MMSE, a Modified MMSE known as 3MS has been developed, which has shown greater reliability and sensitivity for testing early dementia and those with low literacy. Some of the questions from the MMSE have been revised in the 3MS.

Mini-Cognitive Examinations

A rapidly administered, mini-cognitive examination can be used in lieu of the comprehensive MMSE or 3MS. The clinician asks the patient to remember three words, such as "bat," "cow," and "tree." Then the clinician asks the patient to perform the clock drawing test. The clinician supplies a paper for the client and asks the client to draw an arbitrary time on the clock, such as 1:50 (see Fig. 36-2). The clock-drawing test requires a number of cognitive, motor, and perceptual functions for successful completion. After the patient completes drawing the clock, the patient is asked what three words were to be remembered before drawing the clock. Remembering the three words and drawing a completely normal clock suggest that a number of functions are intact and contributes to the weight of evidence that the patient may, for example, be able to continue to live independently. Alternatively, an inability to remember the three words and a grossly abnormal clock are indicators of cognitive impairment warranting further investigation.

Another screening tool that quickly and briefly screens for cognitive impairment is the trail drawing test. The client is provided with a set of consecutive numbers or letters placed on a page in an arbitrary order. The client is asked to connect the numbers or letters from one to another in proper order. This has been shown to test executive functioning in elderly individuals. Executive functioning involves cognitive flexibility, concept formation, and self-monitoring. With impaired executive functioning, instrumental

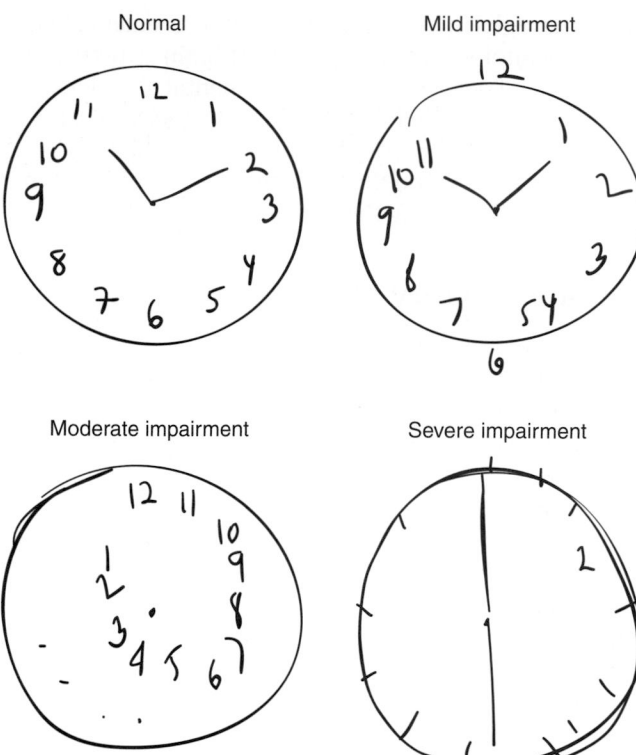

FIGURE 36-2. The clock drawing test for cognitive status. The patient is asked to draw a clock displaying a specific time, such as 1:50. This simple test has been shown to be more sensitive for early Alzheimer's dementia than several other screening tools and can be scored according to standard protocols.

activities of daily living (IADLs), such as accounting, shopping, medication management, and driving, may be beyond the person's capacity even though memory impairment is mild. Executive dysfunction is one element in the *DSM-5* criteria for the diagnosis of dementia.

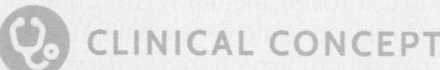 CLINICAL CONCEPT

Screening a patient for the Instrumental Activities of Daily Living (IADLs) is more sensitive for cognitive impairment than ADL screening.

Depression Assessment

Depression is a common psychiatric disorder in adults and the elderly. Persons who are depressed have characteristic symptoms such as feelings of sadness, loneliness, irritability, worthlessness, hopelessness, agitation, and guilt that may be accompanied by an array of physical symptoms. The Beck Depression Inventory and the Geriatric Depression Scale are examples of available screening tools that can be used in the diagnosis of depression. Questions regarding specific symptoms such as appetite, sleep, concentration ability, and anhedonia are answered by the patient. The assessment tool yields a numerical score that indicates mild, moderate, or severe depression.

Psychiatric Treatment

Psychotherapy and psychopharmacology are both involved in the treatment of the majority of mental health disorders. Technological interventions are also available when counseling and medication are ineffective.

Psychotherapy

Successful treatment of mental disorders includes education, psychoactive medication, and psychotherapy. There are different types of psychotherapy, and each focuses on a different aspect of the person's life. Psychodynamic psychotherapy is a therapeutic process that enables the patient to explore feelings and past traumatic experiences. The therapist investigates the patient's background and childhood to look for patterns or significant events that may play a role in the client's current difficulties. Psychoanalysis, the type of therapy associated with Sigmund Freud, is a form of psychodynamic therapy.

Cognitive behavioral therapy (CBT) focuses on specific problems and is commonly used for anxiety and depression. This form of therapy is based on the belief that irrational thinking or faulty perceptions cause psychological dysfunction. A cognitive behavioral therapist often works with a client to change thought patterns and problematic behaviors that have been developed through years of reinforcement.

Interpersonal psychotherapy focuses on the client's interpersonal relationships and skills. It is based on the belief that interpersonal factors strongly contribute to psychological problems, and it aims to change the person's interpersonal behavior by fostering adaptation to current interpersonal roles and situations.

Supportive psychotherapy and education are necessary to assist the patient, family, and others to understand the psychological disorder. Group therapy is a form of supportive psychotherapy where two or more clients work with one or more therapists or counselors. This method is a popular format for support groups, where group members can learn from the experiences of others and offer advice. Group therapy can help clients by providing a peer group of individuals that are currently experiencing the same symptoms or who have recovered from a similar problem. Group members can also provide emotional support and a safe forum to practice new behaviors.

 CLINICAL CONCEPT

CBT and interpersonal therapy are the most commonly used types of psychotherapy.

Psychoactive Medications

Psychoactive medications, also called psychotropic medications, are substances that cross the blood-brain barrier to affect the brain's neurochemistry and alter mood, thoughts, or perceptions. They act by increasing the synthesis of one or more neurotransmitters or reducing its reuptake from the synapses. Alternatively, they can act by decreasing synthesis of one or more neurotransmitters or antagonizing the neurotransmitter at the receptor (see Fig. 36-3). There are six main categories of psychoactive medications:

1. antidepressants, which treat disorders such as clinical depression, dysthymia, anxiety, eating disorders, and borderline personality disorder
2. stimulants, which treat disorders such as ADHD and narcolepsy and suppress the appetite
3. antipsychotics, also referred to as neuroleptics, which treat psychoses such as schizophrenia and augment effects of antidepressants
4. mood stabilizers, which treat bipolar disorder and schizoaffective disorder; some anticonvulsant medications are mood stabilizers
5. anxiolytics, which treat anxiety disorders
6. depressants, which are used as hypnotics, sedatives, and anesthetics.

There are different types of drugs within each category of psychoactive medication (see Table 36-1).

 CLINICAL CONCEPT

Treatment that consists of psychoactive medications in conjunction with psychotherapy is most commonly recommended for mental illness.

ALERT! Most psychoactive medications require 3 to 6 weeks to reach therapeutic level in the bloodstream.

Antidepressants

There are several different types of antidepressant medications, including **selective serotonin reuptake inhibitors (SSRIs), tricyclic antidepressants (TCAs), monoamine oxidase inhibitors (MAOIs), serotonin-norepinephrine reuptake inhibitors (SNRIs),** noradrenergic and specific serotonergic antidepressants (NaSSAs), and dopamine reuptake inhibitors (DRIs).

Selective Serotonin Reuptake Inhibitors. SSRIs are the most widely used medications for the treatment of depression. They are also used for anxiety, insomnia, panic disorder, obsessive-compulsive disorder (OCD), and eating disorders. They inhibit neuronal reuptake of serotonin in the central nervous system (CNS), which increases the concentration of serotonin in the synaptic cleft. This leads to increased serotonergic activity within the brain. It is theorized that serotonin contributes to feelings of well-being, regulation of mood

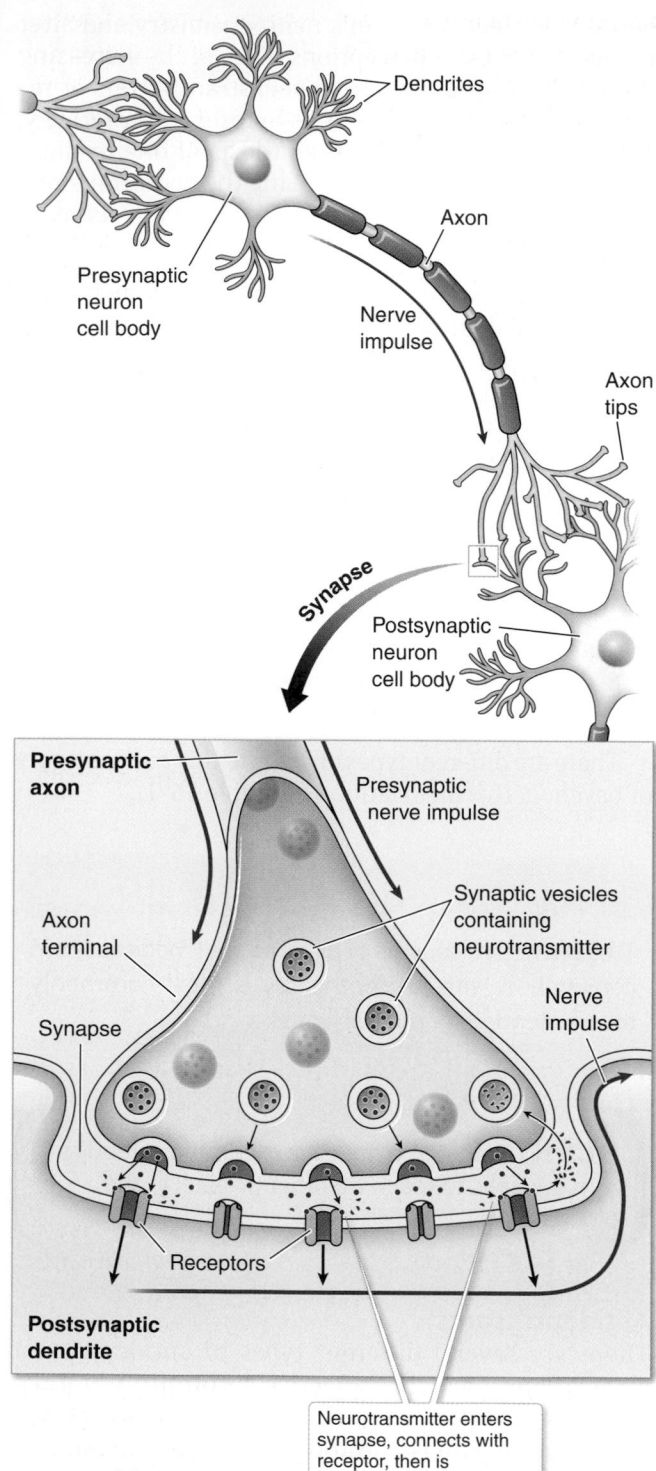

FIGURE 36-3. The process of neurotransmission. The axon of a presynaptic neuron releases chemical neurotransmitters into a synapse. Neurotransmitters include norepinephrine, dopamine, and serotonin. The neurotransmitters stimulate a receptor on the postsynaptic neuron. After the neurotransmitter stimulates the receptor, it may be degraded by enzymes and deactivated. Alternatively, a neurotransmitter can be reabsorbed into the presynaptic neuron for deactivation.

TABLE 36-1. Different Categories and Types of Therapeutic Psychoactive Medications

Classification	Major Types of Therapeutic Drug in Each Category
Antidepressants	DRIs
	MAOIs
	NaSSAs
	SSRIs
	SNRIs
	Tetracyclic antidepressants
	TCAs
Antipsychotics (Neuroleptics)	First generation
	• phenothiazines
	• butyrophenones
	• thioxanthenes
	Second and third generation
	• aripiprazole (Abilify)
	• olanzapine (Zyprexa)
	• quetiapine (Seroquel)
	• risperidone (Risperdal)
	• ziprasidone (Geodon)
Anxiolytics	Benzodiazepines
Mood stabilizers	Anticonvulsants
	Lithium
Psychostimulants	Amphetamines
	Methylphenidate
	Norepinephrine reuptake inhibitors

SSRIs are well tolerated by most patients and have fewer adverse effects than other antidepressants. They do not cause psychological or physiologic dependence. SSRIs lack the anticholinergic and cardiovascular side effects typical of the TCAs, but like many psychiatric medications, they have adverse sexual effects, including decreased libido and anorgasmia. SSRIs are a preferable type of antidepressant because they have a low cardiotoxicity and their lethality is low in suicide attempts compared with other drugs.

SSRIs are useful in patients with substance abuse issues because they do not cause psychological and physiologic dependence. Fluoxetine (Prozac) is the prototypical SSRI medication. When discontinuing an SSRI, one should slowly taper the dose downward. There is a "discontinuation syndrome" that causes anxiety, dizziness, sweating, and insomnia if SSRIs are abruptly stopped.

ALERT! Antidepressants may increase suicidal thoughts in children, adolescents, and young adults during the first few months of therapy.

Tricyclic Antidepressants. TCAs were among the first antidepressants to be developed. In the past, TCAs were the first choice for pharmacological treatment of clinical

and appetite, memory, and sleep. Decreased serotoninergic neurotransmission has been proposed to play a key role in the etiology of depression.

Like most antidepressants, SSRIs require 3 to 6 weeks to reach a therapeutic blood level and beneficial effect.

ALERT! A rare but life-threatening adverse event associated with SSRIs, called serotonin syndrome, is thought to be caused by either too high a dose of the SSRIs or interactions with other drugs, resulting in overactivation of the central serotonin receptors. The clinical presentation of serotonin syndrome includes agitation, confusion, rapid heart rate, loss of muscle coordination, hyperreflexia, diarrhea, high fever, and loss of consciousness.

depression. They have been increasingly replaced by the SSRIs and other newer antidepressants. TCAs' beneficial effects occur because they increase norepinephrine and serotonin in the synapse of brain neurons. They are effective for major depression, particularly treatment-resistant depression. They are also prescribed for chronic pain, generalized anxiety, panic, social anxiety, and obsessive-compulsive and eating disorders. Amitryptiline (Elavil) is the prototypical TCA. Common side effects of TCAs are caused by anticholinergic activity and include dry mouth, blurred vision, tachycardia, constipation, urinary retention, and orthostatic hypotension resulting in dizziness. TCAs also cause sedation and may be given at bedtime to utilize this side effect's benefit for sleep. TCAs are cardiotoxic in overdose and can cause death. Potential adverse reactions include cardiac dysrhythmias, myocardial infarction, and heart block.

ALERT! TCAs cause anticholinergic activity and are contraindicated in patients who have narrow angle glaucoma or prostatic hypertrophy, orthostatic hypotension, or cardiac arrhythmias. Because of possible cardiovascular effects, TCA overdose can be fatal.

Monoamine Oxidase Inhibitors. MAOIs are another class of medications used for the treatment of major depression. These drugs block the activity of monoamine oxidase, the enzyme that destroys norepinephrine, dopamine, and serotonin. Their effect allows the neurotransmitters, particularly norepinephrine, to remain longer in the synapses of the brain. In addition to depression, MAOIs are used for panic disorder, social phobia, atypical depression, bulimia, **posttraumatic stress disorder (PTSD),** and borderline personality disorder. An example of an MAOI inhibitor is phenelzine (Nardil). The major drawback of MAOIs is their possible fatal dietary and drug interactions, as they cannot be taken along with tyramine-containing foods such as dried meats, cheese, and wine. The combination can provoke a malignant hypertensive crisis. MAOIs have potential interactions with many other medications. When changing to another antidepressant medication, there is a 2- to 3-week "washout" period when the patient must slowly taper the dose of MAOI to zero. This

period when there is no antidepressant medication is another drawback of MAOIs. Because of the potential side effects, MAOIs are a last choice of antidepressant therapy. Recently, a transdermal form of MAOI has become available without the unsafe side effects.

Serotonin-Norepinephrine Reuptake Inhibitors. SNRIs are another class of drug used in the treatment of major depression and other mood disorders. They are sometimes also used to treat anxiety, OCD, ADHD, chronic neuropathic pain, fibromyalgia syndrome, and for the relief of premenopausal syndrome. SNRIs increase the levels of serotonin and norepinephrine in the brain synapses. Venlafaxine (Effexor), Duloxetine (Cymbalta), and Desvenlafaxine (Pristiq) are the key drugs in this class. As with SSRIs, the abrupt discontinuation of an SNRI usually leads to withdrawal, or discontinuation syndrome, which could include states of anxiety and other symptoms.

 CLINICAL CONCEPT

To discontinue an MAO inhibitor or SNRI, the patient should slowly taper the dose under the supervision of a professional.

Noradrenergic and Specific Serotonergic Antidepressants. NaSSAs, also called tetracyclic antidepressants, are a class of psychiatric drugs used primarily as antidepressants. They act by antagonizing norepinephrine and serotonin receptors, which allows the neurotransmitters to remain longer in the synapse. Mirtazapine (Remeron) is the main drug within this class.

Dopamine Reuptake Inhibitor. Low dopamine levels are associated with depression. A DRI increases the amount of dopamine that remains in the neural synapse. DRIs are used for major depressive episodes, particularly treatment-resistant depression. DRIs are also used in the treatment of ADHD, narcolepsy, and obesity. They stimulate the narcoleptic individual to maintain wakefulness and assist in management of obesity by suppressing appetite. They are also used for social anxiety disorder and other anxiety disorders. The most common DRI used for therapeutic purposes is bupropion (Wellbutrin).

ALERT! High doses of bupropion increase susceptibility to seizure. Antiseizure medications used in conjunction with bupropion can act to decrease susceptibility to seizure and may be used as a mood stabilizer.

Mood Stabilizers
Lithium has been a standard medication used for many years to prevent the fluctuating mood swings

of depression and mania in bipolar disorder. Anticonvulsant medications, when used in conjunction with antidepressants, can also stabilize mood disorders. Common agents are carbamazepine (Tegretol), divalproex sodium (Depakote), valproic acid (Depakene), and lamotrigine (Lamictal). The exact mechanism of action of lithium and anticonvulsant medications is unknown. However, if lithium is ineffective for a patient, switching to an anticonvulsant is successful in stabilizing mood in many patients.

Psychostimulants

Psychoactive medications that stimulate the central and peripheral nervous system can also be added to a drug regimen if a patient is suffering treatment-resistant depression. Common agents include methylphenidate (Ritalin) and amphetamine/dextroamphetamine (Adderall). The addition of an amphetamine can enhance alertness, endurance, productivity, and motivation. Amphetamines have been used for many years for ADHD and narcolepsy. However, it is important to understand that amphetamines affect the cardiovascular system and increase heart rate and BP. These drugs can cause anxiety and heart failure in some patients. Often, the side effects of appetite suppression and insomnia are reasons to discontinue stimulant medications.

Benzodiazepines

Benzodiazepines (BNZ) are medications that bind with the GABA receptor to decrease neuronal activity. These medications promote muscle relaxation and a decrease in anxiety. Adverse effects include sedation, physical dependence, fatigue, ataxia, memory difficulties, slurred speech, and weakness. Alprazolam (Xanax), diazepam (Valium), clonazepam (Klonopin), and lorazepam (Ativan) are commonly used benzodiazepines.

ALERT! Because of sedating effects, BNZs can increase the risk of fall in the elderly.

ALERT! Used in combination with alcohol, BNZs can create synergistic effects that may cause CNS depression and respiratory arrest in cases of accidental or intentional overdose.

Antipsychotic Medications

Antipsychotic medications block dopamine in the brain, which is theorized as the cause of schizophrenia. These drugs, also called neuroleptics, can inhibit delusions, hallucinations, and disordered thought. They are also used to bolster the antidepressant effects in bipolar disorder.

There are three generations of antipsychotic medications: first, second, and third generation.

First-Generation Antipsychotics. Phenothiazines are first-generation antipsychotic medications that are used in schizophrenia and are extremely sedating. Chlorpromazine (Thorazine), haloperidol (Haldol), thioridazine (Mellaril), and perphenazine (Trilafon) are prototypical antipsychotic agents that have been widely used in the past. These agents have a wide spectrum of side effects and are used infrequently in clinical settings today. Side effects include weight gain, hyperprolactinemia, decreased white blood cell count, glucose intolerance, restlessness (called akathisia), sexual dysfunction, and involuntary movements called tardive dyskinesia. Hyperprolactinemia can cause breast enlargement and milk discharge (called galactorrhea) in both men and women. Tardive dyskinesia, which causes uncontrollable movements of the face, mouth, tongue, and extremities, can occur in long-term users of these medications. At times, patients need an increasing dosage of phenothiazines to prevent breakthrough episodes of psychosis. Patients can experience chemical dependence on these first-generation antipsychotic agents.

Second-Generation Antipsychotics. Second-generation antipsychotic drugs, also called atypical antipsychotic agents, are also used for schizophrenia. These medications are preferred over first-generation antipsychotics because they cause fewer side effects; for example, they do not cause tardive dyskinesia. These medications are commonly used as adjuvant agents in severe mood disorders such as acute mania and bipolar depression. Risperadone (Risperdal), quetiapine (Seroquel), olanzapine (Zyprexa), ziprasidone (Geodon), and lurasidone (Latuda) are second-generation antipsychotic agents.

Third-Generation Antipsychotics. Third-generation antipsychotic medications include aripiprazole (Abilify). The mechanism of action is similar to other antipsychotic medications, although there are fewer side effects.

ALERT! First-generation antipsychotic medications can cause a side effect called tardive dyskinesia, which consists of episodes of involuntary movements of the face, lips, tongue, or extremities. Newer second-generation antipsychotic drugs do not cause tardive dyskinesia.

Pathophysiology of Selected Psychiatric Disorders

Behavioral disorders and psychiatric illness may affect many areas of the brain and, therefore, many areas of the individual's functioning. Some disorders may be primarily biological, whereas others may have a greater component of learned behavior. Studies of psychobiological disorders have strongly relied on neuroimaging studies of the brain and psychopharmacological research. A research base regarding the psychobiology of mental illness is emerging, but there is still a great deal of study needed.

Anxiety Disorders

Anxiety, a vague sense of dread related to an unspecified danger, is a universal human emotion. During periods of anxiety, physiologic stimulation of the SNS causes somatic symptoms such as restlessness and irritability, increased heart rate, hyperventilation, a sense of impending doom, and an inability to process stimuli. Extreme anxiety is called panic; at this level of anxiety, a person is often immobilized and in need of constant monitoring. Anxiety disorders include **generalized anxiety disorder (GAD),** panic attacks, OCD, specific phobias, social anxiety disorder, acute stress disorder, and PTSD.

Generalized Anxiety Disorder

GAD is one of the most common psychiatric disorders. Patients with GAD have fear and worry that are difficult to control. GAD can also lead to physiologic symptoms including fatigue, muscle tension, restlessness, and other somatic complaints. GAD has a prevalence rate of 18% in adults aged 18 and older in the United States. The highest number of cases of GAD occur in persons 45 to 49 years of age, and the lowest rate occurs in persons 60 years and older. Women are almost twice as likely as men to be diagnosed with GAD over their lifetime. Although the prevalence of GAD decreases with age in men, it increases in women.

Etiology. Anxiety is a natural response and a necessary protective mechanism in humans. The emotion of anxiety alerts the individual that there is a threat to safety in the environment. Anxiety is naturally associated with a wide range of physical and affective symptoms as well as changes in behavior and cognition; however, anxiety can also become a pathological disorder when it is excessive, uncontrollable, and triggered by no specific external stimulus.

Genetic risk factors are under investigation, and researchers have found a genetic predisposition for two types of anxiety disorders: a panic-generalized anxiety-agoraphobia group and a specific phobias group. Important risk factors also include comorbid substance abuse and family history. One 20-year study of the offspring of depressed parents found a threefold increase in anxiety disorders, including greater substance abuse, younger onset, and more significant physical health concerns.

Pathophysiology. Anxiety is believed to arise from the neurons in the region of the brain called the amygdala. The amygdala analyzes the emotional significance of environmental stimuli and stores emotional memories. Pathways exiting from the amygdala travel to multiple brain structures, including the parabrachial nucleus,

resulting in dyspnea and hyperventilation; the dorsomedial nucleus of the vagus nerve, activating the parasympathetic nervous system; and the lateral hypothalamus, resulting in SNS activation. The amygdala also sends neuronal signals to the prefrontal cortex, where cognitive experiences of specific anxiety disorders are integrated.

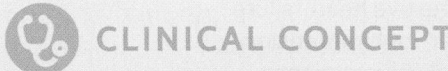

CLINICAL CONCEPT

Chest pain and shortness of breath are common symptoms of anxiety disorder that are mistaken for cardiovascular disease.

Clinical Presentation. Patients with GAD are often overwhelmed by worry about their health, family, work, and finances. Worrying is difficult to control, often negatively affecting relationships and social and occupational activities. Patients with GAD commonly present with physical symptoms of dizziness, hyperventilation, insomnia, headaches, muscle aches, fatigue, and gastrointestinal symptoms. It is important to rule out medical disorders and other psychiatric disorders, particularly depression. GAD and depression are often present together. The clinician should also rule out medications or other substances such as caffeine, alcohol, and amphetamines as a source of anxiety.

Diagnosis. It is important for the clinician to be aware of the medical disorders and medications that can cause anxiety (see Box 36-1). Before diagnosing GAD, it is often necessary to rule out medical disorders with laboratory tests such as complete blood count (CBC), metabolic panel, liver enzymes, serum creatinine, cardiac troponin, and enzymes. It is prudent to perform an electrocardiogram (ECG) when suspecting GAD.

There is a list of criteria for the diagnosis of GAD (see Box 36-2). There is also a self-report questionnaire available to assist clinicians in diagnosing anxiety disorders. The seven-item GAD scale, called GAD-7, is a reliable, valid, and easy-to-use self-report questionnaire for evaluating the presence and severity of GAD.

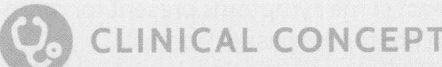

CLINICAL CONCEPT

Anxiety and depression are often present together. SSRIs can be used to treat this combination of disorders.

Treatment. Cognitive behavior therapy and SSRIs, as first-line pharmacological agents, are the treatment for GAD. SSRIs have antianxiety and antidepressant effects. Often, the patient requires a short course of a benzodiazepine to diminish anxiety symptoms. Benzodiazepines promote binding of GABA, a neuroinhibitory transmitter, to GABA receptors. Benzodiazepines have a rapid onset of action, and short- to intermediate-acting agents such as lorazepam (Ativan) are preferred

BOX 36-1. Disorders That Present With Anxiety

CARDIOPULMONARY DISORDERS
- angina pectoris
- cardiac arrhythmia
- cardiomyopathy
- congestive heart failure
- hyper- or hypotension
- mitral valve prolapse
- myocardial infarction
- syncope

ENDOCRINE DISORDERS
- hypercortisolism
- hyperthyroidism
- hypoglycemia
- hypoparathyroidism
- hypothyroidism
- pheochromocytoma

METABOLIC CONDITIONS
- hyperkalemia
- hyperthermia
- hypocalcemia
- hypoglycemia
- hyponatremia

NEUROLOGICAL DISORDERS
- encephalitis
- neoplasms
- Parkinson's disease
- postconcussion syndrome
- seizure
- vertigo

NUTRITIONAL STATES
- anemias
- caffeine overload
- folate deficiency
- pyridoxine deficiency
- vitamin B_{12} deficiency

PSYCHIATRIC DISORDERS
- depression
- panic disorder
- social anxiety disorder
- substance-induced anxiety disorder

RESPIRATORY DISORDERS
- asthma
- chronic obstructive pulmonary disease
- hypoxia
- pneumonia
- pneumothorax
- pulmonary edema

BOX 36-2. Diagnostic Criteria for GAD

A. Excessive anxiety and worry (apprehensive expectation), occurring more days than not for at least 6 months, about a number of vents or activities (such as work or school performance).

B. The person finds it difficult to control the worry.

C. The anxiety and worry are associated with three (or more) of the following six symptoms (with at least some symptoms present for more days than not for the past 6 months).
   NOTE: Only one item is required in children:
   (1) restlessness or feeling keyed up or on edge
   (2) being easily fatigued
   (3) difficulty concentrating or mind going blank
   (4) irritability
   (5) muscle tension
   (6) sleep disturbance (difficulty falling or staying asleep, or restless, unsatisfying sleep).

D. The anxiety, worry, or physical symptoms cause clinically significant distress or impairment in social, occupational, or other important areas of functioning.

E. The disturbance is not attributable to the physiologic effects of a substance (e.g., a drug of abuse, a medication) or another medical condition (e.g., hyperthyroidism).

F. The disturbance is not better explained by another mental condition (e.g., anxiety or worry about having panic attacks in panic disorder, negative evaluation in social anxiety disorder [social phobia], contamination or other obsessions in OCD, separation from attachment figures in separation anxiety disorder, reminders of traumatic events in posttraumatic disorder, gaining weight in anorexia nervosa, physical complaints in somatic symptom disorder, perceived appearance flaws in body dysmorphic disorder, having a serious illness in illness anxiety disorder, or the content of delusional beliefs in schizophrenia or delusional disorder).

(Reprinted with permission from the *Diagnostic and Statistical Manual of Mental Health Disorders*, Fifth Edition. (Copyright 2013). American Psychiatric Association.)

because they are less likely to accumulate and lead to the excessive daytime sedation. Long-acting agents, such as diazepam (Valium), chlordiazepoxide (Librium), and clorazepate (Tranxene), can cause drowsiness and sleepiness. Benzodiazepines should be avoided in patients who have previously demonstrated addictive behavior. Discontinuation should be carried out gradually over several weeks in all patients who have had 4 or more weeks of treatment to avoid withdrawal symptoms such as agitation, insomnia, irritability, and restlessness.

Buspirone (Buspar) is an azapirone that has demonstrated antianxiety effectiveness compared with placebo, but is not as effective as the benzodiazepines. Buspirone is an agonist of the serotonin receptor subtype 5-hydroxytryptamine-1A and is a nonaddictive, nonsedating alternative. However, buspirone requires 1 to 3 weeks to reach therapeutic blood levels and has a short half-life necessitating dosing 2 to 3 times per day.

Stress management is a necessary skill for those who suffer chronic anxiety. Relaxation techniques such as deep breathing, yoga, and meditation are commonly taught to those with GAD. Patients are often asked to keep track of their episodes of anxiety with a log. This log can be used in cognitive-behavioral therapy, which can analyze the triggers of anxiety and teach alternative reactions. The patient also needs education about medications and substances that can cause anxiety.

Panic Disorder

Panic disorder is an anxiety disorder characterized by recurrent, unexpected episodes of extreme anxiety. **Panic attacks** are discrete periods of intense apprehension, fear, and terror, with associated physiologic symptoms of extreme anxiety. Association with the place of the panic attack can result in a pervasive avoidance of places and situations in which a panic attack could occur.

The lifetime prevalence rate of panic disorder is reported to be at 3.5% in the community. However, this is likely a low estimate because many affected individuals do not report these episodes. In clinical settings, the rate is reported to be 10% to 30% in respiratory and neurology clinics and up to 60% in cardiology settings. One-half to one-third of individuals diagnosed with panic attacks in community samples also have agoraphobia, a fear of being outside of the home alone.

Etiology. Panic disorders usually occur in persons of adolescent age through young adulthood up to the mid-30s. Those with first-degree biological relatives with panic disorder are 8 times more likely to develop panic attacks.

Pathophysiology. The central and peripheral neurological systems are involved in panic disorder. Biological theories stress a genetic etiology and argue strongly against the idea that panic is merely a reaction to distressing stimuli. The psychobiology of panic disorder has been extensively investigated in terms of neuroimaging studies and pharmacological evidence.

Sympathetic System Stimulation. Anxiety reactions are associated with increased levels of catecholamines such as epinephrine. The **locus coeruleus** is a part of the brainstem involved in physiologic responses to stress and panic attacks. The locus coeruleus includes 50% of all adrenergic neurons in the CNS and sends projections to many parts of the brain, including the hippocampus, amygdala, limbic system, and the cerebral cortex (see Fig. 36-4). Stimulation of the locus coeruleus causes fear and anxiety. Antianxiety medications inhibit firing of neurons in the locus coeruleus and decrease the noradrenergic response.

GABA-Benzodiazepine System. The GABA receptor complex is involved in panic attacks. Binding of a BNZ to the GABA receptor results in a slowing of neuronal depolarization and neurotransmitter release. Decreased GABA-BNZ binding seen on SPECT scanning is observed in the hippocampus and prefrontal cortex in patients with panic disorder, whereas decreased BNZ binding in the prefrontal cortex and insula has been seen on positron emission tomography (PET) scans of patients with panic disorder.

Neurocircuitry of Fear. The neurocircuitry of fear model proposes that panic attacks are similar to animal fear and avoidance responses. A panic response is

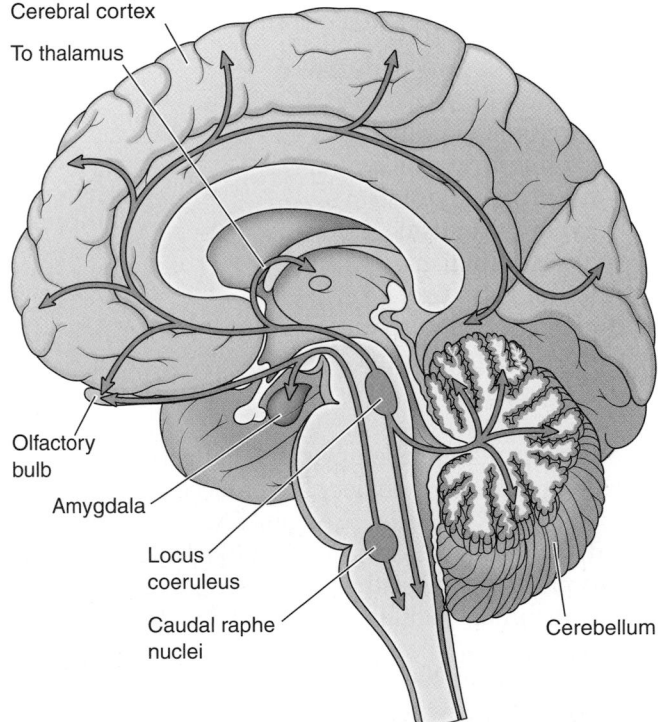

FIGURE 36-4. Locus coeruleus and amygdala. The principal centers for norepinephrine-secreting neurons are the locus coeruleus and the caudal raphe nuclei. The ascending nerves of the locus coeruleus project to the frontal cortex, thalamus, hypothalamus, limbic system, and cerebellum. Nerves projecting from the caudal raphe nuclei ascend to the amygdala and descend to the midbrain. The locus coeruleus is involved in arousal and autonomic activity. The amygdala is involved in memory and emotional reactions.

theorized to originate in the amygdala. Input to the amygdala is modulated by the thalamus and prefrontal cortex. Projections from the amygdala extend to various parts of the brain involved in the fear response, such as the locus coeruleus (arousal), brainstem (respiratory activation), hypothalamus-pituitary-adrenal axis (stress response), and cortex (cognitive interpretation of the stressor).

Clinical Presentation. Symptoms of a panic attack develop quickly, and may include palpitations or increased heart rate, sweating, trembling, shortness of breath, feeling of choking, chest pain, nausea, chills or hot flushes, and paresthesias. In addition, the individual may feel dizzy, detached from oneself, and a sense of unreality. He or she fears losing control and that he or she is dying.

CLINICAL CONCEPT

Commonly, individuals with panic attacks believe they are having a heart attack and go to an emergency department for treatment.

Diagnosis. Although no specific tests exist for panic disorder, several medical conditions can mimic the condition. Medical conditions that should be ruled out before diagnosing a panic disorder include:

- alcohol or drug withdrawal
- angina
- aortic dissection
- cardiac arrhythmias
- hyperparathyroidism
- hyperthyroidism
- hypothyroidism
- mitral valve prolapse
- myocardial infarction
- pheochromocytoma
- vertigo.

Treatment. Psychotherapy can be effective when the disabling aspects of anxiety are reduced with pharmacotherapy. SNRIs, SSRIs, TCAs, and BNZs are comparable in efficacy in the pharmaceutical blockade of spontaneous panic attacks. Other drugs used for treatment of panic disorder include MAOIs and beta-adrenergic blocking agents.

Patients who have co-occurring depression with anxiety disorder will benefit from SSRIs as monotherapy to treat both the panic disorder and depression. Benzodiazepines produce a rapid response in reducing anxiety. They may be preferred alone or in combination with antidepressants in individuals whose anxiety causes functional impairment.

MAOIs are as effective as the TCAs and SSRIs for treatment of panic disorder because they prevent breakdown of norepinephrine by the enzyme monoamine oxidase.

The elevation of norepinephrine reduces depressive symptoms.

Another drug that is effective in the treatment of panic disorder is buspirone (Buspar), a 5HT1a agonist nonbenzodiazepine, antianxiety agent. Buspirone binds to serotonin and dopamine receptors and increases norepinephrine in the brain. However, buspirone requires weeks of treatment before it is effective. Beta-adrenergic blocking agents such as propranolol are effective in specific social situations such as public speaking or musical performances. These agents decrease sympathetic discharge.

Supportive psychotherapy and education are necessary to assist the patient to understand and confront anticipated anxiety. Different techniques may be used to help the patient learn to control the physiologic responses of panic, understand the triggers of the panic disorder, and alleviate stressors.

ALERT! Patients with hypertension on MAOIs should have their BP periodically monitored because MAOIs can incite a hypertensive emergency. MAOIs should not be used with other drugs that can increase BP.

Obsessive Compulsive Disorder

OCD is a chronic illness that has a waxing and waning course; it is characterized by persistent and repetitive thoughts, impulses, or images that are intrusive and inappropriate. They may cause marked distress and anxiety. These thoughts are often related to contamination, the order of objects, or sexual imagery. To relieve the anxiety caused by the obsessions, the patient actively engages in compulsive activities, or rituals, to neutralize the thoughts through actions such as hand washing, praying, cleaning, or putting objects in order. In OCD, a progressive deterioration in an individual's occupational and social functioning may occur.

Lifetime prevalence rate of OCD in community studies is 2.5% in adults and 1% to 2% in children. Age of onset is earlier in males (ages 6 to 15 years) than females (ages 20 to 29 years), but OCD can begin at any time. One-third of first episodes occur between the ages of 10 to 15 years, and 75% develop by age 30 years. The onset of OCD is usually gradual and insidious, and the predisposition to develop OCD is genetically linked.

Pathophysiology. The etiology and pathophysiology of OCD is incompletely understood. Evidence from functional brain imaging studies shows hyperactivity in some cortical and subcortical regions of the brain; specifically, the orbital frontal cortex, limbic system, thalamus, and caudate. There are abnormalities in serotonergic, dopaminergic, and glutamatergic neurotransmission in these regions. Twin studies have supported the idea that heredity is involved in OCD, with a genetic influence of 45% to 65% in studies in children and 27% to 47% in adults. Monozygotic twins are concordant for OCD (80% to 87%), compared with 47% to 50% concordance in dizygotic twins. Interestingly, case reports have revealed OCD arising in children and young adults following acute group A streptococcal infections. Fewer reports cite herpes simplex virus as the apparent precipitating infectious event. It has been hypothesized that these infections trigger a CNS autoimmune response that results in neuropsychiatric symptoms.

Clinical Presentation. OCD is characterized by recurrent obsessions and compulsions that are severe enough to cause social and occupational impairment. Obsessional thinking is repetitive, persistent, intrusive, and distressful to the individual. The individual feels that the obsessions are out of his or her control. A temporary reduction in anxiety results from the completion of a compulsive ritual. If the patient is unable to complete the ritual, anxiety will increase, and physiologic symptoms of anxiety will occur.

CLINICAL CONCEPT

Compulsive rituals such as hand-washing temporarily relieve the distress of obsessions in patients with OCD.

Diagnosis. There are no specific tests for OCD, but two instruments, the Yale-Brown Obsessive Compulsive Scale and the Obsessive-Compulsive Inventory, may be used in addition to the MMSE.

Treatment. CBT and SSRIs are the recommended first-line treatment for OCD. CBT may be focused on changing the patient's response to anxiety-producing situations.

Posttraumatic Stress Disorder

PTSD is a specific type of anxiety disorder that occurs in response to a highly stressful event in a person's life. Symptoms of PTSD follow life-threatening events in which a person perceives actual or threatened death, serious injury, or a threat to physical integrity. The person may have been the victim of, or a witness to, horrific events. PTSD commonly occurs in soldiers, survivors of rape, holocaust survivors, prisoners of war, and physically and emotionally abused children.

Epidemiological studies of the U.S. general population estimate that PTSD will affect 15% to 24% of adults at some time in their lives. The incidence of PTSD depends on the type of stressful event studied. For example, the stressful event of sudden and unexpected loss of a loved one—the most common experience that causes PTSD—accounts for 39% of cases of PTSD in men and 27% of cases of PTSD in women. In general, women have a greater lifetime prevalence of PTSD than men. Persons of all ages are susceptible to PTSD.

The following are risk factors for PTSD:

- being female
- experiencing intense or long-lasting trauma
- having experienced trauma earlier in life
- having other mental health problems, such as anxiety or depression
- lacking a good support system of family and friends
- having first-degree relatives with mental health problems, including PTSD
- having first-degree relatives with depression
- having been abused or neglected as a child.

Pathophysiology. The pathophysiology of PTSD remains relatively unclear with research suggesting the involvement of the HPA axis, ANS, serotonin, and endogenous opioids. It is proposed that individuals with PTSD have higher levels of sympathetic arousal at the time of the trauma than those who do not have PTSD. In persons with PTSD, autonomic responses to both innocuous and harmful stimuli are elevated, but the effects are more noticeable with harmful stimuli.

In the normal response to stress, the body releases catecholamines and cortisol as it attempts to adapt to the stressor. In PTSD, the stress response becomes dysfunctional resulting in chronic autonomic hyperactivity. Stimulation of the ANS causes the hyperarousal and intrusive thoughts seen in patients with PTSD. The patient experiences an increase in heart rate, respiratory rate, and BP. When an individual experiences prolonged and repeated trauma, the SNS is stimulated and endogenous opioids are released by the body. When any stimulus triggers the past trauma, an analgesic effect caused by endogenous opioids develops in the patient with PTSD. This opioid effect is known as psychic numbing. It is theorized that when the levels of natural opioids dwindle, hyperactivity occurs, similar to opioid withdrawal.

Neuroimaging studies are increasing our knowledge base regarding PTSD. MRI of the brain shows a decrease in volume of the hippocampus in those with combat-related PTSD and survivors of childhood abuse. When veterans with PTSD relive mental experiences of combat, PET imaging demonstrates increased blood flow to the amygdala and anterior cingulate and a decrease in blood to Broca's area. Such neuroimaging patterns are beginning to reveal the brain's activity during nonverbal, emotional reactions in PTSD.

ALERT! PTSD can cause suicidal or homicidal actions by the patient.

Clinical Presentation. Individuals who experience PTSD typically have flashbacks, insomnia, hyperarousal, and hypervigilance. An environmental cue can reactivate the traumatic experience, causing the patient to respond in the same way he or she would during the original stressful event. Commonly, such behaviors are socially inappropriate and can lead to legal problems and incarceration.

PTSD can have a chronic course leading to impairment in daily functioning and decreased personal well-being. There may be a reduced capacity to master life skills and impairment of role performance. Chronic stress is associated with dysfunction of the nervous system; hypothalamus-pituitary-adrenal axis; and cardiovascular, metabolic, and immune systems.

Increased arousal in patients with PTSD may affect ANS functioning, with resultant changes in cardiac function. Individuals with PTSD report a significantly greater number of current and lifetime medical conditions than those without PTSD. Medical conditions include anemia, arthritis, asthma, back pain, diabetes, eczema, peptic ulcer, and kidney and lung disease.

Diagnosis. The essential feature of PTSD is the development of characteristic symptoms following exposure to an extreme traumatic stressor. The person's response to the event must involve intense fear, helplessness, or horror.

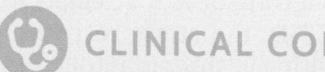

In children, the PTSD response involves disorganized or agitated behavior.

Diagnostic criteria include a strong emotional response that involves fear, helplessness, or horror, as well as impairment in daily functioning and symptoms that begin within 3 months after the trauma. To be diagnosed with PTSD, the individual must demonstrate three types of symptoms:

1. reliving the trauma
2. avoidance
3. hyperarousal.

Persons who relive the traumatic event have distressing images, nightmares, or flashbacks. The individual also demonstrates persistent avoidance of situations associated with the trauma and hyperarousal in the form of insomnia, hypervigilance, or difficulty concentrating. The disorder can be acute, with symptoms lasting fewer than 3 months, or chronic, with symptoms lasting 3 months or more. The full symptom picture causes clinically significant distress or impairment in social, occupational, or other areas of functioning. Delayed onset can occur if symptoms do not erupt until at least 6 months after the traumatic event.

Treatment. Persons with PTSD often self-soothe with alcohol or illicit drugs because the stigma related to mental health problems often prevents them from seeking help. Either disruptions in significant relationships or disproportionate anger may cause an individual to enter treatment for PTSD.

Antidepressants, antipsychotics, benzodiazepine medications, and psychotherapy are used to treat PTSD. The serotonergic system has been implicated in the symptoms of PTSD. Behavioral inhibition and constraint are mediated by serotonergic pathways. The angry and irritable affect seen in patients with PTSD may be related to a deficit in serotonin. This supports the use of the SSRI types of antidepressants in PTSD. Additionally, clonidine or prazosin can be helpful in treating trauma-related nightmares and sleep disruption.

Mood Disorders

Mood disorders are common worldwide and may affect as much as 14% of the world's population. In the United States, more than 20 million people have been diagnosed with a mood disorder. Individuals with mood disorders have an increased risk of self-harm or suicide, as more than 90% of people who commit suicide have been diagnosed with either a mood disorder or substance abuse.

Family studies indicate that if one parent has a mood disorder, the risk that a child will have the disorder is between 10% and 25%. The risk doubles if both parents have a mood disorder. Genetic factors may explain 50% to 70% of the etiology of mood disorders, as predisposition to the disease is inherited.

Major Depressive Disorder

Major depressive disorder (MDD) has the highest lifetime prevalence of any psychiatric disorder at 17%. Women experience MDD twice as frequently as men. This difference in prevalence is thought to be the result of hormonal influences, childbirth, and psychosocial factors. The mean age of onset for MDD is 40 years, although the disorder may be found across the life span. Half of all patients are diagnosed between 20 and 50 years.

ALERT! Suicide is the major complication of mood disorders. The lifetime risk of suicide in mood disorders is 10% to 15%, although two-thirds of depressed individuals have suicidal ideation. Women attempt suicide more often than men, but men are more likely to commit suicide because of utilizing more lethal means.

Major depression occurs most often in persons without close interpersonal relationships, is more common in rural than urban areas, and has no correlation with socioeconomic status. Patients with MDD have an increased risk for having at least one additional psychiatric diagnosis. The most common accompanying psychiatric disorders include alcohol abuse or dependence, panic disorder, OCD, eating disorder, and social anxiety disorder. Men have a high frequency of substance abuse, whereas women have a high frequency of anxiety and eating disorders.

Genetic studies show that many individuals with major depression have a mutation in the serotonin transporter gene. The gene is located at 17q11.1–q12 and controls synthesis of the serotonin transporter protein, which is involved in the recycling of serotonin. Studies show that mutations in the serotonin transporter gene are involved in clinical depression, alcohol abuse, OCD, and social phobia.

Pathophysiology. The underlying pathophysiology of MDD is not clearly understood. Research focuses on disturbances in the neurotransmitters of the CNS: serotonin, norepinephrine, and dopamine. Neuroimaging and pharmacological research have been intricately involved in reaching conclusions about the influence of neurotransmitters in the development of MDD.

The role of CNS serotonergic activity in the pathophysiology of MDD is suggested by the efficacy of SSRIs in treatment. Also, studies show that depressive symptoms can be produced in research subjects when there is tryptophan depletion, which causes a reduction in CNS serotonin levels.

 CLINICAL CONCEPT

Many persons suffer from a type of major depression called seasonal affective disorder (SAD). This disorder is most often seen in the winter months and resolves during the spring and summer. Studies show that SAD is mediated by alterations in CNS levels of serotonin and is likely provoked by alterations in circadian rhythm and lack of sunlight exposure.

Neuroimaging studies show that depression is associated with decreased metabolic activity in the neocortex of the brain and increased activity in the limbic system. By using PET images, researchers have found an area of the prefrontal cortex with abnormally diminished activity in patients with depression compared with nondepressed individuals. This region has widespread connections with areas that regulate dopamine, norepinephrine, and serotonin.

Some endocrine changes are also associated with depression. For example, the postpartum period is a time period of fluctuating hormone levels when women are vulnerable to depression. Menopause, a time of decreasing estrogen, often triggers depression in women, and low testosterone levels are associated with depression in men.

Clinical Presentation. In patients suspected of suffering from MDD, a complete assessment is necessary to rule out any medical illnesses with similar symptoms. Obtaining a list of medications, supplements, and other substances is important because many of these are

associated with the side effect of depression. Table 36-2 and Table 36-3 list medical conditions and medications that are linked to depression. Family history is important because there is a significant genetic role in the development of depression.

TABLE 36-2. Major Medical Conditions That Commonly Cause Depression

Category	Disorder or Condition
Cancer	Lung cancer
	Pancreatic cancer
Cardiovascular	Heart failure
	Myocardial infarction
	Stroke
Endocrine	Hypothyroidism
	Hyperthyroidism
	Addison's disease
	Cushing's disease
Infectious	Acquired immunodeficiency syndrome
	Influenza
	Hepatitis
	Infectious mononucleosis
	Lyme disease
Neurological	Parkinson's disease
	Multiple sclerosis
	Alzheimer's disease
Nutritional deficiencies	Iron deficiency
	Thiamine deficiency
	Vitamin B_{12} deficiency

TABLE 36-3. Common Medications That Can Cause Depression

Classification	Drug
Cardiovascular medications	Clonidine
	Digitalis
	Propranolol
	Reserpine
	Thiazide diuretics
Cancer agents	Chemotherapeutic agents
	Corticosteroids
	Interferon
Endocrine medications	Adrenocorticotropin hormone
	Corticosteroids
	Anabolic steroids
	Oral contraceptives
Gastrointestinal medications	Cimetidine
	Ranitidine
Drugs with abuse potential	Opioids
	Alcohol
	Cocaine
	Marijuana
	Sedative-hypnotics

 CLINICAL CONCEPT

Patients with depression spend more time in bed than patients with diabetes, hypertension, arthritis, or chronic lung disease and have as much functional disability as patients with heart disease.

In addition to the patient's current signs and symptoms, history of prior episodes and treatment for depression (successes and failures) is an important guide to determine current treatment. Psychosocial history of childhood deprivation; abandonment; and physical, emotional, or sexual abuse are important trauma-related data to be assessed because they are contributing factors for depression. A depressed patient should be clearly questioned about suicidal thoughts and plans.

Diagnosis. Diagnosis is based on having at least five of the following symptoms for a minimum of 2 weeks:

- sad mood most of the day, nearly every day
- decreased interest in pleasurable activities (also called anhedonia)
- weight loss or gain
- daily insomnia or hypersomnia
- psychomotor retardation or agitation
- fatigue or loss of energy
- feelings of worthlessness
- inappropriate guilt
- diminished levels of concentration and decisiveness
- recurrent suicidal thoughts and plan.

These symptoms cause significant distress and occupational and social impairment. Objective assessment tools are also used in the diagnosis of depression, including the Hamilton Depression Rating Scale, Zung Self-Rating Depression Scale, Raskin Depression Scale, Beck Depression Inventory, and Geriatric Depression Scale. All of these are valid and reliable self-report questionnaires. The Hamilton Depression Rating Scale has been the gold standard used most often in inpatient populations.

Thyroid testing is recommended in depressed patients to rule out hypothyroidism as a cause of symptoms, because 8% of all patients with depression have a thyroid disorder. The thyrotropin-releasing hormone stimulation test is indicated in patients whose marginally abnormal thyroid test results suggest subclinical hypothyroidism.

The dexamethasone-suppression test (DST) can also be used to help confirm a diagnosis of MDD. With administration of dexamethasone, suppression of cortisol indicates that the HPA axis is functioning properly; nonsuppression indicates HPA axis dysfunction. There is some evidence that patients with a positive DST will respond positively to antidepressant therapy or electroconvulsive therapy (ECT).

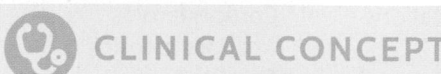

CLINICAL CONCEPT

With DST, false positive and false negative results are common, and medical conditions and medications can interfere with results.

Treatment. Depression can be treated with antidepressant medications, psychotherapy, ECT, transcranial magnetic stimulation (TMS), and vagus nerve stimulation (VNS). Commonly, individuals are prescribed an antidepressant and are referred for psychotherapy. When prescribing an antidepressant, the clinician often uses a trial-and-error approach because different types of medications are therapeutic for different individuals. Most antidepressant medications require 3 to 6 weeks to reach therapeutic blood levels. This waiting period is extremely difficult for the depressed patient. It is important that the depressed patient has psychotherapeutic support during this waiting period.

The SSRIs are the first-line treatment medications for depression, as well as the most commonly used drugs for depression. Fluoxetine (Prozac) is the prototypical SSRI; other common medications used are venlafaxine (Effexor) and duloxetine (Cymbalta), which are SNRIs that block the reuptake of serotonin and norepinephrine. Bupropion (Wellbutrin), another commonly prescribed antidepressant, is a norepinephrine-dopamine reuptake inhibitor. TCAs and MAOIs are commonly used for treatment-resistant depression. Antipsychotic drugs and anticonvulsant medications are often added to the antidepressant regimen. These medications can amplify the antidepressant effect and stabilize mood. Common antipsychotic medications used include quetiapine (Seroquel) and aripiprazole (Abilify). Anticonvulsants include lamotrigine (Lamictal) and carbamazepine (Tegretol).

ECT, which induces a seizure in a well-anesthetized patient, is highly effective in treating depression. The mechanism of ECT is not fully known, but it is suspected that the induced seizure stimulates available neurotransmitters. ECT can be helpful in up to 70% of patients who fail to respond to antidepressants.

VNS was approved by the U.S. Food and Drug Administration in 2005 for treatment-resistant depression. A VNS system is surgically implanted to deliver electrical pulses to the vagus nerve, with mood elevation as the outcome. The device was first used in treating drug-resistant epilepsy. Elevated mood was observed in some of the treated patients, giving rise to use the device in depressed individuals.

TMS, a noninvasive procedure that delivers magnetic impulses to the cortex, can be used for treatment-resistant depression. It uses a stimulating coil placed directly on the head where magnetic impulses pass unimpeded through the skull. Transsynaptic effects depolarize the neurons, leading to increased secretion of growth factors such as brain-derived neurotropic factor. Some studies show that TMS can initiate neuronal reorganization and neurogenesis. Rapid magnetic pulses over the dorsolateral prefrontal cortex have demonstrated antidepressant effects.

Bipolar Disorder

Bipolar disorder is a mood disorder characterized by cyclical episodes of depression and mania; it includes two subtypes. Bipolar I and Bipolar II disorders share similar characteristics, but Bipolar I disorder includes an abnormally and pervasive elevated, expansive, or manic mood of at least 1 week; psychotic features; and potential harm to self or others, frequently requiring hospitalization. In Bipolar II disorder, the expansive, elated, or irritable mood may still occur, but lasts only up to 4 days; in addition, it may be manifested as a less elevated mood, also called hypomania. In Bipolar II there are no psychotic features noted and depression is the major problem; there is also less impairment in social and occupational functioning as compared with patients with Bipolar I disorder.

The annual prevalence of bipolar disorder is 2.6% within the adult population. Out of the 2.6% of affected adults, 2.2% have severe symptoms. Bipolar I disorder is equally prevalent in men and women, but women are more likely to experience mood cycles, defined as four or more episodes per year. Manic episodes are more common in men, whereas women are more prone to mixed depression and mania.

A family history of bipolar disorder conveys a greater risk for mood disorder and bipolar disorder. Patients with bipolar disorders frequently have a substance abuse or anxiety disorder. In both unipolar and bipolar disorders, men are at greater risk to have a comorbid substance abuse problem.

Pathophysiology. Neuroimaging studies have demonstrated that mood regulation is in the prefrontal cortex and the amygdala. In adults with bipolar illness, there is an alteration in connection between the dorsolateral prefrontal cortex and the amygdala, with an increased response by the amygdala to emotional cues. PET and SPECT scans show increased temporal lobe activity and increased amygdala volume. Some structural changes of the brain seem to cause the disorder and some seem to be caused by the disorder.

Bipolar disorder has a strong genetic predisposition. In a landmark study, researchers found a connection between bipolar illness and a genome that encodes for an enzyme called diacylglycerol kinase (DGKH). DGKH is a crucial part of the lithium-sensitive pathway, and lithium is known as the first-line drug to treat bipolar illness. It is also known that chromosomes 13 and 15 are involved in both schizophrenia and bipolar illness.

Clinical Presentation. A patient with Bipolar I disorder may be admitted to an inpatient facility for behavior that is unacceptable in society, because he or she cannot care for him- or herself or is psychotic. A patient in a manic episode of Bipolar I disorder has an elevated, expansive, or irritable mood. The person may be euphoric and have pressured speech and flight of ideas. The patient may talk in rhymes, called clang association, and may attempt to entertain others but instead intrude on conversations. Later, the euphoric mood changes to irritability, after which the patient can become demanding, testing rules and limits on behavior. Early in the manic episode, the patient may not sleep and is hyperactive and hyperverbal. The patient may wear colorful clothes, excessive makeup, and flamboyant hairstyles. Sexual interest and behaviors toward others are common during the manic episode. The patient is typically very impulsive and needs monitoring to avoid aggression or unwanted sexual behaviors toward other patients. Patients in a manic episode demonstrate poor judgment, lack of insight, and can be regressed in their behavior. Attention span may be limited. Patients can be preoccupied with religion, politics, finances, sexuality, or persecution. Paranoid or grandiose delusions are common. Patients may also self-medicate with alcohol or drugs to help themselves sleep or to escape their distress.

In lieu of manic episodes, a patient with Bipolar I or II disorder may exhibit hypomania. Hypomania is similar to mania except the patient has no psychotic symptoms. The individual may be far more productive or outgoing and sociable than usual. This change in functioning and in mood is not subtle—the change is directly noticeable by others (usually friends or family members) during a hypomanic episode. A hypomanic episode is also not severe enough to cause serious impairment in social or occupational functioning, or to necessitate hospitalization.

A major complication of the mania associated with Bipolar I disorder is exhaustion and cardiac collapse caused by lack of rest and sleep. Patients lose weight because they forget to eat as a result of hyperactivity and distractibility. They may also be a danger to themselves or others when they are psychotic, because suicide and homicide are complications of the illness. Social and occupational impairments are complications of not being treated or noncompliance with medications. It can be challenging to help the patient adhere to the treatment regimen because the patient "feels so good" in the manic state and may not want to return to a more euthymic (mood stable) condition. Ups and downs of mood cycling are more common in bipolar I disorder than bipolar II disorder.

Diagnosis. The diagnosis of a bipolar disorder is based on the clinical presentation. The patient may present in either a manic or depressive phase of the disorder. Past medical and psychiatric history need to be obtained, including prior medications and treatment success or resistance. A family history of mental illness, particularly bipolar disorder, is a crucial component of the assessment. Routine blood work such as CBC and serum chemistry should be done to rule out any concomitant illnesses.

Treatment. Treatment for bipolar disorder includes medications and psychotherapy. Categories of medications that are used include mood stabilizers such as lithium, anticonvulsants, and atypical antipsychotic medications. Antipsychotics are used to reduce agitation and to promote rest. Mood stabilizers are one of the most common groups of medications used to treat the symptoms of mania and hypomania. Lithium is included in this class of medications, as well as several anticonvulsant drugs such as carbamazepine, valproic acid, and lamotrigine.

Although it is still considered the ideal mood stabilizer, lithium's mechanism of action remains unclear. It has effects on several neurotransmitter systems: serotonin, dopamine, norepinephrine, and acetylcholine.

> **ALERT!** Lithium has a narrow therapeutic/toxic ratio, so plasma concentrations need to be monitored closely. The signs and symptoms of lithium toxicity include increased tremors, nausea, vomiting, ataxia, and change in mental status. If untreated, lithium toxicity can lead to coma or death.

Antipsychotics may also be used to treat bipolar disorder. This class of medication is often used to control mania or decrease psychotic symptoms that can be present during the manic phase of the illness. Antianxiety medications can also be used during the manic phase.

 CLINICAL CONCEPT

Antipsychotic medications are often added to an antidepressant regimen to boost the effect of the antidepressant.

Schizophrenia

Schizophrenia is a neurobiological disorder considered a **psychosis,** an abnormal condition of the mind where the affected person loses touch with reality. The person often suffers from delusions and hallucinations. In schizophrenia, the individual may express himself or herself in various ways:

- neologisms: using words with special meanings to the individual
- clang associations: rhyming
- word salad: a collection of random words
- echolalia: repeating of others' words
- echopraxia: repeating movements made by another person
- flight of ideas: varied unconnected thoughts.

Individuals often think they are being told to complete certain actions by someone. There is lack of insight and judgment. Often there is bizarre behavior such as wearing inappropriate clothing or having inappropriate social, sexual, or aggressive interactions.

A delusion is a thought that is not grounded in reality. Three specific delusions are classic positive symptoms of schizophrenia:

1. thought broadcasting: thinking one's thoughts are broadcasted so that everyone can hear
2. thought insertion: thinking that others are inserting thoughts into the individual's head
3. thought withdrawal: thinking that thoughts are being drawn out of the person's head by others.

The lifetime prevalence rate of schizophrenia in the United States is approximately 0.5% to 1% of the population. Annual incidence of new cases ranges from 0.5 to 5.0 per 10,000 people per year. Geographical differences exist, as the disorder seems to be more common in urban areas compared with rural areas. Schizophrenia is equally prevalent in both men and women. Peak age of onset for men is age 10 to 25 years; for women, however, the onset of schizophrenia peaks between 25 to 35 years. Approximately 90% of patients in treatment for schizophrenia present to mental health providers between the ages of 15 and 55. Onset before age 10 or after age 60 is extremely rare. Most people who are diagnosed with schizophrenia have their first symptoms and episode in their 20s.

First-degree biological relatives of patients with schizophrenia have a 10 times greater risk for developing the disorder. Substance abuse is a common comorbidity of schizophrenia. This includes alcohol, cannabis, and other street drugs. Drug abuse results in poorer overall functional ability. In addition, 90% of individuals with schizophrenia are prone to have nicotine addiction. Individuals with schizophrenia represent between 15% and 45% of homeless persons; this is attributed to the difficulties these persons have remaining employed and socially functional.

Pathophysiology

The exact cause of schizophrenia is unclear, but a number of theories exist. Many studies have been done using pharmacological agents and neuroimaging to delineate the cause of schizophrenia. There is a genetic component to all forms of schizophrenia, with identical twins having a 50% concordance rate of the illness. The vulnerability-liability theory postulates that genetics lead to vulnerability, but the environment also exerts influence in the cause of schizophrenia. It is also theorized that an individual is at risk for developing schizophrenia if the father is older than age 60 years. This suggests a risk caused by altered sperm development in older men.

The dopamine hypothesis of schizophrenia is derived from the fact that antipsychotic drug treatment is based on antidopaminergic activity. Psychotic symptoms, such as delusions, have been linked to excessive dopamine levels. However, the cause of dopamine excess is unclear. The specific dopamine pathway involved is also unclear, though it is known that dopaminergic neurons project from the midbrain to the limbic system and the cerebral cortex.

Other neurotransmitters are theorized to be involved in schizophrenia. For example, an excess of serotonin has been hypothesized to cause symptoms of schizophrenia. Loss of GABAergic neurons in the hippocampus of some patients with schizophrenia may lead to hyperactivity of serotonin. The serotonin antagonistic activity of clozaril, an atypical antipsychotic drug, in the treatment of chronic schizophrenic patients provides support for this theory. Changes in levels of norepinephrine have been shown to be involved in the symptom anhedonia experienced by patients with schizophrenia. The neurotransmitter glutamate may also be involved based on the fact that phencyclidine, a glutamate antagonist, causes an acute psychosis similar to schizophrenia.

Neuroimaging studies demonstrate a neuropathological basis for schizophrenia, including a loss of brain volume. CT scans note lateral and third ventricle enlargement, as well as reduction in cortical tissue. Reduced symmetry in the temporal, frontal, and occipital lobes has been noted.

On autopsy of persons with schizophrenia, there appears to be a decrease in the size of a number of brain regions, including the amygdala, hippocampus, parahippocampal gyrus, and prefrontal cortex. MRIs show that the hippocampus in individuals with schizophrenia is smaller than normal and has a disturbance in the transmission of glutamate. Disorganized distribution of neurons within the hippocampus of patients with schizophrenia has also been documented.

The basal ganglia and the cerebellum are also of interest to scientists because of movement disorders that occur in schizophrenia. Some researchers believe that instead of discrete brain areas as the focus of the illness, schizophrenia is a disorder of brain neural circuits that are caused by early developmental lesions.

Immune abnormalities seen in schizophrenia include a decreased T-cell interleukin-2 production, a reduced number of peripheral lymphocytes, abnormal cellular and humoral reactivity to neurons, and the presence of antibrain cell antibodies.

Clinical Presentation

Early symptoms of schizophrenia may precede diagnosis. For example, an adolescent with schizophrenia may have not had friends, preferring solitary activities such as watching television or playing on computers, versus group and social activities. The prodromal phase of the illness may begin with vague bodily symptoms and increased emphasis on religious or philosophical ideas, peculiar behavior, changes in affect, and unusual speech, behaviors, and perceptual sensations. The clinical presentation of a patient with schizophrenia varies from someone who is disheveled, aggressive, actively hallucinating, and delusional to someone who is mute and shows lack of spontaneous speech or movement.

Patients with schizophrenia often have a blunted or flattened affect, poverty of speech (alogia), apathy, lack of motivation (avolition), decreased spontaneous movements, and inattention to hygiene/grooming. Inattention, poor problem-solving and decision-making skills, and feelings of dysphoria and hopelessness are common. There may be suicidal feelings. Marked dysfunction occurs in the areas of employment, interpersonal relationships, self-care, and quality of life.

Patients frequently claim to hear voices. These voices may be loud or muffled, and there may be more than one voice in a conversation. The patient may also mumble to himself or herself in response. Command hallucinations tell the person to do something, often to hurt self or others, and are dangerous. Visual hallucinations are possible and are experienced as shadows, waves, or spirits. Patients are often paranoid and lack trust in others such as health-care providers.

Violence, suicide, and homicide are complications of untreated schizophrenia. Patients who are untreated may be violent because of impulsivity and delusions of persecution. Emergency management includes use of antianxiety and antipsychotic medications to control aggression. Suicide is a leading cause of premature death in patients with schizophrenia. Suicide attempts are made by 20% to 50% of patients, which is a 20-fold increase compared with the general population.

Diagnosis

Diagnosis is made based on the clinical presentation and exclusion of any organic causes. A complete psychiatric evaluation, history, and physical examination are needed to rule out any physical or drug-induced psychosis. It is also important to have a complete history of the patient's illness, adherence to treatment, social network, housing, and current medications. Serum lab tests should be performed to rule out medical illness.

Treatment

Although antipsychotic medications are the gold standard treatment for patients with schizophrenia, research has found that psychosocial interventions that include psychotherapy can improve clinical outcomes. Hospitalization may be necessary for safety and to stabilize the patient on antipsychotic medications. Outpatient treatment includes intensive partial hospitalization programs, medication evaluations, and support groups. The recovery model of schizophrenia treatment stresses patient responsibility to manage mental illness and build upon patient strengths so that they may live productive lives. Patients need education about their disease and the importance of adherence to the medication regimen.

Schizophrenia is treated medically through use of both traditional antipsychotics and the newer second generation of atypical antipsychotics. Traditional antipsychotics are dopamine receptor antagonists. Because of the possible motor side effects caused by the typical antipsychotics, such as acute dystonia, akathisia, pseudoparkinsonism, and tardive dyskinesia, patients are prescribed the newer second-generation antipsychotics. Second generation antipsychotic drugs are serotonin-dopamine receptor antagonists. Remission occurs in approximately 70% of those who adhere to treatment.

Attention Deficit-Hyperactivity Disorder

ADHD is the most common psychiatric condition affecting children in the United States. This disorder has a dramatic impact on the child, family, and the community. Approximately 30% of students with ADHD repeat a grade, up to 33% fail to complete high school, and only

5% to 10% complete college. ADHD is also associated with adolescents engaging in antisocial activities in approximately half of the cases. These teens are prone to unintentional injuries as compared with those who do not have ADHD.

The prevalence rates for ADHD range from 1.9% to 14.4%. In school-aged children, the prevalence rate has been estimated to be between 3% and 7%. It is estimated that between 50% and 70% of children with ADHD will continue to have symptoms of the disorder as adults.

Several risk factors for ADHD have been identified. ADHD symptoms have been associated with infection such as meningitis and encephalitis, closed head injury, lead poisoning, hypoxia, and maternal substance abuse during pregnancy. ADHD is more common in low birth weight infants. It can occur with other disabling conditions such as sensory impairment and serious psychological and emotional disturbances. It can also occur in the presence of other extrinsic influences, such as poor socioeconomic background and dysfunctional parenting, though it is not a direct result of these environmental or physical conditions. In the past, ADHD was thought to be related to nutritional intake of sugar or artificial additives; however, there is no scientific evidence to support this.

Pathophysiology

There is no clear etiology in ADHD. Biological and environmental factors, such as genetics, perinatal complications, neurological illness, allergies, and environmental toxins have been correlated with the disorder.

ADHD is a heterogeneous, nonprogressive, neurological condition. Genetic, neurological, and environmental influences play a role in ADHD. The condition is highly inheritable with estimates of 60% to 90% across generations. Twin studies confirm a genetic link between identical twins. ADHD is thought to be a polygenic disorder that interferes with encoding and functioning of the neurotransmitters and the corresponding receptors. Investigations focus on genes responsible for dysregulation of dopamine and norepinephrine, their receptors, and their transporters. These two neurotransmitters influence attention, arousal, impulsivity, and mood. The role of neurotransmitter dysregulation in ADHD is supported in that medications that affect the dopaminergic and noradrenergic systems are successfully used to control symptoms of ADHD. The right prefrontal cortex, caudate nucleus, and globus pallidus appear to be smaller, show less blood flow, and display decreased electrical activity in children with ADHD when compared with those without it. These areas of the brain are usually rich in dopamine receptors.

Perinatal complications, including antepartum hemorrhage, prolonged labor, and low Apgar scores at 1 minute, are more common among children with ADHD. Those infants with low birth weight and injury to the white matter are at increased risk to develop ADHD. The brains of children with ADHD show prefrontal cortex function abnormalities.

Clinical Presentation

Children with ADHD have very high levels of activity that make them look driven, restless, and never tiring in nature. The child may be unable to comply with school routines because of restlessness, causing him or her to become disruptive in the classroom. They may make noise, hum, squirm in their chairs, or tap at their desks.

Children with ADHD cannot filter out extraneous stimuli, and distraction takes the form of an inability to concentrate. This makes completion of class work difficult. At home, children with ADHD have difficulty listening to adults and carrying out multistep instructions. They seem to be in a hurry and rush to complete a task; in addition, they start many activities without completing them. Children with ADHD are impulsive. They may interrupt others and may not have patience to wait their turn, which can result in them becoming disliked by peers. Children with ADHD tend to befriend children who have issues with authority.

Other psychiatric disorders, such as conduct disorder and oppositional defiant disorder, are comorbidities of ADHD. These disorders occur with high frequency in up to 30% to 50% of children with ADHD. Mood and anxiety disorders are also comorbid conditions and affect the degree of impairment and the course of the disorder. Compared with research control subjects, children with ADHD who are followed in adolescence and adulthood show higher rates of antisocial behavior and substance abuse.

Diagnosis

ADHD is suspected in a child who has academic and behavioral problems in preschool or elementary school. No laboratory tests, neurological assessments, or attention assessments have been established as diagnostic in the clinical assessment of ADHD. However, individuals need to be evaluated to rule out any complicating medical illnesses.

Attention-deficit/hyperactivity disorder (ADHD) can be diagnosed in adults. Symptoms include difficulty maintaining attention, as well as hyperactivity and impulsive behavior. Adult ADHD symptoms can lead to a number of problems, including unstable relationships, poor work or school performance, and low self-esteem.

Treatment

Psychostimulant therapy is routinely prescribed to enhance a child's ability to focus on school work and to reduce the child's inattention, impulsivity, and hyperactivity. The medications include methylphenidate, amphetamine preparations, and magnesium pemoline. In persons with ADHD, psychostimulants work in a paradoxical way to increase attention and task-directed behavior while reducing hyperactivity, impulsivity, restlessness, and distractibility. This response is theorized to be the result of the neocortex being stimulated to exert executive control over more impulsive behaviors. There is a risk of substance abuse with the psychostimulants.

Methylphenidate (Ritalin) is the most widely used psychostimulant because of its simplicity of use and safety. Concerta is an extended release version of methylphenidate. There is an amphetamine mixture called Adderall that has proven effective. However, drug abuse has been seen with this prescription medication. Atomoxetine (Strattera), another effective type of medication, is a nonstimulant selective norepinephrine reuptake inhibitor that has the advantage of minimal risk of illicit abuse.

Dementia

Dementia is a decline of reasoning, memory, judgment, and other cognitive functions. The decline in cognition impairs the ability to carry out ADLs, such as household chores, driving, and handling finances and personal care such as bathing, dressing, and feeding. Although common in elderly persons, dementia is not a normal part of aging. It can be caused by reversible or irreversible causes. Dementia is more than age-related forgetfulness; it is a serious illness. Individuals with dementia lose the ability to reason, are unable to solve problems, and cannot think abstractly. They are disoriented to time and place and eventually they cannot identify persons.

Approximately 4 to 5 million people in the United States have some degree of dementia, and that number will increase over the next few decades with the aging of the population. Dementia affects about 1% of people aged 60 to 64 years and as many as 30% to 50% of people older than 85 years. It is the leading reason for placing elderly people in long-term care facilities.

The two main causes of dementia are Alzheimer's disease and vascular disease, also known as multi-infarct dementia. Other causes include Parkinson's disease, metabolic disorders, Creutzfeldt-Jakob disease, and Huntington disease (see Box 36-3).

Pathophysiology

There are different pathological processes for the two major types of dementia: Alzheimer's disease and multi-infarct dementia.

Alzheimer's Disease. Alzheimer's disease, a progressive neurological degenerative disease of the brain, is characterized by significant changes in brain tissue. There is an accumulation of neurofibrillary tangles, senile plaques (also called beta-amyloid plaques), and cerebrocortical atrophy of the brain. Healthy neurons have an internal support structure partly made up of structures called microtubules. These microtubules act like tracks, guiding nutrients and molecules from the cell's body down to the ends of the axon and back. A special kind of protein, tau, makes the microtubules stable. In Alzheimer's disease, tau proteins are changed chemically and become unstable. Tau protein begins to pair with other threads of tau, and they become neurofibrillary tangles. When this happens, the microtubules disintegrate, collapsing the neuron's transport system, resulting in malfunctions in communication

---

BOX 36-3. Causes of Dementia

The following conditions can cause cognitive impairment:

- alcoholism
- AIDS dementia
- Alzheimer's disease
- brain tumor
- Creutzfeldt-Jakob disease
- drug reactions
- Huntington's disease
- infection of brain structures
- Lewy body dementia
- metabolic disorders
- normal pressure hydrocephalus
- nutritional deficiencies
- Parkinson's disease
- Pick disease
- progressive supranuclear palsy
- syphilis
- toxic exposures
- vascular dementia (also called multi-infarct dementia).

---

between neurons. Increasing destabilization of neuronal structures leads to death of brain cells. The tangles and plaques eventually build up and take over normal neural tissue in the brain. There is also oxidative damage in areas of the brain; oxidative stress produces reactive oxygen species, also called free radicals, which cause brain cell damage and cellular apoptosis.

Also in Alzheimer's disease, there is a deficiency of acetylcholine, which is involved in memory functions. Cholinergic deficiency has been implicated in the cognitive decline and behavioral changes of the disease. Activity of the synthetic enzyme choline acetyltransferase (CAT) is significantly reduced in the cerebral cortex, hippocampus, and amygdala in patients with Alzheimer's disease. Loss of cortical CAT and decline in acetylcholine synthesis in biopsy specimens have been found to correlate with cognitive impairment. Because cholinergic dysfunction may contribute to the symptoms of patients with Alzheimer's, drugs that enhance acetylcholine in the brain constitute a rational basis for symptomatic treatment.

Risk factors for Alzheimer's disease include increasing age: after age 65 years, the risk for the disorders doubles every 5 years. Family history increases an individual's chance of acquiring Alzheimer's disease. The strongest genetic risk involves the apolipoprotein e4 (APOE-e4) gene. Other risk genes have been identified, but not conclusively confirmed. Women may be more likely than men to develop Alzheimer's disease, in part, because they live longer. Some evidence suggests that the same factors that increase risk for heart disease also increase risk for Alzheimer's: lack of exercise, smoking, hypertension, high cholesterol, and poorly controlled diabetes. Studies have found an association between lifelong involvement in mentally and socially stimulating activities and reduced risk of Alzheimer's disease. Factors that may reduce the risk of Alzheimer's disease include higher levels of formal education; a stimulating job; mentally challenging leisure activities, such as reading, playing games, or playing a musical instrument; and frequent social interactions.

Vascular Dementia. There are many causes of vascular dementia (also called multi-infarct dementia). Multi-infarct dementia is thought to be an irreversible form of dementia, and its onset is caused by a number of small strokes or, sometimes, one large stroke preceded or followed by other smaller strokes. The main subtypes of vascular dementia are:

- mild cognitive impairment caused by multi-infarct dementia
- vascular dementia caused by a strategic single infarct
- vascular dementia caused by hemorrhagic lesions
- mixed Alzheimer's and vascular dementia.

Vascular lesions can be the result of diffuse cerebrovascular disease or focal lesions—usually both. Mixed dementia is diagnosed when patients have evidence of Alzheimer's disease and cerebrovascular disease, either clinically or based on neuroimaging evidence of ischemic lesions. Vascular dementia and Alzheimer's disease often coexist.

Risk factors for vascular dementia include hypertension, smoking, hypercholesterolemia, diabetes mellitus, cardiovascular disease, and cerebrovascular disease. Arteriosclerosis and hypertension are the major causes of cerebrovascular disease.

Clinical Presentation

The onset of dementia can be subtle at first. **Amnesia** is commonly the first symptom experienced, though language, perceptual skills, reasoning, and personality are affected and may be more noticeable initially. This is especially true in individuals whose symptoms begin before age 65 years. Memory loss can begin with **anomia,** which is the forgetting of names of things and people. Despite being reminded, individuals with this condition often repeatedly forget the same information. Usually memory loss involves short-term memory before long-term memory. For example, persons with dementia often have difficulty remembering events from a few minutes ago or last week but can remember events from childhood. Individuals often can remember and reminisce about the most influential time of their life, such as a time when they were successful in their career or a parent of young children.

Early in dementia, individuals can become disoriented and forget their way home or their original destination. They may not remember the day of the week or month. Reality orientation may frustrate the individual.

The individual with dementia may demonstrate poor judgment, lack of ability to reason, and inability to think abstractly. For example, balancing a checkbook and managing finances become difficult tasks. **Apraxia,** which is difficulty in performing familiar tasks, occurs. The individual may forget how to get dressed properly or forget how to prepare a meal. Often self-hygiene becomes unmanageable. The individual often exhibits **agnosia,** which is forgetting the purpose of familiar items. He or she might exhibit this behavior in subtle ways, such as placing a toothbrush in a sugar bowl or a wrist watch in the refrigerator.

Often the person with dementia exhibits rapid mood swings or personality changes, such as becoming paranoid, angry, or fearful for no apparent reason. It is important for significant others to realize that cognitive impairment and gradual losses of abilities can be extremely anxiety-provoking for the individual with early dementia. Individuals may express this anxiety in a number of ways, including withdrawing from social situations or becoming impatient and irritable when reminded of their lack of cognitive ability.

Apathy or loss of initiative to become involved in activities is common. Individuals with dementia usually do not take part in exercise unless prompted and shown how to perform physical fitness activities. Persons with dementia commonly exhibit insomnia or hypersomnia because of lack of maintaining a proper sleep-wake cycle. **Sundowning,** when the individual shows symptoms of acute confusion, disorientation, hallucinations, and mood swings during late day into night, often occurs. Behavior can become erratic, violent, and difficult to manage. Sedation is frequently employed, which adds to the disruption of circadian rhythms.

With severe dementia, individuals have difficulty recognizing relatives and caregivers. Individuals often also have problems with language. They may experience difficulty with finding the proper words and they often substitute inappropriate words, making sentences incomprehensible. With end stages of dementia, individuals often do not speak or perform activities.

Diagnosis

Individuals suspected of having dementia require a complete history and physical examination. A physical illness should be vigorously sought and ruled out before making the diagnosis of dementia, because there are many possible physical illnesses that can have symptoms that resemble those of dementia. Nutritional deficiencies, metabolic imbalances, drug toxicity, thyroid disease, infection, and heart failure can present with cognitive impairment, confusion, and disorientation in the elderly. Often the patient with cognitive impairment is not a reliable historian and family members need to be interviewed. A complete neurological examination and MMSE should be done. In addition, a depression screening test should be performed, because a "pseudodementia" type syndrome occurs in depression in the elderly.

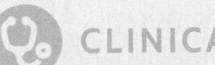
Laboratory tests should be performed to diagnose the cause of dementia. These tests should routinely include a CBC count, erythrocyte sedimentation rate, glucose level, renal and liver function tests, serologic tests for syphilis, vitamin B_{12} and red blood cell (RBC) folate levels, and thyroid function tests. Although not done routinely, blood toxicology tests can detect drug metabolites or heavy metal poisoning.

Neuroimaging studies may include CT and MRI of the brain. The absence of cerebrovascular lesions on CT scanning or MRI is evidence against vascular etiology. The features on CT or MRI that are suggestive of vascular dementia are bilateral multiple infarcts located in the dominant hemisphere and limbic structures, multiple lacunar strokes, or periventricular white matter lesions extending into the deep white matter. PET scans may be useful for differentiating vascular dementia from Alzheimer's disease. Hypoperfusion and hypometabolism can be observed in the frontal lobe, including the cingulate and superior frontal gyri, in patients with vascular dementia; a parietotemporal pattern is observed in patients with Alzheimer's disease. Tests that may be useful for evaluation of stroke and vascular dementia include echocardiography, Holter monitoring, and carotid duplex Doppler scanning.

Specific laboratory tests and neuroimaging studies are available for Alzheimer's disease. On MRI, persons with Alzheimer's disease have a decreased volume of the hippocampus compared with normal controls. On PET scanning, the deposition of beta-amyloid can be found in the brain. On lumbar puncture, the cerebrospinal fluid can demonstrate tau and beta-amyloid proteins. Genetic testing can be done to check for the ApoE gene on chromosome 19, which is associated with Alzheimer's disease.

Treatment

When all physical illnesses have been ruled out and dementia is diagnosed, both nonpharmacological and pharmacological treatments can be used. Medications may be needed to control behavior problems caused by a loss of judgment, increased impulsivity, and confusion. Medications used in dementia include:

- antipsychotics: haloperidol, risperdal, olanzapine
- mood stabilizers: fluoxetine, imipramine, citalopram
- serotoninergic drugs: trazodone, buspirone
- stimulants: methylphenidate.

Certain drugs may be used to slow the rate at which symptoms worsen. These drugs include:

- donepezil (Aricept)
- rivastigmine (Exelon)
- galantamine (Reminyl)
- memantine (Namenda).

Pharmacological approaches involving antipsychotic or sedative medications are often used as first-line treatment in dementia patients. More than 40% of people with dementia in long-term care facilities in the United States are taking antipsychotic drugs. Experts agree that prescription of these medications without attempting nonpharmacological treatment options is of particular concern because of the substantial adverse effects associated with their use. Side effects such as sleepiness, lethargy, falls, and extrapyramidal movement disorders occur with antipsychotic sedating medications.

Behavioral and nonpharmacological approaches are key strategies in the care of the dementia patient. Dementia is commonly the reason for the patient's admission to a long-term care facility. For the patient with dementia, a daily routine that remains stable is important. Having the same caregivers provide the patient with daily care also provides stability. The patient needs familiar items brought from the home environment if transitioning to a long-term care facility. For example, photos can remind the patient of people and places from the individual's past. Likewise, music and artwork that the patient enjoyed provide a sense of constancy.

Reality Orienta.tion. Reality orientation is one of the most widely used management strategies for dealing with people with dementia. It aims to help people with memory loss and disorientation by reminding them of facts about themselves and their environment. It can be used both with individuals and with groups. In either case, people with memory loss are oriented to their environment using a range of materials and activities. This involves consistent use of orientation devices such as signs, labels, calendars, holiday decorations, notices, and other memory aids. Caregivers attempt to bring the patient into the current time. There is debate regarding the efficacy of this approach. Some investigators claim that reality orientation sessions increase people's verbal orientation in comparison with untreated control groups. However, it is also claimed that reality orientation can remind patients of their cognitive deterioration and provoke anxiety.

Validation Therapy. Validation therapy, developed by researcher Naomi Feil, was originated because of studies that showed lack of efficacy of reality orientation. Feil suggested that some of the features associated with dementia, such as retreating into the past, are active strategies on the part of the affected individual to avoid stress, boredom, and loneliness. Feil believes that people with dementia can retreat into an inner reality based on feelings rather than intellect, because they find the present reality too painful. Validation therapists, therefore, attempt to communicate with individuals with dementia by empathizing with the feelings and meanings hidden behind their confused speech and behavior. The caregiver focuses on what is important to the patient and what time period in life was most influential to the patient and uses these memories to motivate the patient. Validation therapists deal with the patient in the time frame that the patient feels comfortable with. If the patient concentrates on past events in life, this is supported. Caregivers assess the patient's reality and work within the patient's world rather than try to reorient the patient to the present. Some investigators assert that validation therapy promotes contentment, results in less negative affect and behavioral disturbance, produces positive effects, and provides the individual with comfort.

Reminiscence Therapy. Reminiscence therapy involves helping a person with dementia to relive past experiences, especially those that might be positive and personally significant, such as family holidays and weddings. This therapy can be used with groups or with individuals. Group sessions tend to use activities such as art and music to provide stimulation.

Reminiscence therapy is seen as a way of increasing levels of well-being and providing pleasure and cognitive stimulation. The therapy also has a great deal of flexibility as it can be adapted to the individual.

Physical Activity and Nutrition. Often, the patient with dementia lacks the initiative to perform physical activities. Caregivers can assist in that role by taking patients on supervised walks. Exercise enhances patient oxygenation, muscle tone, and cardiovascular, gastrointestinal, and mental health. Physical activity is also important for maintenance of the patient's circadian rhythm. For nonambulatory patients, there are some exercise regimens that can be done in a chair. Persons with dementia also need prompting to eat. Because receiving adequate nutrition can be a problem, meals should be prepared consisting of foods easy for the patient to eat. In severe dementia, the patient needs to be fed.

Delirium

Delirium is defined as a transient, usually reversible, cause of cerebral dysfunction. It is manifested by a wide range of neuropsychiatric abnormalities and can be exhibited as a hyperactive or a hypoactive state. For example, drug toxicity often causes impulsive, aggressive delirium behavior, whereas liver failure and renal failure often cause withdrawal and lethargy. Delirium is often mistaken for dementia or depression (see Table 36-4). The clinical hallmarks are decreased attention span and a waxing and waning type of confusion. Hallucinations, delusions, and psychotic behavior are often part of delirium. It is sudden in onset

TABLE 36-4. Differences Between Delirium, Dementia, and Depression			
Features	**Delirium**	**Dementia**	**Depression**
ONSET	Sudden	Gradual	Gradual
COURSE	Fluctuating	Progressive	Progressive
DURATION	Days	Months to years	If untreated, months
CONSCIOUSNESS	Altered level of consciousness	Alert	Alert with possible symptoms of pseudodementia
ATTENTION	Impaired	Normal in early dementia, diminished in late dementia	Alert with possible symptoms of pseudodementia
PSYCHOMOTOR EFFECTS	Increased or decreased	Normal, except in severe dementia can be agitated or retarded	Agitation or retardation
REVERSIBILITY	Fully reversible with treatment	Not reversible	Fully reversible with treatment

and there is usually no apparent inciting event. The patient requires thorough assessment and physical examination to diagnose the reason for delirium. Hospitalization, the postoperative state, electrolyte imbalances, and infection are major causes. Early diagnosis and resolution of symptoms are correlated with the most favorable outcomes.

Delirium has been found in 14% to 56% of elderly patients who are hospitalized. It is present in 10% to 22% of elderly patients at the time of admission, with an additional 10% to 30% of cases developing after admission. Prevalence of postoperative delirium following general surgery is 5% to 10%, and as high as 42% following orthopedic surgery. Delirium has been found in 40% of patients admitted to intensive care units, which commonly have no windows and constant fluorescent lighting that can be disorienting to the elderly patient.

Almost any medical illness, intoxication, or medication can be a risk factor for delirium. Often, delirium is multifactorial in etiology; however, medications are the most common reversible cause. Electrolyte disturbances, metabolic abnormalities, dementia, sleep deprivation, substance abuse, infections, intensive care sensory deprivation, and postoperative states also commonly provoke delirium. Dementia is one of the most consistent risk factors for delirium; underlying dementia is observed in 25% to 50% of patients. The presence of dementia increases the risk of delirium 2 to 3 times. For other risk factors, see Box 36-4.

Pathophysiology

The mechanism of delirium is not fully understood, but studies of delirium focus on the effects of the neurotransmitters acetylcholine, dopamine, and serotonin. It is theorized that decreased levels of acetylcholine are part of the pathogenesis of delirium. In the brain, a reciprocal relationship exists between cholinergic and dopaminergic activities. In delirium, an excess of dopaminergic activity occurs. Other causes of delirium involve disruption of cortisol and beta-endorphin circadian rhythms. This mechanism has been suggested as a possible explanation for delirium caused by exogenous glucocorticoids. Recent studies have suggested a role for inflammatory cytokines, such as interleukin-1 and interleukin-6, in the pathogenesis of delirium. Following a wide range of infectious, inflammatory, and toxic insults, endogenous pyrogen,

---

BOX 36-4. Common Risk Factors for Delirium

Delirium is a state of temporary, transient disorientation or psychotic behavior that can be caused by numerous conditions. The following are the most common conditions associated with delirium:

- alcohol or sedative withdrawal
- cerebrovascular accidents
- closed head injury
- hyperthermia
- hypoxia
- malnutrition
- polypharmacy (particularly in elderly)
- postictal state
- sensory deprivation
- sleep deprivation
- structural lesions of the brain
- unfamiliar environment (mainly in hospitalized elderly)
- use of physical restraints.

METABOLIC CAUSES
- acid-base disturbances
- fluid and electrolyte abnormalities
- hepatic failure
- hypoglycemia
- renal failure
- vitamin deficiency states (especially thiamine and cyanocobalamin)

CARDIOVASCULAR CAUSES
- anemia
- cardiac dysrhythmias

- heart failure
- shock

INFECTIOUS CAUSES
- CNS infections
- human immunodeficiency virus-related brain infections
- pneumonia
- sepsis
- urinary tract infections

DRUG- AND ALCOHOL-INDUCED CAUSES
- illicit drugs, including:
  - alcohol
  - cannabis
  - heroin
  - lysergic acid diethylamide, also known as LSD
  - phencyclidine, also known as PCP
  - substance intoxication.
- medications, including:
  - anticholinergics
  - antiparkinson drugs
  - centrally acting antihypertensives
  - corticosteroids
  - histamine-2 blockers
  - narcotics
  - sedative hypnotics.
- withdrawal from alcohol, opioids, and benzodiazepines

such as interleukin-1, is released from the cells. Head trauma and ischemia, which frequently are associated with delirium, are characterized by brain responses that are mediated by interleukin-1 and interleukin-6. Delirium commonly occurs as a response to infection in the elderly. Clinical studies have found that serotonin is increased in patients with septic delirium.

Clinical Presentation

Delirium always should be suspected when a patient exhibits a sudden deterioration in behavior, cognition, or function, especially in patients who are elderly, demented, or depressed. Delirious patients may have psychotic symptoms such as visual hallucinations or delusions. Some patients with delirium also may become violent, suicidal, or homicidal. Symptoms tend to fluctuate over the course of the day, with some improvement in the daytime and maximum disturbance at night. Reversal of the sleep-wake cycle is common. See Box 36-5 for signs and symptoms of delirium.

In patients with delirium, a careful and complete physical examination, including a mental status examination and neurological examination, is necessary. The clinician should also look for signs of infection. Physical examination is often difficult because patients have difficulty sustaining attention, are disoriented, and have impaired short-term memory and poor insight.

Diagnosis

The diagnosis of delirium is made by the clinical presentation, because no laboratory test can diagnose delirium. Obtaining a thorough history is essential. Delirious patients are unreliable historians, so getting a detailed history from family and caregivers is particularly important. A mini-cognitive test can be administered that asks the patient to draw a clock with a specific time as directed by the examiner. The test can also include a test of the patient's short-term memory by asking the patient to remember three words and then, 5 minutes later, asking the patient to recall them. Other diagnostic instruments are the Delirium Symptom Interview and the Confusion Assessment Method (CAM).

To make an accurate diagnosis, knowledge of the patient's baseline mental status is necessary. The CAM for the Intensive Care Unit (CAM-ICU) offers the clinician the opportunity to identify delirium in critical care patients, especially patients on mechanical ventilation. The CAM-ICU makes use of nonverbal assessments to evaluate the important features of delirium. The *DSM-5* lists specific diagnostic criteria for delirium (see Box 36-6).

Treatment

Components of delirium management include nonpharmacological supportive therapy and pharmacological management.

Nonpharmacological Management. Fluid and nutrition should be provided by the clinician because patients with delirium do not remember to eat or drink. For the patient suspected of having alcohol toxicity or alcohol withdrawal, therapy should include multivitamins, especially thiamine. Environmental modifications that enhance reorientation of the patient should be devised. Memory cues such as a calendar, clocks, and family photos may be helpful. The client should be moved near a window for orientation to daylight. The environment should be stable, quiet, and well-lighted. Family members and staff should explain all procedures, reinforce orientation, and reassure the patient. Sensory deficits should be corrected, if necessary, with eyeglasses and hearing aids. Physical restraints should be avoided. Delirious patients may pull out intravenous lines, climb out of bed, and may not be compliant. Perceptual problems lead to agitation, fear, combative behavior, and wandering. Severely delirious patients require constant observation and should never be left alone or unattended.

Pharmacological Therapy. Delirium that threatens injury to the patient or others should be treated with medications. The most common medications used are antipsychotic drugs such as haloperidol and benzodiazepines such as lorazepam.

Substance Abuse and Addiction

The most common substances of abuse include alcohol, marijuana, cocaine, opiates, amphetamines, and hallucinogens. Although many individuals abuse drugs, not all drug abusers become addicted. Addiction is a compulsive need for and use of a habit-forming substance, such as heroin, nicotine, and alcohol, and is characterized by tolerance and well-defined physiologic symptoms upon withdrawal.

Alcohol, the most commonly used addictive drug, is mainly a CNS depressant. In low doses, alcohol disinhibits the individual, which may lead to out-of-character activities. At higher doses, individuals show irrational thinking, lack of judgment, and absence of motor coordination.

BOX 36-5. Signs and Symptoms of Delirium

The following conditions frequently occur in delirium:

- clouding of consciousness
- difficulty maintaining or shifting attention
- disorientation
- dysarthria
- dysphasia
- fluctuating levels of consciousness
- hallucinations
- illusions
- tremor.

BOX 36-6. Diagnostic Criteria for Delirium

A. A disturbance in attention (i.e., reduced ability to direct, focus, sustain, and shift attention) and awareness (reduced orientation to the environment) is present.

B. The disturbance develops over a short period of time (usually hours to a few days), represents a change from baseline attention and awareness, and tends to fluctuate in severity during the course of a day.

C. An additional disturbance in cognition (e.g., memory deficit, disorientation, language, visuospatial ability, or perception) occurs.

D. The disturbances in Criteria A and C are not better explained by another pre-existing, established, or evolved neurocognitive disorder and do not occur in the context of a severely reduced level of arousal, such as coma.

E. There is evidence from the history, physical examination, or laboratory findings that the disturbance is a direct physiologic consequence of another medical condition, substance intoxication, or withdrawal (i.e., because of a drug of abuse or to a medication), or exposure to a toxin, or is caused by multiple etiologies.

Specify whether:

Substance intoxication delirium: This diagnosis should be made instead of substance intoxication when the symptoms in Criteria A and C predominate in the clinical picture and when they are sufficiently severe to warrant clinical attention.

Substance withdrawal delirium: This diagnosis should be made instead of substance withdrawal when the symptoms of Criteria A and C predominate in the clinical picture and when they are sufficiently severe to warrant clinical attention.

Medication-induced delirium: This diagnosis applies when the symptoms in Criteria A and C arise as a side effect of a medication taken as prescribed.

Delirium caused by another medical condition: There is evidence from the history, physical examination, or laboratory findings that the disturbance is attributable to the physiologic consequences of another medical condition.

Delirium caused by multiple etiologies: There is evidence from the history, physical examination, or laboratory findings that the delirium has more than one etiology (e.g., more than one etiologic medical condition; another medical condition plus substance intoxication or medication side effect).

Specify if:

Acute: lasting a few hours or days
Persistent: lasting weeks or months.

Specify if:

Hyperactive: The individual has a hyperactive level of psychomotor activity that may be accompanied by mood lability, agitation, or refusal to cooperate with medical care.

Hypoactive: The individual has a hypoactive level of psychomotor activity that may be accompanied by sluggishness and lethargy that approaches stupor.

Mixed level of activity: The individual has a normal level of psychomotor activity even though attention and awareness are disturbed. Also includes individuals whose activity level rapidly fluctuates.

(Reprinted with permission from the *Diagnostic and Statistical Manual of Mental Health Disorders,* Fifth Edition. (Copyright 2013). American Psychiatric Association.)

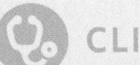 **CLINICAL CONCEPT**

Substance abuse disorder occurs when a person needs alcohol or drug to function normally. Abruptly stopping the substance leads to withdrawal symptoms. Addiction means that a person has a strong urge to use the substance and cannot stop. Tolerance occurs when an individual consistently needs a higher dose of a substance to get the desired effect.

Heroin is a commonly abused opiate that can be injected, ingested, or inhaled. Other drugs of abuse in this category include methadone, morphine, codeine, oxycodone, and fentanyl. Signs of intoxication are diminished respiratory rate and constricted pupils. Acute complications include noncardiogenic pulmonary edema and respiratory failure. Complications of chronic use are primarily infectious and include skin abscess at an injection site, cellulitis, mycotic aneurysms, endocarditis, talcosis, human immunodeficiency virus, and hepatitis. Physiologic and psychological dependence on heroin occurs. Patients can experience withdrawal when they cannot obtain heroin.

Cocaine may be smoked, inhaled, used topically, or injected. Acute cocaine intoxication causes excitation, and the patient often shows agitation, paranoia, tachycardia, tachypnea, hypertension, and diaphoresis. Complications of acute and chronic use can include myocardial ischemia or infarction, stroke, pulmonary edema, and rhabdomyolysis.

Acute intoxication with amphetamines presents with signs of SNS stimulation such as tachycardia and hypertension. Amphetamines cause anorexia, insomnia, and occasionally seizures.

Different hallucinogens present with a variety of organ system effects. Phencyclidine has been known to cause extreme excitation, muscle rigidity, seizures, rhabdomyolysis, and coma.

Prescription drug abuse is common. Narcotics, stimulants, and sedatives are the common prescription drugs of abuse. Deliberate or accidental overdose frequently occurs. Similarly, some over-the-counter medications, such as cough and cold medicines containing dextromethorphan, can also be abused and lead to significant CNS effects.

The abuse of inhalants is increasing across the United States. Abusers, primarily adolescents, inhale chemical vapors from a variety of substances, many of which are common household products. The practice of inhaling these substances is called "huffing." The inhalants give the abuser a euphoric effect, but potential risks include brain damage and death. Some adults also abuse inhalants, particularly nitrites. Adult abusers often inhale substances in order to enhance their sexual experiences. The inhalation of bath salts is becoming a substantial drug abuse problem among teens. Bath salts give the individual a cocaine-like euphoric feeling. The powders sold as "Ivory Snow," "Bliss," "Vanilla Sky," and other brand names contain the ingredient mephedrone, a stimulant that can cause rapid heart rates, seizures, and hallucinations.

The prevalence of substance abuse is difficult to estimate because abusers often do not admit or recognize their habit. Reports indicate that roughly two-thirds of all adults drink alcohol occasionally. Approximately 13% of people in the United States are alcoholics, and 1 person in 5 who uses alcohol for recreational purposes becomes dependent for some period of time. Studies performed in urban emergency departments indicate that up to 20% of patients may have problems with alcohol, with the highest rate in patients who present late at night. Heroin use is on the rise in the U.S. with estimates of heroin users at 750,000. Heavy cocaine use has remained fairly steady since its peak in the late 1980s and early 1990s, with an estimated 600,000 to 700,000 regular users. In rural communities, use of methamphetamine, also known as crystal meth, is on the rise. This drug is easily manufactured from a base ingredient found in over-the-counter cold medications. It is most often abused by those 15 to 25 years old.

Pathophysiology

A dopamine reward system in the brain is hypothesized as a reason for substance abuse.

A specific allele (A1 allele) of the D2 dopamine receptor (DRD2) gene located at 11q23 is associated with addictive behaviors such as alcoholism, drug abuse, smoking, obesity, and compulsive gambling. Studies show that persons with the A1 allele of the DRD2 gene have a diminished number of dopamine receptors and a propensity for addictive behaviors. It is hypothesized that in an effort to compensate for deficiencies in the dopaminergic system, substance abusers may seek to stimulate circuits of the brain involved in behavioral reward and reinforcement. Each drug with abuse potential works on the CNS in a slightly different way (see Table 36-5).

TABLE 36-5. Substance of Abuse and Pathological Mechanism

Drug	Pathophysiologic Mechanism
Alcohol	Psychodepressant
Amphetamines	Psychostimulant
Cocaine	Psychostimulant
Heroin (Opiates)	Psychodepressant/ psychostimulant
Marijuana (THC)	Psychodepressant

Clinical Presentation

Euphoria and sedation are the most common effects of abused drugs. Different kinds of withdrawal symptoms are observed with illicit and prescribed drug abuse.

Alcohol Withdrawal. Many alcoholics experience "the shakes" approximately 12 to 24 hours after their last drink. The shakes are tremors caused by overexcitation of the CNS. These tremors may be accompanied by tachycardia, diaphoresis, anorexia, and insomnia. After 24 to 72 hours, the alcoholic may have seizures. Delirium tremens (DT), which begins 3 to 5 days after the last drink, is characterized by disorientation, fever, tremulousness, and visual hallucinations. This medical emergency should be treated on an inpatient basis.

Opioid Withdrawal. Withdrawal symptoms from opioids may begin just a few hours after their last use, although onset of withdrawal may be delayed in patients abusing long-acting opioids. Along with a strong craving for the drug, opioid withdrawal produces yawning, tears, diarrhea, abdominal cramping, piloerection, and rhinorrhea. Symptoms of withdrawal usually peak around 48 hours and again at 72 hours. Withdrawal usually subsides after 1 week, but some heavily dependent users may have mild symptoms for up to 6 months.

Amphetamine Withdrawal. Amphetamine withdrawal is fairly mild. Patients may complain of depression, increased appetite, abdominal cramping, diarrhea, and headache.

Cocaine and Hallucinogen Withdrawal. Cocaine and hallucinogens do not have a typical withdrawal pattern. These drugs are considered psychologically addicting rather than physically addicting.

Benzodiazepine and Other CNS Depressant Withdrawal. Discontinuing prolonged use or abuse of high doses of CNS depressants can lead to serious withdrawal symptoms such as grand mal seizures. Benzodiazepines are the drug of choice for withdrawal seizures. When BNZ drugs are discontinued after prolonged use, symptoms such as agitation, restlessness, and insomnia are common.

Diagnosis

Individuals interviewed about substance abuse commonly underestimate their consumption and deny their substance abuse. When performing the history, the clinician should question patients about their drug or drugs of choice and the frequency, amount, and method of use. Also, it is important to obtain information about prior detoxifications, concomitant use of other substances, date of first use, and time interval from last use. A short assessment tool for alcohol use is called the CAGE questionnaire (see Box 36-7). A single positive response to the CAGE questions is considered suggestive of an alcohol problem, and 2 or more positive responses indicate the presence of such a problem with a sensitivity and specificity of approximately 90% in most studies.

Several other screening methods exist, with the brief Michigan Alcohol Screening Test the most widely used screen suitable for emergency room use. Another screening tool, the TWEAK screen, has been recommended for use in females (see Box 36-8).

The physical examination should be a complete assessment of the patient, as substance abusers are much less likely to have regular medical care than the general population. In the patient with acute intoxication, a blood and urine toxicology screen for substances of abuse and a blood or breath alcohol level is needed. CBC, serum electrolytes, glucose, blood urea nitrogen, liver enzymes, and serum creatinine are necessary. GI bleeding, anemia, bone marrow suppression, and possible infection are concerns. Complications of cocaine intoxication may require a cardiac or CNS evaluation that may include an ECG and brain CT scan.

Treatment

For opiate addiction, a methadone regimen is commonly administered. Methadone, a synthetic opioid, is used clinically to alleviate opioid dependency. It acts similarly to heroin and morphine, offering very similar effects for a long duration. Oral doses of methadone are used in a clinical setting to stabilize patients and alleviate opioid withdrawal syndrome. Higher doses of

---

BOX 36-7. CAGE Questionnaire

1. Have you ever felt you should **C**ut down on your drinking?
2. Have people **A**nnoyed you by criticizing your drinking?
3. Have you ever felt bad or **G**uilty about your drinking?
4. Have you ever had a drink first thing in the morning to steady your nerves or get rid of a hangover? (**E**ye-opener)?

Scoring: 2 or 3 "yes" answers strongly suggest a problem with alcohol.

(Ewing, J. A. (1984). Detecting alcoholism: the CAGE Questionnaire. *JAMA* 252, 1905–1907.)

BOX 36-8. The TWEAK Questionnaire

The TWEAK Questionnaire involves the following questions:

T olerance (2 points): How many drinks can you hold? (Six or more indicates tolerance.)
W orried (2 points): Have close friends or relatives worried or complained about your drinking in the past year?
E ye openers (1 point): Do you sometimes take a drink in the morning when you first get up?
A mnesia (1 point): Has a friend or family member ever told you about things you said or did while you were drinking that you could not remember?
[K] Cut down (1 point): Do you sometimes feel the need to cut down on your drinking?

Scoring: A 7-point scale is used to score the test. The Tolerance question scores 2 points if (a) the patient reports he or she can hold more than five drinks without falling asleep or passing out, or (b) if it is reported that three or more drinks are needed to feel high. A positive response to the Worry question scores 2 points. A positive response to the last three questions scores 1 point each.

(Russell, M. (1994). New assessment tools for drinking in pregnancy: T-ACE, TWEAK, and others. *Alcohol Health and Research World*, 18(1), 55–61.)

---

methadone can block the euphoric effects of heroin, morphine, and similar drugs. A clinically supervised regimen consisting of a tapered dose of methadone can assist those who are opiate addicted reduce or stop their use of these substances.

Naltrexone is an opioid receptor antagonist used primarily in the management of alcohol dependence and opioid dependence. Naltrexone helps patients overcome urges to abuse opiates by blocking the drugs' euphoric effects. This long-acting antagonist is commonly used as part of a rehabilitation program.

ALERT! Naloxone is a short-acting opioid receptor antagonist that is used in emergency conditions of overdose.

Opioid-receptor antagonists work by modulating the dopaminergic mesolimbic pathway. This area of the brain is theorized to be the major center of reward associated with drugs involved in addiction.

Disulfiram (Antabuse), a drug used to treat chronic alcoholism, allows only partial metabolism of ethanol. Increased levels of serum acetaldehyde concentrations are generated by the partial metabolism of ethanol. High acetaldehyde levels in the bloodstream cause an intense "hangover" type reaction, including headache, nausea, myalgias and postural hypotension. Therefore, if the patient uses alcohol while on disulfiram, he or she becomes intensely ill. The discomfort associated with this syndrome is intended to serve as a negative stimulus, but the reaction may be severe enough to cause hypotension and death. Persons must consent to the use of disulfiram in their rehabilitation and should be clinically monitored.

A patient with an alcohol addiction may require vitamin supplementation with thiamine (200 mg), folic acid (1 mg), and a multivitamin. If the patient develops agitation or tremulousness, short-term use of benzodiazepines may be needed.

All patients with a substance abuse problem require referral to a detoxification clinic for treatment. Substance abuse is a lifelong disease that only can be controlled, not cured. In the detoxification center, treatment initially consists of managing the varied symptoms of withdrawal, which can range from cravings to hallucinations and seizures. Once physical withdrawal is complete, group and individual counseling begins and continues on an inpatient, outpatient, and group support basis with groups such as Alcoholics Anonymous and Narcotics Anonymous.

Chapter Summary

- Statistics show that approximately 26% of the U.S. population suffers from some type of mental illness each year.
- Women and men have the same likelihood of developing mental illness, although women report symptoms and seek treatment more often than men.
- Out of all of those affected by mental illness, only 36% receive treatment.
- The Mini-Mental State Examination is the most commonly used psychiatric test in clinical practice.
- The major neurotransmitters of the brain that are involved in mental illness include serotonin [5-hydroxytryptamine], norepinephrine, dopamine, and GABA.
- A combination of medication and psychotherapy are recommended for most psychiatric disorders.
- Cognitive-behavioral and interpersonal therapy are the most common types of psychotherapeutic treatment.
- Anxiety disorders include GAD, panic attacks, OCD, specific phobias, social anxiety disorder, acute stress disorder, and PTSD.
- MDD is the most common psychiatric disorder in adults and elderly individuals.
- There are various types of antidepressant medications, including SSRIs, TCAs, MAOIs, and SNRIs.
- Antidepressant medications require 3 to 6 weeks to reach therapeutic blood levels.
- Many psychoactive medications have anticholinergic side effects, including dry mouth, blurred vision, tachycardia, constipation, urinary retention, and orthostatic hypotension.
- Schizophrenia is a neurobiological disorder considered a psychosis. A psychosis is an abnormal condition of the mind where the affected person loses touch with reality. The person often suffers from delusions and hallucinations.
- Psychotic symptoms, such as delusions, have been linked to excessive dopamine levels.

- ADHD is the most common psychiatric condition affecting children in the United States. The cause is unknown. Treatment includes psychostimulants such as amphetamines.
- The two main causes of dementia are Alzheimer's disease and vascular disease.
- The characteristics of dementia include amnesia, anomia, agnosia, apraxia, aphasia, and apathy.
- Pharmacological approaches involving antipsychotic or sedative medications are often used as first-line treatment in dementia patients. More than 40% of people with dementia in long-term care facilities in the United States are taking antipsychotic drugs.
- Drugs that enhance acetylcholine neurotransmitters in the brain are used to slow the progression of dementia.
- Delirium is a transient, usually reversible, cause of cerebral dysfunction and is manifested by a wide range of neuropsychiatric abnormalities. Delirium is often caused by drug toxicity, metabolic problems, infection, electrolyte disturbances, renal failure, or liver failure. Delirium is often mistaken for dementia or depression.
- The most common substances of abuse include alcohol, marijuana, cocaine, opiates, amphetamines, and hallucinogens.
- Addiction is a compulsive need for and use of a habit-forming substance characterized by tolerance and well-defined physiologic symptoms upon withdrawal.
- Drug tolerance occurs when a subject's reaction to a specific drug and concentration of the drug is progressively reduced, requiring an increase in concentration to achieve the desired effect.
- Withdrawal symptoms, specific noxious physiologic effects, occur if the addicted individual does not maintain regular use of the drug.
- Alcohol is the most commonly used addictive drug. The CAGE questionnaire is a useful tool in the diagnosis of alcoholism.

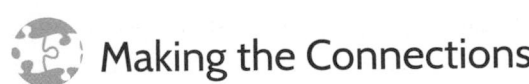 Making the Connections

Disorder and Pathophysiology	Signs and Symptoms	Physical Assessment Findings	Diagnostic Testing	Treatment

GAD | Anxiety is believed to arise from the neurons in the region of the brain called the amygdala. The amygdala analyzes the emotional significance of environmental stimuli and stores emotional memories. Pathways exiting from the amygdala travel to multiple brain structures, including the parabrachial nucleus (resulting in dyspnea and hyperventilation), the dorsomedial nucleus of the vagus nerve (activating the parasympathetic nervous system), and the lateral hypothalamus (resulting in SNS activation). The amygdala also sends neuronal signals to the prefrontal cortex where cognitive experiences of specific anxiety disorders are integrated.

Disorder and Pathophysiology	Signs and Symptoms	Physical Assessment Findings	Diagnostic Testing	Treatment
	Feelings of uncontrollable worry and fear, often accompanied by trembling, hyperventilation, diaphoresis, digestive problems, paresthesias, and palpitations.	Patient may be hyperventilating. Patient may have tachycardia, diaphoresis, and trembling.	Use of GAD assessment tool. Normal CBC, thyroid, cortisol, and serum chemistry lab tests. Normal ECG. Normal toxicology screen.	Benzodiazepine (BNZ), which enhances GABA neuron signals in brain. GABA has an antianxiety effect for use as short-term medication. SSRI, which has antidepressant and antianxiety effects, for long-term management. Buspirone, another antianxiety agent, is an alternative to SSRIs. CBT. Stress management, education, deep breathing, yoga, and meditation.

Panic Disorder | Intense anxiety reactions are associated with increased levels of catecholamines from the locus coeruleus to hippocampus, amygdala, limbic system, and the cerebral cortex. **GABA-BNZ System** Decreased GABA-BNZ binding in the hippocampus and prefrontal cortex. Decreased BNZ binding in the prefrontal cortex and insula. **Neurocircuitry of Fear** Input to the amygdala is modulated by the thalamus and prefrontal cortex. Projections from the amygdala extend to various parts of the brain involved in the fear response, such as the locus coeruleus (arousal), the brainstem (respiratory activation), the hypothalamus-pituitary-adrenal axis (stress response), and the cortex (cognitive interpretation of the stressor).

Disorder and Pathophysiology	Signs and Symptoms	Physical Assessment Findings	Diagnostic Testing	Treatment
	Shortness of breath, palpitations, dizziness, nausea, and feelings of alarm or overwhelming fear.	Hyperventilation, tachycardia, diaphoresis, pallor, and trembling.	Use of GAD assessment tool. Normal CBC, thyroid, cortisol, and serum chemistry lab tests. Normal ECG. Normal toxicology screen.	BNZ, which enhances GABA neuron signals in brain. GABA has an antianxiety effect for use as short-term medication. SSRI, which has antidepressant and antianxiety effects, for long-term management. Buspirone, another antianxiety agent, is an alternative to SSRIs. CBT. Stress management, education, deep breathing, yoga, and meditation.

Continued

Making the Connections—cont'd

Disorder and Pathophysiology	Signs and Symptoms	Physical Assessment Findings	Diagnostic Testing	Treatment
Obsessive Compulsive Disorder | Hyperactivity in some cortical and subcortical regions of the brain; specifically, the orbital frontal cortex, limbic system, thalamus, and caudate. There are abnormalities in serotonergic, dopaminergic and glutamatergic neurotransmission in these regions.				
	Persistent repetitive thoughts and rituals or actions that are inappropriate and may become disabling.	Normal physical exam.	No specific lab tests. Use assessment tool such as Yale-Brown Obsessive Compulsive Scale.	SSRIs keep more serotonin in the synapse of neurons in the brain. Psychotherapy can also be used.
PTSD | Chronic dysregulation of HPA glands. Enhanced SNS responses. Alterations in the medial prefrontal cortex, hippocampus, and visual association cortex.				
	Insomnia and hyperarousal following a life-threatening or traumatic episode. Avoidance of places reminiscent of trauma. Presence of flashbacks or reliving the traumatic experience.	Normal physical exam. If patient is reexperiencing the trauma, patient will have hyperventilation, tachycardia, diaphoresis, and possibly violent impulsive behavior.	No specific lab tests. Use assessment tool PTSD scale.	Clonidine decreases sympathetic neuron activity. Prazosin decreases sympathetic activity. SSRIs prolong serotonin action in the synapses. SNRIs keep serotonin and norepinephrine in the synapse for prolonged time in the brain. Psychotherapy can be used.
MDD | Decreased metabolic activity in the neocortex of the brain and increased activity in the limbic system. Area of the prefrontal cortex with abnormally diminished activity in patients with depression compared with nondepressed individuals. This region has widespread connections with areas that regulate dopamine, norepinephrine, and serotonin.				
	Depressed mood, sadness, loss of pleasure, disturbed sleep patterns, disturbed eating pattern for 2 weeks duration.	Normal physical exam.	Rule out other causes of symptoms. Use an assessment tool such as Zung Self-Rating Depression Scale, Beck Depression Inventory, Raskin Depression Scale, Geriatric Depression Scale, or the Hamilton Rating Scale for Depression. Thyroid-stimulating hormone, cortisol levels are normal. Dexamethasone suppression test.	SSRIs raise serotonin levels in the brain. SNRIs raise both serotonin and norepinephrine levels in the brain. MAOIs prevent breakdown of norepinephrine. TCAs raise norepinephrine levels in the brain. VNS. TMS. Electroconvulsive therapy. Psychotherapy.
Bipolar Disorder | Alterations in the prefrontal cortex and the amygdala. Altered temporal lobe activity.				
	Mood changes such as euphoria, elated mood, or irritable mood alternating with depressive periods.	Normal physical exam.	Lab tests and toxicology screen normal.	Lithium acts as a mood stabilizer. Antiepileptic drugs have mood-stabilizing effects. Psychotherapy is used.

Continued

Making the Connections–cont'd

Disorder and Pathophysiology	Signs and Symptoms	Physical Assessment Findings	Diagnostic Testing	Treatment
Schizophrenia | Increased dopaminergic concentrations in the amygdala and the caudate nucleus. Brain atrophy.				
	Positive symptoms: delusions, hallucinations, disorganized speech, flight of ideas. Negative symptoms: blunted affect, apathy, lack of motivation, lack of speech or spontaneous movement.	Normal physical exam.	Lab tests and toxicology screen normal.	Traditional first-generation antipsychotics such as Haldol are antidopaminergic agents. Second-generation antipsychotic medications such as clozapine or olanzapine are antidopaminergic agents. Psychotherapy is used.
ADHD | Alterations in the neurocircuitry in the prefrontal cortex. Neurotransmitter alterations.				
	Restless, driven, and never tiring in nature. Easily distracted. Both academic and behavioral difficulties.	Normal physical exam.	Normal lab tests and toxicology screen.	Methylphenidate and amphetamine preparations are stimulants that have a paradoxical effect in persons with ADHD. Psychotherapy is used.
Dementia				
Alzheimer's Disease Neurofibrillary tangles, beta-amyloid deposition in brain. Cortical atrophy.				
Vascular Dementia Multiple sites of infarction or single large hemorrhage or ischemia of brain				
	Anomia, amnesia, agnosia, apraxia, apathy. Aphasia. Cognitive impairment. Disorientation to person, place or time.	Poor performance on MMSE. Inability to carry out ADLs independently.	MMSE or clock drawing.	Antiacetyl-cholinesterase drugs allow more acetylcholine to remain in the synapse. Antipsychotics decrease dopaminergic transmission. Attention to nutrition and hydration is needed. Validation therapy, music, art, and reminiscence therapy are utilized.
Delirium | Various causes, such as infection, metabolic imbalances, polypharmacy, or sensory deprivation caused by intensive care unit.				
	Sudden onset of disorientation, confusion, hallucinations, or violent behavior.	Physical exam findings depend on cause of delirium.	Rule out infection and metabolic imbalances. Various lab tests to rule out medical cause of behavior.	Antipsychotic drug such as Haldol has antidopaminergic effects. Attention to nutrition and hydration is required. Reality orientation is needed.

Continued

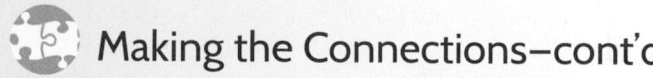

Making the Connections–cont'd

Disorder and Pathophysiology	Signs and Symptoms	Physical Assessment Findings	Diagnostic Testing	Treatment
Substance Abuse and Addiction | Addiction is a compulsive need for and use of a habit-forming substance characterized by tolerance and by well-defined physiologic symptoms upon withdrawal. A dopamine reward system in the brain is hypothesized as a reason for substance abuse. The A1 allele of the DRD2 gene is associated with alcoholism, drug abuse, smoking, obesity, compulsive gambling, and several personality traits.				
	CNS stimulation symptoms or depression symptoms, depending on substance abused.	Findings depend on which substance is abused.	Toxicology screen.	In a detoxification center, treatment initially consists of managing the varied symptoms of withdrawal, which can range from a craving to hallucinations and seizures. Once physical withdrawal is complete, group and individual counseling begins and continues on an inpatient, outpatient, and group support basis.

Bibliography

Arana, A., Wentworth, C. E., Ayuso-Mateos, J. L., & Arellano, F. M. (2010). Suicide-related events in patients treated with antiepileptic drugs. *N Engl J Med*, 363(6), 542–551.

Bateman, J., & Gull, D. (2011). Structural variations in attention-deficit hyperactivity disorder. *Lancet*, 377(9763), 378–379.

Bostwick, J. M. (2010). A generalist's guide to treating patients with depression with an emphasis on using side effects to tailor antidepressant therapy. *Mayo Clin Proceed*, 85(6), 538–550.

Braillon, A. (2013). Care for patients with grave alcohol use disorders. *Lancet*, 382(9908), 1876–1877. doi: 10.1016/S0140-6736(13)62621-5.

Burbach, J. P. (2010). Neuropsychiatric connections of ADHD genes. *Lancet*, 376(9750), 1367–1368.

Caring for older family members with depression. (2011). *Am Fam Phys*, 84(10), 1155–1156.

Chester, J. G., Grande, L. J., Milberg, W. P., et al. (2011). Cognitive screening in community-dwelling elders: performance on the clock-in-the-box. *Am J Med*, 124(7), 662–669.

Cuijpers, P., Beekman, A. T., & Reynolds, C. F., 3rd. (2012). Preventing depression: a global priority. *JAMA*, 307(10), 1033–1034.

Eyre, O., & Thapar, A. (2014). Common adolescent mental disorders: transition to adulthood. *Lancet*, 2014 Jan 15. pii: S0140-6736(13)62633-1. doi: 10.1016/S0140-6736(13)62633-1. Epub ahead of print. No abstract available.

Fagbemi, K. (2011). Q: what is the best questionnaire to screen for alcohol use disorder in an office practice? *Cleveland Clin J Med*, 78(10), 649–651.

Fournier, J. C., DeRubeis, R. J., Hollon, S. D., et al. (2010). Antidepressant drug effects and depression severity: a patient-level meta-analysis. *JAMA*, 303(1), 47–53.

Friedman, M. J. (2010). Prevention of psychiatric problems among military personnel and their spouses. *N Engl J Med*, 362(2), 168–170.

Friedman, R. A. (2012). Grief, depression, and the *DSM-5*. *N Engl J Med*, 366(20), 1855–1857.

Frye, M. A. (2011). Clinical practice. Bipolar disorder—a focus on depression. *N Engl J Med*, 364(1), 51–59.

Guirguis-Blake, J. (2010). Cochrane for clinicians. Aripiprazole vs. other atypical antipsychotics for schizophrenia. *Am Fam Phys*, 81(11), 1335–1336.

Hall, R. C., & Friedman, S. H. (2013). Guns, schools, and mental illness: potential concerns for physicians and mental health professionals. *Mayo Clin Proceed*, 88(11), 1272–1283.

Hamrick, I., Hafiz, R., & Cummings, D. M. (2013). Use of days of the week in a modified Mini-Mental State Exam (M-MMSE) for detecting geriatric cognitive impairment. *J Am Board Fam Med*, 26(4), 429–435. doi: 10.3122/jabfm.2013.04.120300.

Herpertz-Dahlmann, B., Schwarte, R., Krei, M., et al. (2014). Day-patient treatment after short inpatient care versus continued inpatient treatment in adolescents with anorexia nervosa (ANDI): a multicentre, randomised, open-label, non-inferiority trial. *Lancet*, 2014 Jan 16. pii: S0140-6736(13)62411-3. doi: 10.1016/S0140-6736(13)62411-3. Epub ahead of print.

Howes, O. (2014). Cognitive therapy: at last an alternative to antipsychotics? *Lancet*, 2014 Feb 5. pii: S0140-6736(13)

62569-6. doi: 10.1016/S0140-6736(13)62569-6. Epub ahead of print.

Howes, O. D., & Murray, R. M. (2013). Schizophrenia: an integrated sociodevelopmental-cognitive model. *Lancet,* 2013 Dec 5. pii: S0140-6736(13)62036-X. doi: 10.1016/S0140-6736(13)62036-X. Epub ahead of print.

James, B. D., Bennett, D. A., Boyle, P. A., Leurgans, S., & Schneider, J. A. (2012). Dementia from Alzheimer disease and mixed pathologies in the oldest old. *JAMA,* 307(17), 1798–1800.

Jerry, J., Collins, G., & Streem, D. (2012). Synthetic legal intoxicating drugs: the emerging 'incense' and 'bath salt' phenomenon. *Cleveland Clin J Med,* 79(4), 258–264.

Kavan, M. G., Elsasser, G. N., & Barone, E. J. (2012). The physician's role in managing acute stress disorder. *Am Fam Phys,* 86(7), 643–669.

Korsen, N. (2010). Translating a guideline into practice: the USPSTF recommendations on screening for depression in adults. *Am Fam Phys,* 82(8), 891.

Kripke, C. (2010). Risperidone vs. placebo for schizophrenia. *Am Fam Phys,* (9), 1096.

Kuehn, B. M. (2010). Early interventions for schizophrenia aim to improve treatment outcomes. *JAMA,* 304(2), 139–140, 145.

Kuehn, B. M. (2011). Cognitive therapy may aid patients with schizophrenia. *JAMA,* 306(16), 1749.

Kuehn, B. M. (2012). Studies may not provide clear view of antipsychotics. *JAMA,* 307(15), 1572.

Kupfer, D. J., Kuhl, E. A., & Regier, D. A. (2013). Two views on the new *DSM-5: DSM-5:* a diagnostic guide relevant to both primary care and psychiatric practice. *Am Fam Phys,* 88(8), Online.

Kurlansik, S. L., & Ibay, A. D. (2012). Seasonal affective disorder. *Am Fam Phys,* 86(11), 1037–1041.

Libman, H., & Trivedi, N. S. (2012). Update: a 60-year-old woman with mild memory impairment: review of mild cognitive impairment. *JAMA,* 307(17), 1858.

Lin, K. W., & Lam, C. (2010). Screening for depression in adults. *Am Fam Phys,* 82(8), 985–986.

Lyketsos, C. G. (2012). Prevention of unnecessary hospitalization for patients with dementia: the role of ambulatory care. *JAMA,* 307(2), 197–198.

Marcantonio, E. R. (2012). Postoperative delirium: a 76-year-old woman with delirium following surgery. *JAMA,* 308(1), 73–81.

Mayeux, R. (2010). Clinical practice. Early Alzheimer's disease. *N Engl J Med,* 362(23), 2194–2201.

McClellan, J., & King, M. C. (2010). Genomic analysis of mental illness: a changing landscape. *JAMA,* 303(24), 2523–2524.

McDowell, A. K., Lineberry, T. W., & Bostwick, J. M. (2011). Practical suicide-risk management for the busy primary care physician. *Mayo Clin Proceed,* 86(8), 792–800.

McKhann, G. M. (2011). Changing concepts of Alzheimer disease. *JAMA,* 305(23), 2458–2459.

Mitchell, S. L., Teno, J. M., Kiely, D. K., et al. (2012). Effect of telephone-administered vs face-to-face cognitive behavioral therapy on adherence to therapy and depression outcomes among primary care patients: a randomized trial. *JAMA,* 307(21), 2278–2285.

Mitka, M. (2012). CMS seeks to reduce antipsychotic use in nursing home residents with dementia. *JAMA,* 308(2), 119, 121.

Morrison, A. P., Turkington, D., Pyle, M., et al. (2014). Cognitive therapy for people with schizophrenia spectrum disorders not taking antipsychotic drugs: a single-blind randomised controlled trial. *Lancet,* 2014 Feb 5. pii: S0140-6736(13)62246-1. doi: 10.1016/S0140-6736(13)62246-1. Epub ahead of print.

Newman, R. G. (2014). Prescription opioid dependence: the clinical challenge. *JAMA Psych,* 71(3), 338.

Norris, D., & Clark, M. S. (2012). Evaluation and treatment of the suicidal patient. *Am Fam Phys,* 85(6), 602–605.

Okie, S. (2011). Confronting Alzheimer's disease. *N Engl J Med,* 365(12), 1069–1072.

Pelsser, L. M., Frankena, K., Toorman, J., et al. (2011). Effects of a restricted elimination diet on the behaviour of children with attention-deficit hyperactivity disorder (INCA study): a randomised controlled trial. *Lancet,* 377(9764), 494–503.

Petersen, R. C. (2011). Clinical practice. Mild cognitive impairment. *N Engl J Med,* 364(23), 2227–2234.

Phillips, R. L., Jr., Miller, B. F., Petterson, S. M., & Teevan, B. (2011). Better integration of mental health care improves depression screening and treatment in primary care. *Am Fam Phys,* 84(9), 980.

Querfurth, H. W., & LaFerla, F. M. (2010). Alzheimer's disease. *N Engl J Med,* 362(4), 329–3244.

Quinlan, J. D., Guaron, M. R., Deschere, B. R., & Stephens, M. B. (2010). Care of the returning veteran. *Am Fam Phys,* 82(1), 43–49.

Rosenheck, R. A., Krystal, J. H., Lew, R., et al. (2011). Long-acting risperidone and oral antipsychotics in unstable schizophrenia. *N Engl J Med,* 364(9), 842–851.

Roy-Byrne, P., Craske, M. G., Sullivan, G., et al. (2010). Delivery of evidence-based treatment for multiple anxiety disorders in primary care: a randomized controlled trial. *JAMA,* 303(19), 1921–1928.

Schwartz, P. J. (2011). Bipolar disorder—a focus on depression. *N Engl J Med,* 364(16), 1581–1582.

Shultz, E., & Malone, D. A., Jr. (2013). A practical approach to prescribing antidepressants. *Cleveland Clin J Med,* 80(10), 625–631.

Silove, D., & Ward, P. B. (2014). Challenges in rolling out interventions for schizophrenia. *Lancet,* 2014 Mar 4. pii: S0140-6736(14)60085-4. doi: 10.1016/S0140-6736(14)60085-4. Epub ahead of print.

Simmons, B. B., Hartmann, B., & Dejoseph, D. (2011). Evaluation of suspected dementia. *Am Fam Phys,* 84(8), 895–902.

Smith, T., Weston, C., & Lieberman, J. (2010). Schizophrenia (maintenance treatment). *Am Fam Phys,* 82(4), 338–339.

Spoelhof, G. D., Davis, G. L., & Licari, A. (2011). Clinical vignettes in geriatric depression. *Am Fam Phys,* 84(10), 1149–1154.

Unwin, B. K., Goodie, J., Reamy, B. V., & Quinlan, J. (2013). Care of the college student. *Am Fam Phys,* 88(9), 596–604.

Vieweg, W. V., Hasnain, M., & Pandurangi, A. K. (2012). Coordinated medical and psychiatric care in schizophrenia. *Am J Med,* 125(3), 219–220.

Viron, M., Baggett, T., Hill, M., & Freudenreich, O. (2012). Schizophrenia for primary care providers: how to contribute to the care of a vulnerable patient population. *Am J Med,* 125(3), 223–230.

Widera, E. W., & Block, S. D. (2012). Managing grief and depression at the end of life. *Am Fam Phys,* 86(3), 259–264.

Wimbiscus, M., Kostenko, O., & Malone, D. (2011). MAO inhibitors: risks, benefits, and lore. *Cleveland Clin J Med,* 77(12), 859–882.

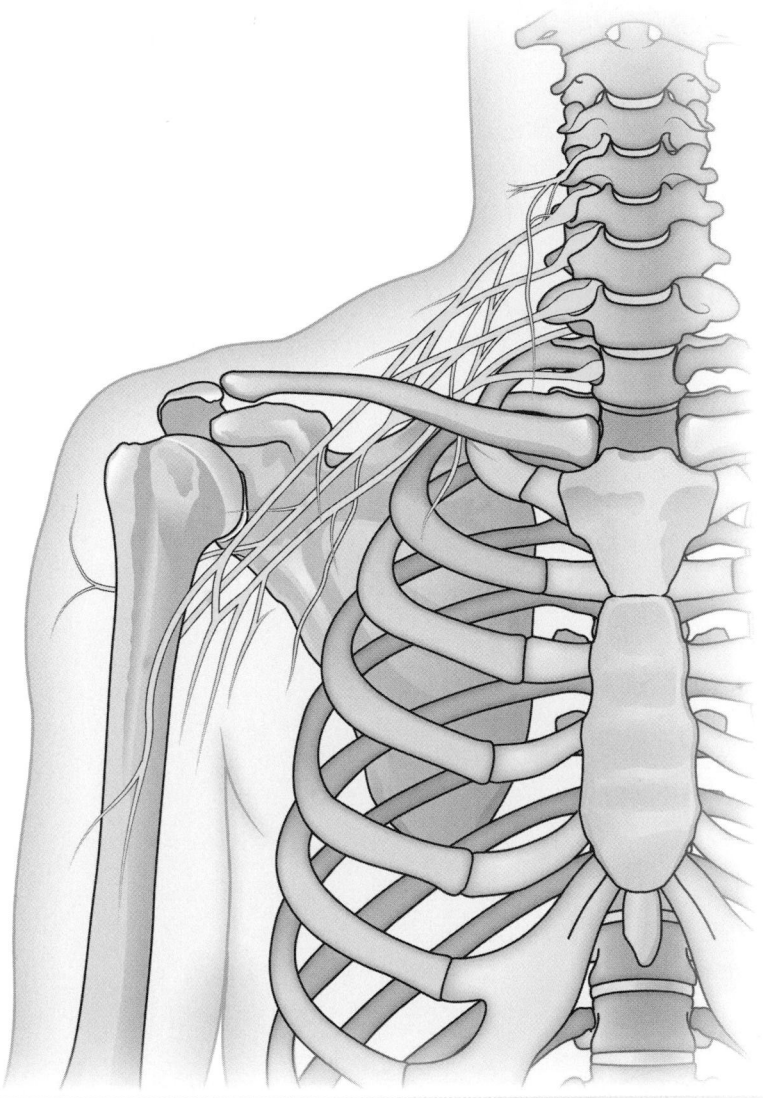

Chapters

MUSCULOSKELETAL DISORDERS

Musculoskeletal Trauma

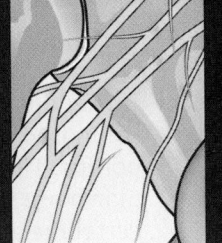

Key Terms

ABCDE of trauma assessment

Adhesive capsulitis

Avascular necrosis (AVN)

Basic multicellular unit (BMU)

Bursa

Callus

Compartment syndrome

Crepitus

Epiphyses

Homans' sign

Kyphosis

Lateral epicondylitis

Malunion

Nonunion

Open reduction and internal fixation (ORIF)

Osteoblasts

Osteoclasts

Osteoprogenitor cells

Pes cavus

Pes planus

Plantar fasciitis

RICE therapy

Temporal mandibular joint (TMJ)

Valgus

Varus

Trauma causes more than 180,000 deaths per year in the United States. It is the leading cause of death for those aged 1 to 44 years and causes more years of lost productivity before age 65 years than coronary artery disease, cancer, and stroke combined. Musculoskeletal disorders, including those acquired from traumatic events, are commonly managed in the outpatient setting. In the United States, 5.6 million fractures occur per year, corresponding to a 2% incidence. Although most musculoskeletal disorders are not life-threatening, they are a frequent cause of work disability and productivity losses in industrialized countries.

Epidemiology

Motor vehicle-related accidents, work-related injuries, sports activities, and fractures related to osteoporosis are common causes of musculoskeletal trauma. These injuries occur frequently, result in significant disability, and consume a major portion of health-care resources. According to the Centers for Disease Control and Prevention (CDC), there were 180,000 injury-related deaths in the United States in 2010. Motor vehicle accidents caused more than 35,000 of the injury-related deaths, and falls caused approximately 27,000 deaths. In 2010, falls among older adults cost the U.S. health-care system $30 billion in direct medical costs, and motor vehicle-related deaths and injuries cost more than $90 billion.

Basic Concepts of the Musculoskeletal System

The musculoskeletal system includes the muscles and bones of the skeleton, including the cartilage, ligaments, and tendons. Muscle and bone provide the framework for body shape and work together to accomplish controlled, precise movements. Contracting muscle fibers use the skeleton for stability and leverage to achieve different postures, positions, and movements.

Bones

The 206 bones in the adult body perform the following five main functions:

1. Structural support of the body: The skeletal system provides structural support for the entire body. Individual bones or groups of bones provide a framework for the attachment of soft tissues.
2. Storage of minerals: Bone is composed of 65% calcium hydroxyapatite, a mixture of mainly calcium and phosphorus, and 35% organic matrix, which includes osteoprogenitor cells, osteoblasts, osteocytes, and collagen. Bone stores 99% of the body's calcium, 85% of the body's phosphorus, and 65% of the body's magnesium and sodium.
3. Production of blood cells: Bone marrow produces red blood cells (RBCs), white blood cells (WBCs), and platelets.
4. Protection of body organs: The skeleton surrounds the soft tissues and organs and helps to protect them from impact injuries.
5. Provide leverage and movement: Many bones function as levers that can change the strength and direction of the forces generated by muscles.

Bone Structure

The skeleton contains two forms of bone: cortical, which is solid, dense bone; and trabecular, also called cancellous, which is nonsolid bone. Trabecular bone is composed of a meshwork of bone that makes the bone porous. The proportion of interior cortical and trabecular bone varies with each bone. The wrist, hip, and vertebrae are composed primarily of trabecular bone.

Bone Development and Growth

Osteogenesis, or bone growth, begins at about 6 weeks after fertilization, and portions of the skeleton continue to grow until about the age of 25 years. Most bones originate as hyaline cartilage; the cartilage is gradually converted to bone through a process called ossification. Bone growth begins at the center of the cartilage. As bones enlarge, bone growth activity shifts to the ends of the bones called **epiphyses**, also called growth plates, which results in an increase in bone length.

There are different types of bone cells:

- **Osteoblasts:** These bone-forming cells secrete osteoid, which forms the bone matrix. They also begin mineralization and are unable to divide.
- Osteocytes: These are mature osteoblasts that maintain metabolism and nutrient and waste exchange; they are unable to divide.
- **Osteoclasts:** These function in resorption and degradation of existing bone, the opposite of osteoblasts.
- **Osteoprogenitor cells:** These are immature cells that differentiate into osteoblasts. These do divide.

Bone Physiology

Osteoblasts and osteoclasts act together and are considered the functional unit of bone called the **basic multicellular unit (BMU)** (see Fig. 37-1). The skeleton grows and enlarges in the process termed modeling, where osteoblastic activity predominates.

Once the bone has reached maturity, breakdown and renewal is caused by osteoclasts in a process called remodeling. Osteoclasts adhere to bone and break it down through acidification and proteolytic enzymes. As osteoclasts leave the site, osteoblasts move in to cover the excavation site and begin the process of new bone formation by secreting osteoid, which is eventually mineralized into bone. The processes of bone formation and resorption occur together, and their balance determines the skeletal mass. In adults, approximately 1 million BMUs are active at one time, causing the remodeling of 10% of the skeleton annually. Peak bone mass is achieved in early adulthood, between ages 30 and 35 years. Bone mass is influenced by many factors, including nutrition, physical activity, age, hormonal status, and vitamin D receptors. Beginning at age 30 or so, the amount of bone resorbed by the osteoclasts exceeds that which is formed by osteoblasts, resulting in a steady decrease in bone mass with age.

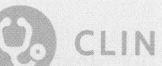 **CLINICAL CONCEPT**

Moderate amounts of physical activity and weight-bearing activities are essential to stimulate bone growth and maintain adequate bone strength.

Skeletal Muscle

Skeletal muscles are composed of tens of thousands of individual muscle fibers, which are arranged in bundles called fascicles. Each fascicle contains approximately 10 to 30 muscle fibers encased in connective tissue called endomysium. Each muscle fiber is made up of myofibrils that are arranged parallel to

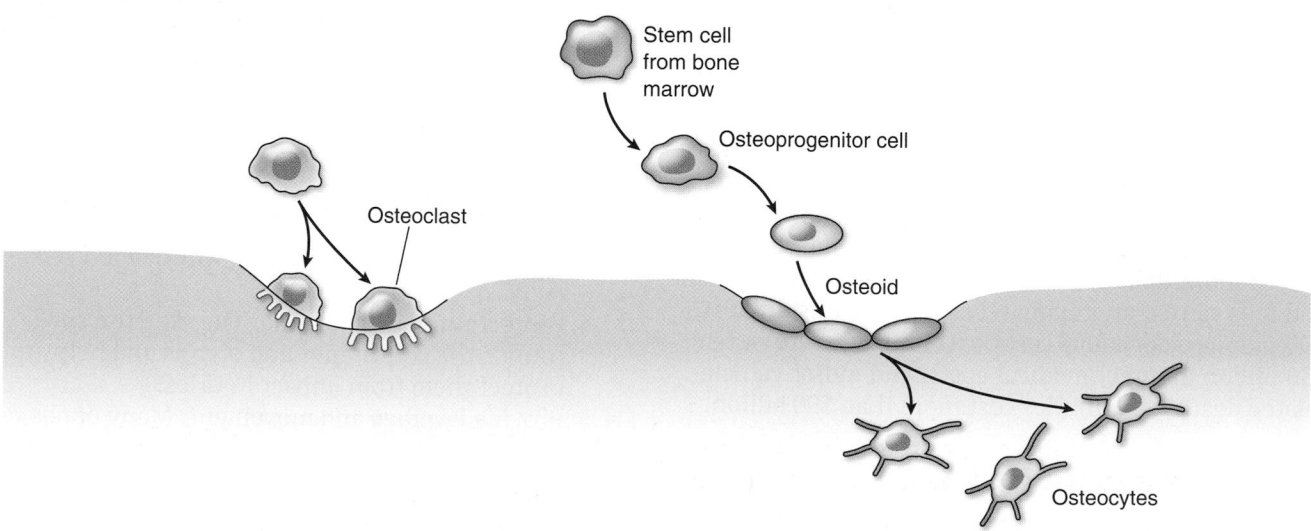

FIGURE 37-1. Bone modeling and remodeling. Bone dynamics encompass continual formation and deterioration (resorption) of bone matrix. The interaction of osteoblasts, osteoclasts, and osteocytes is referred to as a BMU.

each other. Each myofibril consists of sarcomeres, the contractile units of skeletal muscle, which consist of thin and thick filaments that slide over one another to cause contraction of the muscle. The thin filaments are made of the protein actin, whereas the thick filaments are made of the protein myosin. Protein nutrition is important for the development of skeletal muscle.

Skeletal muscle is under voluntary control of the somatic nervous system. Skeletal muscle can become hypertrophied when worked against high resistance. Conversely, muscle can become atrophied if immobile for long periods. Also, loss of neurological stimulation, nutrients, or blood supply can cause atrophy.

 CLINICAL CONCEPT

Casting or immobilization of a bone for a lengthy period of time can cause atrophy of surrounding muscle.

Tendons and Ligaments

Tendons and ligaments are made of tough fibrous connective tissue, parallel arrays of collagen fibers that are closely packed together. Tendons attach muscles to bone and transmit load from muscle to bone, resulting in joint motion. Ligaments attach bone to bone and augment mechanical stability of a joint. Common sites of tendons include:

- rotator cuff of the shoulder
- insertion of the wrist extensors and flexors at the elbow
- patellar and popliteal tendons and iliotibial band at the knee
- posterior tibial tendon in the leg
- Achilles tendon at the heel.

Tendons are subject to many types of injuries. There are various forms of overuse tendon injuries, called tendinopathies. These types of injuries generally result in inflammation and degeneration or weakening of the tendons, which may eventually lead to tendon rupture. Rupture of a tendon requires a complex, prolonged healing process and usually requires surgical intervention.

Alternatively, ligaments connect bones to other bones to form a joint. Capsular ligaments that act as mechanical reinforcements are part of the articular capsule that surrounds synovial joints. Extracapsular ligaments join together and provide joint stability. Cruciate ligaments occur in pairs. Ligaments can gradually lengthen when under tension and return to their original shape when the tension is removed. However, when stretched past a certain point or for a prolonged period of time, they cannot retain their original shape. Like tendons, ligaments can rupture; this also requires surgical intervention. There are

many ligaments throughout the body, but some of the most vulnerable ligaments surround the knee, including the cruciate ligaments, collateral ligaments, and patellar ligament.

When injured, most ligaments heal by a process that is similar to scar formation. Unlike healthy ligaments, healed ligaments consist of a hypertrophic mass of type III collagen. This immature collagen is characterized by smaller diameter fibrils, which result in a mechanically inferior structure compared with normal. A healed ligament often fails to provide adequate joint stability, which can lead to reinjury, a chronically lax joint, or progression to degenerative joint disease. Ligament injuries sometimes require surgical intervention.

Basic Pathophysiologic Concepts of Musculoskeletal Trauma

Musculoskeletal trauma can involve bone fracture, soft tissue injury, skeletal muscle injury, and neurovascular damage. Bone and muscle injury can cause immobility, serious complications, and lasting disability if the healing process is hindered. With bone fracture, soft tissue, and skeletal muscle injury, there is a succession of distinct stages of healing.

Sprains and Strains

Sprains and strains are common injuries that have similar signs and symptoms, but involve different parts of the musculoskeletal system. A sprain is an overstretching of tendons and ligaments with possible tear. The most common location for a sprain is in the ankle. A sprain occurs in response to a quick twist or pull of the muscle. It can be caused by a force that displaces a joint from its normal alignment. Bruising, swelling, instability, and painful movement are common symptoms experienced after a sprain occurs.

There are three grades of sprains:

- Grade I: mild injuries where there is no tearing of the ligament and no lost joint function, although there may be tenderness and slight swelling.
- Grade II: caused by a partial tear in the ligament, these sprains are characterized by obvious swelling, extensive bruising, pain, difficulty bearing weight, and reduced function of the joint.
- Grade III: caused by complete tearing of the ligament where there is severe pain, loss of joint function, widespread swelling and bruising, and the inability to bear weight; have symptoms similar to those of bone fractures.

Strains often occur in the lower back and in the hamstring muscle and result from overuse of muscles, improper use of the muscles, or as the result of injury in another part of the body when the body compensates for pain by altering the way it moves. Pain, weakness, and muscle spasms are common symptoms experienced after a strain occurs.

Muscle Contusions

A bruise, or muscle contusion, can result from a fall or from contact with a hard surface, a piece of equipment, or another player while participating in sports. A bruise results when muscle fiber and connective tissue are crushed; torn blood vessels may cause a bluish appearance. Most bruises are minor, but some can cause more extensive damage and complications.

Bone Fractures

Bone is routinely subjected to a variety of loading forces: tension, compression, bending, torsion, and shear. Usually, these forces are within normal physiologic parameters. When forces exceed physiologic parameters or when a bone abnormality exists, fracture may occur. A fracture is any disruption, complete or incomplete, in the continuity of a bone. There are several common types of fracture (see Table 37-1). Information concerning the mechanism of injury can often help to identify the type of fracture sustained and guide initial treatment until radiological evaluation is obtained.

Soft Tissue Injury

Soft tissue injuries can occur alongside bone fractures, but they can also happen in isolation. The two types of soft tissue, contractile and inert, assist in differentiating the exact site of injury. Contractile tissue includes the structures involved in muscle contraction: the muscle belly, bony insertion, and tendon. Active contraction and passive stretching in the opposite direction will elicit pain if the contractile tissue has been injured. In contrast, inert tissue does not take part in muscle contraction, but plays a supportive role in muscle functioning. Inert tissue includes the joint capsules, ligaments, bursae, fasciae, dura mater, and nerve roots.

To identify inert tissue injuries, clinicians can use clinical signs and symptoms to isolate the structures involved. Generally, passive stretching provokes pain in an inert tissue injury. However, there may also be swelling and erythema, joint instability, weakness, limited motion, and diminished deep tendon reflexes present.

Neurovascular Injury

When musculoskeletal injury occurs, it is important to identify if there is a concomitant neurovascular injury as well. Damage to the brain, spinal cord, nerve roots, and peripheral nerves can cause irreversible dysfunction if left untreated. Injury to the neurological system can cause a loss or decrease in the level of consciousness (LOC),

weakness or paralysis, pain, and paresthesias, as well as other sensory deficits.

When soft tissue and bone are damaged, the integrity of the vascular system may also be compromised, leading to hemorrhage, hematoma formation, and ischemia of tissue and organs. Although it is vital to identify neurovascular injuries during the initial assessment, they may also occur later on in the later stages of healing, which is why it is imperative to routinely assess neurovascular integrity with any type of musculoskeletal injury throughout the course of treatment.

> ## CLINICAL CONCEPT
> Neurovascular integrity should be frequently assessed in an area of musculoskeletal injury. Distal blood flow, pulses, and sensation should be assessed.

Bone Healing

Fracture healing takes place through five stages:

1. Fracture and inflammatory phase: In the inflammatory phase, bleeding initially occurs between the edges of fractured bone, and a hematoma develops during the first few hours and days. Inflammation in the area causes vascular permeability and the attraction of WBCs to the area. Macrophages, monocytes, lymphocytes, and polymorphonuclear WBCs infiltrate the bone area.
2. Granulation tissue formation: In the next phase of healing, fibroblasts are attracted to the area of injury and there is a growth of vascular tissue. Nutrient and oxygen supply during this early process is significant. This stage lasts approximately 2 weeks.
3. Callus formation: During this phase of healing, a **callus** is formed, which consists of osteoblasts and chondroblasts in granulation tissue. These cells synthesize the extracellular organic matrix of woven bone and cartilage, producing newly formed mineralized bone within 4 to 16 weeks.
4. Lamellar bone deposition: This fourth phase is a strengthening phase where ossification is beginning. The meshlike callus of woven bone is replaced by sheets (lamellae) of mineralized bone that are organized parallel to the axis of the bone and are mechanically stronger than the bone of a callus.
5. Remodeling: The final phase involves remodeling of the bone at the site of the healing fracture by osteoclasts and osteoblasts. The formation is sculpted and refined by the mechanical stresses imposed on the bone. Adequate strength commonly occurs in 3 to 6 months.

TABLE 37-1. Types of Fracture

Type	Description	Type	Description
Closed (Complete)	A fracture in which bone fragments separate completely	Incomplete	A fracture in which the bone fragments are still partially joined

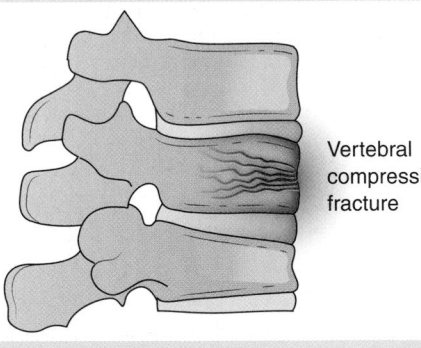

Closed fracture

Intervertebral disc
Vertebral compression fractures
Intervertebral disc

Type	Description	Type	Description
Open (Compound)	A fracture of bone that protrudes to the outside of the body	Compression	A fracture that consists of the crushing of cancellous bone

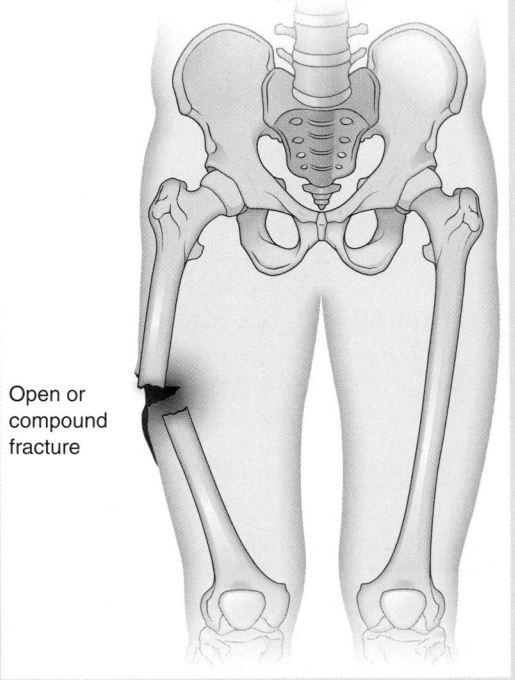

Open or compound fracture

Vertebral compression fracture

Continued

TABLE 37-1. Types of Fracture–cont'd

Type	Description	Type	Description
Transverse	A fracture where parts of the bone are separated but close to each other	Stress fracture	A failure of one cortical surface of the bone, often caused by repetitive activity

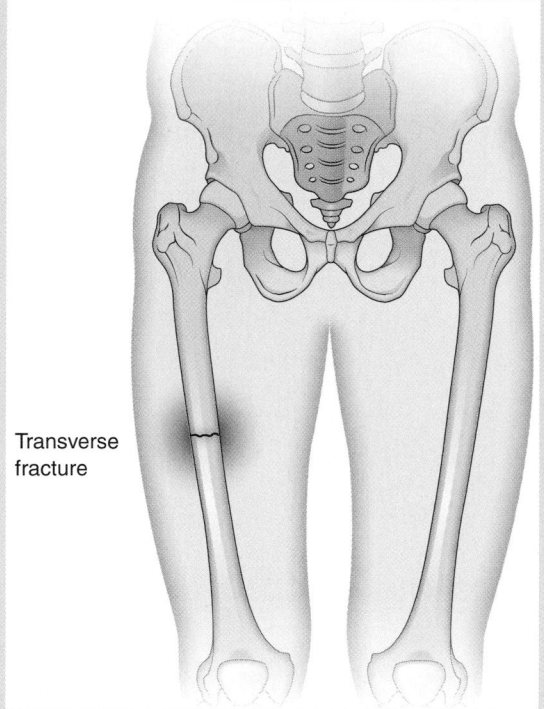

Transverse fracture

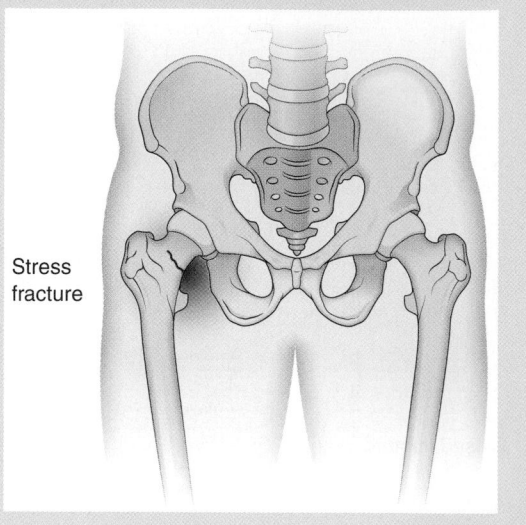

Stress fracture

Type	Description	Type	Description
Comminuted	A fracture with more than one fracture line and more than two bone fragments that may be shattered or crushed	Avulsion	Separation of a small fragment of bone at the site of attachment of a ligament or tendon

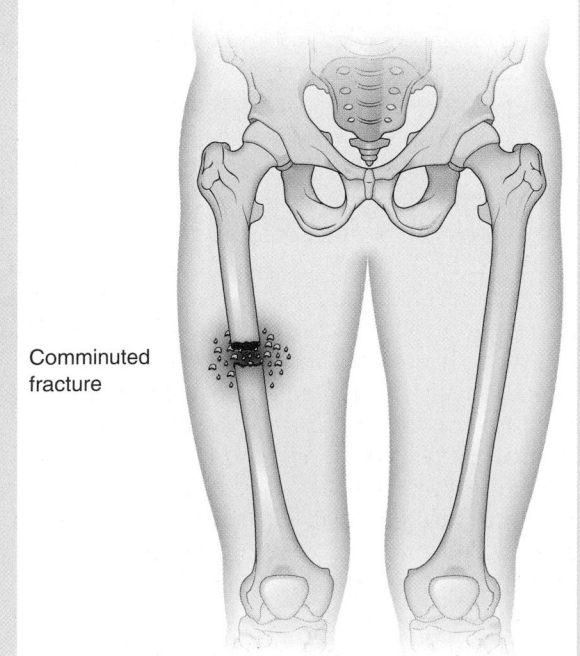

Comminuted fracture

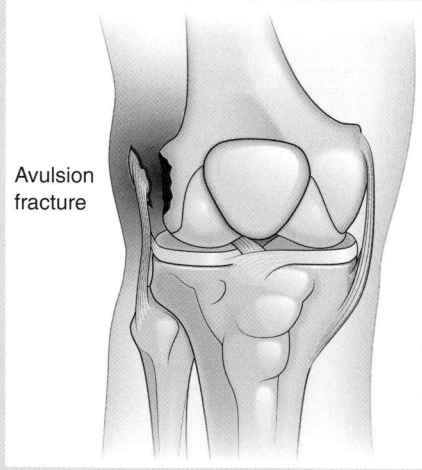

Avulsion fracture

TABLE 37-1. Types of Fracture–cont'd

Type	Description	Type	Description
Greenstick	An incomplete break in the bone with the intact side of the cortex flexed (one side is broken and the other is bent); usually seen in children	Impacted	A fracture in which one part of the fracture is compressed into an adjacent part of the fracture

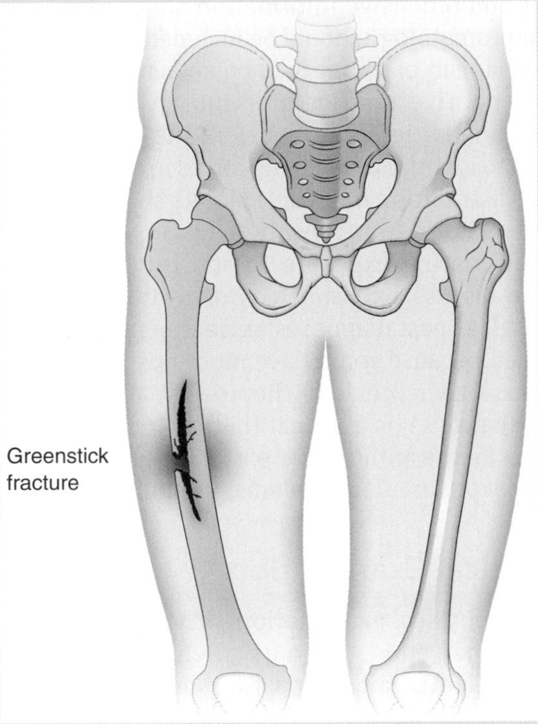

Greenstick fracture

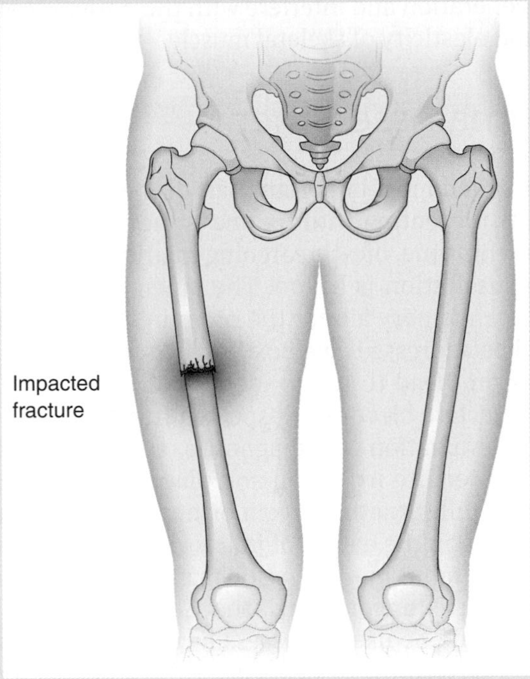

Impacted fracture

Some factors that influence fracture healing include patient age, medication use, nicotine use, and nutrition. Adequate nutrition, especially calcium intake, assists in bone healing. Nicotine delays the healing process. After bone has healed sufficiently, weight-bearing builds bone strength. Other factors that affect fracture healing include the type of fracture, degree of trauma, systemic and local disease, and infection.

CLINICAL CONCEPT

The use of anti-inflammatory or cytotoxic medication such as steroids or immunosuppressive agents during bone's healing process can alter the inflammatory response and inhibit healing.

CLINICAL CONCEPT

After fracture, a bone callus is sufficiently mineralized to show up on x-ray within 6 weeks in adults.

Skeletal Muscle Healing

Skeletal muscle is in a constant state of regeneration, which is heightened in response to injury. When muscle fibers are damaged, several mechanisms work simultaneously to regenerate injured tissue. Initially the inflammation reaction causes the attraction of WBCs to the area of injury. This stage of healing requires an adequate blood supply of the injured area. If blood supply has been significantly damaged, regeneration cannot take place until new blood vessels penetrate the area.

Regeneration of single muscle fibers or entire muscles can then occur with activation of muscle stem cells called satellite cells, which migrate to the area of injury. This process usually takes place within 18 hours of the injury. The muscle stem cells differentiate into muscle fiber cells called myocytes. Within each myocyte, there are bundles of myofibrils that are composed of sarcomeres. There are thick and thin filaments within the sarcomeres of myocytes called actin and myosin; these filaments are the structures involved in muscle contraction. Myoblasts that do not form muscle fibers dedifferentiate back into satellite cells and remain adjacent to a muscle.

The extent of injury to nerves and blood vessels has a clear effect on the maintenance of neurovascular control and how quickly the damaged area can obtain nutrients. Muscle histology is also a factor and can change after injury, as there are fewer numbers of muscle fibers present, with a subsequent reduction in muscle mass. Repaired muscle is not as strong as it was before it was injured, although it may be able to contract just as quickly. Muscle may also heal with fibrous scar tissue instead of with new muscle fibers. Scar tissue is a normal part of the healing process for many injuries, but can obstruct muscle regeneration and interfere with the normal contraction and elasticity of skeletal muscle.

Trauma Assessment

The first and most important part of the assessment of patients presenting with trauma is the primary survey. During this time, life-threatening injuries are identified and resuscitation is begun. The mnemonic **ABCDE** is used as a memory aid for the order in which problems should be addressed (see Box 37-1). Assessment should move from head to toe to identify all wounds and to manage active bleeding. Suspected fractures need immediate evaluation with diagnostic tests, whereas open fractures require irrigation and placement of a sterile dressing while awaiting urgent orthopedic consultation. Depending on the extent of injury, prophylactic antibiotics and tetanus immunization may be administered. If the patient is unconscious, the Glasgow Coma Scale (GCS) should be used to assess level of consciousness (LOC). After treating associated life-threatening injuries, the clinician should perform a thorough secondary survey while obtaining information about the mechanism of the injury and the patient's health history.

Health History

The health history includes information about the individual's age, gender, ethnicity, occupation, current and previous health status, nature of the problem that prompted the individual to seek care, and related effects or changes in the areas of mobility, strength, and activities of daily living. Past medical and surgical history should be obtained along with medications taken on a regular basis, including over-the-counter supplements and herbal therapies. Many medications affect musculoskeletal health: long-term use of steroids can lead to osteoporosis and muscle weakness, and anticoagulant drugs may cause bleeding disorders that contribute to such conditions as hemarthrosis. It is also important to obtain information on any past or present allergies.

Comprehensive information about musculoskeletal symptomatology should be included (see Box 37-2). The mechanism of injury may be an acute event or related to repetitive injuries or trauma. Asking the patient about activities directly before the onset of injury can help to identify the loading forces involved. The number and distribution of involved joints should also be noted. Travel destinations within the past year can be helpful in evaluating exposure to specific diseases, such as Lyme disease. Exposure to sexually transmitted diseases as well as past diagnoses or treatment should be ascertained because some have musculoskeletal manifestations. Other previous therapeutic measures, such as occupational or physical therapy, previous diagnostic tests, joint aspiration, or past injuries related to neurological or vascular problems, should be identified.

Physical Examination

In the physical examination, first note general appearance, body build, contours, alignment, and symmetry. The patient's gait and posture should also be described (see Fig. 37-2).

BOX 37-1. ABCDEs of Acute Trauma Assessment

With major trauma, the following lifesaving measures are instituted first:

- **A**irway with cervical spine protection
- **B**reathing and ventilation
- **C**irculation and hemorrhage control
- **D**isability and neurological evaluation
- **E**xposure and environmental control.

(Source: Initial assessment and treatment with the Airway, Breathing, Circulation, Disability, Exposure (ABCDE) approach. (2012). *Int J Gen Med*, 5, 117–121. Published online Jan 31, 2012. doi: 10.2147/IJGM.S28478.)

BOX 37-2. Signs and Symptoms of Musculoskeletal Trauma

When performing an assessment on a patient with suspected musculoskeletal trauma, make sure to assess for the following:

- color
- deformity
- joint clicking (crepitus)
- joint instability
- joint stiffness
- joint swelling
- muscle strength, 0/5 to 5/5
- pain on a scale of 0–10, with 0 being no pain and 10 being the worst pain imaginable
- paresthesias
- pulse strength
- radiation of pain
- ROM
- sensation
- swelling
- tenderness
- wounds/wound drainage.

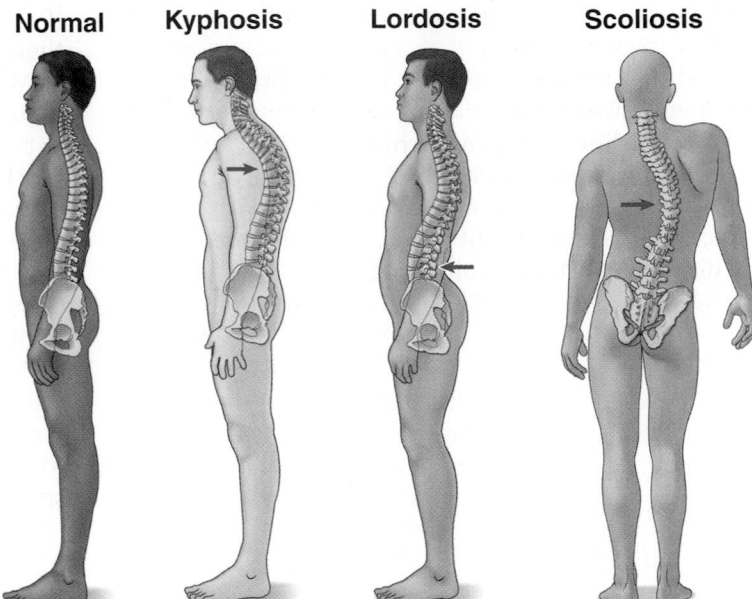

Normal **Kyphosis** **Lordosis** **Scoliosis**

FIGURE 37-2. Types of spine curvature.

Guided by the history, the physical examination helps to distinguish between mechanical problems, soft tissue injury or disease, and inflammatory or noninflammatory joint disease or bone fracture. Sensation should be tested using perception of sharp or dull throughout the dermatomes. Pain or paresthesias caused by irritation of a spinal nerve is exhibited in the corresponding area of dermatome. Paying special attention to the injured tissue, with a comparison of sensation in a noninjured area, can be helpful in ascertaining whether a sensory deficit exists.

Muscle girth should be measured for symmetry to detect atrophy, which indicates a chronic etiology. Assess deep tendon reflexes and circulatory status. When evaluating an extremity after injury, the unaffected side should be checked first and used as the baseline. For an injured extremity, findings distal and proximal to the site of the injury should be compared. To evaluate peripheral vascular integrity, the color, capillary refill time, temperature, presence of peripheral pulses, degree of sensation of the body part, and a pain evaluation should be documented.

Range of Motion
Passive and active range of motion (ROM) should be evaluated. Passive ROM requires that the patient keep the muscles relaxed while the examiner moves the joint, whereas active ROM requires that the patient use his or her muscles for movement. Passive ROM should equal active ROM except when there is paralysis of muscles or a ruptured tendon. As the joint moves through ROM, any stiffness, clicking, or limitation of movement should be noted. **Crepitus,** or joint clicking, may be caused by articular surface abnormalities, joint inflammation, or can be normal. However, when crepitus is present without pain or limited motion, it is generally of no clinical significance.

While putting the muscle through passive ROM, note muscle tone. Muscle should be evaluated for spasticity,

	TABLE 37-2. Lovett Scale of Muscle Strength	
Score	**Grade**	**Description**
0	Zero	No palpable contraction of muscle
1	Trace	Palpable contraction of muscle; no joint motion
2	Poor	Complete ROM with gravity eliminated
3	Fair	Complete ROM against gravity; no added resistance
4	Good	Complete ROM against gravity; some added resistance
5	Normal	Complete ROM against gravity with full resistance

hyperreflexia or fasciculations, with comparison of one side to the other. Muscle strength should be assessed in the injured extremity as well as the normal one. It can be evaluated using the Lovett scale, which is described in Table 37-2.

Signs and Symptoms
The signs and symptoms of traumatic musculoskeletal injury depend on the location, extent of injury, and mechanisms involved. With significant trauma, soft tissue injury, internal derangement, and fracture, there may be significant bleeding, tissue disruption, swelling, and pain. Constitutional signs, such as fever, weight loss, and malaise, are commonly seen with infection, sepsis, or systemic rheumatic disease. If these conditions involve a joint, the joint may become warm, swollen, and painful. Traumatic joint injuries are usually characterized by stiffness or limitation of movement, swelling

or redness, pain or aching, and may have unilateral or bilateral involvement.

Muscular injuries typically involve limitation of movement, weakness or fatigue, paralysis, tremor, spasm, clumsiness, wasting, aching, and pain, whereas skeletal injuries are commonly characterized by numbness, tingling or pressure sensation, pain with movement, crepitus, abnormality or change in bone contour, and difficulty with gait or limping.

Diagnostic Studies

X-rays are used to identify fractures, dislocations, tissue derangement, or bony abnormalities after a traumatic event. They are useful when there is a loss of joint function, when pain continues despite conservative management, when infection is suspected, or when there is a history of malignancy. Ultrasound studies may be useful in the detection of soft tissue abnormalities, specifically synovial (Baker's) cysts, rotator cuff tears, and various tendon injuries. Computed tomography (CT) scan provides an evaluation of the axial skeleton; helical or spiral CT may be used to detect obscured fractures. Magnetic resonance imaging (MRI) or radionuclide bone scanning is useful when specific disorders are suspected, such as rotator cuff tear, spinal stenosis, **avascular necrosis (AVN)** of the bone, or mechanical derangement of the knee. A bone scan is indicated when osteomyelitis, stress fractures, or bony metastases are a concern. Nerve conduction studies such as electromyography (EMG) may be used when neurological abnormalities or paresthesias are present. A dual energy x-ray absorptiometry (DEXA) scan measures bone density. This specialized dual beam scan visualizes the BMD of the hip and lumbar vertebrae and compares that to the BMD of a approximately a 25- to 30-year-old-adult. This scan is used when osteoporosis is suspected.

ALERT! Before any study using contrast dye, the clinician should ask the patient about metal implants, kidney function, medication use (particularly metformin), and allergies to dye. Metformin can cause lactic acidosis in patients injected with contrast dye.

Treatment

Patients presenting with acute trauma should be immediately assessed for the ABCDEs and evaluated using advanced trauma support algorithms. Those with fracture, those with injury to the neurological or vascular system, and those with multiple traumatic injuries require emergent consultation and treatment. Because certain musculoskeletal injuries are a risk factor for deep vein thrombosis (DVT) and pulmonary embolism

(PE), patients may need to be placed on anticoagulant therapy.

Most musculoskeletal injuries are self-limiting and improvement should be expected over a period of weeks. Activity limitations, if appropriate, should be reserved for the most acute period (2 days or fewer) to control spasm and edema. In most cases, the goal is to promote a gradual reintroduction of activities, depending on the patient's symptoms. Pharmacological and nonpharmacological therapies should be used for symptom management. Pharmacological agents include nonsteroidal anti-inflammatory drugs (NSAIDs) or acetaminophen as the first-line choice, topical analgesia, opioids for moderate to severe pain, and skeletal muscle relaxants, which can be given over a 1- to 2-week course to control spasm or tightness.

ALERT! Orthopedic surgery patients are particularly susceptible to DVT and PE. Orthopedic surgery predisposes individuals to DVT because of venous stasis, vessel injury, and hypercoagulability of blood with venous pooling.

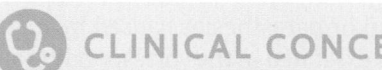
CLINICAL CONCEPT

RICE therapy is used for mild to moderately severe injuries:

- R: rest for initial 24 to 48 hours
- I: ice application on injured region for 20 minutes of each waking hour during the initial 48 hours after injury
- C: compression, with brace or splint, if necessary
- E: elevation above the level of the heart.

Other nonpharmacological therapies may include physical therapy, massage, acupuncture, transcutaneous electrical nerve stimulation (TENS), or chiropractic care. Patients who have progressive symptoms or decreased loss of function may need to be referred to a specialist for evaluation of surgical options. Those with ongoing pain symptoms may benefit from a referral to a pain management specialist.

The process of realigning bones and ancillary structures for maximal healing and restoration of proper function is called reduction. There are two kinds of reduction:

1. Closed reduction: A device is worn outside the musculoskeletal area.
2. Open reduction: An incision is commonly necessary for realignment, with surgical insertion of hardware.

In closed reduction, external devices include splints, casts, and traction devices. With open reduction, fixation

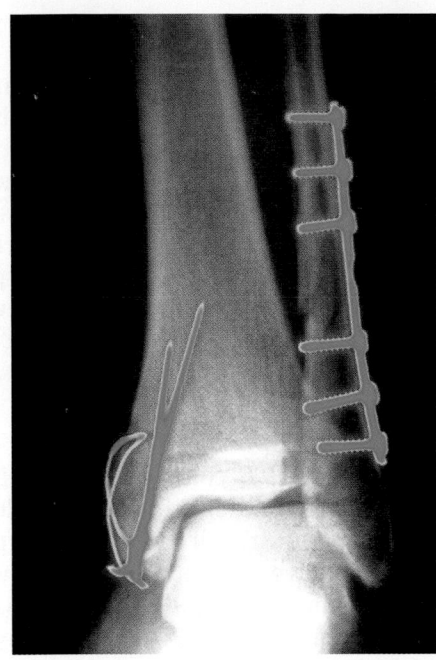

FIGURE 37-3. X-ray showing hardware that reinforces healing of the interior bone. *(From Scott Camazine/Science Source.)*

devices can be inserted inside or outside the body. Internal fixation devices are surgically inserted inside bone. External devices are pieces of hardware that are connected to the internal bone from outside the body. Fixator devices are made of stainless steel or titanium. Commonly, patients undergo **open reduction and internal fixation (ORIF).** Open reduction means that the region of injury was opened for surgical repair. Internal fixation prevents micromotion of bone across fracture lines; this decreases the risk of improper healing (see Fig. 37-3).

Common Complications of Musculoskeletal Trauma

The complications of bone injury include neurovascular damage, infection, and compartment syndrome. To prevent neurovascular damage, periodic assessment of the injured area and distal regions is necessary. Compartment syndrome is an uncommon complication but becomes apparent to the patient because of intense pain. The syndrome causes neurovascular impingement and requires immediate treatment. As in any breach of skin integrity, infection is a possible complication, particularly in compound fracture.

Neurological and Vascular Injury

Neurological and vascular injuries can occur in any fracture, but most likely those that cause a high degree of deformity. Arterial injuries are particularly prevalent in cases of knee dislocation, proximal tibial fracture, and supracondylar humerus fracture. Proper alignment of injured bone, muscle, and ancillary structures is important

for restoration of function. The injured area is susceptible to ischemia and nerve compression caused by edema, inflammation, ruptured vessels, torn nerves, and displaced bone fragments. Patient symptoms that indicate neurovascular injury include weakness, lack of sensation, and pain. The patient will exhibit decreased motor strength, hypoesthesia, or paresthesias and absent or weak pulses. If neurovascular compression is prolonged, severe atrophy of muscle will occur.

An angiogram can demonstrate vascular abnormality, and an MRI or CT scan can exhibit damage to the nerves. In any musculoskeletal injury, there should be frequent and ongoing neurovascular examination.

ALERT! To assess neurovascular status, always check pulses and sensation distal to a musculoskeletal injury.

Compartment Syndrome

In **compartment syndrome,** the patient complains of pain that is out of proportion to the degree of injury. It occurs when tissue pressure exceeds perfusion pressure in a closed anatomical space. This condition can occur in any compartment, such as the hand, forearm, upper arm, abdomen, buttock, or thigh, but it most commonly occurs in the anterior compartment of the leg. Progression of compartment syndrome can cause tissue ischemia, necrosis, and functional impairment. Rhabdomyolysis, the breakdown of skeletal muscle tissue, can also occur in compartment syndrome. The renal excretion of these breakdown products can cause nephron tubule dysfunction. Renal failure and death can occur if the patient is not treated.

Edema, pallor, and paresthesias in the affected area and distally will be apparent. In addition, weak distal pulses or pulselessness can be found. Compartment pressures can be objectively measured as greater than 30 mm Hg. To treat compartment syndrome, surgical fasciotomy is necessary.

ALERT! An immediate surgical evaluation is required at the first sign of compartment syndrome.

Infection

Complications of open wounds and surgical intervention include local infection in the form of cellulitis or osteomyelitis and systemic infection in the form of sepsis. The most common pathogen involved is *Staphylococcus aureus.* Other pathogens that may cause infection are group A streptococci, coagulase-negative staphylococci, and enterococci. The patient with wound infection or sepsis will present with fever, chills, nausea, vomiting, and increased pressure in the affected area. The affected area will be warm, edematous, and erythematous with purulent discharge and foul odor. Blood cultures, complete blood count (CBC) with differential, C-reactive protein, and erythrocyte sedimentation rate (ESR) are necessary lab tests to monitor the infection. Antibiotic treatment and debridement of the wound may also be necessary. Surgical removal of orthopedic hardware is also required.

Deep Venous Thrombosis and Pulmonary Embolism

Injury to a vessel wall, venous stasis, and hypercoagulability of blood are the three conditions, known as Virchow's triad, that increase susceptibility to DVT. After musculoskeletal injury, blood vessels are damaged and blood pools within the damaged area. The sequela of musculoskeletal injury predispose a patient to DVT because of the vessel damage and venous stasis. Within the pooled blood, formation of a venous thrombus is common. From anywhere in the venous system, a venous thrombus can detach from the area and embolize to the pulmonary circulation. Therefore, PE is the dreaded sequel of DVT.

Commonly, a PE will begin as a clot in a leg vein that travels into the inferior vena cava. From the inferior vena cava, the clot reaches the right atrium, right ventricle, and pulmonary arterial circulation. As a PE at that point, it can obstruct blood flow through the lungs and cause hypoxia and possibly death.

Orthopedic surgery carries a high risk of DVT and PE. With any kind of surgery there is vessel damage, and with orthopedic surgery, immobilization is usually needed postoperatively. Therefore, surgical vessel damage and venous stasis caused by immobilization increase the risk of clot formation. Commonly, there are few to no symptoms exhibited by the patient with DVT. The area of DVT may be tender, edematous, and warm, and there can be a palpable ropiness along the course of the involved vein. The patient may exhibit **Homans' sign**, which is pain in the calf with dorsiflexion of the foot. To diagnose DVT, a D-dimer blood test, prothrombin time, partial thromboplastin time, fibrinogen level, and platelet count should be done.

A patient experiencing a PE may exhibit dyspnea, cyanosis, cough, tachypnea, hemoptysis, chest pain, or tachycardia. Most patients who suffer a PE show no symptoms and many suffer rapid cardiovascular collapse. A ventilation-perfusion scan, helical CT scan, or CT pulmonary angiogram can demonstrate a PE.

Prevention of DVT and PE is the therapeutic strategy used for patients undergoing orthopedic surgery. Anticoagulation is the recommended pharmacological approach to prevent DVT and PE. If DVT is strongly suspected, the surgical insertion of a Greenfield filter into the inferior vena cava is recommended. The filter can catch any venous clot that is making its way up to the pulmonary artery. Other therapies for DVT and PE include thrombolysis and pulmonary thrombectomy.

Avascular Necrosis

Avascular vascular necrosis (AVN), deterioration of bone caused by insufficient blood supply, is commonly associated with fractures of the femoral head and neck, scaphoid, talar neck and body, and proximal humerus. The patient with AVN experiences pain and weakness. The examiner will find motor weakness; abnormal gait, if a lower extremity is involved; and lack of rehabilitation progress. An MRI or bone scintigraphy are used to detect AVN. Treatment involves surgical removal of necrotic bone.

Posttraumatic Arthritis

Posttraumatic arthritis is common in intra-articular fractures, particularly in those fractures inadequately reduced. The patient complains of persistent pain and achiness of the involved joint; the examiner will note crepitus in the joint and motor weakness. Diagnostic tests include x-ray and CT scan. Treatment may require arthroscopic debridement, osteotomy, arthroplasty, or arthrodesis.

Delayed Union

When a fracture has not healed after the expected time period, an assessment of union status should ensue. **Nonunion** is defined as a fracture with no possible chance of healing, whereas **malunion** is the healing of bone in an unacceptable position. In either of these conditions, the patient experiences persistent pain and dysfunction of the affected limb. The examiner will note motor weakness, abnormal function of the limb, abnormal gait if it occurs in a lower extremity, and posttraumatic arthritis. Diagnosis is made via x-ray and CT scan. Treatment of nonunion or malunion depends on the cause of the problem. Possible treatments include eradication of infection, stabilization of the fracture, removal of interfering soft tissue, bone grafting, and treatment modifications of comorbidities. Treatment of nonunion and malunion involves surgical correction of anatomical abnormality.

Pathophysiology of Selected Disorders of Musculoskeletal Trauma

There are certain musculoskeletal areas of the body that are susceptible to specific kinds of injury. The following disorders of musculoskeletal trauma are those seen most commonly in the clinical area.

Strains and Sprains

The paravertebral musculature and muscles of the extremities are commonly affected by strains and sprains. Strains occur when muscles or tendons are pulled, small blood vessels tear, and nerve endings are irritated. Sprains occur when ligaments, the connective tissue linking bones together, are stretched and overextended.

Cervical Strain

More than 1 million cases of cervical strain injuries caused by motor vehicle accidents occur annually in the United States. Cervical strain is most often caused by an acceleration-deceleration injury, commonly known as whiplash. It is estimated that the annual incidence of symptoms caused by cervical strain is 3.8 cases per 1,000 population.

Etiology and Pathophysiology. Cervical strain is produced by an injury to the muscles and tendons because of excessive forces placed on the cervical spine. Elongation and tearing of muscles or ligaments occurs with secondary edema and inflammation. The most common cause of cervical strain is whiplash injury caused by a motor vehicle accident. Repetitive stress injuries to the cervical spine or abnormal posture can also cause cervical strain. Such injuries can result from occupational situations that require odd positioning of the neck.

Clinical Presentation. The clinician should elicit a complete history to evaluate how the cervical injury occurred. The most common symptoms of cervical strain are suboccipital headache and motion-induced neck pain. There is difficulty sleeping because of cervical pain. At the time of the accident, neck pain may be minimal, with an onset of symptoms occurring during the subsequent 12 to 72 hours. Shoulder, scapular, and arm pain may also occur.

ALERT! In the acute phase of neck or multitrauma injury, stabilization of the cervical spine is mandatory.

Less common symptoms of cervical strain include visual disturbances, such as blurred vision and diplopia; tinnitus; dizziness; concussion; and disturbed concentration and memory.

In the physical examination, the clinician must exclude cervical spine fracture, herniated disk, and spinal cord injury. If weakness, numbness, or paresthesias of the arms are present there may be cervical spinal nerve impingement, also called cervical radiculopathy.

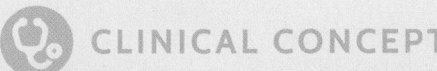
CLINICAL CONCEPT

Cervical radiculopathy is impingement of a cervical spinal nerve; it often occurs because of vertebral bony degeneration and misalignment, disk herniation, and vertebral compression fracture. Neck pain with radiation into the arm, paresthesias, and weakness of the arm are symptoms.

In cervical strain, examination findings include cervical paravertebral muscle spasm and tenderness. There is stiffness of the neck and the posture may show a forward tilt of the head, flexed neck, rounded shoulders, and asymmetry of the neck or shoulders. Palpation may reveal muscle spasm tightness, crepitation, swelling, enlargement of joints, and tenderness. Decreased active and passive ROM of the neck is noted. Deep tendon reflexes of the arms should be normal.

ALERT! Injuries of the cervical spine at or above C4 can cause respiratory failure. The fourth cervical spinal nerve is the phrenic nerve, which innervates the diaphragm. Fatal cervical spine fractures occur in upper cervical levels, either at craniocervical junction C1 or C2.

Diagnosis. Cervical spine x-rays may be normal or show straightening of the normal lordotic curve of the neck. An MRI is the best study for evaluating the status of the vertebral bones, disks, and spinal cord.

Treatment. Early treatment with nonopioid analgesics for pain relief, anti-inflammatory agents, and muscle relaxants for spasms are the main medications used for cervical sprain or strain injuries. A soft cervical collar may be recommended for short-term use.

Lumbar Strain and Sprain

Low back pain is one of the most common reasons patients seek health care. The most common cause is lumbosacral strain and sprain. The lifetime prevalence of low back pain in the United States is 60% to 80%, and it is the most common cause of work-related disability in persons younger than 45 years. Other more serious causes of low back pain that need to be excluded before diagnosing lumbar strain or sprain are herniated disk, vertebral fracture, and spinal cord injury.

Etiology. Sprains are ligamentous injuries that are caused by a sudden contraction, sudden torsion, severe direct blows, or a forceful straightening from a crouched position. Individuals also commonly sustain a low back strain or sprain while lifting heavy objects. During such activities, tremendous loads are placed on the lumbar spine, which may cause a temporary instability and lead to a subsequent injury to the soft tissue that surrounds the spine. Sprain and strain commonly occur when there is lateral bending with flexion-extension or axial rotation with lateral bending of the lumbar spine.

Pathophysiology. Strains are defined as tears, either partial or complete, of the muscles and tendons. Muscle strains and tears most frequently result from a violent muscular contraction during an excessively forceful muscular stretch. Any posterior spinal muscle and its associated tendon can be involved, although the most susceptible muscles are those that span several joints.

The lumbar spine and the hips are responsible for the trunk's mobility. The L4–5 and L5–S1 areas bear the highest loads and tend to undergo the most motion. Consequently, these areas are found to sustain the most spinal strain or sprain injuries. In addition, load-bearing strain and sprain injuries most frequently occur during the strongest coupling patterns.

 CLINICAL CONCEPT

The L4-L5 and L5-S1 segments of the vertebrae are most often involved in lower back strain and sprain. L4-L5 spinal nerves are involved in dorsiflexion of the foot. L5-S1 spinal nerves are involved in plantarfexion of the foot.

Clinical Presentation. Lumbar strain and sprain can present similarly to more serious conditions such as herniated disk or spinal nerve impingement. The clinician has to evaluate the history and perform a comprehensive motor and neurological assessment of the lower extremities. The physical examination findings often cannot make the clear distinction between muscle and nerve damage. Diagnostic testing also often cannot demonstrate the extent of muscle, ligament, and soft tissue damage. However, it can make the necessary distinction of nerve versus muscle involvement.

History. During the history of a patient with low back pain, the following key information needs to be elicited:

- the mechanism of injury, with an exact description of the event leading to the pain
- the exact localization and duration of the pain
- any pain radiation
- movements that aggravate or minimize the pain.

Typical symptoms are sharp pain, tenderness, and spasm over the posterior lumbar paravertebral spinal muscles or at the insertion of the muscle at the iliac crest. ROM, particularly in flexion, is usually painful and decreased.

If the injury is limited to a sprain or strain injury, then structural deformities and neurological symptoms are absent. Any neurological problem, such as

 CLINICAL CONCEPT

Low back pain accompanied by radiating pain down the leg indicates spinal nerve impingement, a syndrome called sciatica.

ALERT! If lumbar pain is accompanied by urinary or fecal incontinence, cauda equina syndrome is probable. Cauda equina syndrome, a medical emergency, occurs when the bundle of nerves at the end of the spinal cord is compressed.

numbness or weakness of the lower extremity, indicates the possible presence of herniated disc or spinal nerve root impingement.

Physical Examination. The clinician should evaluate the patient's back with the patient in a standing position. Assessment should include inspecting the back for obvious deformities or changes in alignment. The patient should be asked to assume changes in position according to full ROM: flexion, extension, lateral flexion, and rotation. The clinician should note restricted ROM. Evaluation of ROM provides clues to muscle spasm and aggravating factors that worsen the patient's pain.

With the patient in the prone position, the clinician should palpate the paravertebral musculature, areas of muscle spasm, and the location of any point tenderness, if present.

Evaluation of the lower extremities should include a motor examination, a sensory evaluation, and reflex testing at the knees and ankles. The patient should be asked to stand on toes and walk on heels, if possible. Standing on toes requires dorsiflexion of the foot and tests the L4 to L5 spinal motor nerve, whereas walking on heels requires plantar flexion of the foot and tests the L5 to S1 spinal motor nerve. Testing of sensation of the patient's lower extremities according to the sensory dermatomes can assist in diagnosis. Also, the patellar and Achilles reflex need to be assessed.

With the patient in the supine position, the clinician should test for the straight-leg raising sign also called Lasègue's sign. The straight-leg raising test helps to evaluate disc involvement, sciatica, or a neurological deficit (see Fig. 37-4). A positive straight-leg raising test indicates sciatica. In addition, the clinician should try to elicit a positive Patrick sign. A positive Patrick test, also called a FABER (flexion, abduction, and external rotation) test,

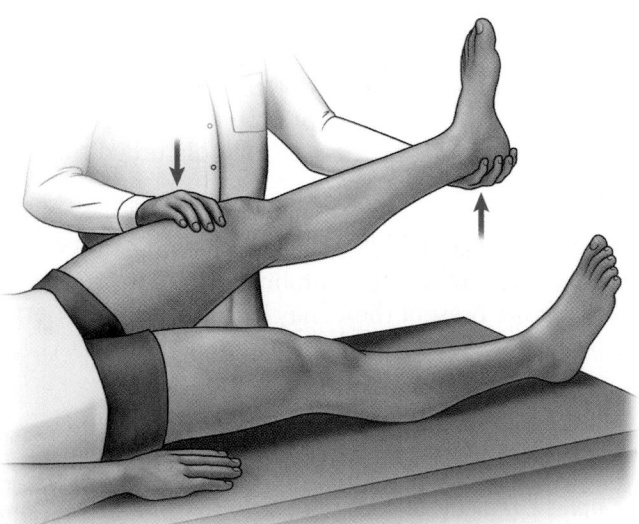

FIGURE 37-4. Straight-leg raising test. The straight-leg test, also called Lasegue's sign, is a test done during the physical examination to determine whether a patient with low back pain has an underlying herniated disk. With the patient lying down on his back on an examination table, the examiner lifts the patient's leg while the knee is straight.

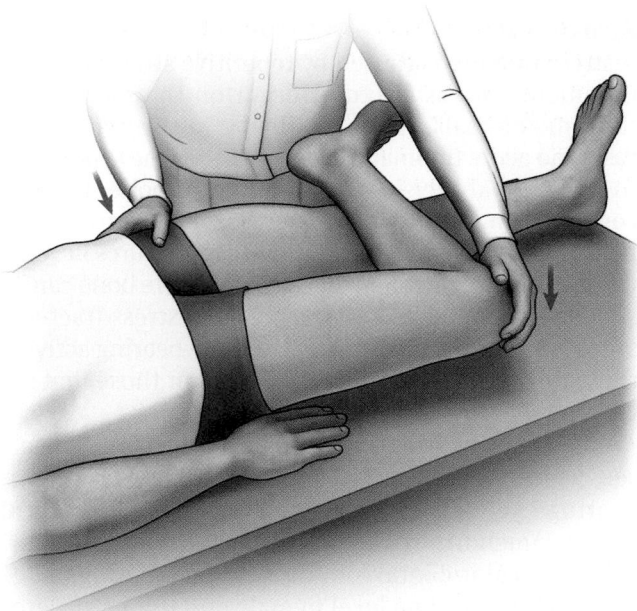

FIGURE 37-5. The Patrick test, also known as the FABER test (Flexion, Abduction, and External Rotation), is performed to evaluate function of the hip joint or the sacroiliac joint. The test is performed by having the tested leg flexed, abducted, and externally rotated. If pain is elicited on the ipsilateral side anteriorly, it is suggestive of a hip joint disorder on the same side. If pain is elicited on the contralateral side posteriorly around the sacroiliac joint, it is suggestive of pathology in that joint.

points to a sacroiliac joint inflammation, but this test should be negative in lumbosacral sprains and strains (see Fig. 37-5).

Diagnosis. Laboratory studies are generally not indicated in the evaluation of lumbosacral spine sprain or strain injuries. Anteroposterior and lateral x-rays of the lumbar spine should be routinely obtained to:

- exclude a fracture, rheumatic disease, or a tumor growth
- evaluate degenerative joint disease as well as overall spinal alignment.

In lumbar strain and sprain there should be no abnormal finding except soft tissue swelling. If neurological signs are present, a CT scan or MRI should be done to evaluate for disc herniation and involvement of the spinal nerve roots.

Treatment. Cold therapy, initially performed for a short period up to 48 hours, can be applied to the affected area to limit the localized tissue inflammation and edema. The patient should maintain a low level of activity. Activities, particularly those involving lifting and extreme ROM of the spine, should be avoided. The patient should be instructed how to perform activities without straining the back muscles. Heat therapy can be applied after the acute phase. Anti-inflammatory agents and muscle relaxants are commonly prescribed. Intramuscular (IM) injections of muscle relaxants or NSAIDs at the site of the pain may help to control muscle spasms. There should be no manipulation of the affected area during the injury's acute phase. A supportive lumbosacral corset may also be used to help control muscle spasms. The patient should be referred to a physical therapist. Abdominal obesity aggravates low back pain; therefore, weight reduction is advised if this is a problem.

Ankle Sprain

Most ankle sprains do not come to the attention of health-care providers because affected individuals often treat themselves. Sprained ankles have been estimated to constitute up to 30% of injuries seen in sports medicine clinics. More than 23,000 people per day in the United States, both athletes and nonathletes, require medical care for ankle sprains. The highest incidence of ankle injuries occurs in football, basketball, and soccer players.

Etiology. Mechanical forces exceeding the tensile limits of the ankle joint capsule and supportive ligaments cause ankle sprains. Risk factors of ankle sprain include lack of physical conditioning, poor proprioception, obesity, and high level of athletic competition.

Pathophysiology. In ankle sprain, the lateral ankle complex, which is composed of the anterior talofibular, calcaneofibular, and posterior talofibular ligaments, is the most commonly injured site. Approximately 85% of sprains are caused by inversion of the foot during plantar flexion of the ankle; most injuries involve the anterior talofibular ligament. Recurrent ankle sprains are common. The cause is unknown, although it is postulated that the scar tissue of healed ligaments creates a weak, unstable joint.

Clinical Presentation. Individuals with ankle sprain complain of severe pain that worsens with weight-bearing. It is most important to exclude ankle fracture; the ability to walk on the foot usually indicates no fracture. The clinician should palpate the ankle for bony point tenderness, especially over the medial malleolus, lateral malleolus, base of the fifth metatarsal, and midfoot bones. Point bony tenderness at one of these areas, as well as bony deformity or crepitus, suggests the possible presence of a fracture. Sensation of the foot should be normal. Palpation of the dorsalis pedis and posterior tibial arterial pulses are necessary. Active ROM must be assessed, because Achilles tendon ruptures can mimic ankle sprains.

There are three grades in the classification of ankle sprains:

- Grade 1: Injuries cause a stretch of the ligament, mild swelling, little or no functional loss, and no joint instability. The patient is able to fully or partially bear weight.
- Grade 2: Injuries cause a stretch of the ligament with partial tearing, moderate-to-severe swelling, ecchymosis, moderate functional loss, and mild-to-moderate joint instability. Patients usually have difficulty bearing weight.

BOX 37-3. The Ottawa Ankle Rules

According to the Ottawa Ankle Rules, an ankle x-ray is only required if there is pain in the malleolar zone and any one of the following:

- bone tenderness along the distal 6 cm of the posterior edge of the tibia or tip of the medial malleolus, OR
- bone tenderness along the distal 6 cm of the posterior edge of the fibula or tip of the lateral malleolus, OR
- an inability to bear weight both immediately and in the emergency department for four steps.

A foot x-ray is only required if there is pain in the midfoot zone and any one of the following:

- bone tenderness at the base of the fifth metatarsal (for foot injuries), OR
- bone tenderness at the navicular bone (for foot injuries), OR
- an inability to bear weight both immediately and in the emergency department for four steps.

(Adapted from Stiell, I. G., McKnight, R. D., Greenberg, G. H., et al. (1994). Implementation of the Ottawa Ankle Rules. *JAMA*, 271, 827–832.)

- Grade 3: Injuries cause complete rupture of the ligament, with severe swelling, ecchymosis, an inability to bear weight, and moderate-to-severe instability of the joint.

Diagnosis. The Ottawa Ankle Rules, a set of conditions that occur in ankle injury, assist in the diagnosis of ankle sprain versus fracture (see Box 37-3). Drawer and talar tilt examination techniques are used to assess ankle instability. X-rays of the ankle are necessary to rule out fracture; in addition, CT scanning may be needed to exclude stress fractures. Electromyographic examinations of individuals with severe ankle sprains have shown that 80% of these patients have some degree of peroneal nerve injury.

Treatment. RICE therapy is the mainstay of acute treatment; more comprehensively, the combination of protection, relative rest, ice, compression, elevation, and support (PRICES) is used. Anti-inflammatory agents can decrease swelling and pain. A compression dressing or splint can be applied to severe sprains. Physical therapy during the recovery phase is aimed at the patient regaining full ROM, strength, and proprioceptive abilities.

Cumulative Trauma Disorders

Cumulative trauma disorders, also referred to as repetitive strain injuries, are caused by constant stresses exerted on a particular body part. The trauma takes place over months to years.

Stress Fracture

A stress fracture is caused by repetitive stress on bone. Commonly, stress fractures occur on the second and third metatarsals, tibia, and fibula. In the majority of cases, no acute traumatic event precedes the symptoms. In the normal physiologic function of bone, there is constant remodeling with osteoclasts and osteoblasts performing opposing activities. Stress fractures develop when extensive microdamage occurs before bone can be adequately remodeled. Bones prone to stress fractures are those constantly involved in weight-bearing activity, those involved in high impact activity, or those that are weakened by osteoporosis.

Risk factors of stress fractures include genetics, female sex, white ethnicity, low body weight, lack of weight-bearing exercise, intrinsic and extrinsic mechanical factors, amenorrhea, oligomenorrhea, inadequate calcium and caloric intake, and disordered eating. A decreased testosterone level in male endurance athletes has also been implicated as a risk factor. Studies show a high incidence of stress fractures in military recruits, distance runners, tennis players, and ballet dancers. The women most at risk for stress fractures are those who restrict their food intake and those who have dysmenorrhea.

The symptom of a stress fracture is localized bone pain that increases with weight-bearing. On physical examination there is tenderness along an involved bone upon palpation and percussion. X-ray, bone scanning, MRI, and CT scanning are the preferred tests for diagnosis, although it is important to note that stress fractures may not be apparent on x-ray for the first 2 to 4 weeks after injury.

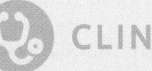 CLINICAL CONCEPT

The triad of disordered eating, amenorrhea, and osteoporosis are conditions that are extremely prevalent in female athletes with low body fat.

Carpal Tunnel Syndrome

Carpal tunnel syndrome (CTS) is a cumulative trauma disorder that causes increased pressure on the median nerve in the wrist. The carpal tunnel is located at the base of the palm, is surrounded by carpal bones, and is wrapped by the transverse carpal ligament. The median nerve runs anteriorly from the forearm into the wrist through the carpal tunnel.

The prevalence of CTS in the United States is estimated at 3.7%, and the annual incidence is estimated at 0.4%. Incidence is probably higher because some persons do not seek health care for CTS. CTS is more prevalent in middle-aged persons and predominately in females. It occurs in persons with occupations that require repetitive strain risk, such as assembly packers, waiters, computer keyboard workers, musicians, or craftspeople. Also, compression of the median nerve can occur during pregnancy or because of oral contraceptive-related edema. There is a strong association between being overweight or obese and the presence of CTS.

Clinical Presentation. Classic CTS is associated with symptoms that affect at least two of the first through third fingers. Wrist pain and radiation of pain proximal to the wrist may also occur. Patients typically complain of an intermittent "pins-and-needles" or paresthesias in the median nerve distribution of the hand. Pain is generally worse at night than during the day. Patients may awaken with a burning pain or tingling that may be relieved with shaking their hands.

Diagnosis. Phalen sign may be elicited by hyperflexion of the wrist for 60 seconds. The patient with CTS experiences paresthesias in the median nerve distribution of the hand. Tinel sign occurs by tapping the anterior surface of the wrist over the median nerve. This produces paresthesias in the median distribution of the hand. Hand and arm x-rays may be needed to rule out other problems; EMG is also sometimes used in the diagnosis.

Treatment. To relieve CTS, rest, splinting, pain management, and surgery may be necessary. Early in the course of the syndrome, the neurological findings are reversible. If untreated, CTS can result in thenar atrophy, chronic hand weakness, and numbness in the median nerve distribution of the hand.

Lateral Epicondylitis

Lateral epicondylitis, also called tennis elbow, occurs in up to 50% of tennis players. However, this condition is not limited to tennis players; it is the result of overuse from many activities. Any activity involving wrist extension or supination can be associated with overuse of the muscles originating at the lateral epicondyle (elbow).

The most important structure involved in epicondylitis is the extensor carpi radialis brevis (ECRB) muscle, which arises from the lateral epicondyle. The etiology of lateral epicondylitis involves inflammatory processes of the radial humeral bursa, synovium, periosteum, and the annular ligament. There is also microscopic tearing with formation of scar tissue in the origin of the ECRB. This microtearing can lead to structural failure of the origin of the ECRB muscle. Patients complain of lateral elbow and forearm pain exacerbated by use. The typical patient is a man or woman aged 35 to 55 years who either is a recreational athlete or one who engages in rigorous daily activities.

Upon examination, the patient has a point of maximal tenderness just distal to the lateral epicondyle in the area of the ECRB muscle, as well as weak muscle grip with painful movement of the forearm. Wrist extension or supination against resistance with the elbow extended should provoke the patient's symptoms. Another helpful test is the chair raise test. The patient stands behind a chair and attempts to raise it by putting his or her hands on the top of the chair back and lifting. In patients with lateral epicondylitis, pain results over the lateral elbow. X-ray, CT scan, and MRI are used to diagnose epicondylitis.

Rest, ice, nonsteroidal analgesics, splinting, steroid injection, and physical therapy are treatment measures for lateral epicondylitis. Approximately 90% to 95% of patients with the disorder recover with conservative measures and do not require surgical intervention. Patients whose condition is unresponsive to 6 months of conservative therapy are candidates for surgery.

Bursitis

Bursa are fluid-filled, saclike structures between skin and bone or between tendons, ligaments, and bone. They act as cushions to lubricate and decrease friction between bone, ligaments, and tendons. Bursitis occurs when the synovial lining produces excessive fluid, leading to localized swelling and pain.

Bursitis accounts for 0.4% of all visits to primary care providers. The incidence of bursitis is higher in athletes, with an incidence of up to 10% in runners. The most common locations of bursitis are the subdeltoid, olecranon, ischial, trochanteric, and prepatellar bursae.

The most common cause of bursitis is repetitive injury or overuse. Repetitive injury within the bursa stimulates the inflammatory cascade, which causes local vasodilatation and increased vascular permeability. Bursitis can also be caused by autoimmune disorders, gout or pseudogout, infection, traumatic events, and hemorrhagic disorders. Systemic diseases such as rheumatoid arthritis, ankylosing spondylitis, psoriatic arthritis, scleroderma, systemic lupus erythematosus, pancreatitis, Whipple disease, oxalosis, uremia, hypertrophic pulmonary osteoarthropathy, and idiopathic hypereosinophilic syndrome have also been associated with bursitis.

Patients complain of pain with motion of a joint and discomfort at rest. There is swelling and decreased ROM of the affected joint. The bursa, which is not normally palpable, becomes enlarged, tender, and painful. Pain is aggravated by movement of the joint, tendon, or both.

On physical examination, patients have tenderness at the site of the inflamed bursa. If the bursa is superficial, physical examination findings are significant for localized tenderness, warmth, edema, and erythema of the skin. Decreased active ROM with preserved passive ROM is suggestive of bursitis, but the differential diagnosis includes tendinitis and muscle injury. A decrease in both active and passive ROM is more suggestive of other musculoskeletal disorders. Patients with septic bursitis may have fever, bursal warmth, tenderness, and associated cellulitis.

In chronic bursitis, the affected extremity may show atrophy and weakness. Tendons may also be weakened and tender. Chronic bursitis leads to continual pain and can cause weakening of overlying ligaments and tendons; ultimately, this can result in rupture of the tendons.

Diagnostic tests include x-ray, ESR, and WBC count. Treatment for pain control includes rest, ice, compression, elevation, and medications (RICEM), which include NSAIDs, acetaminophen, and corticosteroid injections. If no response occurs to other treatments, a mix of corticosteroid and local anesthetic can be injected into each tender site.

Temporomandibular Joint Disorder

The **temporal mandibular joints (TMJ)** connect the jaw to the skull in front of each ear. The joint allows for side-to-side movement and up-and-down motion, as well as protrusion and retraction of the jaw. An estimated 10 million people have TMJ disorders, and roughly 25% of the population has symptoms at some point in their lives. Adults aged 20 to 40 years are most often affected, with a preponderance of females to males.

The pathophysiology of TMJ disorder mainly occurs because of local repetitive injury. Repetitive and cumulative trauma caused by nocturnal jaw clenching, nocturnal bruxism (teeth grinding), and jaw clenching because of stress play a significant role. Irritation of the mandibular branch of the trigeminal nerve results in pain at the TMJ. Conditions such as rheumatoid arthritis, osteoarthritis, and dental malocclusion can also cause the disorder.

Patients complain of pain over the TMJ area, as well as the preauricular region and masseter muscles. Pain is aggravated by chewing and there may be clicking of the TMJ. There is also tenderness and swelling of the muscles surrounding the TMJ.

Diagnostic tests include a dental exam to rule out causes of TMJ that result from malocclusion. X-ray, CT, or MRI of the jaw may be necessary. A diagnostic nerve block of the mandibular branch of the trigeminal nerve can also be helpful in diagnosis. If the patient does not experience pain relief with the nerve block, other causes of facial pain are likely.

Treatment includes pain management with anti-inflammatory agents, physical therapy, and possibly acupuncture. Signs and symptoms of TMJ disorders improve over time with or without treatment for most patients.

Common Fractures

A fracture is a break of the integrity of bone, which is commonly caused by trauma. Pathological fractures occur when there is weakening of the bone by osteoporosis, infection, degeneration, necrosis, or a space-occupying lesion in the bone.

Hip Fracture

A hip fracture is a fracture of the proximal end of the femur. In elderly individuals, the hip can undergo osteoporotic degeneration, a weakness in the hip that often causes a fall. An estimated 340,000 hip fractures occur each year. Furthermore, 9 of 10 hip fractures occur in patients aged 65 years and older, and 3 of 4 occur in women. White females are twice as likely to suffer hip fracture compared with black and Hispanic females. In both men and women, the rate of hip fracture increases with age, doubling each decade after age 50 years. Nearly half of all hip fractures occur in adults older than 80 years.

ALERT! Death after a fall is often caused by the complications that set in after hip fracture and immobility. One out of five elderly hip fracture patients dies within a year of the injury because of complications.

CLINICAL CONCEPT

The hip, wrist, and vertebrae are the most commonly fractured bones in the elderly with osteoporosis.

Etiology. Osteoporosis is a major cause of hip fracture. Osteoporotic fracture usually occurs in the femoral head or neck where there is mainly trabecular (nonsolid) bone. Hip fracture caused by osteoporosis often causes a fall in elderly patients. Young adults can sustain hip fracture because of high-energy trauma caused by accidents or athletic activity. Stress fracture of the hip can also occur in an otherwise healthy person.

Pathophysiology. The hip is a ball-and-socket joint: the acetabulum within the pelvic bone serves as the socket and the head of the femur as the ball. This region is composed of trabecular bone, which is a meshwork of nonsolid bone, which is more susceptible to the degenerative changes of osteoporosis than solid, cortical bone.

In elderly individuals, a common pathological process is osteoporotic degeneration of the hip followed by instability of the joint and consequent fall. The hip becomes unable to bear the individual's weight and gives way, causing a traumatic fall. Femoral neck fractures are common in the presence of osteoporosis, whereas femoral head fractures are more common in younger patients as a result of trauma.

Hip fractures involve fracture of any aspect of the proximal femur, from the head to the first 4 to 5 cm of the subtrochanteric area. Femoral neck fractures often disrupt the blood supply to the head of the femur. Superior femoral head fractures normally are associated with anterior dislocations, whereas inferior femoral head fractures are associated with posterior dislocations. Hip fractures can be classified based on their relation to the hip capsule (intracapsular and extracapsular), location (head, neck, trochanteric, intertrochanteric, and subtrochanteric), and degree of displacement (see Fig. 37-6). Higher-grade displacement implies worse prognosis. Fractures of the femoral

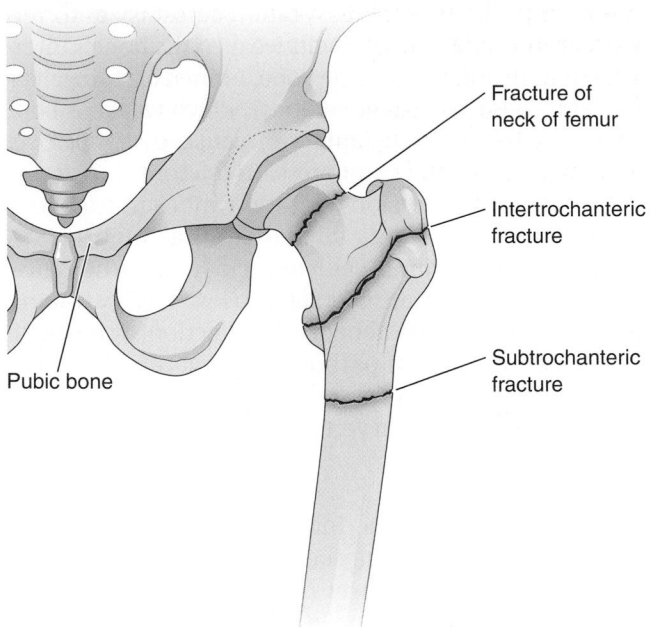

FIGURE 37-6. Sites of hip fracture in femur.

head and neck are intracapsular, whereas those of the trochanteric, intertrochanteric, and subtrochanteric regions are extracapsular. Intracapsular hip fractures frequently have complicated healing. The thick capsule that surrounds these fractures separates them from adjacent soft tissue and capillaries, leading to impaired callous formation. Nonunion necrosis and AVN are frequent complications of these fractures.

Clinical Presentation. The patient usually presents with a history of a fall or extreme trauma. In addition, elderly patients often have a history of osteoporosis and may have a history of vertebral compression or wrist fracture, which are also fractures caused by osteoporosis. Commonly, the patient is a thin, elderly Caucasian woman. Elderly patients should be asked about their current medications, as well as comorbid conditions such as hypertension, diabetes mellitus, and cardiovascular disease. Family history of osteoporosis and other disorders should be elicited.

In younger adults, there is usually trauma that has caused other injuries in addition to hip fracture. Up to 70% of patients with femoral head fractures-dislocations have experienced associated injuries, which include injuries to other extremities, intra-abdominal or intrapelvic injuries, neck injuries, and head injuries. The exact events leading to the trauma need to be investigated to evaluate the risk of associated injuries.

Physical Examination. The patient's vital signs and signs of blood loss should be assessed. The hip and femur position should be inspected, which can provide clues to the type of injury endured. In different types of fractures, the lower extremity assumes different characteristic positions. The abduction or adduction of the leg should be noted as well as the internal or external rotation. Pain and tenderness will be apparent with any motion of the leg. In assessing ROM, first test external and internal rotation with the extremity held in extension. If a fracture exists, especially one that is displaced, ROM will be extremely painful; if this happens, movement of the leg should be discontinued. A neurovascular examination distal to the site of fracture is essential. Pulses, reflexes, sensation, and motor ability should be assessed as tolerated by the patient. If the patient is a trauma victim, the pelvis should be assessed for fractures by stressing the pelvis anteriorly to posteriorly through iliac crests and symphysis pubis, and laterally to medially through iliac crests.

Diagnosis. All x-ray views of the extremities and pelvic bones should be completed. If radiographic findings are ambiguous, CT scan or MRI should be considered. A view of the contralateral hip for comparison is necessary.

Treatment. The patient who complains of hip pain should be immobilized in the supine position. The clinician should perform the **ABCDEs of trauma assessment** and immobilize the patient's cervical spine. Orthopedic as well as neurological or cardiovascular consultations should be sought. If fracture or deformity of the femur is obvious, apply a traction splint and insert an intravenous line for hydration. The patient should be placed on NPO status and have supplemental oxygen. Parenteral analgesia is necessary; in addition, a muscle relaxant also may be necessary. Antibiotics should be administered to cover broad spectrum and tetanus immunization, as necessary, in open fractures. Surgical ORIF or hip replacement is often required. Anticoagulant therapy is necessary because of the high risk for DVT. Calcium and vitamin D supplements are also needed.

Vertebral Compression Fracture

Vertebral compression fractures are pathognomonic of osteoporosis. Osteoporotic vertebral collapse occurs when the body's weight exceeds the bone's ability within the vertebral body to support the load. The interior of the vertebrae consists of trabecular, meshlike bone, which weakens and degenerates in osteoporosis. Consequences include postural changes, particularly kyphosis, loss of height, and pain.

Vertebral compression fractures affect approximately 25% of all postmenopausal women in the United States. Prevalence steadily increases with advancing age, reaching 40% in women 80 years of age. Women diagnosed with a compression fracture of the vertebrae have a 15% higher mortality rate than those who do not experience fractures. Because the elderly age group is the fastest growing segment of the U.S. population, the incidence of vertebral compression fracture will likely increase. More than 700,000 new vertebral compression fractures occur every year, accounting for more than 100,000 hospital admissions and resulting in close to $1.5 billion in annual costs.

Etiology. Vertebral compression fracture often occurs because of a pathological fracture, also called a fragility fracture. A pathological fracture occurs in the vertebrae because of pre-existing disease within the bone that undermines the structural integrity. Osteoporosis is the most common cause of vertebral compression fracture. Cancer, such as prostate, breast, or lung cancer, often metastasizes to the vertebral bones and weakens the inner bone tissue. The fracture of vertebrae can also occur because of a localized infection of the bone caused by osteomyelitis, which may occur in people with diabetes and in those who abuse IV drugs. Tuberculosis of bone, called Pott's disease, can also cause vertebral compression fracture. Ischemia of bone can cause osteonecrosis, which can also lead to fracture. Risk factors for osteoporosis and vertebral compression fracture are categorized as modifiable and not modifiable (see Box 37-4).

Pathophysiology. The vertebrae are composed of trabecular bone, which are horizontal and vertical strands of bone that form a meshwork and appear as scaffolding. Vertebral compression fracture occurs because of the collapse of the internal latticelike meshwork of the vertebral bone. In compression fracture, the vertebral bone becomes thinned and flattened. Osteoporosis, the most common cause of vertebral compression fracture, is a reduction in skeletal mass caused by an imbalance between bone resorption and bone formation. Cancer of the prostate, lung, and breast often metastasizes to vertebral bone and the tumor cells weaken the bone's internal strength. Infection of the bone, termed osteomyelitis, can also cause bone degeneration, which weakens bone strength. Ischemia of bone can cause osteonecrosis, which can also lead to compression fracture.

Vertebral compression fractures can result from low-energy trauma, such as falls, as well as high-energy trauma, such as motor vehicle accidents. Pathological fractures, which occur secondary to low-energy trauma, are characteristic of osteoporosis, infection, or metastatic cancer in bone. In pathological fracture, bone can break when under stress such as weight-bearing. Even minor loads can lead to vertebral compression fractures (see Fig. 37-7).

Clinical Presentation. Individuals with a vertebral compression fracture may be asymptomatic or may experience pain in the lower back, upper back, or neck. Some people may also have hip, abdominal, or thigh pain. A hunched over posture, also called **kyphosis.** is common. There may be numbness, tingling, and weakness of the extremities; such symptoms could indicate compression of the nerves at the fracture site. It is considered a medical emergency if the patient reports incontinence or an inability to urinate, as these symptoms can mean impingement on the spinal cord.

CLINICAL CONCEPT

Osteoporosis of the cervicothoracic vertebrae causes kyphosis in women.

BOX 37-4. Risk Factors for Vertebral Compression Fracture

NONMODIFIABLE RISK FACTORS
- advanced age
- bilateral ovariectomy
- Caucasian or Asian race
- early menopause
- female gender
- history of fractures in adulthood
- history of fractures in a first-degree relative
- premenopausal amenorrhea for more than 1 year
- presence of dementia

MODIFIABLE RISK FACTORS
- alcohol use
- dietary calcium or vitamin D deficiency
- estrogen deficiency
- frailty
- insufficient physical activity
- low body weight
- presence of osteoporosis
- prolonged use of glucocorticoids or anticonvulsants
- tobacco use

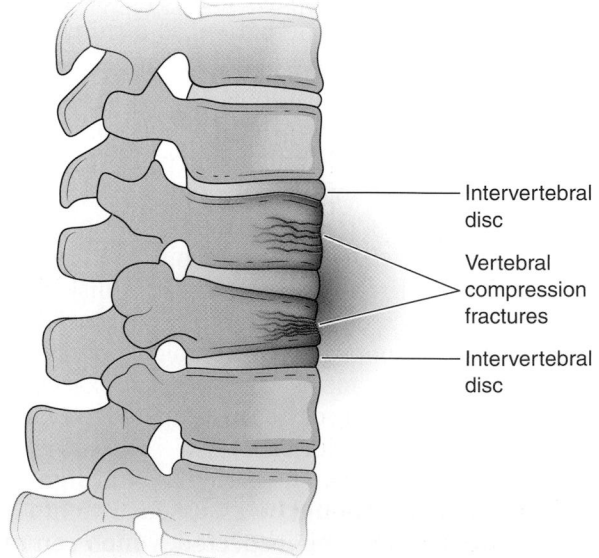

FIGURE 37-7. Vertebral compression fracture. The most common type of fracture in the vertebrae is a compression fracture, commonly in the thoracic spine. The vertebral body is commonly weakened by osteoporosis before a compression fracture occurs.

Diagnosis. Imaging studies such as x-ray can visualize the vertebrae involved in the compression. X-rays demonstrate the wedged appearance of compressed vertebrae; often, more than one vertebrae are involved. CT or MRI scans may be necessary, particularly to exclude impingement on spinal nerves.

Treatment. Calcitonin can relieve the pain of vertebral compression. There may also be a need for muscle relaxants and analgesics. External support devices provide postural stability. The surgical procedures vertebroplasty and kyphoplasty are sometimes recommended. These procedures attempt to build up the compressed area of bone with a surgical type of cement. Calcium and vitamin D supplements as well as bisphosphonates may be necessary to treat osteoporosis.

Femur Shaft Fracture

The femur, the strongest bone in the body, is surrounded by sturdy musculature and rich blood supply. The shaft of the femur, also called the diaphysis, requires a significant amount of force to fracture. Because of the abundant blood supply, fracture of the femur causes a large amount of bleeding. In addition, when fractured, the bone is commonly displaced because of the tension of the musculature that surrounds it.

The incidence of femoral fractures is reported as 1 case per 10,000 population per year. In individuals younger than 25 years and those older than 65 years, the rate of femoral fractures is 3 fractures per 10,000 population annually. Femur shaft fractures are most common in males younger than 30 years because of motor vehicle accidents and sports injury.

Etiology. Fracture of the femur shaft occurs because of a large, high energy force, which may be generated by automobile, motorcycle, or recreational vehicle accidents or gunshot wounds. In these cases, the femoral fracture is often accompanied by other traumatic injuries of the body. The femur is also commonly injured in contact and high-speed sports such as skiing, football, hockey, rodeo, and motor sports. Alternatively, a femoral stress fracture can occur from repetitive forces that overload the bone, causing microfracture. Stress fractures occur most often in repetitive overload sports such as running, baseball, and basketball. Less commonly, a fracture of the femur occurs because of tumor or metabolic disease within the shaft of the bone. The area of the lesion becomes structurally weakened, which leads to fracture.

Pathophysiology. There are three types of femoral shaft fractures:

- Type I, spiral or transverse: A spiral fracture occurs when the injury to the femur causes the bone to twist before it breaks apart; the foot is stable while the leg undergoes torsion. A transverse fracture is a simple break of the bone across the shaft of the femur. The fracture line is perpendicular to the long line of the shaft.
- Type II, comminuted: In a comminuted fracture, the bone is broken into a number of pieces, as occurs in a crushing injury.
- Type III, open: In an open fracture, also called a compound fracture, the break of the bones causes angulation sufficient to protrude through the skin, leaving a wound that is open to the environment; open fractures are extremely vulnerable to infection.

Clinical Presentation. The patient will usually report a high velocity injury, pain, and inability to bear weight on the affected extremity. Patients may be noted to have bruising, shortening of one leg, and a great deal of swelling. Alternatively, stress fractures of the femur are observed with increasing frequency in joggers. The onset of stress fractures is usually gradual, though it may be sudden or severe. Patients may report groin or thigh pain. Symptoms of stress fractures are aggravated by activity and relieved by rest. On physical examination, femoral fracture and associated injuries must be assessed. Advanced cardiovascular life support (ACLS) and the ABCDEs of trauma assessment must be used initially. A head-to-toe examination is indicated. The pelvis, hips, and knees require palpation and any lower extremity deformity should be placed in alignment. An assessment of pulses, circulation of the leg, and sensation distal to the injury is essential. Swelling of the thigh, hematoma, and loss of ROM is common. Blood loss may be severe.

Diagnosis. The clinician should order x-rays of the involved leg, with pelvic and knee views as well. Usually, views of the thorax and opposite leg are important to exclude other traumatic injuries. If x-rays are ambiguous, CT scan may reveal a fracture better. Radionuclide scanning may be needed in cases of stress fracture. An arteriogram is often necessary to assure patency of circulation within the leg.

Treatment. Pain management is necessary for these fractures, and surgical reduction and fixation is commonly required. Traction is also often necessary. Open fractures require antibiotics and tetanus toxoid. Frequent monitoring of distal pulses and sensation is necessary to assure neurovascular integrity.

Clavicle Fracture

Clavicle fractures, the most common of all childhood fractures, account for 5% of all fractures and nearly half of significant injuries to the shoulder girdle. Falls are the most common cause, and the most frequent site of injury is the middle of the clavicle. The annual incidence rate is estimated to be between 30 and 60 cases per 100,000 population. Males are affected twice as often as females, with a high incidence in males younger than 30 years because of sports injuries. A smaller peak of incidence occurs in elderly patients in whom the injury is sustained during low-energy falls.

Pathophysiology. Clavicular fractures are classified according to where the break occurs. Group I fractures, the most common variety, occur in the middle third of the clavicle. Group II fractures involve the distal or lateral third, and Group III fractures occur in the medial third. Clavicle fractures are often greenstick fractures, which means that they splinter when fractured.

The clavicle is vulnerable to fracture because of its protruding, superficial position on the chest. These fractures are common with high-energy force injuries or multiple traumatic injuries. With injury of the clavicle, other important structures are subject to damage. For example, the subclavian artery and vein are both in close proximity to the middle portion of the clavicle. The brachial plexus also passes behind the clavicle posterior to the subclavian vessels and is at risk with displaced fractures of the middle clavicle. The subclavius muscle lies between the clavicle and brachial plexus, though small, it is believed to prevent more frequent damage to the brachial plexus.

With clavicular fractures, the clinician needs to thoroughly examine patients for trauma to other areas in close proximity. Injury to the apices of the lung often occurs with displaced middle third clavicle fractures. There can be rib fractures, scapula fractures, and other fractures about the shoulder girdle; pulmonary contusion; pneumothorax; hemothorax; and closed head injuries.

Clinical Presentation. The patient with clavicular fracture will report some kind of high-energy trauma. Persons often fall onto a shoulder and complain of pain in the region. The clinical examination will reveal a deformed area along the clavicle and extreme tenderness. Often, the fractures become displaced. The clinician needs to complete a physical examination, particularly of the thorax. There can also be damage to the vascular structures in close proximity to the clavicle. Some findings of an injury to the subclavian vessels are hematoma overlying the clavicle, presence of a bruit over the region, diminished or absent pulses in the extremity, first rib fracture, brachial plexus injury, and a wide mediastinum on chest x-ray. The lungs should be auscultated to exclude pneumothorax.

Diagnosis. Chest x-ray is essential in clavicular fracture. X-ray views of the sternoclavicular joint and shoulder girdle should be the focus.

> **ALERT!** Pneumothorax needs to be ruled out with clavicular or rib fractures.

Treatment. Realignment of the clavicle and the use of a sling for 4 to 6 weeks following the injury is the common treatment. During this period, the patient should perform active ROM of the elbow and hand. After 4 to 6 weeks, the patient can begin ROM of the shoulder as tolerated. Use of the sling may be discontinued as pain allows. For more complicated displaced fractures, surgery and fixation may be necessary. The patient may also need treatment for associated injuries.

Distal Radius Fracture

Fractures of the distal radius in the wrist are a very common type of fracture. Peak incidence occurs in persons aged 18 to 25 years, as well as persons older than age 65 years. The mechanism of injury is unique to each group, with high-energy injuries being more common in the younger group and fall injuries being more common in the older group. There are two types:

- Smith's fracture: a fracture of the distal radius most commonly caused by falling onto a flexed wrist or a high-energy force to the lower arm. The distal fracture fragment is displaced ventrally (anteriorly).
- Colles fracture: a similar fracture of the distal radius in the forearm caused by falling onto an extended wrist or a high-energy blow to the lower arm; in Colles fracture, there is dorsal (posterior) displacement of the wrist and hand.

Etiology. Motorcycle or motor vehicle accidents, falls from a height, and similar traumatic situations are common causes for a fracture of the distal radius. Trauma is the leading cause in the 15- to 24-year-old age group. Older patients have much weaker bones and can sustain a fracture of the radius from simply falling on an outstretched hand in a ground-level fall. This type of fracture in an older adult is often caused by osteoporosis. As the population lives longer, the frequency of this type of fracture will increase.

Pathophysiology. The fracture of the distal radius is caused by a high amount of force placed on the bone, more than the bone can sustain. The Smith and Colles fractures are the most common wrist injuries. The wrist is flexed during the trauma, causing the fragmented radius to become displaced anteriorly in a Smith fracture. In contrast, the wrist is extended during the trauma, causing posterior displacement of the fragmented radius in a Colles fracture (see Fig. 37-8). The event that caused the fracture should be thoroughly investigated. If the fracture is caused by a fall in an older adult, the patient should be questioned about the circumstances surrounding the fall and assessed for the cause of the fall. Loss of consciousness, myocardial infarction, transient ischemic attacks, and loss of balance and coordination can be the etiology. These conditions require further investigation and diagnostic testing.

Clinical Presentation. The patient should describe events leading to the fall or trauma. A history of prior fractures should be sought and the patient should be asked about a history of osteoporosis, which can cause reduction of the wrist to be challenging and may require

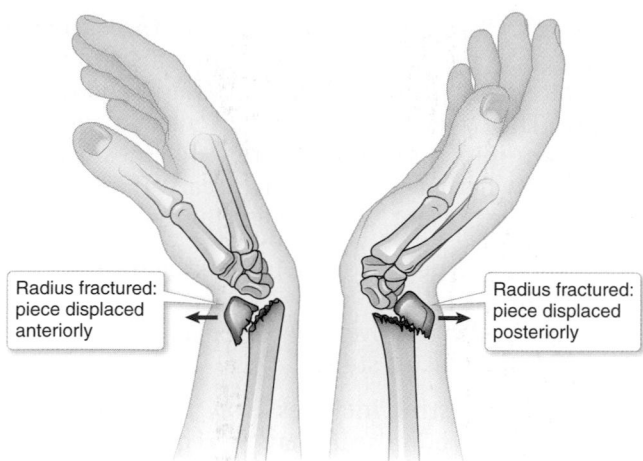

Smith fracture:
commonly due to fall
onto a flexed hand

Colles fracture:
commonly due to fall
onto an extended hand

FIGURE 37-8. Radius fractures: Smith vs. Colles fracture. A Colles fracture, also called an extension fracture of the wrist, is a break in the radius with posterior displacement. A Colles fracture commonly occurs when a patient sustains a fall on an extended hand. A Smith fracture, also referred to as a flexion fracture of the wrist, is a break in the radius with anterior displacement. A Smith fracture commonly occurs when a patient sustains a fall on a flexed hand.

fixation. Pain is present in the wrist, and there may be some deformity and bruising of the wrist's soft tissues. The wrist bones should be examined along with radial and ulnar circulation, development of the hand, ROM, and sensation in the hand. The opposite wrist and hand should be compared. The median nerve function needs to be periodically monitored from the time of the initial examination through treatment. Extreme tenderness and lack of ROM of the wrist will be noted.

Diagnosis and Treatment. X-rays of the wrist and arm should be done. Most fractures can be treated conservatively with a cast or splint. For example, fractures that are not displaced or minimally displaced can be treated in a cast for 6 weeks. If the distal ulna is fractured and unstable, it can be treated in a short arm cast. Fractures in elderly persons that are compressed dorsally can be minimally painful and may appear to be clinically stable; these fractures may be treated with only a splint. Patients with unstable or weak bones may require surgical reduction and internal or external fixation.

Tibia-Fibula Fracture

Fractures of the tibia are the most common long bone fractures. The annual incidence of open fractures of long bones is estimated to be 11.5 per 100,000 persons, with 40% occurring in the lower limb. Lower leg fractures include fractures of the tibia and fibula. Of these two bones, the tibia is the weight-bearing bone. Fractures of the tibia generally are associated with fibula fracture, because there is an interosseous membrane that connects the two bones. Tibia-fibula fractures can occur as a result of low-energy injuries, such as falls, as well as athletic injuries or high-energy injuries, such as motor vehicle accidents and gunshot wounds.

Pathophysiology. The shin, or anterior surface of the tibia, has a very thin layer of subcutaneous tissue, and the bone is easily palpable below the surface. As a result of this, many injuries to the lower leg cause open fractures, which are susceptible to infection.

At the lateral malleolus in the ankle region, the fibula is thinly covered by subcutaneous tissue. It is important to note that the common peroneal nerve, which is susceptible to injury from a fibular fracture, crosses over the fibula and is superficial in this region. In addition, the popliteal artery, which runs along the tibia, is susceptible to injury, which is why neurovascular compromise can easily occur in lower limb fracture.

Diagnosis and Treatment. During the patient history, he or she usually reports a traumatic injury. Associated areas traumatized by the injury also commonly need assessment; treatment should be prioritized. The patient complains of pain, swelling, and inability to bear weight on the leg. The examination commonly shows edema, ecchymosis, and point tenderness. The clinician should perform a neurovascular assessment of the leg; gross deformities should be noted and splinted. Open fractures require emergency orthopedic consultation. Diagnostic testing requires x-ray of the affected leg, as well as the opposite leg for comparison. X-rays of the knee, tibia, fibula, and ankle should be viewed. If widespread trauma occurred to the lower body, the hip and pelvis should be x-rayed as well.

In treating fractures of the lower leg, the patient should be immobilized; in addition, the priority is performing the ABCDEs of trauma assessment. Pain management and lower leg immobilization may require a cast or splint; antibiotics are necessary for an open fracture. Crutches are necessary for patient ambulation; orthopedic consultation is necessary to determine if surgical reduction or fixation is necessary.

Foot Fracture

There are 26 bones of the foot: the calcaneus, talus, navicular, cuboid, 3 cuneiform bones, 5 metatarsal bones, and 14 phalanges. The most common causes of fracture in the foot include a twisting injury as in athletics, trauma directly to the foot, or cumulative trauma that causes a stress fracture.

Several types of fractures occur to the forefoot bone on the side of the little toe (fifth metatarsal). For example, ballet dancers may break this bone during a misstep or fall from a pointe position. An ankle-twisting injury may tear the tendon that attaches to the fifth metatarsal and pull a small piece of the bone away. A more serious injury in the same area is a Jones fracture, which occurs near the base of the fifth metatarsal bone and disrupts the blood supply to the bone. This injury takes longer to heal and may require surgery.

Stress fractures frequently occur in the bones of the forefoot that extend from the toes to the middle of the foot. Stress fractures, tiny cracks in the bone surface, can occur with sudden increases in training, such as running or walking for longer distances or times, improper training techniques, or changes in training surfaces. Toe, tarsal, and navicular fractures are common stress fractures in athletes (see Fig. 37-9).

Dislocation and fracture can occur at the Lisfranc (tarsometatarsal) joint. The Lisfranc joint, found at the base of the second metatarsal, is formed by a 6-bone arch that includes the first, second, and third cuneiforms and first, second, and third metatarsals. Calcaneal (heel) fracture can also occur, usually because of a fall from a lengthy height.

Clinical Presentation. Symptoms of fracture in the foot are pain, deformity, tenderness, and swelling. Bruising and soft tissue injury are common. The patient usually cannot perform ROM or bear weight.

Top view

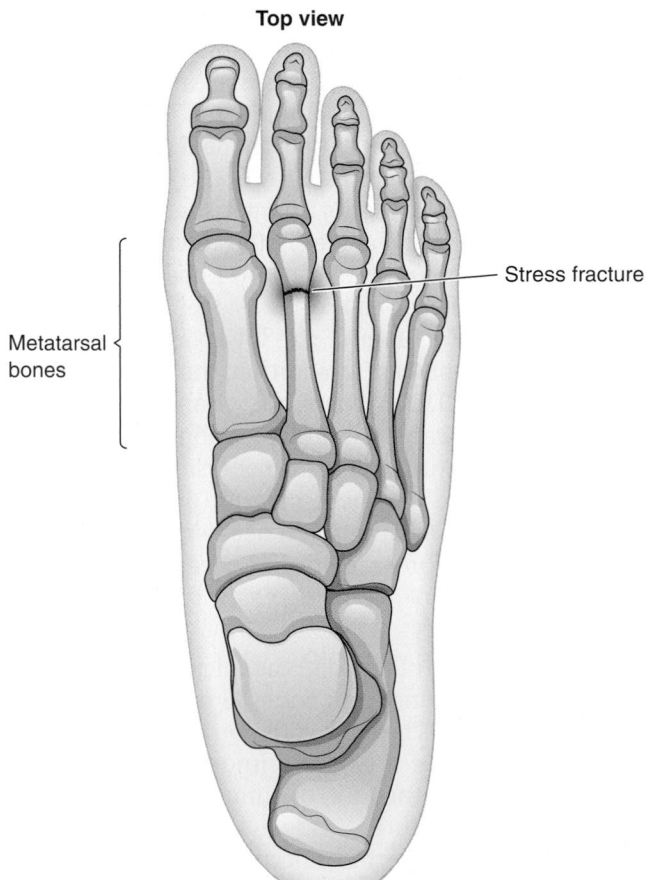

FIGURE 37-9. Stress fracture of the foot. A stress fracture is a small crack in a bone that is often caused by overuse injury. Most stress fractures occur in the weight-bearing bones of the foot and lower leg. When muscles are overtired, they are no longer able to lessen the shock of repeated impact to the foot. When this happens, the muscles transfer the stress to the bones, potentially resulting in small cracks or fractures. The most common sites of stress fractures are the second and third metatarsals of the foot.

Diagnosis. To diagnose foot fracture, the clinician should grasp first and second metatarsals and move them alternately through plantar flexion and dorsiflexion. The Ottawa Foot Rules, a tool that predicts significant midfoot fractures, are guidelines used to determine whether x-rays are necessary. If any of the following are present, an x-ray is required:

- point tenderness over the base of the fifth metatarsal
- point tenderness over the navicular bone
- inability to take 4 steps.

Diagnostic testing includes x-ray, MRI, and ultrasound. A CT or bone scan may be required if a foot fracture is not apparent on plain x-ray. A thorough neurovascular exam is necessary when diagnosing foot injury.

Treatment. Elevation of the leg and analgesics may be necessary until the swelling and pain are relieved. In toe fracture, the procedure of "buddy taping" the toes to each other is used to stabilize the fracture.

Other Common Musculoskeletal Injuries

Rotator cuff injury, shoulder dislocation, brachial plexus palsy, and ulnar nerve injury are other kinds of upper extremity musculoskeletal injuries. Meniscal and ligament tears in the knee are common sports injuries. In the foot, a common inflammatory disorder called plantar fasciitis can cause pain.

Rotator Cuff Injury

Rotator cuff injury or strain is an injury to any of the four rotator cuff muscles in the shoulder. The rotator cuff muscles, a group of muscles that work together to provide stability for the shoulder's glenohumeral joint and control shoulder rotation, include the supraspinatus, infraspinatus, teres minor, and subscapularis. The most commonly injured muscles are the supraspinatus and infraspinatus (see Fig. 37-10). Sports involving constant shoulder rotation, such as baseball pitching or swimming, often cause rotator cuff injury.

There are two major types of rotator cuff injuries:

- tears of the tendons and muscles
- tendonitis, which is inflammation of the tendons.

Clinical Presentation. The patient's chief symptoms are usually pain, weakness, instability, and limited ROM in the shoulder. There may be associated symptoms such as swelling, numbness in the arm, uneven rotation, or "popping" of the shoulder. Pain is often felt over the anterolateral part of the shoulder and is exacerbated by overhead activities. Night pain is a frequent symptom, especially when the patient lies on the affected shoulder.

The patient should be asked about aggravating factors and relieving treatments that have been tried and

View of left shoulder girdle from the front

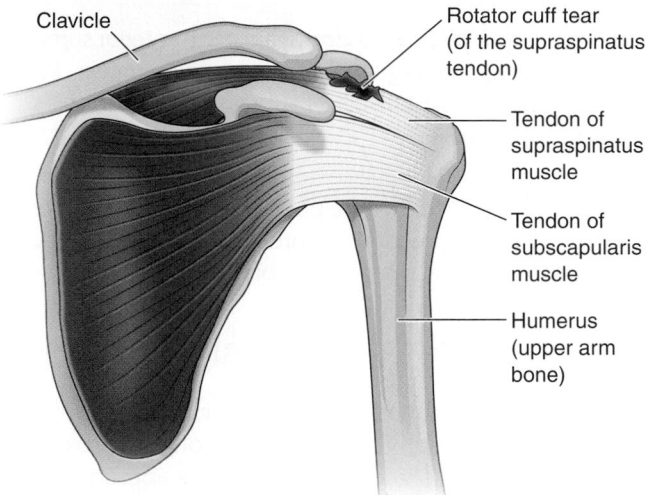

FIGURE 37-10. Rotator cuff injury. The rotator cuff is a group of muscles, tendons, and ligaments around the shoulder joint. The four muscles that form the rotator cuff are the supraspinatus, infraspinatus, teres minor, and subscapularis. A rotator cuff injury includes any type of irritation or damage to the rotator cuff muscles or tendons. Causes of rotator cuff injury may include falling, lifting, and repetitive arm activities.

encouraged to describe the events surrounding any shoulder injuries; previous medical treatment, such as physical therapy; previous injections; and any surgical interventions. The clinician should assess the patient's occupation and sporting activities. In elderly patients, symptoms often are not associated with any specific activity or injury.

The patient requires a thorough physical examination of the shoulder using specific types of maneuvers that assist with diagnosis. Examination should begin with patient observation during the history portion of the evaluation. The clinician needs to carefully inspect the shoulder from the anterior, lateral, and posterior positions. Swelling, atrophy, or asymmetry should be noted. Supraspinatus and infraspinatus muscle atrophy can be observed in rotator cuff tears and in entrapments of the suprascapular nerve. Tenderness is often localized to the greater tuberosity and subacromial bursa. The biceps tendon, which is palpated anteriorly in the bicipital groove, can be inflamed and painful in this condition.

Range of Motion. Total active and passive ROM in all planes and scapulohumeral rhythm should be evaluated. Patients with rotator cuff tears tend to have a decrease in glenohumeral joint motion. Decreased active elevation with normal passive ROM is usually observed in rotator cuff tears secondary to pain and weakness. When both active and passive ROM are decreased, this usually suggests onset of frozen shoulder, also known as **adhesive capsulitis.**

Assess internal rotation by having the patient reach around to his or her back with an extended thumb up the spine. Patients with normal internal rotation reach

the T5–T10 level. Note any accompanying pain and specific pain location in ROM testing.

The impingement syndrome associated with rotator cuff injuries tends to cause pain with elevation ranging from 60° to 120° when the rotator cuff tendons are compressed against the anterior acromion and coracoacromial ligament.

Strength Testing. The clinician should perform strength testing to isolate the relevant muscles individually. The anterior cuff (subscapularis) can be assessed using the lift-off test, which is performed with the arm internally rotated behind the back. Lifting the hand away from the back against resistance tests the strength of the subscapularis muscle. The posterior cuff (infraspinatus and teres minor) is isolated best in 90° of forward flexion with the elbow flexed to 90°, testing external rotation. Significant weakness in external rotation is observed in large rotator cuff tears.

Testing the strength of the supraspinatus muscle can be achieved with the elbow extended, the shoulder in full internal rotation, and the arm in the scapular plane (thumbs down position). Testing of the scapula rotators (trapezius and serratus anterior) is also important. Serratus anterior weakness can be observed by having the patient lean against a wall. Winging of the scapula as the patient pushes against the wall indicates serratus anterior weakness. There are several maneuvers that can be used to assess the strength of the individual muscles of the rotator cuff (see Box 37-5).

Diagnosis. Diagnostic tests include x-ray, MRI, and ultrasound view of the shoulder. It is important that the clinician exclude all other possible causes of shoulder pain, such as angina pectoris and cervical radiculopathy.

Treatment. A physical therapy rehabilitation program is necessary in rotator cuff injury. Pain and inflammation management are required to allow for an active rehabilitation program. A combination of rest; icing for 20 minutes, 3 to 4 times per day; and acetaminophen or an NSAID is advised. The patient should also be advised to sleep with a pillow between the trunk and arm to decrease tension on the supraspinatus tendon and to prevent blood flow. Corticosteroids injected directly into the problem region of the shoulder can facilitate the rehabilitation program.

Shoulder Dislocation

The shoulder is the most commonly dislocated joint in the body. Under normal conditions, the glenohumeral ligaments, the joint capsule, and the rotator cuff muscles maintain shoulder stability. However, a high-energy force from a fall or a striking blow may be sufficient to cause shoulder dislocation, most of which occur anteriorly.

The inferior glenohumeral ligament is commonly injured during an anterior shoulder dislocation. The injury may be a tear of the ligament or capsule off one of its bony attachments, or it may be a stretch injury.

BOX 37-5. Rotator Cuff Assessment Tests

DROP-ARM TEST

Abduct the patient's shoulder to 90° and ask the patient to lower the arm slowly to the side in the same arc of movement. Severe pain or the patient's inability to return the arm to the side slowly indicates a positive test result, which indicates a rotator cuff tear.

NEER IMPINGEMENT TEST

The patient's arm is maximally elevated through forward flexion by the examiner, causing a jamming of the greater tuberosity against the anteroinferior acromion. Pain elicited with this maneuver indicates a positive test result for impingement.

HAWKINS TEST

The examiner forward flexes the arms to 90° and then forcibly internally rotates the shoulder. This movement pushes the supraspinatus tendon against the anterior surface of the coracoacromial ligament and coracoid process. Pain indicates a positive test result for supraspinatus tendonitis.

APPREHENSION TEST

Abduct the arm 90° and fully externally rotate, while placing anteriorly directed force on the posterior humeral head from behind. The patient becomes apprehensive and resists further motion if chronic anterior instability is present.

RELOCATION TEST

Perform the apprehension test with the patient supine and the shoulder at the edge of the table.

In a positive relocation test result indicative of anterior instability, a posteriorly directed force on the proximal humerus causes resolution of the patient's apprehension and usually allows more external rotation of the humerus.

Tears in the rotator cuff muscles or injury to the axillary nerve can also cause shoulder weakness and consequent dislocation.

Clinical Presentation. Patients with a dislocated shoulder complain of severe pain; during a traumatic incident, they may feel the shoulder pop out of its socket. Different shoulder positions during the trauma dislocation cause injury to different ligaments, so the clinician should try to determine the shoulder position at the time of the injury. For example, in an anterior dislocation, the patient reports having the arm abducted and externally rotated.

Some persons have very lax joints; these individuals may report feeling like a joint can roll, rather than pop, out of the socket. However, they are sometimes able to readjust their shoulder joint back into place. Some patients feel numbness and tingling down their arm at the time of the dislocation.

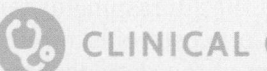 CLINICAL CONCEPT

Patients with previous shoulder dislocations are more apt to redislocate.

In the physical examination, the anteriorly dislocated shoulder is obviously deformed and tender with poor ROM. Posterior shoulder dislocations may not be as obvious because the patient appears to only be guarding the extremity, usually holding the arm against the abdomen.

The clinician needs to complete a detailed neurovascular examination before and after the shoulder has been reduced, because injury to the axillary nerve during shoulder dislocation has been reported to be as high as 40%.

Diagnosis and Treatment. Diagnostic tests include x-ray, CT scan, and MRI scan. Treatment of an acute shoulder dislocation includes maneuvers to reduce the dislocation of the shoulder joint, most commonly the glenohumeral joint. The patient may require conscious sedation or general anesthesia so that there is relaxation of the shoulder musculature. Once reduction has been accomplished, postreduction x-rays are necessary to confirm a normalized joint.

After reduction of the joint dislocation, the arm should be immobilized in a sling for 1 to 3 weeks. The patient should maintain ROM of the elbow, wrist, and hand, and ROM exercises should be continued when the patient comes out of the sling. Rehabilitative therapy that includes active and passive flexion, extension, abduction, and internal and external rotation begins at about the third week, when the patient comes out of the sling. Patients are encouraged to incrementally achieve 10° of improvement in their ROM per week; rehabilitation should restore the ROM over 6 to 8 weeks. In patients who have recurrent shoulder instability, surgery is considered.

 CLINICAL CONCEPT

Immobilization of the shoulder for a lengthy period of time can cause adhesive capsulitis (also called frozen shoulder) (see Box 37-6).

Brachial Plexus Injury

The brachial plexus is a group of nerves that originate at the cervical spinal cord in the neck and run into the axillary region of the arm with branches into the hand and fingers. Nerves within the plexus control the hand, wrist, elbow, and shoulder. The plexus consists of both motor and sensory nerves originating from C5–T1 nerve roots (see Fig. 37-11).

BOX 37-6. Frozen Shoulder

Frozen shoulder is an inflammatory disorder of the shoulder that manifests as stiffness and lack of ROM. Most patients with frozen shoulder have had a period of shoulder immobilization for some reason and then have resulting limited active and passive ROM in the shoulder.

Also called adhesive capsulitis, frozen shoulder commonly affects persons aged 40 to 70 years and is estimated to occur in 2% to 5% of the general population. Females tend to be affected more frequently than males. Frozen shoulder is associated with several conditions, including inactivity; trauma; surgery, including but not limited to shoulder surgery; inflammatory disease; hyperthyroidism; ischemic heart disease; and diabetes. Incidence among patients with insulin-dependent diabetes is 36% with bilateral shoulder involvement.

In the history, information should be gathered regarding the onset and duration of symptoms, trauma or surgery, and affected side. The patient usually complains of pain and stiffness in the shoulder with an inability to stretch the arm above head level. The patient should be asked about any existing conditions. Because frozen shoulder is associated with diabetes, hyperthyroidism, ischemic heart disease, and cervical spinal nerve impingement, these disorders should be excluded using screening tests. Any previous treatments that the patient has received for the shoulder should be documented, as should the individual's current medications. Questions should be directed toward any upper extremity neurological complaints. Any history of cervical pain or radiculopathy should be thoroughly evaluated during the clinical examination to exclude a diagnosis of herniated cervical disc.

The patient's posture should be observed while seated. It should also be noted whether the patient is leaning to one side secondary to pain and whether he or she is holding the neck to one side secondary to spasm or pain. The clinician should try to exclude a cervical condition contributing to the shoulder stiffness.

Diagnostic tests include x-ray, CT scan, and MRI. Treatment involves physical therapy and anti-inflammatory agents, and corticosteroid injection into the shoulder may be necessary. Surgery may be needed if other treatments are unsuccessful.

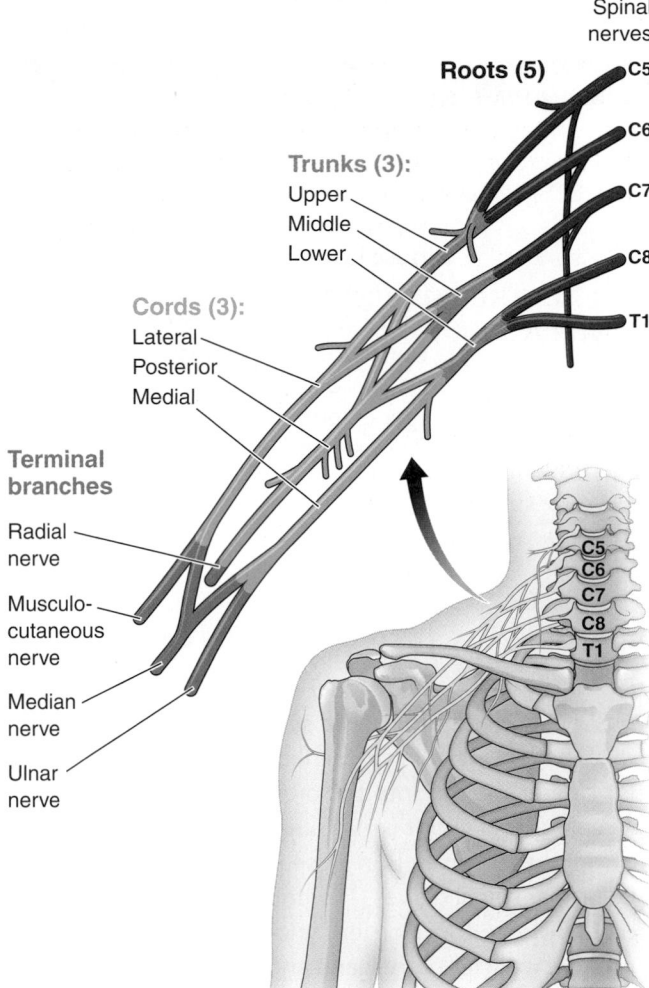

FIGURE 37-11. Brachial plexus. The brachial plexus is a network of nerves that arise from the cervical (C5–C8) and first thoracic spinal nerves. The network consists of the musculocutaneous, radial, ulnar, and median nerves of the arm.

A recent study showed that brachial plexus injuries occur in slightly more than 1% of multitrauma victims. Motorcycle accidents carry especially high risks, with the incidence of injury approaching 5%. Head injuries, thoracic injuries, fractures, and dislocations affecting the shoulder girdle and cervical spine are particularly common associated injuries.

Etiology and Pathophysiology. Most injuries of the brachial plexus involve the spinal nerves C7, C8, or T1.

Pressure, damage, stretching, and crushing injuries can all damage the brachial plexus. A brachial plexus injury, also referred to as Erb's palsy, occurs because of a violent pull of the entire arm and shoulder from the rest of the body. These injuries usually result from high-speed motor vehicle accidents or high-energy forces in activities such as football or wrestling. A fall from a significant height or penetrating injuries such as gunshot wounds can also result in brachial plexus injury. A brachial plexus injury can also occur at birth because of difficult delivery of the newborn's shoulders.

Minor injury occurs when the brachial plexus nerves are stretched. More significant injuries occur with an avulsion, when the nerve root is torn from the spinal cord. The sensory and motor consequences of brachial plexus injury (nerves C5–T1) affect the arm, hand, and fingers (see Table 37-3).

Clinical Presentation. The patient will report a traumatic event that pulled the arm away from the body with high force. Injuries may also be caused by compression

TABLE 37-3. Brachial Plexus Motor Testing

Cervical Root	Clinically Relevant Gross Motor Function
C5	Shoulder abduction, extension, and external rotation; some elbow flexion
C6	Elbow flexion, forearm pronation and supination, some wrist extension
C7	Diffuse loss of function in the extremity without complete paralysis of a specific muscle group, elbow extension, consistently supplies the latissimus dorsi
C8	Finger extensors, finger flexors, wrist flexors, hand intrinsics
T1	Hand intrinsic muscles

TABLE 37-4. Brachial Plexus Sensory Testing

Location of Deep Pressure Test	Affected Spinal Nerve	Nerve
Thumb	C6	Median nerve
Middle finger	C7	Median nerve
Little finger	C8	Ulnar nerve

CLINICAL CONCEPT

Horner syndrome, a disorder of the sympathetic nervous system, causes classic symptoms of autonomic dysfunction, including ptosis (lid droop), enophthalmos (sinking of the eye into the orbit), anhidrosis (dry eye), sweating, and miosis (small pupil). Because the chain of sympathetic nerves is in close proximity to the thoracolumbar spinal nerves, T1 within the brachial plexus is often affected in Horner syndrome. T1 controls the intrinsic muscles of the hand and resultant sensory and motor dysfunction can occur.

between the clavicle and first rib, penetrating injuries, or direct blows. Recognition may be delayed by other injuries, particularly to the spinal cord and head. The patient complains of feeling a shocklike pain or burning sensation, as well as numbness and weakness down the arm. Signs and symptoms of severe injuries can include inability to move the shoulder, elbow, or fingers; complete lack of sensation in the arm; and severe pain.

In brachial plexus injury, there can be swelling in the shoulder region and diminished or absent pulses in the arm. There can also be associated cervical spine, head, and clavicle fractures. It is important for the clinician to examine each cervical nerve root individually for motor and sensory function. Sensory and motor examination according to the sensory and motor dermatomes is important; examination of wrist and finger sensation and motion with respect to the median, ulnar, and radial nerves may help start to locate the lesion within the brachial plexus. Elbow flexion and extension determine radial nerve function, whereas shoulder abduction tests the axillary nerve.

Diagnosis and Treatment. Diagnosis includes clinical examination, x-ray, CT myelogram, MRI, EMG, and nerve conduction studies. The nerves of the brachial plexus can be tested for sensation and motor function to find exactly which brachial nerves are involved in the injury (see Table 37-3 and Table 37-4). Often, brachial plexus injury is a part of multitrauma injuries. Therefore, the ABCDEs of trauma assessment should be followed. After the patient is stabilized, bracing of the arm in the anatomical position is important. Neurological pain often cannot be remedied by traditional analgesics; however, antidepressants and anticonvulsants may ease neurological pain. Transcutaneous nerve stimulation (TNS) and acupuncture have been used for pain control as well. Neurovascular surgery often is necessary; physical therapy and rehabilitation are also required. Prevention of contractures of the arm is a key concern.

Ulnar Nerve Injury

The ulnar nerve, a peripheral branch of the brachial plexus, runs from the axillary region down into the arm and becomes superficial at the elbow's olecranon process. It then continues into the wrist and innervates the ring and small finger. Because of the ulnar nerve's anatomical position, it is subject to entrapment and pressure injury.

Etiology and Pathophysiology. The ulnar nerve is the peripheral branch of the medial cord of the brachial plexus, consisting of fibers C8–T1. Proximally, it is located medial to the axillary artery and then to the brachial artery to the middle of the arm. It pierces the intermuscular septum and follows the medial head of the triceps muscle to the groove between the olecranon process and the medial epicondyle. At this location, ulnar injury commonly occurs because of its superficial location. A blow that strikes the ulnar nerve will cause a sharp pain that radiates into the fingers. The area of the ulnar nerve at the elbow is commonly called "the funny bone" (see Fig. 37-12).

Clinical Presentation. In the history, the patient will complain of symptoms from mild, transient paresthesias in the ring and small fingers to contracture of these digits and severe intrinsic muscle atrophy. The patient usually reports severe pain at the elbow or wrist with radiation into the hand or up into the shoulder and should be tested in the pinch position for Froment sign (see Fig. 37-13).

In ulnar nerve injury, numbness in the arm usually precedes motor loss. Muscle wasting and contracture of the ring and small digits are indicative of a chronic compressive syndrome.

> ### CLINICAL CONCEPT
>
> A positive Froment sign indicates dysfunction of the ulnar nerve motor fibers.

Diagnosis and Treatment. The clinician should obtain x-rays of the neck, chest, elbow, and wrist. Entrapment of the ulnar nerve may occur at more than one level. MRI may be necessary for visualization of soft tissue lesions. EMG tests and nerve conduction studies are indicated to confirm the area of entrapment and examine the extent of the pathology.

Treatment of ulnar neuropathy at the elbow can include splint devices, physical therapy, rehabilitation, or surgery. Nonsteroidal anti-inflammatory medications may relieve nerve irritation. Surgical intervention is indicated if numbness or paresthesias occur despite

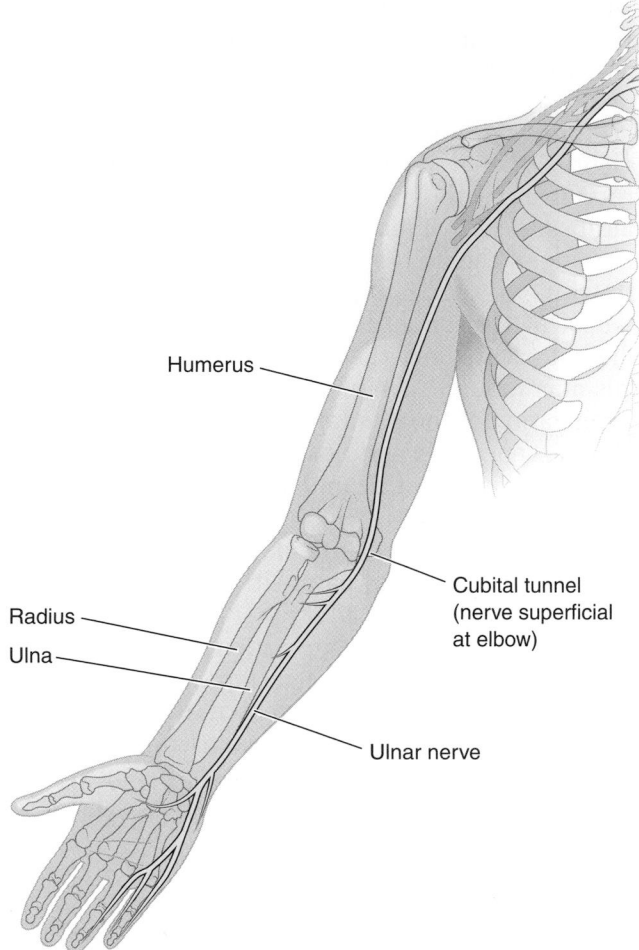

FIGURE 37-12. The distribution of the ulnar nerve. The ulnar nerve originates in the brachial plexus of the axillary region and becomes superficial at the elbow. It continues into the ring finger and little finger of the hand. Common injuries include entrapment of the ulnar nerve or trauma to the ulnar nerve at the elbow. When the ulnar nerve is pinched, the sensation is referred to as "hitting the funny bone."

neck. Patients may report difficulty performing rotation, flexion, and extension of the wrist. When the patient rests on the elbows, numbness and paresthesias down the ulnar side of the arm can occur.

The clinician should examine the neck and shoulder and move down the affected extremity to the elbow. The course of the ulnar nerve should be palpated from the axilla to the forearm and wrist. Pain on neck movement could indicate cervical disc disease or a problem with the brachial plexus. Masses on the ulnar side of the arm could indicate a soft tissue tumor or hematoma compressing the ulnar nerve. At the elbow, deformity and mobility should be assessed. Comparison of the opposite arm is necessary.

The flexor carpi ulnaris and flexor digitorum profundus strength should be assessed by having the patient flex the wrist and make a fist. Intrinsic muscle function is tested by asking the patient to cross the long finger over the index. Only two muscles can be tested accurately in the hand, the abductor digiti quinti and the first dorsal interosseous. The thumb

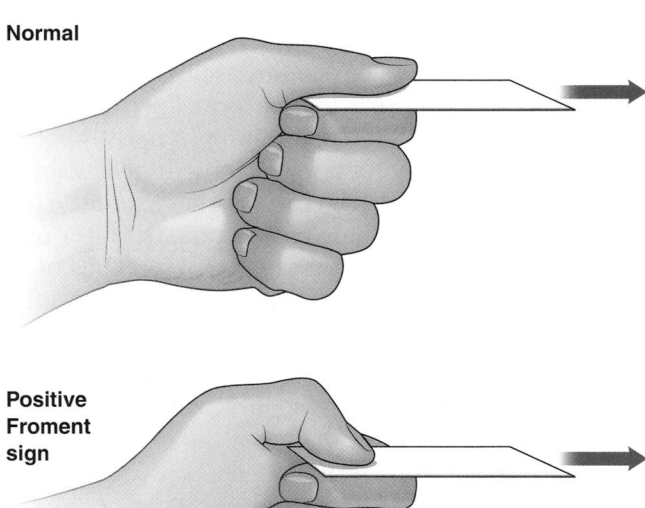

FIGURE 37-13. Froment sign. The Froment test assesses the strength of the adductor pollicis, which is weak with an ulnar nerve palsy. A patient is asked to hold an object, usually a flat object such as a piece of paper, between the thumb and index finger in a pinch grip. The examiner then attempts to pull the object out of the patient's hands. A normal individual will be able to maintain a hold on the object without difficulty. With ulnar nerve palsy, the patient will experience difficulty maintaining a hold and will compensate by flexing the flexor pollicis longus of the thumb to maintain grip pressure, causing a pinching effect.

other treatment and if motor function problems occur. Vitamin B$_6$ supplements may improve neurological function.

Plantar Fasciitis

Plantar fasciitis is an inflammatory degenerative disorder of the connective tissue in the sole of the foot. The plantar fascia originates at the calcaneus (heel bone) and attaches to deep ligaments of the metatarsal heads (see Fig. 37-14). The pain may be substantial, resulting in difficulty walking. There are many causes of heel pain, although plantar fasciitis is the most common cause of heel pain for which medical care is sought. Peak incidence occurs in women aged 40 to 60 years. Women are affected by plantar fasciitis twice as often as men.

> ### CLINICAL CONCEPT
>
> Many individuals mistakenly refer to plantar fasciitis as a heel spur. Although heel spurs can be the cause for the disorder, cumulative trauma is the most common etiology. Approximately 10% of the U.S. population experiences bouts of heel pain, which result in 1 million visits per year to medical professionals for treatment of plantar fasciitis.

Etiology. Most cases of plantar fasciitis are caused by cumulative stress on the foot. Incorrect performance of athletic activities, such as running in nonsupportive shoes, can cause plantar fasciitis. Structural flaws of the leg or foot are also risk factors for the disorder. These anatomical causes include **pes planus** (flat feet), overpronation of the foot, **pes cavus** (high arches of the foot), leg-length discrepancy, excessive lateral tibial torsion, and excessive femoral anteversion. Tightness in the gastrocnemius, soleus muscles, and Achilles tendon are also risk factors for plantar fasciitis.

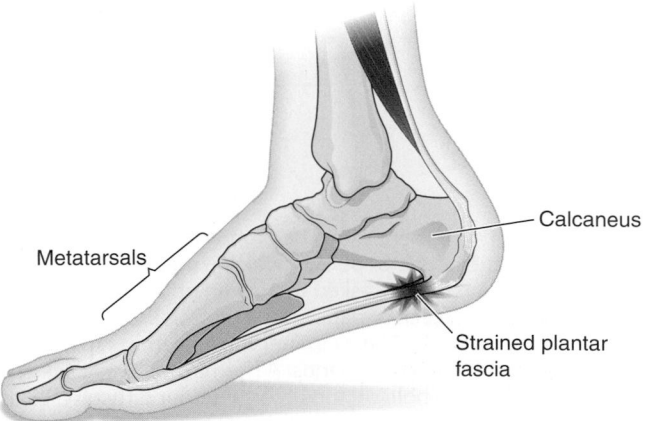

Metatarsals

Calcaneus

Strained plantar fascia

FIGURE 37-14. Plantar fasciitis. Inflammation of the connective tissue that is attached from the metacarpal bones to the calcaneus (heel). It can cause intense pain.

Risk factors that increase susceptibility include obesity, occupations requiring prolonged standing and weight-bearing, and heel spurs.

Pathophysiology. The pathophysiology of plantar fasciitis is believed to be secondary to repetitive microtrauma (microtears), with resulting damage at the calcaneal-fascial interface secondary to repetitive stressing of the arch with weight-bearing. Excessive stretching of the plantar fascia can result in microtrauma of this structure either along its course or where it inserts onto the medial calcaneal tuberosity. This microtrauma, if repetitive, can result in chronic degeneration of the plantar fascia fibers. The loading of the degenerative and healing tissue at the plantar fascia may cause significant foot pain.

Clinical Presentation. Patients with plantar fasciitis complain of sharp heel pain with the first couple of steps in the morning or after other long periods without weight-bearing. Pain is experienced chronically in the sole of the foot. Patients may report that before the onset of pain, they had increased the amount or intensity of athletic activity, such as running. They may have also started exercising on a different type of surface or may have recently changed footwear.

> ### CLINICAL CONCEPT
>
> Plantar fasciitis accounts for about 10% of running-related injuries.

The pain of plantar fasciitis can usually be reproduced by palpating the area of the sole where the plantar fascia inserts into the heel bone. The anteriomedial aspect of the plantar fascia is tender. Less frequently, the pain will localize directly below the heel bone or even in the midsection of the plantar arch. In more severe cases, pain may be reproduced by palpation over the proximal portion of the plantar fascia. A tight Achilles tendon is commonly a secondary finding; ankle dorsiflexion may be limited as a result.

Other maneuvers that may reproduce the pain of plantar fasciitis include passive dorsiflexion of the toes, which is sometimes called the windlass test, and having the patient stand on the tiptoes and toe-walk.

Diagnosis and Treatment. The clinical examination is usually enough to diagnose the condition. However, X-rays can be useful to rule out heel spurs, and CT or MRI may be needed to rule out stress fracture. Traditional treatment usually begins with 6 weeks of consistent and daily icing, stretching, NSAID therapy, strapping and taping, and over-the-counter shoe orthotics. Counseling regarding activity modification, as well as choice of shoe gear, is important. After 6 weeks, some cases require additional treatment with a night splint to keep the foot in dorsiflexion, as well as a possible corticosteroid injection, along with the initial regimen for another 6 weeks. Injection therapy, immobilization in a cast or walker boot, and physical therapy are sometimes needed. For severe cases, fasciotomy, a surgical intervention that cuts the connective tissue to release tension, may be required.

Ligament or Meniscus Injury of the Knee

Knee pain occurs in 20% of the general adult population and accounts for almost 3 million outpatient and emergency department visits per year. Overall, 18.1% of U.S. men and 23.5% of U.S. women aged 60 years and older report knee pain for 6 weeks before seeking medical care. Sixty percent of knee injuries are sports-related, although trauma of the knee is the second most common occupation-related injury.

The knee joint, the largest synovial joint of the body, is a combination of two interdependent joints: the tibiofemoral and the patellofemoral joints. The condyle surfaces of the tibia and the femur come together at the knee. Between these surfaces are cartilaginous structures known as the medial and lateral menisci, which act as shock-absorbers. The knee must support as much as 5 times an individual's body weight, and this force is transmitted through the condyles of the femur and the tibia. A fibrous capsule lined by a synovial membrane composes the knee joint with ligaments surrounding the tibia, femur, and patella bones.

There are two collateral ligaments and two cruciate ligaments that surround the joint capsule. These ligaments consist of the medial collateral ligament (MCL), which counteracts abductive forces coming from the medial side of the knee, and the lateral collateral ligament (LCL), which limits excessive adductive forces coming from the lateral side of the knee. The anterior cruciate ligament (ACL) and the posterior cruciate ligament (PCL) crisscross the joint and brace the knee against excessive anteroposterior forces. The ACL serves as the primary knee stabilizer, preventing forward displacement of the tibia on the femur. Damage to the ACL causes the most joint instability. Also at the knee, the quadriceps muscle fuses into the patellar ligament, which inserts onto the tibial tubercle.

There are many bursae in the knee that cushion the knee and alleviate frictional forces between the susceptible structures. In the back of the knee joint, in the popliteal fossa, are vital neurovascular structures, including the popliteal artery (see Fig. 37-15).

Etiology and Pathophysiology. Valgus- or varus-directed forces and anterior- or posterior-directed

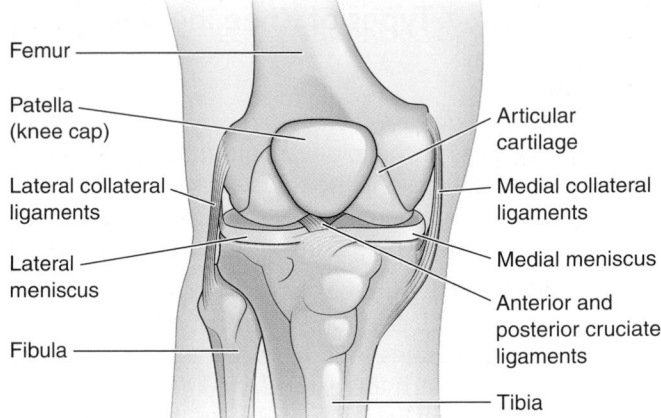

FIGURE 37-15. Knee joint. The structures around the knee joint that are most commonly affected by injury include the menisci and ligaments.

forces can cause injuries to the knee (see Fig. 37-16 and Box 37-7). Direct blows to one side of the knee provoke injury to the contralateral collateral ligaments and patellar dislocation. Pure **valgus** forces, those occurring on the lateral aspect of the knee, are more common than **varus**-directed contact on the medial side of the knee. The MCL is more prone to injury than the LCL. A combination of valgus or varus stress, whether direct or indirect, delivered to a rotated leg accounts for a wide array of injuries. Vulnerable structures include the collateral and cruciate ligaments, the menisci, and the joint capsule.

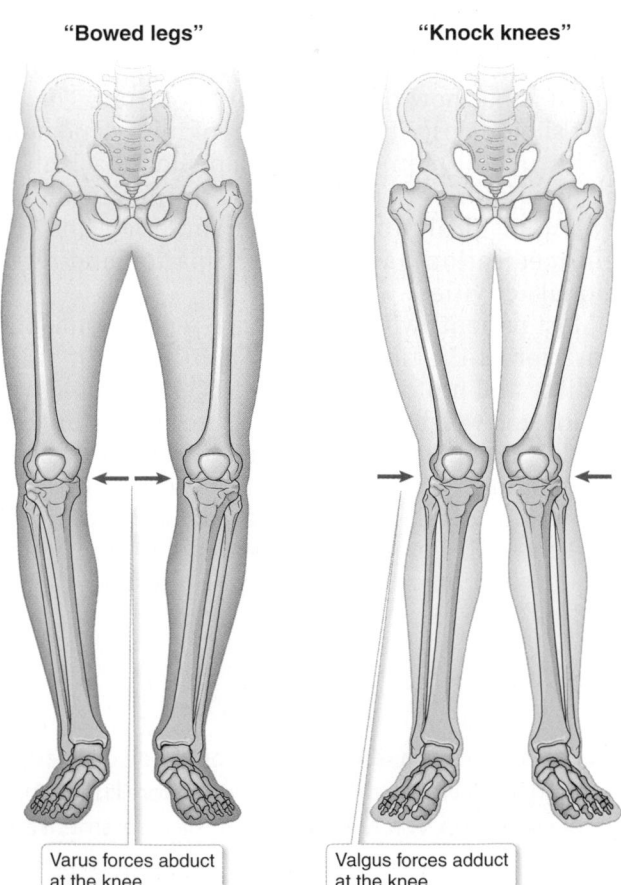

FIGURE 37-16. Valgus vs. varus forces directed at the knee.

 CLINICAL CONCEPT

The medial collateral ligament, medial meniscus, and the anterior cruciate ligament are commonly injured in knee trauma.

BOX 37-7. Types of Knee Injuries

SPRAINS

Sprains to the knee are characterized by the stretching of the ligaments or the joint capsule, whereas a strain refers to stretching along the course of muscles or tendons. Collateral ligament and cruciate ligament sprains, as well as muscular strains, are common in the knee.

RUPTURE OF THE ACL

Rupture of the ACL is among the most serious of the common knee injuries. ACL tears are associated with anterior blows that hyperextend the knee, as well as strong deceleration forces to the knee. Most patients with ACL damage complain of immediate and profound pain, exacerbated with motion, and inability to bear weight on the knee. Disruption of the ACL may occur alone or with other knee injuries, especially a meniscal injury or MCL tear.

MENISCAL TEAR

Rotational movements may cause a meniscal tear. The medial meniscus is firmly fixated compared with the more mobile lateral meniscus. It is attached to the MCL capsule and has less elasticity than the lateral meniscus, which makes it vulnerable to injury. Menisci do not have pain fibers; the tearing and bleeding into peripheral attachments, as well as the traction on the joint capsule, causes the pain.

Clinical Presentation. The patient should be questioned about how the knee injury occurred. The patient should describe the motion of injury and point to the area of pain. The clinician should ask about previous injuries to the knee, and the patient should explain medical problems, past surgeries, and current medications, as well as occupation and recreational activities.

Most patients with ACL damage report a snapping sensation at the time of injury and complain of immediate and profound pain that is exacerbated with motion and weight-bearing. An acute knee injury heralded by a pop or snap, followed by rapidly evolving edema almost always affirms a rupture of the ACL. This injury displaces the tibia backward and pulls apart the PCL. Patellar injury with disruption of normal articulation or fracture may also result.

CLINICAL CONCEPT

In cases of trauma, the patient should be completely examined for life-threatening injuries before knee injury is focused upon. The ABCDEs of trauma assessment are applied to the patient. After the patient has been stabilized, the knee can be the area of concentration.

Focus the initial examination on inspection, palpation, and neurovascular evaluation of the knee. The clinician should examine the injured knee in comparison with the contralateral knee. Observe the patient in a standing position. When an uninjured patient stands with feet together, the medial aspects of both knees and ankles are normally in contact. The knee should be inspected for edema, ecchymosis, masses, patella location and size, muscle mass, erythema, and evidence of local trauma, such as abrasions, contusions, or lacerations. After a knee injury, onset of edema and pain tends to occur within the first 3 hours after injury. The clinician should verify the knee's mechanical trauma by attempting to perform passive ROM. Also, the clinician should observe if the patient can walk or bear weight on the knee. The posterior aspect of the knee should be palpated for the popliteal pulse, abnormal bulges, popliteal thrombophlebitis, or Baker cysts.

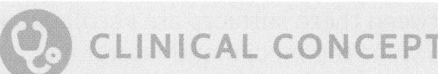 CLINICAL CONCEPT

A Baker cyst, which originates from a herniation of the synovial membrane through the posterior aspect of the joint capsule, tends to be associated with intra-articular disease.

The knee should be palpated in slight flexion. This position can be facilitated by placing a pillow under the popliteal fossa. There also should be stress testing of the knee by applying gentle pressure in various valgus, varus, anterior, and posterior directions. In bursitis, there is tenderness, erythema, warmth, and swelling; however, ROM is usually not restricted.

There are several specific maneuvers that are used in the assessment of the knee (see Box 37-8).

Diagnosis. The clinical examination is an important feature in the diagnosis. Other studies of importance include x-ray, CT, and MRI scan. Ultrasound can be used to diagnose effusions, tendon ruptures, and popliteal cysts. Arthocentesis, the examination of the fluid surrounding the knee, may be necessary.

Treatment. Initial treatment of most knee injuries includes RICE therapy. For the first 1 to 3 days, therapeutic measures are used that minimize tissue damage and reduce pain and inflammation. The knee may be splinted to provide support and to prevent further injury. Intra-articular injection of an analgesic or surgical treatment may be required.

In cases of trauma, the ABCDEs should be applied before focusing on the knee. Stabilization of the lower extremity and monitoring the neurovascular status of the limb are essential. If there is resistance to realignment, this should not be attempted. Wounds should be covered with saline-soaked sterile gauze.

BOX 37-8. Knee Assessment Tests

There are some specific maneuvers used to investigate the individual structures of the knee.

ACL

- Anterior drawer test: The patient assumes a supine position with the injured knee flexed to 90°. The clinician fixes the patient's foot in slight external rotation by sitting on the foot and then placing his or her thumbs at the tibial tubercle and fingers at the posterior calf. With the patient's hamstring muscles relaxed, the clinician pulls anteriorly and assesses anterior displacement of the tibia (positive anterior drawer sign).
- Lachman test: The test is performed with the patient in a supine position and the injured knee flexed to 30°. The clinician stabilizes the distal femur with one hand, grasps the proximal tibia in the other hand, and then attempts to sublux the tibia anteriorly. Lack of a clear endpoint indicates a positive Lachman test.

MCL

- Valgus stress test: This test is performed with the patient's leg slightly abducted. The clinician places one hand at the lateral aspect of the knee joint and the other hand at the medial aspect of the distal tibia. Next, valgus stress is applied to the knee at both 0° (full extension) and 30° of flexion. With the knee at 0°, the PCL and the articulation of the femoral condyles with the tibial plateau should stabilize the knee; with the knee at 30° of flexion, application of valgus stress assesses the laxity or integrity of the MCL.

MENISCAL STABILITY

- McMurray test: Patients with injury to the menisci usually demonstrate tenderness at the joint line. The McMurray test is performed with the patient lying supine. To assess the medial meniscus, the test is performed with the patient supine and the knee flexed to 90°. The examiner grasps the patient's heel with one hand to hold the tibia in external rotation, placing the thumb at the lateral joint line and the fingers at the medial joint line. The examiner flexes the patient's knee maximally to impinge the posterior horn of the meniscus against the medial femoral condyle. A varus stress is applied as the examiner extends the knee.

Chapter Summary

- Trauma is the leading cause of death for persons aged 1 to 44 years.
- Peak bone mass is achieved in early adulthood, around age 30 to 35 years.
- There is a wide spectrum of types of musculoskeletal trauma, from acute, life-threatening injuries to mild sprains and strains.
- Motor vehicle accidents, sports activities, and osteoporosis are major causes of musculoskeletal trauma.
- Whenever musculoskeletal trauma occurs because of high-energy forces, astute assessment skills are necessary. Associated organ trauma, neurovascular damage, and collateral fractures are common.
- A sprain is an overstretching of tendons and ligaments with possible tear. The most common location for a sprain is in the ankle.
- A strain is an overstretching or contraction of muscle. The most common locations for strain are the lower back and hamstring.
- Cumulative trauma disorders occur when the act of performing repetitive movements of parts of the musculoskeletal system cause "wear and tear" injuries.
- There are many different types of bone fractures, and all require immobilization for healing to occur.
- Callus formation takes at least 6 weeks, and by 3 months only 80% of bone strength is regained.

- Initial treatment of most musculoskeletal injuries includes rest, ice, compression, and elevation (RICE).
- To assess neurovascular status, always check pulses and sensation distal to a musculoskeletal injury.
- Compartment syndrome occurs when tissue pressure exceeds perfusion pressure in a closed anatomical space.
- Although immobilization is necessary for healing, it increases the risk of complications, such as deep venous thrombosis, contracture, and muscle atrophy.
- Compound or open fractures are vulnerable to infection.
- The history of how the trauma occurred is an important feature of diagnosis. Physical examination findings often reveal deformity, pain, and limited ROM.
- Vertebral compression fracture is pathognomonic of osteoporosis.
- The hip, wrist, and vertebrae are the most commonly fractured bones in elderly individuals with osteoporosis.
- The shoulder is the most commonly dislocated joint of the body.
- Frozen shoulder is indicated when active and passive ROM of the shoulder are decreased.
- Trauma of the knee is the second most common occupation-related injury. The middle collateral ligament is the most frequently injured ligament in the knee.
- Rupture of the ACL is among the most serious of knee injuries and causes the most joint instability.

Making the Connections

Disorder and Pathophysiology	Signs and Symptoms	Physical Assessment Findings	Diagnostic Testing	Treatment
Cervical Strain | Acceleration-deceleration mechanism of injury causing elongation and tearing of cervical muscles or ligaments with subsequent edema, hemorrhage, and inflammation. Commonly occurs in motor vehicle accidents, while lifting heavy objects, and with abnormal postures.				
	Suboccipital headache; motion-induced neck pain; shoulder, scapular, or arm pain. Visual disturbances, dizziness, difficulty sleeping. Onset of symptoms usually delayed 12 to 72 hours after incident.	Tenderness along cervical spine, paravertebral muscle spasm, swelling.	X-ray shows soft tissue injury.	Short-term use of soft cervical collar, muscle relaxants, heat application to area, possibly steroid injections Pain management.
Lumbar Strain or Sprain | Active strain and sprain of lumbosacral muscles or ligaments with frequent intervertebral disc herniation, causing impingement on spinal nerves.				
	Sharp pain, stiffness, and tenderness in the lumbosacral region, often with pain radiation down into one leg (called radicular pain or sciatica). Numbness and tingling along dermatome into lower extremity. In cauda equina syndrome, bladder and bowel incontinence or saddle paresthesias.	Lumbosacral paravertebral tenderness and swelling. Lack of sensation in dermatome areas of lower extremity. Possibly diminished deep tendon reflexes and weakness in lower extremity. L4-L5 spinal nerve tested with patient's ability to walk on heels. L5-S1 tested with patient's ability to walk on toes.	CBC with differential, ESR, C-reactive protein. Lumbar x-ray, CT, or MRI).	Back support belt, periodic stretching exercises (no prolonged sitting or lying), muscle relaxants, heat application to area, possibly steroid injections. Pain management. Avoidance of heavy lifting, jogging, climbing. Physical therapy, TENS, massage, ultrasound treatments, chiropractic treatments.
Ankle Sprain | Commonly caused by inversion of foot during plantar flexion of ankle; most injuries involve the anterior talofibular ligament.				
	Intense pain, swelling of ankle joint, weakness of foot, inability to bear weight, popping sound during injury.	Tenderness, commonly over either malleolus; edema; ecchymosis; and deformity of ankle. Decreased ROM. Check posterior tibial and dorsalis pedis pulses.	Order ankle x-ray based on Ottawa Ankle Rules.	Rest, ice, compression, elevation (RICE); cessation of weight-bearing may be prescribed. Compression dressing, air stirrup splint, or plaster or fiberglass posterior splint for more severe sprains. Pain management. Physical therapy.
Stress Fracture | Repetitive stress on bone; most commonly tibia, fibula, and second and third metatarsals.				
	Localized bone pain that increases with weight-bearing.	Tenderness along involved bone.	X-ray, bone scanning, MRI, and CT scanning preferred for diagnosis.	Rest with gradual return to increased activity once pain subsides. Pain management.

Continued

Making the Connections–cont'd

Disorder and Pathophysiology	Signs and Symptoms	Physical Assessment Findings	Diagnostic Testing	Treatment
Carpal Tunnel Syndrome | Increased pressure on the median nerve in the carpal tunnel in the wrist.				
	Numbness, tingling, pain in the hand and proximally in the forearm along the distribution of the median nerve.	Wrist pain radiation of pain proximal to wrist. Intermittent paresthesias in the median nerve distribution of hand. Pain worse at night.	Clinical exam, including finding paresthesias in the median distribution of the hand after Phalen sign and Tinel sign.	Rest, splinting, surgery possible. Pain management.
Lateral Epicondylitis | Repeated extension of the wrist and pronation and supination of the forearm.				
	Tenderness of the lateral epicondyle, weak grip strength, painful movement of wrist and forearm.	Tenderness of the lateral epicondyle, weak grip.	X-ray, CT, or MRI.	Rest, ice, nonsteroidal analgesics, splinting, steroid injection, physical therapy. Pain management.
Bursitis | Inflammation of the bursa commonly caused by repetitive. motion injury.				
	Pressure and painful motion of joint.	Swelling, warmth, tenderness of joint.	ESR, x-ray.	Moist heat, immobilization, intrabursal steroid injections, possibly surgery. Pain management.
TMJ Disorder | Repetitive stress on TMJ caused by jaw malocclusion, anterior disc disorder, abnormal chewing patterns, facial trauma, bruxism.				
	Pain over TMJ area, preauricular area, and muscles of mastication, aggravated with chewing or bruxism.	Tenderness, swelling of the masseter, temporalis, medial pterygoid, digastric, and mylohyoid muscles. Clicking of TMJ.	Dental exam to rule out dental etiology.	Physical therapy, patient education, acupuncture possibly. Pain management.
Hip Fracture | Most occur as a fracture through the femoral neck or fracture from greater trochanter to lesser trochanter; intertrochanteric or beneath the trochanters; subtrochanteric. Common sequel of osteoporosis.				
	Pain centered in groin, immobility.	An externally rotated and shortened leg. Motion to the extremity will produce severe pain centered around the affected groin. Edema and ecchymosis possible.	X-ray.	Surgical reduction and fixation, hip replacement sometimes required. Anticoagulant therapy caused by high risk for deep venous thrombosis. Hip fracture indicates osteoporosis is likely; therefore, Ca++/ vitamin D supplements needed. Pain management.

Continued

Making the Connections–cont'd

Disorder and Pathophysiology	Signs and Symptoms	Physical Assessment Findings	Diagnostic Testing	Treatment
Vertebral Compression Fracture | A thinning of the vertebral body. A 15% to 20% or more decrease in vertebral body height. Common sequela of osteoporosis.				
	Back pain, kyphosis, loss of height. Pain worsened by ambulation.	Tenderness over spine Pain with ambulation. Kyphosis. Paravertebral muscle spasm.	X-ray and dual energy x-ray absorptiometry (DEXA) scan of spine.	Calcitonin, muscle relaxants, analgesics, external support devices, vertebral surgery; vertebroplasty, kyphoplasty. Osteoporosis likely in patient; therefore. Ca++/vitamin D supplements needed.
Femur Shaft Fracture | Type I: spiral or transverse. Type II: comminuted. Type III: open.				
	Pain and visible deformity are typical. Extremity may appear shortened. Immobility and thigh swelling.	At site of fracture, tenderness on examination and visible deformity are typical. Extremity may appear shortened, and crepitus is noted with movement. Thigh is often swollen secondary to hematoma formation.	X-ray and neurovascular exam. Arteriogram often needed.	Pain management Surgical reduction and fixation; traction is often necessary. Open fractures require antibiotic and tetanus toxoid.
Clavicle Fracture | Fracture commonly occurs from fall with outstretched hand or direct trauma to shoulder. Middle clavicle most common site.				
	Shoulder pain, swelling, and possible ecchymosis.	Tenderness over clavicular area, edema, ecchymosis.	X-ray. Lung examination.	Sling immobilization or figure-eight bandaging. Pain management.
Colles Fracture | Most common fracture; associated with outstretched hand and arm to prevent fall. Fracture through the distal metaphysis, approximately 4 cm proximal to the articular surface of the radius. Posterior displacement of radius fragment. Often associated with fracture of the ulnar styloid or ulnar neck.				
	Pain in wrist, deformity of wrist, immobility of wrist.	Tenderness over wrist, decreased ROM, edema, and possible ecchymosis.	X-ray, neurovascular exam.	Short arm cast. Pain management.
Smith Fracture | Fracture of the entire thickness of the distal radius, 1 to 2 cm above the wrist with forward and upward displacement of the radius. Anterior displacement of radius fragment. Typically caused by a fall onto a supinated forearm or hand.				
	Pain, immobility, edema, and possible ecchymosis of wrist.	Tenderness, decreased. ROM, deformity, edema, and possible ecchymosis of distal radius.	X-ray. Neurovascular exam.	Short arm cast. Pain management.

Continued

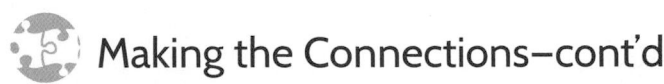

Making the Connections—cont'd

Disorder and Pathophysiology	Signs and Symptoms	Physical Assessment Findings	Diagnostic Testing	Treatment
Tibia or Fibula Fracture | Although the tibia is the only weight-bearing bone, fractures of the tibia are generally associated with fibula fracture.				
	Pain and tenderness over tibial region. Immobility.	Tenderness, edema, diminished weight-bearing ability.	X-ray.	Casting of lower extremity or surgical reduction and fixation. Pain management. If open fracture, antibiotic and tetanus toxoid.
Foot Fracture | Most common causes of foot fracture include fracture from twisting, trauma directly to the foot, and cumulative trauma.				
	Pain, deformity, swelling, difficult weight-bearing on foot.	Tenderness, edema, deformity of foot, diminished weight-bearing.	To facilitate diagnosis, grasp first and second metatarsals and move them alternately through plantar flexion and dorsiflexion. X-ray, MRI, or ultrasound or CT or bone scan if foot fracture occult on plain x-ray. Neurovascular exam.	Nondisplaced fractures are treated with non–weight-bearing short leg cast. ORIF for displaced fractures. Crutch walking. Neurovascular monitoring to prevent compartment syndrome. For toe fracture, common treatment is buddy tape the fractured toe to an adjacent toe and apply a rigid flat-bottom shoe.
Rotator Cuff Injury | A spectrum of disease, ranging from acute reversible tendonitis to massive tears involving the supraspinatus, infraspinatus, and subscapularis muscles. Caused by a history of repetitive overhead activities.				
	Shoulder pain, decreased ROM, shoulder weakness.	Decreased active elevation of arm with passive ROM.	X-ray, MRI, or ultrasound. EMG testing.	Pain management, anti-inflammatory agents, rest, icing. Corticosteroid injections possible. Physical therapy.
Shoulder Dislocation | Anterior dislocation, the most common type of shoulder dislocation, occurs when the humeral head is forced out of the glenohumeral joint, rupturing or detaching the anterior capsule from its attachment to the head of the humerus or from its insertion into the edge of the glenoid fossa.				
	Severe shoulder pain and decreased ROM. Obvious shoulder deformity.	Severe shoulder pain with passive ROM. Severely decreased active ROM.	X-ray, arteriography, EMG.	Conscious sedation when reducing shoulder joint. Shoulder immbolization using a sling and swathe. Neurovascular exam. Postreduction x-ray.
Frozen Shoulder | Shoulder has diminished ROM caused by previous immobilization.				
	Pain and immobility of the shoulder joint.	Decreased active and passive ROM of the shoulder. Tenderness over the deltoid region of the shoulder.	X-ray, ultrasound, MRI, EMG.	Moist heat, anti-inflammatory agents, pain management. Physical therapy.

Continued

Making the Connections—cont'd

Disorder and Pathophysiology	Signs and Symptoms	Physical Assessment Findings	Diagnostic Testing	Treatment
Brachial Plexus Injury | High energy trauma to the upper extremity and neck, causing stretching and injury of the brachial plexus.				
	Pain in neck and shoulder, paresthesias, swelling, weakness or heaviness of the extremity.	Tenderness and weakness of arm. Edema of shoulder. Ptosis of eyelid and miosis of pupil may be present in Horner syndrome, which involves a lower brachial plexus lesion.	X-ray, CT scan, myelography, MRI, angiography, sensory nerve action potentials, EMG testing.	Surgery, nerve grafting, physical therapy.
Ulnar Nerve Injury | Ulnar nerve entrapment. Pressure or injury to the ulnar nerve along its course may cause paralysis of the muscles. One of the most severe consequences is loss of the intrinsic muscle function in the hand.				
	Numbness, motor loss, and possible muscle wasting along course of ulnar nerve.	Motor and sensory losses along course of ulnar nerve.	X-ray of elbow and wrist. MRI or EMG may be necessary. Motor and sensory conduction velocities.	Avoidance of pressure on elbow. Anti-inflammatory agents, oral vitamin B_6. Decompression surgery may be needed.
Plantar Fasciitis | Thickening of plantar fascia caused by overuse and degeneration. Sometimes a calcification at the calcaneus is present (heel spur).				
	Pain, which is intense in morning and lessens with activity.	Anteromedial aspect of plantar fascia is tender. Ankle dorsiflexion is limited secondary to pain. Excessive pronation of foot.	Clinical examination findings, x-ray.	Daily icing, stretching, and NSAID therapy, along with orthotics. Night splints to maintain foot in dorsiflexion during sleep. Corticosteroid injection possible. Plantar fasciotomy may be needed.
Ligamentous or Meniscus Injury of Knee | Knee can suffer acute traumatic injury, infectious injury, chronic overuse injury, or degenerative injury. Knee joint dislocation can occur from high energy trauma.				
	Pain, limited ROM, inability to bear weight, and gait disturbance.	Specific knee maneuvers that stress the joint are used to localize the area of injury. Common maneuvers include the anterior drawer test, Lachman test, and McMurray test.	X-ray, CT scan, MRI, arteriogram, synovial fluid aspiration, and analysis.	RICE, cast, brace, or surgical treatment.

Bibliography

Balagué, F., Mannion, A. F., Pellisé, F., & Cedraschi, C. (2012). Non-specific low back pain. *Lancet*, 379(9814), 482–491. doi: 10.1016/S0140-6736(11)60610-7.

Balogh, Z. J., Reumann, M. K., Gruen, R. L., et al. (2012). Advances and future directions for management of trauma patients with musculoskeletal injuries. *Lancet*, 380(9847), 1109–1119. doi: 10.1016/S0140-6736(12)60991-X.

Berman, B. M., Langevin, H. M., Witt, C. M., & Dubner, R. (2010). Acupuncture for chronic low back pain. *N Engl J Med*, 363(5), 454–461.

Bhangle, S. D., Sapru, S., & Panush, R. S. (2009). Back pain made simple: an approach based on principles and evidence. *Cleve Clin J Med*, 76(7), 393–399. doi: 10.3949/ccjm.76a.08099.

Black, W. S., & Becker, J. A. (2009). Common forearm fractures in adults. *Am Fam Phys*, 80(10), 1096–1102.

Blakeney, W. G. (2010). Stabilization and treatment of Colles' fractures in elderly patients. *Clin Interv Aging*, 5, 337–344.

Borchers, J. R., & Best, T. M. (2012, April 15). Common finger fractures and dislocations. *Am Fam Phys*, 85(8), 805–810.

Buchbinder, R., Osborne, R. H., Ebeling, R. R., et al. (2009). A randomized trial for vertebroplasty for painful osteoporotic vertebral fractures. *N Engl J Med*, 361(6), 557–568.

Carr, A. J., Robertsson, O., Graves, S., et al. (2012). Knee replacement. *Lancet*, 379(9823), 1331–1340. doi: 10.1016/S0140-6736(11)60752-6. Epub 2012 Mar 6.

Casazza, B. A. (2012). Diagnosis and treatment of acute low back pain. *Am Fam Phys*, 85(4), 343–350.

Chou, R., & Shekelle, P. (2010, April 7). Will this patient develop persistent disabling low back pain? *JAMA*, 303(13), 1295–1302. doi: 10.1001/jama.2010.344.

Cimino, F., Volk, B. S., & Setter, D. (2010). Anterior cruciate ligament injury: diagnosis, management, and prevention. *Am Fam Phys*, 82(8), 917–922.

Descatha, A., Godeau, D., & Mediouni, Z. (2014). Physical tests for shoulder disorders. *JAMA*, 311(1), 94. doi: 10.1001/jama.2013.283136.

Eubanks, J. D. (2010). Cervical radiculopathy: nonoperative management of neck pain and radicular symptoms. *Am Fam Phys*, 81(1), 33–40.

Ewald, A. (2011). Adhesive capsulitis: a review. *Am Fam Phys*, 83(4), 417–422.

Gammons, M. (2013). Proper technique for reduction of metacarpophalangeal dislocations. *Am Fam Phys*, 87(3), 160–162.

Girgis, C. M., Sher, D., & Seibel, M. J. (2010). Atypical femoral fractures and bisphosphonate use. *New Engl J Med*, 362(19), 1848–1849.

Goff, J. D., & Crawford, R. (2011). Diagnosis and treatment of plantar fasciitis. *Am Fam Phys*, 84(6), 676–682.

Gourlay, M. L., Fine, J. P., Preisser, J. S., et al. (2012). Bone-density testing interval and transition to osteoporosis in older women. *N Engl J Med*, 366(3), 225–233.

Grady, D. (2013). Spinal augmentation for vertebral fracture. *JAMA Intern Med*, 173(16), 1523. doi: 10.1001/jamainternmed.2013.6761.

Grover, M. (2012). Evaluating acutely injured patients for internal derangement of the knee. *Am Fam Phys*, 85(3), 247–252.

Hermans, J., Luime, J. J., Meuffels, D. E., et al. (2013). Does this patient with shoulder pain have rotator cuff disease?: The Rational Clinical Examination systematic review. *JAMA*, 310(8), 837–847. doi: 10.1001/jama.2013.276187.

Hung, W. W., Egol, K. A., Zuckerman, J. D., & Siu, A. L. (2012). Hip fracture management: tailoring care for the older patient. *JAMA*, 307(20), 2185–2194. doi: 10.1001/jama.2012.4842.

Kallmess, D. F., Comstock, B. A., Heagery, P. J., et al. (2009) A randomized trial of vertebroplasty for osteoporotic spinal fracture, *N Engl J Med*, 361(6), 569–579.

Kane, S. F., Lynch, J. H., & Taylor, J. C. (2014). Evaluation of elbow pain in adults. *Am Fam Phys*, 89(8), 649–657.

Katz, J. N., Brophy, R. H., Chaisson, C. E., et al. (2013). Surgery versus physical therapy for a meniscal tear and osteoarthritis. *N Engl J Med*, 368(18), 1675–1684. doi: 10.1056/NEJMoa 1301408. Epub 2013 Mar 18. Erratum in: *N Engl J Med*. 2013 Aug 15;369(7):683.

Koes, B. (2011). Management of low back pain in primary care: a new approach. *Lancet*, 378(9802), 1530–1532. doi: 10.1016/S0140-6736(11)61033-7. Epub 2011 Sep 28.

Kujawski, E. J., & Morgan, R. L. (2012). Lateral knee pain in a male college student. *Am Fam Phys*, 85(5), 509–510.

LeBlanc, K. E., & Cestia, W. (2011). Carpal tunnel syndrome. *Am Fam Phys*, 83(8), 952–958.

Mallen, C. D., Thomas, E., Belcher, J., et al. (2013). Point-of-care prognosis for common musculoskeletal pain in older adults. *JAMA Intern Med*, 173(12), 1119–1125. doi: 10.1001/jamainternmed.2013.962.

Melton, L. J., 3rd, Christen, D., Riggs, B. L., et al. (2010). Assessing forearm fracture risk in postmenopausal women. *Osteoporos Int*, 21(7), 1161–1169. Epub 2009 Aug 28.

Neal, S., & Fields, K. B. (2010). Peripheral nerve entrapment and injury in the upper extremity. *Am Fam Phys*, 81(2), 147–155.

Patel, D. S., Roth, M., & Kapil, N. (2011). Stress fractures: diagnosis, treatment, and prevention. *Am Fam Phys*, 83(1), 39–46.

Pompan, D. C. (2011). Appropriate use of MRI for evaluating common musculoskeletal conditions. *Am Fam Phys*, 83(8), 83–84.

Salvi, A. E. (2011). The handshake technique: proposal of a closed manual reduction technique for Colles' wrist fracture. *Am J Emerg Med*, 29(1), 115–117. Epub 2010 Apr 2.

Schilcher, J., Michaëlsson, K., & Aspenberg, P. (2011). Bisphosphonate use and atypical fractures of the femoral shaft. *N Engl J Med*, 364(18), 1728–1737.

Shehab, R., & Mirabelli, M. H. (2013). Evaluation and diagnosis of wrist pain: a case-based approach. *Am Fam Phys*, 87(8), 568–573. Erratum in: *Am Fam Phys*. 2013 Oct 1;88(7):427.

Solomon, D. H., Johnston, S. S., Boytsov, N. N., et al. (2014). Osteoporosis medication use after hip fracture in U.S. patients between 2002 and 2011. *J Bone Miner Res*, Feb 18. doi: 10.1002/jbmr.2202.

Tiemstra, J. D. (2012). Update on acute ankle sprains. *Am Fam Phys*, 85(12), 1170–1176.

Tu, P., & Bytomski, J. R. (2011). Diagnosis of heel pain. *Am Fam Phys*, 84(8), 909–916.

Wilson, J. J., & Furukawa, M. (2014). Evaluation of the patient with hip pain. *Am Fam Phys*, 89(1), 27–34.

Degenerative Disorders of the Musculoskeletal System

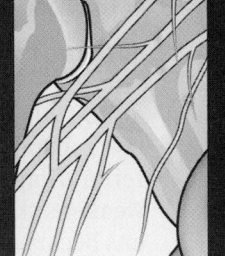

Key Terms

Arthritis
Arthropathy
Bisphosphonates
Bone mineral density (BMD)
Bouchard's nodes
Calcitonin
Cortical bone
Degenerative disc disease (DDD)

Dual-energy x-ray absorptiometry (DEXA)
Heberden's nodes
Lubricin
Osteoarthritis (OA)
Osteocalcin
Osteomalacia
Osteopenia

Osteophyte
Osteoporosis
Radiculopathy
Rickets
Sciatica
Spinal stenosis
Telopeptides
Trabecular bone

Bone health is a critical component of an individual's overall health and quality of life, and bone disease generates pain, anxiety, depression, and a general decline in a person's well-being. Bone density reaches its peak at approximately age 30 years. After age 30, bone deterioration, known as osteoclastic activity, outpaces bone growth, or osteoblastic activity. **Osteoporosis** occurs with aging when osteoclasts cause an increased rate of bone deterioration. **Osteoarthritis (OA)** is the degeneration of joints caused by aging; the joints of the hands and knees are particularly affected.

Epidemiology

Osteoporosis, the most common degenerative disease of bone, is a disorder of bone demineralization that occurs with aging, and prevention is the optimal treatment strategy. The disease is more common in women than men, with over 200 million affected annually worldwide. Among women, 1 in 3 suffer an osteoporotic fracture sometime in their lifetime, with the most common fracture sites being the wrist, hip and vertebrae. Seventy-five percent of women who suffer osteoporotic fracture are older than age 65. With the aging of the population, by the year 2050, it is estimated that the number of women who suffer hip fracture worldwide will increase by 240%. In addition, 1 in 5 men suffer from osteoporosis; by 2050 this number is estimated to increase by 300%.

OA, the deterioration of joints that commonly occurs with aging, is the most common cause of disability in the United States, with approximately 20 million adults diagnosed with OA annually. Obesity and aging are factors that are increasing the incidence of OA in the United States. Obesity, which affects more than 1 in 3 adults, causes excess weight-bearing for the knee and hip joints. It is estimated that 2 out of 3 obese adults in the United

States suffer OA of the knee in their lifetime. By 2030, it is projected that 67 million adults will be suffering from some form of arthritis.

Degenerative disc disease (DDD) is also a very common musculoskeletal problem in the population. The discs between vertebrae become compressed or malaligned, particularly in the lumbar area of the spinal column, causing impingement of spinal nerves. It is the most common cause of back pain in adults throughout the world.

Low back pain is the second most common reason for patient visits to primary care providers in the United States. Vertebral compression and herniated intervertebral discs can cause intractable pain that requires surgery.

Basic Concepts of Healthy Bone and Joint Function

The major structures of the musculoskeletal system—the bones, muscles, tendons, and ligaments—work together to produce flexible, skeletal movement. The skeleton protects the internal organs and tissues and is a storehouse for calcium and phosphorus, which are bound to a matrix made up largely of collagen. In combination, these minerals form calcium hydroxyapatite crystals, $Ca_{10}[PO4]_6[OH]_2$, the major constituent of bone. In addition to providing mechanical support, bone contains hematopoietic cells. Bone marrow is the birthplace of all blood cells—red blood cells (RBCs), white blood cells (WBCs), and platelets.

There are two basic types of bone: trabecular and cortical. **Cortical bone** is solid bone. **Trabecular bone,** also called cancellous, is nonsolid bone with an interior latticelike composition. It is found in high amounts in the upper femur, vertebrae, and wrist. Osteoporosis affects all bones equally, but the areas of trabecular bone display the degeneration first. Osteoporotic deterioration of the latticework of trabecular bone rapidly weakens the nonsolid structure. The bone often weakens because of weight-bearing, and fracture occurs; this is commonly the patient's initial sign of osteoporosis.

Bone Health

Bone is in a constant state of change. The skeleton is sculpted when new bone is formed by osteoblasts and bone resorption is activated by osteoclasts. Osteoblasts secrete alkaline phosphatase, which raises the calcium and phosphorus content of bone. Healthy bone production is directly related to bone's calcium content. There are three calcium-regulating hormones: parathyroid hormone (PTH); calcitriol, which is a form of vitamin D; and calcitonin. The parathyroid glands, found nestled within the thyroid, control calcium levels in the blood. PTH is secreted when calcium concentration in the blood decreases. It acts to bring calcium from bone into the bloodstream and allows phosphates in the blood to enter bone. PTH also acts to stimulate the kidneys to conserve calcium and to stimulate vitamin D production. Ultraviolet light is required to further activate vitamin D, which is needed to absorb calcium from the gastrointestinal tract. **Calcitonin** is a hormone produced by the thyroid gland, which is stimulated by increased calcium levels in the blood; it enhances calcium entry into bone and blocks bone breakdown (see Fig. 38-1).

Sex hormones also have an effect on skeletal health. Estrogen acts to inhibit bone breakdown and stimulates bone formation. Testosterone stimulates muscle growth, which places stress on the bone, thus increasing bone formation. However, because the body's natural production of sex hormones declines with age, it is crucial that maximum bone health is established in the growth years. To build strength, bone requires the stress of weight-bearing exercise such as walking. The stronger the bones are in young adulthood, the better able they are to deal with changes that occur with aging and other health disorders.

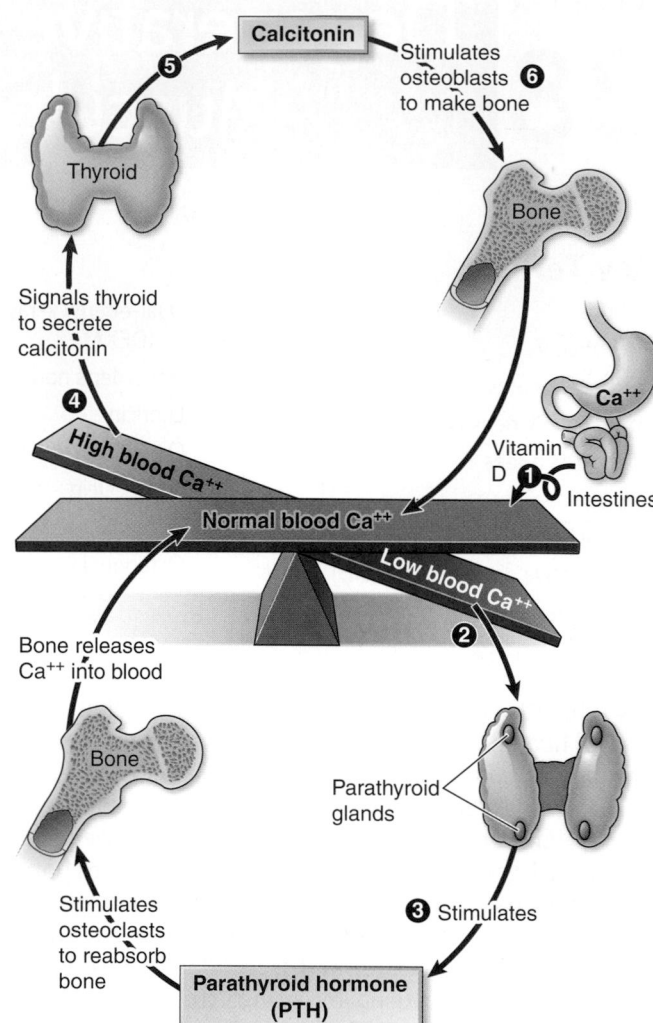

FIGURE 38-1. Calcium balance in the body. (1) Calcium is ingested in the diet, broken down by HCL in the stomach, and absorbed into the bloodstream via the intestine with facilitation by vitamin D. (2) When calcium levels are decreased in the blood, the parathyroid glands are stimulated to release PTH. (3) PTH acts at bone to activate osteoclasts to break down bone and release calcium, which raises the calcium level in the blood. When calcium levels normalize, the parathyroid receives feedback and shuts off. (4) Alternatively, high calcium levels in the blood stimulate the thyroid gland to release calcitonin. (5) Calcitonin activates osteoblasts to build bone.

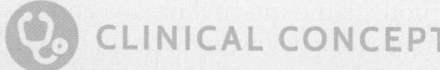

CLINICAL CONCEPT

Overuse of sunblock and cover-ups that block the sun can inhibit activation of vitamin D.

Joint Health

A joint is the location where two or more bones come together. Joints allow mobility and mechanical support, and are classified structurally and functionally. Joints can be classified according to the degree of mobility they allow:

- Synarthrosis: A synarthrosis is a joint where two bones make contact and there is little or

no mobility. Most synarthrosis joints are fibrous joints, such as skull sutures.
- Diarthrosis: A diarthrosis is a joint that allows the most movement. Because all diarthrosis joints are synovial joints, the terms "diarthrosis" and "synovial joint" are interchangeable. Examples include the shoulder, elbow, knee, hip, hand, and fingers.
- Amphiarthrosis: An amphiarthrosis is composed of cartilage and permits slight mobility. Examples include the vertebral joints.

Most joint disorders affect synovial joints. A synovial joint is composed of an outer fibrous capsule, which encases interior synovial membranes, articular cartilage, and synovial fluid. The bones come together and

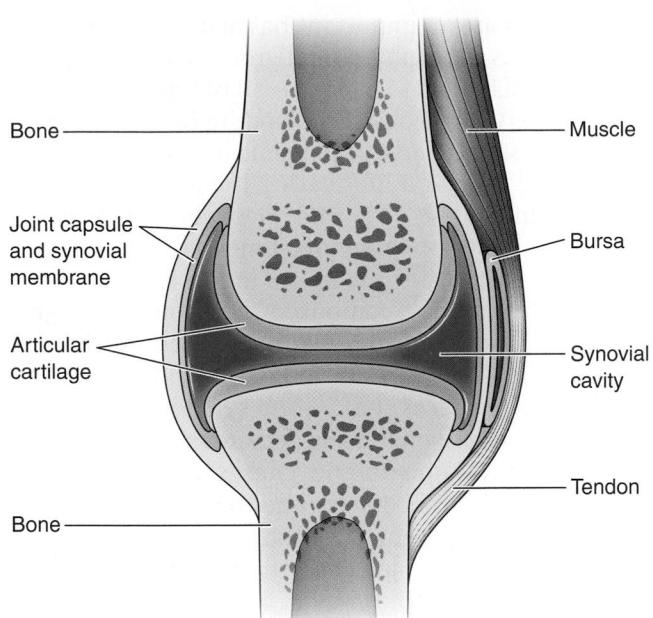

Bone

Joint capsule and synovial membrane

Articular cartilage

Bone

Muscle

Bursa

Synovial cavity

Tendon

FIGURE 38-2. Typical synovial joint.

move easily because of the smooth surfaces of articular cartilage and lubricating synovial fluid (see Fig. 38-2).

A joint disorder is termed an **arthropathy;** when the disorder involves inflammation of one or more joints, the disorder is called **arthritis.** Arthropathies are called polyarticular when involving many joints and monoarticular when involving only one single joint.

Basic Pathophysiologic Concepts of Degenerative Musculoskeletal Disorders

Degenerative musculoskeletal disorders include osteoporosis and OA, which are both related to aging of the skeleton. The pathophysiologic processes of these two diseases differ and cause a great deal of pain and disability for the adult population.

Degeneration of Bone

In adults, bone remodeling—an ongoing process of construction and deconstruction—is the principal metabolic skeletal process. Both osteoblasts and osteoclasts perform bone remodeling, which repairs microdamage of the skeletal architecture and extracts calcium from bone to maintain blood calcium levels. Remodeling is mainly stimulated by excessive or accumulated stresses on bone. Weight-bearing stress and a cadre of circulating factors—including estrogens, androgens, vitamin D, PTH, PTH-related peptide, growth factors, interleukins, prostaglandins, and tumor necrosis factor (TNF)—regulate the rate of bone remodeling. Bone remodeling is a process that consists of bone resorption by osteoclasts, followed by a period of repair during which new bone tissue is synthesized by osteoblasts. Bone is constantly sculpting itself.

Bones contain a certain percentage of solid, cortical bone and a percentage of trabecular bone. Bones that contain a large amount of trabecular bone are the wrist, vertebrae, and upper femur (hip). When osteoclastic activity greatly overtakes osteoblastic activity in trabecular bone, the links of bone within the meshwork disintegrate, leaving it vulnerable to fracture. Microscopic cracks in vertebral bone are some of the first fractures noted when osteoclastic activity is unopposed.

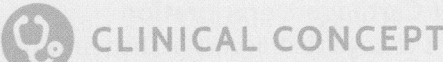

CLINICAL CONCEPT

Bones most susceptible to the effects of osteoporosis include those with a high amount of trabecular bone: hips, wrist, and vertebrae.

Bone formation, which occurs throughout life in the remodeling process, requires adequate calcium in the diet. Insufficient calcium in the diet—which is common among middle age and elderly adults—causes inadequate calcium blood levels that stimulate parathyroid gland activity. PTH regulates blood calcium by stimulating bone remodeling, triggering vitamin D synthesis in the kidney, enhancing gastrointestinal absorption of calcium, and reabsorbing calcium at the kidney. Although all these actions by PTH adjust the blood level of calcium, bone calcium is sacrificed to adjust the blood level. The remodeling of bone is dominated by the osteoclastic activity in calcium deficiency. Although the recommended daily calcium intake for adults is 1,000 to 1,200 mg per day, the average daily intake in the United States is 600 to 800 mg of calcium; this amount is suboptimal, and is one of the major reasons for the high number of adults affected by osteoporosis.

Degeneration of Joints

Osteoarthritis (OA) is the most common type of degenerative joint disease and its pathogenesis has been studied extensively. Interestingly, OA affects certain joints and not others. The commonly affected joints are the cervical and lumbosacral spine, hip, knee, and first metatarsal phalangeal joint. Spared joints include the wrist, elbow, and ankle. According to anthropologists, the joints in the human body were first designed for animals that used four limbs to walk. The center of gravity is widely displaced in a four-legged animal, whereas in a biped, the weight of the body falls mainly on the knees and hips. It is theorized that OA develops in areas that were not designed for walking upright. The knees and the hips take on the majority of the body weight in the upright position; according to Darwinian scientists, this is a relatively new change in the evolution of man from ape. According to evolutionists, the human body is still evolving to accommodate this biped position. The upright position itself predisposes to degeneration of the weight-bearing joints.

The mechanics of the knee have been extensively studied. Under intense activity, it is estimated that the knee bears 5 times the body weight. However, studies reveal that ideal body weight is sustainable, whereas obesity causes excessive loading force on the knees. Anatomical studies reveal that abnormal structural changes of the knee and hip are common in the population. Structural changes exist in persons who suffer joint injury; however, physical and mechanical changes also occur in the joints of asymptomatic persons with age.

Articular Cartilage Deterioration

The major change that occurs in the joints of the body with age is articular cartilage loss. Cartilage is a thin slice of flexible tissue on the surfaces of the ends of two opposing joints. In conjunction with synovial fluid, it provides a cushion upon which two joint surfaces move. Cartilage absorbs the impact of forces affecting the bones across a joint. It is made up of chondrocytes (cartilage cells), which synthesize collagen and aggrecan; this matrix gives cartilage tensile strength. Chondrocytes also produce enzymes that break down the matrix, in concert with cytokines and growth factors that modulate the synthesis of new cartilage. A dynamic equilibrium of cartilage formation and degradation is occurring in cartilage at all times. Healthy cartilage has slow, consistent synthesis of matrix occurring in synchrony with slow breakdown of matrix. Similar to bone, it is in a constant state of modeling and remodeling. However, with excess weight-bearing or injurious force, cartilage becomes metabolically active and chondrocytes are simulated to synthesize more degradative enzymes. The matrix starts to break down with unfurling of the collagen matrix and deteriorated aggrecan. With continued excessive force to bear, the cartilage becomes weak and loses its resilient stiffness and cushioning of the joint surface. Chondrocytes continually exposed to excessive force begin to undergo apoptosis, or programmed degeneration. The excessive force placed on a joint caused by obesity activates the degradation process of cartilage. Although weight-bearing incites metabolic changes leading to joint health, excessive weight acts as a pressure force upon joints, particularly the knees and hips. Similarly, the impact of a traumatic force across a joint incites the enzymatic deterioration process of cartilage. Athletes who sustain repeated injury of a joint undergo cartilage loss with each injury. Repetitive knee injuries suffered by athletes are a particularly common precursor to OA of the knee.

With loss of cartilage comes alterations in subchondral bone, which is bone just below the cartilage layer. Growth factors, cytokines, osteoclasts, and osteoblasts become activated in the subchondral bone, which thickens and develops microscopic cracks. There is some shearing of the microvasculature leading to decreased blood flow to subchondral bone.

At the margin of cartilage loss, osteophytes can form. **Osteophytes** are small bony projections that develop along the rim of bone adjacent to cartilage loss.

Osteophytes are an important hallmark of OA. In malaligned joints, osteophytes will grow larger on the side of the joint subjected to most stress. Osteophytes can impinge on nerves and obstruct blood supply to the joint's components. This nerve impingement will cause pain.

Synovial fluid is a lubricating liquid inside a joint that minimizes shearing force between bones in the joint during motion. A synovial membrane exists between the surfaces of the bones in the joint; this is a very thin membrane composed of fat, macrophages, and fibroblasts. The fibroblasts produce **lubricin,** a mucinous glycoprotein that acts as a lubricant for the joint's bone surfaces. In OA, the synovial membrane often becomes inflamed and edematous. Inflammation of the synovial membrane causes a migration of macrophages into the tissue, and the synovium proliferates and secretes enzymes that further degrade the cartilage within the joint. Also, the concentration of lubricin diminishes with synovial inflammation.

The outer joint protectors include the joint capsule, ligaments, tendons, muscles, and sensory nerves. These joint protectors prevent the joint from malalignment. Muscles, ligaments, and tendons contract at different times throughout joint movement and dissipate joint impact. Edematous fluid that accumulates in a joint with OA stretches the joint capsule, making it less effective as a protector. Sensory nerves are stretched, which causes pain.

Assessment

Assessment of the patient with degenerative bone and joint disease requires a complete history and physical examination. With osteoporosis, the patient does not usually complain of symptoms until the disease process is extensive and fracture has already occurred. A fracture of the wrist, hip, or vertebrae is associated with osteoporosis because these bones have a high amount of trabecular bone. Screening at-risk populations for osteoporosis is the major modality used in the assessment of this disorder.

A patient with OA usually presents to the clinician with physical signs and symptoms, including pain in the joints, physical limitations of the joint's range of motion (ROM), and joint tenderness and deformity. Patients with rheumatoid, psoriatic, gouty, or septic arthritis usually report pain in a joint or joints. As in OA, ROM is limited and there is joint tenderness on physical examination with other types of arthritis. However, systemic symptoms such as fever, myalgias (muscle aches), and fatigue occur in other types of arthritis and not in OA.

Risk Factors

Age, gender, genetics, and certain medications can predispose patients to osteoporosis. Lack of calcium and vitamin D in the diet is also a major risk factor. With OA, obesity, repetitive trauma to a joint, age, and genetic predisposition place a patient at risk.

Signs and Symptoms

In osteoporosis, there are commonly no signs or symptoms until a fracture occurs. In contrast, pain and tenderness are the key signs and symptoms of degenerative joint diseases such as OA. The joints also show the signs of disease through their deformity or swelling; in addition, the patient usually has limited ROM in the joint as well.

Diagnosis

In order to diagnose a patient with osteoporosis, the clinician administers a bone density test. Simple x-rays do not show osteoporosis until the bone is more than 40% deteriorated. Specific blood and urine tests can also show evidence of osteoporosis. However, simple x-rays are usually sufficient to demonstrate OA. In addition, specific laboratory tests can be used to exclude types of arthritis other than OA.

Treatment

There are many treatment options for osteoporosis, including bisphosphonates and calcitonin. However, prevention via the intake of sufficient calcium and vitamin D is the most successful treatment. Once fracture occurs, surgical fixation is usually necessary because osteoporotic bone is fragile.

Different types of arthritis require different treatment modalities depending on the etiology of the disorder. For example, rheumatoid arthritis (RA) requires medications that oppose the immunological destruction of joints. Immunosuppressant drugs, referred to as biological agents, are necessary to relieve the joint damage of RA. OA, in contrast, does not involve the immune system and mainly requires anti-inflammatory medications. Relief of joint pain and inflammation are essential to maintain ROM in all types of arthritis.

Pathophysiology of Selected Degenerative Bone and Joint Disorders

The most common degenerative bone disease, osteoporosis, slowly develops without symptoms until late in the disease. During the process of osteoporosis, the individual is unaware of the bone density breakdown until fracture occurs. OA is also a disease that slowly develops; however, unlike osteoporosis, the development of OA is a painful process. Patients are aware of the joint breakdown because of the tenderness of the joints.

Osteoporosis

Osteoporosis, meaning "porous bone," is a common, yet serious disease, characterized by low bone density

> ### Box 38-1. Consequences of Immobility
>
> Immobility increases patient susceptibility to:
>
> - pressure ulcers, which leads to skin breakdown and, eventually, wound infection
> - slowed bowel peristalsis, which leads to constipation
> - lack of muscle stimulation, which leads to muscle atrophy
> - lack of aerobic exercise, which leads to deconditioning of the cardiovascular system
> - lack of weight-bearing activity, which leads to osteoporosis
> - slowed urinary excretion, urinary stasis, and precipitation of calcium, which leads to kidney stones
> - lack of deep breathing, lack of effective coughing, and stasis of secretions, which leads to pneumonia
> - social isolation and lack of mental stimulation, which leads to depression.

and structural deterioration of bone tissue. This, in turn, leads to bone fragility and an increased risk of fractures, especially of the trabecular bone in the hips, vertebrae, and wrists. **Osteopenia** is the term used for thinning of the trabecular matrix of the bone before osteoporosis, whereas osteoporosis is the term used when actual breaks in this matrix have occurred.

An estimated 10 million Americans suffer from osteoporosis, and another 34 million are determined to be at risk. It is estimated that 1 in 2 women and 1 in 4 men older than age 50 years will suffer an osteoporotic fracture in his or her lifetime.

Osteoporotic hip fractures are specifically linked to an increased risk of mortality. Risk of mortality is 2.8 to 4 times greater among hip fracture patients during the first 3 months after the fracture as compared with nonaffected individuals. Nearly 1 in 4 hip fracture patients will die within 12 months after the injury because of complications related to the injury. Immobility and its many detrimental effects are the cause for a decline in health after hip fracture (see Box 38-1).

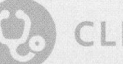 CLINICAL CONCEPT

Only 25% of hip fracture patients will make a full recovery; 40% will require nursing home care, 50% will need a cane or walker, and 24% of those older than age 50 will die within 12 months.

Gender, genetics, age, and nutritional deficiency of calcium or vitamin D are key elements that can affect an individual's risk of osteoporosis. Lack of weight-bearing exercise, alcohol use, and smoking are also major risk factors (see Box 38-2).

Box 38-2. Risk Factors of Osteoporosis

Risk factors of osteoporosis include:

- female gender
- postmenopausal age in female
- lack of estrogen in female
- lack of testosterone in male
- family history
- Asian and Caucasian women
- thin and small-framed women
- lack of recommended daily intake of calcium and vitamin D
- lack of weight-bearing exercise
- excess alcohol consumption
- excess caffeine consumption
- smoking
- long-term use of corticosteroids
- excess carbonated soft drink consumption
- gastric bariatric surgery
- eating disorders such as anorexia
- hyperthyroidism or excessive intake of thyroid medication
- hyperparathyroidism
- anticonvulsant medications.

Etiology

Primary osteoporosis generally results from a prolonged negative calcium balance caused by poor dietary habits, lack of weight-bearing exercise, and lack of daily exposure to natural sunlight. Calcium is absorbed from the intestine with facilitation by vitamin D. If there is insufficient calcium in the diet, then calcium begins to be reabsorbed from bone tissue. Over time, the inner matrix of bone thins and eventually breaks down, often resulting in fractures. Weight-bearing exercise strengthens muscles and stimulates bone modeling and remodeling. A sedentary lifestyle creates a weakened skeleton. In addition to poor diet and exercise patterns, estrogen deficiencies in women and declining gonadal or adrenal function may be factors in primary osteoporosis.

Secondary osteoporosis is caused by disorders that have a direct effect on bone tissue. For example, some hormonal disorders, if not corrected, have a major impact on bone density. Hyperparathyroidism negatively affects serum calcium balance caused by excess secretion of PTH, which reabsorbs calcium from bone to raise the blood levels. This bone resorption from the skeleton leads to weakened bone and increased fracture risk. Hypogonadism in children and young adults causes the loss of the protective effects of estrogen and testosterone, which can result in severe osteoporosis. Exogenous glucocorticoids (corticosteroid medications) taken in excess will cause deterioration of bone tissue. Malabsorption syndrome, celiac disease, and inflammatory bowel disease diminish both calcium and vitamin D absorption from the intestine and therefore increase susceptibility to osteoporosis.

Pathophysiology

The hallmark of osteoporosis is a reduction in bone density caused by an imbalance between osteoclasts and osteoblasts. Under physiologic conditions, bone formation and resorption are in equilibrium. Early childhood nutrition and physical activity are important to the development of bone strength in an adult. Hereditary factors also play a major role in determining an individual's peak bone strength. Genetics account for up to 80% of the variance in peak bone mass between individuals.

Osteoblasts and activated T cells in the bone marrow produce a cytokine that promotes osteoclast formation—in other words, osteoblastic activity provokes osteoclastic activity to keep cellular activity in balance. Osteoclasts require weeks to resorb bone, whereas osteoblasts need months to produce new bone, so any process that increases the rate of bone remodeling results in net bone loss over time.

Bone mass peaks by the third decade of life and slowly decreases afterward. After age 30 years, bone resorption exceeds bone formation and leads to osteopenia and, in severe situations, osteoporosis. Women lose 30% to 40% of their cortical bone and 50% of their trabecular bone over their lifetime, as opposed to men, who lose 15% to 20% of their cortical bone and 25% to 30% of trabecular bone.

Accelerated bone loss can occur in perimenopausal women and elderly men. Loss of gonadal function and aging are the two most important factors contributing to the development of osteoporosis. Studies have shown that bone loss in women accelerates rapidly in the first years after menopause. The lack of the gonadal hormones, estrogen and testosterone, stimulates osteoclast progenitor cells and promotes breakdown of bone. Estrogen deficiency not only accelerates bone loss in postmenopausal women but also plays a role in bone loss in men. Estrogen deficiency sets the stage for intense bone resorption accompanied by inadequate bone formation. T cells and cytokines are activated in the estrogen-deficient environment. In the absence of estrogen, T cells, and cytokines, interleukin-1, interleukin-6, and TNF-alpha significantly promote osteoclast activity. T cells and cytokines also inhibit osteoblast activity and cause premature apoptosis of osteoblasts. Finally, estrogen deficiency sensitizes bone to the bone-deteriorating effects of PTH.

Calcium, vitamin D, and PTH work together to maintain bone homeostasis. Insufficient dietary calcium or impaired intestinal absorption of calcium causes hypocalcemia; this, in turn, stimulates the parathyroid gland to release PTH, which acts on bone tissue to release calcium. This process eventually demineralizes the bone. Other endocrinological conditions, such as Cushing's disease, or medications, such as glucocorticoids, can cause osteoporosis. In Cushing's disease there is hyperadrenal activity that releases an excess of glucocorticoids, which suppress osteoblast function and promote osteoblast apoptosis.

Clinical Presentation

Osteoporosis is known as a silent disease because diagnosis is often made after the individual has already suffered an osteoporotic fracture. Weakening of vertebral bodies results in vertebral compression fractures. Osteoporosis reduces vertebral mass by decreasing the strength of the internal lattice work of bone. Other common osteoporotic fractures are those of the wrist and hip, with the hip defined as the upper femur head and neck. Osteoporotic fractures of the hip often cause the patient to fall when bones are severely weakened and cannot support the patient's weight. Fragility fractures, which occur without trauma, are characteristic of osteoporosis. Alternatively, osteoporotic fractures can be caused by traumatic falls from a lying, sitting, or standing position, or from high-energy trauma, such as a motor vehicle accident. Complaints of back pain that radiate around the trunk are a symptom of vertebral involvement. Increasing deformity, kyphosis, and loss of height are other common symptoms.

Diagnosis

Several diagnostic tests can be utilized to diagnose osteoporosis. **Dual-energy x-ray absorptiometry (DEXA)** measures bone density in the lumbar spine and hips, the areas that most commonly suffer osteoporosis. DEXA is precise and allows for monitoring patients who are being treated for osteoporosis over periods of time. Quantitated computed tomography (CT) provides a true volumetric measurement of trabecular bone density in the spine. Alternatively, ultrasound densitometry uses sound waves to assess bone mass in a variety of peripheral sites, such as the heel or wrist. **Bone mineral density (BMD)** measurement results are compared with a reference population of young, healthy adults of approximately age 30 years; this is called a T score. The World Health Organization (WHO) has established definitions of osteoporosis based on BMD measurements in white women (see Box 38-3).

Blood tests that are helpful in the diagnosis of osteoporosis include blood calcium levels, thyroid function tests, PTH levels, estradiol levels in women, testosterone levels in men, and osteocalcin levels. **Osteocalcin** is a major protein found in bone; when blood levels are high, this indicates bone resorption is occurring. There are also biochemical marker tests that measure the rate at which a person is breaking down or resorbing bone. Urine **telopeptides** are bone-specific collagen breakdown products that also indicate bone breakdown.

Box 38-3. World Health Organization Definitions of Bone Health

According to the World Health Organization (WHO), bone health has the following four definitions:

- **Normal**: BMD is within 1 standard deviation (SD) of the mean bone density for young adult women (T-score at –1 and above).
- **Low bone mass (osteopenia)**: BMD is between 1 to 2.5 SD below the mean for young adult women (T-score between –1 and –2.5).
- **Osteoporosis**: BMD is 2.5 SD or more below the normal mean for young adult females (T-score at or below –2.5).
- **Severe or "established" osteoporosis**: BMD is 2.5 SD or more below the normal mean for young adult females (T-score at or below –2.5) in a patient who has already experienced 1 or more fractures.

The WHO definition applies to postmenopausal women and men aged 50 years or older.

Treatment

Lifestyle changes that are positive for bone health are the first way an individual can take control. This is especially important for prevention of osteoporosis, as well as maintenance if a person has been diagnosed with osteopenia. For the individual with diagnosed osteoporosis, supportive devices such as lumbar supports or other types of bracing may be helpful. At least 1,000 mg of calcium and 400 IU of vitamin D supplements are needed daily. Some pharmaceutical regimens include the use of antiresorptive agents, anabolic medications, and hormonal therapies. **Bisphosphonates,** such as risedronate, are prescribed to suppress osteoclast activity. Calcitonin, which is particularly useful in vertebral compression, is used to prevent bone loss and enhance bone formation. Estrogenlike drugs such as raloxifene act like estrogen on bones but do not have other side effects. Teriparatide, a medication similar to PTH, increases osteoblastic bone formation. Lastly, surgical treatments are available for painful spinal compression fractures. Vertebroplasty involves injecting bone cement into the fractured area of the vertebrae, which reduces pain and helps the person become more active again.

CLINICAL CONCEPT

DEXA scan, which measures BMD in the lumbar spine and hip, is the most commonly used diagnostic imaging study that can diagnose osteoporosis.

CLINICAL CONCEPT

Bisphosphonates have been associated with atypical bone fractures in women. They must be taken with water and the patient should be in the sitting or upright position because they can be extremely irritating to the esophageal and gastric mucosa.

Osteoarthritis

OA commonly occurs in individuals older than age 40 years. Those who have had trauma to joints over the course of their life, such as athletes, are at particular risk. It is the most common form of arthritis and the leading cause of chronic disability in the United States. The disease occurs equally in men and women.

Risk factors of OA include aging, obesity, history of participation in team sports, history of trauma or overuse of a joint, and heavy occupational work. Obesity has become a particularly common risk factor, as excess body weight places excess pressure on the knees and hips. In addition, static or dynamic malalignment of the pelvis, hip, knee, ankle, or foot can contribute to the development of osteoarthritic changes. Muscle weakness, imbalance, and inflexibility can also be risk factors because an individual's risk for injury increases with poor muscle health.

 CLINICAL CONCEPT

The increase in obesity has, in turn, increased the number of orthopedic surgeries related to repair and replacement of weight-bearing joints.

Etiology

OA results from stresses applied to the joints, especially the weight-bearing joints such as the ankle, knee, and hip. Degenerative alterations begin in the articular cartilage as a result of either excessive loading of a healthy joint or relatively normal loading of a previously disturbed joint. It is chronic, with degeneration occurring as a result of the breakdown of chondrocytes and adjacent subchondral bone.

 CLINICAL CONCEPT

Previous joint injury is a major cause of OA. For example, older professional athletes commonly have OA of knees and hips caused by injury during their career.

Pathophysiology

OA is a slowly progressive, degenerative, and inflammatory disease. Excess pressure on a joint gradually wears away the cartilage surface and the subchondral bone is exposed. Inflammation occurs as cytokines, various inflammatory mediators, and metalloproteases are released into the joint and degrade the cartilage. In early OA, chondrocytes synthesize a fluid called proteoglycans in an effort to repair the cartilage. This excess fluid causes swelling of the joint. Proteoglycans and cartilage degeneration can occur for years. As OA progresses,

however, the level of proteoglycans decreases, causing the cartilage to lose elasticity and crack. Microscopically, there is loss of cartilage, resulting in the narrowing of the joint space.

In the weight-bearing joints, a greater loss of joint space occurs because of the great pressures these joints endure. Erosion of the damaged cartilage in an osteoarthritic joint progresses until it exposes the underlying bone.

Bone stripped of the protective cartilage contacts the opposing surface. Eventually, the increasing stresses exceed the bone's strength. The subchondral bone becomes exposed and responds, inflammation increases, and the joint eventually becomes thickened and dense at areas of pressure. The traumatized subchondral bone may also undergo cystic degeneration, caused by either osseous necrosis secondary to chronic impaction or to the penetration of synovial fluid.

Clinical Presentation

The patient history commonly includes complaints of deep, aching joint pain, occurring especially after exercise or weight-bearing. Symptoms may be relieved with rest. Other symptoms include joint pain during cold weather, stiffness when arising in the morning, crepitus of the joint during motion, joint swelling, altered gait, and limited ROM. The patient may report a burning sensation felt in the associated muscles and tendons, or experience muscle spasm and contractions in the tendons with motion. The patient's occupation and recreational activities should be investigated, because these activities often increase susceptibility to OA through repetitive use or injury of certain joints. Family history and past medical history are important features of the history. There is a genetic predisposition to arthritis, and certain comorbidities can increase the risk of OA.

In the physical examination, joint deformity and tenderness may be evident. The involved joints demonstrate decreased ROM. The fingers are often involved in OA, with classic swelling at the distal interphalangeal joint, called **Heberden's nodes.** There is also classic swelling at the proximal interphalangeal joint, called **Bouchard's nodes** (see Fig. 38-3). In OA, regional muscles may atrophy and ligaments may become lax because of decreased movement. Symptoms can be exacerbated by obesity, poor posture, and occupational stress.

Also, in the physical examination, it is important for the clinician to differentiate OA from RA. In early RA, the patient's joints may present similarly with swelling, tenderness, and limited ROM. However, RA is an autoimmune disease that is accompanied by systemic symptoms such as fever, elevated WBC count, and other signs of inflammation. The joints are often not affected symmetrically in RA as in OA, and there is greater joint deformity in RA (see Table 38-1).

Diagnosis

No specific laboratory tests can provide a diagnosis of OA, but biochemical markers such as serum osteocalcin

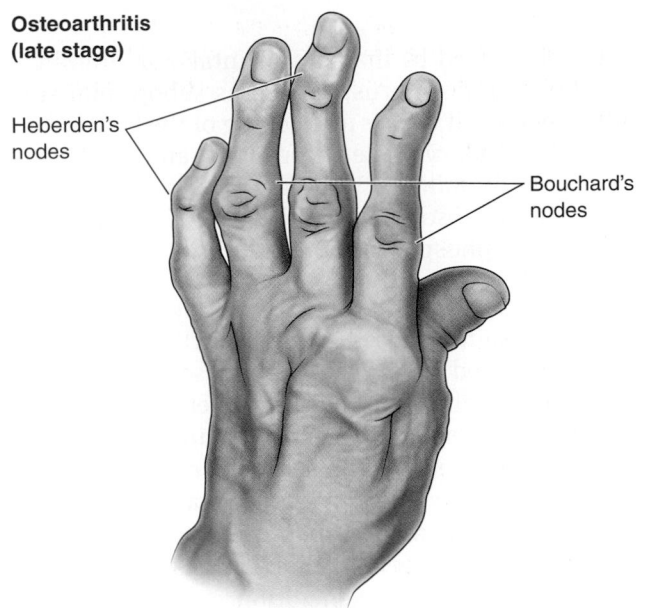

Osteoarthritis
(late stage)

Heberden's
nodes

Bouchard's
nodes

FIGURE 38-3. In OA, the hands can develop two kinds of deformity. Heberden's nodes are swellings in the distal interphalangeal joints. Bouchard's nodes are swellings in the proximal interphalangeal joints.

and hyaluronic acid levels can reflect the presence of synovitis in earlier stages of the disorder. In turn, the biochemical markers can be a valuable tool in evaluating the effects of specific treatments in the course of OA progression. Clinical examination can often provide a diagnosis with reasonable certainty, with actual confirmation of OA made through x-rays. OA is characterized on x-ray by joint space narrowing and with the presence of osteophyte and subchondral sclerosis. Magnetic resonance imaging (MRI) is often only indicated if abnormalities other than OA are expected based on symptomatology and the physical examination.

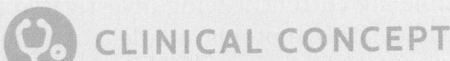

CLINICAL CONCEPT

Osteophytes, which are small bony growths that develop along joints with OA, often impinge upon nerves in the area and cause pain.

Treatment

Treatment goals are to relieve pain, maintain mobility, and minimize disability. Treatment includes exercise and lifestyle modification, use of medications, supportive measures to reduce stress on the affected joint, and, in some cases, surgery. Conservative measures such as weight control and a balance of rest with low impact exercises can be very helpful. Regular exercise, such as daily walking or swimming, is encouraged. These measures alone can relieve joint stress and delay the progression of OA.

Medications include various nonsteroidal anti-inflammatory drugs (NSAIDs). These act by inhibiting the formation of prostaglandins, which are key components in inflammation. Ibuprofen is a common drug used for this purpose.

ALERT! Risks of long-term NSAID use include peptic ulcer with gastrointestinal bleeding and kidney failure.

The use of oral steroids is not recommended for treatment of OA; however, intra-articular injection of glucocorticoids such as hydrocortisone can provide short-term pain relief lasting from a few weeks to a few months. Dietary supplements such as chondroitin sulfate and

TABLE 38-1. **The Differences Between Osteoarthritis and Rheumatoid Arthritis**		
	OA	**RA**
ETIOLOGY	Degenerative joint disease caused by aging or excessive trauma to a joint	Autoimmune disease; antigen unknown; autoantibodies found in joint space
INCIDENCE	10% of population	1% of population
JOINTS MOST COMMONLY AFFECTED	Knee, hip, hand, and proximal interphalangeal and distal interphalangeal joints	Hand; metacarpophalangeal joints
PATHOPHYSIOLOGY	Joint swelling and osteophyte formation	Joint swelling and deformity, intense inflammation with joint erosion
SYMPTOMS	Joint pain, stiffness, and tenderness worst in morning; better as day progresses	Joint pain, stiffness, tenderness, and systemic symptoms such as fever, myalgias, and fatigue
MAJOR TREATMENTS	Acetaminophen, NSAIDs, COX-2 inhibitors, glucosamine chondroitin, cortisone injections, hyaluronic acid injections, joint replacement	Methotrexate and monoclonal antibody biological agents

glucosamine are currently being investigated for their ability to alleviate symptoms and delay progression of OA; however, they do not reverse disease progression. Artificial joint fluid containing hyaluronic acid, such as Synvisc, can also be given via intra-articular injection to provide pain relief for up to 6 months.

Effective treatment also includes reducing stress on the affected joint by supporting or stabilizing the joint with braces and assistive devices, such as a cane or walker. Other supportive measures include the use of moist heat, massage, and low intensity exercises that help to regain or maintain motion and flexibility of the joint and ligaments.

Surgery may be necessary when the disease has progressed in severity and other measures have become ineffective. An osteotomy can be performed to relieve stress on the joint by changing the alignment of bone. This can be done through excision of bone spurs. An osteoplasty, the scraping and removal of deteriorated bone from the joint, can also be performed. Arthrodesis, the surgical fusion of bones, is used primarily in the spine. Lastly, partial or total joint arthroplasty is a common procedure in which the deteriorated bone is removed and replaced with a prosthetic appliance; the knee and hip are the joints most commonly replaced by prostheses. The epidemic of obesity has increased the need for hip and knee replacements.

Rickets

Rickets is a developmental disorder of the bones that occurs in children because of lack of vitamin D, calcium, phosphorus, and sunlight. In the United States and Europe, rickets is uncommon because both infant formula and cow's milk are fortified with 400 IU of vitamin D per liter. Rickets most commonly occurs in pediatric patients with malabsorption syndromes or end-stage renal disease. Breastfed infants who do not receive vitamin D supplementation may also develop rickets.

According to the Centers for Disease Control and Prevention, the incidence of rickets in America is 5 cases per 1 million children aged 6 months to 5 years. However, a retrospective study shows there has been a 6-fold increase in cases of rickets in children between 1990 and 2000. In 1990, incidence of rickets was 3.7 per 100,000, and this number rose to 24.1 per 100,000 children in 2000. Possible reasons include excessive sunscreen use in children while outdoors, thereby blocking the sunlight. Also, there is a tendency for children to spend more time indoors, watching television or playing electronic games, instead of playing outdoors in the sun.

Risk factors for rickets include lactose intolerance, low milk consumption, poor exposure to sunlight, renal disorders, gastrointestinal malabsorption, and vegetarian diet. Infants and children who live in Arctic regions are prone to rickets unless precautions are taken. Individuals with intestinal malabsorption of fats can have difficulty with vitamin D absorption.

Etiology

Rickets is caused by inadequate intake of vitamin D, calcium, or phosphorus, as well as suboptimal sunlight exposure. It causes a softening of the bones, fracture susceptibility, bone deformities, and can lead to permanent disabilities. Without vitamin D in the diet, calcium is not absorbed from the gastrointestinal tract and calcium-phosphorus homeostasis is disrupted.

Pathophysiology

Rickets is mainly caused by deficiency of vitamin D, which is required for proper calcium absorption from the intestine. Sunlight, especially ultraviolet light, is the catalyst for human skin cells to convert vitamin D from an inactive to active state. In the absence of vitamin D, the body only absorbs 5% to 15% of dietary calcium and 50% to 60% of dietary phosphorus, the major minerals that compose bone. Hypocalcemia causes neuromuscular irritability and bone degeneration. A drop in serum-ionized calcium triggers the parathyroid glands to release PTH, which acts on bone to release calcium. The loss of calcium from bones causes the major pathology in rickets—bone weakness, bone deformity, and susceptibility to fracture. Conditions such as fat malabsorption, conditions that interfere with normal small intestine function, and inadequate exposure to sunlight lead to vitamin D deficiency. Patients who take anticonvulsant medications, corticosteroids, or certain cholesterol-controlling medication can also exhibit vitamin D deficiency states.

Clinical Presentation

In the history, malnutrition, intestinal malabsorption, lack of milk products, or lack of sunlight may be reported. Rickets is generally seen in infants between 4 and 12 months of age. Rickets affects bone development in infants because the long bone regions of growth, called the epiphyses and costochondral junctions, are rapidly expanding at this time. Malformation of these bone regions causes protrusion of the sternum and tibial and femoral bowing. Thoracic asymmetry and widening of the thoracic base is a result of muscle traction on the softened rib cage. Delay in fontanelle closure is also a physical sign of this disease. Tooth development may be affected, resulting in delayed tooth eruption, enamel hypoplasia, and early dental caries. Physical deformities become apparent when rickets is present for months to years. These deformities can include low height and weight for age and enlargement at the ends of bones. Carpopedal (wrist) spasms, tetany, seizures, laryngospasms, and hypocalcemic cardiomyopathy can also occur because of the hypocalcemia. Hematologic disorders seen in children with rickets include hypochromic anemia and hypoplastic bone marrow. The spleen and liver can become enlarged because they begin to take over hematopoiesis in bone marrow failure.

Diagnosis

A patient presenting with the symptoms of rickets requires laboratory tests that include serum and ionized calcium levels, bone biopsy, serum alkaline phosphatase, serum phosphorus, PTH levels, and urine calcium. X-rays will show the common changes that occur in rickets such as varus deformity (bowing) of the legs, costochondral swellings called "rickety rosary," lumbar lordosis, and greenstick fractures.

Treatment

The best treatment strategy for rickets is to prevent the vitamin D deficiency. Poor calcium intake by the pregnant mother sets the stage for bone malformations in the infant. Prenatal vitamins with vitamin D and calcium are the norm for optimal maternal child health, as well as increased consumption of fortified daily products.

Vitamin D supplements for those afflicted with rickets should be part of the patient's treatment plan. Most experts agree that 400 to 1,000 IU of vitamin D daily are needed with adequate calcium intake. Daily ultraviolet light exposure of 10 to 30 minutes is also needed for vitamin D metabolism. Special care and consideration should be made for infants who are maintained only on breast milk, in which very little if any vitamin D is expelled. A supplement of 400 IU of vitamin D is recommended for all breastfed infants. Physical therapy is important to strengthen bone and muscle tone. For older children, dairy products should be fortified with vitamin D to assure adequate intake. Children and adolescents should get regular exposure to sunlight and drink at least 500 mL of vitamin D fortified milk daily.

Osteomalacia

Osteomalacia is a disorder of vitamin D deficiency that is similar to rickets, only it occurs in adults. In adults, vitamin D deficiency is not necessarily caused by malnutrition; rather, lack of sufficient exposure to sunlight, renal disorders, cancer, and malabsorption most commonly cause this adult disorder.

The incidence of vitamin D deficiency has largely decreased because of the use of fortified milk and vitamin supplements in the Western world. Despite this, vitamin D-related osteomalacia occurs in certain populations at risk, including the homebound elderly who have little sun exposure, as well as insufficient dietary calcium and vitamin D; patients with malabsorption related to gastrointestinal bypass surgery or celiac disease; and immigrants to cold climates from warm climates, especially women who wear traditional veils or dresses that prevent sun exposure.

Etiology

Osteomalacia can result from low nutritional intake of vitamin D, abnormal vitamin D metabolism, chronic renal failure, tumor-induced osteomalacia, and certain ingested substances such as aluminum or fluoride. Other causes of this condition include cancer, liver disorders, use of anticonvulsant medication, and poor phosphates in diet.

Pathophysiology

The basic problem in osteomalacia is lack of calcium absorption caused by vitamin D deficiency. Hypocalcemia then stimulates the parathyroid gland to secrete PTH, which causes breakdown of bone in order to raise blood calcium levels. Consequently, individuals suffer bone demineralization. Because bones become weakened, ambulation becomes difficult and intense bone pain occurs.

Additionally, with the lack of vitamin D and calcium, the parathyroid glands keep secreting PTH in an attempt to raise blood levels of calcium. As a result, the parathyroid glands become overactive. Therefore, secondary hyperparathyroidism is a feature of osteomalacia. Osteomalacia is often misdiagnosed as fibromyalgia, chronic pain syndrome, or dysthymia (depression).

Clinical Presentation

The patient will often present to the clinician because of lumbar back pain. The patient usually reports that walking—particularly up and down stairs—is difficult. The clinician should investigate the patient's current medications, medical and surgical history, and family history. Renal failure and intestinal malabsorption may be reported in the history. The patient's diet and lifestyle also should be described. The patient may have malabsorption of calcium, lack of sunlight exposure, or lack of fortified dairy products in the diet. Alternatively, ingestion of aluminum or excess fluoride can cause osteomalacia.

Osteomalacia is a difficult diagnosis that is mainly diagnosed via laboratory testing. In a physical exam, the patient with osteomalacia may feel pain when pressure is applied to the sternum or anterior tibia. Symptomatic proximal muscle weakness and diffuse bone pain are also part of the physical findings. With symptomatic proximal muscle weakness, the patient has difficulty rising from a squatting position. The patient may experience diffuse bone pain from stress fractures in the axial skeleton and lower extremities.

Diagnosis

Abnormal blood test results that characterize osteomalacia include low 25-hydroxyvitamin D, elevated PTH level, hypophosphatemia, and elevated alkaline phosphatase. There is usually a normal calcium level until late in the progression of the disease.

Radiological findings for this condition are nonspecific generalized osteopenia noted on x-ray. A DEXA scan can best demonstrate osteopenia. Pseudofracture, also called Looser's zones, can be found along the surfaces and shafts of long bones. A pseudofracture is a band of bone material with decreased density along the surface of bone that gives the appearance of a partial fracture. Subperiosteal resorption, increased cortical thinning, and bone porosity are x-ray findings that occur because of secondary hyperparathyroidism caused by osteomalacia. CT, MRI, or technetium bone scans can confirm diagnosis. In some cases, a bone biopsy may assist in the diagnosis.

Treatment

In osteomalacia, vitamin D deficiency and low phosphate levels require correction. Initial vitamin D supplements would include 50,000 IU of ergocalciferol (vitamin D_2) until normalized. Maintenance doses would be 1,000 IU of vitamin D3 daily. If the underlying etiology is tumor-induced osteomalacia, removal of the tumor would reverse this condition. The patient should get adequate sunlight and increase calcium in the diet.

Increased ingestion of foods high in phosphates helps lessen the hypophosphatemia. In addition, phosphate supplements may be needed. In some incidences parenteral nutrition also may be necessary. Foods such as dairy products, hard cheeses, eggs, bread products that contain baking powder, yeast and beef extracts, herrings, kippers, and sardines can help increase phosphate levels.

Degenerative Disc Disease

DDD is a common cause of pain, motor weakness, and neuropathy. The disorder has effects on the nervous system because anatomically the vertebrae and discs surround the spinal nerves. Motor spinal nerves exit from the spinal cord and travel through narrow openings of the vertebral bone out to the periphery to stimulate muscles of the extremities. Similarly, sensory spinal nerves from the extremities enter the spinal cord through narrow vertebral bone apertures carrying sensory messages from the environment. With age, intervertebral discs and vertebral bone become compressed. The openings in the vertebrae often become so narrow that the bone or discs impinge on the entering and exiting nerves. With impingement on nerves, DDD can cause dysfunction of motor and sensory spinal nerves, impeding movement and sensation in the extremities.

The disorder most commonly occurs in the cervical and lumbar regions of the vertebral column. DDD of the lumbar vertebrae is a common cause of low back pain, which is the second most common reason for patient visits to primary health-care providers. Seventy percent of cases of low back pain are caused by lumbar strain or sprain, 10% are caused by age-related degenerative changes in the intervertebral discs, 4% are caused by herniated discs, 4% are caused by osteoporotic compression fractures, and 3% are caused by spinal stenosis. All other causes account for fewer than 1% of cases.

Back pain is the most common cause of work-related disability in persons younger than 45 years in the United States. Back pain is commonly caused by lumbar DDD, and it affects men and women equally. Lumbar DDD onset most often occurs between ages 30 and 50 years. DDD of the cervical spine also commonly occurs but can be silent; it can be observed with MRI in 25% of asymptomatic individuals aged younger than 40 years and 60% of those aged older than 40 years. The true incidence and prevalence of cervical DDD is uncertain; however, 51% of adults experience neck and arm pain at some time in their lifetime.

Etiology

DDD is a disorder of the intervertebral discs—the fibrocartilaginous cushions that are located between the vertebral bones and allow for vertebral flexibility. The discs, which normally act as spongy shock absorbers for the spine, deteriorate, resulting in malalignment of the spinal column. The intervertebral disc is considered the most critical component of the load-bearing structures of the spinal column. DDD causes malalignment of the vertebral bones which, in turn, increases susceptibility to spinal nerve impingement; this is also called **radiculopathy**.

Risk factors include heavy lifting, sudden traumatic twisting of the torso, obesity, family history, aggressive exercise routine, and poor physical conditioning. There is also a genetic predisposition to DDD.

Pathophysiology

DDD most often occurs in the lumbar region of the vertebral spine. The intervertebral disc consists of a gelatinous center called the nucleus pulposus, which is surrounded by strong cartilage called the annulus fibrosus. Discs flatten and collapse, causing malalignment of the vertebral bones. Discs then become thinner as they dehydrate and change from a supple state to a rigid state that restricts movement. In a herniated disc, the nucleus pulposus is squeezed out of place and herniates through the annulus fibrosus. A herniated disc often causes impingement on a spinal nerve, which can cause motor and sensory problems in the region supplied by the spinal nerve. Weakness of an extremity or paresthesias are commonly found on physical examination.

Osteophyte formation is a common occurrence in DDD; these bony formations can narrow the spinal canal—a condition called spinal stenosis (see Fig. 38-4). Disc degeneration can also lead to disorders such as spondylolisthesis (forward slippage of the disc and vertebrae) and retrolisthesis (backward slippage of the disc and vertebrae).

Clinical Presentation

The patient with lumbar DDD will commonly present to the clinician because of back pain, weakness, or

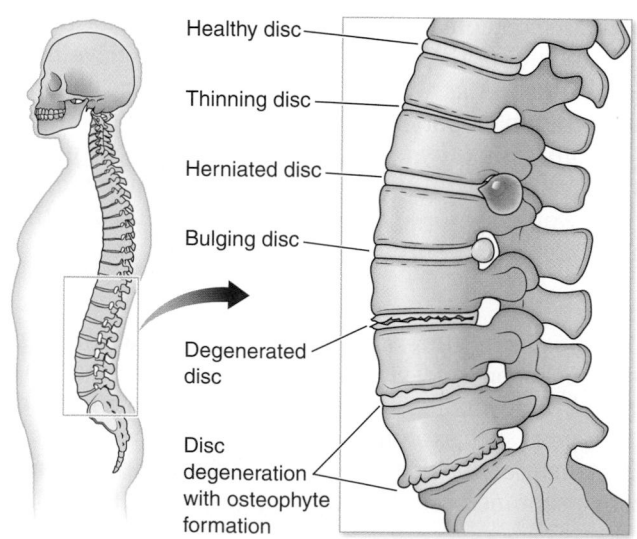

FIGURE 38-4. Degenerative disc disorders include disc thinning and compression, herniated disc, and osteophyte (bone spur) formation. Any of these problems can cause spinal nerve impingement.

numbness in a lower extremity. Cervical DDD causes neck pain, weakness, or numbness in an upper extremity. A history of heavy force trauma, twisting injury, or heavy lifting can provoke the painful event.

The diagnosis of DDD requires a physical examination, with special attention paid to the musculoskeletal and neurological system of the back and extremities. This involves testing muscle strength, deep tendon reflexes, and sensory dermatomes. The dermatomes can give information about which spinal nerve is involved in the disorder. Dermatome maps are helpful in interpreting the level and extent of sensory deficits that are the result of spinal nerve impingement or spinal cord injury.

With a herniated disc, pain is usually intensified with coughing, sneezing, straining, stooping, standing, or jarring motions. Motor weakness, sensory deficit, and decreased deep tendon reflexes can occur in the upper extremities in cervical DDD, whereas motor weakness, sensory deficit, and ambulation problems may occur in lumbar DDD (see Box 38-4).

The most common vertebral discs involved in DDD are the lumbar: L4, L5, and S1. The lumbar spinal nerves L4–S1 make up the sciatic nerve, which arises from the spinal cord and travels down the lower extremity. When lumbar spinal nerve 4 (L4) is involved, the patella reflex may be diminished. When L5 is affected, dorsiflexion of the foot is difficult. When S1 is affected, the Achilles reflex may be diminished and plantar flexion of the foot may be difficult. The most common sensory deficits from spinal nerve impingement are paresthesias, particularly of the leg and foot. Spinal nerve impingement in the L4 through S1 regions is often referred to as **sciatica**.

During the physical examination, the clinician should perform a straight-leg raising test. During this test, the clinician places the patient in the supine position and raises the patient's leg on the affected side. The maneuver applies traction along the sciatic nerve, exacerbating

pain if the nerve is irritated. The test is positive if pain is produced when the leg is raised to 60° or fewer and dorsiflexion of the foot causes pain in the back.

 CLINICAL CONCEPT

Signs of nerve impingement at L4–L5 include weak or absent ability to dorsiflex the foot, sensory loss in lower leg and foot and decreased patella reflex. Signs of nerve impingement at L5–S1 include weak or absent ability to plantarflex the foot, sensory loss in lower leg and foot and decreased Achilles reflex.

Diagnosis

Diagnostic tests useful in diagnosing DDD include x-ray, CT, myelography, and MRI. Electromyography can help identify peripheral neuropathies caused by associated nerve root irritation.

Specific lab tests can be used as a complement to other forms of testing and to screen for causes of spinal pain not related to disc disease or arthritis. These include complete blood count, differential WBC count, serum protein electrophoresis, and erythrocyte sedimentation rate.

Treatment

Treatments for DDD include both conservative and surgical measures; conservative measures are usually tried first. These noninvasive measures include physical therapy, pain management techniques, and alternatives such as chiropractic care. The goal of these measures is to alleviate pain and increase mobility.

Physical Therapy. Physical therapists use a variety of techniques in the treatment of back pain, including the use of heat and cold packs, electrotherapies, massage, biofeedback, traction, and therapeutic exercise. The use of braces limits spinal motion, and therefore enhances healing. Bracing is also used for support following specific spinal surgical procedures, such as fusions. Depending on the problem, there are both rigid and soft braces available. The goal is to provide support to the spine and rest for the spinal muscles.

Pain Management. Traditional drug therapy for those with DDD may include options such as acetaminophen, NSAIDs, muscle relaxants, narcotics, and antidepressants. Narcotics are prescribed for short-term use because of their addictive potential. Antidepressants have analgesic properties and can also improve sleep.

Interventional pain management techniques use injections to an identified area to reduce pain. Of these techniques, epidural steroid injections are the most common. An anti-inflammatory agent, usually cortisone, is injected in the area surrounding a specific nerve or region of the spinal canal. The cortisone reduces swelling in the area, thus reducing pain. These injections can last for weeks to months, depending on the individual, and can help patients benefit from their therapy programs.

Box 38-4. Signs and Symptoms of Degenerative Disc Disease

Signs and symptoms of lumbar DDD include:

- pain in the low back that radiates down the back of the leg (also called "sciatica")
- pain in the buttocks or thighs
- pain that worsens when sitting, bending, lifting, or twisting
- pain that is minimized when walking, changing positions, or lying down
- numbness, tingling, or weakness in the legs
- foot drop.

Signs and symptoms of cervical DDD include:

- chronic neck pain that can radiate to the shoulders and down the arms
- numbness or tingling in the arm or hand
- weakness of the arm or hand.

Chiropractic Care. Chiropractic therapy focuses on adjustment and manipulation techniques of the articulating joints and tissues of the spine. The goal of chiropractic manipulation is to take pressure off sensitive neurological tissue, thereby increasing ROM. This, in turn, will restore blood flow and reduce muscle tension.

Surgery. If conservative treatments are not successful, surgery may be recommended. It is often necessary when back or leg pain limits normal activity and when there is weakness or numbness in the legs, making it difficult to walk or stand. If the lumbosacral spinal nerves are compressed causing bladder or bowel dysfunction, immediate surgery is necessary.

ALERT! Compressed lumbosacral nerves in DDD, which cause loss of bowel or bladder function, is called cauda equina syndrome (CES); this is a medical emergency (see Box 38-5).

Traditional surgical options for DDD include decompression and stabilization surgery. Decompression surgery involves the removal of tissue that is pressing on a nerve. Common decompression options include facetectomy, foraminotomy, laminectomy, and laminotomy.

Following decompression, the spine may be unstable, thus requiring stabilization surgery or a fusion. Often, decompression and stabilization surgery are performed at the same time. As with decompression, spinal fusion can be performed anteriorly or posteriorly, depending on the disease specifics. Spinal fusion surgery involves removal of the intervertebral disc material and then filling in this space with bone graft. Bone grafts are usually autografts, in many cases taken from the patient's pelvic bones. However, allograft or cadaveric bone may be used if the patient has poor bone quality, such as occurs in osteoporosis. Bone graft substitutes are also available, which are biological substances that can stimulate bone growth. In some cases, a surgeon may use spinal instrumentation, such as rods, screws, or wires, to increase spine stability as the bones fuse.

Spinal Stenosis

Spinal stenosis is DDD and degeneration of the lower lumbar vertebrae. An anatomical narrowing of the openings in the vertebrae allows spinal nerves to enter and leave the spinal cord; this narrowing causes nerve impingement and entrapment.

Approximately 250,000 to 500,000 persons in the United States have symptoms of spinal stenosis. This represents about 1 of every 1,000 persons older than age 65 years. Lumbar spinal stenosis is the leading diagnosis for adults older than 65 years who undergo spine surgery. The incidence of spinal nerve entrapment is reported as 8% to 11%. The lower lumbar nerves that are involved most often include L5 (75%), L4 (15%), L3 (5.3%), and L2 (4%).

Box 38-5. Cauda Equina Syndrome

Emerging from the lumbar and sacral nerve roots is the cauda equina. These nerves control sphincter muscles, sexual function, perineal sensation, and sensation and motor function throughout the legs. Damage to this area is known as CES. Causes of CES include fracture or dislocation of the lumbar part of the spine, herniated lumbar discs, spinal stenosis, neoplasms, and inflammatory conditions such as Paget's disease and ankylosing spondylitis. CES causes weakness of the legs, leads to bowel and bladder dysfunction, and requires immediate treatment.

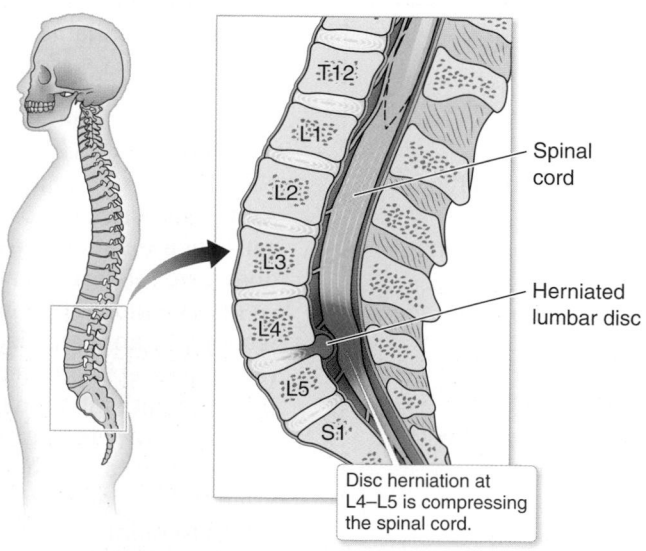

Disc herniation at L4–L5 is compressing the spinal cord.

Etiology

Spinal stenosis is defined as narrowing of the spinal canal, nerve root canal, or intervertebral foramina of the spine. The lumbar and cervical regions are most commonly involved. The narrowing puts pressure on the spinal nerves and causes radiculopathy.

Narrowing of the bony parts of the spinal column can be congenital, acquired, or both. Some people are born with a small spinal canal, but acquired spinal stenosis can occur from trauma or spinal tumors. Aging is often a factor in the formation of spinal stenosis. The intervertebral discs deteriorate with age, and arthritis of the spine commonly occurs. These changes can narrow the nerve root canals and put pressure on the spinal nerves.

Pathophysiology

Spinal stenosis is the narrowing of the lower vertebrae that causes compression on spinal nerves. The patient often has a history of DDD, and spinal stenosis develops over time. It is usually not related to a traumatic event but it is related to gradual spinal degeneration; most commonly, narrowing of the space around the spinal cord is caused by bony overgrowth (osteophytes) from OA or DDD as a result of aging. Osteophytes can compress a spinal nerve and cause pain, sensory disturbances, and motor symptoms.

Clinical Presentation

The first step in diagnosing spinal stenosis is conducting a medical history and a physical exam. Commonly, the compressed nerve causes paresthesias, pain, and weakness of the limbs. Symptoms related to spinal stenosis are similar to those of intervertebral disc herniation. Cervical spinal stenosis causes symptoms in the arms, whereas lumbar spinal stenosis causes symptoms in the legs.

Specific signs and symptoms of spinal stenosis include:

- back pain in lumbar spinal stenosis or neck pain in cervical spinal stenosis
- numbness, weakness, cramping, or pain in the legs or arms in lumbar spinal stenosis or cervical spinal stenosis, respectively, and foot drop in lumbar spinal stenosis
- incontinence in severe spinal stenosis caused by impingement of sacral nerves that control bladder and bowel function.

Diagnosis and Treatment

Diagnostic procedures for spinal stenosis include spinal x-ray, MRI, CT, myelogram, and bone scan. In the majority of patients, symptoms of spinal stenosis respond favorably to nonoperative management. Medical management usually begins with rest, NSAIDs, muscle relaxants, and physical therapy. If there is little relief from the NSAIDs, opioid analgesics and steroid injections may be helpful. Epidural steroid injections and nerve blocks may also relieve the discomfort. In addition, alternative therapies such as acupuncture and chiropractic intervention may be utilized. Nonsurgical treatment is used initially unless the symptoms are intolerable and prevent the patient from normal functioning. For example, a decompressive laminectomy may be performed to relieve pressure on the nerve roots and vertebroplasty used to prevent spinal instability. Problems with bowel or bladder function require immediate decompression surgery.

Chapter Summary

- Osteoporosis is a disorder of bone demineralization that occurs with aging. Lack of calcium or vitamin D in the diet, immobility, age, gender, genetics, and certain medications can predispose patients to osteoporosis.
- Osteoporosis often causes hip, wrist, or vertebral compression fractures.
- A DEXA scan is necessary to visualize BMD in order to diagnose osteoporosis.
- Calcium and vitamin D supplements, bisphosphonates, and calcitonin are used to treat osteoporosis.
- OA commonly occurs with aging.
- Obesity, repetitive trauma to a joint, age, and genetic predisposition place a patient at risk for OA.
- Osteophytes are common outgrowths of osteoarthritic bone surfaces that can impinge on nerves and cause pain.
- DDD often causes impingement on spinal nerves. Cervical and lumbosacral intervertebral discs are most often affected.
- A herniated disc often causes impingement on a spinal nerve, also called radiculopathy. Spinal nerve impingement commonly causes weakness or paresthesias of an extremity.
- The most common DDD is sciatica, impingement on the sciatic nerve that causes pain radiating down the leg.
- Osteomalacia, also called rickets in children, is degeneration of bone caused by hyperparathyroidism, or insufficient calcium or vitamin D in the diet.
- OA can appear like RA; however, RA is an autoimmune disease.
- RA causes systemic symptoms such as fever, elevated WBC count, and other signs of inflammation. In RA, the joints are often not affected symmetrically as in OA, and there is greater joint deformity in RA.
- In degenerative diseases of the musculoskeletal system, diagnostic tests consistently used are plain x-rays. However, x-rays are often insufficient and CT scan, DEXA scan, or MRI are necessary.
- Nonsurgical therapies commonly used in DDD include NSAIDs, epidural steroid or analgesic injections, and muscle relaxants.

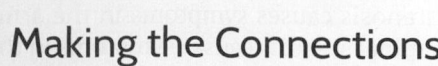 Making the Connections

Disorder and Pathophysiology	Signs and Symptoms	Physical Assessment Findings	Diagnostic Testing	Treatment
Osteoporosis | Bone demineralization caused by greater osteoclastic activity compared with osteoblastic activity. Trabecular bone has high susceptibility to fracture; wrist, upper femur (hip), vertebrae.				
	Loss of height. Kyphosis. Fracture (hip, wrist, vertebrae).	Loss of height. Kyphosis. Fracture (hip, wrist, vertebrae).	DEXA scan; specifically measures bone density in lumbar spine and hip. BMD is 2.5 standard deviations or more below the normal mean for young adult females (T-score at or below −2.5).	Weight-bearing exercise to strengthen bone by stimulating osteoblastic activity. Calcium 1,200 mg/daily to strengthen bone. Vitamin D 400 IU/daily to increase calcium absorption. Bisphosphonates to inhibit osteoclastic activity. Calcitonin to decrease bone loss and diminish pain. Raloxifene, an estrogenlike medication that strengthens bone. Teriparatide (PTH) to strengthen bone. Vertebroplasty to fortify osteoporotic bone.
OA | Slowly progressive, degenerative, and inflammatory disease. Excess pressure on a joint gradually wears away the cartilage surface and the subchondral bone is exposed. Inflammation occurs as cytokines, various inflammatory mediators, and metalloproteases are released into the joint and degrade the cartilage.				
	Pain, stiffness of joints, decreased ROM, and swelling of joints.	Tenderness of joints, decreased ROM, swelling of joints, crepitus heard with joint motion.	X-ray, CT, MRI.	Moist heat to decrease muscle spasm and pain. NSAIDs to decrease inflammation. Intra-articular injection of glucocorticoid decreases pain and inflammation. Supportive devices such as walker or lumbar brace support. Surgery, including osteotomy, osteoplasty, and arthroplasty, that fortifies joints.

Continued

Making the Connections–cont'd

Disorder and Pathophysiology	Signs and Symptoms	Physical Assessment Findings	Diagnostic Testing	Treatment
Rickets | Lack of calcification of bones caused by deficient dietary vitamin D/ calcium in child.				
	Short stature; lack of bone growth. Deformity of bones caused by hypocalcemia. Muscle cramping caused by hypocalcemia. Seizures caused by hypocalcemia. Tooth hypoplasia.	Short stature. Deformity of bones. Muscle cramping. Seizures. Tooth hypoplasia.	X-ray, CT, and MRI can demonstrate the diminished calcification of bones.	Vitamin D to increase absorption of calcium from gastrointestinal tract. Calcium supplement in diet to strengthen bone. Phosphorus in diet to strengthen bone. Sunlight to activate vitamin D.
Osteomalacia | Lack of calcification of bones caused by deficient vitamin D or calcium in adult.				
	Bone pain.	Tenderness of bone. Difficulty with ambulation.	X-ray, vitamin D level, calcium level, phosphate level.	Vitamin D to increase calcium absorption. Calcium supplement to strengthen bones. Phosphorus in diet to strengthen bone. Sunlight to activate vitamin D.
DDD | Intervertebral discs dehydrate and collapse, which causes malalignment of the discs and vertebral bones. In a herniated disc, the central nucleus pulposus tissue of the disc is squeezed out of place and herniates through the annulus fibrosus, which causes impingement on a spinal nerve. Spinal nerve impingement causes inflammation, pain, paralysis, lack of sensation, and paresthesias in region supplied by the spinal nerve.				
	Pain (cervical or lumbar commonly) with radiation (legs or arms commonly), numbness, paresthesias, difficulty walking if DDD in lower spine.	Tenderness of site of DDD, paraspinal muscle spasm, numbness in arms or legs depending on site of DDD.	X-ray, CT, or MRI can demonstrate disc collapse and vertebral malalignment. Electromyography (EMG) can show muscle dysfunction.	Heat to reduce pain and muscle spasm. NSAIDs to decrease inflammation. Short-term narcotic to relieve pain of spinal nerve impingement. Muscle relaxants to reduce muscle spasm. Antidepressants to decrease neuropathic pain. Intra-articular injection of glucocorticoid diminishes inflammation. Physical therapy attempts to realign vertebrae, strengthen muscles, and decrease spasm. Acupuncture is used for pain relief. Chiropractic treatments are used to realign discs.

Continued

Making the Connections–cont'd

Disorder and Pathophysiology	Signs and Symptoms	Physical Assessment Findings	Diagnostic Testing	Treatment
				Supportive devices, such as walker or cervical collar, are used to decrease impingement on spinal nerves. Decompression surgery is used to obliterate the disc impingement on the spinal nerves. Surgical fusion is used to realign discs and vertebrae with supportive hardware.

Spinal Stenosis | Spinal stenosis is DDD and degeneration of the lower lumbar vertebrae. There is an anatomical narrowing of the openings in the vertebrae that allow spinal nerves to enter and leave the spinal cord. The narrowing causes nerve impingement and entrapment. Impingement causes pain, sensory loss, and paralysis.

| | Pain (cervical or lumbar commonly) with radiation (legs or arms commonly), numbness, paresthesias, difficulty walking if in lower spine. | Tenderness of site, paraspinal muscle spasm, numbness in arms or legs, depending on site. | X-ray, CT, or MRI can demonstrate narrowing of vertebral openings and impingement on spinal nerves. EMG can demonstrate muscle dysfunction. | Heat to relieve pain and muscle spasm. NSAIDs to decrease inflammation. Short-term narcotic to relieve pain. Muscle relaxants to decrease muscle spasm. Intra-articular injection of glucocorticoid to decrease inflammation. Physical therapy attempts to realign vertebrae, strengthen muscles, and decrease spasm. Acupuncture may relieve pain. Chiropractic treatment attempts to realign vertebrae, strengthen muscles, and decrease spasm. Supportive devices, such as a walker or cervical collar, are used to decrease nerve impingement. Decompression surgery is used to eradicate nerve impingement. Surgical fusion is used to eradicate nerve impingement and realign vertebrae with supportive hardware. |

Bibliography

Bijlsma, J. W., Berenbaum, F., & Lafeber, F. P. (2011). Osteoarthritis: an update with relevance for clinical practice. *Lancet, 377*(9783), 2115–2126.

Black, D. M., Kelly, M. P., Genant, H. K., et al. (2010). Bisphosphonates and fractures of the subtrochanteric or diaphyseal femur. *N Engl J Med, 362*(19), 1761–1771.

Casazza, B. A. (2012). Diagnosis and treatment of acute low back pain. *Am Fam Phys, 85*(4), 343–350.

Croswell, J. (2011). Screening for osteoporosis. *Am Fam Phys, 83*(10), 1201–1202.

Eubanks. J. D. (2010). Cervical radiculopathy: nonoperative management of neck pain and radicular symptoms. *Am Fam Phys, 81*(1), 33–40.

Favus, M. J. (2010). Bisphosphonates for osteoporosis. *N Engl J Med, 363*(21), 2027–2035.

Fogleman, C. D. (2013). Analgesics for osteoarthritis. *Am Fam Phys, 87*(5), 354–356.

Girgis, C. M., Sher, D., & Seibel, M. J. (2010). Atypical femoral fractures and bisphosphonate use. *New Engl J Med, 362*(19), 1848–1849.

Gourlay, M. L., Fine, J. P., Preisser, J. S., et al. (2012). Bone-density testing interval and transition to osteoporosis in older women. *N Engl J Med, 366*(3), 225–233.

Hauk, L, & American College of Obstetricians and Gynecologists. (2013). ACOG releases practice bulletin on osteoporosis. *Am Fam Phys, 88*(4), 269–275.

Heng, C., Badner, V. M., Vakkas, T. G., Johnson, R., & Yeo, Y. (2012). Bisphosphonate-related osteonecrosis of the jaw in patients with osteoporosis. *Am Fam Phys, 85*(12), 1134–1141.

Hochberg, M. C., Yerges-Armstrong, L., & Mitchell, B. D. (2012). Osteoarthritis susceptibility genes continue trickling in. *Lancet, 380*(9844), 785–787.

Hung, W. W., Egol, K. A., Zuckerman, J. D., & Siu, A. L. (2012). Hip fracture management: tailoring care for the older patient. *JAMA, 307*(20), 2185–2194.

Johnson, G. L. (2012). Denosumab (prolia) for treatment of postmenopausal osteoporosis. *Am Fam Phys, 85*(4), 334–336.

Klazen, C. A., Lohle, P. N., de Vries, J., et al. (2010). Vertebroplasty versus conservative treatment in acute osteoporotic vertebral compression fractures (Vertos II): an open-label randomised trial. *Lancet, 376*(9746), 1085–1092.

Longo, D. L., Fauci, A. S., Kasper, D. L., et al., Eds. (2011). *Harrison's principles of internal medicine.* 18th ed. New York: McGraw-Hill.

Osteoporosis—striking the right balance. (2011). *Lancet, 377*(9784), 2152.

Rao, S. S., Budhwar, N., & Ashfaque, A. (2010). Osteoporosis in men. *Am Fam Phys, 82*(5), 503–508.

Ringdahl, E., & Pandit, S. (2011). Treatment of knee osteoarthritis. *Am Fam Phys, 83*(11), 1287–1292.

Scott, D. (2010). Osteoarthritis of the hip. *Am Fam Phys, 81*(4), 444.

Sinusas, K. (2012). Osteoarthritis: diagnosis and treatment. *Am Fam Phys, 85*(1), 49–56.

U.S. Preventive Services Task Force. (2011). Screening for osteoporosis: recommendation statement. *Am Fam Phys, 83*(10), 1197–1200.

Voelker, R. (2012). Osteoporosis screening may be needed less often than previously believed. *JAMA, 307*(7), 654.

Wardlaw, D., & Van Meirhaeghe, J. (2010). Another chapter for vertebral compression fractures. *Lancet, 376*(9746), 1031–1033.

Weinstein, R. S. (2011). Clinical practice. Glucocorticoid-induced bone disease. *N Engl J Med, 365*(1), 62–70.

Whitaker, M., Guo, J., Kehoe, T., & Benson, G. (2012). Bisphosphonates for osteoporosis—where do we go from here? *N Engl J Med, 366*(22), 2048–2051.

Yu, E. W., & Finkelstein, J. S. (2012). Bone density screening intervals for osteoporosis: one size does not fit all. *JAMA, 307*(24), 2591–2592.

Infection and Inflammatory Disorders of the Musculoskeletal System

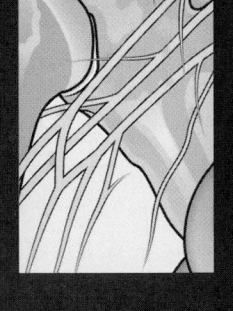

Key Terms

Borrelia burgdorferi

Contiguous spread

Erythema migrans (EM)

Gout

Haversian canal

Hematogenous spread

Hyperuricemia

Lamellae

Myositis

Podagra

Pott's disease

Sacroiliitis

Tophi

Tumor necrosis factor (TNF)

Volkmann canal

Inflammatory disorders of the musculoskeletal system are common in the adult population. The field of rheumatology involves the study of inflammatory muscle, bone, and joint disease. Inflammatory joint disease, or arthritis, is commonly caused by autoimmune disease; it is characterized by inflammatory damage of the synovial membrane or articular cartilage. Inflammation of the skeletal muscles is called **myositis,** a disorder that progressively weakens the muscles. Like arthritis, some forms of myositis are caused by an autoimmune reaction. Inflammatory disorders such as gout, osteomyelitis, and septic arthritis are caused by infection or metabolic disorder.

Epidemiology

The major inflammatory or infectious disorders of the musculoskeletal system include osteomyelitis, rheumatoid arthritis (RA), gout, and septic arthritis. The incidence of osteomyelitis after open fracture is reported to be 2% to 16%, depending on the severity of trauma and type of treatment administered. RA, caused by an autoimmune reaction in the body, is covered in Chapter 11: Disorders of the Immune System. According to the American College of Rheumatology, the incidence of gout has increased over the last decade, from fewer than 1% of the population in 2000 to 4% in 2011. Gout is prevalent in those older than age 40 years and more common in men than in women. The estimated incidence of septic arthritis in industrialized countries is six cases per 100,000 per year. In patients with underlying joint disease or with prosthetic joints, the incidence increases approximately 10-fold, to 70 cases per 100,000 of the population.

Basic Concepts of the Musculoskeletal System Relevant to Inflammation and Infection

The bones and joints are commonly involved in inflammatory or infectious disease. Understanding the normal physiology of these structures is important for the study of musculoskeletal system diseases.

Bone Structure and Susceptibility to Infection

Bone is normally resistant to infection, which occurs if there is exposure to a pathogenic microorganism, if the microorganism is virulent, and if a large number of organisms are present. Although the musculoskeletal system may be infected by any microorganism, the great majority of infections are bacterial. Bacteria can enter bone when a break in bone integrity is exposed to the environment, as in a compound fracture or surgical fixation of a fracture. Alternatively, bone can be infected via the bloodstream. Bacteria invade the cortex of bone via the **Haversian canal** and **Volkmann canal** system located beneath the periosteum. Haversian canals contain the blood vessels, nerves, and lymphatic vessels that travel longitudinally within the bone. Volkmann canals also contain blood vessels and travel horizontally between the Haversian canals to connect them.

The functional unit of bone, called an osteon, consists of concentric layers, or **lamellae,** of compact bone that surround a central Haversian canal. Osteoblasts develop into osteocytes, which occupy small spaces within compact bone called lacuna. Osteocytes make contact with each other via a network of small transverse canals,

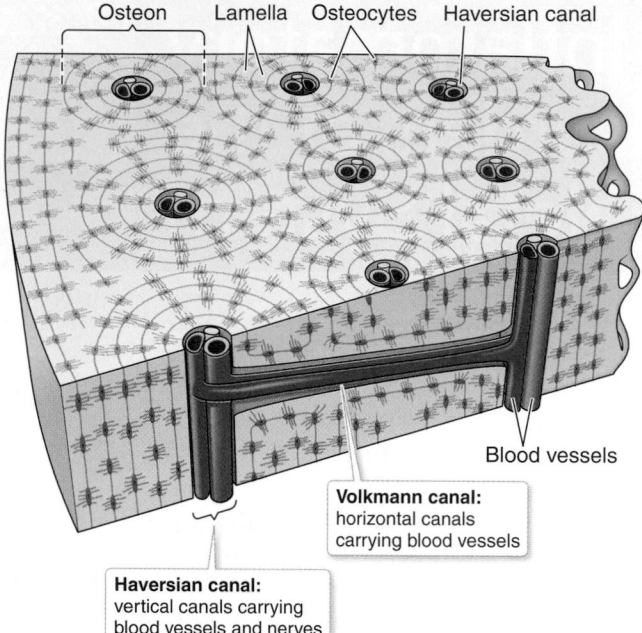

FIGURE 39-1. Haversian and Volkmann canals of compact bone. In compact bone, layers of matrix are arranged in concentric, onionlike rings (called lamellae) around a central canal (called a Haversian or osteonic canal). This basic structural unit is called an osteon (a). Transverse passageways, called Volkmann canals, connect the Haversian canals (b). These canals transport blood and nutrients from the bone's exterior to the osteocytes locked inside.

or canaliculi. This network facilitates the exchange of nutrients and metabolic waste (see Fig. 39-1).

Certain risk factors compromise immunity and make the patient susceptible to bone infection. These risk factors include nutritional deficiency, comorbid diseases such as diabetes, and immunosuppressive medications such as corticosteroids, methotrexate, or tumor necrosis factor inhibitors. In addition, any patient with an implanted synthetic or allograft prosthetic material has an increased risk for musculoskeletal infection. Studies indicate that all biomaterials commonly used for surgical fixation of bone increase incidence of *Staphylococcus aureus* (*S. aureus*) infections. Adherence of bacteria to the surface of implants is promoted by the microorganism's outer capsule, a polysaccharide called glycocalyx. This protective capsule acts as a barrier to immune defense mechanisms and antibiotics. In addition, the capsule makes culture of organisms difficult.

Joints

Cartilage provides a smooth, well-lubricated surface for joints and allows movement between bones with low frictional resistance. Normal articular cartilage is durable and elastic, providing a shock absorber for joints. However, articular cartilage does not have a blood supply; it obtains oxygen and nutrients from the surrounding joint fluid. When a joint is bearing weight, the pressure squeezes fluid, including waste products, from the cartilage; when the pressure is relieved, the fluid seeps back

in together with oxygen and nutrients. An excessively heavy load on a joint is a common cause of injury. Once injured, cartilage has a limited ability to repair itself. Damaged or abnormal cartilage loses its resistance to wear. The two joint surfaces grind together and shed particles of cartilage, which further contribute to joint surface wear. As the joint mechanics deteriorate, the rate of wear increases. The process may continue until most of the joint cartilage is lost.

Synovial Fluid

Synovial fluid contributes significant stabilizing effects as an adhesive seal that freely permits a sliding motion between cartilaginous surfaces. In normal joints, a thin film of synovial fluid covers the surfaces of synovium and cartilage within the joint space. The volume of this fluid increases when disease is present and creates a joint effusion (edema of the joint) that is clinically apparent and may be easily aspirated for study. Because normal articular cartilage has no microvascular supply of its own, it is at risk for ischemia. Chondrocytes or cartilage cells are farther from supporting microvasculature than are any other body cells. Cartilage has limited repair capabilities; damaged cartilage is usually replaced by fibrocartilage scar tissue.

In the synovium, as in all tissues, essential nutrients are delivered and metabolic by-products are cleared by the bloodstream. However, there is limited exchange between the bloodstream and a synovial joint. This limitation hinders the transport of therapeutic agents into inflamed synovial joints. No therapeutic agent is known to be transported into or selectively retained within a joint space. Consequently, intra-articular injection is often needed for medication delivery.

Basic Pathophysiologic Concepts of Musculoskeletal Inflammation and Infections

Compared with other cell types in the body, bone is more resistant to infection. However, certain conditions increase the risk of infection. There are various ways in which a microorganism can come in contact with bone.

Bone Infection and Inflammation

Inflammation of the musculoskeletal tissues occurs via contiguous or hematogenous spread of infection, or via autoimmune disease. **Contiguous spread** is best exemplified by *S. aureus* infection of the musculoskeletal system. *S. aureus* is part of the skin's normal flora but can become pathogenic when it invades interior tissues via contiguous spread. Contiguous spread occurs by invasion of the microorganism via a puncture or wound. *Staphylococcus, Pseudomonas,* and anaerobic bacteria commonly spread to the musculoskeletal system in this manner.

Hematogenous spread occurs when bacteria from tissues within the body spread via the bloodstream to the musculoskeletal system. Pathogens, such as *group A streptococci* or *Streptococcus pneumoniae* that are usually limited to the oropharynx or lung, can be transported within the bloodstream to musculoskeletal tissues.

The infection of bone involves five stages:

1. Inflammation: This stage represents initial inflammation with vascular congestion and increased pressure within the interior bone; obstruction to blood flow occurs with intravascular thrombosis.
2. Suppuration: Infectious material within the bones forces its way through the Haversian system and forms an abscess beneath the bone surface.
3. Sequestrum: Increased pressure, vascular obstruction, and thrombi compromise the periosteal and endosteal blood supply, causing bone necrosis in approximately 7 days.
4. Involucrum: This is new bone formation from the stripped surface of periosteum.
5. Resolution or progression to complications: With antibiotics and surgical treatment early in the course of disease, osteomyelitis resolves without any complications. If there is no resolution, complications can arise such as gangrene, necrotic tissue that becomes infected with bacteria, commonly a clostridium species.

Autoimmune diseases of the musculoskeletal system develop as a result of breakdown in the basic mechanisms regulating the immune system: identifying self versus non-self. For unknown reasons, an immunological reaction develops within the host against its own tissue, with resulting inflammation and injury. The common autoimmune processes include direct T cell-mediated cellular injury, B cell antibody-dependent cellular injury, and antigen or antibody immune complex deposition. Autoimmune diseases can be organ specific, such as ankylosing spondylitis, which affects the sacroiliac joints, or systemic, such as systemic lupus erythematosus (SLE), which causes multiorgan dysfunction.

Systemic autoimmune disorders are commonly characterized by exacerbations and remissions. Despite significant research, there is currently no cure for these diseases; the goal of therapy is to lengthen the time between disease exacerbations.

 CLINICAL CONCEPT

An exacerbation is a period of worsening disease that can be detected by flare-up of patient symptoms and laboratory changes. A remission is a period of diminished apparent disease when symptoms are decreased and laboratory changes often normalize.

Joint Infection and Inflammation

The infection of a joint can occur in different ways:

- via injection or during joint movement through direct colonization
- by direct contact with a neighboring infected site
- by hematogenous or lymphogenous spread of a pathogen.

Bacterial arthritis can be categorized as acute, chronic, or reactive, which differ in type of joint infection and their triggering bacteria. Reactive arthritis (ReA) is a postinfectious complication with no need of the presence of pathogens in the joint. ReA often affects several joints, whereas infection of a joint with bacteria rarely affects more than one joint.

The knee joint is the most common site for a joint infection, and the hip is the second most frequent site. The same types of bacteria can infect the hip joint as well as other large joints. Hip joint infections, however, can exist silently with few symptoms for a long period of time.

An increased rate of infection occurs in a predamaged joint or a joint with a prosthesis. When implanting a prosthesis, the joint is vulnerable to infection because bacteria can enter the joint during surgery. The joint is also vulnerable because the implanted prosthetic material lowers resistance and facilitates infection that enters via the hematogenous route. The prosthetic materials act as binding sites for various bacteria. In addition, the virulence and resistance of the bacteria are involved in the mechanism of infection. Joint infections can also be the starting point of a progressive infection spreading through the contiguous, lymphatic, or hematologic route. In general, the detection and treatment of joint infection (also called infectious arthritis) is an acute situation that requires prompt diagnosis and treatment. A delay can allow progression of the infection and cause sepsis.

Assessment

In the assessment of the patient with any inflammatory or infectious disorder, the clinician should evaluate the following:

- local signs of inflammation including erythema, tenderness, swelling, and discharge
- onset, location, and duration of symptoms
- aggravating factors
- alleviating factors
- severity of pain
- systemic symptoms such as fever, malaise, weakness, or fatigue
- range of motion (ROM) of affected bones or joints, palpating tender areas last.

A comprehensive history and physical examination is necessary with musculoskeletal disorders. It is important to inquire about current medications, medical and surgical history, recent trauma, and family history. The clinician should always compare the extremities for symmetry in physical examination.

In order to gather a thorough history, the patient must be interviewed about any risk factors, including occupation or lifestyle factors, that can lead to the musculoskeletal infection or inflammatory process. Medical disorders such as diabetes, sickle cell anemia, immune disease, and peripheral arterial disease often set the stage for musculoskeletal infection. The patient should also be questioned about past medical history of systemic disorders or infections such as Lyme disease, tuberculosis (TB), gonorrhea, or RA. If Lyme disease is suspected, the patient should be asked about recent travel, outdoor activities, and if the patient has noticed any rashes. Past musculoskeletal injuries should be described in full by the patient. Past surgery, particularly orthopedic surgery and prosthetic implantation, should be noted as these are important risk factors of musculoskeletal infection. In addition, the patient's current medication list should be reviewed because some drugs can change the metabolic profile or decrease immunocompetence.

Signs and Symptoms

During the physical examination, the clinician should note the patient's gait and posture as these can give clues to the location of inflammation or infection and the disability associated with them. Skin rashes should be noted, as these are sometimes related to musculoskeletal disorders. The clinician should ask where exactly pain is located and examine that part of the body last. Examination of the surrounding region for any open wounds, discharge, swelling, or erythema is important. It is critical to evaluate blood flow and sensation in the area around the tender region. The clinician should always examine and compare one area of the body with the opposing area of the body for symmetry. For example, when examining a swollen knee, it should be inspected in comparison to the knee on the opposite leg. The ROM should be examined last because this often causes pain.

Diagnosis

The patient's complete blood count (CBC) with differential, erythrocyte sedimentation rate (ESR), and C-reactive protein (CRP) are important indicators of inflammation or infection. High white blood cell (WBC) count and elevated ESR and CRP are indicative of active inflammation or infection. Analysis of discharge or joint fluid with culture and sensitivity (C&S) can reveal the precise infectious agents in osteomyelitis or septic arthritis. In autoimmune disorders, autoantibodies should be sought in the bloodstream. The most common imaging study is plain x-ray. However, computed tomography (CT) scan and magnetic resonance imaging (MRI) can yield more information because they visualize areas with more detail. Ultrasound examination and dual-energy x-ray absorptiometry (DEXA) scan can be used to investigate bone density and can be abnormal in osteomyelitis. Nuclear bone scans are particularly useful in osteomyelitis and can detect infection earlier than other imaging studies. Blood cultures and bone biopsy are often needed in osteomyelitis.

Treatment

Anti-inflammatory and antibiotic agents are commonly used in infectious or inflammatory musculoskeletal disorders. Anti-inflammatory agents, such as cortisone, may be injected directly into a joint. Osteomyelitis often requires high doses of broad spectrum antibiotics. Septic arthritis often requires intra-articular administration of antibiotic and steroids. In autoimmune disorders, immunosuppressant agents can diminish damage caused by the disease process. Commonly in autoimmune disorders, anti-**tumor necrosis factor (TNF)** inhibitors are used. The inflammatory process in gout requires specific agents that reduce the production of uric acid. Colchicine is a classic drug used in gout. Surgical debridement of necrotic tissue in osteomyelitis is frequently required. Amputation is a last resort but may be the only way to limit the disease process if gangrene is present.

Pathophysiology of Selected Infectious Musculoskeletal Disorders

Infections of the musculoskeletal system can be caused by pathogens that focus their destruction on bones, muscles, or joints. Alternatively, systemic infectious disease can affect the whole body, leaving the musculoskeletal system damaged along with other organs. Osteomyelitis and septic arthritis are diseases where infection is localized in the bone or joint, whereas systemic infections such as Lyme disease affect the whole body and indirectly cause harm to musculoskeletal and neurological systems.

Osteomyelitis

Osteomyelitis is infection of the bone caused by a microorganism, most commonly a bacteria. Although bone is normally resistant to bacterial colonization, events such as trauma, surgery, presence of foreign bodies, or prostheses may disrupt bony integrity and lead to the onset of bone infection.

The incidence of osteomyelitis is 2 in every 10,000 adults. In children, the overall prevalence is 1 case per 5,000. Neonatal prevalence is approximately 1 case per 1,000. The prevalence of osteomyelitis in diabetic patients is 16%; after a foot wound, the risk increases to 30% to 40%. Among individuals who have been treated for an episode of acute osteomyelitis, the prevalence of chronic osteomyelitis is about 5% to 25% in the United States. The presence of a prosthesis increases the risk of osteomyelitis. The incidence of prosthetic joint infection among all prosthesis recipients ranges from 2% to 10%.

Etiology

The most common cause of osteomyelitis for all age groups is *S. aureus*. However, sickle cell disease is often associated with osteomyelitis caused by the *Salmonellae* species. Puncture wounds through athletic shoes have been linked to *S. aureus* and *Pseudomonas* infection. Anaerobes of the bacteroides species and clostridium are also significant pathogens, especially in patients with diabetes mellitus.

There are three basic categories of osteomyelitis: hematogenous, contiguous, and chronic osteomyelitis. Each type is acquired differently and has distinct characteristics.

Hematogenous Osteomyelitis. Hematogenous osteomyelitis arises from a bacterial source within the bloodstream. The infectious process typically has a rapid onset of symptoms within a few days to a week after infection by a pathogen. More than 85% of hematogenous osteomyelitis occurs in children younger than age 17. In adults, thoracic or lumbar vertebrae are typically involved. Regardless of age, males are affected more than females.

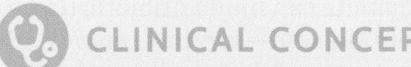

CLINICAL CONCEPT

Children are especially at risk for hematogenous osteomyelitis because of the rapid growth and vascularity of immature bone tissue.

Contiguous Osteomyelitis. Contiguous osteomyelitis results from direct bacterial infection of bone or by extension of an adjacent soft tissue infection. Trauma and surgery are the most common causes of direct bacterial infection in younger individuals. In the older adult, decubitus ulcers or infected joint prostheses are typical sources of infection. Those with peripheral vascular disease (PVD) are especially at risk because of impaired blood flow. Diabetes mellitus also predisposes individuals to osteomyelitis because of impaired blood flow and reduced immunocompetence. Osteomyelitis in diabetes often develops because of a localized foot lesion that becomes infected.

CLINICAL CONCEPT

Older adults, especially those with underlying diseases such as diabetes, are at increased risk for contiguous osteomyelitis.

Chronic Osteomyelitis. Osteomyelitis begins as an acute infection; however, when untreated or undertreated, the destructive process may progress to a chronic disease. Chronic osteomyelitis, which is noted primarily in adults, is defined by the length of time of disease, a lack of response to antibiotic therapy, or presence of necrotic bone. Acute osteomyelitis is considered to be chronic when infection persists longer than 6 to 8 weeks or fails to respond to appropriate antibiotic therapy. The key feature of chronic osteomyelitis is the development of necrotic bone tissue that distinctly separates from the surrounding living bone. Necrotic bone lacks blood supply and cannot attain levels of antibiotic; therefore, it is susceptible to gangrene.

Pathophysiology

Healthy adult bones are normally resistant to bacteremia because bones are not highly vascular, so infection is slow to develop. However, in hematogenous osteomyelitis, bone becomes invaded with bacteria that is present within the bloodstream. The bacteria invade, lodge in bones, and often form an abscess. Because the abscess deprives the bone of its blood supply, the bone tissue dies and becomes necrotic. In adults, the most common region infected is vertebral bone and adjoining intervertebral discs. The infection then commonly spreads into the joint space and adjoining vertebral bodies. Vertebral osteomyelitis at any age is most often a secondary complication of a remote infection. In approximately one-half of vertebral osteomyelitis cases, the source of primary infection is the urinary tract or skin, and in one-third it is endocarditis.

Contiguous osteomyelitis involves direct bacterial invasion through trauma or local extension. The invading pathogen provokes an inflammatory response with vascular engorgement, edema, leukocyte accumulation, and abscess formation. Once the inflammatory process begins, blood vessels thrombose, and exudate extends into the cortex. When the cortex is invaded and disrupted, the bone becomes weaker, predisposing the bone to pathological fracture.

In chronic osteomyelitis, there has been an infection in the bone for a lengthy duration, from weeks to months. The bone is deteriorated and there are no viable blood vessels in the necrotic bone. The avascular, anoxic necrotic bone is a breeding ground for bacteria, particularly anaerobic bacteria. *Clostridia* bacterial species are ubiquitous in the environment and proliferate in areas with low oxygen tension. These resilient, spore-forming bacteria produce toxins that break down surrounding tissue and produce gas. *Clostridium perfringens* is a common type of bacteria that thrives on necrotic tissue, secretes toxins, emits gas, and causes gas gangrene.

Clinical Presentation

The patient history can aid in identifying the mechanism of infection and most likely pathogen. The history obtained from the patient with osteomyelitis should identify present or recent infections of the oropharynx, bladder and kidneys, skin and soft tissue, and musculoskeletal system. The patient should be asked about IV catheter use, IV drug abuse, or hemodialysis. Underlying medical conditions, such as sickle cell anemia, diabetes mellitus, PVD, alcoholism, AIDS, and other forms of immunosuppression should be addressed. The patient should also be asked about any recent trauma such as fracture, animal bite, gunshot wound, puncture wound, or any recent invasive surgical or diagnostic procedure.

The individual with osteomyelitis will often develop generalized symptoms: chills, fever, and malaise. Localized tenderness, erythema, edema, and pain with movement of the infected extremity are common. Loss of ROM can occur as the infection progresses. Postoperative patients, particularly those who have undergone orthopedic surgery or prosthetic implants, may demonstrate delayed wound healing and cutaneous drainage. Those with coexisting diabetes or peripheral arterial disease often lack sensation in the affected extremity and therefore experience less pain. With less pain, the patient is less aware of the infection and will present later in the course of the infection. The patient may not seek health care until infection becomes severe. This is commonly the case with patients who have diabetes: They often seek health care late when there is no chance of saving the limb and amputation is the only way to limit the infection.

Diagnosis

The diagnosis of osteomyelitis is sometimes challenging because laboratory tests and culture may not indicate infection. Laboratory analyses are not diagnostic for osteomyelitis, but provide helpful information. The CBC may reveal an elevation of WBCs, but the WBC count as well as other components of the CBC can be within normal limits. When the WBC count is elevated there is usually an increased number of neutrophils. The ESR is elevated in nearly 90% of cases. CRP rises earlier than ESR rate, but neither of these laboratory values are specific for a diagnosis of osteomyelitis. Blood cultures are positive in only 50% of patients. It is important to recognize that culture or aspiration of infected tissue fails to identify the pathogen in approximately 25% of cases.

Plain x-rays of the affected area often appear unremarkable until late in the osteomyelitis process or abscess formation occurs. Enhanced osteoclastic activity can be seen on radionuclide bone scanning 10 to 14 days before any abnormality appears on x-ray. MRI, CT scanning, and ultrasonography can be used to confirm infection. Although ultrasound can exhibit an effusion of a joint and soft tissue involvement, it is inaccurate in identifying the bone infection. MRI is the most sensitive of these diagnostic tests and is particularly helpful in exhibiting soft tissue involvement. Needle aspiration of bone for culture, commonly under CT guidance, often identifies the causative organism. Bone biopsy for culture should be performed in all patients, except those with hematogenous osteomyelitis who have blood cultures that have positively identified the causative organism.

Treatment

Antibiotic therapy is initially begun intravenously (IV) for 2 to 6 weeks. Most often, a broad spectrum agent is initiated until C&S reports are obtained. Ideally, specific agents are chosen based on the C&S results. Oral therapy follows IV therapy. Debridement of necrotic tissue and debris, as well as surgical drainage of an abscess, may be necessary. Those with prosthetic joints are often treated with the joint prosthesis in place. Hyperbaric oxygen therapy of 100% oxygen at 2 atmospheres of pressure for 2 hours per day for a total of 30 treatments has been shown to be beneficial for those with chronic osteomyelitis. All patients with osteomyelitis should be reevaluated every 3 months for at least 2 years to monitor for relapses, which can occur years after the initial infection.

Complications of osteomyelitis occur as a result of delayed initiation of therapy or failure to respond to therapy. Delayed initiation of therapy most commonly occurs when individuals seek care late in the course of illness or when there is misdiagnosis by the health-care provider. Failure to respond to therapy can result from improper antimicrobial agent selection, dosing, or limited antibiotic penetration. Excessive necrotic tissue, abscess formation, and debris at the infectious site can limit antibiotic tissue penetration. So, debridement—surgical removal of necrotic tissue—is necessary. Additionally, patients with medical conditions, such as immunosuppression or altered sensory and vascular status, are more prone to complications.

Complications can include pathological fractures, especially in weight-bearing bones weakened by infection of the cortex. Removal of the infected joint prosthesis, with mandatory mobility restrictions, may be required in those who develop osteomyelitis postoperatively. Amputation of a digit or distal extremity has been required with advanced, chronic infection.

Septic Arthritis

Septic arthritis, also known as infectious arthritis or pyogenic arthritis, is a direct invasion of the joint space by pathogenic microorganisms: bacteria, viruses, or fungi. Although any infectious agent may cause septic arthritis, bacteria are most common.

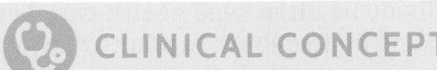

Incidence of septic arthritis ranges from 2 to 10 cases per 100,000 in the general population per year. Gonococcal septic arthritis can occur in the presence of the gonococcal sexually transmitted disease. The incidence of septic arthritis caused by gonococcal infection is 2.8 cases per 100,000 persons per year. Septic arthritis associated with prosthetic implants, which occurs in 2% to 10% of prosthetic recipients, is the most common and challenging form of the disorder. Septic arthritis is also becoming increasingly common in older adults and among those who are immunosuppressed. Of all persons with septic arthritis, 45% are older than 65 years. Those with concurrent disease states are most commonly affected. Fifty-six percent of patients with septic arthritis are male.

Risk factors for septic arthritis include age, underlying medical conditions, and penetrating injury of a joint. Neonates and those older than age 60 are at highest risk for septic arthritis. In children, the epiphyseal growth plate of bones—rich in vascularity—is the region where infection commonly occurs.

In adults, underlying medical conditions that increase the risk of septic arthritis include diabetes, RA, SLE, liver disease, chronic renal failure, IV drug use, organ transplantation, malignancy, and AIDS. Joint-specific factors include puncture wounds, recent joint injection or aspiration, and surgery.

Etiology

Pathogenic microorganisms most commonly invade a joint space via the bloodstream because the synovium of the joint is highly vascular and microbes pass from the blood to the synovial space. Less commonly, organisms enter the joint through direct penetration or contiguous spread from infected surrounding tissue. Direct infection can occur from penetrating or blunt trauma to the joint; this may include diagnostic needle aspiration of the joint or treatments with intra-articular injections of corticosteroids. Prosthetic joint infections are caused by intraoperative contamination in 60% to 80% of cases and bacteremia in 20% to 40% of cases.

Bacterial pathogens have been identified as the most common causes of septic arthritis. Bacterial septic arthritis is often classified as nongonococcal or gonococcal. *S. aureus* remains the most common cause for the vast majority of cases of nongonococcal arthritis in adults and children older than 2 years. Other common pathogens include *Streptococcus* groups A and B, *Streptococcus viridans*, and *S. pneumoniae*. Gram-negative enteric bacilli, such as *E. coli, Salmonella, Proteus*, and *Pseudomonas* species, are common causes of septic arthritis in infants, children, and adults, especially those with recent trauma or abdominal infection. Gonococcal septic arthritis typically occurs in sexually active young adults. *Neisseria gonorrhoeae* is the pathogenic agent in 75% of cases of gonococcal septic arthritis. Gonococcal arthritis is often called ReA.

CLINICAL CONCEPT

Viral infections, such as rubella, hepatitis B, parvovirus B19, and lymphocytic choriomeningitis, can directly infect joints or create antibody-antigen complexes that cause inflammation in joints. With viral infection, multiple joints are usually affected without the formation of purulent exudate; this is also true for the causative agent of Lyme disease, *Borrelia burgdorferi*. Mycobacterial or fungal arthritis typically presents as chronic granulomatous arthritis that affects a single joint.

Pathophysiology

In a healthy joint, synovial fluid has some bactericidal capabilities that allow for resistance of infection. Synovial cells that line the joint can phagocytose microorganisms to protect the joint from bacterial invasion. However, chronic conditions such as RA and SLE decrease the immune defenses in the joints. In hematogenous spread, bacteria are transported from an infectious site in the body into the bloodstream to the arterioles of the bone epiphysis and the synovium. Once the microorganism has invaded the joint space, the microvasculature of the synovial membrane becomes infected. In the infectious process, WBCs synthesize cytokines and other inflammatory products. The end result is the deterioration of essential collagen and intra-articular cartilage. The cytokine and inflammatory products cause joint effusion, which creates swelling that obstructs the delivery of blood and nutrients to the joint. If the inflammatory process continues, the microorganism may invade the adjacent bone.

Clinical Presentation

The history and physical examination for the individual with suspected septic arthritis is similar to that for osteomyelitis. An important focus of the patient history is investigation of underlying medical conditions, such as RA or diabetes, that increase the risk of septic arthritis. The clinician should also investigate any recent problems that may have allowed microorganisms to enter and multiply within the joint structures. The patient should be asked about any recent trauma, invasive procedure, or prosthetic implant. The patient's occupation and lifestyle factors may be related to risk for septic arthritis. Patients should be asked about recent sexually transmitted infection because gonococcus is a common cause of septic arthritis. For other elements of the history, see the Osteomyelitis section.

Patients with septic arthritis often present with inflammation of the synovium with an acutely painful, edematous, and erythematous monoarticular joint. Fever and malaise occur early in the infectious process. Those who have underlying chronic illnesses or are immunocompromised may not present with fever. Individuals often seek health care because of joint pain and limited ROM. In adults, the joints most commonly involved include the knee, hip, elbow, shoulder, and joints of the hand. In children, the hip is the most commonly affected joint.

Diagnosis

Plain x-ray has a limited role in the evaluation of septic arthritis. Soft tissue swelling around the joint, although not diagnostic, is the most common initial finding. Late findings include bone destruction. Ultrasonography can confirm the presence of an effusion, but does not provide clues to the underlying cause. Radionuclide bone scanning is able to localize areas of inflammation through increased dye uptake, but cannot distinguish infectious from noninfectious etiologies. CT scans and MRIs are more sensitive, but also cannot distinguish infectious and noninfectious etiologies.

A definitive diagnosis of septic arthritis requires the detection and identification of bacteria from the blood or synovial fluid by Gram stain or culture. This often requires aspiration of the joint and analysis of the synovial fluid for crystals or microorganisms. For example, the presence of uric acid crystals in synovial fluid would lead to a diagnosis of gout. The presence of more than 50,000 WBCs/mm^3 with more than 75% polymorphonuclear leukocytes in the synovial fluid is common in septic arthritis. Gram stain is less than 60% sensitive for detection of bacteria in synovial fluid, so fluid should also be cultured. Three sets of blood cultures should be obtained to rule out joint infection from bacteremia. If gonococcal infection is suspected, cervical or urethral discharge should be cultured. Elevated ESR and CRP levels are not diagnostic, but can be helpful in monitoring response to therapy.

Treatment

Management of septic arthritis involves drainage of the joint, short-term joint immobilization for pain control, and administration of an antibiotic. Joint aspiration provides fluid for diagnostic analysis and also decreases the joint swelling to relieve pain and allow circulation into the joint. A few aspiration procedures to decrease swelling may be needed during the first 1 to 2 weeks of therapy. Joint immobilization, without weight-bearing, is important while synovitis resolves. The joint should be maintained in a functionally neutral position, with passive ROM exercises scheduled on a regular basis. Once synovitis resolves, physical therapy is used to promote optimal function of the affected joint.

Prompt administration of antibiotic therapy for bacterial infections should be administered to promote complete recovery. The initial antibiotic therapy should cover *S. aureus* and *Streptococcal* species; *Gonococci* should be covered in the sexually active patient. The antibiotic is usually administered IV initially for 2 to 4 weeks. However, a shorter course of IV therapy, with a switch to oral antibiotics, has also proven efficacious in some cases. Oral antibiotic therapy should not be initiated until there are no systemic symptoms and the joint cultures are negative for pathogens.

For those with a prosthetic joint infection, optimal treatment involves removal of the prosthesis and a 6-week course of antibiotics. Replacement of the prosthesis should involve using an antibiotic-impregnated bone cement and new prosthesis.

CLINICAL CONCEPT

Joint dysfunction is the major complication of septic arthritis. In adults, the optimal treatment eradicates bacteria from the synovial fluid within 6 days of initiating antibiotic therapy. *S. aureus* infection, a challenging form of septic arthritis, has been linked to chronic complications such as permanent joint damage with limited ROM or chronic pain in approximately one-half of cases. The mortality rate of *S. aureus* is typically 10%, but can approach 50% in the immunosuppressed patient. In contrast, infection with *N. gonorrhoeae* has a very low mortality rate.

Mycobacterium Tuberculosis

Although pulmonary TB is the most common form of TB, mycobacterium TB can spread to other areas of the body through the bloodstream and can involve multiple organs, particularly the vertebrae. *M. tuberculosis* accounts for 10% to 35% of extrapulmonary TB (EPTB) and most often involves the spine (50%), but may also result in tuberculous arthritis in the hip (15%) or knee (15%) and extraspinal tuberculous osteomyelitis. Studies of the populations of Los Angeles and New York show that musculoskeletal TB primarily affects African Americans, Hispanic Americans, Asian Americans, and foreign-born individuals.

CLINICAL CONCEPT

Immunocompromised individuals, especially those with human immunodeficiency virus (HIV) infection or AIDS, are at greatest risk for rapid spread of TB to extrapulmonary sites, including the bone.

Etiology

M. tuberculosis is an acid-fast, aerobic, slow-growing bacillus. Within the United States, the individual's immunological status is the most important factor in the development of EPTB.

Pathophysiology

Following multiplication of *M. tuberculosis* within the lung (see Chapter 11: Disorders of the Immune System), the bacillus may spread throughout the body via the bloodstream. Although any bone can be infected, infection of the vertebrae is most common.

Vertebral TB is also referred to as tuberculous spondylitis or **Pott's disease.** Pott's disease, a combination of osteomyelitis and arthritis, usually involves more than one vertebra. Compression of spinal nerves that causes pain is common. Thoracic vertebrae are most commonly affected, followed by lumbar and cervical vertebrae. Infection of the vertebral bone most commonly begins in the anteroinferior aspect of the vertebral body with involvement of the intervertebral disc and adjacent vertebrae. Abscesses can develop in the paravertebral muscles with abscess extension into adjacent tissues. Severe kyphosis (cervicothoracic curvature of the spine) can occur in conjunction with destruction of the vertebrae. TB can cause severe destruction of the vertebrae with resulting spinal nerve impingement. If the spinal nerves are severely affected by TB, paralysis can occur.

Clinical Presentation

Exposure to TB is a key component of the patient history. The classic symptoms of pulmonary TB—cough, night sweats, and weight loss—are often *not* present in skeletal TB. The essential history components for the patient with skeletal TB include known or suspected exposure to *M. tuberculosis*. The patient should be asked about recent travel to or from a region where TB is endemic, such as China or underdeveloped countries. Immunosuppression increases susceptibility to TB infection, so patients should be asked about current medications, medical conditions, surgical history, and HIV status.

The patient most commonly complains of chronic back pain. The reported average duration of symptoms at diagnosis is 4 months. The patient may complain of symptoms of spinal nerve impingement such as weakness and numbness of a lower extremity. Some patients report fever and weight loss. Cervical spine TB is less common but is potentially more serious because severe neurological complications can cause breathing problems. Cervical TB symptoms include neck muscle spasm, hoarseness, and dyspnea.

When examining a patient who may have vertebral TB, the clinician should carefully inspect and palpate the vertebrae, as well as carefully observe the patient's posture and gait. The patient should bend over to touch toes with the clinician observing from the back of the patient to look for asymmetry of the paravertebral muscles. The patient's vertebrae should be palpated for tenderness and a comprehensive neurological examination should be done. Neurological deficits may be noted if there is spinal nerve compression. Neurological manifestations can range from single spinal nerve impingement to paralysis of a limb. Clinical manifestations of vertebral TB may vary depending upon the site of skeletal involvement, but the typical presentation of tuberculous arthritis includes pain, joint swelling, and decreased ROM.

Diagnosis

Diagnosing EPTB is difficult because classic signs or symptoms of TB may not be present. It is important to note that a purified protein derivative (PPD) skin test may be negative in EPTB because fewer bacteria are necessary to infect nonpulmonary sites.

Biopsy of bone tissue is the method of diagnosis in vertebral TB. Chest x-ray reveals pulmonary involvement in fewer than one-half of patients with EPTB. X-ray findings of the affected vertebral bone include soft tissue swelling and joint space narrowing. Vertebral lesions cause compressive fractures, exhibited as flattening of the vertebral bone. Joint aspiration and fluid analysis contain mycobacteria in nearly 80% of cases.

Advanced infection and destruction of the vertebrae can lead to spinal deformity with instability, vertebral collapse, and spinal nerve compression. Involved joints may result in joint deformity, chronic pain, and limited ROM.

Treatment

The treatment principles of pulmonary TB also apply to EPTB. A detailed discussion of baseline evaluation, antituberculous therapy, and follow-up can be found in Chapter 20: Respiratory Inflammation and Infection. An extended 12-month regimen is often required for individuals with skeletal TB. When neurological impairment or spine instability is present, surgery may be necessary to drain abscesses, debride infected tissue, stabilize the spine, or relieve spinal cord compression.

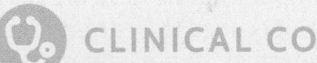 CLINICAL CONCEPT

Vertebral TB usually does not present with the classic signs of pulmonary TB. It is important to assess the patient for spinal nerve compression in vertebral TB, as quadriplegia, paraplegia, or cauda equina can occur.

Lyme Disease

First discovered in Lyme, Connecticut, Lyme disease is caused by the tick-transmitted spirochete *B. burgdorferi*. It is the most common vector-borne disease in the United States.

Lyme disease most often occurs in the late spring and summer months when ticks are most active and human outdoor activity is highest. The disease has been detected more frequently in males than females, with a higher incidence in those 5 to 14 years of age and 50 to 59 years of age. Approximately 20,000 cases are reported annually in the United States. Although most of the states report Lyme disease, more than 95% of cases come from just 12 states: Connecticut, Delaware, Maine, Maryland, Massachusetts, Minnesota, New Hampshire, New Jersey, New York, Pennsylvania, Rhode Island, and Wisconsin. Within these states, incidence can vary from one community to another. In the states where Lyme disease is most common, the average is 34.7 cases per 100,000 persons. However, the incidence is speculated to be much higher because many people do not seek health care and misdiagnosis by health-care providers is common.

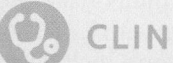

CLINICAL CONCEPT

The greatest risk for Lyme disease is occupational or recreational outdoor exposure in a tick-endemic region. Individuals who live in areas with a high deer population are at increased risk of Lyme disease.

Etiology

Lyme disease bacteria live in mice, squirrels, deer, and other small mammals. In the northeastern and north-central United States, the blacklegged deer tick (*Ixodes scapularis*) is the most common agent of transmission. On the west coast, the western blacklegged deer tick (*Ixodes pacificus*) is the agent of transmission.

Ticks feed on infected animals, resulting in transfer of the spirochete *B. burgdorferi* to a tick. The ticks can become attached to grass or foliage in forested areas; individuals or their pets then can contract the tick when walking through the forested areas. The bacteria *B. burgdorferi* is transferred to a human through a tick bite. Human infection may result when a tick is attached for 24 to 48 hours. Adult ticks are less likely to transmit the disease because they are noticed and removed; nymphs, however, can easily go undetected, especially in hairy areas of the body, because they may be only slightly larger than the period at the end of a sentence (see Fig. 39-2).

The incubation period is typically 7 to 14 days after tick exposure, but can be between 3 and 31 days. Fewer than 50% of individuals recall any tick bite.

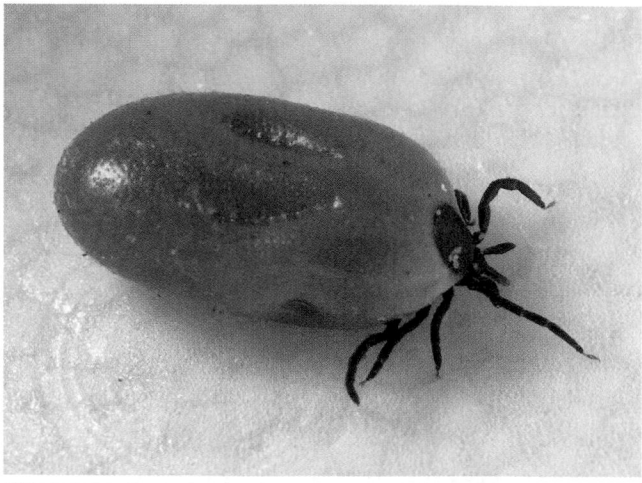

FIGURE 39-2. Deer tick. *(Courtesy of CDC/Gary Alpert–Urban Pests–Integrated Pest Management (IPM).)*

Pathophysiology

Lyme disease pathophysiology is not completely understood. Spirochete infection causes many of the disease manifestations, but the infected individual's immune response is thought to contribute as well. Before the tick delivers the bacteria, the tick injects a substance to inhibit the individual's immune response. Once the bacterium is introduced through the tick bite, the spirochete may be eradicated by the individual's defense mechanisms. However, in many cases the bacterium remains viable, causing a localized rash called **erythema migrans (EM)**. The spirochete secretes enzymes that aid in replication of the bacteria; the infection can be picked up by blood or lymph and disseminated throughout the body. This hematogenous dissemination can occur within days to weeks of initial infection. Once the *B. burgdorferi* spread throughout the body, the bacteria tend to be difficult to detect with laboratory tests. The spirochete has been known to infect the skin, heart, joints, eyes, central nervous system (CNS), peripheral nerves, and other parts of the body.

Clinical Presentation

The clinician who suspects Lyme disease needs to inquire about the patient's occupational or recreational outdoor activities. Particular attention should be given to activities undertaken within the past month. Although the recollection of a tick bite is helpful, it is not essential. The patient should also be asked about any recent rashes. Commonly, the patient presents with a vague combination of arthralgias, myalgias, excessive fatigue, and headache. However, the vague presentation does not give the clinician sufficient clues to suspect Lyme disease. Most patients do not report a tick bite and the rash is often not present. Uniquely, some patients present with facial nerve palsy (also called Bell's palsy) with no recollection of a tick bite or rash.

There are three stages of Lyme disease:

1. early localized
2. early disseminated
3. late disseminated.

Each stage has specific characteristics, but regardless of stage, children may present differently than adults.

Early Localized Disease. Early localized Lyme disease is the most common stage of presentation, occurring 3 to 30 days after a deer tick bite. In 70% to 80% of cases, the individual presents with EM, which often begins as an erythematous macule or papule at the site of the tick bite. The rash enlarges over several days to form a round lesion with a clear area in the middle of the ring, called a "bull's-eye rash" (see Fig. 39-3).

EM can also present as an oval-shaped lesion, with various shades of red, pink, and purple, which can be mistaken for a spider bite or skin infection. The rash is not painful or pruritic (itchy), and the patient may ignore it. Those infected with early Lyme disease often present with skin rash and vague generalized flulike

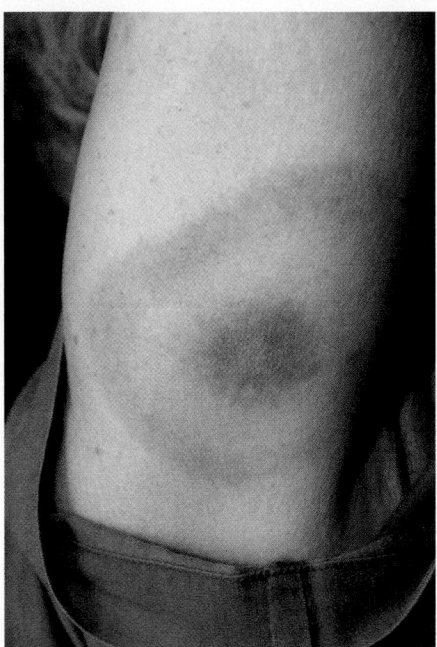

FIGURE 39-3. EM rash of Lyme disease. *(Courtesy of CDC/James Gathany.)*

symptoms: fever (usually low-grade), chills, myalgias, arthralgias, fatigue, and headache. Regional enlargement of lymph nodes (lymphadenopathy) in the area draining the tick bite may be found.

Early Disseminated Disease. Early disseminated Lyme disease occurs from 3 to 12 weeks after the tick bite. The infected individual will usually have one or more EMs and the vague, generalized symptoms as described in early localized disease. *B. burgdorferi* infection can result in lymphocytic meningitis (neck pain and intense headache), cranial neuritis (paralysis of facial nerves), carditis (various degrees of reversible heart block, myocarditis, or pericarditis), and ocular involvement (visual changes or unilateral blindness).

Late Disseminated Disease. When the bacteria are not eradicated, the individual develops late disseminated Lyme disease. This stage occurs months to years following the tick bite. By then, the individual experiences severe joint pain and swelling of large joints, often the knees (in 60% of cases). In a small percentage of patients, CNS involvement can cause subacute encephalopathy, or confusion and difficulty with concentration. If spinal nerves are involved, neural inflammation (polyradiculopathy) can develop with symptoms of shooting pains, numbness, or tingling of the hands or feet.

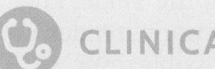

CLINICAL CONCEPT

Fewer than 50% of individuals who develop Lyme disease recall any tick bite.

Diagnosis

The diagnosis of Lyme disease is based on symptoms, physical findings, and a history of exposure to ticks. Lab tests are commonly falsely negative in patients with early disease, though they are more reliable for the later stages of disease.

The Centers for Disease Control and Prevention recommend a two-step process; both tests can be done using the same blood sample. Enzyme-linked immunosorbent assay (ELISA) or immunofluorescent assay (IFA) are the recommended initial laboratory tests. These tests are highly sensitive; the vast majority of those with Lyme disease—and some individuals without the disease—will test positive. Sometimes these tests may provide a result of "indeterminate" or "equivocal," meaning a positive or negative result cannot be determined. For those with positive or indeterminate or equivocal results on ELISA or IFA, Western blot confirmation is the second recommended laboratory test. Western blot is designed to be specific in that it is only positive if the person is truly infected.

Treatment

For those living in an area endemic with Lyme disease and sustaining a known tick bite, the Infectious Disease Society of America recommends a prophylactic single dose of the antibiotic doxycycline. All others who have removed ticks should be closely monitored for signs and symptoms of Lyme disease for 30 days. If EM or generalized symptoms develop, antibiotic therapy is warranted. The treatment of choice is a 21-day course of doxycycline, although alternative antibiotics have been used. The response to antibiotics can vary widely because there are more than 300 strains of *B. burgdorferi* worldwide and greater than 100 strains in the United States alone.

Commonly, Lyme disease is not readily identified in its early stages. However, if antibiotic treatment is begun early, Lyme disease can be cured. Even with antibiotics, a small percent of infected individuals have symptoms that last months, years, or even a lifetime. Patients report neuropathic pain, difficulty concentrating, arthritis, and altered mobility. The cause of these symptoms, called Post-Lyme Syndrome, is not known. It is theorized that the individual has an autoimmune response that remains overactive long after the infection has been eradicated.

Common Musculoskeletal Inflammatory Disorders

Common musculoskeletal inflammatory disorders include RA, gout, SLE, scleroderma, psoriatic arthritis (PsA), ankylosing spondylitis, and dermatomyositis. Most of these disorders occur because of autoimmune reactions triggered by unknown factors. For RA, SLE, and scleroderma, see Chapter 11: Disorders of the Immune System.

Gout

Gout, also termed gouty arthritis, is a disorder of recurrent inflammation triggered by **hyperuricemia,** which is elevated uric acid in the blood, and synovial fluid. For unknown reasons, certain joints of the body, such as the first metatarsal, are specifically affected. Prevalence in the United States has risen over the last 20 years, and the disorder now affects 8.3 million Americans—or 4% of the population. Prevalence of increased uric acid levels (hyperuricemia) also rose, affecting 43.3 million (21%) adults in the United States. Gout often affects the peripheral joints of men older than 30 years of age. Men are four times more likely to develop gout than women. Women are rarely affected until after menopause, as estrogen is believed to be protective against hyperuricemia. Twenty percent of individuals with gout have a family history of the syndrome. Gout is more prevalent in black males; this is thought to occur because black males have a higher incidence of early hypertension and are often treated with diuretics. Diuretics, particularly thiazides, often cause hyperuricemia.

Experts estimate that only 5% of individuals with hyperuricemia develop gout. This leads to questions of why only a small portion of those affected with hyperuricemia progress to symptomatic gout. Many factors are thought to predispose individuals to the syndrome (see Box 39-1).

Etiology

Gout may be designated as primary or secondary. Primary gout, a metabolic disorder, constitutes 90% of cases. The vast majority of individuals with primary gout have a defect in renal excretion of uric acid. A genetic variation has been found that diminishes uric acid transport at the kidney.

Secondary gout can be attributed to a variety of disorders, including myeloproliferative (abnormal growth of bone marrow cells) or lymphoproliferative disease (abnormal production of WBCs), neoplastic disease, glycogen storage disease, psoriasis, and sarcoidosis. Secondary gout is also associated with obesity, lead intoxication, alcoholism, and use of specific medications. In addition, gout can occur in cancer chemotherapy because of the accelerated breakdown of cells. Increased breakdown of cellular deoxyribonucleic acid leads to elevated uric acid levels.

Pathophysiology

Uric acid, a weak acid that remains ionized at the body's normal pH, is a by-product of purine metabolism. Ninety-eight percent of extracellular uric acid is in the form of monosodium urate, which are needlelike crystals that are deposited in connective tissues throughout the body when uric acid levels exceed a concentration of 6.8 mg/dL. Crystallization within synovial fluid results in the acute painful joint inflammation of gouty arthritis. Over time, crystals become deposited in subcutaneous tissue, resulting in the formation of small, white nodules known as **tophi** that are easily visible in the Achilles tendon, joints of the hands, or pinnae of the ears.

Clinical Presentation

Symptoms and frequency of attacks of gout should be described in the history. The patient should be asked about alcohol consumption, current medication use, and dietary intake of meat. Either beer or hard liquor can trigger gout. The patient should also be asked about history of medical conditions such as proliferative or neoplastic disease (cancer), psoriasis, sarcoidosis, or other inflammatory disorders. It is important to ask the patient about recent chemotherapeutic treatments, potential lead exposure, recent weight change, trauma, or surgery. Family history of gout is significant as there is a genetic cause of the disorder.

Signs and Symptoms

Symptoms of gout occur after 15 to 20 years of constant, asymptomatic levels of hyperuricemia. The classic presentation of acute gout is a sudden onset of inflammation and excruciating pain in one joint—the joint of the great toe. **Podagra,** an acute inflammation of the metatarsophalangeal joint of the great toe, is the most common presentation (see Fig. 39-4). Other joints may be affected, including the ankle, knee, wrist, or elbow. Symptoms include a warm, tender, swollen, and erythematous joint with possible fever.

Usually the discomfort of gout begins at night or early in the morning. The affected joint is exquisitely sensitive. Symptoms may subside in a few days to weeks

---

Box 39-1. Risk Factors for Gout

High alcohol consumption increases risk of gout because alcohol stimulates hepatic uric acid production and renal uric acid reabsorption. Specific dietary intake may contribute to the development of gout or exacerbations of primary gout. A diet filled with purine-rich foods, such as meat and seafood, has been linked to exacerbations of primary gout.

The use of medications such as niacin, ethambutol, pyrazinamide, cyclosporine, levodopa, diuretics, or salicylates has been implicated in the development of secondary gout and may contribute to exacerbations in those with primary gout. Chemotherapeutic agents used in the treatment of cancer can also trigger attacks of gout. Chemotherapeutic agents cause the death of high numbers of cells, which yields high amounts of cellular deoxyribonucleic acid; this is made up of purines, which are sources of uric acid. Additionally, trauma or surgery can cause an acute attack of gout. Conditions such as hypertension, diabetes, renal insufficiency, hypertriglyceridemia, hypercholesterolemia, obesity, and early menopause are associated with a higher incidence of gout.

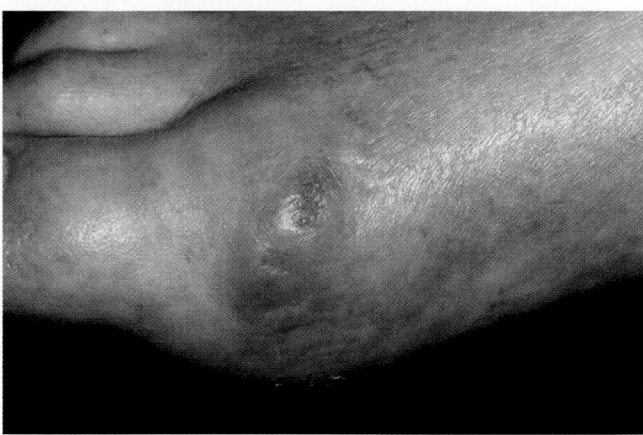

FIGURE 39-4. Podagra of gout. Podagra is an inflamed, reddened area around the joint of the great toe caused by gout, which is an arthritis caused by an excess of uric acid in the bloodstream. Crystals of uric acid collect inside the synovial space within the toe joint, causing inflammation and acute pain. *(From Dr. P. Marazzi/Science Source.)*

without treatment when an interval between attacks occurs, where the individual remains symptom free.

Because chronic gout may involve more than one joint, it can be confused with osteoarthritis and RA. As the disease progresses, asymptomatic intervals shorten, more joints become involved, and attacks last longer. Tophi become visible (see Fig. 39-5) and extra-articular manifestations develop: low-grade fever, nephropathy (kidney disease), and nephrolithiasis (kidney stones).

CLINICAL CONCEPT

The classic presentation of acute gout is a sudden onset of inflammation and excruciating pain in the metatarsophalangeal joint of the great toe; a condition called Podagra.

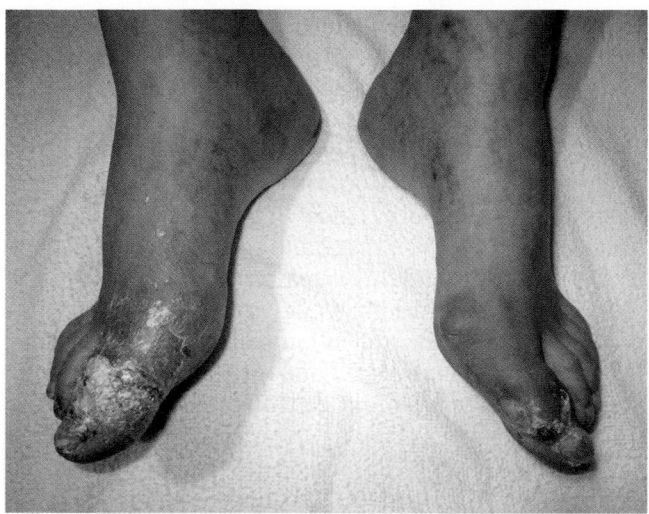

FIGURE 39-5. Tophi of great toe caused by gout. Tophi are swellings that contain uric acid crystals. *(Courtesy of James Heilman, MD.)*

The major complications of gouty arthritis are related to joint and kidney involvement in the disease process. Untreated or undertreated gout can lead to the development of painful, disabling destruction of cartilage and bone. Irreversible joint deformity and loss of motion has been reported. Tophi can grow to significant sizes and require surgical removal. Prolonged hyperuricemia can lead to the formation of renal calculi (kidney stones). Individuals with gout have a 1,000-fold increased incidence of renal calculi; this is especially true when patients excrete more than 1,100 mg of uric acid in a 24-hour urine sample. Forty percent of persons with gout develop kidney stones. Persons with gout can also develop urate nephropathy, in which uric acid crystals are deposited in the tissue of the kidneys and cause renal dysfunction.

Diagnosis

Diagnostic tests should be aimed at ruling out different diagnoses such as pseudogout, cellulitis, septic arthritis, RA, and bunion bursitis. All these disorders resemble gout but are not related. Laboratory tests should include serum uric acid levels, CBC, ESR, CRP, and rheumatoid factor in gout.

A 24-hour urine uric acid of greater than 900 mg suggests overproduction of urate. Serum uric acid level of more than 7 mg/dL in men or 6 mg/dL in women is suggestive of gout, but not diagnostic. Uric acid levels should not be relied upon to provide a diagnosis. Although most individuals with gout have elevated uric acid levels intermittently during the course of the disease, hyperuricemia may not be present during an acute attack. Furthermore, having hyperuricemia alone does not mean that an individual will develop gout. In fact, most individuals with elevated serum uric acid do not develop gout.

X-rays often reveal soft tissue inflammation and asymmetric swelling during the acute phase of gout. As the disease progresses, subtle changes in bony structures on plain x-ray may be noted; yet, these findings do not typically occur until after at least 1 year of uncontrolled disease. Small punched-out lesions can develop within the periphery of affected joints, but may not be detected unless two views of x-ray are obtained. The classic sign of late-stage gout is the development of multiple large tophi. Joint space narrowing will also be apparent on radiological films.

The gold standard of diagnosis is aspiration of joint fluid for culture and urate crystals. The procedure is critical to the diagnosis of gout, in order to rule out other inflammatory or infectious joint disorders. The detection of urate crystals, which are needlelike in appearance under the microscope, establishes a positive diagnosis of gouty arthritis. During acute attacks, the synovial fluid may contain a WBC count of 20,000 to 50,000 cells/mm^3, with a predominance of polymorphonuclear neutrophils.

Box 39-2. Differentiating Gout from Pseudogout

Pseudogout is a form of arthritis that mimics gout in presentation. The inflammation of pseudogout is caused by the formation of calcium pyrophosphate crystals, which have the microscopic appearance of rod-shaped crystals with blunt ends. Pseudogout is also called calcium pyrophosphate disease.

Although anyone can develop pseudogout, risk greatly increases with advancing age. Older adults are more prone to the disease because they have a higher incidence of pre-existing joint disease such as osteoarthritis. Knees are most commonly involved, but ankles, shoulders, elbows, wrists, or hands can be affected. Diagnosis is made with joint aspiration and microscopic evaluation for calcium pyrophosphate crystals.

 CLINICAL CONCEPT

It is important to differentiate gout from pseudogout (see Box 39-2).

Treatment

The management goal in gout is to treat acute attacks and prevent further attacks. It is important to begin administration of medications early in the disease to enhance treatment response. Pain can also be controlled with joint immobilization and decreased weight-bearing.

Nonsteroidal anti-inflammatory drugs (NSAIDs) are first-line agents. Starting doses should be high for the initial 2 to 3 days, with a gradual dose reduction over the next 2 weeks; patients should be asymptomatic for at least 2 days before discontinuation of the NSAID.

 CLINICAL CONCEPT

Only 7% of those with gout remain attack-free for more than 10 years; 78% of those with gout will have a recurrent attack within 2 years; 62% will have one within the first year after diagnosis. Nonpharmacological therapy includes maintaining or obtaining an ideal body weight, avoiding rapid weight loss, limiting overall alcohol and dietary meats (which contain purines that raise uric acid), avoiding binge drinking, intaking a minimum of 2 to 3 liters of fluid per day, and avoiding medications associated with hyperuricemia whenever possible. The medications allopurinol and probenecid are recommended to prevent further attacks of gout. Allopurinol decreases uric acid synthesis and probenecid increases renal excretion of uric acid. The goal is to keep uric acid levels between 5.5 mg/dL and 6.5 mg/dL.

Once an infectious process is ruled out, oral corticosteroids can be initiated as an alternative for those who cannot tolerate NSAIDs. Moderately high doses are used for 1 to 3 days, and tapered over 2 weeks because more abrupt tapering can initiate a rebound flare. Colchicine is the oldest available agent for the treatment of gout. The drug has no analgesic activity but blocks the inflammation caused by uric acid crystals. Colchicine is most effective when initiated during the first 12 to 24 hours of an attack.

Polymyositis and Dermatomyositis

Polymyositis and dermatomyositis are part of a group of musculoskeletal diseases known as idiopathic inflammatory myopathies. These two conditions are both characterized by inflammation and destruction of muscle fibers. Polymyositis is the inflammation of multiple muscle groups in the body. Dermatomyositis is the inflammation of muscle with involvement of the skin.

Polymyositis and dermatomyositis are rare disorders. The prevalence rate of polymyositis ranges from 6 to 10 cases per 1,000,000 individuals. Polymyositis is a disease of adults older than age 20 years; dermatomyositis occurs more commonly in those younger than age 15 years and those older than age 50 years. African Americans have a higher incidence of polymyositis and dermatomyositis than Caucasians, and women are affected by polymyositis nearly twice as often as men.

Etiology

The definitive cause of polymyositis and dermatomyositis is not known, but specific abnormalities within the immune system have been noted. Both polymyositis and dermatomyositis have been linked to the autoimmune disorders RA, SLE, and scleroderma. Dermatomyositis in the adult has also been linked to underlying malignancies. There is also a genetic predisposition, as these disorders are often familial.

Pathophysiology

Although the cause of polymyositis and dermatomyositis is unclear, experts have hypothesized that a viral illness, injury, or microvascular damage leads to the release of muscle proteins that are misidentified as antigens, and an autoimmune process causes inflammation. With both polymyositis and dermatomyositis, autoantigens begin an inflammatory process involving T cells, B cells, interferon gamma, interleukin-2, and tumor necrosis factor-alpha. The WBCs and inflammatory mediators surround muscle fibers and ultimately destroy them. In dermatomyositis, the WBCs and inflammatory mediators also gather around cutaneous blood vessels. This clustering of inflammation around cutaneous vessels causes dermatological changes.

Clinical Presentation

It is important for the clinician to gather information about the patient history. As these disorders are linked to other autoimmune diseases, essential components of the history include a personal or family history of RA, SLE, and scleroderma. Underlying malignancies may also precede the development of polymyositis or dermatomyositis, so the history should focus on previous medical and surgical conditions or potential undiagnosed lung or breast cancer.

The diagnosis of polymyositis or dermatomyositis may be delayed because early signs and symptoms are vague and generalized. Fatigue, weakness, fever, and malaise are often mistaken as a viral illness. The diagnosis is often not made until symmetrically patterned muscle weakness or rash is apparent.

The onset of polymyositis and dermatomyositis is gradual with proximal muscle weakness appearing over a period of weeks to months. The initial signs and symptoms include malaise, fever, myalgias, muscle weakness, muscle pain and tenderness, and lethargy. Polymyositis and dermatomyositis involve striated muscles (voluntary skeletal muscles) simultaneously, resulting in symmetrical muscle weakness.

Although polymyositis spares the dermis, dermatomyositis is associated with a classic skin rash that involves the eyelids, face, chest, and extensor surfaces of the extremities. The presence of a symmetric purplered colored macular skin rash and eyelid edema suggests a diagnosis of dermatomyositis.

Diagnosis

Laboratory tests that indicate inflammation, such as creatinine phosphokinase and ESR, can be elevated 5 to 50 times above the normal range in both polymyositis and dermatomyositis. Other muscle enzymes may be elevated, including lactic dehydrogenase, aspartate aminotransferase, alanine aminotransferase, and aldolase. Additionally, patients may have leukocytosis, a positive rheumatoid factor, or positive antinuclear antibodies. Electromyography studies reveal characteristic muscle changes in nearly all patients with polymyositis or dermatomyositis: muscle membrane irritability and changes of motor unit action potentials.

Muscle biopsy is the most definitive test for polymyositis and dermatomyositis, revealing stages of muscle inflammation. In dermatomyositis, inflammatory cells surrounding blood vessels and atrophy of muscle cells are identified.

Treatment

The goals of treatment are to minimize muscle weakness and improve ability to maintain activities of daily living (ADLs). Corticosteroids, such as prednisone, and immunosuppressive agents are considered first-line treatment. They are often initially administered at high doses and tapered as symptoms subside and creatinine phosphokinase levels decrease to normal range. In patients who fail to respond or develop intolerable side effects, other agents such as azathioprine, cyclosporine, chlorambucil, methotrexate, and cyclophosphamide have resulted in symptom improvement.

Another key treatment component is individually designed physical therapy to prevent contractures and enhance functional ability. Ideally, physical therapy should be initiated early in the disease course so that mobility and strength may be optimized. Most patients improve with treatment; full recovery is accomplished in approximately 50% of patients.

 CLINICAL CONCEPT

Most individuals with polymyositis or dermatomyositis respond to immunosuppressive therapy, and 5-year survival rates have been estimated at more than 80%. Specific complications linked to mortality include advanced muscle weakness, pulmonary involvement, cardiac involvement, dysphagia and aspiration pneumonia, associated malignancies, and adverse effects of immunosuppression.

Psoriatic Arthritis

PsA is a chronic inflammatory disease of the joints and connective tissue that is linked to the skin disorder psoriasis (see Chapter 41: Skin Disorders). In 85% of affected individuals, psoriatic skin disease precedes joint disease. PsA has been linked to other autoimmune disorders, including RA. PsA affects men at a slightly higher rate than women, with the onset of the disease occurring most often between 30 and 50 years of age.

There are five patterns or forms of PsA:

1. Distal interphalangeal (DIP) predominant: known as the "classic" form, DIP occurs in only approximately 5% to 10% of those with PsA
2. Arthritis mutilans: a severe, destructive arthritis that accounts for 5% of those affected by PsA
3. Symmetric arthritis: symmetrical arthritis, which affects fewer than 25% of those with PsA, is similar in appearance and destruction to RA, but has a milder course
4. Asymmetric arthritis: the most common type of PsA, occurring in up to 70% of affected patients
5. Spondylitis: this form, characterized by inflammation of the spinal column, occurs in more than 5% of individuals with PsA.

Although patients can initially present with any one of these forms of arthritis, the patterns of PsA can change during the course of the disease, and up to 60% of patients do not have one permanent pattern of the disease course.

Etiology

The exact etiology is unknown, but PsA is believed to be an autoimmune disorder with T cell–mediated immune response. Like other autoimmune disorders, environmental, genetic, and immunological factors are thought to be key factors in the development of PsA.

Environmental factors include infectious agents and physical trauma. There is a genetic component to the disease, with PsA often present in several members of a family.

Pathophysiology

The pathophysiology of PsA is similar to that of other types of inflammatory arthritis. In psoriasis and PsA, T cells infiltrate the skin and joints. The T cell infiltration sets off a cascade of immune-mediated inflammation. B lymphocytes, also involved in the inflammatory reaction, synthesize immunoglobulins. Immunoglobulins then become deposited in the epidermis and synovial membranes, leading to the classic psoriatic scaly skin lesions and inflammation within joints.

Clinical Presentation

A detailed history should focus on both current and previous skin and nail changes. The patient will often complain of psoriatic skin changes before the development of joint symptoms. Family history of psoriasis should also be investigated.

The symptoms of PsA are similar to those of other arthritic diseases such as RA and gout. There are different patterns of psoriatic involvement of skin and joints. Depending on the pattern or form of the disease, PsA can develop slowly with mild symptoms or quickly with severe symptoms.

PsA typically presents as pain, swelling, and erythema of the affected joints with accompanying extra-articular symptoms: generalized fatigue, redness, and pain of the eye; plaque psoriasis of the skin; and psoriatic nail changes. The nail changes occur in more than 80% of patients: pitting, ridging, and onycholysis (painless separation of nail from the nailbed).

When differentiating between the forms of PsA, signs and symptoms can vary significantly. DIP-predominant PsA primarily involves the distal joints of the fingers and toes. Those with arthritis mutilans suffer from destruction and erosion of the small joints of the hands, feet, and spine. Symmetric PsA usually affects multiple symmetric pairs of joints and can be disabling. Asymmetric arthritis may present with inflammatory changes in both large and small joints and does not occur in the same joints on both sides of the body. These patients may develop dactylitis (inflammation of all the finger joints), with a "sausagelike" appearance of the fingers or toes. The joints may also be warm and red, with periodic joint pain. Spondylitis (inflammation of the vertebral joints) often develops later in the disease and affects men and older patients disproportionately. Often, those with spondylitis have **sacroiliitis,** which is inflammation of the sacroiliac joint, along with complaints of pain, stiffness, and difficulty with movement of the cervical, thoracic, or lumbar spine.

Diagnosis

An individual with PsA may have joint pain before detectable psoriatic skin change. However, a definitive diagnosis of PsA cannot be made without evidence of classic psoriatic skin and nail changes. Health-care providers rely on the history and physical examination to diagnose PsA. Although diagnostic tests are used to rule out other disease processes, there is no specific test to diagnose PsA.

Lab tests can be only somewhat helpful in diagnosing the patient with presumed PsA. Although ESR is elevated in only 40% to 60% of patients with PsA, the degree of ESR elevation often correlates with the severity of skin involvement. A high ESR occurs in severe cases of PsA, whereas low elevation of ESR occurs with mild disease, At least 20% of those with PsA will have an elevated serum uric acid level because of rapid skin turnover, breakdown of the skin's nucleic acids, and metabolism of these nucleic acids to uric acid.

In the early stages of PsA, x-rays do not reveal signs of arthritis and are not usually helpful in making a diagnosis. In the later stages, x-rays may show changes that are characteristic of PsA and not found with other types of arthritis. In those with DIP disease or arthritis mutilans, changes on x-ray of the fingers demonstrate a "pencil and cup" phenomenon where the end of the bone gets whittled down to a sharp point.

Treatment

Treatment goals for the individual with PsA are to control the inflammatory process and improve quality of life. NSAIDs and local corticosteroid injection are the first line of treatment as they decrease inflammation, joint pain, and stiffness. For those with progressive symptoms or treatment resistance, methotrexate has been used. Recently, the standard treatment includes disease-modifying antirheumatic drugs (DMARDs), specifically tissue necrosis factor (TNF) inhibitors. The DMARDs have been shown to relieve more severe symptoms and to slow or halt the joint and tissue damage.

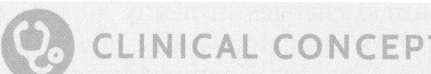

CLINICAL CONCEPT

Early recognition, diagnosis, and treatment of PsA can help to minimize the extensive joint damage that occurs in later stages of the disease. Without adequate treatment, PsA can become disabling. Those with more progressive forms of the disease, such as arthritis mutilans, can suffer from significant impairment early on in the disease process.

Ankylosing Spondylitis

Ankylosing spondylitis is a systemic rheumatic disease that can affect multiple tissues throughout the body, such as the eyes, heart, lungs, and kidneys. Most commonly, ankylosing spondylitis is known as a form of chronic inflammation of the spine and the sacroiliac joints, which results in pain and stiffness in and around the spine. Other problems that can accompany ankylosing spondylitis include arthritis of joints in the extremities, iritis (inflammation of the eyes), and pulmonary fibrosis (scarring throughout the lungs).

Within the United States, the prevalence of ankylosing spondylitis is approximately 0.5% to 1% among Caucasians, 3% to 4% in African Americans, and 18% to 50% in Native Americans. It is more common in males than in females, with symptoms commonly beginning in late adolescence or early adulthood. In women, the sacroiliac joint and joints away from the spine are more frequently affected, and the disease often progresses more slowly than in men.

Etiology

The exact etiology of ankylosing spondylitis remains unknown, though the tendency to develop ankylosing spondylitis is believed to be genetically inherited, as most patients (90% to 95%) with ankylosing spondylitis are born with specific human leukocyte antigen HLA-B27 on the surface of their cells. The genes that promote HLA-B27 increase the tendency of developing ankylosing spondylitis, whereas additional factors, perhaps environmental or infectious, are necessary for disease development.

Pathophysiology

The initial inflammation of ankylosing spondylitis is thought to occur as a result of an activation of the body's immune system by a bacterial infection, possibly *Klebsiella pneumoniae*, or a combination of infectious pathogens. Once activated, the immune system remains chronically stimulated with resulting tissue inflammation, long after the initial bacterial infection has resolved.

The primary site of inflammation for ankylosing spondylitis is the enthesis (the point where tendons and ligaments join the bone around a joint) around the vertebral joints. For unknown reasons, macrophages and lymphocytes infiltrate and erode the enthesis and periosteum. Fibroblasts then proliferate and synthesize collagen to repair the region. However, collagen is fibrous tissue that eventually undergoes calcification and ossification (hardening). Flexibility is lost with ossification. After a period of time, all the cartilage of the spinal joint is replaced by bony scar tissue and the joints become rigid. Simultaneously, the eroded bone undergoes repair with osteoblast activation and proliferation. The osteoblasts lay down callus (new bone), which is eventually replaced by compact, lamellar (stronger, layered) bone. Because of the bone repair, the shape of the bone's surface changes as the new bone grows outward and forms a new enthesis at the end of a deteriorated ligament. As calcification of the spinal ligaments progresses, intervertebral disc fibers, which are normally spongy and elastic, are replaced with bone as well. As the chronic remodeling occurs, the intervertebral discs, bones, and ligamentous tissue fuse, creating a rigid column of vertebrae.

Clinical Presentation

The history for the patient with ankylosing spondylitis needs to focus on identifying the spinal changes that aid in diagnosis. Family history is important because there is believed to be a genetic predisposition.

The symptoms of ankylosing spondylitis are related to inflammation of the spine, joints, and other organs. Classic signs and symptoms of early disease are low back pain and stiffness beginning in young adults in their early 20s. Commonly, the pain is centered over the sacrum and may radiate bilaterally to the buttocks, groin, and down the legs. As a result of inflammation, decreased flexion of the lumbar spine is usually the earliest observed sign. The individual has difficulty bending forward to touch his or her toes. Sacroiliitis is identified by palpation of tender points along the sacroiliac joints. When the disease progresses to involve the cervical spine, flexibility of the neck will also decrease. The extensive spinal changes in severely affected persons can cause kyphosis, inflexible hip, knee, and ankle joints. The individual eventually has ambulatory complications (see Box 39-3).

Diagnosis

In addition to the patient's symptoms and physical examination findings, the diagnosis of ankylosing spondylitis is based on radiological findings and blood tests. X-rays are the single most important imaging technique to detect, diagnose, and monitor patients with ankylosing spondylitis. Early bone and joint changes of calcification and later ossification can be detected on plain x-rays.

ESR and CRP levels are elevated during the acute inflammatory phases of the disease and may be detected

---

Box 39-3. Complications of Ankylosing Spondylitis

Patients with chronic ankylosing spondylitis may have a reduction in pain once the spine has fused, but a complete loss of mobility will result. The fused spine is particularly brittle and vulnerable to fracture when involved in trauma, such as motor vehicle accidents. Patients with involvement of the thoracic spine often develop restricted chest expansion, placing the patient at risk for pneumonia. Ankylosing spondylitis can cause inflammation and scarring of the lungs, demonstrated as apical fibrosis (scarring) and cavitation (formation of a cavity). These processes cause coughing and shortness of breath, especially when the patient exercises or infection develops. Other areas of the body affected by ankylosing spondylitis include the eyes (iritis or anterior uveitis), heart (aortitis, cardiomyopathy, and conduction defects), kidneys (amyloidosis and renal failure), gastrointestinal system (Crohn's disease or ulcerative colitis), and nerves (radiculitis).

in 75% of all patients during their initial presentation. Alkaline phosphatase is elevated in approximately 50% of patients during active ossification (bone hardening). The blood test for genetic marker HLA-B27 is positive in the vast majority of patients.

> **CLINICAL CONCEPT**
>
> When ankylosing spondylitis progresses up the spine, complete fusion of the vertebral bodies results in the x-ray appearance of a "bamboo spine."

Treatment

The treatment of ankylosing spondylitis is targeted at controlling pain and maximizing mobility by reducing inflammation. Treatment plans incorporate physical therapy and home exercise to reduce pain and stiffness, along with medications to decrease inflammation and suppress immunity. NSAIDs are first-line agents to decrease pain and stiffness of the spine and other joints. When NSAIDs fail to provide adequate symptom control, immunosuppressants are considered. Sulfasalazine is often used to suppress inflammation in those with mild to moderate disease. Tissue necrosis factor-blocking medications are extremely effective for halting disease progression, decreasing inflammation, and improving spinal mobility. Methotrexate has been shown to be somewhat effective, but has a significant potential of hepatotoxicity, which can lead to cirrhosis, bone marrow toxicity, and severe anemia.

Polymyalgia Rheumatica

Polymyalgia rheumatica (PMR) is an inflammatory condition characterized by aching and morning stiffness in the cervical neck, shoulder, upper arms, and pelvic girdle (lower back and thighs). It most commonly affects older women, rarely develops before the age of 50 years, and usually occurs after age 60 years. Median age at the time of diagnosis is 72 years. The onset can be abrupt, with patients transitioning from going to bed feeling well to awakening in the morning with pain and stiffness. The average annual incidence in the United States is 52.5 cases per 100,000 persons aged 50 years and older.

Etiology

The etiology of PMR is not known, but individuals with PMR often have elevated interleukin-2 (IL-2) and interleukin-6 (IL-6) levels. There is also a prevalence of elevated antibodies to adenovirus and respiratory syncytial virus in individuals with PMR. Occurrence in close family members suggests a genetic role in the pathophysiology of PMR.

Pathophysiology

The specific cause of PMR is unknown and the pathophysiology is basically a severe inflammatory reaction with immune components. A proposed theory suggests that in a genetically predisposed patient, an environmental factor—potentially a virus—initiates macrophage activation, which results in production of cytokines. The production of the cytokines, along with interleukins and lymphokines, further stimulate a cascade of immune-mediated inflammation that induces the clinical manifestations characteristic of PMR. There is evidence that the affected muscles are infiltrated with T cells around their respective blood vessels. For reasons not completely understood, patients with PMR are commonly affected by giant cell arteritis (also called temporal arteritis).

Clinical Presentation

The history of the patient with PMR does not usually lead the health-care provider to the diagnosis. Other joint and muscle disorders are first ruled out before PMR is considered. The abrupt onset of symptoms and the manifestation of bilateral muscle and joint involvement are key factors in the diagnosis. Family history is also important because of genetic predisposition.

The signs and symptoms of PMR can be nonspecific, however, the abrupt onset of myalgia is a key sign of the disorder. Pain and stiffness are reportedly worse in the morning, lasting at least 1 hour. The shoulder girdle is the first region to become symptomatic in most patients. In the remainder of individuals, the hip or neck is the initial area affected. More rarely, pain occurs in distal joints such as those of the hands and wrists. There may be no remarkable findings on physical examination except muscle tenderness and decreased active ROM caused by pain. Rarely, the affected individual may have systemic symptoms such as low-grade fever, weight loss, malaise, fatigue, and depression.

> **CLINICAL CONCEPT**
>
> Generally, PMR has not been associated with serious medical complications. However, because it has been associated with giant cell arteritis, the patient should immediately seek care if symptoms of headache, changes in vision, or fever arise. In the later stages of PMR, disuse muscle atrophy (atrophy caused by lack of physical activity) with proximal muscle weakness and contractures of the shoulder may lead to limitation of passive and active ROM.

Diagnosis

The diagnosis is based on clinical presentation. Criteria for diagnosis have been suggested (see Box 39-4). Blood tests may assist in ruling out other disease processes, but are not very helpful in confirming a diagnosis of PMR. X-rays of joints are usually not remarkable. ESR is often elevated, but may not be significantly high. There is a rapid positive response to low-dose oral corticosteroids in PMR, which is pathognomonic of the disorder.

Box 39-4. Diagnostic Criteria for Polymyalgia Rheumatica

Diagnostic criteria for PMR include:

- age 50 years or older at onset of symptoms
- bilateral pain or aching with morning stiffness for at least 1 month, which involves at least 2 of 3 areas: neck or torso, shoulders or arms, hips or thighs
- ESR of 40 mm/h or higher
- prompt improvement of symptoms to steroid treatment.

Treatment

Therapeutic goals are to control painful myalgia, improve muscle stiffness, and resolve constitutional symptoms of the disease. The disorder is best treated with anti-inflammatory medications and nonpharmacological therapy. Oral corticosteroids are the first line of treatment. Corticosteroids can completely resolve symptoms rapidly and need to be taken for up to 2 years. Because of the side effects of long-term use of corticosteroids, other drugs have been tried in PMR. NSAIDs have been tried but they are required in high doses that subject the patient to gastrointestinal and renal side effects. Methotrexate has been ineffective, and antitumor necrosis factor agents have been inadequate to treat PMR. A bone mineral density study such as a DEXA scan is recommended at the onset of treatment. Because patients require long-term corticosteroids, bisphosphonate therapy is recommended to prevent corticosteroid-induced osteoporosis.

 CLINICAL CONCEPT

The risk of vertebral fractures is five times greater in women with PMR. Therefore, calcium and vitamin D supplementation should be recommended for all patients taking corticosteroid therapy.

Chapter Summary

- Musculoskeletal infections are uncommon except in situations where there is an open fracture.
- *S. aureus* is the most common bacteria that causes osteomyelitis (infection of bone). Individuals with diabetes mellitus are at particularly high risk for osteomyelitis of the lower extremities because of compromised distal blood flow and immunosuppression.
- Conditions in diabetes mellitus, including lack of sensation and decreased circulation in the lower extremities, favor bacterial invasion; gangrene often necessitates amputation.
- Lyme disease affects persons who live in deer-infested environments. The deer tick carries the bacterium *B. burgdorferi*. Carried by unaffected deer, the tick does not cause pathology until it bites a human and injects the bacteria.
- A classic targetlike rash called erythema migrans often heralds the pathophysiology of Lyme disease, which can cause widespread arthralgias, myalgias, and neurological impairment.
- Septic arthritis is a type of musculoskeletal infection that can arise from staphylococcus that infects a joint. It can also occur in conjunction with a sexually transmitted gonorrheal infection.
- Musculoskeletal inflammatory disease occurs most often because of autoimmune disorders, where the body forms autoantibodies for unknown reasons.
- In RA, scleroderma, SLE, PsA, polymyositis, and dermatomyositis, antibodies against the body's own joints and muscles cause inflammation. Remissions and exacerbations often describe the pattern of autoimmune musculoskeletal inflammatory diseases.
- The individual with PsA usually presents with a red, scaly, patchy rash and pitted nails.
- Gout is one of the inflammatory disorders that can be triggered and exacerbated by certain risk factors and then become controlled when under treatment.
- Ankylosing spondylitis is a disorder caused by calcification and ossification of the intervertebral discs, surrounding ligaments and vertebrae mainly of the sacroiliac joints. Rigidity and inflexibility of the spine occurs.
- PMR is a disorder of inflammation that commonly affects the muscles of the shoulder girdle.

Making the Connections

Disorder and Pathophysiology	Signs and Symptoms	Physical Assessment Findings	Diagnostic Testing	Treatment
Osteomyelitis | Acute or chronic microbial invasion of bone and bony structures. Infectious process results in inflammatory destruction that may be localized or spread through other bony tissues. *S. aureus* is the most common bacterial pathogen.				
	Generalized symptoms of chills, fever, and malaise are common. Limited ROM. Pain.	Localized symptoms include tenderness, erythema, edema, and pain with movement of the affected extremity.	Radionuclide bone scan demonstrates area of infection. Bone biopsy needed for culture of infection.	IV antibiotic therapy for 2 to 6 weeks followed by oral therapy. Debridement of necrotic tissue and debris may be necessary.
Septic Arthritis | Infectious or pyogenic arthritis with direct invasion of the joint space by bacteria, viruses, mycobacteria, or fungi causing effusion. Classified as nongonococcal or gonococcal. Most commonly affects the knee or hip of adults and the hip in children.				
	Fever and malaise; acutely painful, edematous, and erythematous joint. Pain will limit the ROM of the joint.	Acutely tender, edematous, and erythematous joint. Fever.	Definitive diagnosis requires detection and identification of microorganism from blood or synovial fluid.	Treatment focuses on drainage of joint, short-term immobilization for pain control, and administration of appropriate antimicrobial agent. Antibiotics are typically administered IV for 2 to 4 weeks, followed by oral therapy.
Mycobacterium tuberculosis | Extrapulmonary invasion of *M. tuberculosis* into bone and bony structures. Most commonly involves the spine in a condition called "Pott's disease"; less commonly affects the hip or knee.				
	Localized pain, joint effusion, and decreased ROM are common complaints.	Localized pain, joint effusion, decreased ROM, and kyphosis. Abscesses can extend into adjacent tissue.	Purified protein skin derivative (PPD) skin test may be negative in those with extrapulmonary TB). Chest x-ray may reveal lung involvement, but bone x-ray findings are usually nonspecific early in the disease process. Excisional biopsy is the preferred method of obtaining tissue for diagnostic evaluation.	Treated with antitubercular drugs for long-term therapy. A multidrug regimen extended to 12 months is recommended.
Lyme Disease | Most common vector-borne disease in the United States. It is caused by a tick-transmitted spirochete, *B. burgdorferi*, which is often carried by deer. Transmitted by the deer tick to the human, it can affect the heart, joints, eyes, and CNS.				
	Early localized disease occurs 3 to 30 days after tick bite; symptoms include EM	EM "bulls-eye" type rash. Fever, extreme fatigue, joint	Diagnosis based on patient's symptoms, physical examination findings,	A 21-day course of the antibiotic doxycycline is recommended for those

Continued

Making the Connections–cont'd

Disorder and Pathophysiology	Signs and Symptoms	Physical Assessment Findings	Diagnostic Testing	Treatment
	rash, fatigue, fever, chills, myalgias, arthralgias, and headache.	swelling, Bell's palsy are common. Late disseminated disease occurs months to years after tick bite; symptoms can include severe joint pain with edema and chronic cardiac, neuro, musculoskeletal, and CNS effects.	and a history of possible exposure to infected ticks. A two-step lab (ELISA or IFA followed by Western blot) test can assist with the diagnosis.	with early localized disease. Early disseminated disease is treated with a longer course of antibiotic. Late disseminated disease warrants IV antibiotic therapy and should be managed by an infectious disease specialist.

Gout | A syndrome characterized by recurrent inflammation as a result of hyperuricemia in blood and body fluids. An inborn error causes overproduction or inadequate renal excretion of uric acid. Uric acid forms an insoluble precipitate that deposits in joints, as well as connective and subcutaneous tissues.

	Pain, swelling, redness, and tenderness of joint; most commonly, the metatarsalphalangeal joint in the great toe; exquisitely tender.	Sudden onset of a warm, painful, erythematous joint. Podagra, inflammation of the metatarsalphalangeal joint of the great toe, is the most common presentation.	Serum uric acid level of greater than 7 mg/dL in men or 6 mg/dL in women is suggestive of gout. Radiographic studies often reveal soft tissue edema. The gold standard of diagnostics is joint aspiration and fluid analysis for urate crystals.	NSAIDs are first-line agents for acute gout; colchicine may also be used. Recurrent attacks are prevented with medications to decrease uric acid production (e.g., allopurinol) or increase renal excretion (e.g., probenecid).

Polymyositis and Dermatomyositis | Autoantigens begin a series of processes that result in the production of several inflammatory cells. Inflammatory cells surround and ultimately destroy individual muscle fibers and small groups of fibers. In dermatomyositis, the inflammatory cells group around blood vessels and cause damage to the cutaneous vasculature as well as muscles.

	Initial symptoms include malaise, fever, lethargy, and muscle swelling, pain, or tenderness.	Muscle weakness in proximal extremities appears over weeks to months. Classic skin changes include a symmetric purple-red macular rash that affects the eyelids, chest, and extensor surfaces of extremities.	Creatine phosphokinase and ESR can be elevated 5 to 50 times above the normal range. Electromyography is abnormal. Muscle biopsy is the most definitive test.	Immunosuppressants play an important role in limiting the disease process. Corticosteroids are considered first-line agents; they are started at high doses until symptoms improve, then gradually tapered. Physical therapy should be initiated early in the disease to optimize strength and mobility.

Continued

Making the Connections–cont'd

Disorder and Pathophysiology	Signs and Symptoms	Physical Assessment Findings	Diagnostic Testing	Treatment
PsA | A chronic inflammatory disease of joints and connective tissue that is linked to psoriasis. T lymphocytes infiltrate skin and joints and initiate a cascade of immune-mediated inflammation. Immunoglobulins become deposited in the skin and synovial membranes.	Pain and swelling of joints is observed on both sides of the body. Spondylitis usually affects the spine and sacroiliac joint.	Red, scaly, silvery plaque rash (psoriasis) and nail pitting is a key finding for all forms. Swelling over joints.	A definitive diagnosis requires evidence of classic psoriatic skin and nail changes. In later stages, x-rays may reveal characteristic changes: "pencil and cup" phenomenon.	NSAIDs and local corticosteroid injection are first-line agents. Recent management includes DMARDs, primarily antitissue necrosis factor (TNF) agents. Oral corticosteroids and antimalarials should be avoided because they can exacerbate cutaneous psoriasis.
Ankylosing Spondylitis | Systemic rheumatic disease that can affect multiple tissues, but commonly results in chronic inflammation of the spine and sacroiliac joints. Collagen calcifies and ossifies, replacing all cartilage of the affected area with bony tissue. Vertebral bodies become fused with bony bridges to adjacent vertebrae. Inflammation can affect many other organ systems, including the lungs, eyes, heart, kidneys, and gastrointestinal system.	Low back pain (centered over the sacrum) and morning stiffness in young adults. Eyes, heart, lungs, nerves, and gastrointestinal system can be affected.	Limited ROM is common; the thoracic vertebrae develop an inflexible forward curvature. Eyes, heart, lungs, nerves, and gastrointestinal system can be affected.	X-rays are the single most important diagnostic test. A loss of joint space can be detected. More classic signs are the appearance of a "bamboo spine" as the vertebrae fuse. Nonspecific lab tests are often elevated: ESR, CRP, and alkaline phosphatase. Genetic marker for HLA-B27 is positive in the vast majority of cases.	Physical therapy and exercise reduce pain and stiffness and improve posture, joint mobility, and lung capacity. NSAIDs are frequently used first-line; corticosteroids are used as an adjunct. When NSAIDs fail, methotrexate or sulfasalazine have been used. More recently, tissue necrosis factor blocking medications are being used.
PMR | Autoimmune disorder with monocyte activation (potentially by a virus) leading to cytokine production and immune-mediated inflammation. Appears to be related to giant cell arteritis (also called temporal arteritis).	Abrupt onset of myalgia; pain and stiffness are worse in the morning and last more than 1 hour.	Shoulder swelling, pain, limited ROM of other joints.	A presumed diagnosis is based on clinical presentation. Diagnostic tests are not very helpful.	Oral corticosteroids are first-line. NSAIDs are often used, especially during steroid "tapers." Methotrexate, azathioprine, and other immunosuppressants are being used more frequently.

Bibliography

Arias-Santiago, S., Aneiros-Fernández, J., Husein-El-Ahmed, H., et al. (2010). Giant nodules on the hands. *Cleveland Clin J Med*, 77(4), 225, 229.

Ashrith, G., & Arora, R. (2010). Thick skin on the back. *Cleveland Clin J Med*, 77(2), 90–91.

Bailey, J., & Whitehair, B. (2010). Topical treatments for chronic plaque psoriasis. *Am Fam Phys*, 81(5), 596.

Barnett, R. (2012). Bitter medicine: gout and the birth of the cocktail. *Lancet*, 379(9824), 1384–1385.

Burns, C. M., & Wortmann, R. L. (2011). Gout therapeutics: new drugs for an old disease. *Lancet*, 377(9760), 165–177.

Caylor, T. L., & Perkins, A. (2013). Recognition and management of polymyalgia rheumatica and giant cell arteritis. *Am Fam Phys*, 88(10), 676–684.

Dasgupta, B., Cimmino, M. A., Maradit-Kremers, H., et al. (2012). 2012 Provisional Classification Criteria for Polymyalgia Rheumatica: a European League Against Rheumatism/American College of Rheumatology collaborative initiative. *Ann Rheum Dis*, 71(4), 484–492.

de Nijs, R. N. (2011). Spinal tuberculosis. *Lancet*, 378(9807), e18. Epub 2011 Oct 6.

Doghramji, P. P., Edwards, N. L., & McTigue, J. (2010). Managing gout in the primary care setting: what you and your patients need to know. *Am J Med*, 123(8), S2.

Dougados, M., & Baeten, D. (2011). Spondyloarthritis. *Lancet*, 377(9783), 2127–2137.

El-Zawawy, H., & Mandell, B. F. (2010). Managing gout: how is it different in patients with chronic kidney disease? *Cleve Clin J Med*, 77(12), 919–928. Review.

Garcia-Cruz, A., & Garcia-Doval, I. (2010). Images in clinical medicine. Gottron's papules and dermatomyositis. *N Engl J Med*, 363(12), e17.

Gemechu, F. W., Seemant, F., & Curley, C. A. (2013). Diabetic foot infections. *Am Fam Phys*, 88(3), 177–184.

Hardy, E. (2011). Gout diagnosis and management: what NPs need to know. *Nurse Pract*, 36(6), 14–19; quiz 19–20.

Hatzenbuehler, J., & Pulling, T. J. (2011). Diagnosis and management of osteomyelitis. *Am Fam Phys*, 84(9), 1027–1033.

Horowitz, D. L., Katzap, E., Horowitz, S., & Barilla-LaBarca, M. L. (2011). Approach to septic arthritis. *Am Fam Phys*, 84(6), 653–660.

Keller, D. L. (2011). Gout and chronic kidney disease. *Cleveland Clin J Med*, 78(2), 81.

Kermani, T. A., & Warrington, K. J. (2012). Polymyalgia rheumatica. *Lancet*, Oct 5. doi: pii: S0140-6736(12)60680-1 .10.1016/S0140-6736(12)60680-1.

Kumar, V., Abbas, A. K., Fausto, N., & Aster, J. (2010). *Robbins & Cotran pathologic basis of disease*. 8th ed. Philadelphia, PA: WB Saunders.

Landman, G. W. (2010). Vertebral osteomyelitis. *N Engl J Med*, 362(24), 2335; author reply 2335–2336.

Libraty, D. H., Patkar, C., & Torres, B. (2012). *Staphylococcus aureus* reactivation osteomyelitis after 75 years. *N Engl J Med*, 366(5), 481–482.

Longo, D. L., Kasper, D. L., Jameson, J. L., et al. (2011). *Harrison's principles of internal medicine*. 18th ed. New York: McGraw-Hill.

Mandell, B. F., Edwards, N. L., Sundy, J. S., Simkin, P. A., & Pile, J. C. (2010). Preventing and treating acute gout attacks across the clinical spectrum: a roundtable discussion. *Cleveland Clin J Med*, 77 (Suppl 2), S2–25.

Mathews, C. J., Weston, V. C., Jones, A., Field, M., & Coakley, G. (2010). Bacterial septic arthritis in adults. *Lancet*, 375(9717), 846–855.

Osteomyelitis: what you should know. (2011). *Am Fam Phys*, 84(9), 1034.

Richette, P., & Bardin, T. (2010). Gout. *Lancet*, 375(9711), 318–328.

Rider, L. G., & Miller, F. W. (2011). Deciphering the clinical presentations, pathogenesis, and treatment of the idiopathic inflammatory myopathies. *JAMA*, 305(2), 183–190.

Savely, V. (2010). Lyme disease: a diagnostic dilemma. *Nurse Pract*, 35(7), 44–50.

Senior, K. (2012). Chlamydia: a much underestimated STI. *Lancet Infect Dis*, 12(7), 517–518.

Stanek, G., Wormser, G. P., Gray, J., & Strle, F. (2012). Lyme borreliosis. *Lancet*, 379(9814), 461–473.

Tausche, A. K., Panzner, I., Aust, D., & Wunderlich, C. (2010). Disabling gout. *Lancet*, 376(9746), 1093.

Turns, M. (2011). The diabetic foot: an overview of assessment and complications. *Br J Nurs*, 20(15), S19–25.

Weigle, N., & McBane, S. (2013). Psoriasis. *Am Fam Phys*, 87(9), 626–623.

Wright, W. F., Riedel, D. J., Talwani, R., & Gilliam, B. L. (2012). Diagnosis and management of Lyme disease. *Am Fam Phys*, 85(11), 1086–1093.

Zimmerli, W. (2010). Clinical practice. Vertebral osteomyelitis. *N Engl J Med*, 362(11), 1022–1029.

Zychowicz, M. E. (2011). Gout: no longer the disease of kings. *Orthop Nurs*, 30(5), 322–330.

Zychowicz, M. E., Pope, R. S., & Graser, E. (2010). The current state of care in gout: addressing the need for better understanding of an ancient disease. *J Am Acad Nurse Pract*, 22 (Suppl 1), 623–636.

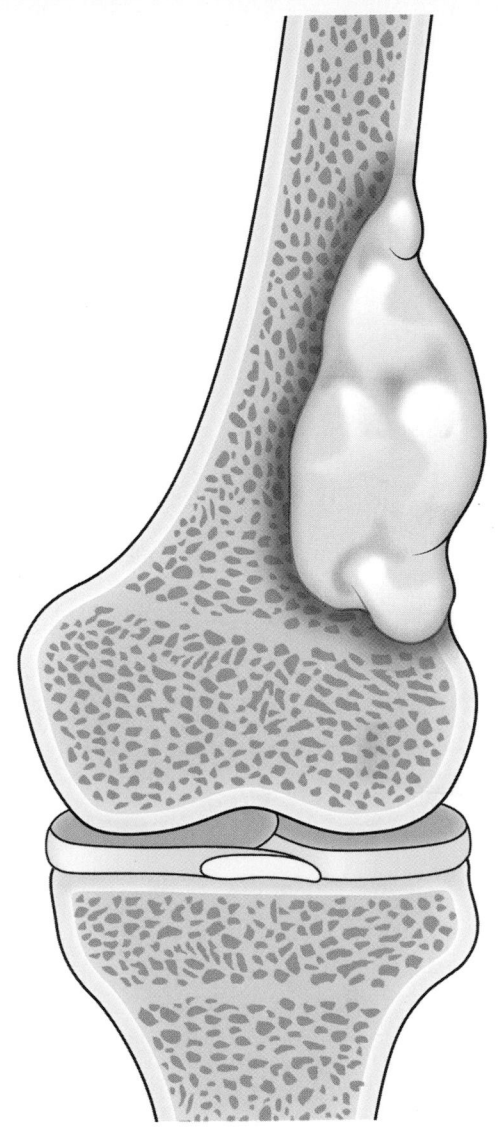

Chapter
Chapter 40. Cancer

Cancer

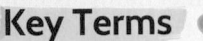

Key Terms

Alpha-fetoprotein (AFP)
Anaplasia
Benign
Brachytherapy
Cachexia
Carcinoembryonic antigen (CEA)

Cell cycle
Defective
Differentiation
Malignant
Metastasis

Oncogene
Paraneoplastic syndrome
TNM system
Tumor suppressor gene
Vascular endothelial growth factor (VEGF)

A cancerous neoplasm is an abnormal mass of tissue that grows in an uncoordinated manner and proliferates independently at a rate greater than normal tissue. Cancerous changes in cells result from sporadic and inherited genetic alterations that persist and perpetuate the growth of cancer cells. For a large number of cancers, there exists a hereditable genetic alteration that originated with either parent of the cancer patient. Other cancers develop because of defective tumor suppressor genes—genes that guard against cancer formation. There are also cancers that develop because of mutated proto-oncogenes, which are genes that control normal cell growth and proliferation. Mutated proto-oncogenes become oncogenes that allow unrestrained cell division. Alternatively, cancer can be caused by faulty cellular apoptosis mechanisms that do not initiate programmed cellular degeneration, as they should.

Regardless of the cause, cancer cells look distinctively different from normal cells. Cancer cells are nonuniform in architecture, disorganized, and misshapen. In addition to looking different, cancer cells fail to function like their normal counterparts. Cancer is an abnormal mass of cells that do not function normally and compete with normal cells for space, blood supply, oxygen, and nutrition. They regenerate, multiply rapidly, and may travel to distant sites in the body where they take up residence and proliferate further. In general, cancer can be seen as a parasite that draws its needs for survival from the human host, gathers strength from surroundings, constantly regenerates, multiplies exponentially, and leaves its victims debilitated.

Epidemiology

Cancer is the second leading cause of death behind heart disease. The most significant risk factor for cancer overall is age: two-thirds of all cancers occur in those older than age 65 years. For persons from birth to age 39 years, 1 in

72 men and 1 in 52 women develop cancer; for those between ages 40 through 59 years, 1 in 12 men and 1 in 11 women develop cancer, and for those between ages 60 and 79 years, 1 in 3 men and 1 in 5 women develop cancer.

In men, the most common cancer is prostate cancer; in women, breast cancer. When rates for men and women are combined, however, the most common cancer is lung cancer, which also happens to be the most common cause of cancer death. Cancers of the lung, female breast, prostate, and colon constitute more than 50% of cancer diagnoses and cancer deaths in the United States. Cancer occurs more often in men than in women, and for reasons that are unclear, African American males have the highest incidence and mortality.

Basic Concepts Related to the Understanding of Cancer

There are basic concepts that pertain specifically to the study of cancer. These concepts include:

- the cell cycle
- immunocompetence as related to tumor development
- tumor classification and staging
- cancer genetics
- role of viruses in cancer
- metastasis and tumor angiogenesis
- paraneoplastic syndromes
- cancer cachexia.

The Cell Cycle

The **cell cycle** is a sequence of growth stages that a cell moves through for mitosis and regeneration. In order for cells to undergo mitosis, the cell must go through stages G0, G1, G2, S, and M (see Fig. 40-1). In stage G0, the cell is at rest and is not actively engaged in the cell cycle. In

Normal cell cycle

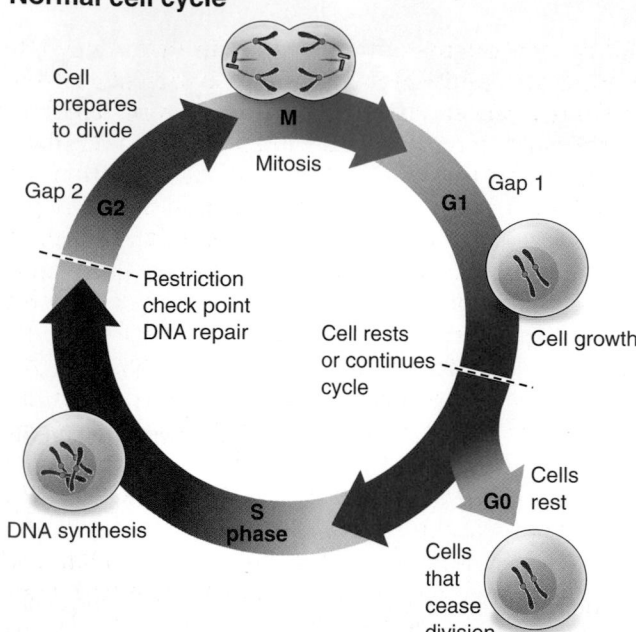

Cancer cell cycle

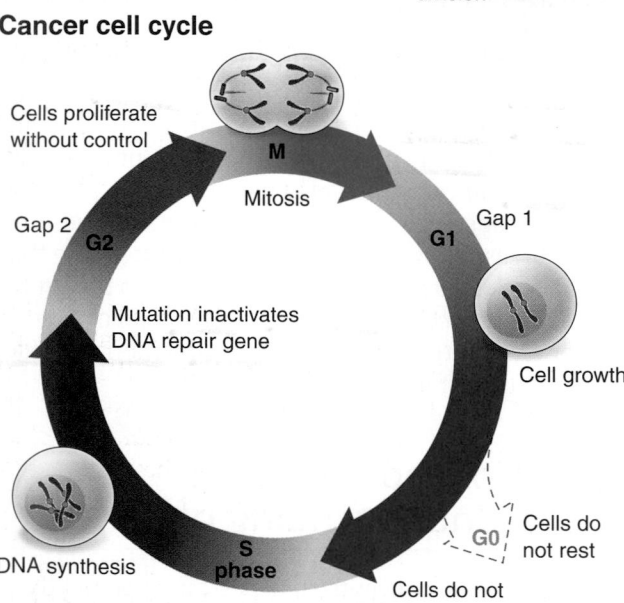

FIGURE 40-1. The normal cell cycle versus the cancer cell cycle. (a) Normal cell cycle. The cell cycle is an ordered sequence of events that occur when cells multiply and regenerate. The specific stages are G0, G1, S, G2, and M. During G0, the cell is quiescent and at rest. In stage G1, enzymes called cyclin-dependent kinases activate the cell to enter the cell stage. In the S stage, the cell is synthesizing new DNA in preparation for mitosis. In stage G2, there is a checkpoint that senses DNA damage and delays the cycle to allow DNA repair before entry into mitosis. In the M stage, mitosis occurs. After mitosis, the cell enters a resting stage (G0) and awaits another signal to enter the cycle. (b). Cancer cell cycle. Cancer cells go through the cell cycle constantly. There are no restrictive checkpoints or resting phases. They are actively proliferating without control.

stage G1, cells enter the cell cycle and prepare for deoxyribonucleic acid (DNA) replication. Proto-oncogenes, genes that control cell replication, are activated. In the G2 stage, DNA replication takes place. During the S stage, synthesis of structures occurs and the structures move to opposite poles in preparation for division into

two separate cells. The 46 chromosomes reorganize as two separate sets of 23 chromosome pairs arranged at opposite poles. Two nuclear membranes develop around the two separate sets of 23 pairs. In the M stage, mitosis is completed and two daughter cells are created.

Cancer cells are constantly moving through the cell cycle stages. During the cell cycle, there are several checkpoints where DNA replication mechanisms can be stopped if errors have occurred in the synthesis of cell parts before mitosis. Cells can undergo repair, recycling, or apoptosis if errors exist. However, cancer cells do not undergo scrutiny at these checkpoints and do not undergo apoptosis, or programmed degeneration. Cancer cells disregard the growth inhibitors released by neighboring cells. As the cancer cells proliferate, they accumulate on top, around, and beside each other, take over boundaries of organs, crowd out normal cells, and may even break free and travel to distant body sites.

Immunocompetence as Related to Tumor Development

Our immune system constantly surveys the body for foreign substances or "non-self" antigens. When a "non-self" antigen is discovered, the immune system initiates an attack to destroy the invading substance. This attack also occurs when our body produces a defective or mutated cell; the body recognizes it as "non-self" and the immune system destroys it. With neoplasm development, once abnormal cells start proliferating, the immune system attacks and destroys these aberrant cells. However, with age, mutated cells can escape immune surveillance, perpetuate themselves, and form tumors. Because immunocompetence declines with aging, older adults are more susceptible to tumor development.

Tumor Classification and Staging

The diagnosis of cancer relies heavily on tissue biopsy and analysis. Compared with normal cells, cancer cells are disorganized and nonuniform in architecture. **Differentiation** refers to the extent that neoplastic cells resemble normal cells both structurally and functionally. Lack of differentiation is called **anaplasia,** a term that indicates total cellular disorganization, abnormal cell appearance, and cell dysfunction. Ordinarily, **benign** tumors are well-differentiated and remain localized, cohesive, and well-demarcated from surrounding tissue. Benign tumors are not invasive, do not destroy surrounding tissue, and do not break away or travel from the tumor cell mass. In general, **malignant** tumors range from well-differentiated to poorly differentiated, but they are invasive and destructive to surrounding tissue. They also lack adhesion to the tumor mass and easily break free to travel to distant sites in a process called **metastasis.** Malignant cells travel via the lymphatic system or bloodstream. For this reason, often the first metastatic site is a lymph node. For the differences between benign and malignant tumors, see Table 40-1.

TABLE 40-1. Differences Between Benign and Malignant Tumors

Characteristic	Benign Tumors	Malignant Tumors
Differentiation	Well-differentiated; resembles tissue of origin	Poorly differentiated; does not resemble tissue of origin
Rate of growth	Progressive, slow	Erratic, slow to rapid
Local invasion	Cohesive cells, well-demarcated tumor	Invasive and infiltrating, surrounding normal tissue
Metastasis	None	Frequent

After establishing that a tumor is malignant, the tumor is examined and classified by grading and staging. Malignant tumors can be graded I through III. Grade I indicates that the cells are well-differentiated, grade II cells are moderately differentiated, and grade III indicates poorly differentiated or anaplastic. Staging classifies the tumor according to size, invasiveness, and spread using a **TNM system.** T is for tumor size, N is for lymph node involvement, and M is for metastasis to distant organs. For example, if a patient has a 2.5 cm tumor in the right breast, palpable lymph nodes, and a CT scan indicative of a metastatic lesion in the liver, it would be staged as T2, N1, M1 breast cancer. See Table 40-2 for an example of staging for breast cancer using a TNM classification system.

TABLE 40-2. TNM Classification System

T (TUMOR)	
Tx	Tumor cannot be assessed
T0	No evidence of primary tumor
Tis	Carcinoma in situ
T1–4	Progressive increase in tumor size or involvement

N (NODES)	
Nx	Regional lymph nodes cannot be assessed
N0	No evidence of regional node metastasis
N1–3	Increasing involvement of regional lymph nodes

M (METASTASIS)	
Mx	Not assessed
M0	No distant metastasis
M1	Distant metastasis present

(Source: http://www.cancer.gov/cancertopics/factsheet/detection/staging. Last accessed on July 8, 2015.)

Cancer Genetics

All cancers originate from changes in DNA. Gene mutations are required for the transformation of a normal cell into a cancer cell. Gene mutations can be hereditary or sporadic. Hereditary gene mutations are passed down from parents to offspring. Sporadic gene mutations are acquired during a person's lifetime due to carcinogen exposure. There are two major classes of cancer genes: **tumor suppressor genes** and **oncogenes.** Tumor suppressor genes normally function to restrain cell growth. However, these genes can also become defective and lose the ability to inhibit cell growth and division, thus allowing cancer formation. The *TP53* gene, the tumor suppressor gene in cells, controls cellular apoptosis natural death of cells with damaged DNA. Approximately half of all cancers have a **defective** *TP53* gene. The *TP53* gene, known as the "guardian of the genome" is located at the short arm of chromosome 17 at region 13.1 (17p13.1). With a defective *TP53* gene, cells with damaged DNA are not destroyed; they proliferate unchecked and progress to malignancy.

Proto-oncogenes are genes that stimulate and regulate a cell's movement through the cell cycle, resulting in cellular growth and proliferation. When mutated, proto-oncogenes become oncogenes that stimulate constant, unrelenting cellular proliferation and cell cycling.

Role of Viruses in Cancer

Certain malignancies are associated with cancer-inducing viruses. For any virus to live and propagate, it must insert its genes into the host cell's genome. The host cell then becomes a manufacturer of the virus. In viral-induced cancer, the mechanisms of action differ among viruses but the mechanisms always involve the activation of growth-promoting pathways or inhibition of tumor suppressors in infected cells. Specific cancers activated by viruses include cervical cancer, Burkitt's lymphoma, and hepatocellular carcinoma (HCC).

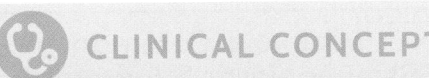

CLINICAL CONCEPT

Cervical cancer is associated with human papillomavirus (HPV), Burkitt's lymphoma is associated with Epstein-Barr virus, and HCC is associated with the hepatitis B and C virus.

Metastasis and Tumor Angiogenesis

Malignant cancer cells are invasive, penetrative, and destructive to surrounding tissue. They penetrate through basement membranes and metastasize from a primary site to a distant site through lymph or blood. Certain tumors have common sites of metastasis, as shown in Table 40-3.

TABLE 40-3. Common Metastatic Sites for Tumors

Cancer	Common Site of Metastasis
Lung	Bone, brain
Colon	Liver
Breast	Bone, brain, liver, lung
Prostate	Vertebrae
Melanoma	Brain

Tumor cells that metastasize must embed where there are sufficient nutrients, blood supply, and oxygen. For establishment in a target organ, the tumor must develop its own blood vessels and connect to the pre-existing blood supply. Cancer cells are suited for this task because they secrete **vascular endothelial growth factor (VEGF),** a substance that gives them the capability to develop new blood vessels.

Paraneoplastic Syndromes

Paraneoplastic syndromes are symptom complexes related to cancer's presence and action on the body. However, these are not symptoms caused by cancer's space-occupying effects nor are they caused by cancer's metastatic effects. A **paraneoplastic syndrome** is an unexpected pathological disorder provoked by the presence of cancer in the body (see Table 40-4). A common type of paraneoplastic syndrome involves the secretion of endocrine hormones unrelated to the cancer tumor. For example, a patient suffering from lung cancer often endures excessive secretion of adrenocorticotropic hormone (ACTH) from the tumor. Another common paraneoplastic syndrome is hypercalcemia. For unclear reasons, in many types of cancers, the body produces a parathyroidlike hormone that stimulates bone breakdown and calcium accumulation in the blood. Cancers most often associated with paraneoplastic hypercalcemia are breast, lung, kidney, and ovary. Another inappropriate hormone

TABLE 40-4. Common Paraneoplastic Syndromes

Cancer	Paraneoplastic Syndrome
Lung	Cushing syndrome, SIADH, hypercalcemia, myasthenia-like syndrome, acanthosis nigricans, dermatomyositis
Breast	Hypercalcemia, disorders of the CNS and peripheral nervous system, dermatomyositis
Pancreas	Venous thrombosis (Trousseau syndrome), carcinoid syndrome, Cushing syndrome
Hepatocellular	Polycythemia, hypoglycemia

secreted during lung cancer is antidiuretic hormone (ADH). A paraneoplastic syndrome is peculiar and unrelated to the cancer that has initiated the condition. However, it can be the cause of the first signs and symptoms of illness, and its investigation can lead to a diagnosis of the cancer that initiated it.

Cancer Cachexia

Patients with cancer commonly develop a progressive loss of body fat and lean body mass known as **cachexia.** The patient suffers profound weakness, unintentional weight loss, fatigue, loss of appetite, and anemia. The cause of the cachexia is theorized to originate with cytokines and mediators released by white blood cells (WBCs) that are attacking the tumor. The cytokines and mediators include tumor necrosis factor-alpha (TNF-alpha), interleukin-1, and proteolysis-inducing factor. These mediators induce the breakdown of muscle and fat and give the patient a wasted (cachectic) appearance.

Assessment

In cancer patients, important information is obtained from every portion of the history and physical examination. Because cancer can present in a variety of ways, various chief complaints may bring the cancer patient to the health-care provider. Patients with cancer often present with general complaints of anorexia, excessive fatigue, and weight loss. The clinician should inquire about any tumor or cancer in the past medical and surgical history. Also, the patient should be asked about the existence of any illnesses that predispose individuals to cancer, such as ulcerative colitis, chronic hepatitis, cervical human papillomavirus (HPV) infection, chronic *H. pylori* gastritis, and breast and skin lesions. Family history may suggest an underlying familial predisposition to cancer. A genogram can map out this family history for a clearer view of susceptibilities. Social history can describe the behaviors, environmental exposures, and lifestyle habits that increase susceptibility to cancer. Behaviors such as smoking, alcohol abuse, unsafe sexual practices, and occupational exposures should be investigated. The review of systems can reveal a spectrum of symptoms, which indicate a paraneoplastic syndrome, metastatic disease, or signs of a primary cancer.

Physical Examination

The clinician should perform a thorough physical examination, which may demonstrate findings consistent with a primary cancer, cancer metastasis, or paraneoplastic syndrome. The clinician should carefully palpate the regions of lymph nodes, such as cervical, axillary, epitrochlear, supraclavicular, infraclavicular, and inguinal. The thyroid should also be inspected and palpated. The breast examination on the female is of particular importance, so the clinician should inspect and palpate all areas of the breast and axilla.

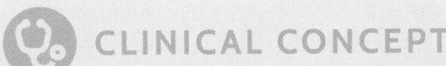

CLINICAL CONCEPT

Virchow's node is the term used for an enlarged left-sided supraclavicular lymph node. This can indicate breast, lung, or abdominal cancer.

Auscultation of the heart and lungs is critical, as is palpation of the abdomen. Paraneoplastic syndromes or metastasis of cancer can present with abnormalities of the heart and lungs. For example, an occult lung tumor or metastasis of cancer to the lungs can present as pulmonary crackles, wheezes, or obstructive atelectasis (collapse of alveoli). The abdominal examination should include palpation of the liver, a common site of metastasis. The patient's skin should be thoroughly inspected for suspicious lesions—those that are asymmetric with irregular borders, varied in color, and larger than a pencil eraser in diameter. The patient should be questioned about any changes in moles or bothersome skin lesions. Wounds that are not healing in a timely manner can also be indicative of cancer. Males should have a digital rectal examination (DRE), which allows palpation of the prostate gland; a fecal occult blood test (FOBT) can be done in conjunction. The male testicles should be palpated for masses or lesions. Females require a pelvic examination and FOBT as well. An anal pap smear is necessary for persons at risk of ano-rectal cancer.

CLINICAL CONCEPT

A hard, nodular prostate gland, which is a sign of prostate cancer, can be palpated through the rectal wall.

Diagnosis

The diagnosis and prevention of cancer relies heavily on specific screening tests that are available for various types of cancer. For example, the Papanicolou (PAP) smear is used in the diagnosis of cervical cancer. Mammograms detect breast cancer, and DREs and blood prostate surface antigen (PSA) tests are used to detect prostate cancer. Magnetic resonance imaging (MRI), computed tomography (CT) scan, and bone scans are other techniques that assist in the diagnosis of cancer. Screening for tumor cell markers is clinically important in identifying and tracking progression of cancers before, during, and after treatment. Tumor cell markers are products of cancer cells such as hormones, enzymes, genes, antigens, or antibodies that are found in blood, spinal fluid, or urine. Some of these tumor markers are called oncofetal antigens because they are normally found during fetal development. Examples of these antigens are **carcinoembryonic antigen (CEA)** and **alpha-fetoprotein (AFP)** (see Table 40-5).

TABLE 40-5. Cancer and Common Tumor Markers

Cancer	Specific Tumor Marker
Colorectal	CEA (carcinoembryonic antigen)
Pancreatic	
Lung	
Breast	
Stomach	
Thyroid	
Liver	
Ovarian	
Breast	CA-15-3 (carcinogenic antigen 15)
Pancreatic	CA-19-9 (carcinogenic antigen 19)
Gall Bladder	
Stomach	
Liver	AFP (alpha-fetoprotein)
Testicular	
Ovarian	CA-125 (carcinogenic antigen 125)
Prostate	PSA (prostate surface antigen)

Treatment

Cancer treatments vary; however, the standard therapies include surgery, radiation, chemotherapy, and immunotherapy, also called biotherapy. Surgery, used for many types of cancers, has the highest cancer cure rate with solid, well-circumscribed tumors. Surgery is also used to reduce the size of tumors that are impinging on neighboring organs or causing pain. Radiation therapy is used to destroy tumor cells; it is most effective during the S and M stages of the cell cycle.

Chemotherapy uses drugs to destroy cells in the S, M, or G stages of the cell cycle. Cancer chemotherapy has a collateral effect on healthy, rapidly multiplying cells such as skin, hair, gastric, and bone marrow cells. The side effects of chemotherapy include anorexia, nausea and vomiting, alopecia (hair loss), and bone marrow suppression. Immunotherapy is commonly used to identify a tumor and sites of its metastasis. Marked fluorescent antibodies are used to localize cancer cells. Immunotherapy can also be used to deliver medications to cancer sites. Monoclonal antibodies have been developed that can deliver chemotherapy to the specific cancer cell area (see Box 40-1).

Pathophysiology of Selected Types of Cancers

Each type of cancer presents in a different way and requires specific treatments. It is important to understand their different nuances.

Lung Cancer

Lung cancer is the leading cause of cancer-related death in both men and women throughout the world;

BOX 40-1. Monoclonal Antibodies

A monoclonal antibody (mAb) is a genetically engineered protein that is designed to bind to cancer cells. The mAb attaches to a specific receptor on the cancer cell and identifies the cancer cell as a target for the patient's natural immune system. The mAb labels the cancer cells and the patient's natural immunoglobulins attack them directly. An mAb can also be used to deliver radiation or chemotherapy directly to cancer cells. The mAb is attached to the therapeutic substance and specifically targets receptors located on the cancer cells. This therapeutic approach allows surrounding healthy tissue to remain unharmed.

(Adapted from http://www.mayoclinic.org/diseases-conditions/cancer/in-depth/monoclonal-antibody/art-20047808. Last accessed July 8, 2015.)

in fact, two-thirds of all cancer deaths are the result of lung cancer. In the United States, the disease causes more deaths than colorectal, breast, and prostate cancers combined. In 2014, approximately 224,000 men and women were diagnosed with lung cancer in the United States. In the same year, there were 159,000 deaths caused by lung cancer. Close to 70% of patients with lung cancer present with locally advanced or metastatic disease at the time of diagnosis. Early diagnosis is the key to effective treatment.

Cancer of the lung occurs most often in persons older than age 65 years, with an average age of 70 years. African American men are 20% more likely to develop lung cancer compared with white men, and African American women have a 10% lower chance of developing lung cancer compared with white women.

Etiology

The leading cause of lung cancer is cigarette smoking: 85% of patients with lung cancer are current or former smokers. Cigarette smoke contains as many as 1,200 potential carcinogens. Risk increases with the total number of cigarettes smoked, expressed by "cigarette pack-year." Asbestos exposure is another risk factor for lung cancer; if the person is a smoker, there is a synergistic risk of developing lung cancer. Having a first-degree family member (parent, sibling, or child) with lung cancer roughly doubles the risk of developing lung cancer. Having a second-degree relative, such as an aunt, uncle, niece, or nephew, with lung cancer raises your risk by around 30%. There are genetic mutations on chromosome 6, 10, and 15 that are associated with lung cancer development. A mutation at the *15q24* gene has been particularly singled out as a risk factor for lung cancer.

Asbestos can cause a specific type of cancer on the pleural membrane, called mesothelioma. Mesothelioma is a relatively rare cancer with approximately 3,000 new cases diagnosed each year in the United States. It occurs more often in men than in women and risk increases with age.

CLINICAL CONCEPT

The rate of mesothelioma was highest in the 1970s through 1990s when asbestos was found as the cause for most cases. Workplaces are now restricted from using asbestos, and asbestos is being removed from older construction. Because of this, the incidence of mesothelioma is decreasing.

Other risk factors for lung cancer include radon exposure, arsenic exposure, history of radiation therapy to the chest, pulmonary fibrosis, and history of chronic obstructive pulmonary disease. Radon is a naturally occurring radioactive material in the ground that is prevalent in certain areas of the United States. It releases a gas that increases the risk of lung cancer and is estimated to cause 12% of lung cancers. Also, frequent exposure to cigarette smoke can affect those in the environment. Passive smoke increases a person's risk of lung cancer by 20% to 30%.

CLINICAL CONCEPT

Smoking history is calculated in pack-years. This is the number of packs of cigarettes smoked multiplied by years smoked. For example, a 60-year-old who smoked two packs of cigarettes per day since age 20 has an (40 x 2) 80 pack-year smoking history.

Pathophysiology

The pathogenesis of lung cancer involves an overload of carcinogens from smoking and other environmental toxins, plus a genetic predisposition acquired from parents. Smoke and other environmental toxins can paralyze the cilia of the respiratory tract's epithelium. Cilia, which would normally sweep away carcinogens, bacteria, and other foreign substances, become less active and accumulation of carcinogens occurs.

On a molecular level, a respiratory tract lesion develops and typically undergoes sequential genetic and structural changes from hyperplasia, an increased mass of cells, to dysplasia, a precancerous mass of cells, to an invasive neoplasia, cancerous mass. There is an activation of oncogenes and a deactivation of tumor suppressor genes that allows the unchecked cell growth and proliferation of cancer. Because there is a lack of cellular apoptosis, the cancer cells multiply rapidly and extensively. The cancer cells also have a capacity for angiogenesis (building of blood vessels) and metastasis. In addition, the cancer causes destructive invasion of surrounding tissue. Lung cancer commonly begins as an area of dysplasia that over time becomes a thickened area of bronchial mucosa. The lesion proliferates and can erode the lining epithelium, grow into the bronchial lumen, or become a mass within the lung tissue. Extension can occur into the pleural surface and then spread to the tracheal, bronchial, or mediastinal lymph nodes.

Lung cancer can develop on bronchial surface epithelium or bronchial mucous glands. It can be divided into two categories: nonsmall cell lung cancer (NSCLC), which makes up about 85% to 90% of all lung cancers, and small cell lung cancer (SCLC). It is important to distinguish between NSCLC and SCLC: SCLC is a rapidly growing tumor that tends to metastasize quickly, whereas NSCLC develops more subtly over a longer period of time.

Nonsmall Cell Lung Cancer. The types of NSCLC include adenocarcinoma, squamous cell carcinoma (SCC), and large cell carcinoma. All have similar treatments but have distinct cellular appearance and clinical characteristics. Adenocarcinoma occurs within bronchial mucosal glands in a peripheral location of the lung. It is the most frequent NSCLC in the United States. Bronchioloalveolar carcinoma is a distinct subtype of adenocarcinoma that arises from alveolar cells and may appear as a solitary peripheral nodule, multiple nodules, or a rapidly progressing pneumonia. SCC accounts for 25% to 30% of all lung cancers. SCC usually occurs in the central parts of the lung as an erosion in a proximal bronchus. Large cell carcinoma accounts for 10% to 15% of lung cancers, appearing as a large peripheral mass on chest x-ray.

Small Cell Lung Cancer. SCLC is also divided into several subcategories, which include pure small cell, mixed small cell, and combined small cell carcinoma. SCLC is a more aggressive form of cancer than NSCLC and occurs as a central lesion with enlargement of the hilar and mediastinal lymph nodes, which are centrally located lymph nodes. Commonly, when first presenting to the health-care provider because of pulmonary symptoms, SCLC already has metastasized to other areas of the body. The most common sites of metastasis of lung cancer are the bones, liver, adrenal glands, pericardium, brain, and spinal cord.

Clinical Presentation

Major presenting complaints of lung cancer include cough, hemoptysis (blood in sputum), wheeze, stridor, chest pain, and dyspnea. Patients may complain of weight loss, excessive fatigue, and weakness. Hoarseness may be a sign if the tumor compresses the recurrent laryngeal nerve. A lung tumor can frequently cause an obstructive accumulation of secretions in the bronchioles that appear as pneumonia. The patient may have symptoms of fever and productive cough, which can lead to a misdiagnosis of pneumonia. Lung cancer patients are often asymptomatic and a tumor may be an incidental finding on a routine chest x-ray. Often, symptoms of a paraneoplastic syndrome may be the first sign of lung cancer (see Box 40-2).

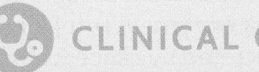

CLINICAL CONCEPT

A common paraneoplastic syndrome involves lung tumor secretion of ACTH. Lung tumors can inappropriately secrete ACTH, which chemically resembles melanocyte-stimulating hormone. Melanocytes are often stimulated, giving the patient with lung cancer a tanned appearance.

Over half the patients diagnosed with lung cancer will have metastatic disease at diagnosis. Patients with metastasis may complain of symptoms related to the spread of the cancer, such as bone pain.

Diagnosis

Diagnostic tests in lung cancer include chest x-ray, CT or MRI scan, cytological examination of sputum, bronchoscopy, and CT-guided tissue biopsy. A spiral CT scan is particularly useful as a diagnostic tool. After a biopsy, the tumor cells are classified according to a stage and TNM system.

CLINICAL CONCEPT

Lung cancer stages range from 0 to 4. A small, localized tumor, referred to as "in situ," is classified as stage 0. A large tumor is classified as stage 1. When a tumor is classified as stage 2 or 3, there is spread to the lymph nodes. Stage 4 lung cancer indicates metastasis has occurred.

Treatment

Treatment depends on the type and the staging of the lung cancer. The earlier the diagnosis, the more effective the treatment. Lung cancer treatment mainly involves surgery, radiation, and chemotherapy. The key treatment for stage 1, 2, and localized NSCLC is surgery. A minimally invasive procedure called video-assisted thoracic surgery may be used, which accesses the chest through small incisions.

A wedge resection is the term used when the patient requires removal of a small section of lung. A segmentectomy is the removal of a segment (part of a lobe) of one lung. A lobectomy—the most common type of surgery for lung cancer—is the removal of an entire lobe of one lung. A sleeve resection involves removal of a lobe of the lung and part of a bronchus. A pneumonectomy is the removal of an entire lung. Radiation treatment is aimed at destruction of rapidly

BOX 40-2. Paraneoplastic Syndromes in Lung Cancer

Lung cancer–SCLC in particular–is the most common cancer to be associated with paraneoplastic syndromes. Paraneoplastic syndromes are disorders that develop because of hormones, enzymes, cytokines, and other chemical mediators secreted by cancer cells. The following are some of the most common syndromes.

ADRENOCORTICOTROPIC HORMONE SECRETION

Adrenocorticotropic hormone (ACTH) is the most commonly produced hormone in lung cancer patients, particularly those with SCLC. Increased levels of ACTH may be detectable in up to 50% of patients with lung cancer. Because of a chemical similarity between ACTH and melanocyte-stimulating hormone, the lung cancer secretion of ACTH causes stimulation of melanocytes and a darkening of the skin. Cushing syndrome, caused by excessive ACTH, is sometimes seen as well.

CACHEXIA

Cachexia, which is the wasting of the body's lean body mass, is perhaps the most common manifestation of advanced malignant disease and is responsible for approximately 25% of cancer deaths. TNF-alpha is one of the chemical mediators that cause this complication. TNF-alpha causes anorexia and other metabolic alterations such as weight loss, muscle loss, anemia, and disorders of carbohydrate, lipid, and protein metabolism. Cancer patients exhibit a relative glucose intolerance, insulin resistance, reduced lipogenesis, and decreased muscle protein synthesis.

CLOTTING AND THROMBOSIS

Tumor cells can directly activate the clotting process through two secreted coagulation factors: tissue factor and cancer procoagulant. A variety of hypercoagulable disorders including Trousseau's syndrome, deep venous thrombosis and thromboembolism, disseminated intravascular coagulation, and others can occur in lung cancer. The incidence of deep venous thromboembolism in cancer sufferers is approximately 40 to 100 per 1,000 persons per year compared with an estimated 1 to 2 cases per 1,000 persons per year in the general population.

HYPERCALCEMIA

Hypercalcemia in lung cancer patients can be caused by cancer metastasis and deterioration of bones or by paraneoplastic syndromes. Cancer tumors can secrete parathyroid hormone peptide, calcitriol, or other cytokines including osteoclast-activating factors. All these act on bone to release calcium into the bloodstream.

NEUROLOGICAL EFFECTS

Autoantibodies are commonly found in neurological syndromes associated with cancer. SCLC is particularly associated with Lambert-Eaton syndrome, which is a weakening of the limbs caused by autoantibodies found in neuromuscular junctions. Similar to myasthenia gravis, it resolves with cancer treatment.

PANCOAST SYNDROME OR HORNER'S SYNDROME

Pancoast syndrome is a disorder caused by a cancerous tumor in the apical region of the lung. The tumor causes destructive lesions of the thoracic inlet and involvement of the brachial plexus and cervical sympathetic nerves. Severe pain of the shoulder radiating down the arm into the hand and atrophy of hand and arm muscles can occur. A disorder called Horner's syndrome, which is caused by cervical sympathetic nerve dysfunction, can occur. It is characterized by ptosis (drooping of the eyelid), miosis (pupil constriction), hemianhidrosis (lack of sweating), and enophthalmos (sinking in of the eyeball within the orbit).

SYNDROME OF INAPPROPRIATE ANTIDIURETIC HORMONE

Elevated levels of ADH occur in 30% to 70% of lung cancer patients. SCLC can secrete excessive amounts of ADH, which causes excess water reabsorption at the nephron. This is termed syndrome of inappropriate antidiuretic hormone (SIADH). ADH stimulates water reabsorption at the collecting duct of the nephron, creating a high water content of the blood. This excess water causes hypo-osmolarity of the bloodstream and dilutes the sodium concentration; this is called dilutional hyponatremia. The ADH also creates a low water content in the tubule fluid, resulting in a highly concentrated urine.

---

dividing cells such as cancer cells. Stereotactic body radiotherapy is used to deliver radiation to a specific region of the tumor while limiting injury to the surrounding healthy tissue.

Patients who have inoperable stage 3 lung cancer and metastatic disease receive chemotherapy. Chemotherapy, which usually requires the combination of different agents, is the main form of treatment for those with SCLC. Recently, targeted molecular chemotherapy has been effective in some patients. For example, the growth of adenocarcinoma has been found to require specific growth factors, enzymes, and signaling pathways. Drugs have been developed that target these specific molecular level cancer components. For example, cancer cells have tyrosine kinase receptors which, when stimulated, trigger massive proliferation of the cells. Pharmaceutical agents that precisely inhibit tyrosine kinase receptors are currently being developed and block the stimulus for cancer growth. Crizotinib is one of these agents used for NSCLC.

Breast Cancer

Breast cancer is the second most common cancer in the United States after lung cancer; 1 in 8 American women will suffer breast cancer in their lifetime. In 2013, an estimated 232,340 new cases of invasive breast cancer were diagnosed among women, as well as an estimated 64,640 additional cases of in situ breast cancer. In 2013, approximately 39,620 women died from breast cancer. Research into effective diagnostic procedures and treatments has increased the survival rate over the last decade; the 5-year survival rate for women diagnosed with breast cancer is now 89%.

Breast cancer incidence increases with age. Seventy-nine percent of new cases and 88% of breast cancer deaths occur in women 50 years and older. Although African American women have lower incidence of breast cancer compared with Caucasian women, African American women have a higher rate of death because of breast cancer. In 2013, the relative 5-year survival rate for African American women was 79% compared with 92% for Caucasian women. This disparity is attributed to the fact that African American women seek care for breast cancer at later stages in the disease compared with Caucasian women.

Etiology

Although the specific etiology of breast cancer is unknown, risk factors are clear: prolonged reproductive life, including early menarche and late menopause; age older than 50 years; obesity, caused by increased levels of estrogen in fat deposits; hormone replacement therapy; personal or family history of breast cancer; having no children or late childbirth after age 30 years; and genetic predisposition. The major risk factors for sporadic (nonhereditary) breast cancer are related to estrogen exposure. Via hormonal action, estrogen can enhance the proliferation of premalignant lesions and cancers with estrogen receptors. However, other mechanisms also play a role, as a significant number of breast cancers are estrogen-receptor negative.

A family history of breast cancer in one first-degree relative, such as a mother or sister, is reported to increase an individual's lifetime risk of breast cancer by 1.8 times. The lifetime risk of breast cancer is up to 3 times higher if two first-degree relatives are affected by breast cancer, particularly if the relative was diagnosed at an early age (50 years or younger). A family history of ovarian cancer in a first-degree relative, especially if the disease occurred at an early age (less than 50 years), has been associated with a doubling of breast cancer risk. Women of Ashkenazi Jewish descent have double the risk of breast cancer compared with other ethnic groups.

Approximately 5% to 10% of breast cancers can be attributed to one of two autosomal dominant genes: BRCA1 and BRCA2. In hereditary cancers, one mutant BRCA allele is inherited and the second allele is affected by a sporadic mutation. The BRCA1 gene locus is 17q21 and the BRCA2 gene locus is 13q12.3. Both BRCA1 and BRCA2 are defective tumor suppressor genes. The estimates of the risk of breast cancer in women with these mutations vary: By age 70 years, up to 78% of women with BRCA 1 mutations develop

breast cancer and up to 56% of women with the BRCA2 mutation will develop the disorder.

CLINICAL CONCEPT

Genetic testing for BRCA1 and BRCA2 can be performed in selected high-risk patients with a strong family history of breast or ovarian carcinoma. Genetic counseling should be available for patients undergoing this test. Many women with these gene mutations opt for preventative mastectomy and oophorectomy, surgical removal of the ovaries.

Pathophysiology

Most breast cancers are epithelial cell tumors that develop from cells lining the ducts or lobules of the breast. Less commonly, cancer of the breast arises from nonepithelial cells such as the supporting connective tissue. In most cancers, a triggering factor, which is unclear, causes the breast epithelial cells to proliferate, grow uncontrollably, and invade surrounding tissue.

Normally estrogen and progesterone act at the breast to stimulate growth and cell proliferation. Estrogen and progesterone receptors are nuclear hormone receptors that promote DNA replication and cell division. In some breast cancers, these estrogen and progesterone receptors are overexpressed; these are called estrogen receptor-positive (ER-positive) breast cancers. Another cellular receptor that promotes breast cell growth is human epidermal growth factor receptor 2 (HER2). This cellular receptor is commonly overexpressed in some forms of breast cancer; these cancers are termed HER2 positive.

Categorizing Breast Cancer. Breast cancers can be categorized based on different characteristics, including molecular subtype and histopathology. There are four basic molecular subtypes of breast cancer: Luminal A, Luminal B, Basal, and HER2 positive. Each different subtype behaves differently and requires specific treatments as follows:

- Luminal A: Slow-growing cancers that have a 90% cure rate and are often found on screening mammogram. Treatment usually includes surgery and radiation.
- Luminal B: Aggressive cancers that invade blood vessels and lymph nodes. The tumor is often difficult to surgically remove from surrounding tissue with clear margins. Often a second surgery is necessary.
- Basal: very aggressive, rapidly growing cancer that lacks estrogen, progesterone, and HER2 receptors. These tumors respond to chemotherapy.
- HER2 positive: These tumors overproduce HER2, which signals breast cancer to grow and spread.

Breast cancers can also be categorized according to the demonstrated changes in the tissue as follows:

- Carcinoma in situ is proliferation of cancer cells within ducts or lobules without invasion of surrounding tissue.
- Lobular carcinoma in situ (LCIS) is a nonpalpable lesion usually discovered via biopsy. LCIS is not malignant, but it indicates an increased risk of future invasive carcinoma in either breast; about 1% to 2% of patients with LCIS develop cancer annually.
- Invasive carcinoma is primarily adenocarcinoma. About 80% of adenocarcinoma is the infiltrating ductal type; most of the remaining cases are infiltrating lobular type.
- Paget's disease of the nipple is a form of ductal carcinoma in situ that extends into the overlying skin of the nipple and areola, manifesting with an inflammatory skin lesion. Characteristic malignant cells called Paget cells are present in the breast epidermis. Rare types of breast cancers are termed medullary, mucinous, and tubular carcinomas.

Breast cancer invades locally and spreads initially through the regional lymph nodes, bloodstream, or both. Metastatic breast cancer may affect almost any organ in the body—most commonly the lungs, liver, bone, brain, and skin. Metastatic breast cancer frequently appears years or decades after initial diagnosis and treatment.

Clinical Presentation

Ninety percent of palpable breast masses are noncancerous; however, all masses require a complete investigation. Most masses that are cancerous are single, nontender, and firm with irregular borders and adherence to the skin or chest wall. The most common place on the breast for a woman to have a tumor is the upper, outer quadrant, where 45% of tumors are found (see Fig. 40-2). By the time a cancer lesion becomes palpable, over half of the patients have metastasis to axillary lymph nodes. Other breast changes associated with cancer include nipple discharge, swelling in one breast, nipple or skin retraction, and a specific type of skin appearance called peau d'orange—a thickening of skin that resembles an orange peel. Paget's disease of the breast, which involves redness, crusting, pruritus, and tenderness of the nipple, is also characteristic of a cancerous change.

Diagnosis

Diagnosis of breast cancer includes a complete history and physical, clinical breast and pelvic examinations, mammogram, breast ultrasound, and biopsy of the lesion. A fine-needle aspiration or excisional biopsy are performed with histology and cytology examination. In some cases, an MRI scan is warranted. The finding of calcifications on a mammogram is associated with breast cancer. In some cases, a ductogram, also called

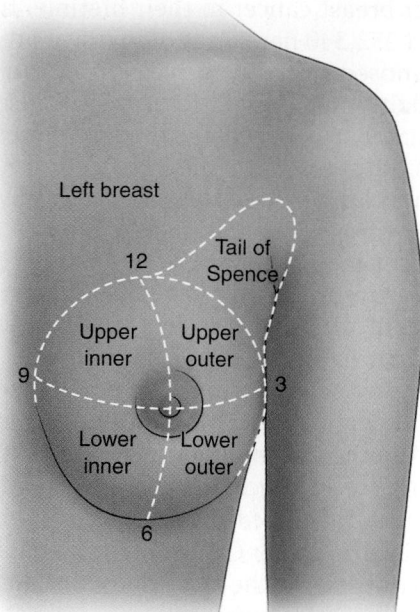

FIGURE 40-2. The breast should be divided into four quadrants when referring to a lesion: upper outer (UO), upper inner (UI), lower outer (LO), and lower inner (LI). Additionally, there is an outer region that includes some of the axilla known as the Tail of Spence. Most breast cancer lesions are found in the UO quadrant.

galactogram, is used to determine the cause of nipple discharge. A fine plastic tube is placed into the opening of the duct in the nipple. A small amount of contrast medium is injected, which outlines the shape of the duct on a mammogram and shows whether a mass is present inside the duct. Scintimammography is a nuclear imaging test that is used when mammography does not show sufficient detail. It is also used to assess high-risk patients, tumor response to chemotherapy, and metastatic involvement of axillary lymph nodes.

Positron emission topography (PET) scanning is the most sensitive and specific of all the imaging modalities for breast disease. Changes in metabolic activity, vascularization, oxygen consumption, and tumor receptor status can be detected.

There are specific tests performed on biopsy samples of cancer tissue. These tests include the following:

- Estrogen and progesterone receptor test: measures the amount of estrogen and progesterone receptors in the breast cancer tissue. Breast cancer tissue with more estrogen and progesterone receptors than normal may grow quickly. About 75% of breast cancers are ER-positive. About 65% of ER-positive breast cancers are also progesterone receptor-positive (PR-positive). Cells that have receptors for one or both of these hormones are considered hormone receptor-positive. Hormone receptor-positive cancer is also called "hormone sensitive" because it responds to hormone therapy such as tamoxifen or aromatase inhibitors. Hormone receptor-negative tumors are referred to as "hormone insensitive" or "hormone resistant." Having this information influences the choice of treatment. Treatments that block estrogen and progesterone may stop the cancer from growing.

- HER2/neu test: measures the number of HER2/neu genes and amount of HER2/neu protein in a sample of cancerous tissue. Cancerous tissue with a high amount of HER2/neu genes or HER2/neu protein is aggressive, grows quickly, and is likely to metastasize. This type of breast cancer can be treated with specific biological drugs that target the HER2/neu protein.
- Oncotype Dx assay: has been used for women with early stage, estrogen-receptor positive, lymph node-negative breast cancer treated with tamoxifen. This assay analyzes 21 genes (16 cancer genes and 5 reference genes). Using a formula based on the expression of these genes, the likelihood of recurrence of the cancer within 10 years can be predicted.

Diagnostic testing also includes histological examination of lymph nodes. Axillary lymph nodes are particularly significant in breast cancer. The staging of breast cancer is highly reliant on spread to axillary lymph nodes and metastasis. There are four stages of breast cancer that are based on the TNM staging system.

Treatment

Treatment of breast cancer usually requires surgery, such as lumpectomy or mastectomy, lymph node biopsy, and adjuvant therapy, which includes radiation, hormonal therapy, chemotherapy, and immunological or biological agents. After surgery, adjuvant therapy is aimed at possible micrometastatic disease. It is possible that surgery does not completely destroy all breast cancer cells in the body. Adjuvant chemotherapy targets breast cancer cells that have escaped the breast and regional lymph nodes but have not yet been identified as metastasis.

Adjuvant therapy is used to reduce the risk of future cancer recurrence. It has been estimated to be responsible for 35% to 72% of the reduction in mortality rate. The presence of specific receptors within the cancer lesion is significant in adjuvant treatment. Selective estrogen receptor modulators (SERMs) can inhibit the estrogen receptors of cancerous tissues. Tamoxifen and raloxifene are SERMs that are equally effective in reducing risk of ER-positive breast cancer in postmenopausal women. Trastuzumab (Herceptin) is an immunotherapeutic agent used to counteract cancers with the HER2 protein. Tyrosine kinase inhibitors target epidermal growth factor receptors that are present in breast cancers. They are commonly combined with other forms of chemotherapy or radiation therapy. Everolimus and lapatinib are examples of tyrosine kinase inhibitors. Aromatase inhibitors, such as Anastrozole, are also used as adjuvant therapy in breast cancer. These agents work by inhibiting aromatase, the enzyme responsible for converting other steroid hormones into estrogen. Bisphosphonates are added to the therapeutic regimen because they may lessen the damage to bone from metastatic disease. Bisphosphonates, such as Zoledronic acid, inhibit osteoclast function and reduce the resorption of bone. Drugs called microtubule inhibitors, such as Eribulin, are also used to interfere with the cell cycle of cancer cells. They inhibit the growth phase of microtubules, leading to disruption of mitotic spindles, and, ultimately, apoptotic cell death. Microtubule inhibitors are indicated for breast cancer patients with metastasis who have previously received at least two chemotherapeutic regimens.

Tumor markers, such as CEA (carcinoembryonic antigen), CA15.3 (carcinoma antigen 15-3), and CA27.29 (carcinoma antigen 27-9), can be used for monitoring patients on therapeutic regimens. CA15.3 and CA27.29 levels correlate with the course of disease in 60% to 70% of patients, whereas CEA levels correlate in 40% of patients. After recovery from breast cancer, if a recurrence develops, it is usually within the first 5 years after treatment.

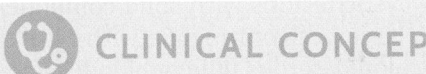

CLINICAL CONCEPT

Individuals with the BRCA1 and BRCA2 genes have an increased risk of breast, ovarian, colon, and pancreatic cancer. Males also have an increased risk of prostate cancer.

Ovarian Cancer

Ovarian cancer is the fifth-leading cause of cancer death in women in the United States, with approximately 22,000 women in the United States developing ovarian cancer annually and 14,000 dying from the disease. It is more common in Caucasian women than African American women, and it is more common in women between ages 55 and 64. Women with advanced disease at diagnosis have an overall 5-year survival rate of 20% to 30%, but those with an early diagnosis have a 90% to 95% probability of successful treatment. Unfortunately, ovarian cancer commonly remains undiagnosed until its advanced stages because of vague presenting symptoms and a lack of screening tests. Frequently, the cancer has already metastasized upon diagnosis.

Etiology

The etiology of ovarian cancer is unclear. Risk factors include older age, nulligravidity (no history of pregnancy), obesity, smoking, estrogen treatment, infertility, family history of ovarian cancer, and Ashkenazi Jewish descent. Family history is a very important risk factor. From 5% to 10% of cases of ovarian cancer occur in individuals with a family history of the disease. Women who have had breast cancer are at higher risk of developing ovarian cancer. The use of talcum powder on the vulva and perineum may be associated with increased risk of ovarian cancer. Women who possess the

BRCA1 or BRCA2 gene, which are defective tumor suppressor genes, have a high risk of developing ovarian cancer. Women with a BRCA1 gene mutation have a 35% to 40% risk of developing ovarian cancer, and those with a BRCA2 gene mutation have a 10% to 30% risk of developing ovarian cancer. Studies show that advanced ovarian cancer is characterized by a mutated tumor suppressor gene (*TP53*) in almost all tumors. The studies also show that ovarian cancer is linked to mutations in nine other genes, including the neurofibromatosis gene and retinoblastoma gene.

Women who have been pregnant have a 50% decreased risk for developing ovarian cancer compared with nulliparous women. Women aged 40 to 59 years who have taken oral contraceptives or undergone tubal ligation also have a reduced risk.

Pathophysiology

More than 90% of ovarian cancer is initiated in the outer epithelial cells of the ovary. Ovarian epithelial tumors are cystic lesions with solid components. The surface may be smooth or irregular with cysts that contain straw-colored, serous fluid or bloody, hemorrhagic fluid. Epithelial ovarian cancer spreads initially within the peritoneal cavity. Metastatic cancerous tissue is often found on the peritoneal surfaces, surface of the liver, outer surface of the small and large bowel and uterus, and para-aortic and pelvic lymph nodes. Outside the peritoneal cavity, the tumors can spread to the pleural cavity, lungs, and inguinal lymph nodes.

Clinical Presentation

Most ovarian cancers cause vague clinical manifestations, which include lower abdominal pain and abdominal enlargement. The patient often complains of abdominal bloating and difficulty eating because of a feeling of fullness. Nausea, vomiting, and constipation also bring the patient to a health-care provider. Urinary frequency, dysuria (difficulty urinating), and pelvic pressure are other symptoms. In advanced disease, anorexia, weight loss, progressive weakness, and cachexia are present, as is characteristic of other malignant tumors. Physical examination in women with ovarian cancer is often normal in the early stages. Later in advanced disease, there may be a solid, irregular, fixed pelvic mass or bowel obstruction.

Diagnosis

There are no screening modalities for ovarian cancer. However, the cancer antigen-125 (CA-125) and transvaginal ultrasound are widely used diagnostic studies. Laparotomy is often the primary procedure used to establish diagnosis and stage of the disease. Cytological analysis of ascites fluid (peritoneal edema fluid), biopsy of the tumor and lymph nodes, and visual inspection of the peritoneum and diaphragm are performed during laparotomy. The staging of disease relies on the acumen of the surgeon performing the laparotomy and the confinement or spread of the tumor. Stage I disease is cancer confined to the ovary or ovaries. Stage II disease is cancer confined to the pelvis. Stage III disease is cancer spread beyond the ovaries and pelvis, but confined to the abdomen. Stage IV disease is cancer spread outside the abdomen.

Treatment

Treatment includes surgical resection of the tumor and chemotherapy. Often the patient requires a total hysterectomy, which includes excision of the other ovary. If metastatic spread is apparent with surgery, surgical excision of all cancerous tissue is necessary. This may require liver resection, bowel excision, and splenectomy. Chemotherapy may be required before surgery to decrease the amount of cancer tissue. Alternatively, chemotherapy is administered after surgery. Standard postoperative chemotherapy is combination therapy with platinum and paclitaxel. These agents interfere with mitosis of cancer cells, thereby inhibiting progression of cancer growth.

A number of different chemotherapeutic agents are being used in platinum-resistant tumors. These alternative agents include tyrosine kinase inhibitors, such as pazopanib, and epithelial growth factor inhibitors, such as pertuzumab. A unique therapeutic approach under investigation is called hyperthermic intraperitoneal chemotherapy, which consists of a heated solution of chemotherapeutic agents instilled directly into the peritoneum. Heat has been found to potentiate the effects of chemotherapy agents. Regardless of the type of chemotherapy used, several cycles of chemotherapy are commonly required. After surgery and chemotherapy, many patients can achieve complete recovery. However, recurrence of ovarian cancer is the most troublesome problem after surgery and chemotherapy are performed. Fifty percent of ovarian cancer patients experience relapse and ultimately die of the disease.

Cervical Cancer

Cervical cancer is the third most common cancer in women worldwide. In industrialized countries with screening programs, the incidence of cervical cancer ranges from 4 to 10 per 100,000 women. Inadequately screened populations such as women older than age 65 years, Hispanic and African American women, and indigent women account for 25% of cervical cancer cases and 41% of deaths caused by the disease. Sixty percent of women who are diagnosed with invasive cervical cancer have not had a Papanicolaou (Pap) smear in the past 5 years.

Etiology

Women at risk for developing cervical cancer include those who smoke, as well as those with a history of sexually transmitted diseases, HPV infection, two or more lifetime sexual partners, or immunosuppression. Cervical cancer most commonly affects women during their forties and fifties. The most significant predisposing conditions to cervical cancer are HPV infection and genetics. HPV is a known human carcinogen, and infection occurs in a high percentage of sexually active women. The prevalence of HPV infection in women is highest in those aged 20 to 24 years. However, approximately 90% of HPV infections resolve on their own with no sequelae of cervical cancer. On average, only 5% of HPV infections develop changes consistent with cervical cancer. There are two major types of HPV, a high-risk and low-risk type. The high-risk type of HPV causes a persistent infection that progresses to cervical cancer. The low-risk type of HPV causes condylomata (genital warts) but does not cause cervical cancer.

Different genetic changes have been linked to cervical cancer. Mutations in the genes *TNFa-8, TNFα-572, TNFα-857, TNFα-863,* and *TNF G-308A* have been associated with a higher incidence of cervical cancer. These genes code for tumor necrosis factor (TNF), a product of WBCs in inflammation, which is involved in cellular apoptosis. Another gene involved in apoptosis and gene repair, *TP53,* has been associated with an increased susceptibility to HPV infection, which progresses to cervical cancer.

Human leukocyte antigen genes, which code for cellular surface antigens, are also involved in susceptibility to cervical cancer. The chemokine receptor-2 gene on chromosome 3p21 and the *Fas* gene on chromosome 10q24.1 predispose an individual to cervical cancer. It is believed these genes diminish the immune response to HPV. Additionally, human immunodeficiency virus (HIV) infection increases susceptibility to cervical cancer, most likely because of an impaired immune response to HPV infection. Cervical cancer is at least 5 times more common in HIV-infected women, and this increased prevalence has remained essentially unchanged with the use of antiretroviral therapy. Women whose mothers used diethylstilbestrol, a medication used to prevent miscarriage during pregnancy, also possess an increased risk of invasive cervical cancer.

Pathophysiology

In cervical cancer, there are two major kinds of cellular changes: SCC, which occurs within epithelial cells, and adenocarcinoma, which involves glandular cells. The earliest preinvasive changes that occur on the cervix are termed squamous intraepithelial lesions. These asymptomatic changes, which are usually diagnosed by Pap smear, are categorized as:

- low-grade squamous intraepithelial lesions
- high-grade squamous intraepithelial lesions
- possibly cancerous (malignant)
- atypical glandular cells of undetermined significance.

The intraepithelial lesions are first limited to the cervical epithelium; as invasion occurs, neoplastic cells penetrate the underlying basement membrane. The squamocolumnar junction, an area of rapid cell turnover

between uterus and cervix, is a very common site of cancerous changes.

If a Pap smear shows abnormal cells, a biopsy is done. Dysplasia that is seen on a biopsy of the cervix is called cervical intraepithelial neoplasia (CIN). It is grouped into three categories:

- CIN I: mild dysplasia
- CIN II: moderate to marked dysplasia
- CIN III: severe dysplasia to carcinoma in situ.

CIN I and CIN II changes can resolve on their own. CIN III indicates early cancerous changes of the cervix.

Almost 100% of cervical cancer cases test positive for HPV. HPV16 is the most carcinogenic HPV genotype and accounts for approximately 55% to 60% of all cervical cancers. Persistent cervical infection with high-risk HPV types is necessary for the development of cervical cancer and its precursor lesion, CIN III. HPV18 is the next most carcinogenic HPV genotype, and accounts for approximately 10% to 15% of cervical cancers. Approximately 10 other HPV genotypes cause the remaining 25% to 35% of cervical cancers. HPV18 causes a greater proportion of glandular cancers, adenocarcinoma, and adenosquamous carcinoma than SCC.

Cervical cancer, both squamous and adenocarcinoma, tends to grow upward to the endometrial cavity, throughout the vaginal epithelium, and laterally to the pelvic wall. It can also invade the bladder and rectum. The common sites for distant metastasis include lymph nodes, liver, lung, and bone.

Clinical Presentation

Cervical cancer has a long asymptomatic period before the disease becomes clinically evident. Commonly, an abnormal Pap test alerts the individual of a problem. The first symptom of cervical cancer may be abnormal vaginal bleeding, commonly after sexual activity. There also may be vaginal discomfort, discharge, and burning on urination. Cervical cancer can invade the rectum and bladder, leading to constipation, hematuria, and ureteral obstruction. The triad of leg edema, pain, and hydronephrosis (swelling of the kidney) suggests pelvic wall involvement. There are usually no abnormal findings in early stage cervical cancer on physical examination. As the disease progresses, the cervix may become abnormal in appearance, with an erosion, ulcer, or mass. These abnormalities can extend to the vagina. Rectal examination may reveal an external mass or gross blood from tumor erosion.

Diagnosis

Pap smears that suggest invasive disease require further evaluation by colposcopy, colposcopic-directed biopsy, and endocervical curettage. Curettage is the scraping of tissue away from a surface of an organ; in this case, the surface of the cervix. Colposcopy is a direct visualization of the cervix where sites of abnormality can be biopsied. Once the diagnosis of cervical cancer is established, the

TABLE 40-6. Stages of Cervical Cancer

Stage	Description
Stage O	Carcinoma in situ. Cervical cells are localized to the inner surface of the cervix.
Stage I	Cancer is found limited to the cervix. It is divided into stage 1A and stage 1B, depending on the amount of cancer cells involved.
Stage II	Cancer has spread beyond the cervix but not to the pelvic wall (the tissues that line the part of the body between the hips) or to the lower third of the vagina. Stage II is divided into stages IIA and IIB, based on how far the cancer has spread.
Stage III	Cancer has spread to the lower third of the vagina, or to the pelvic wall, or has caused kidney problems. Stage III is divided into stages IIIA and IIIB, based on how far the cancer has spread.
Stage IV	Cancer has spread to the bladder, rectum, or other parts of the body. Stage IV is divided into stages IVA and IVB, based on where the cancer is found.

(Adapted from National Cancer Institute (NCI), National Institute of Health (NIH). http://www.cancer.gov/cancertopics/pdq/treatment/cervical/Patient/page2#Keypoint12. Last accessed July 8, 2015.)

disease is clinically staged, which involves assessment of any metastasis. A thorough history and physical examination with emphasis on the pelvic examination is necessary. A rectovaginal examination is also important to identify lymph nodes or locally invasive disease. Use of laparoscopy, chest x-ray, intravenous pyelography, gastrointestinal (GI) endoscopy, CT scan, or MRI of the pelvis and abdomen may be needed to establish the degree of metastatic disease. Cervical cancer is staged from stage 0 to stage IV (see Table 40-6).

Treatment

There are different treatment modalities for the stages of disease. Carcinoma in situ (stage 0) is treated with local excisional measures such as cryosurgery, laser ablation, and loop excision. Loop excision uses an electrified wire that cuts around the tumor to remove it.

The treatment of choice for stage IA disease is surgery. Conization, radical hysterectomy, and total hysterectomy are surgical procedures. Conization is a procedure that removes a wedge of tissue from the cervix. If lymph nodes are involved, radiation therapy is needed. Radical hysterectomy with bilateral pelvic lymphadenectomy and combined external beam radiation with brachytherapy is needed for stage II, III, and IVA. **Brachytherapy** involves imbedding deposits of radioactive material in the cervical tissue. For stage IVB, individualized therapy is used to provide pain relief. Radiation therapy is used for control of bleeding and pain, whereas systemic chemotherapy is used for metastatic disease. For pelvic recurrence after radiation therapy, modified radical hysterectomy or pelvic exenteration is performed. Pelvic exenteration is a radical surgical treatment that removes all organs—the urinary bladder, urethra, rectum, and anus—from a person's pelvic cavity.

Prostate Cancer

The prostate is a small gland that manufactures and secretes semen, which carries sperm. It uniquely increases in size throughout a male's lifetime. Benign prostatic hyperplasia (BPH), which is an increase in the size of the prostate gland caused by excessive proliferation of cells, is a common condition of middle-aged and older adult men. When examining a male older than age 50 years, it is important to exclude the presence of prostate cancer because both BPH and cancer enlarge the size of the gland and present with similar symptoms.

In the United States, the lifetime probability of developing prostate cancer is 1 in 7; this probability increases with age. Approximately 6 out of 10 men aged 65 and older develop prostate cancer. In 2014, there were 233,000 new cases diagnosed and 29,480 deaths attributed to prostate cancer. In 2014, it ranked as the second most common malignancy of men in the United States behind lung cancer. Clinically apparent disease is very rare in men younger than age 40 years; the average age of diagnosis is 66 years. African American men have the highest risk of developing and dying of prostate cancer.

Etiology

The exact etiology of prostate cancer is unknown. However, there are many different risk factors. Having a father or brother who had prostate cancer increases one's risk 2-fold; having a father and a brother with prostate cancer increases one's risk 4-fold. Certain lifestyle factors may also increase the risk of prostate cancer, including consumption of fat, red meat, fried foods, and dairy; high calcium intake; and smoking. African American ethnicity, high alcohol intake, and exposure to Agent Orange and cadmium are also risk factors.

Other factors may decrease the risk of prostate cancer, such as a diet rich in plant-based foods and vegetables, especially lycopene-containing foods such as tomatoes. A diet rich in cruciferous vegetables such as broccoli, Brussels sprouts, cabbage, cauliflower, and kale; soybeans; legumes; carotenoids; antioxidants; and fish oil, along with moderate exercise, all decrease the risk of prostate cancer.

Pathophysiology

Prostate cancer mainly develops in the glandular cells of the organ, so it is referred to as an adenocarcinoma. Prostate cancer is initiated by carcinogenic mutations and its growth is dependent on the male hormone testosterone. Initially, there is an oncogenic or tumor suppressor genetic defect, which causes uncontrolled cellular growth in the gland. As the glandular cells hyperproliferate, further mutations of other genes occur, including the *TP53* gene and *Rb* gene (retinoblastoma). These changes lead to tumor progression and metastasis. The cancer cells proliferate locally and invasively and often spread to the neck of the bladder, ejaculatory ducts, and seminal vesicles. The cancer metastasizes to bone early in the course of the disease, sometimes before any external symptoms are exhibited. Lung, liver, and adrenal metastases can also occur. In early cancer, the tumor grows slowly but becomes more aggressive as the size of the tumor increases.

Clinical Presentation

Early stage prostate cancer has no symptoms. In more advanced disease, the prostate gland can obstruct urine flow from the bladder. This usually causes urinary symptoms such as decreased force of stream and incomplete emptying of the bladder. The patient needs to strain to get urine out and may have frequency of urination. Late-stage symptoms include hematuria, azotemia, anemia, and anorexia. Back pain also is often a late-stage symptom caused by vertebral bone metastasis.

On physical examination, the patient may have no remarkable findings except those on a DRE. The prostate gland can be palpated through the wall of the rectum. The prostate, which is usually a rubbery gland, becomes hard and unmovable in cancer. The inguinal lymph nodes may be enlarged and, if vertebral metastasis has occurred, tenderness over the lumbar region is found.

Diagnosis

Diagnosis of prostate cancer involves a DRE, PSA test, and biopsy. It is important to keep in mind, however, that PSA screening has low specificity, as most men with elevated PSA do not have prostate cancer and lower levels of PSA have been found in men with the disease.

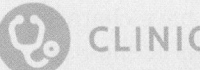 **CLINICAL CONCEPT**

PSA level is influenced by many variables: Men with a higher body mass index have lower PSA levels, there are genetic differences that make some men secrete more PSA than others, and men on statin drugs have lower PSA levels.

The clinician must consider several variables when assessing a patient for risk of prostate cancer: race, age, PSA level, family history of prostate cancer, and findings on DRE. These variables determine which men require a prostate biopsy. Transrectal ultrasound guided-needle biopsy is indicated when DRE or PSA are abnormal.

Classification. There are two classification systems used to determine the pathology and aggressiveness of prostate tumors. The Gleason grading system ranks tumors histologically from 1 (most differentiated) to 5 (least differentiated and most likely to metastasize). The poorer the differentiation of the cancer cells, the worse the prognosis.

The TNM anatomic system (tumor, node, metastasis) characterizes the tumor based on examination of biopsied tissue. The most common site for prostate cancer metastasis is the vertebral column.

ALERT! Back pain is often the presenting symptom of late-stage prostate cancer.

Treatment

Treatment options for prostate cancer include active surveillance, watchful waiting, surgical removal of the prostate, and different types of radiation treatment, cryotherapy, brachytherapy, and hormonal therapy. Prostate cancer is appraised as a low-risk or high-risk disease according to the Gleason score, PSA levels, and the patient's age and life expectancy. For low-risk disease, active surveillance or watchful waiting is increasingly recommended, as prostate cancer is often a slow-growing disease that can be assessed over time. The patient who is a candidate for active surveillance or watchful waiting is usually an elderly man older than age 75 who has other medical disorders. Active surveillance or watchful waiting is preferable because surgery may pose a greater risk to the patient's health and quality of life, so the clinician monitors the progress of the neoplastic growth using repeat PSA levels every 3 months and biopsy every 12 to 24 months. For high-risk disease, radical prostatectomy, radiation, and hormonal therapy are recommended. Treatment of prostate cancer with androgen suppressants remains a cornerstone intervention for advanced disease management.

Colorectal Cancer

Colorectal cancer is the second leading cause of death resulting from cancer. It is a preventable disease if individuals utilize the recommended screening procedures, which include colonoscopy and FOBT. In 2010, the Centers for Disease Control and Prevention reported that 58.6% of adults had undergone some form of colon cancer screening, and 54% of adults had undergone colonoscopy within the last 10 years. Although most cases of colon cancer require surgery, new chemotherapy agents discovered in the last 10 years are lowering the prevalence of the disease.

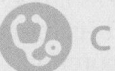 **CLINICAL CONCEPT**

Beginning at age 50, all adults should have a colonoscopy performed every 10 years.

Peak incidence for colorectal cancer is between ages 60 and 79 years. Fewer than 20% of cases develop before age 50 years. There is a disproportionally higher incidence and rate of death from colon cancer in African Americans than in Caucasians. Hispanic persons have the lowest incidence and mortality from colorectal cancer. The incidence of colorectal cancer is about equal for males and females.

Etiology

Current research indicates that genetic factors have the greatest correlation to colorectal cancer. Colon cancer usually starts as a polyp, a tumorous mass that projects into the intestinal lumen. Familial adenomatous polyposis (FAP) is a well-defined hereditary disorder that predisposes an individual to intestinal polyps; it is an autosomal dominant condition caused by a mutation of the gene located at chromosome 5q21, also called the adenomatous polyposis coli (APC) gene. The APC gene is a defective tumor suppressor gene, and it confers an almost 100% likelihood of colon cancer development. In FAP, patients typically develop 500 to 2,500 colonic polyps that cover the mucosal surface of the bowel. Polyps in FAP can become cancerous at an early age; some in childhood. Another similar condition, Hereditary Non-polyposis Colorectal Cancer (HNPCC), is an autosomal dominant familial syndrome characterized by multiple colonic polyps with cancerous potential. There is a smaller number of polyps in HNPCC than in FAP, and HNPCC confers approximately a 40% chance of development of colon cancer.

Although genetic susceptibility is a significant risk factor, most colorectal cancer occurs sporadically in the absence of well-defined familial syndromes. Risk factors include obesity, tobacco use, physical inactivity, insulin resistance, low fiber in the diet, high amount of animal fat in the diet, and diets low in vitamin A, C, and E.

 CLINICAL CONCEPT

Patients with inflammatory bowel diseases such as ulcerative colitis and Crohn's disease have an increased risk of developing colorectal cancer. Although both diseases increase susceptibility, ulcerative colitis seems to be a stronger risk factor. The risk for developing colorectal malignancy increases with the duration of inflammatory bowel disease and the greater extent of colon involvement.

Pathophysiology

Colon cancer most commonly begins as a polyp, which goes through a number of changes to become cancerous (see Fig. 40-3). Polyps with cancerous potential are called adenomatous polyps. Approximately 90% of polyps are small, usually smaller than 1 cm in diameter, and have a small potential for malignancy. The remaining 10% of

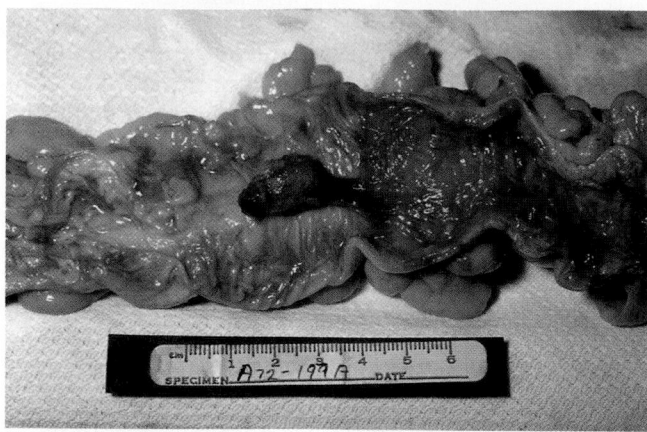

FIGURE 40-3. A colonic polyp. *(Courtesy of CDC/Dr. Edwin P. Ewing, Jr.)*

adenomas are larger than 1 cm and approach a 10% chance of containing invasive cancer. On a molecular level, colon cancer is caused by genetic changes that result in defective tumor suppressor genes, activated oncogenes, or mismatched gene repair. Commonly, an accumulation of multiple genetic mutations results in the progression of normal colonic mucosal cells to benign adenoma to adenomatous polyp to adenocarcinoma. The three types of adenomatous polyps (polyps with cancerous potential)—tubular adenomas, villous adenomas, and tubulovillous adenomas—are characterized as follows.

- Tubular adenomas, also called pedunculated adenomas, have a mass with a stalk coming off the intestinal wall.
- Villous adenomas, also called sessile polyps, have fingerlike projections without stalks that invade the intestinal wall. Villous adenomas are more difficult to remove and have a higher risk of cancerous changes than tubular adenomas.
- Tubulovillous adenomas have characteristics of both tubular and villous adenomas.

Some precancerous lesions are not polyps but flat. A flat area of dysplasia that is confined to the mucosa of the intestinal wall is called carcinoma in situ, which is considered premalignant. When the dysplastic tissue invades the intestinal wall more deeply, it is considered adenocarcinoma.

Clinical Presentation

Colorectal cancer can remain asymptomatic for years. Symptoms develop insidiously and frequently have been present for months before the affected individual seeks medical care. Symptoms include fatigue, weakness, weight loss, iron deficiency anemia, changes in bowel habits, melena (blood in the stool), diarrhea, and constipation. Lower bowel cancers can present with hematochezia (rectal bleeding) and narrowing of stool caliber.

Iron deficiency anemia can be a sign of slow, GI blood loss. Slow GI blood loss occurs in peptic ulcer, esophageal varices, and colon cancer. Colon cancer causes a constant

TABLE 40-7. Staging and Prognosis of Colon Cancer Using Dukes Classification

Stage	Description	Duke's Class	Prognosis/5-year Survival
Stage 0	Carcinoma in situ	N/A	N/A
Stage I	Tumor invades submucosa (muscularis propria)	Dukes A	93%
Stage II	Tumor invades into subserosa, visceral peritoneum, or other organs and structure	Dukes B1, B2	72% to 85%
Stage III	Bowel wall invasion with positive lymph node	Dukes C1/C2	44% to 83%
Stage IV	Distant metastasis	Dukes D	8%

(Adapted from http://www.cancer.gov/cancertopics/pdq/treatment/colon/HealthProfessional/page3. Last accessed July 8, 2015.)

microscopic leakage of blood into the intestine. Blood—an iron source within the body—is slowly depleted. It is important to check for GI blood loss in individuals with iron deficiency anemia. This can be done with performance of an FOBT and colonoscopy to assure that an occult colon cancer is not present.

 CLINICAL CONCEPT

Iron deficiency anemia can be a key sign of GI blood loss from colon cancer.

All colorectal cancers spread by direct extension into adjacent structures and by metastasis through the lymphatics and bloodstream. Spread commonly occurs to regional lymph nodes, liver, lungs, and bones. Staging of colorectal cancers is based on depth of tumor invasion. The TNM anatomic system and the Dukes classification system are used to stage colorectal cancers (see Table 40-7).

Diagnosis

Both diagnostic tests and laboratory tests are used to diagnose colorectal cancer in patients. Diagnostic tests for colorectal cancer include colonoscopy, DRE, FOBT, and barium enema. Virtual colonoscopy involving a CT or MRI scan can be performed for screening. Capsule endoscopy using an ingestible, camera-equipped capsule is available as a means of virtual colonoscopy. However, this procedure has lower accuracy than colonoscopy. Flexible sigmoidoscopy is performed in some settings for colon cancer screening, although this procedure cannot examine the entire colon.

Laboratory tests include complete blood count, serum iron, serum ferritin, CEA, and liver enzymes. Stool DNA tests have been developed that detect mutant, fragmented, and methylated DNA from exfoliated colon tumor cells in stool. Genetic testing of blood samples can detect most cases of HNPCC and FAP.

Treatment

Treatment involves surgical resection of the tumor and evaluation for metastasis. The entire peritoneum should be examined including the liver, pelvis, and diaphragm. Periodic surveillance should take place after surgery. Tests include annual colonoscopy and CEA blood tests every 3 months. Radiation to the pelvis is recommended for patients with cancers of the lower bowel. Chemotherapy is recommended for some patients and has shown modest benefit. Survival rate is related to the stage of the tumor, lymph nodes involved, and presence of metastasis.

Some studies have demonstrated that medical treatment with nonsteroidal anti-inflammatory drugs (NSAIDs) decreases the number and the size of colonic polyps. One study suggests that aspirin may reduce the incidence of recurrent colonic polyps, particularly advanced colonic polyps in patients with a high risk of colon cancer. These drugs are not yet considered preventive medications for colonic polyps.

Liver Cancer

Primary hepatocellular cancer (HCC) or liver cancer is one of the most common tumors in the world and the third most frequent cause of cancer mortality. In a high number of cases, infection with hepatitis B or C is the predisposing condition to liver cancer.

HCC is most common in Asia and sub-Saharan Africa with an annual incidence of 500 cases per 100,000 persons. This high incidence is because of widespread hepatitis B and C infection within the population. In the United States, incidence of HCC has more than doubled over the past 20 years from 2.6 to 5.2 per 100,000 persons per year. It is 3 times more common in men than women. African American males have the highest incidence at 13.1 per 100,000 persons per year.

Etiology

Any agent that contributes to chronic, low-grade liver cell damage is a risk factor for liver cancer. The conditions of hepatitis B or C infection, alcoholic liver disease, alpha-antitrypsin deficiency, hemochromatosis, and nonalcoholic forms of cirrhosis predispose individuals to liver cancer. Other possible causes include long-term androgenic steroid administration, exposure to toxins such as vinyl chloride, or long-term oral contraceptive use.

Pathophysiology

HCC is a primary cancer of the liver and occurs predominantly in patients with underlying chronic liver disease and cirrhosis. It develops when there is a genetic mutation that causes the hepatocytes to proliferate excessively and resist cellular apoptosis. Chronic infections of hepatitis B or C repeatedly provoke the body's own immune system to attack the liver cells. Chronic alcohol abuse repeatedly injures the hepatocytes. A constant cycle of damage followed by cell repair can lead to mistakes during repair, which in turn lead to carcinogenesis. Cancer cells grow and expand locally, spread within the liver, and then leave the organ to cause distant metastases. In general, cancer presents as a single mass lesion or as diffuse growth. On a molecular level, *TP53*, PIKCA, and ß-catenin genes appear to be the most frequently mutated in patients with HCC. There is also inactivation of the tumor suppressor gene *ARID2*. Some investigators speculate that HCC develops from hepatic stem cells that proliferate in response to chronic regeneration caused by viral injury.

Clinical Presentation

The symptoms of liver cancer usually occur when the cancer is in an advanced stage. Symptoms include abdominal pain, weight loss, fever, and sudden onset of symptoms associated with cirrhosis such as ascites, jaundice, or esophageal varices. Esophageal varices are caused by a blockage of the portal vein by a tumor, which causes blood flow to back up into the esophageal veins. On physical examination, the liver is usually enlarged, sometimes tender, and a hepatic artery bruit may be auscultated because of the increased amount of blood flow. In advanced liver cancer, the tumor can spread to nearby tissue or metastasize to distant sites, such as the lungs.

Diagnosis

There is not a specific diagnostic screening test for liver cancer; however, the alpha fetoprotein (AFP) blood test is widely used because it is about 60% accurate in detecting liver cancer. If high levels of AFP (greater than 500 ng/mL) are found, this can indicate primary liver cancer, testicular cancer, ovarian cancer, or metastatic cancer in the liver. Imaging procedures to detect liver tumors include ultrasound, CT scan, MRI, and hepatic artery angiography. Percutaneous liver biopsy can be diagnostic if the sample is taken from an area of cancer cells localized by ultrasound, CT scan, or laparoscopy. The stages of liver cancer are based on the TNM anatomic system.

Treatment

Treatment of liver cancer includes surgical resection of tumor, chemotherapy with hepatic artery embolization (also called chemoembolization), radiofrequency ablation, and liver transplantation. Hepatitis B vaccine has been shown to prevent infection and its sequela, HCC. Interferon has been used for those infected with hepatitis C to reduce the development of HCC.

Brain Tumor

Brain tumors either originate from the neurons or supportive tissue in the brain, or they may be the metastasis of primary tumors elsewhere in the body. Malignant primary tumors of the CNS occur in approximately 16,500 individuals and account for an estimated 13,000 deaths in the United States annually. Metastatic tumors to the brain are more common, with an incidence of greater than 200,000 patients per year in the United States.

Etiology

In adults, most brain cancer affects areas superior to the cerebellum and brainstem. In children, most brain tumors occur inferior to the cerebellum. A prior history of irradiation to the head may increase the chance of primary brain tumor. Some inherited diseases, such as neurofibromatosis, tuberous sclerosis, multiple endocrine neoplasia (type 1), and retinoblastoma, increase the susceptibility to development of brain tumors. Infection with HIV increases susceptibility to CNS lymphoma. Metastatic tumors commonly reach the brain via spread through the bloodstream. Lung cancer is the most common tumor that metastasizes to the brain, followed by breast, melanoma, and colon cancer. Less common sources of metastasis are malignant melanoma, testicular cancer, and renal cell cancer.

Pathophysiology

In general, a benign tumor within an organ has a better prognosis than a malignant tumor. However, benign brain tumors can have similar adverse effects as malignant tumors. Similar to malignant tumors, benign tumors can infiltrate large regions of the brain and cause serious neurological deficits and poor prognosis. Also, whether the brain tumor is benign or malignant, it is difficult to surgically resect large tumors without causing some neurological deficit. In addition, the anatomic site of a brain tumor, whether benign or malignant, can have lethal consequences. Brain tumors increase intracranial pressure (ICP) and place a compressive force on brain tissue. If ICP rises to high levels it can place pressure on the brainstem, affecting vital functions and potentially leading to fatal consequences. Finally, the pattern of spread of primary brain tumors differs from that of other tumors; even the most highly malignant gliomas rarely metastasize outside the CNS.

Brain tumors are classified according to the site of the tumor, the type of tissue involved, and whether they are benign or malignant. In adults, gliomas and meningiomas are most common.

Gliomas. Gliomas come from glial cells, which are nonneuronal supportive cells in the CNS referred to as astrocytes, oligodendrocytes, and ependymal cells. There are three types of gliomas:

1. astrocytic tumors, which include astrocytomas and glioblastomas (most malignant)

2. oligodendroglial tumors, which can vary from less malignant to very malignant
3. glioblastomas, which are the most aggressive type of primary brain tumor.

 CLINICAL CONCEPT

Some primary brain tumors are made up of both astrocytic and oligodendrocytic tumors. These are called mixed gliomas.

Meningiomas. Meningiomas are the other type of brain tumor in adults. These tumors arise from the meningeal tissue and occur most commonly between the ages of 40 to 70 years, more often in women, and are benign 90% of the time.

Other Primary Brain Tumors. Other primary brain tumors in adults are rare. These include:

- ependymomas
- craniopharyngiomas
- pituitary tumors
- primary lymphoma of the brain
- pineal gland tumors
- primary germ cell tumors of the brain.

Clinical Presentation

Most brain tumors cause symptoms because of the pressure they exert on brain tissue. Brain tumors usually present with one of three syndromes:

1. progression of a focal neurological deficit such as weakness of one extremity or cranial nerve dysfunction
2. seizure
3. a nonfocal neurological disorder such as headache (see Box 40-3), visual disturbances, dementia, personality or gait disorders.

Diagnosis

CT or MRI scan is usually a first diagnostic modality in brain tumor. Electroencephalography is a useful test in patients with seizures. Positron emission tomography (PET) and single photon emission tomography may be used in surgical planning to define the tumor's anatomy. Tissue removed from an accessible tumor biopsy or cerebrospinal fluid analysis is sometimes necessary.

Treatment

Treatment modalities used with brain tumors include surgery, chemotherapy, radiation, and glucocorticoids. Glucocorticoids are used frequently to decrease the swelling around the tumor and reduce its pressure on adjacent brain tissue. Treatment depends on the grading of the tumor, which is a I through IV scale. Grade I astrocytomas are well-differentiated, slow growing, and sometimes surgically resectable. Grade II tumors are life-threatening if not removed, slow growing, and may spread to nearby tissue. Grade III are poorly differentiated with many malignant cells, rapidly growing, and require surgery plus radiation or chemotherapy. Grade IV are considered high grade with rapidly growing malignant cells that aggressively spread to adjacent tissue.

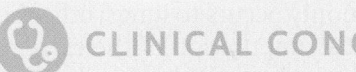 **CLINICAL CONCEPT**

Brain and spinal cord metastasis from other primary sites of cancer is more common than primary CNS tumors.

Bone Cancer

Bone cancer is a tumor that destroys normal bone tissue. The different types of primary bone cancer include osteosarcoma, chondrosarcoma, and Ewing's sarcoma. Often, bone cancer is a metastatic disease from another type of primary tumor in the body.

In the United States, the incidence of osteosarcoma is approximately 750 to 900 cases per year. The majority of affected individuals are younger than 20 years old, and the incidence of osteosarcoma is slightly higher in males than in females. Patients with hereditary retinoblastomas have up to 1,000 times greater risk of subsequently developing osteosarcoma. Mutations in the *Rb* gene (retinoblastoma gene) are also found in 60% to 70% of noninheritable, sporadic osteosarcoma tumors.

Chondrosarcomas, which originate in cartilaginous tissue, have an incidence of 1 per 200,000 population in the United States. Most affected patients are 50 to 70 years old and the majority are male. Ewing's sarcoma tumors are most common in individuals from birth to the age of 20 years, with approximately 250 cases diagnosed per year in the United States. Males are more frequently affected compared with females. The incidence of these tumors in Caucasians is at least nine times higher than it is in African Americans.

Etiology

The cause of primary bone cancer is not clear but there are several risk factors, including use of high doses of

---

BOX 40-3. Headaches Caused by Brain Tumors

Headaches caused by brain tumors may:

- be worse when the person wakes up in the morning, and clear up in a few hours
- occur during sleep
- be accompanied by vomiting, confusion, double vision, weakness, or numbness
- get worse with coughing or exercise, or with a change in body position.

radiation therapy or treatment with some anticancer drugs, hereditary retinoblastoma, bone infarction, chronic osteomyelitis, and a history of Paget's disease, which is a bone remodeling disorder.

Pathophysiology

Osteosarcoma, chondrosarcoma, and Ewing's sarcoma affect different age groups and have slightly different pathological mechanisms.

Osteosarcoma. The most common site for osteosarcoma is in the bone surrounding the knee (see Fig. 40-4). Osteosarcoma develops in areas of greatest bone growth, such as the distal femur, proximal tibia, and proximal humerus. Patients typically present with pain and swelling in the affected area. A sudden pathological fracture can be the first sign of bone cancer.

Osteosarcomas are classified as stage 1, 2, or 3. Stage 1 osteosarcoma is localized and resectable. Stage 2 is more aggressive, causing more tissue necrosis; it may or may not have metastasized to the lymph nodes and lungs. Stage 3 osteosarcoma has lung metastasis. Osteosarcoma has a 50% to 60% survival rate, and metastasis most commonly occurs to lungs, other bones, and the brain. Surgical amputation of the extremity, most commonly above the knee, is the common treatment.

> **CLINICAL CONCEPT**
>
> Retinoblastoma is associated with later development of osteosarcoma.

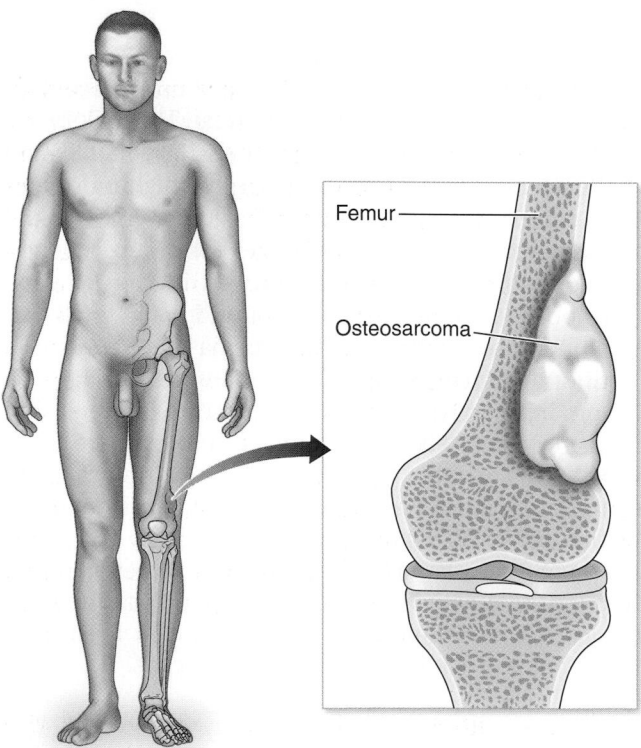

FIGURE 40-4. Osteosarcoma is cancer of the bone. It is commonly located in the leg, close to the knee.

Chondrosarcoma. Chondrosarcoma is a very rare disease. These tumors commonly arise in the central portions of the skeleton, including the pelvis, shoulder, and ribs. They present as painful, progressively enlarging masses. Grade 1 chondrosarcoma grows relatively slowly, has cells with a similar appearance to normal cartilage, and is the least aggressive and invasive. Grades 2 and 3 are increasingly faster-growing cancers, with more varied and abnormal-looking cells, and are much more likely to infiltrate surrounding tissues, lymph nodes, and organs. Grade 4 is the anaplastic and undifferentiated cartilage-derived tumors with worst prognosis.

The most common sites for chondrosarcoma to grow are the pelvis and shoulder, along with the superior metaphyseal and diaphyseal regions of the arms and legs. However, chondrosarcoma may occur in any bone, and are sometimes found in the skull, particularly at its base. Most tumors are low grade and slow growing with a 5-year survival rate of up to 90%. Large tumors are more aggressive than small tumors and metastasis occurs to the lungs and skeleton. Surgical excision and chemotherapy are the treatment modalities used for chondrosarcoma.

Ewing's Sarcoma. Genetic exchange between chromosomes can cause cells to become cancerous. Most cases of Ewing's sarcoma (85%) are the result of a translocation between chromosomes 11 and 22, which fuses the EWS gene of chromosome 22 to the FLI1 gene of chromosome 11. The disease typically involves long bones such as the femur and flat bones of the pelvis. On x-ray, tumors lyse and destroy bone and have a characteristic "onion peel" appearance. Ewing's sarcoma presents as an enlarging, tender, swollen mass and may appear as an infection. Some patients have fever, elevated WBC count, and sedimentation rate. It is an aggressive disease with potential metastasis to the lungs, bones, and bone marrow.

Diagnosis and Treatment

For each type of bone cancer, an x-ray shows a destructive lesion in bone. CT scan, MRI, and bone scan can delineate the tumor and reveal metastases. A biopsy is needed to examine and grade bone cancer cells. Surgery and postoperative chemotherapy are used for limb-salvaging treatment.

Uterine Cancer

Cancers of the female reproductive system account for almost 15% of all cancers in women. The most common of these malignancies is uterine cancer, specifically endometrial cancer. An estimated 52,630 cases of endometrial cancer were diagnosed in 2014, and 8,590 cases were fatal. It is the fourth most common cancer, accounting for 6% of female cancers, following breast, lung, and colorectal cancer. Most patients present with symptoms at an early stage, resulting in only 3% of cancer deaths in women. The chance of a woman being diagnosed with endometrial cancer in her lifetime is 1 in 37. Endometrial cancer affects both premenopausal and postmenopausal women. However, 75% of endometrial cancers occur in postmenopausal women, with the average age of diagnosis at 61 years.

Etiology

Premenopausal women are at increased risk for endometrial cancer if they have risk factors such as obesity, nulliparity, anovulatory menstrual cycles, diabetes, and hypertension. In addition, these younger women are at higher risk (up to 19% to 25%) for primary ovarian cancer. Another group of women at increased risk of premenopausal endometrial cancer are those with hereditary nonpolyposis colon cancer (HNPCC). These women are also at increased risk for cancer of the ovary, stomach, small bowel, hepatobiliary system, pancreas, brain, breast, and ureter or kidney. Incidence of endometrial cancer is higher among Caucasians compared with Asian or African American women; however, mortality is higher among African Americans. Endometrial cancer can occur because of excess estrogen from various sources, either exogenous or endogenous.

Endogenous estrogen sources include obesity, polycystic ovary syndrome, anovulatory cycles, or estrogen-secreting tumors. Obesity has been associated with increased risk of endometrial cancer because, within adipose tissue, androgenic hormones convert to estrogen compounds. This leads to higher levels of unopposed estrogen in obese women. Nulliparity and infertility are also related to chronic anovulation and unopposed estrogen levels. Frequent alcohol use can elevate estrogen levels. Late menopause and early menarche can be associated with more anovulatory cycles and thus more unopposed estrogen.

Pathophysiology

Endometrial cancers are divided into two classes, type I and type II, each with differing pathophysiology and prognosis. More than 80% of endometrial cancers are type I and are caused by unopposed estrogen stimulation. Type I is often found in association with endometrial hyperplasia, which is thought to be a precursor. Type II endometrial cancers are thought to be estrogen independent, occurring in older women. Endometrial cancers are also categorized by grade and stage of disease.

Endometrial cancer may originate in a small area, such as within an endometrial polyp or in a diffuse multifocal pattern. Early tumor growth is characterized by a spreading pattern. Endometrial cancer growth is characterized by fragility of the tissue and spontaneous uterine bleeding. Later tumor growth is characterized by invasion of the uterine muscle layer and growth toward the cervix.

Clinical Presentation

More than 90% of patients with endometrial cancer will present with abnormal vaginal bleeding. Advanced cases may present with abdominal pain and bloating or other symptoms of metastatic disease. Other presenting symptoms may include purulent genital discharge, weight loss, and a change in bladder or bowel habits. Fortunately, most cases of endometrial cancer are diagnosed before this clinical presentation because of the recognition of abnormal vaginal bleeding as a possible early symptom of cancer. About 5% of women may be asymptomatic and diagnosed after abnormal Pap test results.

Diagnosis

Currently, no screening tests for cancer of the uterus are recommended for asymptomatic women. However, a Pap smear can detect preinvasive cervical cancer at early stages which can lead to more intense investigation for uterine cancer. If suspected, endometrial biopsy and transvaginal sonography are used. Although no laboratory tests aid in the diagnosis of uterine cancer, a CA-125 blood level is used to monitor the efficacy of treatment of endometrial cancer. Chest imaging should be obtained in all patients to rule out lung metastases before treatment. A CT scan of the chest, abdomen, and pelvis may be helpful in advanced-stage disease.

Treatment

The mainstay of treatment in endometrial cancer is surgery. Additionally, radiation has an important role in adjuvant treatment of endometrial cancers, as does chemotherapy. Hormonal therapy also has a role in adjuvant therapy in receptor-positive endometrial cancers. Most endometrial cancers are diagnosed as stage I tumors. In fact, most endometrial cancer can be cured with surgery alone, and relatively few patients need adjuvant radiotherapy. Primary radiation therapy is reserved only for patients who are poor surgical candidates or for those with unresectable disease.

Cancer of the Head and Neck

Squamous cell carcinoma (SCC) represents more than 90% of all head and neck cancers. In the United States, SCC of the head and neck comprises about 3% of all malignancies. This corresponds to an estimated 17 per 100,000 persons with newly diagnosed SCC of the head and neck per year. Male-to-female incidence rates are greater than 3:1. The discrepancy in the male-to-female ratio is even more pronounced in laryngeal tumors, in which carcinoma is 4 to 5 times more common in men. African Americans have a higher rate of incidence, more advanced disease on presentation, and greater mortality as compared with Caucasians.

Over the last 30 years, oropharyngeal cancer has decreased in incidence in older adults, which is thought to be caused by successful smoking cessation programs. However, in the last decade, oropharyngeal cancer incidence is increasing in young, nonsmoking adults, which is thought to be related to increased oral HPV infections.

Etiology

There are multiple genetic mutations associated with head and neck cancer. For example, mutations in the *TP53* gene can be attributed to drinking and smoking habits.

CLINICAL CONCEPT

SCC of the head and neck is most commonly associated with the use of alcohol and tobacco, as they act synergistically to raise risk.

Some 15% of patients have a viral etiology. Epstein-Barr virus (EBV) has been implicated in the development of nasopharyngeal carcinoma. HPV infection is another factor implicated in the carcinogenesis of oropharyngeal tumors. In particular, HPV-16 can be isolated in up to 72% of oropharyngeal cancers. Patients who engage in oral sex are at higher risk for HPV oropharyngeal cancer. Environmental exposures to paint fumes, plastic by-products, wood dust, asbestos, and gasoline fumes have been implicated as risk factors. Gastroesophageal reflux is also a significant risk factor for cancer of the larynx. Irritation from poorly fitting dentures as well as vitamin A and iron deficiency are also associated with oral and pharyngeal cancers.

CLINICAL CONCEPT

HPV infection increases the risk of oropharyngeal cancer.

Pathophysiology

It is believed that most malignancies in the oropharynx are caused by constant exposure to carcinogens. Mutations at gene *9p21* have been particularly related to oropharyngeal dysplasia. Mutations in the *TP53* and *Rb* genes are also commonly found in oropharyngeal cancer. Cellular changes in oropharyngeal cancers are commonly SCC, which can range from well-differentiated to poorly differentiated. Poorly differentiated cell changes are found in aggressive tumors with poor prognosis. Head and neck cancers drain into the cervical lymph nodes. Thirty percent of cases are discovered when the lesion is localized and surgically resectable without lymph node infiltration; 60% of cases are found when lymph node infiltration has already occurred. In these lesions, despite spread to the lymph nodes, treatment is usually successful. Fewer than 10% of patients present with metastatic disease that is incurable.

CLINICAL CONCEPT

Concurrent cancer development of the esophagus or lungs is common with head and neck cancer.

Clinical Presentation

When gathering history information, it is important for the clinician to question the patient about use of tobacco and alcohol. The patient's past medical history is important because some disorders can increase susceptibility to oropharyngeal cancer, such as HIV infection, EBV, gastroesophageal reflux, and Fanconi syndrome. The psychosocial history is important because HPV infection of the oropharynx increases the risk of cancer. Occupational exposures should be noted in the history because certain toxins increase risk. Family history is also important because there are several genetic mutations related to oropharyngeal cancers.

When examining the patient, SCCs appear as plaques, nodules, or verrucae (wartlike) lesions. They may be scaly or ulcerated and white, red, or brown. SCCs usually begin as surface lesions with erythema and slight elevation. Early red lesions are asymptomatic and may be either carcinoma in situ or invasive carcinoma. One-third of lesions are white, termed leukoplakia, and only 10% of them are carcinoma in situ or invasive carcinoma.

The most common sites for SCC are the floor of the mouth, the tongue, the soft palate, the anterior tonsillar pillar, and the retromolar region. Cancer of the larynx can occur and present as hoarseness of the voice. Symptoms such as a vague persistent sore throat or ear infection occur. In more advanced cases, enlarged cervical lymph nodes are common and the patient may present with a mass in the neck.

Diagnosis

In order to diagnose SCC, fine-needle aspiration biopsy (FNAB) are performed at the lesion site. CT scans and intravenous contrast are often used to detect the extent of tumor infiltration into deeper tissues and bone. MRI can be used alternatively with similar accuracy, though ultrasound is less sensitive. PET scanning is being used more frequently in patient work-up. Preoperatively, PET scanning can assess a primary tumor and lymph node and distant metastatic disease.

CLINICAL CONCEPT

PET scanning is commonly used to evaluate response to treatment.

Treatment

Factors that influence choice and type of treatment are the site and stage of the primary tumor. The TNM staging system is used for head and neck cancers, similar to the way it is used for lung cancer. Surgery, radiation, and chemotherapy are the treatment modalities used.

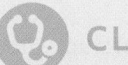

Thyroid Cancer

Approximately 63,000 cases of thyroid cancer were diagnosed in 2014 in the United States. Out of that number, there were fewer than 2,000 deaths. The incidence of thyroid cancer is three times higher in women than in men and peaks in the third and fourth decades of life. Nearly two-thirds of cases occur in adults younger than age 55 years.

Etiology

Radiation exposure of the neck, particularly in childhood, significantly increases the risk for thyroid cancer. However, low-dose radiation exposure from x-ray, CT, or MRI imaging studies has not been found to have a cancer-producing effect. An estimated 5% to 10% of solitary thyroid nodules are malignant. Thyroid nodules are most likely to be malignant in patients older than 60 years and in patients younger than 30 years.

Pathophysiology

Thyroid cancers are categorized as papillary carcinomas, follicular carcinomas, medullary thyroid carcinomas, anaplastic carcinomas, primary thyroid lymphomas, and primary thyroid sarcomas. Among these, 80% of all thyroid cancers are papillary carcinoma. Follicular carcinoma occurs in approximately 10% of cases. Medullary thyroid carcinomas represent 5% to 10% of neoplasms. Anaplastic carcinomas account for 1% to 2% of cases. Primary lymphomas and sarcomas are rare.

Papillary carcinoma, which has the best prognosis, is a slow-growing tumor that arises from the thyroxine (T4) and thyroglobulin-producing follicular cells of the thyroid. The cells are sensitive to thyroid-stimulating hormone (TSH) and take up iodine. They produce a protein called thyroglobulin in response to TSH stimulation. Papillary carcinoma is invasive and grows with fingerlike projections into the gland. Lesions can be unilobular or multilobular. Classic pathological lesions of papillary carcinoma are called psammoma bodies, which are calcifications found in the tumors. Tumors can grow through the thyroid membrane to invade surrounding structures. Growth into the trachea can occur, producing hemoptysis and airway obstruction. The recurrent laryngeal nerves can become involved and cause patients to present with a hoarse, breathy voice and, occasionally, dysphagia. Papillary carcinoma often spreads to the cervical lymph nodes. Clinically evident lymph node metastases are present in approximately one-third of patients at presentation.

Clinical Presentation

Thyroid cancer most commonly manifests as a painless, palpable, solitary thyroid nodule. These nodules are commonly discovered during a routine physical examination of the neck. Rapid growth of a nodule suggests malignancy; malignant thyroid nodules are usually painless. Sudden onset of pain is more strongly associated with benign disease, such as thyroiditis, than with malignancy. Hoarseness suggests involvement of the vocal cords and dysphagia may be a sign of impingement on the esophagus. Family history of thyroid cancer increases the risk of malignancy. Physical examination should include a thorough head and neck examination with careful attention to the thyroid gland and cervical soft tissues, as well as laryngoscopy. Hard and fixed nodules are more suggestive of malignancy than supple, mobile nodules. Cancerous nodules are usually nontender to palpation.

Diagnosis

History taking, physical examination, laboratory evaluation, and fine needle aspiration biopsy (FNAB) are involved in the evaluation of thyroid nodules. Ultrasonographic guidance can help to increase the accuracy of FNAB, with ultrasonography the imaging modality most commonly used. This noninvasive study enables accurate evaluation of the thyroid gland. Microcalcifications noted on sonograms are associated with thyroid malignancy.

Radioiodine imaging can help in determining the functional status of a thyroid nodule. For example, nonfunctional nodules do not take up radiolabeled iodine and appear as cold spots in the thyroid (cold nodules), whereas hyperfunctioning nodules take up radioiodine and appear as hot spots (hot nodules). Cancer usually occurs in cold nodules, but carcinoma cannot be excluded on the basis of radioiodine scans. CT and MRI can be used to evaluate soft-tissue extension of large or suspicious thyroid masses into the neck, trachea, or esophagus and to assess metastases to the cervical lymph nodes.

Treatment

Primary treatment for carcinoma is surgical excision, and total thyroidectomy has been the main treatment modality. Levothyroxine is then needed for life. Thyroglobulin levels are used to monitor recurrences after surgical excision of thyroid cancer.

Kidney Cancer

Cancer of the kidney or renal cell carcinoma (RCC) is an uncommon type of cancer. Among urological tumors, it is third in incidence following prostate and bladder cancer. The peak incidence of RCC is 64 years of age, with 80% of cases occurring in individuals between 40 and 69 years of age. Among urological tumors, RCC carries the worst prognosis because more than 40% of patients die of the disease as compared with the 20% mortality observed in prostate or bladder cancer. In the United States,

639,000 new cases were diagnosed in 2014 and approximately 14,000 patients died. The incidence is greater in men than women, and African Americans have a 10% to 20% higher incidence compared with Caucasians. Most cases of RCC are sporadic, and only 4% are familial. A quarter of patients present with advanced disease; survival for patients with metastatic disease is 13 months.

Etiology and Risk Factors

The cause of RCC is unknown in most patients. However, there are a number of hereditary and environmental risk factors. Hereditary syndromes that increase risk of RCC include von Hippel-Lindau (VHL) syndrome, tuberous sclerosis complex, hereditary papillary renal carcinoma (HPRC), familial renal oncocytoma associated with Birt-Hogg-Dube syndrome, and hereditary renal carcinoma. Other risk factors include smoking, obesity, hypertension, cystic kidney disease, and environmental exposures to asbestos, trichloroethylene, vinyl chloride, cadmium, herbicides, benzene, and other organic solvents. Cigarette smoking is thought to be responsible for one-third of cases and doubles the risk of RCC. Long-term use of NSAIDs is thought to be associated with increased incidence. In patients undergoing long-term renal dialysis, there is an increased incidence of cystic disease of the kidney, which is a risk factor for renal cell cancer.

Pathophysiology

The proximal tubule of the nephron is the origin of most RCC. Renal cancer occurs in a sporadic (non-hereditary) and a hereditary form, and both forms are associated with mutations of the short arm of chromosome 3 (3p), also called the VHL gene. A chromosomal translocation between 3p and chromosome 6 or 8 has also been associated with RCC. RCC consists of malignant epithelial cells with clear cytoplasm that grow along blood vessels in the kidney. It is common for RCC to spread to various locations via the renal vein.

Clinical Presentation

The classic presentation of RCC includes hematuria, flank pain, and palpable abdominal mass. Almost half of RCC cases are asymptomatic and discovered because a renal mass is incidentally detected on x-ray. Other common presenting symptoms include fatigue, weight loss, anemia, and, in the male, varicocele within the scrotum. Hypercalcemia, liver dysfunction, erythrocytosis, and polyneuromyopathy are paraneoplastic disorders in RCC that occur as a result of tumor secretion of inflammatory cytokines. A paraneoplastic disorder may cause the first presenting symptoms in RCC. Up to 30% of patients present with metastatic disease in the kidney from bone, lung, and liver cancers.

Diagnosis

Lab test abnormalities in RCC include hypoalbuminemia, proteinuria, and hypercalcemia. Diagnostic procedures that can be used to outline the renal mass include intravenous pyelogram, arteriogram, venogram, CT scan, MRI, ultrasound, PET, and biopsy. RCC tumors are staged according to the TNM system.

Treatment

Surgical treatment is recommended for localized disease. Radical nephrectomy, or surgical removal of the kidney, is the major form of treatment. Radiation and targeted cancer therapy with immune modulators, such as interferon, are used to treat patients with metastasis. Up to 30% of patients present with metastases, so surgical removal of metastatic tumors is also recommended.

RCC is often a slow growing disease that occurs in an asymptomatic elderly patient. The elderly patient often has other medical disorders that place the patient at high risk for surgery. For these patients, active surveillance is recommended. In active surveillance, the clinician periodically monitors the progress of the tumor and intercedes when the cancer is causing symptoms.

Chapter Summary

- Some cancers develop because of defective tumor suppressor genes, genes that guard against cancer formation. Other cancers develop because of mutated proto-oncogenes, genes that control normal cell growth and proliferation. Mutated proto-oncogenes become oncogenes that allow unrestrained cell division. Alternatively, cancer can be caused by faulty cellular apoptosis mechanisms that do not initiate programmed cellular degeneration, as they should.

- The cell cycle is a sequence of stages that a cell moves through for mitosis and regeneration. In order for cells to undergo mitosis, the cell must go through stages G0, G1, G2, S, and M. At each stage in the cell cycle, normal cells have a checkpoint where they can be repaired or undergo apoptosis if necessary. Cancer cells do not have checkpoints and they constantly cycle through stages.

- Differentiation refers to the extent to which neoplastic cells resemble normal cells both structurally and functionally. Lack of differentiation is called anaplasia.

- In general, benign tumors are well-differentiated and remain localized, cohesive, and well-demarcated from surrounding tissue. Benign tumors are not invasive, do not destroy surrounding tissue, and do not break away or travel from the tumor cell mass.

- In general, malignant tumors range from well-differentiated to poorly differentiated, but they are invasive and destructive to surrounding tissue. They also lack adhesion to the tumor mass and easily break free to travel to distant sites in a process called metastasis.

- Staging classifies a cancer tumor according to size, invasiveness, and spread. Staging uses a TNM system: T is for tumor size, N is for lymph node involvement, and M is for metastasis to distant organs.

- A paraneoplastic syndrome is an unexpected pathological disorder provoked by the presence of cancer in the body. A common type of paraneoplastic syndrome involves the secretion of endocrine hormones unrelated to the cancer tumor.

- Tumor cell markers are products of cancer cells such as hormones, enzymes, genes, antigens, or antibodies that are found in blood, spinal fluid, or urine. Some of these tumor markers are called oncofetal antigens because they are normally found during fetal development.

- Tumor cells are multiplying rapidly, constantly progressing through the cell cycle S and M stages. Radiation has its greatest destructive effect on cells in these two stages. Chemotherapy uses drugs to destroy cells in the S, M, or G stages of the cell cycle. Cancer chemotherapy has a collateral effect on healthy, rapidly multiplying cells such as skin, hair follicles, gastric cells, and bone marrow.

- Lung cancer is the leading cause of cancer-related death in both men and women throughout the world.

- Smoking history is calculated in pack-years. This is the number of packs of cigarettes smoked multiplied by years smoked.

- Individuals with the BRCA1 and BRCA2 genes have an increased risk of breast, ovarian, colon, and pancreatic cancer. Males also have an increased risk of prostate cancer.

- Virchow's node is the term used for an enlarged left-sided supraclavicular lymph node. This can indicate breast, lung, or abdominal cancer.

- A Pap smear can detect preinvasive cervical cancer at the earliest stages. HPV is the cause of cervical cancer in greater than 90% of cases.

- The liver, brain, and bone are frequent sites of metastasis for other primary cancers.

- For women, nulliparity (never being pregnant) is a risk factor for breast, ovarian, and uterine cancer.

- Colorectal cancer should be ruled out in all individuals with iron deficiency anemia.

- Beginning at age 50 years, all adults should have a colonoscopy performed every 10 years.

- Brain and spinal cord metastasis from other primary sites of cancer is more common than primary central nervous system (CNS) tumors.

- Painless hematuria can be a sign of bladder or kidney cancer.

- Prostate cancer commonly spreads to the vertebral bones.

- The risk for oral cancer is up to 40 times greater in users of tobacco and alcohol compared with those who neither smoke nor drink.

- Hepatitis C is a common cause of HCC.

 ## Making the Connections

Disorder and Pathophysiology	Signs and Symptoms	Physical Assessment Findings	Diagnostic Testing	Treatment
Lung Cancer | Small cell and nonsmall cell carcinoma. Begins as cellular dysplasia that develops on bronchial surface epithelium or bronchial mucous glands. Can also develop on the pleura.				
	Cough, hemoptysis, wheeze, dyspnea, unintentional weight loss, stridor. Fatigue, weakness, cachexia, hoarseness.	Cachexia, weight loss. Lungs: wheezes, crackles. Hemoptysis. Supraclavicular enlarged lymph node. Tanned skin often occurs because of tumor secretion of ACTH which stimulates melanocyte-stimulating hormone.	Chest x-ray; CT scan or MRI; tumor biopsy, bronchoscopy, bronchial or transbronchial biopsy, node biopsy, and FNAB by CT guidance.	Surgery to remove tumor and then radiotherapy and chemotherapy to kill any leftover cancer cells.

Continued

Making the Connections–cont'd

Disorder and Pathophysiology	Signs and Symptoms	Physical Assessment Findings	Diagnostic Testing	Treatment
Breast Cancer | Most are epithelial cell tumors that develop from cells lining the ducts or lobules. A triggering factor, which is unclear, causes the breast epithelial cells to proliferate, grow uncontrollably, and invade surrounding tissue. Some breast cancer is attributed to BRCA1 or BRCA2 defective tumor suppressor genes.				
	Breast lump or skin changes, such as nipple discharge, nipple retraction, swelling of breast, "peau d'orange" skin changes, axillary lymph node enlargement.	Breast lump, which is usually hard, nontender, and immovable. Upper outer quadrant most common region of breast tumor. Possible nipple discharge and skin changes, swelling in one breast, nipple or skin retraction, axillary lymphadenopathy, or peau d'orange skin.	Clinical breast examination and annual or biennial mammogram for women 40 to 49 years as decided by physician. Annual mammogram in women 50 to 74 years (American College of Obstetrics and Gynecology). Calcification and densities seen on mammogram indicate breast cancer. Breast ultrasound can be used to examine dense breasts for evidence of cancer. A fine-needle/core needle biopsy; open/excisional biopsy; axillary dissection; and sentinel node biopsy are all performed to stage breast cancer.	Lumpectomy and axillary dissection; sentinel node biopsy and radiation; OR mastectomy; radiation, chemo-hormonal therapy (tamoxifen) for estrogen receptor-positive tumor; and chemotherapy for HER2-positive cancer.
Ovarian Cancer | Unknown cause of proliferation of ovarian cells; risk increased with BRCA1 gene, BRCA2 gene, nulligravity, infertility, family history, Ashkenazi Jewish descent.				
	Vague abdominal pain, bloating, anorexia, weight loss.	A palpable abdominal mass may be present. May present with no significant findings.	Transvaginal ultrasound, blood CA-125 level, laparotomy, biopsy of ovarian tumor.	Surgery to remove ovary or total hysterectomy is commonly performed, as well as chemotherapy.
Cervical Cancer | Abnormal growth of cervical cells, usually in region between uterus and cervix. HPV is a known cervical carcinogen.				
	Abnormal vaginal bleeding.	Abnormal vaginal bleeding. Pelvic examination may show abnormality of cervix.	Pap test, colposcopy, recto-vaginal examination, CT, MRI, intravenous pyelogram, and chest x-ray.	Surgery, usually total hysterectomy, brachytherapy, and radiation may be done.

Continued

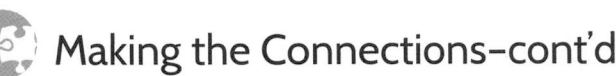

Making the Connections–cont'd

Disorder and Pathophysiology	Signs and Symptoms	Physical Assessment Findings	Diagnostic Testing	Treatment
Prostate Cancer | Cancer that develops in the glandular cells of the prostate. Carcinogenic mutations initiate the cancer, and its growth is dependent on testosterone. Initially, there is an oncogenic or tumor-suppressor genetic defect, which causes uncontrolled cellular growth in the gland. These changes lead to tumor progression and metastasis. The cancer cells proliferate and often spread to the neck of the bladder, ejaculatory ducts, and seminal vesicles. The cancer metastasizes to bone early in the course of the disease.				
	Asymptomatic in early stages. In advanced disease, prostate gland can obstruct urine flow from the bladder, causing urinary symptoms such as decreased force of stream, incomplete emptying of the bladder, and frequency of urination. Late-stage symptoms include hematuria, azotemia, anemia, anorexia, and back pain.	On physical examination, the patient may have no remarkable findings except those on a DRE. The prostate gland can be palpated through the wall of the rectum. The prostate, which is usually a rubbery gland, becomes hard and immovable in cancer. Inguinal lymph nodes may be enlarged; if vertebral metastasis has occurred, tenderness is found over the lumbar region.	Diagnosis of prostate cancer involves a DRE, prostate-specific antigen (PSA) test, and biopsy.	Options include active surveillance, watchful waiting, surgical removal of the prostate, radiation, cryotherapy, brachytherapy, and anti-androgen hormonal therapy.
Colorectal Cancer | Most commonly, an adenomatous polyp has cancer potential. Genetic, environmental, and behavioral causes are noted. Genetic conditions called familial adenomatous polyposis and hereditary nonpolyposis colorectal cancer increase susceptibility to cancerous polyp formation. The APC gene causes multiple polyp formation, which increases susceptibility to cancer.				
	Melena, fatigue, weakness, and changes in bowel habits such as diarrhea or constipation. May be asymptomatic.	Occult blood in the stool appears as black, tarry stool.	Colonoscopy OR flexible sigmoidoscopy shows a polyp, FOBT shows blood, barium enema may outline a polyp. Lab tests: iron deficiency anemia, increase in CEA, increased liver enzymes.	Surgery to remove tumor. Sometimes requires removal of the colon with creation of a stoma and colostomy. Radiation and chemotherapy.
Liver Cancer | Occurs in hepatocytes that undergo chronic inflammation, as in hepatitis B or C or cirrhosis. Cells required to undergo frequent damage repair lose their ability to suppress tumor growth.				
	Jaundice, weight loss, abdominal pain, fever, fatigue, weakness.	Abdominal tenderness, unintentional weight loss, jaundice, fever, hepatic bruit, hepatomegaly possible.	Tumor marker AFP; radiological imaging/ultrasound CT, MRI may show tumor. Liver enzymes abnormal. Possible erythrocytosis, hypoglycemia, hypercalcemia. Liver biopsy or aspiration shows tumor cells.	Liver resection surgery to remove tumor. Chemotherapy to kill all liver cancer cells and any metastasis. Chemoembolization, radiofrequency ablation therapy, proton beam therapy.

Continued

Making the Connections–cont'd

Disorder and Pathophysiology	Signs and Symptoms	Physical Assessment Findings	Diagnostic Testing	Treatment
Brain Tumor | Some tumor growth is related to chromosomal deletions, additions, duplication, and mutations of specific genes. Commonly, a metastatic cancer emerges from another primary cancer.				
	Neurological symptoms common, such as one-sided numbness or weakness. Headache, vomiting, seizure, vision disturbances, gait, or cranial nerve problems.	Neurological deficit may be assessed. Seizures, visual disturbance, headaches, vomiting, unstable gait, and cranial nerve dysfunction.	MRI, CT scan, and cerebral angiography can all show a brain tumor.	Surgery to excise or debulk a tumor. Radiation therapy to decrease size of tumor. Chemotherapy to kill cancerous cells.
Bone Cancer | Three major types: osteosarcoma, chondrosarcoma, and Ewing's sarcoma. Hereditary retinoblastoma is clearly linked to osteosarcoma. This cancer can be a metastasis from another primary cancer.				
	Pain, swelling, and tenderness of an area of bone. Osteosarcoma occurs around the knee region. Bone tumor can cause a pathological fracture.	Localized pain, swelling, and tenderness is present. Osteosarcoma usually is in distal femur, proximal tibia, and humerus. Chondrosarcoma affects flat bones like shoulder and pelvic girdles. Ewing's sarcoma is seen in diaphyseal regions of long bones and flat bones.	X-ray finding, CT scan, or MRI and tumor biopsy.	Treat underlying malignancy with combination of surgery, chemotherapy, and radiation.
Uterine Cancer | Endometrial hyperplasia develops into dysplasia; increased risk because of obesity, nulliparity, anovulatory menstrual cycles, tamoxifen, hormone replacement therapy, polycystic ovary syndrome, alcohol, diabetes, and hypertension; also increased risk in HNPCC.				
	Abnormal vaginal bleeding or discharge, bloating, abdominal pain, change in bladder or bowel habits.	May be asymptomatic. Abdominal mass may be palpable.	Transvaginal ultrasound, pelvic x-ray, CT scan, MRI, chest x-ray, CA-125 blood test.	Surgery, chemotherapy, hormonal therapy, and radiation.
Cancer of the Head and Neck | Commonly is a SCC; linked to tobacco and alcohol use; mutations in *TP53* gene, viral etiology, and gastroesophageal reflux disease.				
	Plaques, nodules, verrucae lesions in mouth, under and side of tongue. Leukoplakia.	Plaques, nodules, verrucae lesions in mouth, under and side of tongue. Leukoplakia.	X-ray, CT scan, MRI.	Surgery, radiation, chemotherapy.
Thyroid Cancer | Unknown cause; papillary carcinoma most common form, increased risk with radiation of neck.				
	Painless, palpable solitary thyroid nodule. Dysphagia possible.	Painless, palpable solitary thyroid nodule.	Ultrasound, FNAB, radioiodine scanning.	Surgery to remove thyroid. Thyroid hormone replacement treatment.

Continued

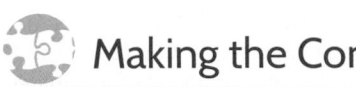 Making the Connections–cont'd

Disorder and Pathophysiology	Signs and Symptoms	Physical Assessment Findings	Diagnostic Testing	Treatment
Kidney Cancer | Unknown cause; increased risk with obesity, smoking, hypertension, cystic kidney disease, environmental toxins, von Hippel-Lindau syndrome gene.				
	Hematuria, flank pain, weight loss, fatigue.	Abdominal mass, costovertebral angle tenderness, hematuria.	Intravenous pyelogram, CT scan, MRI, ultrasound, biopsy.	Surgery, radiation, immunotherapy.

Bibliography

Acheson, L. (2010). Family history and genetic testing for cancer risk. *Am Fam Phys*, 81(8), 934–938.

Andersen, K. N. (2010). Performing digital rectal examination can detect cancers. *Am Fam Phys,* 81(9), 1073.

Breast Cancer Facts and Figures 2011. Retrieved from http://www.cancer.org/acs/groups/content/@epidemiologysurveilance/documents/document/acspc-030975.pdf

Buckler, A., & Luu, P. (2013). Screening for ovarian cancer. *Am Fam Phys*, 87(10), 709–710.

Burns, A., Sanghvi, H., Lu, R., Gaffikin, L., & Blumenthal, P. D. (2011). Saving women's lives from cervical cancer. *Lancet*, 377(9774), 1318.

Buys, S. S., Partridge, E., Black, A., et al. (2011). Effect of screening on ovarian cancer mortality: the Prostate, Lung, Colorectal and Ovarian (PLCO) Cancer Screening Randomized Controlled Trial. *JAMA*, 305(22), 2295–2303.

Croswell, J., & Shin, Y. R. (2013). Screening for prostate cancer. *Am Fam Phys*, 87(4), 283–284.

Croswell, J., & Costello, A. (2012). Screening for cervical cancer. *Am Fam Phys*, 86(6), 563–564.

Davies, L., & Welch, H. G. (2014). Current thyroid cancer trends in the United States. *JAMA Otolaryngol Head Neck Surg*, 140(4), 317–322. doi: 10.1001/jamaoto.2014.1.

Elmore, J. G., & Kramer, B. S. (2014). Breast cancer screening: toward informed decisions, *JAMA,* 311(13), 1298–1299. doi: 10.1001/jama.2014.2494.

El-Serag, H. (2011). Hepatocellular carcinoma. *NEJM,* 365, 1118–1127. doi: 10.1056/NEJMra1001683.

Fontaine, P. L., Saslow, D., & King, V. J. (2012). ACS/ASCCP/ASCP Guidelines for the early detection of cervical cancer. *Am Fam Phys*, 86(6), 501–508.

Forner, A., Llovet, J. M., & Bruix, J. (2012). Hepatocellular carcinoma. *Lancet*, 379(9822), 1245–1255.

Giuffrida, D., Prestifilippo, A., Scarfia, A., Martino, D., & Marchisotta, S. (2012). New treatment in advanced thyroid cancer. *J Oncol*, 2012, 391629. doi: 10.1155/2012/391629.

Goff, B. A., Matthews, B., Andrilla, C. H., et al. (2011). How are symptoms of ovarian cancer managed? A study of primary care physicians. *Cancer*, 117(19), 4414–4423. doi: 10.1002/cncr.26035.

Goldstraw, P., Ball, D., Jett, J. R., et al. (2011). Non-small-cell lung cancer. *Lancet*, 378(9804), 1727–1740.

Hauk, L. (2012). American college of obstetricians and gynecologists updates breast cancer screening guidelines. *Am Fam Phys*, 85(6), 654–655.

Hayes, J. H., & Barry, M. J. (2014). Screening for prostate cancer with the prostate-specific antigen test: a review of current evidence. *JAMA*, 311(11), 1143–1149. doi: 10.1001/jama.2014.2085.

Haymart, M. R., Banerjee, M., Stewart, A. K., et al. (2011). Use of radioactive iodine for thyroid cancer. *JAMA*, 306(7), 721–728.

Heald, B., Church, J., Plesec, T., & Burke, C. A. (2012). Detecting and managing hereditary colorectal cancer syndromes in your practice. *Cleveland Clin J Med*, 79(11), 787–796.

Heuvers, M. E., Stricker, B. H., & Aerts, J. G. (2012). Generalizing lung-cancer screening results. *N Engl J Med,* 366(2), 192–193.

Hyman, D. M., & Spriggs, D. R. (2012). Unwrapping the implications of BRCA1 and BRCA2 mutations in ovarian cancer. *JAMA*, 307(4), 408–410.

Kanjirath, P. P., & Edwards, P. C. (2010). Red and white ulcerated tongue mass. Squamous cell carcinoma. *Am Fam Phys*, 81(6), 785.

Knox, M. A. (2013). Thyroid nodules. *Am Fam Phys*, 88(3), 193–196.

Krishnaiah, P. B., Nunes, N. L., & Safranek, S. (2012). FPIN's clinical inquiries. Screening mammography for reducing breast cancer mortality. *Am Fam Phys*, 85(2), 176–183.

Kumar, V., Abbas, A. K., Fausto, N., & Aster, J. (2010). *Robbins & Cotran pathologic basis of disease.* 8th ed. Philadelphia, PA: WB Saunders.

Ladabaum, U., & Ford, J. M. (2012). Lynch syndrome in patients with colorectal cancer: finding the needle in the haystack. *JAMA*, 308(15), 1581–1583.

Lambert, M. (2012). ACS releases updated guidelines on cancer screening. *Am Fam Phys*, 86(6), 571–576.

Larkin, J., & Gore, M. (2012). Is advanced renal cell carcinoma becoming a chronic disease? *Lancet*, 376(9741), 574–575.

LeFevre, M. L., Calonge, N., Dietrich, A. J., & Melnikow, J. (2010). Mammography screening for breast cancer: recommendation of the U.S. Preventive Services Task Force. *Am Fam Phys*, 82(6), 602, 609.

Lietman, S. A., & Joyce, M. J. (2010). Bone sarcomas: Overview of management, with a focus on surgical treatment considerations. *Cleve Clin J Med*, 77 (Suppl 1), S8–12.

Lin, K. (2011). Screening for the early detection and prevention of oral cancer. *Am Fam Phys*, 83(9), 1047.

Lin, K. W., & Sharangpani, R. (2010). Screening for colorectal cancer. *Am Fam Phys*, 81(8), 1017–1018.

Longo, D. L., Kasper, D. L., Jameson, J. L., et al. (2011). *Harrison's principles of internal medicine.* 18th ed. New York: McGraw-Hill.

McCarthy, A. M., & Armstrong, K. (2014). The role of testing for BRCA1 and BRCA2 mutations in cancer prevention. *JAMA Intern Med,* May 19. doi: 10.1001/jamainternmed .2014.1322.

McIlwain, W. R., Sood, A. J., Nguyen, S. A., & Day, T. A. (2014). Initial symptoms in patients with HPV-positive and HPV-negative oropharyngeal cancer. *JAMA Otolaryngol Head Neck Surg*, 140(5), 441–447.

Mitka, M. (2010). Targeted therapies take aim against lung cancer and melanoma. *JAMA*, 304(6), 624–626.

Morrissey, J. J., London, A. N., Luo, J., & Kharasch, E. D. (2010). Urinary biomarkers for the early diagnosis of kidney cancer. *Mayo Clin Proceed*, 85(5), 413–421.

National Lung Screening Trial Research Team, Aberle, D. R., Adams, A. M., Berg, C. D., et al. (2011). Reduced lung-cancer mortality with low-dose computed tomographic screening. *N Engl J Med,* 365(5), 395–409.

Nichols, C., & Zamudio, A. (2014). Hard decisions about prostate cancer. *Am Fam Phys,* 89(3), 219.

O'Connor, G. T., & Hatabu, H. (2012). Lung cancer screening, radiation, risks, benefits, and uncertainty. *JAMA*, 307(22), 2434–2435.

Pelosof, L. C., & Gerber, D. E. (2010). Paraneoplastic syndromes: an approach to diagnosis and treatment. *Mayo Clin Proceed*, 85(9), 838–854.

Pluta, R. M., & Golub, R. M. (2011). *JAMA* patient page. BRCA genes and breast cancer. *JAMA,* 305(21), 2244.

Pruthi, S., Gostout, B. S., & Lindor, N. M. (2010). Identification and management of women with BRCA mutations or hereditary predisposition for breast and ovarian cancer. *Mayo Clin Proceed*, 85(12), 1111–1120.

Ricard, D., Idbaih, A., Ducray, F., et al. (2012). Primary brain tumours in adults. *Lancet,* 379(9830), 1984–1996.

Roy, H. K., & Khandekar, J. D. (2012). APC gene testing for familial adenomatosis polyposis. *JAMA*, 308(5), 514–515.

Salzman, B., Fleegle, S., & Tully, A. S. (2012). Common breast problems. *Am Fam Phys*, 86(4), 343–349.

Saslow, D., Solomon, D., Lawson, H. W., et al. (2012). American Cancer Society, American Society for Colposcopy and Cervical Pathology, and American Society for Clinical Pathology screening guidelines for the prevention and early detection of cervical cancer. *Am J Clin Pathol,* 137(4), 516–542.

Schauner, S., & Lyon, C. (2010). Bivalent HPV recombinant vaccine (Cervarix) for the prevention of cervical cancer. *Am Fam Phys*, 82(12), 1541–1542.

Shinagare, A. B., Silverman, S. G., Gershanik, E. F., Chang, S. L., & Khorasani, R. (2014). Evaluating hematuria: impact of guideline adherence on urologic cancer diagnosis. *Am J Med*, 2014 Feb 21. pii: S0002-9343(14)00145-4. doi: 10.1016/j.amjmed.2014.02.013. Epub ahead of print.

Shipley, W. U., & Zietman, A. L. (2012). Old drugs, new purpose—bladder cancer turning a corner. *N Engl J Med*, 366(16), 1540–1541.

Smith-McCune, K. (2014). Choosing a screening method for cervical cancer: Papanicolaou testing alone or with human papillomavirus testing. *JAMA Intern Med,* May 5. doi: 10.1001/ jamainternmed.2014.1368.

Tria Tirona, M. (2013). Breast cancer screening update. *Am Fam Phys*, 87(4), 274–278.

van Meerbeeck, J. P., Fennell, D. A., & De Ruysscher, D. K. (2011). Small-cell lung cancer. *Lancet*, 378(9804), 1741–1755.

Wesolowski, R., & Budd, G. T. (2010). A young woman with a breast mass: what every internist should know. *Cleve Clin J Med*, 77(8), 537–546.

Wilkinson, J. E. (2011). Effect of mammography on breast cancer mortality. *Am Fam Phys*, 84(11), 1225–1227.

Wright, J. D., Barrena Medel, N. I., Sehouli, J., Fujiwara, K., & Herzog, T. J. (2012). Contemporary management of endometrial cancer. *Lancet*, 379(9823), 1352–1360.

Yang, D., Khan, S., Sun, Y., et al. (2011). Association of BRCA1 and BRCA2 mutations with survival, chemotherapy sensitivity, and gene mutator phenotype in patients with ovarian cancer. *JAMA*, 306(14), 1557–1565.

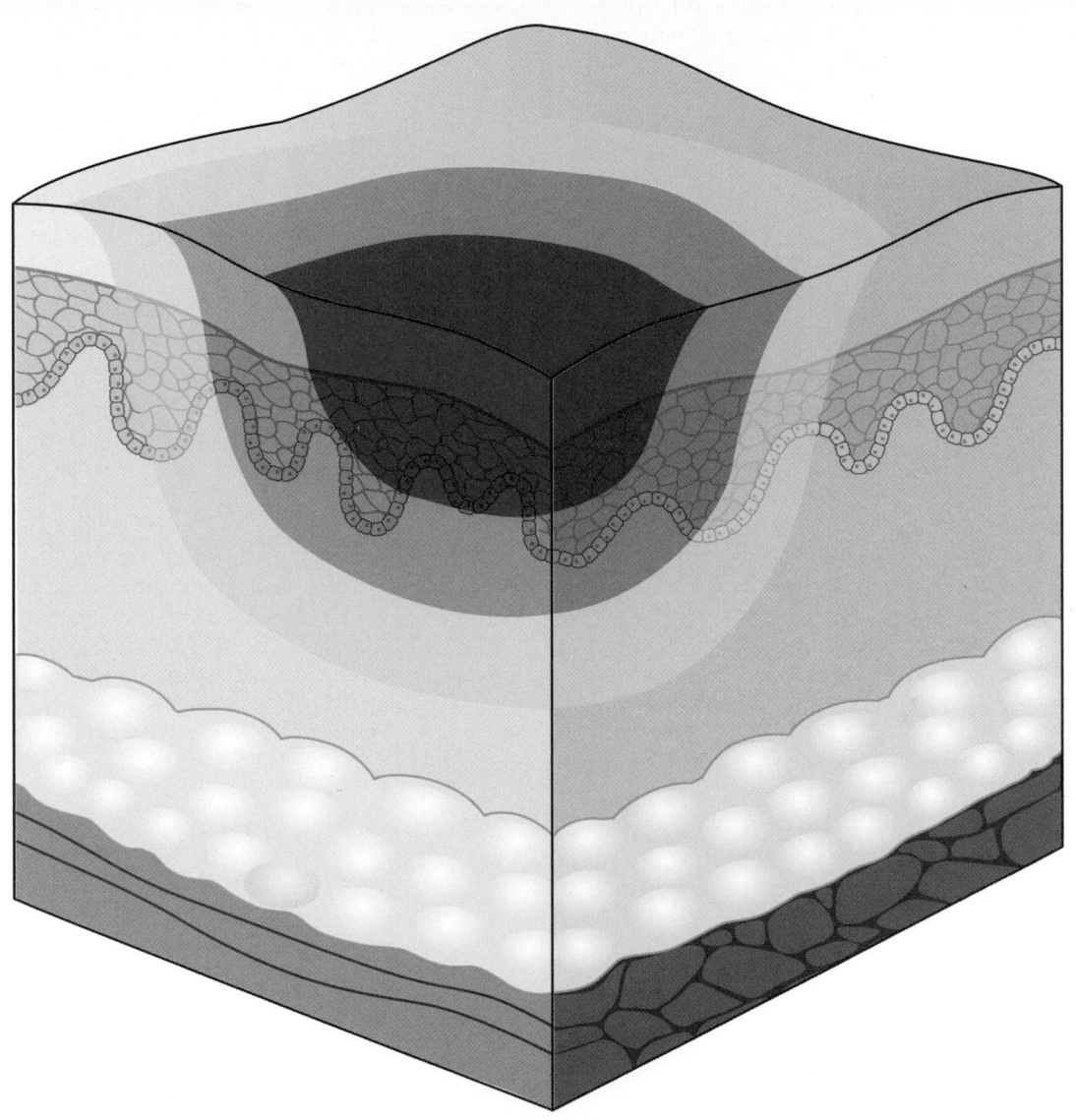

Chapters

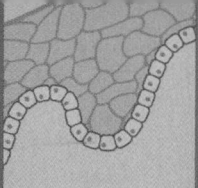

Skin Disorders

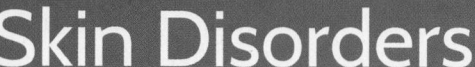

Key Terms

Acne vulgaris	Hymenoptera	Pruritus (itching)
Actinic keratosis	Lentigos	Pulicosis
Angioedema	Lesions	Rash
Basal cell carcinoma	Melasma (chloasma)	Rosacea
Cimex lectularius	Melanoma	Scabies
Comedone	Molluscum contagiosum	Tinea
Dermatophytes	Nevi	Verrucae
Ecchymosis	Onycholysis	Vitiligo
Eczema (atopic dermatitis)	Onychomycosis	Urticaria
Hemangioma	Paronychia	Wood's light
Herald patch	Pediculosis	Xerosis
Hidradenitis suppurativa	Pemphigus	

The integumentary system consists of the layers of the skin—the epidermis, dermis, and subcutaneous tissue—that connect the dermis to muscles and accessory structures. The skin, the body's largest and most visible organ, comprises about 16% of body weight and encompasses about 20 square feet. Its thickness varies from 0.5 mm on the eyelids to 4.0 mm on the soles of the feet. The skin contains many tissues, cell types, and specialized structures, and mediates many aspects of life. It includes associated tissue such as the hair, nails, and sebaceous and sweat glands. The skin reflects ancestral background and expresses genetic structures, race, age, gender, health, and identity. It also gives evidence of environmental exposure, lifestyle, nutrition, and medication use. The skin is a vital organ that establishes identity and maintains boundaries between the person and the environment.

Epidemiology

Approximately 30% of all Americans have a skin condition, ranging from inflammatory and infectious lesions to skin cancers. With age, skin disorders become more likely. For example, it is estimated that more than 90% of older adults have some form of skin disorder.

 CLINICAL CONCEPT

Approximately half of all primary care visits are for skin conditions.

Persons with skin diseases usually seek help from primary care providers or dermatologists in community-based settings.

Basic Concepts Related to the Skin

The skin is accessible and easily biopsied. Health assessments begin with an examination of the skin because the skin provides clinicians with data about health status, age, and systemic disease. Usually skin examinations focus on the top layer of skin, the epidermis, to determine the skin's health, as well as the person's general health.

The Functions of the Skin and Related Tissue

The skin performs vital physiologic functions that correlate with specific properties of the epidermis, dermis, and subcutaneous tissue. These functions include:

- temperature control and regulation
- barrier protection
- secretion and absorption
- vitamin D production
- immunological surveillance.

The skin also acts as a mirror for internal disease processes and serves as an indicator of one's general health.

Temperature Control and Regulation

About 80% of heat loss occurs via the skin. The skin plays a major role in temperature regulation, maintaining a constant body temperature of approximately 98.6°F. Extremes of both heat and cold are very dangerous, increasing the risk of organ failure and death.

Temperature sensors in the skin send information about body temperature to the hypothalamus, the temperature-regulating center in the brain. The brain then "feeds" information to the skin's sweat glands and blood vessels. If the message from the hypothalamus is to cool the body, the sweat glands excrete sweat, a mildly salty substance, onto the skin's surface. As the water in the sweat evaporates, the body cools. In response to hypothalamic stimulation to cool the body, the capillaries, small blood vessels near the surface of the skin, dilate. Heat is lost directly through the skin through radiation and conduction.

If the hypothalamus senses hypothermia, it sends messages to heat the body. The tiny erector muscles of the skin contract, raising small hairs on the skin. This effect traps air and provides insulation that reduces heat loss. Shivering occurs as the body tries to increase its metabolic rate and raise its temperature. Superficial blood vessels also constrict, pulling blood away from the skin's surface and reducing heat loss.

Temperature-regulating systems in the skin can become impaired or overwhelmed by extreme environmental temperature changes. For example, hypothermia occurs after prolonged exposure to frigid water or air. Low environmental temperatures cause severe prolonged constriction of blood vessels that can lead to local ischemia of the skin or frostbite.

Conversely, heat stroke or heat exhaustion can occur because of exposure to high temperatures, such as those greater than body temperature. Heat stroke occurs because of the widespread vasodilation and loss of fluids that occur in extreme heat. As the body tries to cool itself, severe hypotension or shock can occur. Both extremes of temperature challenge the body's restorative powers; if untreated, they can cause death.

Barrier Protection

The skin forms a natural barrier protecting the body from injury and infection, as well as physical, chemical, and environmental hazards. A flora of harmless bacteria coupled with a thin layer of lipid film formed from sweat and sebaceous secretions covers the skin, repels virulent strains of bacteria, and protects the body from infection. The surface film and the thick surface layer called the stratum corneum stop antigens from entering the body and keep the body waterproof even when it is submerged in water.

Excretion and Absorption

By influencing the composition and volume of sweat, the skin influences total fluid volume and the quantity of excreted waste products, notably uric acid, ammonia, and urea. Of course, the skin plays a minor role in excretion when compared with the kidney and the lungs. Primarily, it removes water, heat, salt, carbon dioxide, ammonia, and urea from the body. Although the skin is almost waterproof, it plays a role in absorption. Fat-soluble substances, such as vitamins A, D, E, and K, penetrate the skin. Oxygen, carbon dioxide, and other gases also permeate the skin, along with organic solvents such as acetone; carbon tetrachloride; salts of heavy metals like arsenic, lead, and mercury; and the oils of poison ivy and oak. Medication absorption can occur through the skin because of its permeability to fat-soluble substances.

Vitamin D Production

The interaction of ultraviolet (UV) light with the skin is a major factor in vitamin D synthesis. The first step in the production of vitamin D occurs in the skin when the chemical 7-dehydrocholesterol is converted into a precursor of vitamin D, cholecalciferol. Further synthesis occurs in the liver and the kidney. Vitamin D regulates calcium and phosphorus metabolism, facilitates calcium absorption from the intestine, and affects bone cell development.

Immunological Surveillance

The skin provides the first barrier in the body's immunological defense. It is a major aspect of the innate immunological response offering a nonspecific kind of protection against all antigens. Skin surface enzymes, acids, waxy sebum, and other substances act together to repel pathogens that try to enter the body via the skin. Keratinocytes, surface layer epidermal cells, regulate the immunological response and secrete inflammatory mediators. Langerhans cells detect foreign antigens that have penetrated the epidermis and present antigens to the lymphocytes that take part in the adaptive immunological response.

Mirror for Internal Disease Processes

The skin exhibits the body's internal processes, particularly the body's immunological activity. Urticaria, wheals, blisters, bullae, and various other kinds of inflammatory lesions appear on the skin's surface. These are external signs of the immune response that is actively occurring below the skin's surface.

Some systemic diseases manifest themselves via skin lesions, which are often external signs of disease and can assist in diagnosis. Syphilis is signaled by an asymptomatic rash that resolves; the next lesion, a distinctive chancre, usually appears in the genital area. A Herald patch precedes pityriasis rosea. Kaposi's sarcoma presents as purplish, red-purple-brown plaques and nodules that is an AIDS defining illness. Clinicians closely examine rashes in school-age children to detect the viral exanthems: rubella, measles, chickenpox, or fifth's disease. Rashes on the skin also can indicate drug intolerance, allergic reactions, or communicable diseases.

Indicator of General Health

The skin, the most visible of organs, provides information about itself and the rest of the body. For example, changes in the skin's color and that of the nailbeds reflect circulation and may indicate diseases of the heart, liver, or blood cell synthesis. Persons who lack sufficient oxygen become blue or cyanotic. If bilirubin builds up in the blood, the skin becomes yellow or jaundiced. Erythema, or extreme redness of the skin, reflects capillary engorgement, whereas pallor, extreme paleness of the skin, indicates anemia or shock. A bruise or an **ecchymosis** can exhibit various colors from reddish to brown to yellow green. A diet with high amounts of beta carotene-containing foods like carrots can turn the skin orange.

Assessment

In a comprehensive assessment, the entire skin surface is examined and any evidence of a skin disorder is documented. Initially, the patient's skin should be viewed from a distance of 4 to 6 feet so the distribution and pattern of lesions can be clearly seen. Abnormal skin is compared with normal skin; specific lesions are visualized and palpated with a gloved hand to determine their color, size, texture, consistency, and the presence of scales, inflammation, or edema. Lesions should be described and measured for documentation. A skin lesion can be marked so that the size of the lesion can be measured and monitored throughout treatment. Sometimes lesions are scraped, biopsied, or cultured. These specimens are visualized, perhaps with the assistance of a UV **Wood's light,** or sent to the laboratory for further analysis.

As part of the integumentary examination, it is important to conduct a complete history that elicits information about:

- initial appearance of lesions
- symptoms associated with eruption
- history of allergies
- medication use
- exposure to insects, irritants, or UV light
- other associated systemic symptoms
- current or previous illnesses
- presence of photosensitivity
- remedies the patient has used to treat skin lesions.

Persons with histories of skin diseases, hospitalized patients, and nursing home residents should have frequent skin assessments.

 CLINICAL CONCEPT

It is important that the clinician remembers that no two skin disorders look exactly alike; their classic presentations may be distorted by scratching, swelling, infection, or self-treatment. Skin color also affects the appearance of skin diseases.

A common distinction utilized in describing skin lesions is the difference between a rash and a lesion. A **rash** is a temporary eruption of the skin associated with systemic disease, heat, irritation, allergy, or a response to drug therapy. **Lesions** are traumatic or pathological loss of normal skin continuity, structure, or function.

 CLINICAL CONCEPT

It is important to mark the borders of skin lesions so that changes in the lesions can be measured and therapy can be evaluated.

Clinicians should begin the diagnostic analysis with a graphic description of the presenting skin lesion (see Box 41-1).

Basic Pathophysiologic Concepts of Common Skin Disorders

Skin can be described in terms of color, texture, turgor, tenderness, temperature, moisture, and any secretion that is released. Pathological changes of the skin can

---

BOX 41-1. Terms Commonly Used to Describe Skin Lesions

Terms commonly used to describe skin lesions include the following:

- Atrophy: thinning and loss of skin layers
- Bulla: large blister (greater than 0.5 cm in diameter)
- Crust: dried yellowish and yellow-brown exudate on the skin
- Erythema: reddened skin; area blanches with pressure
- Excoriation: scratch that breaks the skin's surface
- Fissure: crack in the skin that breaks through keratin
- Induration: hardening or thickening of the skin
- Keloid: irregular, elevated scar tissue formed by excessive collagen growth during wound healing
- Lichenification: hardening or thickening of the skin with markings; lichenification develops from repeated trauma such as scratching
- Macule: defined, flat area of altered pigmentation
- Nodule: solid lump greater than 0.5 cm in diameter
- Papule: raised, well-defined lesion, usually smaller than 0.5 cm in diameter
- Plaque: raised, flat-topped lesion, usually greater than 2 cm in diameter
- Purpura: purplish lesion caused by free red blood cells in the skin; does not blanch on pressure and may be nodular
- Pustule: papule filled with pus
- Scale: fragment of dry skin
- Scar: permanent replacement of normal skin with connective tissue
- Telangiectasia: fine, irregular red lines produced by dilatation of the capillaries
- Ulcer: loss of epidermal and dermal tissue
- Vesicle (blister): blister smaller than 0.5 cm in diameter
- Wheals/urticaria: transient pink, itchy, elevated papules that evolve into irregular red maculo-papular patches.

affect all of these qualities. Also, the intactness of the skin is important for full protection from pathogens. Open skin areas are vulnerable to infection. Skin, nails, and hair can develop primary disorders or they can display manifestations of an inner pathological process. Sweat glands beneath the skin cool the body, whereas sebaceous glands secrete sebum that protects the skin. However, both sweat and sebaceous glands can dysfunction, which can create problems for the overlying skin.

Disorders of Skin Color

Skin color may reflect systemic disorders or provide clues to the identity of specific lesions. Several disorders significantly affect skin color, including albinism, vitiligo, and melasma.

Albinism, a genetic disorder, deprives skin, hair, and eyes of pigment. It leaves a person with diminished vision and extreme sensitivity to light and UV rays. Individuals with 1 of the 10 types of albinism have pale or pink skin, yellow hair, and very light or pink eyes. Patients lack the pigment melanin; they should use protection from solar radiation and undergo frequent screening for skin malignancies.

Vitiligo is an acquired skin condition characterized by abnormalities in the production of melanin. It presents as a series of discolored patches on the skin (see Fig. 41-1). Appearing suddenly, these patches present as macules of varying sizes with smooth borders. They commonly appear on the face, neck, axillae, and extremities. The lesions are depigmented, itchy, and easily burned by exposure to the sun or UV rays. The exact cause of vitiligo is unknown and no treatment has yet been effective. Vitiligo often occurs with hypothyroidism or other autoimmune diseases.

Melasma, also called chloasma, by contrast, is characterized by the appearance of dark macules on the face. More common in brown-skinned women, melasma commonly occurs during pregnancy and in women who use oral contraceptives. Sun damage can also cause this skin discoloration. Blue-eyed and fair-skinned people reveal sun damage more dramatically than dark-skinned people. Large pigmented spots, called age spots or **lentigos,** appear on fair, sun-damaged areas of the skin, usually on the hands, forearms, and face. As in other disorders of melanin production, preventative measures include limiting sun exposure through the use of sun screening agents. Skin bleaching agents applied to darkened areas of the skin can be used for cosmetic purposes.

Associated structures of the skin also demonstrate a change in color with age. Genetically programmed graying of the hair often begins in the thirties at the temples and then extends to the top of the scalp. Over time, hair color becomes progressively lighter, eventually turning white. Body and facial hair also turn gray, but usually more slowly than scalp hair. Although the consistency and distribution of hair is determined genetically, hair thinning and loss also occur with age.

Disorders of Skin Texture

Skin texture provides another manifestation of its health and integrity. The skin and related tissue, damaged by repeated infections, overexposure to the sun, trauma, or burns, lose elasticity and functional ability. With age, the skin loses tensile strength and becomes less flexible. Changes in connective tissue reduce the skin's elasticity or turgor. This process of skin aging, called elastosis, is more pronounced in sun-damaged skin.

Some specific diseases—scleroderma and pemphigus, for example—are diagnosed by changes in the skin's texture. Acanthosis nigricans, often associated with diabetes, is characterized by a dark, brownish-black velvety thickening of the skin.

Dry skin, **xerosis,** is a common dermatological complaint. Dry skin appears to be rough, scaly, and wrinkled. Skin dryness can be caused by dehydration of the stratum corneum, changes in sebaceous gland secretions, decreased sweat, and a flattening of the epidermal ridges, which reduce the ability of fluids to move between the skin's layers.

Dry skin is more easily bruised and irritated. Because pruritus is the major symptom of dry skin, excoriation of the extremities, abdomen, back, and waist are found on examination of dry skin. Liberal use of moisturizing agents such as emollients, humectants, and occlusives are the major treatment for dry skin. Each of these substances acts differently by replenishing oil on the skin, drawing water from deeper layers of the skin up to the skin's surface, or preventing water loss from the skin. Lotions or creams, which contain camphor, menthol, or benzocaine, are widely used to decrease pruritus. Temperature control and use of room humidifiers are also helpful.

Pruritus (itching) is a common patient complaint. Sometimes the cause of the itching is localized and associated with a rash or an insect bite. Often persons with severe itching suffer sleep disturbances. At times there are no objective data to explain the itching. This manifestation of itching, which is more difficult to

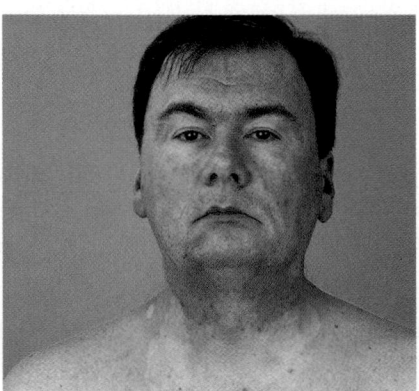

FIGURE 41-1. Vitiligo. (From Dillon, P. (2007). *Nursing health assessment.* 2nd ed. Philadelphia, PA: F.A. Davis Company, with permission.)

diagnose and treat, may be a sign of a systemic illness, such as liver failure, or it may be psychogenic in origin.

Discontinuing drugs known to cause itchy skin or removal of offending agents is usually the first remedy. Treatment addresses the underlying cause of the itching if it can be identified. Local treatment relies on creams, lotions, and antihistamines. Excoriated skin can become infected, so it is important to address pruritus.

Disorders of the Hair

Hair is an extension of the skin that can reflect metabolic changes. For example, hair texture can change with disorders of the thyroid, disruption of sex hormones, nutritional deficiencies, and physiologic aging. Hair loss is the most common disorder of the hair and can be congenital, genetic, or acquired. Four types of hair loss account for 95% of visits to dermatologists:

1. male and female pattern baldness
2. telogen effluvium
3. chemical overprocessing
4. alopecia areata.

Male and Female Pattern Baldness
Male pattern baldness, which can begin at any age, is usually genetic and influenced by male hormones. Typically, the hair loss is on the front, sides, and crown of the head. Female pattern baldness is less common and involves a thinning of hair over the entire head. Conversely, hirsutism, a type of male pattern hair growth, is often seen in women because of increased androgenic hormones.

Telogen Effluvium
Telogen effluvium, a poorly understood condition, affects the growing or resting cycle of hair follicles. In telogen effluvium, the number of resting follicles increases and the number of growing follicles decreases. The result is a generalized thinning of hair over the entire scalp. This reversible type of hair loss is often associated with chronic stress and nutritional deficiencies.

Chemical Overprocessing
Chemical overprocessing, a common cause of hair loss, follows efforts to change the color, quality, texture, and style of hair by curling, straightening, braiding, rinsing, dying, and tinting. Treatment is aimed at discontinuing the processes that stimulated the hair loss.

Alopecia Areata
Alopecia areata is sudden loss of hair in one area of the scalp. The cause is unknown, and usually the hair grows back in several months. A diagnostic tool for hair loss, the hair pull test, provides clues to the amount of hair that is being shed. Often clinicians biopsy the skin in the thin or bald areas or check for fungal or bacterial infections because some hair loss is caused by scalp ringworm.

Although hair loss secondary to radiation or chemotherapy is not identified as a major type of hair loss, it is common in patients undergoing these treatments. Following cessation of treatment, the hair usually returns.

Disorders of the Nails

Nails can be the target of infection or can reflect nutritional status, metabolic changes of the body, or systemic illness. Chronic hypoxia, celiac disease, cirrhosis, malignancies, or inflammatory bowel disease can cause clubbing of the nails where the nails become convex and fingertips thicken. Clubbed fingernails exhibit Schamroth sign: obliteration of the diamond-shaped space at the proximal end of the nail when the distal phalangeal bones are opposed.

Chronic illness can cause pitting of the nails or depressions called Beau's lines. Pitting is commonly associated with psoriasis, whereas Beau's lines are transverse linear depressions across the nail that can also be caused by trauma or Raynaud's syndrome. Spooning of nails, also called koilonychia, can occur in thyroid or liver disorders, cardiovascular disease, or iron deficiency. Splinter hemorrhages of the nails occur in endocarditis. Yellow nail syndrome, where nails thicken and discolor, occurs in rheumatoid arthritis, immunodeficiency, malignancies, or pulmonary problems. Onycholysis, where the nails separate from the nailbeds, can occur in thyroid or autoimmune disease. An obvious black region under the nail can indicate melanoma beneath the nail or subungual hemorrhage caused by trauma. Persons often show short white lines in the nail, called leukonychia, which may be caused by trauma to the nail. Similar to leukonychia are Muehrcke's lines, which are transverse white lines that span the nail width and are indicative of hypoalbuminemia.

Bacterial or fungal infection is the most common cause of nail disease. When the paronychial fold, a seal between the nail plate and the surrounding tissue, is broken, bacteria and fungi can invade the tissue, producing pain, redness, and swelling called a **paronychia**. An acute paronychia is most often caused by *Staphylococcus aureus* and an abscess is commonly present. Chronic paronychias are commonly caused by Candida (yeast) infection.

Onychomycosis is the term for a fungal or yeast infection that involves the proximal and lateral nailfolds. *Pseudomonas* bacteria can also infect the space between the nail plate and the nailbed. Like other organisms that invade the paronychial fold, *Pseudomonas* thrive on moisture. Most infectious agents discolor the nails, causing them to darken; the degree of discoloration indicates the depth of the infection (see Fig. 41-2). A bacterial or fungal invasion may be deep enough to cause the nail plate to separate from the nailbed, a process called **onycholysis**.

Disorders of the Sweat Glands

Two common conditions of the sweat glands are hyperhidrosis, which is excessive sweat production, and

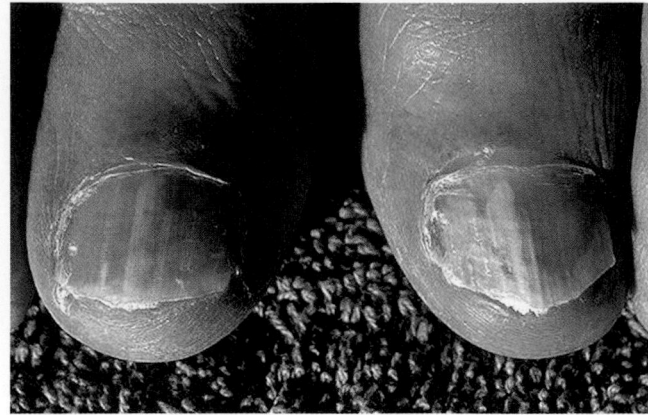

FIGURE 41-2. Finger with onychomycosis infection. *(Courtesy of CDC/Dr. Edwin P. Ewing, Jr.)*

anhidrosis, which is decreased sweat production. Hidradenitis suppurativa is a chronic inflammatory condition affecting sweat glands in the axilla and groin.

Hyperhidrosis

Hyperhidrosis may be related to physiologic, pathological, or endocrine factors; brain trauma; or drug therapy. Often excessive sweat production is localized to the palms, soles, and axilla. Physiologically, sweat is produced in response to emotions; pain; fear and stress; hot, humid environments; work; and exercise. Pathologically, it is associated with febrile diseases, hyperthyroidism, and diabetes. Trauma to the hypothalamus or its tracts can interfere with heat regulation mechanisms and produce excessive sweating. Sympathomimetic (sympathetic stimulant) drugs and drugs that affect the hypothalamus also lead to sweating.

Anhidrosis

It is not uncommon for newborn and premature infants to exhibit anhidrosis for several weeks after birth. In adults, the causes of diminished sweat production include head injuries, tumors, occlusion of the sweat ducts, degeneration of peripheral sympathetic fibers as seen in peripheral neuritis, atrophy caused by burns and radiotherapy, and the use of anticholinergic (antiparasympathetic) drugs.

Hidradenitis suppurativa is a disorder of the apocrine sweat glands, which are present in the axilla and groin areas. In this disorder, there is plugging or clogging of the gland openings onto the skin. The glands become obstructed and inflamed, and tender areas of swelling develop under the arm or in the groin. Bacterial infection is common, causing a purulent exudate that drains from the swollen, erythematous, tender glands onto the skin surface. Hidradenitis suppurativa is often a chronic disorder that occurs as remissions and exacerbations. Obesity, stress, and poor hygiene will make the glandular swellings worse. Chronic exacerbations can cause glandular swellings to develop fibrotic scar tissue.

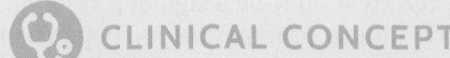

CLINICAL CONCEPT

Antibacterial soap should be used to wash the areas daily, and anti-inflammatory agents such as ibuprofen can be used to decrease the swelling and pain. Shaving of the area should be avoided because this can make the lesions worse.

Medical treatment consists of oral antibiotics as well as topical or intralesional injections of antibiotics. Retin A and Accutane (synthetic forms of vitamin A) have also been used with some success. If medical treatment is ineffective, surgical incision and drainage of the swollen, glandular regions is common.

Disorders of the Sebaceous Glands

Acne vulgaris, a common multifactored inflammatory disorder of the sebaceous glands, affects 85% of the population between the ages of 12 to 25 years. Its lesions are inflammatory papules, pustules, nodules, noninflammatory open or closed comedones, and cysts. A **comedone,** the prototypical lesion in acne, is a plug of sebaceous and necrotic cellular material within the opening of a hair follicle. The follicle may be open (blackhead) or almost closed (whitehead). The lesions most commonly appear on exposed areas of the face, chest, and back.

Acne is more common at puberty because hormones stimulate the sebaceous glands. However, it is not unusual for young adults in their late twenties to develop acne. *Propionibacterium acnes (P. acnes)* colonize the lesions of acne. Topical agents and oral antibiotics are often required to counteract acne. Accutane, a synthetic form of vitamin A, has been very effective in severe acne; however, because of its side effects of depression, it is used with caution.

Acne rosacea, often seen in middle-age adults, appears as erythematous papules and pustules. Usually these lesions, which are associated with inappropriate vasodilation, appear in the middle third of the face but may extend to the forehead and chin. When the inflammatory process of **rosacea** affects the nose, it produces an unsightly, irreversible swelling and inflammation called rhinophyma. Heat exposure and alcohol consumption accentuate the vasodilation and inflammation of this disease. Although the exact cause of acne rosacea is unknown, it is thought that this inflammation of the sebaceous glands results from infection or from an immune-related response. Sunscreen lotions and protective coverings are recommended. In severe cases, oral antibiotic therapy is used.

Birthmarks and Developmental Conditions Affecting the Skin

Birthmarks are skin lesions that are present at birth or develop in infancy. **Hemangiomas,** benign tumors of blood vessels, are apparent in 30% of newborns, with females more likely to be affected. Port-wine stains are permanent blood vessel abnormalities affecting 0.5% of the population. At birth, these lesions look like pink patches; as the child ages, the birthmark darkens and becomes larger. Strawberry hemangiomas, by contrast, are enlarged blood vessels that grow rapidly after birth and resolve by 6 years of age. Spider veins are enlarged blood vessels that grow with age. A Mongolian spot is a benign darkened area of skin commonly on the back or buttocks.

Treatment

Many persons treat their skin problems with over-the-counter preparations before consulting a health-care provider. Treatments are directed at the etiology of the skin eruption as well as its symptoms. Suspicious lesions are biopsied and may be removed or treated with laser surgery. Inflammatory lesions are treated initially with steroidal creams; if the inflammation is severe, short-term oral steroid therapy is used. Skin infections are treated with topical antibiotic creams. If the infection spreads locally or if the patient develops systemic symptoms of infection, oral or intravenous antibiotics are used. Treatment of systemic disease, manifested on the skin, is directed to treating the primary disease. When the skin condition is psychogenic in origin, drugs that treat anxiety or depression, as well as psychotherapy, are combined with treatment of the skin lesions.

Of course, preventive treatment of skin disorders is the first step to maintaining healthy skin. Prevention involves protection of the skin and underlying tissues from environmental hazards, UV rays, injuries, sustained pressure, infections, and bites. One of the key preventive treatments of the skin is protection from the sun. Melanoma, basal cell carcinoma, and squamous cell carcinoma (SCC), the three most serious skin conditions, are all associated with sun overexposure.

Selected Precancerous Skin Disorders

There are several different types of precancerous skin lesions. They are common on the sun-exposed areas of the body, particularly the facial areas. Nevi, actinic keratosis, and lentigos are lesions that should be periodically assessed as these can undergo cancerous changes.

Nevi

Nevi, or moles, are probably the most common benign skin tumors. These lesions, which can be pigmented or depigmented, develop from melanocytes during childhood, usually between 3 to 5 years of age. They present as papules and nodules and vary in size. Atypical or dysplastic nevi are those that are irregular in shape, variegated in color, and have a high susceptibility to cancerous change. These lesions require clinical examination to rule out skin cancer. Persons with a high number of nevi on the body should consult a dermatologist periodically for a whole body skin assessment.

Actinic Keratosis and Lentigos

Actinic keratosis, a premalignant lesion found on skin that has been damaged by the sun's ultraviolet rays, is common in fair-skinned persons. The lesions present as patches of rough, scaly, red plaques. The surrounding tissues are red and may show telangiectasia (branches of delicate capillaries). Lentigos, premalignant skin lesions, usually appear as brown spots on sun-exposed areas. Commonly called solar lentigos, liver spots, or age spots, these lesions are benign, but they bear watching because there is also a lentigo maligna that appears as a freckle on sun-exposed areas. Lentigo maligna are pigmented macules with well-defined borders. Slow growing, they can reach a size of 5 cm. Over time, the lesions may become raised and wartlike in appearance. Persons with a high number of actinic keratosis or lentigos on the body should consult a dermatologist periodically for a whole body skin assessment.

ALERT! Any change in size, color, border, or appearance of a nevus can indicate malignant melanoma. A dysplastic nevus can be considered a premalignant stage of melanoma. The lesions of actinic keratosis should be examined and biopsied because they can progress to SCC, a metastatic disease. Lentigo maligna can become malignant melanoma.

Most Common Skin Cancers

Skin cancer is by far the most common type of cancer. Malignant melanoma, basal cell carcinoma, and SCC are the three types of skin cancer. These lesions can begin as premalignant dysplasia. Periodic dermatological examination is necessary to identify their occurrence.

Malignant Melanoma

Melanoma is the most lethal form of skin cancer, killing about one person per hour in the United States. Over the past 40 years, incidence of melanoma has increased 300%. In 2014, there were more than 76,000 cases of melanoma diagnosed and approximately 9,700 persons died from the disease. Caucasian males have the highest rate of contracting melanoma, with an average age of 61 at diagnosis. Melanoma has a 93% 5-year survival rate.

> ### BOX 41-2. Risk Factors for Melanoma
>
> Risk factors for melanoma include:
>
> - fair, sun-sensitive skin that tans poorly or burns easily
> - red or blond hair, and blue or green eyes
> - having 50 to 100 or more moles
> - having unusual or irregular-looking moles that are typically larger in size (may be referred to as dysplastic or atypical moles)
> - history of sunburns or indoor tanning use
> - blood relatives (parents, children, siblings, cousins, aunts, uncles) who have had melanoma
> - immunosuppression caused by disease, organ transplant, or medication
> - history of previous melanoma or another skin cancer
> - 50 years of age or older.

Etiology

Genetic studies are finding a number of defective tumor suppressor genes that are linked to malignant melanoma. One such gene is located at 9 p 21.

Melanoma originates in melanocytes, the cells that produce the pigment melanin, which colors our skin, hair, and eyes. The majority of melanomas are black or brown, but they can also be skin-colored, pink, red, purple, blue, or white. Approximately 30% of melanomas occur in a nevus. Melanoma begins on the surface, but it penetrates deep into the skin, invades the blood and lymphatic vessels, and then metastasizes throughout the body. There are a number of risk factors, but anyone of any skin color can develop melanoma (see Box 41-2).

It is not clear how all melanomas develop, but exposure to UV radiation clearly plays a role, especially in fair-skinned people. A history of sunburns, especially blistering sunburns as a child or teenager, has been shown to increase the risk of developing melanoma. Some inherited traits increase an individual's risk for melanoma, such as dysplastic nevi (precancerous moles), fair skin, light-colored eyes, freckles, and skin that burns easily or tans poorly. There also is evidence that exposure to UV radiation from indoor tanning equipment increases the risk of melanoma.

Most melanomas develop in areas that have had exposure to the sun, such as the upper back, torso, lower legs, head, and neck. Other factors associated with increased risk include a family history of melanoma, presence of an atypical nevus (mole), and immunosuppression.

Pathophysiology

Malignant melanomas are cancers of the melanocytes, which have a radial and vertical growth phase. During the radial growth phase, malignant cells grow in a radial, spreading manner in the epidermis. With time, melanomas progress to the vertical growth phase, where malignant cells invade deep into the dermis and are able to metastasize.

The types of melanoma are superficial spreading melanoma, lentigo maligna melanoma, acral lentiginous melanoma, and nodular melanoma. Seventy percent of melanoma is the superficial spreading type. The superficial, lentigo, and acral lentiginous types begin with skin surface growth before deeper penetration and spread. The lesion enlarges, its borders widen irregularly, and the lesion attains various pigments. During this time, the melanoma can be cured by surgical excision. Nodular melanoma is the most aggressive type, with deep penetrative growth and early metastasis. Between 10% and 15% of melanomas are of the nodular type, and another 10% to 15% are of the lentigo maligna type.

A set of predictable stages predispose individuals to malignant melanoma:

- benign nevus
- dysplastic nevus
- radial growth phase of melanoma
- vertical growth phase of melanoma
- metastatic malignant melanoma.

Clinical Presentation

Noncancerous moles are generally uniform in color, round to oval in shape, and have a well-defined border. In contrast, melanomas tend to have one or more ABCDE traits:

- A: Asymmetry: one half unlike the other
- B: Border: an irregular, scalloped, or poorly defined border
- C: Color: varied from one area to another; shades of tan, brown, and black; sometimes white, red, or blue
- D: Diameter: usually greater than 6 mm, or the size of a pencil eraser, when diagnosed, but they can be smaller
- E: Evolving: a mole or skin lesion that looks different from the rest or is changing in size, shape, or color.

It is important for the clinician to question the patient about his or her family history of melanoma; approximately 10% of melanoma patients report a family history. Familial pancreatic cancer and astrocytoma are frequently associated with melanoma. In addition, familial atypical mole or melanoma syndrome is a disorder that predisposes the patient to multiple dysplastic nevi.

> **ALERT!** A common warning sign of melanoma is change. A change to the shape, color, or diameter of a mole can be a warning sign of melanoma. Other changes that could indicate melanoma include a mole that becomes painful, or begins to bleed or itch.

Diagnosis

The diagnosis of melanoma begins with examination of a suspicious lesion. Careful inspection of the entire skin surface, including the scalp and mucous membranes, is necessary for diagnosis. Palpation of lymph nodes and abdomen are part of the staging examination for melanoma. Suspicious lesions should be biopsied, evaluated by a specialist, and recorded by chart or photography for follow-up. Computer image analyses are often used to appraise suspicious lesions. If melanoma is diagnosed, chest x-ray, computed tomography (CT) scan, magnetic resonance imaging (MRI) scan of the brain, and ultrasound testing of lymph nodes are necessary to look for any evidence of metastases. Positron emission tomography (PET) scan is also commonly used to look for metastases.

Treatment

Treatment typically begins with complete surgical removal of the melanoma and some healthy skin around the growth. This ensures that all cancerous cells are removed. Treatment for melanoma depends on the stage (see Table 41-1).

To stage melanoma, imaging techniques such as x-ray, ultrasound, CT scan, MRI, PET scan, and radioisotopic bone or organ scan are used. A surgical procedure known as a sentinel lymph node biopsy is also recommended to stage melanoma. In staging melanoma, the thicker the lesion or signs of spread, the worse the prognosis. Stage I and II primary tumors that have not spread have an 85% 5-year survival rate. Stage III melanoma has palpable regional lymph nodes and a 50% 5-year survival rate. Stage IV is distant metastatic disease and has a lower than 5% 5-year survival rate. The distant metastasis of melanoma often occurs in the lungs and brain. If testing indicates that melanoma has metastasized to the lymph nodes or other areas, treatment may include additional surgery to remove the cancer, immunotherapy, radiation therapy, chemotherapy, or a combination of treatments. Various melanoma vaccines are currently under investigation. Melanoma patients have a lifelong risk of developing new melanomas; therefore, follow-up examinations are critical.

Basal Cell Carcinoma

Basal cell carcinoma, the most common form of skin cancer, accounts for more than 90% of all skin cancer in the United States. These cancers rarely metastasize to other parts of the body. They can, however, cause damage by growing deeply and invading surrounding tissue.

Light-colored skin and sun exposure are both important factors in the development of basal cell carcinomas. About 20% of these skin cancers, however, occur in areas that are not sun-exposed, such as the chest, back, arms, legs, and scalp. The face, however, remains the most common location for basal cell lesions. UV radiation from the sun is the main cause of basal cell cancer. Artificial sources of UV radiation, such as tanning beds, can also cause this cancer. Most basal cell cancers appear after age 50 years, but the sun's damaging effects begin at an early age.

A basal cell carcinoma usually begins as a small, dome-shaped bump and is often covered by small, superficial blood vessels called telangiectasias. The texture of the lesion is often shiny and translucent, sometimes referred to as "pearly" (see Fig. 41-3). Basal cell carcinomas grow slowly and deeply, taking months or years to become sizable. Similar to melanoma, a biopsy is necessary for diagnosis. Treatment is also similar to melanoma. However, most cases of basal cell cancer can be cured with surgery alone.

Squamous Cell Carcinoma

Of the more than 1 million cases of skin cancer that will be diagnosed in the United States this year, about 20%

| TABLE 41-1. Stages of Melanoma ||
Stage	Description
Stage O; *in situ*	Melanoma that is confined to the epidermis
Stage I–II	Melanoma that is confined to the skin but has increasing thickness; skin may be intact or ulcerated (top layer of skin is absent)
Stage III	Melanoma that has spread to a nearby lymph node and is found in increasing amounts in one or more lymph nodes
Stage IV	Melanoma that has spread to internal organs, beyond the closest lymph nodes to other lymph nodes, or areas of the skin far from the original tumor

(Adapted from http://www.cancer.gov/cancertopics/pdq/treatment/melanoma/Patient/page2.) accessed July 8, 2015

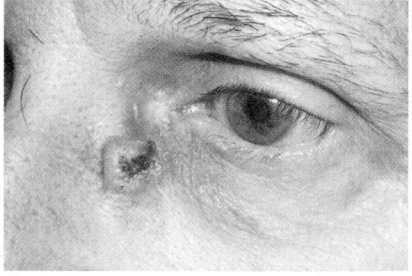

FIGURE 41-3. Basal cell carcinoma. (From Dillon, P. (2007). *Nursing health assessment.* 2nd ed. Philadelphia, PA: F.A. Davis Company, with permission.)

will be SCC. As with melanoma and basal cell carcinoma, most cases of SCC will be caused by exposure to the sun's harmful UV rays. The risk of developing SCC also increases with age because each exposure to UV rays causes more damage to the skin. As this damage accumulates, the risk of developing SCC cancer grows.

SCC appears as a red, crusted, or scaly patch on the skin; a nonhealing ulcer; or a firm red nodule. Some SCCs develop from small, scaly lesions called actinic keratosis, which also are caused by exposure to the sun's UV rays. With early detection and proper treatment, SCC is curable. If allowed to progress, however, SCC can invade and destroy much of the tissue surrounding the cancerous tumor, which can be disfiguring. Some SCCs, such as those that develop on a lip or an ear, can be particularly aggressive. If left untreated, aggressive SCCs have a high risk of metastasis to the lymph nodes and other internal organs. Diagnosis must be confirmed with a biopsy. Treatment options are similar to those of melanoma. Most patients with localized SCC have cure rates that range from 85% to 95% or greater.

Selected Infectious Disorders Affecting the Skin

Bacteria, viruses, fungi, and parasites can cause skin infection. Some microorganisms are normal inhabitants of the skin, such as *Staphylococcus* and *Candida*. With a breach in skin integrity, these organisms, which normally colonize the skin, can cause infection. The most common parasitic infections are caused by lice and scabies. Because these infections commonly do not require medical attention, their incidence and prevalence statistics are difficult to estimate.

Diseases Caused by Fungal Infections

Fungi, or mycoses, are saprophytic plant-like organisms present in the environment and part of the normal skin flora. There are two types of fungi: yeast and mold. Yeast, also known as *Candida albicans*, are single-celled fungi. *Candida* grow in long filaments, called hyphae. All fungi grow in warm, dark, moist areas on animals, plants, and in the soil. Children are often infected by fungi present in the soil, on pets, or by contact with an infected child in day care or school. Hygiene plays a protective role in reducing the incidence of fungal infections, especially in children. Superficial fungi, also called **dermatophytes,** such as **tinea** (ringworm), live on the keratinized tissues of skin, hair, and nails and secrete digestive enzymes that cause skin scaling, nail disintegration, and broken hair (see Box 41-3 and Fig. 41-4).

The pruritus associated with tinea lesions and the associated cosmetic changes in the skin, nails, and hair cause persons to seek diagnosis and treatment. Diagnosis of superficial fungal infections is made clinically by a microscopic examination of scrapings from the

> ### BOX 41-3. **Types of Tinea Infection**
>
> Tinea infections are named for the part of the body they infect:
>
> - Tinea corpora: ringworm of the body
> - Tinea cruris: ringworm of the groin
> - Tinea faciale: ringworm of the face
> - Tinea capitis: ringworm of the scalp
> - Tinea pedis: ringworm of the foot, also called athlete's foot
> - Tinea manus: ringworm of the hand
> - Tinea unguium: ringworm of the nail
> - Tinea versicolor: ringworm of the upper chest, back, or arms.

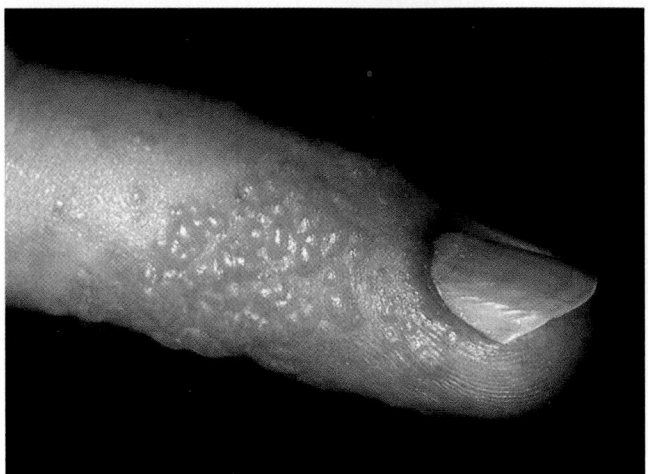

FIGURE 41-4. Tinea. (Courtesy of CDC.)

lesions or by visualizing the lesions with a Wood's light. When viewed under a Wood's light, fungi take on a fluorescent yellow-green appearance. When fungal infections penetrate the keratinized tissue and invade the skin layers, vesicles, redness, and signs of inflammation appear in the affected areas. Invasive fungi can cause septicemia (bloodstream infection) in an immunocompromised individual.

Treatment of superficial fungal infections is simple and involves the use of topical and, in difficult cases, systemic (oral or intravenous) antifungal agents. Most topical agents are over-the-counter preparations. Some persons do not tolerate systemic antifungal agents because these drugs interact with other medications. Toxic reactions to antifungal medication, especially liver toxicity, have also been reported.

Diseases Caused by Viruses

Warts, also called **verrucae,** are benign lesions of the skin caused by the human papilloma virus (HPV). Transmitted by touch, they are round, rough, and gray-colored lesions that can occur anywhere on the body.

Plantar warts, located at pressure points on the feet, usually cause discomfort and are often removed surgically. Genital warts, in contrast, are caused by certain strains of HPV. Seventy-five percent of sexually active adults are infected with genital warts. Women have an 80% chance of contracting HPV genital warts by the time they are 50.

When HPV warts appear on genital areas, they increase the risk of cervical, anal, or rectal cancer. The association between sexual activity, genital warts, and an increased risk of cancer has prompted public health officials to strongly encourage girls to be vaccinated against HPV before the initiation of sexual activity. In 2006, the Food and Drug Administration approved Gardasil, the first vaccine to prevent genital warts and cervical cancer. The vaccine, given in three doses, is licensed for use in individuals aged 13 to 26 years.

Because human immunodeficiency virus (HIV) infections are transmitted sexually, persons with HIV are at risk for HPV warts. In persons with HIV and acquired immune deficiency syndrome (AIDS), warts are large, more numerous, and more uncomfortable than they are in the population that is not HIV-positive. Warts can be prevented, ignored, or removed by freezing, laser treatments or by the application of keratolytics or irritants.

Another viral disease, **molluscum contagiosum,** causes small bumps to appear on the skin. The bumps are smooth, waxy, and small, about the size of a pin, and their central core is filled with a white cheeselike substance. The virus that causes this illness can live in warm water and can be transmitted in spas, baths, and heated swimming pools. In persons with HIV, regardless of their age, the lesions of molluscum contagiosum are more numerous and larger.

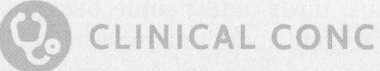

CLINICAL CONCEPT

The vaccine against HPV should be administered to prevent the spread of infection by sexual activity.

Diseases Caused by Arachnoid Bites

Arachnids, which include mites, ticks, and spiders, can cause a number of different skin disorders with their bites, ranging from the benign to the serious.

Mite Bites

Mite bites injure the skin and render it susceptible to other infections. **Scabies,** the disease transmitted by mites, is associated with poverty, malnutrition, and sexual promiscuity around the world. Usually scabies is spread by skin-to-skin contact, but it can also be spread via objects, clothing, and bedding because mites can survive for several days without contact with the skin's blood supply.

Activated by warmth, the female mite finds her way to the bottom of the stratum corneum layer of the skin by creating a tunnel or burrow—a narrow,

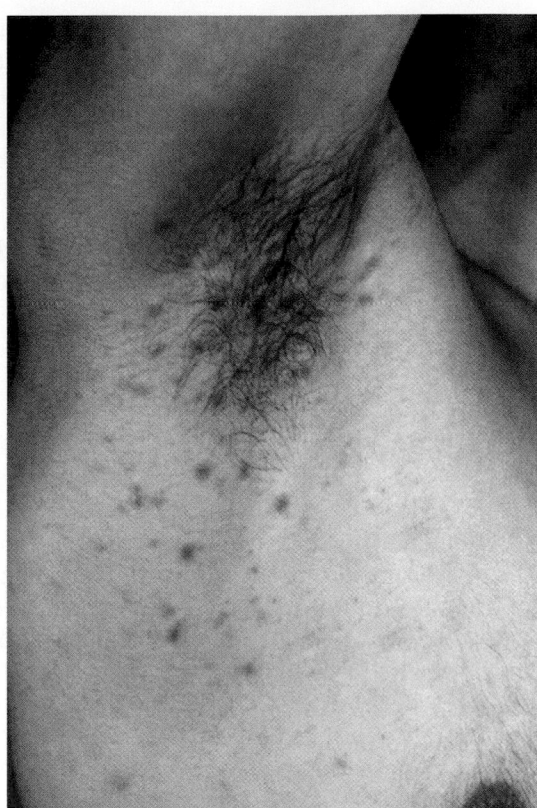

FIGURE 41-5. Scabies. *(Courtesy of CDC/Susan Lindsley.)*

raised irregular channel. Scabies is often suspected when small papules and visible wavy or linear burrows are present on the interdigital webs of the fingers and toes, folds of the skin, nipples, or genitalia. Because the lesions are itchy, the skin around the burrows is usually excoriated (see Fig. 41-5).

Tick Bites

Ticks are insects that live in grasses and bushes, as well as on forest animals, humans, dogs, and cattle. A female tick punctures the skin, sucks blood, and falls to the ground when engorged. Tick bites produce local damage to the skin, which resembles new moles. In some persons, urticarial wheals appear at the site of puncture. A characteristic "bull's eye" type of red rash called erythema migrans, often develops in bites from ticks carrying the microorganism, *Borrelia burgdorferi*. These parasite-carrying ticks can cause Lyme disease after puncturing human skin. Tick bites can produce systemic reactions, such as fever, chills, headache, abdominal pain, and vomiting. It is important to recognize that these symptoms can occur as late as 2 weeks after the original bite. Diseases that tick bites can cause include Lyme disease, Rocky Mountain Spotted Fever, tularemia, and encephalitis. (See Chapter 39: Infection and Inflammatory Disorders of the Musculoskeletal System for more information.)

Spider Bites

Spider bites are common occurrences. They cause pain, redness, itching, swelling, and small puncture wounds.

Although most spider bites are benign, the black widow spider and brown reclusive spider inject toxic substances into the skin. These spider bites present as target marks, pale areas surrounded by red rings. The person who is bitten experiences local itching, rash, and burning and systemic symptoms, which include cramping pain, weakness, fever, sweating, nausea, and vomiting. Severe symptoms include difficulty breathing and increased blood pressure. Children and older adults have more severe symptoms.

Diseases Caused by Insect Bites

Bed Bugs

Bed bugs, known as **cimex lectularius,** are insects associated with a lack of clean mattresses or bedding. They bite children and adults who sleep in unsanitary conditions. Homeless persons are at particular risk of bedbug bites. Although the bite itself is painless, the person awakes to find itchy skin. More careful examination of the skin reveals red wheals arranged in linear patterns (see Fig. 41-6). Because the saliva of bed bugs contains a protein substance, purpuric reactions are not uncommon. Diagnosis of the cause of the skin irritation is made by finding bedbugs in linen or mattresses. Vigorous sanitation of bedding and specific pesticide use are required to kill bed bugs.

Lice

Lice infestation, also called **pediculosis,** is associated with lack of cleanliness. Lice obtain nourishment by attaching themselves to the skin, biting, and sucking blood. They can live on clothing for up to a month. Lice bites produce reddened macules, inflammation, hyperpigmentation, and parallel scratch marks. Although lice bites can cause significant illness—including typhus, relapsing fever, and trench fever—usually they produce itchy skin and social embarrassment.

Lice bites are more common in children, and lice have an affinity for skin that is covered with hair. When lice penetrate the scalp, the hair becomes dry and lacks luster. Scalp itching is a common symptom. Body lice

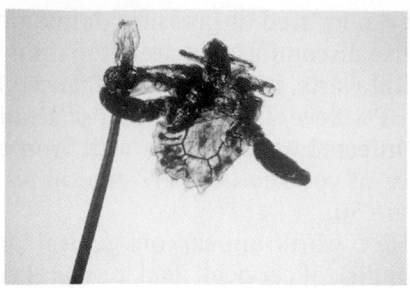

FIGURE 41-7. Head lice. *(Courtesy of Wills Eye Hospital, Philadelphia, PA.)*

is associated with poverty, overcrowding, and poor hygiene. Some lice infections, called pediculosis pubis, are sexually transmitted. If patients have evidence of pubic lice, they should be screened for other sexually transmitted diseases and their sexual contacts should be advised and treated.

Diagnosis of lice is made by finding the lice or lice eggs, called nits, in the clothing, bed linen, or the hair of the person who has been bitten (see Fig. 41-7).

Washing the person, his or her clothing, and the environment is the first step in eradication. Definitive treatment requires the destruction of lice with special soaps, shampoos, and rinses. Fine combs are used to determine if there are nits in hairy parts of the body. Usually this process requires repeated applications of soap, shampoo, or rinse. The eradication process may also require shaving the hair.

Mosquitoes

Mosquito bites are commonly encountered during warm months. The mosquito bite produces a localized, itchy wheal. Sweat attracts mosquitoes, which need protein to produce eggs. Mosquitoes bite horses, cattle, small mammals, birds, and people because of their large skin surface and abundant underlying blood supply. In tropical countries, mosquitoes can carry malaria, yellow fever, dengue fever, and encephalitis. Within the past decade, there have been serious outbreaks of mosquito-borne West Nile viral infections in the United States.

Because mosquitoes can cause serious illness, there are public health initiatives related to eradication of mosquitoes: destruction of breeding grounds, emptying of pools of stagnant water, screening of windows and porches, and spraying of wet lands and grassy breeding areas. In areas where mosquitoes are abundant, mosquito netting, protective clothing, insect repellents, and avoidance of tall grassy areas and stagnant water decrease the incidents of exposure and the number of mosquito bites.

Diseases Caused by Hymenoptera Bites

Hymenoptera bites, which include bites from bees, wasps, and fleas, are another common source of skin injury. These bites cause local inflammation, irritation, swelling, and itching. Some hymenoptera bites trigger

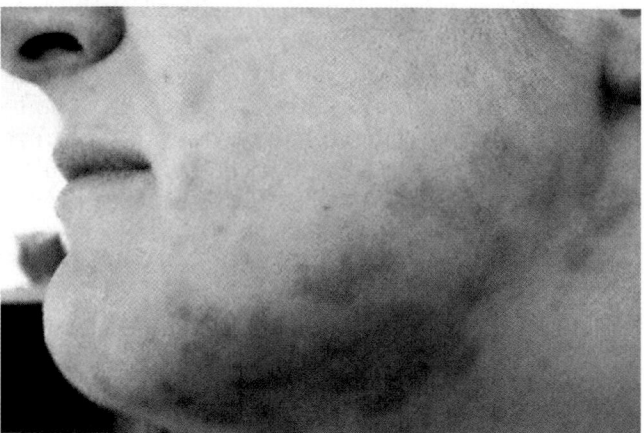

FIGURE 41-6. Bed bug bites. *(Wikipedia: Courtesy of Andy Brookes BSc.)*

the severe allergic reaction termed anaphylaxis. Other reactions result from toxins injected by hymenoptera that penetrate the skin and cause vesicles and bullae formation. Toxins can produce hematologic symptoms, in addition to skin lesions.

Bee and Wasp Stings

Bee and wasp stings are immediately painful, and swelling and itching persist for about a week. A sting can inject poisonous venom into the skin that can reach the blood supply and cause systemic reactions. Serious, even fatal, allergic or anaphylactic reactions can occur immediately or within 1 hour of the sting.

Treatment requires immediate removal of the stinger, if it remains, because it is a source of venom, followed by the application of ice to the area. Persons who continue to have symptoms or show any signs of an anaphylactic reaction, such as hives, should receive prompt medical care.

 CLINICAL CONCEPT

Because a sting is a type of puncture wound, some clinicians recommend tetanus immunization.

ALERT! Persons known to be highly allergic to bee stings should carry self-injectable epinephrine to prevent an anaphylactic reaction.

Flea Bites

Flea bites, known as **pulicosis,** occur when the flea bites its host, most commonly either a human, cat, or dog. Flea bites appear as small, brown lesions, hemorrhagic punctures surrounded by a red, urticarial patch. These bites, which exhibit a zigzag pattern, are usually found around the waist and on the legs. The lesions from the bites are often seen in sets of three (see Fig. 41-8).

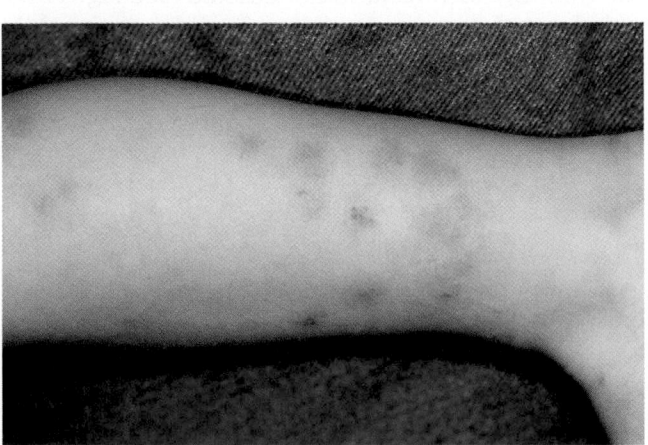

FIGURE 41-8. Flea bites. *(From Scott Camazine/Science Source.)*

Some persons have hypersensitivity responses to flea bites. When disturbed, fleas can jump from one host to another or to rugs, furniture, or bedding and remain in the environment. Pets that go outdoors can transfer fleas to humans. Unsanitary environments are often associated with flea infestation and an increase in bites. Pest control, window screens, removal of garbage and stagnant water, and environmental cleanliness are important modes of preventing flea bites.

Environmental or Physical Injuries Affecting the Skin

Pressure Ulcers

Pressure ulcers, also called decubitus ulcers and bedsores, are the most common of the skin ulcers. Pressure causes diminished blood flow to the skin, especially skin covering bony prominences, which are particularly vulnerable to pressure. If pressure on the skin is released after several hours, the skin is reddened but not damaged. Sustained pressure produces blisters, followed by reddish-blue discoloration, and finally skin breakdown and tissue ulceration, which create opportunities for infection.

Pressure ulcers affect older adults and persons who are immobilized for long periods of time; they are costly, burdensome illnesses. Persons with diabetes are at special risk for all types of skin ulcers because peripheral nerve damage and lack of circulation accompany the disease.

 CLINICAL CONCEPT

Pressure ulcers occur because of sustained pressure on the skin, especially the skin over bony prominences. Change of position and range-of-motion exercises prevent decubitus ulcers.

Stasis Ulcers

Stasis ulcers are also related to diminished circulation and are usually found in the lower extremities. Venous insufficiency, obesity, pregnancy, family history, old age, and blood clotting disorders are factors associated with the development of stasis ulcers.

The process of developing stasis ulcers is subtle; as the valves in the legs become blocked or incompetent, blood flow back to the heart is compromised. As pressure rises in the veins, fluid seeps from the veins into the surrounding tissues. As a consequence of venous blood pooling and accumulation of wastes, the skin in the area becomes darker, thicker, dryer, and itchy. If untreated, these darkened areas of skin become ulcerated and infected.

Loss of sensation, poor circulation, and itching contribute to the development of these easily infected ulcers. Because blood supply is restricted, infected stasis ulcers are difficult to heal.

Tattooing

Tattooing, the practice of placing permanent color into the skin, has been used for centuries in western cultures to decorate the skin. If the tattoo artist uses sterile equipment and aseptic techniques, the procedure is relatively safe. Complications, including secondary infections, are unusual. However, if conditions in the tattoo parlor are unsanitary and equipment is unsterile, infections such as hepatitis B, C, or HIV can be transmitted.

In July 2006, the Centers for Disease Control and Prevention reported 44 cases in three different states of methicillin-resistant *Staphylococcus aureus* (MRSA) skin infections secondary to receiving tattoos. Usually, complications from tattooing present as toxic reactions or immune responses to the pigment in the dye—especially the pigment in red dye. Some persons respond to tattoos by developing granulomas and contact dermatitis. Others find that they experience an exacerbation of existing skin diseases, such as psoriasis or lupus. Tattoo removal is most commonly performed using lasers that break down the ink in the tattoo.

Pattern Injuries

Pattern injuries are bruises, wounds, or those injuries whose shape suggests the instrument that afflicted them, such as belt buckles, irons, or burning cigarettes. These injuries indicate physical abuse. Usually, the history of the injury is inconsistent with its appearance and severity. Clinicians are required to report evidence that a patient has been abused.

> **ALERT!** Patients with suspected pattern injuries should be screened for other signs of physical abuse. Abuse is reportable.

Psychological and Psychiatric Conditions Affecting the Skin

The skin and associated tissues reveal much about the person's emotions and health status. Specialized somatic sensory receptors, located in the dermis, sense and transmit sensations of pain, pressure, touch, and temperature to the brain. When the involuntary erector pili muscles that surround the hair follicles contract, hair literally stands on end. This action conveys fright or adaptation to cold.

Pruritus and purpural (bruising) syndromes are common manifestations of psychogenic skin disease. Often excoriation of the skin from picking, rubbing, scratching, or self-mutilation leads to secondary infections and scarring. A similar manifestation of psychogenic disease is seen in the hair. Trichotillomania is hair loss from repeated urges to pull or twist the hair until it breaks off. Anxiety often reveals itself in obsessive-compulsive behavior such as pulling, twisting, or removing clumps of hair or biting the fingernails.

The sudden appearance of telogen effluvium and alopecia areata, secondary to trauma or surgery, can be psychogenic responses to stress. Persons with psychogenic skin disease seek care for symptoms of skin disease, burning, itching, or pain when there is no clinical, physical, or laboratory evidence to explain these symptoms.

Within the past two decades, biomedical science has enhanced clinicians' understanding of psychogenic skin disease. Often dermatological disorders are manifestations of depression, obsessive-compulsive disorders, anxiety, and pain-prone conditions. Idiopathic pruritus, inflammatory dermatosis, psoriasis, and eczema may also indicate or accompany an underlying emotional disorder. Self-injury, which includes cutting, is often associated with psychological distress.

Treatment of psychogenic skin disorders is aimed at the skin, hair, or nail symptoms, but it is also directed at uncovering and addressing the underlying causes of the skin manifestations. In addition to therapy for the skin disorder, pharmacological agents for depression, anxiety, and obsessive-compulsive behavior; reassurance; psychotherapy; and behavioral and cognitive therapy are helpful.

Eczema and Other Types of Dermatitis

Inflammation or dermatitis characterizes many disorders of the skin, including eczema, contact dermatitis, and seborrheic dermatitis.

Eczema

Eczema, also known as atopic dermatitis, is the most common dermatitis, occurring in two clinical forms: infantile and adult. Vesicle formation, oozing and crusting with excoriation that begins on the cheeks and spreads to the scalp, arms, trunk, and legs, characterizes the infantile manifestation of eczema (see Fig. 41-9). This form of eczema may become milder as the child ages, sometimes disappearing by age 15 years. However,

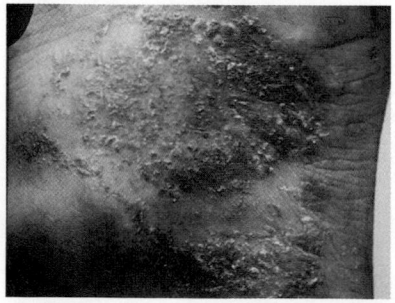

FIGURE 41-9. Eczema. (From Dillon, P. (2007). *Nursing health assessment.* 2nd ed. Philadelphia, PA: F.A. Davis Company, with permission.)

some persons continue to have eczematous lesions and rhinitis throughout their lives. Adolescents and adults with eczema have dry, lichenified lesions that are either hypo- or hyperpigmented; these lesions are usually seen in the antecubital and popliteal areas, spreading to the neck, hands, feet, eyelids, and behind the ears. Because these lesions are itchy, inflammation and infection occur.

Eczema also has a range of clinical presentations: acute, subacute, and chronic. In eczema, there is a recognized interaction among genetic and environmental factors, skin barrier, immune factors, and stress. Persons with eczema often have family histories of asthma or hay fever. The individual has elevated immunoglobulin IgE levels, as it is associated with allergy or type I hypersensitivity reactions. The goal of treatment, usually sought in the acute phase, addresses symptoms such as pruritus, dryness, inflammation, and infection. However, the ultimate therapeutic goal is to keep the eczema in remission. Treatment involves allergen control, good skin care, and avoidance of stress, foods, drinks, and temperature changes that exacerbate the eczema or its symptoms. Topical and occasionally systemic corticosteroids are used. Immune modulators are showing positive results without side effects.

Contact Dermatitis

Contact dermatitis represents delayed hypersensitivity to materials such as metals, chemicals, drugs, and poison ivy. Contact dermatitis affects the head, neck, trunk, arms, hands, abdomen, groin, and lower extremities. This allergic skin reaction usually occurs days after the skin contact with the allergen. Emollients and topical anti-inflammatory medication are standard therapy.

Seborrheic Dermatitis

Seborrheic dermatitis is an inflammation of the skin caused by excessive secretions of the sebaceous glands. Its lesions are red, usually on the face and scalp, and yield yellow to yellow-brown scales known as dandruff. The lesions appear to be greasy, inflamed, and itchy. Removal of scales by frequent washing of the skin and shampooing of the hair provides some relief of this condition.

Papulosquamous Dermatoses

Papulosquamous dermatoses include psoriasis, pityriasis rosea, and lichen planus. They are distinguished by scaling papules and plaques.

Psoriasis

Psoriasis, a genetic, chronic thickening of the epidermis that presents as overlying silver-white scales covering

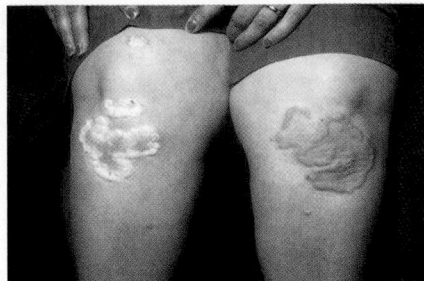

FIGURE 41-10. Psoriasis. (From Dillon, P. (2007). *Nursing health assessment.* 2nd ed. Philadelphia, PA: F.A. Davis Company, with permission.)

red, circumscribed, thickened plaques, is a disease of unknown cause found throughout the world. More common in colder climates, the disease affects fewer than 5% of the American population, although its prevalence increases with age.

Psoriasis is a T cell-mediated autoimmune response to an antigen. Histories of adults with psoriasis reveal that skin trauma, stress, infection, and the use of medications such as plaquenil, angiotensin-converting enzyme inhibitors, and lithium often precede the appearance of psoriasis.

Although the lesions of psoriasis can appear anywhere on the body, they are frequently seen on the extensor surfaces of elbows and knees, as well as on the scalp (see Fig. 41-10). Topical agents, emollients, coal tar products, other agents that soften and hydrate the skin, and steroids are used with varying results. Exposure to sunlight and saltwater baths are known to be helpful. Drugs such as methotrexate, steroids, cyclosporine, and the retinoids are used systemically. Treatment goals center on controlling signs and symptoms of the disease. Treatment varies with the severity of the disease, the age of the patient, and the person's ability to deal with side effects of systemic drug therapy. There is also a link between psoriasis and psoriasis arthritis, a disabling form of arthritis affecting the hands and fingers.

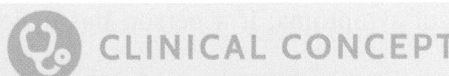

CLINICAL CONCEPT

Psoriasis lesions bleed when the scales are removed. This diagnostic finding, Auspitz sign, differentiates psoriasis from other skin disorders.

Pityriasis Rosea

Pityriasis rosea, an oval, macular, or papular rash surrounded by erythema, appears spontaneously on the skin of young adults. Its cause is unknown, although some infectious agent is suspected because the rash is often found among those who live in close quarters.

The first lesion of pityriasis rosea is a solitary patch, called a **Herald patch,** which usually appears on the neck or trunk. As this lesion enlarges and begins to fade, usually between days 2 and 10, successive patches appear on the neck and trunk. When the patches appear on the back they form a Christmas tree pattern. The patches are itchy, but they clear in 6 to 8 weeks.

Lichen Planus

Lichen planus, from the Greek for tree moss, is a term used to describe flat-topped, small, purple papules with irregular borders, covered with a shiny, white lacelike pattern. It is a common, chronic disease of the skin and mucous membranes, particularly the oral mucosa. The cause is unknown and pruritus is its main symptom when on the skin.

Urticaria and Related Inflammatory Lesions

Acute urticaria is a skin reaction that is commonly caused by allergy. Severe cases of urticaria can include angioedema. Urticaria can also occur as a chronic skin reaction because of an unknown allergen.

Urticaria

Urticaria, or hives, are elevated, pink or red, itchy blotches or plaques of varying size. These lesions, also called wheals, appear suddenly on the skin or mucous membranes and blanch with pressure (see Fig. 41-11). In about 40% of patients, the appearance of urticaria is accompanied by **angioedema,** the swelling of the eyes, face, lips, and the mucous membranes (see Fig. 41-12). Urticaria may occasionally be associated with acute anaphylactic reactions and laryngeal edema.

The release of histamine from the granules of mast cells is the cause of urticaria. Immunological, nonimmunological, physical, and chemical stimuli can cause mast cell degranulation and release histamine into the skin and the circulating blood. The disease classification of either acute or chronic urticaria depends on the duration of symptoms; if a person has urticaria for

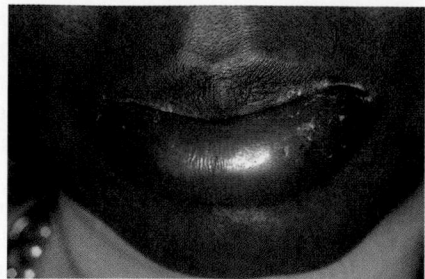

FIGURE 41-12. **Angioedema.** (From Dillon, P. (2007). *Nursing health assessment.* 2nd ed. Philadelphia, PA: F.A. Davis Company, with permission.)

longer than 6 weeks, he or she is considered to have a chronic form of the disease.

Acute urticaria occurs as a discrete, sudden episode often following the ingestion of medicine, food, or drinks, or following insect stings, viral infections, and exposure to dust mites, pollens, and chemicals. Allergy-prone children, especially those with eczema and rhinitis, are particularly susceptible to acute urticaria, which is associated with the ingestion of food or drink. Antihistamines are prescribed in acute urticaria. Injectable epinephrine is used if the swelling is severe, if it involves the mucous membranes, or if it is accompanied by the inability to breathe or by the appearance of shocklike symptoms.

History and allergy testing may determine the trigger of urticaria. Avoidance or discontinuation of the offending agents holds the key to prevention. If the patient's history suggests a food or drink allergy, these substances should be eliminated from the diet immediately. Effort should then be undertaken to discover the chemical or the protein present in the drug, food, or drink that triggered the skin response because this antigen may be the real allergic trigger. In these cases, eliminating one drug or one food or drink may not stop the attacks.

Chronic urticaria affects adults and is twice as common in women as in men. It appears to be an autoimmune disorder, but extensive laboratory work-ups usually fail to identify a causal agent; avoidance of suspect antigens is not helpful. Approximately half of the persons with chronic urticaria have circulating immunoglobulin G antibodies to a subunit of the immunoglobulin E receptor. These antibodies activate the release of histamine from basophils and mast cells. It may manifest an underlying disease, certain cancers, collagen diseases, or hepatitis B.

Physical urticaria is considered to be a chronic form of the disease. These intermittent, short-acting manifestations can be induced by rubbing the skin or by exercise, cold, pressure, sunlight, water, vibration, and heat.

Most types of urticaria are treated with antihistamines that block histamine type 1 and type 2. Leukotriene antagonists may also be prescribed. Local therapy such as oatmeal baths may also be helpful. Persons with histories of angioedema, extreme swelling of the face and throat, should carry injectable epinephrine with them. Oral corticosteroids and antidepressants are used when urticaria persists.

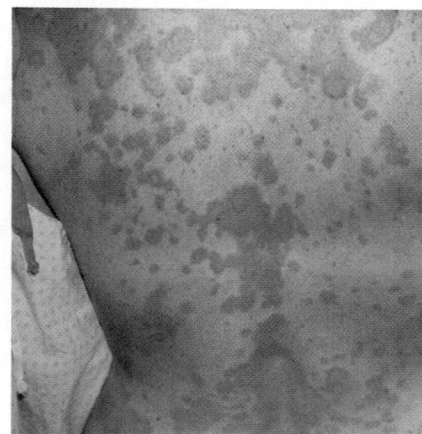

FIGURE 41-11. **Urticaria.** (From Dillon, P. (2007). *Nursing health assessment.* 2nd ed. Philadelphia, PA: F.A. Davis Company, with permission.)

ALERT! Persons with history of angioedema of the airway should carry injectable epinephrine with them.

Disorders Involving the Skin's Blood and Lymphatic Vessels

Vascular lesions are small tumors with chronically dilated blood vessels that arise from the middle to upper dermis. Depending on their size and location, these tumors can be disfiguring.

Senile angiomas are small, asymptomatic, cherry-red, dome-shaped papules that appear on the trunk of elderly individuals. They are a common example of a disorder of the skin's blood vessels.

Telangiectasias appear as a single, dilated capillary. Thought to be genetic, they appear on the face, nose, and other exposed areas likely to be affected by the sun or harsh weather.

Venous lakes appear on exposed areas of the body. They present as small, dark blue papules that resemble the configuration of a lake.

Cutaneous T-cell lymphoma (CTCL), a rare type of non-Hodgkin's lymphoma, presents as either a low-grade or a high-grade lymphoma, based on how rapidly the disease spreads through the lymph system. Unlike other lymphomas in this class, CTCL affects the skin; in 65% of cases, it is caused by a malignant growth of T cells. The cause of CTCL is unknown; diagnosis is made by biopsy. The most common types of CTCL are Mycosis fungoides and Sezary syndrome.

Autoimmune Skin Disorders

Autoimmune diseases are disorders in which the body reacts against itself. The body forms antibodies that attack part of the body. The autoimmune diseases—scleroderma, systemic lupus erythematosus (SLE), pemphigus, and erythema multiforme—have specific dermatological manifestations.

Scleroderma

Scleroderma, an autoimmune disease that occurs more often in women than in men, affects the skin's connective tissue and blood vessels. Beginning as a mild inflammation, the lesions of scleroderma develop into patches of yellow, hardened skin. The disease, which may be localized or generalized, alters the skin's appearance and flexibility and restricts movement. As a systemic disease, scleroderma affects internal organs and can cause cardiac problems. (For more information, see Chapter 11: Disorders of the Immune System.)

Systemic Lupus Erythematosus

SLE, an inflammatory autoimmune disease, can be limited to the skin or become a diffuse multisystem illness. As a skin disease, discoid lupus erythematosus (DLE) is more common in middle-aged women. The lesions of DLE, appearing on exposed areas of the skin, are often seen on the face. Accompanied by photophobia, the classic lesion of DLE presents as a red, plaquelike, asymmetric, butterfly-patterned lesion over the nose and cheeks. Skin biopsies reveal deposits of immunoglobulins, especially IgM in the lesion and surrounding tissues. Lesions last for months, then resolve or atrophy to return again. Persons with DLE often have random hair loss, telangiectasias over the palms and fingers, urticaria, and Raynaud's phenomenon. (For more information, see Chapter 11: Disorders of the Immune System.)

Pemphigus

Pemphigus, a rare, chronic autoimmune disease that is more prevalent between 40 and 50 years of age, causes blisters to form on the epidermis. In some forms of the disease, blisters penetrate deep into the tissues. Caused by circulating IgG auto-antibodies, the blister formation occurs because the auto-antibodies react with intracellular cement, causing a separation in the epidermis. In pemphigus vulgaris, the most common form of the disease, blister formation begins on the oral mucosa or the scalp. As the disease progresses, the flaccid, bullous lesions appear and rupture, leaving crusty, denuded skin.

Erythema Multiforme

Erythema multiforme is an acute, recurring inflammatory disorder of the skin and mucous membranes associated with allergic or toxic reactions to drugs or microorganisms. Erythema multiforme can be a mild or a very serious disease in which immune complex formation and deposits of complement C3, IgM, and fibrinogen develop around superficial dermal vessels, the basement membrane, and keratinocytes. The characteristic "bull's eye" lesion of erythema multiforme appears on the skin as a central, inflamed, red area surrounded by concentric rings of red, swollen tissue. In the vesiculobullous form of the disease, bullae appear on mucous membranes and as plaques on extensor surfaces of the extremities. When these bullae rupture, they leave erosions and crusts. The mouth, airways, esophagus, urethra, and conjunctiva may be involved. Underlying infections need to be treated and the drug or microorganism that triggered the skin's response needs to be identified and eliminated from the patient's life.

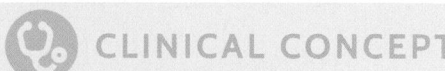

CLINICAL CONCEPT

In children and young adults, erythema multiforme is called toxic epidermal necrolysis or Stevens-Johnson syndrome.

Chapter Summary

- The surface film and the thick surface layer called the stratum corneum stop antigens from entering the body and keep the body waterproof.
- The interaction of UV light with the skin is necessary for vitamin D synthesis.
- A rash is a temporary eruption of the skin associated with childhood diseases, allergies, heat, irritation from clothing, or a response to drug therapy.
- Lesions are traumatic or pathological loss of normal skin continuity, structure, or function.
- Acne is a skin condition caused by propionibacterium.
- Hidradenitis suppurativa is a disorder that causes tender, swollen sweat glands that drain purulent exudate.
- Dysplastic nevi are lesions that are irregular in shape, variegated in color, and have a high susceptibility to cancerous change. These lesions require clinical examination to rule out skin cancer.
- Actinic keratosis, a premalignant lesion found on skin that has been damaged by the UV rays of the sun, is common in fair-skinned persons.
- Malignant melanoma tends to have one or more ABCDE traits: Asymmetry of shape, irregular Borders, Color variation, Diameter more than 6 mm, and a lesion that is Evolving.
- Basal cell carcinoma is the most common form of skin cancer and accounts for more than 90% of all skin cancer in the United States. These cancers, often found on the face, rarely metastasize to other parts of the body. They can, however, cause damage by growing deeply and invading surrounding tissue.
- Light-colored skin and sun exposure are both important factors in the development of malignant melanoma and basal cell carcinomas.
- Superficial fungi live on the keratinized tissues of skin, hair, and nails. When viewed under a Wood's light, fungi take on a fluorescent yellow-green appearance.
- Warts are benign lesions of the skin caused by human papillomavirus (HPV). Plantar warts, located at pressure points on the feet, usually cause discomfort and are often removed surgically. Genital warts are caused by certain strains of HPV.
- Scabies, caused by mites, can be spread by infected clothing, person-to-person contact, or pet-to-human contact.
- A characteristic "bull's eye" type of red rash, called erythema migrans, often develops in bites from ticks carrying the microorganism *B. burgdorferi*. These parasite-carrying ticks can cause Lyme disease after puncturing the skin of humans.
- Bed bugs, known as cimex lectularius, are insects associated with lack of clean mattresses or bedding.
- Lice infestation, also called pediculosis, is associated with lack of cleanliness.
- Bee and wasp stings are associated with anaphylaxis.
- Flea bites occur when the flea bites its host, most commonly either a human, cat, or dog.
- Decubitis ulcers occur because of sustained pressure on the skin, especially the skin over bony prominences.
- Eczema, the most common dermatitis, is characterized by vesicle formation, oozing and crusting with excoriation that begins on the cheeks and spreads to the scalp, arms, trunk, and legs.
- Contact dermatitis represents delayed hypersensitivity to materials such as metals, chemicals, drugs, and poison ivy.
- Psoriasis lesions are erythematous lesions with silvery, white scales that bleed when removed.
- Pityriasis rosea begins as a solitary patch called a Herald patch, which usually appears on the neck or trunk. Successive patches appear on the neck and trunk in a Christmas tree pattern.
- Urticaria (hives) are elevated, pink or red, itchy blotches or plaques of varying size. These lesions can be the first sign of anaphylaxis.
- Urticaria can be accompanied by angioedema, which is swelling of the eyes, face, lips and mucous membranes.
- Erythema multiforme is an acute inflammatory disorder of the skin and mucous membranes associated with allergic or toxic reactions to drugs or microorganisms.
- Scleroderma and SLE are autoimmune diseases, each with characteristic skin changes. Scleroderma causes the skin surface to become extremely tight and shiny.
- SLE causes a characteristic erythematous, "butterfly malar rash" across the cheeks and nose.

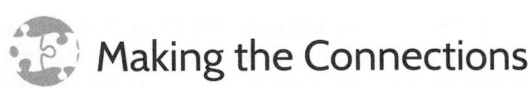
Making the Connections

Disorder and Pathophysiology	Signs and Symptoms	Physical Assessment Findings	Diagnostic Testing	Treatment
Malignant Melanoma | Arises from the melanocytes. Differ in size and shape and may arise from dysplastic nevi or new molelike growths. Slightly raised and brown or black in color. Can appear anywhere on the body and may be slow or rapidly growing.				
	Patient presents with a lesion that has changed in size, shape, and appearance. Lesion is usually asymptomatic, but occasionally pruritus is observed. Cosmetic concerns about appearance of the lesion are frequent. Skin cancers may appear suddenly or develop over time.	Description and comprehensive skin history reveal sun exposure and change of the lesion's appearance in its symmetry, diameter, color, or border. Melanoma **ABCDE** rules: **A:** Asymmetry **B:** Irregular Border **C:** Variable Color **D:** Diameter **E:** Evolving. The general skin examination shows evidence of sun exposure.	Biopsy, with assessment of spread of disease if the biopsy is positive.	Surgery with a wide excision. Cryosurgery, radiation, and chemotherapy. Yearly skin checkup by a dermatologist. Monthly skin self-assessment by patient. Advice about protection from sun rays.
Basal Cell Carcinoma | Arises from the non-keratinizing cells of the basal layer of the epidermis. It is non-metastasizing.				
	Lesion often appears on the face, particularly the nose. Sun-exposed areas are the most common regions of basal cell carcinoma.	Begins as a nodular-cystic, small, pearly, flesh-colored, smooth nodule that enlarges over time.	Biopsy.	Surgery to remove lesion—often needs a very deep excision.
SCC | A more serious epidermal cancer that is aggressive, invasive, and often develops from actinic keratosis.				
	Lesion often appears on face or lips, or can be an oral lesion inside the mouth or on the tongue. Sun-exposed areas are the most common regions of SCC.	Presents as red, scaly, slightly elevated lesions with irregular borders.	Biopsy.	Surgery to remove lesion. Radiation or chemotherapy may be necessary.

Bibliography

Bailey, J., & Whitehair, B. (2010). Topical treatments for chronic plaque psoriasis. *Am Fam Phys*, 81(5), 596.

Bloomquist, L., & Cho, S. (2011). Patient with plaques on lower extremities and systemic symptoms. *Am Fam Phys*, 84(10), 1157–1159.

Bouknight, P., Bowling, A., & Kovach, F. E. (2010). Sunscreen use for skin cancer prevention. *Am Fam Phys*, 82(8), 989–990.

Breen, J. O. (2010). Skin and soft tissue infections in immunocompetent patients. *Am Fam Phys*, 81(7), 893–899.

Dardick, K. (2014). Identifying erythema migrans rash in patients with Lyme disease. *Am Fam Phys,* 89(6), 424.

Davis, M. D., Bundrick, J. B., & Litin, S. C. (2010). Clinical pearls in dermatology. *Mayo Clin Proceed,* 85(9), 855–858.

Dawe, R. S. (2012). Alopecia areata. *N Engl J Med,* 367(3), 279–280.

Drage, L. A., Bundrick, J. B., & Litin, S. C. (2012). Clinical pearls in dermatology. *Mayo Clin Proceed,* 87(7), 695–699.

Durtschi, H. F., & Fargo, M. V. (2010). Infant with vesicular rash. *Am Fam Phys,* 81(9), 1143.

Ely, J. W., & Seabury Stone, M. (2010a). The generalized rash: part I. Differential diagnosis. *Am Fam Phys,* 81(6), 726–734.

Ely, J. W., & Seabury Stone, M. (2010b). The generalized rash: part II. Differential diagnosis. *Am Fam Phys,* 81(6), 735–739.

Firnhaber, J. M. (2012). Diagnosis and treatment of basal cell and squamous cell carcinoma. *Am Fam Phys,* 86(2), 161–168.

Gilhar, A., Etzioni, A., & Paus, R. (2012). Alopecia areata. *N Engl J Med,* 366(16), 1515–1525.

Grotz, T. E., Markovic, S. N., Erickson, L. A., et al. (2011). Mayo Clinic consensus recommendations for the depth of excision in primary cutaneous melanoma. *Mayo Clin Proceed,* 86(6), 522–528.

Halpern, A. C., Marchetti, M. A., & Marghoob, A. A. (2014). Melanoma surveillance in "high-risk" individuals. *JAMA Dermatol.* 2014 Jun 25. doi: 10.1001/jamadermatol .2014.513.

Holland, J., Goldsmith, A., Saitta, P., & Carlson, S. (2011). Arcuate, red plaques with pustules on the trunk. *Am Fam Phys,* 84(12), 1405–1406.

Hsu, W. T., Jones, K., & Peck, J. W. (2011). Rash at the site of a tattoo. *Am Fam Phys,* 84(8), 949–950.

Ivonye, C., Barnes, P., El-Hammali, B., & Nnaji, C. (2012). Generalized red rash. *Am Fam Phys,* 85(3), 271–272.

Jou, P. C., Feldman, R. J., & Tomecki, K. J. (2012). UV protection and sunscreens: what to tell patients. *Cleveland Clin J Med,* 79(6), 427–436.

Kim, A., O'Brien, J., Tseng, L. C., Zhang, S., & Chong, B. F. (2014). Autoantibodies and disease activity in patients with discoid lupus erythematosus. *JAMA Dermatol,* 150(6), 651–654. doi: 10.1001/jamadermatol.2013.8354.

Kumar, V., Abbas, A. K., Fausto, N., & Aster, J. (2010). *Robbins & Cotran pathologic basis of disease.* 8th ed. Philadelphia, PA: WB Saunders.

Kundu, R. V., & Patterson, S. (2013a). Dermatologic conditions in skin of color: part I. Special considerations for common skin disorders. *Am Fam Phys,* 87(12), 850–856.

Kundu, R. V., & Patterson, S. (2013b). Dermatologic conditions in skin of color: part II. Disorders occurring predominately in skin of color. *Am Fam Phys,* 87(12), 859–865.

Lear, J. T. (2014). Evidence-based treatment for low-risk basal cell carcinoma. *Lancet Oncol,* 15(1), 12–13. doi: 10.1016/S1470-2045(13)70582-5. Epub 2013 Dec 11.

Leung, A. K., & Kong, A. Y. (2010). Discrete papules on the thigh of a child. Molluscum contagiosum. *Am Fam Phys,* 81(4), 511.

Lin, K. W., & Sharangpani, R. (2010). Screening for skin cancer. *Am Fam Phys,* 81(12), 1435–1436; quiz 1429.

Longo, D. L., Kasper, D. L., Jameson, J. L., et al. (2011). *Harrison's principles of internal medicine.* 18th ed. New York: McGraw-Hill.

Man, X. Y., & Zheng, M. (2012). Papules, plaques, and nodules in an immunocompromised patient. *JAMA,* 307(4), 404–405.

Margolis, J. S., Abuabara, K., Bilker, W., Hoffstad, O., & Margolis, D. J. (2014, June 1). Persistence of mild to moderate atopic dermatitis. *JAMA Dermatol,* 150(6), 593–600. doi: 10.1001/ jamadermatol.2013.10271.

Mazzarolo, S. S. (2011). Blistering eruption on the leg of an adult. *Am Fam Phys,* 84(2), 231–232.

Melnychuk, I., & Busby, W. (2011). Rash and fever in a college student. *Am Fam Phys,* 84(6), 697–698.

Merchant, F., & Carpenter, T. (2011). Blue-gray discoloration of the skin. *Am Fam Phys,* 84(7), 821–822.

Mulhem, E., & Pinelis, S. (2011). Treatment of nongenital cutaneous warts. *Am Fam Phys,* 84(3), 288–293.

Papp, K., Cather, J. C., Rosoph, L., et al. (2012). Efficacy of apremilast in the treatment of moderate to severe psoriasis: a randomised controlled trial. *Lancet,* 380(9843), 738–746.

Pariser, D. M., Meinking, T. L., Bell, M., & Ryan, W. G. (2012). Topical 0.5% ivermectin lotion for treatment of head lice. *N Engl J Med,* 367(18), 1687–1693. doi: 10.1056/NEJMoa 1200107.

Pickett, H. (2011). Shave and punch biopsy for skin lesions. *Am Fam Phys,* 84(9), 995–1002.

Pluta, R. M., Burke, A. E., & Golub, R. M. (2011). Melanoma. *JAMA,* 305(22), 2368.

Rajan, S. (2012). Skin and soft-tissue infections: classifying and treating a spectrum. *Cleveland Clin J Med,* 79(1), 57–66.

Reamy, B. V., Bunt, C. W., & Fletcher, S. (2011). A diagnostic approach to pruritus. *Am Fam Phys,* 84(2), 195–202.

Reed, K. B., Brewer, J. D., Lohse, C. M., et al. (2012). Increasing incidence of melanoma among young adults: an epidemiological study in Olmsted County, Minnesota. *Mayo Clin Proceed,* 87(4), 328–334.

Robinson, J. K., & Bigby, M. (2011). Prevention of melanoma with regular sunscreen use. *JAMA,* 306(3), 302–303.

Schaefer, P. (2011). Urticaria: evaluation and treatment. *Am Fam Phys,* 83(9), 1078–1084.

Shenenberger, D. W. (2012). Cutaneous malignant melanoma: a primary care perspective. *Am Fam Phys,* 85(2), 161–168.

Silverberg, J. I. (2014, June 1). Persistence of childhood eczema into adulthood. *JAMA Dermatol,* 150(6), 591–592. doi: 10.1001/jamadermatol.2013.10267.

Skin cancer in the USA. (2011). *Lancet,* 378(9802), 1528.

Stern, R. S. (2012). Clinical practice. Exanthematous drug eruptions. *N Engl J Med,* 366(26), 2492–2501.

Thompson, J. F., & Ollila, D. W. (2011). Optimum excision margins for melanoma. *Lancet,* 378(9803), 1608–1610.

Usatine, R. P., & Riojas, M. (2010). Diagnosis and management of contact dermatitis. *Am Fam Phys,* 82(3), 249–255.

Usatine, R. P., & Sandy, N. (2010). Dermatologic emergencies. *Am Fam Phys,* 82(7), 773–780.

Usatine, R. P., & Tinitigan, M. (2011). Diagnosis and treatment of lichen planus. *Am Fam Phys,* 84(1), 53–60.

Villaseñor-Park, J., Wheeler, D., & Grandinetti, L. (2012). Psoriasis: evolving treatment for a complex disease. *Cleveland Clin J Med,* 79(6), 413–423.

West, D. A., & Aires, D. J. (2010). Treatment of actinic keratoses with topical fluorouracil. *Am Fam Phys,* 81(10), 1186.

Wetter, D. A., & Camilleri, M. J. (2010). Clinical, etiologic, and histopathologic features of Stevens-Johnson syndrome during an 8-year period at Mayo Clinic. *Mayo Clin Proceed,* 85(2), 131–138.

Williams, H. C., Dellavalle, R. P., & Garner, S. (2012). Acne vulgaris. *Lancet,* 379(9813), 361–372.

Key Terms

Autografting

Burn shock

Carboxyhemoglobin level

Chemical burn

Debridement

Electrical burn

Eschar

Fasciotomy

Fluid resuscitation

Full-thickness burn

Grafting

Hypermetabolic state

Inhalational injury

Lund and Browder method

Major burn

Minor burn

Moderate burn

Myoglobinuria

Partial-thickness burn

Rad

Rems

Rule of nines

Thermal burn

Total body surface area (TBSA)

Zone of coagulation

Zone of hyperemia

Zone of stasis

Accidental burns, common injuries that can range from mild to life threatening, are the fourth-leading cause of accidental death, after incidents involving falls, motor vehicle accidents and violence.

Although most acute burn injuries are managed on an outpatient basis, severe burns require hospitalization and surgical intervention. They cause a significant amount of pain, scarring, disfigurement, organ dysfunction, and psychological trauma for those affected.

Burns are categorized according to the source that produces the injury, such as thermal, chemical, electrical, or radiation energy. Concern for the harmful effects of radiation injury has increased because of the emerging threat of bioterrorism. Regardless of the etiology, a number of factors determine the magnitude and severity of the burn:

- burn depth
- percentage of the body surface area injured
- age of the patient
- extent of associated systemic involvement.

Prognosis after a burn injury has improved over the last four decades because of an increased understanding of the systemic damage produced by burn trauma and the development of interventions that facilitate wound healing and prevent infection. It is necessary to recognize the clinical features of burn injuries to facilitate prompt treatment, because the quality of care received within the immediate hours after a burn injury is a major determinant of long-term outcome.

Epidemiology

The National Burn Repository is a report based on data from 96 hospitals in 35 states regarding burn injuries between 2004 and 2013. According to the data, approximately 69% of all burn patients were male, and the mean age was 32 years old. Children younger than age 5 years accounted for 19% of burn injuries, and persons 60 years and older accounted for 13%. This is important to note, because children younger than age 5 and adults age 65 and older who suffer a large burn injury are at an increased risk for death.

Among burn injuries reported, 73% occurred in the home; flame or scald burns caused 80% of these cases. Most affected individuals reported burn injuries of less than 10% of **total body surface area (TBSA).** Only a small number of affected individuals reported full-thickness burns and inhalation burns. Deaths from burn injury increased with burn size. Persons with burns of less than 10% TBSA had a 0.6% mortality rate, whereas persons with burns of 50% TBSA had a 37% mortality rate. Those with greater than 90% TBSA had an 84% mortality rate. The most common causes of complications were cellulitis, pneumonia, urinary tract infection, and respiratory failure.

Etiology

Burn trauma can be categorized according to the mechanism of injury, which can be produced by thermal, scald, chemical, electrical, and radiation energy. The etiology is used as a predictor of outcome, but the burn's severity depends upon the degree of heat intensity, duration of contact, and thickness of skin at the point of contact.

Thermal Burns

Thermal burns result after exposure to fire, hot objects, scalding liquids, grease, and steam. They comprise over 90% of all burn traumas and produce damage to the skin and underlying tissues after exposure to temperatures greater than 111.2° F (40°C). Thermal burn injuries can range from superficial, affecting only the epidermis, to full-thickness burns, which injure subdermal tissues.

Flame burns caused by house fires or flammable liquids produce direct tissue injury. If clothing is ignited and composed of synthetic fibers, a full-thickness burn can result as synthetic fibers melt and increase the depth of injury. Flames can create temperatures of thousands of degrees in a confined space, which increases the occurrence of an associated inhalational injury to the airways of the lungs.

Scald Burns

Scald burns occur after exposure from hot liquids or grease and cause tissue necrosis and cellular death within seconds after exposure to temperatures at 158°F (70°C). Because water has a higher specific gravity and is a better conductor of heat than air, a deeper burn can be produced by hot liquids with lower temperatures of 120°F to 130°F. This has prompted many states to mandate that hot water heaters be set below 140°F, which has decreased the incidence of scald burns from hot bath water. The high heat-carrying capacity of steam can also produce significant inhalational injury.

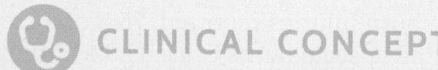

CLINICAL CONCEPT

Accidental scalding from hot liquid produces a characteristic pattern of splashing. A limb that has a circumferential pattern with a demarcation line from the liquid can indicate that the person may have been deliberately burned. Any suspicious history that does not correlate with the appearance of the burn should alert the clinician that abuse might be involved and should be reported.

Chemical Burns

Chemical burns account for fewer than 10% of all burn injuries and generally occur after an industrial accident or ingestion of harsh household chemicals, including strong acids, alkalis, and corrosive materials. Chemical burns induce protein coagulation of tissues (protein breakdown) as chemical energy is converted into thermal energy. This produces a characteristic gray coloring of the skin.

The severity of the response, which can be localized or systemic, is proportional to the type, quantity, and concentration of the chemical, duration of contact, and degree of penetration of the tissues. Chemical agents that are common offenders include sulfuric acid, ammonia, lye, and chemical warfare agents. Exposure to the agent must be halted by removing clothes and vigorously

irrigating the area to decontaminate the patient or neutralizing the chemical agent to limit injury.

Electrical Burns

Electrical burns account for fewer than 10% of all burn trauma and range from mild injury after an electrical shock from a low-voltage household current (110 to 220 volts) to death after exposure to high voltage that exceeds 1,000 volts of energy. The electrical current generates heat when it meets resistance in body tissues and produces damage as the current passes through the body, possibly leaving entrance and exit wounds.

The degree of injury is dependent upon the amount of voltage, length of contact, and pathway of current. Most low-voltage household current produces deep burns at the exit and entrance wounds. High-voltage injury is divided into true high tension and flash injuries produced by a bolt of lightning. Voltage greater than 1,000 volts produces a high-tension injury that causes extensive tissue, muscle, and bone damage and frequently results in loss of limbs. When lightning strikes—a characteristic flash injury lasting only a few milliseconds—it traumatizes the victim. Electricity tends to flow along the path of least resistance toward a natural ground. Nerves and muscles produce less resistance and, therefore, suffer greater damage than tendons, fat, and bones. The pathway of current across the heart is associated with the highest mortality, as the alternating current of the electrical shock disrupts normal cardiac conduction, which can produce cardiac arrest.

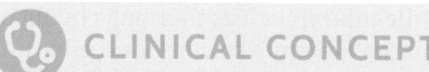

CLINICAL CONCEPT

Electrical injury produces intense tissue damage and cellular death, which can lead to metabolic acidosis. Analysis of arterial blood gases to assess acid-base balance is necessary, and sodium bicarbonate may be needed.

Radiation Burns

The risk of cutaneous injury from radiation burns has increased because of the emerging threat of radiological bioterrorism. Although an emergency response team initially manages this type of disaster, since the September 11, 2001, terrorist attacks against the United States, emphasis has shifted to incorporate the entire hospital in crisis management. Clinicians must be prepared to assess and treat patients who have been exposed to dangerous levels of radiation.

Close proximity to an explosion involving ionizing radioactive material can induce significant harm and produce both thermal burns from the explosion and also internal or external radioactive contamination. External contamination from radioactive material is usually limited to the skin or underlying tissue damage by a layer of clothing, although cutaneous burns might not be immediately visible. It is important to obtain the patient's history to determine the degree of exposure. Some patients may report exposure to radiation or contact with an unknown metal object from industrial exposure, although the onset of visible symptoms can appear weeks after exposure. Radioactive exposure is measured in terms of "rads." A **rad** is a radiation dose of energy absorbed by the tissues, similar to a joule of energy. However, the radiation dose of energy does not indicate the biological risk of the exposure, which is measured in **"rems."** For example, one dental x-ray or chest x-ray causes a biological risk of 4 to 15 millirems, which is considered minor.

Injury to the external and underlying tissues from acute radiation exposure is known as cutaneous radiation injury (CRI). Diagnosis of CRI is based on the scope of visible damage, dose of radiation, and depth of penetration. There are four stages:

1. prodromal stage
2. latent period
3. manifest illness stage
4. third wave of erythema.

The prodromal stage can begin within minutes following intense radiation exposure or can emerge over 2 days with exposure to smaller doses of radiation. Radiation doses as low as 200 rads can damage the hair follicles and basal layer of skin and produce early cutaneous symptoms of pruritis, inflammation, and transient erythema, which might not be evident for days to weeks after initial exposure. This is followed up by the latent period, which is characterized by a lack of symptoms, although cutaneous and systemic damage is still evolving. As the basal cell layer attempts to repair itself, the body enters the manifest illness stage, and severe skin blistering and erythema is observed. If a significant dose of radiation (exposures greater than 1,000 rads) is encountered, then a third phase of cutaneous symptoms known as the third wave of erythema can occur over months or years postexposure. Exposures greater than 1,000 rads produce late effects with permanent damage to hair follicles, sebaceous and sweat glands, and pigment-producing cells. Skin tissue may become fibrotic, then necrotic, and develop ulcers. Usually pain and pigment changes will occur.

Ingestion, inhalation, or entry of radioactive materials via open wounds can induce internal contamination and produce acute radiation syndrome (ARS) if exposure to an excessive dose of penetration radiation occurs over a short time period. Initially, the patient may be asymptomatic, but systemic contamination ensues until treatment is initiated to promote elimination of the radioactive material. Doses of 25 rads produce systemic effects such as bone marrow suppression and the consequent deficient synthesis of blood cells. High doses of radiation can produce aplastic bone marrow, which requires blood transfusion to replace the low blood cell production. Patients exposed to the highest

levels of radiation experience GI symptoms, such as nausea, vomiting, and diarrhea, as well as damage to the central nervous system.

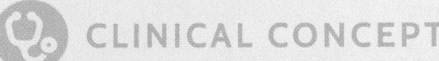

> ### CLINICAL CONCEPT
>
> Initial treatment of ARS focuses on patient decontamination by removing and bagging clothes and shoes, which usually removes greater than 80% of radioactive material.

Gentle irrigation of open wounds helps to minimize internal contamination, whereas irrigation of intact skin helps to decrease further skin abrasion. Localized injuries are treated symptomatically; the Radiation Emergency Assistance Center should be contacted to guide more intensive treatment.

Basic Pathophysiologic Concepts Relating to Burns

Burns cause localized reactions that can be described in terms of three separate zones on the skin. Burns also cause a systemic reaction, which includes hypovolemia and a hypermetabolic state. There are injuries to the pulmonary, gastrointestinal, and renal systems. Persons involved in fire accidents often succumb because of inhalational injury. Burns also impair immunity and increase susceptibility to infection.

Localized and Systemic Responses to Burn Injury

A thermal burn injury produces both a localized and systemic inflammatory response. The localized response consists of three zones of a thermal injury within the skin and subdermal tissues. The deepest point of injury occurs in the **zone of coagulation.** This is the core of the wound with the greatest degree of irreversible tissue necrosis that occurs from protein coagulation and cellular death. The **zone of stasis,** which surrounds the zone of coagulation, is characterized by decreased tissue perfusion with some vascular damage. However, if intervention is aimed at increasing blood flow to this area, minimizing edema and preventing infection, tissue damage is potentially reversible. The outer zone, the **zone of hyperemia,** is reddened from vasodilation and increased blood flow but has minimal tissue damage and heals quickly (see Fig. 42-1).

Normal physiologic organ function is disrupted if the thermal injury is greater than 30% of TBSA. Cellular damage and cell death releases vasoactive substances, including histamine, free radicals, thromboxane, cytokine, and catecholamines, which increase systemic and pulmonary vascular resistance. These vasoactive

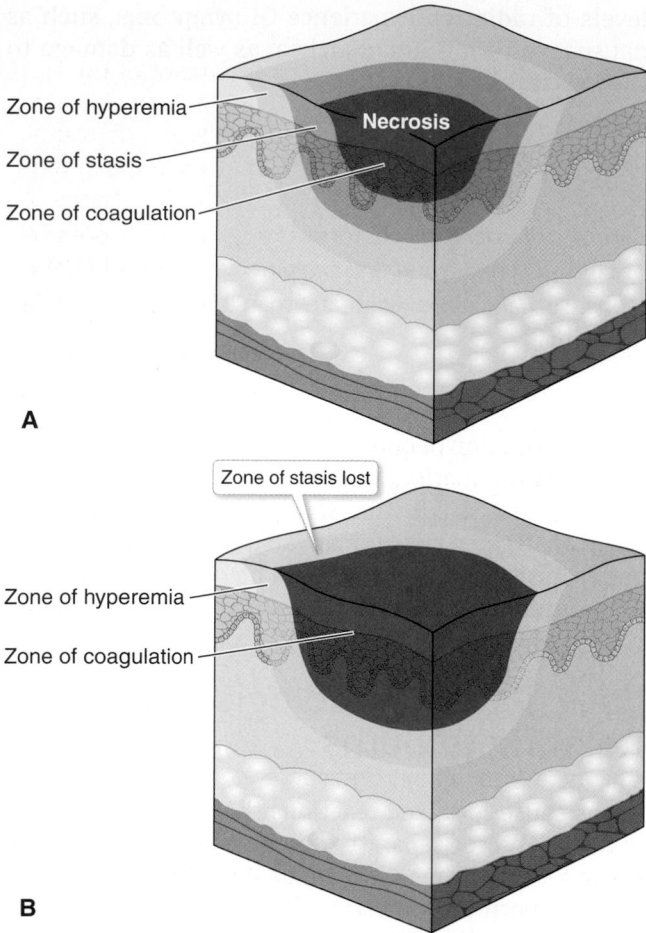

Figure 42–1. Zones of injury in burns. (a) The central part of a burn, called the zone of coagulation, is the worst affected region. The area surrounding the central burn, called the zone of stasis, is characterized by decreased tissue perfusion and can be salvaged with appropriate fluid resuscitation and treatment. (b) If treatment is inadequate, the zone of stasis is lost and the central zone of coagulation expands.

substances increase vascular permeability and hydrostatic pressure, resulting in a massive intravascular to extravascular fluid and protein shift, which is greatest during the first 6 to 8 hours after injury. As albumin continues to leak from the cell, normal colloidal osmotic pressure decreases further, which promotes increased fluid loss into the interstitial space and creates the characteristic tissue swelling seen in burned patients. This, coupled with the tremendous evaporative fluid loss from open burn wounds, significantly decreases intravascular fluid volume. Cellular damage alters normal sodium and potassium ion flow and the large release of potassium into the extracellular fluid increases the risk for hyperkalemia and cardiac arrhythmias.

ALERT! If the patient does not receive adequate fluid resuscitation during the initial resuscitative period of thermal injury, a type of hypovolemic shock termed **burn shock** sets in that compromises organ perfusion.

The stress of a major burn injury causes a hypermetabolic state of the body that is proportional to the percentage of body surface area burned. Resting energy requirements increase 50% to 100% compared with the noninjured adult and averages 1.3 times the basal metabolic rate. A **hypermetabolic state** heightens energy needs, oxygen consumption, body heat production, and body temperature, and causes rapid tissue breakdown. The release of stress hormones such as catecholamines and cortisol activates the mobilization of glycogen, protein, and fat stores, often resulting in a catabolic state, where there is breakdown of lean body mass. To counteract the catabolic state, nutritional supplementation is necessary to meet the increased caloric and protein needs. To calculate the nutritional supplementation required to promote wound healing, the following formula, which is based upon size of the burn and body weight, may be utilized:

$$25 \text{ kcal} \times \text{body weight (kg)} + \% \text{ TBSA}$$

The outpouring of catecholamines also causes peripheral vasoconstriction and, combined with hypovolemia, further compromises cardiac output. This leads to inadequate organ perfusion and oxygenation. Clinically, hypotension, tachycardia, and decreased urine output will be evident as cardiac output is decreased. After adequate fluid resuscitation is administered during the first 24 hours post burn injury, increased blood pressure is seen as cardiac output is restored to normal.

Pulmonary Responses to Burn Injury

After a severe burn, physiologic changes within the pulmonary system are a leading cause of morbidity and mortality. In response to the injury, respiratory rate increases secondary to anxiety or pain, and minute ventilation can increase 2 to 2.5 times the normal rate.

Increased lung capillary permeability and increased pulmonary vascular resistance can affect adequate tissue oxygenation. The two most serious pulmonary complications that develop following a major burn are airway edema of the upper respiratory tract and inhalational injury to the lungs.

Airway Edema of the Upper Respiratory Tract

Exposure to intense heat and flames produces mucosal damage, erythema, and edema of the upper airway. Edema of the upper airway tissues progresses rapidly, so if the patient manifests signs such as stridor, which is indicative of upper airway edema, the patient should be intubated immediately to prevent total airway obstruction.

Inhalational Injury

Inhalational injury should be suspected in people trapped in an enclosed space exposed to smoke, noxious fumes, and steam inhalation. It should also be suspected in individuals who lose consciousness, because the protective reflex of the vocal cords that protects the lungs from injury is lost, resulting in damage to the lower airway. Depending upon the type of burning material, injury of the respiratory tract mucosa from the oropharynx to the alveoli can occur. Damage includes loss of bronchial cilia, decreased alveolar surfactant, interstitial edema, and release of inflammatory substances that increase pulmonary vascular resistance and narrow small airways. All these factors impair the diffusion of oxygen from the alveoli into the pulmonary capillaries and create a mismatch of ventilation and perfusion, as well as the potential for hypoxemia. It is also important to realize that overhydration from excessive fluid resuscitation can cause accumulation of fluid in the interstitial space, because increased capillary permeability allows the shifts of fluid from the intravascular to interstitial space. This can cause chest wall edema, which will decrease total lung compliance, promote atelectasis (collapse of alveoli), and perpetuate hypoxemia.

The risk of inhalational injury and carbon monoxide (CO) poisoning is increased if the patient is burned in an enclosed space. CO is contained in the smoke and fumes of a fire. In the body, CO binds to hemoglobin and pushes oxygen off, which leads to hypoxia. The initial chest x-ray may be normal and the patient may be asymptomatic for up to 24 hours before respiratory distress develops. If the patient is demonstrating signs or symptoms indicative of respiratory distress, such as stridor, hoarseness, use of accessory muscles, and increased work of breathing, the patient should be intubated immediately to prevent total airway obstruction.

Gastrointestinal Responses to Burn Injury

Patients with burns greater than 25% of TBSA have decreased circulating blood flow to the gastrointestinal tract (GI) secondary to hypovolemia. This can impair GI motility, interfere with absorption of nutrients, and lead to paralytic ileus. Hypovolemia and reduced cardiac output can promote ischemia and sloughing of the gastric mucosa. Interventions to increase perfusion to the GI tract include adequate fluid resuscitation and the use of positive inotropic medications such as dopamine to support blood pressure. Additionally, the combination of early enteral feedings and the use of proton pump inhibitors (PPIs) and H_2 blockers are needed to prevent damage to the gastric mucosa. This has virtually eliminated the development of Curling's ulcer, a gastric stress ulcer that occurred in severely burned patients years ago before the availability of PPIs.

 CLINICAL CONCEPT

A Curling's ulcer is a gastric ulcer that develops in individuals who are severely burned. PPIs are commonly used to treat this disorder.

Effects of Burn Injury on Immunity

A thermal injury causes massive impairment of the immune system; therefore, any prior immunological abnormality has a profound impact on morbidly and mortality. Serum levels of immunoglobulins and complement activation are reduced, and the production and function of white blood cells such as neutrophils, monocytes, and macrophages are suppressed. Decreased interleukins-1 and interleukins-2, decreased T-helper cells, and overstimulation of suppressor T cells impair cellular immune response. An increased risk of infection is promoted by loss of the skin barrier, by excessive nutritional needs induced by the hypermetabolic state, and by increased release of mediators at the wound site that causes suppression of the immune response. Additionally, an open burn wound provides excellent conditions to support bacterial growth: Dead cell debris provides nutrients for the bacteria, and burns reduce blood flow and inflammatory response to invasion of organisms. Thus, aggressive early surgical **debridement** is advocated to improve blood flow to the burned area. This stimulates tissue regeneration and restores phagocytic activity to fight invading organisms while decreasing the risk of opportunistic infection. Opportunistic infections can lead to rejection of skin grafts and delayed wound closure; despite improvement in antimicrobial therapy, sepsis continues to be a leading cause of death in burn patients.

Renal Responses to Burn Injury

After the initial burn injury, reduced blood flow to the kidneys is proportional to the degree of hypovolemia. Diminished renal blood flow activates the renin-angiotensin-aldosterone system and stimulates the release of antidiuretic hormone, which causes retention of sodium and water, as well as major loss of potassium, calcium, and magnesium. If fluid resuscitation is inadequate to restore intravascular volume, renal ischemia can develop and lead to acute renal failure. Laboratory findings include elevated serum creatinine and decreased creatinine clearance. Intervention is aimed at restoring intravascular volume and avoidance of nephrotoxic medications such as aminoglycoside antibiotics and vancomycin. In addition, an electrical burn injury causes significant muscle breakdown and the release of myoglobin into the bloodstream. Because of the large size of myoglobin, mechanical obstruction of the renal tubules can develop and lead to acute tubular necrosis and renal failure if fluid resuscitation is inadequate. Therefore, it is recommended to maintain urine output at 50 to 100 mL per hour until laboratory studies indicate that myoglobin levels are normal.

Assessment

During the assessment of a burn patient, determining the size and depth of the burn is important because it:

- provides information about the severity of the injury

- guides fluid resuscitation
- determines the need for surgical intervention
- acts as a strong predictor of mortality.

The depth of the burn injury also impacts long-term cosmetic appearance and degree of functional impairment. The traditional classification of burns as first, second, third, and fourth degree have been replaced by categories that describe the depth of destruction of the cellular layers of the skin: superficial, partial thickness, and full thickness.

Superficial Burns

Superficial burns, also known as first-degree burns, damage only the epidermal layer. They result from severe sunburn, hot liquid splash, or a brief flash burn. The skin is dry, as blistering does not occur, but vasodilatation of the blood vessels produces a characteristic redness of the skin. Although initially painful, these burns usually heal in less than a week without long-term scarring. It is not necessary to calculate the percentage of body surface area affected for a superficial burn.

Partial-Thickness Burns

Partial-thickness burns, also known as second-degree burns, can be either superficial partial thickness or deep partial thickness, depending upon the degree of tissue necrosis of the dermal layer. Superficial partial-thickness burns char the epidermis and papillary dermal layer with resultant edema and formation of epidermal blisters. Burned skin is wet, raw, and pink or cherry red in color that blanches with pressure. These burns are quite painful and usually result from hot liquid scalding or direct skin contact with chemicals, flash, or open flame. Although superficial partial-thickness burns can spontaneously heal within 3 to 6 weeks without surgical intervention, some degree of scarring and change in skin pigmentation is possible. However, if the potential for infection is a concern, excision and skin grafting may be necessary.

A deep partial-thickness burn injury extends from the epidermis through the papillary and reticular layers of the dermis. The appearance of the skin is similar to a superficial partial-thickness burn, although skin color may be more mottled depending upon the degree of blood flow to the area. Nerve endings are damaged, so the patient tends to describe more discomfort.

Full-Thickness Burns

Full-thickness burns, also known as third-degree burns. damage the epidermis, dermis, hair follicles, and all underlying structures. Pain is rare because of the destruction of nerve endings. The skin's appearance is white, brown, black, or red, and the surrounding tissue is very edematous. These burns are caused by prolonged exposure to intense heat, open flames, electrical currents, or chemical agents. In children or older adults, a hot liquid scald can produce a full-thickness burn.

Diagnosis

Diagnosis of a burn requires assessment of the extent and depth of the burn injury; this also determines the appropriate treatment. The extent of injury is expressed as a percentage of TBSA burned and must be established before developing a plan of care.

There are various methods for determining the extent of the burn wound, including the rule of nines, the Lund and Browder method, and the American Burn Association Classification of Burn Injury.

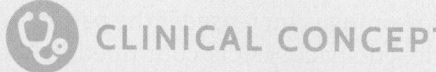

> **CLINICAL CONCEPT**
>
> The diagnosis of burns entails the thickness of involved body layers and percentage of body surface area.

Rule of Nines

The **rule of nines** is a rapid method used during the prehospital and emergent phase of care. The body is divided into regions that present 9% or multiples of nine, with the exception of the perineum, which is 1% body surface area. The face and back of the head are 4.5% each, so the entire head is 9%. The anterior and posterior portion of the arm is 9%, and the total for each leg is 18%.

The rule of nines is fairly accurate for adults; however, for children it must be modified because of the differences in body surface area between an adult and child. For example, a child's head comprises 18% of his or her TBSA, because a child's head is large in proportion to the child's body, whereas in the mature adult the head comprises only 9% of the TBSA. The patient's total area of burn is estimated by adding the percentages of surface area burned (see Fig. 42-2).

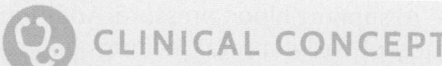

> **CLINICAL CONCEPT**
>
> In adults, the rule of nines is most commonly used to estimate TBSA involved in a burn.

Lund and Browder Method

The **Lund and Browder method** of assessing burns is a more accurate estimation of affected body surface. It divides the body into smaller sections of TBSA and evaluates the percentages of these areas. Again, the patient's total area of burn is estimated by adding the percentages of surface area burned.

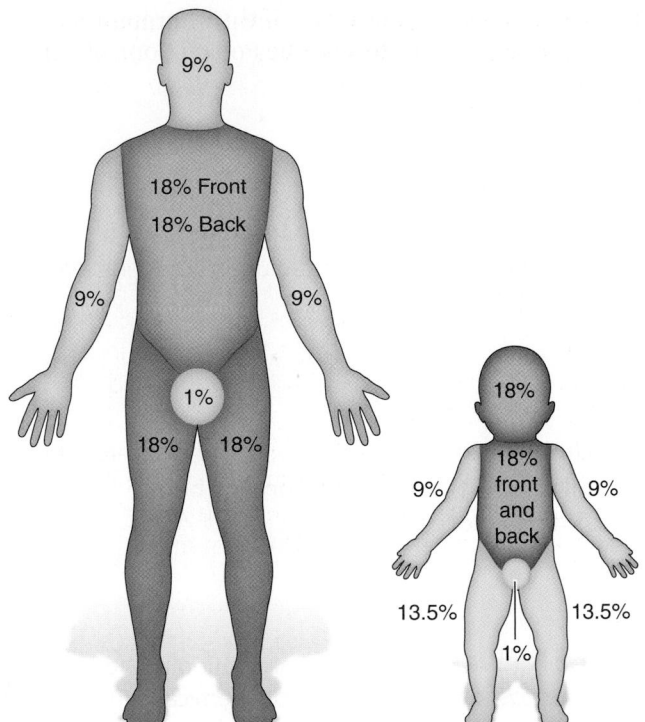

Figure 42–2. Rule of nines. The rule of nines is a standardized method used to quickly assess how much body surface area has been burned on a patient. This rule is only applied to partial-thickness (second-degree) and full-thickness (third-degree) burns. The diagrams depict BSA percentages for adults (a) and infants of 1 year or younger (b).

American Burn Association Classification of Burn Injury

The American Burn Association Classification of Burn Injury uses both the extent and the depth of burns to classify burns as minor, moderate, or major. A **minor burn** injury is described as:

- a partial-thickness burn of less than 15% TBSA in adults and less than 10% TBSA in children
- a full-thickness burn of less than 2% TBSA not involving special care areas, such as the eyes, ears, face, hands, feet, perineum, or joints.

A **moderate burn** injury, or uncomplicated burn, is described as:

- a partial-thickness burn of 15% to 25% TBSA in adults or 10% to 20% in children
- a full-thickness burn of less than 10% TBSA not involving special care areas.

A **major burn** injury is described as:

- a partial-thickness burn exceeding 25% TBSA in adults or 20% in children
- all full-thickness burns exceeding 10%
- all burns involving eyes, ears, face, hands, feet, perineum, and/or joints
- all burns involving inhalation injury, electrical injury, concurrent trauma, and poor-risk patients.

Significant Laboratory Parameters in Burn Injury

There are some basic laboratory tests to obtain when treating a patient with burn injury. Upon admission, baseline labs should be obtained, which includes a complete blood count (CBC), electrolyte level, urinalysis, arterial blood gas, and a **carboxyhemoglobin level** if the burn injury occurred in a closed space and inhalation injury is suspected. A CBC is monitored routinely to assess the degree of hemoconcentration and the elevation of white blood cells if infection is present. Electrolytes are monitored to evaluate sodium concentration, which decreases secondary to fluid shifts and potassium levels, which are initially elevated as a result of fluid shifts into the extracellular space. Potassium levels return to normal as the burn shock resolves. Creatine phosphokinase (CPK) is measured in electrical burns to indicate the severity of muscle damage. Renal function tests, including blood urea nitrogen (BUN) and serum creatinine, are routinely measured; elevation of BUN indicates dehydration and elevation of creatinine indicates renal insufficiency. A urinalysis is used to monitor the adequacy of renal perfusion and the patient's nutritional status. **Myoglobinuria**, or dark brown urine, signals development of tubular necrosis. The breakdown of plasma proteins and dehydration are indicated through spilling protein in the urine (proteinuria) as nitrogen is excreted in large amounts in catabolic states. Arterial blood gases indicate the presence of hypoxia, as well as acid-base disturbances.

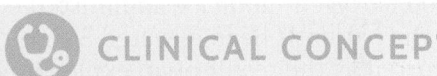

CLINICAL CONCEPT

In severe burns, muscle breakdown causes myoglobinuria. Myoglobinuria causes acute tubular necrosis, which leads to acute renal failure.

Treatment

Treatments of burns vary from outpatient application of topical antiseptics to the multidisciplinary team approach of the burn center. Individuals who sustain a major burn injury will require the specialized care of a burn center. However, most burns are minor and are treated in the emergency department. Burn care occurs in three phases:

1. emergent phase
2. acute phase
3. rehabilitation phase.

Emergent Phase

The emergent phase begins with the onset of the injury and continues until completion of fluid resuscitation.

During this phase, the estimation of the extent of the burn, first aid measures, and fluid resuscitation are accomplished. The goal is to prevent shock and respiratory distress and to assess and treat additional injuries. The initial focus of care addresses the ABCDEF (airway, breathing, circulation, disability, exposure, and fluid resuscitation) of trauma care, because the systemic injuries, if present, pose a threat to life.

Thermal Burns

All prehospital interventions are aimed at eliminating the heat source, stabilizing the patient's condition, identifying the type of burn, preventing heat loss, and preparing to transport. At the scene of thermal burn injury, the flames must be extinguished so the rescuers can assure both their own and the victim's safety. The burn wound is then irrigated with cool water to halt the burning process; this gives immediate relief from the pain and limits edema and tissue damage.

> **ALERT!** It is important to never use ice on a large burn area because it may induce blood vessel constriction, worsen tissue damage, and cause hypothermia.

The next step is to quickly assess the airway and initiate oxygen therapy based on the type and location of injury. Maintain a patent airway or intubate if the patient is demonstrating signs and symptoms of respiratory compromise. If no respiratory distress is present, 100% oxygen should be administered by facemask and the patient's head elevated 30°. If the burn injury occurred as the result of an explosion or in an enclosed space, there is a higher likelihood of inhalation injury; supplemental oxygen is the treatment of choice to reverse the systemic effects of CO poisoning. No fluids are given by mouth because of a potential for vomiting and aspiration related to stress. A large bore IV will be started, preferably in a nonburned area, to initiate fluid resuscitation and prevent burn shock in patients with a TBSA greater than 20%. **Fluid resuscitation** is initiated with lactated Ringer's solution, which is a fluid that is similar to the composition of blood. A cardiac monitor will be connected to the patient to evaluate for hemodynamic stability including the presence of dysrhythmias. Vital signs will be monitored to assess the circulatory system, as well as the patient's response to fluid resuscitation. Burned extremities are elevated above the level of the heart to facilitate circulation.

Chemical Burns

When the injury is related to chemical exposure, brush off the dry chemical agent, remove all clothing, and irrigate with copious amounts of water immediately for approximately 20 minutes to interrupt the chemical's contact with the skin. There may be chemicals that require specialized treatment; if the information is not readily available on site, call the Poison Control Center for information.

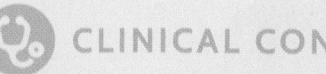

> In patients with a burn of greater than 20% of TBSA, intravenous lactated Ringer's solution is administered.

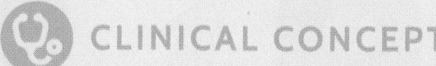

> Health-care providers must wear chemical-resistant clothing and protective equipment before initiating treatment for chemical burns.

> **ALERT!** Acid or alkali contamination to the eyes is the most detrimental type of chemical burn and requires immediate and copious irrigation.

Electrical Burns

For electrical burns, first ensure the source of electrical current has been disconnected. Assess the patient for responsiveness, and initiate cardiopulmonary resuscitation (CPR) if indicated.

All patients injured with an electrical burn, including those injured by lightning, have an increased risk for trauma and fractures caused by intense muscle contraction from the electrical current, from a fall, or from the hazardous flash of the electricity. The major concern is the increased risk for cervical spine injury. So, it is imperative that the patient not be moved until the cervical spine has been immobilized with the application of a semirigid collar. This places the cervical spine in a neutral position and reduces the risk of spinal cord compression.

Radiation Burns

For radiation burns resulting from an industrial accident, trained personnel will render the contaminated areas safe for entry. Interventions are focused on shielding, distance, and limiting the time of exposure. Specific conditions exist for a patient to be transferred to a specialized burn center (see Box 42-1).

> **ALERT!** Compartment syndrome occurs when there is an increase in pressure in a limited space, causing restriction or decreased circulation to muscles and nerves. Early manifestations include pain and decreased peripheral pulses. Later signs include numbness, tingling, and severe pain.

Acute Phase

The acute phase begins 48 to 72 hours after the burn injury; it includes the start of diuresis (loss of water from the body) and ends with closure of the burn wound. Continued assessment of respiratory and circulatory status, related to edema and fluid shifts, nutritional support, infection prevention, and burn wound care, are priorities during this phase. Hydrotherapy, excision, and early **grafting** (surgical implantation of new skin) of full-thickness wounds are performed as soon as possible after the injury. Infection is combated through application of topical antimicrobial agents to the burn surface areas in addition to daily wound cleansing. Enteral (tube feedings) or total parenteral nutrition feedings will be initiated as necessary to meet the caloric needs for healing and the hypermetabolic state of the burn patient. Pain management continues to be a priority in the plan of care for the burn patient, especially before procedures such as dressing changes and wound debridement.

During this time frame, there is a shift of fluids from the interstitial to the intravascular space and diuresis begins as capillaries regain integrity. There must be continued caution with fluid administration because of the fluid loss from large burn wounds. In older adult patients and in patients with inadequate cardiac or renal function, fluid overload occurs with the resulting signs and symptoms of congestive heart failure (CHF). Early detection and intervention with vasoactive medications, diuretics, and fluid restriction may prevent CHF and pulmonary edema.

The burn patient is at high risk for sepsis related to the immunosuppression that accompanies extensive burn injuries. Monitoring of the patient's temperature is important for early detection of bacteremia or septicemia. It is not uncommon for burn patients to have a low-grade fever for several weeks after the burn injury. In order to reduce the metabolic stress and oxygen requirements of the tissue, the patient may be given acetaminophen and a cooling blanket to maintain a temperature of 99°F to 101°F (37.2°C to 38.3°C).

The burn wound is an excellent site for bacterial growth, such as *E. coli*, the primary source being the patient's own intestinal tract; it is also an excellent site for fungi such as *Candida albicans* to grow. Tissue specimens are obtained routinely for culture and sensitivity to monitor for colonization by microbes. Antibiotics are not prescribed routinely unless a specific organism has been identified because of the risk of promoting resistant organisms. The exception to this is preoperatively and postoperatively; the patient is given systemic antibiotics because of the increased risk of exposure to the surface bacteria during the debridement.

ALERT! Infection is the major cause of death in the burn patient who survives a major burn.

The environment is a secondary source of microbes. So, when providing wound care, use clean technique when caring directly for burn wounds. Burn wounds are cleansed daily at a minimum and by a variety of methods, including immersion in a hydrotherapy tub. Treatments can be metabolically and psychologically stressful for the patient, so paying attention to the patient's physiologic and emotional comfort will enhance his or her ability to participate. Topical antimicrobial agents are the best method of local wound care in extensive burn injuries. The most common broad-spectrum antibiotic agents are silver sulfadiazine (Silvadene), silver nitrate, and mafenide acetate (Sulfamylon). The topical agent is applied in a thin layer to the burn wound and then covered with gauze dressings. Fingers and toes are each wrapped separately to promote mobility and ability to heal. Facial burns may be left open to air, but are observed closely to prevent drying that may cause conversion to a deeper burn. Circumferential burns are dressed from the distal portion to the proximal portion with attention paid to the joints to allow for motion.

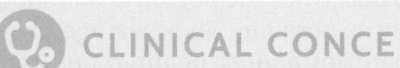
CLINICAL CONCEPT

Acticoat Antimicrobial Barrier Dressing is a new silver-coated dressing approved for burn wound and donor site treatment. This particular dressing may be left in place for up to 7 days and is remoistened every 3 to 4 hours with sterile water.

Dressings are changed on a schedule that is dependant on the topical agent used. Patients must be premedicated approximately 20 minutes before the treatment. The staff performing the dressing change wears gown, gloves, and hair and eye protection for their protection, as well as the patient's protection. Dressings are usually cut, removed, and disposed of according to the procedure established for contaminated materials. If the dressing adheres to a burn wound it may be moistened with saline or it may be soaked off in the hydrotherapy tub.

Wounds are initially debrided and cleansed by the patient, which gives the patient some control over this painful procedure. Later, the trained staff may use scissors and forceps to remove devitalized tissue. The conditions of the wounds are carefully documented, with special attention noted related to color, odor, exudates, and any signs of re-epithelialization. Debridement removes contaminated and necrotic tissue, also called **eschar.** Debridement enhances healing and prepares a site for grafting.

Natural debridement occurs when the dead tissue separates from the underlying tissue spontaneously. The body's natural enzymes cause this separation of burn tissue from the underlying viable tissue. Mechanical debridement involves scissors and forceps to remove the eschar, usually done with the dressing changes. Dressings themselves may be used as a debridement agent, as in the instance of wet to dry dressings that remove tissue as the dressing is removed. However, this method of wet to dry can be extremely painful to the patient and cause damage to granulation tissue.

Surgical interventions include escharotomy, surgical debridement, and autografting. Escharotomy is a surgical procedure to prevent circumferential constriction of a limb or chest. Surgical debridement is an operative procedure as opposed to natural debridement. It consists of removing tissue to the level of the viable tissue at the fascia level, also called **fasciotomy.** This procedure is reserved for patients with full-thickness burns because it removes potentially viable fat and lymph tissues.

Autografting is a procedure performed in the operating room to provide early wound coverage. In this procedure, healthy skin is removed from nonburned areas, known as donor sites, on the patient and transferred to burn areas.

In patients with large burn areas, it may be necessary to use biosynthetic dressings to provide temporary coverage. These dressings contain animal-derived components and synthetic polymers and should be applied as early as possible. The coverage of the wound decreases pain, promotes healing, and reduces the incidence of infection.

Most graft sites are covered with an occlusive dressing to immobilize the graft. Depending on the graft's site, occupational therapy may construct a splint to assist in preventing the graft from dislodging. The occlusive dressing will be left in place for 2 to 5 days after surgery. Great care is taken in positioning and turning the patient to prevent dislodging of the graft or placing pressure to the graft site. The donor site will be painful if not covered, because it is a partial-thickness wound.

The site must be observed for excess drainage and signs of infection. It is usually covered with a moist gauze dressing and heals within 7 to 14 days.

Rehabilitation Phase

The rehabilitation phase may extend for years after the injury, and actually begins during the emergent phase with the application of splints and the initiation of physical therapy. Active and passive range-of-motion exercises are initiated as soon as possible to prevent the development of contractures (inflexible contracted musculature). Scar tissue formation can be modified with pressure dressings, such as ace wraps over the burn dressings, especially when the patients are ambulating. As the burn wounds are grafted, specialized tubular support bandages are applied to supply an equal amount of pressure to the wounds to prevent or decrease the amount of scar formation.

Pain Management in Burn Injuries

Pain management is one of the most difficult challenges of burn care. Not only does the burn injury produce severe pain, but wound care modalities induce a significant amount of discomfort above the baseline pain experienced at rest. Yet, despite these complications, pain must be treated aggressively to keep it controlled.

In burn care, there are different types of pain depending on the extent and depth of the burn area. A partial-thickness burn causes constant pain when exposed to air because the nerve endings are exposed. Full-thickness burns are not painful in the areas of the deep burn because the nerve endings are damaged, but they are painful at the edges of the burn.

Pain management is initiated during the emergent phase. The patient's degree of pain must be routinely assessed and medicated appropriately to manage the intensity. Pharmacological treatment options include intravenous opioid agents, which provide the most rapid and efficacious relief of pain. Oral, intramuscular, and subcutaneous routes are avoided until the patient is hemodynamically stable and has full tissue perfusion. Patient-controlled analgesia using intravenous opioid agents enhances the patient's ability to cope with the pain, because the patient has control of the medication. Severe pain is usually treated with morphine, hydromorphone, fentanyl, or meperidine.

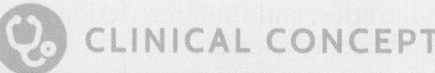

CLINICAL CONCEPT

Premedication with analgesics is necessary before dressing changes in severe burn injuries. Opioid agents are usually required to relieve the pain.

Chapter Summary

- Burns are the third leading cause of accidental death in the United States and can result in injuries that are mild to life-threatening.

- Burns are categorized as thermal, chemical, electrical, or radiation injuries.

- The severity of a burn depends upon the degree of heat intensity, duration of contact, and thickness of skin at the point of contact.

- Inhalation injury and CO poisoning occur when individuals suffer burns in a closed space. The patient requires measurement of the CO level.

- Ingestion, inhalation, or entry of radioactive materials via open wounds can induce internal contamination and produce ARS.

- High doses of radiation can produce bone marrow suppression or aplastic bone marrow, which requires blood transfusion to replace the low blood cell production. Patients exposed to the highest levels of radiation experience gastrointestinal symptoms (nausea, vomiting, and diarrhea) and damage to the central nervous system.

- Treatment of ARS focuses on patient decontamination by removing and bagging clothes and shoes, which usually removes greater than 80% of radioactive material.

- Electrical shock can cause cardiac conduction abnormalities including cardiac arrest.

- Thermal injury causes three zones of tissue damage: Zone of coagulation, zone of stasis, and zone of hyperemia.

- The traditional degree classification of first-, second-, third-, and fourth-degree burns has been replaced by categories that describe the depth of destruction of the cellular layers of the skin, termed superficial, partial thickness, and full thickness.

- A common method of assessing the extent of burn injury involves the rule of nines, in which the body is divided into regions that present 9% or multiples of nine.

- Normal physiologic organ function is disrupted if thermal injury is greater than 30% of TBSA.

- The American Burn Association Classification of Burn Injury uses both the extent and the depth of burns to classify burns as minor, moderate, or major.

- The focus of care in burns involves the ABCDEF (airway, breathing, circulation, disability, exposure, and fluid resuscitation) aspects of trauma care.

- A tetanus booster is recommended with burn injuries of partial or full thickness.

- Aside from localized destruction of tissue, an extensive burn injury can cause pulmonary, renal, and gastrointestinal complications.

- Myoglobinuria can cause acute tubular necrosis, which leads to acute renal failure.

- Burns cause a hypermetabolic state and fluid shifts that require IV fluids.

- Contractures can occur if the burn patient remains immobile; active and passive range of motion exercises are required.

- Compartment syndrome can occur if there is excess swelling or fluid accumulation within the musculoskeletal compartments.

- Infection is the major cause of death in the burn patient who survives a major burn.

- Silver nitrate and other silver preparations are often used as antibiotic treatment in burns.

- Debridement is the removal of dead, necrotic, or infected tissue to improve the healing potential of the remaining viable tissue. Debridement causes pain, and premedication with opioid medication is necessary.

Making the Connections

Disorder and Pathophysiology	Signs and Symptoms	Physical Assessment Findings	Diagnostic Testing	Treatment
Superficial Burns | Injury is limited to the outermost layer of the skin (epidermis). Tissue damage is minimal; protective barrier is not impaired. Overexposure to the sun is the most common cause of injury.				
	Painful erythema of the skin. Extremely tender to the touch.	Skin is tender and appears pink, red, and dry. Blisters common. Peeling skin. No break in the epidermal layer of the skin.	None.	Treatment limited to analgesics and moisturizers. The area heals within 3 to 5 days, no scarring.
Superficial Partial-Thickness Burns | The injury involves the epidermis and limited dermis. Protective barrier is impaired, causing heat and fluid loss. Scalds or brief contact with hot objects is the usual cause of injury.				
	Painful redness of the skin and exposure of dermal tissue beneath the epidermis. Blisters.	Skin is bright red, pearl-pink, painful, wet, or blistered. Dermis is exposed. Extremely tender.	Depending on how much body surface area is involved, CBC, electrolytes, urinalysis, arterial blood gas, CPK, and carboxyhemoglobin level may be needed. If infection occurs, one may need to culture the exudate.	Topical agents used on the wound area. Debridement. Skin grafting may be needed. Burn heals in 10 days to 2 weeks. Monitor for infection. Tetanus booster. Depending on how much of the body is involved, IV fluids may be needed. Antibiotic treatment may be needed. Pain control.
Deep Partial-Thickness Burns | Injury involves the epidermis and most of the dermis. Wound is not painful, as the nerve endings are destroyed.				
	Deep area of exposed tissue. The area appears dry, pale, or whitish-yellow in color. May be nontender if nerves are destroyed.	Deep area of exposed tissue. The area appears dry, pale, or whitish-yellow in color. May be nontender if nerves are destroyed.	Depending on how much surface area is involved, CBC, electrolytes, urinalysis, BUN, serum creatinine, arterial blood gas, CPK, and carboxyhemoglobin level may be needed. Increased risk for infection. If infection occurs, may need to culture the exudate.	Topical agents on wound area. Healing occurs within 3 to 5 weeks. Debridement. Skin grafting may be necessary for injuries within the deeper layers of the dermis. Pain control. Tetanus booster. IV fluids or enteral feedings may be needed, depending on surface area involved. Antibiotic treatment may be needed.

Continued

Making the Connections–cont'd

Disorder and Pathophysiology	Signs and Symptoms	Physical Assessment Findings	Diagnostic Testing	Treatment
Full-Thickness Burns	Injury involves the entire epidermis, dermis, and underlying subcutaneous tissues. Common causes are direct contact with flames or hot liquids, or steam. Fluid and heat loss are related to the loss of the protective layer.			
	Acutely, the layers beneath the epidermis and dermis are totally exposed. Red, raw appearing wound. No pain sensed.	Skin exhibits a dry, leathery, and white or yellow color that does not blanche with pressure, which indicates it is avascular. Nontender because nerves are destroyed.	CBC, electrolytes, urinalysis, BUN, serum creatinine, arterial blood gas, CPK, and carboxy-hemoglobin level. There is an increased risk for infection. Culture of exudate may be needed.	Tetanus booster. Topical agents and wound dressing. Burns heal within weeks to months. Wounds usually require surgical intervention. Debridement and skin grafting. Depending on percentage of body surface involved, IV fluids or enteral feedings may be needed. Antibiotic agents may be needed. Pain control.

Bibliography

Angelotti, M. (2010). A burn that keeps hurting. *Am Fam Phys*, 81(7), 829.

Burns. (2012). WHO violence and injury prevention. Retrieved from http://www.who.int/violence_injury_prevention/other_injury/burns/en/index.html

CDC. (2012a). Burns environmental preparedness and response. (2012). Retrieved from http://www.cdc.gov/masstrauma/factsheets/public/burns.pdf

CDC. (2012b). Fire death and injuries. Retrieved from http://www.nsc.org/safety_home/HomeandRecreationalSafety/Pages/Burns.aspx

Davis, C. S., Janus, S. E., Mosier, M. J., et al. (2012). Inhalation injury severity and systemic immune perturbations in burned adults. *Ann Surg*, Nov 15[C4].

Hemington-Gorse, S. J., Slattery, M. A., & Drew, P. J. (2010). Burns related to sunbed use. *Burns*, 36(6), 920–923.

Kraft, R., Herndon, D. N., Al-Mousawi, A. M., et al. (2012). Burn size and survival probability in paediatric patients in modern burn care: a prospective observational cohort study. *Lancet*, 379(9820), 1013–1021.

Lloyd, E. C., Michener, M., & Williams, M. S. (2012). Outpatient burns: prevention and care. *Am Fam Phys*, 85(9), 25–32.

Raz-Pasteur, A., Hussein, K., Finkelstein, R., Ullmann, Y., & Egozi, D. (2012). Blood stream infections (BSI) in severe burn patients—early and late BSI: a 9-year study. *Burns*, Nov 15. doi: pii: S0305-4179(12)00304-X. 10.1016/j.burns.2012.09.015.

Sheridan, R. L., Schaefer, P. W., Whalen, M., et al. (2012). Case records of the Massachusetts General Hospital. Case 36-2012. Recovery of a 16-year-old girl from trauma and burns after a car accident. *N Engl J Med*, 367(21), 2027–2037. doi: 10.1056/NEJMcpc1200088.

Tompkins, R. G. (2012). Survival of children with burn injuries. *Lancet*, 379(9820), 983–984.

WHO. (2012a). Burn prevention and care. Retrieved from http://whqlibdoc.who.int/publications/2008/9789241596299_eng.pdf

WHO. (2012b). Media centre. Burns. Retrieved from http://www.who.int/violence_injury_prevention/other_injury/burns/en/index.html

Yang, H. T., Hur, G., Kwak, I. S., et al. (2012). Improvement of burn pain management through routine pain monitoring and pain management protocol. *Burns*, Nov 22. doi: pii: S0305-4179(12)00360-9. 10.1016/j.burns.2012.10.025.

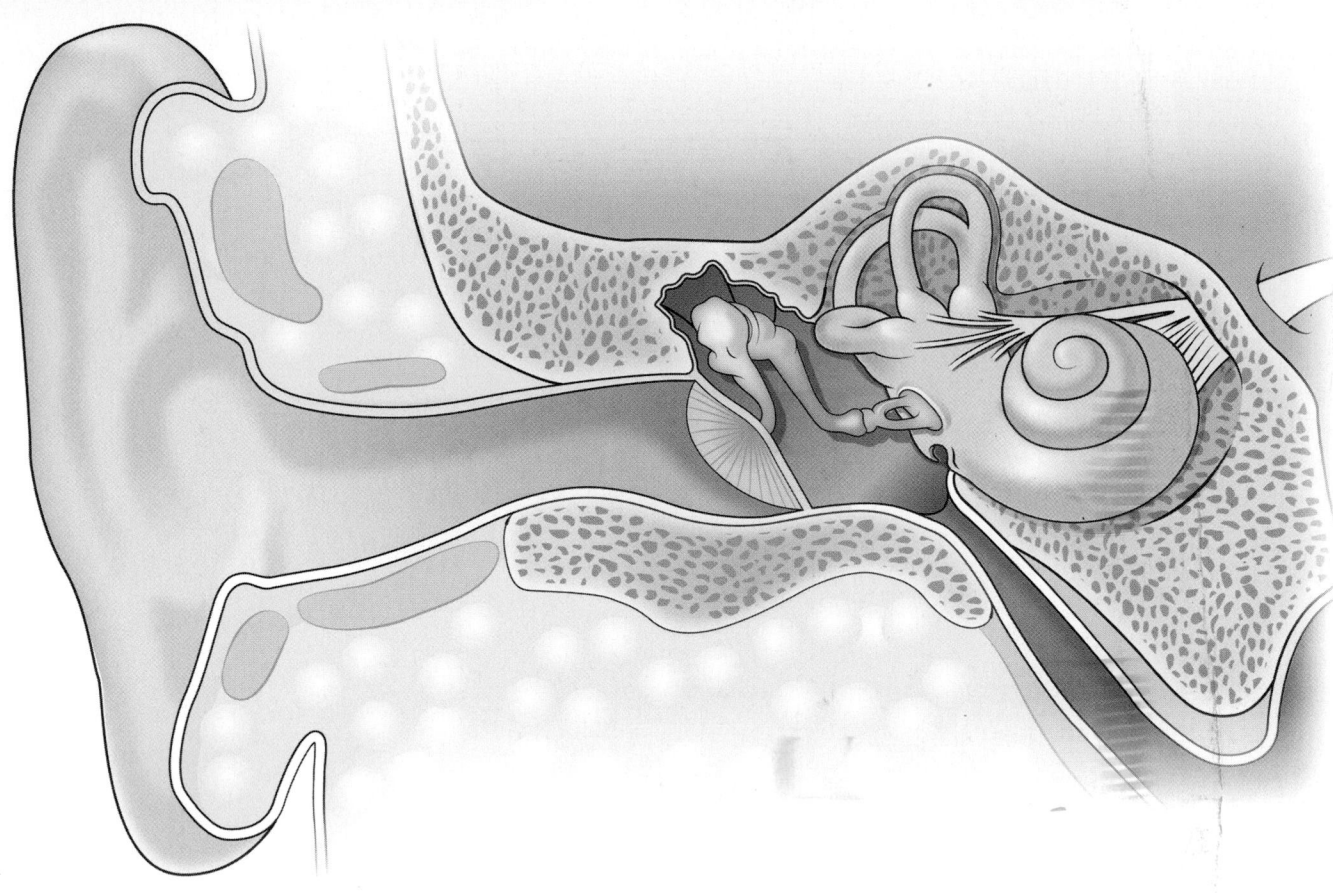

SENSORY DISORDERS

Chapters

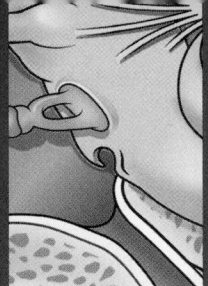

Key Terms

Amblyopia

Aqueous humor

Astigmatism

Canal of Schlemm

Cataracts

Ciliary muscle

Conjunctivitis

Drusen

Extraocular movements (EOMs)

Glaucoma

Hordeolum

Hyperopia

Keratoconjunctivitis

LASIK

Macula

Myopia

Optic cup

Optic disc

Papilledema

Retinal detachment

Strabismus

Trachoma

Vision acuity

Vitreous humor

More than 3 million people in the United States are visually impaired; with the aging of the population, this number is estimated to double by the year 2030. Visual impairment may be caused by a number of eye diseases, including age-related macular degeneration (AMD), diabetic retinopathy, glaucoma, and cataracts. The increasing incidence of diabetes is one of the major reasons visual impairment is rising in the population. Per some estimates, fewer than two-thirds of people with diabetes obtain regular visual examinations. Persons with vision loss are more likely to report depression, falls, cognitive decline, and premature death.

To understand the definition of visual impairment, it is necessary to know how vision is measured. **Vision acuity** is measured using an eye chart and results are recorded as a pair of numbers. Normal sight is scored as a ratio of 20/20; the numerator indicates that the object to be visualized is at a distance of 20 feet, whereas the denominator indicates how far away the object seems to the patient. Someone with a visual acuity of 20/20 can see letters at a distance of 20 feet away as if he or she is 20 feet away. Someone with a visual acuity of 20/60 sees letters at 20 feet as if he or she is 60 feet away. The higher the denominator of visual acuity, the worse the individual's vision. A person is considered blind if his or her vision is 20/200 or worse.

Having good vision is important to safety, independent living, and self-confidence. By comprehending the various eye disorders, clinicians should be able to recognize the signs of impending eye problems and chronic eye conditions to adequately assist patients with visual disturbances.

Epidemiology

According to the World Health Organization (WHO), 285 million people are visually impaired worldwide: 39 million are blind and 246 million have low vision. About 90% of the world's visually impaired live in underdeveloped countries. About 65% of all people who are visually impaired are aged 50 and older. Globally, uncorrected refractive errors are the main cause of visual impairment. In middle and low income countries, cataracts are the leading cause of blindness. In underdeveloped regions of the world, *Chlamydia trachomatis* is a major cause of blindness. The WHO is leading an international alliance of governments and private sector and civil society organizations aiming to eliminate *C. trachomatis* from the world by the year 2020.

According to U.S. Census data, blindness or low vision affects approximately 1 in 28 Americans older than 40 years. The specific causes of visual impairment, and especially blindness, vary greatly by race/ethnicity. An estimated 937,000 (0.78%) Americans older than 40 years are blind. An additional 2.4 million Americans (1.98%) have low vision. The leading cause of blindness among Caucasians is age-related macular degeneration AMD (54.4% of the cases), whereas among African Americans, cataracts and glaucoma account for more than 60% of blindness. Cataracts, the leading cause of low vision, are responsible for approximately 50% of bilateral vision worse than 20/40 among Caucasians, African Americans, and Hispanic Americans.

Basic Concepts of the Structure and Function of the Eye

The eye is a sensory organ with complex structure and function. It allows us to constantly interpret our environment by bringing images to the brain. It is not until a structure of the eye dysfunctions that we understand the significance of this sensory organ.

Structure of the Eye

The eye consists of the eyeball, or globe, that sits in the orbit of the skull. The eyeball is a fluid-filled sphere composed of three layers: the sclera, choroid, and retina. The fluid is **aqueous humor.** The sclera is the white outermost layer of the eye. Within the sclera is the cornea, the transparent section through which light enters the eye. The choroid is the thin vascular layer between the sclera and the retina. The iris, the colored part of the eye, is located in the choroid layer. The pupil is an opening in the center of the iris. Light waves enter the eye through the pupil and are transmitted to the brain for interpretation. The body of the eyeball behind the lens is a clear, gel-like substance called **vitreous humor.** Refraction of light occurs as rays move from the pupil through the aqueous and vitreous humors to the retina, the innermost layer of the eye (see Fig. 43-1 and Fig. 43-2).

The retina is the sensory portion of the eye that changes light waves into neuro-impulses that travel to the brain for interpretation (see Fig. 43-3). On funduscopic examination, the optic nerve is visualized as a bright, yellow, round structure located medially on the retina. It consists of a lighter colored **optic cup** in the center, surrounded by the darker yellow **optic disc.** The disc should have a clear and distinct border, and the optic cup diameter should be less than 1/3 the disc diameter. Blood vessels, both arterial and venous, lead out of the optic disc and perfuse the retina. Blood vessels should have clear, smooth borders. The ratio of artery-to-vein diameter should be approximately 2 to 3. The retina is the only place in the body where active blood vessels are directly visible. Approximately two-and-a-half disc diameters to the left of the optic disc is the **macula,** a slightly oval-shaped, blood vessel-free, dark red area. The central region of the macula is called the fovea which is responsible for sharp central vision.

Attached to each eyeball are four rectus muscles and two oblique muscles that are innervated by cranial nerves III, IV, and VI (see Fig. 43-6). Normally, the eyeballs move symmetrically with six possible positions of gaze, also called the six cardinal fields of gaze. CNs III, IV, and VI control **extraocular movements (EOMs)** (see Fig. 43-4).

The conjunctiva is a mucous membrane with two parts. The palpebral portion of the conjunctiva is a pink membrane that lines the eyelid, whereas the bulbar conjunctiva is colorless and it covers the eyeball except for the cornea.

Protecting the anterior portion of the eye are the eyelids, which consist of smooth and striated muscles covered by thin skin. The lateral portion of the eyelids contains eyelashes that protect the eye from dust and other small particles. Other accessory structures that

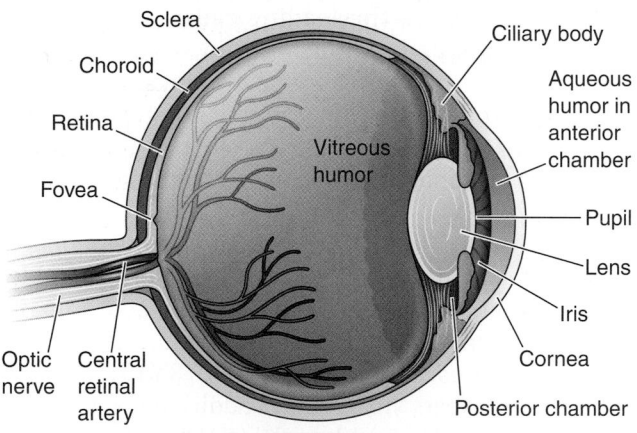

FIGURE 43-1. Cross section of the eye.

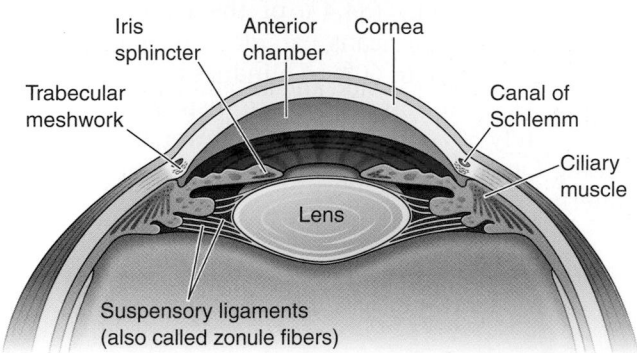

FIGURE 43-2. Alternate view of cross section of the eye.

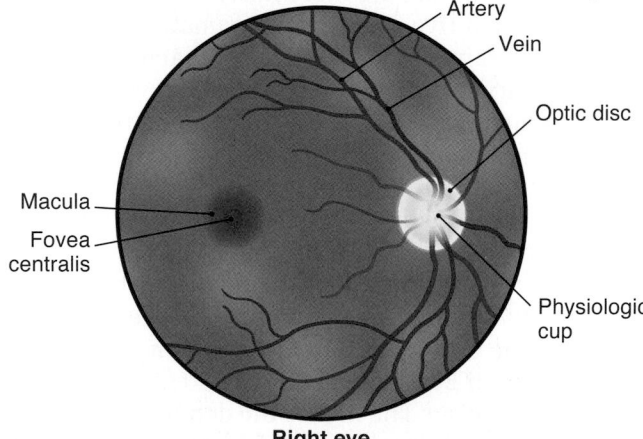

Right eye

FIGURE 43-3. Normal retina. (From Dillon, P. (2007). *Nursing health assessment.* 2nd ed. Philadelphia, PA: F.A. Davis Company, with permission.)

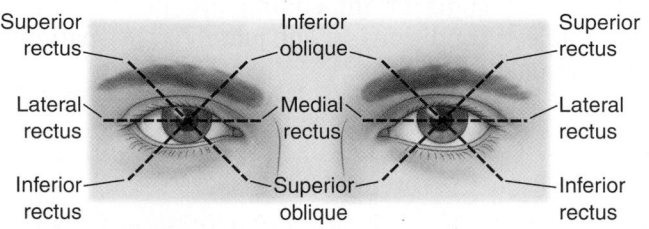

FIGURE 43-4. Six cardinal fields of gaze.

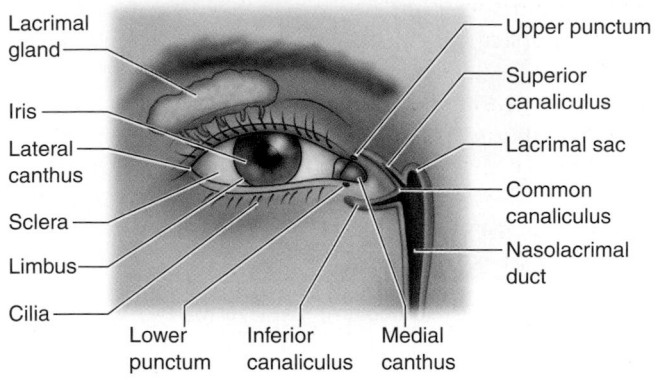

Lacrimal gland
Iris
Lateral canthus
Sclera
Limbus
Cilia
Lower punctum
Inferior canaliculus
Medial canthus
Upper punctum
Superior canaliculus
Lacrimal sac
Common canaliculus
Nasolacrimal duct

FIGURE 43-5. Lacrimal apparatus.

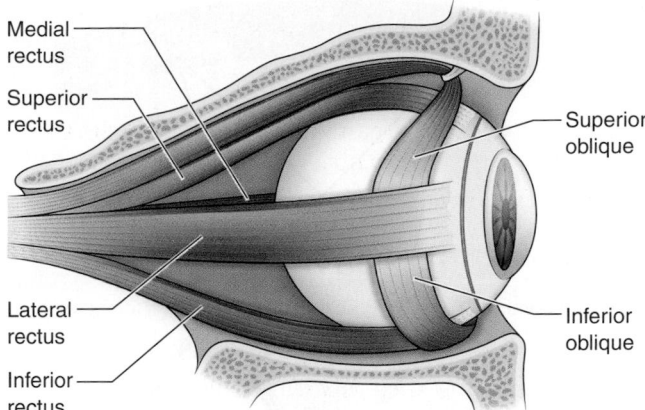

Medial rectus
Superior rectus
Lateral rectus
Inferior rectus
Superior oblique
Inferior oblique

FIGURE 43-6. Extraocular muscles.

protect the eye include the brows, lashes, meibomian glands, and lacrimal apparatus. The meibomian glands are sebaceous glands located at the rim of the eyelids, which secrete an oily substance. The lacrimal apparatus consists of the lacrimal gland, lacrimal sac, and duct. The lacrimal gland produces tears and is located in the upper lateral region of the orbit under the brow. Tears pass over the eye surface to the lacrimal puncta, tiny openings found at the medial corner of the eyelids. From there, tears collect in the lacrimal sac and then flow into the nasolacrimal duct, which empties into the nose (see Fig. 43-5).

Function of the Eye

In order to visualize an object, light rays pass through the cornea, anterior chamber, pupil, lens, and posterior chamber to the retina. The retina is the gateway where the optic nerve enters the brain. Blood vessels, optic nerves, and the macula can be seen on the retina with an ophthalmoscope. Changes in blood vessels associated with arteriosclerosis, hypertension, and diabetes can be exhibited on the retina. The optic nerve can be visualized on the retina as a yellow, circular, clearly defined disc. When there is increased intracranial pressure, the optic disc becomes swollen with irregular borders, a condition termed **papilledema.**

Vision requires the pupil to dilate and constrict, which allows the appropriate amount of light into the retina. The lens focuses the light rays on the retina. The ciliary muscle is attached to zonular fibers that are attached to the lens. The **ciliary muscle** is a smooth muscle controlled by the autonomic nervous system that changes the shape of the lens for accommodation; near versus far vision. Sympathetic nervous system stimulation causes relaxation of the ciliary muscle, which places high stress on the zonular fibers attached to the lens that flattens its shape. Conversely, parasympathetic nervous system stimulation causes ciliary muscle contraction, which allows the zonular fibers to relax; in response, the lens bulges. The change of the lens' shape changes how light converges on the retina.

The ciliary muscle also regulates the flow of aqueous fluid through the **canal of Schlemm**—an important structure that regulates intraocular pressure (IOP) (see Fig. 43-6). Sympathetic stimulation causes relaxation of the ciliary muscle, which blocks drainage of the canal of Schlemm. Consequently, aqueous fluid can accumulate within the eye. Parasympathetic stimulation causes contraction of the ciliary muscle, which opens the way for the canal of Schlemm to drain.

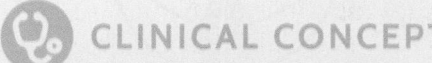

CLINICAL CONCEPT

Sympathetic or anticholinergic drug action on the ciliary muscle blocks the canal of Schlemm, causing accumulation of aqueous fluid, thereby increasing IOP; high IOP can trigger or worsen glaucoma.

The retina contains specialized nerve cells called rods and cones, also called photoreceptor cells, that further focus images, allow visualization of color, and carry impulses to the optic disc. Nerve fibers from the optic disc form the optic nerve, which sends impulses to the optic tracts, optic radiations, and visual cortex of the brain. Nerve fibers from the nasal portion of each eye cross over at the optic chiasm and travel to the contralateral, or opposite, side of the brain. Nerve fibers from the temporal portion of each eye do not cross over and remain on the ipsilateral, or same, side of the visual (occipital) cortex (see Fig. 43-7).

Basic Pathophysiologic Concepts of the Structure and Function of the Eye

The basic pathophysiologic processes that occur in the eye are caused by infection and inflammation, or structural changes, though any pathophysiologic process has the potential to cause visual impairment. Blindness is the most severe complication of any dysfunctional process in the eye.

Infection and Inflammation of the Eye and Surrounding Area

Infection and inflammation can occur in various parts of the eye and surrounding structures. Accurate diagnosis

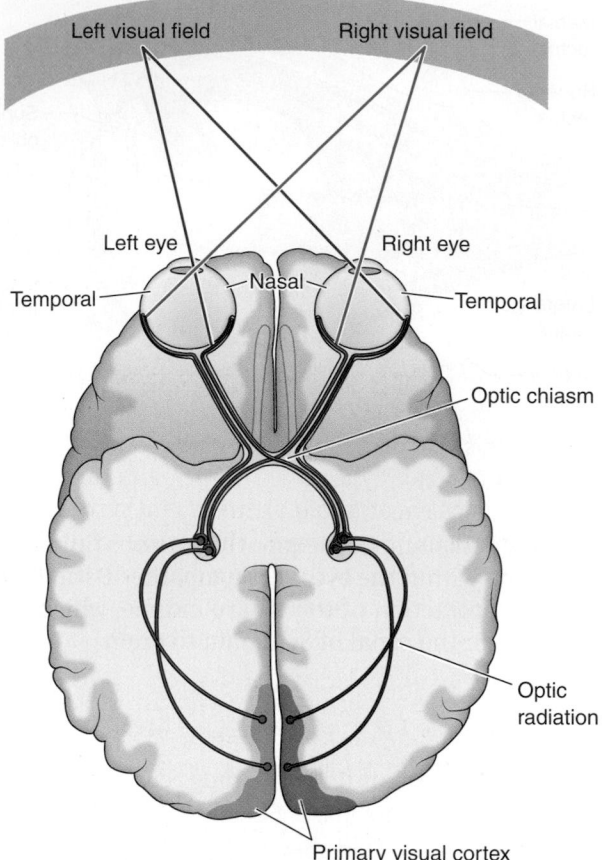

FIGURE 43-7. Optic pathways into the brain.

of the cause of the infection or inflammation is crucial in order to choose the correct treatment.

Blepharitis

Inflammation of the eyelids, called blepharitis, is also referred to as granulated eyelids. Symptoms of blepharitis include red, watery eyes; dry, gritty sensation of the eyes, burning sensation in the eye; itchy eyelids; erythematous, swollen eyelids; flaking of the skin around the eyes; crusted eyelashes upon awakening; photophobia; excessive tearing; abnormal eyelash growth; and loss of eyelashes. The eyelids may also appear greasy and crusted with scales that cling to the lashes. Acne rosacea and seborrheic dermatitis are skin disorders associated with blepharitis of the eyelids. Blepharitis can be difficult to treat. Good eye hygiene is key to effectively treating this eye infection.

Stye

A stye, also known as a **hordeolum**, is a bacterial infection that develops near the root of an eyelash and appears on the outside of the eye (see Fig. 43-8). Pain, swelling, and redness of the conjunctiva and eyelid are symptoms. *Staphylococcus aureus* is the most common pathogenic etiology. Physical examination of a stye reveals swelling, erythema, and tenderness to touch. Treatment includes antibiotics and warm compresses with diluted boric acid solution.

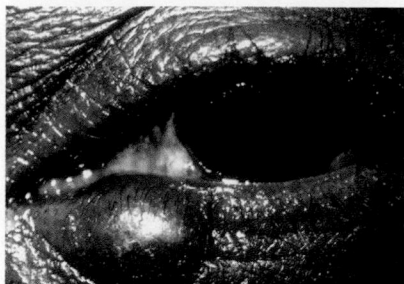

FIGURE 43-8. Stye (Hordeolum). *(Courtesy of Wills Eye Hospital, Philadelphia, PA.)*

Chalazion

A chalazion is a blockage in one of the small meibomian oil glands at the margin of the eyelid (see Fig. 43-9). Symptoms include eyelid tenderness, increased tearing, painful swelling on the eyelid, and sensitivity to light. Warm compresses, steroid injection, and surgical excision are the treatments.

Conjunctivitis

Conjunctivitis occurs when the conjunctiva of the eye becomes infected or inflamed. There are viral, bacterial, and allergic causes of conjunctivitis (see Fig. 43-10). The conjunctiva becomes red, swollen, and the eye feels itchy to the affected individual. There may be a purulent or watery discharge from the eye. Bacterial or viral conjunctivitis, commonly called pinkeye, is highly contagious. Persons can spread the bacteria or virus through touching the eye and then contacting the hands of another individual. Contaminated objects or bedding can transmit the microorganism as well.

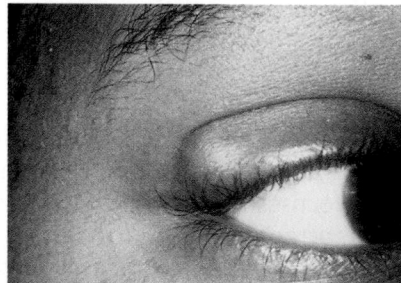

FIGURE 43-9. Chalazion. *(Courtesy of Wills Eye Hospital, Philadelphia, PA.)*

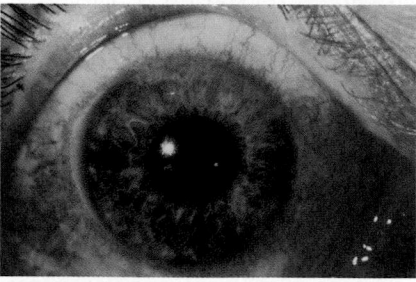

FIGURE 43-10. Conjunctivitis. *(Courtesy of Wills Eye Hospital, Philadelphia, PA.)*

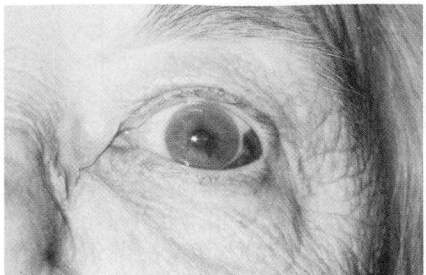

FIGURE 43-11. Subconjunctival hemorrhage. *(Courtesy of Wills Eye Hospital, Philadelphia, PA.)*

Keratitis

Inflammation of the cornea, called keratitis, is commonly caused by herpes simplex virus type 1. The infection usually begins by affecting the outer layer of the cornea, but it can go deeper into the cornea, increasing the risk of impaired vision. Other viruses that cause keratitis include varicella zoster and the adenoviruses. More rarely, keratitis is caused by other infections such as bacteria, parasites, and fungi. The term **keratoconjunctivitis,** meaning corneal and conjunctiva inflammation, is often used.

Keratoconjunctivitis sicca, commonly called dry eye, is seen in many autoimmune disorders. In keratoconjunctivitis sicca, tear production is inadequate. A number of systemic medications can cause this condition, including antihistamines, anticholinergics, and psychotropic drugs. Sarcoidosis, Sjogren's syndrome, and lesions affecting cranial nerve V or VII can also cause dry eye, which is treated with artificial tears. Antibiotics may be needed with bacterial keratoconjunctivitis. Acyclovir is the treatment for herpes simplex or varicella zoster.

Dacryocystitis

Dacryocystitis, an inflammation of the lacrimal sac, is often caused by an obstruction of the nasolacrimal duct. Incomplete canalization of the nasolacrimal duct or infection is the cause. The most common organisms include *Staphylococcus aureus*, *Haemophilus influenzae*, beta-hemolytic streptococci, and pneumococci. Newborns frequently have dacryocystitis caused by obstruction of the nasolacrimal duct.

When dacryocystitis infection is present, the area around the lacrimal sac is painful, red, and swollen. The eye becomes red and watery and oozes purulent exudate. Slight pressure applied to the lacrimal sac may push exudate through the opening at the inner corner of the eye, near the nose. Fever is also common.

Dacryocystitis is typically diagnosed by physical examination. Additionally, blood cultures may be necessary. Standard treatment consists of antibiotics and warm compresses. However, if conservative measures are ineffective, this condition is treated surgically.

Scleritis

Scleritis, or inflammation of the sclera, causes severe eye pain that may radiate to the eyebrow, temple, or jaw. Other symptoms include photophobia, tearing without discharge, eye tenderness, and purplish-red, edematous, engorged blood vessels. Inflammation of the sclera is usually associated with autoimmune diseases such as rheumatoid arthritis and systemic lupus erythematosus. Sometimes the cause is unknown. Treatment involves corticosteroid drops and oral nonsteroidal anti-inflammatory drugs.

Subconjunctival Hemorrhage

Blood vessels can become apparent in the sclera in a subconjunctival hemorrhage (see Fig. 43-11). A subconjunctival hemorrhage occurs when a small blood vessel breaks open and bleeds near the surface of the white of the eye. Alternatively, pinpoint subconjunctival hemorrhage is exhibited by red blood vessels in the sclera; sometimes this is referred to as "injected sclera" or "bloodshot eyes." Sudden increases in pressure such as violent sneezing or coughing can cause a subconjunctival hemorrhage. The hemorrhage may also occur in persons with high blood pressure or those who take blood thinners. A bright red patch appears on the white of the eye, but it does not cause pain or discharge. Vision does not change. No treatment is needed; eventually, the body absorbs the blood.

Uveitis

Uveitis is inflammation of the uveal tract, which includes the iris, choroid, and ciliary body. Common causes include infection or autoimmune disorders, such as rheumatoid arthritis or ankylosing spondylitis; inflammatory disorders, such as Crohn's disease or ulcerative colitis; infections, such as syphilis, toxoplasmosis, and tuberculosis; and eye injury. Symptoms, which can develop quickly, include eye redness and irritation, blurred vision, eye pain, photophobia, and floaters. Uveitis is diagnosed with a thorough examination of the eye with a slit lamp microscope and ophthalmoscopy. Treatment of active inflammation usually involves corticosteroids and antibiotics.

Structural Disorders of the Eye

A corneal abrasion is the most common type of eye injury. This usually benign condition heals within 24 hours. Other structural eye disorders include entropion and ectropion, which are abnormalities of the eyelids that can cause irritation of the eye. These benign conditions can be surgically treated. A more serious condition is exophthalmos, which is an eye condition that occurs in hyperthyroidism. The eye bulges and the cornea can dry out, causing irritation or injury that can be surgically corrected. A pterygium and pinguecula are benign growths on the eye that usually do not affect vision.

Corneal Abrasion

Corneal abrasion, which is the most common type of structural eye trauma, is damage to the epithelial surface of the cornea, usually caused by a foreign body that comes into contact with the eye. It can also be caused by either physical or chemical trauma. Contact lens wearers are more vulnerable to corneal abrasions because foreign bodies may become trapped between the cornea and the contact lens, causing scratching of the corneal membrane. Also, persons who play sports are more prone to corneal abrasions because of the increased risk of foreign bodies entering the eyes.

Often, persons with a corneal abrasion present with the following: foreign body sensation of the eye, gritty eye sensation, unilateral eye watering pain, photophobia, and mild erythema of the conjunctiva. Minor corneal abrasions may be asymptomatic. In cases of a significant abrasion, slit lamp examination reveals a defect in the corneal epithelium. This defect can be confirmed by placing a drop of fluorescein dye in the eye. The fluorescein dye flows into the defect and glows under the light of a Wood's lamp (see Fig. 43-12).

Treatment includes topical antibiotic ointments to prevent bacterial growth. Untreated corneal abrasions are susceptible to infections that may cause corneal ulcerations and blindness.

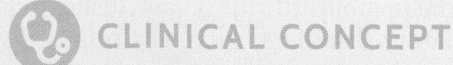

CLINICAL CONCEPT
Most cases of corneal abrasion heal within 24 hours.

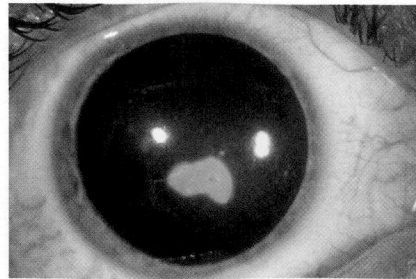

FIGURE 43-12. Corneal abrasion with fluorescein dye. *(Courtesy of Wills Eye Hospital, Philadelphia, PA.)*

Entropion and Ectropion

Entropion and ectropion are benign conditions of the eye. Entropion occurs when the eyelid turns inward and irritates the eye, whereas ectropion occurs when the eyelid turns outward, revealing the pink, conjunctival membrane. Both of these conditions can cause eye irritation, excessive tearing, and corneal dryness. Artificial tears and surgery are the treatments.

Exophthalmos

Exophthalmos, also called proptosis, is a bulging of the eye out of the orbit; hyperthyroidism or ocular tumor are the most common causes. Dryness and irritation of the eyes can occur. The cornea becomes inflamed because of the friction that occurs when the patient blinks. Some patients may experience compression of the optic nerve or ophthalmic artery, which can eventually affect the patient's vision, leading to blindness. Corticosteroid drops and surgical treatment are necessary.

Enophthalmos

Enophthalmos is the recession of the eyeball within the orbit. It may be a congenital anomaly or acquired as a result of trauma, collapse of the facial sinuses, Horner's syndrome, or other disorders. Treatment is aimed at the disorder's etiology; surgery may be necessary.

Benign Growths

A pinguecula is a benign, yellowish growth that forms on the conjunctiva (see Fig. 43-13a). A pterygium is another benign growth that resembles a pinguecula; however, it encroaches on the corneal surface (see Fig. 43-13b). Exposure to ultraviolet light is thought to cause the abnormality. These remain on the eye unless surgically removed; however, neither requires treatment unless they interfere with vision.

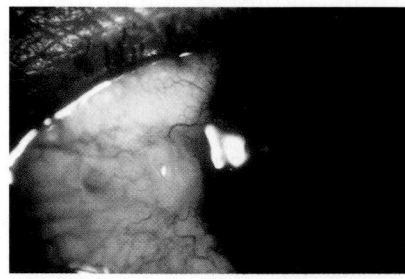

FIGURE 43-13a. **Pinguecula.** *(Courtesy of Wills Eye Hospital, Philadelphia, PA.)*

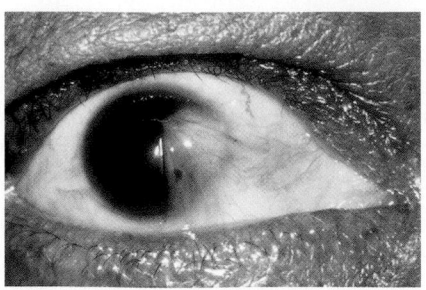

FIGURE 43-13b. **Pterygium.** *(Courtesy of Wills Eye Hospital, Philadelphia, PA.)*

Types of Vision Impairment

The different types of visual impairment include myopia (nearsightedness), hyperopia (farsightedness), presbyopia, astigmatism, amblyopia, and color blindness.

Myopia

Normally, light enters the eye via the pupil and contacts the lens, which causes bending of the light. The lens is important because it projects an image on the retina. **Myopia,** or nearsightedness, occurs when the eyeball becomes elongated and visual images are focused in front of the retina (see Fig. 43-14). In other words, individuals with myopia see better when objects are close up; hence, the further away an object moves, the blurrier it becomes.

Myopia is very common, affecting approximately one-third of Americans, with aging adults being most affected. Symptoms include blurry distal vision, headache, squinting, and eyestrain. Visual acuity examinations are used to diagnosis myopia. Treatment includes corrective lenses via eyeglasses or contact lenses, or corrective surgery such as laser-assisted in situ keratomileusis (**LASIK**) surgery. If left untreated, myopia may worsen with age.

Hyperopia

Hyperopia, or farsightedness, occurs when visual objects are focused behind the retina because of shortening of the eyeball. Individuals with hyperopia see better when objects are farther away. The closer an object moves, the blurrier it becomes. Aging adults are most commonly affected with hyperopia. Treatment includes corrective lenses or surgery. If untreated, hyperopia tends to worsen with age.

Presbyopia

Presbyopia, a common disorder in aging adults caused by the decreased elasticity of the lens with age, is a vision defect exhibited as a gradually diminished ability to focus on close objects. This begins around the age of 40 years, which is why some individuals start to require reading glasses at this age.

As with hyperopia, individuals need to have objects held at a distance to see clearly. Individuals may first notice that the ability to read small print is more difficult. Treatment for presbyopia includes corrective lenses such as contacts and glasses with bifocals.

Astigmatism

In normal vision, light rays focus directly on the retina. With **astigmatism,** the rays are diffusely spread about the retinal area, resulting in blurred vision.

The cause of astigmatism is the shape of either the lens or the cornea. The eyeball is often referred to as having a football shape rather than its normal spherical shape. These changes in shape distort the light rays entering the eye so that the rays do not center on the retina.

Although some individuals may be asymptomatic, people with astigmatism may experience blurred vision, headaches, and eyestrain. Keratoscope and videokeratoscope are ophthalmic devices to measure and assess the curvature of the cornea to diagnose astigmatism. Treatment for astigmatism includes use of corrective lenses or refractive surgery such as LASIK.

Amblyopia

Amblyopia, also known as lazy eye, affects just 2% to 3% of the population. In this condition, central vision fails to develop properly, usually in one eye, which is called amblyopic. **Strabismus,** commonly called crossed eyes, is a related condition where the visual axes of the eyes are not parallel and the eyes appear to be looking in different directions (see Fig. 43-15). Strabismus often causes amblyopia.

Amblyopia generally develops in children before the age of 6 years; parents, caregivers, or health-care professionals often note the symptoms. These symptoms include eyestrain, poor visual acuity, squinting, or completely closing one eye to see.

Trauma to the eye at any age can cause amblyopia, as well as a strong uncorrected refractive error (myopia and hyperopia) or strabismus. When amblyopia occurs in a child, the visual cortex of the brain will neglect to interpret images from the amblyopic eye as the child grows. It is important to correct amblyopia as early as possible, before the brain learns to entirely ignore vision in the affected eye.

Myopia (nearsightedness)

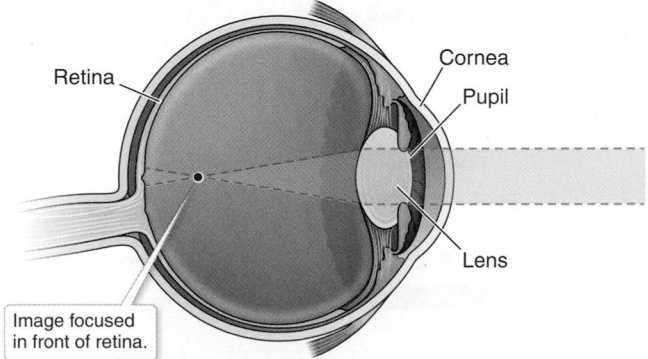

FIGURE 43-14. Refraction of light in myopia.

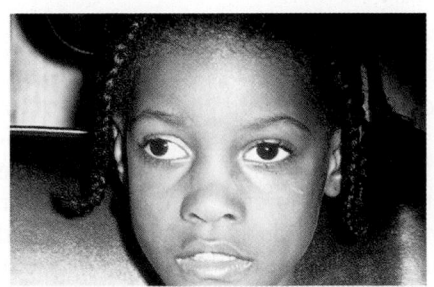

FIGURE 43-15. Strabismus. *(Courtesy of Wills Eye Hospital, Philadelphia, PA.)*

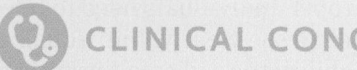

CLINICAL CONCEPT

To treat amblyopia, the eye with good vision is patched in order to strengthen the weaker eye.

ALERT! Untreated amblyopia may lead to functional blindness in the affected eye. Although the amblyopic eye has the capability to see, the brain turns off this eye because vision is very blurred and the brain elects to see only with the stronger eye.

Color Blindness

Color blindness is a condition that impairs an individual's ability to distinguish certain colors. It occurs in about 8% to 12% of males and in about 0.5% of females. Red/green color blindness, in which the individual has problems distinguishing between reds and greens, is the most common type. The red and green objects in the environment appear grey in color. The disorder, inherited from the mother, is a dysfunction of the rods and cones within the retina. The gene for color blindness is carried on the X chromosome; males have a higher incidence than females because X chromosome traits are dominant over Y chromosome traits. Color blindness is normally diagnosed through clinical testing using the Ishihara color chart. There is no treatment for color blindness, and most persons compensate well for their defect.

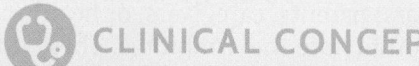

CLINICAL CONCEPT

The colorblind individual cannot decipher words or numbers on the Ishihara color chart.

Blindness

A person with vision that cannot be corrected to better than 20/200 in the best eye, or who has 20 degrees (diameter) or less of visual field remaining, is considered to be "legally blind," meaning he or she suffers from blindness.

Assessment of the Eye

Assessment of the eye and vision is part of every comprehensive physical examination. Examination of the pupil and extraocular movements (EOMs) are key features of the neurological examination. Examination of the eyes and eyelids yield results about the optic, oculomotor, trochlear, abducens, and facial cranial nerves. It is also important to assess the eyelids and

orbital region for infection, inflammation, and structural disorders. If the eyes are not accurately evaluated, vision can be permanently affected.

Physical Examination

The structures around the eye, including the eyelashes, eyebrows, and eyelids, should be carefully inspected. The clinician should note any apparent inflammation, swelling, seborrheic debris along lashes and brows, or entropion, ectropion, or ptosis of the eyelids. The patient's eyes should be inspected for exophthalmos, enophthalmos, lesions, deformities, and asymmetry. The conjunctiva, sclera, cornea, iris, and pupil should be examined for color, discharge, and lesions.

Visual acuity should be assessed before proceeding with the rest of the eye examination. The patient should use his or her corrective lenses and be positioned 20 feet from a Snellen chart (see Fig. 43-16). The Snellen chart is printed with 11 lines of block letters. The first line consists of one very large letter, "E." Subsequent rows have increasing numbers of letters that decrease in size. A patient should cover one eye and read the letters of each row, beginning at the top. The smallest row that can be read accurately indicates the visual acuity in that eye. Alternatively, the patient's vision can be tested with a Rosenbaum chart, which has lines of numbers. The patient holds this pocket-sized chart at approximately 14 inches from the face. The

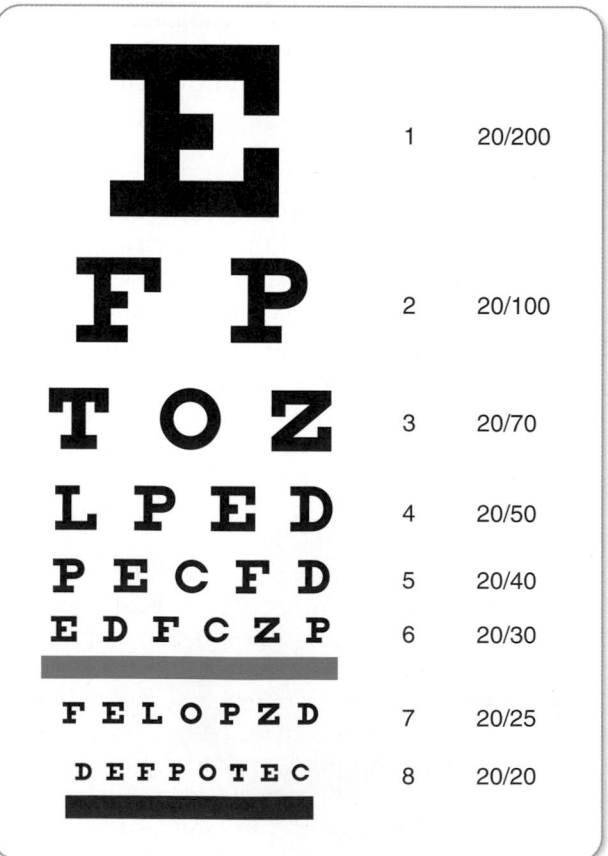

FIGURE 43-16. Snellen chart.

first line consists of one very large number. Subsequent rows have more lines of numbers that decrease in size. Each eye should be tested one at a time. The smallest row that can be read accurately indicates the visual acuity in that eye.

The clinician should shine a penlight on the pupil of each eye; both pupils should be equally round and reactive to light. A light reflex in one eye should occur consensually in the other eye. To assess the eye's ability to accommodate, observe the patient's pupils as you bring your finger toward the patient's nose. The pupils should constrict as the eyes follow your finger toward the nose. The term PERRLA indicates that the pupils are equally round and reactive to light and accommodation.

The clinician should observe the six cardinal fields of gaze to assess the EOMs. During this examination, the conjugate movement of the eyes should be observed, demonstrating function of the extraocular muscles. The extraocular muscles are the medial, inferior, and superior rectus muscles, as well as the superior and inferior oblique and the levator palpebrae muscles. The extraocular muscles are controlled by the oculomotor nerve (cranial nerve III), trochlear nerve (cranial nerve IV), and abducens nerve (cranial nerve VI). To test the EOMs, the clinician should form an "H" or "star" with the index finger in the air, as the patient observes using only his or her eyes and not moving the head. At the end of EOM assessment, the clinician should bring his or her finger toward the patient's nose to test convergence of eyes.

The corneal reflection can be used to assess functional symmetry of extraocular muscles. A penlight can be used to shine a light directly in front of the patient; the reflection of this light on the cornea should appear on both eyes at symmetrical locations. Asymmetry suggests extraocular muscle pathology.

The patient's peripheral vision can be assessed with the clinician standing approximately 2 feet from the patient. The patient should look straight into the clinician's eyes. The clinician then has to bring his or her own hands around to the sides of the patient. The clinician should slowly move his or her hands in an arc from back to front toward the front of the patient. Without head movement, the patient needs to report when the hands come into view peripherally. When the clinician's hands are approximately half way around the patient, the he or she should report peripheral visualization of the clinician's hands.

For a complete examination of the eye, the clinician should complete a funduscopic examination of the patient's retina. This examination requires an ophthalmoscope that shines a bright beam of light through the patient's pupil to examine the retina. For easier inspection, a clinician will often dilate the patient's pupils with application of an optic mydriatic agent. The patient needs to focus on an object in the distance without changing position of the eyes or head throughout the examination. The clinician needs to shine the ophthalmoscope light on the eye from a distance and observe the pupil's red reflex. After capturing the red reflex, the clinician needs to slowly advance toward the patient; finally, when head to head, the clinician looks into the patient's pupil for a blood vessel. This blood vessel should be followed medially to the optic disc, where its borders and color can be visualized. The retinal vessels should be examined for color, continuity, and lesions. The retina is the only place on the body where active, live blood vessels can be seen directly. Specific changes of the blood vessels can indicate hypertension, arteriosclerosis, and diabetes mellitus (DM). The ophthalmoscope should be moved laterally on the retina for observation of the macula, a red area without any blood vessels. The macula is an area of central vision that can undergo degeneration with age. The fovea is the central region of the macula.

Diagnosis

Tonometry

A tonometer, a handheld device that measures the pressure within the eye, is similar in shape to a pencil. Once placed on the numbed exterior eye, it can instantly record eye pressure. More often, a tonometer within a slit lamp apparatus shoots a small puff of air into the eye and measures IOP, which is a test to screen for glaucoma.

Slit Lamp Examination

The slit lamp, an instrument with a high-intensity light source, shines a thin beam of light into the eye. A microscope is also contained within the instrument. The slit lamp examination provides a three-dimensional, magnified view of the eye structures in detail. The instrument facilitates an examination of the eye's anterior structures, which include the sclera, conjunctiva, iris, lens, and cornea. The instrument facilitates diagnosis of a variety of eye conditions.

Other Diagnostic Procedures

Other diagnostic procedures used in ophthalmology include plain x-ray and contrast-media procedures such as orbital venography and angiography. Other imaging techniques include computed tomography (CT) scan, ultrasonography, and magnetic resonance imaging (MRI). For more specific diagnostic methods, see the section on Selected Disorders of Vision.

Treatment

Corrective lenses are the major forms of treatment for vision impairment. Alternatively, some patients can be treated with LASIK surgery in lieu of their use of lenses. There are many different classes of ophthalmic medications used in treatments of various eye disorders. For specific medications, see the section on Selected Disorders of Vision.

Laser coagulation is used in diabetic retinopathy. Many different surgical procedures are also used in ophthalmology.

Corrective Lenses

Corrective lenses are used to treat myopia (nearsightedness), hyperopia (farsightedness), or astigmatism (abnormal shape of the eyeball). Lenses are pieces of transparent material (glass or plastic) that are shaped to bend light rays.

Myopia Correction

Myopic individuals have impaired distance vision. In myopia, the eyeball is elongated and visual images fall in front of the retina. Concave lenses are used in myopia because they spread the light out before it reaches the lens of the eye; this lets the image focus directly on the retina (see Fig. 43-17).

Hyperopia Correction

Hyperopic individuals cannot see objects in close range, such as reading material. In hyperopia, the eyeball is shortened and visual images fall behind the retina. Convex lenses are used in hyperopia because they focus the light on the lens of the eye, making the image land directly on the retina (see Fig. 43-18).

Myopia

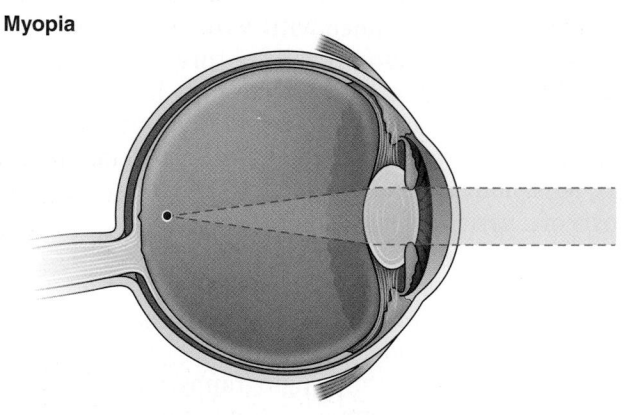

Myopia corrected

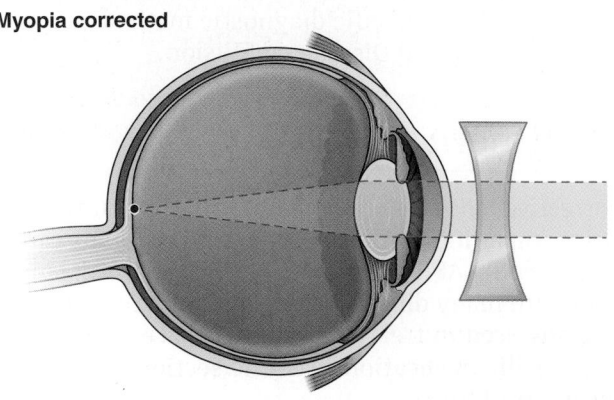

FIGURE 43-17. How corrective lenses change light refraction in myopia.

Hyperopia

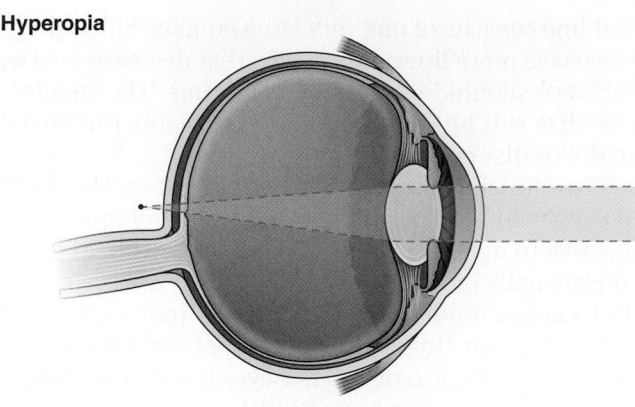

Hyperopia corrected

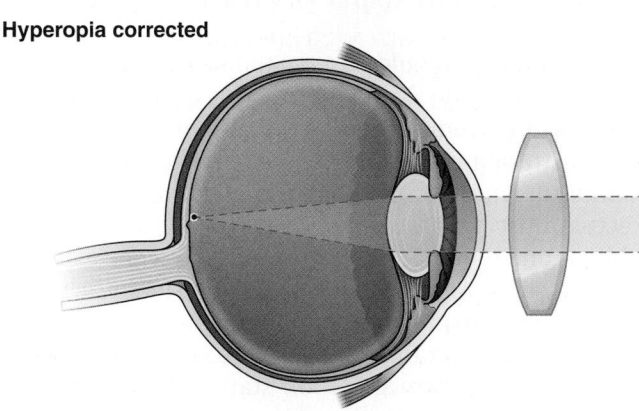

FIGURE 43-18. How corrective lenses change light refraction in hyperopia.

Astigmatism Correction

Astigmatism is the result of an irregularly shaped cornea or lens. The eye is shaped like a football instead of a baseball. The eye's shape in astigmatism makes the light rays focus on two spots instead of one on the retina. The cornea has a steep, flat curve that can be corrected with lenses. A cylindrical curve in the corrective lens compensates for the eye's abnormal shape.

LASIK and PRK Surgery

LASIK, commonly referred to as laser eye surgery, is a procedure that can correct myopia, hyperopia, and astigmatism. LASIK is performed by using a laser to reshape the cornea to enhance vision. This relatively safe procedure has a low incidence of complications. Other surgical corrective procedures include photorefractive keratectomy (PRK), also called advanced surface ablation. These procedures also reshape the cornea to correct vision. Both LASIK and PRK are advanced technological procedures that have replaced past use of radial keratotomy; they offer alternatives to wearing corrective eyeglasses or contact lenses for many patients.

Selected Eye Infections and Inflammatory Disorders

Various infection and inflammatory disorders affect the eye. *C. trachomatis*, the most common cause of blindness worldwide, is highly contagious. Although uncommon in the United States, it is prevalent in underdeveloped regions. In the United States, bacterial and viral conjunctivitis are more common, especially among children. Allergic conjunctivitis is a problem for many individuals in the United States because of environmental antigens such as pollen, dust, or pollutants.

Bacterial and Viral Conjunctivitis

The term **conjunctivitis,** often referred to as pinkeye, describes any inflammatory process that involves the bulbar conjunctiva, which covers the sclera, and the palpebral conjunctiva, which lines the eyelids. The bulbar conjunctiva is a colorless membrane, whereas the palpebral conjunctiva is a deep pink mucous membrane that keeps the eye moist and protected.

Conjunctivitis is one of the most common nontraumatic eye complaints that presents to the emergency department (ED) or primary care clinician. Three percent of all ED visits are ocular related, and conjunctivitis is responsible for approximately 30% of all eye complaints. Two percent of all visits to primary care clinicians are for eye conditions, with 54% of these being either conjunctivitis or corneal abrasion. Bacterial conjunctivitis is more common in children, and viral conjunctivitis is more common in adults.

Etiology

Bacteria, viruses, parasites, fungi, chemicals, and environmental allergens are the possible etiologies of conjunctivitis. Viral conjunctivitis represents up to 50% of all acute conjunctivitis in primary care. A foreign body in the eye and contact lenses increase an individual's risk of bacterial or viral conjunctivitis. Exposure to others with conjunctivitis is the most significant risk factor, and the common mode of transmission is hand-to-eye transmission.

Pathophysiology

In conjunctivitis, both the palpebral and bulbar conjunctiva undergo inflammation because of a pathogen, allergen, or toxin. *Streptococcus*, *Staphylococcus*, and *Haemophilus aegyptius* are the most common bacterial organisms that cause conjunctivitis. Viral conjunctivitis is more common than bacterial conjunctivitis, with adenovirus being the most common etiologic agent. Adenovirus conjunctivitis, usually accompanied by rhinitis or upper respiratory infection, is relatively benign and self-limited.

Herpes viral infection of the conjunctiva is a more problematic disorder than adenovirus. Herpes viruses remain dormant in the body and can become active at unpredictable times of life. The types of herpes viruses that can affect the eye are herpes zoster and herpes simplex I or II.

Herpes zoster conjunctivitis, also called herpes zoster ophthalmicus, not only affects the conjunctiva but can also cause keratitis, or corneal inflammation. Herpes zoster infection is actually a reactivation of latent varicella zoster. When an individual contracts varicella zoster, the virus becomes dormant and remains in the body; it reactivates as herpes zoster, commonly called shingles. This disorder usually presents as painful blisters on the skin that follow a linear path of a nerve. When this virus is activated along the trigeminal nerve, blisters along the ophthalmic branch affect the eye's cornea. Complications can occur in the form of keratitis, erosion of the cornea, corneal ulceration with keratoconjunctivitis, and bacterial superinfection. Corneal scarring can occur without treatment.

Herpes simplex virus I or II can also cause conjunctivitis. These viruses, which commonly cause either oral or genital lesions, can infect the eye as well. Similarly to herpes zoster infection, herpes simplex causes blisters of the skin along a nerve's path. If the virus infects the trigeminal nerve, then corneal lesions are possible. Corneal ulceration, keratitis, and keratoconjunctivitis can occur.

Clinical Presentation

Bacterial conjunctivitis produces a mucopurulent exudate, whereas viral infection causes a watery discharge of the eye. In both bacterial and viral conjunctivitis, the patient has a sensation that a foreign body is in the eye, a red teary eye, or photophobia. The eye may be "glued" shut because of discharge, and is usually itchy and edematous with pinpoint subconjunctival hemorrhages. The patient rubs the eyes and blinks frequently, trying to resolve the discomfort with no result. Visual acuity is only slightly affected.

Diagnosis

The diagnosis of conjunctivitis is usually based on the clinical symptoms. Culture of exudate is done with severe infections. Slit lamp examination is necessary if corneal involvement is present.

Treatment

A broad spectrum, topical, ocular antibiotic is commonly prescribed for bacterial infection. Oral and topical antiviral preparations are used with herpes conjunctivitis. In both bacterial and viral conjunctivitis, patients should be discouraged from touching their eyes and should limit direct contact with others until treatment is underway. All bed linens should be thoroughly laundered in hot water. Frequent hand washing is essential.

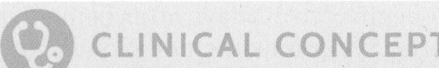

CLINICAL CONCEPT

Topical corticosteroid drops can provide relief in bacterial infection; however, corticosteroids will worsen a herpes zoster infection.

Chlamydia Trachomatis

C. trachomatis, a bacterial organism, is the leading cause of eye infection worldwide. The most common cause of blindness in underdeveloped countries, it causes an infection called chronic keratoconjunctivitis, commonly referred to as **trachoma.** In keratoconjunctivitis, both the conjunctiva and cornea undergo inflammation.

Trachoma is endemic in parts of Africa, Asia, the Middle East, Latin America, the Pacific Islands, and aboriginal communities in Australia. Worldwide, an estimated 84 million people in 55 endemic countries have active trachoma. Approximately 1.3 million people across the world are blind because of trachoma.

Etiology

Trachoma, a severe eye infection caused by *C. trachomatis* serotypes A, B, Ba, and C, occurs mostly in rural settings where sanitation is poor. Although trachoma is rare in the United States, certain populations marked by poverty, crowded living conditions, or poor hygiene are at high risk for this eye disorder. Trachoma is spread through direct contact with the secretions from an infected eye, nose, or throat, or by contact with contaminated objects, such as towels or clothes. Flies can also spread the bacteria. Disease transmission occurs primarily between children and the women who care for them. Repeated episodes of reinfection within a family is common.

Pathophysiology

Active trachoma is characterized by a mucopurulent keratoconjunctivitis that mainly affects the conjunctival surface of the upper eyelid and cornea. There is intense conjunctival inflammation, which leads to conjunctival fibrosis and scarring. Also, there are obvious corneal abrasions, corneal scarring, and opacification. Ultimately, these conditions lead to blindness. Infection concurrently occurs in extraocular mucous membranes, commonly the nasopharynx, leading to a nasal discharge. These nasal secretions commonly cause the spread of infection.

Clinical Presentation

When taking the patient's history, the clinician should include questions regarding recent travel to regions of the world where trachoma is endemic. The patient's current living situation should be investigated because crowded, unsanitary living conditions increase susceptibility. In addition to questions about the discomfort experienced in the eyes, the patient should be asked about family infection. Symptoms of trachoma begin 5 to 12 days after being exposed to the bacteria. Symptoms include cloudy cornea, discharge from the eye, swelling of preauricular lymph nodes, swollen eyelids, and entropion formation. The patient endures eye discomfort and tends to rub the eyes, which allows secretions to spread to others from the hand.

Diagnosis

The patient is often diagnosed based on the clinical manifestations in endemic regions. The best laboratory techniques to confirm diagnosis of *C. trachomatis* infection is the nucleic acid amplification test referred to as the polymerase chain reaction. This test amplifies the deoxyribonucleic acid (DNA) of the pathogen which, in turn, identifies the specific organism.

Treatment

The key to treating trachoma is the SAFE strategy developed by the WHO:

S – surgery
A – antibiotics
F – facial cleanliness
E – environmental improvement.

Two antibiotics are used for trachoma control: oral azithromycin and tetracycline eye ointment. Infection occurs in the nasopharynx as well as the eyes; oral antibiotics are necessary for this reason. If a topical eye antibiotic is used alone, patients can reinfect themselves from their nasal secretions.

The promotion of sanitation, hygienic living conditions, and clean water is key to diminishing contagion among persons. Regions affected by *C. trachomatis* infection require safe drinking water and sanitary disposal of human feces. Improvements in personal and community hygiene are associated with significant reduction in the prevalence.

Allergic Conjunctivitis

Often mistaken for infectious conjunctivitis, allergic conjunctivitis is extremely common. Airborne antigens, such as pollen, pet dander, dust mites, cockroach debris, cigarette smoke, weeds, and grass, are the most frequent cause of allergic conjunctivitis. Seasonal conjunctivitis occurs during specific times of the year. In spring, trees are the usual stimulus of allergic response. In summer, grasses provoke allergy; in fall, weeds often trigger allergy. People with seasonal conjunctivitis also have allergic rhinitis. In addition, conjunctivitis can occur in atopic individuals—persons with asthma or eczema.

The palpebral conjunctiva becomes inflamed and swollen with a cobblestone appearance. Individuals have tearing and redness of the eye with intense itching. Diagnosis is made from the clinical examination and history. Symptoms are alleviated by the avoidance of allergens; cold compresses, topical vasoconstrictors, and antihistamines can reduce the symptoms. Topical nonsteroidal anti-inflammatory agents are also used for immune-mediated forms of conjunctivitis. Corticosteroids provide relief, but long-term use can lead to complications such as glaucoma, cataracts, and secondary infection.

Selected Disorders of Vision

Glaucoma, diabetic retinopathy, AMD, papilledema, and cataracts are among the most common eye disorders that can cause blindness. Each disorder has a distinct pathophysiology and characteristic signs and symptoms. Structural eye disorders such as vitreous hemorrhage and retinal detachment cause unique visual symptoms and can also cause blindness without treatment. Optic neuritis, retinitis pigmentosa, retinoblastoma, and melanoma of the eye are less common disorders, but can also cause blindness if untreated.

Glaucoma

Glaucoma—one of the leading preventable causes of blindness in the world—is caused by elevated IOP, which leads to pressure on the optic nerve with consequent nerve damage and blindness (see Fig. 43-19). There are two main types of the disorder: primary open-angle glaucoma (POAG) and acute angle-closure glaucoma (AACG). Open angle glaucoma is usually silent and slowly progressive, whereas acute angle glaucoma occurs suddenly and is an emergency situation. With appropriate screening and treatment, glaucoma usually can be identified and its progress arrested before significant effects on vision occur.

Ninety percent of glaucoma patients have POAG and 10% have AACG. Primary open-angle glaucoma affects more than 2 million individuals in the United States. With the aging of the U.S. population, this number will increase to more than 3 million by 2020. It is estimated that 1% to 2% of people older than 40 years of age have POAG, with 25% of cases undetected. Glaucoma has been called the "silent thief of sight" because the loss of vision is gradual over a prolonged time, and symptoms only occur when the disease is quite advanced.

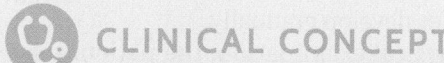

> ### 🩺 CLINICAL CONCEPT
>
> Glaucoma is the most common cause of blindness among African Americans. They are more likely to develop glaucoma early in life, and they tend to have a more aggressive form of the disease. Prevalence of POAG is three to four times higher in African Americans than in Caucasians, and African Americans are up to six times more susceptible to optic nerve damage than Caucasians.

AACG is an acute emergency and its outcome is dependent on duration from onset to treatment. For unknown reasons, AACG is common in persons of Asian

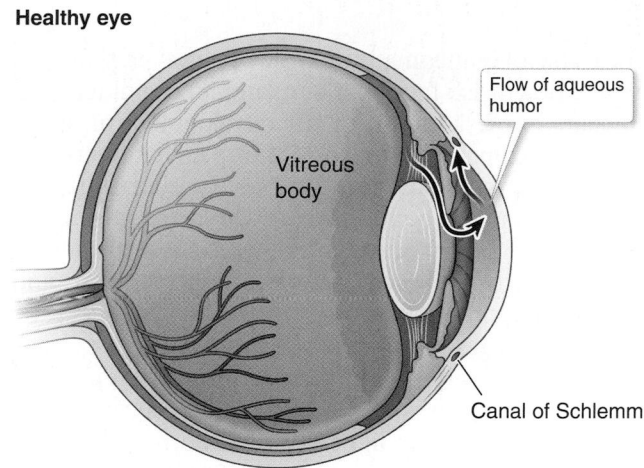

Healthy eye

Vitreous body

Flow of aqueous humor

Canal of Schlemm

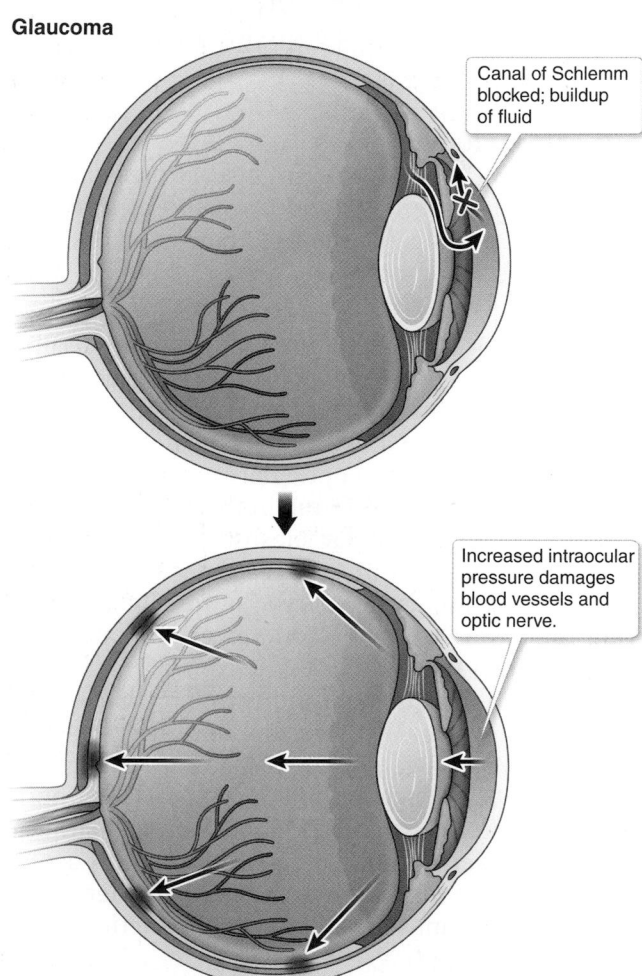

Glaucoma

Canal of Schlemm blocked; buildup of fluid

Increased intraocular pressure damages blood vessels and optic nerve.

FIGURE 43-19. Structures involved in glaucoma.

American descent. AACG occurs in 1 of 1,000 Caucasians, but about 1 in 100 Asian Americans. In addition, Asian Americans with AACG are difficult to treat because medical management often fails. Despite treatment, they often suffer a progressive increase in IOP and deterioration in visual acuity. AACG predominately affects females because of their shallower anterior chamber. Older adult patients in their sixth and seventh decades of life are at greatest risk.

Etiology

The cause of glaucoma is unknown; however, there are many known risk factors. For example, age older than 40 years is a risk factor for the development of open-angle glaucoma, with up to 15% of people affected by age 70. As previously noted, ethnicity is a risk factor. Other risk factors include genetic predisposition, myopia, and a history of migraine headaches, cardiovascular disease, diabetes, systemic hypertension, and systemic hypotension.

Specific drugs can precipitate AACG, such as sympathomimetics, anticholinergics, serotonin receptor inhibitor antidepressants, sulfonamides, cocaine, and botulinum toxin. Dim light and rapid correction of hyperglycemia can also trigger AACG. Studies have identified AACG associated with carotid artery-cavernous sinus fistula, trauma, prone surgical positioning, and giant cell arteritis.

Pathophysiology

POAG and AACG have different disease mechanisms. Although they are triggered by different etiologic factors, they basically require treatment that decreases IOP.

Primary Open-Angle Glaucoma. The pathophysiology of glaucoma is not completely understood. There are known structural changes that occur in glaucoma; however, there are many different theories about the cause of retinal cell and optic nerve damage. Significant structural changes found in the eyes involve the ciliary muscle, trabecular meshwork, and canal of Schlemm. The ciliary muscle is attached to a trabecular meshwork that allows free flow of aqueous fluid from the anterior chamber to posterior chamber of the eye. When the ciliary muscle contracts, it allows the drainage of aqueous fluid through the canal of Schlemm; however, with muscle relaxation there is obstruction of the canal. The ciliary muscle is innervated by both the sympathetic and parasympathetic nervous system. Stimulation of parasympathetic nerves contract the ciliary muscle, allowing ocular fluid drainage. Stimulation of sympathetic nerves relaxes the ciliary muscle and causes obstruction of ocular fluid drainage.

🩺 CLINICAL CONCEPT

Drugs or conditions that enhance anticholinergic activity have the same effect as sympathetic nerve activation—both cause relaxation of the ciliary muscle and obstruction of fluid drainage. This is particularly important for clinicians to recognize when prescribing drugs with anticholinergic effects. For example, many antidepressants have anticholinergic side effects, so glaucoma can be initiated or worsened by antidepressants.

When ocular fluid drainage is obstructed, the high level of fluid raises IOP and places pressure on the junction of the optic nerve and the retina at the back of the eye. The optic cup in the center of the optic disc enlarges under high IOP. Until recently, it was believed that elevated IOP was responsible for optic nerve damage in glaucoma. However, studies show that only 30% to 50% of all glaucoma patients have elevated IOP; up to 50% do not have high IOP. So, elevated IOP is now believed to be an important—but not the only—factor responsible for optic nerve damage. Other mechanisms of glaucoma are under investigation. Regardless of the mechanisms involved, the outcome of glaucoma is the death of retinal and optic nerve cells, leading to irreversible visual field loss.

Acute Angle-Closure Glaucoma. AACG can occur in people who were born with a narrow angle between the iris and the cornea. This type of glaucoma is more common in people who are hyperopic. In AACG, the ciliary muscle is relaxed and the canal of Schlemm is obstructed. Relaxation may occur because of sympathetic or anticholinergic activity or other etiology. With ciliary muscle relaxation, there is obstructed drainage of aqueous fluid, resulting in a sudden increase of IOP within the eyes. Consequently, there is a sudden loss of peripheral or central vision.

Clinical Presentation

When gathering information for the history, the clinician should focus on age, use of lenses, past eye problems, family history of glaucoma, ethnicity, and medications. The use of anticholinergic medications is a common trigger of glaucoma. It is important for the clinician to recognize that many medications—including antidepressants, antipsychotics, antihistamines, specific anticholinergic bronchodilators, and muscle relaxants, as well as gastrointestinal and some cardiac drugs—have anticholinergic side effects. The patient with glaucoma complains of eye pain, eye redness, nausea, halos around lights, and vision loss. In AACG, these symptoms develop suddenly and rapidly, whereas in POAG symptoms may be silent or develop gradually.

On physical examination, the patient may show no signs of illness. Redness of the eye and blood vessels in the sclera may be apparent. Funduscopic examination is necessary. The clinician should inspect the retina, particularly the optic nerve.

ALERT! Anticholinergic drugs and drugs with anticholinergic side effects are contraindicated in glaucoma.

Diagnosis

An examination of the optic nerve is essential to look for an increase in the cup-to-disc ratio. The optic cup is the portion of the optic disc not occupied by nerve fibers. Located in the center of the optic disc, the optic cup-to-disc ratio is normally 0.3 or lower. With glaucoma, there is a progressive increase in optic nerve damage, which increases the optic cup area. Patients with glaucoma have an increased cup-to-disc ratio from 0.7 to 1.0. The greater the optic nerve damage, the greater the vision loss. The patient should be referred to an ophthalmologist for slit lamp examination. Computerized optic nerve imaging is needed if there is any suspicion of damage to the optic nerve.

Treatment

The treatment of glaucoma is aimed at reducing IOP by improving aqueous fluid outflow, reducing the production of aqueous fluid, or both. Treatments available for glaucoma include topical eye medication, oral medications, laser procedures, and incisional surgery. Major drug classes for medical treatment of POAG include the following: alpha-2 agonists, beta blockers, carbonic anhydrase inhibitors, miotic agents, and prostaglandin analogs. Research continues to investigate pharmacological sites of action in glaucoma, including nitric oxide and cannabinoid pathways, although no topical product has been evaluated in U.S. Food and Drug Administration trials. Medical marijuana lowers IOP minimally and its duration of action is very short. If glaucoma is left untreated, blindness will occur.

Papilledema

Papilledema is a swelling of the optic nerve caused by an increase in intracranial pressure. Patients with papilledema may report headache, intermittent diplopia (double vision), vomiting and nausea, and tinnitus. Papilledema is a critical sign of intracranial hypertension, a potentially life-threatening situation. On funduscopic examination, the borders of the optic disc are unclear and undefined (see Fig. 43-20). Treatment is tailored to the underlying pathological process that caused the elevated intracranial pressure, such as a brain tumor. Untreated papilledema eventually may lead to permanent blindness.

ALERT! Papilledema is indicative of increased intracranial pressure (ICP), which requires immediate medical intervention.

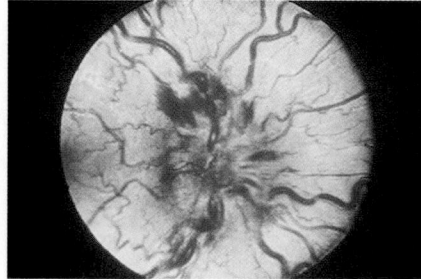

FIGURE 43-20. Papilledema. *(Courtesy of Wills Eye Hospital, Philadelphia, PA.)*

Diabetic Retinopathy

Diabetic retinopathy is a change in the retina that occurs in individuals with type 1 or type 2 diabetes. Before the diagnosis of either type of diabetes, vascular changes occur that are caused by periodic high blood glucose levels. Retinopathy, one of these vascular changes, is often present upon the diagnosis of diabetes.

There are 25.8 million people living with diabetes in the United States, accounting for 8.3% of the population. It is theorized that 45% of adults with diabetes in the United States have some degree of diabetic retinopathy at diagnosis. With the epidemic of diabetes worldwide, there will be an increase in diabetic retinopathy in the future.

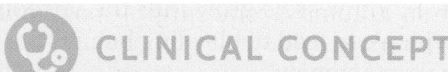

CLINICAL CONCEPT

Diabetic retinopathy is the most frequent cause of blindness among adults aged 20 to 74 years.

Etiology

There are various risk factors for diabetes (see Chapter 25: Diabetes Mellitus and the Metabolic Syndrome). High glucose levels are the major cause for vascular changes that lead to diabetic retinopathy. It is theorized that before the initial diagnosis of DM, there are intermittent periods of high glucose levels that are asymptomatic, unmonitored, and untreated. During these times, the damage of the retina probably starts to occur. After diagnosis, if the patient has poor blood sugar regulation, this leads to retinal blood vessel changes.

Pathophysiology

There are two forms of diabetic retinopathy: nonproliferative and proliferative. Early in diabetes, nonproliferative retinopathy occurs. On funduscopic examination, tiny aneurysms and hemorrhages are seen. Areas of ischemia of the retina, microinfarcts, and areas of nerve damage called "cotton wool spots" are also seen.

The exact pathophysiologic mechanism of retinal vessel aneurysms and hemorrhages in nonproliferative diabetic retinopathy is incompletely understood, but there are many theories. Platelet and red blood cell abnormalities are seen in diabetes, such as increased erythrocyte aggregation, increased platelet aggregation, and increased platelet adhesion. These changes predispose the patient to sluggish circulation, endothelial damage, and capillary occlusion within the retinal blood vessels. This leads to retinal ischemia which, in turn, contributes to the development of diabetic retinopathy.

Another theory involves the high glucose levels that occur in DM. Increased levels of blood glucose are thought to cause endothelial injury throughout the body, including the retinal blood vessels. This renders the blood vessel walls susceptible to arteriosclerosis, aneurysm, and rupture.

Other researchers assert that high blood glucose levels stimulate a process called the aldose reductase pathway in certain tissues, which converts sugars into sorbitol. The walls of retinal blood vessels are directly damaged by this increased level of sorbitol, eventually leading to weakness and aneurysms.

Later in the course of diabetes, proliferative retinopathy occurs. In this stage, diabetes stimulates vasoactive growth factors that cause neovascularization. This is called a proliferative retinopathy because the retina has many more blood vessels than normal. The new blood vessels grow throughout the retina and are seen on funduscopic examination. The new blood vessels have very weak walls, which leads to aneurysms and hemorrhages. Also, new blood vessels grow into the vitreous of the eyeball, which can lead to bleeding behind the vitreous and retinal detachment.

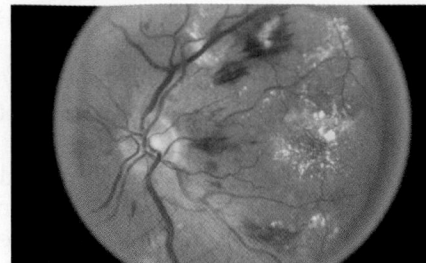

FIGURE 43-21. Diabetic retinopathy. *(Courtesy of Wills Eye Hospital, Philadelphia, PA.)*

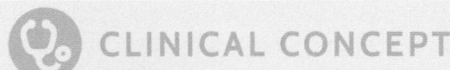

CLINICAL CONCEPT

When an individual is diagnosed with diabetes, a funduscopic examination should be done to rule out diabetic retinopathy.

Clinical Presentation

The patient history should contain information about the duration of diabetes and daily glucose control. The history should document the patient's current medications and last ophthalmic examination. The history should also contain current medical or surgical disorders such as cardiovascular or peripheral vascular disease. Details about the patient's vision are necessary, so a vision test should be done. Initially, diabetic retinopathy may be asymptomatic or cause only mild vision problems. As the condition progresses, symptoms may include floaters, blurred vision, poor night vision, and vision loss. It usually affects both eyes. Proliferation of new blood vessels is indicative of a poor prognosis.

Diagnosis

In diabetic retinopathy, the retina often shows lesions such as microaneurysms, hemorrhages, hard exudates (lipid residues), cotton wool spots (areas of nerve destruction), and proliferation of fragile, new blood vessels (see Fig. 43-21). A thorough slit lamp examination is necessary with an ophthalmologist.

Treatment

Blood glucose control is necessary to slow the progression of retinal changes. Photocoagulation laser technology is used to destroy new, fragile vessels, as well as hemorrhages. Treatment of diabetic retinopathy can decrease the risk of vision loss by over half.

Cataracts

Cataracts, a major cause of blindness worldwide, cause visual impairment because of excessive growth of the epithelial layers of the eye lens (see Fig. 43-22). The lens becomes thickened with less transparency and flexibility. It commonly affects older adults because lens thickening is a physiologic change associated with advancing age. Approximately 20.5 million (17.2%) Americans older than 40 years have a cataract in either eye. With the rising number of older adults in the population, this number is expected to increase to 30.1 million people by 2020.

There are different types of cataracts; this section discusses senile and congenital cataracts.

Etiology

Risk factors for senile cataract development include advancing age, cigarette smoking, obesity, diabetes, kidney disorders, musculoskeletal disorders, trauma, long-term steroid use, and exposure to ultraviolet light. In addition to steroids, other drugs associated with increased risk of cataract development include alfluzosin and tamsulosin, which are used to treat benign prostatic hyperplasia.

Congenital cataracts develop in the fetus because of infection contracted during pregnancy. Infections such as rubella, syphilis, toxoplasmosis, and cytomegalovirus are associated with congenital cataract. Other causes of congenital cataract include Down syndrome, Marfan syndrome, and Alport syndrome, as well as many other genetic disorders.

Pathophysiology

Multiple mechanisms contribute to the progressive loss of transparency of the lens in senile cataract formation.

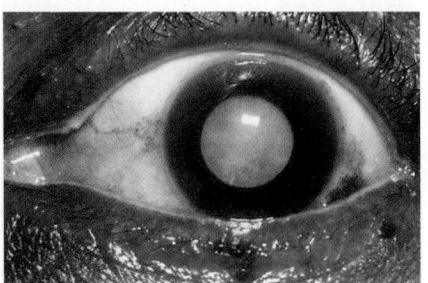

FIGURE 43-22. Cataract. *(Courtesy of Wills Eye Hospital, Philadelphia, PA.)*

As a consequence of normal aging, the lenses in the eyes develop excessive layers of epithelium. The epithelial cells lose the ability to degenerate as new layers of cells proliferate and accumulate. The increased thickness of the lens makes it less able to accommodate. Also, the water solubility of the lens diminishes, making it more inflexible. Protein fibers are normally arranged in a precise manner that makes the lens clear and allows light to pass through without interference. With aging, there is accumulated damage of the protein fibers of the lenses by free radicals. Protein fibers degenerate, begin to clump together, and clouding of small areas of the lens occurs. As the cataract continues to develop, the clouding becomes denser and involves a greater part of the lens.

Clinical Presentation

A patient with a cataract often presents with a history of gradual loss of vision. Individuals with cataracts develop blurry vision and have cloudiness in the lens of the eye. Many people see halos at night around bright objects or they become more sensitive to glare. The patient's eyes have an opacity covering the center of their eyes.

The progression of cataracts frequently creates changes in the lens that result in myopia. Presbyopia can be counteracted by the myopic effect of cataracts. Patients often report an improvement in their near vision and less need for reading glasses as they experience this phenomenon of second sight. However, this is temporary because the lens increases in excessive thickness with time, which undermines this effect.

A complete ocular examination must be performed beginning with visual acuity for both near and far distances. When the patient complains of glare, visual acuity should be tested in a brightly lit room. The patient's extraocular muscles should be assessed in all directions of gaze and it is important to rule out any other causes for the patient's visual symptoms.

Diagnosis

Ocular imaging studies such as ultrasound, CT scan, and MRI are often needed for an adequate view of the back of the eye. If macular involvement or glaucoma is suspected, specialized tests are done as well.

Treatment

Treatment involves surgical removal of the cataract and replacement with an artificial lens called an intraocular lens. If cataracts go untreated, the individual will have worsening of vision and possible blindness.

Age-Related Macular Degeneration

AMD is a deterioration of the macula, a specific area on the retina that provides central vision. As the macula degenerates, central vision deteriorates and the patient develops a blind spot in the center of the visual field. AMD usually produces a slow, painless loss of vision.

AMD is the most common cause of vision loss in the United States in those 50 years or older, and its prevalence increases with age. It occurs in approximately 10% of the population aged 65 to 74 years and in 25% of the population older than age 74. As the population of individuals older than 85 years is projected to increase by the year 2020, the prevalence of AMD is expected to increase from 1.75 million individuals to 2.95 million individuals.

Etiology

AMD is caused by a combination of genetic, behavioral, and environmental factors. Advanced age and family history are nonmodifiable risk factors associated with AMD. Genetic mutations on chromosomes 1, 6, and 10 are associated with the disorder. Genetic factors contribute to approximately 50% of the sibling risk of developing AMD. Smoking, hypertension, obesity, and dietary fat intake are the modifiable risk factors.

Pathophysiology

AMD involves two layers of the eye: the retina, which contains the nerves, and the choroid, which contains the blood supply. There are two types of AMD: nonexudative, also called "dry" macular degeneration, and exudative, also called "wet" macular degeneration. The pathophysiologic mechanism of each type is different. Greater than 90% of patients diagnosed with AMD have the nonexudative type.

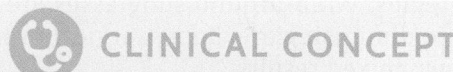

CLINICAL CONCEPT

Nonexudative AMD can progress over the course of decades, whereas exudative AMD can result in visual loss over the course of months.

The pathophysiology of both types of AMD involves the retinal pigmented epithelium (RPE), a metabolically active layer of cells that support the retina's function. RPE cells normally phagocytose degenerated retinal cells and continually recycle and process the cellular materials. However, as the RPE cells age, they become less able to process accumulated cellular debris. The RPE cells excrete the cellular debris for removal by the vessels of the choroid layer, but changes in the permeability of the choroid membrane lead to deposition of material between the RPE and choroid. The deposited material is called **drusen.** The capillaries of the choroid also become less able to absorb extracellular material; this also contributes to drusen formation. Drusen appear as yellow-white accumulations of material in the macula region of the retina.

In the nonexudative form, drusen accumulate between the retina and the choroid layers of the eye; this can separate the layers, leading to retinal detachment. In the wet form, which is more severe, blood vessels grow from the choroid layer to behind the retina and separate the layers; this leads to retinal detachment.

Clinical Presentation

Patients with AMD usually report a family history of decreased vision late in life, including difficulty with night vision or low light conditions. Commonly, patients with AMD report fluctuations in vision, with some poor vision days and other days when it appears improved. Patients also report difficulty with reading and seeing faces. Central vision is affected with peripheral vision intact. The clinician can see areas of yellow-white drusen in the macula region on funduscopic examination.

Diagnosis

Age-related macular degeneration is usually diagnosed by using an Amsler grid to measure central vision. Individuals with macular degeneration will notice black spots in their central vision when looking through the Amsler grid; slit lamp examination is also necessary. Fluorescein angiography is a procedure that can highlight the retinal epithelium.

Treatment

To prevent AMD, consumption of antioxidants, including vitamin A, vitamin E, zinc, and lutein, is recommended, as is a supplement consisting of folic acid, pyridoxine, and vitamin B_{12}. A low-fat diet and cessation of smoking, if applicable, are also preventive strategies. Wrap-around sunglasses are recommended to diminish glare. Some surgical procedures have shown mixed results.

Retinal Detachment

Retinal detachment occurs when the retina is pulled away from its normal position in the back of the eye. It can occur at any age, but it is more common in people older than 40 years of age. It affects men more than women, and Caucasians more than African Americans.

Etiology

As the vitreous gel of the eyeball ages it liquefies. As it liquefies, it places traction on the retinal layer, which lies beneath and pulls away, causing a tear. Risk factors for retinal detachment include myopia, prior intraocular surgery, aphakia (absence of the lens), some inflammatory conditions, and genetic susceptibility. Prior intraocular surgery for cataract removal, inflammation caused by cytomegalovirus, and Marfan syndrome are conditions that increase the risk of retinal detachment.

Retinal detachment is also more likely to occur in people who have had a retinal detachment in the other eye, a positive family history of retinal detachment, and a history of eye injury. In young children and teenagers, eye trauma can cause this condition.

Pathophysiology

Retinal detachment occurs when the inner layers of the retina break away from the retinal epithelial cells. This is often caused by fluid accumulation in between the layers from liquefied vitreous, inflammatory conditions of the choroid layer, hypertensive retinopathy, proliferative diabetic retinopathy, sickle cell disease, or penetrating trauma.

Clinical Presentation

Initial symptoms commonly include the sensation of photopsia, accompanied by floaters and vision loss. Over time, the individual may report a shadow in the peripheral visual field, which may spread rapidly to involve the entire visual field in a matter of days. Vision loss may be described as filmy, cloudy, irregular, or curtainlike.

Diagnosis and Treatment

Ophthalmoscopic examination is used to diagnose retinal detachment. Treatment depends on the type, location, and size of the detachment. Retinal tears are usually treated with laser surgery or cryotherapy to reseal the retina to the back wall of the eye. Retinal detachments do not improve without treatment.

ALERT! Prompt treatment and repair of retinal detachment is necessary to prevent permanent vision loss.

Retinoblastoma

Retinoblastoma is a malignant tumor of the retina caused by genetic mutation that generally affects children younger than the age of 6 years. Incidence is 1 in every 15,000 to 20,000 live births. In 60% of cases, the disease is unilateral, and the median age at diagnosis is 2 years. Retinoblastoma is bilateral in about 40% of cases. Survival rates are between 86% and 92%, although many individuals suffer another cancer later in life.

Etiology

The etiology of retinoblastoma is a mutation in the gene located at 13q14, referred to as the *Rb* gene. At the time of initial examination, the clinician should obtain a careful family history and ask specific questions about the occurrence of retinoblastoma, eye problems, or malignancy in any family members. Approximately 5% of patients who develop this disease have a positive family history.

Pathophysiology

Retinoblastoma is a cancerous development in the optic nerve. The tumor arises in the retina and can invade the brain. The tumor cells have an immature appearance and are referred to as retinoblasts. Often the tumor presents as a white mass seen with the ophthalmoscope.

Clinical Presentation

Signs and symptoms of retinoblastoma include white spots in the pupil, strabismus, redness of the eye, pain, and poor vision. Often the abnormality is discovered while viewing photographs of the child. Instead of the typical "red reflex" from the camera flash, the pupil may appear white or distorted. During the examination with the ophthalmoscope, the clinician can see that the red reflex is absent.

Diagnosis and Treatment

An examination of the retina under general anesthesia leads to diagnosis of the eye tumor. If the cancer is in one eye and the tumor is large, treatment is usually removal of the eyeball, a procedure known as enucleation. If the cancer is in one eye and it is expected that vision can be saved, treatment may include radiation therapy, cryotherapy, and chemotherapy. If the cancer is in both eyes, treatment may include the enucleation of the eye with the most cancer, and radiation therapy to the other eye, or chemotherapy followed by local treatment. Enucleation surgery is done when vision cannot be saved.

The prognosis and treatment options depend on the stage of the cancer and the likelihood of restoring vision in one or both eyes. Without treatment, the cancer will spread through the optic nerve to the brain and cause death in 98% of patients. As previously indicated, treatment often means blindness—including the loss of one or both eyes; patients who survive treatment of retinoblastoma are at risk for second nonocular cancers.

Chapter Summary

- Vision is measured using an eye chart and results are recorded as a pair of numbers called visual acuity. Normal sight is scored as a ratio of 20/20. The numerator indicates that the object to be visualized is at a distance of 20 feet. The denominator indicates how far away the object seems to the patient.
- The leading cause of blindness among Caucasians is AMD; among African Americans, cataract and glaucoma account for more than 60% of blindness. Trachoma, an infection caused by Chlamydia, is a leading cause of blindness in undeveloped countries.
- The WHO has specific parameters that categorize vision impairment and blindness. The different types of visual impairment include myopia, hyperopia, presbyopia, astigmatism, amblyopia, and color blindness. Different lenses are used to correct vision.
- According to the American Medical Association, vision that is worse than 20/200 in the best eye with correction is considered blindness.
- LASIK, commonly referred to as laser eye surgery, is a procedure that can correct myopia, hyperopia, and astigmatism.
- Infection of the eyelid, termed a stye or hordeolum, is most often caused by *Staphylococcus aureus.*
- Conjunctivitis, which is inflammation of the conjunctiva, is a common disorder; it is bacterial, viral, or allergic in origin.

- Corneal abrasion, the most common type of structural eye trauma, is damage to the epithelial surface of the cornea, usually caused by a foreign body that comes into contact with the eye. Diagnosis requires fluorescein dye instillation in the eye and inspection with a blue cobalt light, which highlights the area of trauma.
- Diabetic retinopathy is the most frequent cause of blindness among adults aged 20 to 74 years.
- Glaucoma is one of the leading preventable causes of blindness in the world. It is caused by elevated IOP, which leads to pressure on the optic nerve with consequent nerve damage and blindness.
- Papilledema is the swelling of the optic disc caused by increased intracranial pressure.
- A cataract is clouding of the cornea of the eye caused by overgrowth of the lens. Cataracts commonly affect older adults because lens thickening is a physiologic change associated with advancing age.
- AMD is a deterioration of the macula, a specific area on the retina that provides central vision. As the macula degenerates, central vision deteriorates and the patient develops a blind spot in the center of his or her visual field. It is the most common cause of vision loss in the United States in those 50 years or older, and its prevalence increases with age.

Making the Connections

Disorder and Pathophysiology	Signs and Symptoms	Physical Assessment Findings	Diagnostic Testing	Treatment
Bacterial and Viral Conjunctivitis | Infection or allergy that causes inflammation of the palpebral portion of the conjunctiva. Exudative discharge may be present in bacterial infection.				
	Mild foreign body in the eye and photophobia. Visual acuity slightly affected.	Red, swollen conjunctiva. Bacterial conjunctivitis yields mucopurulent exudates, whereas viral infection and allergy cause a watery discharge.	Culture of exudate if present.	Topical antibiotic. Anti-inflammatory topical drops prevent contagion with bacterial infection.
C. Trachomatis | A bacterial infection that causes mucopurulent keratoconjunctivitis. There is intense conjunctival inflammation, which leads to conjunctival fibrosis, scarring, corneal abrasions, corneal scarring, and opacification. Ultimately, these conditions lead to blindness.				
	Symptoms include discharge from the eye, swelling of preauricular lymph nodes, and swollen eyelids. The patient endures eye discomfort and tends to rub the eyes, which allows secretions to spread to others from the hand.	Patient's eyes demonstrate cloudy corneas, discharge from the eyes, swelling of preauricular lymph nodes, swollen eyelids, and entropion formation.	Nucleic acid amplification test, referred to as the polymerase chain reaction. This test amplifies the DNA of the pathogen which, in turn, identifies the specific organism.	The key to treating trachoma is the SAFE strategy developed by the WHO: **S** – surgery **A** – antibiotics **F** – facial cleanliness **E** – environmental improvement. Two antibiotics are used: oral azithromycin and tetracycline eye ointment.
Allergic Conjunctivitis | In allergic conjunctivitis, both the palpebral and bulbar conjunctiva undergo inflammation because of an allergen irritant such as pollen or animal dander.				
	The patient has a sensation that a foreign body is in the eye, a red teary eye, and photophobia. The eye may be "glued" shut because of discharge. The eye is usually itchy and edematous. Visual acuity is slightly affected.	Redness and tearing of the eye, swelling of the eyelid and surrounding tissue. Watery, nonpurulent discharge from the eye. Pinpoint subconjunctival hemorrhages.	The diagnosis of conjunctivitis is usually based on the clinical symptoms. Culture of exudate is done with severe infections. Slit lamp examination is necessary if corneal involvement is present.	Avoidance of allergen. Antihistamine eye drops.
Glaucoma | Elevated IOP caused by the obstruction of drainage of aqueous humor.				
	Painful, red eye; blurry vision.	Optic cup-to-disc ratio greater than 0.3.	Ophthalmoscopic examination. Tonometry.	Medications that reduce IOP. Possible surgical intervention.

Continued

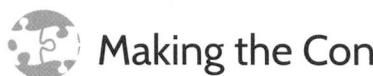 ## Making the Connections—cont'd

Disorder and Pathophysiology	Signs and Symptoms	Physical Assessment Findings	Diagnostic Testing	Treatment
Papilledema | Swelling of the optic disc, which is a sign of pressure on the optic nerve, a sign of increased intracranial pressure.				
	Headaches, which are worse upon awakening and exacerbated by coughing, holding breath, or other maneuvers that increase intracranial pressure. Nausea and vomiting. Changes in vision, such as temporary and transient blurring, graying, flickering of light, and double vision.	Swelling of optic disc; has become blurred with nondiscrete borders.	Dilated visual examination of eye with ophthalmoscope.	Treatment of underlying condition, causing high intracranial pressure.
Diabetic Retinopathy | Proliferation of new blood vessels in the retina. Blood vessels are fragile; can cause blindness.				
	Floaters, blurred vision, poor night vision, and vision loss. Usually affects both eyes.	Visualization of the retina through funduscopic examination shows lesions such as hemorrhages, microaneurysms, hard exudates, dilatation and beading of retinal veins, cotton wool spots, and proliferation of fragile, new blood vessels.	Funduscopic examination and diagnostic tests related to diabetes such as fasting serum glucose or HgbA1c.	Laser photocoagulation of blood vessels.
Cataract | Excess protein layers and irregular clumping of proteinaceous substances within the lens. May be a change of physiologic aging.				
	Blurry vision and cloudiness in lens of eye. Halos at night around bright objects such as light sources. Sensitivity to glare.	Cloudy lens of the eye.	Visual acuity test. Slit lamp and tonometry; an instrument within the slit lamp measures IOP (pressure inside the eye).	Antiglare sunglasses. Surgical removal of cataract.
Age-Related Macular Degeneration | RPE cells of the macula region of the retina age and become less able to process accumulated cellular debris. The RPE cells excrete the cellular debris for removal by the vessels of the choroid layer, but changes in the permeability of the choroid membrane lead to deposition of material between the RPE and choroid. The deposited material is called drusen.				
	Patients with AMD report fluctuations in vision, with some poor vision days and other days when it appears improved. Patients also report difficulty with reading and seeing faces. Central vision is affected with peripheral vision intact.	The clinician can see areas of yellow-white drusen in the macula region on funduscopic examination.	Amsler grid to measure central vision; individuals notice black spots in their central vision when looking through the Amsler grid. Slit lamp examination is necessary. Fluorescein angiography is a procedure that can highlight the retinal epithelium.	Consumption of antioxidants, including vitamin A, vitamin E, zinc, and lutein, is recommended, as is a supplement consisting of folic acid, pyridoxine, and vitamin B_{12}. A low-fat diet and cessation of smoking are preventive strategies.

Continued

Making the Connections—cont'd

Disorder and Pathophysiology	Signs and Symptoms	Physical Assessment Findings	Diagnostic Testing	Treatment
				Wraparound sunglasses are recommended to diminish glare. Surgical interventions are sometimes used.

Retinal Detachment | Retina peels away from its underlying layer of support tissue. Initial detachment may be localized, but without rapid treatment entire retina may detach, leading to vision loss and blindness.

	Symptoms include a sudden or gradual increase in either the number of floaters or light flashes. Appearance of a curtain over field of vision.	Abnormal retina; holes or peeling away of retina from vitreous apparent on ophthalmoscopic examination.	Slit lamp ophthalmoscopic examination.	Emergency laser photocoagulation.

Retinoblastoma | A cancerous development of the optic nerve. The tumor arises in the retina and can invade the brain. The cells of the tumor have an immature appearance and are referred to as retinoblasts.

	Strabismus, redness of the eye, pain, and poor vision.	White spots are seen in the pupil; strabismus of eye and redness of the eye are apparent. Absent "red reflex" of the pupil during the examination with the ophthalmoscope.	An examination of the retina under general anesthesia leads to diagnosis of the eye tumor.	If the cancer is in one eye and it is expected that vision can be saved, treatment may include radiation therapy, cryotherapy, and chemotherapy. If the cancer is in both eyes, treatment may include the enucleation of the eye with the most cancer, and radiation therapy to the other eye, or chemotherapy followed by local treatment. Enucleation surgery of both eyes is done when vision cannot be saved.

Bibliography

ACCORD Study Group, ACCORD Eye Study Group, Chew. E. Y., Ambrosius, W. T., Davis, M. D., et al. (2010). Effects of medical therapies on retinopathy progression in type 2 diabetes. *N Engl J Med, 363*(3), 233–244. Epub 2010 Jun 29.

American Family Physician. (2011). Patient information. Allergic conjunctivitis. *Am Fam Phys, 83*(4), 476.

Antonetti, D. A., Klein, R., & Gardner, T. W. (2012). Diabetic retinopathy. *N Engl J Med, 366*(13), 1227–1239.

Bieler, B. M. (2010). Quality of life after LASIK: the picture remains hazy. *Am Fam Phys, 82*(9), 1044–1046.

Bradfield, Y. S. (2013). Identification and treatment of amblyopia. *Am Fam Phys, 87*(5), 348–352. Erratum in: *Am Fam Phys.* 2013 Aug 1;88(3):159.

Cheung, N., Mitchell, P., & Wong, T. Y. (2010). Diabetic retinopathy. *Lancet, 376*(9735), 124–136. Epub 2010 Jun 26.

Chew, E. Y., Clemons, T. E., Agrón, E., et al. (2014). Ten-year follow-up of age-related macular degeneration in the age-related eye disease study: AREDS report no. 36. *JAMA Ophthalmol, 132*(3), 272–277. doi: 10.1001/jamaophthalmol.2013.6636.

Cronau, H., Kankanala, R. R., & Mauger, T. (2010). Diagnosis and management of red eye in primary care. *Am Fam Phys,* 81(2), 137–144.

Dimaras, H., Kimani, K., Dimba, E. A., et al. (2012). Retinoblastoma. *Lancet.* 2012 Mar 9. Epub ahead of print.

Fiore, D. C., Pasternak, A. V., & Radwan, R. M. (2010). Pain in the quiet (not red) eye. *Am Fam Phys,* 82(1), 69–73.

Gelston, C. D. (2013). Common eye emergencies. *Am Fam Phys,* 88(8), 515–519.

Gower, E. W. (2012). Solving the trachoma elimination puzzle, one piece at a time. *Lancet,* 379(9811), 102–103. Epub 2011 Dec 20.

Han, D. P. (2014). The ForeSeeHome Device and the HOME Study: a milestone in the self-detection of neovascular age-related macular degeneration. *JAMA Ophthalmol.* 2014 Jul 24. doi: 10.1001/jamaophthalmol.2014.1405. Epub ahead of print.

Jacobson, S. G., & Cideciyan, A. V. (2010). Treatment possibilities for retinitis pigmentosa. *N Engl J Med,* 363(17), 1669–1671.

Liew, G., Mitchell, P., Wong, T. Y., Rochtchina, E., & Wang, J. J. (2013). The association of aspirin use with age-related macular degeneration. *JAMA Intern Med,* 173(4), 258–264. doi: 10.1001/jamainternmed.2013.1583.

Lin, K. W., & Hollis, E. M. (2011). Screening for impaired visual acuity in older adults. *Am Fam Phys,* 83(2), 189–190.

Meltzer, D. I. (2013). Painless red eye. *Am Fam Phys,* 88(8), 533–534.

Mishori, R., McClaskey, E. L., & WinklerPrins, V. J. (2012). *Chlamydia trachomatis* infections: screening, diagnosis, and management. *Am Fam Phys,* 86(12), 1127–1132.

Pfeiffer, K. J., Ropers, S. K., & Short, M. W. (2010). Diplopia and ptosis. Diagnosis: diabetic third nerve palsy. *Am Fam Phys,* 82(2), 187–188.

Quigley, H. A. (2011). Glaucoma. *Lancet,* 377(9774), 1367–1377.

Schneider, K. (2013). Caring better for patients who are blind or visually impaired. *Am Fam Phys,* 88(11), 774.

Schwartz, S. D., Hubschman, J. P., Heilwell, G., et al. (2012). Embryonic stem cell trials for macular degeneration: a preliminary report. *Lancet,* 379(9817), 713–720. Epub 2012 Jan 24.

Sheffield, V. C., & Stone, E. M. (2011). Genomics and the eye. *N Engl J Med,* 364(20), 1932–1942.

Sloan, F. A., & Hanrahan, B. W. (2014). The effects of technological advances on outcomes for elderly persons with exudative age-related macular degeneration. *JAMA Ophthalmol,* 132(4), 456–463. doi: 10.1001/jamaophthalmol.2013.7647.

Strandberg, T. E., & Tarkkanen, A. (2014). Cataracts and statin use: cause and effect not confirmed. *JAMA Ophthalmol,* 132(3), 365. doi: 10.1001/jamaophthalmol.2014.23.

Tran, K. T., Qualm, A. S., & Shannon, M. A. (2010). Retinal changes and visual impairment. *Am Fam Phys,* 81(1), 73.

Weinreb, R. N., Aung, T., & Medeiros, F. A. (2014). The pathophysiology and treatment of glaucoma: a review. *JAMA,* 311(18), 1901–1911. doi: 10.1001/jama.2014.3192.

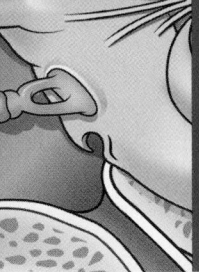

Key Terms

Bony labyrinth
Central hearing impairment
Cochlea
Conductive hearing loss (CHL)
Decibels (dB)
Endolymph
Eustachian tube
Labyrinthitis

Membranous labyrinth
Ménière's disease
Myringotomy tubes
Organ of Corti
Ossicles
Pneumatic otoscope
Presbycusis
Semicircular canals

Sensorineural hearing loss (SNHL)
Tinnitus
Tympanic membrane
Tympanotomy
Umbo
Vertigo
Vestibular caloric reflex
Vestibular schwannoma

The ears are a pair of organs made up of the external, middle, and inner ear compartments. The functions of the external and middle ear include collecting, amplifying, transmitting, and receiving sound. The inner ear consists of sensory organs that are stimulated by sound waves, which are transmitted through a delicate, integrated circuit of structures and transformed into neural impulses sent to the brain via the auditory nerve. The inner ear is also stimulated by the position and movement of the head, which is involved in the maintenance of balance and equilibrium.

Epidemiology

Hearing loss occurs in approximately 5 to 10 of every 1,000 children in the United States; roughly 1 to 3 children of every 1,000 are born with profound hearing loss, and 3 to 5 children of every 1,000 are born with mild-to-moderate hearing loss. As the individuals age, incidence of hearing loss increases: approximately 17% of adults aged 20 to 69 years suffer hearing loss from excessive noise, and 50% of adults older than age 75 years suffer hearing loss of old age, called presbycusis. Data from the U.S. Census show that almost 3% of the population in the workforce reports having some hearing loss.

Basic Concepts Related to Ear Anatomy and Function

The design of the human ear consists of three separate compartments; the external, middle, and inner ear. The external ear is made up of structures that gather sound and deliver it to a delicate tympanic membrane, which changes sound waves into vibrations. The middle ear takes the vibrations and amplifies them via a triad of delicate bones. The delicate bone vibrations then cause movement of fluid and fine hair cells within the inner ear. Within the inner ear, signals are sent to the auditory nerve, which then takes its impulses to the auditory cortex.

The External Ear

The external ear, which is shaped like a funnel, conducts sound waves through the ear canal to the **tympanic membrane,** commonly known as the eardrum. The lining of the ear canal consists of a thin layer of epidermis with fine hairs, sebaceous glands, and glands that produce cerumen, or earwax. The function of the external ear is altered when there is blockage, inflammation, or drainage within the canal or disruption of the tympanic membrane.

The Middle Ear

The middle ear transmits sounds to the auditory organ called the **cochlea,** a small fluid-filled area located in the temporal bone. The middle ear contains three tiny bones called the auditory **ossicles.** These ossicles, which hang from the roof of the middle ear, are the connection between the tympanic membrane and the oval window, which is an opening into the vestibule of the inner ear. The first of the three bones is called the malleus or the "hammer." The handle of the malleus connects to the upper portion of the tympanic membrane and can be seen through the membrane as the **umbo.** The head of the malleus attaches to the incus, also known as the "anvil," which attaches to the stapes, a stirrup-shaped bone. The stapes, in turn, attaches and is sealed into the oval window by the annular ligament. Sound waves

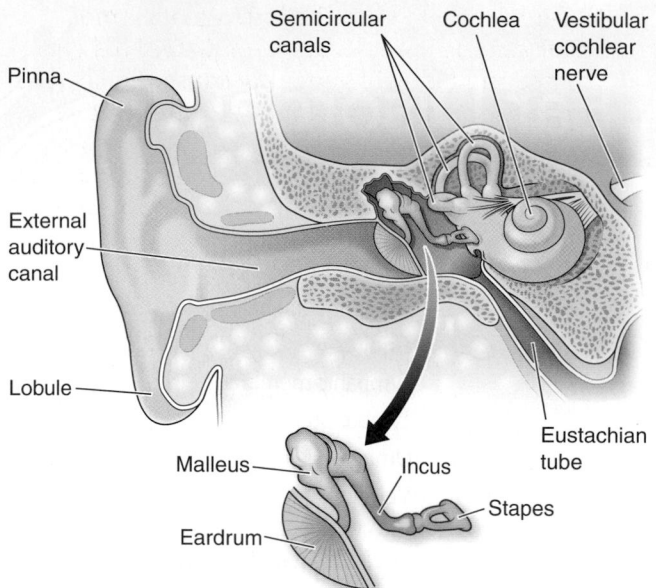

FIGURE 44-1. Anatomy of the ear.

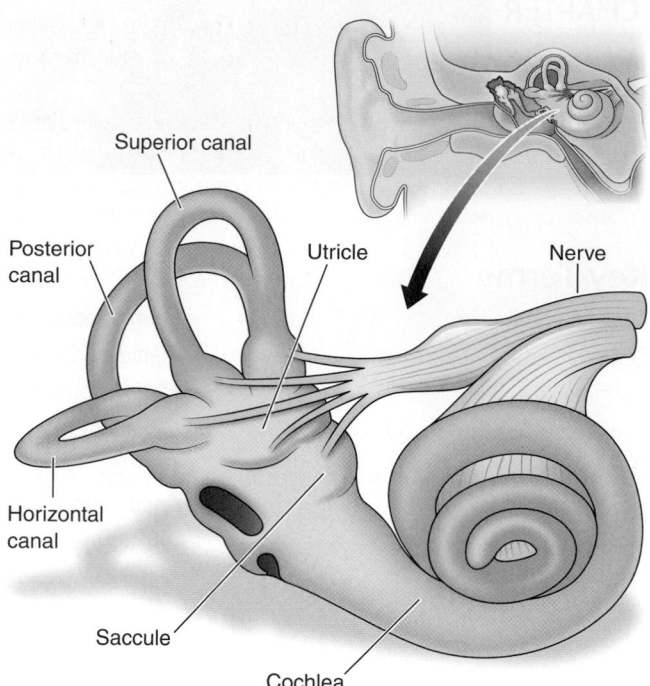

FIGURE 44-2. Inner ear anatomy; demonstrating the anatomic relationships of the cochlea, utricle, saccule, and semicircular canals.

cause vibrations of the tympanic membrane, which moves the ossicles and, in turn, vibrates the oval window and fluid in the inner ear. The two tissue-covered openings—the oval and the round windows—located in the medial wall of the inner ear are responsible for transmission of sound from the middle ear to the inner ear. Vibrations are amplified as they travel from the ossicles in the middle ear to the membrane of the oval window in the inner ear (see Fig. 44-1).

The middle ear is connected to the nasopharynx by means of the **eustachian tube.** The eustachian tube usually remains closed unless yawning or swallowing occurs, which allows equalization between the pressure of the inner ear and the outside atmosphere. This mechanism of equalizing pressure prevents rupture of the tympanic membrane when there is a sudden pressure change, such as during airplane travel.

The Inner Ear

The inner ear is the most complex portion of the ear, containing many important parts for both balance and hearing. These parts include the labyrinth, cochlea, and spiral organ of Corti. Balance depends upon vision, vestibular function from the ear, and proprioception (neurological position sense).

Balance

The inner ear has a system of communication channels called a labyrinth as well as receptors for hearing and position sense. They are part of the vestibular system of the inner ear, which regulates movement and balance. There are two parts to the labyrinth, an outer bony wall called a **bony labyrinth** that encases a thin-walled **membranous labyrinth** that floats inside. These comprise the portion of the inner ear referred to as the **semicircular canals.** The utricle and saccule are organs that are part of the membranous labyrinth (see Fig. 44-2).

Two separate fluids are found in the inner ear. The periotic fluid, also known as perilymph, separates the two labyrinths from each other. The second fluid is otic fluid, also known as **endolymph,** which fills the membranous labyrinth. The periotic fluid has a similar composition to cerebral spinal fluid, whereas the otic fluid is comparable to intracellular fluid because of its potassium content.

During physical movement, the flow of the endolymph fluid fluctuates. This movement is sensed by the auditory nerve, also called CN VIII. Coordinated responses of this nerve provide a sense of balance and stability of movement.

Hearing

The cochlea and the organ of Corti are special sensory areas in the membranous labyrinth. The cochlea is housed in a snail-shaped bony tubule; the center of this tubule contains the cochlear duct. The cochlea is divided into three parts by the cochlear duct and the spiral lamina, which is a thin, shelflike extension. The three chambers of the cochlea are the scala vestibule, scala tympani, and scala media. Contained within the cochlear duct is the **organ of Corti,** the spiral-shaped, receptor organ used for hearing. The organ of Corti is made up of supporting cells and many long rows of cochlear hair cells: one row of inner hair cells and three outer rows, all resting on the basilar membrane in the scala media. Afferent sensory nerve fibers from the cochlear nerve are wrapped at the base of the cochlear hair cells. The stapes deliver sound waves to the oval window, which are then transmitted to the scala vestibule and the scala tympani where the periotic fluid is located. The transmission of sound occurs when the trapped cilia of the hair cells in the organ of Corti are bent by the movement of sound of the basilar membrane.

Level of hearing is measured in terms of **decibels (dB),** a logarithmic unit that describes loudness of sound, with 0 being the threshold for sound perception of people with normal hearing. A soft whisper is approximately 0 to 20 dB. Normal conversation is approximately 60 dB. Sounds louder than 85 dB can cause hearing loss.

 CLINICAL CONCEPT

Audiometric tests, or hearing tests, evaluate the ability to hear sounds based on both frequency and loudness. The results are utilized to determine if the individual can hear normal levels of speech.

Basic Pathophysiologic Concepts of Common Ear Disorders

Common pathophysiologic conditions that affect the ear include conductive and sensorineural hearing loss, tinnitus, and vertigo. **Conductive hearing loss (CHL)** is caused by a problem with any of the structures involved in bringing sound waves to the auditory nerve. **Sensorineural hearing loss (SNHL)** is caused by any disorder that damages the auditory nerve. Tinnitus, a constant ringing or hum heard in the ear, is commonly caused by Ménière's disease. **Vertigo,** the feeling of spinning and imbalance, is the result of labyrinthitis.

Hearing Loss

Hearing loss is marked by the inability to either detect or perceive sound. It affects over 30 million people in the United States, including people of all ages and walks of life. Hearing loss can be described as mild, moderate, severe, or profound. These categories are based on the range of sounds that cannot be heard in terms of dB hearing levels.

- Mild hearing loss: The individual cannot hear sounds lower than 26 to 40 dB. Symptoms of mild hearing loss include difficulty following conversations if people are not close to the patient, and complaints that others are whispering or mumbling.
- Moderate hearing loss: The individual cannot hear sounds that are lower than 41 to 55 dB. A patient experiencing moderate hearing loss would experience difficulty hearing clearly with background noise and will generally need to wear hearing aids to hear normal conversation clearly.

- Severe hearing loss: The individual cannot hear sounds lower than 60 to 90 dB. This type of hearing loss will generally cause the patient to be able to hear someone speaking, but he or she usually cannot make out the words unless he or she is watching the lips of the person talking. Without the significant assistance of hearing aids, someone with severe hearing loss may not be able to follow even loud conversations.
- Profound hearing loss: The individual cannot hear sounds that are lower than 90 dB. This type of patient typically can only hear extremely loud sounds and has difficulty hearing or following conversations. New types of digital hearing aids for profound losses can help. Additional assistance, such as lip reading or sign language training, would also be indicated for patients with profound hearing loss.

Hearing loss may be congenital and discovered in infancy or acquired in later life. It can be described as genetic, acquired, sudden, progressive, unilateral, bilateral, partial, complete, reversible, or irreversible. Most types of hearing loss fit into the categories of conductive, sensorineural, or mixed deficiencies.

Conductive Hearing Loss

CHL is related to disorders of sound transmission from the outer or middle ear to the receptors in the middle ear. One of the most common causes of CHL is impacted cerumen (earwax). Other possible causes of CHL include impaction of foreign bodies, trauma, otitis media (OM), and otosclerosis, which is the hardening of the ossicles.

Sensorineural Hearing Loss

SNHL occurs because of disorders of the inner ear, auditory nerve, or auditory pathways within the brain. It is commonly caused by loss of hair cells from the organ of Corti within the inner ear, but it can also occur because of damage to cranial nerve VIII or, more rarely, the auditory cortex of the brain, which is located within the temporal lobe. When there is damage to this area of the brain, sounds may be heard but not understood. This type of SNHL is referred to as **central hearing impairment.**

ALERT! Excessive levels of aminoglycoside antibiotics, such as gentamicin, tobramycin, and amikacin, can cause dysfunction of CN VIII. Patients on high doses of these antibiotics are at risk for permanent damage to their hearing and balance.

SNHL may also be caused by genetic disorders or infections while the fetus is in utero. Trauma, tumors, vascular disorders, infection, Ménière's disease, acoustic neuroma, and multiple sclerosis also can cause SNHL. Hearing loss can occur because of noise trauma, which is exposure to excessively loud noises for a prolonged period of time. Noise trauma can diminish the individual's ability to hear high frequency sounds. Eventually, this loss can progress to more severe loss, including the inability to hear the sound frequency of normal speech. Noise injury commonly occurs in the workplace, but also with recreational and social exposure to loud noises. This includes the use of personal music devices and attendance at concerts with excessively loud sound systems.

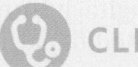 **CLINICAL CONCEPT**

Noise levels of greater than 85 dB are associated with injury to the cochlea.

Mixed Hearing Deficiency

Individuals can suffer both SNHL and CHL concurrently, a combination referred to as mixed hearing deficiency. Causes of mixed hearing deficiency include barotrauma (pressure changes), otosclerosis, cholesteatoma, and temporal bone fractures.

Tinnitus

Tinnitus is the perception of abnormal sounds in the head or the ear, often described as ringing in the ears. Some patients describe the noise they hear as buzzing, ringing, humming, or hissing in nature. Tinnitus can be continuous or intermittent, unilateral or bilateral, and high, medium, or low pitch. It can occur because of CN VIII disorders, injury from prolonged noise exposure, infection, or medications such as aminoglycosides and aspirin.

To resolve tinnitus, it is first necessary to find its cause. Sometimes there are triggers such as red wine, caffeine, or the food additive monosodium glutamate (MSG). Ménière's disease is a common cause of tinnitus that can be treated with medication or surgery.

Vertigo

Patients with vertigo have the sensation that the room is spinning around them, when in fact there is no movement. Additionally, patients report an exaggerated sense of motion with any self-initiated movement. Episodes of vertigo usually last minutes to hours and are often associated with severe nausea and vomiting. This may be because of Ménière's disease or alterations in the labyrinth of the inner ear. It is important to distinguish vertigo from dizziness. In dizziness, the patient reports incoordination and a feeling that he or she is going to "black out" or fall. Nausea and vomiting do not necessarily accompany dizziness as they do with vertigo.

Assessment

As with any patient assessment, history taking is important when examining for hearing and balance-related disorders. Assess for history of head trauma, exposure to loud noise, and history of aminoglycoside use. Ask the patient to fully explain associated symptoms.

If the patient is a child, ask about family history, genetic disorders, congenital infection, OM, history of meningitis, and speech problems. Healthcare providers should understand that normal speech volume is between 30 and 50 dB and that children with hearing loss in this range cannot develop normal speech. Speech problems may be the first manifestation of hearing impairment in children.

 CLINICAL CONCEPT

The American Academy of Pediatrics recommends hearing screening in all infants by the age of 1 month. If a newborn fails the initial test, then a thorough audiological evaluation should be performed by the age of 3 months, with appropriate intervention by the age of 6 months.

Initially, in the physical examination of the outer ear, there should be no discharge or tenderness of the auricle. A painful outer ear is often present in otitis externa (OE). During a general physical examination, a whisper test can be used to get a general sense of the patient's hearing ability. The patient closes his or her eyes, then the clinician whispers into the patient's ear. The patient is asked which ear is able to hear the whisper.

Assessment of balance can be done with the Romberg test. The clinician performs this test by asking the patient to stand upright with feet together and then close his or her eyes. If the patient is unable to maintain this position with eyes closed and begins to sway or fall, the test is considered to be positive. A positive test can be indicative of impaired vestibular function caused by damage to CN VIII or the membranous labyrinth.

Physical examination also includes use of the otoscope, which enables direct view of the patient's tympanic membrane. The normal tympanic membrane has a number of key features, including the umbo, pars flaccida, and cone of light. Cerumen impaction, foreign body, erythema of the ear canal and membrane, or fluid located behind the tympanic membrane can be seen with an otoscope.

A puff of air propelled against the tympanic membrane from a **pneumatic otoscope** can demonstrate movement of the tympanic membrane. A healthy tympanic membrane is slightly movable when air pressure is propelled against it. In middle ear infection, the tympanic membrane will be immobile and bulging without demonstration of the key features. Pneumatic otoscopy should be performed to detect current or chronic infections, perforation or scarring of the tympanic membrane, cholesteatoma, or fluid behind the tympanic membrane.

Diagnosis

Genetic testing may be useful to determine the etiology of hearing impairment. There are many different genetic syndromes that can trigger hearing loss. Blood tests to search for evidence of thyroid and renal disease are also suggested. Thyroid function, blood urea nitrogen (BUN), serum creatinine levels, and urinalysis should be done.

A specific blood test can identify the presence of connexin-26, a marker for genetic deafness. The test indicates the presence of the *DFNB1* gene, which codes for GJB2, a protein that regulates the composition of the fluid in the cochlea known as endolymph. There are more than 150 distinct mutations of this gene that can cause hearing impairment.

Magnetic resonance imaging (MRI) and computed tomography (CT) scan can uncover abnormalities such as head trauma, tumors, or malformation of the cochlea or the auditory nerve. Other specific tests for hearing loss include audio brainstem response, otoacoustic emissions (OAEs), and audiometry.

Audio brainstem response testing is similar to an electroencephalography. When a hearing ear is given a stimulus, there is resulting electrographic activity that can be followed from the ear to central areas of the brain. In OAE, there are certain sounds that are generated by the inner ear that can be recorded. These sounds are present in normal functioning ears and likely reflect the presence and function of structures responsible for hearing. The sounds may be spontaneous or evoked. How they are produced is unclear. Audiometry is performed by placing headsets over the patient's ears and instructing them to raise the corresponding hand when a sound is heard. Pure tone sounds can be presented so that specific volumes at specific frequencies can be documented. CHL and SNHL can be differentiated, and speech recognition can also be tested.

Treatment

Treatment of ear disorders involves removal of anything that blocks the ear canal, such as impacted cerumen or a foreign body. Antibiotics are prescribed for middle ear infections. Children with persistent chronic or recurrent OM with resultant effusions may benefit from the placement of **myringotomy tubes**. These tubes are inserted into the tympanic membrane to allow drainage of discharge from the middle-ear space. If otitis results in the destruction or fixation of the ossicles, surgery on the ossicles may improve hearing function. Hearing aids can be used to increase the sound that is transmitted to the affected ear. Bone-anchored hearing aids may be useful in some patients. Cholesteatoma and vestibular schwannoma, also called acoustic neuroma, are tumors that can be eradicated surgically. In addition, SNHL can be treated with cochlear implantation.

Pathophysiology of Selected Disorders of the Ear

There are different disorders that can interfere with the ear's function. External ear infection, cerumen impaction, middle ear infection, and tumor of CN VIII are the most common disorders.

Disorders of the External Ear

This section discusses the disorders of the auricle and the ear canal. The auricle is easily inspected and the ear canal requires use of an otoscope.

Cerumen Impaction

The most common cause of reversible hearing loss is impacted cerumen. Cerumen can build up and narrow—or even occlude—the canal despite the ear's ability for self-cleaning. This condition is usually asymptomatic until complete occlusion of the ear canal occurs. The complaints patients report most often include hearing loss, tinnitus, and a feeling of fullness or coughing.

Most often, cerumen is removed by irrigation with warm tap water and a bulb syringe. Some health-care providers may choose to use a wire loop or blunt curette to remove excess cerumen. It is best to use warm water as an irrigant to avoid disruption of equilibrium that may occur because of stimulation of the **vestibular caloric reflex**. The vestibular caloric reflex occurs when the ear's vestibular system is disrupted by cold water placed in the ear canal. Nystagmus, a horizontal movement of the eyes, is a sign of the vestibular caloric reflex.

Otitis Externa

OE, also called swimmer's ear, is identified by mild to severe inflammation of the external ear. This condition can vary from mild pain when the external ear is manipulated to severe erythematous, or tender cellulitis of the external ear. The most common causes are associated with infectious agents, external irritants, and allergic responses. Some predisposing factors include water in the ear canal after swimming or bathing. The canal has excess moisture, which is an environment conducive to microbial growth. Common etiologic organisms include *Pseudomonas*, *Staphylococcus aureus*, and *Candida*.

Clinical Presentation. OE is diagnosed most frequently during the summer months and is usually identified by redness, itching, tenderness, and narrowing of the ear canal because of inflammation. Swelling of the auricle and external canal makes moving the external ear extremely painful. A clear to purulent drainage may be observed depending on the inflammation's severity. There may be temporary CHL secondary to the canal's inflammation.

Diagnosis and Treatment. Diagnosis of OE is usually based on clinical examination. Culture of discharge can identify the pathogen responsible for the infection. Treatment options usually include an antibiotic or antifungal agent specific to the causative agent in conjunction with a corticosteroid to aid in decreasing the inflammation. Instruct the patient to avoid exposing the ear to water until the condition has cleared and to use ear plugs while swimming once the infection has resolved.

Disorders of the Middle Ear

Disorders of the middle ear occur within the area behind the tympanic membrane. Often upper respiratory infections of the pharynx will cause middle ear infections because of the eustachian tube's involvement.

Otitis Media

OM is the most common disorder to affect the middle ear. This infection results from fluid accumulation in the middle ear. Even though OM can occur at any age, it is most commonly seen in children; peak incidence is usually between the ages of 6 and 24 months.

Etiology. The most common causative bacteria of OM in children are *S. pneumoniae*, *H. influenzae*, and *Moraxella catarrhalis*. More than one bacterium may be responsible for acute OM, and a resistant strain of one of the bacteria listed above may be the reason that there is an increase of failed treatment attempts.

OM is most often diagnosed in the winter months secondary to the increase in respiratory tract infections. Infants and toddlers are at highest risk because of their frequent supine position and the anatomical location of their eustachian tube, which is on the same horizontal plane as the middle ear.

Risk factors for OM include male sex, bottle feedings, pacifier usage, day care attendance, exposure to tobacco smoke, family history of OM, allergic rhinitis, and immune deficiencies.

Pathophysiology. Anatomically, the mucosa of the nasopharynx continues into the eustachian tube of the

---

Box 44-1. Otitis Media With Effusion

OM with effusion occurs when there is an intact tympanic membrane with an accumulation of fluid in the middle ear without signs and symptoms of an infection. People with OM with effusion do not have a fever or other manifestations of an OM infection. Many cases resolve spontaneously in about 3 months. Management includes observation, antibiotics, and corticosteroids. A hearing evaluation may be required if the effusion persists longer than 6 months. A hearing loss of 20 dB or greater may require tympanostomy with tube placement.

---

throat and then into the middle ear. Bacteria of the nasopharynx easily enter the eustachian tube and the middle ear. Infants and children are at highest risk for OM because their eustachian tubes are shorter, wider, and more horizontal in relation to the middle ear, which develops inflammation; an effusion accumulates behind the tympanic membrane. OM can be seen as acute, recurrent, or OM with an effusion. Effusion related to OM can be serous (clear, watery), mucoid (thick and mucuslike), or purulent (puslike) fluid (see Box 44-1).

Clinical Presentation. Frequent complaints associated with OM include earache, fever, and hearing loss. In infants and toddlers, nonspecific symptoms may include ear tugging, poor feeding, night waking, and irritability. Older children and adults may have rhinorrhea, vomiting, and diarrhea. Pain will increase as an effusion accumulates behind the tympanic membrane. Tympanic membrane rupture is possible when there is too much pressure behind the membrane. Rupture can occur suddenly, resulting in decreased pain and discharge from the ear.

Diagnosis. Diagnosis of OM is made by reviewing the signs and symptoms, as well as performing an otoscopic examination, which is usually conducted with a pneumatic otoscope to test the tympanic membrane's mobility. Upon physical examination, the tympanic membrane will be reddened.

A puff of air from a pneumatic otoscope will demonstrate decreased movement of the tympanic membrane. In severe cases of OM, the tympanic membrane will be nonmobile and bulging outward.

Treatment. Treatment for OM varies depending on the individual. Children at high risk, usually those younger than 2 years of age, should be given antibiotics judiciously. Older children that do not present with a fever usually do not require antibiotic therapy, but they do require follow-up in 1 to 3 days. All individuals with acute OM should have supportive therapy such as analgesics, antipyretics, and localized heat, whether or not antibiotics are prescribed.

When accumulation of fluid is excessive, a tympanotomy may be necessary. A **tympanotomy** is an incision in the tympanic membrane to promote drainage that has accumulated behind it. This procedure also helps to relieve pain, prevent further hearing loss, and prevent spontaneous rupture of the tympanic membrane, which can lead to scarring. A tube is often inserted into the tympanic membrane to maintain an opening for release of discharge in the procedure referred to as a tympanostomy.

If OM goes untreated or is poorly treated, complications can develop (see Box 44-2).

Labyrinthitis

Labyrinthitis is inflammation of the labyrinth of the inner ear. It occurs as a sudden episode of vertigo that may last several days, and is often associated with hearing loss and tinnitus. It may occur in conjunction with a bacterial or viral infection or autoimmune disorder. Symptoms of labyrinthitis occur when infectious microorganisms or inflammatory mediators invade the membranous labyrinth and damage the vestibular and auditory end organs. Symptoms often resolve as the infection is treated with antibiotics. Meclizine has been used to reduce the sensation of movement produced by the vestibular system of the inner ear.

Box 44-2. Complications of Otitis Media

Complications of OM include hearing loss, middle ear problems, and infection of the mastoid process, temporal bone, or the intracranial structures. Hearing loss associated with OM is usually temporary, conductive, and resolves as the effusion resolves. Permanent hearing loss is often related to damage to the tympanic membrane or structure of the middle ear. Tinnitus is another potential complication related to chronic OM.

Adhesive OM is a chronic inflammatory condition characterized by occlusion of the eustachian tube and adhesions in the middle ear because of abnormal healing of an infected middle ear. Often the result of poorly treated or chronic OM, it causes irreversible immobilization of the ossicles, causing CHL. Cholesteatoma, another problem associated with OM, is a mass with white keratin debris that may erode the surrounding tissue and the temporal bone, causing intracranial complications. This condition may be linked to a genetic predisposition or be secondary to chronic OM.

Severe OM can lead to an infection that can extend into the intracranial cavity as well as mastoiditis, which is inflammation of the bone posterior to the auricle.

Ménière's Disease

Ménière's disease, a disorder of the inner ear, was named for the French physician who first described the condition's symptoms. The symptoms are the result of changes in the fluid volume of both the bony and membranous labyrinth of the inner ear. In Ménière's disease, there is an increase in the endolymph that fills the membranous labyrinth, resulting in distension of this portion of the inner ear. Over time, this disorder is associated with progressive hearing loss and tinnitus. Although head trauma is one of the major causes of this disorder, there is frequently no known etiology. Ménière's disease most commonly affects persons ages 40 to 50 years old.

The clinical presentation for Ménière's disease includes episodic vertigo associated with SNHL, tinnitus, and a feeling of pressure within the ear. Because there is no specific diagnostic test for this disorder, it is diagnosed by the clinical symptoms. However, a complete history and physical examination must be performed to rule out other causes. Treatment includes a low-salt diet, diuretics, and steroids. Transtympanic administration of aminoglycosides is sometimes effective in treatment-resistant Ménière's disease. A Meniett device is also used for treatment-resistant disease. The device delivers pulses of pressure to the inner ear via a tympanostomy tube. Some patients have symptomatic relief when the device is used on a daily basis. The precise mechanism that provides relief is unclear.

A destructive surgical procedure may be necessary in treatment-resistant Ménière's disease. Because a high volume of endolymph in the inner ear sends abnormal signals to the auditory nerve, destruction of these structures may be the last resort to relieve symptoms. Destruction of the inner ear structures, the auditory nerve, or both prevents abnormal signals from reaching the brain. As long as the opposite inner ear and vestibular apparatus function normally, the brain eventually will compensate for the loss of one labyrinth over the following weeks to months.

Vestibular Schwannomas

Vestibular schwannomas, also called acoustic neuromas, are benign tumors that develop from the Schwann cells that surround CN VIII. About 5% are associated with a genetic disorder called neurofibromatosis. The clinical incidence is about 10 to 15 individuals per million people per year. It is most often diagnosed in adults ranging in age from 46 to 58 years.

The symptoms result from compression of CN VIII; these symptoms include tinnitus and decreased hearing with loss of speech discrimination in the affected ear. There is also a persistent loss of balance. The definitive diagnosis is made with an MRI. If symptoms interfere with activities of daily living, it can be removed with microsurgical techniques or with gamma knife radiosurgery.

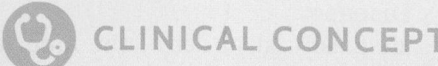

CLINICAL CONCEPT

Removal of the schwannoma may not be necessary unless the symptoms increase in severity.

Hearing Loss in Older Adults

Older adults suffer from **presbycusis** or degenerative changes that diminish hearing. The changes begin around age 50 years and may remain undetectable for a decade or so. The symptoms are caused by gradual loss of hair cells in the cochlea.

In older adults, it is important to assess both high- and low-frequency sounds. High-frequency sounds are lost first, with a frequent complaint of being unable to hear in a crowded room. One of the best ways to assess for high-frequency loss is to use a ticking watch, whereas low-frequency sounds are best assessed by speaking vowel sounds.

Patients with hearing loss need to consult an audiologist who can prescribe the patient with the correct type of hearing aid. Most hearing aids amplify sounds using computer/digital technology.

Chapter Summary

- The functions of the external and middle ear include collecting, amplifying, transmitting, and receiving sound.
- The inner ear consists of sensory organs that are stimulated by sound waves. Sound waves are transmitted through a delicate integrated circuit of structures and transformed into neural impulses sent to the brain via the auditory nerve, also called CN VIII.
- The inner ear is also stimulated by position and movement of the head, which is involved in the maintenance of balance and equilibrium.
- Level of hearing is measured in terms of dB. A soft whisper is approximately 0 to 20 dB. Normal conversation is approximately 60 dB. Sounds louder than 85 dB can cause noise trauma and hearing loss.
- CHL is related to disorders of sound transmission from the external or middle ear to the receptors in the middle ear. CHL is commonly caused by OM or cerumen impaction. SNHL occurs because of disorders of the inner ear, auditory nerve, or auditory pathways within the brain. SNHL is commonly caused by loss of hair cells from the organ of Corti within the inner ear.
- Tinnitus is the perception of abnormal sounds in the head or the ear, often described as ringing in the ears. Some patients describe the noise they hear as buzzing, ringing, humming, or hissing in nature.
- Vertigo is the sensation that the room is spinning around you.
- Newborns should undergo a hearing screening examination before 3 months of age, and intervention before 6 months of age.

- Excessive levels of aminoglycoside antibiotics can cause dysfunction of CN VIII.
- A specific blood test can identify the presence of connexin-26, a biomarker for genetic deafness. The test indicates the presence of the *DFNB1* gene, which codes for GJB2; this protein regulates the composition of endolymph.
- OE is inflammation of the external ear. The most common causes are infectious agents, external irritants, and allergic responses. Predisposing factors include water in the ear canal after swimming. Common etiologic organisms include *Pseudomonas*, *Staphylococcus aureus*, and *Candida*.
- OM, the most common disorder to affect the middle ear, is an infection that results from fluid accumulation in the middle ear. Even though OM can occur at any age, it is most commonly seen in children.
- Labyrinthitis is a sudden episode of vertigo that may last several days; it is often associated with hearing loss and tinnitus.
- Ménière's disease is caused by an increase in the endolymph that fills the membranous labyrinth, resulting in distension of this portion of the inner ear. This disorder is associated with progressive hearing loss, vertigo, and tinnitus.
- Vestibular schwannomas, also called acoustic neuromas, are benign tumors that develop from the Schwann cells that surround CN VIII. CN VIII becomes compressed and dysfunctional.
- Older adults suffer from presbycusis or degenerative changes that diminish hearing. The changes begin around age 50 and may remain undetectable for a decade or so. The symptoms are caused by gradual loss of hair cells in the cochlea.

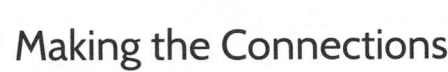
Making the Connections

Disorder and Pathophysiology	Signs and Symptoms	Physical Assessment Findings	Diagnostic Testing	Treatment
Cerumen Impaction | Earwax within the ear canal that impairs sound conduction from the external ear to the inner ear. CHL.				
	Hearing difficulty. Sense of "fullness" or itching in the ear.	Hearing impairment. Yellow-brown colored earwax buildup in the ear canal seen with otoscope.	None.	Removal of impacted cerumen using irrigation technique or curette.
Otitis Externa | Infection of the auricle and ear canal. Common microorganisms include *Pseudomonas*, *Staphylococcus*, and *Candida*.				
	Pain and tenderness of the auricle, fullness and itching of the ear canal. Discharge from ear canal common. Hearing difficulty.	Tenderness, erythema, and edema of the auricle and ear canal. Purulent or serous discharge from the ear canal.	None.	Antibiotic and steroid treatment. Ear plugs when in water.
Otitis Media | Infection of the middle ear region. Discharge accumulation in middle ear. Common microorganisms include *Streptococcus pneumonia* and *Haemophilus influenza*.				
	Earache. Hearing difficulty, sense of fullness. Fever, nausea, and vomiting possible. Children are extremely irritable, tug at ear, do not feed, and may have vomiting.	Bulging, red tympanic membrane. Erythema and edema of the ear canal. Hearing impairment. Often pharyngeal erythema, edema, and rhinorrhea present.	Pneumatic otoscope will demonstrate decreased movement of the tympanic membrane. Throat culture may be needed.	Antibiotic treatment. Antipyretics and analgesic may be needed. Tympanostomy may be necessary in chronic OM.
Labyrinthitis | Inflammation of the membranous labyrinth of the inner ear.				
	Dizziness. Loss of balance. Hearing difficulty and tinnitus possible.	Hearing loss. Romberg test may be positive.	None.	Antibiotic and meclizine.
Ménière's Disease | Increased volume of endolymph in inner ear.				
	Tinnitus, hearing loss, and vertigo.	Hearing loss. Romberg test: may be positive.	None.	Low salt diet, diuretics, and steroids. Aminoglycosides may relieve symptoms. Meniett device or destructive surgery may be necessary.
Vestibular Schwannoma | Tumor of the auditory nerve that compresses nerve and causes hearing impairment.				
	Hearing loss, tinnitus, and loss of balance.	Hearing loss. Romberg test may be positive.	MRI.	Surgery.

Bibliography

Basner, M., Babisch, W., Davis, A., et al. (2014). Auditory and non-auditory effects of noise on health. *Lancet*, 383(9925), 1325–1332. doi: 10.1016/S0140-6736(13)61613-X. Epub 2013 Oct 30.

Darby-Stewart, A., Graber, M. A., & Dachs, R. (2011). Antibiotics for acute otitis media in young children. *Am Fam Phys*, 84(10), 1095–1097.

Ebell, M. H. (2011). Short course of antibiotics for acute otitis media treatment. *Am Fam Phys*, 83(1), 37.

Harmes, K. M., Blackwood, R. A., Burrows, H. L., et al. (2013). Otitis media: diagnosis and treatment. *Am Fam Phys*, 88(7), 435–440.

Johns, C., & Zuromskis, T. (2012). The sound of silence. *Lancet*, 380(9854), 1712. doi: 10.1016/S0140-6736(12)61331-2.

Knight, S., Sams, R., & Foster-Harper, S. (2012). Infectious etiologies of acute otitis media. *Am Fam Phys*, 86(10), Online.

Kral, A., & O'Donoghue, G. M. (2010). Profound deafness in childhood. *N Engl J Med*, 363(15), 1438–1450. doi: 10.1056/NEJMra0911225.

Liao, Y. J., & Liu, T. C. (2013). Images in clinical medicine. Mastoiditis. *N Engl J Med*, 368(21), 2014. doi: 10.1056/NEJMicm1205007.

Lomen-Hoerth, C., & Messing, R. O. (2010). Nervous system disorders. In S. J. McPhee & G. D. Hammer, *Pathophysiology of disease: an introduction to clinical medicine*. 6th ed. New York: McGraw-Hill/Lange Medical.

McPhee, S. J., Papadakis, M. A., & Rabow, M. W. (2011). *Current medical diagnosis & treatment*. 50th ed. New York: McGraw-Hill/Lange Medical Series.

Post, R. E., & Dickerson, L. M. (2010). Dizziness: a diagnostic approach. *Am Fam Phys*, 82(4), 361–368, 369.

Schaefer, P., & Baugh, R. F. (2012). Acute otitis externa: an update. *Am Fam Phys*, 86(11), 1055–1061.

Schreiber, B. E., Agrup, C., Haskard, D. O., & Luxon, L. M. (2010). Sudden sensorineural hearing loss. *Lancet*, 375(9721), 1203–1211. doi: 10.1016/S0140-6736(09)62071-7.

Shaikh, N., Hoberman, A., Kaleida, P. H., Ploof, D. L., & Paradise, J. L. (2010). Videos in clinical medicine. Diagnosing otitis media—otoscopy and cerumen removal. *N Engl J Med*, 362(20), e62. doi: 10.1056/NEJMvcm090439.

Shargorodsky, J., Curhan, G. C., & Farwell, W. R. (2010). Prevalence and characteristics of tinnitus among US adults. *Am J Med*, 123(8), 711–718. doi: 10.1016/j.amjmed.2010.02.015.

Tapiainen, T., Kujala, T., Renko, M., et al. (2014). Effect of antimicrobial treatment of acute otitis media on the daily disappearance of middle ear effusion: a placebo-controlled trial. *JAMA Pediatr*, May 5. doi: 10.1001/jamapediatrics.2013.5311. Epub ahead of print.

van Dongen, T. M., van der Heijden, G. J., Venekamp, R. P., Rovers, M. M., & Schilder, A. G. (2014). A trial of treatment for acute otorrhea in children with tympanostomy tubes. *N Engl J Med*, 370(8), 723–733. doi: 10.1056/NEJMoa1301630.

Vergison, A., Dagan, R., Arguedas, A., et al. (2010). Otitis media and its consequences: beyond the earache. *Lancet Infect Disease*, 10(3), 195–203. doi: 10.1016/S1473-3099(10)70012-8.

Walling, A. D., & Dickson, G. M. (2012). Hearing loss in older adults. *Am Fam Phys*, 85(12), 1150–1156.

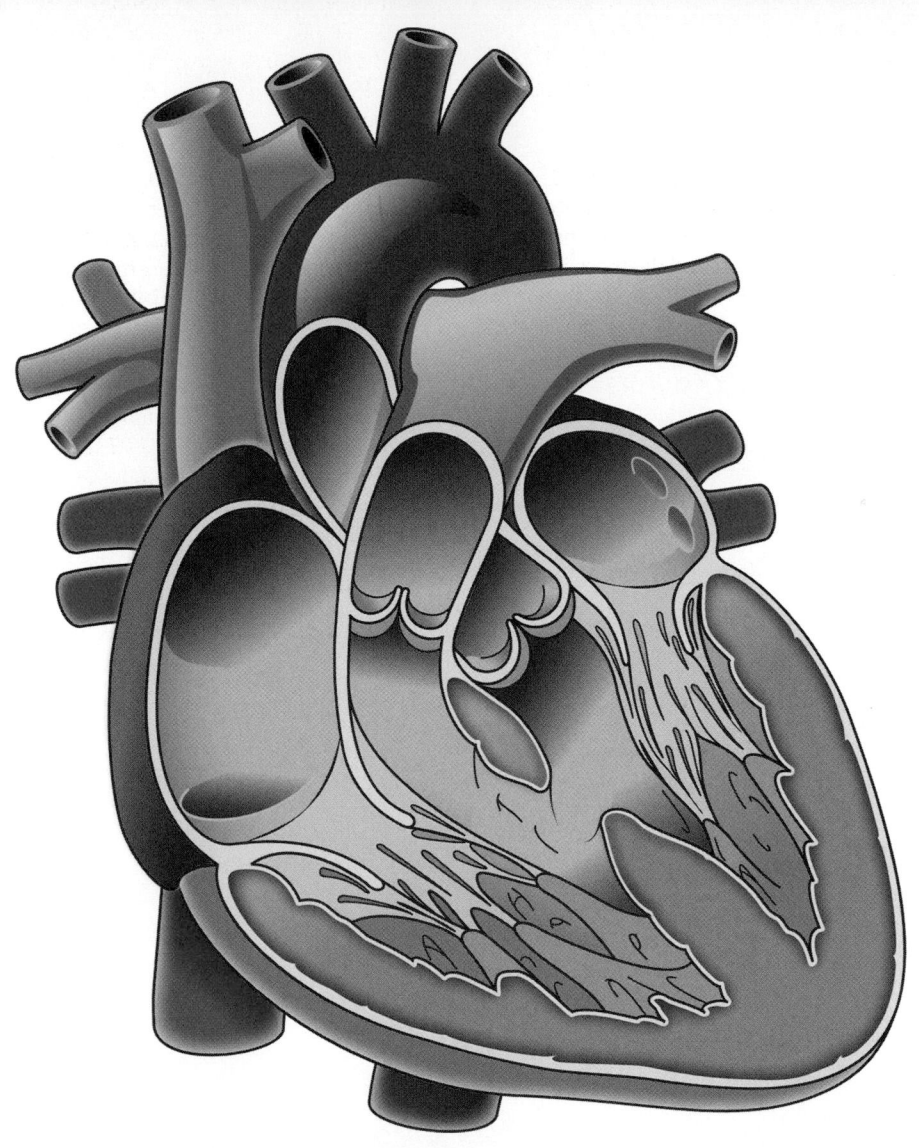

UNIT 16
DISEASE ACROSS THE LIFE SPAN

Chapters

Pediatric Disorders

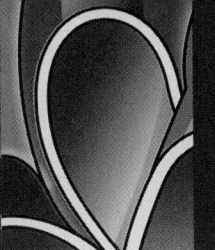

Key Terms

Atrial septal defect (ASD)

Cerebral palsy (CP)

Cleft lip and palate

Coarctation of the aorta (COA)

Croup

Fetal alcohol syndrome (FAS)

Gastroschisis

Hydrocephalus

Meckel's diverticulum

Meningocele

Myelomeningocele

Necrotizing enterocolitis (NEC)

Omphalocele

Patent ductus arteriosus (PDA)

Spina bifida

Spontaneous abortion

Talipes equinovarus (TEV)

Teratogens

Tetralogy of Fallot (TOF)

TORCH infections

Tracheoesophageal fistula (TEF)

Transposition of the great vessels (TGV)

Ventricular septal defect (VSD)

Pediatrics is the branch of medicine that deals with the health care of infants, children, and adolescents. Pediatric illnesses are markedly different from adult disorders. Children obviously have smaller body size than adults, but they also endure and express disease differently. A child's body is less resilient than an adult's body—it has less ability to withstand changes and fight disease. The adult has the advantage of years of exposure to the environment and the consequent development of immunity. The child's body has more susceptibilities, greater metabolic needs, and higher nutritional demands. Events that occur during the fetus's gestational period affect the newborn's health. The mother's health during pregnancy impacts the newborn's condition and the child's future. Pediatricians need to consider maternal health when making diagnoses in the newborn.

As children mature, different levels of growth and development influence the diagnosis of illness. Common illnesses and causes of death vary according to the child's age. Because of advances in health-care technology, many children who would not have survived infancy in the past now have the chance for a normal life span. At times, however, longer life span comes with health challenges. Some disorders that originate in childhood carry over into adulthood and can cause complications later in life. Pediatrics is not health care of a small adult; it is a specialty that is distinctly different from adult medicine.

Basic Concepts of the Gestational Period

The newborn's health greatly depends on a healthy gestational period. The gestational period, which is the time frame when the fetus develops in utero, can be divided into three trimesters, each of which is 3 months long (see Fig. 45-1):

- First trimester: from the last menstrual period to the 13th week
- Second trimester: from the 14th week to the 27th week
- Third trimester: from the 28th week to the 42nd week.

Birth normally occurs at a gestational age of about 40 weeks, although a normal range is from 37 to 42 weeks. The term *embryo* is used to describe the developing offspring during the first 8 weeks following conception; after 8 weeks, the term *fetus* is used until birth.

First Trimester

The first 3 to 4 weeks of gestation is a critical time when initial cellular growth and differentiation of tissues occur in the embryo. Critical foundational structures are beginning to develop. The embryo is significantly susceptible to teratogens during these first few weeks

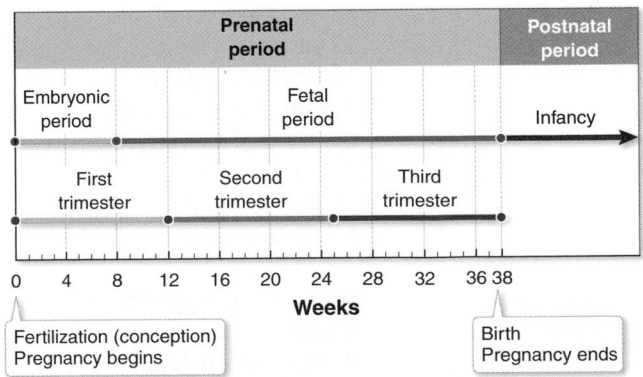

FIGURE 45-1. Prenatal (gestational) development time line.

after conception. **Teratogens** are substances that cause malformations of the fetus. Some drugs and chemicals are known to be teratogenic to the fetus. The Food and Drug Administration (FDA) categorizes drugs based on their safety during pregnancy.

Environmental factors and teratogens account for 10% of all birth defects. Maternal infections, maternal chronic disease, and drug exposure are other causes. Teratogen exposure early in pregnancy causes organ and structural defects. Teratogen exposure after 12 weeks of gestation usually affects growth and cognitive development.

Aside from drugs, there are other known substances that pose a significant hazard to a fetus during development. Alcohol use during pregnancy can cause fetal alcohol spectrum disorder, which causes a wide range of physical, developmental, and neurological abnormalities. Children exposed to prenatal cigarette smoke may experience a broad range of behavioral, neurological, and physical difficulties. Smoking increases risk of preterm delivery, intrauterine growth retardation, respiratory distress syndrome, cardiovascular defects, cleft lip and palate, and sudden infant death syndrome (SIDS). Exposure to air pollution during pregnancy is related to adverse birth outcomes, including low birth weight, premature delivery, and heart malformations. The heavy metals lead and mercury are toxic to the growing embryo's nervous system, especially brain development. Table 45-1 lists examples of prescription medications and substances that, if taken by women in early pregnancy, may affect the newborn.

The fifth week of the embryonic period is when the embryo's brain, spinal cord, heart, and other organs begin to form. At this point, the embryo is made up of three layers: ectoderm, mesoderm, and endoderm. The ectoderm will give rise to the embryo's outermost layer of skin, central and peripheral nervous systems, eyes, inner ear, and connective tissues. The mesoderm, or middle layer, initiates creation of the heart and the beginning of the circulatory system, as well as the bones, muscles, and kidneys. The endoderm, the inner layer of the embryo, serves as the starting point for the development of the lungs, intestine, and bladder.

In the sixth week, the embryo will be developing basic facial features and the arms and legs start to grow. In the following week, the brain, face, and arms and legs quickly develop. In the eighth week, the embryo starts moving, and in the next 3 weeks, the embryo's toes, neck, and genitals develop as well.

During the first trimester, birth defects can occur because of maternal illness, exposures, or unhealthy behaviors. Miscarriage, also called **spontaneous abortion,** can also occur during the first trimester. Often the reason for miscarriage is not determined; however, many are thought to occur because of genetic anomalies, which are incompatible with life. Once pregnancy moves into the second trimester, risks of miscarriage and birth defects drop drastically.

Second Trimester

Weeks 13 to 27 of the pregnancy are called the second trimester. At this time, movement of the fetus, often referred to as quickening, can be felt. This typically happens in the 20th to 21st week. The fetus takes on a definite human form with reproductive organs distinguished as male or female. The placenta is fully functioning at this time.

Third Trimester

The fetus grows significantly during this stage and moves into a downward position ready for birth. Movement of the fetus becomes stronger and more frequent. Neurological, cardiovascular, and gastrointestinal systems, as well as bone and muscle, undergo further development to prepare the fetus for birth. During this time, a baby born prematurely may survive.

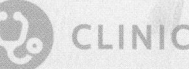

CLINICAL CONCEPT

Premature infants born at 24 weeks are viable outside the uterus with use of technology in neonatal intensive care. However, premature birth remains a major threat to fetal viability and may result in health challenges after birth and later in life.

Malformations of the Cardiovascular System

The development of the cardiovascular system begins with a beating heart at 5 weeks gestation. By the end of the first trimester, the placenta and umbilical vein are

TABLE 45-1. Teratogen Exposure and Infant Health	
Teratogen	**Possible Outcome**
Tobacco smoking	Low birth weight
Ethanol/alcohol (substance abuse)	Cardiac septal defects
	Fetal alcohol syndrome
	Microcephaly
	Patent ductus arteriosus
Isotretinoin (anti-acne medication)	Congenital heart defects
	Facial abnormalities
	Malformed ears
Streptomycin (antibiotic)	Hearing loss
Tetracycline (antibiotic)	Altered bone growth
	Discolored teeth
Phenytoin (anticonvulsant)	Cleft lip and palate
	Intrauterine growth retardation

formed. Fetal blood is oxygenated via the placenta and returns to the fetus via the umbilical vein. Oxygenated blood flows through the ductus venosus—which is the fetal structure between the umbilical vein and inferior vena cava—to the right atrium. Another fetal structure called the foramen ovale, an opening between the right and left atrium, allows the oxygenated blood to flow from the right atrium to the left atrium, then to the left ventricle, and on to general circulation. Fetal blood returning to the heart from the head and upper extremities enters the superior vena cava. Once in the right atrium, some returning blood flows into the right ventricle and then to the pulmonary artery. Most of the returning blood will pass through a fetal structure called the ductus arteriosus, which is a vessel that takes blood from the pulmonary artery to the descending aorta and general circulation. Only a small amount of blood circulates to the lungs from the pulmonary artery during fetal life. The lungs are not functioning and oxygenation of the fetal blood occurs via the placenta. The pattern of fetal circulation is depicted in Figure 45-2.

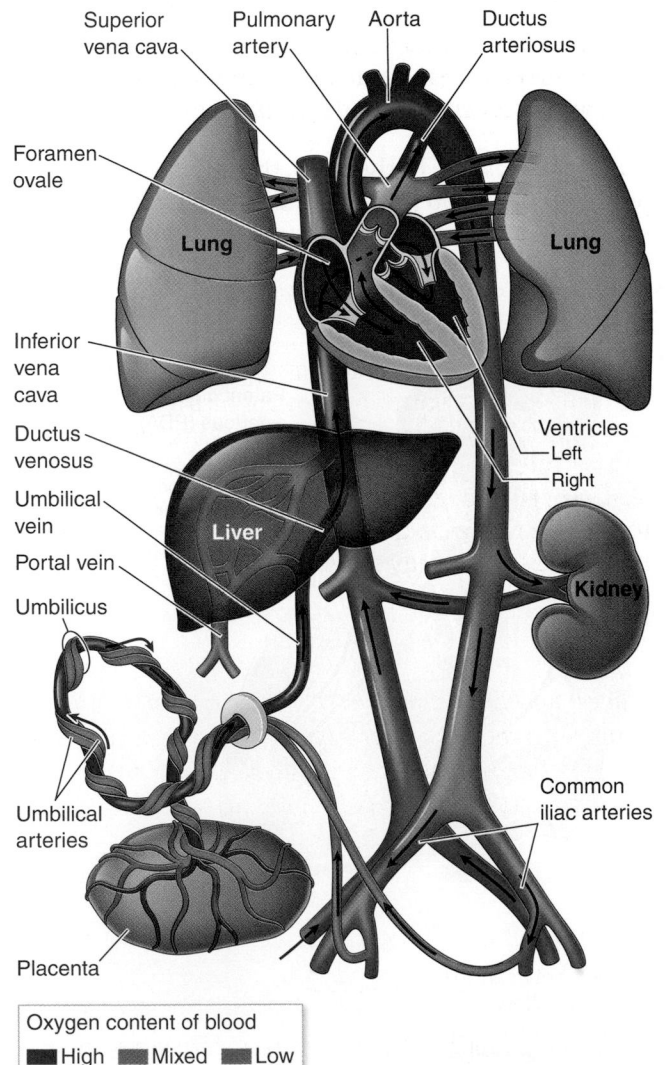

FIGURE 45-2. Fetal circulatory system.

Superior vena cava
Pulmonary artery
Aorta
Ductus arteriosus
Foramen ovale
Lung
Lung
Inferior vena cava
Ductus venosus
Ventricles
— Left
— Right
Umbilical vein
Liver
Portal vein
Umbilicus
Kidney
Umbilical arteries
Common iliac arteries
Placenta

Oxygen content of blood
■ High ■ Mixed ■ Low

Upon birth, when the newborn takes a breath, the blood that was passing through the ductus arteriosus is redirected to the lungs to be oxygenated. The ductus venosus collapses once the umbilical cord is cut and blood stops flowing via the umbilical vein to the infant. Pressure in the left atrium increases as a larger blood volume flows to the left atrium via the pulmonary veins from the lungs. This atrial pressure causes the foramen ovale to close. Although closure of the foramen ovale occurs quickly after birth, closure of the ductus arteriosus takes longer. Full closure occurs within 10 to 15 hours after birth with permanent closure in 10 to 21 days. These postbirth circulatory changes are shown in Figure 45-2.

Congenital Heart Defects

A congenital heart defect (CHD) is a malformation in the structure of the heart or great vessels that is present at birth. Many types of heart defects exist; some obstruct blood flow in the heart or great vessels, whereas others cause an abnormal pattern of blood flow through the heart. Heart defects are among the most common birth defects and are the leading cause of birth defect-related deaths. Approximately 9 persons in 1,000 are born with a congenital heart defect.

Some CHDs occur because the necessary postbirth circulatory changes do not occur. For example, once the newborn takes a breath, the lungs should begin to function and this changes pressures within the chambers of the heart and circulatory system. The pressure changes give rise to the newborn cardiovascular system

Patent Ductus Arteriosus

A **patent ductus arteriosus (PDA)** is an example of a CHD that occurs because of failure of postbirth circulatory changes. PDA accounts for 10% of all CHDs. There is a higher incidence among premature infants and female infants. On average, PDA occurs in 8 out of every 1,000 premature infants, and 2 out of every 1,000 full-term newborns.

Etiology. PDA is common in premature infants because of a high number of circulating prostaglandins in gestation that keep the duct open. There is some evidence suggesting that there is a genetic cause: As many as one-third of cases are caused by a PDA1 gene mutation on chromosome 12. There are also some teratogens known to cause PDA in the newborn. These include maternal rubella viral infection, fetal alcohol spectrum disorder, maternal amphetamine use, and maternal phenytoin use.

Pathophysiology. The ductus arteriosus in the fetus brings blood from the pulmonary artery into the aorta; it diverts blood flow away from the lungs because the fetal lungs are not functioning. The ductus arteriosus is supposed to be functional only in utero, when pulmonary arterial blood flows into the aorta. After birth, this channel should close off so that all blood flows into the pulmonary artery and into the lungs. The ductus arteriosus normally closes within the first 2 weeks of life. If it remains open, some blood from the aorta will flow via the pulmonary artery into the lungs because of the pressure gradient (see Fig. 45-3). If left untreated, the child will develop high pulmonary vascular pressure, also known as pulmonary hypertension. Eventually, there will be right-sided heart failure.

Clinical Presentation. Newborns with PDA are often asymptomatic at birth. Three-week to 6-week-old infants often present with poor feeding, low weight gain or weight loss, diaphoresis, and tachypnea. A cough, hoarse cry, and pneumonia are common. A systolic heart murmur is heard in the first few days to weeks of life. It is described as a continuous machinery murmur. The point of maximal impulse is laterally displaced. Peripheral pulses are bounding and there may be high systolic blood pressure.

Diagnosis. The size of the PDA determines whether the child has symptoms at birth. Sometimes there is partial closure of a PDA, which causes few symptoms. A large PDA will cause a continuous heart murmur heard at birth. If not diagnosed at birth, a large PDA may be diagnosed later in the newborn period as part of an evaluation for failure to thrive and growth retardation. Chest x-rays indicate an enlarged pulmonary artery with increased pulmonary vascularity in PDA. If other CHDs are suspected along with PDA, a cardiac catheterization may be done.

Treatment. Indomethacin, an NSAID that blocks prostaglandin formation, is given to premature infants to initiate closure of a PDA. If the PDA does not close in full-term infants during the first year of life, spontaneous closure is unlikely. Transcatheter surgical PDA closure is performed.

Atrial Septal Defect

An **atrial septal defect (ASD)** is an opening in the septum between the heart's right and left atria. The defect allows left-to-right shunting of oxygenated blood from the left atrium into the right atrium (see Fig. 45-4). ASD is a common type of CHD and is found more frequently in females. Approximately 0.67% to 2.1% of 1,000 live births have an ASD, but most are not apparent until late childhood, adolescence, or adulthood.

Etiology. Atrial septal defect has a genetic etiology in many cases. Genetic mutations that lead to ASD occur in Trisomy 21, Trisomy 18, Klinefelter syndrome, Holt-Oram syndrome, Williams syndrome, and others. Genetic mutations on chromosomes 1, 4, 5, 6, 10, 11, 13, 17, 18, and 22 are associated with ASD. Maternal risk factors that can cause ASD in the newborn include diabetes, phenylketonuria, fetal alcohol spectrum disorder, and influenza. Medications such as anticonvulsants and nonsteroidal anti-inflammatory drugs (NSAIDs) have also been associated with development of ASD.

Pathophysiology. In the fetus, there is an opening between the right and left atria, called the foramen ovale.

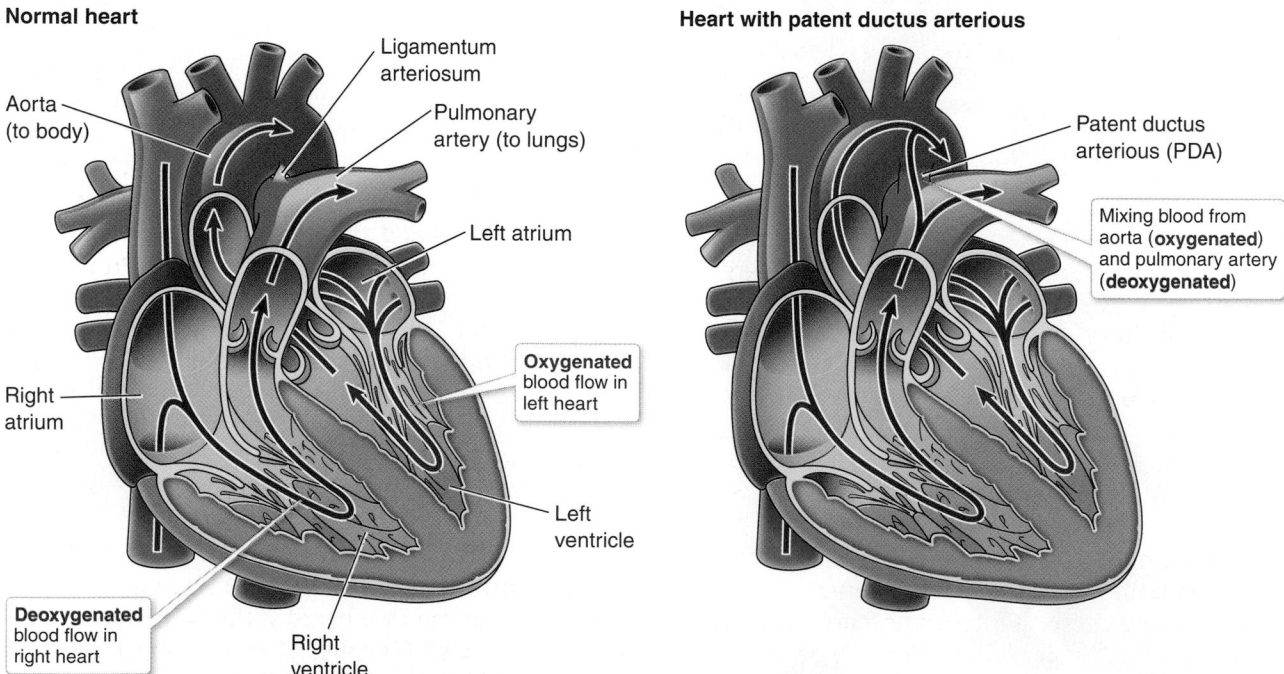

Normal heart

- Aorta (to body)
- Ligamentum arteriosum
- Pulmonary artery (to lungs)
- Left atrium
- **Oxygenated** blood flow in left heart
- Right atrium
- Left ventricle
- **Deoxygenated** blood flow in right heart
- Right ventricle

Heart with patent ductus arterious

- Patent ductus arterious (PDA)
- Mixing blood from aorta (**oxygenated**) and pulmonary artery (**deoxygenated**)

FIGURE 45-3. Patent ductus arteriosus. In fetal circulation, there is a connection between the aorta and the pulmonary artery called the ductus arteriosus. The ductus arteriosus allows for blood to bypass the nonfunctioning lungs in the fetus. After birth, the ductus arteriosus is supposed to close and degenerate. If the ductus arteriosus remains patent, congenital heart disease known as patent ductus arteriosus results in the newborn; this causes mixing of deoxygenated blood from the pulmonary artery with oxygenated blood from the aorta.

Atrial septal defect (ASD)

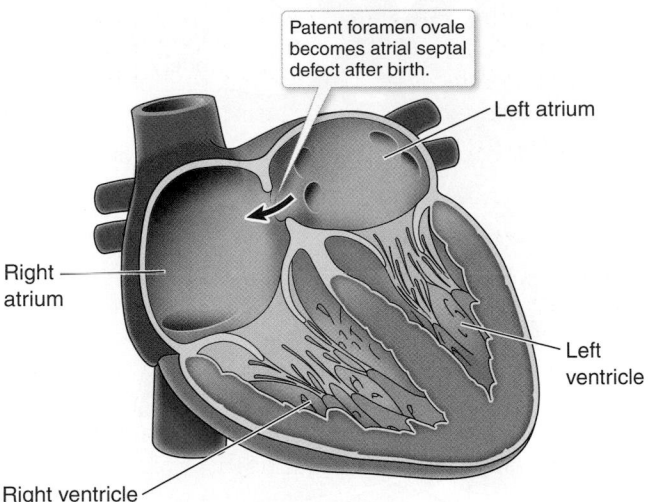

Patent foramen ovale becomes atrial septal defect after birth.

Left atrium

Right atrium

Left ventricle

Right ventricle

FIGURE 45-4. Atrial septal defect. In the fetal heart, the foramen ovale is an opening between the right and left atria. This opening is supposed to close after birth. When it remains open, it is called an atrial septal defect and allows deoxygenated and oxygenated blood to mix in the atria.

This opening allows blood to bypass the lungs and go from the right atrium directly into the left atrium during fetal circulation. In the fetus, the foramen ovale serves a purpose, but in the newborn the foramen should close, because upon birth the newborn takes his or her first breaths through the lungs. The lungs open and the pulmonary artery resistance decreases. This diminished resistance changes the pressures in the atria. As lung circulation increases, blood from the right atrium flows into the right ventricle and pulmonary artery to enter the lungs. However, in patients with ASD, the foramen ovale remains open and left to right shunting of blood occurs from the left atrium into the right atrium. This extra blood flow into the right side of the heart can cause heart failure.

Clinical Presentation. Signs and symptoms of ASD depend on the size of the septal opening. The patient with a small defect can be asymptomatic, whereas a large defect can cause right-sided volume overload and symptoms associated with right-sided heart failure. Children with a large ASD will develop enlargement of the right side of the heart as they age, which can be seen on x-ray and ultrasound images. Right-sided atrial arrhythmias and increased pulmonary vascularity can occur as the child matures. An ASD is often present with no symptoms from birth and throughout childhood, and there may be no signs on physical examination. However, later in adult life, the ASD may become evident by causing exercise intolerance, arrhythmias, or signs of right ventricular failure. Seventy percent of congenital ASDs are first detected in adulthood.

Diagnosis. On chest x-ray, there is an enlargement of the right side of the heart. Electrocardiogram (ECG) will demonstrate right axis deviation. Doppler transthoracic echocardiography can be used to visualize the

ASD; transesophageal echocardiography is also sometimes used to better visualize the ASD. Cardiac magnetic resonance imaging (MRI) and computed tomography (CT) angiography are other studies that can be used to visualize an ASD.

Treatment. Cardiac catheterization is used as a diagnostic and interventional technique for ASD. After the age of 2 years, children with ASD may be candidates for a transcatheter occlusion device that is inserted into the defect during cardiac catheterization. Heart tissue then grows around the device and fills in the ASD. If heart failure is present, digoxin, which strengthens heart contractility, and diuretics, such as furosemide (Lasix), are safe for use in children.

Ventricular Septal Defect

Ventricular septal defect (VSD) is one of the most common congenital heart defects, accounting for about 20% of all CHDs. It occurs in 2 to 6 out of every 1,000 newborns and often occurs with other CHDs.

Etiology. A VSD occurs at 4 to 8 weeks gestation when the ventricles of the heart are developed. The cause of the malformation is a combination of hereditary and environmental factors. Maternal diabetes and alcohol abuse are risk factors for development of VSD in the fetus. Family history of a congenital cardiac defect is a major risk factor. There are a number of chromosomal abnormalities associated with VSD, which is known to occur in Trisomy 13, Trisomy 18, and Trisomy 21. There are many genetic deletions associated with development of VSD, including deletions at 4q, 5p, and 22q11.

Pathophysiology. In VSD, there is an opening in the septum between the left and right ventricle. Whenever the left ventricle contracts, oxygenated blood is shunted from the left ventricle to right ventricle (see Fig. 45-5). Excessive pulmonary blood flow occurs as left ventricular blood shunts into the right ventricle and then into the pulmonary artery. Pulmonary edema commonly occurs in VSD. A VSD also shunts blood out of the left ventricle, decreasing cardiac output. The diminished cardiac output activates the baroreceptor compensatory mechanism that causes tachycardia and triggers the renin-angiotensin-aldosterone system. In newborns, a VSD can undergo spontaneous closure or can lead to heart failure.

Clinical Presentation. Children with small VSDs are asymptomatic, whereas children with large VSDs have a harsh systolic murmur heard at the mid to lower sternal border. Large VSDs cause excess volume in the right ventricle, enlargement of the right side of the heart, and eventual right ventricular failure. Physical examination at birth may indicate the presence of a murmur that is heard continuously and sounds like rolling thunder. Newborns frequently exhibit problems with feeding, failure to thrive, and respiratory infection.

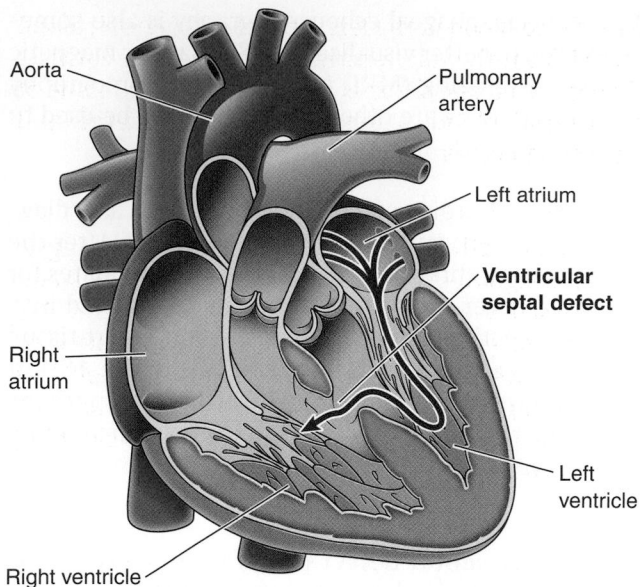

FIGURE 45-5. Ventricular septal defect. An opening between the ventricles in a ventricular septal defect allows deoxygenated and oxygenated blood to mix. Blood from the left ventricle is shunted into the right ventricle.

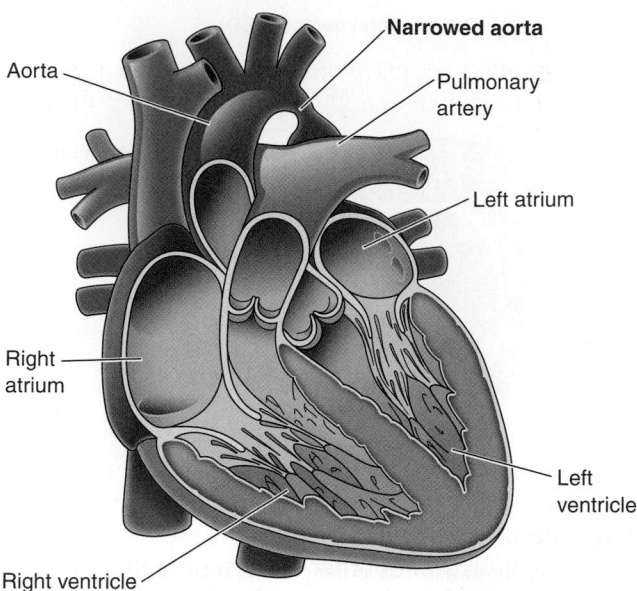

FIGURE 45-6. Coarctation of the aorta. The narrowing of a section of the aorta causes excessive pressure to back up and place high workload on the left ventricle. The narrowing of the aorta also diminishes full arterial blood flow into the aorta.

Exercise intolerance, cyanosis, dyspnea, and syncope occur in early childhood.

Diagnosis and Treatment. An x-ray will show cardiomegaly and increased pulmonary vasculature. Echocardiography can demonstrate the defect. MRI will often demonstrate the defect if echocardiography is not able to show the VSD. Small VSDs may close without intervention, whereas large VSDs require surgical closure. Heart failure is treated with digoxin, diuretics, and ACE inhibitor drugs.

Coarctation of the Aorta

Coarctation of the aorta (COA) is a narrowing of the aorta at the descending curve, just past the ductus arteriosus site (see Fig. 45-6). COA accounts for 5% to 8% of all cases of CHD, and occurs more frequently in boys than girls. When COA occurs in a girl, the clinician should rule out the possibility of Turner's syndrome, which is a genetic disorder that involves COA among other anomalies.

Etiology. COA involves a segment of the aorta that is constricted, usually below the origin of the left subclavian artery. Other cardiovascular defects, such as patent ductus arteriosus, bicuspid aortic valve, transposition of the great vessels, and VSD, commonly accompany COA.

Pathophysiology. COA creates high resistance in the first section of the aorta, which exerts stress on the left ventricle with resulting left ventricular hypertrophy. Low arterial pressure occurs in the segment of aorta that is distal to the narrowed region of aorta. Because of the low arterial blood volume and high afterload against the left ventricle, cardiac output diminishes. The diminished cardiac output triggers compensatory mechanisms that include activation of the renin-angiotensin-aldosterone system. Also, baroreceptors sense the low arterial blood pressure and stimulate the sympathetic nervous system. The low blood pressure also stimulates secretion of antidiuretic hormone. The triggered compensatory mechanisms cause hypertension and can lead to heart failure.

Clinical Presentation. The infant with COA may be asymptomatic or be irritable, feed poorly, and appear to have failure to thrive. Femoral pulses are weak or delayed compared with brachial pulses. Coarctation causes buildup of blood pressure proximal to the narrowed portion of the aorta and decreased blood pressure distal to the narrowed area of the aorta. This causes a marked difference in blood pressure, with pressure in the upper extremities much higher than that of the legs.

Diagnosis and Treatment. Chest x-ray can demonstrate an "inverted 3 sign" where the coarctation is located. The ribs near the COA develop a notched appearance on chest x-ray as well. Echocardiography can show the pressure changes in the heart chambers and the region of coarctation. ECG can demonstrate left ventricular hypertrophy. CT or MRI imaging can also demonstrate the coarctation.

The preferred treatment for COA is surgery. Interventional balloon dilation angioplasty and stent placement are some types of surgical interventions. A significant number of children require surgical revisions later in life.

Tetralogy of Fallot

Tetralogy of Fallot (TOF) accounts for 7% of all CHDs and consists of a combination of four cardiac defects (see Fig. 45-7):

1. pulmonary artery stenosis (narrowing of the pulmonary artery)
2. right ventricular hypertrophy
3. VSD
4. overriding large ascending aorta.

Etiology. TOF has been linked to a genetic mutation at the gene locus 22q11. Other risk factors include maternal rubella infection, maternal diabetes, maternal alcohol abuse, poor maternal nutrition, and older maternal age. Newborns with Down syndrome or DiGeorge syndrome often have the TOF defects. It is also associated with a constellation of other congenital defects called "CATCH 22," which include cardiac defects, abnormal facies, thymic hypoplasia, cleft palate, and hypocalcemia.

Pathophysiology. In TOF, pulmonary stenosis and VSD are the major causes of blood flow disruption. Blood return to the right side of the heart is normal; however, as the right ventricle contracts, not all of the deoxygenated blood can flow into the lungs because of pulmonary artery stenosis. Some of the blood in the right ventricle is shunted into the left ventricle through a VSD. So, some deoxygenated blood mixes with the

Tetralogy of Fallot

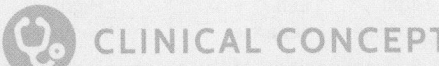

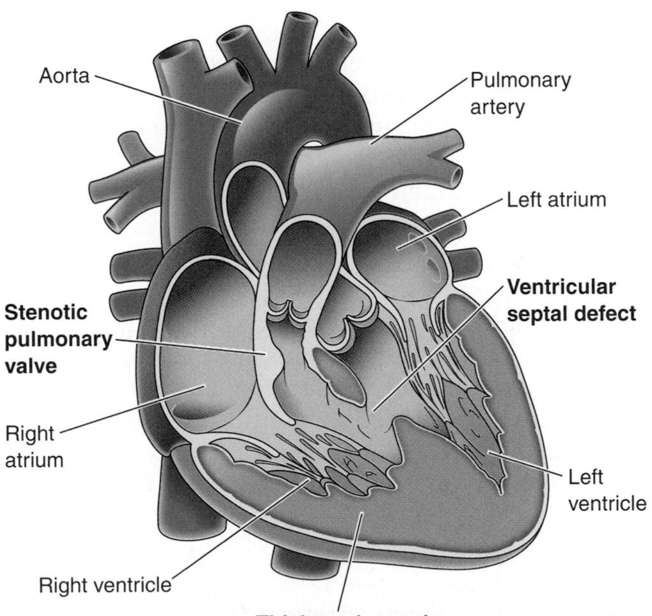

FIGURE 45-7. Tetralogy of Fallot. Tetralogy of Fallot occurs when there are four specific conditions occurring in the heart at the same time: pulmonary stenosis, ventricular septal defect, overriding aorta, and right ventricular hypertrophy. Together, these conditions create a state in which there is not enough blood flow to the lungs; in turn, this means that there is not enough oxygen in the blood, and the child appears blue.

oxygenated blood in the left ventricle. Therefore, blood ejected from the left ventricle into the aorta consists of oxygenated and deoxygenated blood. Thus, some of the arterial blood is inadequately oxygenated and hypoxemia occurs.

Clinical Presentation. Infants born with TOF are cyanotic at birth because of right-to-left shunting of blood through the VSD and decreased pulmonary blood flow caused by the narrowed pulmonary artery. The newborn will exhibit failure to thrive and difficulty with feeding. The child's symptoms include spells of cyanosis, rapid breathing, and agitation known as "tet" spells. Children with chronic hypoxia develop clubbing of the fingers.

CLINICAL CONCEPT

The squatting position provides some relief of dyspnea in children, because in this position peripheral vascular resistance against the left ventricle is increased. This enhanced resistance decreases the shunting of blood from right to left through the VSD.

Diagnosis and Treatment. Chest x-ray indicates an abnormal cardiac silhouette referred to as a boot-shaped heart. The left ventricle is misshapen and dilated because of blood flow into the left ventricle from the VSD. There is a lack of pulmonary circulation on the chest x-ray because of pulmonary valve stenosis. The diagnosis is made by cardiac catheterization and echocardiogram that will demonstrate the abnormal structures.

Immediate treatment includes keeping the ductus arteriosus open, which will allow some blood to enter the pulmonary artery from the aorta. This will improve oxygenation of the blood. Surgical insertion of a pulmonary stent from the aorta to the pulmonary artery will keep the ductus arteriosus open. Surgical repair of the VSD will keep right deoxygenated blood separated from left oxygenated blood. Pulmonary stents may need to be replaced in later life as the child grows.

Transposition of the Great Vessels

Transposition of the great vessels (TGV) accounts for 5% to 7% of all CHDs. The overall incidence is 20 to 30 per 100,000 newborns per year, and it is found more often in male infants than female infants.

Etiology. The cause for TGV is unknown, but it arises because of an embryonic malformation of the heart. The only known risk factor is maternal diabetes.

Pathophysiology. In TGV, the aorta abnormally arises from the right ventricle and the pulmonary artery abnormally arises from the left ventricle (see Fig. 45-8).

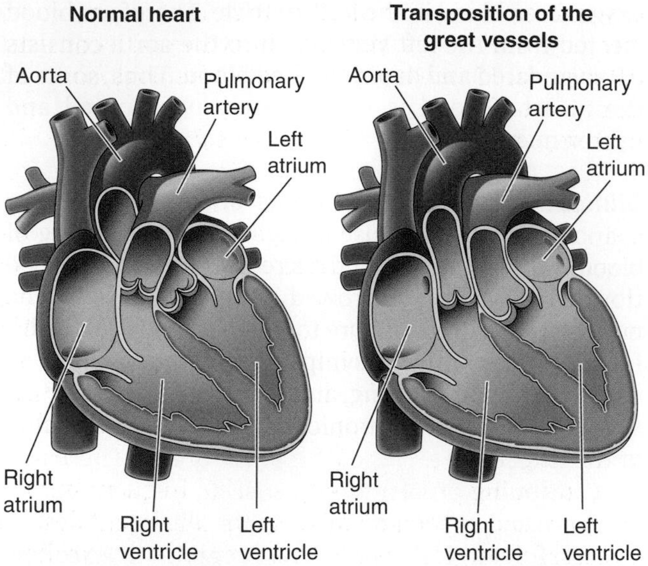

Normal heart

Transposition of the great vessels

FIGURE 45-8. Transposition of the great vessels. In this congenital heart disorder, the major arteries are reversed; the aorta arises from the right ventricle and the pulmonary artery arises from the left ventricle. Deoxygenated blood flows into the aorta and oxygenated blood is pumped into the pulmonary artery. The patient experiences low blood oxygen levels and cyanosis in the first few weeks of life.

Because of these abnormalities, oxygenated blood enters the lungs and deoxygenated blood goes into the arterial circulation.

Clinical Presentation. In TGV, there is marked cyanosis at birth and murmurs from the various defects are audible. Newborns may develop signs of heart failure and fail to gain weight. Tachycardia, tachypnea, and diaphoresis are usually evident, particularly during exertion and when the newborn cries.

Diagnosis. Chest x-ray indicates cardiomegaly and increased pulmonary vascularity. An ECG will indicate right axis deviation caused by right ventricular hypertrophy as the right side of the heart is supplying systemic circulation. After administration of 100% oxygen for 10 minutes, newborns demonstrate hypoxemia on an arterial blood gas test. An echocardiogram demonstrates a pulmonary artery arising from the left ventricle. A cardiac catheterization with angiography is used to examine the heart for other abnormalities.

Treatment. Mixing of oxygenated and deoxygenated blood is needed for survival, and this is accomplished by keeping the ductus arteriosus open with a prostaglandin medication, PGE1. Other defects at birth, such as ASD and VSD, also help to produce mixing and are left unrepaired until surgical reversal of the blood vessels takes place. A procedure to temporarily keep the openings between the two sides of the heart open is done in the cardiac catheterization lab immediately after birth to increase the mixing of oxygenated and deoxygenated blood. Surgery to switch the vessels is done within a few days of birth.

Malformations of the Gastrointestinal System

Many different problems with the gastrointestinal (GI) system and the associated organs can develop in the prenatal period. They occur in as few as 1 per 10,000 births to as frequently as 1 per 1,000 depending on the specific malformation. Boys and girls are affected at different rates by these malformations. GI malformations include tracheoesophageal fistula, cleft lip and palate, biliary atresia, diaphragmatic hernia, gastroschisis, and omphalocele.

Tracheoesophageal Fistula (TEF)

Tracheoesophageal fistula (TEF) is a rare structural defect that affects fewer than 1 out of 2,000 to 4,000 neonates. If untreated, a TEF can lead to severe, life-threatening pulmonary complications.

Etiology
TEF, an abnormal connection of the esophagus and trachea, is associated with the maternal risk factor of polyhydramnios, meaning excessive amniotic fluid. It is also common in newborns with Trisomy 13, 18, and 21. Approximately 17% to 20% of newborns with TEF have additional congenital abnormalities, including congenital heart disease, lack of normal GI development, malformation of the kidneys, and musculoskeletal disorders.

Pathophysiology
Abnormal trachea development occurs in a 4- to 6-week-old embryo. Esophageal atresia, or the absence of part of the esophagus, may also be present. The connection between the trachea and esophagus permits passage of oral secretions and feedings into the trachea and lungs.

Clinical Presentation
TEF is usually detected shortly after birth with the first few feedings. The newborn may appear to have a poor suck, gag during the feeding, and have respiratory distress if the feeding continues. Some infants seem asymptomatic for several months but have a chronic cough and pneumonia until a diagnosis is determined.

Diagnosis
When an infant demonstrates feeding problems, an attempt is made to pass a nasogastric tube into the stomach. If esophageal malformation is present, a chest x-ray with the feeding tube in place will show a coiled-up tube. The fistula between the esophagus and trachea may be confirmed by CT scan, or direct visualization through bronchoscopy. Some instances are detected throughout the prenatal period by fetal ultrasound.

Treatment

Surgical repair is necessary, and is usually scheduled soon after birth. If the newborn has other health problems, or weighs fewer than 1,500 g, surgical repair may be delayed. In that case, the newborn will be fed by a gastrostomy tube inserted directly into the stomach until surgery can take place. The goal of care is to prevent aspiration of secretions and feedings into the trachea.

Cleft Lip and Palate

Cleft lip and palate are abnormalities that occur because of incomplete closure of the maxillary facial bones. Cleft lips are more common in boys than girls, and occur in 1 out of 500 births. Cleft palates are not always present with cleft lips and occur more often in females. Caucasians have a higher incidence than African Americans.

Etiology

There is a strong family history of cleft lip and cleft palate. Many genes play a role in craniofacial development, and many different genetic mutations are being studied related to these malformations. Newborns with fetal alcohol syndrome are found to have a high rate of cleft lip and palate. Maternal diabetes, rubella infection, smoking, and use of some medications increases risk. Newborns with Trisomy 13, 18, and 21 also have a higher risk of orofacial clefts.

Pathophysiology

A cleft lip is formed during gestation in utero, when facial bone development occurs. Early in pregnancy, between 4 and 7 weeks, a cleft lip or palate forms when the two sides of the face fail to completely fuse together, leaving a crevasse. This produces a defect that may appear as only a dimple of the upper lip or as a complete cleft through the lip into the nares, the most severe form of this defect. Cleft palate can occur in the soft palate, hard palate, and uvula and extend to the upper jaw.

Clinical Presentation

The appearance of the newborn's face is the major symptom. Cleft lip and palate are easily seen upon inspection. Feeding and respiratory difficulties may arise from the defects before repair.

Diagnosis

In utero, ultrasound can demonstrate orofacial abnormalities in the fetus. In the newborn with cleft lip or palate, x-ray studies are done to ensure that there are not more facial cranial abnormalities to be considered.

Treatment

Surgical repair of the lip is done shortly after birth so that feeding issues are resolved and the child has no problem with vocalization. Some cleft lip and palate specialists use a rule of 10 to determine when to do surgery; this means that the infant should be at least 10 pounds, 10 weeks old, and have a hemoglobin level of at least 10.

Temporary feeding difficulties can be resolved by holding the infant on the unaffected side for feeding and using a soft nipple with an enlarged opening. Breastfeeding should be encouraged if the mother desires, but the infant may not be able to feed sufficiently because of the abnormal lip and palate. Breastfeeding mothers should be referred to a lactation consultant for assistance, and may need to use a combination of at-the-breast and bottle feeding of pumped breast milk.

Cleft palates are repaired at a much later time than cleft lip, usually at 12 to 24 months of age. There may be continuing problems with speech, frequent ear infections, and upper jaw and teeth misalignment despite successful surgical repair. The prognosis is excellent following surgery, and cosmetic surgery is usually not needed later in life, because the scar is not obvious in most cases. In economically developing countries, children often live for years with no surgical intervention. In these circumstances, the lip and palate are repaired in the same surgery. The quality of life for the child will be improved, but the cosmetic results may not be equal to those obtained with surgeries performed earlier in life.

Biliary Atresia

Biliary atresia, the absence of some or all of the liver bile ducts, appears in 1 out of 10,000 to 20,000 births, and is associated with neonatal hepatitis (inflammation of the liver). Some cases of biliary atresia develop in the postnatal period.

Etiology

The cause for biliary atresia is unknown. Many premature infants are born with the disorder in conjunction with neonatal hepatitis. After birth, infants with biliary atresia show a progressive inflammation of the liver and bile duct destruction. Infectious microorganisms that may cause the progressive deterioration have been under investigation. Some studies have revealed that 25% or more newborns with biliary atresia have cytomegalovirus infection. Researchers have also linked rotavirus and reovirus type 3 to biliary atresia.

Pathophysiology

During gestation, there is a failure in the embryonic development of the bile duct. Obliteration of either the distal segment of the bile duct or the entire extrahepatic biliary tree causes an impairment of bile excretion. After birth, the liver shows evidence of progressive inflammation. Bile obstruction raises the serum bilirubin level, which causes jaundice. The failure of bile excretion can also lead to bile plugs, hepatic fibrosis, and liver failure.

Clinical Presentation

The first symptoms are usually seen as inadequate digestion and malabsorption of fat and fat-soluble vitamins. Fat in the stool, called steatorrhea, appears as clay-colored stools. An enlarged liver is often present early in the disease. When bile is obstructed, bilirubin backs up in the liver and accumulates in the blood; this causes hyperbilirubinemia, which leads to jaundice. Because of poor digestion and malabsorption, growth failure eventually occurs.

Diagnosis

The infant will demonstrate elevated liver enzymes and serum bilirubin levels. Nuclear liver scintiscan, called a DISIDA scan, is used to diagnose biliary atresia. Abdominal ultrasound, exploratory laparoscopy, and liver biopsy are also used to diagnose biliary atresia. Alpha 1 antitrypsin deficiency and cystic fibrosis must be ruled out because these disorders often present with obstructed bile flow.

Treatment

If the lesions causing the atresia are correctable, as in the case of problems limited to the distal segment of the bile duct, several surgical procedures may be done. If the affected bile ducts and biliary epithelium appear necrotic, a liver transplant is the best treatment option. Liver transplants for children have undergone major changes since they were first performed.

 CLINICAL CONCEPT

In the past, a child had to wait for a donor organ harvested from a child cadaver. Now, it is possible for an adult cadaver-donated liver to be split into lobes for two pediatric transplants. It is also possible to transplant a single lobe of a liver from a live donor who is compatible. Liver tissue regenerates if healthy. The transplanted lobe will grow with the child and the live donor will have new tissue growth to take the place of the donated lobe.

Prognosis is poor for children with biliary atresia who are not candidates for corrective surgery or a transplant, with eventual outcomes of hepatic coma and death.

Congenital Diaphragmatic Hernia

Congenital diaphragmatic hernia (CDH) is a structural defect whereby the abdominal organs protrude into the chest and inhibit pulmonary development and function. The severity of CDH depends on the size and exact location of the hernia, the degree of respiratory distress, and the presence of other associated anomalies. Congenital diaphragmatic hernia occurs twice as often in females than males. The incidence is 1 out of 2,000 to 3,000 births, and the survival rate is 40% to 62%.

Etiology

CDH is often seen in combination with several chromosomal abnormalities and is a part of many congenital syndromes. It is seen in Turner syndrome and Trisomy 13, 18, and 21. Specific chromosomal mutations are seen at 1q, 8p, and 15q. Vitamin A deficiency is also associated with CDH.

Pathophysiology

In CDH there is defective formation of the diaphragm and lack of complete lung development. CDH is more common on the left side of the abdomen where the stomach protrudes through the defect in the diaphragm. The pulmonary blood vessels are underdeveloped and there is deficient surfactant, which increases susceptibility to respiratory distress.

Clinical Presentation

The child with CDH may experience respiratory distress immediately after birth, although some infants may not have respiratory distress for up to 48 hours after birth. The child may present with vomiting, intestinal obstruction, and respiratory distress. Bowel sounds may be heard in the chest because intestinal loops are able to enter the thorax through the hernia, and breath sounds are diminished.

Diagnosis and Treatment

Prenatal ultrasound can detect CDH by 16 to 24 weeks of gestation. After birth, chest x-ray can demonstrate the stomach or loops of bowel above the diaphragm. A cardiac shift to the right and pneumothorax are common findings. Echocardiogram often demonstrates cardiac anomalies. Ultrasound can also show if renal abnormalities are present. An MRI of the brain should be done to check for neural tube defects.

If prenatal diagnosis is made, fetal surgical repair is possible. The ideal time to perform surgical repair of CDH is controversial. If the defect is small and has only minor protrusion of abdominal organs into the chest, surgery is not an emergency. If the defect is large and fetal lung development is compromised, fetal surgery is recommended.

Gastroschisis and Omphalocele

Gastroschisis is a weakness in the abdominal wall that allows the intestines to protrude into the umbilical cord opening, forming an **omphalocele** (or umbilical hernia). The omphalocele is covered by the peritoneum, but not by abdominal muscle and skin. Gastroschisis occurs in 1 out of every 2,000 births. Omphalocele occurs in 1 out of every 4,000 births. The conditions are more prominent in males than females with a ratio of 1.5 to 1.

Etiology

The causes of gastroschisis and omphalocele are unknown. This defect is often seen with chromosomal disorders and cardiac defects. Maternal polyhydramnios (excessive amniotic fluid in the mother) and lack of development of the intestine in the fetus often accompany gastroschisis and omphalocele. Premature birth and Trisomy 13, 18, and 21 are often associated with the defects.

Pathophysiology

Gastroschisis and omphalocele occur during the development of the embryo in the 6th to 10th week of gestation. The exact trigger of the condition is unclear. Usually a section of the intestine is apparent protruding through the umbilicus. The stomach, intestines, liver, and bladder may also be exposed. Intestinal underdevelopment and malabsorption are common as well as gastroesophageal reflux. The lungs are commonly underdeveloped and the liver may be located high in the mid epigastric-thoracic region. The liver in this position is susceptible to injury.

Diagnosis

In fetal gastroschisis and omphalocele the maternal bloodstream contains a high level of alpha-fetoprotein (AFP). High AFP indicates that fetal ultrasound should be done. Gastroschisis and omphalocele are visible on ultrasound (see Fig. 45-9).

Treatment

The size of the gastroschisis varies, but it is a serious emergency in the newborn because of the potential for infection and rupture. The treatment is surgical repair, either during the prenatal period or immediately after birth. Fetal surgery has improved survival rates. If the defect is not repaired in the prenatal period, the child is delivered by Cesarean section (C-section) to prevent further injury. Immediately after birth, surgery is done.

Malformations of the Neural Tube

Defects such as spina bifida and related spinal cord malformations, as well as hydrocephalus, may arise during the development of the neural tube of the fetus in utero. The incidence of neural tube defects has decreased dramatically in the United States because of a public health campaign from the Centers for Disease Control and Prevention (CDC) to encourage pregnant women to take folic acid supplements. Neural tube defects are the most common congenital defects second to congenital heart disease.

Spina Bifida and Related Spinal Cord Malformations

Spina bifida refers to an opening in the lining of the spinal canal. The contents of the canal may then bulge out between the vertebrae. A **meningocele** is the protrusion of the meninges outside of the spinal cord, whereas **myelomeningocele** is the protrusion of both neural and meningeal tissue. Myelomeningocele is the most common type of neural tube defect. The protrusions are seen at birth in the lumbosacral area (see Fig. 45-10). When no protrusions are seen outside the skin, a birthmark, dimple, or hairy tuft at the base of the spine may indicate the presence of a defect, known as spina bifida occulta. The incidence of spina bifida is 1 to 2 cases per 1,000 live births. The disease is more common in Caucasians compared with African Americans, as well as more common in females compared with males.

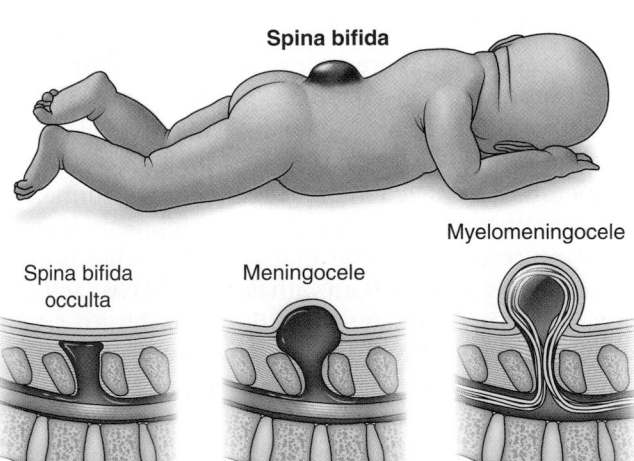

FIGURE 45-10. Spina bifida. In spina bifida, there is incomplete closure of the membranes over the spinal cord, which exposes the spinal cord to injury. In general, there are three types: (1) In spina bifida occulta, there is an opening in one or more of the vertebrae (bones) of the spinal column without apparent damage to the spinal cord. (2) In meningocele, the meninges protrude through an opening in the vertebrae. However, the spinal cord remains intact. This form can be repaired with little or no damage to the nerve pathways. (3). In myelomeningocele, the most severe form of spina bifida, a portion of the spinal cord itself protrudes through the back.

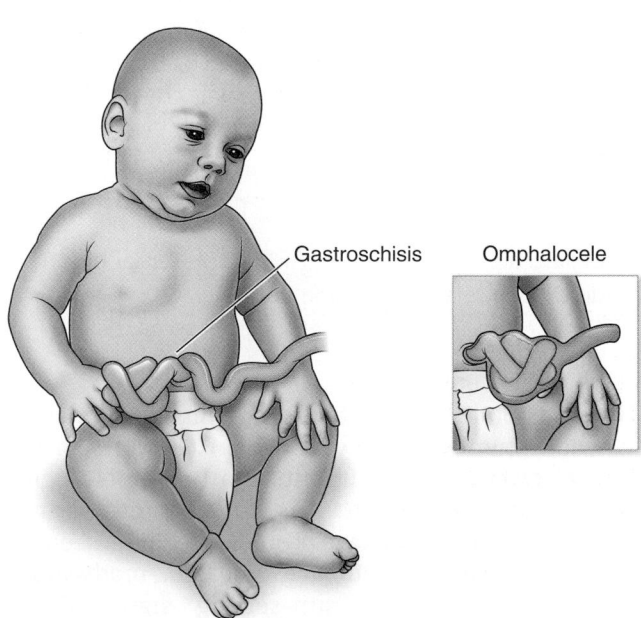

FIGURE 45-9. Gastroschisis and omphalocele. In gastroschisis, the newborn has intestines protruding from the abdomen. In an omphalocele, the protruding intestines are in a sac.

Etiology

Before 1980, folic acid deficiency was the major risk factor for neural tube defects. However, since 1988, the U.S. Public Health Service has required mandatory food fortification with folic acid. The folic acid fortification of foods and an increased awareness of the importance of maternal vitamins have dramatically decreased the incidence of neural tube defects.

Myelomeningocele is more common in newborns with Trisomy 13, 18, and 21. Women with diabetes have a 2- to 10-fold increased risk of having a child with myelomeningocele. Also, maternal obesity, hyperthermia (hot tub use, tanning beds, or febrile illness), and antiseizure medications increase the risk of myelomeningocele.

Pathophysiology

Neural tube defects occur between the 17th and 30th day of gestation. At this point in a pregnancy, many women are unaware of their pregnancy and may be exposed to teratogens. Myelomeningocele and anencephaly are thought to occur at this time in gestation. In myelomeningocele, the lumbosacral end of the spinal cord is uncovered and exposed in a sac above the skin. This exposure causes dysfunction of the spinal nerves at the level of the defect. In some cases, the cranial neural tube is also underdeveloped with varying degrees of cerebral and cerebellar defects. If the flow of cerebrospinal fluid is obstructed, hydrocephalus will also be apparent. Hydrocephalus occurs in more than 90% of newborns with myelomeningocele.

Clinical Presentation

The newborn with myelomeningocele is born with obvious exposed neural tissue exposed in the lumbosacral region of the spinal cord. Some newborns have spina bifida occulta where there is no apparent exposure of the spinal cord; however, a lipoma, dimple, pigmentation, or patch of hair may be apparent in the lumbosacral region. Infants with hydrocephalus have an enlarged head diameter. Infants born anencephalic have formation of the brainstem but do not have development of cerebrum or cerebellum. The majority of newborns with myelomeningocele are born with flaccid paralysis and lack of sensation in the lower extremities. Some have a spastic paralysis of the extremities and upper extremity paresis or paralysis as well. Scoliosis, lordosis, and other musculoskeletal abnormalities are common.

Diagnosis

Prenatal testing of maternal blood between 16 to 18 weeks of gestation can be done to screen for risk of spinal bifida. Elevated alpha-fetoprotein in the mother's blood is associated with spina bifida, although there can be both false negatives and positives with the screening test. An amniocentesis for AFP and acetylcholinesterase can diagnose 99% of myelomeningoceles in utero. This is then followed up with fetal ultrasound, which is also diagnostic.

Treatment

The defects are closed as soon as possible after birth to prevent infection and further damage to the spinal cord. Paraplegia and lack of sensation in the lower body are the results of spina bifida. The kidneys may not develop normally and serum creatinine and urinalysis are necessary. These children may require long-term care for problems with mobility, as well as bowel and bladder control. Fetal surgery to correct the defect before birth is available in major pediatric centers but does not prevent long-term problems associated with this defect. The advantage of fetal surgery is to lower the risk of infection postbirth and to allow a vaginal delivery without danger to the child.

Hydrocephalus

Hydrocephalus occurs when there is excess volume of cerebrospinal fluid (CSF) that circulates around the brain and spinal cord and the skull enlarges to accommodate the excess CSF within the cranium. The incidence of congenital hydrocephalus is 3 per 1,000 live births.

Etiology

Although hydrocephalus is usually associated with a neural tube defect and is a comorbidity of spina bifida, it may also occur from infection and brain tumors. Toxoplasmosis, cerebral hemorrhage caused by prematurity, achondroplasia, astrocytoma, and medulloblastoma are causes of hydrocephalus. Bacterial meningitis is a common etiology, and occurs in preschool and school-aged children. Children with decreased immunity because of human immunodeficiency virus (HIV) or immunosuppressant therapy are at increased risk of meningitis.

Pathophysiology

Hydrocephalus occurs if there is either excessive CSF produced or diminished CSF excreted. Tumor, edema, or inflammation can block the normal excretion of CSF, which then accumulates and increases the diameter of the developing cranium in the fetus or newborn.

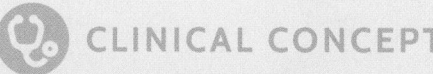 CLINICAL CONCEPT

Elevated alpha-fetoprotein (AFP) in maternal blood is indicative of fetal neural tube defect.

Clinical Presentation

The first notable sign of hydrocephalus is an increase in head circumference beyond what is expected on the normal growth curve. Infants may exhibit bulging fontanelles, dilated scalp veins, and disjointed cranial sutures; they may also have problems feeding, seem irritable and lethargic, and have apnea and bradycardia. The infant may exhibit "sun-setting" sign, which is characteristic of increased intracranial pressure (ICP). Ocular globes are deviated downward, the upper lids are retracted, and the white sclerae may be visible above the iris (see Fig. 45-11). Older children may have the same symptoms along with complaints of a headache, nausea, projectile vomiting, and problems with vision.

Diagnosis

A CT scan is the gold standard for diagnosis when clinical signs indicate possible hydrocephalus. In a young infant, a cranial ultrasound may be used instead. Fetal ultrasound is able to measure the head circumference as well.

Treatment

Treatment is surgical intervention with the placement of an internal shunt to drain the cerebral spinal fluid to the peritoneal cavity. Excess length of the shunt is coiled in the peritoneal cavity and expands as the child grows taller. Shunts can remain in place for decades and are usually only replaced if they become infected or blocked, and thus stop working. Without shunt placement, the prognosis is poor, with resulting developmental delays, blindness, impaired mobility, cognition, and eventual death.

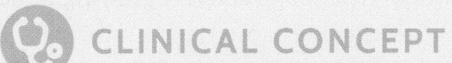 CLINICAL CONCEPT

In the infant, "sun-setting" sign of the eyes is an indication of increased intracranial pressure.

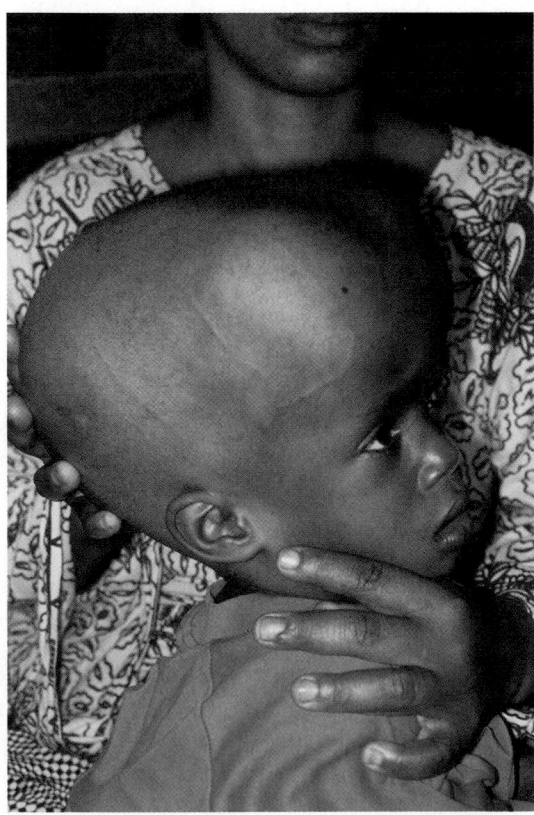

FIGURE 45-11. High intracranial pressure of hydrocephalus. *(From Scott Camazine/Science Source.)*

Malformations of the Genitourinary System

A variety of malformations may affect the genitourinary tract. Some are transient, whereas others may require corrective surgery.

Ambiguous Genitalia

Ambiguous genitalia is a rare condition seen in newborns who have other structural defects of the genitourinary system. It is referred to as a disorder of sexual development (DSD). Infants may seem to have both male and female genital organs, but the genetic karyotype can clearly define one sex or the other. Genetic testing of a buccal smear via a cheek cell sample is usually sufficient to determine a child's sex. In the past, an infant born with ambiguous genitalia was called a hermaphrodite.

The most common cause of DSD is congenital adrenal hypoplasia (CAH), which has an incidence of 1 per 15,000 live births. Sixty percent of newborns with ambiguous genitalia have CAH. In boys with hypospadias and cryptorchidism, there is a 50% incidence of DSD.

Etiology

In CAH, the most common etiology of DSD, there is an excess of androgens because of an enzyme deficiency that produces a virilized (masculine) female. The female genitalia are not clearly distinguished as male or female. There is hirsutism, infertility, and male pattern baldness.

Pathophysiology

During the first trimester of pregnancy, reproductive organs are developed according to the influence of the Y chromosome, which has a sex-determining region that, when present, causes nondescript gonads to develop into testes. When this Y region is absent, as in females, the gonads develop into ovaries. However, there are other genes on other chromosomes that influence the sex of the fetus. On the X chromosome there is the DAX 1 gene that contributes to the development of testicular tissue. Other important genes that influence male development are at 9q33, 11p13, 17q 24-25, and 19q13.3. After formation of the testicular tissue, the production of testosterone stimulates the formation of vas deferens, epididymis, and seminal vesicles. Therefore, there are multiple genetic mutations that can cause DSD.

Clinical Presentation

In DSD, the external genitalia may be neither identifiably female nor male. The clitoris may be enlarged and resemble a phallus. Labial folds can resemble a scrotum. The testes may be undescended and located within the abdomen and mistaken for ovaries. In congenital adrenal hyperplasia, a female can be significantly virilized to resemble a male newborn at birth.

Diagnosis

A karyotype is the necessary test to determine the newborn's sex. An ultrasound can demonstrate enlarged adrenal glands that occur in CAH. Genitourography is an x-ray procedure that can highlight the reproductive system to determine the presence of a uterus, fallopian tubes, and ovaries.

Treatment

Surgical intervention and hormonal medications can give a child the physical appearance of a male or female. Because of the other presenting abnormalities, there has been a tendency in the past to assign the gender identity of the predominant structure, or the gender most easily created by drugs and surgery. The goal of current treatment focuses on surgical and pharmacological intervention to retain genetic gender identity. The urinary system can be repaired so that voiding takes place via a penis or female urethra. Advances in plastic surgery have created a functional penis or a vaginal vault for sexual intercourse. At this time, creation of functional testes or ovaries and uterus in a child not born with these parts is not possible.

Malformations and Disorders of the Musculoskeletal System

Any portion of the skeleton may be affected by malformation in the prenatal period. Corrective surgical treatment dramatically improves the quality of life for affected children.

Congenital Talipes Equinovarus

Talipes equinovarus (TEV), one of the most common orthopedic conditions in newborns, is a foot deformity that causes the foot's bones and tendons to turn inward, resembling a golf club, hence the name club foot. This malformation includes medial rotation of the tibia, inversion of the foot, fixed plantar flexion at the ankle, and adduction of the forefoot. TEV is seen in 1 out of 1,000 births, and can affect one or both feet. It is more common in males than in females, and has some genetic link. The incidence of TEV is 1 in 4 among children who have a parent and a sibling with the defect; 1 in 7 children born with TEV have other congenital anomalies.

Etiology

The etiology of TEV is unknown; however, there are several theories, including restricted position of the fetus in utero, disrupted ossification of the foot in utero, and abnormal vascular perfusion of the foot in utero. Often, TEV is one of the characteristics associated with a syndrome because of genetic or chromosomal abnormalities. However, the majority of newborns with TEV do not have a syndrome associated with genetic mutations.

Pathophysiology

Talipes equinovarus is a foot and ankle deformity that prevents the child from walking on his or her feet. The deformity includes medial rotation of the tibia, inversion of the foot, fixed plantar flexion at the ankle, and adduction of the forefoot.

Clinical Presentation

Physical examination at birth reveals the deformity when the newborn's legs are extended at the hip and knee. The feet appear to turn inward or medially and the plantar surfaces of the feet face each other.

Diagnosis and Treatment

Radiographic studies are done to determine the extent of the bone misalignment. Nonoperative treatment is started soon after birth with progressive braces or casts to gradually move the feet and ankles into correct position. The bracing or casts are readjusted weekly until the feet are well aligned. Residual deformities are common, and surgery is required later in childhood to release the heel cord, reposition the joints, and lengthen the muscles. Compliance with wearing a splint is key to successful treatment. The Ponseti method, with long-term bracing only at night while the child sleeps, has been developed for the child who has residual deformities in childhood. Nighttime splints need to be used for at least 5 years while the child is actively growing in height.

Congenital Hip Dysplasia

Congenital hip dysplasia, also known as developmental dysplasia of the hip, is a common orthopedic condition in the newborn. It is more common in girls, first-born children, and children born during breech deliveries. As many as one-third of children with congenital hip dysplasia have relatives who also are affected by this disorder. The global incidence is 1 to 1.5 out of 1,000 births.

Etiology

The etiology of congenital hip dysplasia is unclear, although theories include breech positioning of the fetus in utero; lack of sufficient amniotic fluid in utero, which causes fetal malposition; and the method of carriage of the baby after birth. For example, the rate of congenital hip dysplasia is much lower in Asia and Africa where newborns are carried in shawls against their mother's body, which forces their hips to be flexed and abducted. The rate is much higher in Native Americans and Eastern Europeans, where the newborn is swaddled in clothes and infant carriers that bring their hips into extension.

Pathophysiology

In congenital dysplasia of the hip, the head of the femur is not in functional alignment with the acetabulum, and the joint is unstable. There are varying degrees of dysplasia, from partial dislocation and dislocatable on exam to fully dislocated. Laxity of the hip ligaments is also part of the pathology.

Clinical Presentation

During the newborn exam, the appearance of asymmetry in the gluteal folds is a sign that hip dysplasia is present. The exam includes the Ortolani maneuver of abduction. During this maneuver, the infant's legs are abducted then adducted. The Ortolani sign is considered positive for dysplasia if the examiner feels a click as the head of the femur relocates into the joint.

Diagnosis and Treatment

If there is a positive Ortolani sign in the newborn, pelvic ultrasound and x-ray are done to confirm hip instability. Partial and dislocatable hips will usually stabilize within the first month of life without intervention. For easily dislocated hips, a first line of treatment is to use a removable brace called a Pavlik harness to keep the hips abducted and flexed. In rare situations, surgery is used to perform either a closed reduction (repositioning without an incision) or an open reduction (with an incision to manipulate the joint), followed by casting with a special molded plaster cast that is called a hip spica cast.

Treatment is best initiated before 6 months of age. If the defect is not corrected, the child will walk with a limp, the leg on the affected side will appear shorter, and the child will walk on the toes of the affected side.

CLINICAL CONCEPT

A positive Ortolani sign is an indication of hip dysplasia in the infant.

Osteogenesis Imperfecta

Osteogenesis imperfecta (OI) is a group of genetic disorders characterized by fragile and brittle bones. The incidence is 1 out of 20,000 births.

Etiology

Osteogenesis imperfecta is caused by a genetic mutation at chromosome 17 that causes abnormal composition of the patient's collagen. Collagen is widespread in the body and is a main constituent of bone, muscle, and skin. There are different forms of the disease; they range from a mild, nondeforming condition to a severely debilitating and deforming disease.

Pathophysiology

In this syndrome, the bone matrix contains abnormal collagen, and the bones break down similarly to osteoporotic bones. Instead of a strong bone matrix of collagen fibrils with calcium deposits along the long axis of the fibrils, the bone lacks structural density to support the extremities or spine. Bones easily fracture because of abnormal composition.

Clinical Presentation

Newborns with OI demonstrate short stature and have a bowlegged appearance. There may be evidence of multiple rib fractures and the thorax appears deformed. The sclerae of the eyes are dark blue-gray in color.

Hearing impairment is common in OI. In the mild form of the disease, the individual can survive with multiple episodes of fractures over his or her lifetime. The severe form of the disease can be lethal and the newborn does not survive infancy.

Diagnosis

The diagnosis is made by clinical inspection and bone biopsy that demonstrates abnormal collagen biochemical composition. Genetic testing is also done to determine the type of OI (I, II, III, or IV). Types are based on the condition and amount of abnormal collagen present in the bones. Children with Type I OI have normally formed collagen, but insufficient quantities of it. Those with Types II to IV OI have both abnormally formed collagen and a deficiency of it. Radiographic studies are used to confirm the diagnosis and locate fractures. Another characteristic sign is a "popcornlike" appearance of the growth plates in the long bones.

Treatment

There is no cure for OI. Mild forms have the best prognosis with use of braces and physical therapy to strengthen muscles and prevent fractures. No nutritional supplements have shown to have a positive effect; however, some success has been seen with administration of growth hormone during childhood in order to improve bone growth. The child treated with growth hormone will have increased bone volume although the bone will still contain defective collagen.

CLINICAL CONCEPT

A characteristic sign of osteogenesis imperfecta is blue sclerae.

Neoplasms Specific to Childhood

Several cancers are found only in children, including neuroblastoma and Wilms' tumor. Other cancers common in childhood are also found in adults, such as leukemia, Hodgkin's lymphoma, non-Hodgkin's lymphoma, and brain tumors. Those cancers found in both children and adults are discussed in Chapter 40: Cancer.

Neuroblastoma

Neuroblastoma is the most common solid tumor seen in infants, and accounts for 7% of all childhood cancers. The prevalence is 1 out of 7,000 births, and approximately 500 new cases are seen each year in the United States. Boys are affected slightly more frequently than girls, and the average age of diagnosis is 19 months. Diagnosis before the age of 12 months is associated with an improved survival rate, and most children are diagnosed by 5 years of age.

Etiology

The cause for neuroblastoma in a child is unknown, although a deletion of the short arm of chromosome 1 is found in 70% to 80% of patients. There is also some evidence that the genetic mutation responsible for this cancer is related to parental occupational exposure to chemicals, farming, or electronic work.

Pathophysiology

Neuroblastoma, a tumor that develops from the sympathetic nervous system, is embryonic in nature. The event that triggers tumor growth is unknown. The disease most often presents as an abdominal tumor in the adrenal gland, but primary tumors can develop in the thoracic cavity, head, or neck.

Clinical Presentation

The signs and symptoms depend on the location of the tumor. Abdominal tumors are hard masses often found displacing the kidney. Respiratory distress is seen with thoracic tumors. Most children will be asymptomatic until the tumor causes pain. Metastasis often has taken place before diagnosis, and symptoms such as weight loss, fever, enlarged liver, or back pain may be the first indication that a child is ill.

Diagnosis

Following a health history and physical, CT scan is used to confirm the suspected presence of a mass. Tumor cells from a biopsy of the mass or from a bone marrow specimen are used to confirm that the mass is a neuroblastoma.

Treatment

Treatment involves surgery and, later, chemotherapy to eradicate metastases. On occasion, radiation therapy may also be used to treat any residual tumor tissue. Neuroblastoma may also spontaneously regress, although it is unclear how or why this happens.

For extensive disease, full body irradiation with bone marrow transplant is the treatment plan if surgical and chemotherapy are not successful. Survival rates range from 90% in children of any age with localized disease to only 20% in children with extensive disease who are older than 1 year.

 CLINICAL CONCEPT

Neuroblastoma is the most common solid tumor that occurs in infancy.

Wilms' Tumor

Wilms' tumor, also known as nephroblastoma, is the most common abdominal tumor in children. It originates as an embryonic neoplasm of the kidney and develops into an abdominal mass during early childhood. The incidence rate is 10 cases out of 1 million children in the United States. It usually is diagnosed in children who are between the ages of 2 and 5 years.

Etiology

Chromosomal studies have linked Wilms' tumor to a wide number of gene mutations. There are gene mutations at chromosome 11p13 and 11p15. Genes at 16q, 1p, 7p, and 17p are also involved in the process of tumor formation. Despite the number of genes that appear to be involved in the development of Wilms' tumor, hereditary cases are uncommon, with approximately only 2% of patients having a positive family history. Siblings of children with Wilms' tumor have a low likelihood of developing the tumor.

Pathophysiology

The genetic changes found in Wilms' tumor cause an abnormal development of the genitourinary system. Common abnormalities found in conjunction with Wilms' tumor are cryptorchidism (undescended testes), horseshoe kidney, a double collecting system, and hypospadias (abnormal urethral opening under the penis). Wilms' tumor can progress through five stages of growth. In stage I the tumor is limited to the kidney, whereas in stages II and III the tumor invades more than the kidney and involves the lymph nodes and peritoneum. In stages IV and V there is bilateral renal involvement and metastasis.

Clinical Presentation

The child with Wilms' tumor is often asymptomatic and the abdominal mass is found by a parent while bathing or dressing the child. Abdominal pain, hematuria, and hypertension are signs that the tumor has enlarged or invaded the kidney.

Diagnosis

Wilms' tumor is differentiated from other tumors by a specific tumor marker that can be analyzed in the blood. Ultrasound, CT scans, and MRIs are used to image the location of the tumor.

Treatment

Preoperative chemotherapy and radiation are used in treatment because of the high incidence of metastasis. Surgical excision of the involved kidney is common. Surgery does not always involve removal of the kidney if the tumor is small, there is no intravascular invasion, or no evidence exists of lymph node metastases.

Infectious and Inflammatory Disorders

Infants and children are particularly at risk for certain infectious and inflammatory disorders. Some infections that occur in utero can cause congenital defects in the infant.

TORCH Infections

TORCH infections are some of the most common infections associated with congenital defects. Most of the TORCH infections cause mild maternal morbidity, but have serious fetal consequences; treatment of maternal infection frequently has no impact on fetal outcome. TORCH infections can be called teratogenic infections. Screening for TORCH infections is part of routine care during pregnancy. **TORCH** is an acronym for:

Toxoplasmosis (spread by domestic cat feces) and **T**reponema pallidum (Syphilis)
Other
Rubella
Cytomegalovirus
Herpes simplex and **H**uman immunodeficiency virus.

The *other* group is an expanding group of viruses and bacteria that includes hepatitis B and Group B streptococci. Other viruses now known to cause congenital infections include parvovirus B19 (B19V), varicella-zoster virus (VZV), West Nile virus, measles virus, enteroviruses, adenovirus, and hepatitis E virus. Recently, lymphocytic choriomeningitis virus has been found to be a teratogenic virus carried by rodents. For a more detailed explanation of infections, see Chapter 10: Infectious Diseases.

Maternal history and history of any recent exposures to ill individuals is important when TORCH infections are suspected in the newborn. The maternal immunization history is also extremely important. Physical examination and diagnostic testing can indicate the source of infection.

Toxoplasmosis

Toxoplasmosis is an infection caused by the protozoan *Toxoplasma gondii* (*T. gondii*) that can threaten the health of an unborn child. *T. gondii* is a parasitic organism found in soil and cat feces. It can also be found in undercooked meat from animals infected with the parasite or from uncooked foods that have come in contact with contaminated meat. Toxoplasmosis causes a flulike illness in the infected patient.

In pregnancy, the rate of transplacental infection has been estimated to be 50% for untreated mothers and 25% for treated mothers. The most vulnerable time for infection of the fetus is the first or second trimester. Congenital *T. gondii* infection can cause chorioretinitis, blindness, seizures, microcephaly, anemia, and encephalitis in the fetus.

Rubella

Rubella, previously known as German measles, is a virus that most commonly affects young children. Clinical manifestations and severity of illness vary with age. Infection in younger children is characterized by flulike symptoms, lymphadenopathy, and an erythematous, maculopapular rash that spreads from head and trunk out to the extremities. In older children, adolescents, and adults, rubella can present as arthralgia, arthritis, and thrombocytopenic purpura.

In the pregnant woman, rubella virus has teratogenic effects on the fetus, especially in the early weeks of gestation. The virus can be transmitted to the fetus through the placenta and is capable of causing serious congenital defects, spontaneous abortions, and stillbirths. Congenital rubella syndrome (CRS) is associated with four common problems: deafness, central nervous system (CNS) abnormalities, cataracts, and cardiac defects. At birth, many infants with CRS exhibit growth limitations, bone disease, and hepatosplenomegaly. Because of the severity of effects on the fetus, young children are given the measles, mumps, and rubella (MMR) immunization. This prevents children from transmitting the rubella virus to pregnant women. The MMR immunization is also important for health-care providers.

Cytomegalovirus Infection

Cytomegalovirus (CMV) infection presents with symptoms similar to infectious mononucleosis: fever, fatigue, and lymphadenopathy. CMV infection is common among young children. Toddlers or preschool-aged children, day care workers, or health-care workers are at a high risk for CMV infection.

Most newborns with congenital CMV infection are asymptomatic at birth. Congenital CMV infection occurs in 5% to 10% of fetuses. After birth, complications of CMV become evident. Complications include hepatosplenomegaly, petechiae, respiratory distress, jaundice, and neurological problems. Neurological involvement may include microcephaly, motor delay, cerebral calcifications, lethargy, and seizures.

Herpes Simplex Virus

Herpes simplex virus (HSV) is a virus that causes blisters on mucous membranes. There are two types: herpes simplex I (HSV 1) and herpes simplex II (HSV 2). Herpes viruses remain dormant in the body for life and can reactivate at times when the patient is immunosuppressed. In the history of the pregnant patient, it is important for the clinician to ask about previous genital HSV infection. However, approximately 70% of women who have been exposed to HSV do not know they are infected. One-third of patients with HSV infection have multiple painful vesicular eruptions (blisterlike rash) on the outer genitalia and perineum.

Most infants exposed to HSV during gestation appear healthy at birth. However, complications appear in early infancy. HSV infection presents with fever or temperature instability, respiratory distress, lethargy, and poor feeding. HSV infection can also cause CNS infection, sepsis, and septic shock in the newborn. The classic skin findings of vesicular lesions may be absent or may appear late.

Syphilis

Syphilis is a disease caused by *Treponema pallidum* (*T. pallidum*), a spiral-shaped bacterium called a spirochete. Syphilis can be transmitted to the fetus from the mother transplacentally or during passage through the birth canal by contact of the newborn. *T. pallidum* can gain access to the fetus as early as 9 to 10 weeks. Syphilis can seriously complicate pregnancy and result in spontaneous abortion, stillbirth, intrauterine growth restriction, and perinatal death, as well as serious sequelae in infected children.

Screening in the first trimester includes rapid plasma reagin (RPR) or the venereal disease research laboratory (VDRL) test combined with confirmation of reactive individuals with treponemal tests such as the fluorescent treponemal antibody absorption assay. Those at risk of syphilis should be retested in the third trimester. At birth, infants with congenital syphilis can have rash, fever, hepatosplenomegaly, anemia, and jaundice. Later symptoms of congenital syphilis include delays in development, seizures, and damage to the bones, teeth, eyes, ears, and brain. Classic symptoms of congenital syphilis in the child include:

- blunted upper incisor teeth known as Hutchinson's teeth
- inflammation of the cornea known as interstitial keratitis
- deafness from auditory nerve disease
- frontal bossing (prominence of the brow ridge)
- saddle nose (collapse of the bony part of the nose)
- hard palate defect
- swollen knees
- short maxillae
- protruding mandible
- snuffles (rhinitis).

Treatment with penicillin early in congenital syphilis, before the development of late symptoms, is essential. For more detailed discussion of syphilis, see Chapter 28: Sexually Transmitted Diseases.

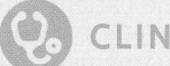 **CLINICAL CONCEPT**

A common group of symptoms in the infant with congenital syphilis is Hutchinson's triad, which consists of Hutchinson's teeth (notched widespread incisors), keratitis, and deafness.

Human Immunodeficiency Virus

Transmission of HIV from mother to baby may occur during intrauterine life, delivery, or breastfeeding. Approximately 50% of infants born to HIV-positive mothers develop HIV infection. The greatest risk factor for intrauterine transmission is high maternal HIV viral load.

Because of anti-retroviral therapy (ART), delivery by C-section, and counseling regarding restricted breastfeeding, the mother-to-infant transmission of HIV has decreased to fewer than 200 cases per year in the United States.

A variety of signs and symptoms should alert the clinician to the possibility of HIV infection in a child. The presentations include recurrent bacterial infections, unrelenting fever, relapsing thrush, recurrent pneumonia, chronic parotitis (inflammation of the parotid gland), generalized lymphadenopathy, delay in development with failure to thrive, and significant pruritic dermatoses. *Mucocutaneous candida* may be the first sign of HIV infection and may vary in presentation, depending on the child's immune status.

The CDC recommends routine prenatal HIV testing as the standard of care for all pregnant women in the United States, with repeat screening in the third trimester recommended in certain jurisdictions with elevated rates of HIV infection among pregnant women. Diagnosis of HIV infection in infants is aided by HIV culture or deoxyribonucleic acid/ribonucleic acid (RNA) polymerase chain reaction (PCR); positive results are confirmed by repeating the test. In suspected cases, HIV testing should occur before the infant is 48 hours old, at age 1 to 2 months, and again at age 3 to 6 months.

According to studies, there may be a higher incidence of premature delivery with use of the protease inhibitor type of anti-retroviral therapy (ART). There is also a possible association between anti-retroviral therapy (ART) and preeclampsia. The development of glucose intolerance may be more common in pregnant women with HIV. Originally thought to be associated with protease inhibitors, gestational diabetes appears to be somewhat increased regardless of the medication regimen. As such, during pregnancy, women should be screened and monitored for glucose intolerance.

Erythema Infectiosum

Erythema infectiosum, also known as fifth disease, is a common infectious disorder in children that is caused by parvovirus B19. Children who develop erythema infectiosum have a characteristic slapped-cheek appearance and usually have mild illness that resolves within a week. More than 50% of pregnant women have immunity to parvovirus B19, and most women who develop infection during pregnancy have no complications. In most cases, the infection can resolve, leaving the fetus or infant unaffected. For more information see Chapter 10: Infectious Diseases.

 CLINICAL CONCEPT

Approximately 5% of women who develop erythema infectiosum develop complications that may include spontaneous abortion, stillbirth, hydrops fetalis, and myocarditis in the fetus. Hydrops fetalis is a condition of widespread edema in the fetus, which presents as pleural effusion, ascites, skin edema, hydropic placenta, pericardial effusion, cardiomegaly, or heart failure. In most cases, parvovirus B19 infection can resolve, leaving the fetus or infant unaffected.

Varicella Zoster Virus

The varicella zoster virus (VZV) causes the clinical syndrome varicella, which is more widely known as chicken pox. Varicella is largely a childhood disease, with more than 90% of cases occurring in children younger than 10 years old. As with measles, mumps, and rubella, varicella is becoming a less common disease because of immunization programs. The disease is benign in the healthy child, whereas increased morbidity is seen in adults and in patients who are immunocompromised.

 CLINICAL CONCEPT

Adults who contract VZV are more prone to complications than children.

If the pregnant woman contracts VZV, the fetus can be affected. Manifestations of congenital VZV in infants may include multiple, reddish, pigmented areas; limb abnormalities; chorioretinitis; optic nerve atrophy; and failure to thrive. Most of these cases occur if the mother was infected between 8 and 20 weeks' gestation. Later in gestation, when the mother has been infected within 2 weeks of delivery, the infant may exhibit fever and a vesicular eruption. Some infants can develop herpes zoster infection, which is commonly known as shingles, if the mother had VZV during pregnancy. For more information see Chapter 10: Infectious Diseases.

Rheumatic Fever

Rheumatic fever (RF) is an autoimmune inflammatory syndrome that can develop 3 to 4 weeks after group A beta-hemolytic streptococci (GABHS) pharyngitis. Rheumatic fever is uncommon in the United States because of widespread antibiotic use. In underdeveloped countries, however, RF affects 300 to 500 children per 100,000. Globally, approximately 470,000 persons are diagnosed with RF annually. Rheumatic fever most commonly occurs in school-age children, and is uncommon in children younger than 3 years. Approximately 60% of persons with RF go on to develop rheumatic heart disease (RHD).

Etiology. Rheumatic fever occurs after an untreated streptococcal infection of the throat in susceptible individuals. It is unclear why some persons develop RF after strep throat and others do not. Risk factors include crowded living conditions and lack of proper sanitation, particularly in underdeveloped countries.

Pathophysiology. In RF, GABHS organisms stimulate antibody formation in the body. The antibodies attack the strep microorganism; for unknown reasons, they damage cardiac valve tissue as well, resulting in RHD. Long-term inflammatory damage to the mitral and aortic heart valves commonly occurs.

Clinical Presentation. Classic symptoms of RF include fever, dyspnea, chest pain, cardiac murmur, carditis, polyarthritis, and the development of subcutaneous nodules over bony prominences. All the heart's layers are affected by RF, and myocarditis, endocarditis, and pericarditis occur. Most commonly, the mitral and aortic heart valves are damaged. Heart failure can also occur as a result of carditis. Arthritis classically affects the knees, ankles, elbows, and wrists, and subsides after 2 to 4 weeks. An erythematous rash, known as erythema marginatum, may occur. Sydenham's chorea, a movement disorder, occurs in 25% of patients with RF. The average duration of untreated RF is 3 months.

Diagnosis. Diagnosis is based on a recent history of a sore throat, physical examination, elevated C-reactive protein levels in the serum, ECG abnormalities, and a positive test for GABHS. Echocardiogram commonly shows abnormalities of the aortic or mitral valve.

Treatment. Treatment for RF includes antibiotics, anti-inflammatory drugs, and bedrest.

 CLINICAL CONCEPT

Group A beta-hemolytic streptococcus is also called *Streptococcus pyogenes*. In patients with pharyngitis, a throat culture is necessary to rule out GABHS infection.

Kawasaki Disease

Kawasaki disease is a systemic vasculitis that is more prevalent in boys than girls and in persons of Asian ancestry. It is exclusively seen in infants and young children. The cause is unknown, but it is probably autoimmune. The disease is an inflammatory vasculitis that can affect the coronary arteries and cause aneurysms. There are approximately 3,000 cases per year in the United States.

Etiology. Kawasaki disease, a rare disease with unknown etiology, involves an environmental agent and a genetic susceptibility. It has recently been suggested to be caused by an RNA virus that probably enters the body through the inhalation route. An infectious pathogen is theorized as the probable cause because the disease affects persons in an epidemiclike manner, with many persons ill during late winter and spring. Genetic factors are likely because Kawasaki disease is more common in persons with a gene mutation at 19q13.2.

Pathophysiology. Kawasaki disease causes inflammation of small- and medium-sized arteries. The coronary arteries are most frequently affected; however, any of the body's blood vessels can be involved. The tunica intima and tunica media of the blood vessels become edematous. White blood cells, plasma cells, and CD8 cells attack the inner lining of the blood vessels and release cytokines, causing widespread damage of arteries. Eventually, the vessel walls become fibrotic and infiltrated by connective tissue. These arterial wall changes cause stenosis and formation of aneurysms. Platelets are drawn to the damaged regions of the artery wall and create thrombi that can cause ischemia and infarction of tissue.

Clinical Presentation. The classic symptoms of Kawasaki disease include fever, lymphadenopathy, bilateral conjunctivitis, and color changes of the lips and mouth, described as strawberry tongue. Also present will be edema of the hands and feet, a polymorphous rash on the trunk, and swelling of cervical lymph nodes. In the late stage, symptoms include arrhythmias, myocardial infarctions, and congestive heart failure.

Diagnosis. There is no definitive laboratory test for Kawasaki disease. A clinical diagnosis may be made based on elevations in leukocyte count, erythrocyte sedimentation rate, C-reactive protein level, or platelet count, as well as characteristic physical examination findings of fever, lymphadenopathy, conjunctivitis, and strawberry tongue.

Treatment. Treatment of Kawasaki disease includes intravenous immune globulin, as well as aspirin in high doses, as an antiplatelet treatment while the disease resolves.

ALERT! Aspirin is administered to the child with Kawasaki disease even though its use is usually avoided in children because of the risk of Reye syndrome.

Juvenile Rheumatoid Arthritis

Juvenile rheumatoid arthritis (JRA) is one of the most common chronic diseases of childhood. There are many subtypes of this disorder based on different genetic etiologies, and so the term *juvenile idiopathic arthritis* (JIA) is increasingly being used in order to define the disease. The incidence rate for JIA ranges from 4 to 14 cases per 100,000 children annually. JIA can occur at all ages across the span of childhood. The disorder affects girls more than boys.

Etiology. The precise etiology of JIA is unclear; however, many experts consider it an autoimmune disorder. Both humoral (B cell) and cell-mediated (T cell) immunity are involved in the pathogenesis of JIA.

Pathophysiology. T cells and B cells are both stimulated by an unknown antigenic trigger and involved in inflammation of the synovial linings of joints. T lymphocytes release proinflammatory cytokines such as prostaglandins, tumor necrosis factor, and interleukins. B cells produce autoantibodies, especially antinuclear

antibodies, and these form circulating immune complexes that are deposited in joint linings.

Clinical Presentation. Arthritis must be present for 6 weeks before the diagnosis JIA can be made. Disease onset can be gradual or sudden, with the child complaining of joint stiffness in the morning or after long periods of inactivity. The child may exhibit a limp that improves with increasing use of the joint. Typically, children may not complain of pain, though they stop using the affected joints and, in turn, become less mobile. JIA may cause spiking fevers, typically occurring once or twice each day, at about the same time of day, with temperature returning to normal or below normal. JIA is a disease of remissions and exacerbations.

Diagnosis. Laboratory studies of leukocytosis, elevated erythrocyte sedimentation rate, and high C-reactive protein indicate inflammation. However, the diagnosis may be delayed because laboratory values are often normal. As many as 70% of children with JIA have positive antinuclear antibody (ANA) assays. However, a positive ANA can occur in other autoimmune diseases, and these need to be excluded. Joint x-rays may not show signs of joint damage. CT scan and MRI are superior for showing signs of joint inflammation and soft tissue swelling. Some clinicians prefer to use ultrasound to detect cartilage erosions and effusions because this does not cause exposure to radiation.

Treatment. Treatment is based on the extent of joint involvement. Main goals include keeping the patient mobile, limiting joint damage, and decreasing pain. NSAIDs are the first line of medications used. If NSAIDs are inadequate for complete relief, methotrexate, sulfasalazine, and tumor necrosis factor-alpha inhibitors such as etanercept are used. Joint injection or oral corticosteroids are sometimes needed. Exercises and physical therapy help to keep joints mobile. In severe disease, surgical treatments such as hip and knee replacement may be necessary.

Respiratory Disorders

In infancy, apnea is a potentially fatal condition that is often associated with prematurity and sudden infant death syndrome (SIDS). Common respiratory disorders in childhood include bronchiolitis, bronchopulmonary dysplasia, and asthma, which all cause bronchoconstriction. Cystic fibrosis is a common hereditary disease that affects the lungs and pancreas. Croup is common in young children with a characteristic "barking" like cough; it can deteriorate into the medical emergency called epiglottitis.

Apnea

Apnea, which is the cessation of respiration, is associated with prematurity, but it can also occur in full-term and otherwise healthy infants. Apnea may be rooted in alteration of CNS regulation, airway clearance, or a combination of the two. SIDS, also known as crib death, is an extreme example of apnea, and the causes of it are poorly understood. Apneic episodes that last longer than 20 seconds, or shorter periods of apnea with cyanosis, decreased responsiveness, choking, gagging, or bradycardia are potentially fatal conditions in infants (see Box 45-1).

Many tests are performed to rule out causes of the apnea. Blood analysis may indicate the presence of infection or metabolic disorders. An electroencephalogram may be used to determine if the problem is related to seizures. Airway obstruction or aspiration from gastroesophageal reflux can be investigated by bronchoscopy and swallowing studies. An ECG will indicate if there are cardiac arrhythmias.

Treatment of apnea is directed at the underlying disease process. However, often there is no apparent cause. Infants can be managed at home and in day care with the use of a home apnea monitor. The monitors are easy to use, and all caregivers should be instructed on how to apply the monitor, interventions to take if the alarm is activated, and infant cardiopulmonary resuscitation. The monitor should be in place at all times except for bath time. Home sleep studies are usually performed at intervals to determine continued need for apnea monitoring. Most healthy full-term infants seem to outgrow apnea by the age of 6 months. For older children with recurring apnea during sleep, home pulse oximeters can be used. In most situations, gentle stimulation of the child is enough to end the apnea episode; the noise of the apnea alarm or pulse oximeter frequently arouses the child enough to stimulate normal breathing. In extreme cases of sleep apnea, the child may need to be on assisted ventilation for sleep.

Bronchiolitis

Bronchiolitis—a disorder unique to children—is a viral infection of the lower respiratory tract. This seasonal disease, with the highest incidence seen in colder months, is most often caused by respiratory syncytial virus (RSV) and sometimes referred to as RSV bronchiolitis. Almost 100% of infants and children contract RSV infection at some point in their first 3 years of life. Bronchiolitis or pneumonia occurs in 25% to 40% of infants exposed to RSV. The younger the infant, the more severe the infection. Peak incidence of RSV infection occurs at 2 to 8 months old. Most recover without complications; however, 1% to 2% require hospitalization. Most children who are hospitalized are younger than 6 months old.

Etiology

RSV causes more than 65% of bronchiolitis cases. Influenza, human metapneumovirus, and rhinovirus account for the rest of the cases of bronchiolitis. Infants born prematurely and those with chronic lung disease are at higher risk for complications such as apnea and pneumonia. Other risk factors include:

- prematurity, small body weight lower than 1,500 g
- age younger than 3 months
- crowded living conditions
- day care
- parental smoking
- congenital heart disease
- immunodeficiency syndrome
- neurological disease.

Pathophysiology

RSV, the major cause of bronchiolitis, is an RNA virus that has an incubation period of 2 to 8 days. It is spread by droplet infection from the nasopharynx. The virus invades the smaller bronchioles and lower respiratory tract epithelium; therefore, infection is termed bronchiolitis. It incites small airway constriction, edema, and mucus production. Mucus and cellular debris obstruct the narrowed airways, and oxygen and carbon dioxide exchange are impaired.

> ### BOX 45-1. Sudden Infant Death Syndrome
>
> SIDS is diagnosed when an infant younger than age 1 year dies unexpectedly from an unknown cause after complete investigation of the possible etiologies and autopsy. Approximately 4,000 infants die each year from SIDS, and it is the most common cause of death in infants between 1 and 12 months old. It occurs most commonly in infants between 2 to 3 months of age, and occurs more in male infants than female infants. Family history of SIDS increases susceptibility. It is more common in African Americans, Native Americans, and Eskimo infants than Caucasian infants.
>
> It is important to follow the recommendations to prevent SIDS:
>
> - Always place infants in the supine position during naps and sleep.
> - Do not allow an infant to sleep with an adult, in an adult bed, on a couch, or a chair.
> - Do not use old cribs or bassinets or modify crib assembly. Only use cribs with certification of U.S. Consumer Product Safety regulations.
> - Use a firm sleep surface without use of pillows, toys, or bedding.
> - Make sure you cannot insert more than two fingers between the crib and its mattress.
> - Never place a crib near window blind cords, curtain cords, or baby monitor cords.
> - Do not expose the infant to smoke.
> - Give the infant only a pacifier that has no string attached.
> - Do not allow the infant to become overheated during sleep.

Clinical Presentation

The child with bronchiolitis first appears to have an upper airway respiratory infection with fever, cough, and rhinorrhea. Infants may initially present with crying and irritability. Symptoms progress to tachypnea, wheezing, rhonchi, and crackles heard in the lung fields. A serious sign of respiratory distress is the use of accessory muscles for breathing, with noticeable nasal flaring and substernal and intercostal retractions. Stridor, a harsh, high-pitched sound on inspiration, and grunting with respiration are also indications of serious distress. Later signs of distress include lethargy, lung hyperinflation, and decreased respiratory rate as the child becomes critically ill. The mortality rate for hospitalized infants is 1%.

Diagnosis

There are rapid assays for RSV and influenza from nasal washings. Chest x-rays are used to determine if the patient has pneumonia and also to rule out foreign body aspiration. Lateral neck x-ray can rule out epiglottitis.

Treatment

Most treatment is supportive with supplemental oxygen and fluids. Secondary bacterial infections are treated with antibiotics. Ribavirin, a nebulized antiviral medication, has shown to help improve respiratory function in hospitalized children. There is no vaccine for RSV; however, anti-RSV immunoglobulin can provide passive immunity. Because of the short-term duration of immunity offered by anti-RSV immunoglobulin, it must be given monthly. The yearly vaccine for seasonal influenza can be given to all infants older than 6 months unless there is an allergy to eggs. The initial year of influenza vaccine for a child requires two doses 1 month apart. Once the child has received the two doses of yearly vaccine the first year, he or she needs only one dose in each subsequent year.

Bronchopulmonary Dysplasia

Bronchopulmonary dysplasia (BPD) affects 25% of all premature infants whose birth weight is lower than 1,500 grams. This chronic lung disease results from long-term respiratory support by mechanical ventilation and high levels of supplemental oxygen. Infants with BPD are at high risk for mortality during the first 2 years of life.

Etiology

Mechanical ventilation, prematurity, and body weight lower than 1,500 grams are risk factors for BPD in infants. Premature infants born between 22 and 30 weeks' gestation are at highest risk.

Pathophysiology

In the premature infant, mechanical ventilation can damage areas of the lung and cause squamous cell metaplasia and hypertrophy of the small airways. The alveoli may collapse, significantly reducing the surface area available for oxygen and carbon dioxide exchange. BPD may also be the result of immature lung development in utero. Alveoli do not develop appropriately; instead of multiple small alveoli, fewer large alveoli form. The few large alveoli cannot supply sufficient oxygenation as the child grows.

ALERT! Children with BPD are at greater risk for SIDS, although the mechanism is unclear.

Clinical Presentation

Initially, the infant suffers tachypnea, tachycardia, and obvious respiratory distress with use of accessory muscles to breathe. Nasal flaring and grunting are obvious signs of breathing difficulty. The infant usually loses weight during first 10 days of life.

Diagnosis

BPD is most common in premature infants. Chest x-ray shows atelectasis, areas of hyperinflation, pulmonary edema, and pneumonia. Arterial blood gases are abnormal, demonstrating decreased arterial oxygen saturation, low PO_2 and high PCO_2. Pulmonary function tests show high residual volume in the lungs.

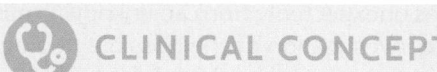

CLINICAL CONCEPT

CT or MRI scan may be better able to show lung findings than x-ray.

Treatment

Infants with BPD require mechanical ventilation shortly after birth. Infants have respiratory distress syndrome caused by low surfactant levels in the lungs. Low surfactant causes alveolar collapse and widespread atelectasis. Supplemental surfactant is administered within the first 6 hours of birth. Synthetic surfactant is administered via an endotracheal tube. Oxygen therapy via mechanical ventilation is necessary. Low pulmonary volumes are critical to avoid trauma to the infant's delicate alveoli. Continuous positive airway pressure is sometimes used instead of endotracheal intubation. Vitamin A supplements have been found to prevent BPD in premature infants. Diuretics, bronchodilators, and methylxanthines can decrease pulmonary bronchial and vascular resistance. Inhalation of nitrous oxide relaxes the pulmonary vasculature. Caffeine is used to stimulate breathing. Corticosteroids are sometimes used to diminish inflammation. Enteral and parenteral nutrition supports the infant's growth.

Asthma

Asthma is a chronic disease of airway inflammation and obstruction in reaction to a respiratory irritant, commonly called a trigger. Examples of triggers include pet dander, cigarette smoke, dust mites, mold, chemical fumes, perfumes and fragrances, cleaning products, exercise, cold air, emotions, respiratory infections, pollen, and some foods. The smooth muscles of the bronchi constrict, producing bronchospasm, and bronchial goblet cells produce excessive mucus.

Asthma rates are on the increase in the United States. The highest rates of childhood asthma are found in urban areas, areas of poverty, and in homes where children are exposed to cigarette smoke. There is a higher prevalence of asthma in the African American population, but it is unclear if the rate is caused by genetic differences or an urban environment. Despite advances in the science of management, the mortality rate from asthma for children has risen over the past 20 years because of nonadherence to treatment and delay in seeking treatment during severe attacks.

Etiology

Asthma is most commonly caused by a combination of genetic susceptibility and environmental antigen. Asthma susceptibility is associated with gene mutations at 17q21 and 11q13.5. There are multiple known triggers for an asthma attack. In an infant, RSV bronchiolitis is the most common cause of bronchoconstriction and wheezing. As the child matures, other viruses or microorganisms can trigger asthma. Allergens such as pollen, dust, molds, or animal dander are common stimulants. Cold air and exercise are also known to incite bronchospasm.

Pathophysiology

After exposure to a stimulant, the bronchioles constrict, mucus secretion increases, and bronchial inflammation obstructs the airways. Bronchial inflammation occurs because of a combination of T cells, cytokines, and immunoglobulin E. Air is retained in the lungs because of a lack of expiratory ability, and hyperinflation of the lungs often occurs. As inhaled air decreases, the alveoli lack oxygen and hypoxia develops, which stimulates pulmonary vessel constriction. Inadequate ventilation capacity develops, and various regions of the lungs demonstrate arteriolar constriction. Ventilation-perfusion mismatching occurs within the lungs. Alveolar-capillary exchange of oxygen and carbon dioxide diminish.

Clinical Presentation

Asthma is classified according to the severity and frequency of attacks. Asthma can be classified as mild intermittent asthma, in which symptoms occur fewer than 2 times per week, to severe persistent asthma with continual symptoms that limit the child's physical activity. An attack is an acute, reversible hyperactive response to a trigger, leading to bronchospasm. During an attack, the child will experience wheezing, coughing, and respiratory distress. The child may complain that the chest feels tight.

Diagnosis

Diagnosis is based on history and symptoms. Pulmonary function tests are diagnostic studies that can determine severity of asthma; a peak flow meter can be used at home for this purpose. Arterial blood gases will commonly reveal low pH, low PO_2, and elevated PCO_2. Chest x-ray during an asthma attack may show hyperinflation of the lungs. Adjunctive testing for allergies with skin scratch testing can determine the child's specific triggers.

Treatment

Treatment for asthma consists of prevention, as well as early intervention when attacks do occur to reverse the reactive airway. Most children receive a combination of maintenance therapy to prevent attacks and rescue medication to treat acute attacks. Maintenance medications include inhaled corticosteroids, leukotriene antagonists, long-acting beta-2 sympathetic agonists, and cromolyn. The most common rescue medication is albuterol, a rapid-acting beta-2 sympathetic agonist. Corticosteroid and sympathetic agonists are delivered via metered dose inhalers.

Important to the treatment is the avoidance of triggers, including environmental changes at home. Children need to be a partner in the management of asthma as soon as they are mature enough to cooperate with daily peak flow monitoring and the use of metered dose inhalers. Infants and toddlers need their medications in nebulizer form. When using metered dose inhalers, all children should be given a spacer or aero chamber to help administer the dose. For more information see Chapter 21: Restrictive and Obstructive Pulmonary Disorders.

Cystic Fibrosis

Cystic fibrosis (CF) is an inherited disease from an autosomal recessive gene. Over 1,000 different gene mutations exist that lead to CF, and there is a wide variation in the disorder's severity. It occurs in 1 out of 3,500 births in Caucasian children, and 1 out of 17,000 births in African American children. The current life expectancy for individuals with CF in the United States is 37.4 years; in 2000, it was 32 years, and 50 years ago, children with CF did not usually survive to attend kindergarten.

Etiology

Cystic fibrosis is an autosomal recessive disorder caused by a disruption of exocrine gland function and chloride excretion in the epithelial cells of the respiratory tract, pancreas, sweat glands, salivary glands, intestines, and reproductive system. A mutation at the CFTR gene 7q31 impairs chloride transport across epithelial cells at mucous membrane surfaces.

Pathophysiology

In CF there is disruption of chloride channels in cells located at mucous membranes. This leads to a disturbance in the sodium-chloride levels at the body's epithelial mucosal surfaces. A state of dehydration occurs at the cell surfaces, which creates conditions for secretion of thick, viscous, mucous secretions. Mucous secretions, particularly within the lungs and GI tract, are denser than normal. This adversely affects airway clearance and digestion. Accumulation of retained, dense mucous secretions in the bronchioles impedes effective oxygen and carbon dioxide exchange in the alveoli. The stasis of mucus also promotes the growth of viral and bacterial pathogens, leading to pneumonia.

The pancreatic ducts are particularly obstructed by excessive mucus which leads to deficiency of pancreatic enzymes. Lack of pancreatic enzymes causes deficient protein, carbohydrate, and fat digestion.

Clinical Presentation

The signs and symptoms of CF are most commonly seen as respiratory or GI alterations. Cough, excessive sputum, chronic infections, wheezing, air trapping, sinus disease, and pallor all indicate impaired respiration. Failure to thrive, fat-soluble vitamin deficiencies, edema, pancreatitis, rectal prolapse, and loose and fatty stools indicate GI alterations.

Diagnosis

When CF is suspected from the presenting symptoms, a skin test is performed for the sweat chloride concentration. If the sweat chloride is elevated, genetic testing can be used to determine the presence of the CF genotype. Prenatal testing is now available for CF.

Treatment

There is no cure for CF; treatment is focused on symptom management. Impaired respiratory function can be improved by chest physical therapy, exercise, and medications to produce bronchodilation, decrease inflammation, and prevent infections. Treatment to support nutritional needs includes pancreatic enzyme replacement, fat-soluble vitamin supplements, and high caloric/protein diets. Tube feedings may be used if oral intake is insufficient to keep the child above the 25th percentile in height and weight. When death occurs, it is usually the result of treatment-resistant pneumonia or pneumothorax.

Croup

Croup, also called laryngotracheobronchitis, results from a viral infection that produces inflammation in the upper airway. Croup affects approximately 5 out of every 100 children per year in the United States, and occurs in infants and young children up to the age of 3 years. Peak incidence occurs during the colder winter months. More male children are affected than females. Croup does not occur in older children, as the airway below the vocal cords is wider and significant narrowing is unlikely to occur.

Etiology

Croup is mainly caused by a parainfluenza virus that spreads from the nasopharynx by droplet infection.

However, influenza, mycoplasma, adenovirus, rhinovirus, and RSV can also cause croup. A cough, sneeze, contaminated hands, or surfaces can spread the infection. The virus initially affects the trachea and then invades the bronchioles.

Pathophysiology

Croup is an inflammation of the trachea and bronchioles. The inflammation causes narrowing of the airway just below the vocal cords and can progress to complete obstruction. The involved area is edematous and infiltrated by lymphocytes and neutrophils. Edema causes narrowing of the small diameter of the trachea under the cricoid cartilage. Airflow limitation occurs and breathing becomes difficult.

Clinical Presentation

Croup gets its name from the hoarse noises made by the child while trying to breath. The sound has been compared with barking sounds made by ocean seals. Croup first presents as a typical upper respiratory infection with fever and rhinorrhea but clear breath sounds. Within 24 hours, the child appears to be more seriously ill with irritability, agitation, an inability to calm down, and labored breathing. Breath sounds include stridor, a harsh, high-pitched sound heard on inspiration. The child has signs of increasing respiratory effort, including tachycardia, hypoxia, nasal flaring, and retractions.

Diagnosis

The diagnosis is determined from the history of the symptoms and physical exam. Chest x-ray is unlikely to add useful diagnostic information and will delay intervention. However, lateral neck x-ray is in order if epiglottitis is suspected. The "steeple sign" on neck x-ray is pathognomonic of epiglottitis, which is an emergency.

Treatment

Treatment must be prompt to prevent severe respiratory distress. Cool and humidified air, such as a nebulizer treatment with saline, or steam from a shower, often brings relief. If the croup persists, epinephrine via a nebulizer is given; however, the child must be taken to the emergency department for this treatment. Oral or parenteral steroids may be used in extreme cases to decrease swelling of the respiratory tract. Most children with croup recover in a few days.

Epiglottitis

Epiglottitis is inflammation and edema of the epiglottis and aryepiglottic folds. It is usually secondary to an upper respiratory infection such as croup. It occurs during the cold months, targeting children between the ages of 3 and 5. The development of *H. influenza* type B vaccine has dramatically reduced incidence of epiglottitis. The incidence is 0.63 cases per 100,000 children.

Etiology

Epiglottitis is most often caused by *H. influenzae*, *H. parainfluenzae*, *S. pneumoniae*, or group A beta-hemolytic streptococcus. Often a viral infection will lead to a bacterial superinfection that results in epiglottic inflammation. Other causes include thermal injury, such as throat burns from high temperature bottle feeding; swallowing of caustic substances; and foreign body ingestion.

Pathophysiology

The epiglottis is a membrane that covers the trachea when an individual is swallowing in order to prevent food from entering the trachea. In epiglottitis, this membrane is swollen and obstructs air from entering the trachea.

Clinical Presentation

The child initially presents with symptoms of upper respiratory infection such as fever, sore throat, hoarseness, and cough. As respiratory distress increases, the child will appear pale and anxious and will lean forward when sitting in order to reduce the effort needed to move air in and out of the lungs. Stridor is a sign of the need for immediate treatment such as endotracheal intubation.

Diagnosis

Diagnosis is made based on history, symptoms, and the physical exam. During the physical exam, use of a tongue depressor to view the airway can stimulate complete airway closure. Therefore, the clinician should be prepared to intubate when examining the child. A chest x-ray is of no diagnostic value; however, a lateral neck x-ray can show "steeple sign," which is indicative of epiglottitis.

Treatment

Endotracheal intubation or tracheotomy is necessary if the patient cannot breathe. Antibiotic treatment is usually required. Antipyretics such as acetaminophen or ibuprofen are used as well.

> **ALERT!** Epiglottitis is considered a medical emergency, as the airway can become completely obstructed in a matter of seconds.

Disorders of Nutrition, Digestion, and Elimination

There are some common GI disorders that occur in infancy. Disorders that can be treated medically include colic, necrotizing enterocolitis, Hirschsprung disease, and gastroesophageal reflux disease. Other disorders, such as pyloric stenosis. Meckel's diverticulum, and intussusception, require surgery.

Colic

Colic is a poorly understood pediatric phenomenon thought to be related to GI distress. It is one of the most common reasons parents seek the advice of a clinician during early infancy. It occurs in 10% to 30% of infants, both breastfed and formula-fed, though this is likely a low estimate because many parents do not report episodes of colic. It occurs equally in males and females and is self-limited and benign. Etiology is unknown and there are no known risk factors for colic.

Pathophysiology

Numerous theories exist about the cause of colic. It has been hypothesized that colic may be caused by large amounts of air entering the gastric lumen as the infant feeds, which causes accumulation of intestinal gas. Another theory asserts that colic is caused by fermentation of substances in the intestine that release gas, which causes GI distress. Some studies show that infants with colic have a food allergy involving an adverse reaction to cow's milk. Other studies have focused on intestinal bacteria and its association with colic. Lower counts of intestinal lactobacilli have been observed in infants with colic compared with infants without colic. Some investigators assert that irritability and crying may be caused by esophagitis and gastroesophageal reflux disease in infants. Another theoretical cause of colic has been inexperienced parenting. Parental anxiety and parental stress has been a subject of many studies. Smoking during pregnancy has also been correlated with colic in infants. No one theory has been established as a definite cause of colic.

Clinical Presentation

Colic is a common syndrome of infancy characterized by excessive, sudden bouts of crying that most often occur in the evenings. It occurs without any identifiable cause in an otherwise healthy infant aged 2 weeks to 4 months. The technical definition of colic is a periodic bout of infant crying lasting greater than 3 hours per day for more than 3 days per week with no pathological cause.

Diagnosis

The infant should have a physical examination to rule out other possible causes of periodic infant irritability and crying. Laboratory studies are usually not indicated unless the clinician suspects another condition. If the infant's stools are excessively watery, testing for lactose intolerance and fecal occult blood can be done to rule out cow's milk allergy.

Treatment

Although no one treatment has proven successful, there are numerous suggested remedies for colic. In breastfed infants, a maternal low-allergen diet that is low in dairy, soy, egg, peanut, wheat, and shellfish may offer relief from excessive crying in some infants. Simethicone is a nonabsorbable medication used for GI gas that some pediatricians recommend. Some mothers suggest feeding the infant glucose in sterile water for relief of colic. Although probiotics may have some role in colic, advice should be sought from a pediatrician regarding any over-the-counter remedy used for colic. More research is needed about probiotic use and herbal remedies. Many parents find that the vibrations of a car ride with the infant in a car seat are often soothing. Parents should not exhaust themselves regarding the infant's periodic irritability caused by colic. Medications should not be given for colic. Parental education and reassurance regarding the benign nature of colic is necessary.

Meckel's Diverticulum

Meckel's diverticulum, the most common congenital abnormality of the small intestine, is caused by incomplete obliteration of the embryonic structure called the vitelline duct. Meckel's diverticulum is present in approximately 2% of persons. Out of that number, approximately 40% are asymptomatic and the diverticulum is discovered incidentally when investigating another disorder. It is usually discovered in toddlers younger than 2 years old, and is more common in males than females.

Etiology
The vitelline duct, which transports nutrition from the yolk sac to the embryo, should undergo atrophy by 7 weeks' gestation. When the duct fails to fully atrophy, the remaining tissue is known as Meckel's diverticulum—a small outpouching of the intestinal wall (see Fig. 45-12).

Pathophysiology
Meckel's diverticulum is most commonly composed of all the same layers of tissue as the ileum. This blind

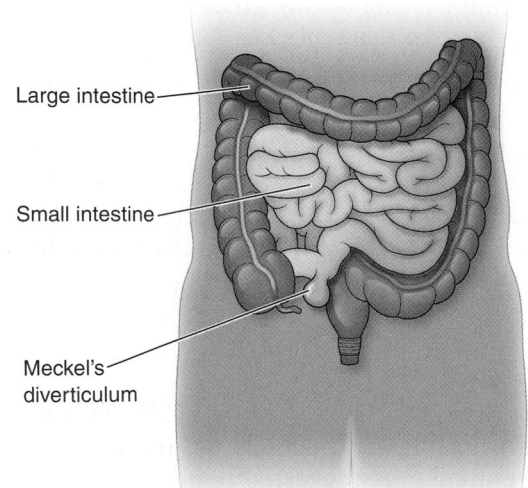

FIGURE 45-12. Meckel's diverticulum. A Meckel's diverticulum is a weakness in the wall of the small intestine that forms a pouch. It is a remnant of the omphalomesenteric ducts, also called the vitelline duct.

pouch, which is usually 40 to 60 cm proximal to the ileocecal valve, is usually 3 cm long and 2 cm wide. The diverticulum can be lined by ileal or gastric mucosa. Gastric mucosa can develop ulceration or perforation, which can cause bleeding. The diverticulum can also become filled with intestinal contents and become obstructed.

Clinical Presentation
Usually asymptomatic, Meckel's diverticulum is often not discovered until adulthood. The classic presentation is painless hematochezia (rectal bleeding) in a toddler younger than 2 years. The clinical presentation includes abdominal pain in the periumbilical area that radiates to the right lower quadrant, which is sometimes mistaken for appendicitis. Possible complications of Meckel's diverticulum include bowel obstruction (35%), hemorrhage (32%), diverticulitis (22%), umbilical fistula (10%), and other umbilical lesions (1%).

Diagnosis and Treatment
A Meckel's scan, a nuclear study called a technetium scintiscan, can reveal the diagnosis. Radioactive isotope will be taken up by the mucosa of the diverticulum and highlighted via a specialized camera. Sometimes a mesenteric arteriogram is needed to highlight the vascularity associated with diverticulum. CT scan, ultrasound, magnetic resonance enterography, and capsule endoscopy have also been used to visualize the diverticulum. Laparoscopic surgery is the most common treatment. Antibiotics are also administered.

Necrotizing Enterocolitis

Necrotizing enterocolitis (NEC) is an acute, inflammatory disease characterized by intestinal tract injury ranging from mucosal ischemia to full wall necrosis and perforation. It develops in 25% of all premature and low birth weight infants and can develop any time from birth until 6 weeks of age. Incidence of the disease is 0.3 to 2.4 cases per 1,000 births. Studies show that up to 50% of infants weighing fewer than 1,000 grams develop NEC.

Etiology
The etiology is unknown but is thought to be multifactorial; a combination of the immaturity of the premature infant's intestine, specific maternal prenatal health disorders, and possibly microbial infection. Gram-positive and gram-negative bacteria, fungi, and viruses have all been isolated from affected infants; however, many infants have negative culture findings. Associated prenatal risk factors, in addition to prematurity, include maternal age above 35 years, maternal infection, premature rupture of the membranes, and maternal cocaine use. Neonatal risk factors are low Apgar scores at 5 minutes of age, comorbidities from congenital heart defects, use of the umbilical cord for IV access, and blood transfusions. Both breast- and bottle-fed neonates are susceptible.

Pathophysiology

Although the etiologic agent that triggers NEC is unknown, the disease's pathogenesis involves severe inflammation of the intestine. It is unclear if bacteria are the trigger for NEC; however, the following have been found in blood cultures of newborns with NEC: *E. coli*, *Klebsiella pneumoniae*, *Proteus mirabilis*, *Staphylococcus aureus*, *Clostridium perfringens*, *Enterococcus*, and *Pseudomonas*.

An infectious etiology is theorized because of epidemic-like occurrences in nurseries. The damaged portion of the intestinal wall is nonfunctional, leading to obstruction. The abdomen becomes distended from the buildup of gas, and bacterial toxins create further damage to the intestine. In the most severe cases, the intestine may perforate and release its contents into the peritoneum, resulting in sepsis.

Clinical Presentation

Infants with NEC present with early symptoms of feeding distress, occult blood in the stool, and abdominal distention. The stool becomes grossly bloody, the abdomen becomes discolored, and the child exhibits symptoms of hyperglycemia, metabolic acidosis, difficulty maintaining body temperature, and impaired oxygenation.

Diagnosis

The stools of any neonate at risk for NEC are tested for occult blood. Changes in blood counts and acid-base balance are indicators of changes in the neonate. Abdominal x-rays are done to determine if the bowel is dilated from gas or if there is free air in the abdomen. Blood cultures are done as another measure to determine the risk for sepsis as a complication. Once NEC is suspected, abdominal x-rays are done frequently to monitor possible perforation of the intestinal wall exhibited by the escape of free air into the abdomen.

Treatment

Treatment begins with immediate discontinuation of any feedings. A nasogastric tube is used to decompress the stomach and intestine. IV therapy maintains fluid and electrolyte balance. If there is no free air seen in the abdomen, treatment includes a 2-week rest of the bowel and administration of antibiotics. Bowel rest requires that no food or fluids are introduced to the GI system; therefore, the infant is restricted from any oral intake. If free air is seen on x-ray, surgery is performed to remove the diseased portion of the intestine that is allowing gas to escape into the abdomen. A partial colectomy with colostomy may be necessary until the intestine is healed.

Pyloric Stenosis

Pyloric stenosis, an obstruction of the gastric outlet, presents in the first 2 to 3 months of life. Most children are diagnosed within 2 to 4 weeks of life, as the infant increases feeding volume and the stomach contents cannot empty into the small intestine. Baby boys are at higher risk for developing pyloric stenosis, and a family history is also associated with increased risk. The incidence is 1 in 500 live births.

Etiology

In pyloric stenosis there is a contracted pyloric sphincter of the stomach that prevents fluid and food from passing into the duodenum. Both environmental and hereditary factors are involved in the development of the condition. Studies have found that the neurons in the pyloric sphincter muscle lack an important enzyme, called nitric oxide synthase, that relaxes muscle. In addition to neurological problems in the GI tract, infants are found to have high gastrin levels, which stimulates acid production in the stomach. It is proposed that the high acidity triggers pyloric muscle contraction. Some studies link use of macrolide antibiotics, such as Erythromycin, to pyloric stenosis in the infant.

Pathophysiology

In pyloric stenosis there is a hypertrophic pyloric sphincter muscle at the opening of the stomach to the duodenum. For unknown reasons, there are abnormalities found in the neurons that supply the muscle.

Clinical Presentation

The main symptom of pyloric stenosis is projectile vomiting shortly after feeding. The emesis will be curdled feeding, with no blood or bile seen. A small olive-sized mass can be palpated in the epigastric area.

Diagnosis

Diagnosis is based on history and physical exam, and is confirmed by ultrasound. Upper GI series or feeding studies are usually not done if the ultrasound confirms the diagnosis, as these studies themselves will cause more vomiting.

Treatment

Treatment for pyloric stenosis involves surgical opening of the constricted muscle at the pyloric outlet. The success rate is almost 100%. While waiting for surgery, the infant may be fed by a nasogastric tube that is advanced beyond the pylorus. Optimum fluid and electrolyte balance must be established before surgery. If treatment is delayed, the infant will develop dehydration and failure to thrive.

Gastroesophageal Reflux Disorder

Gastroesophageal reflux disorder (GERD) is the regurgitation of stomach contents and peptic acids into the esophagus, which is caused by the failure of the esophageal sphincter to close completely after a feeding. A small degree of GERD exists in all infants and it improves in most infants once they start eating solids foods at approximately 6 months. It is difficult to estimate how many infants are affected by the disorder, because many caregivers do not recognize the difference between true GERD and spitting up. Approximately 85% of newborns exhibit some GERD in the early 1 to 3 months; by 6 months, 60% of infants still exhibit GERD, but by 8 to 10 months the problem is resolved in 90% of infants.

Etiology

Anatomically, the angle between the esophagus and stomach is wide in infants, which causes easy reflux during feedings. In the majority of infants, growth within the first month or so narrows the angle between the lower esophagus and stomach, which resolves reflux. In a small number of infants, GERD may be present because of pathological conditions. In premature infants, GERD is common because of small gastric capacity, decreased lower esophageal sphincter tone, and decreased peristalsis.

Pathophysiology

As the stomach contracts to begin digestion, it is normal for a small amount of gastric content to reflux up into the esophagus in the young infant. If an infant is lying supine, for instance, reflux occurs because of the shallow angle between the stomach and esophagus. Also, it is normal for an infant to have transient episodes of lower esophageal sphincter relaxation. However, some disorders can include reflux as a symptom. These disorders include pyloric stenosis, Hirschsprung disease, and neurodevelopmental disorders such as cerebral palsy. Regardless of the cause, if a child has failure to thrive, poor weight gain, gags on feedings, becomes cyanotic during feedings, or seems to be averse to being fed, the infant may have GERD that should be treated.

Diagnosis

Mild GERD is diagnosed by history. Lab studies to determine GERD include pH probes in the esophagus and an upper GI series such as a barium swallow. Endoscopies are rarely used to diagnose GERD in infants because it is usually not necessary to confirm the diagnosis with such an invasive procedure. Abdominal ultrasound is used to rule out more serious pathology such as a tumor. If aspiration is suspected, chest x-ray is done.

Treatment

Treatment, in most cases, relates to feeding. Smaller and more frequent feedings help to reduce the number of episodes and their severity. The infant should be maintained in a sitting position at a 45° angle for 20 minutes after each feeding. Infant car seats provide the ideal position and angle, and often work well as infant seats in the home. Thickening of feedings with rice cereal is a controversial treatment strategy. If GERD does not improve with these measures, medication to increase gastric emptying time is used. If esophagitis is present, use of a histamine-2 blocker or proton pump inhibitor may be used in the treatment. These medications reduce the production of gastric acid, minimizing

damage to the esophageal tissues. In severe cases of GERD and when the disorder is related to other comorbidities, a surgical intervention called the Nissan fundoplication is done. In this procedure, the gastric fundus is wrapped around the distal end of the esophagus to improve esophageal sphincter tone.

Hirschsprung Disease

Hirschsprung disease is a structural obstruction of the large intestine caused by lack of neurons within the colonic muscle wall. In utero, the ganglion cells of the myenteric plexus do not develop along the colon; thus, the neonate is born with a constricted distal colon. Some infants with the disorder will not pass meconium within the first 24 hours of life. However, some infants do pass meconium, appear healthy, and are discharged, only to be readmitted in a week or two with symptoms of obstruction, such as poor feeding, vomiting, and abdominal distention. Hirschsprung disease occurs in approximately 1 of every 5,000 births in the United States. Males are affected more than females by a ratio of 4 to 1. The disorder is 3 times more common in Asian Americans compared with Caucasians.

Etiology

Multiple gene mutations are involved in the etiology of Hirschsprung disease. Mutations are noted in 13q22, 21q22, and 10q. The disorder is strongly associated with Down syndrome, Waardenburg syndrome, congenital deafness, and multiple endocrine neoplasia. An infant is commonly diagnosed with Hirschsprung disease within the first year of life.

Pathophysiology

Hirschsprung disease arises in the 8th to 12th week of gestation when neurons within the colon should be developing. The colon and rectum lack the necessary neurons that are involved in peristaltic contractions. Dilation of the colon and obstruction of the colon develop because of lack of movement of bowel contents.

Diagnosis

A rectal exam of the infant with no feces present despite the initiation of feeding is suggestive of the disease. Normal barium enemas do not rule out the disease, but may be done to rule out other diagnoses. Abdominal x-ray will show the presence of stool above the obstruction and no air or gas in the rectum. Rectal biopsy determines whether there are ganglion cells and nerves in the rectum.

Treatment

Treatment is surgical intervention in two stages: First, a colostomy is done above the level of the diseased bowel, enabling the healthy bowel containing ganglion cells and nerves to empty and allowing the infant to resume feeding. Once the infant is 12 months old, a second surgery is performed to remove the bowel segment that is missing ganglion cells as well as to reconstruct a functional bowel and rectum. Most surgeries are successful in establishing normal bowel functioning. In some cases, the colostomy may need to remain in place throughout the child's life.

Intussusception

Intussusception is the telescoping of one part of the intestine into another, resulting in bowel edema, tissue ischemia, necrosis, and possible bowel perforation (see Fig. 45-13). Incidence of the disease is 1.5 to 4 out of every 1,000 births. The disease most commonly occurs in infants 9 months to 24 months with a male to female ratio of 3 to 1.

Etiology
The etiology of intussusception is unclear, but it is theorized that lymphoid tissue within the intestine becomes inflamed and edematous because of adenovirus or rotavirus infection. Other conditions associated with intussusception are Meckel's diverticulum, viral infections, lymphoma, polyps, and foreign body ingestion.

Pathophysiology
In intussusception, a segment of intestine shifts into a more distal segment of intestine; it is commonly described as an invagination of one part of the intestine into another. The most common area for intussusception is at the junction of the ileum and colon. This region becomes inflamed and edematous, and arterial obstruction can cause ischemia and necrosis of the bowel segment. Intussusception causes intestinal obstruction when intestinal contents cannot move forward in the affected region. Obstruction of bowel can result in intestinal perforation, peritonitis, and widespread sepsis.

Clinical Presentation
Children with intussusception present with lethargy, irritability, vomiting, and pain. The symptoms are transient. The child feels better at times, only to feel sick again. Rectal bleeding is seen in 80% of the cases, and the discharge that is characteristic of intussusception is called currant jelly stools, as they are a mixture of blood and mucus. A painful mass can be palpated in most patients, but muscle rigidity of the abdomen may make the mass difficult to detect. Bowel sounds may be normal.

 CLINICAL CONCEPT

In Meckel's diverticulum and intussusception a child often passes maroon, tarry, gel-like stool referred to as "currant jelly" stool.

Diagnosis
The diagnosis of intussusception is made based on symptomatology. Abdominal x-ray indicates an obstruction and no evidence of gas in the lower right quadrant. Barium enemas determine if the bowel has a coiled spring appearance and may also be used for intervention. The flow of barium as it is introduced in the rectum is often enough to release the intussusception and resolve the obstruction.

Air enema may also be used to diagnose the disorder. Air is introduced into the rectum and lower bowel via a catheter. The air becomes blocked at the region of intussusception. Abdominal x-ray can then be used to look for the obstructed pattern of air in the bowel.

Ultrasound and CT scan of the abdomen may also be used for diagnosis. Open abdominal surgery or laparotomy technique is used to release the intussusception. However, if signs of bowel perforation are present, the only accepted intervention is open surgical repair of the perforated bowel segment. The surgeon can manually untangle the telescoping section of the bowel and irrigate the abdominal cavity.

Central Nervous Disorders of Childhood

Epilepsy, brain tumors, cerebral palsy (CP), and attention deficit hyperactivity disorder (ADHD) are common central nervous system disorders in children. For information on epilepsy, see Chapter 34: Chronic and Degenerative Neurological Disorders and for brain tumor see Chapter 40: Cancer.

Cerebral Palsy

Cerebral palsy (CP) is a chronic disorder of muscle tone and coordination that begins in infancy to early childhood, many times without obvious causes. The incidence of CP is 2 to 2.5 children per 1,000 live births per year in the United States. In underdeveloped

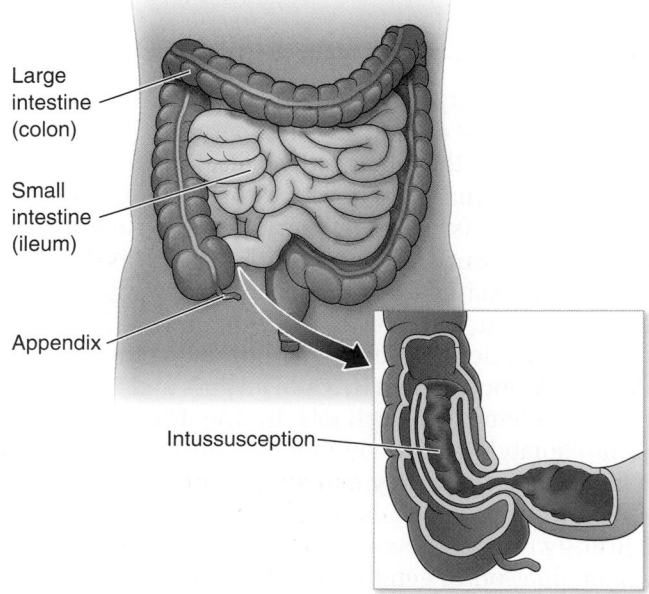

FIGURE 45-13. Intussusception of the intestine. Intussusception is a condition where a portion of the intestine collapses into another portion. This fold causes a painful obstruction.

Large intestine (colon)

Small intestine (ileum)

Appendix

Intussusception

countries, incidence is as high as 6 children per 1,000 live births per year.

Etiology

The prevailing theory of causation of CP is trauma at birth or episodes of fetal hypoxia that cause immature brain development. The exact etiologic cause of hypoxia can occur at any time between the prenatal period through age 3. The following are considered etiologic agents of CP: fetal or neonatal vascular insufficiency, infection, toxins, and pathological disorders related to premature birth. There are numerous risk factors for development of CP in the infant (see Box 45-2), though in many infants, CP has no one exact etiology and is assumed to be caused by a combination of factors.

Pathophysiology

Neurological development begins at approximately 3 to 4 weeks gestation and continues throughout the pregnancy. Postnatally, myelination of neurons continues into the second year of childhood. The many physiologic stresses of premature infants can cause vascular insufficiency of the brain. Intracerebral hemorrhage is also a common occurrence in premature infants, which can result in CP. Insults that cause vascular insufficiency of the newborn's brain most frequently occur in the region of the middle cerebral artery. This arterial circulation affects the sensorimotor

---

> ## BOX 45-2. Risk Factors for Cerebral Palsy
>
> **FETAL AND NEONATAL FACTORS**
> - birth asphyxia of fetus
> - congenital abnormalities
> - low Apgar score at 5 minutes postnatally
> - multiple gestation pregnancy
> - postmature birth
> - premature birth
> - prenatal stroke in the fetus
>
> **MATERNAL FACTORS**
> - bleeding in the third trimester
> - hypertension and proteinuria
> - intrauterine infection
> - iodine deficiency
> - mental retardation
> - mercury poisoning
> - polyhydramnios
> - previous birth of child with mental retardation or sensory or motor dysfunction
> - previous loss of a newborn
> - seizure disorder
> - thyroid abnormalities
> - treatment with thyroid supplement, estrogen, or progesterone

---

cortex and often involves speech. In CP, children often present with problems in motor function of the extremities and speech. Cognitive functioning is not necessarily impaired; children with CP may be of high intelligence but may be unable to communicate appropriately, leading some to assume they are intellectually impaired. Speech can be a problem, as children may not be able to coordinate the movements in order to produce recognizable sounds.

Clinical Presentation

Cerebral palsy is not a progressive condition and it is not usually diagnosed until after the age of 1 year. The first symptom is usually the appearance of hypotonia (lack of muscle tone) in a newborn. The hallmark symptoms are developmental delays: failure to meet milestones such as head control, rolling over, sitting up, and crawling. Seizures and hydrocephalus are also common. Spasticity of the extremities is commonly apparent as the child approaches his or her first birthday.

Diagnosis

Diagnosis is made based on the presenting symptoms. Usually, an interdisciplinary team approach is used to determine the diagnosis, as all activities of daily living and functioning need to be assessed.

Treatment

Treatment also needs to be interdisciplinary, as children with CP have many problems related to quality of life and independent functioning. The team should consist of the family, nurse, developmental pediatrician, physical therapist, occupational therapist, speech-language therapist, nutritionist, school officials, and social services. Children with suspected CP and developmental delays should be referred for infant stimulation and early intervention programs in their communities.

Attention Deficit Hyperactivity Disorder

Attention deficit hyperactivity disorder (ADHD) is a syndrome of inattention, hyperactivity, and impulsiveness. It is thought to be a biochemical malfunction in the brain and may coexist with other behavioral syndromes, such as lower IQ, pervasive developmental disorder, and autism. Coexisting learning disabilities such as dyslexia, auditory processing deficit, visual processing deficit, and sensory integration dysfunction make the clinical picture of ADHD more complex. The disorder is documented in 5% of all girls and 10% of all boys in elementary schools in the United States. Approximately 70% of children diagnosed with ADHD will continue to have symptoms in adulthood.

Etiology

A combination of genetic susceptibility and environmental influences most likely causes ADHD, as family, adoption, and twin studies show a high hereditary component in ADHD. Also, ADHD has been associated with poor child care during infancy, prenatal alcohol consumption by the mother, and exposure to lead or other heavy metals.

Pathophysiology

Numerous studies of the brain structure and neurotransmitters in ADHD have been done and continue to reveal more about the disorder. The brain's frontal lobes control functions that require judgment and inhibition of impulses. Studies of the brain in persons with ADHD show decreased activation of the frontal lobes during tasks that require inhibition of impulses. A 10-year study by the National Institute of Mental Health showed that the brains of children with ADHD are 3% to 5% smaller than those who do not have ADHD. Also, the more severe the ADHD, the smaller the frontal lobes. Another study has shown that there is thinning of the cortex in the brain in children with ADHD.

Clinical Presentation

The symptoms of ADHD are behaviors that are seen in two or more settings, such as school and home, which were present before the age of 7 years. The behaviors may include inattentiveness to a task, forgetfulness, disorganization, feelings of restlessness, having difficulty participating in a quiet activity such as reading, and interrupting others. The child cannot control the need to fidget or talk excessively, and may have difficulty paying attention. Academic performance as well as social relationships may be affected because of the child's behavior.

Diagnosis

Diagnosis of ADHD is based on observation, parent and teacher report, and several available rating scales. A comprehensive physical exam should be part of the diagnostic workup so that vision, hearing, and neurological causes of the behaviors can be ruled out.

Treatment

ADHD treatment is best given in an interdisciplinary approach between the health-care team, family, and school. Psychostimulant medication such as methylphenidate (Ritalin) and mixed amphetamine salts (Adderall) have been used by many children with great success. However, these medications are controlled substances and have side effects such as insomnia and anorexia. Because of this, there has been a great deal of debate on the appropriateness of medications for the treatment of ADHD, and some professionals believe that they are overprescribed in the United States.

Family and school staff should observe and evaluate children who are given a trial on medication for several months to determine the medication's effectiveness. Dosing is individualized and titrated according to

behavior changes. Many families see a beneficial effect from the medication, and choose to continue it. It is equally important to ask the child about the response to the medication.

Behavior modification techniques and academic support help the child to learn to cope with ADHD. The learning plan at school should be modified to include tutoring, extended time for testing, coaching with life skills, and organization. These interventions will help to prevent issues the children may have with self-concept and feelings of failure.

Pediatric Musculoskeletal Disorders

Common pediatric musculoskeletal disorders include muscular dystrophy, Osgood-Schlatter disease, Legg-Calve-Perthes disease, and scoliosis.

Muscular Dystrophy

Muscular dystrophy (MD) is a collective group of inherited, noninflammatory, progressively degenerative muscle disorders. Duchenne muscular dystrophy (DMD) is the most common form of the disorder, with a prevalence rate of 1 per 3,500 male infants. Other forms of MD include Becker MD, a milder form affecting 1 case per 30,000 male births, and facioscapulohumeral MD and limb-girdle MD, both of which are rare.

Etiology

DMD, the most common form of MD, is an X-linked recessive genetic disorder with a defect found at Xp21. Half of the number of cases of DMD are caused by a sporadic mutation; the other half are caused by a hereditary mutation. The X chromosome carries the gene for DMD, so females can carry the disease but not be affected. However, males are affected by DMD if they inherit the mutation from their mother.

Pathophysiology

There is a genetic basis underlying all types of MD: defects in the genetic code for dystrophin, a protein present in skeletal, smooth, and cardiac muscle and brain tissue. Although muscle damage in MD is not thought to be immunologically mediated, T cells attack the membranes of dystrophic muscles. The muscle cell gradually dies and macrophages invade. Over time, the dead muscle is replaced by a fibrous, fatty infiltrate, which clinically appears as pseudohypertrophy (enlargement) of the muscle. The lack of functioning muscle units causes weakness, poor muscle postures, spasms, and eventually contractures.

Clinical Presentation

MD is a disorder that presents in early childhood with progressive muscle weakness without obvious causation.

Usually, there is little indication that it is present in infancy. The child's motor milestones may be slightly delayed; children usually do not walk until 18 months or later and commonly exhibit difficulty with ambulation. A waddling, wide-based gait with hyperlordosis (concavity) of the lumbar spine and toe walking are classic signs of MD. This usually occurs between the ages of 7 and 13 years, with some patients becoming wheelchair bound by the age of 6 years. Other clinical findings in MD include Gower's sign, absent deep tendon reflexes in the upper extremities and patella, pain in the calves with activity, and pseudohypertrophy of the calves (see Fig. 45-14).

 CLINICAL CONCEPT

Gower's sign, which is caused by weakness of proximal hip muscles, is a physical examination finding in MD. The patient uses his hands and arms to "climb" up from a squatting position because of a lack of hip and thigh muscle strength.

Diagnosis
Genetic testing, muscle creatinine phosphokinase (CPK) elevation, PCR testing, electromyography, ultrasound of muscles, and muscle biopsy can be used to diagnose the disease.

Treatment
Care of the patient consists of supportive treatments to maintain independence and quality of life. Physical therapy, occupational therapy, and surgical interventions for contractures are common forms of treatment. DMD is a terminal disease; death usually occurs by the third decade of life because of respiratory failure or cardiac insufficiency.

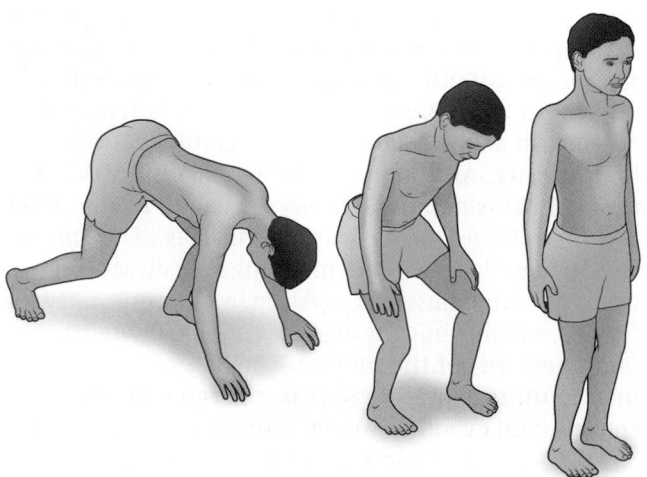

FIGURE 45-14. Gower's sign. Gower's sign describes how a patient with lower limb muscle weakness has to use his or her hands and arms to "walk" up the body to rise from a squatting position because of a lack of hip and thigh muscle strength.

Osgood-Schlatter Disease

Osgood-Schlatter disease (OSD) is a disorder caused by traction of the quadriceps muscle on the tibial tubercle. It is a very common cause of knee pain in children aged 8 to 15 years. Girls and boys are both affected, particularly athletic adolescents. The incidence of OSD can be as high as 21% among athletic adolescents, compared with 4.5% in nonathletic adolescents. Males are affected 3 times more than females.

Etiology
The etiology of OSD is unknown; however, the condition is a result of repetitive quadriceps tension on the tibial tubercle. The tibial tubercle is in an immature, cartilaginous phase of development and tension on it causes tiny breaks in the bone. Athletes who run, jump, and perform gymnastics are at highest risk. Fifty percent of patients report a precipitating traumatic event, although the disorder can arise without trauma. The disorder is bilateral in 20% to 50% of patients.

Pathophysiology
Normally, the large quadriceps thigh muscle inserts onto a bony protuberance on the head of the tibia. The area of bone at the top of the tibia, called the tibial tubercle, is in a preossification phase of development. During adolescence, the tibial tubercle bone tissue is delicate and bone cells are immature. During trauma or repetitive exercise, the patella tendon of the quadriceps muscle pulls on the tibial tubercle. With strain on the tubercle, small microfractures develop; these trigger repetitive repair of bone which, in turn, creates a protruberant tibial tubercle.

Clinical Presentation
Knee pain occurs with activities such as running, jumping, and stair climbing. Rest can relieve the pain. On physical examination, the patient has point tenderness over the tibial tubercle, and there is usually enlargement or prominence of the tibial tubercle as well. There is no knee instability and range of motion is normal. Neurovascular examination of the extremity is also normal.

Diagnosis
Usually diagnostic testing is not necessary; however, a knee x-ray may be done to exclude other disorders.

 CLINICAL CONCEPT

The clinician should always rule out a hip disorder because in hip conditions radiation of pain to the knee is common.

Treatment
Treatment includes the application of ice for 20 minutes every 2 to 4 hours if the knee is tender. Analgesics and

NSAIDs may be given for pain relief and reduction of local inflammation. A knee brace or supportive bandage also can be used. The patient needs to rest the knee for a few days. For long-term treatment, quadriceps stretching exercises may be performed to reduce tension on the tibial tubercle. Stretching exercises for the hamstrings may also be recommended because commonly they are tight. If there is severe pain or evidence of tibial fracture, surgery is necessary. There is no long-term disability associated with OSD except some tenderness at the tubercle with kneeling.

Legg-Calve-Perthes Disease

Legg-Calve-Perthes disease (LCPD) is a condition that causes necrosis of the femoral head of the hip because of inadequate blood supply. It usually occurs during a child's growth spurt between ages 4 and 10 years old. It occurs in 4 out of 100,000 children per year in the United States. For unknown reasons, males are four times more likely to exhibit this disease compared with females. Both hips are involved simultaneously in fewer than 10% of cases, but each hip joint can be involved at different times.

Etiology

The exact cause of LCPD is unknown. However, it is most common in children with delayed bone growth and short stature. Trauma, congenital dislocation of the hip, steroid use, sickle cell disease, and slipped femoral capital epiphysis are associated with LCPD. Slipped femoral capital epiphysis occurs when there is a structural malposition of the femur as it sits in the acetabulum of the hip.

Pathophysiology

The disease process occurs when the head of the femur of one leg undergoes rapid growth and outgrows its blood supply temporarily. The result is ischemia and necrosis of the head of the femur. The necrotic area exists temporarily until blood supply can be reestablished by therapeutic strategies. Bone healing and bone replacement may be so perfect that completely normal bone may result. Because of the lack of blood supply, one limb may be shorter than the other if there is no treatment. Therapeutic strategies can assist in new bone growth.

Clinical Presentation

Usually, the only symptom is a painless limp with no history of an associated injury. Hip pain may develop, however, as the result of necrosis of the involved bone; the pain may be referred to the knee or lateral thigh. If therapy is not instituted, quadriceps muscles and adjacent thigh soft tissues may atrophy, and the hip may develop adduction flexion contracture. The patient may develop an abnormal gait with limited hip motion.

Diagnosis

Radiography and bone scans are diagnostic, as they can visualize the bone defect. There are different stages of the disease exhibited on x-ray. Stage 1 shows lack of growth of the head of the femur with decreased bone density and swelling of the joint. Stage 2 reveals a collapse of the femoral head with obvious bone resorption. Stage 3 shows healing ossification of the center of the femur. In stage 4, healing is completed.

Treatment

Orthotic bracing or surgery is used to keep the head of the femur in the acetabulum. The bracing should remain during growth of the leg. As the child grows, the head of the femur will reossify and keep its round shape, thereby maintaining the hip joint's normal range of motion.

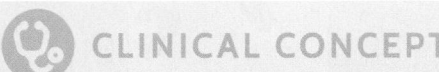

CLINICAL CONCEPT

Osgood-Schlatter and LCPD are osteochondroses, a term used to describe skeletal disorders that arise because of growth.

Scoliosis

Some degree of curvature of the spine is seen in all children, but children with scoliosis have a lateral curvature that exceeds normal variation. Studies of 16,000 children in the United Kingdom show a prevalence rate of scoliosis in 1.2% to 4.5%. Children 12 to 14 years old are most affected. Scoliosis is seen more often in females, and all school-age children should be screened annually.

Etiology

The exact cause of scoliosis is unknown. However, studies reveal there may be a muscle condition that predisposes individuals to scoliosis, as there are high levels of a skeletal muscle constituent called calmodulin in individuals with scoliosis. There is also abnormal fibrillin metabolism in the elastic connective tissues in many individuals with scoliosis. A likely genetic predisposition to the disorder also exists, as there are noted genetic mutations in chromosomes 6, 10, and 18.

Pathophysiology

In addition to the initial curve of the vertebrae in scoliosis, there is a compensatory curvature to the other side (see Fig. 45-15). The degree of curve in the vertebrae increases as the child approaches adolescence and a period of rapid linear growth.

Clinical Presentation

Most children with scoliosis complain of the back deformity but usually do not have pain. A school nurse or primary care clinician is often the first to find the deformity and refers the child to an orthopedic clinician. There are different levels of the shoulders and protruding scapula. The most common curve pattern involves a right thoracic curve with the right shoulder

Scoliosis   **Normal spine**

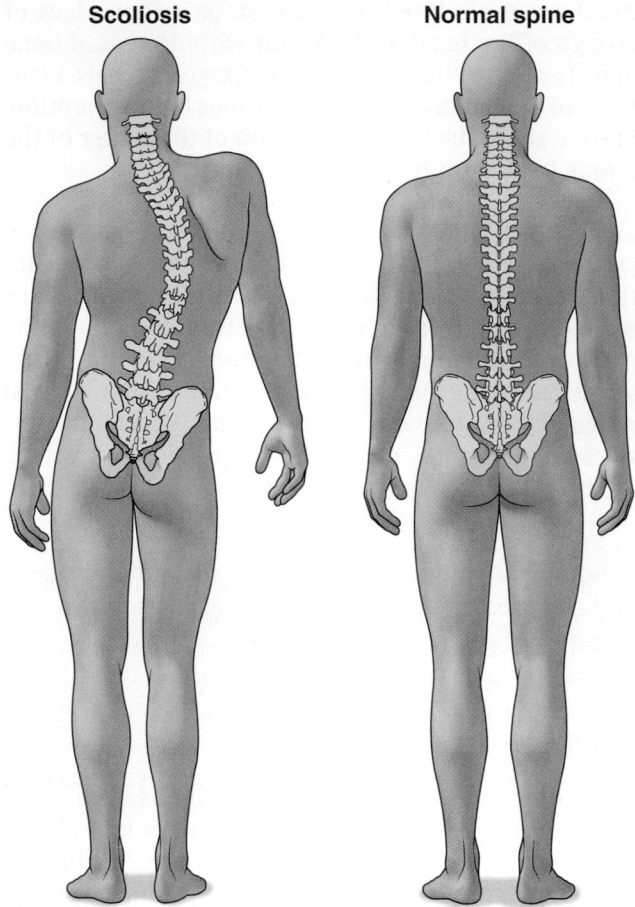

FIGURE 45-15. Scoliosis. Scoliosis is curvature of the spinal column.

Scoliosis   **Normal spine**

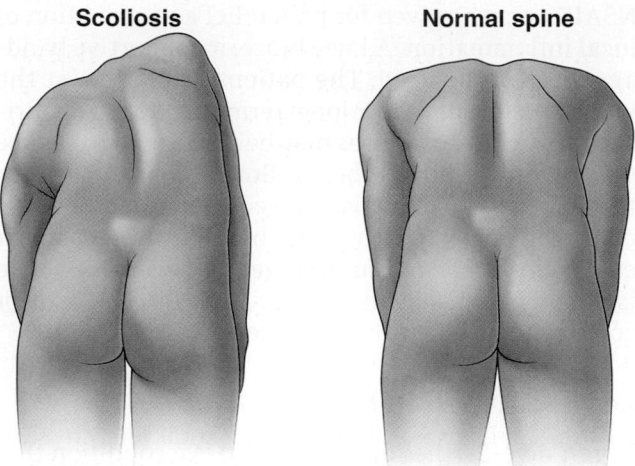

FIGURE 45-16. Forward bending test for scoliosis. To assess for scoliosis, ask the patient to bend forward. Note the asymmetry of the paravertebral musculature.

rotated forward and the medial edge of the scapula protruding posteriorly.

Diagnosis

There is no pain or difficulty with ambulation noted, and physical exam is the primary diagnostic test. The child should be examined by first looking at the scapulas and iliac crests from the back to determine symmetry and identical height. The child's back should also be viewed in the forward bending position (see Fig. 45-16). Scoliosis is measured by degrees of curvature, and any curvature greater than 11° is considered diagnostic.

 CLINICAL CONCEPT

The forward bend test is the most frequently used screening test for scoliosis. The child is asked to bend forward with arms hanging straight toward the floor. The examiner looks for spinal alignment and symmetrical height of the ribs.

Treatment

Bracing, which is indicated for curves of 25° to 45°, halts curvature progression while the child is actively growing, but bracing does not repair the curvature already

present. Curvatures of fewer than 25° do not usually merit active intervention, other than periodic monitoring. Surgical intervention is usually required for curvature greater than 45°, as the curvature typically worsens as the child grows.

Curvatures of greater than 50° can cause major shifts of the abdominal organs, as well as compromise respiratory function and cardiac output. If severe scoliosis in a girl is not corrected, problems during pregnancy and childbirth may ensue because of anatomical limitations.

Toxic Exposures of Children

Toxic exposures of children can interfere with growth and development. Maternal alcohol abuse is known to cause **fetal alcohol syndrome (FAS),** which is a combination of congenital abnormalities. Lead exposure, common in the past, is now a less frequent cause of toxicity. Reye syndrome is a disorder of early childhood involving ingestion of aspirin.

Fetal Alcohol Syndrome

FAS is a disorder that is present in the child who was exposed to excess maternal alcohol consumption while in utero. It occurs in 1 to 2 infants per 1,000 births, although the exact incidence is unknown because many pregnant women do not report use of alcohol.

Etiology

Children born with this syndrome have varying degrees of the syndrome components, depending on the mother's level of alcohol intake and the timing of the intake during the pregnancy. Greater exposure, through intake of large amounts or consuming alcohol early in pregnancy, results in more congenital anomalies as compared with infants with lower exposure. Social determinants of FAS include advanced maternal age, habits of binge drinking, and lower socioeconomic status.

Pathophysiology

FAS may occur from the effects of the blood alcohol levels or from the metabolism of the alcohol. There has been some evidence in animal studies that maternal alcohol intake blocks the transfer of essential amino acids and zinc across the placenta. Another factor to consider is the quality of the maternal diet during pregnancy. Often persons who habitually drink alcohol have a poor diet. If the woman is not consuming enough nutrients to support a healthy pregnancy, the infant may have poorer outcomes.

Clinical Presentation

Infants with FAS are born with retarded physical growth, intellectual disabilities, cardiac defects, and musculoskeletal abnormalities. They are also born smaller than normal in length, weight, and head circumference. Facial abnormalities may not be present in all children with FAS, but thin upper lips, a flat midface, low nasal bridge, a short upturned nose, and an elongated philtrum (space between nose and lips) are characteristic findings. Children with FAS have lifelong health problems with failure to thrive, poor coordination, and low cognitive skills.

Diagnosis

Diagnosis is based on physical findings and the prenatal health history of maternal alcohol intake. Many cases of FAS are undiagnosed at infancy and the diagnosis becomes clearer as the child grows and demonstrates developmental deficits. Many children diagnosed with FAS demonstrate attention deficit disorder (ADD) and other learning disabilities as their brain develops.

Treatment

Current practice guidelines recommend no alcohol intake at any point during pregnancy, and there is no treatment to reverse the effects of alcohol exposure during pregnancy. Special education and therapy may be of some benefit to help the child develop to his or her full potential.

Reye Syndrome

Reye syndrome is a hepatic disorder that follows a viral infection in children, most commonly an upper respiratory illness. It is also associated with administration of aspirin to young children. The incidence of Reye syndrome has decreased from 6 cases per 100,000 children in 1980 to 1 or 2 cases per year in 2014. This is largely because of the CDC warnings that discourage use of aspirin in children.

Etiology

Reye syndrome is a disorder that follows a viral infection such as varicella, influenza, coxsackievirus, or Epstein-Barr virus—common causes of upper respiratory infection in children. In addition to occurring after a viral infection, it is also associated with the administration of aspirin to young children.

Pathophysiology

The pathophysiology of Reye syndrome appears to involve mitochondrial dysfunction in the cells of a virus-infected host. The host has usually been exposed to mitochondrial toxins, most commonly salicylates (greater than 80% of cases). Cellular changes include fatty infiltration of hepatocytes, cerebral edema, loss of neurons in the brain, and edema and degeneration of the kidneys. All cells have swollen mitochondria that are in reduced number, along with glycogen depletion and inflammation. Hepatic mitochondrial dysfunction results in high ammonia levels in the blood, which is thought to induce cerebral edema and increased ICP.

Clinical Presentation

A child with Reye syndrome will present with lethargy and sleepiness, as well as vomiting. The child may appear to be confused and delirious. An enlarged liver may be palpated. As the syndrome progresses, the child may abruptly become comatose and have seizures. Death occurs from increased intracranial pressure, which causes brainstem dysfunction. Brainstem dysfunction causes cardiorespiratory failure.

Diagnosis

Diagnosis of Reye syndrome is based on physical assessment, a recent history of a viral illness, and ingestion of aspirin. Lab data will indicate that blood glucose levels are below normal and prothrombin time is longer than normal. Liver enzymes will be elevated, although serum bilirubin remains normal. At times, a liver biopsy is performed to confirm a diagnosis made from physical assessment and lab data.

Treatment

Children with Reye syndrome require hospitalization in an intensive care unit so that their level of consciousness can be monitored. Once a child is in a coma, the pulmonary system requires mechanical ventilation. Treatment is supportive and consists of surveillance to assess further deterioration. Maintenance of fluid and electrolyte balance and blood glucose within normal limits is paramount to the child's survival. Physical therapy during the comatose phase and in recovery can offset the hazards of immobility. Long-term monitoring of the child's development and neurological functioning is indicated at discharge.

Lead Poisoning

Lead poisoning can occur at any age, but it is seen more often in children ages 1 to 3 years because of hand-to-mouth behavior. Incidence is difficult to estimate because many children go untested for lead exposure. However, the incidence of lead toxicity has significantly diminished since the 1970s when the CDC warned about the sources and effects of lead poisoning. Out of 1.5 million children tested in 1997, 8% were found to have high blood lead levels. In 2012, 4% out of 2.5 million children tested had high blood lead levels. No safe blood level of lead is known, but the CDC considers > 5 ug/ml as elevated blood lead levels. It is estimated that 4 million homes have children living in them that are exposed to high levels of lead.

Etiology

Lead can be inhaled, ingested, or absorbed via transdermal application. There is increased risk if the child lives in housing older than 1977 because of lead-based paint. The banning of lead gasoline in the United States has reduced the incidence, but considerable environmental contamination exists from lead paint and gas residue in the soil. Exposure from the environment can arise from beauty products, toys, jewelry, batteries, lead-based plumbing, imported canned food, ceramic pottery, folk remedies, painted household surfaces, and painted metal snaps/zippers on clothing.

Lead poisoning is a significant public health problem in underdeveloped countries. In general, children with heavy environmental exposure to lead have high levels of lead in the bloodstream. Nutritional deficiencies such as iron, calcium, zinc, copper, and protein deficiencies result in greater lead absorption. Physiologic uptake rates of lead in children are higher than those in adults. Children are rapidly growing, and their systems are not fully developed, rendering them more susceptible to the effects of lead.

Pathophysiology

Once ingested, lead remains in the bloodstream and tissues for 30 to 70 days. Some is deposited in the brain and sequestered in bone for several years. Lead also interferes with hematopoiesis, causing less heme synthesis and the accumulation of toxic products. Less heme synthesis leads to diminished hemoglobin levels and decreased synthesis of red blood cells in the bone marrow. The red blood cells that form in the presence of lead toxicity appear smaller and paler than normal. Microcytic hypochromic anemia is a result of long-term lead poisoning. High levels of lead in the bloodstream can also cause brain damage.

Clinical Presentation

Children often have mild cases of lead poisoning and remain asymptomatic. However, cognitive impairment and hyperactivity have been linked to lead toxicity. Research has demonstrated that cognitive defects may occur at levels below the currently accepted blood lead level of 5 μg/dL. Studies have shown the higher the blood–lead concentration, the lower the cognitive function scores; this result was observed in math and reading scores for concentrations as low as 2.5 μg/dL.

Severe lead toxicity affects the brain; symptoms include increased intracranial pressure, vomiting, ataxia, and confusion. If not treated, the child becomes semicomatose, has seizures, and can die.

Diagnosis

A blood lead level of 5 mcg/dL or higher is considered lead poisoning. Fingerstick capillary lead level has been most commonly used for screening. Properly collected capillary samples have a 10% false positive rate. Once an elevated lead level is detected, a venous lead level is assessed for confirmation. Hair samples can also be used to measure lead level.

Treatment

The primary treatment of lead poisoning is eliminating or abating the source of exposure. Chelation with IV edetate calcium-disodium (EDTA) is often used. IM dimercaprol is given with EDTA for children with very high levels.

Chapter Summary

- Events that occur during the gestational period of the fetus affect the newborn's health. The normal pregnancy lasts 38 to 42 weeks. Pregnancy is divided into three trimesters.

- Teratogens, which include some drugs and chemicals, are substances that cause malformations of the fetus. Environmental factors and teratogens account for 10% of all birth defects.

- A congenital heart defect is a malformation in the structure of the heart or great vessels that is present at birth.

- Transesophageal fistula, an abnormal connection of the esophagus and trachea, is a common birth defect. The connection between the esophagus and trachea permits passage of oral secretions and feedings into the trachea and lungs.

- Gastroschisis is a weakness in the abdominal wall that allows the intestines to protrude into the umbilical cord opening, forming an omphalocele.

- Spina bifida refers to an opening in the lining of the spinal canal. The contents of the canal may then bulge out between the vertebrae, usually the lumbosacral region.

- Meningoceles are the protrusion of the meninges outside of the spinal cord, whereas myelomeningoceles are protrusions of both neural and meningeal tissue. These disorders can cause paraplegia and other neurological deficits.

- Hydrocephalus occurs when there is excess volume of cerebrospinal fluid that circulates around the brain and spinal cord.

- Common musculoskeletal congenital defects include talipes equinovarus, also known as clubfoot, and congenital hip dysplasia. Congenital hip dysplasia occurs when the head of the femur is not in functional alignment with the acetabulum, and the joint is unstable.
- Osteogenesis imperfecta is a group of genetic disorders characterized by fragile and brittle bones.
- Neuroblastoma is a common tumor of the sympathetic nervous system in children.
- Wilms' tumor, also referred to as nephroblastoma, is the most common abdominal tumor in children.
- TORCH infections cause congenital defects in the fetus. TORCH is an acronym for:

  Toxoplasmosis and **T**reponema pallidum (syphilis), **O**ther, **R**ubella, **C**ytomegalovirus,

  Herpes simplex and **H**uman immunodeficiency virus.
- An exanthem is a rash-producing infection. Childhood exanthems include measles, rubella, roseola, erythema infectiosum, scarlet fever, and varicella zoster infections.
- Rheumatic fever can develop 3 to 4 weeks after group A beta-hemolytic streptococci pharyngitis.
- Kawasaki disease is a systemic vasculitis exclusively seen in infants and young children. The disease is an inflammatory vasculitis that can affect the coronary arteries and cause aneurysms.
- Apnea—the cessation of respiration—is associated with prematurity, but it can also occur in full-term and otherwise healthy infants.
- Bronchiolitis is an infection of the lower respiratory tract in children, usually caused by respiratory syncytial virus.
- Bronchopulmonary dysplasia affects 50% of all premature infants whose birth weight is lower than 1,000 g. BPD is a chronic lung disease that results from long-term respiratory support, which can damage areas of the lung and cause squamous cell metaplasia and hypertrophy of the small airways.
- Cystic fibrosis is an inherited disease that causes a disorder in exocrine gland function, as well as chloride excretion in the epithelial cells of the respiratory tract, pancreas, sweat glands, salivary glands, intestines, and reproductive system.
- Croup results from a viral infection that produces inflammation in the upper airway and causes stridor and a "barking" cough. This inflammation can progress to complete obstruction. Epiglottitis, which can occur with croup, is a medical emergency.
- Colic is a common syndrome of infancy characterized by excessive, sudden bouts of crying that often occur in the evening. It occurs without any identifiable cause in an otherwise healthy infant aged 2 weeks to 4 months of age.
- Meckel's diverticulum, the most common congenital abnormality of the small intestine, is caused by incomplete obliteration of the vitelline duct.

- Necrotizing enterocolitis is an inflammatory disease of the intestine characterized by mucosal ischemia to full wall necrosis and perforation. The damaged portion of the intestinal wall is nonfunctional, leading to obstruction.
- Pyloric stenosis, an obstruction of the gastric outlet, presents in the first 2 to 3 months of life.
- Gastroesophageal reflux disorder, the regurgitation of stomach contents and peptic acids into the esophagus, is caused by the failure of the esophageal sphincter to close completely after a feeding.
- Intussusception is the "telescoping" of one part of the intestine into another, resulting in bowel edema, tissue ischemia, necrosis, and possible bowel perforation.
- Hirschsprung disease is a structural obstruction of the large intestine. In utero, the ganglion cells of the myenteric plexus do not develop along the colon, and the neonate is born with a constricted distal colon.
- Cerebral palsy is a chronic disorder of muscle tone and coordination that begins in childhood, often without obvious causes. The prevailing causation seems to be trauma at birth or episodes of fetal hypoxia.
- Attention deficit hyperactivity disorder (ADHD) is a syndrome of inattention, hyperactivity, and impulsiveness. ADHD is thought to be a biochemical malfunction in the brain.
- Duchenne muscular dystrophy (DMD) is an X-linked recessive genetic disorder with a defect found at Xp21 that causes severe muscle weakness. There is a defect in the genetic code for dystrophin, a protein present in skeletal, smooth, and cardiac muscle, as well as brain tissue. Gower's sign, which is caused by weakness of proximal hip muscles, is a physical examination finding in MD.
- Osgood-Schlatter disease (OSD) is a disorder caused by traction of the quadriceps muscle on the tibial tubercle. OSD is a very common cause of knee pain in children ages 8 to 15.
- Legg-Calve-Perthes disease is spontaneous avascular necrosis of the femoral head. The disease process occurs when the head of the femur of one leg undergoes rapid growth and outgrows its blood supply temporarily.
- Scoliosis is lateral curvature of the spine that occurs more commonly in girls than boys during growth.
- FAS is a disorder that is present in the child who was exposed to excess maternal alcohol consumption while in utero.
- Reye syndrome is a disorder that follows a viral infection such as varicella, influenza, coxsackievirus, or Epstein-Barr virus, which are common causes of upper respiratory infection in children. It is also associated with the administration of aspirin to young children.
- Lead poisoning is seen most often in children ages 1 to 3 years because of hand-to-mouth behavior. Lead can be inhaled, ingested, or absorbed via transdermal application. It can cause cognitive impairment and anemia.

Bibliography

Adzick, N. S., Thom, E. A., Spong, C. Y., et al. (2011). A randomized trial of prenatal versus postnatal repair of myelomeningocele. *N Engl J Med*, 364(11), 993–1004.

Atanda, A., Shah, S. A., & O'Brien, K. (2011). Osteochondrosis: common causes of pain in growing bones. *Am Fam Phys*, 83(3), 285–291.

Bucher, B. T., & Keller, M. S. (2010). Images in clinical medicine. Meckel's diverticulum. *N Engl J Med,* 363(21), 2045.

Bush, A., & Saglani, S. (2010). Management of severe asthma in children. *Lancet*, 376(9743), 814–825.

Busse, W. W., Lemanske, R. F. Jr., & Gern, J. E. (2010). Role of viral respiratory infections in asthma and asthma exacerbations. *Lancet,* 376(9743), 826–834.

Corbyn, Z. (2012). Promising new era dawns for cystic fibrosis treatment. *Lancet*, 379 (9825), 1475–1476.

Davis, P. B. (2011). Therapy for cystic fibrosis—the end of the beginning? *N Engl J Med,* 365(18), 1734–1735.

Dawson-Caswell, M., & Muncie, H. L., Jr. (2011). Respiratory syncytial virus infection in children. *Am Fam Phys*, 83(2), 141–146.

Del Pizzo, J. (2011). Focus on diagnosis: congenital infections (TORCH). *Ped Rev*, 32(12), 537–542.

Ege, M. J., Mayer, M., Normand, A. C., et al. (2011). Exposure to environmental microorganisms and childhood asthma. *N Engl J Med*, 364(8), 701–709.

Graham, L. (2011). AAP revises policy statement on the use of postnatal corticosteroids for bronchopulmonary dysplasia. *Am Fam Phys*, 83(12), 1501.

Grover, C. (2011). Images in clinical medicine. "Thumb sign" of epiglottitis. *N Engl J Med*, 365(5), 447.

Hall, C. B. (2010). Respiratory syncytial virus in young children. *Lancet*, 375(9725), 1500–1502.

Johnston, S. C. (2012). Patent foramen ovale closure—closing the door except for trials. *N Engl J Med,* 366(11), 1048–1050.

Kliegman, R. M., Berhrman, R. E., Jenson, H. B., & Stanton, B. E. (Eds.). (2011). *Nelson's textbook of pediatrics.* 19th ed. Philadelphia, PA: Saunders Elsevier.

Kumar, M. (2010). Childhood mortality due to respiratory syncytial virus. *Lancet*, 376(9744), 872; author reply 872–873.

Larson, H. J., Cooper, L. Z., Eskola, J., Katz, S. L., & Ratzan, S. (2011). Addressing the vaccine confidence gap. *Lancet,* 378(9790), 526–535.

Laumbach, R. J. (2010). Outdoor air pollutants and patient health. *Am Fam Phys*, 81(2), 175–180.

Lemanske, R. F., Jr., Mauger, D. T., Sorkness, C. A., et al. (2010). Step-up therapy for children with uncontrolled asthma receiving inhaled corticosteroids. *N Engl J Med*, 362(11), 975–985.

Lin, H. C., Wu, S. F., & Underwood, M. (2011). Necrotizing enterocolitis. *N Engl J Med*, 364(19), 1878–1879.

Lindell, A., Kelsberg, G., & Safranek, S. (2011). FPIN's clinical inquiries. Antibiotics for viral upper respiratory tract infections in children. *Am Fam Phys*, 83(6), 747–752.

Maris, J. M. (2010). Recent advances in neuroblastoma. *N Engl J Med,* 362(23), 2202–2211.

Melendez, E., Goldstein, A. M., Sagar, P., & Badizadegan, K. (2012). Case records of the Massachusetts General Hospital. Case 3-2012. A newborn boy with vomiting, diarrhea, and abdominal distention. *N Engl J Med*, 366(4), 361–372.

Neu, J., & Walker, W. A. (2011). Necrotizing enterocolitis. *N Engl J Med*, 364(3), 255–264.

Penny, D. J., & Vick, G. W., 3rd. (2011). Ventricular septal defect. *Lancet*, 377(9771), 1103–1112.

Poland, G. A., & Jacobson, R. M. (2011). The age-old struggle against the antivaccinationists. *N Engl J Med,* 364(2), 97–99.

Pollart, S. M., Compton, R. M., & Elward, K. S. (2011). Management of acute asthma exacerbations. *Am Fam Phys*, 84(1), 40–47.

Respiratory syncytial virus infection. (2011). *Am Fam Phys*, 83(2), 149–150.

Seehusen, D. A., & Yancey, J. R. (2011). Effectiveness of bronchodilators for bronchiolitis treatment. *Am Fam Phys*, 83(9), 1045–1047.

Servey, J. T. (2010). Addition of long-acting beta agonists for asthma in children. *Am Fam Phys,* 81(5), 598.

Sidani, M., & Murray, J. (2011). Croup: an overview. *Am Fam Phys*, 83(9), 1067–1073.

Simpson, J. L., & Greene, M. F. (2011). Fetal surgery for myelomeningocele? *N Engl J Med*, 364(11), 1076–1077.

Sosenko, I. R., & Bancalari, E. (2010). Nitric oxide for preterm infants at risk of bronchopulmonary dysplasia. *Lancet,* 376(9738), 308–310.

Tageja, N. (2010). Prognostic indicators for Ewing's sarcoma. *Lancet,* 376(9737), 232.

Tarnow-Mordi, W. O., Wilkinson, D., & Trivedi, A. (2011). Necrotizing enterocolitis. *N Engl J Med*, 364(19), 1877–1879.

von Mutius, E., & Drazen, J. M. (2010). Choosing asthma step-up care. *N Engl J Med,* 362(11), 1042–1043.

Weiss, L. N. (2008). The diagnosis of wheezing in children. *Am Fam Phys*, 77(8), 1109–1114.

Welsh, M. J. (2010). Targeting the basic defect in cystic fibrosis. *N Engl J Med,* 363(21), 2056–2057.

Zoorob, R., Sidani, M., & Murray, J. (2011). Croup: an overview. *Am Fam Phys*, 83(9), 1067–1073.

Pathophysiologic Concepts of Aging

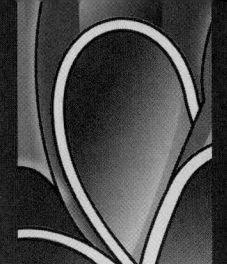

Key Terms

Apoptosis

Immunosenescence

Life expectancy (LE)

Maximum life span (MLS)

Multicausality

Physiologic reserve

Polypharmacy

Presbycusis

Presbyesophagus

Presbyopia

Reactive oxygen species

Senescence

Telomerase

Telomere

Approximately 13% of the U.S. population is older than age 65 years, and that number is climbing: In fact, the number of older adults is increasing by 2.6% every year, more than double the rate of general population growth. This pattern is expected to continue through 2020 as the "Baby Boomer" generation reaches old age. By the year 2030, the older population is projected to double from 35 million to 72 million, representing nearly 20% of the total U.S. population. Among older adults, people aged 85 years and older are the fastest growing segment of the aged population. This growth in one segment of the population is unprecedented in the United States.

Only a small number of older Americans are infirmed or disabled. Although the majority of older Americans admit having a chronic condition, only 20% report a disability. A very low number of elderly Americans live in nursing homes. Most live in a variety of community settings, with only 4.3% living in extended care facilities.

The United States is not the only country with increasing numbers of older adults. In fact, the United States ranks 43rd in the world in terms of percent of the population older than age 60 years (17.2%). Japan has the largest aged population, with 27.9% of all Japanese being older than age 60. Although the developed countries have the largest proportion of adults older than the age of 65, all countries, in every stage of development, are experiencing rapid growth in their older populations.

Older adult individuals are categorized in three different groups according to age:

- young-old: individuals aged between 65 and 74 years
- middle-old: individuals aged between 75 and 84 years
- old-old: individuals older than age 85.

Maximum Life Span Versus Life Expectancy

Study of the aging process involves the concepts of maximum life span and life expectancy. The **maximum life span (MLS)** is the maximum potential years of survival for a species. The MLS for humans has changed over the past century, and is approximately 125 years. This is to say that, barring accident, illness, or other biological catastrophe, the human body can function for about 125 years. MLS is contrasted to the concept of **life expectancy (LE),** the expected number of years an organism may live from a particular point in time. Studies of the U.S. population demonstrate that the average life span for women is 81 years; for men, it is 76 years.

Although MLS may remain constant for long periods of time, LE fluctuates based on the ability of the environment to support life. Major improvements in LE have been noted in response to public works initiatives, such as improved food and water supplies and waste disposal. The LE for Americans has nearly doubled since 1900, reflecting the aforementioned improvements in public works, as well as enhanced health-care quality and quantity. It may be helpful to think of MLS in terms of successful aging, and LE in regard to usual aging. Because of research in regenerative medicine and advancing biotechnology, our nation is gaining 1 year of longevity every 6 years.

Basic Concepts of Physiologic Aging

Many different disciplines are involved in the study of how and why we age. Although each discipline may research specific phenomena, there are some that are shared by all. When studying why we age, a comprehensive view of all the theories is necessary because aging is thought to be a complex and multifactorial process.

Senescence

Senescence refers to the cell's progressive loss of the ability to replicate over time. The changes in the human body that take place throughout adulthood are toward decrements in function, and make the human organism more vulnerable to challenges from disease, injury, or environmental factors. In gerontology and geriatrics, senescence refers to the biological, intrinsic phenomena of aging, including the characteristic patterns of change that are specific to a species and lead to a gradual loss of function of body systems. Senescent changes are universal and easily recognized within a species based on physical appearance and behavior.

Loss of Physiologic Reserve

As organisms age, the ability to repair damage and adapt to physiologic stressors decreases. This decreased ability is referred to as loss of **physiologic reserve.** In humans, physiologic reserve is correlated with an individual's functional status. Loss of physiologic reserve is part of the reason that older adults are more impacted by infectious disease than younger adults, and may have poorer outcomes from surgery and its complications. Although older adults may be able to function adequately in daily life, they are less resilient to stress compared with the younger adult. For example, a urinary tract infection (UTI) is usually a minor inconvenience that is easily resolved for a young adult. In older adults, however, UTIs can lead to urosepsis, a severe body-wide infection. Similarly, in a young adult, influenza is a disorder that resolves within a week, whereas in the older adult, it often leads to pneumonia.

Multicausality

Physiologic and pathophysiologic changes that occur with aging have many etiologies. Both internal processes and influences from the environment cause senescent cell changes; this combination of factors is referred to as **multicausality.** Biological, epidemiological, and demographic data have generated a number of theories that attempt to identify a process to explain aging. However, in recent years, the search for a single cause of aging, such as a single gene or the decline of a key body system, has been replaced by the view of aging as an extremely complex, multifactorial process. Several processes may interact simultaneously to cause aging.

Theories of Aging

Most researchers believe that different theories of aging are not mutually exclusive and may adequately describe features of the normal aging process in combination.

Programmed Aging of the Cell. The programmed aging of the cell theory asserts that cells have a

---

Box 46-1. Genetics of Healthy Aging Study (GEHA)

The 5-year GE (for GEHA) of Healthy Aging (GEHA) Project, constituted by 25 partners (24 from Europe plus the Beijing Genomics Institute from China), has identified a number of genes involved in healthy aging and longevity. It is believed that these genes allow individuals to survive to advanced old age in good cognitive and physical function and in the absence of major age-related diseases. Genes related to healthy aging were found by studying selected elderly individuals who survive over the age of 90 years. The study focused on 2,118 ninety plus-year-old Caucasian sibling pairs. The analyses demonstrated four regions that show linkage to longevity: chromosome 14q11.2, chromosome 17q12-q22, chromosome 19p13.3-p13.11, and chromosome 19q13.11-q13.32. Although these genes have been identified, it remains difficult to differentiate the effect of the shared environment and that of genetics in the sibling subjects of the study.

---

programmed schedule for aging and degeneration. According to the programmed theories, aging depends on biological clocks regulating the timetable of the life span through the stages of growth, development, maturity, and old age. This regulation would depend on genes sequentially switching on and off signals to the nervous, endocrine, and immune systems responsible for maintenance of homeostasis and for activation of defense responses. For example, the female ovary has a programmed time span of function. In most females, at age 55 years or so, the ovary undergoes **apoptosis,** a programmed degeneration of function. The question asked by many gerontologists is: Like the ovary, do all cells replicate a finite number of times before they die? Some scientists are studying the telomeres of chromosomes to answer this question (see Box 46-1).

Telomere Shortening Theory. A **telomere** is a region of repetitive nucleotide sequences at the end of a chromosome. It has been observed that with each mitotic division of a cell, the telomere regions of its chromosomes shorten. This observation has led to the question: As human telomeres shorten, do cells eventually reach their replicative limit and progress into senescence or old age? The telomere shortening theory focuses on the enzyme telomerase, which allows for replacement of telomeres, which are otherwise shortened when a cell divides via mitosis. It is known that embryonic stem cells express **telomerase,** which allows them to divide repeatedly. With the presence of telomerase, a dividing cell can replace the lost bit of deoxyribonucleic acid (DNA) at the end of the chromosome, and then divide in uninhibited fashion. Although this unbounded growth property is an exciting finding, caution is warranted regarding this property, as this exact same uninhibited growth enables cancerous growth. Currently, the question is: If telomerase is used to block chromosomal shortening, will this, in turn, prevent aging of the cell?

Damage-Based Theory of Aging. The damage-based theory of aging asserts that cellular damage occurs over time, either because of toxic by-products of metabolism or inefficient cellular repair systems. Cumulative damage to DNA occurs with age and eventually causes errors in metabolism and protein malfunction, leading to cell death. This is true for many types of cells; however, cumulative damage has also been observed in cells that have longevity. Because cumulative damage is not correlated with senescence in all cells, the theory is questionable. In the aforementioned theories, cellular changes do occur, but it is not clear if these changes *cause* aging or are a *result* of aging. As such, there are other theories regarding the etiology of aging: the free radical accumulation, immunosenescence, and calorie restriction theories.

Free Radical Accumulation Theory. Free radicals are highly reactive chemical compounds; sometimes they are referred to as **reactive oxygen species,** because they contain a free electron on an oxygen atom that endows the free radical with chemical instability and a strong affinity to bind to other molecules. Free radicals are referred to as oxidizing agents because they react with other compounds and cause damage. Free radicals target cellular structures, especially DNA, proteins, and the fatty acids in the cell membrane. For example, cigarette smoke contains free radicals that cause cell damage.

Free radicals cause cross-linkages and biochemical bonds to form between cell proteins and other molecules. The bonds make proteins less flexible, particularly those in muscle and collagen. For example, with free radical damage, muscles lose contractility, skin loses elasticity, and cartilage becomes rigid. Free radicals also injure the endothelial membranes of the arteries and create conditions that are conducive to the formation of arteriosclerotic plaque. Free radicals cause cell damage that produces some of the characteristic changes of aging. With cumulative free radical effects, cells and tissues are irreparably damaged and organs eventually are unable to function properly.

Immunosenescence. **Immunosenescence** refers to the weakening of both the innate and adaptive immune system with increasing age. Natural killer cells, part of the innate system, become more numerous with increased age, but become less functional. T lymphocytes, major participants within the adaptive system, are similarly affected, with a decreased ability to recognize and attack the antigens.

New T lymphocytes are essentially not produced in older adults, severely impairing the older adult's ability to combat previously unencountered antigens. B lymphocytes continue to be produced, but become less effective in producing antibodies to pathogens. In the population of T and B cells, there is a smaller pool of "naïve" cells that can be programmed for a specific antigen. Cytokine secretion, particularly of tumor necrosis factor, also declines in old age, with concomitant degeneration of the entire process of inflammation. There is a diminished inflammation reaction with decreased external signs and symptoms. With infection, white blood cell (WBC) numbers do not rise to the same level as in younger adults and fever is commonly absent. This is problematic because health-care providers rely on diagnostic clues such as high WBC levels and fever as signs of infection.

Other factors that diminish an individual's ability to mount a fever include poorer thermoregulation by the central nervous system (CNS), less responsiveness of the hypothalamus, decreased production of endogenous pyrogens (fever-producing substances), decreased ability to produce and conserve body heat, and less vasodilation and subcutaneous fat.

Immunizations may be less effective in the older adult because the immune system does not respond as vigorously as a younger adult to a newly introduced vaccine. Antibody levels do not rise as robustly as in the younger person. This may be particularly true with immunization for influenza, when unique strains of the virus are present each season.

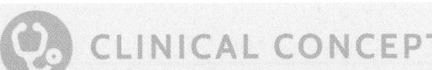

CLINICAL CONCEPT

Signs of infection are blunted in the older adult; there is less rise in WBCs, reduced ability to mount a fever, and less sensation of pain. Behavioral changes, such as confusion and disorientation, may be the only symptoms expressed during infection.

ALERT! Recommended immunizations for the older adult include yearly flu vaccine, one time pneumovax after age 65 years, and varicella zoster (shingles) vaccine.

Life-Prolonging Calorie-Restricted Diets. It has been recognized for quite some time that limiting daily calories to as few as 60% of normal extends the life span of mice up to 40%. In lab experiments, calorie-restricted (CR) older adult mice are similar to young mice physiologicly in many ways. The CR mice maintain youthful appearances and activity levels longer than non-CR mice and show delays in age-related diseases. The learning ability of CR older aged mice is more like that of younger adult mice. Reduction in calories in mice is associated with reduced free radical activity, less biological waste accumulation, and fewer numbers of damaged mitochondria.

Detractors of the CR diets assert that the quality of the diets consumed by the low-body mass index individuals are difficult to assess, and may lack nutrients important to longevity. Calorie restriction in mice has been reported to hinder their ability to fight infection. Also, CR diets cannot support the caloric demands of exercise in athletics. CR diets increase morbidity and mortality in children and adolescents and should not be emulated by the young. Even though there has been research on CR for more than 70 years, the mechanism by which CR works is still not well understood. Currently, CR diets are being studied in monkeys. An ongoing study on rhesus macaques, funded by the National Institute on Aging, was started in 1989. Results to date have also found a trend toward a reduced overall death rate; however, results are not of statistical significance (see Box 46-2).

Functional Consequences of Physiologic Aging

All systems of the human body are affected by aging. The nature and extent of the changes vary from system to system, as well as from person to person. Lifestyle and environment play a large part in the human aging process.

Box 46-2. Calorie Restriction and Aging

A small research study investigated the effects of a calorie-restricted diet with 10% to 25% lower calorie intake than the average "Western" diet. There was a calorie-restricted (CR) group of subjects and a control group of subjects on a typical Western diet. The age range of the control and CR group was 35 to 82. Mean body mass index (BMI) was 19.6 in the CR group; the matched control group BMI was 25.9, comparable to the BMI for middle-aged people in the United States. Adjusting for age, the average total cholesterol and low-density lipoprotein (bad) cholesterol levels in the CR group were below those seen in the majority of control subjects. The average high-density lipoprotein (good) cholesterol levels were in the 85th to 90th percentile range for normal middle-aged American men. The CR group also fared much better than the control group in terms of average blood pressure (100/60 vs. 130/80 mm Hg), fasting glucose, fasting insulin (65% reduction), BMI, body fat percentage, and C-reactive protein. The CR group had triglyceride levels as low as the lowest 5% of Americans in their twenties. Systolic and diastolic blood pressure levels in the CR group were about 100/60, a level more typical of 10-year-olds. Fasting plasma insulin concentration was 65% lower. Fasting plasma glucose concentration was also lower.

Cardiovascular System

Changes in the cardiovascular system may represent the most widely varied manifestations of aging and pathology found in humans. In addition, cardiopathology represents the single largest cause of death in the United States, as well as a major source of morbidity, and advanced age is the greatest risk to cardiovascular health. One out of 4 adults dies from heart disease each year in the United States; one-half of these deaths are in persons older than age 65 years.

Atherosclerosis, the development of cholesterol-laden plaques within the endothelial lining of arteries and increased connective tissue in the walls of the vessels, is common in young and older adults. Although atherosclerosis is considered to be a disease, because of the universal presence in humans and animals, it may be more correct to attribute it to aging.

The elastic blood vessels—particularly the aorta, carotid, subclavian, and renal arteries—become stiffer with age. Free radical damage of cell membranes causes protein cross-linking that diminishes elasticity and decreases the ability of arteries to vasodilate. The heart itself also undergoes changes with age; mainly, increased amounts of fibrous and calcified tissues infiltrate muscle and conductive tissue. The heart of an older adult is less compliant and has some degree of diastolic dysfunction because the chambers cannot expand as widely as in youth. On the other hand, systolic function—contraction of the left ventricle of the heart—is preserved, although systolic blood pressure increases with advanced age. There is connective tissue infiltration of the conductive tissues in the heart, notably in the sinoatrial and atrioventricular nodes, as well as in the bundle of His. This change in conductive tissue increases the risk of arrhythmias. Changes in the conductive tissue causes increased refractory periods for the heart muscle and decreased responsiveness to sympathetic nervous system stimulation. These factors lead to markedly smaller increases in heart rate in the face of stress or exercise. Maximum achievable heart rate decreases linearly with age, and may be calculated with the formula 220 − age = maximal heart rate (beats per minute). Baroreceptors in the arterial walls, which sense changes in blood pressure, are slower to respond. There is less ability to raise blood pressure with position changes, causing increased susceptibility to orthostatic hypotension. The heart's reaction to sympathetic nervous system stimulation is blunted, and the increase in heart rate in response to lower blood pressure is limited.

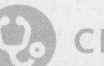 CLINICAL CONCEPT

It is important to observe for the signs of orthostatic hypotension when changing the position of an older adult from lying to sitting or sitting to standing. The older patient requires a few minutes to adjust to the new position before attempting to walk.

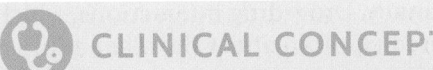

ALERT! Antihypertensive medications can increase susceptibility to orthostatic hypotension.

ALERT! Orthostatic hypotension is a common cause of falls in the older adult.

Respiratory System

The main function of the respiratory system is to provide the cells with adequate oxygenation. The aerobic capacity for older adults decreases about 10% per decade, with peak performance in the early to mid-twenties. Men have a slightly greater loss of capacity than women. The changes are related to normal aging, and are not indicative of damage from smoking or poor fitness levels. Older adults do not respond as briskly to hypoxia or hypercapnia as younger adults. The usual response of increased respiratory rate, depth, and inspiratory pressure to changing partial pressures of oxygen or carbon dioxide are blunted, although the mechanism is poorly understood. Older adults with serious respiratory conditions, such as pneumonia, may not exhibit the "early warning signs" of tachypnea and dyspnea, thus delaying diagnosis. Older individuals cannot mount the same maximum heart rate in reaction to hypoxia. Furthermore, aging is accompanied by earlier transition from aerobic to anaerobic metabolism in the body cells, further decreasing respiratory adaptation to exercise.

The elasticity of the thoracic rib cage and lung tissue decreases with age, which causes the resistance to expansion of the chest to increase. In addition, strength of the respiratory muscles decreases, which creates less vital capacity and tidal volume. Residual volume in the lungs, however, increases by as much as 50% from young adulthood. The alveoli lose surface area, and less oxygen is diffused into the pulmonary capillaries. The diameter of the bronchioles and smaller airways also decrease with advancing age. These changes may be caused, in part, by exposure to atmospheric air, with its many damaging pollutants and free radicals. Remember that aging is related to accumulation of free radical damage from the environment and the lungs are in constant contact with the inspired air.

The rib cage and vertebrae undergo changes with age that affect respiratory function. Specifically, the costal cartilage becomes calcified, thereby increasing the stiffness of the chest wall. Kyphosis, related to both osteopenia in the vertebrae and collapse of the intervertebral discs, leads to an increased anteroposterior diameter, or barrel chest. The diaphragm becomes less important in ventilation, and the abdominal muscles take on a greater role, resulting in an increased effort in both inspiration and expiration. Accordingly, pulmonary function tests are adjusted based on age.

CLINICAL CONCEPT

The cough reflex in the older adult is weaker than in the younger adult, which increases stasis of secretions in the lungs. Stasis of secretions increases susceptibility to pneumonia.

Renal System

The renal function in an 85-year-old person is only about 50% of that of a 30-year-old person, which is attributed to loss of nephrons and decreased activity of the nephron tubules. Blood flow to the kidney decreases as a result of atrophy of the arterial blood vessels, particularly in the renal cortex. In addition, the proximal tubules of nephrons decrease in number and length. Although these changes start around the age of 40 years, they do not become significant until an individual reaches old age. At that time, there will be noticeable decreases in the ability to respond to a fluid overload and to concentrate urine. The older adult will usually demonstrate a lower creatinine clearance than a young adult, indicating less filtration ability of the kidney. The older person will typically excrete lower levels of glucose, acid, and potassium, and the specific gravity of the urine will be lower. The response of the nephrons to antidiuretic hormone is less than in younger adults, and so the ability to concentrate urine is diminished. The kidney in the older adult will not respond to atrial natriuretic peptide as briskly as in the younger adult. This causes less excretion of water from the bloodstream as well. In addition, excretion of hydrogen ions to maintain acid-base balance will not occur as rapidly as the individual ages. The serum creatinine level and the blood urea nitrogen rises in healthy older adults, with a concomitant decrease in glomerular filtration rate (GFR). The older kidney, in contrast to the kidneys in younger adults, excretes more fluid and electrolytes at night than in the daytime. More urine is formed at night, potentially interrupting sleep patterns.

ALERT! Serum creatinine should be checked before administering medications that are excreted by the kidney. Less filtration ability of the kidneys increases susceptibility to medication toxicity.

The ability to respond to a fluid overload by increasing urine production is also decreased in the older adult. One of the consequences of these changes is impairment in the excretion of drugs and their metabolites, making older adults extremely susceptible to drug toxicity and other adverse medication effects, even within a normal dose range. Often, older adults are on five or more medications, a phenomenon called

polypharmacy. Drug-drug interactions, which are difficult to predict, often affect the older adult.

Another consequence is an increased probability of hyperkalemia, particularly when certain cardiac or analgesic drugs are used. The changed ability to concentrate urine makes the older adult more susceptible to dehydration, a problem that is further complicated by a diminished thirst response; therefore, the older adult will not feel thirsty even when significantly dehydrated.

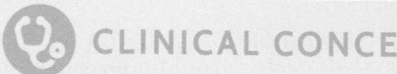 **CLINICAL CONCEPT**

Dosages of prescribed medication should start low and be increased slowly in the older adult.

Gastrointestinal System

Changes in the digestive system in older adults may have major influences on their quality of life. Motility of the gastrointestinal (GI) tract slows and becomes less coordinated with increasing age, as the nerves that supply the system change in function. The autonomic nerves in the entire GI tract decline, beginning in middle age, and continuing on throughout old age. The denervation is most severe in the distal portion of the tract. The lack of neural strength in the wall of the large bowel and rectum causes decreased peristalsis and constipation.

There is diminished function of the taste and olfactory senses which, in turn, changes release of saliva and other digestive enzymes. Also, most older adults experience loosening of the teeth (because of osteopenia in the mandible and maxilla), loss of dentin, gingival recession, and narrowing of the root canal. The muscles involved in swallowing become weaker with age and may not work in concert, increasing susceptibility to dysphagia. The lack of synchronization may be related to loss of cholinergic neurons in the esophagus. **Presbyesophagus** is the term used for age-related changes in the esophagus. In presbyesophagus, there is some loss of strength of the lower esophageal sphincter (LES). With less strength of the LES, acid refluxes up from the stomach into the esophagus. This causes esophagitis and increases susceptibility to gastroesophageal reflux disease.

The stomach lining atrophies with age and produces less hydrochloric acid (HCl) and intrinsic factor (IF). Lack of IF causes decreased absorption of vitamin B_{12}, which causes decreased red blood cell production in the bone marrow, a condition called pernicious anemia. If untreated, pernicious anemia can lead to neurological consequences. Lack of vitamin B_{12} can cause gait disturbance and paresthesias in the lower extremity. Severe vitamin B_{12} deficiency can cause dementia-like symptoms.

Diminished HCl leads to less absorption of calcium and iron. Lack of calcium increases bone breakdown, and lack of iron can cause lack of hemoglobin synthesis, which leads to decreased red blood cell production. In other words, iron deficiency leads to anemia. Although older adults produce less HCl, they are at greater risk of hyperacidity, because the gastric mucosa atrophies in aging.

The intestinal wall has decreased muscle and increased collagen and fibrous tissue, whereas the interior lining has villi that become somewhat flattened. The change in the villi makes less surface area available for transport of nutrients into the bloodstream.

The microbes that normally inhabit the intestines change in their proportion to each other, with an increase of enterobacteria in comparison to other bacteria. There is decreased immunity of the GI tract in older adults, which may be related to the change in composition of the intestinal flora. The change in flora predisposes the older adult to GI infections, particularly with *Clostridium difficile*. There is also a diminished amount of the enzyme lactase in the intestine. Lactase breaks down lactose; with lack of lactase, lactose intolerance occurs; this causes indigestion, gas accumulation, and diarrhea.

Constipation occurs because of the loss of innervation of the intestinal wall, particularly in the colon and rectum. Loss of innervation decreases the motility of the intestinal tract. In addition, the muscle layer of the intestine becomes weaker with age, predisposing individuals to the formation of weakenings in the wall called diverticula. Diverticula are tiny sacs that develop along the intestinal wall and fill with intestinal contents. The syndrome is called diverticulosis. These diverticula can become inflamed, in which case diverticulitis develops, causing pain in the left lower quadrant of the abdomen.

Two hormones related to digestion, insulin and thyroxine, also undergo changes with advancing age. The pancreatic beta cells that secrete insulin become less active as a normal part of aging, and this is coupled with the body's overall increased insulin resistance. Older adults are less physically active than their younger counterparts, and have a higher percentage of body fat; both of these factors increase insulin resistance. Older adults also secrete less insulin in response to a glucose load, which is manifested by higher postprandial (after meal) blood glucose levels. These changes predispose the older adult to glucose intolerance and diabetes.

The thyroid gland shrinks with increasing age, and the hormone thyroxine does not convert to triiodothyronine to the same extent in older adults that it does in younger adults. This makes the older adult susceptible to hypothyroidism. As a result, the basal metabolism rate is lower, and fewer calories are required to maintain body weight.

Integumentary System

The most commonly visible characteristics of aging are seen in the integumentary system. The skin is affected by environmental free radicals and sun exposure, which cause cross-linkages in proteins, leading to decreased elasticity. Replacement of epidermal cells slows dramatically with age, and the typical "thin" skin of older adults reflects this slow replacement. Skin breakdown can occur easily. Discoloration of the skin is related to decreased function of melanocytes, and the dryness of older skin is a result of fewer sebaceous glands. The decrease in subdermal fat not only exacerbates the wrinkled appearance of the skin, but removes an important layer of protection; this is involved in the older adults' inability to conserve body heat. The loss of sweat glands, hair follicles, and sensory end organs in the skin are related to difficulties in thermoregulation.

The small blood vessels in the skin become more fragile with age, so they are more likely to rupture, producing purpura and other lesions. Fewer mast cells and fibroblasts are found in the skin of older adults; the junction between the dermis and epidermis is flattened, creating a more tenuous bond between the two layers, as well as fewer nutrients being passed into the epidermis. This may explain the propensity for older adults to experience injuries to the skin.

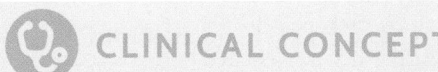

CLINICAL CONCEPT

The skin is delicate and can be sheared off easily. The loss of subdermal fat contributes to the fragility of the skin; increasing susceptibility to pressure sores.

Musculoskeletal System

Human aging is also marked by changes in muscle mass, strength, and oxygen uptake. Much of the lean muscle mass is replaced by intramuscular fat and connective tissue. For example, the area of lean muscle mass in a cross section of the human thigh decreases dramatically from age 30 years to age 80 years. Older adults who maintain higher levels of physical activity lose less muscle mass. The loss of muscle mass is accompanied by diminished strength and aerobic capacity of the remaining muscle. These losses appear related to decreased myosin heavy chain and mitochondrial proteins in skeletal muscle. Although muscle protein may be increased with aerobic exercise, once muscle mass is lost, it cannot be regenerated. So, an older adult cannot increase the amount of muscle present, but can increase the strength of the remaining muscle.

Both men and women experience age-related loss of bone, particularly in the trabecular (nonsolid) bones of the vertebrae, hip, and wrist. The bone loss becomes most apparent 10 years after menopause in women, and sometime after age 65 years in men. In women, estrogen keeps osteoblasts viable; however, after the dramatic decrease of estrogen in menopause, bone resorption outpaces bone formation. Calcium lost from bone enters the extracellular tissues, and the kidneys increase the excretion of calcium to prevent hypercalcemia. The parathyroid gland becomes more active in older age, and may be related to bone loss. It also appears that changing levels of estrogen in aging men cause bone loss. In both men and women, the loss of skeletal muscle mass is involved in bone loss, as the decreased stress placed on bone by weakened muscles leads to bone loss.

Nervous System

Older adults are frequently characterized as forgetful, senile, confused, or childish, leading one to expect major changes in the aging nervous system. Although it is true that there is a small decrease in brain weight—6% to 11%—in some healthy older adults, there is tremendous individual variation in this; furthermore, it is offset by the large numbers of neurons that compensate for each other. There are changes in the actions of neurotransmitters, as well as in the balance among them. Serotonin, norepinephrine, dopamine, b-endorphins, glutamate, and gamma-aminobutyric acid (GABA) all show decreases in either production or reception with increased age. Behaviors related to sleep pattern and mild memory loss may be related to changes in neurotransmitters. In the peripheral nervous system, loss of myelin accompanies increased age, and is likely related to the decrease in nerve conduction velocity. These changes take place at different rates, and in different areas of the nervous system.

Neurological health also involves proper nutrition and vitamin absorption. Pernicious anemia, caused by lack of gastric intrinsic factor, is common in the older adult. Gastric atrophy also causes decreased secretion of HCl in the stomach. Diminished intrinsic factor and HCl lead to decreased absorption of vitamin B_{12}. Low vitamin B_{12} levels have neurological consequences. In untreated vitamin B_{12} deficiency there is demyelination of the dorsal columns of the spinal cord, causing gait instability and paresthesias in the lower extremities. Vitamin B_{12} supplements may be necessary. Intranasal or injectable Vitamin B_{12} is required because patients cannot absorb B_{12} via the intestinal mucosa with decreased intrinsic factor and HCl.

One of the important sequelae of the changes in the nervous system is that older adults have pain thresholds that are higher than those found in younger adults. The higher threshold is consistent for many stimuli, such as mechanical and thermal injury, although there is some evidence that older adults experience greater levels of visceral pain. Higher pain thresholds may interfere with protective actions, such as pulling away from the source of pain, and may be related to poorer tissue repair. Length of the stimulus is an important variable to consider, as older adults experience a lowered pain threshold if the stimulus is present over a long period of time, such as occurs in chronic pain.

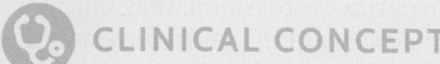

CLINICAL CONCEPT

Older adults may not be aware of an injury because they have less pain sensitivity than younger adults.

Plasticity persists in the nervous system well into old age. The decrements in neurotransmitters and neurons can be delayed, inhibited, or reversed. The current popular notion of "use it or lose it" has a physiologic basis. Studies with rats and mice have demonstrated that interesting and enriched environments can increase the levels of neurotransmitters present, as well as functional performance.

The sense organs also undergo age-related changes. The aging eye contains fewer rods and cones than are found in the younger adult's eye, with concomitant losses in color vision, visual acuity, need for increased contrast, and need for increased ambient lighting. Furthermore, the lens becomes more opaque and stiffer, causing blurring of vision, increased glare, and decreased ability to accommodate. These combined defects are known as **presbyopia,** literally meaning "old vision." Cataracts are also common among older adults.

Hearing is also affected by normal aging, with losses in the ability to detect both low and high frequency sounds. The result is that the older adult is not able to interpret some speech sounds. Deterioration of the organ of Corti, ganglia, hair cells, and basement membranes are all implicated in **presbycusis,** age-related hearing loss.

Older adults also have less ability to taste salt, sweet, bitter, and sour, and this is likely related to a time lag in the turnover of taste buds, rather than a decrease in the total number.

Thermoregulation

Thermoregulation is a function of both the autonomic nervous system and behavioral adaptation. Older adults tend to have lower basal temperatures and often do not produce fevers in response to even overwhelming infection. Fever in older adults is defined as a rise of 2°F (1.1° C) over baseline, or repeated findings of oral temperature of 99°F (37.2°C) or higher, or rectal temperature of 99.5°F (37.5°C) or higher. Even with these lowered criteria, only about 55% of older adults in nursing homes with infections ever demonstrate any fever. The reasons for this are a combination of the fewer antigen-specific antibodies that are produced by older adults, poorer thermoregulation by the CNS, less responsiveness of the hypothalamus, and a decreased production of endogenous pyrogens. Changes in the body, including less subcutaneous fat and less vasodilation, render the body less able to produce and conserve body heat. These changes also lead to lack of fever and increased likelihood of hypothermia. In addition, older adults may be less able to recognize loss of body heat and take the appropriate actions, such as adding more clothing.

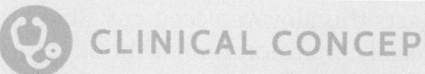

CLINICAL CONCEPT

Older adults are prone to hypo- and hyperthermia.

Common Age-Related Diseases

Older adults have increased rates of disease and disability. Most disease is not a consequence of normal aging, but rather of lifestyle choices, injury, and genetics. In addition, most older adults have more than one existing disease, greatly complicating both diagnosis and treatment of new conditions. Furthermore, the many physiologic changes of aging lead to unusual presentations of disease. Disease then often causes subtle changes in the older adult's behavior. Frequently, a change in mental status will be the first indication of a pathological process, particularly an infectious one.

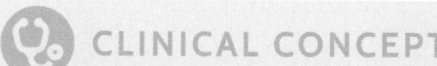

CLINICAL CONCEPT

Disease in the older adult, particularly infection, often presents with mental status or behavioral changes, such as confusion and irritability.

It is critically important to remember that treatment goals may be different for older adults. Comorbidities and frailty may dictate less aggressive goals and treatment guidelines.

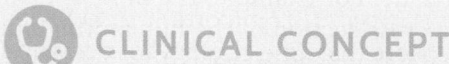

CLINICAL CONCEPT

Quality of life and functional independence, rather than cure, are the treatment goals with older adults.

Chronic Pain

Chronic pain is too often a factor in the lives of older adults; common types of pain include joint pain, neuralgias, and cancer pain. Undermedication of pain is common, as many older adults presume that pain is a part of aging, whereas health-care providers are concerned about addiction. Overall, slightly more than 3% of patients treated with opioids for chronic pain will demonstrate addiction or substance abuse, but among patients with no prior history of abuse or addiction, that number drops to 0.19%. Chronic pain has serious health consequences for older adults, including loss of functional ability, depression, and structural brain changes. The gray matter in the posterior parietal cortex and white matter in the middle cingulated region are most affected, with subsequent deficits evident in attention and mental flexibility.

Chronic Renal Failure

Chronic renal failure (CRF) is caused by irreversible damage to the kidney and is more common in older adults than in younger adults. Adults older than age 65 years are the fastest growing patient population that require dialysis; it is estimated that 60% of persons aged 65 years and older have renal impairment compared with 7% in adults ages 40 to 65 years.

Atherosclerosis and diabetes are the most common causes of CRF in older adults. Most older adults who require assisted living support because of frailty have advanced kidney disease (Stage 3 or greater), but very few have been diagnosed with renal impairment. Calculating the patient's estimated GFR is important before administering medications that are metabolized in the kidney. The definitive treatment for CRF is renal replacement therapy, either through dialysis or through renal transplant. For more information regarding CRF, see Chapter 22: Renal Disorders.

Dementias

Dementia is defined as a syndrome of loss of cognitive function and memory that is progressive and impedes the functions of daily living, although level of consciousness is not affected until late in the disease process. There are many different causes of dementia, with Alzheimer's disease (AD) being the most common etiology, followed by vascular dementia, dementia with Lewy bodies (DLB), frontotemporal dementia (FTD), and dementias related to specific diseases such as Parkinson's disease or acquired immune deficiency syndrome (AIDS). It is important to note that people can have more than one etiology for dementia, such as comorbid vascular dementia and AD. Each dementia has different early behavioral manifestations, risk factors, and disease courses.

Alzheimer's Disease

Alzheimer's disease is discussed in further detail in Chapter 36: Psychobiology of Behavioral Disorders, but a few points are important to cover in this chapter. It is absolutely critical to remember that cognitive impairment is not a part of normal aging and must be thoroughly investigated when symptoms first appear. Only 6% to 7% of older adults have dementing illnesses, although the percentage increases to nearly 38% in those aged 90 years and over. The average time from diagnosis of dementia to death from dementia is 7 to 10 years, depending upon the type of dementia.

The etiology of AD is unknown; however, the pathophysiologic processes are the subject of recent research.

Genetic mutations within chromosome 21, 14, 19, and 1 are seen in AD. The APOE 4 gene on chromosome 19 increases susceptibility to AD. Neuron degeneration, accumulation of abnormal proteins, and lack of acetylcholine occur in AD; this is particularly true in the hippocampus and medial temporal lobe, which control memory, thinking, and decision making.

Alzheimer's disease is mainly diagnosed by symptoms and clinical examination. Imaging studies such as computed tomography (CT), magnetic resonance imaging (MRI), and positron emission tomography (PET) scans are also used to diagnose AD. Treatment involves medications, such as acetylcholinesterase inhibitors, which can slow the development of AD and psychosocial support.

> **ALERT!** Cognitive changes are never normal in the older adult and must always be thoroughly assessed.

Vascular Dementia

Vascular dementia, formerly called multi-infarct dementia, is similar to stroke in that a blood vessel is damaged and the tissues beyond it receive no oxygenation. Unlike stroke, however, there are no physical deficits, and cognitive deficits may not be apparent until several infarcts have occurred. The prevalence of vascular dementia is unknown because many cases are unreported; however, it is estimated that 40% of persons with dementia have vascular dementia.

Chronic hypertension and diabetes mellitus, particularly when poorly controlled, put an older adult at higher risk for developing vascular dementia because of the level of damage caused to the microvasculature. The degree of cognitive impairment and behavioral manifestations are dependent upon the area of the brain that is affected by ischemia; because of this, symptoms are quite varied. Imaging studies such as CT, MRI, and PET scans are used to diagnose vascular dementia. Acetylcholinesterase inhibitors, antiplatelet medications, antihypertensives, and antilipidemia medications are used to manage the cognitive decline in vascular dementia.

Dementia With Lewy Bodies

Dementia with Lewy bodies (DLBs) occurs in 10% to 20% of persons with dementia. Incidence and prevalence are difficult to estimate because diagnosis is difficult. It may share etiologic factors with Parkinson's disease, in that both demonstrate abnormalities in the substantia nigra, which is part of the basal ganglia in the midbrain. Lewy bodies are abnormal protein clusters that accumulate in the synapses of the basal ganglia, and the number of them does not coincide with the severity of symptoms.

Pathophysiology. In DLB, there are inclusion bodies, called Lewy bodies, seen inside the cells of many sections of the brain, including the substantia nigra, locus ceruleus, dorsal raphe, and cranial nerve X. The primary constituent in Lewy bodies is alpha-synuclein, a protein with unknown activity. In DLB, acetylcholine is also diminished. Certain regions of the brain with DLB have been studied under single photon emission computed tomography (SPECT) to show different areas of perfusion. In DLB, hypoperfusion of the parietal and occipital regions are seen in patients who have visual hallucinations. Hyperperfusion occurs in the frontal cortex, which is thought to be related to delusional behaviors.

Clinical Presentation. A key feature of DLB, and one that differentiates it from other dementias, is fluctuation of symptoms. An older adult with DLB may be quite demented on one day, but significantly less so on the next day, although the average level of cognitive impairment is progressive. DLB causes visual hallucinations, delusions, and vivid, frightening dreams. Parkinsonian-like motor symptoms can occur where the patient suffers resting tremor, impaired balance, slowed movements, uncontrollable muscle jerks, and freezing episodes when they cannot move.

Diagnosis and Treatment. Clinical examination of the patient will exhibit signs of dementia, whereas SPECT shows decreased perfusion in the occipital region of the brain. Acetylcholinesterase inhibitors, antipsychotic drugs, antidepressants, and levodopa/carbidopa may all help control symptoms. Clonazepam and melatonin are helpful for sleep.

Frontotemporal Dementia

Frontotemporal dementia (FTD), also known as Pick's disease, is a less common type of dementia than AD or vascular dementia. The incidence of FTD is unknown; however, it is thought to be the cause for 10% of cases of dementia. Most patients are affected after age 50 years with a peak incidence at 64 years old.

Etiology. The etiology of FTD is unknown. There is a strong genetic risk factor: As many as 50% of persons with FTD have a family history of the disease. Mutations are found at 17q21-22, which is the gene that controls the production of the tau protein; tau proteins build up in the brain in FTD. Other genetic mutations on chromosome 17 cause decreased production of the progranulin protein and excess production of the ubiquitin protein.

Pathophysiology. Cerebral atrophy is evident in the frontal or temporal lobes of one or both hemispheres of the brain in FTD. Commonly, there is loss within the brain's language area. Some patients will show motor neuron atrophy.

Clinical Presentation. Persons with FTD demonstrate loss of social skills, the hallmark of this disease. Persons with FTD also become increasingly antisocial and disinhibited, oftentimes using crude language and sexual acting-out, as well as being unconcerned about the needs of others. Furthermore, patients with FTD may manifest compulsive oral behaviors, such as overeating, sucking on objects, or eating nonfoods. These behaviors may be extremely upsetting to family members, who may need reassurance that the behaviors are symptoms of the disease. This may be difficult for families to understand, as patients with FTD do not have memory losses or difficulties speaking, symptoms that most people connect with diagnoses of dementia. Additionally, FTD seems to have a strong genetic link within some families, and family members may worry that they, too, will develop the disease. It is important to remind families that the mechanisms of developing FTD are still being investigated, and having a relative with FTD does not guarantee that others in the same family will develop it.

Diagnosis and Treatment. MRI and PET scanning of the brain demonstrate cerebral atrophy and hypometabolism in specific areas of frontal and temporal lobes. Language and neuropsychological tests are commonly administered. Unfortunately, there are few treatment options for FTD, and most are used to control problematic behavior. Antidepressants are commonly prescribed. Trazodone is given to induce sleep.

Diabetes Mellitus, Type 2

Nearly 40% of adults aged 65 years and older meet the diagnostic criteria for diabetes mellitus type 2 (T2DM). Older adults are at increased risk for developing T2DM because of increased cellular resistance to endogenous insulin and pancreatic beta cell dysfunction. Even without diagnosed T2DM, older adults tend to have postprandial glucose levels that are above 200 mg/dL, a condition known as isolated postchallenge hyperglycemia. An elevated glucose level is a risk factor for depression, cognitive impairment, urinary incontinence, falls, persistent pain, and gastroparesis. Older adults, as with all other adults, are also at risk of both microvascular and macrovascular complications from DM. The management of blood glucose in older adults, however, is more challenging than with other population groups because of comorbidities, aging changes, and potential injury from falls brought on by hypoglycemia.

Damage from persistent hyperglycemia is more appropriately controlled by attending to other cardiovascular risk factors, such as smoking cessation, weight control, lipid management, blood pressure control, and aspirin therapy. Glycemic control remains important, but will not yield microvascular benefits nearly as quickly as controlling blood pressure and lipids. Taking the older adult's life expectancy into consideration, a more modest HgbA1c goal of 8%, an average blood glucose level of 183 mg/dL, is often targeted for frail older adults, whereas healthy older adults have the same target of lower than 7% as do younger adults.

Furthermore, many older adults have impaired renal function, and medications such as metformin and angiotensin-converting enzyme (ACE) inhibitors may be contraindicated. Because of alterations in medication metabolism among older adults, it is important to be particularly alert for changes in peak action times of insulins. It may be wise to consider insulin with a very predictable peak of action, such as lispro, over regular insulin or aspart, which have a wider variation in peak and duration of action. For more information about T2DM, see Chapter 25: Diabetes Mellitus and the Metabolic Syndrome.

 CLINICAL CONCEPT

When working with older patients who have T2DM, it is important to monitor blood pressure and lipid levels with the same vigilance as glucose levels.

Geriatric Syndromes

Geriatric syndromes are health conditions that are common among older adults, and which have many causative factors. Urinary incontinence, falls, pressure wounds, delirium, and functional decline are some common examples of geriatric syndromes. Frail older adults are more likely to have geriatric syndromes, which lead to increased frailty.

Frailty in an older adult is described as a constellation of symptoms that include weakness, weight loss, decreased balance and physical activity, slowness, social withdrawal, cognitive impairments, and fatigue. The frail older adult has increased vulnerability to stressors, and is less able to maintain or regain homeostasis after physiologic or psychosocial threat. For example, some frail older adults would not be able to endure the stress of surgery and so are treated with medications whenever possible. A frail older adult with coronary artery disease could not endure angioplasty or coronary bypass surgery; therefore, long-acting nitrate medications are used instead.

The factors that lead to frailty include many of the normal changes of aging, plus diseases that are common to older adults. Specifically, changes in the musculoskeletal, neurological, and immune systems, as well as molecular and genetic changes, predispose some older adults to a heightened vulnerability to stressors. Surgery, either emergent or elective, may be the event that precipitates a cascade of events that lead to greater neuromuscular instability, then to a fall, then to new injuries. Subclinical problems that may have been just beneath the surface of the older adult's functional status begin to appear.

It is extremely difficult to treat geriatric syndromes because of the many contributing factors, but it is important to foster maintenance of function and independence.

Heart Failure

Heart failure (HF) occurs most commonly in older adults because of age-related changes in the cardiovascular system, as well as the high survivorship of ischemic heart disease in the United States. Almost 10% of all older adults have HF, and among all patients with HF, 70% are more than 80 years old. With the predicted increase in the population of older adults in the future, HF will become a very prevalent disease.

Older adults are much more likely to have diastolic HF—a stiff left ventricle with decreased compliance and impaired relaxation. As a group, it is common for the older HF patient to receive substandard treatment as compared with younger adults. For more information, see Chapter 17: Heart Failure.

Hypertension

Not many years ago, isolated systolic hypertension was considered a normal aspect of aging, and older adults were not offered treatment. Some believed that if high blood pressure was treated in older adults, dementia would ensue because blood would not effectively circulate in the brain. Now, although age-related changes clearly may predispose older adults to increased blood pressure, it is recognized that hypertension among older adults is a disease and must be treated, just as hypertension in a middle-aged adult must be treated. Sixty-four percent of male adults older than age 65 years have hypertension, and almost 70% of women older than age 65 years have the disorder. African Americans have a higher prevalence of hypertension than Caucasian adults. Recently, the American Heart Association/American College of Cardiology have recommended different blood pressure guidelines and medical management for the older adult. See chapter 15; Arterial Disorders.

Blood vessels become stiffer with advancing age and contain atherosclerotic plaques. These changes narrow the diameter of blood vessels and increase peripheral vascular resistance. This is most noticeable in the systolic blood pressure of older adults. The older adult's body becomes adjusted to a higher systolic blood pressure for adequate cerebral perfusion. Commonly, 120 mm Hg systolic is too low for the older adult and leaves the older adult susceptible to orthostatic hypotension.

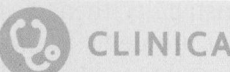

CLINICAL CONCEPT

The risk of hypotensive episodes and concomitant risk of falls are significant issues for the older adult. It is important to measure blood pressure in at least two positions (standing, sitting, and lying down) on older adults to detect orthostatic hypotension. It has been known anecdotally by many practicing clinicians that blood pressure targets in older, frail adults should be higher than in younger adults. A systolic BP of 140 to 145 mm Hg is now considered acceptable in older adults.

Also, a significant decrease in GFR is common in the older adult and this condition has important indications for choice of antihypertensive therapy. The patient's GFR should be calculated before administering medications. Also, it is important to consider the patient's use of alcohol and nonsteroidal anti-inflammatory drugs, which can raise blood pressure in older adults.

Diuretic antihypertensive therapy commonly causes electrolyte disturbances in older adults. Diuretic therapy also causes frequent urination, which may be problematic in older adults. Calcium channel blockers have been shown to cause ankle edema and reflux esophagitis in some older adults. ACE inhibitors sometimes worsen symptoms of dementia. Different medications have different side effects, particularly in the older adult who is routinely on 6 or 7 medications, which is why older adults on blood pressure medications require periodic assessment and need careful monitoring. Patient education regarding weight loss, exercise, and a low sodium diet are an important component of treatment.

Infections

Older adults have alterations in their immune systems that make them more susceptible to infections. They also have changes in their neurological and metabolic systems that may lead to unique manifestations of infection. Older adults do not run high fevers and often do not mount a high WBC count. Also, pain sensitivity is decreased in the older adult, and signs of inflammation are blunted. Uniquely, the older adult with an infection may show changes in behavior or disorientation as the only symptoms of infection.

CLINICAL CONCEPT

Behavioral or mental status changes should increase suspicion of a covert infection in the older adult.

Many older adults have significant levels of bacteria in their urine all the time, referred to as asymptomatic bacteriuria. In fact, older adults who have indwelling catheters have a 100% rate of bacteriuria; yet, many of these individuals are without symptoms. So, in the absence of typical UTI symptoms such as dysuria, frequency, urgency, and flank pain, or sudden onset behavioral change, routine urinalysis for older adults is contraindicated. Asymptomatic bacteriuria in the older adult does not require treatment. Treatment does not improve the morbidity or mortality in affected older persons, and exposes them to adverse drug effects without any benefit.

Pneumonia is also a common infection in the older adult; its prevalence is caused by a combination of age-related changes in the lungs, immune system, and gastrointestinal system. The thoracic cage becomes stiffer, which decreases the expansion and capacity for deep breathing. The cough and gag reflexes in the older adult weaken, which increases susceptibility to aspiration. In addition, stasis of pulmonary secretions is common because of the sedentary behavior common in elders. Pneumonia occurs frequently after an upper respiratory infection such as influenza; for this reason, flu vaccine and pneumonia vaccine are recommended for the elderly adult.

CLINICAL CONCEPT

Gerontologists use the mnemonic "wind, water, wounds" to remember that when an older adult has a sudden change in mental status, infections of the respiratory, urinary, or integumentary systems may be the cause.

Altered Medication Effectiveness

Changes that occur in the kidney, liver, intestine, muscle, and subcutaneous fat of older adults have important implications for the pharmacokinetics and dynamics of medications. Absorption, distribution, metabolism, and excretion may all be affected by changes related to aging. Intramuscular injections may be faster absorbed because of the decreased muscle mass, but that is offset by decreased peripheral blood flow that may decrease absorption. Because older adults generally have more overall body fat in comparison to lean muscle, fat-soluble medications such as diazepam will remain in the body longer, leading to a possible overdose if adjustments in timing and dose are not made. Water-soluble medications such as gentamycin, in contrast, will be metabolized much more rapidly because of the relative lack of free water. The loss of lean muscle mass means that older adults have less protein in their bodies, so the amount of free drug will circulate in higher quantities. Clinicians who work with older adults should become familiar with the Beers criteria for potentially inappropriate medication use in older adults, and the most recent update. The list includes 48 medications that should always be avoided in older adults, and 20 problematic medication-disease combinations.

The liver becomes less effective with increased age, which particularly affects medication metabolism. With age, there is less blood flow to the liver and diminished detoxification capacity. Standard liver function tests, such as aspartate transaminase (AST) and alanine transaminase (ALT), often do not accurately reflect pharmacokinetics. The kidney also becomes less effective in excretion of drug metabolites. The combination of the decreased functioning of these two organs means that older adults are at risk for accidental overdose.

Conversely, immunosuppression in older adults dictates that antimicrobials be used in doses that are large enough to be effective, while also carefully monitoring for adverse drug effects. Macrolides such as azithromycin do not concentrate well in older adults, but the acidic anti-infectives such as penicillin, ceftriaxone, sulfonamides, and clindamycin may reach concentrations higher than in younger adults. When possible, culture and sensitivity (C&S) testing should be done to ensure that infections are completely treated.

Chapter Summary

- Population studies show that the average life span for women in the United States is approximately 81 years; for men, 76 years.

- People aged 85 years and older are the fastest growing segment of older Americans.

- Older adult individuals are categorized in three different groups according to age: young-old, individuals aged between 65 and 74 years; middle-old, individuals aged between 75 and 84 years, and old-old, individuals older than age 85 years.

- As organisms age, the ability to repair damage and adapt to physiologic stressors decreases. This decreased ability is referred to as loss of physiologic reserve.

- Although older adults may be able to function adequately in daily life, they are *less resilient* to stress, compared with younger adults.

- In the telomere shortening theory of aging, telomeres–the end segments of chromosomes–diminish each time the cell divides in mitosis. Telomerase is an enzyme under intense study because it prevents the shortening of telomeres, thereby counteracting aging.

- The damage-based theory of aging asserts that cellular damage occurs over time, either because of toxic by-products of metabolism or inefficient cellular repair systems.

- Limiting total calories to as few as 60% of the recommended daily allowance extends the life span of mice up to 40%. In lab experiments, calorie-restricted older adult mice are similar to young mice physiologically in many ways.

- Cardiovascular changes in the older adult include development of atherosclerosis, stiffening of the elastic blood vessels, development of diastolic dysfunction in the heart, and connective tissue infiltration of the conductive tissues in the heart.

- Respiratory changes in the older adult include a less elastic thoracic cage, which limits lung expansion with inhalation, as well as diminished cough reflex, which increases stasis of secretions in the lungs.

- Renal changes in the older adult include decreased ability of the kidney to filter waste from the blood and a decreased glomerular filtration rate, which lends to medication toxicity.

- Gastrointestinal changes in the older adult include decreased peristaltic activity, which increases susceptibility to constipation; atrophy of the stomach lining and intestinal villi; and decreased strength of lower esophageal sphincter, allowing for acid reflux.

- Integumentary changes in the older adult include the loss of sweat glands, hair follicles, and sensory end organs, which can lead to difficulties in thermoregulation. Skin also becomes less elastic and thinner, increasing susceptibility to breakdown.

- Musculoskeletal changes in the older adult include an increased susceptibility to osteoporosis because osteoclastic activity begins to outpace osteoblastic activity. Lean muscle mass diminishes and body fat increases.

- Nervous system changes in the older adult include an increased pain threshold, which can interfere with protective actions, as well as increased problems with sight, hearing, and taste.

- A majority of older adults with infections demonstrate no fever, and older adults are more susceptible to hypothermia and hyperthermia than younger adults.

- Cognitive changes are never normal in the older adult and must always be thoroughly assessed. Vascular dementia, Alzheimer's disease, and frontotemporal disease are common causes of cognitive impairment.

- Geriatric syndromes are health conditions common among older adults. These conditions have many causative factors. Urinary incontinence, falls, pressure wounds, delirium, and functional decline are common examples of geriatric syndromes.

- Frailty in an older adult is described as a constellation of symptoms that includes weakness, weight loss, decreased balance and physical activity, slowness, social withdrawal, cognitive impairments, and fatigue. The frail elder has increased vulnerability to stressors, and is less able to maintain or regain homeostasis after physiologic or psychosocial threat.

- Clinicians who work with older adults should become familiar with the Beers criteria for potentially inappropriate medication use in older adults.

Bibliography

Ahlskog, J. E., Geda, Y. E., Graff-Radford, N. R., & Petersen, R. C. (2011). Physical exercise as a preventive or disease-modifying treatment of dementia and brain aging. *Mayo Clin Proceed*, 86(9), 876–884. doi: 10.4065/mcp.2011.0252.

Alpert, J. S. (2011). The importance of being elderly—some thoughts on the care of geriatric patients. *Am J Med*, 124(10), 889–890. doi: 10.1016/j.amjmed.2011.05.016.

Alpert, J. S., & Chen, Q. M. (2012). So, you want to live to 120? The genie in the bottle. *Am J Med*, 125(7), 621–622. doi: 10.1016/j.amjmed.2012.02.002. Epub 2012 May 8.

American Geriatrics Society 2012 Beers Criteria Update Expert Panel. (2012, April). American Geriatrics Society updated Beers Criteria for potentially inappropriate medication use in older adults. *J Am Geriatr Soc*, 60(4), 616–631. doi: 10.1111/j.1532-5415.2012.03923.x. Epub 2012 Feb 29.

Anonymous. (2014, May 1). Unintentional weight loss in older adults. *Am Fam Phys*, 89(9): Online.

Anversa, P., & Leri, A. (2013). Innate regeneration in the aging heart: healing from within. *Mayo Clin Proc*, 88(8), 871–883. doi: 10.1016/j.mayocp.2013.04.001.

Beekman, M., Blanché, H., Perola, M., et al. (2013). Genome-wide linkage analysis for human longevity: Genetics of Healthy Ageing Study. *Aging Cell*, Jan 3. doi: 10.1111/acel.12039. Epub ahead of print.

Brown, N. A., & Zenilman, M. E. (2010). The impact of frailty in the elderly on the outcome of surgery in the aged. *Adv Surg*, 44, 229–249.

Buchner, D. M. (2010). Promoting physical activity in older adults. *Am Fam Phys*, 81(1), 24.

Cayea, D., Eckstrom, E., & Christmas, C. (2012). Update in geriatric medicine. *J Gen Intern Med*, 27(3), 371–375. doi: 10.1007/s11606-011-1876-5. Epub 2011 Oct 25.

Chakravarty, E. F., Hubert, H. B., Krishnan, E., et al. (2012). Lifestyle risk factors predict disability and death in healthy aging adults. *Am J Med*, 125(2), 190–197. doi: 10.1016/j.amjmed.2011.08.006.

Chronic disease management in ageing populations. (2012). *Lancet*, 379(9829), 1851. doi: 10.1016/S0140-6736(12)60790-9.

Clegg, A., Young, J., Iliffe, S., Rikkert, M. O., & Rockwood, K. (2013). Frailty in elderly people. *Lancet*, 381(9868), 752–762. doi: 10.1016/S0140-6736(12)62167-9. Epub 2013 Feb 8.

Elsawy, B., & Higgins, K. E. (2010). Physical activity guidelines for older adults. *Am Fam Phys*, 81(1), 55–59.

Elsawy, B., & Higgins, K. E. (2011). The geriatric assessment. *Am Fam Phys*, 83(1), 48–56.

Fried, T. R., Vaz Fragoso, C. A., & Rabow, M. W. (2012). Caring for the older person with chronic obstructive pulmonary disease. *JAMA*, 308(12), 1254–1263.

Fyhrquist, F., & Saijonmaa, O. (2012). Telomere length and cardiovascular aging. *Ann Med*, 44 (Suppl 1), S138–S142. doi: 10.3109/07853890.2012.660497.

Gaddey, H. L., & Holder, K. (2014). Unintentional weight loss in older adults. *Am Fam Phys*, 89(9), 718–722.

Gitlin, L. N., Kales, H. C., & Lyketsos, C. G. (2012). Nonpharmacologic management of behavioral symptoms in dementia. *JAMA*, 308(19), 2020–2029. doi: 10.1001/jama.2012.36918.

Hallan, S. I., Matsushita, K., Sang, Y., et al. (2012). Age and association of kidney measures with mortality and end-stage renal disease. *JAMA*, 308(22), 2349–2360.

Hess, B. J., Lynn, L. A., Conforti, L. N., & Holmboe, E. S. (2011). Listening to older adults: elderly patients' experience of care in residency and practicing physician outpatient clinics. *J Am Geriatr Soc*, 59(5), 909–915. doi: 10.1111/j.1532-5415.2011.03370.x. Epub 2011 Apr 21.

Hohensinner, P. J., Goronzy, J. J., & Weyand, C. M. (2011). Telomere dysfunction, autoimmunity and aging. *Aging Dis*, 2(6), 524–537. Epub 2011 Dec 2.

Hubbard, R. E., & Rockwood, K. (2011). Frailty in older women. *Maturitas*, 69(3), 203–207. doi: 10.1016/j.maturitas.2011.04.006. Epub 2011 May 13.

Jacobs, E. G., Epel, E. S., Lin, J., Blackburn, E. H., & Rasgon, N. L. (2014). Relationship between leukocyte telomere length, telomerase activity, and hippocampal volume in early aging. *JAMA Neurol*, 71(7), 921–923. doi: 10.1001/jamaneurol.2014.870.

Jacobs, J. M., Cohen, A., Ein-Mor, E., Maaravi, Y., & Stessman, J. (2011). Frailty, cognitive impairment and mortality among the oldest old. *J Nutr Health Aging*, 15(8), 678–682.

Jeffery, C. A., Shum, D. W., & Hubbard, R. E. (2013). Emerging drug therapies for frailty. *Maturitas*. 74(1), 21–25. doi: 10.1016/j.maturitas.2012.10.010. Epub 2012 Nov 7.

Kanasaki, K., Kitada, M., & Koya, D. (2012). Pathophysiology of the aging kidney and therapeutic interventions. *Hypertens Research*, 35(12), 1121–1128. doi: 10.1038/hr.2012.159. Epub 2012 Oct 18.

Kolovou, G. D., Kolovou, V., & Mavrogeni, S. (2014). We are ageing. *Biomed Res Int*, 808307. Epub 2014 Jun 22.

Lang, P. O., Govind, S., Michel, J. P., Aspinall, R., & Mitchell, W. A. (2011). Immunosenescence: implications for vaccination programmes in adults. *Maturitas*, 68(4), 322–330. doi: 10.1016/j.maturitas.2011.01.011. Epub 2011 Feb 12.

Lee, J. S., Auyeung, T. W., Leung, J., et al. (2011). Physical frailty in older adults is associated with metabolic and atherosclerotic risk factors and cognitive impairment independent of muscle mass. *J Nutr Health Aging*, 5(10), 857–862.

Leibowitz, D., Jacobs, J. M., Stessman-Lande, I., et al. (2011). Cardiac structure and function and dependency in the oldest old. *J Am Geriatr Soc*, 59(8), 1429–1434. doi: 10.1111/j.1532-5415.2011.03534.x. Epub 2011 Aug 8.

Lin, J. S. (2010). Encouraging physical activity among frail older adults. *Am Fam Phys*, 82(3), 230.

Lloyd-Sherlock, P., McKee, M., Ebrahim, S., et al. (2012). Population ageing and health. *Lancet*, 379(9823), 1295–1296. doi: 10.1016/S0140-6736(12)60519-4. Epub 2012 Apr 4.

Loeser, R. F. (2013). Aging processes and the development of osteoarthritis. *Curr Opin Rheumatol*, 25(1), 108–113. doi: 10.1097/BOR.0b013e32835a9428.

Mithal, A., Bonjour, J. P., Boonen, S., et al. (2012). Impact of nutrition on muscle mass, strength, and performance in older adults. *Osteoporos Int*, Dec 18. Epub ahead of print.

Moncada, L. V. (2011). Management of falls in older persons: a prescription for prevention. *Am Fam Phys*, 84(11), 1267–1276.

Odden, M. C., Coxson, P. G., Moran, A., et al. (2011). The impact of the aging population on coronary heart disease in the United States. *Am J Med*, 124(9), 827–833.e5. doi: 10.1016/j.amjmed.2011.04.010. Epub 2011 Jun 30.

Pahor, M., Guralnik, J. M., Ambrosius, W. T., et al. (2014). Effect of structured physical activity on prevention of major mobility disability in older adults: the LIFE study randomized clinical trial. *JAMA*, 311(23), 2387–2396. doi: 10.1001/jama.2014.5616.

Perissinotto, C. M., & Valcour, V. (2011). Preventing dementia: is there hope for progress? *Am Fam Phys,* 83(9), 1034–1035.

Resnick, B., & Fick, D. M. (2012, July-August). 2012 Beers criteria update: how should practicing nurses use the criteria? *Geriatr Nurs,* 33(4), 253–255. doi: 10.1016/j.gerinurse.2012.06.001.

Robinovitch, S. N., Feldman, F., Yang, Y., et al. (2012). Video capture of the circumstances of falls in elderly people residing in long-term care: an observational study. *Lancet,* doi: pii: S0140-6736(12)61263-X. 10.1016/S0140-6736(12)61263-X.

Salzman, B. (2010a). Encouraging physical activity among frail older adults. *Am Fam Phys,* 82(1), 61–68.

Salzman, B. (2010b). Gait and balance disorders in older adults. *Am Fam Phys,* 82(1), 61–68.

Sánchez, E., Vidán, M. T., Serra, J. A., Fernández-Avilés, F., & Bueno, H. (2011). Prevalence of geriatric syndromes and impact on clinical and functional outcomes in older patients with acute cardiac diseases. *Heart,* 97(19), 1602–1606. doi: 10.1136/hrt.2011.227504. Epub 2011 Jul 27.

Shioi, T., & Inuzuka, Y. (2012). Aging as a substrate of heart failure. *J Cardiol,* 60(6), 423–428. doi: 10.1016/j.jjcc.2012.07.015. Epub 2012 Oct 12.

Simmons, B. B., Hartmann, B., & Dejoseph, D. (2011). Evaluation of suspected dementia. *Am Fam Phys,* 84(8), 895–902.

Singh, B., Parsaik, A. K., Mielke, M. M., et al. (2013). Chronic obstructive pulmonary disease and association with mild cognitive impairment: the Mayo Clinic Study of Aging. *Mayo Clin Proceed,* 88(11), 1222–1230. doi: 10.1016/j.mayocp.2013.08.012.

Singh, I., Gallacher, J., Davis, K., et al. (2012). Predictors of adverse outcomes on an acute geriatric rehabilitation ward. *Age and Ageing,* 41(2), 242–246. doi: 10.1093/ageing/afr179. Epub 2012 Feb 1.

Sinha, S. K., & Detsky, A. S. (2012). Measure, promote, and reward mobility to prevent falls in older patients. *JAMA,* 308(24), 2573–2574. doi: 10.1001/jama.2012.68313.

Spoelhof, G. D., Davis, G. L., & Licari, A. (2011). Clinical vignettes in geriatric depression. *Am Fam Phys,* 84(10), 1149–1154.

Strandberg, T. E., & O'Neill, D. (2013). Dementia—a geriatric syndrome. *Lancet.,* 381(9866), 533–534. doi: 10.1016/S0140-6736(13)60275-5.

Tonelli, M., & Riella, M. (2014). Chronic kidney disease and the ageing population. *Lancet,* 383(9925), 1278–1279. doi: 10.1016/S0140-6736(14)60155-0. Epub 2014 Mar 13.

Tümpel, S., & Rudolph, K. L. (2012). The role of telomere shortening in somatic stem cells and tissue aging: lessons from telomerase model systems. *Anns New York Acad Science,* 1266, 28–39. doi: 10.1111/j.1749-6632.2012.06547.x.

Unützer, J., & Park, M. (2012). Older adults with severe, treatment-resistant depression. *JAMA,* 308(9), 909–918. doi: 10.1001/2012.jama.10690.

Unwin, B. K., Porvaznik, M., & Spoelhof, G. D. (2010). Nursing home care: part I. Principles and pitfalls of practice. *Am Fam Phys,* 81(10), 1219–1227.

Unwin, B. K., Porvaznik, M., & Spoelhof, G. D. (2011). Nursing home care: part II. Clinical aspects. *Am Fam Phys,* 81(10), 1229–1237.

van der Jagt-Willems, H. C., van Hengel, M., Vis, M., et al. (2012). Why do geriatric outpatients have so many moderate and severe vertebral fractures? Exploring prevalence and risk factors. *Age and Ageing,* 41(2), 200–206. doi: 10.1093/ageing/afr174. Epub 2012 Jan 4.

Verrill, M. M., Hall, M. N., & Loven, B. (2012). FPIN's clinical inquiries. Evaluation of hip pain in older adults. *Am Fam Phys,* 86(4), 1–2.

Virdis, A., Ghiadoni, L., Giannarelli, C., & Taddei, S. (2010). Endothelial dysfunction and vascular disease in later life. *Maturitas,* 67(1), 20–24. doi: 10.1016/j.maturitas.2010.04.006. Epub 2010 May 8.

Walling, A. D., & Dickson, G. M. (2012). Hearing loss in older adults. *Am Fam Phys,* 85(12), 1150–1156.

What is it to grow old? (2012). *Lancet,* 380(9844), 779. doi: 10.1016/S0140-6736(12)61431-7.

Yen, Y. C., & Lung, F. W. (2012). Older adults with higher income or marriage have longer telomeres. *Age and Ageing,* Sep 4. Epub ahead of print.

Zekry, D., Krause, K. H., Irminger-Finger, I., et al. (2012). Telomere length, comorbidity, functional, nutritional and cognitive status as predictors of 5 years post hospital discharge survival in the oldest old. *J Nutr Health Aging,* 16(3), 225–230.

SIRS, Sepsis, Shock, MODS, and Death

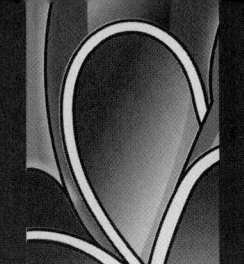

Key Terms

Abdominal compartment syndrome (ACS)

Acute kidney injury (AKI)

Acute lung injury (ALI)

Adult respiratory distress syndrome (ARDS)

Anaphylactic shock

Brain death

Compensatory anti-inflammatory response syndrome (CARS)

Disseminated intravascular coagulation (DIC)

Intra-abdominal hypertension (IAH)

Microthrombi

Multiple organ dysfunction syndrome (MODS)

Sepsis

Septic shock

Septicemia

Shock

Systemic inflammatory response syndrome (SIRS)

Patients that are suffering severe illnesses such as **systemic inflammatory response syndrome (SIRS),** sepsis, septic shock, and **multiple organ dysfunction syndrome (MODS)** are commonly treated in intensive care settings. Patients with these disorders require minute-to-minute monitoring of vital signs and organ function. Through the use of advanced technology, health-care providers can continuously monitor many of the critical parameters and lab values that influence the patient's condition. As technology has progressed, so has our knowledge of the cellular basis of disease. There is more information about inflammation and infection on a molecular basis than ever before, and this allows for specific targets of treatment. Pharmacological agents can aim directly at the biochemical, molecular, and genetic components of disease. These discoveries are reshaping our understanding of the biology of the very ill patient and introducing new treatment modalities. Critical illness can lead to recovery or multiple system failure; often, there is a sequential decline in body function before death. Clinicians can recognize these early signs and symptoms of lethal conditions and stave off death.

Epidemiology

It is estimated that more than 750,000 people develop sepsis annually in the United States. The disease is often fatal, with an overall mortality rate of 30%. Mortality rates range from 20% to 52% in severe sepsis and 82% for patients with septic shock. In MODS, there is a 20% increase in mortality with each additional organ dysfunction. In the presence of **acute kidney injury (AKI),** the mortality rate increases to 70%.

SIRS occurs in 82% of hospitalized children, with 23% experiencing sepsis, 4% with severe sepsis, and 2% with septic shock. Eighteen percent of children with sepsis develop MODS, which increases the mortality rate.

Basic Concepts of Critical Systemic Illnesses

Infection, burn, trauma, hemorrhage, and major surgery can trigger SIRS, sepsis, septic shock, MODS, and shock. MODS is the cause of death in 50% to 80% of intensive care patients. It is commonly a terminal stage of a deteriorating process triggered by an insult to the body.

Systemic Inflammatory Response Syndrome

SIRS is an overwhelming inflammatory reaction of the body initiated by a severe insult to the body. It is an intense immunological and cytokine response in the body. The precise reason for SIRS is not entirely understood, but it has the potential to do significant damage to body tissues and organs. There are specific criteria for a diagnosis of SIRS (see Box 47-1).

During SIRS, the cardiac, hepatic, respiratory, digestive, and renal systems attempt to compensate for an insult to the body. There is also a large sympathetic nervous system (SNS) and endocrine reaction similar to the alarm stage in the stress response. Heart rate, cardiac output, and respiratory rate increase. Gastrointestinal (GI) activity and urine output are reduced. There are increased levels of catecholamines, glucocorticoids, mineralocorticoids, antidiuretic hormone (ADH), and angiotensin II.

BOX 47-1. Criteria for SIRS

The criteria for diagnosing SIRS is the presence of any two of the following four signs:

- tachycardia (heart rate greater than 90/min)
- tachypnea (respiratory rate greater than 20/min)
- hyperthermia or hypothermia (temperature greater than 100.4°F (38°C) or lower than 96.8°F (36°C)
- leukocytosis (greater than 12,000/mm³), leukopenia (lower than 4,000/mm³), or greater than 10% immature forms.

Systemic infection, also referred to as sepsis, often follows SIRS. Following the intense SIRS reaction, there is a period where the immune system is markedly less active (see Fig. 47-1). This period of reduced immunity and increased susceptibility to infection is called the **compensatory anti-inflammatory response syndrome (CARS).** Even if the initial, precipitating insult is not infectious, the intense inflammatory response to the insult is followed by a period of immunological suppression during which the patient is highly susceptible

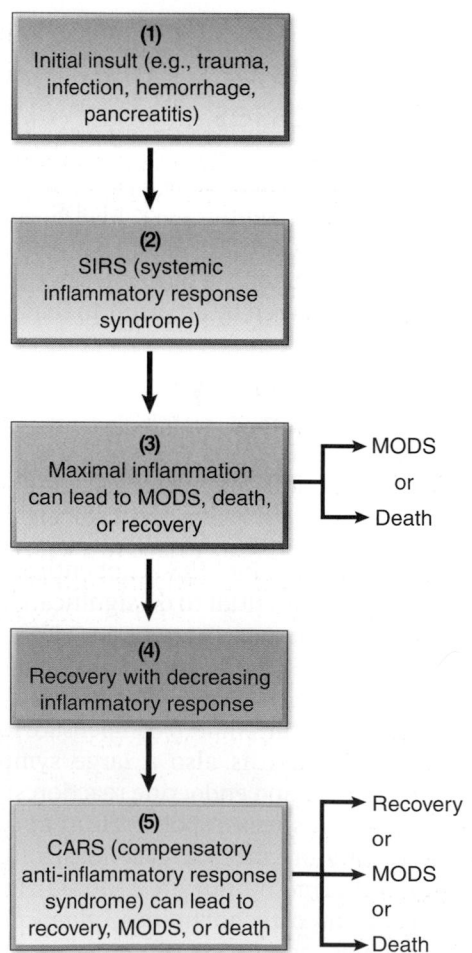

FIGURE 47-1. Mechanism of SIRS. An initial insult leads to SIRS followed by maximal inflammation, which can lead to MODS, death, or recovery with CARS, during which there is decreased immunity. CARS can lead to MODS, death, or full recovery.

to nosocomial (hospital-acquired) infection. The immune response of the patient is muted and the source of infection is not obvious. Frequently, the infection is caused by common skin or bowel microbes that normally are not pathogenic.

The majority of patients who manifest a SIRS reaction recover. However, for some, the nature of the initial insult is so severe that prompt recovery does not occur. Pre-existing conditions such as cardiac disease, chronic obstructive pulmonary disease (COPD), and renal disease can render the patient unable to withstand the metabolic demands of SIRS. These patients are likely to develop early MODS or die.

An example of the progression of SIRS, CARS, sepsis, septic shock, and MODS can be seen in the following patient scenario: A patient in status asthmaticus (unrelenting asthma) is admitted to the emergency department for life-threatening hypoxemia and severe pulmonary atelectasis. The patient is promptly treated with endotracheal intubation to stabilize ventilation. However, despite the stabilization of the patient, SIRS develops in response to the overwhelming stress on the body. CARS, which is a period of low immunity and high susceptibility to infection, follows. During this period the patient is particularly susceptible to infection from nosocomial microorganisms such as methicillin-resistant *Staphylococcus aureus*, which often causes pneumonia in intubated patients. The infection starts in the lungs but overwhelms the immunosuppressed patient and leads to infection of the bloodstream, called sepsis. Sepsis often progresses to septic shock. During the period of shock, MODS can develop and lead to death.

Sepsis

Sepsis, also called **septicemia,** is a bodywide infection that overwhelms the immune system and causes severe multiorgan compromise. Although bacteria are the most common cause of sepsis, any organism—viral, fungal, or parasite—can cause the infection. Bacterial sepsis is the active multiplication of bacteria in the bloodstream that results in an overwhelming infection; the term *bloodstream infection* is also commonly used.

Immunosuppressed persons, older adults, and infants are most susceptible to sepsis. Infection usually begins in one organ system and then spreads into the bloodstream, causing sepsis. For example, a common cause of sepsis is a urinary tract infection in older adults; this is termed *urosepsis.* Pneumonia, abdominal infections, and postoperative infections can also lead to sepsis. Sepsis is sometimes described as SIRS with an infectious origin. There are specific criteria that describe sepsis (see Box 47-2). Severe sepsis is defined as sepsis complicated by end-organ dysfunction, as demonstrated by altered mental status, an episode of hypotension, renal insufficiency, or evidence of **disseminated intravascular coagulation (DIC)**—failure of the coagulation system.

BOX 47-2. Criteria for Sepsis

With sepsis, at least one of the following manifestations of inadequate organ function/perfusion is typically included:

- alteration in mental state
- hypoxemia (arterial oxygen tension lower than 72 mm Hg and overt pulmonary disease not the direct cause of hypoxemia)
- elevated plasma lactate level
- oliguria (urine output lower than 30 mL or 0.5 mL/kg for at least 1 h).

Septic Shock

Septic shock is defined as a state of severe sepsis with persistent life-threatening hypotension that is refractory to fluid replacement and vasopressors. Intravenous fluids and vasoconstrictor medications cannot elevate the blood pressure in septic shock. The presence of septic shock indicates an infection of great severity, which is the result of a very virulent microbe. Certain pathogens, such as some *Clostridia*, *S. aureus*, *Streptococci A*, *Yersinia pestis*, and *Meningococci*, can produce potent toxins that rapidly produce septic shock. Infection with one of these pathogens is overwhelming and mortality is considerable. Microbial exotoxins or endotoxins can stimulate potent vasodilation.

Septic shock most often develops in people who are immunologically compromised. This group includes older adults, infants, postoperative patients, and patients with diabetes, pulmonary disease, renal insufficiency, and cancer, especially if the cancer is advanced or the patient is taking chemotherapy. Other predisposing factors are chronic corticosteroid therapy, transplants, human immunodeficiency virus infection, trauma, and being in an intensive care unit (ICU). Patients who have long-term indwelling catheters, endotracheal tubes, or IV lines are also at risk. These patients can develop sepsis with microbes that are not usually pathogenic or that cause milder infections in people with normal immune systems.

At times, the etiology of septic shock is not readily apparent. Blood cultures are positive for bacteria or microbes less than 50% of the time.

Toxins and inflammatory mediators, such as interleukins (Ils), nitric oxide (NO), thromboxane A2, prostacyclin, and tumor necrosis factor-alpha (TNF-alpha), cause widespread arterial vasodilation. Capillary permeability is greatly increased with plasma entering the tissues. Inflammatory mediators also activate the coagulation pathway, which leads to formation of small blood clots called **microthrombi.** Sepsis causes injury to the capillary bed endothelium and leads to initiation of the coagulation cascade. It also inhibits the activation of protein C, a naturally occurring anticoagulant, and activation of the plasmin fibrinolysis system. Some exotoxins interfere with the coagulation cascade, producing coagulopathy, which is a lack of ability to clot.

There is an outpouring of epinephrine and cortisol that accompanies sepsis, severely reduces insulin sensitivity, and incites glycogenolysis. Blood sugar becomes elevated and difficult to control with insulin. The hyperglycemia impairs the white blood cells' (WBCs)? ability to phagocytose and lyse offending microbes. The mortality of patients with severe sepsis and hyperglycemia is elevated and control of glucose levels plays an important part in the treatment of severe sepsis.

The vasodilation and intravascular fluid loss causes increased cardiac activity. This is a hypermetabolic state and fever usually develops. The widespread vasodilation, inflammation, and microthrombi can lead to extensive tissue hypoperfusion with ischemia, leading to MODS. The patient may appear pink and the skin may be warm despite the onset of shock. This is the stage of so-called "warm shock."

ALERT! Septic shock is a medical emergency and has a high death rate—up to 60% mortality.

Multiple Organ Dysfunction Syndrome

MODS is a clinical syndrome characterized by progressive and potentially reversible dysfunction in two or more organs or organ systems that is induced by a variety of acute insults, commonly sepsis. It is the leading cause of death in the ICU. There is a common continuum in the critically ill patient that begins with infection, which leads to sepsis, septic shock, and MODS. The exact pathophysiology of MODS in patients with sepsis is not fully understood. However, there are some theories and proposed mechanisms.

Hypoxia–Microvascular Theory

It is proposed that sepsis or severe inflammatory reactions can initiate MODS, as these conditions cause endothelial dysfunction and microvascular abnormalities. Inflammatory mediators, free radicals, lytic enzymes, and vasoactive substances lead to microcirculatory injury. Erythrocytes cannot navigate through the disrupted microvasculature of different organs, which ultimately leads to cellular hypoxia.

Gut Theory

During severe sepsis, blood flow to the GI system decreases, causing mucosal ischemia and liver dysfunction. Mucosal ischemia leads to increased permeability of the GI wall. The mucosal permeability allows normal bacterial flora of the GI tract to escape into the bloodstream. These bacteria provoke a large immune reaction, resulting in tissue injury throughout the body.

Endotoxin Theory

It is believed that gram-negative bacteria are largely responsible for septic shock and MODS. These bacteria

BOX 47-3. Four Clinical Phases of MODS

There are four clinical phases of MODS:

- **Stage 1:** The patient has increased volume requirements and mild respiratory alkalosis, which is accompanied by oliguria, hyperglycemia, and increased insulin requirements.
- **Stage 2:** The patient is tachypneic, hypocapneic, and hypoxemic. There is moderate liver dysfunction and possible hematologic abnormalities.
- **Stage 3:** The patient develops shock with azotemia and acid-base disturbances. There are significant coagulation abnormalities.
- **Stage 4:** The patient is vasopressor dependent and oliguric or anuric. Ischemic colitis and lactic acidosis follow.

release endotoxins that stimulate a widespread inflammatory reaction involving interleukins, TNF, thromboxane A2, prostacyclin, and NO. These inflammatory actions take place in multiple organ systems.

The pathophysiology of MODS is most likely caused by a combination of the theoretical mechanisms. In MODS, it is common to see respiratory failure occur early in the course of illness, followed by liver failure, GI bleeding, and renal failure. There are four clinical phases of MODS (see Box 47-3).

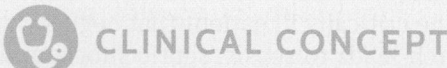

CLINICAL CONCEPT

Mortality of MODS increases by about 20% for each additional organ involved. If AKI is involved, the mortality increases to 70%.

Shock

Shock is the inability of the heart and lungs to satisfy the metabolic and oxygen requirements of the peripheral tissues. Commonly, shock occurs when blood pressure falls below a systolic measurement of 90 mm Hg or drops 40 mm Hg below the patient's normal BP. Shock can be thought of as severe hypotension. However, it is important to understand that blood pressure does not define shock. Although a decrease in blood pressure is commonplace in shock, it is not always present, at least not at first. Similarly, heart rate is commonly elevated in shock but not always.

For example, a hypertensive patient with usual BP measurements of 150/90 can go into shock with a BP that seems normal, such as 100/70. This low BP, in a person with chronic hypertension, may not be able to deliver blood to the peripheral and cerebral arterial vessels. In chronic hypertension, the body commonly adjusts to a high BP, so that high pressure becomes necessary for arterial perfusion throughout the body. In

this way, a patient with chronic hypertension can have inadequate cerebral perfusion and lose consciousness with a BP of 100/70.

Similarly, tachycardia is not always found in a patient with shock. For example, a patient with complete heart block may have a pulse of 25 beats per minute, which does not permit delivery of adequate cardiac output to meet the needs of the periphery. This patient is in shock without compensatory tachycardia because his heart is dysfunctional and not capable of a rate increase. Mental changes, acidosis, renal failure, and death will follow if the heart rate is not raised.

Types of Shock

Shock is classified into five broad categories based on etiology:

- cardiogenic shock
- hypovolemic shock
- septic shock
- anaphylactic shock
- neurogenic shock.

It is important to realize that all five categories of shock converge onto the same pathophysiologic pathway of cellular hypoxia, which triggers anaerobic metabolism and lactic acidosis (see Fig. 47-2).

Once shock has occurred, prompt reversal of the situation is necessary. This requires treating the cause as well as the signs and symptoms. If shock cannot be

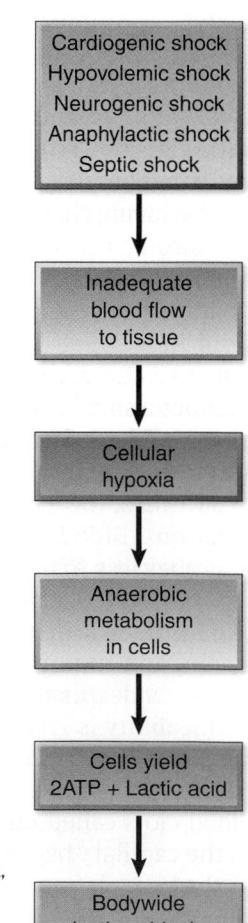

FIGURE 47-2. Mechanism of shock. All types of shock lead to inadequate blood flow to the tissues and cause widespread cellular hypoxia. In hypoxia, anaerobic metabolism occurs in cells. Each cell yields 2 ATP and lactic acid, resulting in widespread lactic acidosis.

reversed quickly, the body suffers the consequences of inadequate perfusion and ischemia.

Stages of Shock

Shock has three stages: initial, progressive, and irreversible. There are specific pathophysiologic changes and patient symptoms in each stage.

Initial Stage. In the initial stage of shock, when there is a sudden drop in tissue perfusion, the SNS and renin-angiotensin-aldosterone system (RAAS) are triggered. The SNS stimulates tachycardia as a compensatory mechanism. The RAAS system increases blood volume and stimulates peripheral vasoconstriction in efforts to bring up BP. However, in shock these compensatory mechanisms cannot normalize BP and medical intervention is necessary. The patient is anxious, pale, and his or her extremities are cold and clammy.

Progressive Stage. If shock is not corrected promptly, a progressive stage ensues in which the lungs, kidneys, gut, pancreas, and liver suffer decreased perfusion. All available blood is conserved for the heart and brain. The patient may begin to show signs of MODS. Commonly, if the kidneys suffer ischemia for 20 to 30 minutes, they begin to fail. The kidneys cannot filter blood of wastes; therefore, waste products accumulate. The liver and GI system also suffer ischemia. The GI system undergoes ileus, a state of no peristalsis. The liver dysfunctions and cannot clear the blood of toxins, so toxins accumulate in the bloodstream.

Irreversible Stage. Failure to terminate shock during the progressive stage produces the irreversible stage of shock. In this stage, the heart and brain begin to sustain decreased perfusion. Myocardial and cerebral ischemia occur. If ischemia is prolonged, myocardial infarction (MI) or cerebral infarction (stroke) can occur.

During this stage, there is widespread cellular hypoxia with extensive anaerobic metabolism occurring throughout the body. Anaerobic metabolism utilizes glucose to produce a small amount of energy (2 adenosine triphosphate [ATP]) and lactic acid. Energy stores are rapidly depleted and not replenished. Cellular ATP is insufficient and the mitochondria do not receive adequate oxygen to make more ATP. Lactic acid builds up in the bloodstream, and the cell's ATP pump fails. Sodium and water enter the cell and potassium exits the cell. The organelles within the cell begin to fail. As cells die, lysosomes break open and release digestive enzymes that break down cellular debris. This is the final step in a downward spiral.

Inflammatory Response in Shock

The release of the necrotic contents of the cellular matrix and membrane is a powerful stimulant of the immune system. The resulting chemotaxis increases the influx of neutrophils, macrophages, and killer T cells. Their action increases the local demand for oxygen and energy that cannot be fulfilled.

The intestine, the home of many bacteria, is always in a state of hypoxia when the body is in shock. The normal intestinal barrier to microbes and their toxins breaks down. The release of microbes and their toxins into the general circulation results in a systemic inflammatory response syndrome (SIRS) that causes injury to organs distant from the original insult.

Shock, of any cause, initiates a SIRS with the production of cytokines, bradykinin, and histamine. These chemicals have a profound influence on all organs, including the capillary endothelial cells. WBCs adhere to the endothelium and their output of cytokines causes endothelial injury and dysfunction. Increased capillary permeability causes the accumulation of interstitial edema. Clearly, SIRS plays a large role in the multiple organ dysfunction syndrome (MODS) seen following shock.

Lactic Acidosis in Shock. A result of anaerobic metabolism is lactic acid production. Because of hypoperfusion, the liver is unable to convert the lactic acid back to sugar compounds. Renal hypoperfusion causes decreased filtration of the blood and excretion of wastes, which diminishes elimination of lactic acid. As long as a state of shock persists, lactic acidosis will persist and worsen. This lactic acidosis adversely affects cardiac, respiratory, neurological, and brain function. As the lactic acidosis worsens, neurological activity, oxygen and carbon dioxide transport, and cellular enzyme activity become increasingly impaired. Impaired mentation with eventual loss of consciousness, as well as impaired cardiac efficiency and arrhythmias, follow. Cardiac output diminishes despite the powerful stimulus of endogenous catecholamines.

Gastrointestinal Consequences of Shock. In shock, there is severe vasoconstriction of the splanchnic arteries that perfuse the intestine. If hypoxia of the abdominal contents persists, the abdominal organs do not function and the following occurs:

- Toxins and microbes that normally inhabit the bowel lumen enter the circulation and generate a powerful systemic inflammatory response.
- The pancreas is unable to make sufficient quantities of insulin.
- Secretion of incretins—intestinal hormones such as gastric inhibitory polypeptide (GIP) and glucagonlike peptide (GLP-1) that increase cellular sensitivity to insulin—are reduced.
- Endothelium of the capillaries of the abdominal organs becomes markedly more permeable. Intestinal edema ensues with loss of intravascular and extracellular fluid into the bowel wall, bowel lumen, and mesentery. This phenomenon is commonly referred to as intestinal third space fluid loss, which can sequester many liters of fluid.

Hormonal Release During Shock. Epinephrine and cortisol are secreted in large quantities during the stress of shock. Both hormones inhibit the effects of insulin.

Glycogen stores in the liver are broken down and converted to glucose. Glucose uptake in the periphery is blocked by the effects of high cortisol and epinephrine levels and by reduced levels of incretins and insulin. The ensuing hyperglycemia reduces the immune system's ability to resist infection by interfering with the neutrophils' ability to phagocytose and kill microbes.

Activity of the Coagulation System in Shock. In shock, the blood is susceptible to clot formation. There is extensive secretion of thromboxane A$_2$ and thromboplastin by the endothelium, activation of the coagulation cascade, and inhibition of activated protein C and other fibrinolytic pathways. The blood is susceptible to forming clots that the body cannot break up. Spontaneous intravascular microthrombi form in the capillaries, lodge in the capillaries, block blood flow, and cause ischemia of tissues. Prolonged ischemia causes tissue hypoxia, which leads to cell death; this leads to cellular necrosis (see Fig. 47-3).

Prevention Versus Treatment of Shock

Clearly, prevention of shock is better than the perfect treatment. Unfortunately, shock often cannot be prevented and it is important to initiate appropriate therapy without delay. It has been shown that prompt treatment of acute MI prevents cardiogenic shock. Likewise, large volume fluid infusion in the bleeding patient before shock appears is more effective than after shock occurs. The prevention of sepsis by strict adherence to hand washing and instrumentation protocols has been shown to significantly reduce sepsis in the ICU setting.

The treatment of shock is very complicated and depends on its etiology. Treatment often requires the expertise of several specialists, including an intensivist, surgeon, cardiologist, infectious disease specialist, pulmonologist, and nephrologist.

Specific Shock States

There are different types of shock based on etiology of the condition. Cardiogenic shock is caused by failure of the heart. Hypovolemic shock is caused by a large depletion of blood or fluids from the body. Anaphylactic shock is triggered by a severe allergic reaction. Most often, neurogenic shock occurs because of spinal cord or brain injury. Both anaphylactic and neurogenic shock involve widespread vasodilation, which causes extensive hypoperfusion of tissues.

Cardiogenic Shock

Cardiogenic shock is defined as severe hypotension—lower than 90 mm Hg systolic for 30 minutes, despite adequate fluid status. Cardiogenic shock causes significant decrease in aortic perfusion, which leads to loss of circulation in the systemic arteries. The low circulation

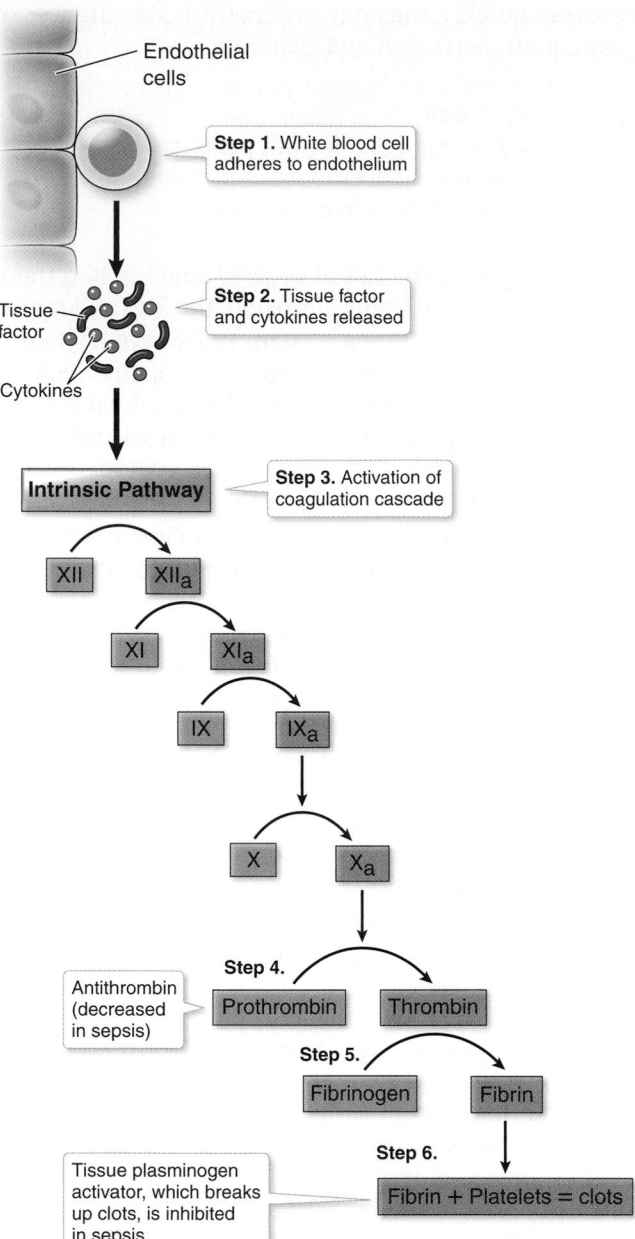

FIGURE 47-3. Microthrombi formation in sepsis. In sepsis, WBCs adhere to the endothelial cells and release cytokines, which damage the endothelial cells. When endothelial cells are damaged, tissue factor (thromboplastin) is activated, which stimulates the coagulation cascade. In the last steps of the coagulation cascade, prothrombin is converted to thrombin, which in turn converts fibrinogen to fibrin. Antithrombin is inhibited by sepsis and clots form without inhibition. Fibrin binds with platelets to form small clots. Any time clots are formed in the body, the process of fibrinolysis by tissue plasminogen activator should occur. Sepsis, however, inhibits formation of tissue plasminogen activator.

leads to low urine output, peripheral cyanosis, and altered mental status. The most common cause of cardiogenic shock is severe acute MI. A severe acute MI can cause an extensive loss of myocardial muscle and lead to heart failure. Cardiac tamponade, a state where the heart is restricted from pumping blood to the periphery, can also induce a state of shock. Also, severe tachyarrhythmias and bradyarrhythmias can cause shock. In the very rapid arrhythmias, the heart's ventricles cannot fill with adequate blood volume. Cardiac output is low and reduced blood is pumped forward with each contraction. In the very slow arrhythmias, the heart is beating at a very low rate, which causes low cardiac output. Low cardiac output cannot supply the tissues with adequate circulation.

Shock Caused by Acute Myocardial Infarction

Cardiogenic shock develops in about 10% to 15% of patients with acute MI who arrive alive at a hospital. Early thrombolytic therapy, intra-aortic balloon counterpulsation, and early myocardial revascularization (by coronary angioplasty and stenting or coronary artery bypass surgery), are associated with mortalities of 35% to 65%.

In the past, it was thought that cardiogenic shock would occur if an MI destroyed 40% or more of the ventricle. Cardiogenic shock was common with anterior or anterior lateral infarctions. It was thought that the destruction of such a significant amount of myocardium could explain the symptoms of cardiogenic shock on a purely mechanical basis. However, cardiogenic shock can be seen after infarctions that involve less than 40% of the myocardial muscle. Complications of an MI—such as acute mitral valve regurgitation as a result of the necrosis and rupture of the papillary muscles, acute rupture of the ventricular septum, or cardiac tamponade from cardiac perforation—can cause cardiogenic shock. In addition, elements of SIRS play an important role in the development of cardiogenic shock. Elevated temperature, elevated levels of WBCs, and release of inflammatory mediators commonly accompany MIs. Inflammation increases the body's need for oxygen and nutrients, and the heart works harder to supply the body with sufficient blood. This extra work increases the heart's muscle damage.

In cardiogenic shock, the heart is unable to meet the circulation needs of the peripheral tissues. Systemic arterial blood flow decreases. This low arterial blood flow is sensed by the arterial baroreceptors, which in turn stimulate the SNS. The SNS stimulates the peripheral arteries to vasoconstrict. At the same time, the kidney senses low circulation and releases renin, which sets off the RAAS. The RAAS causes release of angiotensin II, which further vasconstricts the arteries. It also triggers release of aldosterone which increases sodium and water reabsorption into the bloodstream and increases blood volume. The resistance against the heart is increased because of peripheral artery vasoconstriction. The blood volume is enhanced. Together, the increased arterial resistance and enhanced blood volume intensify the workload on the failing heart, which causes widening of the infarction area; as a result, more cardiac muscle dies.

Shock Caused by Cardiac Tamponade

Cardiac tamponade occurs when there is an increased amount of fluid in the pericardial sac that surrounds the heart. The fluid within the pericardial sac compresses the heart and restricts the heart's ability to fill with blood. There are various causes of cardiac tamponade, including bleeding into the pericardium caused by trauma, ascending aortic dissection, cardiac perforation following MI, and postoperative bleeding following open heart surgery. Cardiac tamponade can also occur from the accumulation of fluid in the pericardium caused by uremic pericarditis, lupus pericarditis, and metastatic cancer to the pericardium.

Normally, the pericardial space contains a very little amount (20 to 50 mL) of clear serous fluid, which does not cause any restriction on the heart. In cardiac tamponade, there is an excess of fluid in the pericardial sac and the atria cannot fill because of the external compression. The reduced filling of the atria causes low blood volume in the ventricles. Cardiac output drops, and the heart compensates by increasing the heart rate.

A sign of cardiac tamponade is pulsus paradoxus, which is exhibited by the jugular veins. Under normal conditions, during inspiration the thoracic cage expands and the jugular venous pressure decreases. However, in pulsus paradoxus, there is an increase in jugular venous pressure during inspiration. The heart is compressed in tamponade; with inhalation, there is further pressure placed around the heart. The pressure on the right atrium causes backflow of pressure into the superior vena cava which, in turn, causes backflow of blood into the jugular veins. Consequently, the patient exhibits jugular venous distension with inhalation.

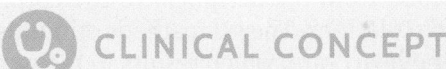

CLINICAL CONCEPT

Beck's triad is a key sign of cardiac tamponade: distant heart sounds, low BP, and high jugular venous pressure.

In the case of bleeding into the pericardium, the increase in pericardial pressure compressing the heart is very rapid. Small amounts of fresh blood (100 to 200 mL) can cause significant signs of tamponade, as there is no time to allow for the stretching of the pericardium. Death ensues quickly unless the pericardium is decompressed. This requires emergently opening the chest and making an incision into the pericardial membrane to let the blood escape. Such drastic actions are commonly unsuccessful in saving the patient.

In the case of an inflammatory pericarditis, the fluid accumulation is much slower (over weeks) and the pericardium can stretch out to relieve pressure. By the time tamponade occurs, 1 or more liters of fluid have accumulated and the pericardium is very large and tautly filled. These patients present with a history of a chronic underlying disease such as renal insufficiency, lupus erythematosus, or other autoimmune disorder, tuberculosis, chest wall radiation therapy, or cancer. The presence of chest pain is variable. Tachycardia and hypotension are always present, as are the signs of catecholamine secretion, including cyanosis, tremor, anxiety, and diaphoresis.

Hypovolemic Shock

In hypovolemic shock, the amount of blood in the body's vasculature is reduced. The low blood volume causes low blood pressure. Commonly, hypovolemic shock is caused by extensive loss of blood, as occurs in hemorrhage. Hypovolemic shock can also be caused by loss of extracellular fluid volume through diarrhea (especially in children), vomiting, ascites, or severe burns. Less commonly but significant, loss of adequate venous return can cause hypovolemic shock. Lack of venous return to the heart lowers blood volume in all the heart's chambers. Therefore, less blood is pumped out of the ventricles and into the arterial circulation.

Hypovolemic shock creates conditions that reduce coronary artery blood flow. With severely diminished blood pressure, the aorta suffers low volume; the coronary arteries that come off the aorta will then demonstrate low blood volume. Low coronary artery blood flow can cause myocardial ischemia or infarction.

Compensatory Mechanisms in Hypovolemia

In hypovolemic shock, two major compensatory mechanisms are triggered by reduced BP. There is a stimulation of the arterial baroreceptors, which are sensors of BP in the walls of the arteries. There is also a trigger of the RAAS. In hypovolemic shock, low blood volume is sensed by the arterial baroreceptors, which then stimulate the SNS. The sympathetic stimulus causes peripheral arterial vasoconstriction, which raises BP and directs blood from the periphery to the coronary and cerebral circulations. The sympathetic stimulus also increases the heart rate, which results in tachycardia.

As hypovolemic shock continues, the kidneys sense a drop in circulation and release renin. Renin stimulates the liver to release angiotensinogen, which becomes angiotensin I. Angiotensin I is transformed into angiotensin II by the angiotensin-converting enzyme (ACE). Angiotensin II directly stimulates peripheral arterial vasoconstriction and triggers the adrenal gland to release aldosterone. Under the influence of aldosterone, the kidneys increase water and salt reabsorption to restore intravascular fluid volume. Therefore, the body compensates for hypovolemic shock by vasoconstricting all the peripheral arteries, bringing in more volume of water into the blood and increasing heart rate.

Hypovolemic Shock Caused by Loss of Blood or Fluids

A normal person can lose up to 20% of his or her blood volume (approximately 1 liter) without exhibiting any sign of hypovolemic shock. In healthy, young individuals, the blood loss can even be greater because the intensity of vasoconstriction and the efficiency of cardiac performance can dramatically hide the signs of shock. The normal BP can fool the caregiver into believing that the patient is stable. However, shock is present and is demonstrated by the signs of inadequate tissue perfusion: cyanosis, tachycardia, reduced urine output, confusion or agitation, poor skin turgor, and thirst.

These signs may be missed; only after exhaustion of the ATP that is allowing constriction of the vascular smooth musculature does the blood pressure fall. In these cases, the drop in blood pressure is sudden and death follows quickly if the blood volume is not restored immediately.

Hypovolemic Shock Caused by Diminished Venous Return

Hypovolemic shock can be caused by the lack of venous return to the heart. For example, victims of disasters who are pinned under fallen structures often suffer lack of venous return from the lower extremities up to the heart. The low pressure on the venous side of the circulation leads to inadequate filling volumes in the heart's ventricles and a drop in cardiac output. Consequently, there is a drop in tissue perfusion. The tissues resort to anaerobic metabolism. Production of lactic acid results and a metabolic acidosis ensues. If the situation is not reversed, depletion of ATP occurs, lysosomes break open, and cellular death follows. Cell death releases a host of chemotactic elements and activates the immune system sharply. The SIRS that follows cellular injury is intense and can lead to MODS. Hypovolemic shock induces renal tubular dysfunction and eventual renal tubular necrosis if not reversed. This renal tubular necrosis can be permanent.

Hypovolemic Shock and Coronary Ischemia

Hypovolemic shock can unmask pre-existing coronary artery disease. When there is a drop in blood pressure, aortic pressure is reduced. With reduced aortic pressure, there is diminished coronary artery blood flow. If the coronary arteries are already compromised by arteriosclerosis, low aortic blood volume will further diminish low coronary artery perfusion. In addition, the heart, in hypovolemic shock, is stimulated by the SNS to increase cardiac contractility and heart rate. Higher heart rate and contractility requires more coronary artery blood flow in the heart muscle. Thus, the drop in coronary artery perfusion by hypovolemic shock is accompanied by an increased demand for more coronary artery blood. This lack of sufficient coronary blood flow can precipitate an acute MI. The MI complicates the picture enormously because some heart muscle dies, heart failure begins, and cardiogenic shock ensues. Cardiogenic shock combined with hypovolemic shock carries a very high mortality.

Anaphylactic Shock

Anaphylactic shock, also known as anaphylaxis, is the extreme manifestation of an allergic reaction. It is unknown why anaphylaxis occurs; it can occur at any time in a person's life, and it is known that prior exposure to an allergen prepares the immune system for repeat exposure. Immunoglobulin E develops memory for a specific antigen, which makes it ready to attack when re-exposure occurs. However, the attack on the antigen creates a bodywide reaction. Only a miniscule amount of antigen is necessary, and IgE stimulates the eosinophils, basophils and mast cells to degranulate, which releases large amounts of histamine, bradykinin, complement, and prostaglandins. Massive vasodilatation with increased capillary permeability throughout the body leads to a hypoperfusion of tissues and hypotension. Shock and bronchospasm occurs. Bronchospasm, increased respiratory secretions and edema of the airways cause respiratory distress. Stridor and wheezing are heard and laryngospasm can be fatal. The same responses in the skin cause erythema and edema of the dermis (hives and angioedema). If untreated, this reaction is often fatal.

Almost anything can cause anaphylaxis. Frequent substances include penicillin and other medications, food allergies (shellfish and peanuts are common), iodinated radiological contrast media, and hymenoptera (wasps and red ants) bites.

Neurogenic Shock

Neurogenic shock can occur when the SNS is disrupted by spinal cord injury, brain injury, or during anesthesia. The underlying cause of neurogenic shock is widespread vasodilation that reduces venous return to the heart; this reduces the volume of blood that can be pumped out of the ventricles. Low blood volume causes widespread hypotension. If the spinal cord injury is in the upper thoracic area or higher, there is lack of sympathetic tone; unopposed parasympathetic nervous system (PSNS) discharge then takes over. Parasympathetic stimulation causes bradycardia and cardiac output becomes very low. Unless corrected, widespread hypoperfusion causes extensive tissue ischemia, which leads to cell death.

CLINICAL CONCEPT

Tachycardia is the expected compensatory response in shock. However, bradycardia occurs in neurogenic shock because of the shutdown of the SNS and unopposed influence of the PSNS.

Assessment of the Critically Ill Patient

A complete history and physical exam is necessary in the critically ill patient. Often the history cannot be given by the patient; instead, family members or significant others can supply important information. The clinician needs to be aware that critically ill patients demonstrate distinctive signs and symptoms in the different stages of the illness. To establish the level of risk to the patient, the clinician uses various assessment tools.

History

A thorough history is important when dealing with a critically ill patient. Often the etiology of the critical illness is not readily apparent. For example, hypovolemic shock can occur without obvious blood or fluid loss. Septic shock often develops without fever or positive blood culture. Previous medical history plays a pivotal role. Patients who have recently had chemotherapy or who have a major immunodeficiency disease such as AIDS or leukemia have a much worse prognosis than previously healthy patients. Age is important, with higher mortality in older patients.

Signs and Symptoms

Most critically ill patients develop common signs of generalized systemic inflammation, such as fever, increased pulse, rapid respirations, and hypotension. Tachycardia persists despite the correction of fluid deficits. Tachypnea is present despite the correction of acidosis. Abnormal temperature readings may be present without a known infection. Leukocytosis or leukopenia may also be present. Multiple investigations to demonstrate a source of infection are often negative. Blood cultures may be positive or negative in sepsis and septic shock.

Shock, no matter what the cause, is the body's inability to supply adequate oxygen and nutrition to vital organs. The following signs and symptoms of inadequate perfusion are some of the parameters clinicians use to diagnose shock:

- tachycardia or bradycardia
- tachypnea
- cyanosis
- metabolic acidosis
- changes in mentation or consciousness
- low urine output
- electrocardiographic changes
- cardiac output, either reduced or increased
- central venous pressure, either high or low
- total peripheral resistance, either markedly increased or reduced
- blood pressure is usually low, but not necessarily.

The parameters vary depending on the etiology of shock (see Table 47-1).

MODS can result from such disorders as MI, major trauma, burns, hemorrhage, infection, pancreatitis, or major surgery. The SIRS that follows these events can lead immediately to MODS, or there can be a delay of several days to a week between SIRS and the onset of MODS. In that case, there is usually a "second hit" in the form of infection during the period of CARS. Major infection during this period of immunocompromise can manifest subtly without the usual signs of fever, tachycardia, or tachypnea. Alteration of mental status in this setting is ominous.

Diagnosis

In an effort to predict a level of risk of the critically ill patient, several scoring models have been developed. The APACHE II (Acute Physiology And Chronic Health Evaluation system) scoring model is an example (see Table 47-2). It assesses the probability of survival of an ICU patient based on standard physiologic parameters, standard blood tests, Glasgow Coma Scale

TABLE 47-1. Parameters of Shock

	Hypovolemic	Cardiac	Septic	Anaphylactic	Neurogenic
BLOOD PRESSURE	↓	↓	↓	↓	↓
RESPIRATORY RATE	↑	↑	↑	↑	↑
HEART RATE	↑	↑ or ↓	↑	↑	↑ or ↓
TEMPERATURE	↔	↔	↑ or ↓	↔	↔
SKIN COLOR	Pale	Cyanotic	Flush or cyanotic	Flush or hives	Variable
MENTAL STATUS	Anxious, thirsty	Anxious	Confused or obtunded	Anxious	Anxious or obtunded to comatose
CARDIAC OUTPUT	↓	↓	↑ or ↓	↓	↓
URINE OUTPUT	↓	↓	↓	↓	↓
ACIDOSIS	Present	Present	Present	Present	Present
CVP	↓	↑	↓ or ↔	↓	↓

(GCS) score (see Table 47-3), and medical history in the first 24 hours after admission. There are several, easily linked online sites and downloadable programs for personal data assistants where the data is easily entered and the calculations automatic. The scores correlate to the statistically expected mortality.

The Simplified Acute Physiology Score (SAPS II), Sepsis-related Organ Function Assessment score (SOFA) and the Multiple Organ Dysfunction Score are similar assessment tools. In all these scoring systems, the higher the score, the higher is the probable mortality. Although it is useful to have the information afforded by the

TABLE 47-2. APACHE II Score

Use the value for each parameter that is the most abnormal during the first 24 hours after admission to the ICU.

Physiologic Variable	Point Score								
	+4	+3	+2	+1	0	+1	+2	+3	+4
Temperature rectal (°C)	≥41°C	39°C–40.9°C	–	38°C–38.9°C	36°C–37.9°C	34°C–35.9°C	32°C–33.9°C	30°C–31.9°C	<30°C
Heart rate	≥179	140–179	110–139	–	70–109	–	55–69	40–54	<40
Mean arterial pressure (mm Hg)	≥159	130–159	110–129	–	70–109	–	50–69	–	<50
Respiratory rate, nonventilated	≥49	35–49	–	25–34	12–24	10–11	6–9	–	<6
Arterial pH	≥7.69	7.60–7.69	–	7.50–7.59	7.33–7.49	–	7.25–7.32	7.15–7.24	<7.15
Oxygenation if $FIO_2 \geq 0.5$, use A-aDO_2	≥500	351–499	–	200–350	<200	–	–	–	–
Oxygenation if $FIO_2 <50\%$, use PO_2	–	–	–	–	>70	61–70	–	55–60	<55

TABLE 47-2. APACHE II Score–cont'd

Physiologic Variable	Point Score								
	+4	+3	+2	+1	0	+1	+2	+3	+4
Serum sodium	≥180	160–179	155–159	150–154	130–149	–	120–129	111–119	<111
Serum potassium	≥7.0	6–6.9	–	5.5–5.9	3.5–5.4	3–3.4	2.5–2.9	–	<2.5
Creatinine (mg/dL) – *double point score for acute renal failure*	≥3.5	2–3.4	1.5–1.9	–	0.6–1.4	–	<0.6	–	–
Hematocrit	≥59.9	–	50–59.9	46–49.9	30–45.9	–	20–29.9	–	<20
WBC (10³ cells/mm³)	≥39	–	20– 38.9	15–19.9	3–14.9	–	1–2.9	–	<1

AGE

0 points if younger than 44 years
2 points if between 45 and 54 years
3 points if between 55 and 64 years
5 points if between 65 and 74 years
6 points if older than 74 years.

HISTORY OF ORGAN DYSFUNCTION OR IMMUNOCOMPROMISE

5 points if yes and emergency postop or nonresponsive
2 points if yes and elective postop
0 points if no

NEUROLOGICAL EVALUATION

Score = 15 – actual GCS

ICU MORTALITY AS PREDICTED BY APACHE II SCORES

APACHE II score = Physiologic Variable Points + Age Points + History of Organ Dysfunction or Immunocompromise Points + Neurological Evaluation Points

Score	Mortality
0–4	4%
5–9	8%
10–14	15%
15–19	25%
20–24	40%
25–29	55%
30–34	75%
>34	85% or higher

Source: Knaus, W. A., Draper, E. A., & Wagner, D. P. (1985). APACHE II: a severity of disease classification system. *Crit Care Med*, 13(10), 818–829. PMID 3928249.

scoring systems to determine the chances of survival from critical illness, it cannot dictate care.

All of these scoring systems correlate statistically with mortality in the ICU, but they refer to the ICU population as a group. The APACHE and other scores represent a level of risk for the group of patients with a particular score, but do not accurately predict outcome for the individual patient with that score. The score is useful when discussing possible outcomes and probabilities of cure or death with family members. The scoring systems are also useful in evaluating the quality of care in an ICU based on the observed mortality versus the expected mortality.

TABLE 47-3. Glasgow Coma Scale

Areas of Response	Points
EYES OPENING	
Eyes open spontaneously	4
Eyes open in response to voice	3
Eyes open in response to pain	2
No eye opening response	1
BEST VERBAL RESPONSE	
Oriented (e.g., to person, place, time)	5
Confused, speaks but is disoriented	4
Inappropriate, but comprehensible words	3
Incomprehensible sounds but no words are spoken	2
None	1
BEST MOTOR RESPONSE	
Obeys command to move	6
Localized painful stimulus	5
Withdrawals from painful stimulus	4
Flexion, abnormal decorticate posturing	3
Extension, abnormal decerebrate posturing	2
No movement or posturing	1
TOTAL POSSIBLE POINTS	3–15
MAJOR HEAD INJURY	≤ 8
MODERATE HEAD INJURY	9–12
MINOR HEAD INJURY	13–15

Treatment of the Critically Ill Patient

There is no one universal treatment used for shock. Different types of shock require distinctive treatment modalities. Therefore, treatment relies on the accurate diagnosis of the type of shock that is occurring.

Treatment of Cardiogenic Shock

Cardiogenic shock is most commonly caused by extensive MI. The left ventricle is often involved, which weakens the forward pumping of blood into the aorta and systemic arterial circulation. The treatment goal of MI is reduction of the heart's oxygen needs, support of cardiac output, and revascularization of the myocardium. Beta blockers, given early, reduce the heart's work and oxygen consumption. If there is profound cardiogenic shock, beta blockers may be contraindicated. Aspirin inhibits platelet activation and reduces extension of the infarction. It may also play a role as an anti-inflammatory agent. Dobutamine and dopamine increase cardiac output, but the increase in contractility and heart rate from these drugs increases cardiac work and oxygen demands, which may not be desirable.

BOX 47-4. Intra-Aortic Balloon Counterpulsation

An IABP is a useful device for cardiogenic shock. This catheter, which has an inflatable balloon on the tip, is inserted into the femoral artery and threaded up the aorta. During diastole of the heart, the balloon is inflated and pressure is created by the open balloon in the aorta. This increased pressure in the aorta increases blood flow into the coronary arteries. During systole of the heart, the balloon is deflated, and there is a suction effect that assists in the drive to push blood forward into the arterial circulation.

An intra-aortic balloon pump (IABP) device can provide a lifesaving treatment in cardiogenic shock. The procedure, called IABP counterpulsation, enhances coronary blood flow, reduces afterload, and decreases the heart's work (see Box 47-4).

Early reperfusion of the myocardium after MI can reduce extension of the infarcted muscle tissue. Revascularization procedures include thrombolytic medications, angioplasty, stenting, or coronary artery bypass. These procedures significantly reduce the incidence of cardiogenic shock after an MI.

Acute mitral valve regurgitation, cardiac tamponade, and acute ventral septal defect are surgical emergencies that can occur after MI with a high mortality. If the pericardial sac surrounding the heart has fluid that is constricting the heart (cardiac tamponade), it is necessary to relieve pericardial pressure. This can be accomplished with a surgical procedure called percutaneous, subxiphoid pericardiocentesis. In the procedure, the clinician uses a #18 gauge needle (large bore needle) that is inserted through the chest under the sternum into the pericardial sac. This incision into the pericardial sac relieves the constriction around the heart; however, it is associated with a mortality of 4% and a serious complication rate of 17%. The same procedure performed with ultrasonic guidance is much safer and a catheter can be left in place to ensure further drainage of fluids.

🩺 CLINICAL CONCEPT

Cardiogenic shock caused by acute mitral insufficiency, acute ventricular septal defect, or acute ventricular perforation requires emergency surgery.

Treatment of Hypovolemic Shock

The treatment of hypovolemic shock requires rapid, adequate replacement of the fluid loss. At the same time, every effort should be made to stop the fluid loss, which is not always immediately apparent.

If fluids are replaced before hypotension occurs, shock may be avoided. The initial type of fluids administered is controversial, but most practitioners agree that 1 or 2 liters of normal saline, 5% dextrose in normal saline, or Ringer's lactate solution should be given immediately. These solutions are volume expanders and have a similar ratio of solute and solvent as blood. Persistent bleeding will require blood transfusions; before transfusion, the patient needs to be tested for blood type. Some practitioners advocate using mostly crystalloid solutions for hypovolemic shock, such as Ringer's lactate, with transfusions used sparingly. Others recommend the use of colloid solutions, such as Dextran, instead of crystalloids. All practitioners agree on the need for rapid fluid resuscitation. However, there is controversy about how much is appropriate. The amount of resuscitation should be gauged by urine output because this is a true measure of tissue perfusion.

Treatment of Sepsis and Septic Shock

The treatment of septic shock is clearly very complex and may involve multiple specialists, including an infectious disease specialist, a pulmonologist, a surgeon, an intensivist, a cardiologist, and nephrologists. It requires the use of appropriate antibiotics, support of cardiac output, the use of vasoconstrictors, respiratory support, and sometimes surgery to treat the source of infection. Renal failure is frequent and dialysis may be necessary. Respiratory failure is also frequent, requiring intubation with mechanical ventilator support.

Control of hyperglycemia with continuous IV insulin and hourly blood sugar determinations reduce mortality. Hypoglycemia must be avoided. The administration of glucocorticoids is controversial. There appears to be a subgroup of patients with inadequate cortisol secretion that may benefit from it. In general, the administration of glucocorticoids to septic patients increases overall mortality. Despite the amount of high tech equipment found in modern ICUs and the advances in the pharmacological treatment of septic shock, mortality remains very high.

 CLINICAL CONCEPT

Septic shock is associated with a significant increase in capillary permeability so that a large part of the fluids used in resuscitation end up in the subcutaneous tissues, making the patient seem very bloated.

Treatment of Anaphylactic Shock

Anaphylactic shock is treated with IM or IV epinephrine, antihistamines, and glucocorticoids. Intravenous saline administration is necessary because anaphylaxis causes a large shift of fluid from the bloodstream into the tissues. Intubation may be necessary if bronchoconstriction is severe. The antigen that triggered

the severe allergic reaction should be identified. Patients need to carry an EpiPen with them at all times.

Treatment of Neurogenic Shock

The treatment for neurogenic shock consists of IV vasoconstrictors and fluid administration. Atropine, an anticholinergic agent, may be needed to counteract the parasympathetic-driven bradycardia. The treatment of the underlying central nervous system injury is essential. In cases of spinal injury, stabilization of the injury is key.

Pathophysiology of Selected Types of Organ Dysfunction

In critically ill patients, organ failure can occur. Adult respiratory distress syndrome (ARDS), renal failure, and DIC are the major disorders involved in MODS that can be lethal. Each organ system failure will present with different signs and symptoms and require different management.

Adult Respiratory Distress Syndrome

Adult respiratory distress syndrome (ARDS) is caused by widespread injury of the alveoli that often occurs in the presence of shock or MODS. This acute condition is characterized by bilateral pulmonary infiltrates and severe hypoxemia. It is important to differentiate ARDS from pulmonary edema caused by heart failure. Both of these disorders cause pulmonary infiltrates; however, in ARDS, there is no heart failure. ARDS is sometimes referred to as the most severe form of **acute lung injury (ALI).**

ARDS may occur in people of any age; however, it is most common in older adults. The annual incidence of ARDS in the United States increases with advancing age, ranging from 16 cases per 100,000 persons in those aged 15 to 19 years to 306 cases per 100,000 persons in those between the ages of 75 and 84 years.

Etiology

The most common risk factor for ARDS is sepsis. Other risk factors include lung injury (most commonly, aspiration of gastric contents), systemic illnesses, and traumatic injuries; however, approximately 20% of patients with ARDS have no identified risk factor. Advanced age, cigarette smoking, and alcohol use increase susceptibility to ARDS. Many conditions can increase the risk of developing ARDS (see Box 47-5).

Pathophysiology

ARDS can result from different mechanisms:

1. direct lung injury and local inflammation, such as from pneumonitis, aspiration, heat, or chemical inhalation injuries

BOX 47-5. Major Risk Factors for ARDS

The major risk factors for ARDS include:

- aspiration
- bacteremia
- burns
- drug overdose
- fat embolism
- fractures, particularly multiple fractures and long bone fractures
- massive transfusion
- near drowning
- pancreatitis
- pneumonia
- postperfusion injury after cardiopulmonary bypass
- sepsis
- trauma, with or without pulmonary contusion.

2. indirect lung injury from an intense inflammatory reaction elsewhere in the body with systemic inflammatory mediators such as cytokines and microbial toxins damaging the lung
3. cardiogenic pulmonary edema.

Any injury to the lungs is followed by the secretion of cytokines, superoxidases, and other deleterious substances by the pulmonary macrophages and the neutrophils that rush to the site of injury by chemotaxis. The capillaries of the lungs are particularly rich in neutrophils; migration of these neutrophils occurs quickly after the onset of any pulmonary injury. The presence of inflammatory substances increases the permeability of the alveolar capillaries and fluid from the bloodstream infiltrates the lung tissue.

Both type I and type II alveolar epithelial cells are injured in ARDS. The loss of type I cells increases alveolar epithelial permeability, leading to increased fluid in the alveoli. Injury of type II cells reduces the production of surfactant. Surfactant is a lubricating substance that lines the alveoli to keep them from completely collapsing. Loss of surfactant decreases pulmonary compliance and causes alveolar collapse. The increased fluid in the alveoli impedes the diffusion of oxygen into the bloodstream. The combination of alveolar collapse and reduced diffusion of oxygen decrease the arterial partial pressure of oxygen (PaO_2) in the bloodstream. Alveolar carbon dioxide diffusion is much less affected because CO_2 is 20 times more soluble in water than oxygen. The lack of oxygen cannot be overcome by hyperventilating or by administering high oxygen concentration.

Clinical Presentation
ARDS presents with acute dyspnea and hypoxemia within hours to days of an inciting event, such as trauma, sepsis, drug overdose, massive transfusion, acute pancreatitis, or aspiration. In many cases, the inciting event is obvious; in others, such as drug overdose, it may be difficult to identify.

Patients who develop ARDS are critically ill, often with multisystem organ failure, and they may not be capable of providing a history. In this situation, a history should be sought from family or significant others. The clinician should inquire about recent infection, trauma, drug use, recent surgery, and pancreatitis because these are key preceding conditions. Typically, the illness develops within 12 to 48 hours after an inciting event, although, in rare instances, it may take up to a few days.

Signs and Symptoms. Patients are typically short of breath at rest. They are breathing rapidly, feeling anxious, and need increasingly high concentrations of inspired oxygen. Despite the increase in oxygen administration, the patient's condition does not improve.

In the physical examination, there is tachypnea, tachycardia, and the need for high concentrations of oxygen to maintain oxygen saturation. The patient may be febrile or hypothermic. Older adult patients are often hypothermic. If ARDS is occuring in the presence of sepsis, hypotension, peripheral vasoconstriction with cold extremities, and cyanosis of the lips and fingertips may be apparent. Auscultation of the lungs may reveal bilateral crackles.

Manifestations of the underlying etiology may be present, such as acute abdominal findings in the case of ARDS caused by pancreatitis. If sepsis is the cause of ARDS, the clinican should try to identify the cause of infection.

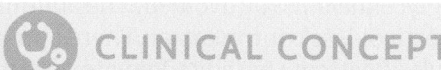 CLINICAL CONCEPT

In cases of ARDS caused by sepsis, acute abdomen, surgical wounds, intravascular lines, and decubitus ulcers are commonly the source of infection.

ARDS should be differentiated from pulmonary edema caused by heart failure because the pulmonary findings are similar in both disorders. However, the disorders have different etiologies and require different treatments. The clinician needs to examine the patient to rule out signs of heart failure, which include jugular venous distension, hepatosplenomegaly, ankle edema, or ascites.

Diagnosis
Chest x-ray is the first diagnostic procedure used in ARDS. ARDS is defined by the acute onset of bilateral pulmonary infiltrates, which is evident on chest x-ray. Computed tomography scan can be used if x-ray is not sufficient. It can be difficult to differentiate between pulmonary edema caused by heart failure and ARDS.

An echocardiogram is often done to exclude the possibility of heart dysfunction. The echocardiogram can show left ventricular ejection fraction and valvular dysfunction. Another way to differentiate ARDS from cardiogenic pulmonary edema is to obtain a B-type natriuretic peptide (BNP) level. BNP levels are elevated in heart failure. A BNP level of lower than 100 pg/mL in a patient with bilateral pulmonary infiltrates and hypoxemia favors the diagnosis of ARDS rather than heart failure. BNP levels are commonly 400 pg/mL or greater in heart failure.

Another diagnostic procedure that can differentiate ARDS from heart failure is hemodynamic monitoring, also called the Swan-Ganz procedure, with a pulmonary artery catheter. Pressure measurements can be taken in the right side of the heart with this specialized catheter. Heart failure can be excluded based on these measurements.

In ARDS, there is severe hypoxemia apparent in arterial blood gases (ABGs). A low PO_2 will be demonstrated on ABGs. In addition to hypoxemia, ABGs often initially show a respiratory alkalosis caused by hyperventilation. Hyperventilation diminishes carbon dioxide in the lungs, which in turn decreases H+ concentration in the blood and creates alkalotic (high pH) blood. However, if ARDS occurs because of sepsis, a metabolic acidosis with or without respiratory compensation may be present. In ARDS, as the condition worsens, the respiratory rate decreases; carbon dioxide is retained in the lungs and rises to high levels, which results in H+ accumulation in the bloodstream, creating respiratory acidosis.

In septic patients, leukopenia (low WBC count) or leukocytosis (high WBC count) may be noted. Thrombocytopenia (low platelet count) may be observed in the presence of DIC. Acute tubular necrosis often develops in the course of ARDS, probably from ischemia to the kidneys. Serum creatinine should be closely monitored, and liver function abnormalities may be noted. Multiple cytokines, such as IL-1, IL-6, and IL-8, are elevated in the serum of patients with ARDS.

Treatment

Thus far, the only treatment found to improve survival in ARDS is mechanical ventilation using low tidal volumes (6 mL/kg based upon ideal body weight). Numerous pharmacological therapies, including the use of steroids, inhaled synthetic surfactant, IV antibody to endotoxin, ketoconazole, and ibuprofen, have been tried and have been proven ineffective in ARDS. However, a randomized, clinical trial recently determined that simvastatin, a hydroxymethylglutaryl-coenzyme A reductase inhibitor, which is usually used to lower cholesterol, improved oxygenation and respiratory mechanics in patients with ALI. Other trials suggest a potential role for antibody to tumor necrosis factor TNF and recombinant IL-1 receptor antagonist. More research is necessary before these agents become standard therapies for ARDS.

Treatment of the etiology is most important in ARDS; supportive care, mechanical ventilation, and conservative fluid management are currently the major treatments used. Because infection is often the etiology, early administration of broad spectrum antibiotic therapy is essential, as is meticulous patient assessment for sources of infection. Removal of intravascular lines, drainage of infected fluid collections, surgical debridement, or resection of an infected site may be necessary.

CLINICAL CONCEPT

In patients with critical illness, family and friends are under stress and likely have many questions and concerns. It is important to communicate with the family and significant others. Clinicians and caregivers should assume that even though sedated, the patient may be capable of hearing and understanding all conversations in the room and may experience pain. Therefore, all conversation at the bedside should be appropriate and all procedures should be performed with local anesthesia and pain medication.

Acute Kidney Injury

In the setting of shock, sepsis, SIRS, or MODS, AKI frequently occurs. Thirty percent of patients in intensive care develop AKI, and there is a high mortality rate in these patients compared with those without AKI.

Etiology

The most common causes of renal injury are renal ischemia and renal toxicity, also called nephrotoxicity. Renal ischemia occurs because of reduced renal perfusion, which in turn causes ischemic injury of the nephron tubules. This is usually caused by large blood loss from the body or large water deficit in the blood. Renal toxicity commonly occurs because of the toxic effects of drugs such as antibiotics, aspirin, nonsteroidal anti-inflammatory drugs, chemotherapeutic agents, ACE inhibitors, illicit drugs, and iodinated IV contrast dye used in diagnostic tests. Many other drugs are also nephrotoxic.

A combination of ischemic injury and medication nephrotoxicity is often seen in the patient with sepsis. The septic patient often receives combinations of potentially nephrotoxic antibiotics with other drugs or iodinated contrast dye needed for diagnosis. Newer types of contrast dyes are noniodinated, nonallergenic, and nonnephrotoxic.

Pathophysiology

The kidney is responsible for the elimination of nitrogenous waste, non-nitrogenous waste and nonvolatile acids, as well as the maintenance of electrolyte and water balance. In sepsis, shock, and MODS, caused by hypotension, the kidney has to conserve water and maximally concentrate urine. In the adult, the daily average amount of waste the kidney excretes is about 600 mOsm of solutes. In order to excrete this amount of solute, the urine output has to be at least 400 mL/day. Oliguria is defined as a urine output of less than 400 mL/day, whereas anuria is defined as a urine output of 100 mL/day or lower. In patients with pre-existing renal disease, the added stress of sepsis or MODS can precipitate complete acute renal failure.

In MODS and sepsis, renal ischemia can occur because of several distinct mechanisms:

- Hypotension reduces glomerular perfusion directly.
- The hormonal responses to shock, epinephrine, norepinephrine, vasopressin, and angiotensin II depress glomerular perfusion by vasoconstriction.
- Microthrombi associated with the procoagulant state of shock block the glomerular capillaries.

The nephron tubules are exquisitely sensitive to hypoperfusion. The glomerular capillaries cannot endure extreme drops in blood pressure. Shock for only 15 minutes causes dysfunction of the nephron tubules; longer periods of time cause tubular necrosis. When there is tubular dysfunction, the tubular cells are unable to excrete a concentrated urine. Nephron tubule dysfunction also causes diminished excretion of potassium and less reabsorption of sodium. Hyperkalemia and hyponatremia often occur in AKI. In tubular necrosis, the epithelial cells that line the nephron tubules slough off and clog the tubules. No urine can be excreted from these clogged nephrons; oliguria or anuria exists. Nitrogen wastes such as blood urea nitrogen (BUN) and creatinine accumulate in the bloodstream as nephron tubules continue to dysfunction. High serum creatinine and BUN are signs of kidney injury.

Clinical Presentation

An accurate history is crucial for diagnosing AKI. People with the following comorbid conditions are at an increased risk for developing AKI:

- hypertension
- chronic heart failure
- diabetes
- multiple myeloma
- chronic infection
- myeloproliferative disorder (excessive growth of bone marrow cells)
- connective tissue disorders
- autoimmune diseases.

When the patient has a critical illness such as sepsis or MODS, it is important to review the patient's medications because these can be nephrotoxic. Also, it is important to note if any iodinated dye has been used in diagnostic procedures. Blood loss or transfusions can also cause AKI. The patient's urine output may indicate oliguria or anuria. The patient's mental status may be stuporous because of the accumulation of nitrogenous wastes—a syndrome called uremic encephalopathy.

Diagnosis

Serum creatinine and BUN are elevated in renal injury. Findings of granular, brown casts are highly suggestive of tubular necrosis. Casts are cellular debris that come from the nephron tubules and appear in urine. Reddish brown or cola-colored urine suggests the presence of myoglobin or hemoglobin, especially in the setting of a positive dipstick for heme and no red blood cells (RBCs) on the microscopic examination. The urine dipstick test may reveal significant proteinuria as a result of tubular injury.

Treatment

The development of AKI in ICU patients considerably increases the risk of death. Because renal failure can be treated by dialysis, it is rare today for a patient to die of renal failure itself; however, the presence of renal failure does increase the overall mortality.

Abdominal Compartment Syndrome and Intra-Abdominal Hypertension

In **abdominal compartment syndrome (ACS),** the pressure within the abdominal cavity increases to a point that exceeds the perfusion pressure of the capillaries. This causes ischemia and necrosis of the tissues supplied by the abdominal arterial vessels and capillaries.

The abdominal compartment is contained by the retroperitoneum posteriorly and a fibromuscular wall anteriorly and laterally. The retroperitoneum is not distensible and the fibromuscular wall is only somewhat distensible. The normal intra-abdominal pressure (IAP) is usually 0 to 5 mm Hg and when it increases above 8 mm Hg, **intra-abdominal hypertension (IAH)** exists. IAH causes decreased perfusion of the GI organs. This lack of GI perfusion can lead to ischemia and tissue necrosis, at which time it is called ACS. ACS affects the intra-abdominal viscera, such as the intestine, liver, and pancreas, as well as the retroperitoneal viscera (kidneys).

Etiology

The cause of acute ACS is increased capillary permeability of the intestinal vasculature associated with SIRS. Circulating cytokines increase endothelial permeability, and protein-rich fluid escapes into the bowel walls and lumen, the mesenteric walls, and into the peritoneal cavity. The fluid in the peritoneal cavity is an example of third space edema. Peristalsis ceases and the edematous bowel becomes distended with gas. This accumulation of fluid and gas causes a rapid increase of intra-abdominal volume that exceeds the abdominal wall's ability to distend.

Pathophysiology

As IAP increases, it exceeds the pressure in the inferior vena cava; as a result, the vessel collapses. The venous return to the heart drops, as does cardiac output. The decrease in cardiac output exacerbates the hypoperfusion in all tissues, including the intra-abdominal organs; this reinforces the mechanism by which the IAH was initiated.

This positive feedback loop, if unchecked, can lead to death. Increased IAP has multiple adverse consequences:

- Compression of the inferior vena cava reduces cardiac output.
- Renal perfusion is reduced, increasing the likelihood of acute tubular necrosis.
- The barrier between the bowel wall and the bowel content with its myriad pathogenic microbes and their toxins breaks down. There is diffusion of microbes and toxins into the bloodstream. This phenomenon then leads to sepsis, shock, and MODS.
- The increased IAP pushes up the diaphragm. This compresses the bases of the lungs and causes decreased ventilation.
- The increased intrathoracic pressure is transmitted upward via the jugular veins. There is jugular vein distension and increase in the pressure of the cerebral vasculature; this leads to an increase in intracranial pressure, which causes decreased level of consciousness.

 CLINICAL CONCEPT

In SIRS, IAP can rise to levels that compress the inferior vena cava, restrict venous return to the heart, and cause death.

Clinical Presentation

The patient usually experiences abdominal pain in ACS; the patient feels weak and systemic BP decreases, causing the patient to lose consciousness. Difficulty breathing or decreased urine output may be the first signs of IAH. Furthermore, patients who develop ACS may be unable to communicate, because they are often intubated and critically ill.

Signs and symptoms of ACS and IAH can include the following:

- increased abdominal girth
- difficulty breathing
- decreased urine output
- syncope
- melena
- nausea and vomiting.

ACS may be obscured in patients with critical injuries. Many disease processes can contribute to ACS. IAH should be considered in the following patients:

- intubated patients who are difficult to ventilate
- patients who have GI bleeding or pancreatitis and are not responding to IV fluids, blood products, and vasopressor medications
- patients who have severe burns or sepsis with decreasing urine output and are not responding to IV fluids and vasopressors
- any patient with contradictory Swan-Ganz readings.

Diagnosis

One must distinguish between increased IAP, which can be treated conservatively, and full-blown ACS, which is a surgical emergency. Monitoring of IAP is appropriate in patients at risk of IAH. In order to evaluate the abdominal perfusion pressure (APP), subtract intraabdominal pressure (IAP) from mean arterial pressure (MAP).

$$APP = MAP - IAP$$

Abdominal compartment syndrome (ACS) is present when abdominal perfusion pressure (APP) is low, mean arterial pressure (MAP) is low and intra-abdominal pressure (IAP) is high. Normal IAP is approximately 5 to 7 mm Hg. An IAP in excess of 15 mm Hg is associated with significant end-organ dysfunction and failure.

 CLINICAL CONCEPT

In order to measure IAP, you need to monitor the pressure in the urinary bladder. Specialized Foley catheters can automatically transduce this value to a patient monitor.

Treatment

In patients at risk for IAH, hourly determination of IAP is appropriate. A trend of increasing IAP requires intervention before compartment syndrome develops. Conservative treatment for increasing IAP includes:

- restriction of fluid resuscitation
- removing any object that may press on the patient's abdomen, such as an abdominal binder
- aggressive pain management to relax the abdominal musculature
- colloid infusions such as albumin to increase intravascular oncotic pressure
- nasogastric tube suction to remove air and fluid from the stomach and small intestines
- hemodialysis or hemofiltration to remove excess edema fluid
- rectal tube to evacuate colonic gas
- catecholamine support of cardiac output to improve perfusion of the intra-abdominal organs.

 CLINICAL CONCEPT

The goal in measuring and treating IAP is to keep APP greater than 60 mm Hg.

Hepatic Failure

In conditions of sepsis, MODS, and IAH, liver function is at risk; these conditions all can decrease the blood supply to the liver. The liver receives about two-thirds of its blood supply from the portal vein and about one-third from the hepatic artery.

Etiology

Arterial blood supply to the liver is reduced whenever there is decreased cardiac output and splanchnic vasoconstriction, as occurs in MODS. The venous perfusion of the liver is compromised when IAH reduces portal vein blood flow. Decreased arterial or venous blood flow to the liver will result in ischemia of hepatocytes and liver dysfunction.

Liver damage can also result from total parenteral nutrition (TPN), the IV infusion of a high-protein, carbohydrate, fat, and electrolyte solution. TPN is used when a patient is NPO (not allowed oral feedings) for an extended period of time. Although it can support the patient nutritionally for a lengthy period of time, TPN has possible hepatic complications.

Pathophysiology

In sepsis, shock, and MODS, hepatic arterial flow is diminished in order to conserve blood supply for the heart and brain. Also, splanchnic blood supply to the intestine decreases, which leads to intestinal ischemia. In intestinal ischemia, there is translocation of bacteria from the gut lumen into the portal vein. This portal vein bacteremia leads to direct bacterial infection of the liver. Bacterial toxins poison the mitochondria of hepatocytes and ATP production in the liver is markedly reduced. This reduced energy then impairs the liver's role of processing wastes.

In addition, TPN treatment can cause liver injury. When a patient is treated with TPN, fatty infiltration of the liver can occur from the administration of too many calories or the administration of too many carbohydrates. This fatty infiltration is a precursor of cirrhosis, which further depresses liver function.

Clinical Presentation

Jaundice, abdominal distension, and decreased level of consciousness will occur with liver failure (for more information, see Chapter 31: Infection, Inflammation, and Cirrhosis of the Liver).

Diagnosis and Treatment

Most patients with acute liver failure tend to develop some degree of circulatory dysfunction. The patient needs IV fluids, airway support, and possibly intubation. Monitoring of metabolic parameters such as liver enzymes, coagulation, and bilirubin are necessary. Maintenance of nutrition and prompt recognition of GI bleeding are crucial.

Disseminated Intravascular Coagulopathy

DIC is the impairment of the coagulation cascade, which causes episodes of bleeding alternating with bouts of clotting. DIC is exhibited when the entire, complex, regulatory feedback mechanism of coagulation goes awry.

Etiology

DIC is frequently part of sepsis and MODS. It is known to occur in gram-negative sepsis, major incompatibility transfusion reactions, after placement of peritoneovenous shunts, and in amniotic fluid emboli.

Pathophysiology

In DIC, there is major, widespread intravascular clotting and clotting factor depletion. There is also widespread activation of the fibrinolytic (clot-dissolving) mechanisms. Transient episodes of excessive clotting are interspersed with episodes of extreme fibrinolysis, which causes bleeding. Uncontrolled bleeding from all orifices, any wounds, and any IV sites is possible. This characterizes DIC, a syndrome with prohibitively high mortality. Brain injuries with significant, permanent neurological damage frequently occur because of the widespread coagulation of intracerebral vessels.

Clinical Presentation

Bleeding from at least three unrelated sites—such as gingiva, nose, and IV sites—is suggestive of DIC. DIC often presents with petechiae and ecchymosis, along with blood loss from IV lines and catheters. In postoperative DIC, bleeding can occur from surgical sites externally and internally. Patients with pulmonary involvement can present with dyspnea, hemoptysis, and cough. Comorbid liver disease or hemolytic reactions can lead to jaundice. Neurological changes such as coma are also possible.

 CLINICAL CONCEPT

In patients enduring major surgery under general anesthesia, the most common presentation of a transfusion reaction is DIC. The patient will suddenly start to bleed profusely from all cut surfaces.

Diagnosis

Patients with DIC can present with a wide range of abnormalities in their laboratory values. Typically, prolonged coagulation times, thrombocytopenia, high levels of fibrin degradation products, elevated D-dimer, and schistocytes (misshapen RBCs) on peripheral smears are suggestive findings. Lab tests need to be frequently done because of the rapidly changing conditions of clotting and bleeding in DIC.

Treatment

Treatment of DIC is controversial and is under current investigation. Hemorrhage caused by DIC requires rapid treatment; initially, treatment of hemorrhage usually occurs with crystalloid solutions, which have the same solute/solvent concentration as normal blood.

 CLINICAL CONCEPT

Ringer's lactate is an example of a crystalloid solution that can temporarily replace lost blood.

After the patient's blood type is determined, transfusions of typed RBCs are administered. It is important to recognize that transfusions of RBCs and crystalloid solutions are devoid of clotting factors. Therefore, after the patient is stabilized with crystalloid solutions and receives transfusions of RBCs, a substance containing coagulation factors should be administered.

CLINICAL CONCEPT

Fresh, frozen plasma contains coagulation factors and should be part of the treatment plan in DIC.

CLINICAL CONCEPT

Blood transfusions contain citrate which binds calcium. Therefore, treatment with multiple blood transfusions requires calcium supplementation.

CLINICAL CONCEPT

Multiple transfusions can cause drop in patient core temperature, therefore blood warmers are necessary.

The rapid administration of multiple transfusions introduces large amounts of citrate into the bloodstream. This chemical is used as an anticoagulant in banked blood because it binds calcium, an element necessary in almost every step of the coagulation cascade. With multiple transfusions there is a decrease in the amount of calcium in the blood. Decreased calcium can worsen hemorrhage and reduce cardiac contractility. Therefore, every treatment plan for severe hemorrhage needs to include calcium administration.

The administration of crystalloid, packed RBCs, and fresh frozen plasma in large quantities drops the core body temperature. The coagulation pathways, which are temperature dependent, are impaired in hypothermia. Blood warmers are commercially available and should be used when large amounts of IV fluid are rapidly administered.

Concepts Related to Death

Because of the advances in technology and emergence of critical care medicine, the concept of what defines death has been debated for almost 50 years. Death was initially defined as the cessation of respiration and circulation. However, because of increased knowledge in the area of neurology, mechanical ventilation, and cardiovascular support, death is currently defined by brain death. Certain neurological criteria must be met in order for a patient to be classified with brain death.

Determination of Death

The gold standard for the determination of **brain death** is the neurological exam. However, before this exam, other morbid conditions must first be ruled out. These include severe electrolyte, acid-base, and endocrine

abnormalities; core temperature lower than 89.6°F (32°C); hypotension; and possibility for drug intoxication, poisoning, or neuromuscular blockade. The neurological exam of patients with locked in syndrome, which is stroke involving the brainstem, hypothermia, or drug intoxication, could mimic that of brain death and lead to misdiagnosis.

Determining Brain Death

The clinical neurological exam assesses the patient for coma, absence of brainstem reflexes, and apnea. A positive exam for the evaluation of brain death includes:

- presence of coma
- absence of motor responses
- absence of pupillary responses to light and pupils at midposition with respect to dilatation (4 to 6 mm)
- absence of corneal reflexes
- absence of caloric responses
- absence of gag reflex
- absence of coughing in response to tracheal suctioning
- absence of sucking and rooting reflexes
- absence of respiratory drive at a $PaCO_2$ that is 60 mm Hg or 20 mm Hg above normal base-line values.

There should be two examinations performed; the interval between the two examinations is determined by the patient's age. The recommended intervals are 48 hours for term to 2-month-old newborns, 24 hours for infants older than 2 months to younger than 1 year, and 12 hours for children older than 1 year to younger than 18 years. The interval is optional for adults older than 18 years.

Assessment of Coma and Brainstem Reflexes. During the neurological exam, presence of coma is determined first, followed by the depth of coma, which is established by the presence or absence of motor response to painful stimulus. The patient's reaction to pain can be determined by pressing on a supraorbital nerve, pinching the sternum, or pressing on the nailbed of a finger. The GCS can be used to establish depth of coma; the GCS is based on certain criteria: eye opening, motor response, and verbal output (see Table 47-3).

After coma and depth of coma are established, the exam proceeds to evaluate for the presence or absence of brainstem reflexes. Absence of brainstem reflexes includes round or oval pupils in midposition and dilated 4 to 6 mm with no response to bright light. Rapid turning of the head normally elicits eye movements called oculocephalic movements. Oculocephalic movements are absent in brain death. This is confirmed by a procedure called cold caloric stimulation, which is done by irrigating the ear canal with ice water after tilting the head to 30°. In the coma patient, no neck or eye deviation toward the cold stimulus should be noted. Corneal reflex is evaluated by touching the edge of the cornea with a cotton swab; there should be no blinking in response to this stimulus in the coma patient. Bronchial suctioning is the best stimulus for a cough reflex and no coughing occurs in the coma patient.

The procedure to determine the lack of independent respiratory drive in coma patients is called apneic diffusion oxygenation. In healthy persons, stimulation of the respiratory center in the brainstem occurs when pressure of CO_2 in blood (PCO_2) reaches 60 mm Hg (in patients with COPD, the value is greater). During the procedure, the mechanical ventilator is turned off and preoxygenation is given through an oxygen catheter in the trachea to eliminate stores of respiratory nitrogen. The PCO_2 will increase at approximately a rate of 3 mm Hg per minute; there will be no spontaneous respirations in a patient with brain death.

Confirmatory Tests for Brain Death. Confirmatory tests are optional in patients who are older than 1 year of age. For term infants to those up to 2 months of age, two confirmatory tests are needed. From 2 months to 1 year, one confirmatory test is required. Confirmatory tests include:

- Cerebral angiography: performed by an injection of dye in the aortic arch in order to visualize anterior and posterior cerebral circulation of the brain. A positive exam indicating brain death would be lack of flow at the foramen magnum in posterior circulation and lack of flow at the petrous portion of the carotid artery in the anterior circulation.
- Electroencephalography: readings are obtained for at least 30 minutes. A minimum of eight scalp electrodes must be used with a distance of 10 cm between each. In the patient who is brain dead, electrical activity is absent at levels higher than 2 μV per millimeter.
- Transcranial Doppler ultrasonography: a diagnostic test in which a portable 2-HZ pulsed-wave instrument evaluates middle cerebral and vertebral arteries. The probe may be placed at the temporal bone above the zygomatic arch or the vertebrobasilar arteries through the suboccipital window. In the patient who is brain dead, transcranial Doppler ultrasonography would reveal a lack of diastolic flow and small systolic peaks in early systole.
- Nuclear imaging: in this test, technetium is injected within 30 minutes and x-ray images are

obtained immediately, between 30 and 60 minutes, and at 2 hours. Determination of brain death is made if there is no uptake of the technetium.

Postmortem Changes

After death, postmortem changes progress along an approximate timeline. Putrefaction and autolysis are the two processes that start to alter the body immediately after death. Putrefaction involves the action of bacteria on the body's tissues. There is discoloration of the body, gas production with associated bloating, and a foul odor. Autolysis is the breakdown of the body's cells. Upon cell death, lysosomes open within the cell and release the lysozymes that digest dead tissue. In most circumstances, autolysis and putrefaction occur together. In warm climatic conditions, they can result in rapid degradation of the tissues.

Some of the more well-known postmortem changes, such as rigor mortis, livor mortis, and algor mortis, occur in a progressive manner. However, climate, cause of death, and environmental conditions affect their development.

Postmortem changes include:

- Rigor mortis: the postmortem stiffening of the body's muscles. Some muscles may be contracted and remain in position. In most cases, rigor mortis begins within 1 to 2 hours after death; it begins to pass after 24 hours.
- Livor mortis: a purple-red discoloration that appears on dependent portions of the body after the heart stops. It results from the settling of the blood because of gravity.
- Tardieu spots: petechiae and small hemorrhages that occur in dependent areas of the body because of rupture of degenerating blood vessels.
- Algor mortis: the cooling process of the body after death. Cooling takes place only if the environmental temperature is cooler than body temperature at the time of death.
- Purge fluid: exudative fluid from cellular decomposition released from the oral and nasal passages as well as other body cavities.

Chapter Summary

- SIRS is the term used to describe a severe physiologic response to inflammation. This inflammation can occur from any source, whether infectious or noninfectious.
- Sepsis is diagnosed when a patient meets SIRS criteria, and has a documented or suspected source of infection. The infection can be caused by bacteria, fungi, viruses, or parasites. Common diagnostic procedures include blood culture, urine culture, sputum culture, imaging showing pneumonia or a perforated viscus, and

the existence of WBCs in normally sterile fluid. Sepsis is the most common cause of death.

- Severe sepsis is diagnosed when a patient meets sepsis criteria and has signs of end-organ damage or hypoperfusion. Signs of end-organ damage include ARDS, GI ischemia causing ileus, renal insufficiency causing decreased urine output, liver dysfunction causing increased total bilirubin, and DIC.

- Septic shock is diagnosed when a patient meets severe sepsis criteria, and has sepsis-induced vascular instability demonstrated by hypotension that is refractory to fluid resuscitation. Hypotension is defined as a systolic blood pressure lower than 90 mm Hg, a mean arterial pressure lower than 60 mm Hg, or a decrease in systolic blood pressure greater than 40 mm Hg.

- MODS is a state of progressive dysfunction of two or more major organ systems in a critically ill patient that cannot maintain homeostasis without medical intervention. In the presence of MODS, there is a 20% increase in mortality with each additional organ dysfunction. In the presence of acute renal failure, the mortality rate increases to 70%.

- Shock is classified into five broad categories: cardiac shock, hypovolemic shock, septic shock, anaphylactic shock, and neurogenic shock. It is important to realize that all five categories of shock converge onto the same pathophysiologic pathway of cellular hypoxia, cellular metabolic exhaustion and dysfunction, and death.

- Shock has three stages. In the initial stage of shock, there is a rapid drop in tissue perfusion. If this is not corrected promptly, a progressive stage of shock ensues in which the lungs, kidneys, gut, pancreas, and eventually the protected areas of the heart and brain suffer cellular injury and no longer function properly. Failure to terminate shock during the progressive stage produces the irreversible stage of shock.

- During MODS, respiratory failure is referred to as ARDS or ALI. Because of alveolar injury, the lungs become inflamed, edematous, less compliant, and less able to oxygenate the blood.

- AKI is most commonly caused by hypoperfusion of the kidney or by medications necessary to treat sepsis, including aminoglycosides, vancomycin, and iodinated IV radiological contrast media.

- IAH causes decreased perfusion of the GI organs, which can lead to ischemia and tissue necrosis, also called ACS. The intra-abdominal viscera–such as the intestine, liver, pancreas, and retroperitoneal viscera (kidneys)– are affected by ACS.

- Arterial blood supply to the liver is reduced whenever there is decreased cardiac output and splanchnic vasoconstriction as occurs in MODS and shock. The venous perfusion of the liver is compromised when IAH reduces portal vein blood flow. Decreased arterial or venous blood flow to the liver will result in ischemia of hepatocytes and liver dysfunction. Liver damage can also result from TPN, the IV infusion of a high-protein, carbohydrate, fat, and electrolyte solution.

- DIC is the impairment of the coagulation cascade, which causes episodes of bleeding alternating with bouts of clotting.

- Death is defined by brain death. Certain neurological criteria must be met in order for a patient to be classified with brain death. The gold standard for the determination of brain death is the neurological exam.

- Postmortem changes occur in a progressive manner: rigor mortis, livor mortis, algor mortis.

 ## Making the Connections

Disorder and Pathophysiology	Signs and Symptoms	Physical Assessment Findings	Diagnostic Testing	Treatment
SIRS	Overwhelming inflammatory reaction of the body initiated by a severe insult to the body, such as major trauma, burns, hemorrhage, infection, or major surgery. The inflammation reaction, coagulation system, and immune system work in an exaggerated mode to synergistically defend the body.				
	Dependent upon the source of SIRS reaction: pain, tenderness, cough, shortness of breath (SOB), fatigue, headache, neck stiffness, dysuria, abdominal pain, flank pain, fever, and chills are all possible.	To establish the presence of SIRS, any two of the following criteria should be present: • Heart rate: >90/min. • Respiratory rate: > 20/min (or need for mechanical ventilation). • Temperature: 38°C or < 36°C.	Chest x-ray. ABGs. Blood lactate. WBC with differential showing leukocytosis or leukopenia. Urine analysis. Gram stain of blood, sputum, purulence, and urine (perhaps cerebrospinal fluid [CSF]). Culture and sensitivity of blood, sputum, purulence, and urine (perhaps CSF).	***Respiratory, if not intubated*** Assess airway. Administer O_2 by mask or nasal cannula. ***Respiratory, if ventilated*** Administer O_2 at lowest level to maintain PO_2 greater than 60. ***Circulatory*** Administer fluids, vasopressors, or blood as appropriate to keep: mean arterial pressure greater than 65 mm Hg and central

Continued

Making the Connections–cont'd

Disorder and Pathophysiology	Signs and Symptoms	Physical Assessment Findings	Diagnostic Testing	Treatment
			Ultrasonography or computed tomography (CT). Electrolytes, BUN, creatinine, glucose coagulation, platelet count, partial thromboplastin time (PTT), international normalized ratio (INR). Liver function testing, including bilirubin, alanine aminotransferase (ALT), aspartate aminotransferase (AST), and alkaline phosphatase. Measurement and continued assessment of IAP and APP. Blood glucose monitoring.	venous pressure between 8 and 12 cmH$_2$O. ***Renal*** Administer sufficient fluids to keep urine output at 0.5 mL/kg/hr or greater. If infection is present, broad spectrum antibiotics are used unless gram stains allow identification of the specific organism. Drainage of abscess or wounds, if present. Treatment of organ dysfunction is based on symptomology and is given as needed. May include: • dialysis or hemofiltration • continuous insulin drip • mechanical ventilation • platelet transfusions • fresh frozen plasma.

Sepsis | An infection that begins locally; through hematogenous spread, it becomes a bodywide infection that overwhelms the immune system and causes severe multiorgan compromise.

Disorder and Pathophysiology	Signs and Symptoms	Physical Assessment Findings	Diagnostic Testing	Treatment
	Alteration in mental state. Fever or hypothermia. Other symptoms depend on the source of sepsis: pain, tenderness, cough, SOB, fatigue, dizziness, headache, neck stiffness, dysuria, abdominal pain, flank pain, fever, and chills are all possible.	Alteration in mental state: Heart rate: > 90/min. Respiratory rate: > 20/min (may need for mechanical ventilation). Temperature: > 38°C or < 36°C. Hypotension or normal BP.	Chest x-ray may show pneumonia. ABGs show hypoxemia. Blood lactate elevated. WBC with differential showing leukocytosis or leukopenia. Urinalysis may show bacteria. Low urine output. Gram stain of blood, sputum, purulence, and urine (perhaps CSF). Culture and sensitivity of blood, sputum, purulence, and urine (perhaps CSF). Ultrasonography or CT may show source of infection.	***Respiratory, if not intubated*** Assess airway. Administer O$_2$ by mask or nasal cannula. ***Respiratory, if ventilated*** Maintain tidal volume (T.V.) at 6 mL/kg of body weight (BW). Assess for the need for positive end expiratory pressure (PEEP). Maintain FIO$_2$ at lowest level to maintain PO$_2$ greater than 60 mm Hg. ***Circulatory*** Administer fluids, vasopressors, blood as appropriate to keep: MAP > 65 mm Hg.

Continued

Making the Connections—cont'd

Disorder and Pathophysiology	Signs and Symptoms	Physical Assessment Findings	Diagnostic Testing	Treatment
			Electrolytes, BUN, creatinine, glucose coagulation, platelet count, PTT, INR.	Central venous pressure (CVP) between 8–12 cmH$_2$O. Hemoglobin levels adequate. ***Renal*** Administer sufficient fluids to keep urine output ≥ 0.5 ml/kg/hr. If infection, broad spectrum antibiotics unless gram stains allow identification of specific organism. Drainage of wounds or abscesses, if present.

Septic Shock | Septicemia with vasomotor instability; widespread capillary permeability, and hypotension.

Disorder and Pathophysiology	Signs and Symptoms	Physical Assessment Findings	Diagnostic Testing	Treatment
	Alteration in mental state. Fever or hypothermia. Other symptoms depend on the source of sepsis: pain, tenderness, cough, SOB, fatigue, dizziness, headache, neck stiffness, dysuria, abdominal pain, flank pain, fever, and chills are all possible.	Alteration in mental state: Heart rate: > 90/min. Respiratory rate: > 20/min (may need for mechanical ventilation). Temperature: > 38°C or < 36°C. Hypotension < 90 systolic or 40 mm Hg below patient's normal BP.	Chest x-ray may show pneumonia. ABGs showing hypoxemia. Blood lactate elevated. WBC with differential showing leukocytosis or leukopenia. Urinalysis may show bacteria. Low urine output. Gram stain of blood, sputum, purulence and urine (perhaps CSF). Culture and sensitivity of blood, urine, sputum, and purulence (perhaps CSF). Ultrasonography or CT may show source of infection. Electrolytes, BUN, creatinine, glucose coagulation, platelet count, PTT, INR.	***Respiratory, if not intubated*** Assess airway. Administer O$_2$ by mask or nasal cannula. ***Respiratory, if ventilated*** Maintain administered O$_2$ at lowest level to maintain pO$_2$ > 60. ***Circulatory*** Administer fluids, vasopressors, blood as appropriate to keep: MAP > 65 mm Hg. CVP between 8–12 cmH$_2$O. Hemoglobin levels adequate. ***Renal*** Administer sufficient fluids to keep urine output ≥ 0.5 ml/kg/hr. If infection, broad spectrum antibiotics unless gram stains allow identification of specific organism. Drainage of wounds or abscesses if present.

MODS | State of progressive dysfunction of two or more major organ systems in a critically ill patient that cannot maintain homeostasis without medical intervention. It can result from such disorders as MI, major trauma, burns, hemorrhage, infection, pancreatitis, or major surgery.

Disorder and Pathophysiology	Signs and Symptoms	Physical Assessment Findings	Diagnostic Testing	Treatment
	Alteration in mental state. Fever or hypothermia. Variable symptoms depending on the organ that is	Alteration in mental state: Heart rate: > 90/min. Respiratory rate: > 20/min (may need for mechanical ventilation).	Chest x-ray may show pulmonary infiltrates. ABGs show hypoxemia. Blood lactate elevated.	***Respiratory, if intubated*** Assess airway. Administer O$_2$ by mask or nasal cannula.

Continued

Making the Connections–cont'd

Disorder and Pathophysiology	Signs and Symptoms	Physical Assessment Findings	Diagnostic Testing	Treatment
	failing: pain, tenderness, cough, SOB, fatigue, dizziness, headache, neck stiffness, dysuria, abdominal pain, flank pain, and chills are all possible.	Temperature: > 38°C or < 36°C. Hypotension < 90 systolic or 40 mm Hg below patient's normal BP.	WBC with differential may show leukocytosis or leukopenia. Electrolytes, BUN, creatinine, glucose coagulation, platelet count, PTT, INR. Urinalysis may show bacteria. Low urine output. Gram stain of blood, sputum, purulence, and urine (perhaps CSF). Culture and sensitivity of blood, urine, sputum, and purulence (perhaps CSF). Ultrasonography or CT may show source of infection.	***Respiratory, if ventilated*** Maintain administered O_2 at lowest level to maintain pO_2 > 60. **Circulatory** Administer fluids, vasopressors, blood as appropriate to keep: MAP > 65 mm Hg. CVP between 8-12 cmH_2O. ***Renal*** Administer sufficient fluids to keep urine output ≥ 0.5 ml/kg/hr. If infection, broad spectrum antibiotics unless gram stains allow identification of specific organism. Drainage of wounds or abscesses if present.

ARDS | Acute failure of the lungs caused by widespread injury of the alveoli that often occurs in the presence of shock or MODS. Condition causes pulmonary infiltrates and inability of lungs to oxygenate blood. Sometimes referred to as the most severe form of ALI.

Disorder and Pathophysiology	Signs and Symptoms	Physical Assessment Findings	Diagnostic Testing	Treatment
	Respiratory distress. Possible alteration in mental state.	Possible alteration in mental state. Heart rate: > 90/min. Respiratory rate: > 20/min (need for mechanical ventilation). Hypotension < 90 systolic or 40 mm Hg below patient's normal BP.	Chest x-ray shows pulmonary infiltrates. ABGs show hypoxemia. WBC with differential may show leukocytosis or leukopenia. Electrolytes, BUN, creatinine, glucose coagulation, platelet count, PTT, INR. Low urine output.	***Respiratory, if not intubated*** Assess airway. Administer O_2 by mask or nasal cannula. ***Respiratory, if ventilated*** Maintain administered O_2 at lowest level to maintain pO_2 > 60. ***Circulatory*** Administer fluids, vasopressors, blood as appropriate to keep: MAP > 65 mm Hg. CVP between 8–12 cmH_2O. ***Renal*** Administer sufficient fluids to keep urine output ≥ 0.5 ml/kg/hr.

Continued

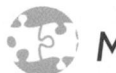 Making the Connections–cont'd

Disorder and Pathophysiology	Signs and Symptoms	Physical Assessment Findings	Diagnostic Testing	Treatment
ACS | Pressure within the abdominal cavity increases to the point that it exceeds the perfusion pressure of the capillaries, causing ischemia and necrosis of the tissues supplied by the abdominal arterial vessels and capillaries.				
	Increase in abdominal girth. Difficulty breathing. Decreased urine output. Syncope. Melena. Nausea and vomiting.	Increase in abdominal girth. Difficulty breathing. Decreased urine output. Syncope. Melena. Nausea and vomiting. Hypotension.	Monitoring of IAP via bladder. APP calculated by MAP less the IAP: APP = MAP-IAP. Compartment syndrome present when APP remains low with refractory acidosis and hypotension despite appropriate conservative intervention. Abdominal x-ray or CT scan or ultrasound. WBC with differential may show leukocytosis or leukopenia. ABGs show respiratory acidosis. Liver function tests. Serum electrolytes, BUN, glucose, coagulation, platelet count, PTT, INR.	Restriction of fluid. Removing any object that may press on the patient's abdomen, such as an abdominal binder. Pain management. Colloid infusions such as albumin to increase intravascular oncotic pressure. Nasogastric tube suction to remove air and fluid from the stomach and small intestines. Hemodialysis or hemofiltration to remove excess edema fluid. Rectal tube to evacuate colonic gas.

Bibliography

Angus, D. C. (2012). The acute respiratory distress syndrome: what's in a name? *JAMA*, 307(23), 2542–2544. doi: 10.1001/jama.2012.6761.

Boomer, J. S., To, K., Chang, K. C., et al. (2011). Immunosuppression in patients who die of sepsis and multiple organ failure. *JAMA*, 306(23), 2594–2605. doi: 10.1001/jama.2011.1829.

Brodie, D., & Bacchetta, M. (2011). Extracorporeal membrane oxygenation for ARDS in adults. *N Engl J Med*, 365(20), 1905–1914. doi: 10.1056/NEJMct1103720.

Christensen, M., & Chen, F. (2012). Advanced arterial blood gas analysis in septic shock: A Singaporean nursing case review. *Int Crit Care Nurs*, Sep 18. doi: pii: S0964-3397(12)00078-X. 10.1016/j.iccn.2012.08.002.

Dechert, R. E., Haas, C. F., & Ostwani, W. (2012). Current knowledge of acute lung injury and acute respiratory distress syndrome. *Crit Care Nurs Clin N America*, 24(3), 377–401. doi: 10.1016/j.ccell.2012.06.006.

Donnino, M. W., Salciccioli, J. D., Dejam, A., et al. (2012). APACHE II scoring to predict outcome in post-cardiac arrest. *Resuscitation*. 2012 Nov 20. doi: pii: S0300-9572(12)00882-9 .10.1016/j.resuscitation.2012.10.024. Epub ahead of print.

Dushianthan, A., Cusack, R., Goss, V., Postle, A. D., & Grocott, M. P. (2012). Clinical review: exogenous surfactant therapy for acute lung injury/acute respiratory distress syndrome—where do we go from here? *Crit Care*, 16(6), 238.

Fourrier, F. (2012). Severe sepsis, coagulation, and fibrinolysis: dead end or one way? *Crit Care Med*, 40(9), 2704–2708. doi: 10.1097/CCM.0b013e318258ff30.

Funk, D. J., Jacobsohn, E., & Kumar, A. (2013). The role of venous return in critical illness and shock: part I–physiology. *Crit Care Med*, 41(1), 250–257. doi: 10.1097/CCM.0b013e3182772ab6.

Funk, D. J., Jacobsohn, E., & Kumar, A. (2013). Role of the venous return in critical illness and shock: part II–shock and mechanical ventilation. *Crit Care Med*. 2012 Dec 19. Epub ahead of print.

Guillamet, M. C., Rhee, C., & Patterson, A. J. (2012). Cardiovascular management of septic shock in 2012. *Curr Infect Dis Rep*, 14(5), 493–502. doi: 10.1007/s11908-012-0279-z.

Hai-peng Shi, Dao-miao Xu, & Guo-en Wang. (2010). Prognostic indicators of patients with acute kidney injury in intensive care unit. *World J Emerg Med*, 1(3), 209–211.

Hall, J. B., & Kress, J. P. (2011). The burden of functional recovery from ARDS. *N Engl J Med*, 364(14), 1358–1359. doi: 10.1056/NEJMe1101057.

Hibbert, K., Rice, M., & Malhotra, A. (2012). Obesity and ARDS. *Chest*, 142(3), 785–790. doi: 10.1378/chest.12-0117.

Hotchkiss, R. S., & Opal, S. (2010). Immunotherapy for sepsis—a new approach against an ancient foe. *N Engl J Med*, 363(1), 87–89. doi: 10.1056/NEJMcibr1004371.

Isotani, E. (2012). Pathophysiology of acute respiratory distress syndrome. *Crit Care Med*, 40(7), 2233–2234. doi: 10.1097/CCM.0b013e3182514a29.

James, M. M., & Beilman, G. J. (2012). Mechanical ventilation. *Surg Clin N America*, 92(6), 1463–1474. doi: 10.1016/j.suc.2012.08.003. Epub 2012 Oct 13.

Knaus, W. A., Draper, E. A., & Wagner, D. P. (1985). APACHE II: a severity of disease classification system. *Crit Care Med*, 13(10), 818–829. PMID 3928249.

Kobayashi, L., Costantini, T. W., & Coimbra, R. (2012). Hypovolemic shock resuscitation. *Surg Clin N America*, 92(6), 1403–1423. doi: 10.1016/j.suc.2012.08.006. Epub 2012 Oct 5.

Kumar, V., Abbas, A. K., & Aster, J. C. (2013). *Robbins basic pathology*. 9th ed. Philadelphia, PA: Saunders Elsevier.

Lee, W. L., & Slutsky, A. S. (2010). Sepsis and endothelial permeability. *N Engl J Med*, 363(7), 689–691. doi: 10.1056/NEJMcibr1007320.

Longo, D., Fauci, A., Kasper, D., & Hauser, S. (2011). *Harrison's principles of internal medicine: volumes 1 and 2*. 18th ed. New York: McGraw-Hill.

Mann, A., & Early, G. L. (2012). Acute respiratory distress syndrome. *Mole Med*, 109(5), 371–375.

Matthay, M. A., Ware, L. B., & Zimmerman, G. A. (2012). The acute respiratory distress syndrome. *J Clin Invest*, 122(8), 2731–2740. doi: 10.1172/JCI60331. Epub 2012 Aug 1.

New hope for sepsis. (2012). *Lancet*, 379(9825), 1462. doi: 10.1016/S0140-6736(12)60614-X.

Perner, A., Haase, N., Guttormsen, A. B., et al. (2012). Hydroxyethyl starch 130/0.42 versus Ringer's acetate in severe sepsis. *N Engl J Med*, 367(2), 124–134. doi: 10.1056/NEJMoa1204242. Epub 2012 Jun 27. Erratum in: *N Engl J Med*. 2012 Aug 2; 367(5):481.

Pulido, J. N., Afessa, B., Masaki, M., et al. (2012). Clinical spectrum, frequency, and significance of myocardial dysfunction in severe sepsis and septic shock. *Mayo Clin Proceed*, 87(7), 620–628. doi: 10.1016/j.mayocp.2012.01.018. Epub 2012 Jun 8.

Ranieri, V. M., Thompson, B. T., Barie, P. S., et al. (2012). Drotrecogin alfa (activated) in adults with septic shock. *N Engl J Med*, 366(22), 2055–2064. doi: 10.1056/NEJMoa1202290. Epub 2012 May 22.

Rimmer, E., Kumar, A., Doucette, S., et al. (2012). Activated protein C and septic shock: a propensity-matched cohort study. *Crit Care Med*, 40(11), 2974–2981. doi: 10.1097/CCM.0b013e31825fd6d9.

Russell, J. A. (2012). How much fluid resuscitation is optimal in septic shock? *Crit Care*, 16(4), 146. Epub ahead of print.

Sugita, H., Kinoshita, Y., & Baba, H. (2012). The duration of SIRS before organ failure is a significant prognostic factor of sepsis. *Int J Emerg Med*, 5(1), 44.

Teasdale, G., & Jennett, B. (1974). Assessment of coma and impaired consciousness. *Lancet*, 81–84 vol 2 issue 7872.

Teasdale, G., & Jennett, B. (1976). Assessment and prognosis of coma after head injury. *Acta Neurochir*, 34, 45–55.

Thiele, H., Zeymer, U., Neumann, F. J., et al. (2012). Intraaortic balloon support for myocardial infarction with cardiogenic shock. *N Engl J Med*, 367(14), 1287–1296. doi: 10.1056/NEJMoa1208410. Epub 2012 Aug 26.

Venkataraman, R., & Kellum, J. A. (2013). Sepsis: update in the management. *Advances Chronic Kidney Dis*, 20(1), 6–13. doi: 10.1053/j.ackd.2012.10.013.

von Dossow-Hanfstingl, V. (2012). Advances in therapy for acute lung injury. *Anesthes Clin*, 30(4), 629–639. doi: 10.1016/j.anclin.2012.08.008. Epub 2012 Sep 1.

Ward, P. A. (2011). Immunosuppression in sepsis. *JAMA*, 306(23), 2618–2619. doi: 10.1001/jama.2011.1831.

Watkins, T. R., Nathens, A. B., Cooke, C. R., et al. (2012). Acute respiratory distress syndrome after trauma: development and validation of a predictive model. *Crit Care Med*, 40(8), 2295–2303. doi: 10.1097/CCM.0b013e3182544f6a.

Wenzel, R. P., & Edmond, M. B. (2012). Septic shock—evaluating another failed treatment. *N Engl J Med*, 366(22), 2122–2124. doi: 10.1056/NEJMe1203412. Epub 2012 May 22.

Index